THE MOSES H. CONE MEMORIAL HOSPITAL
GREENSBORO, NORTH CAROLINA

THE HEART

With the Editorial Assistance of

ROBERT C. SCHLANT, M.D.

Associate Professor of Medicine, Emory University
School of Medicine, and Director of Cardiac Research
Laboratory, Grady Memorial Hospital, Atlanta, Georgia

NANETTE KASS WENGER, M.D.

Assistant Professor of Medicine, Emory University
School of Medicine, and Director of Cardiac Clinic,
Grady Memorial Hospital, Atlanta, Georgia

RUTH JESSEE STRANGE, A.B.

Administrative Assistant, Department of Medicine,
Emory University School of Medicine, Atlanta, Georgia

THE HEART

ARTERIES AND VEINS

Editors

J. WILLIS HURST, M.D.

Professor and Chairman, Department of Medicine,
Emory University School of Medicine, and
Chief of Medicine, Grady Memorial Hospital,
Atlanta, Georgia

R. BRUCE LOGUE, M.D.

Professor of Medicine,
Emory University School of Medicine, and
Chief of Medicine, Emory University Hospital,
Atlanta, Georgia

The Blakiston Division

McGRAW-HILL BOOK COMPANY

New York   Toronto   Sydney   London

THE HEART

To

our wives,

Nelie Wiley Hurst and Carolyne Clements Logue

and the many other people who have helped

in the creation of this book

CONTRIBUTORS

ARTHUR C. BEALL, Jr., M.D.
Assistant Professor, Cora & Webb Mading Department of Surgery, Baylor University College of Medicine, Houston, Texas

S. GILBERT BLOUNT, Jr., M.D.
Professor of Medicine, University of Colorado School of Medicine, Denver, Colorado

ALBERT N. BREST, M.D.
Head, Section of Vascular Diseases and Renology, and Associate Professor of Medicine, Department of Medicine, Hahnemann Medical College and Hospital, Philadelphia, Pennsylvania

DOROTHY BRINSFIELD, M.D.
Assistant Professor of Pediatrics, Emory University School of Medicine, Atlanta, Georgia

HOWARD B. BURCHELL, PH.D., M.D.
Consultant, Section of Medicine, Mayo Clinic; Professor of Medicine, Mayo Graduate School of Medicine, University of Minnesota, Rochester, Minnesota

J. SCOTT BUTTERWORTH, M.D.
Associate Professor of Medicine, New York University School of Medicine and Post-Graduate Medical School, New York, New York

B. WOODFIN COBBS, M.D.
Associate Professor of Medicine, Emory University School of Medicine, Atlanta, Georgia

ELIOT CORDAY, M.D.
Associate Clinical Professor of Medicine, University of California, Los Angeles, California

MICHAEL E. DE BAKEY, M.D.
Professor and Chairman, Cora & Webb Mading Department of Surgery, Baylor University College of Medicine, Houston, Texas

LEWIS DEXTER, M.D.
Clinical Professor of Medicine, Harvard Medical School; Physician, Peter Bent Brigham Hospital, Boston, Massachusetts

EDWARD R. DORNEY, M.D.
Associate Professor of Medicine, Emory University School of Medicine, Atlanta, Georgia

JOSEPH THEOBALD DOYLE, M.D.
Professor of Medicine and Head of the Sub-Department of Cardiovascular Medicine; Director, Cardiovascular Health Center, Albany Medical College, Albany, New York

JAMES W. DuSHANE, M.D.
Head of Section of Pediatrics, Mayo Clinic; Professor of Pediatrics, Graduate School of Medicine, University of Minnesota, Rochester, Minnesota

E. E. EDDLEMAN, Jr., M.D.
Professor of Medicine, Medical College of Alabama; Associate Chief of Staff for Research and Education, Veterans Administration Hospital, Birmingham, Alabama

F. KATHRYN EDWARDS, M.D.
Associate Professor of Pediatrics, Emory University School of Medicine, Atlanta, Georgia

JESSE E. EDWARDS, M.D.
Director of Laboratories, The Charles T. Miller Hospital, St. Paul, Minnesota; Professor of Pathology, Graduate School, University of Minnesota, Minneapolis, Minnesota

ROBERT S. ELIOT, M.D.
Assistant Professor of Medicine, University of Minnesota School of Medicine, Minneapolis, Minnesota; Research Associate in Cardiovascular Pathology, Department of Pathology, The Charles T. Miller Hospital, St. Paul, Minnesota

E. HARVEY ESTES, Jr., M.D.
Professor of Medicine, Duke University Medical Center, Durham, North Carolina

NOBLE O. FOWLER, M.D.
Professor of Medicine, University of Cincinnati College of Medicine, Cincinnati, Ohio

ROBERT H. FRANCH, M.D.
Associate Professor of Medicine, Emory University School of Medicine, Atlanta, Georgia

JOHN T. GALAMBOS, M.D.
Associate Professor of Medicine, Emory University School of Medicine, Atlanta, Georgia

BRIT B. GAY, JR., M.D.
Associate Professor of Radiology, Emory University School of Medicine; Radiologist, Henrietta Egleston Hospital for Children, Atlanta, Georgia

PETER C. GAZES, M.D.
Associate Professor of Medicine (Cardiology), The Medical College of South Carolina, Charleston, South Carolina

RAY W. GIFFORD, JR., M.D.
Cleveland Clinic Foundation, Division of Medicine, Cleveland, Ohio

LEON I. GOLDBERG, PH.D., M.D.
Associate Professor of Medicine (Clinical Pharmacology) and Associate Professor of Pharmacology, Emory University School of Medicine, Atlanta, Georgia

RICHARD GORLIN, M.D.
Assistant Professor of Medicine, Harvard Medical School; Senior Associate in Medicine, Peter Bent Brigham Hospital, Boston, Massachusetts

ROBERT F. GROVER, PH.D., M.D.
Assistant Professor of Medicine, University of Colorado School of Medicine, Denver, Colorado

E. GARLAND HERNDON, JR., M.D.
Associate Professor of Medicine, Emory University School of Medicine, Atlanta, Georgia

J. WILLIS HURST, M.D.
Professor and Chairman, Department of Medicine, Emory University School of Medicine; Chief of Medicine, Grady Memorial Hospital, Atlanta, Georgia

THOMAS N. JAMES, M.D.
Chairman, Section of Cardiovascular Research, Henry Ford Hospital, Detroit, Michigan

HERBERT R. KARP, M.D.
Professor of Medicine (Neurology), Emory University School of Medicine, Atlanta, Georgia

JOHN W. KIRKLIN, M.D.
Chairman, General Surgical Sections, Mayo Clinic; Professor of Surgery, Mayo Foundation Graduate School, University of Minnesota, Rochester, Minnesota

TZU-WANG LANG, M.D.
Research Adjunct, Cedars of Lebanon Hospital, Los Angeles, California

R. BRUCE LOGUE, M.D.
Professor of Medicine, Emory University School of Medicine; Chief of Medicine, Emory University Hospital, Atlanta, Georgia

RICHARD P. LYNCH, M.D.
Associate Pathologist, The Charles T. Miller Hospital, St. Paul, Minnesota

MARVIN M. McCALL, M.D.
Charlotte Medical Clinic, Charlotte, North Carolina; formerly Instructor in Medicine, Emory University School of Medicine, and Chief Resident in Medicine, Grady Memorial Hospital, Atlanta, Georgia

THOMAS W. MATTINGLY, M.D.
Chairman, Department of Medicine and Cardiology, Washington Hospital Center, Washington, D.C.; formerly Chief of Medicine and Cardiology, Walter Reed General Hospital

JAMES METCALFE, M.D.
Professor of Medicine, Oregon Heart Association Chair of Cardiovascular Research, University of Oregon Medical School, Portland, Oregon

JOHN H. MOYER, M.D.
Professor and Chairman, Department of Medicine, Hahnemann Medical College and Hospital, Philadelphia, Pennsylvania

ROBERT E. OLSON, PH.D., M.D.
Professor of Biochemistry and Nutrition, Graduate School of Public Health; Lecturer in Medicine, School of Medicine, University of Pittsburgh, Pittsburgh, Pennsylvania

EDWARD S. ORGAIN, M.D.
Professor of Medicine, and Director, Cardiovascular Disease Service, Duke University Medical Center, Durham, North Carolina

LOREN F. PARMLEY, JR., M.D.
Colonel, Medical Corps, Department of the Army; Chief of Medicine, Walter Reed General Hospital, Washington, D.C.

E. ALAN PAULK, JR., M.D.
Georgia Heart Association Fellow in Cardiology, Department of Medicine, Emory University School of Medicine, Atlanta, Georgia

HERBERT D. PROCTOR, M.D.
Director of Medical Education, St. Mary's Hospital, Huntington, West Virginia; formerly Instructor in Medicine, Emory University School of Medicine, and Chief Resident in Medicine, Grady Memorial Hospital, Atlanta, Georgia

WILLIAM L. PROUDFIT, M.D.
Department of Cardiovascular Disease, Cleveland Clinic Foundation, Cleveland, Ohio

C. THORPE RAY, M.D.
Professor and Chairman, Department of Medicine, University of Missouri Medical Center, Columbia, Missouri

EDMUND H. REPPERT, M.D.
Assistant Professor of Medicine, and Director, Cardiac Catheterization Laboratory, University Hospital, New York University School of Medicine and Post-Graduate Medical School, New York, New York

ROYAL S. SCHAAF, M.D.
Associate Medical Director, Prudential Insurance Company of America, Newark, New Jersey

ROBERT C. SCHLANT, M.D.
Associate Professor of Medicine, Emory University School of Medicine; Director of Cardiac Research Laboratory, Grady Memorial Hospital, Atlanta, Georgia

THOMAS F. SELLERS, JR., M.D.
McAlister Professor and Chairman of Preventative Medicine and Community Health, Associate Professor of Medicine, Emory University School of Medicine, Atlanta, Georgia

WADE H. SHUFORD, M.D.
Associate Professor of Radiology, Emory University School of Medicine, Atlanta, Georgia

F. MASON SONES, JR., M.D.
Head, Department of Pediatric Cardiology and Cardiac Laboratory, Cleveland Clinic Foundation, Cleveland, Ohio

HOWARD B. SPRAGUE, M.D.
Past President, American Heart Association; Former Lecturer in Medicine, Harvard Medical School; Member of the Board of Consultation, Massachusetts General Hospital, Boston, Massachusetts

JOHN E. STEINHAUS, PH.D., M.D.
Professor and Chairman, Department of Anesthesiology, Emory University School of Medicine; Chief of Anesthesiology, Grady Memorial Hospital, Atlanta, Georgia

W. JAPE TAYLOR, M.D.
Professor of Medicine and Chief, Division of Cardiology, University of Florida Teaching Hospital and Clinics, Gainesville, Florida

ELBERT P. TUTTLE, JR., M.D.
Associate Professor of Medicine, Georgia Heart Association Chair of Cardiovascular Research, Emory University School of Medicine; Director of Renal Laboratory, Grady Memorial Hospital, Atlanta, Georgia

KENT UELAND, M.D.
Instructor, Department of Obstetrics and Gynecology, University of Washington School of Medicine, Seattle, Washington

ROBERT B. WALLACE, M.D.
Section of Surgery, Mayo Clinic, Rochester, Minnesota

JAMES V. WARREN, M.D.
Professor and Chairman, Department of Medicine, Ohio State University College of Medicine, Columbus, Ohio

WILLIAM C. WATERS III, M.D.
Assistant Professor of Medicine, Emory University School of Medicine, Atlanta, Georgia

H. STEPHEN WEENS, M.D.
Chairman, Department of Radiology, and Charles Howard Candler Professor of Radiology, Emory University School of Medicine; Chief of Radiology, Grady Memorial Hospital, Atlanta, Georgia

ARNOLD M. WEISSLER, M.D.
Associate Professor, Department of Medicine, Ohio State University College of Medicine, Columbus, Ohio

NANETTE KASS WENGER, M.D.
Assistant Professor of Medicine, Emory University School of Medicine; Director of Cardiac Clinic, Grady Memorial Hospital, Atlanta, Georgia

EDWIN O. WHEELER, M.D.
Clinical Associate in Medicine, Harvard Medical School; Associate Physician, Massachusetts General Hospital, Boston, Massachusetts

JOSEPH A. WILBER, M.D.
Clinical Assistant Professor of Medicine, Emory University School of Medicine, Atlanta, Georgia

A. CALHOUN WITHAM, M.D.
Professor of Medicine, and Chief, Division of Cardiology, Medical College of Georgia, Augusta, Georgia

J. EDWIN WOOD, M.D.
Professor of Medicine, Virginia Heart Association Research Professor of Cardiology, University of Virginia School of Medicine, Charlottesville, Virginia

PREFACE

As long ago as 1955 it was obvious that the discipline of cardiology, the largest subspecialty of medicine, was growing so rapidly that to prepare a book authored by one or two average men would be a very difficult task. *Medical giants such as Paul D. White, M.D., Samuel Levine, M.D., Charles Friedberg, M.D., and Paul Wood, M.D. are few in number.* (The debt the medical profession owes these men for their contribution is enormous.) Accordingly, it was obvious that we would need the help of many contributing authors. We then faced the problem of how to proceed.

It was 5 years after the original idea that the form and general content of the book were finally crystallized. First, the objectives of the book had to be clearly defined. The book would be as complete as possible and yet be contained within one volume; it would include discussions of the heart, arteries, and veins; the material in the book would encompass and blend the knowledge recently acquired in physiology, pathology, chemistry, and pharmacology with the practical matters of diagnosis and treatment. The book would be written for all who were interested in the field, including internists, cardiologists, pediatricians, cardiovascular surgeons, students, interns, and residents. Since we, the editors, are basically teachers and clinicians, we hoped to develop a book that had considerable communicative value. To do this we needed to include numerous illustrations, some of them in color. The bibliography and index would be extensive in order for the book to serve as a source of reference.

Secondly, the contributing authors would be carefully chosen. The editors, of course, have certain views regarding cardiovascular problems, and the object of a book created by us would be to express these views. The contributing authors were chosen because they generally agree in our views. In fact, many of the authors, through their writing and teaching, have taught us much that we know and believe. The contributors have had extensive experience in the field of heart disease and many have written books themselves. Thus, with the agreement of the contributing authors, the book was conceived and the period of gestation had begun.

Thirdly, after the manuscripts were written, they could not merely be compiled and stacked together to form the book. Each manuscript was carefully reviewed by the editors. There was frequent communication with the contributors in order to standardize the text, avoid confusion, prevent unnecessary repetition, and ensure completeness while striving for brevity. And so through the months the book grew and developed!

We thank each author for his contribution. This word of thanks is a mere token for his work, for as he gathered and wrote his material he gave not only of his knowledge, time, and effort but truly of himself. To each we are indebted.

The editors cannot type—we do not have time to attend to the details of keeping order—we are not artists or photographers or librarians. Accordingly, we wish to express our recognition of the genius of Ruth Strange, Administrative Assistant in the Department of Medicine, Emory University School of Medicine, who is able to get things done in an extraordinary fashion. The book would never have been completed had it not been for her. We express our thanks to those who did most of the typing of manuscripts—Nancy Bivins, Marie Sadler, Marie Corn, and Mary Kate Riha. We also express our appreciation for the work done by Miriam Caldwell, Trena Graf, Johanna Heath, Ellen Lynn, Catherine Macris, Alison Brown, Sally Lanford, Mae Hall, Anne Webb, Carol Miller, Allene Robbins, Marthelle Cherry, and all the other typists and secretaries who worked with the contributors. We are grateful to McClaren Johnson, Jr., M.D., Fellow in the Department of Medicine, Emory University, who conceived and executed many of the diagrams in the chapters written by Emory University faculty members; to Miss Kathleen Mackay, Medical Illustrator, who prepared some of the illustrations; to Mr. Joe Jackson and Mr. Bob Wynne, Medical Photographers at Emory University, and their staff who worked for countless hours in order to present the photographs in the best possible manner; and to the medical artists and photographers who helped each of the contributing authors. We thank Neil Kelley and Anne Alexander, Medical Librarians at Emory University, for their help with the bibliography.

The editors believe that the index of a book is

as important as the contents. Dr. Nanette Wenger worked for months in the preparation of a preliminary outline of an index. She was later joined by Dr. Robert C. Schlant and Polly Young who worked for 2 months to complete the indexing. Each contributing author was asked to indicate the portions of his material that should be indexed. This was then considered when the complete index was made. Each paragraph of the book was discussed in detail by the two physicians involved and the following questions were asked and answered: What has the paragraph contributed? How many possible ways could a reader look up and find this material? During the process of indexing we frequently insisted that some one *try* the index. It works!

We express our gratitude to the Blakiston Division of the McGraw-Hill Book Company. The publishers joined the editors and contributors in desiring the production of an excellent book. We wanted an extensive bibliography, and the publishers allowed us to have two—one at the end of a chapter specifically supporting the matter con-

tained in the body of the chapter and, in some instances, a second list giving selected references supplying additional information related to the subject material being considered. We wanted to use numerous illustrations. The publishers allowed this and even permitted us to have a number of these illustrations in color. Throughout the entire period—the conception and gestation of the book —the publishers exhibited faith in the project.

We have tried to give proper credit to everyone involved in the preparation of this book and to those authors and journals whose work has been reproduced. Despite our efforts to do this, some may have been overlooked. We will try to avoid this in the next edition.

At the time of delivery of the book we realize it is not perfect although we would like to have it so. We are determined to continue our efforts to improve it and to strive toward perfection. We will welcome the readers' help.

J. Willis Hurst, M.D., and R. Bruce Logue, M.D.

CONTENTS

Color Plates

PART I
General Considerations

1 GENETICS AND THE CARDIOVASCULAR SYSTEM

W. Jape Taylor, M.D.

Recent revelations of the molecular mechanisms by which like begets like have enveloped the field of genetics in an aura of excitement. The deductions of the structure of the ultimate genetic material, deoxyribonucleic acid (DNA), and of a portion of the triplet code of bases by which it transmits directions for protein synthesis to cytoplasmic ribosomes via messenger ribonucleic acid (RNA) have stimulated clinical interest in less basic and more directly applied aspects of inheritance.[1] The development of new techniques in cytogenetics has led to the recognition of gross chromosomal aberrations as a cause of disease and new understanding of such common entities as mongolism, thus providing a further impetus for a new look at clinical genetics.

Realizing that the total organism is the sum of genetic and environmental influences and their interactions, the author of this section will approach the topic primarily by emphasizing instances in which genetic determinants appear to have a major role. With full acknowledgment that a small portion of the total of congenital heart anomalies is caused solely by specific gene effects, emphasis will be put on this segment in the belief that just as small a sector is related to environmental teratogens alone. A similar statement may be made about all other types of heart disease. By examination of these relatively undiluted effects subsequent delineation of the more complex interrelationships between genetic and environmental effects may be simplified. If it can be demonstrated that a myocardium or pulmonary vascular bed or set of coronary arteries of specific genetic constitution becomes diseased under normal environmental stresses, it can hardly be doubted that genetic attributes may similarly govern responses to increased loads.

CONGENITAL HEART DISEASE

Evaluation of a possible genetic role in the etiology of congenital heart disease has been hampered by many factors. Deaths in early life have interrupted sequences in pedigree study, often at ages when the cardiac defect either was not recognized or was improperly diagnosed. Hospital records often contain inadequate family histories because physicians at large attach little significance to them. The stigma that some parents feel is associated with a congenital anomaly has compounded this problem so that several interviews are often required to obtain information of which the family is well aware. Finally, most investigators have grouped all forms of congenital heart disease as one; inherent in this approach is the possibility that lesions with a strong genetic tendency may be masked by others in which environmental teratogens are more important.

Despite the objection to consideration of all types of congenital heart disease as a single group, such studies have the advantage of allowing compilation of information from large numbers of patients. From such efforts, Polani and Campbell, who notably also have reported smaller groups of patients with specific lesions, have demonstrated that the incidence of congenital cardiac lesions in the siblings of patients with congenital heart defects is 2 per cent, which is twenty times the usual expectancy in the population which they were investigating.[2] Although this may be interpreted as due to a continuing effect of a teratogen, it is more likely to be an expression of a genetic defect. Lamy and his colleagues have reported the largest study of this type, involving 1,188 families, and have come to comparable conclusions in regard to incidence rates.[3] Most writers have commented that when multiple cases of congenital heart disease are found in one family, usually the defects are either identical or similar; Lamy is the major dissenter from this view. Consanguineous marriages have been found more frequently in the families with congenital heart disease as compared with a comparable controlled population. Although the medical literature is replete with the reports of multiple cases of congenital heart disease within a family, frequently the material is so limited that it does not submit to any genetic analysis. A more profitable approach has been presented by a few authors who have analyzed the family histories of a large group of patients with the same anomaly. In such a study Anderson determined that the incidence of patent ductus arteriosus in the later siblings of index patients with this entity had a 1.4 per cent incidence of this lesion and a 2 per cent risk of having some other type of congenital heart disease.[4] These findings are remarkably similar to those of investigators who have analyzed the pedigrees of children with diverse types of congenital heart disease.

It should be noted that in most large studies of this nature monozygotic twins have frequently not been concordant for congenital heart disease in that one member of these single-egg twins would have a cardiac anomaly and the other would be normal. This is evidence against a genetic factor in the causation of congenital heart disease. In this regard, it is of note that identical twin mongols have been reported in which only one of the twins was said to have congenital heart disease although the electrocardiogram was abnormal in the other.[5] Mongolism is a disease which involves an aberration of a whole block of genes during the meiotic process, and in this situation it cannot be denied that the congenital heart disease is of a genetic origin. Still, however, only one of this identical mongol twin pair had heart disease, indicating the importance of some additional factor. It is widely accepted that environment may determine the degree to which certain specific genetic disorders become manifest after birth, but both factors undoubtedly begin their interactions in utero. Fraser has demonstrated, for example, that in a strain of mice with a genetic propensity towards the development of cleft palate, the actual incidence can be modified upward by the administration of cortisone during pregnancy.[6] The incidence of this anomaly is also related to the fetal uterine position.[7] It is probable that the degree of expression of genes which govern embryonic development of cardiac as well as other tissues is influenced by the intrauterine environment. It should be mentioned that most studies in relationship to congenital anomalies in twins have reported inadequate information as to whether the twins were monochoriate or dichoriate monozygotic. Such information has a bearing on the interpretation of twin data in congenital anomalies since it is likely that inequities of fetal blood supply occur more often in monochoriate twins.

In recent years the occurrence of cardiovascular anomalies in certain inbred strains of animals has provided additional information on the genetics of such defects. Patterson has reviewed this evidence, as well as reported his experiences on the incidence of congenital heart disease in dogs.[8] Heart anomalies are more prevalent in purebred dogs than in mongrels, suggesting the possible importance of recessive genetic factors in the purebred strains. Subaortic stenosis is rarely seen in dogs except in boxers and German shepherds, indicating an even higher degree of genetic specificity.

Recessive Inheritance in Congenital Heart Disease

The increased incidence of congenital heart disease in siblings of affected patients without a striking increase of incidence in more distant kin is suggestive of a recessive genetic effect, but the proof that some trait is due to a recessive gene may be difficult. To be manifest to a significant degree a completely recessive gene must be the only genetic determinant of a specific effect. In the case of an autosomal recessive gene, an offspring usually receives the gene from each parent, who bears no overt evidence of the trait but is a heterozygous carrier. Quantitative divergences from normal can be detected in many of these heterozygotes and probably exist in all of them, but sufficiently precise methods of detection have not led to their definition. Classically, the occurrence of multiple affected members of a single generation with normal preceding and following generations has suggested recessive inheritance. If large groups are analyzed, the mathematic ratio of one homozygous recessive demonstrating the trait to three apparently normal individuals should be found. Numerous authors have emphasized, however, that in relatively small families, such as are now the rule in the United States and Europe, the number of isolated cases will outnumber those with a familial incidence. From a simple mathematic formulation Lenz has pointed out that 66 per cent of recessively determined cases will appear as single nonfamilial cases in families consisting equally of two or three children.[9]

Common ancestry obviously can increase the likelihood that recessive genes may be present in both marriage partners, and evaluation of consanguinity has been widely applied to the study of recessive inheritance. At the present this method is of limited value in the United States, where the incidence of consanguineous marriage is estimated at 0.05 per cent, and in most areas of the world where racial isolates are breaking up under a variety of social forces. Two diseased parents, whether related or not, must produce affected offspring, but this event is uncommon with relatively rare recessive genes or those producing severe illness. Special circumstances, such as albinism or deaf-mutism where the nature of the illness has tended to increase social contacts between affected individuals, have led to pedigrees with homozygous recessive parents producing diseased children. If recessive inheritance is responsible for many congenital cardiac lesions, the various forces which act to bring together patients who have survived surgery for such defects similarly may produce such matings.

On the basis of the increased familial incidence, a high rate of consanguineous marriages, and the occurrence of the defect in both members of monozygotic twins, Cockayne postulated that complete transposition of the viscera is inherited via a single autosomal recessive gene.[10] The study was based on an analysis of 115 cases; a high incidence of associated defects, including congenital heart disease, was noted. This mode of inheritance has been challenged by subsequent authors and accepted by others, but Cockayne's study remains, after 25 years, as one of the more authoritative comments on a specific congenital cardiac defect.

All the common congenital cardiac lesions and

most of the uncommon ones have been described in two or more siblings but not in such numbers as to have much relevance in considering the possible contribution of genetics to the causation of these lesions.

Dominant Inheritance of Atrial Septal Defect

If one considers that the reproductive capacities of patients with the more severe cardiac anomalies have been severely limited before the present era of surgery, it would seem unlikely that a dominant gene could be responsible for many of such lesions. On the other hand, a defect which is generally well tolerated through early adult life, such as the secundum type of atrial septal defect, theoretically could have this mode of inheritance.

Several kinships with atrial septal defects in multiple involved members have been reported. In general they have involved marriages between heterozygous individuals manifesting the defect and normal mates, with the production of approximately 50 per cent of patients with the disorder. Involved offspring have had at least one parent with an atrial septal defect, except in a few instances where incomplete expression of the gene may be present (possibly a patent foramen ovale). A representative pedigree, such as that published by Zuckerman et al.[11] (Fig. 1-1), does not indicate the proportion of atrial septal defects which are the result of genetic influence, but certainly it indicates that a gene which is transmitted in classical autosomal dominant fashion can result in this defect. In such a family one can state that the odds are 50:50 that further children from affected members will be involved, rather than using the less precise

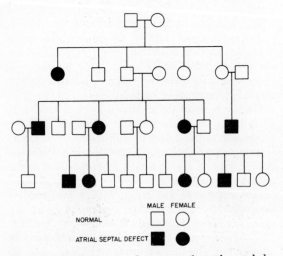

Fig. 1-1. The dominant inheritance of atrial septal defects in this family is demonstrated by its multiple occurrence in both sexes for three generations. (*Adapted from Zuckerman et al., Am. J. Cardiol.* 9:515, 1962.)

figure derived from studying groups of all types of congenital anomalies. In addition to those cases with a dominant type of inheritance, an increased rate of consanguinity in the ancestry of some patients with atrial septal defects led Campbell and Polani to postulate that recessive inheritance may be acting in these cases.[12]

Transmission of interventricular septal defect or patent ductus arteriosus through two or more generations has also been reported by several authors; other lesions have rarely been diagnosed in consecutive generations. These rare cases have not been present in most large surveys of congenital heart disease, indicating a lack of quantitative significance.

Chromosomal Aberrations

The remarkable process of meiosis, which appears deceptively simple, generally is successful in assuring that each ovum or sperm receives 22 autosomes and either the X or Y sex chromosome so that the fertilized egg contains its full complement of 44 autosomes and 2 sex chromosomes. However, the techniques of the past decade, which allowed Tjio and Levan in 1956 to determine that the correct human chromosome constitution is 46, have permitted the definition of a number of diseases as being due to abnormalities of chromosome distribution.[13] In relationship to cardiac disease, as well as historically, mongolism is the most important of these disorders.

The human chromosomes are classified generally into seven groups on the basis of their size and the position of the centromere, which appears as a constriction of the arms of the chromosome (Fig. 1-2). Only a matter of months after the determination of the correct human chromosome number it was demonstrated by Lejeune, Gautier, and Turpin that one of the smallest of the chromosomes appeared in triplicate in a patient with mongolism.[14] Ready availability of material from patients led to quick confirmation of this discovery in many laboratories, and a fruitful search was on for other conditions with gross chromosomal aberrations.

Two other syndromes of relatively frequent occurrence have been described in which a triplication of chromsomes (trisomy) is associated with cardiac defects as well as with a number of other malformations. In one of the entities, microphthalmia, cleft palate, polydactyly, hemangiomas, and ventricular septal defects are present; in the other, anomalies of the ear, micrognathia, deformities of the feet, spasticity, and intracardiac defects are seen[15] (Fig. 1-3). In general, abnormalities of the autosomes create widespread anomalies, but syndromes involving abnormalities of only the sex chromosomes have also appeared and are not

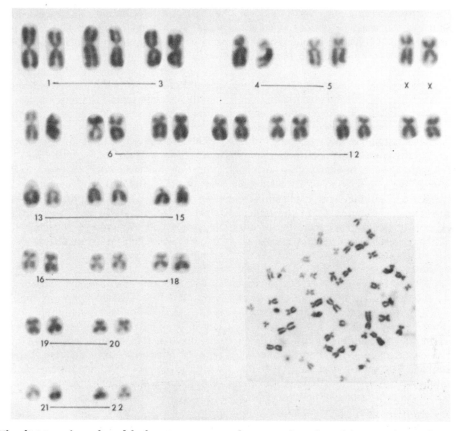

Fig. 1-2. The division of a cultured leukocyte was arrested in metaphase by colchicine. The application of a hypotonic solution and squashing leads to a spread of chromosomes such as this from a normal female; classification of the chromosomes is then possible. (*Courtesy of Dr. J. R. Green, Jr.*)

associated with such disastrous effects. In this group gonadal dysgenesis (Turner's syndrome) is of particular interest to the cardiologist; here the autosomes appear normal but only one sex chromo-some, an X, is present, giving a total complement of 45. The patient develops as a female without ovarian function, and with varying combinations of other defects, including webbing of the neck, hyper-

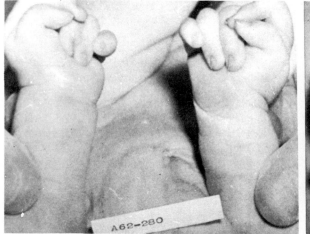

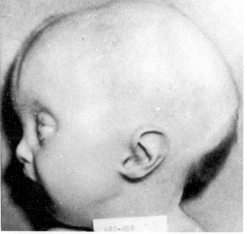

Fig. 1-3. The clinical diagnosis of a trisomy of chromosome 18 was made on the basis of the bizarre hand position, low-set ears, micrognathia, and patent ductus arteriosus. (*Courtesy of Dr. D. R. Shanklin.*)

telorism, an increased carrying angle of the elbows, and congenital heart disease (Fig. 1-4). Coarctation of the aorta is one of the more frequent cardiac associations in this entity but is by no means the only one.

The common denominator in the genesis of the above syndrome appears to be nondisjunction of a chromosome during meiosis. In this circumstance a gamete (either egg or sperm) may be formed which has two of a given chromosome while the other gamete formed in that particular meiotic division is devoid of this chromosome. In mongolism an egg containing two of the chromosome 21 is fertilized by a normal sperm, resulting in a triplication of this small acrocentric chromosome and the typical clinical syndrome. If fertilization occurs between a gamete which has been deprived of its sex chromosome by this process and a gamete with an X chromosome, the typical gonadal dysgenesis arises. It is felt that a more frequent occurrence of nondisjunction in the ovarian tissues of aging mothers accounts for the increasing incidence of mongolism in older mothers.

Reported families in which mongolism has been present for three or more generations could not readily be explained by such a disaster of gametogenesis. Subsequent observations have indicated that one parent of these mongol children has a translocation of chromosome 21 on to either chromosome 15 or another small chromosome.[16] Accordingly this parent is monosomic for chromosomes 15 and 21 and has an abnormal translocation chromosome for a total count of 45; however, the total genetic composition is normal, as is the carrier of this aberration in regard to phenotype. Half the children will end up with the equivalent of the trisomy of 21 and will be mongols if a gamete containing the abnormal chromosome as well as the normal chromosomes 15 and 21 becomes the fertilized zygote.

The frequency of congenital heart disease in mongolism is quite high, with most large series indicating its occurrence in approximately 50 per cent of mongol children. Although the figures have been variable, depending primarily on the mode of selecting patients, Berg and his coworkers reported that about 50 per cent of the congenital cardiac defects in mongolism are some type of endocardial cushion defect, while transposition, hypoplastic aorta, and coarctation were not found in their study of 131 autopsies.[17] It appears that the incidence of congenital heart disease is approximately the same in the translocation and trisomy types of mongolism, but it is regretable that the published papers to date have not been sufficiently specific about the type of heart disease which has been associated with the chromosomal aberrations in the specific cases to allow a definitive conclusion.

Syndromes with Distinctive Noncardiac Anomalies

In many well-defined syndromes anomalies at other sites may be clues to the diagnosis of congenital heart disease. The dominant inheritance of atrial septal defects with associated bony abnormalities of the upper extremities was traced through four generations by Holt and Oram.[18] The skeletal aberration, although moderately variable, usually consists of loss of apposition of the thumb which now lies in the same plane as the other fingers (or may be absent) and is so distinctive as automatically to suggest an associated atrial septal defect. The relationships are not always so clearly defined as in the Holt-Oram syndrome, but patients with congenital heart disease have a greatly increased incidence of defects outside the cardiovascular system. The comprehensive study by Lamy and coworkers reports that 17.9 per cent of patients with congenital heart disease have other anomalies, most commonly cleft palate, skeletal defects of the thorax or upper extremities, and angiomatosis, but encompassing a wide variety of lesions. A partial list of frequently coexisting malformations is presented in Table 1-1. These associated defects should strongly suggest the possibility of congenital cardiac anomalies and may be helpful in the differential diagnosis of known heart disease.

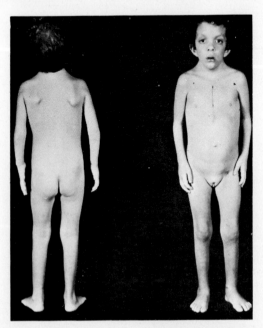

Fig. 1-4. Webbing of the neck and an increased carrying angle of the elbows led to the diagnosis of ovarian agenesis (Turner's syndrome) in this girl.

Table 1-1. ABNORMALITIES ASSOCIATED WITH CARDIOVASCULAR SYNDROMES

Syndrome	Usual cardiovascular anomaly	Associated abnormality
Holt-Oram	Atrial septal defect	Nonapposed or absent thumb and other upper-extremity defects
Ellis-van Creveld	Single atrium, ventricular septal defect (variable)	Chondroectodermal dysplasia and polydactylism
Horseshoe kidney[19]	Ventricular septal defect	Horseshoe kidney
Supravalvular aortic stenosis[20]	Supravalvular aortic stenosis, pulmonary artery stenosis	Hypertelorism, hypoplasia of mandibles, pouting lips, and mental retardation
Mongolism	Endocardial cushion defect (variable)	Skeletal and mental retardation and mongoloid facies
Turner's	Coarctation	Female with absent sexual maturation, web neck, and skeletal changes
Trisomy syndromes	Ventricular septal defect, patent ductus arteriosus (variable)	Multiple: micrognathia, harelip, polydactylism flexion of fingers, and neurologic defects
Marfan's	Aortic insufficiency (variable)	Arachnodactyly, kyphoscoliosis, and subluxation of lens
Hurler's	Myocardiopathy, mitral valve deformity	Dwarfism, deafness, hepatosplenomegaly, and mental retardation
Ehlers-Danlos	Mitral regurgitation	Hyperelastic skin, hyperextensible joints, and friable connective tissue
Tuberous sclerosis	Rhabdomyoma	Adenoma sebaceum, epilepsy, and mental retardation
Rubella*	Patent ductus arteriosus	Microphthalmos, cataracts, deafness
Situs inversus	Dextrocardia with simple noncyanotic or complex cyanotic lesions	Bronchiectasis, variable skeletal and intestinal defects
Absent spleen[21]	Complex intracardiac lesions—single ventricle, single atrium	Absent spleen, partial situs inversus, organ symmetry, and multiple defects; changes in red-cell structure
Laurence-Moon-Biedl[22]	Variable	Obesity, mental retardation, retinitis pigmentosa, hypogonadism, and polydactylism

* See Fig. 1-5. The postrubella syndrome is in reality secondary to an environmental factor but is included here because of its distinctive noncardiac features. It is congenital but is not genetically determined.

MYOCARDIAL DISEASE

In recent years the genetics of a number of diseases with severe myocardial manifestations has been defined. Association with easily recognized neurologic or systemic syndromes, or a dominant type of inheritance has been the factor which facilitated recognition of these entities. Only in endocardial fibroelastosis, which is set apart by a distinctive clinical and pathologic picture, has it been

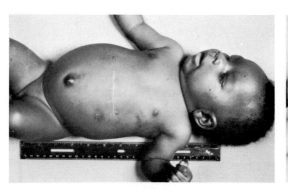
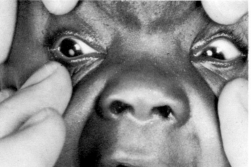

Fig. 1-5. Dense cataracts and microphthalmos are clearly seen in this infant with the postrubella syndrome. A patent ductus had been repaired because of heart failure in the first months of life. (*Courtesy of Dr. G. L. Schiebler.*)

possible to recognize a recessive inheritance of any disease in which cardiac muscle disturbance is the major defect. Many genes influence various facets of myocardial contractility either structurally or metabolically. The degree to which these polygenic effects may influence the myocardial responses to stress (hypertension, valvular heart disease, etc.) is unknown and will be difficult to determine.

Isolated Myocardiopathies

In the 15 years since Evans used the term *familial cardiomegaly* to describe the condition of a group of patients with severe manifestations of myocardial disease, a number of families and literally hundreds of patients have been described in whom the genetic transmission of myocardial disease can be demonstrated.[23]

A striking hemodynamic alteration aided in the recognition of one of these defects, at the same time leading to a variety of names ranging from "hypertrophic subaortic stenosis" to "obstructive cardiomyopathy." Brent and his colleagues outlined the genetic mechanism of this entity by demonstrating that it was inherited as an autosomal dominant trait in three generations of two families.[24] Although many isolated cases have been described, approximately one-half the known cases have occurred as familial cases. In any patient who presents clinically with aortic stenosis and a family history of cardiac disease, this entity is immediately suspect. The pitfalls of family histories can be emphasized by the fact that the matriarch of the kinship reported by Brent et al. was well aware that serious cardiac disease existed in her husband's family but the initial hospital record of the index patient mentioned only a brother who had died of "stroke" and a nephew who had been operated on for congenital heart disease.

Familial muscular subaortic stenosis may become manifest at any age and is probably progressive. The symptoms of syncope, angina, and sudden death are identical to those of aortic stenosis from any cause; congestive heart failure usually does not occur before angina or syncope but may be present and persist for a few years in some patients. Angiographic studies demonstrate that a massively hypertrophied interventricular septum and free wall of the left ventricle produce an obstruction to systolic emptying of the left ventricle after allowing a brisk initial ejection of blood into the aorta. A very characteristic pulse contour is produced by this combination of rapid initial ejection and subsequent obstruction. In some stages of the disease inotrophic stimuli, such as isopropyl norepinephrine (Isuprel), are necessary to induce this pressure gradient across the outflow tract of the left ventricle, which probably advances with age in an individual patient. The pathologic picture of this entity with its massive ventricular hypertrophy and little fibrosis or other change is quite distinctive (Fig. 1-6).

Other myocardial entities with symptoms punc-

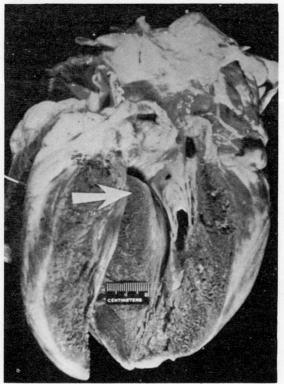

Fig. 1-6. A single syncopal episode had preceded the sudden death of the 55-year-old man whose heart demonstrates the extreme bulk of the left ventricular musculature which generally accompanies muscular subaortic stenosis. (*From Brent et al., Circulation,* **21**:167, 1960; *by permission of the American Heart Association, Inc.*)

tuated by syncope and sudden death appear to be inherited as autosomal dominant traits. Cardiac arrhythmias are prominent in this group of illnesses, and a characteristic hemodynamic derangement is absent. In one group of these patients vacuolization and glycogen deposits have been prominent in the myocardium; in another, diffuse fibrosis has been the major alteration.[25] Congestive heart failure is a major manifestation of both these groups, and some overlap appears between the two. Quite possibly the variations in pathologic findings represent different stages of the same disease rather than different diseases.

Isolated endocardial fibroelastosis has been considered by some investigators to be a genetic illness, but this has been hotly disputed by others. In contrast to the above myocardial syndromes, transmission from one generation to the next has not been reported. On the basis of multiple incidence in one generation of some families and of concordance in monozygotic twins, Rosahn postulated that isolated endocardial fibroelastosis is the result of a single autosomal recessive gene.[26] Similar observations have been made by other investigators and appear to support this concept. The biochemical mechanisms by which a genetic alteration results in the pathologic defect in fibroelastosis is unknown.

Neuromuscular Syndromes[27]

The muscular dystrophies produce cardiac disease by two mechanisms. Muscle weakness and accompanying thoracic deformity can result in ventilatory difficulties which are analogous to those of other types of kyphoscoloisis or the alveolar hypoventilation of the extremely obese subject. The typical syndrome of right ventricular failure can result from this pathophysiologic alteration. From the genetic standpoint the myocardial disease which is seen in many forms of muscular dystrophy is of more interest, representing as it does a single gene defect which in all likelihood induces a very localized biochemical disturbance of both peripheral and cardiac muscle metabolism or structure.

The Duchenne type of muscular dystrophy is characterized by its early age of onset, rapid progression, pseudohypertrophy, and incidence primarily in males with transmission by apparently healthy females. The latter feature is characteristic of a sex-linked recessive trait. In this type of genetic defect the phenotypically normal mother carries the abnormal recessive gene on one of her X chromosomes but does not manifest the disease because of the normal dominant gene on her other X chromosome. However, one-half her male prodigy receive the X chromosome bearing the mutant gene

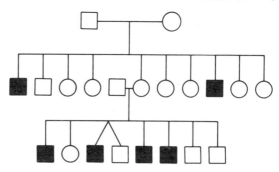

○ FEMALE

□ NORMAL MALE

■ DISEASED MALE

Fig. 1-7. The transmission of muscular dystrophy from healthy females to diseased males is demonstrated in this pedigree, which is characteristic of a sex-linked recessive disorder. (*Adapted from Walton and Nattrass, Brain,* **77**:169, 1954.)

and have the disorder since the only other sex chromosome is a Y which does not have the gene; the remaining male offspring are normal genetically as well as phenotypically (Fig. 1-7). This particular gene has a rather high mutation rate so that all patients do not have a family history but may appear as sporadic cases. Cardiac enlargement with varying degrees of heart failure due to atrophy and fibrosis of the myocardium are commonly seen in this disease.[28]

Myotonia dystrophia, in contrast, is inherited as an autosomal dominant trait with appearance in both sexes and with transmission through several consecutive generations since its onset is generally later. Cataracts, testicular atrophy, and baldness, as well as mental deficiency, combine with involvement of skeletal and cardiac muscle to aid in the recognition of patients with myotonia dystrophia. Rhythm disturbances are particularly common, with a high percentage of the patients having first-degree AV block.[29] Occasionally the electrocardiographic changes simulate myocardial infarction.

Cardiovascular involvement has long been recognized as part of Friedreich's ataxia, with the uncoordination which is a dominant neurologic feature of the illness leading to confusion with acute rheumatic fever. In a few families a dominant type of genetic grouping can be traced, but more frequently it is seen as an isolated disease within one sibship, suggesting an autosomal recessive inheritance. It appears that cardiovascular anomalies may be a part of the entity in either of the genetic varieties, although the literature is not entirely clear in this regard. The theories of the genesis of the cardiovascular involvement in Friedreich's ataxia are varied, ranging from considerations that it is a vascular disease with secondary cardiac involvement to the postulation that it is a cardiac myopathy. Boyer, Chisholm, and McKusick review the cardiovascular manifestations of this disease, as well as reporting cardiomegaly and electrocardiographic changes in 55 per cent of 33 patients with this disease whom they examined.[30]

Generally it has been stated that the other types of muscular dystrophy which may be classified according to their mode of inheritance (as either an autosomal dominant or a recessive trait), and myotonia congenita (an autosomal dominant characteristic) are not associated with cardiac manifestations. However, both clinical and pathologic evidence in this regard is scanty, and the issue should not be considered completely closed.

Conduction Defects

Rhythm disturbances have been reported in multiple members of certain families with sufficient frequency to suggest a genetic basis. In some pedigrees, such as that published by Combrink and his associates, bundle branch block or complete heart block appears to have been inherited as a Mendelian dominant because of the number of affected individuals in three generations.[31] More commonly multiple cases of complete heart block have appeared in a single generation.[32] Similarly the pre-excitation syndrome (Wolff-Parkinson-White) occurs in multiple family members in both single and subsequent generations.[33] Unfortunately in these situations detailed pathologic examinations of the conduction system have not been reported.

A familial incidence of tachycardias has been noted less frequently, but Gould reported a five-generation pedigree with 22 members in whom atrial fibrillation without other evidence of heart disease was well tolerated.[34] A similar suggestion of a dominant inheritance of nodal rhythm has been made by Bacos, Eagen, and Orgain[35] and of multifocal premature ventricular contractions by Böhn and Lampen.[36]

VASCULAR DISORDERS

Arteriosclerosis

Elucidation of a genetic contribution to the causation of a disease which is variable and late in its age of onset, and which is influenced by multiple environmental conditions, is a monumental task, for which available evidence remains inadequate. Environmental factors such as diet, emo-

tional tension, cigarette smoking, and exercise are undoubtedly important in the development of arteriosclerosis and its symptoms. Evidence for a familial concentration of arteriosclerotic patients is also available, despite the fact, as Schweitzer and his colleagues have pointed out, that good studies of the genetic factors in coronary artery disease have been few.[37]

Diabetes is the most important genetically determined known contribution to the incidence of arteriosclerosis. The concept that diabetes mellitus predisposes both to the severity of arteriosclerosis and to an earlier appearance in life is widely accepted, despite lack of knowledge of the exact mechanism by which these effects are mediated. A high incidence of diabetes in parents and siblings of diabetic patients and the degree of concordancy in monozygotic twins has led to agreement that a genetic predisposition of diabetes exists, but the type of inheritance has been the subject of much debate. The predominant view, as summarized excellently by Steinberg, is that diabetes mellitus is inherited via a single autosomal recessive gene.[38] Population genetic studies indicate that the frequency of this gene is in the neighborhood of 20 to 25 per cent, which corresponds to an incidence of diabetes in the general population of about 5 per cent. On a quantitative basis, this single autosomal recessive gene must be high on any etiologic list for arteriosclerosis.

Other clear-cut genetic diseases which lead to arteriosclerosis are familial hypercholesteremia and familial hyperlipemia. Familial hypercholesteremia is the more common of the two conditions and several large kinships with this disease have been reported. In addition to being characterized by elevated levels of serum cholesterol and β-lipoproteins, this entity consists of tendinous and tuberous xanthomas, xanthelasma, and arteriosclerosis. Disagreement exists as to whether this condition is inherited as a complete or incomplete dominant trait—i.e., whether the heterozygote and homozygote have identical manifestations. Wilkinson suggested that only the homozygotes have xanthomas whereas the heterozygotes have the remaining manifestations with a less severe degree of hypercholesteremia.[39] Piper and Orrild reported in 1956 on a follow-up of 12 Danish families which had been originally studied in 1948 and which present evidence that familial hypercholesteremia is transmitted as a complete dominant trait, with the xanthomas conditioned more by age and cholesterol levels than by degree of zygosity.[40]

A striking milky lactescence of serum, related primarily to elevated levels of neutral fats, is characteristic of familial hyperlipemia, in which abnormally high levels of low-density β-lipoproteins, and, to a lesser degree, cholesterol, are present also. In this entity xanthomas are more likely to be tuberous than tendinous, and a high association with diabetes and pancreatitis is seen. Evidence has been presented by Aldersberg that this, too, is transmitted as an autosomal dominant trait.[41] In some families which he described, members presented either hyperlipemia or hypercholesteremia, raising the possibility that these two disorders may represent variants of one. At any rate they both constitute clear-cut evidence of a genetic role in the origin of arteriosclerosis in some patients.

Pseudo-xanthoma elasticum is a genetic disease of connective tissue which predisposes to arteriosclerosis, providing further evidence that disturbances in lipid metabolism are not the only factors in this disease. Genetically determined differences in vessel branching or other anatomic characteristics likewise may be important, but data are inadequate for evaluation.

Systemic Hypertension

Since essential hypertension is diagnosed only after all known causes of an elevated blood pressure are excluded, it is likely that it does not represent a homogeneous population. However, evidence is accumulating that a major portion of this disease may be due to a single biochemical defect. The evidence for this concept is examined in Chap. 38.

Pheochromocytoma was one of the earliest recognized causes of elevated systemic blood pressure. This hormone-producing tumor may occur in association with neurofibromatosis, a disorder with well-known genetic transmission. As an isolated lesion it has been described in multiple members of several kinships, although the exact mode of inheritance is unclear because of lack of uniformity in these reported kinships.[42]

Hypertension is present in the rarest of the adrenogenital syndromes, in which the error appears to be an enzymatic defect in 11-hydroxylation of the steroid molecule. Many of the facets of this intriguing entity, seemingly inherited as an autosomal recessive characteristic, are discussed by Wilkins.[43]

Pulmonary Hypertension

Generally elevations of pressure in the lesser circulation are secondary to elevations of pulmonary venous pressure, left-to-right shunts with large increases in lung blood flow, or to alterations in the vascular bed due to intrinsic lung disease. However, the rise in pulmonary vascular resistance which causes this pulmonary hypertension is by no means uniform from individual to individual in response to apparently identical stimuli.

A genetic basis for primary, or essential, pulmonary hypertension, in which pulmonary vascular resistance becomes elevated without a known stimulus, suggests that the responses to an abnormal load may be governed, at least in part, by inheritance. This relatively infrequent illness has been reported in more than one member of a family many times. In one of the more recent reports the family Bible and old autopsy reports authenticated its presence in three nonconsanguineous generations studied by Melmon and Braunwald.[44] In this kinship the reactivity of the pulmonary vessels seems to have been related to a dominant gene.

Genetic disorders such as mucoviscidosis and a rare metabolic syndrome described by Rosenberg et al. may lead to elevations of pulmonary artery pressure and failure of the right side of the heart from repeated pulmonary infections.[45]

Familial Telangiectasia

Pulmonary arteriovenous fistulas are often a part of familial telangiectasia, a well-established dominant genetic disorder. The variable expression of this disease and its ramifications in many spheres of family life are described by Hodgson and co-workers in a six-generation survey of 91 afflicted members.[46] In this large kinship pulmonary arteriovenous fistulas were found in 15 per cent of the involved members. Cyanosis in a patient with lesions such as those demonstrated in Fig. 1-8 is sufficient to make this diagnosis.

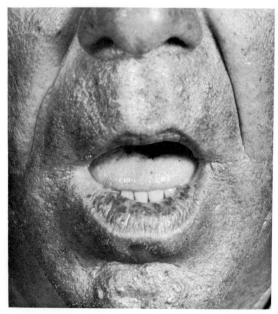

Fig. 1-8. The clue to the source of gastrointestinal bleeding in this man was provided by the clusters of characteristic telangectasia on the lips.

SYSTEMIC DISORDERS

Connective-tissue Disorders

The precise biochemical defects which lead to widely distributed inadequacies of these tissues have not been defined. It is likely that isolated biochemical errors in the formation of various types of connective tissue lead to the production of pathologic tissues, allowing these disorders to be fitted into the one gene–one enzyme (or protein) scheme. The entire group, including those in which cardiovascular manifestations are not prominent, is examined in detail by McKusick.[47]

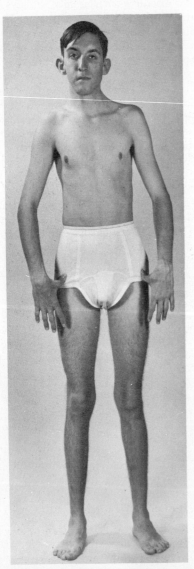

Fig. 1-9. Absence of subcutaneous tissue, frail muscular development, and scoliosis in this young man with aortic insufficiency and cleft palate are characteristic of Marfan's syndrome.

Marfan's syndrome is the best known of this group of disorders and is characterized, from the cardiovascular standpoint, by aortic dilatation and dissecting aneurysm. A variety of skeletal defects, related in part to lack of support by diseased ligaments and fascia, aids in the recognition of this syndrome (Fig. 1-9). A similar laxity of the suspensory ligaments of the lens is generally present and may be of varying severity, often producing subluxations or dislocations of this structure within the eye. Several pedigrees from a large number of involved patients are on record with involvement of a high percentage of members of both sexes for three or more generations. Although the severity of expression of the disease may vary even within the same family, sometimes leading to a lack of recognition of a mildly involved patient, the clearcut pattern of an autosomal dominant disorder is easily recognized, although sporadic cases are often seen.

Hurler's syndrome has been of particular interest because of the demonstration that patients with this heritable disorder excrete large quantities of mucopolysaccharides in their urine. Not only does this aid in the differential diagnosis, but it provides an area on which to focus research for the specific biochemical defect which leads to an overproduction of these chemicals. Considerable evidence points to two genetic forms of this disease, but clinical distinctions between the two have not been apparent. Skeletal deformity, growth retardation, hepatosplenomegaly, variable degrees of mental retardation, and cardiovascular abnormalities are seen in both varieties (Fig. 1-10). Heart failure is present in many patients with Hurler's syndrome. Pathologically a thickening of the intima of arteries of all dimensions has been described, as well as endocardial changes which are frequently associated with valvular deformity. An increased rate of consanguinity and involvement of multiple siblings from normal parents without regard to sex provide the typical features of autosomal recessive type of inheritance in the pedigrees of most patients. A lesser number of cases appears as a sex-linked recessive condition with the same genetic pattern as described above for muscular dystrophy.

Cardiovascular involvement is common in pseudoxanthoma elasticum, which is inherited as an autosomal recessive disorder. Thickening of the endocardium and the valves is occasionally seen in this disease and may lead to the presence of an opening snap on auscultation, although physiologic derangement of valve functioning ordinarily does not occur. The more dominant cardiovascular changes involve the peripheral arteries, where degeneration and calcification may occur prematurely and may lead to occlusive vascular disease.

In the autosomal dominant Ehlers-Danlos syndrome, heart disease is less clearly defined, although cardiomegaly and evidence of valvular insufficiency are occasionally seen. Generally the skin manifestations, which have led to the synonym of "rubber man syndrome," hyperextensibility of the joints, and friability of the gastrointestinal tract are more striking.

Diseases of the Immune Mechanism

Although the prime importance of an environmental factor, group A streptococcal infection, in the causation of rheumatic fever is unchallenged, considerable interest persists in the possible role of genetic susceptibility since only a small portion of persons with the appropriate streptococcal infection develop active rheumatic fever. Before the role of the streptococcus had been elucidated, a large number of studies of family groups was reported in an effort to support or deny some type of specific genetic framework for the disease. Although investigations such as those by Gould and Read demonstrate that the attack rate is higher among the siblings of rheumatic patients from rheumatic parents than in siblings of similarly affected children from nonrheumatic parents, it is not possible to fit the data into any specific genetic pattern.[48] Other evidence for a genetic background for rheumatic fever has been sought through an association with other genetically determined traits. Attempts have been made to correlate a susceptibility to the rheumatic diathesis with physical features, such as light reddish-blonde complexion, and, more objectively, with specific blood group antigens. Buckwalter and associates recently reported a mild increase in susceptibility to rheumatic fever in persons with blood groups A_1, A_2, A_1B, A_2B, while group O lends a degree of resistance to the disease.[49] Similarly it has been felt by Glynn, on the basis of extensive studies in rheumatic and nonrheumatic patients, that all rheumatic fever patients carry the nonsecretor gene which, in the homozygous state, inhibits the secretion of blood group substance A into the saliva.[50]

In the related rheumatic diseases such as systemic lupus erythematosus, polyarteritis, rheumatoid arthritis, and scleroderma, similar epidemiologic surveys have been applied in an attempt to assay the roles of genetic as well as environmental factors. In a study of the families of patients with systemic lupus erythematosus, Siegel and his coworkers found that 4.9 per cent of the immediate family members of the propositi had antinuclear antibodies while 3.5 per cent of them had false-positive serologic tests for syphilis; these contrast with figures of 0.7 per cent and 0 for the respective tests in the group of control families.[51] Blumberg

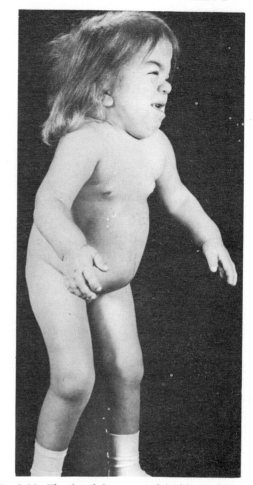

Fig. 1-10. The facial features and bodily configuration of this child are characteristic of Hurler's syndrome, a hereditary disease of mucopolysaccharide metabolism. (*Courtesy of Dr. L. J. Krovetz.*)

has reviewed the information regarding the possible role of genetics and the etiology of rheumatoid arthritis.[52] Most studies demonstrate an increased incidence of rheumatoid arthritis (including positive serologic tests) in the families of patients with this illness. Little other genetic information is available in this disease, and Blumberg is careful to point out that the data, although consistent with a genetic susceptibility, do not constitute proof of one.

Miscellaneous

Cardiovascular manifestations are found in a diverse group of illnesses which are related, in varying degrees, to genetic factors. These include the hemoglobinopathies, systemic amyloidosis, hemochromatosis, and tuberous sclerosis.

The genetically determined chronic hemolytic anemias frequently produce severe cardiomegaly

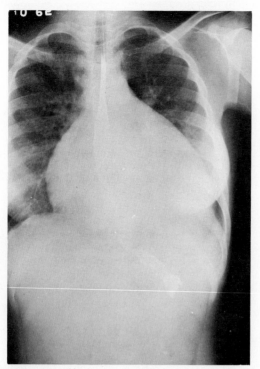

Fig. 1-11. A variety of murmurs may accompany the massive generalized cardiomegaly which frequently characterizes sickle-cell anemia, as in this 18-year-old girl.

and heart failure. Large increases in the iron storage of the body with deposits in the myocardium and the long-continued severe anemia may be factors in the production of cardiac disease (Fig. 1-11). No biochemical abnormalities of myocardial tissue, either in energy metabolism or protein structure, have been demonstrated.

The precise genetic defect in sickle-cell anemia has been defined at the biochemical level to a greater degree than any of the other defects which are discussed in this chapter.[53] The two alpha chains and the two beta chains of the adult hemoglobin molecule are under the control of separate genes. The mutant gene for sickle hemoglobin has been demonstrated to cause a substitution of valine for glutamic acid in the number four peptide of the beta chain of the hemoglobin molecule. The gene for hemoglobin C is an allele of those for hemoglobin S and A and results in another simple amino acid substitution. A codominant expression of the hemoglobin gene is seen, meaning that an individual who is heterozygous for the genes of hemoglobin A and hemoglobin S will produce both hemoglobins in almost equal quantities but is minimally symptomatic because of the protective presence of the hemoglobin A. Only in the homozygous

state when all the hemoglobin contains the abnormal beta chains with the valine substitution does sickle-cell anemia exist. This substitution of 2 in roughly 500 of the amino acids of the globin moiety of hemoglobin (1 in each beta chain) results in profound changes in hemoglobin solubility, which in turn produces the abnormally shaped erythrocytes and alterations in viscosity of these cells. These physiochemical changes produce effects on the cardiovascular system which are additive to those of iron deposition of severe anemia mentioned above and a tendency towards thrombosis which may result in pulmonary thrombi and occasional cor pulmonale as well as other occlusive vascular lesions.

In the thalassemia group of anemias no unique cardiovascular findings are observed, merely those common to all severe hemolytic anemias. In this group of illnesses increasing evidence is developing for the concept of a repressor gene action so that the rate of the synthesis of the hemoglobin polypeptide chains is altered.

In systemic amyloidosis cardiovascular manifestations may be the dominant feature of the illness in some patients. Often the cardiac findings mimic those of constrictive pericarditis, as in the 5 patients among 12 siblings of a family reported by Frederiksen and his coworkers.[54] In this family, evidence for an abnormality of serum globulins in members of the next generation was found. Depositions of amyloid tissues are often widespread in vascular structures throughout the body and undoubtedly contribute to the neuropathy, nephropathy, and retinal vascular changes which are seen in some of these patients. Sohar[55] has presented evidence that the amyloidosis associated with familial Mediterranean fever is inherited as an autosomal recessive disorder, but other studies, such as that by Frederiksen, appear to indicate a dominant type of inheritance. At the present time the precise biochemical defect which produces amyloidosis is not clear. The characteristic abnormal deposits of this disease may be the end result of different metabolic errors; this might explain the variations in clinical picture as well in genetic transmission. Although many cases of systemic amyloidosis appear not to have a familial incidence, in all instances thorough family studies are indicated until the exact role of genetic factors in this illness is better defined.

Hemochromatosis is another disorder of variable expression in which excess of iron deposits in the myocardium may lead to cardiomegaly and congestive heart failure. A number of studies, such as that by Frey and his fellow workers, have indicated that studies of serum-iron levels and liver biopsies may detect asymptomatic individuals with this illness.[56] From such studies these workers have demonstrated its occurrence in members of three generations of a family, which suggests an autosomal dominant type of inheritance. The role of genetics in this disease appears attractive, since it may well be related to a single enzymatic defect leading to excessive iron absorption from the gastrointestinal tract. Certainly there is sufficient evidence in this regard that family investigations are indicated in all such patients, even though reported familial cases are still in the minority.

Tuberous sclerosis is of note in regards to the cardiovascular system primarily because of its association with rhabdomyomas of the myocardium. Malformations of the brain, which led to the designation of tuberous sclerosis, result in the mental deficiency and epilepsy which characterize the illness. Adenoma sebaceum of the skin may appear earlier than the cardiovascular or neurologic manifestations, leading to its recognition quite early in life. From the genetic standpoint it is of some interest that the gene which is responsible for this entity must be associated with a relatively high mutation rate. The reproductive capacity of affected patients is retarded, and it would be expected to become extinct if it were not for the appearance of additional mutant genes since it is inherited as an autosomal dominant disorder.

REFERENCES

1. Crick, F. H. C.: On the Genetic Code, *Science,* **139**:461, 1963.
2. Polani, P. E., and Campbell, M.: An Aetiological Study of Congenital Heart Disease, *Ann. Human Genet.,* **19**:209, 1955.
3. Lamy, M., De Grouchy, J., and Schweisguth, O.: Genetic and Non-genetic Factors in the Etiology of Congenital Heart Disease: A Study of 1188 Cases, *Am. J. Human Genet.,* **9**:17, 1957.
4. Anderson, R. C.: Causative Factors Underlying Congenital Heart Malformations. I. Patent Ductus Arteriosus, *Pediatrics,* **14**:143, 1954.
5. Young, R. J.: Mongolism in Both of Monozygotic Twins, *Arch. Dis. Childhood,* **29**:55, 1954.
6. Fraser, F. C., Kalter, H., Walker, B. E., and Fainstat, T. D.: Symposium on Effects of Radiation and Other Deleterious Agents on Embryonic Development: The Experimental Production of Cleft Palate with Cortisone and Other Hormones, *J. Cell. & Comp. Physiol.,* **43**:237, 1954.
7. Trasler, D. G.: Influence of Uterine Site on Occurrence of Spontaneous Cleft Lip in Mice, *Science,* **132**:420, 1960.
8. Patterson, D. F.: Clinical and Epidemiological Studies of Congenital Heart Disease in the Dog, *Scientific Proceedings of the 100th Annual Meeting Am. Vet. Med. Assoc.,* 1963.
9. Lenz, W.: "Medical Genetics," The University of Chicago Press, Chicago, 1963.
10. Cockayne, E. A.: The Genetics of Transposition of the Viscera, *Quart. J. Med.,* **7**:479, 1938.
11. Zuckerman, H. S., Zuckerman, G. H., Mannen, R. E., and Wassermil, M.: Atrial Septal Defect: Familial Occurrence in Four Generations of One Family, *Am. J. Cardiol.,* **9**:515, 1962.
12. Campbell, M., and Polani, P. E.: Factors in the Aetiology of Atrial Septal Defect., *Brit. Heart J.,* **23**:477, 1961.
13. Tjio, J. H., and Levan, A.: The Chromosome Number of Man, *Hereditas,* **42**:1, 1956.
14. Lejeune, J., Gautier, M., and Turpin, R.: Etude des chromosomes somatiques de neuf enfants mongoliens, *Compt. Rend.,* **248**:1721, 1959.
15. Smith, D. W., Patau, K., Therman, E., and Inhorn, S. L.: A New Autosomal Trisomy Syndrome: Multiple Congenital Anomalies Caused by an Extra Chromosome, *J. Pediat.,* **57**:338, 1960.
16. Carter, C. O., Hamerton, J. L., Polani, P. E., Gunlap, A., and Weller, S. D. V.: Chromosome Translocation as a Cause of Familial Mongolism, *Lancet,* **2**:679, 1960.
17. Berg, J. M., Crome, L., and France, N. E.: Congenital Cardiac Malformations in Mongolism, *Brit. Heart J.,* **22**:331, 1960.
18. Holt, M., and Oram, S.: Familial Heart Disease with Skeletal Malformations, *Brit. Heart J.,* **22**:236, 1960.
19. Mehrizi, A.: Congenital Malformation of the Heart Associated with Congenital Anomalies of the Urinary Tract; Including a Syndrome of Ventricular Septal Defect, Pulmonary Hypertension, Mental Retardation, and Skeletal Deformity, *J. Pediat.,* **61**:582, 1962.
20. Beuren, A. J., Apitz, J., and Harmjanz, D.: Supravalvular Aortic Stenosis in Association with Mental Retardation and a Certain Facial Appearance, *Circulation,* **26**:1235, 1962.
21. Ruttenberg, H. D., Neufeld, H. N., Lucas, R. V., Jr., Carey, L. S., Adams, P., Jr., Anderson, R. C., and Edwards, J. E.: Syndrome of Congenital Cardiac Disease with Asplenia: Distinction from Other Forms of Congenital Cyanotic Cardiac Disease, *Am. J. Cardiol.,* **13**:387, 1964.
22. McLoughlin, T. G., Krovetz, L. J., and Schiebler, G.: Heart Disease in the Laurence-Moon-Biedl-Bardet Syndrome: A Review and a Report of Three Male Siblings, *J. Pediat.,* **65**:388, 1964.
23. Evans, W.: Familial Cardiomegaly, *Brit. Heart J.,* **11**:68, 1949.
24. Brent, L. B., Aburano, A., Fisher, D. L., Moran, T. J., Myers, J. D., and Taylor, W. J.: Familial Muscular Subaortic Stenosis: An Unrecognized Form of "Idiopathic Heart Disease" with Clinical and Autopsy Observations, *Circulation,* **21**:167, 1960.
25. Barry, M., and Hall, M.: Familial Cardiomyopathy. *Brit. Heart J.,* **24**:613, 1962.

26. Rosahn, P. D.: Endocardial Fibroelastosis: Old and New Concepts. *Bull. New York Acad. Med.,* 31:453, 1955.

27. Walton, J. W., and Nattrass, F. J.: On the Classification, Natural History and Treatment of the Myopathies, *Brain,* 77:169, 1954.

28. Levin, S., Baens, G. S., and Weinberg, T.: The Heart in Pseudohypertrophic Muscular Dystrophy, *J. Pediat.,* 55:460, 1959.

29. Fisch, C.: The Heart in Dystrophia Myotonica, *Am. Heart J.,* 41:525, 1962.

30. Boyer, S. H., IV, Chisholm, A. W., and McKusick, V. A.: Cardiac Aspects of Friedreich's Ataxia, *Circulation,* 25:493, 1962.

31. Combrink, J. M., Davis, W. H., and Suyman, H. W.: Familial Bundle Branch Block, *Am. Heart J.,* 64:397, 1962.

32. Lynch, R. J., and Engle, M. A.: Familial Congenital Complete Heart Block: Its Occurrence in Two Children with Another Genetically Determined Anomaly, *Am. J. Dis. Child.,* 102:210, 1961.

33. Westlake, R. E., Cohen, W., and Willis, W. H.: Wolff-Parkinson-White Syndrome and Familial Cardiomegaly, *Am. Heart J.,* 64:314, 1962.

34. Gould, W. L.: Auricular Fibrillation: Report on a Study of Familial Tendency, 1920–1956, *A.M.A. Arch. Int. Med.,* 100:916, 1957.

35. Bacos, J. M., Eagen, J. T., and Orgain, E. S.: Congenital Familial Nodal Rhythm, *Circulation,* 22:887, 1960.

36. Böhn, C., and Lampen, H.: Familial Disturbances of Heart Rhythm, *Deutsche med. Wchnschr.,* 87:876 1962.

37. Schweitzen, M. D., Clark, E. G., Gearing, F. R., and Perera, G. A.: Genetic Factors in Primary Hypertension and Coronary Artery Disease: A Reappraisal, *J. Chron. Dis.,* 15:1093, 1962.

38. Steinberg, A. G.: Heredity in Diabetes Mellitus, *Diabetes,* 10:269, 1961.

39. Wilkinson, C. F., Hand, E. A., and Fliegelman, M. T.: Essential Familial Hypercholesterolemia, *Ann. Int. Med.,* 29:671, 1948.

40. Piper, J., and Orrild, L.: Essential Familial Hypercholesterolemia and Xanthomatosis: Follow-up Study of Twelve Danish Families, *Am. J. Med.,* 21:34, 1956.

41. Aldersberg, D.: Inborn Errors of Lipid Metabolism: Clinical, Genetic, and Chemical Aspects, *A.M.A. Arch. Path.,* 60:481, 1955.

42. Carma, C. T., and Brashear, R. E.: Pheochromocytoma as an Inherited Abnormality, *New England J. Med.,* 263:419, 1960.

43. Wilkins, L.: Adrenal Disorders. II. Congenital Virilizing Adrenal Hyperplasia, *Arch. Dis. Childhood,* 37:231, 1962.

44. Melmon, K. L., and Braunwald, E.: Familial Pulmonary Hypertension, *New England J. Med.,* 269:770, 1963.

45. Rosenberg, L. E., Mueller, P. S., and Watkin, D. M.: A New Syndrome: Familial Growth Retardation, Renal Aminoaciduria and Cor Pulmonale. II. Investigation of Renal Function, Amino Acid Metabolism and Genetic Transmission, *Am. J. Med.,* 31:205, 1961.

46. Hodgson, C. H., Burchell, H. B., Good, C. A., II, and Clagett, O. T.: Hereditary Hemorrhagic Telangiectasia and Pulmonary Arteriovenous Fistula: Survey of a Large Family, *New England J. Med.,* 261:625, 1959.

47. McKusick, V. A.: "Heritable Disorders of Connective Tissue," The C. V. Mosby Company, St. Louis, 1960.

48. Gould, R. L., and Read, F. E. M.: Studies of Rheumatic Disease. III. Familial Association and Aggregation in Rheumatic Disease. *J. Clin. Invest.,* 19:393, 1940.

49. Buckwalter, J. A., Naifeh, G. S., and Aver, J. E.: Rheumatic Fever and the Blood Groups, *Brit. M. J.,* 2:1023, 1962.

50. Glynn, A. A., Glynn, L. E., and Holborow, E. J.: Secretion of Blood-group Substances in Rheumatic Fever: A Genetic Requirement for Susceptibility, *Brit. M. J.,* 2:266, 1959.

51. Siegel, M., Lee, S. L., Widelock, D., Reilly, E. B., Wise, G. J., Zingale, S. B., and Fuerst, H. T.: The Epidemiology of Systemic Lupus Erythematosus: Preliminary Results in New York City, *J. Chron. Dis.,* 15:131, 1962.

52. Blumberg, B. S.: Genetics and Rheumatoid Arthritis, *Arthritis & Rheumatism,* 3:178, 1960.

53. Ingram, V. A.: Biochemical Genetics at the Molecular Level, *Am. J. Med.,* 34:674, 1963.

54. Frederiksen, T., Gotzsche, H., Harloe, N., Kiser, W., and Mellemgaard, K.: Familial Primary Amyloidosis with Severe Amyloid Heart Disease, *Am. J. Med.,* 33:328, 1962.

55. Sohar, E., Prass, M., Heller, J., and Heller, H.: Genetics of Familial Mediterranean Fever (FMF): A Disorder with Recessive Inheritance in Non-Ashkenazi Jews and Armenians, *Arch. Int. Med.,* 107:529, 1961.

56. Frey, W. G., Milne, J., Johnson, G., and Ebaugh, F. G.: Management of Familial Hemochromatosis, *New England J. Med.,* 265:7, 1961.

2 NORMAL ANATOMY AND FUNCTION OF THE CARDIOVASCULAR SYSTEM

Robert C. Schlant, M.D.

The basic transport functions of the cardiovascular system are to provide oxygen and other nutrients to the cells of the body, to remove the metabolic waste products from the cells, and to carry substances such as hormones from one part of the body to another. This chapter provides an introduction to some of the mechanisms by which these ends are accomplished in the normal circulatory system.

FUNCTIONAL ANATOMY OF THE CARDIOVASCULAR SYSTEM

Ventricles

Most of the force for the circulation of the blood is produced by the left and right ventricles. The two ventricles share the common interventricular septum and many of the muscle bands which continue from one ventricle to the other. In the adult the left ventricle is larger and has an outer wall which is 8 to 12 mm thick; the outer wall of the right ventricle is usually 3 to 4 mm. The shape of the right ventricular cavity differs considerably from that of the left (Fig. 2-1). In the right side of the heart, the ventricular cavity is crescent-shaped and the pumping action of the right ventricle resembles that of a bellows pump. In contrast, the left ventricular cavity is more nearly spherical, and the pumping action resembles a rapid peristaltic squeezing or wringing out of the blood.

Atria

The atria are thin-walled structures which act as booster pumps for the ventricles. At rest, they contribute about 15 to 25 per cent of ventricular filling by their contraction, although they may double or even triple their contribution during tachycardia or extreme exertion. In addition, the atria may be considered as "reservoirs" for blood storage during ventricular systole. As a result, there is a large amount of blood available to flow into the ventricles at the onset of ventricular diastole. During normal contraction the thin, interlacing atrial muscle fibers reduce the size of the atria in all dimensions. The "valves" at the openings of the superior vena cava and of the coronary sinus into the right atrium are rudimentary and frequently incompetent. There are no definite valves at the openings of the four pulmonary veins into the left atrium; however, the left atrial musculature frequently forms sphincter valves around these openings which usually prevent significant back flow of blood into the pulmonary veins during left atrial systole but which allow the retrograde transmission of the left atrial pressure pulse.

Cardiac Valves

There are two important types of heart valves: semilunar and atrioventricular (Fig. 2-2). Both semilunar valves (aortic and pulmonic) are basically the same in design. Each semilunar valve consists of a fibrous valve ring at the base of a major arterial vessel (aorta and pulmonary artery) and three valve leaflets, each of which occupies approximately 120° of the closed valve orifice. Each valve leaflet is a thin, delicate structure with some thickening along the free edges of the leaflet and a small tendinous tubercle (*corpus Arantii*) at the midpoint of the free edge of each valve leaflet. In both the pulmonic and aortic valves there is a small recess (sinus of Valsalva) above each leaflet. These are much more prominent above the aortic valve, and the coronary arteries normally originate from two of these sinuses of the aortic valve.

The atrioventricular valves are of the same basic design. Each valve has an incompletely closed valve ring, or annulus, which is part of the fibrous skeleton of the heart. Most of the ventricular bands of muscle connect to the tricuspid or mitral valve rings, which become smaller during ventricular systole. The atrioventricular valve between the

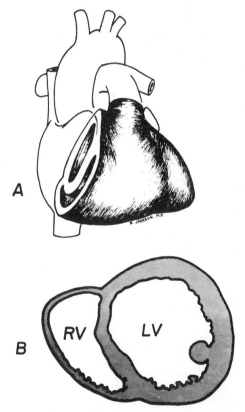

Fig. 2-1. Schematic drawing of the heart to illustrate the differences in shape of the right and left ventricles. In *A* the ventricles are shown in approximate anatomic position; *B* represents a cross section to illustrate the more nearly circular dimensions of the left ventricle.

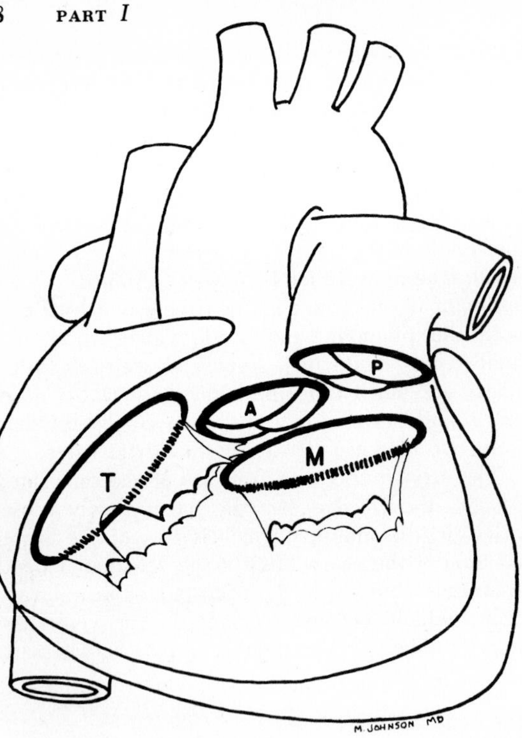

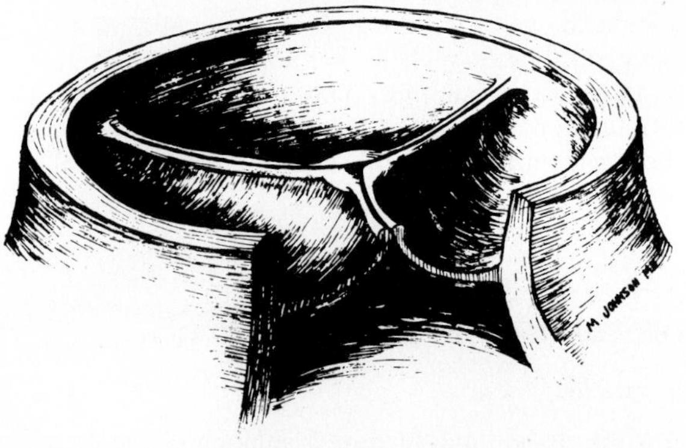

Cusps in closed position.

B

A

Fig. 2-2.*A.* Schematic drawing to illustrate the approximate positions of the two semilunar valves (aortic *A* and pulmonic *P*) and of the two atrioventricular valves (tricuspid *T* and mitral *M*) during ventricular diastole. The attachments of the AV valve leaflets to the chordae tendinae and papillary muscles are not shown. *B.* Drawing of semilunar valve in the closed position illustrating the thickening along the edges of the valve cusps and the thickening (*corpus Arantii*) at the center of the free margin of each cusp. The recesses above each valve are the *sinuses of Valsalva*. In the aortic valve the right and left coronary arteries originate from two of the sinuses of Valsalva.

right atrium and ventricle consists of three valve leaflets, or cusps, and is named the *tricuspid valve*. The *mitral valve* between the left atrium and the left ventricle usually has two valve leaflets, of which the anteromedial is larger. In both the tricuspid and the mitral valve, the valve leaflets descend into the ventricular cavity somewhat in the form of a funnel. The edges of the valve leaflets are attached to *chordae tendinae,* which are connected to papillary muscles within the ventricles. Usually each valve leaflet is connected to more than one papillary muscle. These connections of the valve leaflets to the papillary muscles, which contract early in the sequence of ventricular systole, help to prevent regurgitation across the atrioventricular valves.

Conduction System

The normal pacemaker of the heart is the sinoatrial (SA) node, which is composed of specialized cells with the capability of rhythmic electrical excitation impulse formation (Fig. 2-3). It lies at the lateral margin of the junction of the superior vena cava and the right atrium and is about 2 cm long. In man it is uncertain whether the major conduction from the sinoatrial node to the atrioventricular node occurs through special conducting fibers or bands, or whether it occurs generally through the atrial musculature as such. The sinus node artery originates from the right coronary artery in 60 per cent of human beings and from the left circumflex artery in 40 per cent.

The atrioventricular (AV) node is located at the base of the interatrial septum just beneath and slightly anterior to the coronary sinus. The bundle of His is a continuation of the specialized conduction system from the AV node. It begins at the anterior margin of the AV node, crosses the junction of the interatrial and interventricular septums, and then passes along the inferior margin of the membranous portion of the interventricular septum. At about the level of the muscular portion of the interventricular septum it divides into two separate bundles which pass down the endocardial surface of each side of the septum toward the apex of the heart. On the left side, the main bundle usually divides into several branches; on the right side there is usually one main branch. These branches ramify in the subendocardium of both ventricles as the Purkinje system, which distributes the excitation throughout the subendocardium. Purkinje fibers pass from the endocardium more or less perpendicularly into the myocardium. As they penetrate, these fibers gradually lose their identity and merge in staining characteristics with those of the ordinary myocardial cells. The blood supply to the atrioventricular node and the initial portion of the bundle of His is from the posterior descending artery, which is a branch of the right coronary artery in approximately 90 per cent of human beings (see Chaps. 28 and 29).

Innervation of the Heart

Although the SA node, AV node, and specialized conduction system of the heart possess the inherent ability for spontaneous, rhythmic initiation of the cardiac excitation impulse, the autonomic nervous system has an important role in the regulation of the rate of impulse formation. In addition, the autonomic nervous system influences the rate of

spread of the excitation impulse and influences the contractility of both the atria and the ventricles. It is probable that sympathetic nerve fibers supply all areas of the atria and the ventricles whereas vagal nerve fibers are primarily found in the SA node, atrial muscle fibers, and the AV node and are insignificant in the ventricular conduction system or the ventricular myocardium.

The efferent sympathetic innervation of the heart originates in the upper thoracic spinal cord and reaches the heart via the *superior, middle,* and *inferior cervical ganglions,* from which come the *superior, middle,* and *inferior cardiac nerves* (Fig. 2-4). These nerves contribute to the cardiac plexus surrounding the root and arch of the aorta. The major areas to which the cardiac plexus sends fibers are the sinoatrial node, the atrioventricular node, and the main trunks of the right and left coronary arteries. The efferent parasympathetic innervation originates in the medulla oblongata and passes by way of the vagus nerves to join the sympathetic fibers in the cardiac plexus. The sympathetic fibers generally produce an acceleration of the rate of discharge in the sinoatrial node, a faster AV nodal

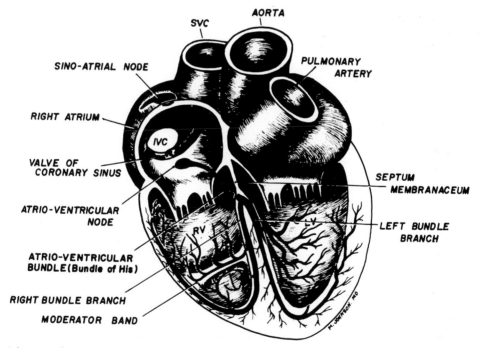

Fig. 2-3. Schematic drawing of the heart to illustrate the location of the major components of the conduction system in the heart. The impulse originates at the sinoatrial (SA) node near the orifice of the superior vena cava and spreads through the atria to the atrioventricular (AV) node. The impulse is carried from the AV node in the atrioventricular bundle (bundle of His), which penetrates the fibrous AV ring and runs in the posterior membranous septum, branching into the right and left bundle at this side or in the upper muscular septum. The right bundle is solitary in its course through the septum to the base of the moderator band; the left bundle subdivides into many branches. The terminations of each bundle form many fine fasciculi, intimately applied to the endocardium before merging with the contractile myocardium.

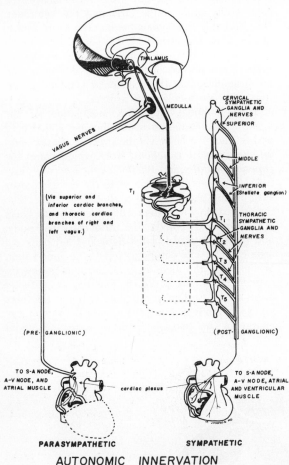

**AUTONOMIC INNERVATION
OF THE HEART**

Fig. 2-4. A simplified, diagrammatic representation of the efferent autonomic innervation of the heart. The parasympathetic and sympathetic nerves to the heart, many of which closely accompany each other in and through the various cardiac and coronary plexuses, have been separated for illustrative purposes. The parasympathetic innervation of the heart originates in the medulla and passes through the right and left vagus nerves. Two sets of cardiac nerves arise from each vagus nerve: the *superior* (superior and inferior cervical) *cardiac nerves,* which arise from the vagi in the neck, and the *inferior* (thoracic) *cardiac nerves,* which arise from either the vagus nerves or the recurrent branches of the vagi. The sympathetic innervation of the heart passes from the spinal cord to the upper four or five thoracic ganglions. Some fibers from the upper thoracic ganglions pass up the cervical sympathetic to the superior, middle, or inferior cervical ganglions. The *superior* (cervical), *middle* (cervical), and *inferior* (cervical) *cardiac nerves* originate from their respective ganglions and pass downward through the deep and superficial parts of the cardiac plexus to the heart. When the inferior cervical and first thoracic ganglions are fused together, the resulting ganglion is known as the *stellate ganglion.*

Additional cardiac branches arise from the upper four or five thoracic ganglions and pass to the cardiac plexuses or to the aorta. The cardiac and coronary plexuses are formed by cardiac branches from both the sympathetic and parasympathetic systems. Both sympathetic and parasympathetic fibers are thought to terminate in the SA node, AV node, and atrial muscle, whereas only the sympathetic fibers are thought to terminate in the ventricular muscle.

conduction, and an increase in the contractile force of both the atrial and ventricular musculature. Parasympathetic stimulation produces some cardiac slowing and has an inhibitory effect on atrioventricular conduction. Vagal stimulation decreases atrial contractility but has no significant direct effect on ventricular contractility.

Afferent impulses from the pain-sensitive areas in the pericardium, connective tissue, adventitia, and walls of the heart pass by peripheral sensory axons through sympathetic plexuses and through the lower two cervical and upper four thoracic sympathetic ganglions to thoracic dorsal ganglions where the cell bodies of the neurons are located. The impulses are carried by the central axon of this neuron through the dorsal roots to the posterior gray column of the spinal cord, where the fibers synapse with the second-order neuron. From this neuron, fibers cross the median plane, ascend in the ventral spinothalamic tract, and terminate in the posteroventral nucleus of the thalamus. Some afferent vagal ganglions have been found in the

left coronary artery system. Impulses passing through these neurons and ganglions are thought to be important in the Bezold-Jarisch reflex.

Pericardium

The heart is anchored in the mediastinum by the attachments of the pericardium superiorly to the pretracheal layer of the deep cervical fascia, anteriorly to the posterior surface of the sternum, and inferiorly to the diaphragm. The inner serous layer of the pericardium serves as a lining membrane for the outer fibrous layer and is normally in contact with the surface of the heart. In the pericardium, there is normally about 10 to 15 ml^3 of serous fluid, which functions as a lubricant. Acutely, the amount of distension of the pericardium which is possible is rather limited; under chronic conditions, however, the pericardium can be distended to great degrees without producing significant limitations to the diastolic filling of the ventricles. It is possible that the inability of the pericardium to dilate acutely may contribute to failure of the heart as a whole under conditions in which one chamber acutely dilates; however, the degree of such chamber dilatation would have to be extremely massive. In some patients with heart disease, particularly diffuse myocardial disease, the pericardium does act to prevent excessive dilatation of the cardiac chambers. In many instances, this is probably to the advantage of the heart.

Systemic Circulation

Aorta and Great Vessels

The origins of the aorta and pulmonary artery are similar in that they are both derived from the division of the embryonic truncus arteriosus. Although at birth the walls of these vessels are of approximately equal thickness, in adult life, the wall of the aorta is considerably thicker than that of the pulmonary artery. This is presumably a result of the decreased pulmonary artery pressure in the adult state. The aorta has many elastic fibers which allow it to function as a compression chamber or reservoir for blood during the rapid ejection from the left ventricle. The term *Windkessel* (the German word for the air compression chamber in water pumps which converts pulsatile flow to nearly continuous flow) is customary in the literature for this function.

Arteries

The systemic arteries originate from the aorta and its branches, and they branch successively to become individually smaller. As the total cross-sectional area of the arteries, arterioles, and capillaries increases, the average velocity of blood flow decreases. The arteries eventually branch into small arterioles, which have become identified as the major areas of resistance in the systemic circulation (Fig. 2-5). At the junction of the arterioles and the capillaries, there are often vascular sphincters for the local regulation of blood flow. In addition, there may be small vascular shunts between small arterioles and venules which are capable of shunting blood past the capillary bed.

Capillaries

The capillaries are small vessels, usually consisting of single endothelial cells. At times the capillaries seem capable of holding several red cells transversely; at other times the red cells appear to pass singly through the capillaries. In a given capillary bed, there is frequently a stasis of flow in some capillaries and at the same time there is an active flow in other capillaries. This periodic flow through different capillary beds is thought to have a normal physiologic function of increasing nutrition in these

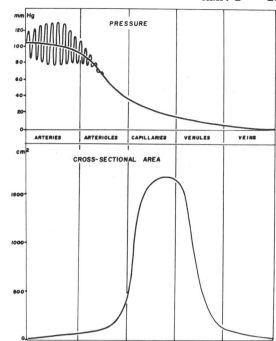

Fig. 2-5. Schematic illustration of the peripheral vascular system, showing that most of the fall in systemic pressure occurs at the level of the arterioles. Note that the systolic pressure is higher in the peripheral arteries than in the aorta near the heart. The large increase in cross-sectional area of the vascular bed at the level of the small arteries, capillaries, and venules is associated with a marked slowing of blood flow.

areas. Under conditions of maximal flow the entire capillary bed may be maximally dilated. Under normal flow conditions, there may be some gravitational layering of red cells, white cells, and plasma in the capillaries. Under certain conditions, such as acute stress, shock, or toxemia, or uncontrolled diabetes, there may be a sludging or congregation of red blood cells in the capillaries. The normal capillary pressure in the systemic circulation is estimated to be approximately 25 to 35 millimeters of mercury (mm Hg). In contrast, the normal pulmonary capillary pressure is 7 to 10 mm Hg. It is estimated that the systemic capillary bed, under basal resting conditions, has a volume of approximately 5 per cent of the total blood volume.

Veins

The veins of the body collect the blood from the capillaries and successively join one another to form progressively larger vessels which return the blood to the heart by way of the superior and inferior venae cavae. There is normally a slight pressure gradient between the systemic veins and the right atrium. In addition, the flow of blood returning to the heart is aided by the presence of valves in many of the larger veins, particularly those of the legs. This allows the muscular contraction of the arms and legs and the normal pressure changes in the thoracic and abdominal cavities to contribute to the return of blood to the heart. Since they are normally subjected to less pressure than arteries, veins are considerably thinner walled. Their pressure-volume characteristics are also significantly different from those of arteries. As a result, veins are capable of accommodating much larger volumes of blood with very slight changes in pressure. The veins, as well as the arteries, are capable of changing their pressure-volume characteristics in response to hormonal or neural stimulation. At times this change in venomotor "tone" enables the veins to increase the return of blood to the heart and to make available blood needed in other areas. In a sense, such shifts in the distribution of blood volume are a type of internal blood transfusion. At rest, about 50 to 65 per cent of the blood volume is located in the venous portions of the circulation.

Lymphatic Vessels

Although the cardiovacular system is sometimes considered to be a closed fluid system, there is a large volume of fluid with small amounts of protein filtered in the renal glomeruli and a considerable quantity of similar filtration through the systemic capillaries into the interstitial spaces.

Fluid and protein filtered from blood capillaries into the interstitial fluid must return to the heart either by way of the veins or by way of the lymphatic circulation. Generally, the smallest lymphatic vessels in the tissues are closed, permeable vessels similar to blood capillaries. The major terminal vessel of the lymphatic system is the *thoracic duct*. The thoracic duct usually terminates by joining the left brachiocephalic vein at the junction of the internal jugular and left subclavian veins. Occasionally, it may end in branches of the left brachiocephalic vein or may even subdivide into branches ending separately in various great veins. On the right side there are three major lymphatic vessels: the right jugular, right subclavian, and right mediastinal lymphatic ducts. Although they usually enter the right internal jugular, subclavian, and brachiocephalic veins respectively, occasionally the right jugular and right subclavian unite to form a *right lymphatic duct,* which usually enters the right brachiocephalic vein. The right mediastinal lymphatic vessel almost always enters the right brachiocephalic vein separately. The significance of other lymphaticovenous connections, such as those present in the abdomen, is uncertain at present.[1]

Some of the importance of the lymphatic system becomes apparent when one realizes that in 24 hr the thoracic duct alone returns to the circulation a volume of fluid about equal to the total plasma volume and contining 50 to 100 per cent of the total circulating plasma protein.

The importance of the myocardial lymphatic vessels in the maintenance of normal myocardial nutrition and in the response to injury of the heart, particularly the endocardium and heart valves, has recently been emphasized.[2,3] Undoubtedly, a more significant role will be shown for the lymphatic system in many other conditions, particularly pulmonary edema[4,5] and rheumatic and bacterial valvulitis.

Pulmonary Circulation

The basic function of the pulmonary circulation is the uptake of oxygen and the liberation of carbon dioxide by the blood. This function is efficiently accomplished by the pulmonary circuit, which normally carries all the cardiac output through the lungs at a pressure in the adult approximately one-sixth that of the systemic circulation. It is obvious, therefore, that its resistance to blood flow (the ratio of pressure difference across the pulmonary circuit to flow through the pulmonary circulation) is one-sixth that of the systemic circulation.

The pulmonary circulation differs from the systemic circulation in several important ways. The pulmonary arterial vessels have thinner walls and less medial muscle than their counterparts in the systemic circulation with the same luminal cross-sectional area. The main pulmonary artery, which in the fetus is histologically similar to the aorta, becomes much thinner walled than the aorta after birth. There is normally a conspicuous fragmentation of the elastic fibers in the pulmonary artery following birth, unless there is a congenital heart defect which allows pulmonary hypertension to persist. In general, the pulmonary circulation may be said to be relatively passive. In comparison with systemic vessels, its blood vessels in most instances react relatively less to neural, humoral, or pharmacologic agents. In some instances the reactions are opposite those produced in systemic vessels, e.g., arterial hypoxia and hypercapnia may both produce vasoconstriction in the pulmonary circulation, whereas in the systemic circulation their effect is generally vasodilatation. Although pulmonary vasoconstriction has been demonstrated experimentally to occur under autonomic nervous system stimulation and as a result of carotid sinus and carotid body reflexes, the importance of these mechanisms in the normal control of the pulmonary circulation is uncertain. Two mechanisms which help to maintain the normal relationship between pulmonary ventilation and blood flow in different areas of the lung are local regional vasoconstriction produced by alveolar hypoxia and local bronchoconstriction in underperfused areas, possibly produced by a lack of normal carbon dioxide concentration.

In the normal person at rest in the upright position, there is relatively little perfusion of the upper segments of the lung and consequently there is little exchange of oxygen and carbon dioxide in these areas. This pattern of blood flow is the result of the relatively low pulmonary artery pressure, which is barely adequate to perfuse the upper areas of the lungs. When an individual lies on one side, there is correspondingly a greater flow of blood to the dependent parts of the lung.

In contrast to systemic capillaries, which have a pressure of 25 to 35 mm Hg, the pulmonary capillaries at rest have a pressure of only 7 to 10 mm Hg. This is of distinct advantage, since pulmonary capillary pressure must be elevated to 25 to 30 mm Hg before pulmonary edema occurs if the serum proteins, capillary walls, and lymphatic drainage are normal ("pulmonary capillary reserve"). Actually, the net effect of the low pressure in the pulmonary capillaries combined with a normal oncotic pressure of blood causes the pulmonary circulation to keep the interstitial tissues of the lung in a relatively "dehydrated" state.

The total pulmonary blood volume is probably about 500 ml. As in the systemic circulation, about 50 to 65 per cent of this volume is on the venous side. Normal pulmonary capillary blood volume at rest is about 100 ml. The total surface area of the pulmonary capillaries is estimated to be 50 to 100 m^2.

The flow through the lungs of a normal person can increase about threefold before there is a significant increase in the required driving pressure, or pressure gradient, between the main pulmonary artery and the left atrium. This is usually attributed to the utilization of vascular channels not used at rest and to dilatation of other vessels. In the presence of pulmonary vascular disease or lung disease, this reserve may be markedly diminished.

Coronary Circulation

There is considerable variation among individuals in the anatomic pattern of their coronary arteries. This variability accounts for some of the diversity in the responses of patients to similar forms of heart disease. It is probable that genetic factors are important in determining the pattern of coronary arteries possessed by an individual.

There are normally two coronary ostiums. The *right coronary artery* arises from the sinus of Valsalva above the anterior cusp of the aortic valve, and the *left coronary artery* arises from the sinus of Valsalva above the left posterior cusp of the aortic valve. Not infrequently, there is a very small third coronary artery called the *conus artery*, which arises

separately from the aorta near the right coronary ostium and supplies a region of the pulmonary conus. The right coronary artery enters the right atrioventricular sulcus and curves to the right around the border of the heart. In more than 90 per cent of human hearts it gives rise to the *posterior descending coronary artery*. The right coronary artery also supplies the region of the pulmonary conus if there is no separate conus artery. In approximately 60 per cent of human beings, the right coronary artery supplies the artery to the sinoatrial node by a branch which comes off within the first few centimeters of the origin of the right coronary artery.

The left coronary artery varies from 5 to 30 mm in length and then divides into the *anterior descending coronary* and the *left circumflex* arteries. The anterior descending artery curves anteriorly around the base of the main pulmonary artery and enters the anterior interventricular sulcus. In about 80 per cent of subjects, it extends around the ventricular apex to ascend in the posterior interventricular sulcus to meet the end branches of the posterior descending coronary artery. The circumflex artery curves to the left in the atrioventricular sulcus and terminates as the *left marginal artery*. Rarely it continues as the *posterior descending artery*. The anterior descending coronary artery supplies most of the blood to the interventricular septum and supplies some branches to the right ventricle. In the posterior one-third of the interventricular septum, branches of the anterior descending coronary artery anastamose with branches from the posterior descending coronary artery. The terminal branches of the anterior descending coronary artery supply the posterior apical portions of both the right and left ventricles.

The left circumflex coronary artery supplies the anterior and lateral walls of the left ventricle, and, in approximately 40 per cent of human beings, a branch of either this artery or of the main left coronary artery supplies the sinoatrial node. In only approximately 10 per cent of human beings does the left circumflex coronary artery continue posteriorly to supply the atrioventricular node.

Approximately 75 to 80 per cent of coronary blood flow to the left ventricle occurs during diastole. This fact is particularly important in conditions such as tachycardia in which the total period of diastole per minute may be significantly curtailed. During systole there is relatively more coronary blood flow to the right ventricle than to the left ventricle; this is probably related to the lower intramyocardial systolic pressure of the right ventricle.

There are extensive anastamoses between the branches of the right and left coronary arteries and their branches throughout the normal heart. There is some evidence that normal hearts occasionally may have relatively large anatomic anastamoses; however, it is difficult to prove that all anatomic communications are able to function as collateral vessels.

SEQUENTIAL PHASES OF THE CARDIAC CYCLE

The successive mechanical events of the cardiac cycle may be described by a modification (Plate 1) of Wiggers's classical diagram, which divided the cardiac cycle into periods of systole and diastole and subdivided these periods into phases of cardiac activity. In the following discussion, the cardiac cycle is divided according to events on the left side of the heart. Corresponding periods and phases may also be described for events on the right side of the heart, with some differences (see below).

The first phase of ventricular systole is *isovolumetric contraction*. This phase begins with the first detectable rise in left ventricular pressure after the Z point; it is associated with the sound of mitral "closure" (MC) and the beginning of the isovolumetric contraction (IC) wave of the apex cardiogram. The end of the isovolumetric contraction phase and the beginning of the succeeding *rapid ventricular ejection* phase are indicated by the opening of the aortic valve (AO), a rise in aortic pressure, a decrease in ventricular volume, and the peak of the ejection (E) wave of the apex cardiogram. The onset and termination of the succeeding *reduced ventricular ejection* phase are less well defined. This phase may be said to begin when the shape of the ventricular volume curve indicates a significant decrease in the rate of ejection. This normally occurs prior to the peak systolic pressure in the left ventricle and aorta. The phase of reduced ejection lasts until actual ejection from the ventricle ends at the beginning of diastole, just prior to the recording of the incisura on the aortic pressure tracing. The very brief initial phase of diastole, referred to as *protodiastole*, represents the time required for the reversal of flow in the aorta and for closure of the aortic valve (AC), which is responsible for the incisura of the aortic pressure tracing. The beginning of the next phase of *isovolumetric relaxation* of the left ventricle is signified by the closure of the aortic valve (AC) and by an inward isovolumetric relaxation (IR) wave of the apex cardiogram. This phase lasts until the left ventricular pressure falls below the left atrial pressure and blood begins to flow into the ventricle. The left ventricular pressure usually falls below the left atrial pressure tracing slightly after the peak of the left atrial V wave, since there is a slight fall in left atrial pressure caused by a decrease in the upward bulging of the atrioventricular valve structures during ventricular isovolumetric relaxation. In a sense, this is the opposite of the mechanism thought to produce the C wave in the atrium during early ventricular systole. The end of the *isovolumetric relaxation* phase and the beginning of the *rapid ventricular filling* phase are indicated by an increase in the ventricular volume curve, by the O point of the apex cardiogram, and by opening of the mitral valve (MO). If the mitral valve is diseased, the opening of the valve may be audible as an "opening snap" (OS). The rapid ventricular filling phase is associated with a continuation of the decrease in atrial pressure (the Y descent) begun during isovolumetric relaxation, a rapid increase in ventricular volume, and an outward rapid-filling wave (RFW) in the apex cardiogram. The end of the *rapid ventricular filling phase* and the beginning of the *slow ventricular filling phase* are evidenced by a change in the slope of the ventricular volume curve, which indicates a change in the rate of ventricular filling. At times the end of rapid ventricular filling is associated with a valvular sound (S_3 or ventricular gallop), which occurs very shortly before the nadir of the Y descent of the atrial pressure tracing. The end of the rapid ventricular filling phase (and the identification of S_3) is indicated on the apex cardiogram at the moment when a change in slope, at times indicated by an F peak or wave, occurs at the transition from the rapid-filling wave (RFW) to the slow-filling wave (SFW).

During the period of slow ventricular filling phase, or diastasis, the pressures in the left atrium and left ventricle slowly increase until the next atrial systole produces the A wave in the left atrial pressure tracing. Atrial contraction and the increased ventricular filling produced by atrial contraction are reflected in an increase in ventricular pressure, an increase in ventricular volume, and an outward atrial A wave of the apex cardiogram. At the end of the atrial A wave there may be a sound (S_4) produced by the atrioventricular valve, particularly if there is a vigorous atrial contraction and relaxation. After the A wave of atrial contraction and relaxation, there is a very brief period or point (Z point) when atrial and ventricular pressures are essentially equal in normal individuals. The next cardiac cycle begins when the next ventricular contraction causes a definite sharp rise in pressure from the Z point.

Although contraction of the left ventricle begins prior to contraction of the right ventricle, the beginning of ejection of blood into the pulmonary artery slightly precedes ejection into the aorta,

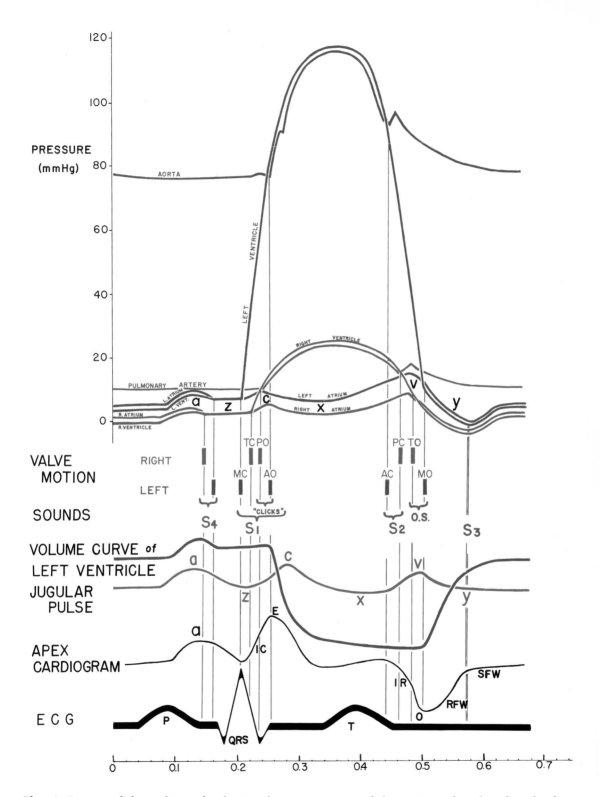

Plate 1. Diagram of the cardiac cycle, showing the pressure curves of the great vessels and cardiac chambers, valvular events and heart sounds, left ventricular volume curve, jugular pulse wave, apex cardiogram (Sanborn piezo crystal), and the electrocardiogram. For illustrative purposes, the time intervals between the valvular events have been modified and the Z point has been prolonged. Valve motion: *MC* and *MO*, mitral "closure" and opening; *TC* and *TO*, tricuspid "closure" and opening; *AC* and *AO*, aortic "closure" and opening; *PC* and *PO*, pulmonic "closure" and opening; *O.S.*, opening snap of atrioventricular valve(s). Apex cardiogram: *IC*, isovolumetric contraction wave; *IR*, isovolumetric relaxation wave; *O*, opening of mitral valve; *RFW*, rapid-filling wave; *SFW*, slow-filling wave. See text for details.

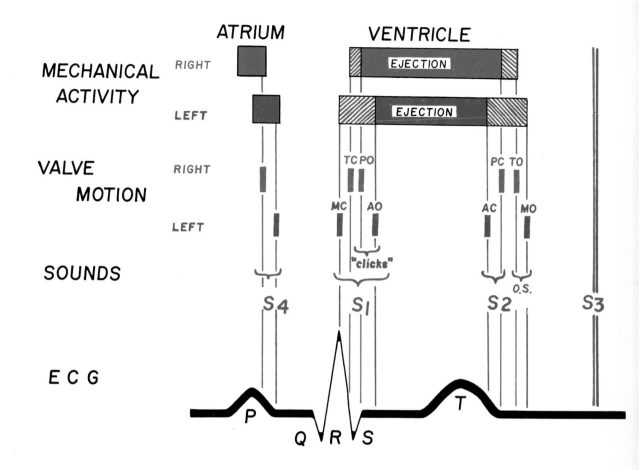

Plate 2. Schematic presentation of the relationship between electrical and mechanical events and heart sounds. The sequence and duration of mechanical activity is indicated for each chamber. The periods of isovolumetric contraction and isovolumetric relaxation are indicated for each ventricle. Valve motion is depicted, indicating the order of events: *MC*, mitral "closure"; *TC*, tricuspid "closure"; *PO*, pulmonic opening; *AO*, aortic opening; *AC*, aortic "closure"; *PC*, pulmonic "closure"; *TO*, tricuspid opening; and *MO*, mitral opening.

Although the sounds produced by the opening of the cardiac valves are normally not audible, in disease states the opening of the tricuspid or mitral valve may produce an "opening snap," and tensing and opening of the aortic and pulmonic valves may produce some ejection "clicks" or sounds analogous to the opening snaps of the AV valves. The sound occurring at the end of the rapid-filling phase of the ventricle is referred to as a ventricular filling sound (S_3) or ventricular gallop; it is produced by the atrioventricular valve of the involved ventricle. Similarly, the atrial gallop (S_4) sound at the end of atrial systole is probably produced by the atrioventricular valve of the involved ventricle. The principal components of the first heart sound (S_1) are produced by acute tensing of the mitral and tricuspid valve structures. Actual hemodynamic or functional closure of heart valves may at times occur very slightly prior to the production of "closure."

since the pressure in the right ventricle does not have to increase to such a high level before ejection begins. (Plate 2). In contrast, right ventricular ejection lasts beyond left ventricular ejection, producing the normal interval between aortic valve closure (A_2) and pulmonic valve closure (P_2). The shorter period of ejection of the left ventricle is also related to the greater contractile force of the left ventricle and to the differences in the compression-chamber effect of the aorta and the pulmonary artery. Contraction of the right atrium and opening of the tricuspid valve occur slightly before the corresponding events on the left side.

THE ARTERIAL PULSE

The arterial pressure pulse is produced by the ejection of blood from the left ventricle into the aorta and great vessels at a rate faster than its run-off into the peripheral circulation. In man, an average left ventricular stroke volume of 60 to 100 ml is ejected in about 0.25 sec, and of this volume approximately two-thirds is ejected during the rapid ejection phase. Although the highest rate of ejection of blood occurs prior to the peak pressure in the left ventricle or aorta, the pressure continues to rise in the aorta as long as blood is ejected into

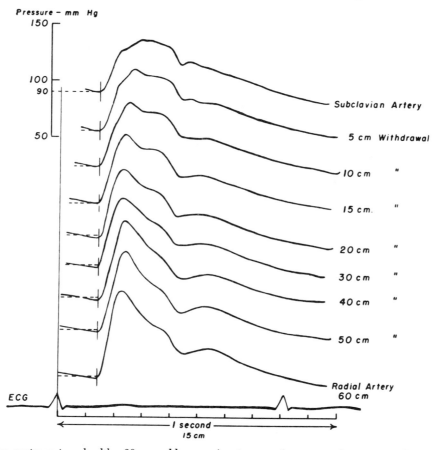

Fig. 2-6. Pulse contours in a healthy 30-year-old man, showing transformation of pressure pulse in subclavian-radial system. Pressure pulses were recorded consecutively during withdrawal of tip of arterial catheter from sub-clavian artery near aorta to radial artery in left arm. Onsets of pressure pulses are aligned for purposes of comparison. As pulse wave moves peripherally, initial wave steepens and increases in magnitude, dome-shaped systolic maximum becomes peaked, and dicrotic halt moves down and to right and becomes slurred. Low-amplitude, central postdicrotic wave is not seen after catheter has been withdrawn 10 cm or more. Prominence of radial dicrotic wave is due, in part, to change in position of dicrotic halt. Horizontal broken line intersecting onset of each pulse contour is calibration reference point (90 mm Hg). Interval of time from peak of R wave of electrocardiogram to onset of systolic upswing of each pulse wave is indicated by duration of each tracing to left side of short vertical lines, which mark onset of systole for each pulse. (*From H. W. Marshall, H. F. Helmholz, Jr., and E. H. Wood, Physiologic Consequences of Congenital Heart Disease, in "Handbook of Physiology: Circulation," American Physiological Society, Washington, 1962, sec. 2, vol* **I**, *pp. 417–488.*)

the aorta faster than it runs off into the peripheral arteries. There is sometimes a slight notch in the central arterial pulse wave during or toward the end of the rapid ejection phase. This is referred to as the *anacrotic notch* or *shoulder;* it is accentuated in valvular aortic stenosis. At the end of ventricular ejection (and after the very brief phase of protodiastole) the aortic valve closes. In central aortic pressure tracings, this event is reflected by a sharp downward deflection on the descending limb of the pressure curve referred to as the *incisura,* which is followed by an upward deflection of the pressure tracing and a gradual fall during diastole. At times atrial contraction causes a slight positive deflection in central arterial tracings just prior to the onset of the main arterial pulse wave.

As the arterial pressure pulse wave passes to the periphery, there are very marked changes in its form (Fig. 2-6). As the pulse moves away from the heart, the initial upstroke of the pulse becomes steeper, there is normally no anacrotic pause on the ascending limb, and the systolic maximum becomes peaked and increased in magnitude. The *dicrotic notch,* or halt, which corresponds to the incisura recorded more centrally, tends to occur later and lower and to be smoother in contour than the incisura. The positive wave which follows the dicrotic notch is referred to as the *dicrotic wave* and is normally much more prominent than the slight upward deflection recorded centrally following the incisura. Although the systolic pressure increases as the wave moves to the periphery, the diastolic and mean arterial pressures decrease slightly. The major factors responsible for these changes in the arterial pulse contour are (1) distortion of the components of the pulse waves as they travel peripherally, (2) different rates of transmission of various components of the pulse wave, (3) amplification or distortion of different components of the pulse by standing or reflected waves, (4) differences in elastic behavior and in caliber of the arteries, and (5) conversion of some kinetic energy to hydrostatic energy.

THE VENOUS PULSE

The form of the venous pressure pulse is determined by the rate of return of the blood from the peripheral tissues into the venous segment, the pressure-volume characteristics of the segment of vein, the nature of the resistance to flow offered by the right atrium and ventricle at the different phases of the cardiac cycle, and, to a slight degree, by the tissues overlying the veins at the point of observation. Although the venous pressure pulse wave travels peripherally away from the heart

there is at the same time a venous flow of blood in the opposite direction toward the heart.

The *A wave* of the venous pressure pulse is related to contraction of the right atrium and is followed by the *Z point* immediately preceding ventricular systole. In the jugular venous pulse, the *C wave* is predominantly produced by the systolic impulse in the adjacent carotid artery. Following the C wave, there is a rapid venous inflow into the heart during the first part of ventricular systole. The descent of the tricuspid valve ring and the rapid inflow of blood to the heart during early ventricular systole produce a fall in the venous pulse called the *X descent.* As the inflow continues into the atria after the X descent, the pressure in the atria and in the veins builds up, producing the *V wave.* At the end of ventricular systole and after isovolumetric relaxation of the right ventricle and opening of the tricuspid valves, the venous system is in direct continuity from the large veins to the right atrium and to the right ventricle. The opening of the tricuspid valve shortly after or at the peak of the V wave produces the *Y descent* of the peripheral venous pulse wave. The venous pulse wave is somewhat damped when recorded externally, and even when recorded directly, the waves are usually less steep in rise and descent than the corresponding waves in the atria. This is in part because of the damping effect of the large veins, which can accommodate markedly different volumes of blood without a marked change in pressure.

NORMAL PRESSURES AND FLOW RATES IN THE CARDIOVASCULAR SYSTEM

In general, the pressures in the systemic arteries are about five or six times greater than in the pulmonary arteries, while the amount of blood flowing in each unit is essentially the same. The left ventricular output may be slightly greater than the right ventricular output because of the small amount of bronchial flow. In order to compare measurements between individuals of different sizes, measurements of flow and resistance are often expressed in terms of square meters of body-surface area, i.e., instead of comparing cardiac output in absolute number of liters per minute, the output of the heart is expressed as the *cardiac index,* in liters per minute per square meter of body-surface area. There is still a need for additional data to establish the limits of "normal" for vascular pressures and flow for all ages of "normal" individuals under conditions of rest, exercise, or emotional stress. Furthermore, some of the slight differences in normal values reported from different laboratories are related to the use of different methods of measure-

Table 2-1. HEMODYNAMIC VALUES OF
NORMAL RECUMBENT ADULTS

	Mean	Range
Cardiac index, L/min/m²	3.4	2.8–4.2
Arteriovenous oxygen difference,		
ml/L blood	38	30–48
Arterial saturation, %	98	94–100
Pressures,* mm Hg		
Brachial artery		
Systolic	130	90–140
Diastolic	70	60–90
Mean	85	70–105
Left ventricle		
Systolic	130	90–140
End-diastolic	7	4–12
Left atrium		
Maximum	13	6–20
Minimum	3	−2–+9
Mean	7	4–12
Pulmonary artery wedge		
("PC")		
Maximum	16	9–23
Minimum	6	1–12
Mean	9	6–15
Pulmonary artery		
Systolic	24	15–28
Diastolic	10	5–16
Mean	16	10–22
Right ventricle		
Systolic	24	15–28
End-diastolic	4	0–8
Right atrium		
Maximum	7	2–14
Minimum	2	−2–+6
Mean	4	−1–+8
Venae cavae		
Maximum	7	2–14
Minimum	5	0–8
Mean	6	1–10
Resistances, dyne-sec-cm⁻⁵		
Total systemic	1,150	900–1,400
Systemic arteriolar	850	600–900
Total pulmonary	200	150–250
Pulmonary arteriolar	70	45–120

* Base line for pressure measurements one-half of anteroposterior chest diameter.

ment or different base lines for measurement of pressure. Table 2-1 lists the mean and range of hemodynamic measurements for normal resting adults.

MECHANISMS OF CARDIAC RESERVE

The normal homeostatic mechanisms regulate cardiac output to meet the demands of the body and enable the heart to vary its output five- to six-fold. It is not possible to separate sharply those mechanisms by which the cardiovascular system is normally controlled and those mechanisms of *cardiac reserve* which the heart may utilize to meet increased demands on the normal heart and/or to maintain cardiac function in the presence of disease of the heart or circulatory system. It is true that many of these homeostatic and regulatory mechanisms act synergistically in the intact organism; others, such as the sympathetic and parasympathetic nervous control of the heart, are in a state of constantly varying balance. Although it is often possible to separate and even quantify the relative contribution of each mechanism in the experimental animal, it is at present difficult, if not impossible, to separate the possible mechanisms functioning at any one instant in an individual. Indeed, the demonstration of mechanisms during physiologic experiments indicates only potential mechanisms of reserve or control, not what actually happens in the intact organism. In the following discussion we will consider some of these mechanisms from the standpoint of their being utilized as forms of *cardiac reserve*, although many of these same mechanisms are utilized in the *normal circulatory regulation*.

The two basic mechanisms of cardiac reserve by which the heart or any other pulsatile pump can increase its minute output in the face of increased demands (or attempt to maintain output in the presence of myocardial disease) are (1) change in rate and (2) change in stroke volume.

Change in Rate

A change in pulse rate is one of the simplest and most effective ways of increasing cardiac output. It is probably the most important mechanism for effecting rapid changes in cardiac output, particularly in untrained individuals under conditions of moderately increased demands. An increase in heart rate by itself may increase cardiac output about threefold; however, above a certain rate (probably about 170 to 180 for most normal young individuals but lower in the presence of myocardial disease), cardiac output may actually begin to decrease with further increases in rate. This decrease is thought to be due to the shortening of the diastole, limiting the time for adequate filling of the ventricles and for coronary blood flow, which occurs predominantly during diastole, particularly in the left ventricle. Most changes in pulse rate are effected by decrease in vagal inhibition and/or by sympathetic stimulation of the sinoatrial pacemaker of the heart. In addition to increase in cardiac output produced by a change in pulse rate itself, there is evidence that an increase in pulse rate may in itself increase ventricular contractility (Bowditch effect). The latter response, which takes several beats to develop fully, has been referred to by Sarnoff and Mitchell [6] as a form of *homeometric autoregulation* (see p. 000).

Change in Stroke Volume

As indicated by Fig. 2-7, the ventricle may increase stroke volume by utilizing *systolic reserve volume* (i.e., greater emptying) or *diastolic reserve volume* (i.e., greater filling) or both. The various mechanisms by which these can be accomplished are complex and interrelated. There is still a large gap in current knowledge of these mechanisms and their interrelationships in both the normal and the diseased cardiovascular system. Undoubtedly, this will continue to be a fruitful area for investigation,

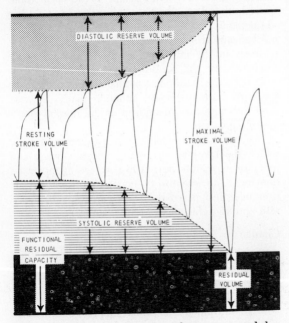

Fig. 2-7. Scheme of ventricular volume at rest and during exercise or sympathetic stimulation. The "systolic reserve volume" is that additional amount of blood which is not ejected under resting conditions but can be ejected with a more forceful contraction. This corresponds to the expiratory reserve volume of the lungs. The "diastolic reserve volume" defines the maximal amount of blood which the ventricle can receive and then eject in addition to the normal diastolic inflow. This volume corresponds to the inspiratory volume of the lungs. The "residual volume" is that volume remaining, in the ventricle after maximal ejection. The heart may increase stroke volume by utilizing either systolic or diastolic reserve volume or both, in addition to increases in heart rate. (*From G. A. Brecher and P. M. Galletti, Functionary Anatomy of Cardiac Pumping, in "Handbook of Physiology: Circulation," American Physiological Society, Washington, 1963, sec. 2, vol. II, pp. 759–798.*)

as it has for the past 200 years since Stephen Hales.

The Frank-Straub-Wiggers-Starling principle describes one of the most important characteristics of the heart. Since this principle is so important, a brief review of its development is warranted. In 1871 H. P. Bowditch[7] showed that if the condition of the heart muscle remains unaltered, contractions remain equal in strength, regardless of the strength of stimuli applied. This principle, which has become known as the "all-or-none" law of the heart, implies that cardiac muscle either does not contract at all or responds to the fullest extent, but that the magnitude of the all-or-none response is determined by the inherent "condition" of the muscle. In 1884 Howell and Donaldson[8] presented unequivocal evidence that the heart itself has intrinsic mechanisms by which the output of the heart is adjusted to the venous input. Using a heart-lung preparation, they found that increasing the venous return increased cardiac output and stroke output as well as right atrial pressure. In 1895 O. Frank[9] published his classic studies on "the dynamics of heart muscle." His object was to correlate the reactions of cardiac muscle with the responses of skeletal muscle, which had been previously shown by A. Fick, J. von Kries, and Blix to be related to the force of contraction and the initial length and tension. Frank studied the frog atria and ventricle and showed that, within limits, stepwise increases in diastolic volume and pressure just before contraction—the *presystolic* or *end-diastolic* volume and pressure—determine the magnitude of the all-or-none response. His studies emphasized the dependence of the cardiac response on hemodynamic events preceding excitation. In 1914 Wiggers[10] reported experiments which were the first to demonstrate that the reactions established by Frank for the frog's ventricle are also applicable to the naturally beating right ventricle of dogs. He concluded that the rate of isometric pressure rise and the peak systolic pressure are determined by changes in the initial tension, as long as marked changes in inherent contractility are not simultaneously produced by experimental procedures. Also in 1914 Straub[11] and Starling and associates[12,13] independently reported their studies of the effect of changes in initial tension and length on the response of isolated hearts. The studies of Starling and associates have received the greatest amount of attention in the English-speaking areas of the world, and the general principle is often referred to as *Starling's law of the heart.*[14] Starling and associates, on the basis of highly suggestive, but not quite conclusive, studies on the heart-lung preparation, concluded that "the mechanical energy set free on passage from the resting to the constricted state depends on the area of chemically active surfaces; i.e., on the length of the muscle fibers." Wiggers[15] has pointed out that although there is a general impression that the often reproduced representation of the law by Starling and associates was based on data from their own experiments, the careful reader will discover that the published curves were acknowledged to be reproductions of graphs previously published by Blix and by O. Frank. From the earlier studies of Frank, Straub, and Wiggers, it was not certain whether the responsiveness of the heart was fundamentally related to changes in presystolic pressure (initial tension) or to changes in volume (initial length). The conclusion by Starling that cardiac responsiveness was primarily related to presystolic fiber length has been validated by nearly all investigators. Wiggers[15] has emphasized the importance of other factors affecting the responsiveness of the myocardium and has stressed that the statement of the law of the heart, in which the energy of contraction is a function of the length of the muscle fiber, should be modified by the phrase "under equivalent states of responsiveness." Sarnoff and Berglund[16,17] have demonstrated this principle by showing that a "family of curves" exists for each ventricle and that many other factors, such as humoral agents, neural influences, and metabolic condition of the myocardium determine which particular "curve" the ventricle is operating on at a given moment. The studies of Braunwald and associates[18–21] have shown the applicability of the law of the heart in both the normal and the diseased heart.

Although the primary importance of initial fiber length rather than intraventricular pressure is now generally accepted, these two factors are usually, though not always, related to each other. Since it usually is not possible to measure initial fiber length in clinical studies, end-diastolic pressure is often measured in its place. It should be mentioned that it is also possible that the fundamental factor controlling the strength of muscular contraction is tension *within* the muscle fiber rather than fiber length per se.

An additional concept of importance in the application of the law of the heart to the ventricle as a whole concerns the sequence of ventricular activation and contraction. Since the ventricular myocardial fibers do contract sequentially, the strength of contraction of the later-contracting myocardial fibers is influenced by the strength and rate of contraction of the fibers which begin to contract earlier. Since one aspect of increased contractility is a faster rate of contraction, an increased contractility of the initially contracting fibers may, by increasing the end-diastolic fiber length or tension within the

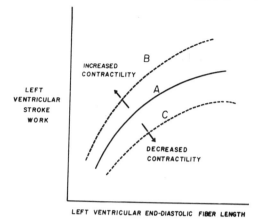

LEFT VENTRICULAR END-DIASTOLIC FIBER LENGTH

Fig. 2-8. Relationship between left ventricular end-diastolic fiber length and left ventricular stroke work. Curve A represents the normal function; curve B illustrates the "shift to the left" of the original curve associated with increased contractility, such as might result from sympathetic stimulation of the ventricle or the infusion of epinephrine or norepinephrine. Curve C represents a "shift to the right" of the original curve associated with decreased contractility, such as might result from ventricular failure from ischemia or myocardial depressant drugs. A ventricle functioning on curve C might be restored to curve A by the action of digitalis or inotropic drugs, such as levarterenol (norepinephrine) or epinephrine. Similar but not indentical curves are obtained when left ventricular stroke work is plotted against left ventricular end-diastolic pressure or volume, and in most instances, against left atrial mean pressure. "Function curves" such as these may be obtained for both ventricles and both atria.

myocardial fibers which have not yet begun to contract, directly increase the contractility of those fibers which contract later.

Starling's law, or principle, of the heart is probably the major mechanism by which the right and left ventricles maintain their minute outputs at equal rates of flow even though their stroke outputs may vary considerably. Thus, if the right ventricle temporarily pumps more blood into the pulmonary circulation than the left ventricle pumps into the systemic circulation, the proper balance between the two pumps is soon achieved, since the venous return to the left atrium and ventricle causes the left ventricular end-diastolic fiber length to be greater, increasing left ventricular stroke output. In addition, a decreased left ventricular stroke output would eventually lead to decreased return of blood to the right atrium and ventricle, producing a decrease in right ventricular stroke output. By this mechanism the two ventricles, which function as two pumps in series, are able to balance their outputs and prevent pulmonary edema despite marked variations in stroke volumes.

Figure 2-8 represents a schematic left ventricular "function curve" in which left ventricular work is plotted against left ventricular myocardial fiber length. Although similar curves may be obtained by plotting work against left ventricular end-diastolic pressure or left atrial mean pressure (which are more easily measured) or left ventricular volume (which is difficult to measure), the basic factor is probably fiber length or, possibly, tension within the myocardial fiber. Because end-diastolic fiber length and intraventricular pressure are normally related to each other, it is common in clinical situations to measure left ventricular end-diastolic pressure, since fiber length is difficult to determine in patients. In Fig. 2-8, curve A represents a hypothetical normal left ventricular pressure curve. Curve B represents a "shift to the left" of the function curve of the same ventricle under the influence of sympathetic stimulation or the infusion of epinephrine, norepinephrine, or any of numerous other catecholamines. Curve C represents a "shift to the right" of curve A, such as might occur with myocardial depression from hypoxia or cardiodepressant drugs or in myocardial "failure." Note that under normal conditions (curve A) very slight changes in fiber length, which can be produced by even smaller changes in filling pressure, are associated with significant increases in cardiac work. Sarnoff and Mitchell[6] have referred to this form of intrinsic autoregulation described by the Frank-Starling principle and such ventricular function curves as *heterometric autoregulation*, since they employ a change in initial fiber length. As mentioned above, it is one of the major mechanisms by which the two ventricles balance their outputs equally over any period of time even though their stroke outputs may vary considerably from beat to beat, particularly during the respiratory cycle. It should be emphasized that sympathetic stimulation may increase cardiac output, not only by producing an increase in pulse rate but also by increasing the contractile force of the atria and of the ventricles. The increase in ventricular contractile force produced by sympathetic stimulation may be shown graphically by a "shift to the left" of the ventricular function curve. Thus, sympathetic impulses can produce an increase in ventricular stroke work without the necessity of a change in end-diastolic fiber length or pressure.

The term *homeometric* ventricular autoregulation has been used by Sarnoff and Mitchell[6] in reference to the increased *myocardial contractility**° oc-

curring after an increase in ventricular activity such as that associated with an increase either in heart rate (Bowditch effect) or in aortic pressure (Anrep effect). Unlike heterometric autoregulation, which occurs immediately as a result of increased fiber length, homeometric autoregulation requires at least several beats to develop fully. It has been experimentally demonstrated that several seconds after acute increases in heart rate or aortic pressure are produced, the left ventricular end-diastolic pressure and fiber length may return to or toward the control values despite the increased work of the ventricle. It is thought that this occurs as a result of an increase in ventricular contractility during this period of time. The actual mechanisms by which *homeometric ventricular autoregulation* is accomplished are unknown; however, Sarnoff and Mitchell have noted its relationship to the ventricular *tension-time index* (area under the systolic portion of the curve per minute). They also suggested that tachycardia, by shortening the total period of diastole per minute, may allow less opportunity for "re-entry of potassium relative to efflux" and thus "lower the intracellular potassium in the new equilibrium state, a condition known to increase contractility." They further considered the possibility that increased ventricular activity (tension developed) either increases the locally available norepinephrine or facilitates its utilization during homeometric regulation. A particular advantage to the organism of homeometric autoregulation is the ability of the ventricle to eject the same stroke volume against a wide range of resistances without requiring an increase in ventricular end-diastolic pressure or fiber length.

When an increase in myocardial contractility is produced by an increase in heart rate, it is of particular advantage that the increase in myocardial contractility is associated with an increase in the rate of rise of ventricular pressure as well as an increase in the rate of ventricular relaxation. Both these effects shorten the relative proportion of the cardiac cycle occupied by each systole, while protecting the vital period of diastole during which ventricular filling and most coronary flow occur. If such a shortening of the duration of systole of

---

° The expression *myocardial contractility* is used according to the following definition of Sarnoff and Mitchell: "When, from any given end diastolic pressure or fiber length, the ventricle produces more external stroke work and more external stroke power (stroke work per systolic second) an increase in ventricular contractility is said to have taken place, and vice versa. Implicit in this definition is an increased rate of development of tension when contractility increases. Specifically excluded is any increased work that may be performed as the result of afterload from the same end diastolic length since the rate of development of tension is not increased under such circumstances prior to the application of the afterload." [6]

each beat did not occur with an increase in heart rate, tachycardia of even moderate degree would have profound effects on the total period of diastole available per minute.

An additional intrinsic mechanism by which the heart adjusts to increased return and to increased resistance is related to ventricular relaxation and diastole. When the heart contracts with greater contractility, not only is the contraction more forceful and more rapid, but the relaxation and elastic recoil of the ventricular musculature are also more rapid. This in itself tends to increase stroke volume and contractility in the next beat, since the diastolic filling period will be longer and since with the more rapid elastic recoil, the ventricular diastolic pressure will be lower earlier, and possibly lower absolutely, than it would otherwise be. Since flow into the ventricles is related to the pressure difference between atria and ventricle, any lowering of ventricular pressure will tend to increase ventricular filling. It is uncertain how much this mechanism, sometimes referred to as *diastolic suction*, plays in the normal cardiovascular control system.

When the ventricular stroke volume suddenly increases by the occurrence of a beat utilizing the systolic reserve volume, there is an additional intrinsic mechanism contributing to greater filling on the next beat. At the onset of ventricular filling

after such a beat the average ventricular fiber length will be shorter than otherwise because of the greater emptying of the ventricle. Accordingly, at the beginning of ventricular filling, the ventricle will have greater distensibility and will be able to fill with a greater volume at a lower filling pressure. Fig. 2-9B illustrates this important characteristic, by which very slight increases in venous pressure markedly increase fiber length when operating at this point on the ventricular pressure–fiber length curve.

A major extrinsic mechanism regulating myocardial performance consists of neural reflexes, particularly from the carotid sinus. When the pressure in the carotid sinus diminishes, there is a reflex decrease in venous distensibility, producing an increase in venous return and a resultant increase in ventricular end-diastolic fiber length with a subsequent increase in ventricular contractility. At the same time, carotid sinus hypotension produces a reflex increase in peripheral vascular (arteriolar) resistance, which may also increase ventricular contractility by the homeometric autoregulatory mechanism described above. Furthermore, carotid sinus hypotension elicits the *carotido-ventricular reflex*, by which the reflex sympathetic nerve stimulation of the ventricle produces an increase in contractility (a "shift to the left" in the ventricular function

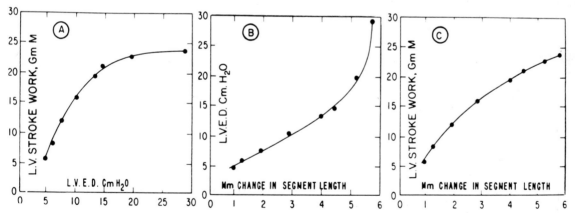

Fig. 2-9. Panel *A* shows the relation between left ventricular end-diastolic pressure and stroke work. Panel *B* shows the relation between left ventricular segment length and left ventricular end-diastolic pressure. Panel *C* shows the relation between changes in left ventricular segment length and stroke work. In Panel *A* it is apparent that large changes in ventricular stroke work are obtained without extensive changes in the pressure necessary to fill the ventricule or the pressure in the atrium and veins behind it when the ventricle is functioning on the initial steep portion of the curve, as it probably is normally during the various phases of the respiratory cycle. In curve *B* it is apparent that at low segment lengths, such as might occur after greater emptying of the ventricle, relatively large changes in fiber length are brought about by small pressure changes in the ventricle and hence in the atrium and veins behind it. In panel *C* it is apparent that there is a more nearly ·1:1 relationship than in the other panels. This supports the opinion that end-diastolic fiber length is the most appropriate factor in the analysis of ventricular function even though other values (e.g., end-diastolic pressure) are more readily determined experimentally. (*From S. J. Sarnoff and J. H. Mitchell, The Control of the Function of the Heart, in "Handbook of Physiology: Circulation," American Physiological Society, Washington, 1962, sec. 2, vol. I, pp. 489–532.*)

curve) and a slightly increased synchronicity of ventricular contraction, both of which result in a more complete emptying of the ventricle from a given ventricular end-diastolic fiber length or pressure. When the pressure in the carotid sinus decreases and the carotid sinus is less stretched, there is also a reflex increase in heart rate which occurs as the result of both increased sympathetic stimulation and decreased vagal inhibition of the SA pacemaker node. The release of catecholamines from the adrenal medulla as a result of emotions, exercise, or carotid sinus hypotension also produces a significant increase in both ventricular and atrial contractility. The release of catecholamines from the heart itself may also play a role in the regulation of peripheral vascular tone during periods of stress.

In addition to the above mechanisms, which primarily concern the ventricles, the atria have a significant role in the control of overall cardiac function. Like the ventricles, the atria possess a heterometric autoregulatory mechanism by which an increase in atrial end-diastolic pressure, volume, or fiber length produces an increase in atrial contractility and a "shift to the left" in their function curves. Not only does this cause an atrium to pump a greater amount of blood forward into the ventricle, but the resulting greater elongation of the end-diastolic fiber length of the ventricle in turn produces increased ventricular contractility. In addition, the atria are influenced by neural mechanisms which influence the pulse rate by varying degrees of vagal inhibition and sympathetic stimulation of the sinoatrial pacemaker node. Atrial contractility is directly influenced by the autonomic nervous system. Sympathetic stimulation increases whereas vagal stimulation decreases atrial contractility. Since both types of nerve fibers reach the atrial musculature, the net effect is the balance between the two opposing neural influences. At times an increase in atrial contractility may be produced by decreasing the inhibitory vagal influences on the atria. Thus, carotid sinus hypotension elicits the *carotido-sympatho-atrial reflex* and the *carotido-vago-atrial reflex,* both of which increase atrial contractility. In contrast, stimulation of the carotid sinus nerve, as might occur with carotid sinus hypertension, produces a depressant effect on the atria.

When the tissue requirements for oxygen increase, the tissues may, up to a point, extract more oxygen from each volume of blood passing through the tissue. This is a major mechanism of reserve utilized by the tissues of the body acutely during extreme exertion or chronically when the cardiac output is diminished. This reserve mechanism is of less value to the myocardium, which even normally extracts about two-thirds of the oxygen carried to it. Many tissues may also utilize anaerobic metabolism. In a normal individual during moderate exercise this may account for about 5 per cent of the energy utilized; patients with congestive failure may obtain 30 per cent of their immediate energy requirements by anaerobic metabolism during exercise.

Dilatation and hypertrophy may be considered forms of myocardial reserve, although they are also swords of Damocles for the heart. They are discussed in Chap. 11.

The normal person constantly utilizes the above mechanisms not only to maintain the average output of the two ventricles at the same level but also to help meet the changing total and local requirements for increased blood flow. Unfortunately, it is not possible to quantify the relative contributions of each mechanism in the intact human being. Not only are many of the variables difficult to measure, but most of the mechanisms are interrelated and affect one another, so that the contribution of any one mechanism depends upon and changes with the contribution of the other mechanisms. Despite these limitations and the dirth of additional studies upon normal individuals, it would appear that most "normal" individuals, at least in the present American culture, respond to mild or moderate exercise by increasing their cardiac output mainly by an increase in pulse rate rather than in stroke volume. With more extreme exercise even this type of individual will increase stroke volume. In normal persons who are more accustomed to physical exertion, there is perhaps an earlier increase in stroke volume. In trained athletes, the resting pulse rate is often slow and there may even be mild hypertrophy and dilatation of the heart as a consequence of the chronic increased work requirements upon the heart. There is no evidence that this "physiologic" hypertrophy is detrimental to the individual.

REGULATION OF REGIONAL BLOOD FLOW

The amount of blood flowing to an individual organ of the body is determined by the difference between the arterial and venous pressures in the vessels supplying the organ and by the vascular resistance of the organ. Although the arterial and venous pressures change in situations such as exercise, eating, or emotional stress, most of the alterations in the distribution of blood flow are the consequences of changes in vascular resistance of the organ.

The major mechanisms by which decreases in organ vascular resistance are effected are a increase in caliber of the vessels and an opening of new vascular channels. Since most of the vascular resistance appears to be located at the level of the small arteries and arterioles, it is probable that most of the regulation occurs by changes in caliber of these vessels, although changes in the capillaries and veins may at times play an important role.

In a consideration of the local control of blood flow, several fundamental relationships and definitions should first be introduced.

The *resistance* to blood flow through a given portion of the circulation is expressed by the ratio of pressure difference (gradient) between two points in the vascular system to the amount of blood passing from one point to the other. It is usually calculated using mean pressures and flows, although most vascular flow is pulsatile. If it were possible to measure instantaneous pressure gradients and flow values, it would be theoretically more proper to calculate resistance from these measurements. Vascular resistance may be expressed in various units, i.e., *peripheral resistance units* (PRU), pressure gradient (mm Hg) per unit of blood flow (ml per sec); by Aperia's formula to give results in absolute (cgs, or cm-Gm-sec) units by multiplying PRU units by a conversion factor of 1,332 to express resistance in terms of dyne-sec-cm⁵; or by the ratio of pressure gradient (mm Hg) to blood flow expressed in liters per minute to give R units. R units may be approximately converted to dynes-sec-cm⁵ by multiplying by 80. Minor changes in calculated resistance are usually of no significance, not only because of possible errors in pressure or flow measurements but also since changes in apparent resistance may result from the distending effect of inflow or exit pressure, or, conversely, alteration in the distending force may mask changes in the vascular bed. Because of such considerations and the nonlinear relationship between pressure and flow of most vascular beds, changes in calculated resistance cannot be equated simply with vasoconstriction or vasodilatation.

The relationship of the various factors affecting the resistance to fluid flow in rigid tubing is expressed by *Poiseuille's equation:*

$$\text{Fluid flow} = \frac{(\text{pressure difference})(\text{radius})^4 \, \pi}{(\text{vessel length})(\text{fluid viscosity}) \, 8}$$

Since the experiments from which the equation was derived were performed in straight, rigid tubes with steady, streamlined flow of an ideal, viscous fluid, it is not possible to apply this relationship directly to the vascular system, in which the vessels are neither straight nor rigid, the blood is not a simple viscous fluid, and the flow is not always streamlined. Nevertheless, the predominant influence of the radius of the vessel (radius is raised to the *fourth* power in the above equation) on flow

is apparent. Of the other factors, changes in vessel length are thought to be ordinarily unimportant, but changes in viscosity related to changes in hematocrit and serum proteins are often of marked significance, particularly in small blood vessels. It should also be noted that in most vascular beds, most of the blood vessels are connected in parallel rather than in series. The total resistance of vessels connected in parallel is calculated by adding the *conductance* of each individual vessel ($1/R$, the reciprocal of the individual resistance) to obtain the total conductance of all the vessels (Fig. 2-10). Generally, the resistance of vessels in parallel is much less than that of any single vessel, and if they are all about equal size, the total resistance is equal to the resistance of a single vessel divided by the number of vessels in parallel.

Since all normal blood vessels are at least to some extent distensible, it follows that increasing the *intraluminal pressure* will increase the *transmural pressure* on the vessel wall and increase the diameter and radius of the vessel. This in itself will decrease the resistance of the vessel. This effect is seen in Fig. 2-11, which illustrates the pressure-flow and pressure-resistance curves of an isolated peripheral vascular bed. Note that as pressure is increased from 20 to 40 mm Hg there is a marked decrease in calculated resistance (Fig. 2-11*B*), associated with an increase in flow (Fig. 2-11*A*). The pressure at about 20 mm Hg, at which flow ceases entirely, has been sometimes referred to as the *critical closure pressure*; however, it is better referred to as the *critical flow pressure*, since it is unlikely that there is often complete anatomic closure of the vessels.

The amount of distension present in an individual

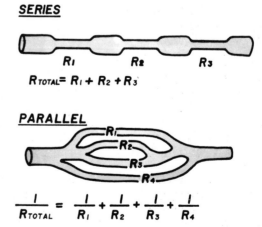

SERIES

R_1 R_2 R_3

$R_{TOTAL} = R_1 + R_2 + R_3$

PARALLEL

R_1
R_2
R_3
R_4

$$\frac{1}{R_{TOTAL}} = \frac{1}{R_1} + \frac{1}{R_2} + \frac{1}{R_3} + \frac{1}{R_4}$$

Fig. 2-10. Comparison of the calculation of vascular resistance of vessels in series and in parallel. In most vascular beds most of the blood vessels of the same size are connected in parallel.

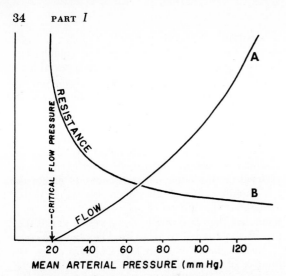

Fig. 2-11. Relationships between pressure, flow, and resistance of a peripheral vascular bed. In *A* it is seen that no flow is apparent below about 20 mm Hg, the critical flow pressure ("critical closure pressure"). At pressures above this value the flow increases progressively more for each unit of pressure rise as the resistance of the vascular bed is decreased by the pressure within the vessels. The marked decrease in calculated resistance is illustrated in *B*. (*Adapted from Guyton.*[22])

blood vessel is dependent on the stiffness or *tone* of the vessel and on the *distending* or *transmural pressure*, i.e., the difference between the intraluminal pressure, which tends to expand the vessel, and the external pressure, which tends to compress the vessel. The tone or stiffness of a blood vessel is determined by the geometry of the vessel and the mechanical properties of the vessel wall. Important relationships between the distending pressure and the tension in the wall of a blood vessel are expressed in the following form of the *law of Laplace*:

$$\text{Wall tension} = \text{distending pressure} \cdot \frac{\text{vessel radius}}{\text{wall thickness}}$$

From this equation it is apparent that the tension in the wall of a blood vessel tending to expand it is greater if the radius of the vessel is greater or if the blood vessel wall is thinner. Thus, veins, with greater radii and thinner walls than their arterial counterparts, have a greater wall tension than their arterial counterparts *at the same pressure*. The degree of stretching of the vessel wall produced by wall tension depends upon the elastic stiffness of the vessel wall. The term *distensibility* is usually defined by the pressure-volume characteristics of a given vessel and is dependent on the above and other factors.

The regulation of vascular stiffness achieved by alterations in the physicochemical-mechanical prop-

erties of vascular smooth muscle is referred to as *vasomotion*. The major mechanisms by which changes in vasomotion and changes in vessel caliber are accomplished are (1) metabolic, chemical, and hormonal substances carried in the blood and/or locally produced, and (2) the activity of fibers from the autonomic nervous system innervating the blood vessels and locally releasing norepinephrine or acetylcholine. The relative importance of these two mechanisms varies markedly from one vascular bed to another. Although it was formerly thought that the release of epinephrine and norepinephrine from the adrenal medulla played an important role in the normal physiologic control of vascular tone, this mechanism is not currently thought to be important except under conditions of extreme stress when the adrenal medulla does release significant quantities of these substances.

Most systemic arteries, and probably veins, respond to hypoxia and/or an increase in pCO_2 with vasodilatation. Whether or not substances such as lactic acid, histamine, or unknown "metabolic products" are also important in the local control of vasomotion is still uncertain. The cerebral vessels are particularly sensitive to pCO_2, whereas the coronary vessels respond strikingly to changes in pO_2, although qualitatively similar changes are found in most other systemic vessels. In most organs, the effects of pO_2 and pCO_2 work synergistically with the autonomic nervous system to regulate regional blood flow. In contrast to systemic vessels, the pulmonary vessels seem to respond in the opposite manner to changes in pCO_2 and pO_2. In addition to their regional effects, pO_2 and pCO_2 in the mixed venous blood returned to the heart appear to be involved, through poorly understood mechanisms, in the control of the total output of the heart.

Three types of nerve fibers are important in the control of blood vessels: (1) sympathetic vasoconstrictor fibers, (2) sympathetic vasodilator fibers, (3) parasympathetic vasodilator fibers.

Sympathetic vasoconstrictor fibers are found in both arteries and veins throughout the body, but not in capillaries. These fibers appear to effect vasoconstriction by the release of levarterenol (norepinephrine) at the nerve-fiber endings. Vasodilatation may be produced by inhibition of the discharge rate of these nerve fibers. These fibers are important in responding to local or regional stimuli of many types. In addition, they are the major pathways for reflex changes in peripheral resistance secondary to changes in carotid sinus and aortic stretch receptors. They are thought to be the principle mechanism by which impulses from the cortical and subcortical areas of the brain influence total and regional peripheral resistance. The effect of these nerve fibers on the coronary and cerebral blood vessels is ordinarily very slight, being overshadowed by the influence of pO_2 and pCO_2.

Sympathetic vasodilator fibers appear to be of importance mainly in skeletal muscles, although it is possible that some cutaneous blood vessels and coronary vessels also receive this type of fiber. It is probable that these fibers are not normally tonically active and that they are not significantly influenced by the carotid sinus or aortic arch stretch receptors. They are thought to be important in increasing blood flow to muscles during exercise. The effector agent at the nerve-fiber ending is thought to be acetylcholine.

Parasympathetic vasodilator fibers are restricted to the tongue and salivary glands and to the sacral area, particularly the erectile vessels of the genital organs. In the sacral area these nerves take part in the local regulation of blood flow according to the needs of local activity, but they are not thought to play an important role in the reflex control of major cardiovascular functions. The transmitter substance at their nerve-root endings is acetylcholine. Parasympathetic stimulation of the salivary glands causes the release of an enzyme which acts on proteins in the tissue fluid to produce a polypeptide, *bradykinin*, which has powerful vasodilator properties. There is also evidence that the sweat glands of the skin, innervated by sympathetic cholinergic fibers, may also liberate bradykinin.

In general, vasoconstriction occurs as the result of increased activity of the sympathetic nervous system, which effects an increase in levarterenol (norepinephrine) of the nerve-fiber endings in blood vessels, and vasodilatation is produced by inhibition of sympathetic vasoconstrictor impulses and/or by local environmental conditions (pO_2, pCO_2, etc.). Localized vasodilatation may also be produced in exercising muscle by sympathetic vasodilator fibers and in the sacral area and salivary glands by parasympathetic fibers. In some areas vasodilatation may be produced by the formation of polypeptides under autonomic system influence.

It is not possible to present a succinct but accurate description of the anatomic pathways by which the central nervous system helps to control cardiovascular function. Even more impossible is a description of the mechanisms by which the nervous system is able to integrate impulses from all levels —the cortex and limbic system, reticular system, diencephalon, mesencephalon, medulla oblongata, spinal cords, etc.—and to synthesize these impulses in order to provide the organism with responses varying from the massive sympathetic discharge associated with shock to very discrete vasomotor changes. It is becoming increasingly apparent that the concept of a "vasomotor center" in the medulla oblongata was an oversimplification and that the central internuncial system possesses extremely complex interconnections and feedback mechanisms at many levels by which integrative regulation of the cardiovascular system may be carried out. It is also apparent that impulses from high levels at times bypass lower integrative areas. There is unfortunately little information regarding the nature of the processes by which conditioning involving the autonomic nervous system occurs.

REFERENCES

1. Paldino, R. L., and Hyman, C.: Alternative Pathways for the Return of Lymph, *Am. Heart J.*, **67**:280, 1964.
2. Miller, A. J., Pick, R., and Katz, L. N.: Ventricular Endomyocardial Changes after Impairment of Cardiac Lymph, *Brit. Heart J.*, **25**:182, 1963.
3. Miller, A. J., Pick, R., and Katz, L. N.: The Importance of the Lymphatics of the Mammalian Heart: Experimental Observations and Some Speculations, *Circulation*, **29**:485, 1964.
4. Uhley, H., Leeds, S. E., Sampson, J. J., and Friedman, M.: Some Observations on the Role of the Lymphatics in Experimental Acute Pulmonary Edema, *Circulation Res.*, **9**:688, 1961.
5. Uhley, H., Leeds, S. E., Sampson, J. J., and Friedman, M.: Role of Pulmonary Lymphatics in Chronic Pulmonary Edema, *Circulation Res.*, **11**:966, 1962.
6. Sarnoff, S. J., and Mitchell, J. H.: The Regulation of the Performance of the Heart, *Am. J. Med.*, **30**:747, 1961.
7. Bowditch, H. P.: Ueber die Eigenthümlichkeiten der Reizbarkeit, welche die Muskelfasern des Herzens zeigen, *Verh. Ber. Kgl. Sachs. Ges. d. Wsch. Leipzig, Math. Physische. Cl.*, **23**:652, 1871.
8. Howell, W. H., and Donaldson, F., Jr.: Experiments upon the Heart of the Dog with Reference to Maximum Volume of Blood Sent Out by Left Ventricle in a Single Beat, *Philosophical Tr.*, London, pt. 1, 154, 1884.
9. Frank, O.: Zur Dynamik des Herzmuskels, *Ztschr. Bio.*, **32**:370, 1895. Trans. by C. B. Chapman and E. Wasserman, *Am. Heart J.*, **58**:282, 467, 1959.
10. Wiggers, C. J.: Some Factors Controlling the Shape of the Pressure Curve in the Right Ventricle, *Am. J. Physiol.*, **33**:382, 1914.
11. Straub, H.: Dynamik des Säugetierherzens. I. *Deutsche Arch klin. Med.*, **115**:531, 1914. II. *Ibid.*, **116**:409, 1914.
12. Patterson, S. W., and Starling, E. H.: On the Mechanical Factors Which Determine the Output of the Ventricles, *J. Physiol.*, **48**:357, 1914.
13. Patterson, S. W., Piper, H., and Starling, E. H.: The Regulation of the Heart Beat, *J. Physiol.*, **48**:465, 1914.
14. Starling, E. H.: "The Linacre Lecture on the Law of the Heart," Longmans, Green, and Co., Ltd., London, 1918.

15. Wiggers, C. J.: Determinants of Cardiac Performance, *Circulation*, 4:485, 1951.
16. Sarnoff, S. J., and Berglund, E.: Ventricular Function. I. Starling's Law of the Heart Studied by Means of Simultaneous Right and Left Ventricular Function Curves in the Dog, *Circulation*, 9:706, 1954.
17. Sarnoff, S. J.: Myocardial Contractility as Described by Ventricular Function Curves; Observations on Starling's Law of the Heart, *Physiol. Rev.*, 35:107, 1955.
18. Braunwald, E., and Frahm, C. J.: Studies on Starling's Law of the Heart. IV. Observations on the Hemodynamic Functions of the Left Atrium in Man, *Circulation*, 24:633, 1961.
19. Braunwald, E., Frahm, C. J., and Ross, J., Jr.: Studies on Starling's Law of the Heart. V. Left Ventricular Function in Man, *J. Clin. Invest.*, 40:1882, 1961.
20. Braunwald, E., and Ross, J., Jr.: Applicability of Starling's Law of the Heart to Man, in J. R. Evans (guest ed.), Symposium: Structure and Function of Heart Muscle, *Circulation Res.*, 15 (Supp. 2): 169, 1964.
21. Braunwald, E.: The Control of Ventricular Function in Man, *Brit. Heart J.*, 27:1, 1965.
22. Guyton, A. C.: "Textbook of Medical Physiology," 2d ed., W. B. Saunders Company, Philadelphia, 1961, p. 347.

SUGGESTED READING

Functional Anatomy

General Anatomy

Barry, A., and Patten, B. M.: The Structure of the Adult Heart, in S. E. Gould (ed.), "Pathology of the Heart," 2d ed., Charles C Thomas, Publisher, Springfield, Ill., 1960, p. 93.
Evans, J. R. (guest ed.): Symposium: Structure and Function of Heart Muscle, *Circulation Res.*, 15 (Supp. 2): 1–224, 1964.
Gardner, E. D., Gray, D. J., and O'Rahilly, R. I.: "Anatomy," W. B. Saunders Company, Philadelphia, 1960.
James, T. N.: Anatomy of the Heart: Normal and Pathologic, as Related to Cardiac Function, in B. L. Gordon (ed.), "Clinical Cardiopulmonary Physiology," 2d ed., Grune & Stratton, Inc., New York, 1960, p. 8.
Kisch, B. (translated from German by A. I. Kisch): "Electron Microscopy of the Cardiovascular System," Charles C Thomas, Publisher, Springfield, Ill., 1960.
Licata, R. H.: Anatomy of the Heart, in A. A. Luisada (ed.), "Cardiology, An Encyclopedia of the Cardiovascular System," McGraw-Hill Book Company, New York, 1959, Vol. 1, p. 30.

Robb, J. S., and Robb, R. C.: The Normal Heart: Anatomy and Physiology of the Structural Units, *Am. Heart J.*, 23:455, 1942.
Spalteholz, W.: "Hand Atlas and Textbook of Human Anatomy," rev. by R. Spannder, Little, Brown and Company, Boston, 1954.
Spiro, D., and Sonnenblick, E. H.: Comparison of the Ultrastructural Basis of the Contractile Process in Heart and Skeletal Muscle, in J. R. Evans (guest ed), Symposium: Structure and Function of Heart Muscle, *Circulation Res.*, 15 (Supp. 2): 14, 1964.

Innervation of the Heart

Hirsch, E. F.: The Innervation of the Human Heart, *Arch. Path.*, 75:378, 1963.
Mitchell, G. A. G.: "Cardiovascular Innervation," The Williams & Wilkens Company, Baltimore, 1956.
White, J. C.: Cardiac Pain: Anatomic Pathways and Physiologic Mechanisms, *Circulation*, 16:644, 1957.

Lymphatic Circulation

Mayerson, H. S.: Lymphatic Vessels and Lymph: Physiology, in D. I. Abramson (ed.), "Blood Vessels and Lymphatics," Academic Press Inc., New York, 1962, p. 709.
Mayerson, H. S.: The Physiologic Importance of Lymph, in W. F. Hamilton and P. Dow (eds.), "Handbook of Physiology," sec. 2, "Circulation," vol 2, American Physiological Society, Washington, D.C., 1963, p. 1035.
Mayerson, H. S.: On Lymph and Lymphatics, *Circulation*, 28:839, 1963.
Miller, A. J., Pick, R., and Katz, L. N.: Lymphatics of the Mitral Valve of the Dog: Demonstration and Discussion of the Possible Significance, *Circulation Res.*, 9:1005, 1961.
Miller, A. J.: The Lymphatics of the Heart, *Arch. Int. Med.*, 112:501, 1963.
Miller, A. J., Ellis, A., and Katz, L. N.: Cardiac Lymph: Flow Rates and Composition in Dogs, *Am. J. Physiol.*, 206:63, 1964.
Patek, P. R.: The Morphology of the Lymphatics of the Mammalian Heart, *Am. J. Anat.*, 64:203, 1939.
Rusznyák, I., Földi, M., and Szabó, G.: "Lymphatics and Lymph Circulation," Pergamon Press, New York, 1960.
Trapnell, D. H.: The Peripheral Lymphatics of the Lung, *Brit. J. Radiol.*, 36:660, 1963.
Yoffey, J. M., and Courtice, F. C.: "Lymphatics, Lymph and Lymphoid Tissue," Harvard University Press, Cambridge, Mass., 1956.

Pulmonary Circulation

Adams, W. R., and Veith, I. (eds.): "Pulmonary Circulation: An International Symposium, 1958," Sponsored by Chicago Heart Association, Grune & Stratton, Inc., New York, 1959.

Aviado, D. M., Jr., Ling, J. S., and Schmidt, C. F.: Effects of Anoxia on Pulmonary Circulation: Reflex Pulmonary Vasoconstriction, *Am. J. Physiol.*, **189:** 253, 1957.

Cournand, A.: Some Aspects of the Pulmonary Circulation in Normal Man and in Chronic Cardiopulmonary Diseases, *Circulation*, **2:**641, 1950.

Dexter, L., Dow, J. W., Haynes, F. W., Whittenberger, J. L., Ferris, B. G., Goodale, W. T., and Hellems, H. K.: Studies of the Pulmonary Circulation in Man at Rest: Normal Variations and the Interrelations between Increased Pulmonary Blood Flow, Elevated Pulmonary Arterial Pressure, and High Pulmonary "Capillary" Pressure, *J. Clin. Invest.*, **29:**602, 1950.

Euler, U. S. v., and Liljestrand, G.: Observations on the Pulmonary Arterial Blood Pressure in the Cat, *Acta. physiol. scandinav.*, **12:**301, 1946.

Fishman, A. P., Fritts, H. W., Jr., and Cournand, A.: Effects of Acute Hypoxia and Exercise on the Pulmonary Circulation, *Circulation*, **22:**204, 1960.

Fishman, A. P.: Respiratory Gases in the Regulation of the Pulmonary Circulation, *Physiol. Rev.*, **41:**214, 1961.

Fishman, A. P.: Dynamics of the Pulmonary Circulation, in W. F. Hamilton and P. Dow (eds.), "Handbook of Physiology," sec. 2, "Circulation," vol. 2, American Physiological Society, Washington, D.C., 1963, p. 1667.

Gordon, B. L.: "Clinical Cardiopulmonary Physiology," 2d ed., Grune & Stratton, Inc., New York, 1960.

Motley, H. L., Cournand, A., Werkö, L., Himmelstein, A., and Dresdale, D.: The Influence of Short Periods of Induced Anoxia upon Pulmonary Pressures in Man, *Am. J. Physiol.*, **150:**315, 1947.

Rapaport, E., and Severinghaus, J.: Pulmonary Circulation: Physiology, in D. I. Abramson (ed.), "Blood Vessels and Lymphatics," Academic Press Inc., New York, 1962, p. 306.

Reuck, A. V. S. de, and O'Connor, M. (eds.): "Problems of Pulmonary Circulation," Ciba Foundation Study Group no. 8, Little, Brown, and Company, Boston, 1961.

Coronary Circulation

Berne, R. M.: Regulation of Coronary Blood Flow, *Physiol. Rev.*, **44:**1, 1964.

Gregg, D. E.: "The Coronary Circulation in Health and Disease," Lea & Febiger, Philadelphia, 1950.

Gregg, D. E., and Fisher, L. C.: Blood Supply to the Heart, in W. F. Hamilton and P. Dow (eds.), "Handbook of Physiology," sec. 2, "Circulation," vol. 2, American Physiological Society, Washington, D.C., 1963, p. 1517.

James, T. N.: "Anatomy of the Coronary Arteries," Paul B. Hoeber, Inc., New York, 1961.

Smith, G. T.: The Anatomy of the Coronary Circulation, *Am. J. Cardiol.*, **9:**327, 1962.

Hemodynamics

General

Abbott, B. C., and Mommaerts, W. F. H. M.: A Study of Inotropic Mechanisms in the Papillary Muscle Preparation, *J. Gen. Physiol.*, **42:**533, 1959.

Abramson, D. E. (ed.): "Blood Vessels and Lymphatics," Academic Press Inc., New York, 1962.

Badeer, H.: Effect of Heart Size on the Oxygen Uptake of the Myocardium, *Am. Heart J.*, **60:**948, 1960.

Badeer, H.: Contractile Tension in the Myocardium, *Am. Heart J.*, **66:**432, 1963.

Bargmann, W., and Doerr, W. (eds.): "Das Herz des Menschen," Georg Thieme Verlag, Stuttgart, 1963, 2 vols.

Barratt-Boyes, B. G., and Wood, E. H.: Hemodynamic Response of Healthy Subjects to Exercise in the Supine Position While Breathing Oxygen, *J. Appl. Physiol.*, **11:**129, 1957.

Barratt-Boyes, B. G., and Wood, E. H.: Cardiac Output and Related Measurements and Pressure Values in the Right Heart and Associated Vessels, Together with an Analysis of the Hemodynamic Response to the Inhalation of High Oxygen Mixtures in Healthy Subjects, *J. Lab. & Clin. Med.*, **51:**72, 1958.

Bayliss, L. E.: The Rheology of Blood, in W. F. Hamilton and P. Dow (eds.), "Handbook of Physiology," sec. 2, "Circulation," vol. 1, American Physiological Society, Washington, D.C., 1962, p. 137.

Bing, R. J., and Michal, G.: Myocardial Efficiency, *Ann. New York Acad. Sci.*, **72:**555, 1959.

Braunwald, E., Fishman, A. P., and Cournand, A.: Time Relationship of Dynamic Events in the Cardiac Chambers, Pulmonary Artery and Aorta in Man, *Circulation Res.*, **4:**100, 1956.

Brecher, G. A.: "Venous Return," Grune & Stratton, Inc., New York, 1956.

Brecher, G. A., and Galletti, P. M.: Functional Anatomy of Cardiac Pumping, in W. F. Hamilton and P. Dow (eds.), "Handbook of Physiology," sec. 2, "Circulation," vol. 2, American Physiological Society, Washington, D.C., 1963, p. 759.

Burch, G. E., Ray, C. T., and Cronvich, J. A.: Certain Mechanical Peculiarities of the Human Cardiac Pump in Normal and Diseased States, *Circulation*, **5:**504, 1952.

Burch, G. E.: Theoretic Considerations of the Time Course of Pressure Developed and Volume Ejected by the Normal and Dilated Left Ventricle during Systole, *Am. Heart J.*, **50:**352, 1955.

Burton, A. C.: On the Physical Equilibrium of Small Blood Vessels, *Am. J. Physiol.*, **164:**319, 1951.

Burton, A. C.: Relation of Structure to Function of the Tissues of the Wall of Blood Vessels, *Physiol. Rev.*, **34:**619, 1954.

Burton, A. C.: The Importance of the Size and Shape of the Heart, *Am. Heart J.*, **54:**801, 1957.

Burton, A. C.: Hemodynamics and the Physics of the Circulation, in T. Ruch and J. F. Fulton (eds.),

"Medical Physiology and Biophysics" (18th ed. of Howell's "Textbook of Physiology"), W. B. Saunders Company, Philadelphia, 1960, p. 643.

Burton, A. C.: Physical Principles of Circulatory Phenomena: The Physical Equilibria of the Heart and Blood Vessels, in W. F. Hamilton and P. Dow (eds.), "Handbook of Physiology," sec. 2, "Circulation," vol. 1, American Physiological Society, Washington, D.C., 1962, p. 85.

Chapman, C. B., Fisher, J. N., and Sproule, B. J.: Behaviour of Stroke Volume at Rest and during Exercise in Human Beings, *J. Clin. Invest.*, **39**:1208, 1960.

Dexter, L., Whittenberger, J. L., Haynes, F. W., Goodale, W. T.. Gorlin, R., and Sawyer, C. G.: Effect of Exercise on Circulatory Dynamics of Normal Individuals, *J. Appl. Physiol.*, **3**:439, 1951.

Donald, K. W., Bishop, J. M., Cumming, G., and Wade, O. L.: The Effect of Exercise on the Cardiac Output and Circulatory Dynamics of Normal Subjects, *Clin. Sc.*, **14**:37, 1955.

Evans, C. A. L., and Matsuoka, Y.: The Effect of Various Mechanical Conditions on the Gaseous Metabolism and Efficiency of the Mammalian Heart, *J. Physiol.*, **49**:378, 1915.

Fishman, A. P. (guest ed.): The Myocardium—Its Biochemistry and Biophysics, Symposium of the New York Heart Association, *Circulation*, **24**:321–542, 1961.

Fry, D. L., Griggs, D. M., Jr., and Greenfield, J. C., Jr.: Myocardial Mechanics: Tension-Velocity-Length Relationships of Heart Muscle, *Circulation Res.*, **14**:73, 1964.

Gauer, O. H., Henry, J. P., and Sieker, H. O.: Cardiac Receptors and Fluid Volume Control, *Progr. Cardiovasc. Dis.*, **4**:1, 1961–1962.

Gauer, O. H., and Henry, J. P.: Circulatory Basis of Fluid Volume Control, *Physiol. Rev.*, **43**:423, 1963.

Gerola, A., Fineberg, H., and Katz, L. N.: Role of Catecholamines on Energetics of the Heart and Its Blood Supply, *Am. J. Physiol.*, **196**:394, 1959.

Green, H. D., and Kepchar, J. H.: Control of Peripheral Resistance in Major Systemic Vascular Beds, *Physiol. Rev.*, **39**:617, 1959.

Green, H. D., Rapela, C. E., and Conrad, M. C.: Resistance (Conductance) and Capacitance Phenomena in Terminal Vascular Beds, in W. F. Hamilton and P. Dow (eds.), "Handbook of Physiology," sec. 2, "Circulation," vol. 2, American Physiological Society, Washington, D.C., 1963, p. 935.

Green, H. D.: Circulation: Physical Principles, in O. Glasser (ed.), "Medical Physics," The Year Book Medical Publishers, Inc., Chicago, 1944, vol. 1, p. 208.

Gregerson, M. I., and Rawson, R. A.: Blood Volume, *Physiol. Rev.*, **39**:307, 1959.

Guyton, A. C.: "Textbook of Medical Physiology," 2d ed., W. B. Saunders Company, Philadelphia, 1961.

Guyton, A. C.: Venous Return, in W. F. Hamilton and P. Dow (eds.), "Handbook of Physiology," sec. 2, "Circulation," vol. 2, American Physiological Society, Washington, D.C., 1963, p. 1099.

Guyton, A. C.: "Circulatory Physiology: Cardiac Output and Its Regulation," W. B. Saunders Company, Philadelphia, 1963.

Hamilton, W. F.: The Lewis A. Conner Memorial Lecture: The Physiology of the Cardiac Output, *Circulation*, **8**:527, 1953.

Hamilton, W. F., and Dow, P. (ed.): "Handbook of Physiology," sec. 2, "Circulation," vols. 1–3, American Physiological Society, Washington, D.C., 1962–1964.

Hardung, V.: Propagation of Pulse Waves in Viscoelastic Tubings, in W. F. Hamilton and P. Dow (eds.), "Handbook of Physiology," sec. 2, "Circulation," vol. 1, American Physiological Society, Washington, D.C., 1962, p. 107.

Harrison, T. R., Dixon, K., Russell, R. O., Jr., Bidwai, P. S., and Coleman, H. N.: The Relation of Age to the Duration of Contraction, Ejection, and Relaxation of the Normal Human Heart, *Am. Heart J.*, **67**:189, 1964.

Hawthorne, E. W.: Instantaneous Dimensional Changes of the Left Ventricle in Dogs, *Circulation Res.*, **9**:110, 1961.

Haynes, R. H., and Rodbard, S.: Arterial and Arteriolar Systems: Biophysical Principles and Physiology, in D. I. Abramson (ed.), "Blood Vessels and Lymphatics," Academic Press Inc., New York, 1962, p. 26.

Hertzman, A. B.: Vasomotor Regulation of Cutaneous Circulation, *Physiol. Rev.*, **39**:280, 1959.

Heymans, C., and Neil, E.: "Reflexogenic Areas of the Cardiovascular System," Little, Brown and Company, Boston, 1958.

Huxley, H. E.: The Contractile Structure of Cardiac and Skeletal Muscle, *Circulation*, **24**:328, 1961.

Johnson, P. C. (guest ed.): Symposium: Autoregulation of Blood Flow, *Circulation Res.*, **15** (Supp. 1): 1–291, 1964.

Kahler, R. L.. Goldblatt, A., and Braunwald, E.: The Effects of Hypoxia on the Systemic, Venous and Arterial, Systems and on Myocardial Contractile Force, *J. Clin. Invest.*, **41**:1553, 1962.

Katz, L. N., and Feinberg, H.: The Relation of Cardiac Effort to Myocardial Oxygen Consumption and Coronary Flow, *Circulation Res.*, **6**:656, 1958.

Luisada, A. A., and Liu, T. C.: "Intracardiac Phenomena in Right and Left Heart Catheterization," Grune & Stratton, Inc., New York, 1958.

Luisada, A. A. (ed.): "Cardiology: An Encyclopedia of the Cardiovascular System," McGraw-Hill Book Company, New York, 1959–1961, vols. 1–5.

Lundin, G.: Mechanical Properties of Cardiac Muscle, *Acta physiol. scandinav.*, **7** (Suppl. 20), 1944.

McDonald, D. A.: "Blood Flow in Arteries," The Williams & Wilkins Company, Baltimore, 1960.

McDowall, R. J. S. (ed.): "The Control of the Circulation of the Blood, Dawson & Sons, London, 1956, 2 vols.

Markwalder, J., and Starling, E. H.: On the Constancy of the Systolic Output under Varying Conditions, *J. Physiol.*, **48**:348, 1914.

Messer, J. V., and Neill, W. A.: The Oxygen Supply of the Human Heart, *Am. J. Cardiol.*, **9**:384, 1962.

Mommaerts, W. F. H. M., and Langer, G. A.: Fundamental Concepts of Cardiac Dynamics and Energetics, *Ann. Rev. Med.*, **14**:261, 1963.

Olson, R. E.: The Contractile Proteins of Heart Muscle, *Am. J. Med.*, **30**:692, 1961.

Olson, R. E.: Physiology of Cardiac Muscle, in W. F. Hamilton and P. Dow (eds.), "Handbook of Physiology," sec. 2, "Circulation," vol. 1, American Physiological Society, Washington, D.C., 1962, p. 199.

Peterson, L. H.: The Dynamics of Pulsatile Blood Flow, *Circulation Res.*, **2**:127, 1954.

Peterson, L. H.: Regulation of Blood Vessels, *Circulation*, **21**:749, 1960.

Peterson, L. H.: Vascular Tone, *Mod. Concepts Cardiovas. Dis.*, **31**:725, 731, 1962.

Peterson, L. H.: Properties and Behaviour of Living Vascular Wall, *Physiol. Rev.*, **42** (Suppl. 5):309, 1962.

Physiology Society Symposium on Mechanical Aspects of Cardiac Muscle, *Fed. Proc.*, **21**:954–1005, 1962.

Podolsky, R. J.: The Mechanism of Muscular Contraction, *Am. J. Med.*, **30**:708, 1961.

Remington, J. W.: The Physiology of the Aorta and Major Arteries, in W. F. Hamilton and P. Dow (eds.), "Handbook of Physiology," sec. 2, "Circulation," vol. 2, American Physiological Society, Washington, D. C., 1963, p. 799.

Remington, J. W.: Introduction to Muscle Mechanics, with a Glossary of Terms, *Fed. Proc.*, **21**:954, 1962.

Renkin, E. M.: Eighth Bowditch Lecture: Transport of Large Molecules Across Capillary Walls, *Physiologist*, **7**:13, 1964.

Rodahl, K., and Horvath, S. M.: "Muscle as a Tissue," McGraw-Hill Book Company, New York, 1962.

Rushmer, R. F., and Thal, N.: The Mechanics of Ventricular Contraction: A Cineflurographic Study, *Circulation*, **4**:219, 1951.

Rushmer, R. F., Crystal, D. K., and Wagner, C.: The Functional Anatomy of Ventricular Contraction, *Circulation Res.*, **1**:162, 1953.

Rushmer, R. F.: "Cardiovascular Dynamics," 2d ed., W. B. Saunders Company, Philadelphia, 1961.

Rushmer, R. F., Citters, R. L. v., and Franklin, D. L.: Some Axioms, Popular Notions, and Misconceptions Regarding Cardiovascular Control, *Circulation*, **27**:118, 1963.

Sarnoff, S. J., Braunwald, E., Welch, G. H., Jr., Case, R. B., Stainsby, W. N., and Macruz, R.: Hemodynamic Determinants of Oxygen Consumption of the Heart with Special Reference to the Tension-time Index, *Am. J. Physiol.*, **192**:148, 1958.

Sarnoff, S. J.: Certain Aspects of the Role of Catecholamines in Circulatory Regulation, *Am. J. Cardiol.*, **5**:579, 1960.

Sonnenblick, E. H.: Force-Velocity Relations in Mammalian Heart Muscle, *Am. J. Physiol.*, **202**:931, 1962.

Spencer, M. P., and Denison, A. B., Jr.: Pulsatile Blood Flow in the Vascular System, in W. F. Hamilton and P. Dow (eds.), "Handbook of Physiology," sec. 2, "Circulation," vol. 2, American Physiological Society, Washington, D.C., 1963, p. 839.

Symposium on the Physiology of Cardiac Muscle, *Am. P. Med.*, **30**:649–771, 1961.

Wallace, A. G., and Sarnoff, S. J.: Effects of Cardiac Sympathetic Nerve Stimulation on Conduction in the Heart, *Circulation Res.*, **14**:86, 1964.

Wang, Y., Marshall, R. J., and Shepherd, J. T.: The Effect of Changes in Posture and of Graded Exercise on Stroke Volume in Man, *J. Clin. Invest.*, **39**:1051, 1960.

Warren, J. V., Brannan, E. S., Weens, H. S., and Stead, E. A., Jr.: Effect of Increasing the Blood Volume and Right Atrial Pressure on the Circulation of Normal Subjects by Intravenous Infusions, *Am. J. Med.*, **4**:193, 1948.

Wells, R. E., Jr.: Rheology of Blood in the Microvasculature, *New England J. Med.*, **270**:832, 889, 1964.

Wetterer, E.: Flow and Pressure in the Arterial System: Their Hemodynamic Relationship and the Principles of Their Measurement, *Minnesota Med.*, **37**:77, 1954.

Wiggers, C. J.: Studies on the Consecutive Phases of the Cardiac Cycle. I. The Duration of the Consecutive Phases of the Cardiac Cycle and the Criteria for Their Precise Determination, *Am. J. Physiol.*, **56**:415, 1921.

Wiggers, C. J.: "The Pressure Pulses in the Cardiovascular System," Longmans, Green & Co., Inc., New York, 1928.

Wiggers, C. J.: "Circulatory Dynamics," Grune & Stratton, Inc., New York, 1952.

Cardiac Control, Cardiac Reserve, Starling's Law

Aviado, D. M., Jr., and Schmidt, C. F.: Reflexes from Stretch Receptors in Blood Vessels, Heart and Lungs, *Physiol. Rev.*, **35**:247, 1955.

Aviado, D. M., Jr.: Some Controversial Cardiovascular Reflexes, *Circulation Res.*, **10**:831, 1962.

Beznak, M.: Hormonal Influences in Regulation of Cardiac Performance, in J. R. Evans (guest ed), Symposium: Structure and Function of Heart Muscle, *Circulation Res.*, **15** (Supp. 2): 141, 1964.

Blix, M.: Die Länge und die Spannung des Muskels, *Skandinav. Arch. Physiol.*, **5**:173, 1895.

Braunwald, E., and Ross, J., Jr.: Applicability of Starling's Law of the Heart to Man, in J. R. Evans (guest ed.), Symposium: Structure and Function of Heart Muscle, *Circulation Res.*, **15** (Supp. 2): 169, 1964.

Braunwald, E.: The Control of Ventricular Function in Man, *Brit. Heart J.*, **27**:1, 1965.

Brecher, G. A.: Experimental Evidence of Ventricular Diastolic Suction, *Circulation Res.*, 4:513, 1956.

Bruce, T. A., Chapman, C. B., Baker, O., and Fisher, J. N.: The Role of Autonomic and Mycardial Factors in Cardiac Control, *J. Clin. Invest.*, 42:721, 1963.

Burch, G. E.: The Dilated Heart, in K. Rodahl and S. M. Horvath (eds.), "Muscle as a Tissue," McGraw-Hill Book Company, New York, 1962, p. 233.

Chapman, C. B., Baker, O. B., and Mitchell, J. H.: Left Ventricular Function at Rest and during Exercise, *J. Clin. Invest.*, 38:1202, 1959.

Eichna, L. W., and McQuarrie, D. G. (eds.): Proceedings of a Symposium on Central Nervous System Control of Circulation, *Physiol. Rev.*, 40 (Suppl. 4): part 2, 1960, pp. 1–311.

Folkow, B.: Nervous Control of the Blood Vessels, *Physiol. Rev.*, 35:629, 1955.

Folkow, B.: Role of the Nervous System in the Control of Vascular Tone, *Circulation*, 21:760, 1960.

Gleason, W. L., and Braunwald, E.: Studies on Starling's Law of the Heart. VI. Relationships between Left Ventricular End-Diastolic Volume and Stroke Volume in Man with Observations on the Mechanism of Pulsus Alternans, *Circulation*, 25:841, 1962.

Hamilton, W. F.: Role of the Starling Concept in Regulation of Normal Circulation, *Physiol. Rev.*, 35:161, 1955.

Hemingway, A.: The Circulation in Muscular Exercise, in R. J. S. McDowell (ed.), "The Control of the Circulation of the Blood," W. M. Dawson & Sons Ltd., London, 1956, suppl. vol., pp. 205–223.

Henderson, Y., and Prince, A. L.: The Relative Systolic Discharges of the Right and Left Ventricles and Their Bearing upon Pulmonary Congestion and Depletion, *Heart*, 5:217, 1914.

Katz, L. N.: Analysis of the Several Factors Regulating the Performance of the Heart, *Physiol. Rev.*, 35:91, 1955.

Katz, L. N.: The Performance of the Heart, *Circulation*, 21:483, 1960.

Katz, L. N.: Recent Concepts of the Performance of the Heart, *Circulation*, 28:117, 1963.

Linden, R. J., and Mitchell, J. H.: Relation between Left Ventricular Diastolic Pressure and Myocardial Segment Length and Observations on the Contribution of Atrial Systole, *Circulation Res.*, 8:1092, 1960.

Mitchell, J. H., Linden, R. J., and Sarnoff, S. J.: Influence of Cardiac Sympathetic and Vagal Nerve Stimulation on the Relation between Left Ventricular Diastolic Pressure and Myocardial Segment Length, *Circulation Res.*, 8:1100, 1960.

Mitchell, J. H., Gilmore, J. P., and Sarnoff, S. J.: The Transport Function of the Atrium: Factors Influencing the Relation between Mean Left Atrial Pressure and Left Ventricular End Diastolic Pressure, *Am. J. Cardiol.*, 9:237, 1962.

Mitchell, J. H., Wallace, A. G., and Skinner, N. S., Jr.: Intrinsic Effects of Heart Rate on Left Ventricular Performance, *Am. J. Physiol.*, 205:41, 1963.

Nickerson, M.: Adrenergic Regulation of Cardiac Performance, in J. R. Evans (guest ed.), Symposium: Structure and Function of Heart Muscle, *Circulation Res.*, 15 (Supp. 2): 130, 1964.

Patterson, S. W., Piper, H., and Starling, E. H.: The Regulation of the Heart Beat, *J. Physiol.*, 48:465, 1914.

Peterson, L. H.(guest ed.): Symposium on Regulation of the Cardiovascular System in Health and Disease, *Circulation*, 21:739–768, 1176–1192, 1960.

Pickering, G.: Starling and the Concept of Heart Failure, *Circulation*, 21:323, 1960.

Pieper, H. P., and Ogden, E.: Determinants of Stroke Work in the Dog Heart-Lung Preparation, *Am. J. Physiol.*, 206:43, 1964.

Ross, J., Jr., Frahm, C. J., and Braunwald, E.: Influence of Carotid Baroreceptors and Vasoactive Drugs on Systemic Vascular Volume and Venous Distensibility, *Circulation Res.*, 9:75, 1961.

Rushmer, R. F.: Applicability of Starling's Law of the Heart to Intact, Unanesthetized Animals, *Physiol. Rev.*, 35:138, 1955.

Rushmer, R. F.: Anatomy and Physiology of Ventricular Function, *Physiol. Rev.*, 36:400, 1956.

Rushmer, R. F.: Autonomic Balance in Cardiac Control, *Am. J. Physiol.*, 192:631, 1958.

Rushmer, R. F., Smith, O., and Franklin, D.: Mechanisms of Cardiac Control in Exercise, *Circulation Res.*, 7:602, 1959.

Rushmer, R. F., and Smith, O. A., Jr.: Cardiac Control, *Physiol. Rev.*, 39:41, 1959.

Rushmer, R. F.: Regulation of the Heart's Function, *Circulation*, 21:744, 1960.

Rushmer, R. F., Smith, O. A., Jr., and Lasher, E. P.: Neural Mechanisms of Cardiac Control during Exertion, *Physiol. Rev.*, 40 (Suppl. 4):27, 1960.

Rushmer, R. F., Clitters, R. L. v., and Franklin, D. L.: Some Axioms, Popular Notions and Misconceptions Regarding Cardiovascular Control, *Circulation*, 27:118, 1963.

Rushmer, R. F.: Effects of Nerve Stimulation and Hormones on the Heart; The Role of the Heart in General Circulatory Regulation, in W. F. Hamilton and P. Dow (eds.), "Handbook of Physiology," sec. 2, "Circulation," vol. 1, American Physiological Society, Washington, D.C., 1962, p. 533.

Sarnoff, S. J., Mitchell, J. H., Gilmore, J. P., and Remensnyder, J. P.: Homeometric Autoregulation in the Heart, *Circulation Res.*, 8:1077, 1960.

Sarnoff, S. J., Brockman, S. K., Gilmore, J. P., Linden, R. J., and Mitchell, J. H.: Regulation of Ventricular Contraction: Influence of Cardiac Sympathetic and Vagal Nerve Stimulation on Atrial and Ventricular Dynamics, *Circulation Res.*, 8:1108, 1960.

Sarnoff, S. J., Gilmore, J. P., Brockman, S. K., Mitchell, J. H., and Linden, R. J.: Regulation of Ventricular Contraction by the Carotid Sinus: Its Effect on

Atrial and Ventricular Dynamics, *Circulation Res.,* 8:1123, 1960.

Sarnoff, S. J., and Mitchell, J. H.: The Control of the Function of the Heart, in W. F. Hamilton and P. Dow (eds.), "Handbook of Physiology," sec. 2, "Circulation," vol. 1, American Physiological Society, Washington, D.C., 1962, p. 489.

Siegel, J. H., and Sonnenblick, E. H.: Isometric Time-Tension Relationships as an Index of Myocardial Contractility, *Circulation Res.,* 12:597, 1963.

Sonnenblick, E. H., Siegel, J. H., and Sarnoff, S. J.: Ventricular Distensibility and Pressure-Volume Curve during Sympathetic Stimulation, *Am. J. Physiol.,* 204:1, 1963.

Starling, E. H.: On the Circulatory Changes Associated with Exercise, *J. Roy. Army M. Corps,* 34:258, 1920.

Starling, E. H., and Visscher, M. B.: The Regulation of the Energy Output of the Heart, *J. Physiol.,* 62:243, 1927.

Stead, E. A., Jr., and Warren, J. V.: Cardiac Output in Man: An Analysis of Mechanisms Varying the Cardiac Output Based on Recent Clinical Studies, *Arch. Int. Med.,* 80:237, 1947.

Symposium on the Regulation of the Performance of the Heart, *Physiol. Rev.,* 35:91–168, 1955.

Uvnäs, B.: The Vasodilator Nerves, *Am. Heart J.,* 62:277, 1961.

Uvnäs, B.: Central Cardiovascular Control, in J. Field (ed.), "Handbook of Physiology," sec. 1, "Neurophysiology," vol. 2, American Physiological Society, Washington, D.C., 1960, p. 1131.

Warner, H. R., and Toronto, A. F.: Regulation of Cardiac Output through Stroke Volume, *Circulation Res.,* 8:549, 1960.

Wiggers, C. J., and Katz, L. N.: Contour of the Ventricular Volume Curves under Different Conditions, *Am. J. Physiol.,* 58:429, 1922.

Wiggers, C. J.: The Dominant Control of Mammalian Ventricular Dynamics by Initial Length, *Rev. Soc. argent biol.,* Suppl. 10:546, 1934.

PART II

The Examination of the Cardiovascular System

Section A: History and Physical Examination

3 THE APPROACH TO THE PATIENT

J. Willis Hurst, M.D.

It is the doctor's job to collect and to interpret medical data. If he knows the normal range, he can then identify various abnormalities. From these abnormalities he can synthesize a reasonable diagnosis and institute treatment. Throughout this process—known as the "work-up and disposition of the patient"—the doctor must employ the deductive reasoning of a pure scientist and have the understanding and compassion of a true physician.

The approach to the patient with cardiovascular disease fits exactly into this scheme. The techniques used to gather data include the *medical history*, the *physical examination, electrocardiography, radiography,* and *special diagnostic procedures.* These five techniques of study have been likened by Dr. Proctor Harvey[1] to the fingers of the hand (Fig. 3-1A).

The diagnostic clues of cardiovascular disease

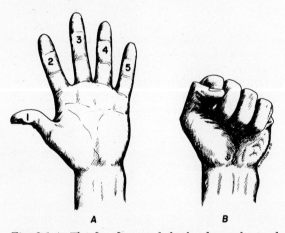

A   **B**

Fig. 3-1.*A.* The five fingers of the hand may be used to illustrate the techniques utilized in studying a patient with possible heart disease. The thumb, 1, is the history, which is frequently the most important technique. Finger 2 represents the physical examination; finger 3, the electrocardiogram; finger 4, the chest x-ray; finger 5, "other diagnostic procedures." (*After Harvey.*[1]) *B.* The clenched fist suggests that the best diagnostic tool is developed when all the diagnostic techniques are correlated, one with the other, and welded together into a single diagnostic unit.

are sometimes found only in the medical *history,* with all other methods of examination revealing no abnormality. For example, angina pectoris due to coronary atherosclerosis can be diagnosed by history and history alone. Clues to the diagnosis of heart disease revealed by a patient's symptoms are discussed in Chap. 4.

The cardiovascular abnormality may be found on *physical examination.* For example, slight diastolic hypertension may be found by sphygmomanometry before other evidence of this disease is apparent. An important cardiac murmur such as aortic regurgitation may be found on physical examination, and no other evidence of rheumatic heart disease may be found. Clues to the diagnosis of heart disease found on physical examination are discussed in Chap. 5.

An abnormality may be found on the *electrocardiogram,* and all other methods of study may reveal no other abnormality. For example, evidence of myocardial infarction may be present in the electrocardiogram, and the remainder of the examination, including the history, may be negative. The Wolff-Parkinson-White syndrome may be noted with no other clues being apparent. Left ventricular hypertrophy in a cyanotic child may offer the first clue to the diagnosis of congenital tricuspid atresia. Electrocardiography and vectorcardiography are discussed in Chap. 6.

Diagnostic clues may be present in the *roentgenogram* of the chest and no other clues may be elicited. For example, congestive heart failure may not be diagnosed by history and physical examination but may be readily identified on the x-ray of the chest. Roentgenographic examination of the heart is discussed in Chap. 7.

As a general rule, the chief complaint of a patient should stimulate the examiner to consider various possibilities. The remainder of the history should add or subtract certain possibilities. At the end of the history, a list of reasonable diagnoses should be in mind. A complete physical examination is then performed with these diagnostic possibilities under consideration. Approached in this manner, the physical examination becomes more than a routine procedure. The examiner specifically searches for certain abnormalities suggested to him by his interpretation of the patient's symptoms. What a pleasure it is to observe the expert who, on history, identifies paroxysmal nocturnal dyspnea in a young female and then listens specifically for mitral stenosis. He does not always find it but often does after a number of other physicians have missed it. Following the physical examination the diagnostic possibilities are then revised. At this point the examiner must attempt to weld the clues found on history and physical examination into a reasonable diagnosis.

The electrocardiogram is then surveyed. The findings there should fit the possibilities already under consideration, and new clues should be sought. For example, suppose that definite left ventricular hypertrophy is detected on the electrocardiogram when this abnormality was not previously suspected. Go back to the patient and find a cause for left ventricular hypertrophy. Perhaps aortic stenosis was overlooked; it often is.

As a rule, the roentgenogram of the chest should complete the diagnostic study. Here again, the findings on x-ray should support the diagnosis already suspected, but other clues may be present. For example, slight rib notching may be found on the chest x-ray of a patient with undiagnosed coarctation of the aorta. The diagnosis might have been missed on physical examination because the patient had mitral stenosis which captured everyone's attention. The determination of the blood pressure in the legs of such a patient, who could also be normotensive, might not have seemed necessary; accordingly, a diagnosis usually made on physical examination might not be made until the chest x-ray has been carefully studied.

The majority of cardiovascular diagnoses will be made after careful consideration of the patient's symptoms, the findings on physical examination, analysis of the electrocardiogram, and study of the routine chest roentgenogram. As stated earlier, the diagnostic clue may be found in only one of these parameters of study, but as a rule diagnostic clues can be identified in the same patient by several of these methods of study. Frequently the diagnostic thread can be picked up by many of the diagnostic techniques. When it is found in only one area of examination, go back, look carefully; it may be found in other areas of study also. The findings based on the history, the findings at physical examination, the information provided by the electrocardiogram and x-rays must be welded into a reasonable diagnosis. If all pieces of the diagnostic jigsaw puzzle fit together and make a clear picture, then you are on the road to a correct diagnosis. If the picture is not complete, you should know it. In such a case, more work, study, and thought may be needed.

In some patients, it is necessary to employ other methods of study in order to delineate the type of heart disease that is present, or to determine its severity. For example, discovery of the cause of pulmonary hypertension may depend on the results of cardiac catheterization. The cause of systemic hypertension may depend on selective renal arteriography. Left atrial angiography may be needed to prove that a left atrial myxoma is present. The point is, however, that the special diagnostic procedures selected will depend on and be determined by a careful analysis of the history, physical examination, electrocardiogram, and x-rays. It is not possible to do all things to all patients. Accordingly, it is necessary to have some idea of what to look for and how to look for it when selecting special diagnostic procedures. Special diagnostic procedures are discussed in Chaps. 8, 9, and 10. When they have been performed, the study is complete. An attempt has been made to explain all the abnormalities. The diagnostic thread has been followed to its end. The five diagnostic fingers are now correlated, each with the others, and are welded together into a clenched fist (Fig. 3-1B). The fist symbolizes the final diagnostic tool, which is far more powerful than any of the individual units.

Once the evidence of heart disease has been collected it is necessary to make a *complete diagnosis*. In order to make a complete diagnosis it is necessary to determine the etiologic cardiac diagnosis, the anatomic cardiac diagnosis, the physiologic cardiac diagnosis, and the physical capacity of the patient. The New York Heart Association has emphasized this approach to the problem for many years. The Criteria Committee of this organization has recently completed the sixth edition of *Diseases of the Heart and Blood Vessels*.[2] This book stresses the nomenclature and criteria used in the diagnosis of heart disease. Everyone interested in heart disease should be familiar with the concepts promoted by this book. Adherence to the principles set forth in it will ensure complete cardiovascular diagnoses based on accepted diagnostic criteria. The following brief case report illustrates the harmful result of an incomplete diagnosis and the value of a correct, complete one.

Mrs. Brown, age 41, began to experience progressive dyspnea on effort and palpitation. She could walk only one block without symptoms. The physical examination revealed a normal blood pressure, expiratory wheezes in the lungs, no edema, and normal neck veins at the time of examination. The heart rate was 80 beats per minute and was regular. The heart was not definitely large. The first heart sound was loud. The electrocardiogram was normal except for broad-notched P waves. The x-ray of the chest showed the heart to be normal in size, and it showed an increase in pulmonary "markings."

The *careless* observer might possibly make a diagnosis of chronic bronchitis or bronchial asthma or even "some sort of emotional disturbance." He might diagnose heart failure without any other qualifying statements. The *careful* observer would be stimulated by the first sentence to consider mitral stenosis. He would make additional inquiry regarding the dyspnea and palpitation. He would detect that the anterior portion of the chest lifts the hand with systole, suggesting right ventricular hypertrophy. He would feel the apex impulse carefully and would listen for the rumble of mitral stenosis. He would search for the opening snap of the mitral valve and for the loud pulmonic component of the second heart sound. The broad-notched P wave in the electrocardiogram would mean far more in the patient with such a history who had the murmur of mitral stenosis. The x-ray of the chest really showed many things—the left atrium was large, the atrial appendage was visible, the pulmonary artery was large, and Kerley lines were present. This observer would make the following complete diagnosis of heart disease:

1. Etiology: Rheumatic heart disease
   (The etiologic diagnosis refers to categories such as hypertensive, rheumatic, congenital, coronary atherosclerosis, etc. It does not refer to the many theories regarding the causation of coronary atherosclerosis, rheumatic fever, hypertension, etc.)
2. Anatomy: Mitral stenosis, right ventricular hypertrophy, and left atrial enlargement
   (The anatomic diagnosis should indicate all the abnormalities that can be seen when the heart is viewed directly.)
3. Physiology: Congestive heart failure, normal sinus rhythm with possible history of atrial fibrillation, and hemodynamic significant mitral stenosis
   (The physiologic diagnosis should indicate all the cardiac diagnoses that are not determined by viewing the anatomic features of the heart. These include the heart rhythm, the competence of the ventricles, angina pectoris, etc.)
4. Physical capacity
   a. Functional: Class III
      (Class I refers to patients with heart disease who have no symptoms of any kind. Ordinary physical activity does not cause fatigue, palpitation, dyspnea, or anginal pain. Class II refers to patients who are comfortable at rest but have symptoms with ordinary physical activity. Class III refers to patients who are comfortable at rest but have symptoms with less than ordinary effort. Class IV refers to patients who have symptoms at rest.)

   b. Therapeutic: Class C
      (The functional capacity of a patient does not always determine what is best for the patient. Accordingly the therapeutic classification is a prescription for the amount of activity the physician believes wise in the individual case. Class A applies to patients whose physical activity need not be restricted. Class B refers to patients whose ordinary activity need not be restricted but who should be advised against severe activity. Class C applies to patients whose ordinary activity should be restricted. Class D applies to patients whose ordinary activity should be markedly restricted. Class E applies to patients who should be at complete rest in the bed or chair.)

The physician who makes this complete diagnosis is in the proper position to consider both the medical and surgical management of the case. The careless observer might not even recognize the problem as being due to severe heart disease. If he did recognize heart failure, he might leave it at that and deny the patient surgical treatment.

After a complete cardiac diagnosis has been made on a patient, it is necessary to look for precipitating or aggravating conditions. For example, *acute* congestive heart failure associated with mild systemic hypertension is rare and it is wise to look for myocardial infarction or pulmonary infarction in such cases. The pulmonary edema encountered with mitral stenosis may be due to the development of uncontrolled atrial fibrillation. Chronic congestive heart failure due to coronary atherosclerosis may be caused by recurrent pulmonary emboli or by unrecognized urinary tract obstruction resulting from an enlarged prostate. Angina pectoris may become worse because of slow gastrointestinal bleeding or thyrotoxicosis. The precipitating and aggravating factors are often treatable and must not be ignored.

After a complete diagnosis has been made and precipitating and aggravating factors have been sought, the proper therapy can be initiated. The sensitive and sagacious physician dispenses his opinion and therapy in an understanding manner. The truth is stated. In most cases the patient has a darker view of the situation than the facts justify. Beware of creating "disease" when none is present or of producing an invalid when slight disease is present. Many electrocardiographic "abnormalities" are harmless, and many murmurs are unimportant.

Finally, although this book deals with the cardiovascular system, it is obvious that this system of the body cannot be viewed as isolated. To illustrate, a patient treated for a cardiovascular problem is scarcely better off if a rectal carcinoma is missed. A patient should not be allowed to leave the office or hospital without some thought being given to his total health problems.

REFERENCES

1. Dr. W. Proctor Harvey: Personal communication.
2. Criteria Committee of the New York Heart Association, Inc.: "Diseases of the Heart and Blood Vessels" (Nomenclature and Criteria for Diagnosis), 6th ed., Little, Brown and Company, Boston, 1964.

4 SYMPTOMS DUE TO HEART DISEASE

J. Willis Hurst, M.D.

HISTORY TAKING

An enormous amount of valuable diagnostic information can be found in the medical history of a patient. The importance of the history is perhaps realized most when one attempts to understand an illness in the comatose patient, the psychotic patient, or the very young child.

The medical history may accomplish the following:

1. Many diagnostic clues may be found. For example, the patient may relate the typical story of angina pectoris or give a history of paroxysmal rapid heart action. The remainder of the examination may be negative.

2. The severity of the heart disease may be ascertained. For instance, the mere presence of a diastolic rumble of mitral stenosis is not sufficient evidence to recommend immediate surgical correction of the abnormality if the patient's exercise tolerance is truly excellent. On the other hand, if there is a story of dyspnea on effort, hemoptysis, or peripheral embolism, then surgery is indicated. Another example is as follows: the presence of chronic complete heart block is not sufficient reason for the surgical implantation of a cardiac pacemaker if the history reveals no episodes of syncope and an excellent tolerance to effort.

Two causes of error must not be overlooked when the history is said to be negative. First, the history may only "seem" negative because the subtle clues have been overlooked. For example, a patient might deny the existence of chest pain but recall the repeated presence of substernal "pressure" characteristic of angina pectoris. Secondly, patients may gradually do less and therefore have fewer symptoms. For example, the patient with mitral stenosis may complain of few symptoms but when the exact amount of activity is determined, it becomes clear that he is doing less. The patient may be less active and not be aware of it until the proper inquires have been made. This sequence of events may not be recognized by the patient initially.

3. The personality of a patient may be assessed. Medical clues gathered by the physician during history taking must be interpreted in the light of the patient's personality and emotional status. A second-hand history given in the hallway will not give the true picture of a patient's problem. The significance of a complaint may, at times, be determined by *how* a patient relates a story rather than by the exact content of the story. The therapeutic action of the physician may depend on the assessment of a patient's personality and emotional status. For example, if mitral valve surgery is clearly indicated but is not urgent at the moment and the patient abhors the idea of surgery because her neighbor died on the operating table, then it is prudent to see the patient several times and gently lead her toward the treatment that is really needed. On the other hand, if another patient with the same degree of disability due to mitral stenosis is emotionally prepared for surgical correction because her neighbor was well rehabilitated by the same operation, then surgery may be planned for the near future. The different management of these two patients with the same disease was based entirely on a certain aspect of the history.

4. The proper doctor-patient relationship may be established. The interview with a patient has two purposes, (1) to collect useful medical information, and (2) to make friends with the patient. When the period of history taking is over the patient should realize that the physician *is* his friend, is concerned about his problem, is honest, and will make every effort to help him. If these facts are not transmitted to the patient, he may refuse a badly needed special diagnostic procedure such as cardiac catheterization, or he may refuse the surgery recommended for patent ductus arteriosus. This possibility is highlighted frequently in the medical school environment, where the patient may feel emotionally closer to the intern, resident, or medical student and may agree to a special test only when one of them assures him that it is needed for his proper care, even though the "senior wheel" has recommended the procedure repeatedly.

It is much easier to teach physical diagnosis and the other methods of diagnosis than it is to teach history taking. History taking involves three acts: talking, listening, and thinking. Of these three, talking is the easiest to teach; listening and thinking are not easy to do or to teach. Talking is divided into that done by the patient and that done by the doctor. While the patient is talking, the doctor should listen and think. He does not simply record what the patient says. He does not function as a court recorder who passively records but does not interpret the statements of a witness. Everything the patient says has significance and must be interpreted properly in order for it to be meaningful. The first sentence uttered by the patient may be the major diagnostic clue. It has been said that patients eventually tell you their symptoms and that *all* the doctor has to do is to listen and think. Although this statement makes a point and emphasizes that the doctor must listen and think, it does not describe a realistic approach to history taking. Patients do not always tell all the ramifications of their complaints unless the physician prompts them a bit, and the exact sequence of events may not be appreciated unless there is some organized approach to the problem. The physician must learn to lead a patient but not to mislead him—and not to be misled himself.

The words used by a doctor as he inquires about a complaint may vary from patient to patient and will be determined by understanding the patient's background, including his education, occupation, and environment. He must be certain that the patient really understands what he is asking and further that he understands what the patient is trying to say. The examiner must not only understand the ramifications of each complaint, but he must establish the sequence of events with as much certainty as possible. Some diagnoses are made by analyzing a single complaint; other diagnoses are established by identifying a particular sequence of events.

The ability to determine the significance of a patient's complaints improves as the examiner learns more about people in general, about physiology, pathology, various clinical conditions, and the natural history of disease. History taking does not, however, improve without effort. Improvement depends on the effort spent in constantly correlating the patient's complaints with the abnormalities found on physical examination, electrocardiograms, x-rays, special diagnostic procedures, and autopsy findings. Such correlation cannot be accomplished unless all observations are recorded in the patient's chart, in order that the medical data will be available for subsequent review.

Finally, it must be emphasized that iatrogenic heart disease may have its inception during the interview known as history taking. The words used by the physician and his facial expressions are powerful tools—whether for good or bad.

The history, then, assumes great importance. It takes years to master the technique of communicating with a patient. It also takes years to learn to interpret properly every word the patient utters.

The patient with heart disease may have no symptoms whatsoever. The symptoms ordinarily considered to be due to heart disease may in reality be arising from another system of the body. For example, dyspnea may be due to pulmonary disease, not to heart disease. The symptoms ordinarily attributed to noncardiovascular disease may, in reality, be arising in the heart. For example, pain in the jaw may be considered to be a toothache when it is actually due to angina pectoris secondary to coronary atherosclerosis.

A general survey of the symptoms expressed by patients who have cardiovascular disease will be considered in the following pages. Complaints suggesting heart disease but due to other conditions will also be considered. The symptoms will be discussed in greater detail in the chapters dealing with specific diseases.

PAIN

The ability to evaluate pain and discomfort is a direct index of the expertise of the physician. This is especially true of the pain and discomfort related to cardiovascular disease. In order to evaluate pain, it is necessary to determine its location, its radiation, its quality, its duration, the factors that produce it, and the factors that relieve it.

Pain may be due to ischemic heart disease. The most common cause of myocardial ischemia is coronary atherosclerosis. Pain and discomfort occur when the disease reaches a critical degree of severity and the lumen of the coronary arteries becomes sufficiently narrow to cause ischemia of the cardiac muscle. Angina pectoris may develop when the coronary flow is adequate at rest but is not adequate when the demands of the heart are increased. The diagnosis of angina pectoris may be missed if the physician inquires only about pain. Many patients with angina pectoris deny pain but complain of an aching, heavy, or squeezing sensation, pressure, tightness, dyspnea, or indigestion in the chest. The discomfort occurs during effort, is precipitated by emotions, especially anger, and by exposure to cold, and may follow meals. The unpleasant sensation is usually located in the substernal region of the chest or across the anterior portion of the upper part of the chest. The discomfort usually affects an area about the size of a clenched fist; as a matter of fact, the patient frequently clenches his fist and places it on the region of the chest where the discomfort is located. It is always useful to have the patient delineate the extent of the pain by indicating the location, using a single finger. The pain may radiate to the neck, jaw, hard palate, tongue, left arm, right arm, elbow, wrist, back, or upper part of the abdomen. On rare occasions the discomfort may be more pronounced in these areas or may be felt only in one or more of the areas mentioned. The pain usually lasts from 1 to 3 min if the provoking effort is discontinued. The duration of angina pectoris provoked by anger is perhaps longer; it may be as much as 20 min. It is usually relieved promptly after nitroglycerin is placed under the tongue. The development of angina pectoris for the first time, or an increase in frequency or intensity of angina pectoris, is quite a different problem from that of stable angina and is frequently the result of recent coronary thrombosis or small myocardial infarction. Angina pectoris may be aggravated by many other medical conditions and may, on rare occasions, occur in the absence of coronary atherosclerosis.

Myocardial infarction frequently develops when a clot forms in an atherosclerotic coronary artery. The pain of myocardial infarction differs from that of angina pectoris in several respects. The discomfort may develop when the patient is doing very little. In fact, it may awaken him from sleep. It is usually, but not always, more severe and as a rule lasts much longer than the discomfort of angina. The pain of infarction usually lasts from ½ hr to many hours. The location and radiation of the pain of myocardial infarction are similar to those of angina pectoris. Whereas the pain of acute myocardial infarction is rarely aggravated by deep breathing or turning, the pain related to pericarditis secondary to myocardial infarction, including the "postmyocardial infarction syndrome," may be aggravated by such movements.

Coronary insufficiency is a clinical syndrome said to be "between" angina pectoris and myocardial infarction. Most patients said to have this condition have had a coronary thrombosis, and many of them, in reality, have experienced a small myocardial infarction.

Acute dissection of the aorta is usually associated with excruciating pain. The pain is usually located in the anterior portion of the chest, lasts for hours, and is frequently of maximum intensity at the onset. More than the usual amount of opiates may be needed to offer relief. This pain tends to radiate into the thoracic portion of the back more often than that due to myocardial infarction, and may be felt predominantly in the back. It is not aggravated by deep breathing or turning. It may be located in the abdomen if the arteries of the abdominal viscera are involved. Occasionally, the pain seems to shift from one area in the chest to a lower portion as the dissection progresses.

The pain of acute *pericarditis* is not related to effort but is usually aggravated by deep breathing at the very beginning of the illness. It is sharp, is usually located in the precordial area, and may radiate to the upper portion of the shoulders or sides of the neck. The patient tends to avoid deep breaths or even normal respiration because of the intense aggravation of the discomfort associated with the activity. Turning the body from side to side may aggravate the pain, as may swallowing. Leaning forward may occasionally relieve the discomfort. Pericarditis must be considered whenever a patient complains of chest pain in order that a search may be made for other clinical clues.

The majority of small *pulmonary emboli* produce no chest pain. In fact, the patient may not identify any symptoms that are directly due to pulmonary emboli. This is why the majority of emboli are not diagnosed. The pain of pulmonary embolism may, at times, be similar to that of myocardial infarction. Acute, distressing dyspnea may be the only clue to pulmonary embolism. The diagnosis is frequently based on circumstantial evidence. When pulmonary infarction develops, then pleuritis may be identified. The pain in such cases is located in the lateral portion of the chest and is aggravated by breathing.

The most common cause of chest pain is not related to cardiovascular disease but is associated with anxiety. The discomfort is usually located in the inframammary region, rarely radiates to other locations, does not occur *during* effort but may occur *after* effort, and is not related to breathing but is related to other signs of anxiety such as periodic deep-sighing respiration, hyperventilation, sinus tachycardia, fatigue, and a fear of "closed places." The discomfort may be characterized as a series of short sticks and stabs lasting no longer than it takes one to "snap" his fingers, or it may be a dull ache lasting for hours to days at a time. This type of discomfort may be disabling to the patient and may consume his every waking thought. Since angina pectoris and the discomfort associated with anxiety may—and frequently do—coexist, great care and skill are needed to clarify such problems. The medical history offers the major diagnostic clues in such a situation.

The pain associated with pulmonary hypertension, the shoulder-hand syndrome, esophageal dysfunction, esophageal rupture, disease of the spine, shoulder girdle, pleura, lung, mediastinum (including mediastinal emphysema), hiatal hernia, stomach and duodenal disorders, gallbladder disease, thrombophlebitis of the chest wall, herpes zoster, and other chest-wall pain must be considered in differential diagnosis.

Intermittent claudication of the lower extremities is frequently overlooked because the physician demands that the discomfort be localized in the calf of the leg. Whenever discomfort develops in the arch of the foot, calf of the leg, thighs, hips, or gluteal region as a result of effort, then peripheral arterial vascular disease must be considered. The symptoms associated with acute arterial occlusion of the lower extremities may at the onset be no more than hypesthesia (interpreted by the patient as "the leg going to sleep"). These symptoms and others related to arterial and venous diseases of the extremities will be discussed in Chap. 56.

DYSPNEA

One of the most common and distressing symptoms is dyspnea. The patient complains of "shortness of breath" or that he "can't get enough breath."

There are many causes of dyspnea. The details of the disease states responsible for this complaint will be discussed in the text that follows. The history must include the factors that precipitate and relieve dyspnea and must identify the body position associated with the complaint.

Dyspnea on effort is a common complaint. It is usually due to congestive heart failure or chronic pulmonary disease. It is necessary to establish the degree of activity required to produce dyspnea. This may be done by inquiring about the daily activity of each patient. It is useless to ask, "Do you get short of breath climbing stairs?" when the patient never climbs stairs. The patient may, however, climb a hill near his work every day. It is also valuable to determine when the patient began to notice increasing dyspnea. For example, if the patient has only recently had difficulty climbing a hill near his home, the dyspnea is more likely to be due to heart failure than to lung disease. On the other hand, the dyspnea could be related to chronic lung disease, but it would then be wise to look for recent complications such as pneumothorax, atelectasis, and asymptomatic pulmonary infection in order to explain the recent increase in symptoms.

When a patient complains of *wheezing* associated with dyspnea, he may have lung disease or heart disease. If the patient is an adult, especially over 40 years old, heart failure should be foremost in the mind of the physician and this clue should prompt him to search for other clues indicating heart disease. When the wheezing is due to heart disease, the patient is said to have cardiac asthma. If there is a history of periodic wheezing and dyspnea since childhood, then, of course, bronchial asthma and lung disease are more likely to be the cause. Wheezing on effort may be due to either heart failure or chronic lung disease. Wheezing due to the latter becomes apparent because the effort evokes deeper respiratory excursions.

Orthopnea is a special type of dyspnea. It im-

plies that the patient has less dyspnea when the trunk is elevated to the sitting position as compared with when he is lying down. The patient relates that he must use two or three pillows in order to have a restful night. This symptom is often associated with congestive heart failure but may also be associated with severe lung disease. The fatigue associated with the exertion of breathing seems to be less when the dyspnea is due to pulmonary disease as compared with that of heart failure.

Paroxysmal nocturnal dyspnea is a very important variety of shortness of breath. It is almost specific for congestive heart failure due to disease of the left side of the heart. Characteristically, the patient goes to bed and has little difficulty going to sleep in the recumbent position. One or two hours later he is awakened from sleep with acute shortness of breath. He seeks relief by sitting upright, perhaps on the side of the bed, or he even sits in a chair. He occasionally goes to the open window searching for air. After a time, he becomes comfortable and returns to bed. He may then sleep comfortably the remainder of the night. The only other causes for this unusual sequence of events are hyperventilation syndrome due to anxiety and pulmonary emboli. It would be most unusual for pulmonary emboli to occur for very many nights at the same hour. The hyperventilation syndrome due to anxiety is not so clearly relieved by sitting up and is associated with other signs suggesting this syndrome, such as tingling of the arms and hands and other evidence of anxiety.

Acute pumonary adema is usually due to disease of the left ventricle or to mitral valve disease. The patient experiences the sudden development of dyspnea and cough, and he may produce "frothy," blood-tinged sputum. This symptom may occur without previous warning, as in myocardial infarction, or it may be preceded by cardiac asthma or dyspnea on effort.

A dry, *nonproductive cough* may be related to the pulmonary congestion associated with heart failure. It may develop with effort but may also occur at rest. Although dyspnea is usually present, cough may dominate the clinical picture.

Cheyne-Stokes breathing is characterized by periods of hyperpnea which alternate with periods of apnea. This type of breathing usually occurs in older patients with heart failure. The patients usually have cerebral vascular disease and the heart disease is on the left side of the heart. Patients with Cheyne-Stokes respiration rarely complain of dyspnea, perhaps because they are so sick. They are occasionally aware of acute shortness of breath during the hyperpneic phase of the cycle. The type of breathing associated with the hypoventilation syndrome of obesity, or the Pickwickian syndrome, may be periodic in nature but is not identical with Cheyne-Stokes breathing.

Obviously, an infant or small child does not complain of shortness of breath, and, of course, does not climb a hill near its home. Therefore, other clues to respiratory distress are required. The rate of breathing is greatly increased in this age group when there is heart failure or acute lung disease. The respiratory rate of adults with heart failure is not so greatly increased as would be expected from the complaint of dyspnea.

The shortness of breath associated with *anxiety* assumes two forms. Both may be terrifying to the patient. The patient may simply feel as though the air "does no good," or "the air does not go down far enough," or "I can't get a good satisfying breath." Normal breathing is interrupted by deep sighs. Some patients experience an element of claustrophobia. Fatigue, palpitation, and precordial "aching" or "sticks" may also be present. The patient may develop prolonged periods of hyperventilation which are frequently associated with numbness of the arms, hands, and lips, tetany, and unreal sensation. This type of dyspnea may occur in patients with pulmonary or heart disease, thereby testing the diagnostic acumen of the physician.

Acute dyspnea may be, and frequently is, the only clue to *pulmonary embolism.*

Severe *anemia* may be the sole cause of dyspnea on effort and is a frequent contributing factor. *Methemoglobinemia* may also be responsible for dyspnea of effort. *Thyrotoxicosis* may be the cause of dyspnea on effort and, like anemia, may be a contributing factor.

The full-term *pregnant* female may "huff and puff" with effort but has a curious reaction to the audible respiratory effort. She seems quite conscious of her labored breathing but is rarely, if ever, alarmed by it. Accordingly, it is not truly dyspnea. The patient with *metabolic acidosis* due to diabetes mellitus or uremia rarely complains of his enormous breathing problem.

PALPITATION

The term *palpitation* is sometimes used by patients to describe a disagreeable awareness of the heart beat. The patient may use some other term and report "pounding," "stopping," "jumping," or "racing." The mother may observe an abnormal heart rhythm as she looks at or feels the precordium of her child.

The sensitiveness of the nervous system determines which patients complain of palpitation. The complaint is not directly related to the seriousness of the heart disease or to the exact type of arrhythmia. For example, one patient may feel every ectopic beat when there is no evidence of heart disease; another patient may not detect ventricular tachycardia associated with serious heart disease. Patients may complain when the heart beat is slow or fast and when the heart beat is regular or irregular. The patient may detect whether the onset and offset of the rapid heart is regular or irregular. He may complain of forceful, regular heart beat. Conditions associated with an increased stroke output may be associated with a feeling of forceful contraction of the heart. The best example of this is perhaps found in aortic regurgitation. Ectopic beats, atrial fibrillation, and other arrhythmias are perhaps more troublesome to patients with aortic regurgitation, because in such cases the variations of the stroke output are so radically different from normal. On rare occasions a patient may be aware of his heart beat after digitalis medication has been given because of an increased force of contraction induced by the drug. When this occurs, ectopic beats due to digitalis intoxication are frequently noted by the patient.

Patients may therefore complain of palpitation of the heart when the rhythm and rate are entirely normal or when the regular cadence of the rhythm is interrupted by ectopic contractions, paroxysmal rapid heart beat, or extreme bradycardia, including complete heart block. The rhythm responsible for the palpitation may not be present when the patient is seen. Accordingly, it is valuable to have the patient mimic his normal heart action with his finger and then request that he simulate the event responsible for the palpitation. At times, he will give a dramatic reproduction of an ectopic beat or paroxysmal atrial tachycardia.

Patients may hear or feel other worrisome cardiovascular events. Patients with really severe tricuspid regurgitation may feel the expanding pulse in the neck. Some feel the pulse wave hit the ear, and others note that their collar is "too tight" when the heart beats. A loud heart murmur may be heard by a patient or a member of the family. For example, the murmur of interventricular septal defect is often heard by the patient, who may even time an event with great precision. A patient with intermittent retroversion of an aortic valve due to syphilis may hear the typical mumur each time it occurs. Some noises emanating from the chest can even be heard at a good distance. It is not uncommon for an individual to become aware of his heart beat by hearing an arterial bruit or even heart sounds when the side of his head is placed on a pillow at night. The murmur of an arteriovenous fistula located near the head may be heard, thrills may be felt, and ballistic forces of the body may be seen. For example, a patient with severe aortic regurgitation may detect that his head "bobs."

Most patients are accustomed to this, but when placed in the hospital, they may detect that the chain on the overhead bed light moves with each heart beat.

Ordinarily, the term *palpitation* refers to the discomfort felt within the chest and neck associated with the heart movement. Other sensations felt, seen, or heard by patients—all drawing attention to the heart and circulation—are discussed in this section merely because it is convenient to do so at this point.

EDEMA

Patients may give a history of "swelling of the legs," weight gain, and enlarging girth, and edema may be found on physical examination. The patient may be unaware of its existence. On the other hand, there may be a history of "swelling," and edema may not be found at the time of examination.

Ages ago generalized edema, "heart dropsy," was required before a diagnosis of heart failure could be made. Although this extreme degree of edema is not required today, it is still unfortunate that many physicians demand the presence of at least some edema before seriously considering the diagnosis of congestive heart failure. Of course, patients are seen today with considerable peripheral edema due to heart failure, but it must be stated emphatically and underscored that edema is a *late* sign of congestive heart failure. Many other subtle signs of heart failure are usually present before the appearance of edema.

Considerable weight gain due to retention of extracellular fluid may occur without associated edema. This may, at times, be as much as 10 to 15 lb. On the other hand, there are numerous causes of edema other than congestive heart failure, and its presence is not specific for congestive heart failure. If the diagnosis of heart failure is delayed until edema develops, or if heart failure is diagnosed merely because edema is present without other considerations, then it is safe to say that the approach to the problem is superficial.

Local factors play a major role in determining the distribution of fluid in the body. Pulmonary edema due to mitral stenosis provides a good illustration of the importance of local factors. When ventricular diastole is shortened to a critical point, pulmonary edema develops because the right ventricle continues to pump more blood into the lungs than can pass the stenosed mitral valve. Here there has been no weight gain but the body fluid has been redistributed. Patients with pulmonary edema may exhibit thin, watery, frothy, blood-tinged sputum associated with profound dyspnea and wheezing. The patient with chronic congestive heart failure who has gained weight because of retention of sodium and water secondary to altered renal function may detect edema during the day and note that it subsides during the night. This occurs partly because of local hydrostatic factors related to the upright position.

It is important to ascertain whether edema of the extremities preceded or followed dyspnea on effort. Although there are many exceptions, edema due to heart disease secondary to disease of the left ventricle, mitral stenosis, or cor pulmonale is usually preceded by dyspnea.

Edema of one leg only is usually due to local factors such as varicose veins, thrombophlebitis, or lymphedema. When there is bilateral leg edema, there may be more on one side than the other if local factors are also present. Edema may shift from the extremities to the sacral region when a patient is confined to bed.

Periorbital edema is more common in children than in adults. Although this finding on history or physical examination is more often due to renal disease, it also occurs in heart failure. It is, on rare occasion, due to trichinosis.

Ascites may be recognized by the patient as an increase in girth or swelling of the abdomen. Ascites due to congestive heart failure is uncommon today and invariably follows peripheral edema. A local factor, such as cirrhosis, is also suggested when ascites, associated with heart failure, seems to be out of proportion to edema. Constrictive pericarditis, though rare today, should also be thought of in this setting.

The distribution of extracellular fluid is somewhat different in the child as compared with the adult. The child with heart failure forms ascites more readily than does the adult.

SYNCOPE

Syncope is defined as the transient loss of consciousness due to an inadequate cerebral blood flow. Although epilepsy may produce similar symptoms, cerebral vascular disease is a more common problem in differential diagnosis.

Although some patients seek medical advice because of frequent episodes of syncope, many others do not give such a history spontaneously. In such cases the patient has either forgotten the episodes or has been unaware of their occurrence. Also it is not uncommon for the physician to forget to inquire about the occurrence of syncope while interviewing the patient and the family.

Syncope may occur in many types of heart disease and circulatory states, including aortic stenosis, aortic regurgitation, mitral stenosis, left atrial tumor, primary pulmonary hypertension, pulmonary arteriolar disease secondary to left-to-right shunts, pulmonary stenosis, tetralogy of Fallot, paroxysmal rapid heart beat, sinus arrest, ventricular standstill or fibrillation related to atrioventricular block (Stokes-Adams attacks), carotid sinus syncope, cough syncope, micturition syncope, vagovagal syncope, vasodepressor syncope, acute blood loss, pulmonary embolism, etc.

BLOODY SPUTUM

When a patient gives a history of "coughing blood," it is necessary to ascertain the exact nature of the sputum. When a patient is seen during such an episode, the sputum must be examined grossly and microscopically as part of the complete examination of the patient.

It is well to determine whether the material being coughed up contains large volumes of liquid blood, which would indicate brisk bleeding, or whether it contains smaller quantities of dark or clotted blood, which would indicate slow bleeding from low-pressure vessels, or subsiding bleeding. Brisk bleeding, for example, is commonly associated with specific focal ulceration of a vessel of considerable size, and may well reflect an ulceration of the bronchus, such as a bronchogenic carcinoma, foreign body, or bronchiectasis. Slow bleeding, on the other hand, strongly suggests venous bleeding and is more likely to be the result of increased pulmonary vascular resistance, with secondary increase in flow through the bronchial venous system. This may occur as a result of mitral stenosis or bronchiectasis, and these possibilities should be considered carefully.

It is also particularly helpful to notice whether the expectorated blood is intimately admixed with sputum or pus, because this is a valuable clue as to possible site of origin of the bleeding. Intimate admixtures of blood and pus are eloquent signs pointing to a deep-seated site of pulmonary suppuration such as pyogenic lung abscess.

At times, posterior epistaxis associated with systemic hypertension may simulate "bloody sputum." On rare occasions localized disease of the nose may give a similar clinical picture. As a rule, however, epistaxis is obvious and is not confused with bloody sputum.

Pink, frothy sputum is frequently associated with acute pulmonary edema. Blood-streaked sputum may occur with acute pulmonary congestion when the classic findings of acute pulmonary edema are not fully developed. In these clinical states the blood comes from pulmonary capillaries which have ruptured under high intravascular pressure. This type of sputum may also be associated with bronchitis and pulmonary infection.

Hemoptysis means "coughing up blood." The term should not be used to refer to blood-streaked sputum. Frank hemoptysis may be due to pulmonary tuberculosis, pneumonia, bronchiectasis, bronchogenic carcinoma, primary pulmonary hemosiderosis, and necrotic pulmonary arterial lesions due to periarteritis nodosa and lupus erythematosus.

Two conditions must never be overlooked as causes of frank hemoptysis: (1) mitral stenosis, and (2) pulmonary infarction.

1. Mitral stenosis. Hemoptysis due to mitral stenosis is frequently induced by physical exercise, sexual intercourse, or marked excitement. It may be the first symptom of mitral stenosis and may occur during pregnancy. The blood comes from a break in the pulmonary veins which have ruptured under very high pressure. The bleeding often occurs from bronchopulmonary venous varicosities. Episodes of pulmonary hemorrhage of this type tend to subside as the veins adapt to the high pressure and as pulmonary arteriolar disease develops.

2. Pulmonary infarction. Many pulmonary emboli do not lead to pulmonary infarction, but when they do, frank hemoptysis occurs in the minority of instances. Despite this, when hemoptysis occurs in a patient with heart failure, pulmonary infarction is likely. The bloody sputum usually appears from a few hours to a day after the embolus.

Two additional rare causes of pulmonary hemorrhage should be remembered: (1) the rupture of a pulmonary arteriovenous fistula, and (2) the rupture of a syphilitic aneurysm of the aorta into the trachea or bronchus.

FATIGUE

There are many causes of fatigue, and therefore this complaint is far from specific as a symptom of heart disease. When a patient is waterlogged or when there is pulmonary congestion, he is likely to complain primarily of dyspnea. Now, with modern therapy, this complaint may actually be supplanted by fatigue.

The actual physiologic mechanism of the fatigue associated with heart failure is not definitely known, but it is associated with an inadequate cardiac output. The heart fails in its prime objective to nourish adequately all the tissues and organs of the body, including the muscles. The muscular weakness associated with heart failure is usually related to effort. The signs of heart failure are usually present but may be in subtle form.

CYANOSIS

Cyanosis may be detected by the patient or by the patient's family. This abnormality will be discussed in the chapters dealing with congenital heart disease, congestive heart failure, and cor pulmonale. The following points are emphasized here. Many patients are cyanotic and are unaware of it. A mother may not be aware of cyanosis in her child; on the other hand, cyanosis at birth may be due to lung disease and be misinterpreted as being due to heart disease. Doctors are not able to detect minor degrees of cyanosis. This explains why errors are made when congenital heart disease is divided into cyanotic and noncyanotic groups. Such a division may be useful when cyanosis is definitely present, but lesser degrees of arterial oxygen unsaturation are not recognized with regularity. A bluish tint to the skin may be due to argyria and methemoglobinemia. Cyanosis in the patient with chronic congestive heart failure should suggest the possibility of associated pulmonary embolism.

The symptoms of pain, dyspnea, palpitation, edema, syncope, bloody sputum, fatigue, and cyanosis make up the majority of complaints due to cardiovascular disease.The physiologic mechanisms responsible for these findings will be discussed in the chapters that follow. The purpose of presenting the material in this section is to direct attention toward the type of information that must be collected from patients who are suspected of having cardiovascular disease.

5 THE PHYSICAL EXAMINATION

INTRODUCTION

J. Willis Hurst, M.D.

The photographs of Sir William Osler are shown at the outset of this section because they provide a reminder of how physicians learned to practice medicine at the turn of the century (Fig. 5-1). Having carefully examined the patient by inspection, palpation, and auscultation, Osler then *contemplated.* Let us be presumptuous and guess what he was thinking. Without a doubt, he was contemplating his clinical findings in the light of his previous experience in pathology, since he grew up professionally in that discipline. How would Osler learn the practice of medicine today if we were fortunate enough to have him with us? He would, without a doubt, have a cardiac catheterization

laboratory, he would use the phonocardiograph, he would record arterial, venous, and precordial pulsations. He would study the records made by the finest of instruments, but—more than that—he would correlate the findings from the graphic records with the patients' symptoms and physical abnormalities. Today, after *contemplating* the physical findings of the cardiovascular system of a patient, Osler would think in terms not only of pathology but also of the physiologic abnormalities responsible for the findings. In fact, he would have a mental image of the curves shown in Plate 1.

True it is that proficiency in physical examination requires skill and this demands practice, but we must now recognize that physical diagnosis of the cardiovascular system has a scientific basis. In fact, the renaissance in physical examination has been made possible because of scientific advances in modern instrumentation.

The physical examination will be divided into general inspection of the patient, examination of the arteries, examination of the veins, percussion versus inspection and palpation of the heart, inspection and palpation of the precordium, auscultation of the heart, and examination of the retinal fundi.

GENERAL INSPECTION OF THE PATIENT WITH CARDIOVASCULAR DISEASE

R. Bruce Logue, M.D., and *J. Willis Hurst, M.D.*

Although a careful history remains the most important diagnostic tool in general medicine, many tell-tale *clues* may be identified by mere *inspection* of the patient. These clues are meaningful only to the receptive and trained observer. They may help unravel difficult diagnosis or aid in the understanding of some obvious and simple disorder. They aid in diagnosis by tipping the scale as one balances probabilities. Many medical disorders will go unrecognized unless certain diagnostic clues are identified at the initial examination of the patient.

Marfan's syndrome[1,2] of the classical type is usually apparent on inspection. The long, tapering fingers with webbing, dislocation of the lens, high, narrow-arched palate, scoliosis, pectus carinatum and excavatum, relaxation of fascia and ligaments, and genu valgum and recurvatum are well known (Fig. 5-2). Enlargement of the great toe, prognathism, and congenital cystic disease of the lung have been noted. The *forme fruste* variety may lack many of the features, and the asethenic habitus may be replaced by the sthenic habitus. Marfan's

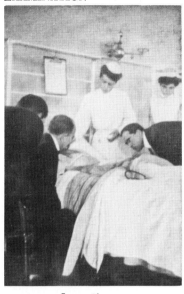

Inspection

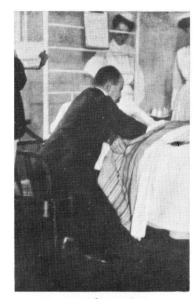

Palpation

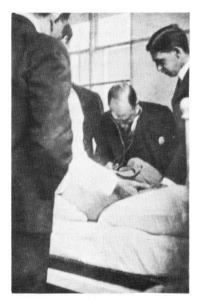

Auscultation

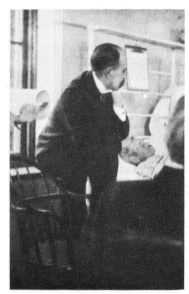

Contemplation

SNAPSHOTS OF OSLER AT THE BEDSIDE

Fig. 5-1. "Sir William Osler at the Bedside." (*Reprinted with permission from "The Life of Sir William Osler," by Harvey Cushing, M.D., Oxford University Press at Clarendon, 1925.*)

syndrome is often associated with medial cystic necrosis of the aorta or pulmonary arteries and may result in aneurysm formation, either saccular or dissecting. Patients with this disorder may also have atrial septal defect, degeneration of the heart valves, and myocardial disease. Aortic insufficiency due to dilatation of the aorta is common in such patients. The incidence of dissecting aneurysm is also more common in patients with scoliosis but without other features of Marfan's syndrome than it is in the normal population.[3]

Dissecting aneurysm may be a complication of the *Ehlers-Danlos syndrome* as well as of the Marfan syndrome.[1] The clinical features of this disorder of connective tissue are hyperelasticity and fragility of the skin and hyperextensibility of the joints. The ordinary types of congenital heart disease and valve disease occur. Ocular abnormalities, mediastinal

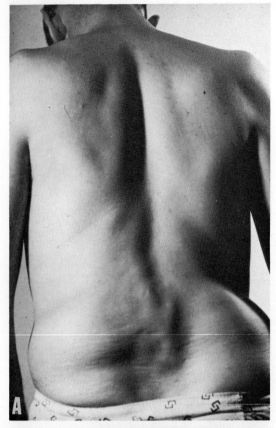

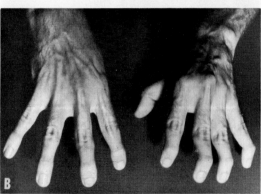

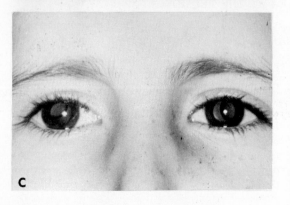

emphysema, pneumothorax, hernias, and other intestinal diseases also occur.

Osteogenesis imperfecta, a connective-tissue disorder, is expressed clinically as brittle bones, deafness, blue sclerae, thin skin, loose jointedness, and hernia. Aortic insufficiency may develop in this syndrome.[1]

Patients with *pseudo-xanthoma elasticum* have abnormalities of the skin, especially in the areas of wear and tear (Fig. 5-3). The skin is "crepe-like," lax, redundant, and inelastic. Angioid streaks are noted in the ocular fundi (see "Examination of Retinal Fundi," further on in this chapter). Arterial degeneration with calcification may occur. Hypertension and gastrointestinal hemorrhage are common.[1]

In the presence of congenital heart disease, one should suspect *coarctation of the aorta* when confronted with unusual muscular development in the upper part of the body, particularly in the male.[4] Conversely, one should suspect a large *left-to-right shunt*, especially atrial septal defect, in the female with underdevelopment of musculature and the so-called "gracile habitus."[5] The range of normal limits the value of these observations. Patients with congenital heart disease who have right-to-left shunts and decreased pulmonary blood flow may *sweat* in a characteristic manner after slight exertion. Children with left ventricular failure, such as occurs with endocardial fibroelastosis, also sweat abnormally. Tetralogy of Fallot is the most common disorder associated with squatting in children (see Chap. 20).

The presence of "pouting" lips, full cheeks, strabismus, prominent chin and nose, and dull expression may suggest *supravalvular aortic stenosis*[6] (see Chap. 20).

Hypertelorism and "moon facies" have been noted with severe valvular *pulmonary stenosis*. Pulmonary stenosis has been observed in children who have small stature, hypertelorism, mild mental retardation, and in some instances ptosis, undescended testes, and skeletal malformations.[7]

Turner's syndrome of gonadal agenesis is often associated with coarctation of the aorta or pulmonary stenosis[8] (Fig. 5-4). Patients with typical features show webbing of the neck, short stature, increased carrying angle, shield chest, and absence

Fig. 5-2. Marfan's syndrome. The patient experienced painless dissection of the aorta with aortic regurgitation following a vigorous game of basketball. (*A*) Note scoliosis. Not all patients with this syndrome are asthenic; note the muscular build of this patient. (*B*) Long, tapering fingers (arachnodactyly of same patient). (*C*) Dislocation of lens of the eye in another patient with Marfan's syndrome.

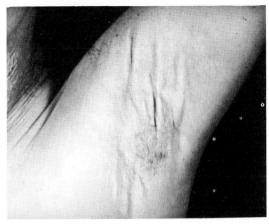

Fig. 5-3. Pseudo-xanthoma elasticum. The skin is crepe-like, lax, redundant, and inelastic. Arterial calcification, hypertension, and gastrointestinal hemorrhage occur in these patients.

of breast development with retained pubic and axillary hair. It is likely that Turner's syndrome will be further clarified in the future.

Mongolism (Down's syndrome), with slant eyes,

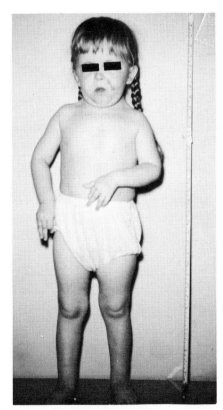

Fig. 5-4. Turner's syndrome. Note the "webbed" neck and shield chest. (The eyes had an anti-Mongol appearance.) These patients have a high incidence of coarctation of the aorta and pulmonary stenosis.

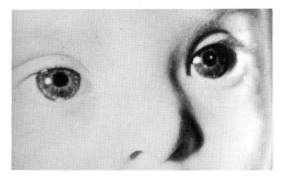

Fig. 5-5. Mongolism (Down's syndrome). Brushfield's spots in the iris and epicanthal folds are apparent. Atrial septal defect and endocardial cushion defects may be present in such patients.

epicanthal folds, Brushfield spots in the iris, shortening of the middle phalanx of the fifth fingers, characteristic cry, typical movements of the mouth, and protruding tongue, is readily recognized [9] (Fig. 5-5). This condition is assciated with a high incidence of atrial septal defect and abnormalities of the endocardial cushion, including the atrioventricularis communis and anomalies of the mitral and tricuspid valves. Mongolism is genetically determined, and some patients have 46 chromosomes, but the majority have 47 with trisomy of chromosome 21.

The *Gregg-Swan syndrome* following rubella, or German measles, in the first 2 months of pregnancy is characterized by cataracts, eighth-nerve deafness, and congenital heart disease[10] (Fig. 5-6). Patent ductus arteriosus, often associated with pulmonary stenosis, is common in this group of patients. Coarctation of the pulmonary artery also occurs.

Deaf-mutism may be accompanied by prolonged Q-T interval in the electrocardiogram and a tendency to sudden death.[11]

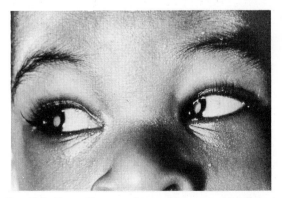

Fig. 5-6. Gregg-Swan syndrome. Note cataracts. Patent ductus arteriosus with or without pulmonary stenosis is common in these patients. Coarctation of the pulmonary artery may occur.

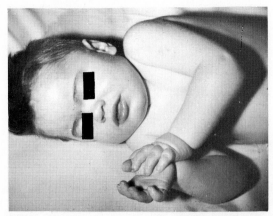

Fig. 5-7. Hurler's syndrome. Note the coarse features, bushy eyebrows, and short, stubby hands. Abnormal amounts of mucopolysaccharides may be deposited in the heart valves, coronary arteries, and aorta of such patients.

Gargoylism, or Hurler's syndrome,[1] is associated with dwarfism, coarse features, clouding of the cornea, mental deficiency, hepatosplenomegaly, multiple deformities of the skeleton, and a high incidence of cardiovascular lesions (Fig. 5-7). Acid mucopolysaccharide is deposited in the aorta and in the coronary arteries and valves, particularly the mitral and tricuspid, with nodular thickening which may produce stenosis or insufficiency.

Anomalies in the E_1-*trisomy (group 16 to 18) syndrome* include malformations of the heart, gastrointestinal tract, and kidneys.[12] Cardiovascular defects thus far reported include ventricular septal defect, patent ductus arteriosus, patent or fenes-

trated foramen ovale, valvular deformities, and many others. Patients with this syndrome show micrognathia, low-set ears, short neck, flexion deformity of arms, and characteristic posturing of the hands (Fig. 5-8).

Relapsing polychondritis is characterized by redness, swelling, and destruction of the cartilaginous structures.[13] The ears may have a "cauliflower" appearance, and the bridge of the nose may collapse (Fig. 5-9). Interstitial keratitis may be present. Aortic insufficiency has been noted.[14]

Acromegaly, due to excessive liberation of growth hormone, may be associated with cardiac enlargement and heart failure.[15] The classic features of prognathism and "spade" hands are readily recognized on inspection.

Cushing's syndrome as a cause of curable hypertension and heart failure may be suspected because of the moon facies, "buffalo hump" obesity, thin atrophic skin, purplish striae of the trunk, hirsutism, and acne[16] (Fig. 5-10). Of course, it is common today for these features to be due to corticosteroid administration.

Muscular dystrophy of the classic type is recognized by the large calves and infraspinatus muscles with thin thighs and wasted triceps and trapezius muscles. There may be progressive, symmetric involvement of the muscles of the pelvic girdle, resulting in a waddling, steppage gait, loose shoulders, and inability to attain an erect position without bracing of the upper extremities. The myocardium may be involved, with death due to congestive heart failure.[17]

Friedreich's ataxia may be associated with cardiac enlargement, congestive heart failure, and electrocardiographic abnormalities.[18] The disorder may be suspected from the characteristic gait, and kyphoscoliosis may develop (Fig. 5-11).

The presence of tower skull and leg ulcers are

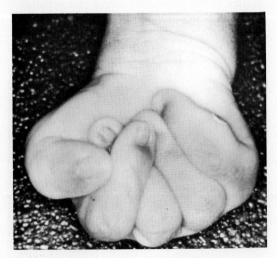

Fig. 5-8. E₁ trisomy (group 16 to 18) syndrome. Typical posturing of the hands occurs in these patients. A variety of cardiac abnormalities has been reported with this syndrome.

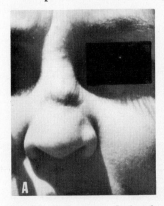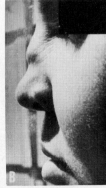

Fig. 5-9. Relapsing polychondritis. Note collapse of the bridge of the nose. This patient developed aortic regurgitation.[14] (*Courtesy of Dr. Warren Sarrell Anniston, Alabama.*)

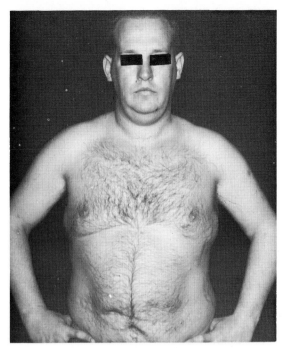

Fig. 5-10. Cushing's syndrome. Note the absence of typical "moon facies." The striae on the lateral aspects of the upper portion of the abdomen suggest the diagnosis.

such late manifestations of *sickle-cell disease* as to be of little help in the evaluation of an enlarged heart and murmurs which closely simulate rheumatic heart disease.[19]

Kyphoscoliosis, regardless of cause, may produce severe cardiorespiratory failure.[20]

Thyrotoxicosis as a sole or aggravating factor of heart failure with atrial fibrillation is obvious in its common form, but in the cardiac form the manifestations are unfortunately more subtle[21] (Fig. 5-12). The fine texture of the skin, warm edema, wide pulse pressure, inability to slow the rate satisfactorily with digitalis, refractory heart failure, intolerance to heat, absence of constipation despite inactivity, weight loss with good appetite, and occasionally weakness due to myopathy may force consideration of this disease. Advanced aortic stenosis, aortic insufficiency, and tuberculosis may simulate thyrotoxicosis.

Myxedema as a cause of pericardial effusion and cardiomegaly is still overlooked[22] (Fig. 5-13). The slow release of tendon reflexes may be most helpful.

The *demeanor* of the patient may provide information. The patient with some atypical or indescribable chest distress, who, observed during an attack, presents the "clenched-fist sign" over the sternum, with pallor and sweating, supports the diagnosis of

coronary disease.[23] (Dr. Samuel A. Levine in many years of teaching has emphasized this clue.)

Aldosteronism may be suspected when profound weakness is noted.[24] (One patient seen by us was so weak she could not comb her hair. This was the first clue that the cause of her hypertension was an aldosteroma.)

The observation of a typical "epinephrine reaction" with pallor, sweating, tremulousness, and elevated blood pressure may prompt a diagnosis of *pheochromocytoma. Café au lait* spots and neurofibromatosis are occasionally seen.[25]

Dyspnea, cyanosis, drowsiness, and heart failure may develop in the *obese* patient with *pulmonary hypoventilation.*[26]

Insufficient attention is paid to the *respiratory rate* and the character of the respirations. Although the patient with chronic heart failure may have a normal respiratory rate, the early evidence of interstitial edema of the lungs may be manifested by tachypnea and a rising pulse rate. These signs may occur when there are no rales, no ventricular gallop, and no venous distension. The infant with heart failure may show tachypnea and tachycardia without rales in the lungs on auscultation. The char-

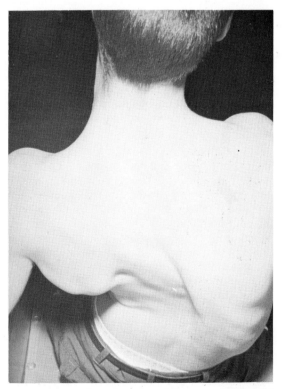

Fig. 5-11. Kyphoscoliosis secondary to Friedreich's ataxia. This young boy developed marked cardiac enlargement of the type seen in Friedreich's ataxia before kyphoscoliosis developed.

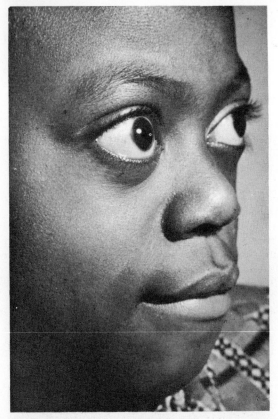

Fig. 5-12. Thyrotoxicosis. Thyrotoxicosis may occur at any age. This photograph shows typical exophthalmos in a young boy. Thyrotoxicosis in the older age group may not be so obvious. Atrial fibrillation is frequently due to thyrotoxicosis. Thyrotoxicosis may precipitate or aggravate heart failure and angina pectoris.

acter of the respirations may be helpful. For example, the initial suspicion that symptoms are due to anxiety may be aroused by the frequent *sighing respirations* associated with the hyperventilation syndrome.[27] The clue to troublesome insomnia aggravated by sedatives and opiates may be the observation of *Cheyne-Stokes respirations*. At times this type of breathing may be an early symptom of left ventricular failure.

Dyspnea or *syncope* occurring in the *sitting* position should suggest the possibility of left atrial myxoma.

Edema of the eyelids may occur in adults with heart failure who are able to sleep in the recumbent position. Edema of the eyelids is common in children with heart failure, when it may be erroneously attributed to renal disease.

The skin may furnish significant clues to the presence of cardiovascular disease. One need only mention *erythema marginatum*, the evanescent erythematous circinate lesions occurring particularly on the trunk in about 10 per cent of patients with acute rheumatic fever. The *subcutaneous nodules* are more specific but are less common, appearing in 3 to 4 per cent of patients and always in association with active myocarditis. They may appear in crops, are nontender, and have predilection for the region of the scapulae, dorsal spine, extensor surfaces of the elbows, wrists, knees, or ankles. They may appear on the forehead (Fig. 5-14).

Though most patients with acute disseminated lupus erythematosus do not have a *butterfly type of rash*, its appearance may give ready explanation of the cause of myocarditis or pericarditis[28] (Fig. 5-15).

A history of *Raynaud's syndrome* may antedate other evidence of lupus erythematosus for many years; this syndrome is, of course, common with scleroderma and at times is seen with primary pulmonary hypertension and aortic arch syndrome. In patients with *scleroderma* the characteristic changes of the skin of the fingers, face, and neck may clarify the cause of heart failure due to diffuse myocardial involvement.[29]

Skin lesions are common in *periorteritis nodosa*, but they lack specificity. (The initial suspicion of periarteritis in one patient seen by us with hypertension and unexplained fever was aroused by the presence of a pea-sized pulsating nodule at the angle of the left scapula.) It is not widely recognized that the testicles are frequently involved in the course of this disease. Painful swelling of the epididymis or testicle may follow vascular involvement. Baggenstoss noted testicular involvement in 86 per cent of 38 male patients with periarteritis; he suggested that testicular biopsy should be done when this disease is suspected and there is no clinical involvement of the skin or muscles.[30]

Today it is deplorable to depend in any degree on skin manifestations for the diagnosis of bacterial endocarditis. However, if the physician is rusty and has a low index of suspicion for the disease, he may be rudely awakened ultimately by the presence of *Osler's nodes, Janeway lesions, petechiae,* and *splinter hemorrhages*[31] (Fig. 5-16). Of these, Osler's nodes are most characteristic; they are painful pea-sized, reddish-purple nodules which appear on the pads of the fingers, toes, or palms and disappear after 2 to 3 days. Janeway lesions are erythematous, nontender macular lesions on the soles or palms. Splinter hemorrhages under the nails may occur with subacute bacterial endocarditis but are also seen in trichinosis, infectious mononucleosis, blood dyscrasias, cryoglobulinemia, and occasionally in patients with mitral stenosis without infection, and they may be due to trauma (Fig. 5-16). Late during the course of endocarditis, mycotic aneurysms may present as reddened, tender, pulsa-

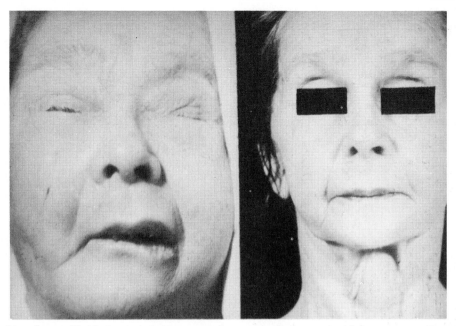

Fig. 5-13. Myxedema. (*Left*) Patient in near-coma shows typical facies. (*Right*) Some months after thyroid therapy. Pericardial effusion is common in this group and is the major cause of the large cardiac silhouette seen on the x-ray.

tile nodules along the course of small or medium-sized arteries.

The petechiae and purpura of *fat emboli* may be diagnostic clues in the patient with sudden onset of hypoxia, cyanosis, dyspnea, and collapse within 24 hours after fracture or surgical incision of bone.[32] Anxiety, restlessness, delirium, and coma may develop.

The skin lesions of amyloidosis may become hemorrhagic when stroked with the hand or traumatized by clothing.[33] (One of our patients had *purpura* in a necklace distribution over the upper trunk. He also had angina pectoris, cardiomegaly, heart failure, and Q-S deflections in leads V_1, V_2,

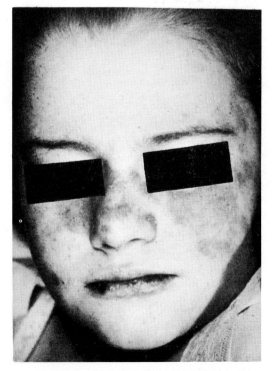

Fig. 5-15. Young girl with lupus erythematosus. Typical "butterfly" rash of the face. The rash may not be so obvious or may not be present at all. Patients with lupus erythematosus may have "myocarditis" and pericarditis.

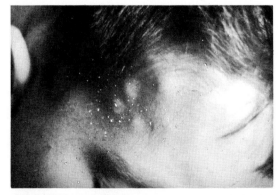

Fig. 5-14. Subcutaneous nodules on the forehead in a child with acute rheumatic fever.

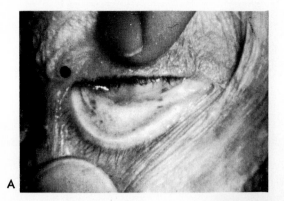

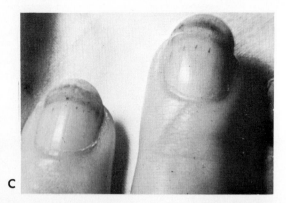

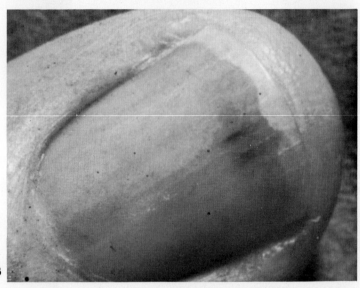

Fig. 5-16. Bacterial endocarditis.
A. Petechial hemorrhages of the
lower eyelid of a patient with bacterial endocarditis. B. Splinter
hemorrhages beneath the nails may
occur in bacterial endocarditis but
also may be due to other conditions. The splinter hemorrhage
shown here occurred in a *normal*,
healthy medical school professor.
The splinter hemorrhages shown in
C were due to trichinosis.

and V_3 of the electrocardiogram. The diagnosis was
thought to be coronary atherosclerosis, and the purpura was attributed to anticoagulants. Amyloidosis
was found at autopsy. The amyloid deposits in the
myocardium gave a dead-zone effect in the electrocardiogram, and there was no significant atherosclerosis.[34,35]

Spider angiomas over the upper trunk and extremities are common in cirrhosis and may lead to
the solution of rare, puzzling instances of high-
output failure due to liver disease.[36]

Hemochromatosis may cause myocardial failure;
it may be suspected in the diabetic patient with
brownish-gray pigmentation due to hemosiderin
and melanin distributed particularly in the folds and
creases of the skin. Hepatosplenomegaly, testicular
atrophy, and diminished axillary and pubic hair are
common in this condition.[37]

Carcinoid of the small intestine with metastasis
to the liver produces an unusual and dramatic clinical picture. The patient may experience intense
abdominal cramps, severe diarrhea, bronchial

asthma, and episodes of intense flushing of the skin.
In time the flushing may become persistent. There
may be marked telangiectasis of the face and trunk.
The clinical picture is produced by the serotonin
liberated by the tumor. Abnormalities of the pulmonary and tricuspid valves are common in such
patients. Heart failure may occur, and lesions have
been noted on the left side of the heart.[38,39] Tumors
other than carcinoid may produce flushing of the
skin (Plate 3). Pancreatic neoplasms have been
reported to produce symptoms suggesting the carcinoid syndrome.[40]

Familial hypercholesterolemia may be readily
recognized by the presence of *xanthomatous* deposits in the Achilles tendons and in the extensor
tendons of the fingers (Fig. 5-17). There are usually, but not always, associated high levels of serum
cholesterol and a strong family history of coronary
disease at a young age. Aortic stenosis may also
occur in patients with this disorder.[41]

Patients with *pulmonary arteriovenous fistulas* frequently have *hereditary hemorrhagic telangiectasis*.

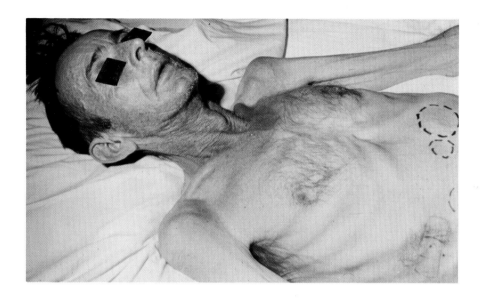

Plate 3. Flushing of the skin may be due to certain tumors. Intense flushing of the skin may occur in patients with carcinoid of the small intestine with metastasis to the liver. Such patients may have lesions on the right side of the heart and heart failure. The patient shown had severe diarrhea, episodes of intense abdominal pain, and persistent cutaneous flushing of the face and neck. He noted attacks of increased flushing and "general stimulation" after smoking a cigarette. His skin was too sensitive to permit shaving. Large amounts of 5-hydroxyindole acetic acid were excreted in the urine. This particular case of "carcinoid syndrome" was due to cancer of the tail of the pancreas.

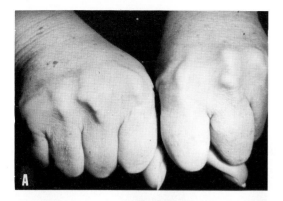

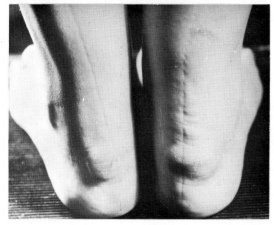

Fig. 5-17. Xanthomatosis. (A) Xanthomatous nodules located on the tendons of the hands. (B) Large xanthomatous masses located in the Achilles tendons. This patient was a middle-aged female with aortic stenosis and coronary atherosclerosis.

Therefore, telangiectasis of the lips, tongue, nasal mucosa, and fingertips should stimulate one to consider this disorder. Pulmonary arteriovenous fistula may mimic congenital heart disease.[42]

Clubbing of the fingers and toes occurs as a familial abnormality in otherwise normal persons.[43] It may be a late finding in bacterial endocarditis.[31] When clubbing of the fingers and toes is associated with cyanosis, congenital heart disease with a right-to-left shunt or a pulmonary arteriovenous fistula should be considered (Fig. 5-18). Clubbing of the great toes and thumbs may become apparent in small children before the abnormality is obvious in the other toes and fingers. Painful clubbing of the fingers does not occur as a result of congenital heart disease; it suggests the possibility of bronchogenic carcinoma, lung abscess, or bronchiectasis. Clubbing has also been noted in patients with cirrhosis of the liver, ulcerative colitis, and regional enteritis. Unilateral clubbing occurs with congenital arteriovenous fistulas, superior sulcus tumor, aortic

or subclavian aneurysm, and chronic dislocation of the shoulder. Clubbing of the toes and fingers of the left hand, but not of the right, may be seen in patients with patent ductus arteriosus with reversed shunt.

Scars on the extremities secondary to trauma and at old operative sites may stimulate one to think of acquired systemic arteriovenous fistula.[44] The scar may be small, no larger than would be made by an ice pick, and may be hidden deep in the axilla. A laminectomy scar is very suspect. Having found a scar, one must listen over the scar with a stethoscope for the continuous murmur of an *arteriovenous fistula*. When the fistula is located in the extremities, it is often possible to see a large, pulsating mass and huge, tortuous veins. A systemic arteriovenous fistula may produce a hyperkinetic circulation, cardiac enlargement, and heart failure. The pulse rate usually slows when the fistula is occluded.

Asymmetric lengthening and overgrowth of an extremity or digit associated with varicose veins and perhaps with distal ulceration due to ischemia are common in *congenital peripheral arteriovenous fistulas* of the part.[45] Many of the patients with this condition have port-wine stains and hemangioma of the skin (Fig. 5-19).

Macroglossia may occur with primary systemic amyloid disease,[34,35] glycogen-storage disease, myxedema, and acromegaly. Patients with amyloid may be suspected of having tumors of the submaxillary glands because of enlargement of the base of the tongue, which depresses these glands (Fig. 5-20). Vitreous opacities are common in familial amyloidosis.

Patients with *rheumatoid arthritis* of the spine, psoriasis, and iritis may have *aortic insufficiency*.[46]

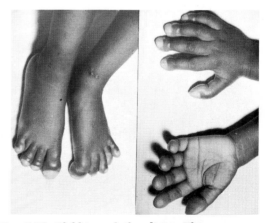

Fig. 5-18. Clubbing of the digits. There are many causes of clubbing of the digits. Congenital heart disease with right-to-left shunt associated with cyanosis is the most common cause.

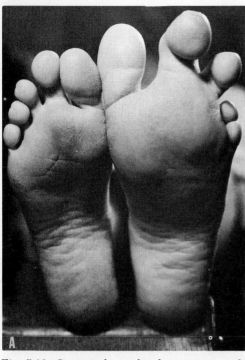
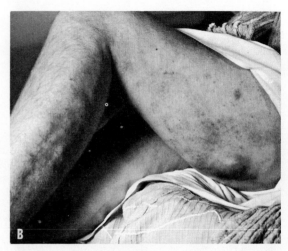

Fig. 5-19. Congenital peripheral arteriovenous fistulas. Asymmetric enlargement of an extremity or digit associated with unusual varicose veins may occur in patients with congenital peripheral arteriovenous fistulas. (A) The grotesque enlargement of the toes and foot on the right is obvious. (B) Note the peculiar location of the "masses" due to dilatation of the veins on the lateral aspect of the lower leg and on the posterior surface of the upper leg. In addition, this young female had multiple pulmonary emboli.

Pericarditis may also occur in patients with rheumatoid arthritis.[47]

The notation of *pectus excavatum* may alert one to the probability of a functional murmur in the patient with a loud ejection type of murmur over the outflow tract of the right ventricle. This type of chest abnormality may not be appreciated on the

frontal-view x-ray of the chest, and the heart in such cases may be thought to be enlarged.

The detection of obstructive emphysema may give a clue to the cause of dyspnea and edema.

Cyanosis, as detected by the doctor's eye, is not a reliable guide to arterial oxygen unsaturation.[48] The arterial oxygen saturation may be as low as 85 per cent before cyanosis is detected. A bluish color of the skin is noted when at least 5 Gm of reduced hemoglobin is present, whereas only 1.5 Gm of methemoglobin or 0.5 Gm of sulfhemoglobin is required. Cyanosis due to methemoglobinemia or sulfhemoglobinemia is usually a consequence of drug administration and should be suspected when no cardiorespiratory disease is present. If the skin is bluish but the mucous membranes are of normal color, argyria is the likely cause. Cyanosis of the feet and left hand, with absence of cyanosis of the right hand and face, indicates that patent ductus arteriosus with reverse flow is likely.[49,50] Patent ductus arteriosus may be the only abnormality; however, many other associated abnormalities may be present.

Signs of high-output cardiac failure have been observed in patients with widespread psoriasis and eczema. The signs of failure disappear as the skin improves. It seems likely that the high cardiac out-

Fig. 5-20. Amyloidosis. Macroglossia may be due to amyloid infiltration of the tongue. This young woman had amyloid deposits in the base of the tongue. This depressed the submaxillary glands that are seen in the photograph.

put may be the result of increased blood flow through vasodilated skin.[51]

Certain abnormalities of the arterial, venous, and precordial *pulsations* may be seen at a distance; they will be discussed subsequently. *Buckling* of the right common carotid artery is often mistaken as an aneurysm. This condition is more common in the elderly female with hypertension and atherosclerosis and may be responsible for cerebral ischemic attacks. Some patients also have a kinked innominate artery. Distension, due to kinking, of the left innominate vein may develop when the aorta becomes enlarged and sclerotic, compressing the vein against the sternum.[52] Unilateral distension of the neck veins may lead to a diagnosis of mediastinal tumor; bilateral distension of veins, plus evidence of collateral venous circulation over the upper part of the chest, suggests superior vena cava obstruction.

Sounds may be heard at a distance from the patient.[53] The "dove-coo" murmur of aortic regurgitation secondary to eversion (syphilis), laceration, or rupture (endocarditis and trauma) of one or more aortic cusps may be heard at a great distance from the chest. Other murmurs that have been heard a distance from the heart include aortic stenosis and mitral stenosis. "Splashing" noises due to air and water in the pericardial space may be heard at a distance.

This section could be expanded to the length of a large book. These few comments serve only to make a single point. *The first glance at a patient is extremely important. When diagnostic clues are missed, they are likely to be missed entirely—even after days of observation.*

The photographs shown in Figs. 5-2, 5-3, 5-9, 5-10, 5-11, 5-13, 5-14, 5-16, 5-17, 5-19, and 5-20 are of patients seen on the medical services of the Department of Medicine of Emory University School of Medicine (Emory University Hospital and Grady Memorial Hospital). The photographs shown in Figs. 5-4, 5-5, 5-6, 5-7, 5-12, 5-15, and 5-18 were kindly supplied by the Department of Pediatrics of Emory University and Grady Memorial Hospital. The photograph shown in Fig. 5-8 was supplied by the Department of Gynecology and Obstetrics, Emory University School of Medicine and Grady Memorial Hospital. The Photograph in Plate 3 was made on the medical service of Grady Memorial Hospital, and the autopsy was performed by Dr. Alan Clepper and Dr. Earl Barton of the Department of Pathology of Emory University School of Medicine at Grady Memorial Hospital. (This case will be reported in detail elsewhere.)

REFERENCES

1. McKussick, V. A.: "Heritable Disorders of Connective Tissue," 2d ed., The C. V. Mosby Company, St. Louis, 1960.

2. Papaevannon, A. C., Agustsson, M. H., and Gosul, B. M.: Early Manifestations of the Cardiovascular Disorders in Marfan's Syndrome, *Pediatrics,* **58:**255, 1961.

3. Bean, W. B., and Ponseti, I. V.: Dissecting Aneurysms Produced by Diet, *Circulation,* **12:**185–192, 1955.

4. Fowler, N. O.: "Physical Diagnosis of Heart Disease," The Macmillan Company, New York, 1962.

5. Taussig, H. B., Harvey, A. M., and Follis, R. H., Jr.: The Clinical and Pathological Findings in Interauricular Septal Defects, *Bull. Johns Hopkins Hosp.,* **63:**61–89, 1938.

6. Morrow, A. G., Waldhausen, J. A., Peters, R. L., Bloodwell, R. D., and Braunwald, E.: Supravalvular Aortic Stenosis: Clinical Hemodynamic and Pathological Observation, *Circulation,* **20:**1003, 1959.

7. Noonan, J. A., and Ehmke, D. A.: Associated Noncardiac Malformations in Children with Congenital Heart Disease, *J. Pediat.,* **63:**468–470, 1963.

8. Ranier-Pope, C. R., Cunningham, R. D., Nadas, A. S., and Crigler, J. F., Jr.: Cardiovascular Malformations in Turner's Syndrome, *Pediatrics,* **33:**919, 1964.

9. Rowe, R. D.: Cardiac Malformation in Mongolism, *Am. Heart J.,* **64:**567, 1962.

10. Lundstrom, R.: Rubella During Pregnancy; Its Effect upon Perinatal Mortality, Incidence of Congenital Abnormalities and Immaturity, Preliminary Report. *Acta pediat.,* **51:**583, 1952.

11. Levine, S. A., and Woodworth, C. R.: Congenital Deaf-Mutism, Prolonged QT Interval, Syncopal Attacks and Sudden Death, *New England J. Med.,* **259:**412–417, 1958.

12. Rohde, R. A., Hodgman, J. E., and Cleland, R. S.: Anomalies in E₁-trisomy (Group 16–18) Syndrome, *Pediatrics,* **33:**258, 1964.

13. Pearson, C. M., Kline, H. M., and Newcomer, V. D.: Relapsing Polychondritis, *New England J. Med.,* **263:**51, 1960.

14. Logue, R. B., and Sarrell, W.: Personal observations.

15. Hejtmancik, M. R., Bradfield, J. Y., and Herman, G. R.: Acromegaly and the Heart: A Clinical and Pathologic Study, *Ann. Int. Med.,* **34:**1945, 1951.

16. Albright, F.: Cushing's Syndrome. Harvey Lectures, series 38, Science Press Printing Co., Lancaster, Pa., 1943.

17. Gailani, S., Danowski, T. S., and Fisher, D. S.: Muscular Dystrophy: Catheterization Studies Indicating Latent Congestive Heart Failure, *Circulation,* **17:**583–588, 1958.

18. Hartman, J. M., and Booth, R. W.: Friedreich's Ataxia, a Neurocardiac Disease, *Am. Heart J.,* **60:**716–720, 1960.

19. Shubin, H., Kaufman, R., Shapiro, M., and Levinson, D. C.: Cardiovascular Findings in Children with Sickle Cell Anemia, *Am. J. Cardiol.,* **6:**875–885, 1960.

20. Bergofsky, E. H., Turino, G. M., and Fishman,

A. P.: Cardiorespiratory Failure in Kyphoscoliosis, *Medicine*, **38**:263, 1959.

21. Abrahamsen, H. M., Haarstad, J., and Onlie, C.: Haemodynamic Studies in Thyrotoxicosis, *Acta med. scandinav.*, **174**:463, 1963.

22. Aber, C. P., and Thompson, G. S.: Factors Associated with Cardiac Enlargment in Myxoedema, *Brit. Heart J.*, **25**:421, 1963.

23. Levine, S. A. (Attributed to).

24. Conn, J. W. Aldosteronism and Hypertension, *Arch. Int. Med.*, **107**:813, 1961.

25. Krale, W. F., and Roth, G. M.: Some Aspects of Pheochromocytoma, *Circulation*, **21**:161, 1960.

26. Hackney, J. D., Crane, M. G., Collier, C. C., Rokaw, S., and Griggs, D. E.: Syndrome of Extreme Obesity and Hypoventilation: Studies of Etiology, *Ann. Int. Med.*, **51**:541, 1959.

27. Wood, P. H.: Differential Diagnosis of Da Costa's Syndrome, *Proc. Roy. Soc. Med.*, **34**:543, 1941.

28. Schoenfield, M. R., and Messeloff, C. R.: Cardiac Tamponade in Systemic Lupus Erythematosus, *Circulation*, **27**:98, 1963.

29. Bergelman, P. M., Baylis, T. B., and Goldner, F.: Progressive Systemic Sclerosis (Scleroderma), *New England J. Med.*, **249**:45, 1953.

30. Rose, G. A., and Spencer, H.: Periarteritis Nodosa, *Quart. J. Med.*, **26**:43, 1957.

31. Libsman, E., and Friedberg, C. K.: "Subacute Bacterial Endocarditis," Oxford University Press, Fair Lawn, N.J., 1941.

32. Love, J., and Stryker, W. S.: Fat Embolism: A Problem of Increasing Importance to the Orthopedist and the Internist, *Ann. Int. Med.*, **46**:342, 1957.

33. Hurley, H. J., and Weinberg, R.: Induced Intralesional Hemorrhage in Primary Systemic Amyloidosis, *Arch. Dermat.*, **89**:678–681, 1964.

34. Cassidy, J. T.: Clinical Manifestations of Cardiac Amyloidosis, *Am. Heart J.*, **64**:136, 1962.

35. Conter, W. T., and Reichert, R. E.: Primary Systemic Amyloidosis Mimicking Chronic Constrictive Pericarditis, *Circulation*, **2**:441, 1950.

36. Bean, W. B.: "Vascular Spiders and Related Lesions of the Skin," Charles C Thomas, Publisher, Springfield, Ill., 1958.

37. Lewis, H. P.: Cardiac Involvement in Hemochromatosis, *Am. J. M. Sc.*, **227**:554, 1954.

38. Mattingly, T. W., and Sjoerdsma, A.: The Cardiovascular Manifestations of Functioning Carcinoid Tumors, *Mod. Concepts Cardiovas. Dis.*, **25**:337–341, 1956.

39. Roberts, W. C., and Sjoerdsma, A.: The Cardiac Disease Associated with Carcinoid Syndrome (Carcinoid Heart Disease), *Am. J. Med.*, **36**:5, 1964.

40. Peart, W. S., Porter, K. A., Robertson, J. I. S., Sandler, M., and Baldock, E. I.: I. M. L. T. Carcinoid Syndrome Due to Pancreatic-duct Neoplasm Secreting 5-hydroxytryptophan and 5-hydroxytryptamine, *Lancet*, **1**:239–242, 1963.

41. Lever, W. F., Smith, P. A. J., and Hurley, N. A.: Idiopathic Hyperlipemic and Primary Hypercholesterolemic Xanthomatosis, *J. Dermat.*, **22**:23, 1954.

42. Husson, G. S.: Pulmonary Arteriovenous Aneurysm in Childhood, *Pediatrics*, **18**:871–878, 1956.

43. Fischer, D. S., Singer, D. H., and Feldman, S. M.: Clubbing: A Review with Emphasis on Hereditary Acropachy, *Medicine*, **43**:459, 1964.

44. Rowe, G. C., Castillo, C. A., Alfonso, S., and Crumpton, C. W.: The Systemic and Hemodynamic Effects of Arteriovenous Fistulas, *Am. Heart J.*, **64**:44, 1962.

45. Hurst, J. W.: Some Disconnected Odds and Ends of Cardiology, *Tr. Am. Clin. & Climatol. A.*, **72**:159–167, 1960.

46. Lebowitz, W. B.: The Heart in Rheumatoid Arthritis (Rheumatoid Disease): A Clinical and Pathological Study of Sixty-two Cases, *Ann. Int. Med.*, **58**:102, 1963.

47. Lietman, P. S., and Byrvaters, E. G. L.: Pericarditis in Juvenile Rheumatoid Arthritis, *Pediatrics*, **32**:855, 1963.

48. Comroe, J. H., Jr., and Botelho, S.: The Unreliability of Cyanosis in the Recognition of Arterial Anoxemia, *Am. J. M. Sc.*, **214**:1, 1947.

49. Campbell, M., and Hudson, R.: Patent Ductus Arteriosus with Reverse Shunt Due to Pulmonary Hypertension, *Guy's Hosp. Rep.*, **100**:26, 1951.

50. Huetgren, H., Selzer, A., Purdy, A., Holmon, E., and Gerbode, F.: The Syndrome of Patent Ductus Arteriosus with Pulmonary Hypertension, *Circulation*, **8**:15, 1953.

51. Shuster, S.: High Output Cardiac Failure from Skin Disease, *Lancet*, **1**:1338–1340, 1963.

52. Smith, K. S.: The Kinked Innominate Vein, *Brit. Heart J.*, **22**:110, 1960.

53. Groom, D., and Boone, J. A.: The "Dove-coo" Murmur and Murmurs Heard at a Distance from the Chest, *Ann. Int. Med.*, **42**:1214–1226, 1955.

EXAMINATION
OF THE ARTERIES *

*J. Willis Hurst, M.D., and
Robert C. Schlant, M.D.*

Palpation of the peripheral arteries may yield the following information: the frequency and regularity of the pulsations, the condition and patency of the peripheral arteries, and the characteristics of the arterial pressure pulse wave. The purpose of this section is to discuss the arterial pressure pulse wave in the normal and abnormal states.

During the transmission of the arterial pulse wave, the normal peripheral arteries expand but very slightly. Although this expansion may be vis-

* Grateful acknowledgment is made to Dr. Gerhard A. Brecher, Professor and Chairman of the Department of Physiology of Emory University School of Medicine, for his assistance in the preparation of this manuscript.

ualized, particularly when it is increased in disease states, much of the apparent expansion which one may visualize is the result of partial straightening in addition to actual diameter changes. The pressure-volume characteristics of arterial vessels are complex. Accordingly, "pulse" recordings of volume changes (the *volume pulse*) or of flow changes (the *flow pulse*) are not identical with *pressure pulse* recordings. Furthermore, many external recordings of the carotid artery pulse, particularly those made using piezoelectric or other so-called linear microphones, do not faithfully register all components of the true carotid arterial pressure pulse curve. The wave form of the pressure wave—the *pressure pulse*—should be distinguished from the *pulse pressure*, which is the pressure difference between the maximum systolic pressure and the minimum diastolic pressure.

Although some local distortion of the pressure pulse curve is produced by the arterial compression necessary to palpate an arterial pulse, much valuable clinical information may be obtained by this simple means. In order for one to palpate the arterial pressure pulse, it is necessary to apply pressure to the wall of the vessel. This pressure is applied by the examining finger through the overlying skin and subcutaneous tissue. The applied pressure may completely or partially compress the peripheral artery. When one palpates a peripheral artery and applies pressure to compress the lumen of the artery partially, the arterial pressure pulse wave is sensed by the pressure receptors in the fingers as a pressure pulse wave superimposed on the base-line pressure produced by the examiner's finger.

CONTOUR CHANGES OF THE ARTERIAL PULSE DURING TRANSMISSION

The arterial pressure pulse undergoes characteristic changes in contour as it passes from the ascending aorta to the peripheral arteries (Figs. 5-21 and 5-22 and 2-6). The major factors which are responsible for these changes in contour as the pulse wave is transmitted peripherally are (1) distortion and damping of components of the pulse wave, (2) different rates of transmission of various components, (3) distortion or amplification by reflected, resonance, or standing waves, (4) conversion of kinetic energy into potential or hydrostatic energy, and (5) differences in elastic behavior and caliber of the arteries.

In normal persons the arterial pulse wave in the ascending aorta is characterized by a fairly rapid anacrotic rise to a somewhat rounded peak. An *anacrotic shoulder* or pause is frequently present on the ascending limb at about the moment when the peak of ejection is maximal, which occurs just before the peak pressure is reached. The descending limb of the pressure pulse is usually less steep than the ascending limb. It is interrupted by the *incisura*, a sharp downward deflection produced by closure of the aortic valve. Following the incisura, the pulse wave rises slightly and then falls more gradually until the next pulse occurs. A small wave

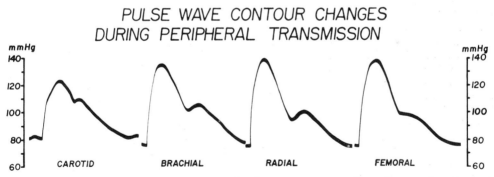

PULSE WAVE CONTOUR CHANGES DURING PERIPHERAL TRANSMISSION

Fig. 5-21. Pulse wave contour changes during peripheral transmission. As the pulse is palpated or recorded more peripherally, note that the ascending limb becomes steeper and the systolic pressure becomes higher, whereas the diastolic and mean pressures are lower. The anacrotic shoulder present in central recordings cannot ordinarily be felt, and it is not present normally in the peripheral pulses. In central pulses, the nadir of the incisura occurs very slightly after the closure of the aortic valve; therefore, the incisura is commonly used to identify A_2. As the pulse wave travels peripherally, there is a progressive "transition" of the incisura to a deeper and smoother dicrotic notch. The dicrotic notch occurs at a lower pressure and later in the pulse wave than the incisura. It is followed by a dicrotic wave which is largely produced by reflected or resonance waves. In the femoral artery, the dicrotic notch and dicrotic wave may be indistinct or even imperceptible. In the brachial-radial system there may normally be a slight suggestion of a positive wave in late systole just prior to the dicrotic notch. This is not normally palpable. A small presystolic arterial wave produced by atrial systole may be present in arterial pulse recordings but is not palpable. It tends to be less prominent peripherally.

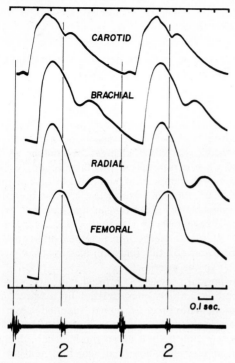

Fig. 5-22. Pulse wave contour changes during peripheral transmission arranged to indicate the transmission delay in various arteries. The onset of the carotid pulse occurs about 80 msec after closure of the mitral valve. This time interval is occupied by isovolumetric contraction of the left ventricle and the interval for the pulse to be transmitted from the ascending aorta to the carotid artery. The intervals between the onset of the carotid pulse and the onset of the pulse wave in various other peripheral arteries are as follows: 60 msec (brachial), 80 msec (radial), and 75 msec (femoral). Note that the pulse wave normally arrives at the radial and femoral arteries virtually simultaneously. As the pulse wave is transmitted peripherally, the systolic upstroke time (from onset of pulse to peak pressure) becomes shorter, whereas the measured systolic ejection period (from onset of pulse wave to incisura or dicrotic notch) becomes slightly longer.

produced by atrial systole immediately prior to the main pressure pulse is frequently recorded centrally but less frequently peripherally.

As the pulse wave is transmitted into the periphery, the initial upstroke characteristically becomes steeper and the anacrotic shoulder becomes barely visible or disappears. The systolic summit becomes increased in magnitude and sharper. The incisura becomes smoother in the peripheral pulse and is gradually replaced by a *dicrotic notch* or *halt*. The dicrotic notch usually occurs at a lower level than the incisura. The interval between the onset of the pulse wave and the dicrotic notch is greater than

the interval in the central pulse between the onset of the pulse wave and the incisura. The dicrotic notch is followed by a positive *dicrotic wave,* which is mainly produced by reflected waves from the periphery. The dicrotic wave is usually more prominent than the slight positive wave following the incisura in central tracings. At times, particularly in recordings from the femoral artery, the dicrotic notch and dicrotic wave are barely perceptible. As the pulse wave is transmitted to the brachial, radial, or femoral arteries, the systolic peak pressure increases about 10 per cent, whereas the diastolic pressure and the mean pressure decrease slightly. The pulse pressure is considerably increased. The brachial-radial system may develop a small second wave in the late systole which is usually not found in tracings from the carotid arteries or the femoral–dorsal pedis system.

Since the central arterial pressure pulse is progressively deformed as it travels peripherally, the peripheral pulse often reveals less information than the central pulse concerning alterations in left ventricular ejection or in aortic valve function. Accordingly, the carotid artery is generally preferable to more peripheral arteries for the bedside evaluation of the arterial pulse. On the other hand, certain types of pulse waves may be altered in such a way that the characteristic pulse abnormalities become accentuated rather than obscured in more peripheral vessels. This is particularly likely to occur with the large, bounding pulse of aortic regurgitation, with pulsus bisferiens, and with pulsus alternans. Accordingly, examination of the pulse should include all the major arteries, both for patency and for pulse wave form.

TECHNIQUE OF EXAMINING THE ARTERIAL PULSE

The arterial pulses are ordinarily examined while the patient is reclining with the trunk of the body elevated about 15 to 30°. In order to examine the carotid arteries the sternocleidomastoid muscles should be relaxed and the head rotated slightly toward the ipsilateral side. The examiner places either his forefinger or his thumb (depending on individual preference) lightly over the artery. *It is necessary to listen to the heart with the stethoscope in order to identify the first and second heart sounds while simultaneously palpating the carotid artery* (Fig. 5-23). The heart sounds are used as reference points for the examination not only of the arterial pulse but also of the jugular venous pulse. While listening to the heart sounds, the examiner carefully and slowly applies more and more pressure to the carotid artery until the maxi-

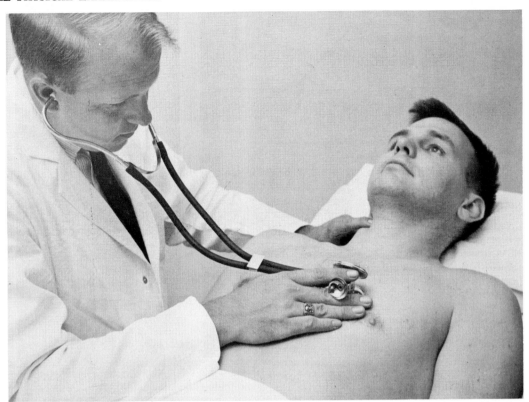

Fig. 5-23. Palpation of the carotid artery. The examiner palpates the common carotid artery while simultaneously listening to the heart sounds. In most instances, the heart sounds are the most satisfactory reference points for timing venous and arterial pulsations in the neck.

mum pulse is felt. The examiner should then slowly release the pressure on the artery while attempting to form a *mental image* of the pulse wave. It is best to divide the pulse wave into three parts: ascending limb, peak, and descending limb. While palpating, the examiner should concentrate on one part at a time, in a fashion corresponding to that used in cardiac auscultation. In most instances, a better appreciation of different parts of the curve can be gained by the application of varying amounts of pressure. For example, it may be possible to detect an anacrotic notch or a mild bisferiens pulse more easily with light pressure than with heavier pressure. In patients with evidence of diseased carotid arteries, palpation of the vessels should obviously be extremely gentle.

Further information should be obtained by simultaneously palpating the radial and femoral arteries and noting the relative time of onset of the pulse at the two locations. Normally, the pulse wave arrives in these locations virtually simultaneously; in coarctation of the aorta, both the onset and the peak of the weak femoral pulse are delayed. One may obtain an impression of the thickness and hardness of the walls of the brachial, radial, and dorsalis pedis arteries by "rolling" the compressed vessel against the underlying tissue.

THE NORMAL ARTERIAL PULSE

The normal carotid arterial pressure pulse wave is illustrated in Fig. 5-24, with the heart sounds as reference points. The upstroke of the carotid tracing begins about 80 milliseconds (msec) after the initial component of the first heart sound. This interval is variable and represents the phase of isovolumetric contraction and the short period required for actual transmission of the pulse wave in the aorta and the carotid artery. The upstroke or ascending limb is rapid and smooth. The anacrotic notch is not palpable in most normal persons although it can often be recorded from the aorta and the carotid artery. The summit of the carotid pressure pulse is smooth and dome-shaped. At rest the peak pressure usually occurs about 100 msec (range 60 to 140 msec) after the onset of the recorded pulse wave, when the measurement is corrected for heart rate by dividing the measured interval by the square root of the cycle length in

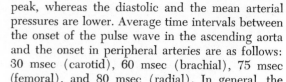

Fig. 5-24. The normal carotid artery pulse wave and heart sounds. The anacrotic shoulder is seen as a change in slope of the ascending limb shortly before the systolic peak. It is not normally palpable. The summit of the pulse is smooth and rounded. The sharp incisura, produced by closure of the aortic valve, is usually palpable as a change in downslope and less frequently as a distinct notch. Note that the ascending limb of the pulse wave is normally steeper than the descending limb. The first heart sound commences very slightly before the onset of the pulse wave, and the closure of the aortic valve (A_2) occurs at or very slightly prior to the nadir of the incisura. Closure of the pulmonic valve (P_2) normally occurs after closure of the aortic valve.

seconds.* The descending limb from the systolic peak is usually less steep than the ascending limb. In most normal individuals the carotid incisura or dicrotic notch is not palpable as a definite notch; however, one can usually sense a change to a less steep downslope. Occasionally in normal subjects, a definite dicrotic notch and dicrotic wave can be felt in the carotid pulse. These are particularly accentuated in young persons with fever, at times of excitement, or following exercise. In the carotid artery of normal subjects at rest, the incisura or dicrotic notch usually occurs about 300 msec (range 260 to 340 msec) after the onset of the pulse wave when the measurement is corrected for heart rate.

As noted above, in more peripheral vessels the pulse wave arrives later and is characterized by a steeper initial wave which reaches a higher systolic

* Several investigators have used various formulas utilizing the square root of the cycle length in attempts to adjust for the effect of heart rate on varying electrocardiographic and hemodynamic intervals.[1-4] Although the large number of variables affecting the systolic upstroke time and the systolic ejection period [2-5] obviously precludes the use of any simple formulas to correct accurately for heart rate, the clinical usefulness of these measurements from pulse recordings does appear to be enhanced when they are "corrected" by dividing by the square root of the cycle length in seconds.[6-9]

peak, whereas the diastolic and the mean arterial pressures are lower. Average time intervals between the onset of the pulse wave in the ascending aorta and the onset in peripheral arteries are as follows: 30 msec (carotid), 60 msec (brachial), 75 msec (femoral), and 80 msec (radial). In general, the systolic upstroke time is shorter but the systolic ejection period is longer in peripheral pulse tracings as compared to central pulse recordings. In the brachial artery, the rate-corrected systolic upstroke time is about 120 msec (range, 90 to 160 msec) and the systolic ejection time is about 320 msec (range, 280 to 360 msec).

Although the skilled examiner can detect many abnormalities by palpation of the peripheral arterial pulse, it is not possible to estimate the systemic blood pressure or cardiac output by palpating an artery.

THE ABNORMAL ARTERIAL PULSE

General Abnormalities of the Arterial Pulse

The apparent size of the arterial pulse is an important characteristic. It is determined by many factors, including the left ventricular stroke volume and rate of ejection, the distensibility of the systemic arterial bed, the peripheral resistance, the pulse rate, the systolic and diastolic pressures, the size and pressure-volume characteristics of the vessel being palpated, and the distance between the vessel and the heart. Despite the obvious complexities of the many factors influencing the peripheral arterial pulse, one may clinically divide abnormalities of pulse size into two groups: *small, weak* pulses and *large, bounding* pulses. While palpating an artery, one may obtain an impression of both the height of the pressure pulse and the rate of pressure change. Accordingly, patients who have a wide pulse pressure with a very rapid rate of pressure rise are easily distinguished from patients with a narrow pulse pressure and a slow rate of rise. One should also concentrate separately on the descending limb of the pulse wave and attempt to characterize its downslope in addition to the presence of absence of an incisura or dicrotic notch or dicrotic wave.

Small, Weak Pulse

A small, weak pulse is often found in conditions with a low stroke volume of the left ventricle, a narrow pulse pressure, and an increased peripheral vascular resistance. Common causes are left ventricular failure due to myocardial infarction, diffuse myocardial disease, cardiac tamponade or constrictive pericarditis, and stenosis of the mitral, pulmonic, or tricuspid valve. In many instances of left ventricular "failure," not only is the stroke volume diminished but the rate of ejection is decreased. In most of these conditions the increased peripheral vascular resistance is produced by a compensatory peripheral arteriolar vasoconstriction. Aortic stenosis may also be associated with a small, weak pulse. Since the cardiac output and stroke volume in pure aortic stenosis are usually well maintained (until the preterminal state is reached), the small, weak pulse in this instance is the result of the mechanical obstruction to left ventricular discharge. In aortic stenosis the peak rate of left ventricular ejection is limited and there is a compensatory prolongation of the duration of ejection. The special characteristics of the arterial pulse in aortic stenosis will be discussed subsequently.

Large, Bounding Pulse

When the arterial pulse is large and strong and the contour is normal, it is called a bounding pulse. When the large, bounding pulse, with fairly normal contour, becomes more extreme, depending on the severity of the clinical state, it may blend into the abnormalities known as *water-hammer* or *collapsing* pulses. These terms refer to an extremely rapid and high upstroke or ascending limb (water-hammer pulse) and to an extremely rapid downstroke or descending limb (collapsing pulse). (Fig. 5-25). In both instances the peak or crest of the pulse wave is sharp and of short duration. Usually the dicrotic notch is very low, and often no definite dicrotic notch or dicrotic wave can be felt. Most patients who have an abnormally steep upstroke also have an abnormally rapid downstroke and the terms used to describe the pulse are a matter of individual preference. The rapid upstroke and rapid downstroke tend to be exaggerated as the pulse wave is transmitted peripherally. Accordingly, these abnormalities are often better appreciated by palpating the brachial or radial arteries than by palpating the carotid artery.

In an occasional patient with aortic regurgitation, the large, rapidly ascending pulse wave is followed by a downward dip and a second, "tidal" wave during sytole. This produces a type of *bisferiens pulse*. Rarely, this type of pulse is followed by an accentuated and palpable dicrotic wave in early diastole, thereby producing a *triple beat.*

A very large, bounding pulse of the water-hammer or collapsing variety is usually associated with an increased stroke volume of the left ventricle, a wide pulse pressure, and a decrease in peripheral resistance. Most of the conditions responsible for a bounding, water-hammer, or collapsing pulse may be considered as "hyperkinetic circulatory states." These may be considered in three main categories:

1. In the normal person, a hyperkinetic circulation may develop in response to anxiety, exercise, or fever. Normal females may develop a hyperkinetic state during pregnancy, secondary to the arteriovenous shunt in the placenta. Otherwise normal subjects may develop a hyperkinetic condition related to hyperthyroidism or anemia. Gorlin, Brachfeld, Turner, Messer, and Salazar[10] have described a hyperkinetic state of unknown cause which may even precipitate heart failure. Although the cause of the syndrome is not clear, it may be related to an increased sensitivity of the tissues, including the heart, to normal circulating catecholamines.

2. A hyperkinetic state may be present in the aorta and arteries when there is an abnormally rapid runoff of blood from the arterial system. This may occur by shunting of blood from the aorta (patent ductus arteriosus, aorticopulmonary septal defect, or rupture of a sinus of Valsalva into the right atrium or other chambers), through a large peripheral arteriovenous fistula (congenital, traumatic, mycotic, or in a tumor), or through multiple small arteriovenous fistulas (Paget's disease of bone or cirrhosis of the liver). In severe aortic regurgitation the pulse is classically described as water-hammer and collapsing (Fig. 5-25). In this situation not only is the total discharged volume of the left ventricle tremendously increased, but the left ventricle accomplishes this ejection at a very rapid rate although the total duration of systole is also usually somewhat prolonged. As a result, the upstroke of the arterial pulse rises steeply to a high

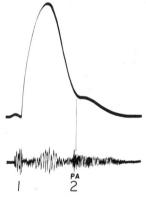

Fig. 5-25. Carotid artery pulse and heart-sound tracings in severe aortic regurgitation. The large, bounding arterial pulse wave has a steep ascent, a high systolic peak, and a rapid descent. Note that the "collapse" occurs during systole prior to the second sound. The dicrotic notch in severe aortic regurgitation is often indistinct. The term "water-hammer pulse" is used in reference to the very rapid-ascending limb of the pulse, and the expression "collapsing pulse" is used in reference to the rapid descent from the peak pressure.

peak; however, during late systole the rate of ejection decreases rapidly. This decreased rate of ejection in late systole contributes to much of the palpable "collapse" of the arterial pulse. Accordingly, in aortic regurgitation, there is predominantly a "systolic collapse," since most of the pressure fall from the peak pressure occurs during systole, not, as commonly thought, during diastole. An increase in peripheral arteriolar vasodilatation contributes to the arterial collapse during both systole and diastole. The volume of blood regurgitated into the left ventricle can contribute only to the diastolic collapse, which follows the incisura or aortic component of the second heart sound if these are still present. In some patients with severe aortic regurgitation who develop a marked elevation of the left ventricular diastolic pressure and left ventricular "failure," the hyperkinetic state may disappear. This may be associated with a decreased total volume and rate of left ventricular ejection, a diminished volume of regurgitation secondary to the elevation of left ventricular diastolic pressure, and a decrease in peripheral vasodilatation. Occasionally, patients with mitral regurgitation or an interventricular septal defect without left ven-

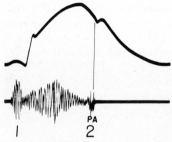

Fig. 5-26. Carotid artery pulse and heart-sound tracings showing a characteristic *parvus et tardus* pulse produced by severe valvular aortic stenosis. The initial upstroke is moderately steep but is interrupted by an early *anacrotic shoulder*, or *notch*, which may be palpable in the carotid artery. In more peripheral arteries, the anacrotic shoulder occurs later and is less pronounced, or even absent. Coarse vibrations are frequently present between the anacrotic shoulder and the delayed peak pressure. The pulse pressure is characteristically somewhat small. The central *incisura* and the peripheral *dicrotic notch* both tend to be diminished or absent. The systolic upstroke time, which is measured from the onset of the pulse to the peak pressure, and the systolic ejection time, which is measured from the onset of the pulse wave to the incisura or the dicrotic notch, are both prolonged in valvular aortic stenosis. Supravalvular and fixed subaortic stenosis are associated with similar arterial pulse-contour changes. In general, pulsus parvus et tardus is more readily recognized by palpation of the carotid artery than by palpation of more peripheral arteries.

tricular failure may appear to have a bounding pulse. In these patients, the vigorous left ventricular ejection produces a rapid upstroke in the arterial pulse even though the duration of systole and the aortic stroke volume may be diminished.

3. A hyperkinetic pulse may be present in complete heart block with bradycardia secondary to the markedly increased stroke volume. A similar situation may be present in tetralogy of Fallot, in which both ventricles eject into the aorta. The pulse pressure may also be wide and the pulse may appear to be bounding in patients with systolic, but not diastolic, hypertension.

Specific Abnormalities of the Arterial Pulse

Pulsus Parvus et Tardus

This term describes a small pulse with a delayed systolic peak. Such a pulse is characteristic of moderate or severe valvular aortic stenosis (Fig. 5-26). It may be possible to palpate an anacrotic notch on the upstroke of the carotid pulse wave. Although this notch usually occurs earlier when the stenosis is more severe, it is seldom possible to time its occurrence with sufficient accuracy at the bedside for this to be of value. In most instances of severe aortic valvular stenosis, no incisura or dicrotic notch is palpable in peripheral arterial pressure pulses. Coarse systolic vibrations or a thrill may be palpable and recorded on the carotid pulse wave. These usually occur between the anacrotic notch and the peak of the pulse wave. These vibrations are frequently absent when the stenosis is extremely severe. The vibrations are usually not palpable in the femoral, brachial, or radial pulses. The systolic upstroke time (from the beginning of the pulse wave to the peak pressure) is prolonged in aortic stenosis, as is the systolic ejection phase [from the beginning of the pulse wave to the (recorded) incisura or to the aortic component of the second heart sound]. Unfortunately, while the typical parvus et tardus (or, alternately, *plateau* or *anacrotic pulse*) pulse is found in almost all patients with uncomplicated severe valvular aortic stenosis, the finding of this characteristic pulse does not enable one to estimate the severity of the stenosis. Patients with mild stenosis may have normal carotid artery pulsations. Conversely, patients with severe aortic stenosis may have relatively normal pulse waves when the stroke volume is markedly reduced by ventricular failure or by coexisting mitral stenosis.

When *subvalvular aortic stenosis* is produced by a discrete fibrous ring or diaphragm, it may also be associated with a parvus et tardus pulse. In addition, severe left ventricular failure from various causes may produce a small, weak pulse which may be difficult at the bedside to distinguish from that of aortic stenosis. Patients with *supravalvular aortic stenosis* have carotid pulse abnormalities similar to those observed in valvular aortic stenosis. In most patients, however, the blood pressure is significantly higher in the right arm than in the left arm. In addition, the characteristic facies in this syndrome offers a strong diagnostic clue (Fig. 20-20).

The Twice-beating Pulse (Double-beat)

The terms "twice-beating" pulse or "double-beat" are applied to the pulse when two waves are palpated during each cardiac cycle (Fig. 5-27). The additional wave which is felt may occur during either diastole or systole.

Dicrotic Pulse. When the double beat is produced during diastole by an accentuated and palpable dicrotic wave following the second heart sound, the pulse is referred to as a dicrotic pulse (Fig. 5-27). This may be palpated in the peripheral vessels as well as the carotid arteries. It is especially likely to be present when the peripheral resistance and the diastolic pressure are low, as with fever. Aortic regurgitation, when only mild or moderate, may be associated with an accentuated and palpable dicrotic wave.

Anacrotic Pulse. A palpable twice-beating pulse with both impulses occurring during systole before the second heart sound is most commonly produced by pulsus bisferiens. Rarely, the anacrotic notch in severe valvular aortic stenosis may be so marked that it is possible to feel the initial portion of the pulse wave and the main pulse wave as separate waves. This is referred to as an anacrotic pulse (Fig. 5-27) and is usually felt only in the carotid arteries.

Bisferiens Pulse. Pulsus bisferiens may be produced by *functional hypertrophic subaortic stenosis*. This characteristic pulse (Figs. 5-27 and 5-28) is quite different from the typical parvus et tardus pulse of valvular aortic stenosis (Fig. 5-26) and may be the first diagnostic clue to the correct diagnosis. In pulsus bisferiens produced by functional hypertrophic subaortic stenosis, the upstroke or ascending limb of the pulse wave initially rises very rapidly. This initial systolic wave is referred to as the *percussion wave*. It produces the first systolic peak of the pulse and is followed by a short dip in pressure, presumably associated with a sudden decrease in the rate of left ventricular ejection as the obstruction becomes effective or significant. Following this trough, there is a second, slower-rising and late positive pulse wave referred to as the *tidal wave*. This second systolic wave is produced by continued but slower ventricular ejec-

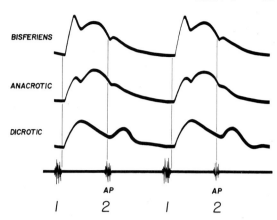

Fig. 5-27. Diagrammatic representation of some of the more common types of *double beats. Pulsus bisferiens* is characterized by a steep initial "percussion" wave, which is followed by a downward dip or trough. The second palpable wave is referred to as the "tidal" wave. The ascending limb of this wave is usually not so steep as that of the "percussion" wave, particularly in functional hypertrophic subaortic stenosis. The systolic ejection period is prolonged. Pulsus bisferiens is characteristic of functional hypertrophic subaortic stenosis. It is also frequently found in patients with combined aortic regurgitation and stenosis. In these patients, it signifies that the regurgitation is at least moderate in severity. Less commonly, it may be found in patients with pure aortic regurgitation or, rarely, in normal subjects with very rapid ventricular ejection. An *anacrotic pulse* may also produce two palpable impulses during systole. In this type of pulse wave, an accentuation of the normal *anacrotic shoulder* produces an *anacrotic notch*. An anacrotic pulse is typical of severe valvular aortic stenosis. A prolongation of the upstroke time to the main peak and a prolongation of the systolic ejection period are also characteristic of an anacrotic pulse. This type of pulse is better felt (or recorded) in the carotid arteries, since damping and distortion may eliminate the anacrotic phenomena in peripheral arteries. In contrast to the previous pulses, a *dicrotic pulse* has its second beat after the second heart sound. This type of double beat is produced by an accentuation of the dicrotic notch and dicrotic wave. It may be seen in patients with mild or moderate aortic regurgitation or occasionally in normal persons during exercise or fever. In some instances, it is better felt in the carotid arteries; in other individuals, it may be felt better more peripherally. A *bigeminal pulse* (Fig. 5-30) may also simulate a double beat when the regularly occurring premature beat follows the normal beat very closely. The rhythm disturbance producing a bigeminal pulse may usually be detected readily by cardiac auscultation. On rare occasions a *triple beat* may be produced by the combination of a prominent dicrotic wave (dicrotic pulse) and two systolic waves (bisferiens pulse).

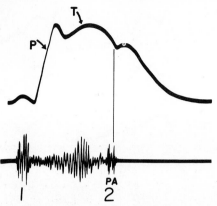

Fig. 5-28. Carotid artery and heart-sound tracings in *pulsus bisferiens* produced by functional hypertrophic subaortic stenosis. The first systolic wave, referred to as the "percussion" (P) wave, has a very rapid and uninterrupted ascending limb. The peak of the P wave is followed by a negative or downward dip. This is followed by a second systolic wave, known as the "tidal" (T) wave. The ascending limb of the tidal wave characteristically has a slow ascent in functional hypertrophic subaortic stenosis; however, the tidal wave may have a normal or rapid ascent when pulsus bisferiens is produced by pure aortic regurgitation or by combined aortic regurgitation and stenosis if the aortic stenosis is quite mild. The total duration of systole is prolonged in pulsus bisferiens.

tion, in addition to reflected waves from the periphery. In most instances, the height of the percussion wave is greater than the tidal wave, although this is not always true. The duration of ejection is prolonged if one measures from the onset of the pulse wave to the incisura or dicrotic notch or to the aortic component of the second heart sound. It is essential to establish that both peaks or humps occur during systole by listening to the heart sounds while palpating the carotid pulse. Occasionally, the bisferiens character of the pulse wave may be more easily palpated in the brachial than in the carotid artery. The latter finding is related to the normally greater pulse pressure in peripheral vessels and to the peripheral augmentation of either the percussion or the tidal wave by reflected or resonance waves.

In some patients the functional obstruction or the characteristic pressure pulse is present only intermittently. In such instances it may be possible to bring out the characteristic bisferiens pulse by administering nitroglycerin, amyl nitrite, or inotrophic catecholamines (isoproterenol or levarterenol), by performing a Valsalva maneuver, or by having the patient exercise.

An additional feature of the arterial pulse which may be helpful in diagnosing functional hyper-

trophic subaortic stenosis is the character of the pulse wave produced by the first beat following a premature beat. In a normal individual or a patient with valvular aortic stenosis, the first beat following a premature beat is *larger* than normal because the long diastolic period results in greater ventricular filling. As a result the stroke volume and pressure pulse of the next beat are larger. On the other hand, in patients with hypertrophic subaortic stenosis, the increased contractility of the beat following the longer period of filling causes the hypertrophic ("muscle-bound") segment to contract with greater force and therefore to produce a greater amount of obstruction. Consequently, the peripheral pulse beat following the premature beat may be paradoxically *smaller* than normal.

Pulsus bisferiens may also be found in patients with combined aortic regurgitation and stenosis in whom regurgitation is at least moderately severe. Less commonly, pulsus bisferiens may be found in patients with apparently pure aortic regurgitation. In some apparently normal persons, a bisferiens pulse wave may be felt in the carotid pulse when systolic ejection is extremely rapid, as during exercise or during the administration of sympathomimetic amines. In some normal individuals, it may be possible to palpate a bisferiens pulse in the radial artery which is not present in central or carotid pulse waves. Usually in this instance, the main pulse wave is normal and the second systolic wave is smaller and occurs just prior to the dicrotic notch.

Pulsus Alternans

Pulsus alternans refers to a characteristic pulse pattern in which the beats occur at regular intervals but in which there is a regular alternation of the height of the pressure pulses (Fig. 5-29). It is produced by an alternation in left ventricular contractile force associated with an alternation of left ventricular fiber length. There may or may not be alternation of end-diastolic pressure. This valuable sign should be searched for diligently by palpating the carotid, femoral, brachial, and radial arteries. In most instances, the weak pulses are only slightly weaker than the strong beats. On rare occasions the weak beat may be so small that no palpable pulse is detected at the periphery. This has been *total alternans*. Very rarely pulsus alternans may appear to be irregular to palpation. This is caused by a slight delay in sensing the weak beat by the palpating finger. Pulsus alternans is a very valuable sign of left ventricular "failure." In most instances, it is found in association with an abnormal ventricular gallop or filling sound (S_3); conversely, some, but not all, patients who have an abnormal S$_3$ have pulsus alternans by palpation. In apparently normal persons, pulsus alternans may occur during paroxysmal tachycardia or for several beats following a premature beat. In such circumstances, it does not necessarily signify left ventricular "failure" although a failing ventricle is more likely to have this sign following a premature contraction.

Pulsus alternans is frequently associated with left ventricular failure produced by severe hypertension, aortic valve disease, coronary atherosclerosis, or diffuse myocardial disease. It is more readily identified in patients with hypertension or aortic regurgitation, since the magnitude of the pulse makes it easier to identify. In contrast to many pulse abnormalities, pulsus alternans is usually easier to identify in a peripheral (femoral) artery than in the aorta or the carotid artery. This is related to the fact that the femoral artery has a greater pulse pressure than the central aorta in normal subjects at rest.

Pulsus alternans associated with ventricular failure may disappear following improvement of myocardial function with therapy. Conversely, pulsus alternans occasionally disappears when heart failure becomes much worse. Patients may have *latent* pulsus alternans, which can be produced or exaggerated by decreasing venous return to the heart, e.g., by assuming an upright position or by taking nitroglycerin. Occasionally, exercise may produce failure of the left side of the heart and pulsus alternans which was not present at rest. In contradistinction, pulsus alternans which is present at rest may be abolished by exercise, presumably because the effect of increased venous return on the pulsus alternans predominates over the effect of increased myocardial stress.

Right ventricular and pulmonary artery alternans at times occurs simultaneously with peripheral pulsus alternans. When this condition is present and the strong beats and the weak beats from the two ventricles occur synchronously, the alternans is said to be *concordant*. Very rarely, the weak beat of one ventricle occurs with the strong beat of the other ventricle and vice versa. This is referred to as *discordant alternans*. The physical signs of right ventricle alternans are currently being investigated.

The alternation of the force of ventricular contraction in pulsus alternans may be associated with alternation in intensity of heart sounds and murmurs, producing *auscultatory alternans*. The murmur of aortic stenosis is particularly apt to exhibit this sign. Occasionally, the left ventricle and aorta may pulsate with alternating displacement when viewed fluoroscopically, producing *visual alternans*. Pulsus alternans is only rarely associated with *electrical alternans* on the electrocardiogram.

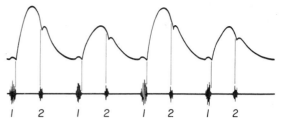

Fig. 5-29. Carotid artery and heart-sound tracings in *pulsus alternans*. The cardiac rhythm is regular but there is an alternation of the strength of the beats produced by left ventricular systole. This valuable sign of left ventricular "failure" may be detected by sphygmomanometry or by palpation, particularly of the femoral or radial arteries. When marked pulsus alternans is palpated in a peripheral artery, one may occasionally have the impression that the weak beat occurs slightly late even though the heart sounds are regular. This is related to differences in the transmission and distortion of the smaller pulse wave. In addition, it may take slightly longer for the palpating finger to perceive the onset or arrival of the weak pulse beat. Pulsus alternans may be associated with an alternation of the intensity of the heart sounds or heart murmurs. This is referred to as *auditory alternans*.

Bigeminal Pulse

Bigeminal pulse is the most common cause of peripheral arterial pulsations which alternate in size from beat to beat. It is usually produced by a small premature ventricular ectopic beat which regularly occurs after a larger normally conducted beat (Fig. 5-30). The large pulsation occurs after the long diastolic filling phase following the premature beat. In contrast to pulsus alternans, the irregularity of the heart beat is readily detected by arterial palpation or cardiac auscultation.

Pulsus Paradoxus

In normal persons the systolic blood pressure may decline 3 to 10 mm Hg during inspiration (Fig. 5-31). This change in systolic pressure is best identified by careful measurement of the blood pressure, but it may be barely perceptible by palpation of a peripheral artery. This normal variation of blood pressure with respiration is thought to be predominantly the result of relative pooling of blood in the pulmonary vasculature during inspiration as the result of lung expansion and of the more negative intrathoracic pressure. Transmission of the negative intrathoracic pressure to the aorta and great vessels may also contribute to a lesser degree. Although inspiration increases venous return to the right side of the heart, the effect of pulmonary vascular pooling normally predominates during the active phase of inspiration. The net result is a decrease in return of blood to

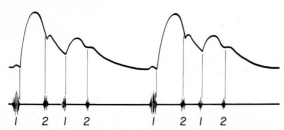

Fig. 5-30. Carotid artery and heart-sound tracings in *bigeminal pulse*. The strong beat is usually produced by a normally conducted impulse following a long diastolic filling period; the weak beat is produced by a premature beat coupled to the normal beat. If the premature beat occurs very shortly after the normal beat, the premature beat may not produce a palpable peripheral pulse. If it occurs slightly later, the peripheral pulse may resemble a double beat (see Fig. 5-27). Simultaneous cardiac auscultation will enable one to make the proper diagnosis at the bedside. At the other extreme, if the bigeminal pulse is produced by a mechanism in which the interval between the normal beat and the premature beat is relatively long, a bigeminal pulse may initially feel like pulsus alternans (Fig. 5-29). This resemblance is particularly likely to occur when there is tachycardia. Simultaneous cardiac auscultation will almost always allow one to distinguish between these two conditions.

the left atrium and left ventricle and a subsequent decrease in left ventricular output and decrease in arterial blood pressure. When the systolic blood pressure falls more than is normal during inspiration—i.e., more than 10 mm Hg—the pulse is (mistakenly) referred to as pulsus paradoxus (Fig. 5-31). This may be produced by conditions which (1) limit the inspiratory increase in blood flow to the right ventricle and the pulmonary artery; (2) cause a greater than normal amount of inspiratory pooling of blood in pulmonary vasculature; (3) cause the intrathoracic pressure to have wide extremes of pressure during inspiration and expiration; or (4) interfere with venous return to either atrium relatively more during inspiration, e.g., by an abnormal increase in pericardial pressure produced during inspiration by the change in shape of a distended pericardium from semiglobular to semielliptical.

Many different conditions may produce pulsus paradoxus. Often the major mechanism responsible for its production differs in these varying conditions, although common mechanisms may play a minor role. In superior vena cava obstruction the major mechanism is a limitation of the normal inspiratory increase in return of blood to the right atrium. In asthma, emphysema, and airway obstruction, the wide fluctuations in intrathoracic pressure are prob-

ably transmitted to the aorta and great vessels and, in addition, may cause a greater than normal respiratory variation in pulmonary vascular volume. In patients with severe congestive heart failure, with marked increase in venous pressure, with cardiac tamponade due to pericardial effusion, or with constrictive pericarditis, there are probably several important mechanisms. If the pericardium is distended by fluid or by a huge heart, it tends to assume a globular shape. During inspiration, the diaphragm tends to pull the pericardium downward and to change the shape of the pericardium to more nearly elliptical. This is thought to raise the intrapericardial pressure and thereby to hinder venous return to the right and left atria. The hyperpnea associated with heart failure tends to exaggerate this mechanism and may also increase the variations in intrathoracic pressure. In contrast to the above mechanisms it has recently been suggested by Dornhorst, Howard, and Lethart[11] that in cardiac tamponade the *right* ventricle may actually become overdistended during inspiration and thereby interfere with *left* ventricular filling

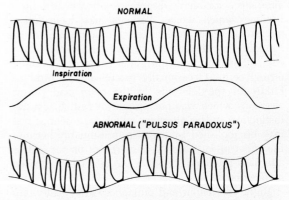

Fig. 5-31. Schematic representation of the normal variation in blood pressure during the respiratory cycle. During active inspiration, the blood pressure may fall 3 to 10 mm Hg from its level during or following expiration. The pulse rate often increases during inspiration and decreases during expiration. The inspiratory decrease in systolic pressure is usually greater than the decrease in diastolic pressure. This causes the pulse pressure to decrease slightly during inspiration. The expression "pulsus paradoxus" is a misnomer, since it refers not to a truly paradoxic response but to an exaggeration of the normal response. In general, variations greater than 10 mm Hg are referred to as *pulsus paradoxus*. The exact relationship between the cyclical changes in blood pressure and the respiratory cycle may vary somewhat. This variation depends on the particular disease process producing the abnormal response, as well as on differences between individual patients.

and hemodynamics, presumably by causing further elevation of intrapericardial pressure or by actually compressing the left ventricle.

Pulsus paradoxus does not always accompany cardiac tamponade. The reasons for this are obscure, but it is likely that other compensatory mechanisms are brought into play in order to maintain a normal systemic blood pressure. It seems possible that severe aortic regurgitation may prevent pulsus paradoxus from occurring. Patients with severe rheumatoid spondylitis or other severe disease of the bony thorax may not have pulsus paradoxus even with proved cardiac tamponade caused by pericardial effusion. In these patients, the movements of the thorax may be so limited that respiratory efforts are not associated with significant changes in intrathoracic pressure and in the respiration variation of venous return.

On rare occasions pulsus paradoxus may simulate pulsus alternans when the respiratory rate is half the pulse rate in patients with cardiac tamponade. Usually, the differentiation can be made by having the patient hold his breath.

Patients with cardiac tamponade who have pulsus paradoxus of the arterial system may have *Küssmaul's sign* (a *truly* paradoxic finding), which is an *increase* in peripheral venous distension and pressure during inspiration. The major mechanism is probably the inspiratory change in the shape of the pericardium, which raises intrapericardial pressure and obstructs venous return to the heart. In contrast to this *inspiratory* increase in jugular venous distension, which is seen in patients with cardiac tamponade, patients with pulmonary disease (e.g., asthma, emphysema, or obstructive emphysema) may have an *expiratory* increase in venous pressure. This diagnostic point is of value since both groups of patients may have pulsus paradoxus.

REFERENCES

1. Bazett, H. C.: An Analysis of the Time-Relation of Electrocardiograms, *Heart*, 7:353, 1918–1920.
2. Katz, L. N.: Factors Modifying the Duration of Ventricular Systole, *J. Lab. & Clin. Med.*, 6:291, 1921.
3. Katz, L. N., and Feil, H. S.: Clinical Observations on the Dynamics of Ventricular Systole. I. Auricular Fibrillation, *A.M.A. Arch. Int. Med.*, 32:672, 1923.
4. Katz, L. N., and Feil, H. S.: Clinical Observations on the Dynamics of Ventricular Systole. III. Aortic Stenosis and Aortic Insufficiency, *Heart*, 12:171, 1925.
5. Braunwald, E., Sarnoff, S. J., and Stainsby, W. N.:

Determinants of Duration and Mean Rate of Ventricular Ejection, *Circulation, Res.*, 6:319, 1958.
6. Wood, P.: Aortic Stenosis, *Am. J. Cardiol.*, 1:553, 1958.
7. Dexter, L., Harken, D. E., Cobb, L. A., Jr., Novack, P., Schlant, R. C., Phinney, A. O., Jr., and Haynes, F. W.: Aortic Stenosis, *A.M.A. Arch. Int. Med.*, 101:254, 1958.
8. Kraus, W. L., Schlant, R. C., Moore, C. B., Dock, D. S., Woodward, E., Jr., Haynes, F. W., and Dexter, L.: The Hemodynamic Results of Surgery for Aortic Stenosis, *Am. Heart J.*, 58:174, 1959.
9. Epstein, E. J., and Coulshed, N.: Assessment of Aortic Stenosis from the External Carotid Pulse Wave, *Brit. Heart J.*, 26:84, 1964.
10. Gorlin, R., Brachfeld, N., Turner, J. D., Messer, J. V., and Salazar, E.: The Idiopathic High Cardiac Output State, *J. Clin. Invest.*, 38:2144, 1959.
11. Dornhorst, A., Howard, P., and Leathart, G.: Pulsus Paradoxus, *Lancet*, 1:746, 1952.

SUGGESTED READING

General

Alexander, R. S.: Factors Determining the Contour of the Pressure Pulses Recorded from the Aorta, *Fed. Proc.*, 11:738, 1952.

Alexander, R. S.: Transformation of the Arterial Pulse Wave between the Aortic Arch and Femoral Artery, *Am. J. Physiol.*, 158:287, 1949.

Bedford, D. E.: The Ancient Art of Feeling the Pulse, *Brit. Heart J.*, 13:423, 1951.

Bergel, D. H.: The Static Elastic Properties of the Arterial Wall, *J. Physiol.*, 156:445, 1961.

Bergel, D. H.: The Dynamic Elastic Properties of the Arterial Wall, *J. Physiol.*, 156:458, 1961.

Bramwell, C.: Arterial Pulse in Health and Disease, *Lancet*, 2:239, 301, 366, 1937.

Chlebus, H.: Value of Examination of Carotid Pulse by Means of Resonance Electrosphygmographs in Relation to Intra-arterial Pressure Tracings, *Am. Heart J.*, 64:22, 1962.

Dontas, A. S.: Comparison of Simultaneously Recorded Intra-arterial and Extra-arterial Pressure Pulses in Man, *Am. Heart J.*, 59:576, 1960.

Dontas, A. S., and Cottas, C. S.: Arterial Volume and Pressure Pulse Contours in the Young Human Subject, *Am. Heart J.*, 61:676, 1961.

Dow, P., and Hamilton, W. F.: An Experimental Study of the Velocity of the Pulse Wave Propagated through the Aorta, *Am. J. Physiol.*, 125:60, 1939.

Feinberg, A. W., and Lax, H.: Studies of the Arterial Pulse Wave, *Circulation*, 18:1125, 1958.

Fenn, W. O., and Marsh, B. S.: Muscular Force at Different Speeds of Shortening, *J. Physiol.*, 85:277, 1935.

Fleming, P. R.: The Mechanism of the Pulsus Bisferiens, *Brit. Heart J.*, 19:519, 1957.

Frank, O.: Die Grundform des arteriellen Pulsus, *Ztschr. Biol.*, **19**:483, 1898–99.

Green, H. D.: Circulatory System: Physical Principles, in O. Glasser (ed.), "Medical Physics," The Year Book Medical Publishers, Inc., Chicago, 1950, vol. 2, pp. 228–251.

Hamilton, W. F., and Dow, P.: An Experimental Study of the Standing Waves in the Pulse Propagated through the Aorta, *Am. J. Physiol.*, **125**:48, 1939.

Hamilton, W. F.: The Patterns of the Arterial Pressure Pulse, *Am. J. Physiol.*, **141**:235, 1944.

Heyman, F.: Comparison of Intra-arterially and Extra-arterially Recorded Pulse Waves in Man and Dog, *Acta med. scandinav.*, **157**:503, 1957.

Hill, A. V.: Work and Heat in a Muscle Twitch, *Proc. Roy. Soc., London, Ser. B*, **136**:220, 1949–50.

Howarth, S.: Atrial Waves on Arterial Pressure Records in Normal Rhythm, Heart Block and Auricular Flutter, *Brit. Heart J.*, **16**:171, 1954.

Kroeker, E. J., and Wood, E. H.: Comparison of Simultaneously Recorded Central and Peripheral Arterial Pressure Pulses during Rest, Exercise and Tilted Position in Man, *Circulation Res.*, **3**:623, 1955.

Kroeker, E. J., and Wood, E. H.: Beat-to-Beat Alterations in Relationship of Simultaneously Recorded Central and Peripheral Arterial Pressure Pulses during Valsalva Maneuver and Prolonged Expiration in Man, *J. Appl. Physiol.*, **8**:483, 1956.

Lawton, R. W.: Some Aspects of Research in Biological Elasticity, in "Tissue Elasticity," papers arising from a conference held at Dartmouth College, Sept. 1–3, 1955, J. W. Remington (ed.), American Physiological Society, Washington, D.C., 1957, pp. 1–11.

Levine, S. A.: "Clinical Heart Disease," 5th ed., W. B. Saunders Company, Philadelphia, 1958.

Lewis, T.: "The Mechanism and Graphic Registration of the Heart Beat," 3d ed., Shaw & Sons, Ltd., London, 1925.

Luchsinger, P. C., Sachs, M., and Patel, D. J.: Pressure-Radius Relationship in Large Blood Vessels of Man, *Circulation Res.* **11**:885, 1962.

McDonald, D. A.: "Blood Flow in Arteries," The Williams & Wilkins Company, Baltimore, 1960.

McDonald, D. A.: Relation of Pulsatile Pressure to Flow in Arteries, *J. Physiol.*, **127**:533, 1955.

McDonald, D. A., and Taylor, M. G.: The Hydrodynamics of the Arterial Circulation, *Progr. Biophys.*, **9**:105, 1959.

McLean, C. E., Clason, W. P. C., and Stoughton, P. V.: The Peripheral Pulse as a Diagnostic Tool, *Angiology*, **15**:221, 1964.

Okino, H.: Measurement of Intraluminal Pressure from External Pressure with Strain Transducers, *J. Appl. Physiol.*, **19**:546, 1964.

Patel, D. J., and Fry, D. L.: In Situ Pressure-Radius-Length Measurements in Ascending Aorta of Anesthetized Dogs, *J. Appl. Physiol.*, **19**:413, 1964.

Patel, D. J., Greenfield, J. C., Jr., and Fry, D. L.: "In Vivo Pressure-Length-Radius Relationship of Certain Blood Vessels in Man and Dog," (In press).

Peterson, L. H.: The Dynamics of Pulsatile Blood Flow, *Circulation Res.*, **2**:127, 1954.

Peterson, L. H., Jensen, R. E., and Parnell, J.: Mechanical Properties of Arteries in Vivo, *Circulation Res.*, **8**:622, 1960.

Peterson, L. H.: Regulation of Blood Vessels, *Circulation*, **21**:749, 1960.

Remington, J. W., and Wood, E. H.: Formation of the Peripheral Pulse Contour in Man, *J. Appl. Physiol.*, **9**:433, 1956.

Remington, J. W.: Contour Changes of the Aortic Pulse During Propagation, *Am. J. Physiol.*, **199**:331, 1960.

Remington, J. W.: The Physiology of the Aorta and Major Arteries, in W. F. Hamilton and P. Dow (eds.), "Handbook of Physiology," sect. 2, "Circulation," vol. 2, American Physiological Society, Washington, D.C., 1963, p. 799.

Robinson, B.: The Carotid Pulse. II. Relation of External Recordings to Carotid, Aortic, and Brachial Pulses, *Brit. Heart J.*, **25**:61, 1963.

Rushmer, R. F.: Pressure-Circumference Relations in the Aorta, *Am. J. Physiol.*, **183**:545, 1955.

Ryan, J. M., Stacy, R. W., and Watman, R. N.: Role of Abdominal Aortic Branches in Pulse Wave Contour Genesis. *Circulation Res.*, **4**:676, 1956.

Spencer, M. P., and Denison, A. B. Jr.: Pulsatile Blood Flow in the Vascular System, in W. F. Hamilton and P. Dow (eds.), "Handbook of Physiology," sect. 2, "Circulation," vol. 2, American Physiological Society, Washington, D.C., 1963, p. 839.

Van Citters, R. L., and Rushmer, R. F.: Longitudinal and Radial Strain in Pulse Wave Transmission, *Am. J. Physiol.*, **200**:732, 1961.

Wehn, P. S.: Pulsatory Activity of Peripheral Arteries, *Scand. J. Clin. Lab. Invest.*, **9** (Supp. 30), 1957.

Weissler, A. M., Peeler, R. G., and Roehll, W. H., Jr.: Relationships between Left Ventricular Ejection Time, Stroke Volume, and Heart Rate in Normal Individuals and Patients with Cardiovascular Disease, *Am. Heart J.*, **62**:367, 1961.

Wetterer, E.: Die Wirkung der Herztätigkeit auf die Dynamik des Arteriensystems, *Verhandl. deutsch. Gesellsch. Kreislaufforsch.*, **22**:26, 1956.

Wetterer, E.: Flow and Pressure in the Arterial System, Their Hemodynamic Relationship, and the Principles of Their Measurement, *Minnesota Med.*, **37**:77, 1954.

Wiggers, C. J.: "The Pressure Pulses in the Cardiovascular System," Longmans, Green & Co., Inc., New York, 1928.

Wiggers, C. J.: Dynamics of Ventricular Contraction under Abnormal Conditions, *Circulation*, **5**:321, 1952.

Wright, J. L., and Wood, E. H.: Value of Central and Peripheral Intra-arterial Pressures and Pulse Contours in Cardiovascular Diagnosis, *Minnesota Med.,* **41**:215, 1958.

Aortic Valve Disease
(See References, Chaps. 24 and 25.)

Alexander, R. S.: Arterial Pulse Dynamics in Aortic Insufficiency, *Am. J. Physiol.,* **158**:294, 1949.

Bergeron, J., Abelmann, W. H., Vazquez-Milan, H., and Ellis, L. B.: Aortic Stenosis: Clinical Manifestations and Course of the Disease, *A.M.A. Arch. Int. Med.,* **94**:911, 1954.

Buteler, B. S.: The Relation of Systolic Upstroke Time and Pulse in Aortic Stenosis, *Brit. Heart J.,* **24**:657, 1962.

Corrigan, D. J.: On Permanent Patency of the Mouth of the Aorta, or Inadequacy of the Aortic Valves, *Edinburgh M. & Surg. J.,* **37**:225, 1832.

Daoud, G., Reppert, E. H., Jr. and Butterworth, J. S.: Basal Systolic Murmurs and the Carotid Pulse Curve in the Diagnosis of Calcareous Aortic Stenosis, *Ann. Int. Med.,* **50**:323, 1959.

Dow, P.: The Development of the Anacrotic and Tardus Pulse of Aortic Stenosis, *Am. J. Physiol.,* **131**:432, 1940.

Doyle, A. E., and Neilson, G. H.: The Valsalva Manoeuvre in Aortic Valve Disease, *Brit. Heart J.,* **19**:525, 1957.

Duchosal, P. W., Ferrero, C., Leupin, A., and Urdaneta, E.: Advance in the Clinical Evaluation of Aortic Stenosis by Arterial Pulse Recordings in the Neck, *Am. Heart J.,* **51**:861, 1956.

Duroziez, P.: Du double souffle intermittent crural, comme signe de l'insuffissance aortique, *Arch. gén. méd., Paris,* (Ser. 5) **17**:417, 588, 1861.

Epstein, E. J., and Coulshed, N.: Assessment of Aortic Stenosis from the External Carotid Pulse Wave, *Brit. Heart J.,* **26**:84, 1964.

Feil, H. S., and Gilder, M. D. D.: Pulse in Aortic Disease as Felt and Graphically Inscribed, *Heart,* **8**:4, 1921.

Feil, H. S., and Katz, L. N.: The Transformation of the Central into the Peripheral Pulse in Patients with Aortic Stenosis, *Am. Heart J.,* **2**:12, 1926.

Gorlin, R., McMillan, I. K. R., Medd, W. E., Matthews, M. B., and Daley, R.: Dynamics of the Circulation in Aortic Valvular Disease, *Am. J. Med.,* **18**:855, 1955.

Gorlin, R., and Case, R. B.: Clinical Diagnosis of Aortic Valve Disease, *New England J. Med.,* **255**:368, 1956.

Gupta, T. C., and Wiggers, C. J.: Basic Hemodynamic Changes Produced by Aortic Coarctation of Different Degrees, *Circulation,* **3**:17, 1951.

Hancock, E. W., and Abelmann, W. H.: A Clinical Study of the Brachial Arterial Pulse Form, with Special Reference to the Diagnosis of Aortic Valvular Disease, *Circulation,* **16**:572, 1957.

Katz, L. N., Ralli, E. P., and Cheer, S. H.: The Cardio-

dynamic Changes in the Aorta and Left Ventricle Due to Stenosis of the Aorta, *J. Clin. Invest.,* **5**:205, 1927.

Mason, D. T., Braunwald, E., Ross, J., Jr., and Morrow, A. G.: Diagnostic Value of the First and Second Derivatives of the Arterial Pressure Pulse in Aortic Valve Disease and in Hypertrophic Subaortic Stenosis, *Circulation,* **30**:90, 1964.

Matthews, M. B., Medd, W. E., and Gorlin, R.: Aortic Stenosis: A Clinical Study, *Brit. M. J.,* **2**:759, 1955.

Mitchell, A. M., Sackett, C. H., Hunzicker, W. J., and Levine, S. A.: The Clinical Features of Aortic Stenosis, *Am. Heart J.,* **48**:684, 1954.

Raber, G., and Goldberg, H.: Left Ventricular, Central Aortic, and Peripheral Pressure Pulses in Aortic Stenosis, *Am. J. Cardiol.,* **1**:572, 1958.

Robinson, B.: The Carotid Pulse. I. Diagnosis of Aortic Stenosis by External Recordings, *Brit. Heart J.,* **25**:51, 1963.

Segal, J., Harvey, W. P., and Hufnagel, C.: A Clinical Study of 100 Cases of Severe Aortic Insufficiency, *Am. J. Med.,* **21**:200, 1956.

Smith, J. E.: A Technique for Recording Carotid Artery Pulsations with Special Reference to Aortic Stenosis, *Am. Heart J.,* **49**:428, 1955.

Smith, J. E., Hsu, I., Evans, J. M., and Lederer, L. G.: Aortic Stenosis: A Study with Particular Reference to an Indirect Carotid Pulse Recording in Diagnosis, *Am. Heart J.,* **58**:527, 1959.

Tjong, O. S., and Verheugt, A. P. M.: Peripheral and Central Arterial Pressure Pulse in the Estimation of the Severity of Aortic Stenosis, *Am. Heart J.,* **62**:180, 1961.

Wiggers, C. J., and Maltby, A. B.: Further Observations on Experimental Aortic Insufficiency. IV. Hemodynamic Factors Determining the Characteristic Changes in Aortic and Ventricular Pressure Pulses, *Am. J. Physiol.,* **97**:689, 1931.

Wood, P.: Aortic Stenosis, *Am. J. Cardiol.,* **1**:553, 1958.

Wright, J. L., Toscano-Barboza, A., and Brandenburg, R. O.: Left Ventricular and Aortic Pressure Pulses in Aortic Ventricular Disease, *Proc. Staff Meet. Mayo Clin.,* **31**:120, 1956.

Pulsus Bisferiens, Functional Hypertrophic Subaortic Stenosis
(See References, Chaps. 24 and 25.)

Pulsus Alternans

Cooper, T., Braunwald, E., and Morrow, A. G.: Pulsus Alternans in Aortic Stenosis: Hemodynamic Observations in 50 Patients Studied by Left Heart Catheterization, *Circulation,* **18**:64, 1958.

Ferrer, M. I., Harvey, R. M., Cournand, A., and Richards, D. W.: Cardiocirculatory Studies in Pulsus Alternans of the Systemic and Pulmonary Circulation, *Circulation,* **14**:163, 1956.

Friedman, B., Daily, W. M., and Sheffield, R. S.: Orthostatic Factors in Pulsus Alternans, *Circulation,* **8:**864, 1953.

Gleason, W. L., and Braunwald, E.: Studies on Starling's Law of the Heart. VI. Relationships between Left Ventricular End-diastolic Volume and Stroke Volume in Man with Observations on the Mechanics of Pulsus Alternans, *Circulation,* **25:**841, 1962.

Hering, H. E.: Das Wesen des Herzalternans, *München. med. Wchnschr.,* **55:**1417, 1908.

McIntosh, H. D.: Discordant Pulsus Alternans, *Circulation,* **21:**214, 1960.

Mitchell, J. H., Sarnoff, S. J., and Sonnenblick, E. H.: The Dynamics of Pulsus Alternans: Alternating End-diastolic Fiber Length as a Causative Factor, *J. Clin. Invest.,* **42:**55, 1963.

Ryan, J. M., Schieve, J. F., Hull, H. B., and Oser, B. M.: The Influence of Advanced Congestive Heart Failure on Pulsus Alternans, *Circulation,* **12:**60, 1955.

Straub, H.: Dynamik des Herzalternans, *Deutsch. Archiv. klin. Med.,* **23:**403, 1917.

Traube, L.: Ein Fall von Pulsus Bigeminus, nebst Bemerkungen über die Leberschwellungen bei Klappenfehlern und über acute Leberatrophie, *Berlin. klin. Wchnschr.,* **9:**185, 1872.

Constrictive Pericarditis, Cardiac Tamponade, Pulsus Paradoxus, Küssmaul's Sign

Beck, W., Schire, V., and Vogelpoel, L.: Splitting of the Second Heart Sound in Constrictive Pericarditis with Observations on the Mechanism of Pulsus Paradoxus, *Am. Heart J.,* **64:**765, 1962.

Berglund, E.: Ventricular Function. VI. Balance of Left and Right Ventricular Output. Relation between Left and Right Atrial Pressures, *Am. J. Physiol.,* **178:**381, 1954.

Berglund, E., Sarnoff, S. J., and Isaacs, J. P.: Ventricular Function. Role of the Pericardium in Cardiovascular Hemodynamics, *Circulation Res.,* **3:**133, 1955.

Burwell, C. S., and Ayer, G. D.: Constrictive Pleuritis and Pericarditis, *Am. Heart J.,* **22:**267, 1941.

Dock, W.: Inspiratory Traction on the Pericardium: The Cause of Pulsus Paradoxus in Pericardial Disease, *Arch. Int. Med.,* **108:**837, 1961.

Dock, W.: Some Paradoxes in the History of Pulsus Paradoxus, *Am. J. Cardiol.,* **11:**569, 1963.

Dornhorst, A. C., Howard, P., and Leathart, G. L.: Pulsus Paradoxus, *Lancet,* **1:**746, 1952.

Eliasch, H., Lagerlöf, H., and Werkö, L.: Diagnosis of Adhesive Pericarditis, with Special Consideration of Heart Catheterization, *Nord. med.,* **44:**1128, 1950.

Fowler, N. O., Shabetai, R., and Braunstein, J. R.: Transmural Ventricular Pressures in Experimental Cardiac Tamponade, *Circulation Res.,* **7:**733, 1959.

Gauchat, H. W., and Katz, L. N.: Observations on Pulsus Paradoxus (with Special Reference to Pericardial Effusion). I. Clinical, *Arch. Int. Med.,* **33:** 350, 1924.

Gibson, R.: Atypical Constrictive Pericarditis, *Brit. Heart J.,* **21:**583, 1959.

Golinko, R. J., Kaplan, N., and Rudolph, A. M.: The Mechanism of Pulsus Paradoxus during Acute Pericardial Tamponade, *J. Clin. Invest.,* **42:**249, 1963.

Hansen, A. T., Eskildsen, P., and Götzsche, H.: Pressure Curves from the Right Auricle and the Right Ventricle in Chronic Constrictive Pericarditis, *Circulation,* **3:**881, 1951.

Hitzig, W. M.: On Mechanisms of Inspiratory Filling of the Cervical Veins and Pulsus Paradoxus in Venous Hypertension, *J. Mt. Sinai Hosp. New York,* **8:**625, 1942.

Isaacs, J. P., Berglund, E., and Sarnoff, S. J.: Ventricular Function. III. The Pathologic Physiology of Acute Cardiac Tamponade Studied by Means of Ventricular Function Curves, *Am. Heart J.,* **48:**66, 1954.

Katz, L. N., and Gauchat, H. W.: Observations on Pulsus Paradoxus (with Special Reference to Pericardial Effusion). II. Experimental, *Arch. Int. Med.,* **33:**371, 1924.

Kuno, Y.: The Significance of the Pericardium, *J. Physiol.,* **50:**1, 1915.

Küssmaul, A.: Über schwielige Mediastino-Pericarditis und den paradoxen Puls, *Berl. Klin. Wchnschr.,* **10:**433, 445, 461, 1873.

Lauson, H. D., Bloomfield, R. A., and Cournand, A.: The Influence of the Respiration on the Circulation in Man, *Am. J. Med.,* **1:**315, 1946.

Lewis, Sir T.: Studies on the Relationship between Respiration and Blood Pressure. Part I. The Effect of Changes of Intra-pericardial Pressure on Aortic Pressure, *J. Physiol.,* **37:**213, 1908.

Lindell, S. E., Swanborg, A., Soderholm, B., and Westling, H.: Haemodynamic Changes in Chronic Constrictive Pericarditis during Exercise and Histamine Infusion, *Brit. Heart J.,* **25:**35, 1963.

McGuire, J., Kotte, J. H., and Helm, R. A.: Acute Pericarditis, *Circulation,* **9:**425, 1954.

McKusick, V. A.: Chronic Constrictive Pericarditis. I. Some Clinical and Laboratory Observations, *Bull. Johns Hopkins Hosp.,* **90:**3, 1952.

Metcalfe, J., Woodbury, J. W., Richards, V., and Burwell, C. S.: Studies in Experimental Pericardial Tamponade: Effects on Intravascular Pressures and Cardiac Output, *Circulation,* **5:**518, 1952.

Sawyer, C. G., Burwell, C. S., Dexter, L., Eppinger, E. C., Goodale, W. T., Gorlin, R., Harken, D. E., and Haynes, F. W.: Chronic Constrictive Pericarditis: Further Considerations of the Pathologic Physiology of the Disease, *Am. Heart J.,* **44:**207, 1952.

Schuler, R. H., Ensor, C., Cunning, R. E., Mon, W. G., and Johnson, V.: The Differential Effects of Respiration on the Left and Right Ventricles, *Am. J. Physiol.,* **137:**620, 1947.

Sealy, R. D.: Dynamic Effect of Inspiration on the Simultaneous Stroke Volumes of the Right and Left Ventricles, *Am. J. Physiol.,* **154:**273, 1948.

Shabetai, R., Fowler, N. O., Braunstein, J. R., and Gueron, M.: Transmural Ventricular Pressure and

Pulsus Paradoxus in Experimental Cardiac Tamponade, *Dis. Chest*, **39**:557, 1961.

Shabetai, R., Fowler, N. O., and Gueron, M.: The Effects of Respiration on Aortic Pressure and Flow, *Am. Heart J.*, **65**:525, 1963.

Sharp, J. T., Bunnell, I. L., Holland, J. F., Griffith, G. T., and Greene, D. G.: Hemodynamics during Induced Cardiac Tamponade in Man, *Am. J. Med.*, **29**:640, 1960.

Trimby, R. H., and Nicholson, H. C.: Some Observations on the Nature of the Respiratory Waves in Arterial Blood Pressure, *Am. J. Physiol.*, **129**:289, 1940.

Williams, C., and Soutter, L.: Pericardial Tamponade: Diagnosis and Treatment, *A.M.A. Arch. Int. Med.*, **94**:571, 1954.

Wilson, R. H., Hoseth, W., Sadoff, C., and Dempsey, M. E.: Pathologic Physiology and Diagnostic Significance of the Pressure Pulse Tracings in the Heart in Patients with Constrictive Pericarditis and Pericardial Effusion, *Am. Heart J.*, **48**:671, 1954.

Wood, P.: Chronic Constrictive Pericarditis, *Am. J. Cardiol.*, **7**:48, 1961.

Yu, P. N., Lovejoy, F. W., Joos, H. A., Nye, R. E., and Mahoney, E. B.: Right Auricular and Ventricular Pressure Patterns in Constrictive Pericarditis, *Circulation*, **7**:102, 1953.

EXAMINATION
OF THE VEINS *

J. Willis Hurst, M.D., and
Robert C. Schlant, M.D.

The venous return of blood to the right side of the heart is primarily accomplished by the "left ventricular pump" (*vis a tergo*). Auxiliary forces are contributed by the skeletal "muscle pump" and the "respiratory pump." Whether or not under normal conditions blood is also attracted to the heart by a systolic and diastolic "ventricular suction force" (*vis a fronte*) is not yet fully established. Venous blood returning from the capillaries has a nonpulsatile flow. Changes in volume flow created by the muscle and respiratory pump are nonsynchronous with the pulsatile activity of the heart. However, the changes in flow and pressure, caused by discontinuous atrial and ventricular filling, give rise to pulsations in the central veins which are transmitted toward the peripheral veins opposite to the direction of blood flow. Thus, except for the carotid arterial impact (*c wave*), the venous pulsations observed at the bedside are produced by right atrial and ventricular activity. Although often

* Grateful acknowledgement is made to Dr. Gerhard A. Brecher, Professor and Chairman of the Department of Physiology of Emory University School of Medicine, for his assistance in the preparation of this manuscript.

neglected, the bedside study of these pulsations is the clinical key to the dynamics of the right side of the heart.

TECHNIQUE OF STUDYING
THE NECK VEINS

There are two main objectives in the bedside observation of neck veins: the study of the wave form of the venous pulsations, including the determination of cardiac rhythm, and the estimation of venous pressure. In an individual patient it is necessary to examine both the internal and external jugular veins on both sides of the neck, as well as the venous pulsations which may be visible in the suprasternal notch or in the supraclavicular fossa. In most patients, however, the *right internal jugular vein* is superior for accurate evaluation of venous wave form, although occasionally one of the other locations may be preferable.

Since the internal jugular vein lies beneath the sternocleidomastoid muscle adjacent to the carotid artery, the visible pulsations are transmitted movements of the overlying subcutaneous tissue produced by pressure-volume changes within the vein. In examining the jugular veins, the position of the patient is extremely important. The neck muscles, particularly the sternocleidomastoid muscles, should be relaxed by placing a small pillow under the neck. The head should not be rotated more than a few degrees, if at all, since rotation may tense the sternocleidomastoid muscle and obscure the transmission of the venous pulsations. The trunk of the body should be elevated until maximum pulsation is noted. *The degree of trunk elevation necessary for maximum venous pulsation varies from subject to subject and must be established for each person.* In most normal persons, maximum pulsation of the internal jugular vein is usually observed when the trunk is inclined less than 45°, usually about 15 to 30°. In patients with elevated venous pressure, it may be necessary to elevate the trunk more than 45° to visualize maximum venous pulsation. At times, the pulsations are best seen with the patient upright at 90°. On the other hand, if the venous pressure is greatly elevated or the veins are markedly distended, pulsations of the internal jugular veins may not be apparent even when the trunk is elevated to 90°. The administration of vasoconstrictor drugs, such as levarterenol (norepinephrine or Levophed), may produce marked venous vasoconstriction and obscure the venous pulsations. At the bedside, internal jugular venous pulsations may be highlighted by shining a beam of light tangentially across the skin overlying the vein. This technique may cast a shadow of neck vein pulsations on the pillow or bedsheet behind the neck. In some patients, particularly those with marked tricuspid regurgitation and chronic elevation of venous pressure, venous pulsations may occasionally be seen better in the external jugular veins, although in most subjects the presence of competent venous valves at the lower end of these veins prevents a satisfactory retrograde transmission of the venous pulse wave. In patients with marked tricuspid regurgitation and chronic elevation of venous pressure, it may even be possible to detect the large, regurgitant wave during systole in the veins of the arms or legs.

The venous pulsations in the neck must be separated from carotid arterial pulsations. The differentiation may be made by several means: (1) differences in contour and different relationships to the carotid activity on the other side of the neck and to the heart sounds, (2) application of slight pressure below the point of observation to block the venous pulsations, and (3) differences between the effects of changes in body position, of respiration, and of abdominal pressure.

In most instances the visible venous pulse waves are slower and more undulating than the brisk, forceful arterial pulse waves. In patients with visible neck pulsations suspected of being arterial in origin, the arterial pulses in the arms and legs are usually large and bounding. It is possible to feel the carotid pulse on one side of the neck and to study simultaneously the venous pulsation on the other side of the neck. When this is done, one may feel the rapid upstroke of the arterial pulse with one hand and simultaneously observe the slow, less forceful venous pulsations. Occasionally, even venous pulsations may become palpable; this usually signifies that the venous pressure is 250 mm water or higher.

Generally, internal or external jugular venous pulsations may be eliminated by applying gentle pressure below the point of observation. This maneuver blocks the retrograde transmission of the venous pulse wave to the jugular vein, leaving only arterial pulsations. It should be noted that this procedure also may produce increased distension of the vein by blocking the flow of blood to the heart.

At times, venous pulsations may be distinguished from arterial pulsations by changing the patient's *position,* which produces a more marked effect upon the relative pressure, volume, and pulsations of veins than of arteries. Venous pulsations of the internal jugular vein which are visible at 15 or 30° may diminish or disappear when the trunk is further elevated. Occasionally, a more upright position may increase the amplitude of the visible venous pulsations in lower areas such as the in-

ferior jugular bulb, the suprasternal area, or the supraclavicular area. In patients with extremely high venous pressure and engorged jugular veins, significant pulsations may not be visible when the patient is lying flat or even when he is elevated to 45°. In fact, venous pulsations may not be seen even when the patient's trunk is elevated to 90°.

Respiration may also produce marked changes in venous pulsations, whereas arterial pulses normally change relatively little. Under normal circumstances, inspiration decreases intrathoracic pressure and increases the return of bood to the heart from the peripheral veins. The result of this is to lower or decrease the mean *level* of venous pulsation and distension during inspiration; the opposite occurs during expiration. Although the mean *level* of venous pulsations is normally *decreased* by inspiration, the *amplitude* of venous pulsation is often *increased* by full inspiration. Patients with severe heart failure with greatly increased venous pressure or with constrictive pericarditis may have a paradoxic *increase* in jugular venous distension during inspiration. This is known as *Küssmaul's sign.* The performance of a *Valsalva maneuver* by the patient increases intrathoracic pressure, impeding the return of blood to the heart and increasing the pressure and the distension of the peripheral veins. The effects of the Valsalva maneuver on the visible arterial pulse are usually less marked.

Abdominal pressure is also useful to distinguish venous from arterial neck pulsations. This test is best performed with the patient lying comfortably in bed at the optimal angle for bringing out the internal jugular venous pulsation. The patient is instructed to continue his normal breathing pattern in order to avoid performance of a Valsalva maneuver. Moderately firm pressure is then slowly applied for about 30 sec with the palm of the hand to the abdomen, usually on the right side ("over the liver") although other areas are frequently almost as satisfactory. Normally, this maneuver produces no visible change in the arterial pulses. In normal persons there is slight, if any, increase in the prominence of the jugular venous pulsations, but if there is "failure" of the right side of the heart, the jugular venous distension and pulsations may markedly increase. It is thought that the abdominal compression increases venous return to the heart and that the "failing" heart is not able to increase its output in a normal manner to accommodate the increased load. As a consequence the pressure and volume in the jugular venous system increase. This maneuver may also be used in place of exercise to bring out typical jugular venous waves of tricuspid regurgitation which may be absent under normal resting conditions. This test, known as the *hepatojugular reflux test*,* is useful not only in distinguishing the venous from arterial pulses but also in the diagnosis of "heart failure" (see subsequent discussion).

THE NORMAL VENOUS PULSE

Proper evaluation of venous pulsations is possible only when they are correlated with all events of the cardiac cycle. Although the carotid pulse may be used to time venous pulsations, the heart sounds generally are preferable for timing of venous pulsations at the bedside (Fig. 5-32). Despite the slight and variable transmission delay—about 0.02 sec—between pressure events in the right atrium and pulsations as usually recorded in the neck, the heart sounds are remarkably good reference points for venous pulsation at the bedside. In fact the jugular venous pulsations are often of great value in the timing and identification of normal and abnormal heart sounds. It should be noted that various techniques for recording the external jugular

* The term *reflux* is probably preferable for this test, although it is possible that abdominal compression at times might initiate additional "reflex" mechanisms.

venous pulsations (the *jugular phlebogram*) may reveal some venous pulsations which are not detectable by visual inspection at the bedside. On the other hand, some of these recording techniques may introduce instrumentation artifacts which distort the time relationships between the jugular pulsations and intracardiac events.

The normal visible jugular venous pulse wave consists of three positive pulse waves (*a, c, v*) and two negative pulse waves (*x* and *y*) (Fig. 5-33). It should be noted that the portion of a pulse wave connecting the summit of a positive wave to the trough of a negative wave may be looked upon as either the terminal part of the positive wave or the initial part of the negative wave.

The positive *a* wave is produced by right atrial contraction and the retrograde transmission of the pressure pulse so generated to the jugular veins. During right atrial systole there is frequently a brief backward flow of blood from the right atrium to the caval veins. In normal subjects the *a* wave is often the largest positive wave visible, particularly during inspiration, although the degree of elevation of the subject may alter the prominence of the *a* wave in relation to that of the *c* and *v* waves.

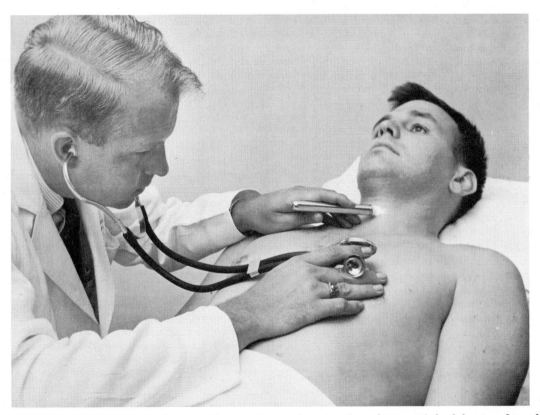

Fig. 5-32. Examination of the neck veins. The examiner is observing the pulsations of the left internal jugular vein while listening to the heart sounds. In most instances, the heart sounds are the most satisfactory reference points for timing of venous and arterial pulsations in the neck.

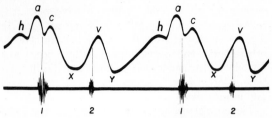

Fig. 5-33. Normal jugular venous and heart-sound tracings. The relative and absolute magnitude of the venous waves depend on many variables, including the position of the patient, the phase of respiration, the P-R interval, and the heart rate. The precise relationship between intracardiac events and recordings of the jugular venous waves varies with the particular recording system used. In this diagrammatic illustration, the first heart sound is synchronous with the end of the *a* wave and the beginning of the *c* wave. When the P-R interval is very short, the *a* wave may be fused with the *c* wave to form a ·larger *a-c* wave, which may also be seen in nodal rhythm. During ventricular systole, the "systolic collapse" is produced by the negative *x* wave. The second heart sound occurs shortly prior to the summit of the *v* wave, which marks the opening of the tricuspid valve. The *y* descent (or *v* descent) follows the peak of the *v* wave and coincides with the rapid-filling phase of ventricular diastole. The normal third heart sound, which originates from the left side of the heart, usually occurs either during the *y* descent shortly before the *y* trough, while a third heart sound from the right side of the heart usually occurs at the *y* trough. Following the *y* ascent, there may be a small *h* wave or plateau representing the jugular venous prior to the *a* wave produced by atrial systole. It is usually not possible to distinguish a discrete *h* wave at the bedside, although it is not infrequently recorded when diastole is long. In general, inspiration decreases the mean level of pressure but increases the relative amplitude of the *a* wave. The *x* wave is usually lower than the *v* wave during full inspiration but may not be so low as the *v* wave during expiration.

The *a* wave begins before the first heart sound and reaches its peak either just before or during the first heart sound. If an atrial gallop (S_4) is heard, it ordinarily occurs at the moment the peak of the *a* wave is recorded.

As the result of atrial relaxation, the venous pulse descends from the summit of the *a* wave. Depending on the P-R interval, this descent may continue until a plateau (often called the "*z* point") is reached just prior to ventricular systole. More frequently, the descent is interrupted by the occurrence of a second positive venous pulse wave, the *c* wave.* The *c* wave in the neck is probably pro-

---

* The term *c* wave was originally suggested by Mac-Kenzie for the "carotid impact" wave in the jugular

duced by two events: (1) the impact of the carotid artery adjacent to the jugular vein, and (2) the retrograde transmission of a positive wave in the right atrium produced by right ventricular systole and the bulging of the tricuspid valve into the right atrium. The *c* wave normally begins at the end of the first heart sound and reaches its peak shortly after the first heart sound.

Following the summit of the *c* wave, the venous pulse contour declines, forming a negative wave, the *x* wave. The initial portion of this wave, following the *c* wave summit, is referred to as the *x* descent because it is sometimes rather steep. The forces responsible for the production of the negative *x* wave result in the normal "systolic collapse" of the jugular venous pulsations. The *x* wave in the neck is produced by (1) downward displacement of the base of the ventricles, including the tricuspid valve, during ventricular systole and the resultant fall in right atrial pressure, and (2) continued atrial relaxation. That atrial relaxation is not solely responsible for the genesis of the *x* wave is apparent from the presence of distinct *x* waves in right atrial or jugular venous pulse tracings of patients with atrial fibrillation in the absence of tricuspid regurgitation. During inspiration the *x* wave is usually lower than the *y* wave; during expiration, the *y* wave may be as low as the *x* wave or lower. In the right atrium, the trough or nadir of the *x* wave occurs in early or midventricular systole; in the jugular vein, it usually occurs in late systole, shortly before the second heart sound.

As blood continues to fill the caval veins and the right atrium during ventricular systole when the tricuspid valve is closed, the increasing volume in these structures leads to a pressure increase. Thus, the pressure rises from the trough of the *x* wave to another peak, the *v* wave. After this peak is reached, the pressure in the right atrium begins to fall as a result of (1) opening of the tricuspid valve, and (2) decreased bulging of the tricuspid valve into the right atrium associated with isovolumetric relaxation of the right ventricle. The opening of the tricuspid valve normally occurs either at the peak of the *v* wave or very shortly afterward. The opening snap of mitral stenosis often occurs shortly prior to the peak of the jugular *v* wave.

Following the summit of the *v* wave, the descending limb of the pulse wave is ordinarily referred to as the *y* descent, less frequently as the *v* descent. The *y* descent forms the initial portion of the normal jugular venous "diastolic collapse" produced

---

pulse. Later the nearly simultaneously occurring positive wave in the atrial pulse, although not produced by the carotid arterial distensions, was also labeled *c* wave.

by the forces responsible for the negative *y* wave. In the jugular venous pulse the *y* wave is produced mainly by the opening of the tricuspid valve and the subsequent rapid inflow of blood from the right atrium and caval veins into the right ventricle. The initial *y* descent corresponds to the phase of rapid filling of the right ventricle. If the patient has a right-sided diastolic filling sound (S_3), it usually occurs at the trough or nadir of the recorded *y* wave, whereas a filling sound from the left side of the heart often occurs earlier during the descending limb of the *y* descent, shortly before the trough. The exact relationship of these events to recordings of the jugular venous pulse tracing depends on the particular recording techniques employed. In most patients the nadir, or trough, of the *y* wave occurs in early diastole and is followed by the ascending limb of the *y* wave, which is produced by continued diastolic inflow of blood into the great veins, right atrium, and right ventricle (which are all essentially in "free" communication during diastole). The rate of rise of the ascending limb of the *y* wave depends on the rate of venous return to these structures and the distensibility of these chambers and vessels. When diastole is long, the ascending limb of the recorded *y* wave may be followed by a rather small, brief positive wave, the *h* wave, which marks the ends of slow filling of the right ventricle and occurs prior to the succeeding *a* wave. At times there is a plateau phase, which represents the base line of the jugular venous tracing, rather than a distinct positive *h* wave. With increasing heart rate, the *y* depression and *y* ascent are followed immediately by the *a* wave of the next cycle and no *h* wave or plateau is present. (With very fast heart rates, even the *y* depression may be eliminated by fusion of the *v* wave with the following *a* wave. Constrictive pericarditis and tricuspid regurgitation are particularly likely to have prominent and early *h* waves, but even in these instances the *h* wave is much better appreciated when electronically recorded, since it is usually not possible to detect *h* waves at the bedside.

In most instances it is possible to discern the three major positive waves (*a*, *c*, *v*) and the two negative waves (*x*, *y*) if the pulse rate is below 85 to 90 beats per minute. With faster heart rates there is often a fusion of some of the pulse waves and accurate analysis of wave form is more difficult. In circumstances associated with significant tachycardia, however, the neck veins may reveal clues regarding the nature of the tachycardia, e.g., irregularly occurring "cannon waves" in ventricular tachycardia (see below). In children, the jugular pulsations are difficult to study, not only because of the faster heart rate, but also because the short neck makes examination difficult.

ABNORMALITIES OF THE VENOUS PULSE

Abnormalities of the *a* Wave. Most of the significant abnormalities of the *a* wave which may be observed involve their *timing* and *amplitude*. The *a* wave is usually the highest venous wave, particularly during inspiration, which, like abdominal compression, tends to increase venous return to the heart and to enhance the force of right atrial contraction. Even though the mean *level* of venous pressure is normally decreased by inspiration, the *amplitude* of the *a* wave is usually increased.

No *a* wave is found in atrial fibrillation (Fig. 5-34); however, in certain other conditions the *a* wave may not be apparent. In sinus tachycardia, the *a* wave may be fused with the preceding *v* wave, particularly if the P-R interval is prolonged. In some patients with sinus tachycardia, the *a* wave may occur during the *v* or *y* descent (reflecting the phase of rapid ventricular filling) and be diminutive or even absent. On the other hand, if the P-R interval is very short or if there is nodal rhythm, the *a* wave may be fused with the following *c* wave. Such *a-c* waves are usually very large and are one type of regularly occurring cannon waves (see below). The *a-c* waves are large, not only because they represent the fusion of two events during which pressure rises, but also because the *a* wave itself is frequently "giant" since the tricuspid valve is closed by ventricular systole before or soon after the onset of atrial systole.

When a discrete *a* wave with ascending and descending limbs is clearly completed prior to the first heart sound, the P-R interval is likely to be prolonged (Fig. 5-35). This finding may be the first indication that one should search carefully for other evidence of first-degree heart block, e.g., faint

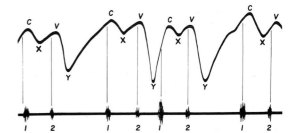

Fig. 5-34. Atrial fibrillation: jugular venous and heart-sound tracings. Note the absence of *a* waves and the somewhat decreased amplitude of the negative *x* wave during ventricular systole. The predominant wave is the negative *y* wave during diastole. When diastole is sufficiently long, an *h* wave may be recorded following the *y* ascent in late diastole. When atrial fibrillation is associated with tricuspid regurgitation, as it frequently is, the *x* wave may become even smaller or may even be completely obscured by a positive regurgitant *s* wave during systole (see Fig. 5-38).

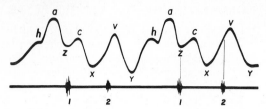

Fig. 5-35. Prolonged P-R interval: jugular venous and heart-sound tracings. Note the relatively prominent *a* wave produced by atrial systole. The *a* wave is clearly completed before the first heart sound, and there is a definite interval between the *a* wave and the *c* wave. This interval corresponds to the *z* point in atrial pressure tracings. The *h* wave in late diastole is more likely to be present with long diastolic periods, and at times is merely a horizontal plateau prior to the *a* wave. It is usually not possible to discern *h* waves at the bedside, although they may be recorded. When the P-R interval is markedly prolonged, particularly with tachycardia, the *a* wave may occur during the *y* descent or the *y* wave and may be small or even obliterated. With even faster heart rates and prolonged P-R intervals, the *a* wave may even fuse with the preceding *v* wave.

first heart sound or an atrial gallop, with or without a palpable presystolic impulse at the apex.

Very large *a* waves are of considerable diagnostic value. When such large or giant *a* waves are present with each beat, one should suspect that the right atrium is contracting against an increased resistance (Fig. 5-36). This may be an increase in resistance at the tricuspid valve (tricuspid stenosis or atresia) or to right ventricular filling. The latter may be associated with pulmonary stenosis, primary or secondary pulmonary hypertension, or acute pulmonary embolism. A truly giant *a* wave is more likely to occur when the interatrial and interventricular septums are both closed and right atrial contraction can therefore more easily produce a very high pressure. Accordingly, giant *a* waves are likely to be seen in patients with pure pulmonary stenosis. They are less often noticed in patients with pulmonary stenosis associated with either an atrial septal defect (trilogy of Fallot) or a ventricular septal defect (tetralogy of Fallot) or in patients with pulmonary hypertension secondary to a ventricular or atrial septal defect.

A different type of large positive venous pulse wave produced by atrial contraction is the *cannon wave*. It occurs when the right atrium happens to contract while the tricuspid valve is closed by right ventricular systole. The resultant jugular venous cannon wave is the result of fusion of the giant *a* wave with some part (*c*, *x*, or *v*) of the usual jugular venous pulse waves occurring during ventricular systole.

Cannon waves may occur either regularly or ir-

regularly. One type of regularly occurring cannon wave is produced by nodal rhythm, as described above. Cannon waves occurring with each ventricular systole may also be seen at times in patients with 2:1 atrioventricular block, with or without tachycardia. In these persons every other atrial contraction occurs during the latter part of ventricular systole, thereby producing a large cannon wave. At times in such patients it may be possible to see the other, smaller *a* wave which occurs during ventricular diastole.

Irregularly occurring cannon waves are the most common type and are frequently of great diagnostic importance. The most common cause of irregularly occurring cannon waves is an ectopic beat, whether it originates in the atria, the AV node, or the ventricles. An atrial or a nodal ectopic beat which is premature may cause a cannon wave if the ectopic beat occurs during ventricular systole while the tricuspid valve is closed. Nodal beats, even if not premature, may be associated with large *a* waves or cannon (*a-c*) waves, since the tricuspid valve is closed by ventricular systole either before or soon after the onset of atrial systole. A ventricular ectopic beat may also be associated with a large *a* wave or cannon wave if a premature ventricular contraction occurs during or just after the peak of atrial contraction.

Perhaps the best example of irregularly occurring

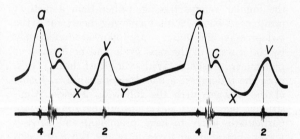

Fig. 5-36. "Giant" *a* waves: jugular venous tracings and heart-sound tracings. If a right atrial sound (S_4) is present, it is usually synchronous with the peak of the *a* wave, although some sound vibrations may at times be recorded during the *a* descent. When the P-R interval is very short or with nodal rhythm, the *a* wave and the *c* wave may be fused to produce a very large *ac* wave. "Giant" *a* waves may be associated with any conditions associated with increased resistance to emptying of the right atrium, e.g., tricuspid stenosis or right ventricular hypertrophy secondary to pulmonic stenosis, primary pulmonary hypertension, or pulmonary hypertension secondary to mitral stenosis, cor pulmonale, pulmonary embolism, or left ventricular failure. In this illustration, the relatively normal downslope of the *y* descent, following opening of the tricuspid valve at the summit of the *v* wave, favors a diagnosis other than tricuspid stenosis.

cannon waves is seen in patients with complete heart block without atrial fibrillation (Fig. 5-37). In these patients with a slow ventricular rate, it is particularly easy to identify the giant cannon wave produced when atrial systole happens to occur when the tricuspid valve is closed by ventricular systole. Such cannon waves are likely to be even larger than the often prominent carotid arterial impacts associated with complete heart block. Not infrequently such a cannon wave visibly moves the ear lobe. It should be noted that cannon waves in the jugular venous pulse occur when atrial systole occurs *during* ventricular systole, whereas the *cannon sound* of an accentuated first heart sound occurs in complete heart block when atrial systole occurs slightly (0.10 to 0.14 sec) *before* ventricular systole.

Irregularly occurring cannon waves are of great diagnostic value in the examination of patients with tachycardia. At times one may be able to make the tentative diagnosis of ventricular tachycardia by finding cannon waves which occur at irregular intervals. In ventricular tachycardia the cannon waves usually occur irregularly since the cause of their production—concomitant atrial and ventricular systole, with a closed tricuspid valve—is not present with each beat.

Abnormalities of the Normal "Systolic Collapse" (x Wave). The most important alteration of the normal negative "systolic collapse" x wave of the jugular pulse contour is that the collapse becomes obliterated or even replaced by a positive wave. The common denominator in most instances is the presence of tricuspid regurgitation. Although atrial relaxation may contribute to the normal x descent, the development of atrial fibrillation does not obliterate a distinct x wave except in the presence of tricuspid regurgitation. Accordingly, the occurrence of a positive jugular venous pulse wave during ventricular systole is strong evidence of tricuspid regurgitation.

The effects of mild, moderate, and severe tricuspid regurgitation are diagrammatically illustrated in Fig. 5-38. It is seen that mild regurgitation merely lessens and shortens the downward x wave. It is thought to be caused by the regurgitation of blood from the right ventricle into the right atrium, producing a positive wave which lessens the usual systolic fall in right atrial and venous pressures. In some patients with moderate degrees of regurgitation, it may be possible to record (but not see) this regurgitant s (s = systolic) wave as a fairly distinct positive venous wave during ventricular systole between the c and v waves. The s wave may completely obliterate the x wave or may leave only a small notch in its place. When the regurgitation is severe, the regurgitant s wave completely obliterates the negative x wave and fuses

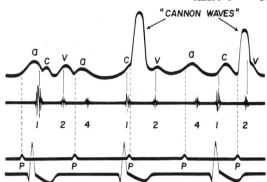

Fig. 5-37. "Cannon waves" in complete heart block: schematic jugular venous and heart-sound tracings and electrocardiogram. Note the irregularly occurring cannon waves produced by atrial systole when atrial contraction occurs with the tricuspid valve closed by ventricular systole. Whenever atrial systole occurs during the phase of rapid ventricular filling (the y descent), the a waves are smaller than usual.

with the c and v waves to produce a venous pulse wave similar to that found in the ventricles, i.e., so-called *ventricularization* of the atrial or venous pulse wave. In such patients the large positive systolic venous pulse wave may be so prominent as to be confused with an arterial pulse. The ear lobe is frequently moved by such deep jugular systolic pulses. In some patients with severe tricuspid regurgitation and very high venous pressure with marked distension of the jugular veins, it may not be possible to discern an isolated systolic jugular pulse. Rather, the only apparent wave may be the rapid deep y descent in early diastole. This is especially likely to occur when the right atrial and venous pressures have been markedly elevated for a long period of time, with marked dilatation of the right atrium and the great veins. In such patients the jugular venous pulse wave often increases rapidly following the precipitous y descent. This type of sharp, deep y wave reflects the pressure-volume characteristics of the failing right ventricle, which is usually dilated and has an increased end-systolic residual volume.

In patients with a jugular venous pulse suggestive of insignificant or only mild tricuspid regurgitation, it is often possible to produce significantly more regurgitation and a clearly abnormal jugular pulse wave by exercise or by abdominal compression. At times even deep inspiration may make a borderline venous pulse clearly abnormal. It should be noted that atrial fibrillation, which in itself only lessens the negative x wave to a slight degree (Fig. 5-34), is often associated with tricuspid regurgitation, which may produce additional changes in the venous wave form during systole (Fig. 5-38).

TRICUSPID   REGURGITATION

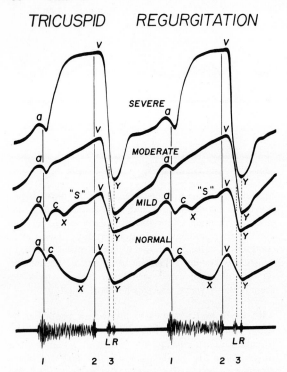

Fig. 5-38. Tricuspid regurgitation: diagrammatic jugular venous and heart-sound tracings to illustrate the changes from normal associated with mild, moderate, or severe tricuspid regurgitation. With mild tricuspid regurgitation, the *x* descent and *x* wave are briefer and more shallow than normal, while the *v* wave and *y* descent are somewhat more prominent than normal. With moderate regurgitation the *x* descent and *x* wave are even more abbreviated and may even be completely obliterated. Between the *c* wave and the moderately accentuated *v* wave it may be possible to record the regurgitant *s* wave as a faintly demarcated wave. At the bedside, however, the pulse wave is seen merely as a positive wave during systole. With severe tricuspid regurgitation, the huge regurgitant *s* wave completely obliterates the *x* descent and fuses with the smaller *c* and *v* waves to produce a single large positive systolic wave "ventricularization" of the venous wave form. Note that the *y* descent becomes progressively more prominent as the severity of tricuspid regurgitation increases. If a third heart sound from the right side of the heart is present, it characteristically is synchronous with the *y* trough, whereas the normal third sound from the left side of the heart often occurs during the *y* descent shortly before the *y* trough, although it may occur synchronously with the *y* trough.

Occasionally, in patients with constrictive pericarditis the negative *x* wave during a systole may be more prominent than the early diastolic *y* wave (Fig. 5-39). This finding seems to be more frequently found in patients with associated acute pericarditis. On the other hand, the finding of a

markedly positive systolic wave decreases the possibility of constrictive pericarditis. In this evaluation, however, one should be careful to distinguish between patients whose predominant venous pulse wave is a large positive wave during systole (as in tricuspid regurgitation) and patients who have distended veins and a high venous pressure and whose predominant wave is a deep negative *y* wave during early diastole. At times the latter type of pulse wave may initially appear to be a positive wave during systole.

Abnormalities of the Normal "Diastolic Collapse" (*y* Wave). Shortly after the second heart sound, the tricuspid valve opens and the rapid-filling phase of ventricular diastole begins. The onset of this phase occurs at or very slightly after the peak of the right atrial and venous *v* wave. The downslope of the *y* descent (or *v* descent) depends on several factors, including the height of the right atrial and venous pressure at the summit of the *v* wave, the pressure-volume characteristics of the right atrium and great veins, the rate of venous return from more peripheral veins during this phase, the resistance to forward flow across the tricuspid valve and the pressure-volume characteristics of the right ventricle. Important factors influencing the rate and volume of right ventricular filling include the amount of residual blood left in the ventricle after the preceding systole ("functional residual capacity"), the rate of ventricular relaxation, and the impedance of the ventricular myocardium and of the pericardium.

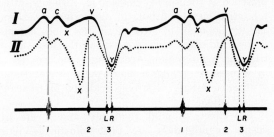

Fig. 5-39. Constrictive pericarditis: jugular venous and heart-sound tracings to illustrate two types of pulse-wave forms. In both types the level of venous pressure is markedly elevated. In type I, illustrated by the solid line, the predominant wave is a sharp, deep *y* descent and *y* wave in early systole, which is followed by a brisk *y* ascent. Frequently it is possible to record (but not to see) a small positive *h* wave at the end of the rapid *y* ascent. In the type II, the negative *x* wave during systole is prominent and may be deeper than the *y* wave. A third heart sound from the right side of the heart is usually synchronous with the trough of the *y* wave, whereas a third heart sound from the left side of the heart may occur either slightly earlier during the *y* descent or synchronously with the *y* trough. If atrial fibrillation develops, the *a* waves are absent.

The finding of a slow y descent of the jugular venous tracing shortly after the second heart sound suggests the presence of an obstruction to right atrial emptying, i.e., tricuspid stenosis (Fig. 5-40). On the other hand, a very rapid y descent is strong evidence against the presence of tricuspid stenosis. A rapid y descent from a high v point is characteristic of tricuspid regurgitation. At times this may be the predominant pulsation observed, particularly if the positive venous wave during ventricular systole is obscured by a very high venous pressure and marked distension of the caval veins and right atrium.

A venous pulse characterized by a sharp y descent, a deep y trough, and a rapid y ascent is seen both in patients with constrictive pericarditis (Fig. 5-39) and in patients with severe heart failure in whom the venous pressure is extremely high. In both these conditions, the sharp, exaggerated negative y wave occurring shortly after the second heart sound may be the predominant wave. In both situations, the rapid inflow of blood into the right ventricle causes the intraventricular pressure to rise precipitously following the sharp y dip. Since the right ventricle, right atrium, and great veins essentially form a common cavity during diastole, this rise in pressure is also apparent in the pulse of the right atrium and jugular veins. At times, a distinction between constrictive pericarditis and heart failure may be made by finding a large positive systolic venous wave due to tricuspid regurgitation (Lancisi's sign). This finding is very common in severe heart failure but is against the diagnosis of constrictive pericarditis.

VENOUS PRESSURE

In addition to the information that can be gained from the study of the jugular venous pulse contour, it is also possible to obtain information about the level of venous pressure from the bedside examination of peripheral veins. The veins which are most useful in the estimation of venous pressures are the arm and hand veins, the external jugular veins, and the internal jugular veins. In the examination of any vein, one should keep in mind the distinction between venous distension and venous pressure. At times, veins may be large and dilated with only slight elevation of pressure. At other times one may encounter patients with very high venous pressure but without significant visible distension. These extremes reflect the diverse pressure-volume characteristics which different venous beds may have.

Venous pressure may be estimated from examining the veins on the dorsum of the hand. To perform this estimation the patient should be in either

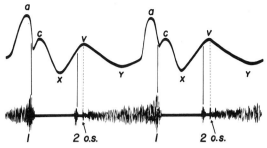

Fig. 5-40. Tricuspid stenosis: jugular venous and heart-sound tracings. Note the "giant" a waves and the slow y descent produced by the obstruction to flow from the right atrium to the right ventricle. The y depression is shallow, and the y ascent also has a decreased slope. The h wave is late or absent. Note that the peak of the v wave is synchronous with the opening of the tricuspid valve.

a sitting or lying position at a 30° elevation or greater, and the hand should be kept below the level of the heart long enough for the veins on the dorsum of the hand to become distended. The arm is then slowly and passively raised while the physician observes the veins. Care should be taken that the arm is not flexed excessively at either the shoulder or the elbow and that the upper arm is not constricted by clothing. Normally, the veins will be seen to collapse when the level of the dorsum of the hand reaches the sternal angle of Louis or the level of the suprasternal notch. If the veins do not collapse until the hand is raised still higher, the pressure in the veins may be considered to be elevated. The *vertical distance above the sternal angle* at which the veins do collapse should be recorded, as well as the position of the patient during the test. An elevated pressure in the veins on the dorsum of the hand may also be produced by any type of local obstruction to venous return, such as constriction of the upper part of the arm, marked subcutaneous edema produced by infiltration of administered fluids, or even by partial venous obstruction at the thoracic inlet. On the other hand, the increased peripheral venous vasoconstriction associated with heart failure or the administration of vasoconstrictor agents may alter the pressure-volume characteristics of these veins and make it difficult to discern a definite level at which there is a significant change in the amount of venous distension. For these reasons, this method for the estimation of venous pressure is less accurate than other methods. It is usually employed when it is impossible to examine the neck veins satisfactorily, e.g., in patients with short, very fat necks.

The external jugular vein may also be used to estimate venous pressure. The technique is to place the patient with the trunk elevated about 30 to 60°.

The head is rotated only slightly away from the external jugular vein being examined. The examiner's forefinger is placed just above and parallel to the clavicle. It is then gently pressed inward against the neck, occluding the external jugular vein. After waiting 15 to 45 sec for this vein to fill and become somewhat distended, the examiner suddenly withdraws the finger and observes the apparent height of the distended fluid column within the vein. Normally this level, if visible at all, will be only a few millimeters above the superior border of the clavicle or less than 3 cm above the sternal angle of Louis. If the venous pressure is markedly elevated, it may be necessary to perform the test with the patient's trunk at a 90° elevation. Rarely, the pressure will be so high that even in this position no definite upper level of distension is apparent after the compressing finger is removed. The external jugular veins are likely to be obstructed by local venous obstructions or kinking at the base of the neck. Whenever possible this estimation of venous pressure should be compared with other bedside estimations or, preferably, with direct measurements of venous pressure (see Chap. 10 for technique).

The internal jugular veins may be used to estimate venous pressure as well as to evaluate venous pulse wave form. The technique is similar to that for examination of internal jugular venous pulses, i.e., the patient is examined at the optimum degree of trunk elevation for inspection of the venous pulse. While the patient is breathing gently or, preferably, is at the end of a normal expiration, the highest point of visible pulsation of the internal jugular vein is determined. The *vertical* distance between this level and the level of the sternal angle is then recorded, together with the degree of elevation of the patient. Normally this distance is not greater than 3 or 4 cm. The sternal angle (of Louis) is chosen as the reference point for convenience at the bedside. It does not have a constant relationship in all positions to the midpoint of the right atrium (the ideal reference level for venous pressure measurements), nor are the distances sometimes used for this relationship consistently accurate.

The most common cause of an elevated venous pressure is failure of the right ventricle secondary to failure of the left ventricle. Other causes of right ventricular failure include cor pulmonale and pulmonary stenosis. Pressure in the jugular veins may also be increased by cardiac tamponade, tricuspid stenosis, superior vena cava obstruction, certain hyperkinetic circulatory states, and at times, increased blood volume. At times patients with pulmonary disease associated with severe obstruction to expiration, e.g., asthma or obstructive emphy-

sema, may have a marked expiratory increase in intrathoracic pressure, which may elevate the jugular venous pressure during expiration. Careful observation will usually enable one to distinguish this type of expiratory elevation from elevation due to cardiac causes.

Not infrequently patients are seen who are suspected of having failure of the right ventricle but in whom the venous pressure at rest is normal. In this situation, as in many other clinical evaluations of organ or system function, abnormalities may be brought out by applying *stress* in order to test the reserve capacity of the organ in question. One of the better simple methods of evaluating the function of the right ventricle is to measure the venous pressure in a medial antecubital vein during leg exercise. An even quicker and simpler method—though perhaps not quite so accurate or quantitative—is to employ the *hepatojugular* (or *abdominojugular*) *reflux* test. The trunk of the patient should be elevated to about 30 to 45° above the horizontal, in which position venous pulsations are normally seen only at or just above the level of the clavices if the resting pressure is normal. The patient is instructed to continue his normal breathing during the test in order to avoid performing a Valsalva maneuver, the most common cause of false-positive tests. After the examiner has identified the upper level of internal jugular pulsation, he places the palm of his hand over the right upper quadrant of the abdomen and applies firm but not painful pressure for about 30 to 60 sec. In the normal subject the level of jugular venous distension and pulsation is not significantly altered; in patients with right-sided heart failure the upper level of venous pulsation in the internal jugular vein, and the amount of its distension, may significantly increase. It is thought that the increased abdominal pressure enhances venous return to the right side of the heart and that a right ventricle with latent "failure" is unable to accept this extra stress, causing pressure in the great veins to rise. Abdominal compression may also be used to bring out the typical jugular venous pattern of tricuspid regurgitation in patients in whom the resting pulse wave is not definitely abnormal. It should be noted that there is no special advantage to applying the abdominal compression to the right upper quadrant of the abdomen, "over the liver"; however, since examination of the heart is best performed from the right side of the patient and since pulsations of the right internal jugular vein are usually better seen than those of the left, it is merely more convenient at the bedside to apply the right hand to the upper right quadrant.

Occasionally abdominal compression is inadvertently produced by the patient himself when he sits up from a lying position in bed and slumps forward, increasing intraabdominal pressure. The increased intraabdominal pressure may usually be relieved when the patient sits more erect. This modification of the hepatojugular reflux test is more likely to be seen in a patient with a large abdominal girth.

SUGGESTED READING

General

Altman, R.: "Der Venenpuls," Urban & Schwarzberg, München, 1956.

Bloomfield, R. A. Lauson, H. D., Cournand, A., Breed, E. S., and Richards, D. W., Jr.: Recording of Right Heart Pressures in Normal Subjects and in Patients with Chronic Pulmonary Disease and Various Types of Cardio-circulatory Disease, *J. Clin. Invest.*, 25:639, 1946.

Brecher, G.: "Venous Return," Grune & Stratton, Inc., New York, 1956.

Burch, G. E.: "A Primer of Venous Pressure," Lea & Febiger, Philadelphia, 1950.

Burch, G. E., and Ray, C. T.: Mechanism of the Hepatojugular Reflux Test in Congestive Heart Failure, *Am. Heart J.*, 48:373, 1954.

Cossio, P., and Buzzi, A.: Clinical Value of the Venous Pulse, *Am. Heart J.*, 54:127, 1957.

Feder, W., and Cherry, R. A.: External Jugular Phlebogram as Reflecting Venous and Right Atrial Hemodynamics, *Am. J. Cardiol.*, 12:383, 1963.

Fowler, N. O., and Marshall, W. J.: Cardiac Diagnosis from Examination of Arteries and Veins, *Circulation*, 30:272, 1964.

Gibson, A. G., Oxon, M. B., and Land, M. R. C. P.: The Significance of a Hitherto Undescribed Wave in the Jugular Pulse, *Lancet*, 2:1380, 1907.

Groedel, F. M.: "The Venous Pulse and Its Graphic Recording," Brooklyn Medical Press, New York, 1946.

Hartman, H., and Snellen, H. A.: Die klinische Bedentung des Venenpulses, *Arzneimittel-Forsch.*, 13:404, 1959.

Hartman, H.: The Jugular Venous Tracing, *Am. Heart J.*, 59:698, 1960.

Hering, H. E.: Zur Analysis des Venenpulses, *Deutsche med. Wchnschr.*, 33:1895, 1907.

Hirschfelder, A. D.: Some Variations in the Form of the Venous Pulse, *Bull. Johns Hopkins Hosp.*, 18:265, 1907.

Hochstein, E., and Rubin, A. L.: Pressure and Pulses, in "Physical Diagnosis," McGraw-Hill Book Company, New York, 1964, pp. 248-274.

Hussey, H. H., and Jeghers, H.: Practical Considerations of Venous Pressure, *New England J. Med.*, 237:776, 812, 1947.

Landis, E. M., and Hortenstein, J. E.: Functional Significance of Venous Blood Pressure, *Physiol. Rev.*, 30:1, 1950.

Levine, S. A.: "Clinical Heart Disease," 5th ed. W. B. Saunders Company, Philadelphia, 1958.

Lyons, R. H., Kennedy, J. A., and Burwell, C. S.: The Measurement of Venous Pressure by the Direct Method, *Am. Heart J.*, 16:675, 1938.

MacKay, I. F. S.: An Experimental Analysis of the Jugular Pulse in Man, *J. Physiol.*, 106:113, 1947.

MacKenzie, J.: "The Study of the Pulse, Arterial, Venous and Hepatic and of the Movements of the Heart," Young J. Pentland, Edinburgh, 1902.

Mathews, M. B., and Hampson, J.: Hepatojugular Reflux, *Lancet*, 1:873, 1958.

White, P. D., and Cooke, W. T.: Recognition and Significance of Marked and Chronic Systolic Pulsation of Deep Jugular Veins, *Tr. A. Am. Physicians*, 54:199, 1939.

White, P. D.: "Clues in the Diagnosis and Treatment of Heart Disease," Charles C Thomas, Publisher, Springfield, Ill., 1955.

Wiggers, C. J.: "Pressure Pulses in the Cardiovascular System," Longmans, Green & Co., New York, 1928.

Wiggers, C. J.: "Circulatory Dynamics," Grune & Stratton, Inc., New York, 1952.

Winsor, T., and Burch, G. E.: Phlebostatic Axis and Phlebostatic Level: Reference Levels for Venous Measurements in Man, *Proc. Soc. Exper. Biol. & Med.*, 58:165, 1945.

Wood, P.: "Diseases of the Heart and Circulation," 2d ed., J. B. Lippincott Company, Philadelphia, 1956.

Tricuspid Valve Disease

Aceves, S., and Carral, R.: The Diagnosis of Tricuspid Valve Disease, *Am. Heart J.*, 34:114, 1947.

Cooke, W. T., and White, P. D.: Tricuspid Stenosis, with Particular Reference to Diagnosis and Prognosis, *Brit. Heart J.*, 3:147, 1941.

Ferrer, M. I., Harvey, R. M., Kuschner, M., and Richards, D. W., Jr.: Hemodynamic Studies in Tricuspid Stenosis of Rheumatic Origin, *Circulation Res.*, 1:49, 1953.

Gibson, R., and Wood, P.: The Diagnosis of Tricuspid Stenosis, *Brit. Heart J.*, 17:552, 1955.

Killip, T., III, and Lukas, D. S.: Tricuspid Stenosis: Physiologic Criteria for Diagnosis and Hemodynamic Abnormalities, *Circulation*, 16:3, 1957.

Killip, T., III, and Lukas, D. S.: Tricuspid Stenosis: Clinical Features in Twelve Cases, *Am. J. Med.*, 24:836, 1958.

McCord, M. C., and Blount, S. G., Jr.: The Hemodynamic Pattern in Tricuspid Valve Disease, *Am. Heart J.*, 44:671, 1952.

McCord, M. C., Swan, H., and Blount, S. G., Jr.: Tricuspid Stenosis: Clinical and Physiologic Evaluation, *Am. Heart J.*, 48:405, 1954.

Messer, A. L., Hurst, J. W., Rappaport, M. B., and Sprague, H. B.: A Study of the Venous Pulse in Tricuspid Valve Disease, *Circulation*, 1:388, 1950.

Müller, O., and Shillingford, J.: Tricuspid Incompetence, *Brit. Heart J.*, **16**:195, 1954.

Perloff, J. K., and Harvey, W. P.: Clinical Recognition of Tricuspid Stenosis, *Circulation*, **22**:346, 1960.

Salazar, E., and Levine, H.: Rheumatic Tricuspid Regurgitation: The Clinical Spectrum, *Am. J. Med.*, **33**:111, 1962.

Smith, J. A., and Levine, S. A.: The Clinical Features of Tricuspid Stenosis, *Am. Heart J.*, **23**:739, 1942.

Vesell, H.: Tricuspid Stenosis; A Simple Diagnostic Sign, *Am. J. Med.*, **7**:497, 1949.

Yu, P. N., Harken, D. E., Lovejoy, F. W., Jr., Nye, R. E., Jr., and Mahoney, E. B.: Clinical and Hemodynamic Studies of Tricuspid Stenosis, *Circulation*, **13**:680, 1956.

Zeh, E.: Die Diagnose der Trikuspidalinsuffizienz, *Arch. Kreislaufforsch.*, **30**:127, 1959.

Constrictive Pericarditis, Cardiac Tamponade, Küssmaul's Sign
(See References Chap. 49.)

PERCUSSION VERSUS INSPECTION AND PALPATION OF THE HEART

J. Willis Hurst, M.D.

In most instances inspection and palpation of cardiac pulsations give all the information made available by the technique of expert percussion. In addition, a great deal of additional information can be obtained by these techniques. Therefore, percussion of the heart will not be discussed in this text. Instead, we choose to emphasize inspection and palpation as superior methods of examining the heart. The reasons supporting this view are discussed below.

In years past it was customary to determine the outer limit of cardiac dullness by the technique of percussion and to compare it with the left midclavicular line. When the outer limit of cardiac dullness was found to be within the midclavicular line, the heart was said to be of normal size. The expert learned to determine the outer limit of pulmonary artery dullness and could, on occasion, identify a large left atrial appendage or a large right atrium. Certain exceptions to the rules were always obvious. For example, when the diaphragm was higher than normal, the outer limit of cardiac dullness could be located outside the left midclavicular line without necessarily indicating enlargement. On the other hand, slight left ventricular enlargement could be missed, since the outer limit of dullness might not extend beyond the midclavicular line. This was especially true when the left ventricular hypertrophy was due to aortic stenosis. In certain clinical situations, such as obesity and pulmonary emphysema, percussion was known to be especially poor because extracardiac factors interfered with the technique of percussion.

It became obvious that the technique of percussion merely gave information regarding the outer limits of cardiac dullness.

Obviously, no one will percuss the outer limit of cardiac dullness outside or beyond a prominent visible and palpable apex impulse; just as obviously, inspection and palpation of the precordium are difficult or impossible when there is considerable obesity or pulmonary emphysema. A vigorous pulsation of the sternoclavicular joint on the right may indicate a right-sided aortic arch. An abnormal pulsation of either the right or left sternoclavicular joint may be due to dissecting aneurysm in a patient with chest pain or to an aortic aneurysm of another cause. The main pulmonary artery is often visible and palpable. This may be normal in children or in adults with hyperkinetic circulations. With practice, it is possible to identify abnormal pulsation of a prominent pulmonary artery. When the pulsation is vigorous, it is prudent to consider that the right ventricle has ejected a large volume of blood, such as occurs with an atrial septal defect. This type of pulsation occurs, but to a lesser degree, with ventricular septal defect and patent ductus arteriosus. Pulmonary regurgitation augments the finding considerably. When the pulmonary artery is large and the pulsation is sustained, it is proper to consider that the pressure is elevated and that the blood flow is normal. This occurs with mitral stenosis of moderate degree. Pulmonary regurgitation may also change this finding to a more hyperkinetic state. When there is poststenotic dilatation of the pulmonary artery, secondary to valvular pulmonary stenosis, the pulmonary artery may also be prominent and the pulsation becomes slow and sustained. The right ventricle is really an anterior structure, and when it is enlarged, it lifts the anterior portion of the chest, including the sternum. In the normal excited child and in the thin adult, a slight pulsation is found in this area. When the right ventricle ejects a large volume of blood, as it does with an atrial septal defect, there is likely to be a vigorous anterior lift of the sternum and precordium. When there is right ventricular hypertrophy due to an obstructive lesion, such as mitral stenosis or pulmonary stenosis, there may be a sustained but forceful lift to the precordium and sternum. Pulmonary emphysema may obscure the usual findings of right ventricular hypertrophy. Accordingly, pulsations due to enlargement of the right ventricle in these patients may be detected by sliding the finger up under the rib cage just beneath the sternum. The large right ventricle strikes the ends of the fingertips, whereas aortic pulsations are felt by the palmar surface of the fingers. The normal apex impulse is located somewhere near the left midclavicular line. The size of the normal apex impulse is less than 3 cm in diameter. The normal

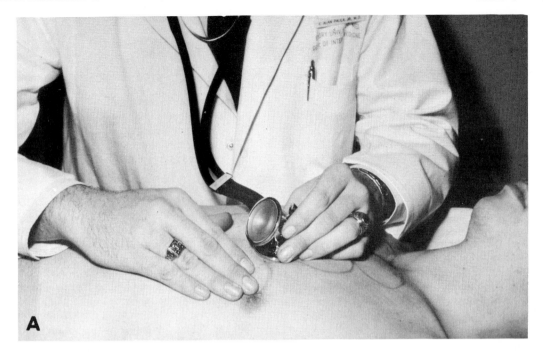

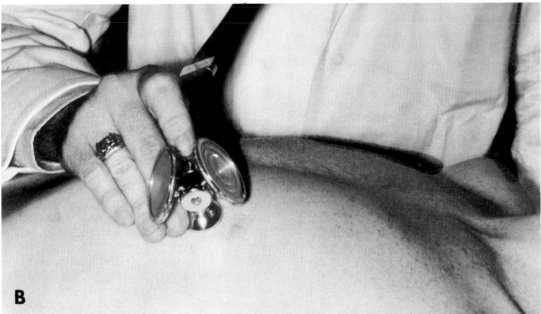

Fig. 5-41. Technique of inspecting and palpating precordial cardiac pulsations. In order to time precordial pulsations, it is necessary to identify heart sounds at the same time that cardiac pulsations are observed. A. The cardiac apex is palpated with the fingertips. At the same time, heart sounds are identified with the stethoscope. B. With practice, it is possible to identify the movement of the stethoscope. At the same time, heart sounds are identified.

apex impulse is not sustained. The outward thrust lasts about one-third of systole, and no diastolic pulsations are palpable. When there is left ventricular hypertrophy, the apex impulse may be outside the midclavicular line and larger than normal. The nature of the apical pulsation may be more important than its location and size. When there is left ventricular hypertrophy, there may be a sustained forceful thrust occupying one-half or more of systole. The thrust may be more forceful when there is aortic regurgitation, as compared with aortic stenosis, systemic hypertension, and myocardial disease (including coronary atherosclerosis), in which the impulse is sustained but not so vigorous. Abnormal pulsations due to myocardial infarction and associated with angina pectoris may be felt at the apex, the anterior precordium, and in "ectopic" positions such as the area between the pulmonary artery region and the apex.

Subaudible diastolic cardiac events may be seen and felt. For example, atrial and ventricular gallop movements may be detected.

In order to time the systolic and diastolic cardiac movements, it is essential to use the heart sounds as reference points. Therefore, it is necessary to inspect and palpate the movements while actually listening to the heart (Fig. 5-41). With experience, it is possible to watch the movements of the stethoscope while listening to the heart sounds.

The thrills associated with heart murmurs can be palpated. The diastolic rumble of mitral stenosis and the systolic murmur of mitral regurgitation may be palpated at the cardiac apex. The thrill of aortic stenosis cuts across the palm of the hand toward the right side of the neck, while the thrill of pulmonary stenosis cuts across the palm of the hand to the left side of the neck. The thrill due to a ventricular septal defect is usually located in the third and fourth intercostal spaces near the left sternal border.

Heart sounds may be palpable. The loud first sound of mitral stenosis may be palpated at the apex and at times all over the precordium, including the second right intercostal space adjacent to the sternum. The opening snap of mitral stenosis is occasionally felt. Pulmonary and aortic ejection clicks may be palpable. The loud second sound associated with pulmonary hypertension may be palpable in the second and third left interspace adjacent to the sternum.

To restate: in determining the heart size, percussion of the chest is not so useful as inspection and palpation of the cardiac movements and events. The technique of inspection and palpation gives all the information that can be obtained by percussion but also yields much additional information. Just as the phonocardiogram has taught us auscultation, the kinetocardiogram and apex cardiogram have taught us inspection and palpation. These topics are discussed in the section that follows.

INSPECTION AND PALPATION OF THE PRECORDIUM

E. E. Eddleman, Jr., M.D.

Contraction and relaxation of the heart result in a wide spectrum of vibrations that are transmitted to the anterior chest wall. The vibrations that are very slow (low frequency, 0 to 30 cycles per second) and large in amplitude are often visible or palpable. These are primarily due to the movements and shape changes of the heart (Fig. 5-42). The vibrations of higher frequency (30 cps and above) are in general associated with valve closures or function and are audible but rarely palpable unless of marked intensity (thrills) (Fig. 5-42). The present chapter deals with the low-frequency group. Palpation and inspection will be considered together, since these two types of physical examination detect the same phenomena.

Specific cardiac diagnoses can seldom be made from inspection and palpation of the precordium alone, but when these observations are correlated with other findings, considerable clinical information is often added. For example, a systolic lift of the lower parasternal region of the chest in a patient with severe congestive heart failure may indicate not right ventricular hypertrophy but a dilated heart; however, in a patient with mitral stenosis, a parasternal lift is diagnostic of right ventricular hypertrophy. Similarly, an outward localized movement at the V_3 precordial electrocardiographic position may have varying significance, depending on the clinical situation. In patients with hypertension and no evidence of ischemic heart disease, the impulse is probably due to left ventricular hypertrophy. However, if the patient has never had any cardiac lesion that could result in left ventricular hypertrophy, and has a history of chest pain, compatible with that noted in patients with myocardial infarctions, the paradoxic pulsation probably indicates the presence of an ischemic "bulge" due to an infarction. In addition, the precordial findings often yield clues that point toward coexisting disorders. For example, a localized, sustained systolic outward apical impulse in patients with mitral stenosis may suggest enlargement of the left ventricle and thus lead to a successful search for an associated mitral insufficiency or aortic valvular lesion. Thus, the information obtained by inspection and palpation must be correlated with the findings by other methods. With these limitations the physical examination of chest-wall motion is useful and important, especially in recognizing specific ventricular enlargement.[1-3]

TECHNIQUES OF THE EXAMINATION

Generally, it is best to palpate and inspect the precordium with the patient supine. When the patient is turned on his left side, the apical region of the heart is displaced against the lateral chest wall and distortion of the movements occurs. For

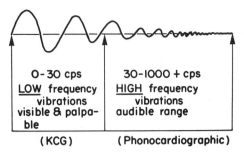

Fig. 5-42. Diagram illustrating the types of precordial movements or vibrations that can be encountered over the precordium. In general, the vibrations fall into two groups: (1) low-frequency vibrations which are of large amplitude and are both visible and palpable; (2) higher-frequency vibrations, which are audible. The demarcation line as drawn obviously is not so sharp as that presented on the graph. The lower labels represent the two types of graphic methods used in recording the various vibrations. Note that as the frequency of the movements becomes higher, the amplitudes of the movements become smaller.

example, the normal brief outward impulse of the apex in normal subjects may become a sustained thrust which may mimic the impulse of left ventricular hypertrophy. On the other hand, the dyspneic patient cannot comfortably lie flat and some elevation of the chest and head is necessary. Usually, a slight degree of elevation (not over 45°) is not sufficient to alter the chest-wall movements from those noted in the supine position. However, in the sitting position or with the patient slightly bent forward, the heart is displaced anteriorly against the chest wall and normal movements may be interpreted as abnormal. In these instances, a recheck of the findings should be made after the patient is comfortable and can be placed in the proper position for examination.

AREAS OF PALPATION

Limiting the examination to the apical region of the chest wall is the most common mistake made in palpating the precordium. With this type of procedure, only left ventricular hypertrophy is usually detected and abnormal movements due to ischemic heart disease or right ventricular hypertrophy are easily missed. Figure 5-43 presents the principal areas where abnormal movements are encountered over the precordium. These include the apical, midprecordial, parasternal, pulmonic, and epigastric areas. In addition, specific locations will, for convenience, be referred to as follows.* K will

* Kinetocardiographic (graphic representation of

indicate the "position" or point in the chest wall. The first subnumeral will refer to the vertical line comparable to the precordial electrocardiographic position, and the second numeral will refer to the intercostal space. For example, K_{14} will indicate a position in the right parasternal line and in the fourth intercostal space. Similarly, K_{45} denotes a point in the left midclavicular line and in the fifth intercostal space.

It is important to inspect not only by looking down at the chest but also by looking from the side or at a right angle to the various areas under question. Small localized inward movements or even diffuse movements (movements distributed over a large area) of minimal amplitude often can be detected better by inspection than by palpation. Inspection, though superior to palpation for detecting inward movements, is much inferior for recognizing outward movements. Since systolic outward movements are more clinically significant, palpation of the precordium in general is more important than inspection. The movements over a wide area of the precordium can be best felt with the palm of the hand flat against the chest; localized movements are often more easily detected with the tips of the fingers. The following are the factors to be considered about any precordial movement that can be felt or seen:

1. Amplitude. Most outward movements of large amplitude are abnormal; however, physical characteristics of the chest wall should be considered when judging the amplitude of any movement.

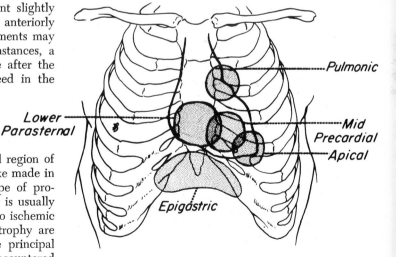

Fig. 5-43. Areas over the precordium where significant vibrations are usually detected. These include the lower parasternal regions, midprecordial, apical, epigastric, and pulmonic areas.

low-frequency movement) nomenclature for positions will be used because of its simplicity.

Table 5-1. CHARACTERISTIC FEATURES OF VARIOUS TYPES OF PRECORDIAL IMPULSES

Impulse	Direction of movement	Time in cardiac cycle	Duration of impulse	Location	Amplitude and quality	Diffuse or localized
Normal left ventricular impulse (PMI) (apex impulse)	Outward	Very early part of ejection	Brief—not over 0.08 sec above base line*	K_{34}, K_{45}; rarely at K_{55}	Tapping, not forceful	Localized 2–3 cm in diameter
Left ventricular hypertrophy	Outward	Systolic	Sustained—0.09–0.30 sec above base line	K_{34}, K_{45}, K_{55}; rarely elsewhere (lower intercostal spaces)	Sustained "thrust"	Localized 3–5 cm in diameter
Right ventricular hypertrophy	Outward	Systolic	Sustained in pressure loads	K_{14}, K_{24}, K_{35}; rarely at K_{45}	Sustained parasternal lift	Diffuse lifts lower parasternal area
"Bulge" due to myocardial infarction	Outward	Pansystolic	Sustained	K_{24}, K_{34}, K_{45}, K_{55} and epigastric areas	Sustained thrusting	Usually localized but may be diffuse in large infarctions
"Bulge" due to angina	Outward	Usually early systolic, few late systolic	Sustained	K_{24}, K_{34}, K_{45}, K_{55}, and epigastric areas	Sustained impulse	Usually localized

* Base line arbitrarily defined as a horizontal line placed at a point on the kinetocardiogram trace 0.04 sec after the onset of the QRS complex to the electrocardiogram.

Also, all movements are exaggerated in amplitude in hyperkinetic states.

2. Duration of the impulse. A sustained outward movement is usually pathologic; a brief nonsustained movement is often normal.

3. The direction of the impulse. During systole, outward movements are in general abnormal, inward movements are usually normal.

4. The time of the impulse in relation to the cardiac cycle. This is important in separating filling movements from those associated with ventricular contractions. The most frequent abnormal movements occur during systole.

5. Location of the impulse. A sustained, outward, and exaggerated systolic impulse near the apical region usually indicates left ventricular hypertrophy if ischemic heart disease is excluded. A similar impulse in the left parasternal region may signify right ventricular hypertrophy.

6. Distribution. Whether or not the impulse is diffuse and present in several areas or is localized to one point is often a help in interpreting the findings. For example, the impulse is usually diffuse with right ventricular hypertrophy but localized with left ventricular hypertrophy.

The importance of the above points will be dis-cussed subsequently in more detail in the description of the various types of movements. Table 5-1 presents some of the characteristics of the various precordial movements frequently encountered.

NORMAL FINDINGS

Apex Impulse (Left Ventricular Thrust). The apex impulse (probably the term *left ventricular thrust* is preferable) is the point of maximum outward movement (PMI) in a normal person. The movement is a tapping early systolic outward thrust, brief in duration and of minimal amplitude.[4,5] This outward movement usually occurs in the fifth intercostal space in the midclavicular line (K_{45}) and is localized to one point or to a small area not more than 2 to 3 cm in diameter. The movement is mainly due to a recoil of the heart as blood is ejected. However, it is possible that other factors are involved, such as a slight rotation of the heart anteriorly and to the right which tips the apex of the heart lightly against the chest wall. Figure 5-44 is the kinetocardiogram* of the left

* Kinetocardiograms are low-frequency displacement records of precordial motion and represent a graphic

Fig. 5-44. Photograph of a low-frequency tracing (kinetocardiogram) of the apex beat in a normal person. The upper trace is the carotid pulse, the lower trace is the kinetocardiogram. The arrow marked QRS indicates the onset of the QRS complex in the electrocardiogram. The curved arrows point to the normal apex thrust. Note that it is a small nonsustained early systolic impulse that to the fingers would feel tapping in quality.

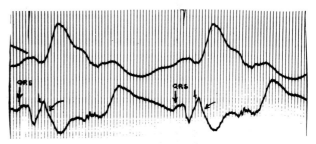

ventricular thrust which is characteristic of the normal apex impulse that one feels at the bedside. Note that the duration is brief and the outward movement is not particularly prominent. The duration above the base line seldom exceeds 0.08 sec.* The thrust of maximum amplitude is located at the K_{45} (V_4) area in about 50 per cent of the subjects but does occur at the K_{34} (V_3) in about one-third. The remaining persons have the maximum impulse at the K_{55} (V_5) position. Thus, three-fourths of the normal left ventricular thrusts occur in the K_{34} (V_3) or K_{45} (V_4) areas.

The chief differences between a normal left ventricular thrust (apex beat) and that of left ventricular hypertrophy are the duration, amplitude, and size of the area where the impulse is felt. In other words, if the impulse is sustained throughout systole or is exaggerated in amplitude and distribution, it is abnormal.

Parasternal Retraction. The lower parasternal region of the chest in normal individuals usually retracts (moves inward) during ejection and is sustained throughout most of ejection systole. It is best noted by looking at the chest from the side. In this position it is easy to visualize an abrupt inward systolic movement with each heart beat. This inward movement is probably due to a volume change in the underlying heart as ejection of blood occurs. The lower parasternal region of the chest retracts as the heart volume becomes smaller. Abnormal movements in this area are paradoxic or outward during systole.

LEFT VENTRICULAR HYPERTROPHY

Left ventricular hypertrophy results in an exaggeration of the normal left ventricular thrust, both in amplitude[5,6] and in duration. Figure 5-45 is the graphic representation of the outward movement

record of the movements felt or seen over the precordium. These traces differ from apex cardiograms in that they represent absolute chest-wall movements, not relative interspace motion.

* A base line can be arbitrarily set at a point on the curve 0.04 sec after the onset of the QRS complex. This serves as a useful reference in measuring durations and in comparing curves from various patients.

associated with left ventricular hypertrophy. It is systolic in time and is usually localized to an area about 5 or 6 cm in diameter and often detected in an adjacent intercostal space. This abnormal left ventricular thrust, when considered carefully, can be one of the most reliable guides as to the presence of left ventricular enlargement. Table 5-2 compares standard electrocardiographic findings with studies which evaluate the abnormality in the left ventricular thrust. The maximum impulse is noted in the K_{55} position in 13 per cent of the patients, K_{45} (V_4) position in 73 per cent, K_{34} (V_3) position in 13 per cent, and in other adjacent areas in about 1 per cent of the patients (these figures exclude patients with severe heart failure and markedly enlarged hearts). The location of the maximum thrust is of some help in distinguishing left ventricular hypertrophy from other cardiac ab-

*Table 5-2.** INCIDENCE OF ABNORMAL LEFT VENTRICULAR THRUSTS AND ELECTROCARDIOGRAPHIC FINDINGS IN 115 PATIENTS WITH HYPERTENSIVE AND AORTIC VALVULAR DISEASE

	No. of patients abnormal	Percentage of patients abnormal
Left ventricular impulses of abnormal left ventricular thrust as determined by an abnormally prolonged duration (hypertensive and aortic valvular disease, KCG)	100	87
Left ventricular hypertrophy by voltage (40 mm R + S in any V lead — Grant criterion)	53	46
Left ventricular hypertrophy by Sokolow criteria (using only one criterion)	81	70
Left axis deviation	21	11
Prolonged intrinsicoid deflection (0.05 sec or greater)	28	25

* SOURCE: Davie et al.[5]

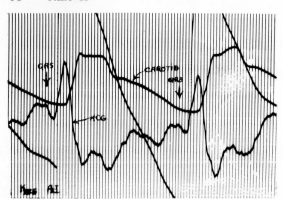

Fig. 5-45. Apex beat of a patient with left ventricular hypertrophy due to aortic insufficiency. Upper trace, carotid pulse; lower trace, kinetocardiogram. The arrow indicating the onset of a QRS complex of the electrocardiogram is labeled in each complex. The left ventricular thrust or apex impulse begins shortly after the onset of the QRS complex in the electrocardiogram and is characterized by a large outward movement which is larger and more sustained than the normal impulse.

normalities. For example, the maximum impulse of right ventricular hypertrophy rarely if ever occurs in the anterior axillary line, and conversely left ventricular hypertrophy does not result in a maximal impulse in the parasternal region. Contrary to what is generally thought, left ventricular hypertrophy can be present without the largest impulse being displaced left or laterally and to a lower intercostal space. Left ventricular hypertrophy without dilatation in patients with left ventricular pressure loads such as hypertension or aortic stenosis may have the largest outward movement at the K_{34} (V_3) position. Left ventricular flow loads, such as occur in aortic insufficiency which results in

ventricular dilatation, more frequently displace the impulse laterally and to a lower interspace. Consequently, palpation offers a crude means by which one can obtain some idea as to the degree of ventricular dilatation present. Differentiation of the movement from a normal impulse depends on detecting an exaggerated amplitude to the thrust and a more sustained impulse and to a lesser extent the location.

All types of heart disease that can cause left ventricular hypertrophy may result in a similarly exaggerated left ventricular impulse as described; however, there are a few differentiating features, related to the type of heart disease. Left ventricular flow load such as occurs in aortic insufficiency is associated with an impulse that is exaggerated in amplitude but not so sustained as that noted in patients with left ventricular pressure loads[5,7] (Figs. 5-45 and 5-46). Although the differences seem minute, it is often possible with practice to distinguish these two types of impulses at the bedside. Patients with "pure" mitral insufficiency may have a prominent late systolic outward movement that can be detected also at the bedside with practice. It may occur both in the apical region of the chest as well as in the midprecordial area.[5] This outward movement is of aid in deciding whether or not a given systolic murmur is the result of mitral insufficiency or of a hemic murmur. In the latter type (hemic or functional murmur) this abnormally late systolic outward movement is not found and only normal pulsations occur.

RIGHT VENTRICULAR HYPERTROPHY

Right ventricular hypertrophy results in a sustained systolic lift of the lower parasternal region of

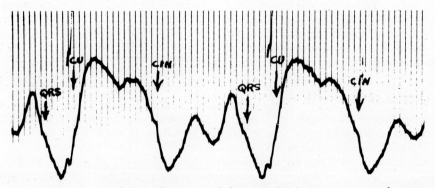

Fig. 5-46. Kinetocardiographic record from the region of the apex (K_{45}) in a patient with aortic stenosis. The timing of the onset of the QRS complex in the electrocardiogram is noted by the arrows: *CU*, upstroke in the carotid pulse; *CIN*, upstroke in the incisural notch. Beginning shortly after the onset of the QRS complex there is a slow, sustained outward movement through most of systole. Patients with left ventricular pressure loads usually show a sustained exaggerated movement. In contrast, patients with left ventricular flow loads have a much greater degree of retraction (inward movement) during mid- and late systole, although the initial portion of the impulse is exaggerated over normal both in amplitude and in duration.

the chest (Fig. 5-47).[5,8,9] Although the outward movement can be detected over a wide area, the point of maximum impulse is most frequently located at the K_{24} (V_2) area. This outward, or paradoxic, movement is probably due to a shape change of the heart. It is best detected by placing the hand over the lower parasternal region of the chest and noting a sustained systolic lift to the entire hand. The parasternal lift is present in patients with mitral stenosis and in those with cor pulmonale. Such a lift is infrequent in chronic lung disease in the absence of right-sided heart failure (cor pulmonale). The parasternal systolic lift is present in approximately 96 per cent of the patients with mitral stenosis (Table 5-3) and probably offers the most reliable evidence of right ventricular hypertrophy. The comparison with the electrocardiogram in a group of patients with mitral stenosis is given in Table 5-3. Note that diagnostic features of the electrocardiogram were present in only approximately 56 per cent of the same group. In general, the higher the pulmonary artery pressure, the more pronounced is the "lift." Interatrial septal defects (right ventricular flow loads) usually have a move-

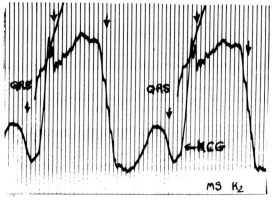

Fig. 5-47. Graphic representation of the K_{24} (V_2) kinetocardiogram from a patient with marked mitral stenosis and right ventricular hypertrophy. The first arrow in each complex indicates the onset of the QRS complex in the electrocardiogram; the second arrow, the onset of ejection, is determined by the upstroke of the carotid pulse; the third arrow, the end of systole, is determined by the carotid incisural notch. Note the marked sustained systolic outward movement. This is a graphic representation of the parasternal lift that can be felt in patients with mild-to-severe right ventricular hypertrophy.

Table 5-3. COMPARISON OF AN ABNORMAL PARASTERNAL LIFT WITH ELECTROCARDIOGRAPHIC FINDINGS IN 57 PATIENTS WITH PURE MITRAL STENOSIS

	No. of patients abnormal	Percentage of patients abnormal
KCG findings:		
Abnormal parasternal lift:		
By pattern*	54	95
By measurement†	53	93
ECG findings:		
Atrial fibrillation	24	42
Right axis deviation	7	
Notched P waves	14	42% of
(33 patients)		those with normal sinus rhythms
R = S (V_1)	14	25
RR¹ (V_1)	7	12
qR (V_1)	12	21
R = S, RR¹, qR (V_1)	33	58
RR¹ or qR (V_1)	19	33
Right bundle branch block	1	2

* Kinetocardiograms were inspected for a right ventricular hypertrophy pattern.

† The outward movements (right ventricular) in the kinetocardiograms were measured. When movements were abnormally prolonged in the K_{24} record (over 0.08 sec) they were interpreted as indicating right ventricular hypertrophy.

ment that is exaggerated but not so sustained as in patients with right ventricular pressure loads.[10] It has been commonly thought that patients with chronic obstructive emphysema and with right ventricular hypertrophy have an impulse that is more easily palpable in the epigastric area. Although epigastric pulsations are often exaggerated, they are not so reliable as the parasternal lift in diagnosing right ventricular hypertrophy.

A few patients (about 8 per cent) with "pure" mitral stenosis have a maximum impulse at the K_{45} (V_4) position, which may be confused with left ventricular hypertrophy. However, on careful inspection and palpation it can be noted that the outward movement is part of the same movement as the parasternal lift and not an isolated thrust as occurs in left ventricular hypertrophy. This usually is sufficient to distinguish left from right ventricular hypertrophy in these few patients.

ISCHEMIC HEART DISEASE

Wiggers and Tennant demonstrated that after ligation of a coronary artery an area of the myocardium becomes ischemic, fails to contract, and balloons out during systole.[11] Since then Vakil has reported palpating these abnormal pulsations at the bedside.[12] Similarly, patients with myocardial infarctions and those with angina pectoris may have an outward paradoxic precordial movement which

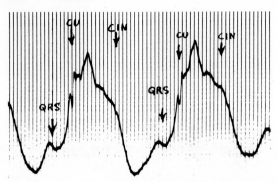

Fig. 5-48. Kinetocardiogram of a bulge taken from a patient with an old anterior myocardial infarction. The first arrow in each complex represents the onset of the QRS complex in the electrocardiogram; *CU*, the upstroke in the carotid pulse; *CIN*, the end of ejection systole, as determined by the carotid incisural notch. Note the early systolic outward movement which continues throughout most of ejection. These bulges are usually sustained and in many aspects resemble the apex impulses seen in patients with left ventricular hypertrophy. The clinical features and the clinical aspects of the patient's condition should be considered before the interpretation of these movements.

often can be palpated or seen at the bedside (Fig. 5-48), and these movements occur in approximately 68 per cent of the patients with myocardial infarctions when graphic methods are used.[5,13] Table 5-4 presents the incidence of bulges in patients with known myocardial infarctions. Not all these bulges are palpable, but in many instances they can be easily felt. Most "bulges" occur in the K_{24}, K_{34}, and K_{45} areas or in the midprecordial area; however, a few occur in the epigastric positions (primarily in those patients with posterior or diaphragmatic myocardial infarctions). The impulse is usually sustained throughout systole and by palpation alone; the impulse is difficult to distinguish from that of left ventricular hypertrophy. Consequently, some clinical information must be available for the proper interpretation of these paradoxic outward movements. For example, if the patient has never had any causes for left ventricular hypertrophy but has had a history of chest pain compatible with an infarction, and a paradoxic pulsation occurs in one of these areas, a presumptive diagnosis of a bulge due to an infarcted myocardium can be made. In addition to the use of the other clinical findings, in the interpretations of these impulses, the location is of some distinguishing value. A sizable number (35 per cent) of patients with myocardial infarction may have the maximum impulse or bulge at the K_{34} area, in contrast to only 13 per cent of patients with left ventricular hypertrophy. Thus, a sustained outward movement in this area is much more likely to be due to an infarct than to left ventricular hypertrophy. In addition, if one can exclude right ventricular hypertrophy by other clinical findings, a maximum outward movement in the K_{24} is usually a "bulge" as no patients with left ventricular hypertrophy so far have been noted to have a PMI at this area. Thus, the proper consideration of other clinical findings and location of the maximum impulse often makes it possible to diagnose an infarct or an ischemic area in the myocardium by palpation. However, a paradoxic outward movement, or "bulge," in the K_{45} and K_{55} areas cannot be distinguished at the bedside from left ventricular hypertrophy with any assurance. It should be noted that a "bulge" may be physiopathologic (functional) and may not be a true myocardial aneurysm. Autopsy correlation so far has shown that both infarctions with and without true anatomic aneurysms may be associated with bulges.

About one-third of the patients with angina pectoris will have a paradoxic outward movement ("bulge") present at rest and in the absence of pain. A considerably higher percentage of patients will have a bulge (about 75 per cent) during pain, either spontaneous or induced by exercise. Thus, the palpation of the precordium in patients with angina often offers some ancillary clinical evidence in confirming the diagnosis of angina pectoris.

Table 5-4. INCIDENCE OF BULGES THAT CAN BE RECORDED (KCG TECHNIC) ON PATIENTS WITH MYOCARDIAL INFARCTIONS

Infarction	No. of patients	No. with bulges by KCG	Percentage with bulges
Anterior myocardial infarctions (acute and old)	57	41	72
Diaphragmatic myocardial infarctions (acute and old)	45	28	62
All infarctions	102	69	68

Source: Davie et al.[5]

CONGENITAL HEART DISEASE

Inspection or palpation in patients with congenital heart disease primarily reflects the underlying ventricular abnormality; e.g., right or left ventricular hypertrophy. Occasionally the findings may be misleading, probably because the position and architecture of the heart in these patients may vary considerably from those in patients with acquired heart disease. For example, a patient with pulmonic stenosis may exhibit an apex impulse characteristic of left ventricular hypertrophy. The reasons for this are obscure. Often patients with large pulmonary arteries and/or increased pulmonary blood flow will have a palpable systolic pulsation in the pulmonic area (second and third intercostal spaces on the left). In patients with atrial septal defects and large pulmonary blood flows, it is possible actually to palpate the systolic impulse from pulmonary ejection.

MISCELLANEOUS FINDINGS

Patients with combined left and right ventricular hypertrophy often present findings of an isolated, exaggerated, thrusting left ventricular impulse as well as parasternal lift. However, marked dilatation of the heart and biventricular heart failure will produce the same findings. In fact, it is difficult to interpret any precordial pulsations in the presence of large dilated hearts and marked congestive heart failure (class IV cardiacs).

Only low frequency precordial movements have been discussed; however, there are many other significant phenomena that can be felt at times such as thrills, clicks, palpable sounds, and friction rubs. A discussion of the latter group is beyond the scope of this chapter.

REFERENCES

1. Harrison, T. R.: Palpation of the Precordial Impulses, *Stanford M. Bull.*, **13**:385, 1955.
2. Dressler, W.: Pulsations of the Chest Wall as Diagnostic Signs, *Mod. Concepts Cardiovas. Dis.*, **26**: 421, 1957.
3. Hurst, J. W., and Blackard, E.: Inspection and Palpation of Pulsations on the Front of the Chest, *Am. Heart J.*, **56**:159, 1958.
4. Eddleman, E. E., Jr., Hefner, L., Reeves, T. J., and Harrison, T. R.: Movements and Forces of the Human Heart, *A.M.A. Arch. Int. Med.*, **99**:401, 1957.
5. Davie, J. C., Langley, J. O., Dodson, W. H., and Eddleman E. E., Jr.: Clinical and Kinetocardiographic Studies of Paradoxical Precordial Motion, *Am. Heart J.*, **63**:775, 1962.
6. Beilin, and Mounsey, P.: The Left Ventricular Impulse in Hypertensive Heart Disease, *Brit. Heart J.*, **24**:409, 1962.
7. Eddleman, E. E., Jr.: Kinetocardiographic Findings in Aortic Insufficiency, *Am. Heart J.*, **53**:530, 1957.
8. Eddleman, E. E., Jr., Yoe, R. H., Tucker, W. T., Knowles, J. L., and Willis, K.: The Dynamics of Ventricular Contraction and Relaxation in Patients with Mitral Stenosis as Studied by the Kinetocardiogram and Ballistocardiogram, *Circulation*, **11**:774, 1955.
9. Dressler, W., Kleinfeld, M., and Ripstein, C. B.: Physical Sign of Tight Mitral Stenosis, *J.A.M.A.*, **154**:49, 1954.
10. Eddleman, E. E., Jr., and Thomas, H. D.: The Recognition and Differentiation of Right Ventricular Pressure and Flow Loads, *Am. J. Cardiol.*, **4**:652, 1959.
11. Tennant, R., and Wiggers, C. J.: The Effect of Coronary Occlusion on Myocardial Contraction, *Am. J. Physiol.*, **112**:351, 1935.
12. Vakil, R. J.: Ventricular Aneurysms of the Heart: Preliminary Report on Some New Clinical Signs, *Am. Heart J.*, **49**:934, 1955.
13. Eddleman, E. E., Jr., and Langley, J. O.: Paradoxical Pulsation of the Precordium in Myocardial Infarction and Angina Pectoris, *Am. Heart J.*, **63**: 579, 1962.

AUSCULTATION OF THE HEART

*J. Scott Butterworth, M.D., and
Edmund H. Reppert, M.D.*

HISTORICAL

Auscultation, which is the auditory perception of sounds made by the heart, and phonocardiography, which is the graphic recording of these sounds, have evolved through several eras. These eras have resulted from the development of new methods or instruments to improve the ability to hear or record the heart sounds.

The first era dates from early civilization and lasts to the time of Laennec in about 1816. During this period auscultation was practiced by placing the ear directly on the precordium and was called *immediate or direct auscultation*. Hippocrates is believed to have used this method, and Harvey is reported to have recognized the first heart sound in 1628.

Modern auscultation, however, began with the development of the stethoscope when Laennec[1] rolled a sheaf of paper into a tight, hollow tube and found that by placing one end on the chest and the other to his ear he could hear heart sounds more distinctly than by immediate auscultation. He subsequently developed the wooden monaural stethoscope, varieties of which are still used today in certain parts of the world. The binaural stethoscope, now commonly used, has been the outgrowth of designs by Leared[2] in 1851 and Camman[3] in 1885.

It is remarkable that with simple instruments such as the monaural and early binaural stethoscopes fundamental clinical observations were made in the nineteenth century. For example, respiratory splitting of the second heart sound was described by Potain[4] in 1866; yet little significance was attached to this description, even with the development of better recording instruments, until it was reemphasized by Leatham.[5] It would appear that clinical recognition and application have not kept pace with instrumentation.

The next era was introduced at the turn of the century with the introduction of the capillary electrometer and string galvanometer by Einthoven,[6] and the segment capsule by Frank[7] for the graphic recording of the sounds produced by the heart. With the discovery of the vacuum tube it became possible to design amplifiers for both amplifying and selectively filtering the heart sounds. A very good amplifier of this type was developed by the engineers of the Western Electric Company in 1924.[8] The recording of these amplified sounds was further improved by the construction of high-frequency optical galvanometers and subsequently by the development of the cathode-ray oscilloscope.

The perfection of long-lasting coatings for oscilloscopes during World War II enabled easy visualization of the sounds, and the discovery of magnetic tape recording during this same period also contributed to present-day instrumentation in this field. Finally, the application of the transister has enabled engineers to reduce the size and increase the portability of instruments, and thereby making it possible to monitor the physiologic phenomena of individuals anywhere in space.

Today's methods of auscultation and phonocardiography[9] permit the physician to hear the heart sounds and simultaneously to view them on an oscilloscope. At the same time tape recordings can easily be made for future reference.

THE USE OF THE STETHOSCOPE

The stethoscope has become the trademark of the physician; yet it is probably the least well-used or understood instrument in the hands of physicians today.

There are many reasons for this, one of which is that physicians have the impression that all necessary information can be obtained by ordering a phonocardiogram. Let us emphasize that though the phonocardiogram is a useful instrument, its primary purpose is to teach the physician how to recognize the sounds heard through his stethoscope (as evidenced by the phonocardiograms used to illustrate this chapter). Auscultation is taught far better by actual listening at the bedside, or even better by listening and looking at the sounds simultaneously. However, the latter method has not been generally utilized.[10]

One must learn to develop a routine or technique

for performing auscultation and to follow it rigidly until it becomes a habit. The actual routine is perhaps not so important as the discipline.

Our own practice is to listen first at the base of the heart over the aortic and pulmonic areas for the purpose of recognizing the first and second heart sounds and more particularly to listen carefully for either physiologic or pathologic splitting of the second heart sound.

One can usually recognize the second sounds easily because of their shorter duration and higher pitch as compared with the first sounds. However, a finger on the carotid artery will sense the systolic thrust which is coincident with the first heart sound.

Once one has identified the second sounds, one concentrates on this period and, watching respiration (or listening to the inspiratory sounds in the background), notes any splitting or changes in the character of the second sound with inspiration and expiration. The area in which splitting is best heard is variable, but it encompasses the pulmonic area to the lower-left sternal border.

If there is difficulty in identifying the two components of the second sound, one should remember that normally (except in infants and children) the aortic component is louder than the pulmonic. Also, the second sound heard at the apex is the aortic component, so that by starting at the apex and "inching" [11] toward the base one can usually identify the two components.

From the base of the heart one proceeds to listen to the apex and over the tricuspid area to the right of the lower sternum. The open bell of the stethoscope, being better for low frequencies, is used to advantage here where low-frequency gallop sounds and rumbling murmurs are heard.

The first sound is of longer duration and lower pitch than the components of the second sound. This probably stems from the larger area of the mitral and tricuspid valves and the lower closing velocity. These valves close at a pressure of 0 to 5 mm Hg; the aortic and pulmonic valves close at much higher pressures.

The first sound is a fusion of the mitral and tricuspid components and is loudest at the apex or inside the apex. One listens carefully for variations from the normal which may be difficult to quantitate. These variations include various degrees of splitting of the two components and an increased or decreased intensity of the sound. Although these changes may be most useful in certain states, variations in the second sound are usually a more useful diagnostic aid.

Changing the position of a patient from sitting to supine to left lateral, and occasionally to the prone position, may accentuate sounds and murmurs either by bringing the heart closer to the chest wall or, more probably, by acceleration of blood flow due to the exertion.

And finally, let us not forget that the stethoscope can be most useful over other areas of the body such as the skull, the eyes, the carotids, the lumbar areas, the abdomen, and over scars. The purpose of these examinations, of course, is to identify noise produced by abnormal arteriovenous communications or by stenosis or kinking of arterial segments.

HEART SOUNDS

Importance and Significance

Too frequently, the major objective of cardiac auscultation is the recognition and identification of murmurs, little or no attention being given the heart sounds. There is no question that murmurs are important in cardiac diagnosis; however, the heart sounds are also of diagnostic value, and effort spent in their recognition and interpretation will frequently be more rewarding than the identification of murmurs. Furthermore, unless one can certainly identify the first and second heart sounds (and this can almost always be done by paying attention to their pitch and duration), one cannot always be certain whether a murmur is systolic or diastolic in time by auscultation alone.

Terminology

It is common to refer to heart sounds as "normal" (the first, second, third, and fourth sounds) or "abnormal" (all other heart sounds), e.g., the opening snap of the mitral valve, gallops, etc. This is confusing, in that not all "normal" sounds, e.g., the fourth, are always heard in normal persons, and certain "abnormal" sounds, e.g., the systolic click, are not necessarily related to an abnormal cardiac condition. Furthermore, some of the "abnormal" sounds, e.g., gallops, are simply alterations of the "normal." This problem in terminology may be resolved if it is accepted that the first through fourth sounds are those produced by normal hemodynamic events, although the third and fourth sounds may be inaudible. Any of these sounds may be altered by abnormal hemodynamic situations, and additional sounds may occur in pathologic as well as in nonpathologic states (e.g., the opening snap of the mitral valve and the systolic click, respectively).

An additional problem is the terminology of the individual sounds. It has long been customary, for example, to refer to the second sound in the aortic area as A_2 and to the second sound in the pulmonary area as P_2. Since the second sound consists of

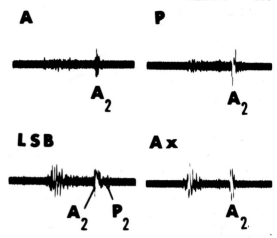

Fig. 5-49. Stethogram from a patient with systemic hypertension showing that the aortic component (A_2) of the second sound is louder in the pulmonic than in the aortic area. To state here that P_2 is greater than A_2 would be misleading. (All recordings made at exactly the same frequency and intensity settings.)

two components, each produced by a distinct hemodynamic event (see below), it is important to identify each component properly. It is cumbersome to say "aortic valve closure sound" or "pulmonary valve closure sound," and it is our feeling that the terms A_2 and P_2 should be retained but should be used to refer to the specific component of the second heart sound, regardless of the anatomic area in which the sound is heard (Fig. 5-49). The same line of reasoning applies to the components of the first heart sound, T_1 referring to the tricuspid valve closure sound and M_1 to the mitral valve closure sound.

Hemodynamic Events Responsible for Heart Sounds

The timing and relation to hemodynamic events of the various heart sounds are depicted schematically in Fig. 5-50.

First Sound

It is generally accepted that the audible portions of the first heart sound [5,12-16] are related to closure of the mitral and tricuspid valves (Fig. 5-51). Since under usual conditions, left and right ventricular contraction, and hence mitral and tricuspid valve closure, are asynchronous, the first heart sound is often split. It is probable that mitral valve closure (M_1) precedes tricuspid valve closure (T_1). Both components are of lower frequency and longer duration than are the components of the second sound and hence usually are easily differentiated from the latter. Because of the lower frequencies and longer duration of M_1 and T_1 as com-

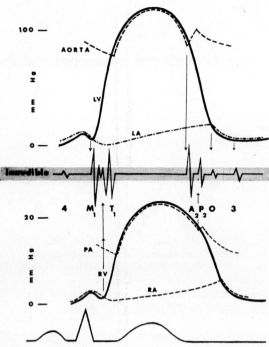

Fig. 5-50. The upper portion of the diagram shows the pressure curves of the aorta, left ventricle, and left atrium; the lower portion represents those of the pulmonary artery, right ventricle, and right atrium on an expanded pressure scale. The pressure changes which result in the production of heart sounds are indicated. Thus, the mitral component (M_1) of the first heart sound occurs at the point when left ventricular pressure exceeds left atrial pressure, resulting in closure of the mitral valve. The tricuspid component (T_1) of the first sound is the result of closure of the tricuspid valve when the pressure in the right ventricle exceeds that in the right atrium. Similarly the aortic (A_2) and pulmonic (P_2) components of the second sound result from sudden closure of the aortic and pulmonic valves, respectively, when the ventricular pressures fall below the pressures in the aorta and pulmonary artery. The third heart sound (3) occurs at the end of rapid diastolic filling of the ventricles and is usually below the limits of audibility in adults. The fourth sound (4), also usually inaudible, follows shortly after atrial contraction. 0 represents the point at which the left ventricular pressure falls below the left atrial pressure and the mitral valve opens. This is inaudible, but when mitral stenosis is present it frequently becomes audible and is called an opening snap of the mitral valve. (*From J. S. Butterworth, M. R. Chassin, R. McGrath, and E. H. Reppert.*[10])

pared to A_2 and P_2, splitting of the first sound is less easily recognized than that of the second sound; however the mechanism of the splitting is probably similar (see below). Wider degrees of splitting may occur in right bundle branch block, while pre-

sumably left bundle branch block and situations causing delay in mitral valve closure should result in reversed splitting. The degree of splitting is of little clinical significance, however, except that a widely split sound may be confused with a presystolic murmur or an ejection sound. The intensity of the components of the first heart sound may be of clinical significance, being louder in mitral stenosis or in conditions which produce an increased cardiac output, and decreased in conditions with diminished cardiac output.

Ejection Sounds

Ejection sounds (Fig. 5-52) have a sharp clicking quality and occur in early systole, approximately 0.08 to 0.12 sec after the onset of electrical ventricular activity. These sounds may be either aortic or pulmonic in origin; whether they actually result from distension of the great vessels or from abnormalities of the semilunar valves is not clear. Although frequently considered to represent hypertension of either circuit, in our experience they occur whenever either great vessel is significantly dilated, irrespective of the presence of hypertension. The pulmonic ejection sound is best heard at the pulmonic area and is common in mild valvular pulmonic stenosis, idiopathic dilatation of the pulmonary artery, and pulmonary hypertension when the latter is accompanied by a dilated pulmonary artery. The aortic ejection sound is often best heard at the apex and may be present in any condition

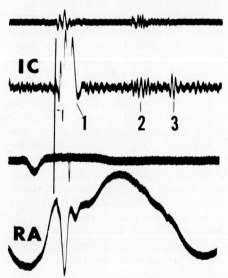

Fig. 5-51. Amplified right atrial pressure curve (*RA*) showing the deflection on the pressure curve coincident with tricuspid valve closure and the first heart sound, recorded with the Telco intracardiac manometer. *IC*, sound from the right atrium.

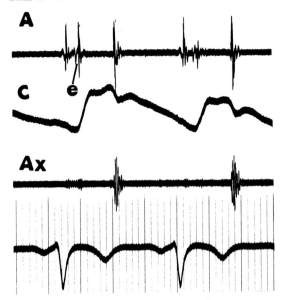

Fig. 5-52. Ejection sound (*e*) recorded from the aortic area (*A*) of a patient with dilatation of the aorta. Note the relation of the ejection sound to the upstroke of the carotid pulse wave (*C*), indicating that it occurs with opening of the aortic valve, or soon after. (Time lines, 0.04 sec.)

associated with a dilated aorta, e.g., aortic stenosis, tetralogy of Fallot, coarctation of the aorta, and systemic hypertension. When hypertension is present in either circuit, the ejection sound tends to be later than in normotensive conditions.[17]

By auscultation alone it is difficult to differentiate an ejection sound from a split first sound. Whenever distinct splitting of the first sound is present one should consider conditions producing ejection sounds as the cause.

Systolic Clicks

These are systolic sounds having a character similar to ejection sounds, and are often confused with them. Indeed the latter sounds are sometimes referred to as "ejection clicks," which compounds the confusion. However, the true clicks tend to occur in mid- or late systole and frequently move appreciably with respiration, being closer to the first sound in inspiration and approaching the second sound in expiration (Fig. 5-53). They may be multiple. These sounds have no known clinical significance, although some investigators[14,18] relate their occurrence to a previous pericarditis; our experience has not borne this out.

Second Heart Sound

Probably no single factor is more rewarding in clinical auscultation than proper analysis of the sec-

ond heart sound. This sound consists normally of two components having their origins in vibrations set up by abrupt closure of the aortic and pulmonary valves. Normally, aortic valve closure (A_2) precedes pulmonary valve closure (P_2) by 0.02 to 0.04 sec during expiration, while with inspiration the two components may be split 0.04 to 0.06 sec, rarely 0.10 sec (Fig. 5-54). The variation of the degree of splitting with respiration was described in 1866 by Potain,[4] but was neglected until reemphasized by Leatham.[5] *The respiratory or physiologic variation of the split is felt to be due largely to delayed pulmonary valve closure secondary to increased flow into the right side of the heart occurring with inspiration.* The contribution of the drop in pulmonary artery pressure with inspiration should not be neglected. Some movement of the aortic valve closure sound also occurs with respiration, but this contribution to the degree of splitting is relatively insignificant.[19,20]

The splitting of the second sound is best appreciated at the pulmonary area or left sternal border, since the pulmonary component is normally louder in this area. The degree of splitting may be greater in those conditions resulting in increased pulmonary flow, e.g., atrial septal defects, or decreased pulmonary pressure, e.g., pulmonary stenosis. Splitting may also be wide in situations resulting in early aortic valve closure, e.g., mitral insufficiency

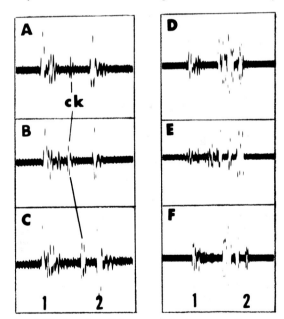

Fig. 5-53. Systolic clicks recorded at or near the apex. *A*, *B*, and *C*, normal respiration, inspiration, and expiration in the same person, showing movement of the click with the respiratory phase. *D*, *E*, and *F*, from different individuals, are examples of multiple clicks which may frequently be mistaken for murmurs.

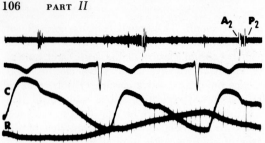

Fig. 5-54. Physiologic splitting of the second heart sound recorded from the pulmonic area. Note the separation of A₂ and P₂ by approximately 0.06 sec at the end of inspiration, indicated by the high peak of the respiratory curve (R). (Time lines, 0.04 sec.) (*From J. S. Butterworth, M. R. Chassin, R. McGrath, and E. H. Reppert.*[10])

or ventricular septal defect (Fig. 5-55). Reversal of the time of occurrence of the two components (paradoxic splitting) may occur in conditions causing delay in aortic valve closure, e.g., aortic stenosis or systemic hypertension. Delay in ventricular conduction of the complete bundle branch block type will also alter the split, right block (Fig. 5-56)

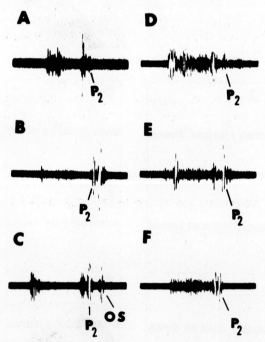

Fig. 5-55. Splitting of the second heart sound as recorded from the pulmonary area in a patient with A, complete right bundle branch block; B, complete left bundle branch block, showing paradoxic splitting; C, mitral stenosis, showing narrow splitting as well as the opening snap of the mitral valve (OS); D, mitral insufficiency; E, atrial septal defect; and F, ventricular septal defect. A₂ is not labeled but immediately preceded P₂ except in B.

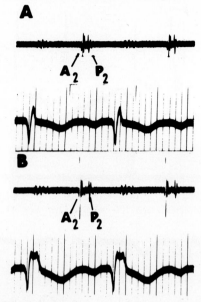

Fig. 5-56. Splitting of the second heart sound in complete right bundle branch block B which developed during cardiac catheterization. The split is slightly wider than during the immediately preceding normal conduction A. (Time lines, 0.04 sec.) (*From J. S. Butterworth, M. R. Chassin, R. McGrath, and E. H. Reppert.*[10])

causing wider splitting and left block (Fig. 5-57) causing paradoxic splitting.

The intensity of either component also has diagnostic importance, a loud component suggesting hypertension or increased flow, and a soft component suggesting hypotension in the respective circuit. However, it is extremely important to remember that the pulmonary component is normally loud in children and in persons with thin chest walls.

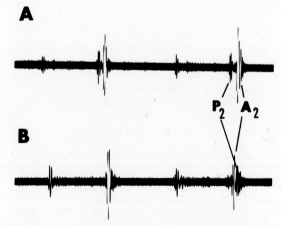

Fig.. 5-57. Paradoxic splitting of the second heart sound in a patient with intermittent left bundle branch block A and in normal conduction B. (Time lines, 0.04 sec.)

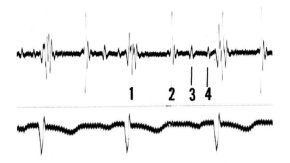

Fig. 5-58. Stethogram recorded just inside the cardiac apex, showing the third and fourth heart sounds. (Time lines, 0.04 sec.)

Third and Fourth Heart Sounds

The third and fourth heart sounds are diastolic sounds of low frequency and low intensity and are generally felt to be due to vibrations initiated by abrupt limitation of ventricular distensibility which may produce tensing of the valve or its chordae.[21,22] The third sound occurs during early ventricular filling, approximately 0.12 to 0.16 sec after the second sound; the fourth or atrial sound occurs prior to the first sound and is related to atrial contraction (Fig. 5-58). Both sounds are best heard at the apex with the patient supine. The third is present in most children and occasionally in adults; the fourth is rarely heard normally. The initial appearance of a third heart sound in the adult with heart disease is abnormal. The third sound may be augmented in conditions which alter the distensibility of the ventricle, e.g., dilated left ventricle in mitral insufficiency. The fourth sound may be augmented in situations of increased atrial pressure along with altered distensibility of the ventricle, e.g., systemic hypertension or pulmonary stenosis. There is also some evidence to suggest that the diastolic sound of constrictive pericarditis is an augmented third heart sound.[23] It is presumed that the third or fourth sound may originate from either ventricle or both ventricles, depending on the hemodynamic situation.

Gallop Sounds

It seems best to restrict the term *gallop rhythm* to a three-sound sequence resulting from the intensification of the normal third (Fig. 5-59) or fourth heart sounds occurring usually, but not invariably, with a rapid ventricular rate. Hence, one may have a protodiastolic gallop (third sound) (Fig. 5-60), a presystolic gallop (fourth sound), or a summation gallop (both third and fourth sounds). They may arise from the left ventricle and be heard best at the apex. Gallops of right ven-

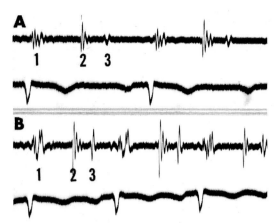

Fig. 5-59. Normal third heart sound in a young healthy nurse A. Following exercise B there is an increase in rate, and the third sound becomes intensified and could be called a gallop. (Time lines, 0.04 sec.) (*From J. S. Butterworth, M. R. Chassin, R. McGrath, and E. H. Reppert.*[10])

tricular origin are maximal near the sternal border. Gallops generally occur in patients with an inefficient myocardium, but with present-day therapy they do not necessarily have the grave prognosis formerly attributed them.

Sounds Due to Opening of the AV Valves

These sounds are normally inaudible (Fig. 5-50), but under pathologic conditions they may become

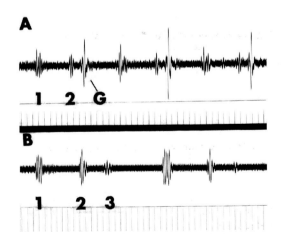

Fig. 5-60. A. Protodiastolic gallop sound G recorded at the apex in an adult male with congestive heart failure. In B, after treatment of the patient with diuretics, the heart rate is slower, and the sound now has the characteristics of a normal third heart sound. (*Time lines,* 0.04 sec.) (*From J. S. Butterworth, M. R. Chassin, R. McGrath, and E. H. Reppert.*[10])

accentuated and are then referred to as the opening snap of the mitral or tricuspid valve (see Chap. 25).

Alteration of Sounds in Arrhythmias and Conduction Disturbances

It is obvious that accuracy of diagnosis of arrhythmias and conduction disturbances is best accomplished with the electrocardiogram, but information may also be gained by auscultation. Reference has already been made to the splitting of the second sound in bundle branch block. Premature ventricular contractions tend to have widely split first and second heart sounds; premature atrial contractions do not. Indeed the ventricular site of a premature contraction may be identified by noting the relationship of the two components of the second heart sound (Fig. 5-61). In arrhythmias characterized by an inconstant relationship between atrial and ventricular contraction, variation in intensity of the first sound may result. In some instances, e.g., atrial fibrillation, the variable first sound is largely related to previous diastolic filling, whereas in ventricular tachycardia and complete heart block (Fig. 5-62) the first sound is more intense when atrial and ventricular contraction occur in close approximation. For example, when the P-R interval is less than 0.16 sec, the first sound is usually loud; when it is 0.20 to 0.26 sec, the first heart sound is usually faint. In any degree of atrioventricular block, and in some cases of atrial flutter, audible atrial sounds may occur.

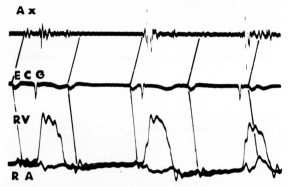

Fig. 5-62. Recording from the cardiac apex of a patient with complete heart block. Straight lines are drawn to show the interrelationship of P waves on the electrocardiogram (*ECG*), atrial sounds on the stethogram (*Ax*), and pressure deflections on the right atrial pressure curve (*RA*). The latter curve was recorded simultaneously with the right ventricular pressure curve (*RV*). Note that the first sound is louder whenever atrial and ventricular contraction occur in close approximation even though atrial contraction occurs after atrioventricular valve closure (last complex).

MURMURS

The term *murmur* comes from the Latin *murmur*, meaning "whispering." The heart sounds which have been discussed in a previous section are more accurately described as "heart noises," since they are often a combination of sounds of unrelated frequencies; the same is true of murmurs. A murmur is difficult to define, but it is a noise which is of longer duration than the heart sounds. (If one takes tape recordings of heart sounds and, by splicing the tape properly, puts two or three first sounds together, this combination has all the characteristics of a murmur.)

As blood flows through the chambers of the heart and great vessels it normally does not produce sufficient sound to be heard on the surface of the body; this type of flow is referred to as laminar or silent.

If, however, flow through the vessel exceeds a certain critical value, or if the walls of the vessel are uneven, or if there is a change in the diameter of the vessel, the flow pattern is suddenly deranged and a chaotic type of flow results (Fig. 5-63). This type of flow produces a noise or murmur. The exact way in which noise is produced is not known, although the mechanism of sound generation within a fluid may involve (1) turbulence, (2) eddy formation or vortex shedding, and possibly (3) cavitation.[24-26] If the sound generated is sufficiently loud it is transmitted through the tissues to the body surface, where it is appreciated as a murmur.

Although the exact mechanism of noise forma-

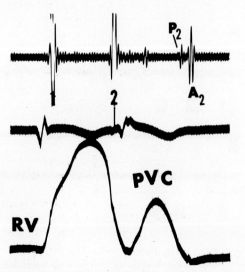

Fig. 5-61. Paradoxic splitting of the second heart sound with a premature ventricular contraction (*PVC*), produced with a cardiac catheter in the right ventricle. *RV*, right ventricular pressure curve. P_2 and A_2 are evidently fused in the first beat. (Time lines, 0.04 sec.)

tion may not be clearly understood, present empirical knowledge and the correlation of the noises (murmurs) with hemodynamic data give murmurs considerable clinical value. Actually it is probable that noise is normally produced at certain portions of the cardiovascular system where velocity of flow is high. Examples of this may be the aorta and the pulmonary artery just beyond the valves. Even though the noise produced normally in these areas may be minimal, increased velocity of flow produced by exercise, hyperthyroidism, pregnancy, and the like may make the noise (murmur) audible on the surface of the body.

From the clinical standpoint, whenever there is an increase in the diameter of the structure into which blood flows and if a sufficient pressure gradient exists along the course of blood flow, a murmur is likely to result. In the presence of a change in diameter or a pressure gradient, an increase in velocity of blood flow increases the probability of noisy flow. The intensity (loudness) and character of a murmur are dependent on many factors but are most intimately related to the prevailing hemodynamics (velocity of blood flow and pressure gradient), the time of occurrence of the murmur in the cardiac cycle, and the adjacent anatomic structures. For example, the murmur of mitral stenosis would be similar in configuration to that of aortic stenosis if it were not interrupted by the first heart sound; furthermore, its intensity and character would probably resemble that of the murmur of aortic stenosis if the pressure gradient and flow across the valves were similar.

Classification of Murmurs

No general system of classification of murmurs has been entirely satisfactory although various descriptive terms have been applied. The important features in the analysis and classification of any murmur are (1) the timing and duration in relation to hemodynamic events, and (2) the intensity and changes in intensity in various phases of the cardiac cycle. Other factors, probably of less importance, are the pitch and quality of the murmur and the area of maximal intensity.

Murmurs are usually either systolic or diastolic in time, although occasionally they may be both. The beginning of systole may be defined in several ways, but for clinical purposes it begins when the pressure in the ventricles exceeds that in the atria, causing sudden closure of the mitral and tricuspid valves, producing the first heart sound (Fig. 5-50). The end of systole is indicated by aortic and pulmonic valve closure, resulting in the components of the second sound. Diastole is, therefore, the interval from the second sound to the next first sound. Systole and diastole may be divided into

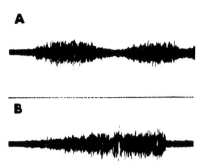

Fig. 5-63. This figure shows noise generated in a plastic tube attached to a water faucet. The sound was picked up by a microphone on a catheter introduced downstream to the obstruction and placed 1 to 2 cm distal from the constriction of the tube. In A the tube was partially constricted and the flow was varied by the valve on the water faucet. The greater the flow the more noise generated beyond the constriction. In B the flow was kept constant and the constriction was gradually increased and then suddenly released, causing the abrupt end to the noise.

three parts: early, mid-, and late. A systolic murmur may begin with or after the first sound, it may be limited to early, mid- or late systole or may persist throughout systole (holosystolic), and it may reach maximum intensity in any of these periods. The same is true of diastolic murmurs, although early diastole is frequently called *protodiastole* and late diastole is called *presystole*.

The intensity of a murmur is difficult to define in precise units and indeed is dependent on many factors which vary from person to person. If one is to use a classification other than faint, moderate, and loud, that of Levine and Harvey[11] is probably the most satisfactory. In this system there are six levels of intensity. Grade I is the faintest audible murmur; a grade VI murmur can be heard with the stethoscope just removed from contact with the chest wall. The intensity of a murmur also determines whether or not the palpable manifestation (thrill) will be present.

When a murmur increases in intensity after its onset, it is termed a "crescendo murmur"; if it decreases in intensity after its onset it is a decrescendo murmur. If a crescendo murmur decreases in intensity the complex is termed a crescendo-decrescendo murmur,[27] and this form is frequently referred to as a "diamond-shaped" murmur.[11]

The quality of a murmur is difficult to define but seems to depend on an interrelation of intensity and pitch. With increasing experience one learns the meaning of such terms as blowing, harsh, musical, rumbling, and the like. Most murmurs are a combination of unrelated frequencies and thus are

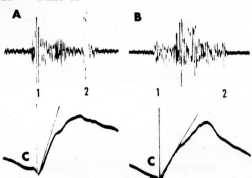

Fig. 5-64. Stethograms from the aortic area in two cases: *A*, mild aortic stenosis (aortic systolic gradient, 30 mm Hg); *B*, severe aortic stenosis (pressure gradient, 90 mm Hg). Note the late onset and the late peak of intensity of the murmur in the more severe case. Note also the greater distortion of the carotid pulse *C* in *B*.

noises, but at times in the production of a murmur some structure is set into rapid vibration and this produces a loud fundamental frequency and various harmonics. Murmurs of this type sound more like musical instruments and hence are termed "musical murmurs." Examples of this type of murmur result when a valve cusp or chordae tendinae are set into vibration in some manner (Fig. 5-69).

In general most pathologic murmurs are constant, although they may become louder with increased blood flow such as occurs after exercise or when the body is in certain positions.

The point of maximal intensity of a murmur is also useful, and murmurs arising from specific areas in the heart are usually heard best in specified areas on the surface of the body. Thus the murmur of mitral stenosis is generally heard best at the apex, and the murmur of aortic stenosis is loudest over the upper sternum, but exceptions are not uncommon, and in general the experienced physician recognizes specific valvular lesions by their character and position in the cardiac cycle.

Murmurs Originating at the Semilunar Valves

Aortic Stenosis. In this abnormality blood is forced, under increased pressure, through a narrow valve orifice into the aorta, whose diameter greatly exceeds that of the valve opening. Hence two factors, viz., high velocity of flow and flow through a narrow orifice into a dilated structure, combine to produce disturbances in flow, giving the clinically appreciated murmur. In addition, because of the anatomic distortion and calcification of the valve and the lengthening of systole due to the stenosis, the aortic component of the second sound tends to be diminished in intensity and delayed in time.

The murmur is systolic in time, beginning shortly after the first heart sound and ending just before the aortic component of the second sound. It is usually maximal in the aortic area but radiates widely to the neck, back, and apex. It usually has a characteristic crescendo-decrescendo character first described by Leatham[27] and later given the term "diamond-shaped" by Levine and Harvey.[11] In severe stenosis, with systolic pressure gradients in excess of 50 mm Hg, the point of maximal intensity of the murmur tends to occur at mid-systole or later, whereas in mild stenosis the peak intensity occurs in early systole.[27] However, more important in judging the severity of the stenosis is the late onset of the murmur in the more severe cases (Fig. 5-64).

Alterations of heart sounds, as well as additional sounds, are common in aortic stenosis. In mild cases, an aortic ejection sound is commonly heard. Absence of appreciable physiologic splitting or inspiration or actual paradoxic splitting of the second sound is common, the latter occurring in the more severe cases (Fig. 5-65). The presence of third and/or fourth heart sounds is fairly common in the more severe cases; however, this finding is of value only in adults, since children may have such sounds normally.

The murmur is loud and harsh and, therefore, is not only accompanied by a thrill but tends to radiate widely, especially to the apex. However, it retains its crescendo-decrescendo character

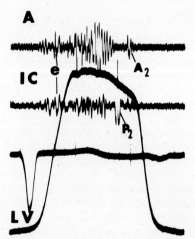

Fig. 5-65. Severe aortic stenosis. Left ventricular pressure (*LV*), 210 mm Hg. Note the late onset and late peak of intensity of the murmur recorded from the aortic area (*A*). An ejection sound (*e*) is also present. An intracardiac sound recording (*IC*) from the pulmonary artery shows that P_2 precedes A_2 (paradoxic splitting). (Time lines, 0.04 sec.) (*From J. S. Butterworth, M. R. Chassin, R. McGrath, and E. H. Reppert.*[10])

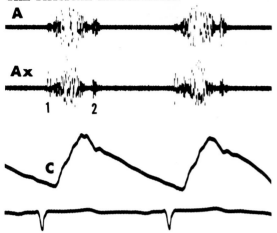

Fig. 5-66. Aortic stenosis. Note that the murmur is nearly as loud at the apex (*Ax*) as at the aortic area (*A*) but that it retains its characteristic crescendo-decrescendo configuration, which differentiates it from the murmur of mitral insufficiency.

wherever heard (Fig. 5-66). In general, the auscultatory findings are similar whether the stenosis is congenital or acquired.[28]

Muscular Subvalvular Aortic Stenosis. This less common form of aortic stenosis results in a murmur similar in configuration and character to the murmur of valvular aortic stenosis;[29] however, in these instances the murmur tends to start later in systole, perhaps because of the late contraction of the hypertrophied outflow tract.[30] In addition, it is usually maximal at the lower left sternal border and does not radiate well to the neck. There is often a prominent atrial gallop sound which may be palpable as well as audible.

Aortic Insufficiency. When the aortic valve cusps do not close completely the pressure gradient across the valve causes regurgitaton of blood from the aorta back into the left ventricle, producing a murmur. The latter is diastolic in time, of relatively high frequency, begins abruptly after the second sound, and, because of the gradually decreasing pressure gradient across the valve during diastole, has a descrescendo character (Fig. 5-67). It is usually maximal at the second to fourth left intercostal spaces. The second heart sound is usually intensified, for reasons not well understood.

Aortic insufficiency is usually an acquired valvular deformity secondary to rheumatic fever, syphilis, endocarditis, aortic dissection, or trauma. A similar murmur can be heard in the absence of valvular deformity because of a dilated valve ring in systemic hypertension or dilatation of the ascending aorta due to any cause.

Occasionally a rumbling late diastolic or presystolic murmur[31] may be heard at the apex in

patients with marked aortic insufficiency. This simulates the murmur of mitral stenosis (Fig. 5-68) but occurs in the absence of a pressure gradient across the mitral valve (Austin Flint murmur). It probably results from the expulsion of blood from the left atrium into the ventricle dilated by regurgitant flow through the aortic valve.

Quite frequently the murmurs of aortic stenosis and insufficiency are combined, and in such cases the predominance of either lesion may be appreciated by timing the onset as well as the peak intensity of the systolic murmur, recording the carotid pulse wave,[32] or palpating the carotid pulsations.

Ruptured Aortic Cusp. Rupture, retroversion, or fenestration of one or more of the aortic valve cusps results in aortic insufficiency of variable degree. The resultant murmur is similar in timing and location to the usual murmur of aortic insufficiency, but in these cases the murmur frequently has a musical quality that is due to its pure frequency (Fig. 5-69).

Pulmonary Stenosis. The hemodynamics resulting in the auscultatory findings of pulmonary stenosis are similar to those described above in aortic stenosis and result in a crescendo-decrescendo systolic murmur[33] maximal at the pulmonary area. It should be recognized, however, that the right ventricle is normally a low-pressure chamber (relative to the left ventricle) and, consequently, until the pulmonary stenosis is sufficiently severe to result in significant elevation of right ventricular pressure, the murmur may lack the crescendo-decrescendo character and have a rather nondescript form. Furthermore the time of peak intensity of the murmur is a more accurate indication

LSB

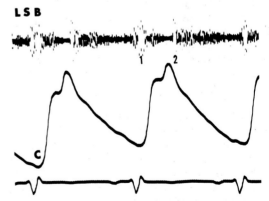

Fig. 5-67. Aortic insufficiency. Recorded from the left sternal border (*LSB*) of a 38-year-old male. The diastolic murmur begins immediately after the aortic component of the second sound and continues in descrescendo fashion throughout most of diastole. The carotid pulse contour (*C*) is typical of aortic insufficiency.

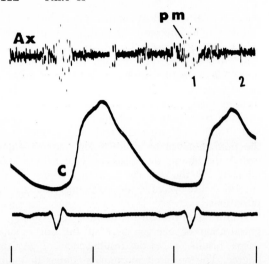

Fig. 5-68. Austin Flint murmur. Recording from the apex (*Ax*) of the same patient as in Fig. 5-67. Note the presystolic vibrations (*pm*) of rather low frequency. Although this murmur suggests mitral stenosis, no opening snap of the mitral valve is present. At cardiac catheterization, no pressure gradient across the mitral valve was present and the valve was normal at the time of surgery. (Time lines, 0.1 sec.)

of the severity of the stenosis than it is in aortic stenosis. Indeed one can usually quite accurately estimate right ventricular pressure from the contour of the murmur and the appearance of the pulmonic component of the second sound[33] (Fig. 5-70). The prolonged right ventricular systole is directly proportional to the severity of the stenosis, and hence the peak intensity of the murmur occurs later in

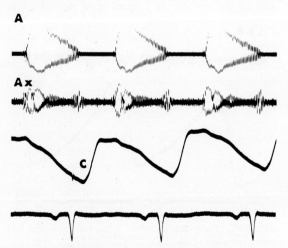

Fig. 5-69. Recording from the aortic area (*A*) of a 13-year-old male showing a relatively pure-frequency, musical, diastolic murmur. This appeared abruptly, and aortic insufficiency was demonstrated by cineangiography. (Time lines, 0.04 sec.)

systole and the pulmonary component is more delayed in the more severe cases. In addition the intensity of the pulmonary component is indirectly proportional to the severity of the stenosis. (This concept applies only to pulmonary stenosis with intact ventricular system.) Additional sounds are frequently present in pulmonary stenosis, a pulmonary ejection sound being common in mild cases while a fourth heart sound may be heard in quite severe stenosis.

Pulmonary stenosis of the infundibular variety, when associated with an intact ventricular septum, results in similar auscultatory findings to those noted above, although the murmur may be maximal lower down the left sternal border,[34] and an ejection sound is rarely present. However, when pulmonary stenosis, either valvular or infundibular, is associated with a ventricular septal defect (Fallot's tetralogy), the auscultatory findings are quite different.[35] Because of the presence of the ventricular septal defect, the right ventricular pressure rarely exceeds that of the left ventricle, and consequently right ventricular contraction is not markedly delayed. Hence the murmur tends to

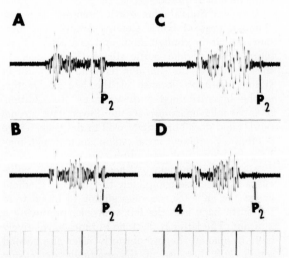

Fig. 5-70. Recordings from the pulmonary area of four patients with variable degrees of pulmonary stenosis. In *A*, with mild pulmonary stenosis (right ventricular systolic pressure 40 mm Hg), the systolic murmur does not have the typical crescendo-decrescendo configuration, and the pulmonary component of the second sound, although widely split, has normal intensity. *B*, from a patient with right ventricular pressure of 60 mm Hg, shows a more typical configuration of the murmur. With more severe stenosis (*C*, right ventricular pressure of 150 mm Hg, and *D*, right ventricular pressure of 200 mm Hg), the murmur is displaced to late systole and P_2 is markedly delayed in time and diminished in intensity. *D* also shows a fourth heart sound, which is heard in the more severe cases. (Time lines, 0.1 sec.)

begin earlier and reaches its peak intensity before mid-systole. The second heart sound in these cases is single and represents the aortic component; the pulmonary component is rarely heard but may be recorded with intracardiac sound technique (Fig. 5-71).

Pulmonary Insufficiency. This is a relatively uncommon valvular abnormality, usually due to bacterial endocarditis, occasionally of congenital origin. If pulmonary hypertension is absent, the regurgitant flow is of low velocity because of a relatively low pressure gradient, and consequently the murmur has a lower frequency than its counterpart in aortic insufficiency.[36,37] Furthermore, since it begins with the pulmonic component of the second sound, which may be of low intensity and difficult to hear, it gives the impression of starting late after the second sound (aortic component).

A more common form of pulmonary insufficiency is the relative pulmonary incompetence (Graham Steell murmur[38]) associated with pulmonary hypertension of any cause. In these instances the auscultatory findings are usually similar to those in aortic insufficiency, since the pulmonary hypertension causes a high-velocity regurgitant flow and at the same time causes early appearance of the pulmonary component of the second sound, often merging it with the aortic component. Even this form of pulmonary insufficiency is relatively uncommon as compared to aortic insufficiency.

Postoperative Findings. Repair of aortic valve disease at present is usually accomplished by valve replacement, most frequently with a type of ball-valve prosthesis, and the auscultatory findings are dominated by the artificial valve sounds. Following repair of pulmonary stenosis, either by closed or open technique, the change in auscultatory findings depends on the degree of relief of the pressure gradient. A good result is indicated by the appearance of the peak intensity of the murmur earlier in systole and movement of the pulmonary component closer to the aortic component.[39] In addition, the diastolic murmur of pulmonary insufficiency often appears after valvulotomy.[40]

Murmurs Originating at the Atrioventricular Valves

Mitral Insufficiency. This murmur is produced by regurgitation of blood from the left ventricle into the left atrium through an insufficient mitral valve. There are several findings but they are by no means constant. A typical case presents a murmur which begins with the first sound, since this is when left ventricular pressure exceeds left atrial pressure, and continues throughout systole, going even beyond the aortic component of the second sound, since at this point the pressure in the left

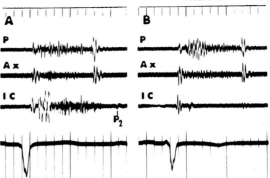

Fig. 5-71. Tetralogy of Fallot. *A,* intracardiac sound recording (IC) from within the pulmonary artery at the time of catheterization, showing a late pulmonary component of the second heart sound (P_2), which was not heard on the chest wall *P.* Note also in *B,* recording (IC) from within the right ventricle, that the murmur is absent, suggesting that in this case the systolic murmur was due to the pulmonary stenosis, rather than to the ventricular septal defect. (Time lines, 0.04 sec.) (*From J. S. Butterworth, M. R. Chassin, R. McGrath, and E. H. Reppert.*[10])

ventricle is still above that in the left atrium. The murmur ends abruptly when the left ventricular pressure falls below that in the left atrium; this is usually after both aortic and pulmonic closure, so that both second sounds are apt to be lost in the murmur. Following the murmur there is often a third heart sound, which is frequently so loud that it may be mistaken for the second sound when the latter is lost in the murmur. In addition to the above features, the duration of left ventricular systole is shortened, resulting in increased splitting of the second sound, best heard at the left sternal border or in the pulmonic area (Fig. 5-72). This may be because the left ventricle now has an additional exit of lesser resistance into the left atrium.

The variations from this type of murmur are several (Fig. 5-73), for reasons not well understood.

One variation is that the murmur may occupy only early systole, starting with the first sound and lasting from one-half to two-thirds of systole.

Another variation is that the murmur does not start until well after the first sound and often near mid-systole.[41] It may be introduced by a sharp sound resembling a systolic click, and the murmur itself has late accentuation. There may or may not be increased splitting of the second sound. In our experience this late systolic murmur usually represents a relatively mild degree of insufficiency, as demonstrated by left ventricular cineangiograms.

Still another variation is represented by changes in early diastole. An opening snap of the mitral valve may be heard,[42] as well as a third heart

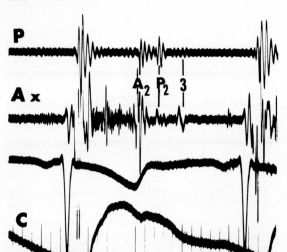

Fig. 5-72. Mitral insufficiency. Stethogram from the apex (*Ax*) of a young male shows a holosystolic murmur and a third heart sound. The second sound is widely split, as noted in the recording from the pulmonic area (*P*). (Time lines, 0.04 sec) (*From J. S. Butterworth, M. R. Chassin, R. McGrath, and E. H. Reppert.*[10])

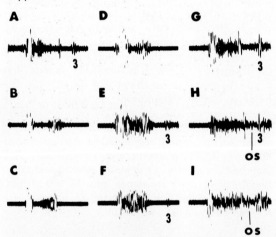

Fig. 5-73. Examples of various murmurs associated with mitral insufficiency recorded at the cardiac apex supine. *A* shows an early systolic murmur and a third sound. *B*, *C*, and *D* are examples of late systolic murmurs or show late accentuation of the murmurs. *B* shows a sound similar to a midsystolic click. *E* and *F* are examples of holosystolic murmurs with third heart sounds. *G*, *H*, and *I* show holosystolic murmurs combined with diastolic rumbles which often incorporate a third heart sound and sometimes an opening snap (*OS*), as in *H* and *I*. Note in all of the examples that the intensity of the first heart sound varies rather markedly, and also that the components of the second sound are difficult to identify in many of the tracings, being "lost" in the terminal portion of the systolic murmur.

sound (Fig. 5-74). The latter, in this instance, is often not discrete but part of a low-pitched series of vibrations, constituting a short early diastolic murmur (Fig. 5-73). In some instances this is probably due to some degree of actual stenosis, as well as insufficiency, of the mitral valve. In others, this murmur may represent a relative mitral stenosis due to the dilatation of the left ventricle and to an increased diastolic flow across the mitral valve. Indeed, it has been shown that a pressure gradient may exist, in such cases, between the left atrium and ventricle in early diastole.[43]

Nothing has been said about the intensity of the first heart sound in this condition, but in our experience this is not of great help and tends to be variable.

Tricuspid Insufficiency. The murmur of insufficiency of the tricuspid valve is very similar to that of mitral insufficiency, and the two may be very difficult to separate. Tricuspid insufficiency is less common and is usually secondary to dilatation of the right ventricle and the tricuspid ring. A useful means of clinical differentiation, when present, is the increase in intensity of the murmur of tricuspid insufficiency on inspiration[44] (Fig. 5-75); the murmur of mitral insufficiency remains unchanged or diminishes.

Mitral Stenosis. Pressure in the left atrium rises (Fig. 5-76) when the valve becomes stenotic because of fibrosis and frequently calcification. The thickened valve then acts like a rigid diaphragm with a small opening. This change in the physical character of the valve is thought to account for two of the clinical findings commonly present in mitral stenosis; i.e., the accentuation of the first sound and the opening snap of the mitral valve.

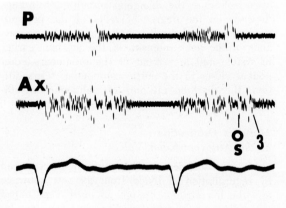

Fig. 5-74. Mitral insufficiency. The apex stethogram (*Ax*) shows the holosystolic murmur and the third heart sound. In addition, an opening snap of the mitral valve is seen, even though no mitral stenosis was present at the time of surgery. (Time lines, 0.04 sec.)

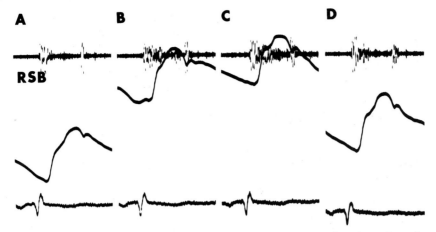

Fig. 5-75. Tricuspid insufficiency. Representative cycles from a continuous recording from the right sternal border (RSB) during inspiration. The carotid pulse curve and ECG are also shown. A, B, C, and D represent various phases of the respiratory cycle. C shows the maximum inspiratory phase, at which time the systolic murmur is the loudest.

Accentuation of the first sound is usually marked and occurs when left ventricular pressure exceeds left atrial pressure and the rigid diaphragm snaps toward the atrium, producing more sound than normal. The sound may be slightly delayed in onset,[45] but this can be determined only by comparing with the electrocardiogram or other timing function (Fig. 5-76). Because other conditions may produce a similar delay, this is not of particular diagnostic value.

Fig. 5-76. Mitral stenosis. This figure shows left ventricular and aortic pressure curves at the top. The dotted lines in the lower portion represent two different elevated left atrial pressures as the result of mitral stenosis. The normal left atrial pressure is indicated by the solid line below these dotted lines. Note that the mitral component of the first sound (M_1) normally occurs at the time that left ventricular pressure exceeds left atrial pressure, causing the mitral valve to close. When, however, the left atrial pressure is abnormally elevated, the left ventricular pressure exceeds the left atrial at a later time and the mitral component of the first sound is delayed (indicated by the sound in broken line just after the normal M_1). Likewise, the opening of the mitral valve, which is normally silent (0), occurs when the pressure in the left ventricle falls below that in the left atrium. With stenotic disease of the mitral valve, this sound becomes audible as the opening snap, and the higher the left atrial pressure, the earlier the left ventricular pressure falls below the left atrial pressure, hence the earlier the opening snap (indicated by the broken-line figures between A_2 and 0). Thus, the more severe the mitral stenosis, the higher the left atrial pressure and the closer the opening snap approaches the second sound. (From J. S. Butterworth, M. R. Chassin, R. McGrath, and E. H. Reppert.[10])

When the ventricle relaxes and its pressure falls below that in the left atrium, the rigid mitral valve, which can no longer open normally, snaps toward the ventricle, producing the opening snap of the mitral valve. There is a relationship between the left atrial pressure and the time of the opening snap.[46,47] The higher the left atrial pressure, the closer the opening snap to the aortic second sound (Fig. 5-76). In atrial fibrillation the interval will usually vary from beat to beat, because of variations in cardiac filling.

The opening snap is widely heard but is more easily identified at the left sternal border or base, where the diastolic murmur, which follows immediately, is less intense.

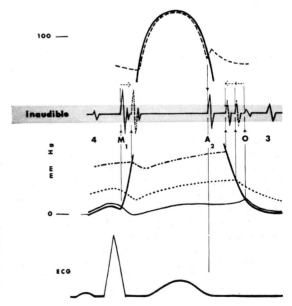

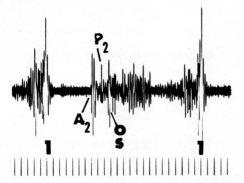

Fig. 5-77. Mitral stenosis. Apex stethogram showing the accentuated first heart sound, closely split second sound, opening snap of the mitral valve (*OS*), and a holodiastolic murmur. The latter is loudest in early diastole and presystole, corresponding to the times of greatest ventricular filling in a patient with sinus rhythm. (Time lines, 0.04 sec.) (*From J. S. Butterworth, M. R. Chassin, R. McGrath, and E. H. Reppert.*[10])

The murmur of mitral stenosis is diastolic in time, low-pitched, and rumbling in character. The classical murmur is loud in early diastole, less intense during mid-diastole, and accentuated again in late diastole (presystole) (Fig. 5-77). This is not unexpected if one remembers that maximal ventricular filling occurs in early and late diastole. The murmur, however, is variable (Fig. 5-78) and may be only presystolic or early diastolic in time, and occasionally the opening snap and the loud first sound are the only auscultatory signs of mitral stenosis. If atrial fibrillation is present the presystolic accentuation of the murmur is lost. With a long P-R interval the atrial contraction is early and the murmur becomes discrete and does not fuse into the following first heart sound.

Although it is possible to have both an opening snap and a third heart sound with combinations of mitral stenosis and insufficiency, the third sound is not present in severe mitral stenosis.

Tricuspid Stenosis. Tricuspid stenosis seldom exists as a single valvular abnormality and is usually associated with mitral valve disease. The murmur and opening snap produced by tricuspid stenosis are indistinguishable from the findings of mitral stenosis, with the possible exception that the tricuspid murmur may be accentuated by inspiration[44] and is usually more intense near the sternum. Although clinical suspicion may be present, the actual determination must be made by special techniques.

The murmur of tricuspid stenosis is also encountered in conditions in which there is rapid blood flow through a normal tricuspid valve into a dilated right ventricle, such as occurs with an atrial septal defect.

Changes Following Surgery on the Atrioventricular Valves. Changes may or may not occur in the auscultatory findings following surgical attacks on the valve structures. With simple finger fracture of the mitral valve in suitable cases the diastolic murmur may almost completely disappear, although an opening snap usually remains. A marked diminution of the murmur and/or an opening snap that is later than before the operation (Fig. 5-79) usually mean a good clinical result. On the other hand good clinical results may be seen without much change in the murmurs. If mitral insufficiency should be produced by the manipulations, then a systolic murmur, usually early, becomes audible.

Plastic surgical repair of an insufficient mitral valve under direct vision usually results in marked

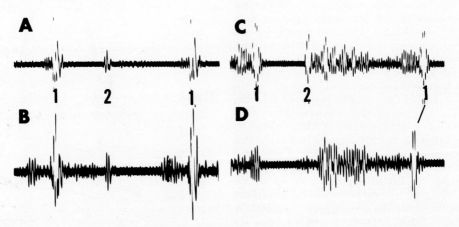

Fig. 5-78. The diastolic murmur of mitral stenosis. *A* shows a rather faint presystolic murmur and a minimal diastolic rumble. In *B* the presystolic murmur is separated from the first sound because of a long P-R interval. *C* shows a holodiastolic murmur with maximal intensity in early diastole and presystole in a patient with sinus rhythm. In *D* the presystolic accentuation is absent because of the presence of atrial fibrillation.

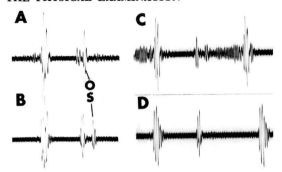

Fig. 5-79. Mitral stenosis, pre- and postoperatively, from two patients. Preoperative recording A from the left sternal border shows the opening snap (OS) close to the second sound. B shows later opening snap (OS) postoperatively. Recording in another patient from the apex (Ax) after surgery: D shows disappearance of the diastolic murmur seen preoperatively. C. The opening snap is still present but extremely faint.

diminution of the intensity and duration of the systolic murmur previously present.

When prosthetic devices of the ball-valve type have been used, the valve sounds dominate the auscultatory findings (Fig. 5-80).

Murmurs Resulting from Nonvalvular Deformities

Atrial Septal Defect. In the secundum type of this congenital abnormality, the auscultatory findings result almost entirely from the effects of altered hemodynamics at sites distal to the anatomic deformity. The excessive left-to-right shunt through the defect produces a prolongation of right ventricular systole,[48] resulting in marked delay of pulmonary valve closure with wide splitting of the second heart sound, often with little respiratory variation. Similarly, the excessive flow across the pulmonary valve into the dilated pulmonary artery produces disturbed flow, which results in a systolic murmur maximal at the pulmonary area (Fig. 5-81). This murmur is usually crescendo-decrescendo in character but begins almost immediately after the first sound and ends before the second sound, thus differing from the murmur of significant pulmonary stenosis. The same torrential flow across the normal tricuspid valve into the dilated right ventricle often results in a rumbling diastolic murmur at the apex. Occasionally, in patients with pulmonary hypertension, the murmur of pulmonary incompetence may be present at the left sternal border. Because of the dilated pulmonary artery, a pulmonary ejection sound may be present, but this is not so frequent as in mild pulmonary stenosis.

The second heart sound is of considerable value in the diagnosis of atrial septal defect, but it must

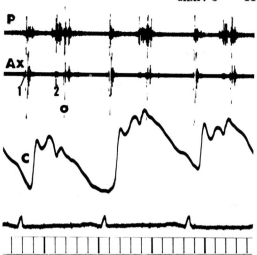

Fig. 5-80. Stethogram of patient with Starr-Edwards mitral valve replacement. The valve sounds dominate the picture, O probably representing opening of the ball valve. Following this is an additional sound, suggesting that on opening the ball may "bounce." (Time lines, 0.1 sec.)

be interpreted with care. Generally speaking, the wider degrees of splitting with the least respiratory variation[49] are associated with the greater left-to-right shunts, but this is not invariable. The intensity of the pulmonary component is usually increased, and it must be recognized that this does not necessarily signify pulmonary hypertension, as increased flow alone can cause a more intense pulmonary second sound. Indeed, the degree of splitting is frequently a better indication of the presence of pulmonary hypertension, since when the latter is present, splitting of the second sound is minimal or absent, even in the presence of significant left-to-right shunt (Fig. 5-82).

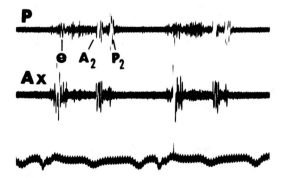

Fig. 5-81. Atrial septal defect. Stethogram showing an early crescendo-decrescendo systolic murmur which is not of great intensity and is maximal in the pulmonary area (P). More diagnostic is the widely split second heart sound. An ejection sound (e) is probably also present. (Time lines, 0.04 sec.)

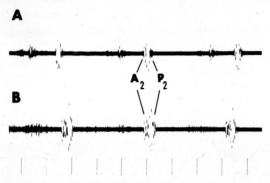

Fig. 5-82. Atrial septal defect with pulmonary hypertension. Stethogram from the pulmonary area preoperatively *A* shows single loud second sound representing fusion of A_2 and P_2. Pulmonary artery pressure was 75/30 mm Hg. In *B*, 3 years after surgical closure, the components of the second sound are separated because of the drop in pulmonary artery pressure. (Time lines, 0.04 sec.)

In the less common form of atrial septal defect of the primum type, all the above findings may be present, but in addition there is often a holosystolic murmur of even intensity throughout systole, maximal at the apex. This represents the murmur of mitral or tricuspid insufficiency due to the frequent presence of cleft atrioventricular valves in this entity.

Ventricular Septal Defect. In this congenital abnormality the auscultatory findings are related to the degree and direction of shunt through the

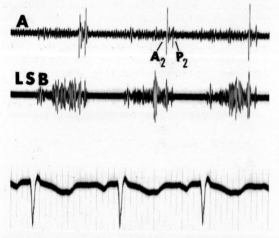

Fig. 5-83. Ventricular septal defect. Stethogram showing holosystolic murmur maximal at left sternal border recording (*LSB*). The murmur is of even intensity throughout systole (first cycle) but is variable in the other two cycles. The second heart sound is split but may be hard to identify if the murmur is loud. (Time lines, 0.04 sec.) (*From J. S. Butterworth, M. R. Chassin, R. McGrath, and E. H. Reppert.*[10])

defect, which is controlled primarily by the level of the pulmonary vascular resistance.[50,51] With large left-to-right shunt and normal pulmonary vascular resistance, a medium-frequency holosystolic murmur is present along the lower-left sternal border (Fig. 5-83). Most frequently this murmur is of even intensity throughout systole and resembles the murmur of mitral insufficiency. Occasionally smaller defects may act as a stenotic orifice and produce a crescendo-decrescendo systolic murmur or may close during ventricular contraction and produce only an early systolic murmur. The second heart sound is split more widely than normal but retains its respiratory variation, the abnormal splitting presumably being due both to early aortic valve closure and to late pulmonary valve closure.[52] In the presence of large left-to-right shunts with or without pulmonary hypertension but with relatively normal pulmonary resistance, the pulmonary component becomes accentuated but the split of the second sound remains. As pulmonary resistance increases, however, flow diminishes and the pulmonary component becomes extremely loud and occurs early, often merging with the aortic component. At the same time the systolic murmur diminishes in intensity and may entirely disappear.

In cases with large left-to-right shunt, an early rumbling diastolic murmur is usually present at the apex, resulting from the excessive blood flow across the mitral valve.[53] A Graham Steell murmur of pulmonary incompetency is occasionally heard in patients with severely increased pulmonary vascular resistance.

Patent Ductus Arteriosus and Other AV Fistulas. Flow from the high-pressure aorta through a patent

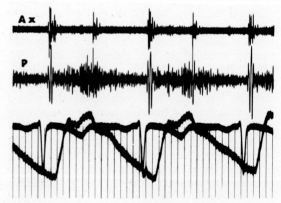

Fig. 5-84. Patent ductus arteriosus. The lower tracing *P* is from the pulmonic area and shows the murmur to be continuous throughout systole and diastole, often obscuring the heart sounds. The murmur is typically most intense in late systole. The electrocardiogram and carotid pulse curve are also shown.

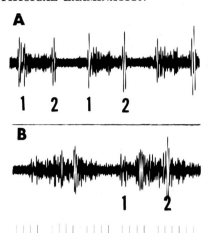

Fig. 5-85. Patent ductus arteriosus. A shows the recording from the pulmonary area in a child at age 3 months. Only a systolic murmur is present. In the same child at age 1 year (B) the typical continuous murmur has appeared. The diastolic component of the murmur may be absent in any case of patent ductus arteriosus associated with pulmonary hypertension. (Time lines, 0.04 sec.)

ductus into the low-pressure pulmonary artery occurs both in systole and diastole and produces the well-known continuous (machinery) murmur (Fig. 5-84). This is loudest in the pulmonary area or under the left clavicle. The maximal pressure gradient between aorta and pulmonary artery is in systole, while the maximal intensity of the murmur occurs at the time of the second heart sound; the lateness of the murmur is probably due to the distance of its origin from the site of origin of the heart sounds. The second heart sound is often obscured by the murmur, but when identified it may be physiologically split or, in patients with large left-to-right shunt, paradoxically split.

With severe pulmonary hypertension at any age the murmur may lose its continuous character; frequently it is only systolic in time.[54,55] In these patients the pulmonary component of the second sound is accentuated and occurs early, often merging with the aortic component. Similar auscultatory findings are frequently present in infants with patent ductus, even though pulmonary artery pressure is normal; the characteristic continuous murmur may not appear until 1 or 2 years of age (Fig. 5-85).

Arteriovenous fistulas at any site may produce a continuous murmur similar to that described in patent ductus, the exact character being related to the pressure gradient and velocity of flow between the two vessels. When these occur in the chest, e.g., coronary or pulmonary AV fistula, they may be mistaken for patent ductus arteriosus. Other conditions which may simulate the murmur of patent ductus are combined aortic stenosis and insufficiency, dilated pulmonary artery with pulmonary insufficiency, and coarctation of the pulmonary artery.

Venous Hum. Disturbance of laminar flow in the venous system, particularly in the jugular veins, may produce sound. This is usually continuous throughout the cardiac cycle and may be mistaken for the murmur of patent ductus arteriosus or other AV fistula. However it tends to be of higher pitch and can be obliterated by changes in position or by compression of the jugular veins (Fig. 5-86).

Coarctation of the Aorta. In the usual coarctation of the aorta, the constricted area is followed by a dilated portion of the aorta, and there is a variable pressure gradient across the constriction. These factors result in increased velocity of flow through a narrow area into a more dilated chamber, producing disturbance of laminar flow. This is heard as a rather nondescript murmur, loudest in the back but also prominent on the precordium, beginning shortly after the first heart sound and having variable length, depending on the severity of the constriction; in the more severe cases the murmur extends into early diastole (Fig. 5-87), simulating a continuous murmur.[56] A systolic bruit may also

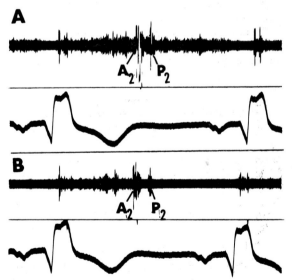

Fig. 5-86. Venous hum. Recordings from the left supraclavicular area. The upper tracing shows the hum which occupies both systole and diastole and may simulate the murmur of patent ductus arteriosus. However, the hum may be obliterated by jugular compression, and the bottom tracing was taken during this maneuver. The hum disappears, but a systolic murmur and splitting of the second sound due to right bundle branch block remain. (From J. S. Butterworth, M. R. Chassin, R. McGrath, and E. H. Reppert.[10])

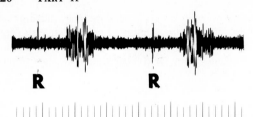

Fig. 5-87. Coarctation of the aorta. This recording is from the interscapular area, and the sharp deflections indicated by R were introduced electronically at the peak of the QRS complex of the electrocardiogram for timing. The loud delayed murmur probably results from turbulence at the site of coarctation, but there is also a continuous low-pitched hum, which is probably the result of blood flow through dilated intercostal arteries. (Time lines, 0.04 sec.) (*From J. S. Butterworth, M. R. Chassin, R. McGrath, and E. H. Reppert.*[10])

be heard over the collateral arterial vessels, particularly in the back. On the precordium the systolic murmur may be mistaken for the murmur of aortic stenosis which accompanies coarctation in approximately 10 per cent of cases. In addition, the diastolic murmur of aortic insufficiency may be present in about one-third of the cases. The second heart sound may be paradoxically split, and the aortic component is usually intensified.

Coarctation of the Pulmonary Artery. Constrictions of the pulmonary arteries may be single or multiple and may cause murmurs in a manner similar to that described for coarctation of the aorta. The location of the murmur varies, depending on the location of the constriction. When this murmur is continuous in nature, it may be mistaken for that of patent ductus arteriosus.

Dilatation of Aorta and Pulmonary Artery. These situations result in disturbance of flow as blood passes through the normal valve area into the dilated vessel. The murmurs produced are usually crescendo-decrescendo in character but are early in systole and hence should not be mistaken for significant stenosis of either semilunar valve. In addition an ejection sound is almost invariably present.

Pericardial Rubs and Sounds

Mention has already been made of the diastolic sound of constrictive pericarditis (p. 107) and of the questionable relationship of systolic clicks to a previous episode of pericarditis (p. 105). In addition, acute pericarditis from any cause may result in a series of sounds or rubs. These sounds are produced by the rubbing together of the roughened surfaces of the epicardium and inner pericardium during movement of the heart. Consequently the sounds or rubs may be present in atrial systole,

ventricular systole, and ventricular diastole. Rubs are variable and may resemble the sounds produced by rubbing together two pieces of sandpaper or leather. They may be faint or loud and tend to have a higher pitch than most murmurs. They are usually maximal along the left sternal border, are variable in intensity, and often transitory. The presence of sufficient fluid in the pericardial cavity to separate the two pericardial surfaces precludes the production of a rub.

With inflammation of the pleura adjacent to the pericardium, a similar pleuropericardial rub may be produced which is recognized by its variation with respiration.

Murmurs Occurring in the Absence of Cardiac Disease

In most instances there is nothing about the intensity, character, or pitch of a murmur which allows it to be categorized unequivocally as innocent or functional. Final classification of a murmur as innocent depends on the absolute demonstration of the absence of any cardiac abnormality, and this is not always possible. Innocent murmurs are systolic in time and can generally be divided into three types.

The innocent pulmonary systolic murmur occurs in early systole and is maximal at the pulmonary area. It tends to be crescendo-decrescendo in configuration but rarely extends beyond mid-systole. It may be due to a relative increase in velocity of blood flow, and hence will have increased intensity following exercise or during the febrile state. Perhaps some of these murmurs are due to some dilatation of the pulmonary artery which is not sufficiently marked to be considered abnormal. It is apparent that the mechanism of production of this murmur is not unlike that of the murmur of an atrial septal defect or a mild pulmonary stenosis; consequently close attention should be directed to the second heart sound. If the latter is normally split, such a murmur is more likely to be innocent.

Another type of innocent murmur is the vibratory early systolic murmur described by Still in 1909.[57] This murmur has a distinct "twanging" or vibratory character and is maximal between the lower-left sternal border and the apex. It tends to be of relatively pure frequency and is somewhat different in pitch from the murmurs of mitral insufficiency or ventricular septal defect, with which it is often confused.

Most difficult to categorize as innocent are the systolic murmurs occurring at the cardiac apex.[58] When a systolic murmur in this area is limited to very late systole, and even occasionally to very early systole, it is tempting to call it an innocent murmur. This is all the more true if the murmur is introduced by a systolic click. However, we have demonstrated mitral insufficiency by left ventricular angiography in patients presenting such a murmur (Fig. 5-73B) even in the absence of other abnormal parameters. It is probable that such murmurs, particularly the late systolic type, should be considered innocent if other parameters, such as heart sounds, electrocardiogram, and cardiac fluoroscopes, are normal. However, it is apparent that some of these cases may in time have to be reclassified as mitral insufficiency.[41]

Effect of Certain Drugs on Sounds and Murmurs

Any condition which makes the heart beat faster and increases the velocity of blood flow will generally increase the intensity of heart sounds and murmurs, whether these be on a normal or pathologic basis. Examples of this are provided by simple exercise, hyperthyroidism, and high-output states. However, it is stated that the inhalation of amyl nitrite,[59] by producing differential changes in the dynamics of the right and left circulation, simplifies the recognition and separation of certain clinical entities. This is accomplished by lowering the peripheral resistance and hence the left ventricular pressure. Thus the murmurs of small ventricular septal defect, mitral insufficiency, etc., may disappear or become less intense for a few seconds following the inhalation of amyl nitrite (Fig. 5-88). It should be pointed out that these changes are evanescent and may be difficult to quantitate with the stethoscope alone. The cardiac rate increases at the same time, which further complicates the problem. However, by continuous recording of the sounds on tape it may be possible to make the necessary comparisons more accurately.

AUSCULTATORY FINDINGS FOLLOWING MYOCARDIAL INFARCTION

With acute myocardial infarction the heart sounds have frequently been described as distant or muffled and as having a "tic-tac" character. Many factors, including the cardiac rate, the cardiac output, and the velocity of ventricular contraction, enter into the intensity and character of the sounds under these conditions. We have the general impression, without being able to document it, that the heart sounds do become less intense following myocardial infarction, but this seems rather directly related to the severity of infarction and to be true whether or not a shocklike state develops. On the other hand it would be difficult to say that one can recognize changes in the sounds when there has been little encroachment on the cardiac function as a result of the infarction.

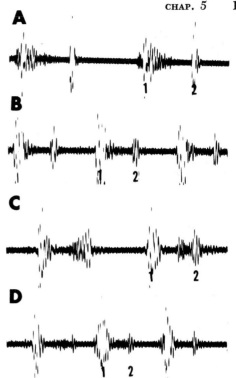

Fig. 5-88. Effect of the inhalation of amyl nitrite on murmurs. These recordings were selected from continuous tape recording of the sounds at constant amplification and frequency settings. A represents the early systolic murmur recorded over the aortic area in a 56-year-old man with mild aortic stenosis (gradient 35 mm Hg). Note how early the murmur is in systole. In B, 30 sec after amyl nitrite, the rate is accelerated and the first heart sound is much louder but the intensity of the murmur and the second heart sound are diminished. These are not the usual findings,[59] since the murmurs of aortic stenosis are said to increase after amyl nitrite. C is the late systolic murmur of mild mitral insufficiency (proved by left ventricular cineangiography) recorded at the apex in the supine position. D represents the findings 30 sec after amyl nitrite and again shows the increase in rate without too much change in the first heart sound. The murmur is much less intense, and the aortic component of the second sound (which was incorporated in the murmur in C) is now easy to identify.

In addition to changes in the first and second sounds, one may hear audible third and fourth sounds (gallop rhythms) following myocardial infarction, but again this is usually directly related to dilatation of the left ventricle or the presence of cardiac failure and is similar to these sounds heard under other circumstances of ventricular dilatation or failure.

One may also, following myocardial infarction, hear low-frequency diastolic rumbles, as in a number of other conditions where there is dilatation of the ventricle.

During the acute phase of myocardial infarction several auscultatory findings may develop. One of these is pericardial friction rub in patients who have no epicardial involvement. These rubs do not differ from rubs caused by other factors.

Perforation of the interventricular septum is a relatively rare complication; it produces a loud systolic murmur of sudden onset and usually maximal in the fourth left intercostal space.

Rupture of a papillary muscle with subsequent mitral insufficiency is another situation in which the onset of the murmur is usually abrupt and dramatic. It may be difficult to differentiate from perforation of the interventricular septum, and there seems to be a wide latitude as to the type of murmurs produced as well as the character and point of maximum location. In addition, individual chordae may separate, giving a somewhat similar picture.[60] Again, the type of murmur is not specific and may at times be confused with the murmur of aortic stenosis.[61] In many instances a chorda or valve leaflet is set into high-frequency vibration by a jet of blood; the murmur produced is usually loud and of higher and relatively pure frequency, which gives it a musical character. This musical quality is not specific for any type of either systolic or diastolic murmur but is generally due to the perforation of a valve cusp or a chorda set into vibration.

Recently a syndrome of papillary muscle dysfunction[62] secondary to myocardial infarction has been described; it is characterized by the clinical combination of an apical systolic murmur with the electrocardiographic features of infarction of the anterolateral papillary muscle. This murmur is delayed in onset after the first sound and frequently has a diamond-shaped configuration.

Murmurs may be heard in association with ventricular aneurysms secondary to myocardial infarction. These are usually diastolic in time and are of the type described as a diastolic rumble associated with a dilated ventricle.

Rupture of the ventricle produces a loud systolic murmur, but this is seldom heard[63] because of the rapid development of cardiac tamponade and death.

LIMITING FACTORS IN AUSCULTATION

Several factors limit the ability of a physician to practice good auscultation. Naturally the degree of previous training or skill acquired is of great importance, as is the environment in which the act is practiced. Almost any environmental noise will interfere with the interpretation of the sounds heard through the stethoscope.

The degree of transmission of sounds from their origin in the heart through the various tissues of the body to the surface varies from patient to patient. Bone and blood are reasonably good conductors of sound energy, but lung tissue and adipose tissue are poor conductors. Hence, in the emphysematous or obese patient, sounds that are of normal intensity at their origin may be faint by the time they reach the skin. Sounds in children are usually loud because of the thin chest wall and the close proximity of the heart to the anterior chest wall. Pneumothorax, pleural effusions, pericardial effusions, etc., may likewise change the normal transmission of cardiac sounds.

Although the stethoscope is useful, it has certain drawbacks related to the collecting and transmitting of sound energy to the ear. Many studies[64-66] have been conducted on this subject, but we will mention only general principles to be followed: (1) The instrument should have an open bell at least 2.5 cm in diameter. (2) The diaphragm should be at least 3.5 cm in diameter, should be of material supplied by the manufacturer, and should have no cracks or holes. (3) The total length should be as short as possible consistent with ease of use—20 in. or less from endpiece to ear tips. (4) The earpieces should fit well and not impinge on the walls of the external auditory canal, nor should they be obstructed by wax.

The diaphragm endpiece transmits higher-frequency murmurs better; the open bell is better for very low-frequency murmurs. In order for the open bell to function efficiently and pick up the low-frequency vibrations from the skin it must be applied with the lightest possible pressure to avoid tensing the skin, making the latter act as a diaphragm. Increasing pressure damps the intensity, particularly of the low frequencies (Fig. 5-89).

Perhaps the factor which is most limiting in auscultation of the heart is the human hearing mechanism. Figure 5-90 illustrates the average threshold of audibility at various frequency ranges and indicates the area of heart sounds and murmurs. The human hearing mechanism is so poor in this range that perhaps only 10 per cent or less of the total sound energy produced by the beating heart falls above the threshold of audibility. It thus behooves us to use the utmost care and concentration in practicing auscultation.

AUSCULTATION, PHONOCARDIOGRAPHY, AND AUDIOVISUAL ANALYSIS

Of the several methods of evaluating the sounds produced by the heart, the first is auscultation with an ordinary stethoscope, which has the values of simplicity and low cost but has the limitations mentioned previously.

A second method is phonocardiography, in which the heart sounds are translated into electrical energy and recorded by an instrument with the proper frequency response for heart sounds. A reference timing tracing such as the electrocardiogram, the carotid pulse curve, or the apex cardiogram is recorded simultaneously. This gives permanent visual recording along with a timing reference which is necessary for measuring time intervals and correlating timing of various hemodynamic events. A variation of this technique is the spectrophonocardiogram,[14,67] which correlates frequency, intensity, and timing of sounds and murmurs. A disadvantage in most instruments is that the recordings are on photographic paper and the results cannot be seen until the film is developed. Moreover, the eye cannot easily translate this pattern into the sound.

The third method, or audiovisual analysis, combines auscultation and phonocardiography.[9,10] This is accomplished by amplifying and filtering the heart sounds so they can be heard well in various frequency ranges and at the same time feeding the signal into an oscilloscope with a long-persistence screen so that the examiner both hears and sees

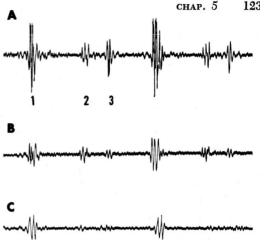

Fig. 5-89. Recordings at constant intensity and frequency from the cardiac apex with the bell of the stethoscope. In A, light pressure of the bell against the chest wall accentuates the low frequencies and the third heart sound is easily apparent. B and C represent increasing degrees of pressure of the bell against the chest, with almost complete disappearance of the low-frequency third heart sound as well as attenuation of all sounds.

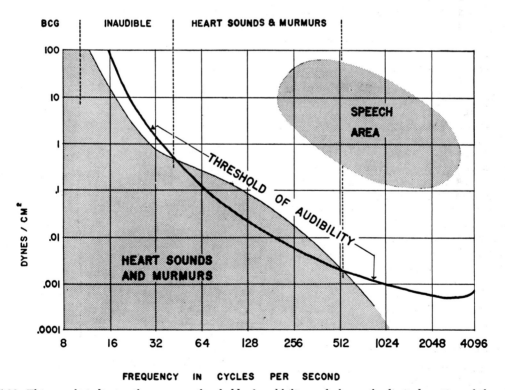

Fig. 5-90. This graph indicates the average threshold of audibility and shows the limited portion of the vibratory spectrum of the heart which lies above the threshold. Since there may be considerable variation in the threshold from person to person, this is another variable in auscultation, causing differences of opinion when sounds are near the threshold of audibility. (*From J. S. Butterworth, M. R. Chassin, R. McGrath, and E. H. Reppert.*[10])

the sound at the same time. Tape recordings can be made for future reference. A timing reference is not usually necessary when the sounds can be visualized, but if it is desired, the sounds can be superimposed via a direct writing electrocardiograph on either the electrocardiogram or the carotid pulse curve. The electrocardiogram is a poor reference since only the first sound can be identified, but a pressure wave such as the carotid pulse, which can be easily obtained, is intimately related to the production of the sounds and is useful both for timing of the first sound and identification of the aortic component of the second sound.

In our experience the audiovisual combination has advantages in that certain murmurs, such as those of faint aortic insufficiency, are much better recognized by the human ear than by phonocardiography. On the other hand certain low-frequency and low-intensity sounds and murmurs may often be more easily seen than heard.

RECENT DEVELOPMENTS IN AUSCULTATION AND PHONOCARDIOGRAPHY

Many advances have been made in recent years which have contributed to our knowledge in this field. These have been mainly the result of progress in technology. Microphones on the tips of catheters are now available for recording sound from vessels, chambers of the heart, esophagus, etc. Although not of routine clinical usefulness, they have proved to be a helpful research tool and have stimulated interest in clinical cardiology by demonstrating the relationship of sound to the hemodynamic events in the cardiac cycle.

It is difficult to predict what the future will bring, but with improved recording equipment and experience the analysis of heart sounds by computers is a distinct possibility.

However, the future progress that will contribute most to the diagnosis and thus to the care of the patient will be the communication to all physicians who use the stethoscope of the accumulated information which is *presently* available.

REFERENCES

1. Läennec, R. T. H.: De l'auscultation médiate ou traité du diagnostic des maladies des poumons et du coeur, fondé principalment sur ce nouveau moyen d'exploration, J. A. Brosson et J. S. Chaude, Paris, 1819.
2. Leared, A.: Quoted by Camman, D. M., ref. 3.
3. Camman, D. M.: An Historical Sketch of the Stethoscope, *New York J. Med.*, 43:465, 1886.
4. Potain, C.: Note sur les dédoublements normaux des bruits du coeur, *Bull. et mém. Soc. méd. hôp.* 3:138, Paris, June 22, 1866.
5. Leatham, A.: Splitting of the First and Second Heart Sounds, *Lancet*, 2:607, 1954.
6. Einthoven, W.: Die Registrierung der menschlichen Herztöne mittels des Saitengalvanometers, *Arch. ges. Physiol.*, 117:461, 1907.
7. Frank, O.: Die unmittelbare Registrierung der Herztone, *München. med. Wchnschr.*, 51:953, 1904.
8. Frederick, H. A., and Dodge, H. F.: The Stethophone: An Electrical Stethoscope, *Bell System Tech.* J., 3, Oct. 1924.
9. Butterworth, J. S., and Poindexter, C. A.: Visual and Auditory Educational Aids in Cardiology, *J. M. Educ.*, 27:258, 1952.
10. Butterworth, J. S., Chassin, M. R., McGrath, R., and Reppert, E. H.: "Cardiac Auscultation," 2d ed., Grune & Stratton, Inc., New York, 1960.
11. Levine, S. A., and Harvey, W. P.: "Clinical Auscultation of the Heart," 2d ed. W. B. Saunders Company, Philadelphia, 1959.
12. Dock, W.: Mode of Production of the First Heart Sound, *Arch. Int. Med.*, 51:737, 1933.
13. Wolferth, C. C., and Margolies, A.: The Influence of Varying A-V Intervals on Split First Heart Sounds: Its Bearing on the Cause of Split Sounds and the Mechanism of the First Sound, *J. Clin. Invest.*, 14:605, 1935.
14. McKusick, V. A.: "Cardiovascular Sound in Health and Disease," The Williams & Wilkins Company, Baltimore, 1958.
15. Braunwald, E., and Morrow, A. G.: Origin of Heart Sounds as Elucidated by Analysis of the Sequence of Cardiodynamic Events, *Circulation*, 18:971, 1958.
16. Rappaport, M. D., and Sprague, H. B.: The Graphic Registration of the Normal Heart Sounds, *Am. Heart J.*, 23:591, 1942.
17. Leatham, A.: Auscultation of the Heart, *Lancet*, 2:703, 1958.
18. McKusick, V. A., Webb, G. N., Humphries, J. O'N., and Reid, J. A.: On Cardiovascular Sound: Further Observations by Means of Spectral Phonocardiography, *Circulation*, 11:849, 1955.
19. Boyer, S. H., and Chisholm, A. W.: Physiologic Splitting of the Second Heart Sound, *Circulation*, 18:1010, 1958.
20. Shafter, H. A.: Splitting of the Second Heart Sound, *Am. J. Cardiol.*, 6:1013, 1960.
21. Dock, W., Grandell, F., and Taubman, F.: The Physiologic Third Heart Sound: Its Mechanism and Relation to Protodiastolic Gallop, *Am. Heart J.*, 50:449, 1955.
22. Nixon, P. G. F.: The Genesis of the Third Heart Sound, *Am. Heart J.*, 65:712, 1963.
23. Dunn, F. L., and Dickerson, W. J.: Third Heart Sound: Possible Role of Pericardium in Its Production, *Circulation Res.*, 3:51, 1955.

24. Symposium on Cardiovascular Sound, *Circulation,* **16:**270, 1957.

25. Meisner, J. E., and Rushmer, R. F.: Eddy Formation and Turbulence in Flowing Liquids, *Circulation Res.,* **12:**455, 1963.

26. Bruns, D. L.: A General Theory of the Causes of Murmurs in the Cardiovascular System, *Am. J. Med.,* **27:**360, 1959.

27. Leatham, A.: The Phonocardiogram of Aortic Stenosis, presented to British Cardiac Society, 1959.

28. Braunwald, E., Goldblatt, A., Aygen, M. M., Rockoff, S. D., and Morrow, G. M.: Congenital Aortic Stenosis, *Circulation,* **27:**426, 1963.

29. Goodwin, J. F., Hollman, A., Cleland, W. P., Aygen, M. M., and Teare, D.: Obstructive Cardiomyopathy Simulating Aortic Stenosis, *Brit. Heart J.,* **22:**403, 1960.

30. Braunwald, E., Morrow, A. G., Cornell, W. P., Aygen, M. M., and Hilbisk, T. F.: Idiopathic Hypertrophic Aortic Stenosis: Clinical, Hemodynamic and Angiographic Manifestations, *Am. J. Med.,* **29:**924, 1960.

31. Flint, Austin: On Cardiac Murmurs, *Am. J. M. Sc.,* **44:**29, 1862.

32. Daoud, G., Reppert, E. H., and Butterworth, J. S.: Basal Systolic Murmurs and the Carotid Pulse Curve in the Diagnosis of Calcareous Aortic Stenosis, *Ann. Int. Med.,* **50:**323, 1959.

33. Leatham, A., and Weitzman, D.: Auscultatory and Phonocardiographic Signs of Pulmonary Stenosis, *Brit. Heart J.,* **19:**303, 1957.

34. Blount, S. G., Jr., Vigoda, P. S., and Swan, H.: Isolated Infundibular Stenosis, *Am. Heart J.,* **57:** 684, 1959.

35. Vogelpoel, L., and Schrire, V.: The Role of Auscultation in the Differentiation of Fallot's Tetralogy from Severe Pulmonary Stenosis with Intact Ventricular Septum and Right-to-Left Interatrial Shunt, *Circulation,* **11:**714, 1955.

36. Sloman, G., and Wee, K. P.: Isolated Congenital Pulmonary Valve Incompetence, *Am. Heart J.,* **66:**532, 1963.

37. Runco, V., and Booth, R. W.: Basal Diastolic Murmurs, *Am. Heart J.,* **69:**697, 1963.

38. Steell, Graham: The Murmur of High Pressure in the Pulmonary Artery, *M. Chron.,* Manchester, 9: 182, 1888-1889.

39. Vogelpoel, L., and Schrire, V.: Pulmonary Stenosis with Intact Ventricular Septum and Fallot's Tetralogy: Assessment of Postoperative Resutls by Auscultation and Phonocardiography, *Am. Heart J.,* **59:** 645, 1960.

40. Talbert, J. L., Morrow, A. G., Collins, N. P., and Gilbert, J. W.: The Incidence and Significance of Pulmonic Regurgitation after Pulmonary Valvulotomy, *Am. Heart J.,* **65:**590, 1963.

41. Barlow, J. B., Pocock, W. A., Marchand, P., and Denny, M.: The Significance of Late Systolic Murmurs, *Am. Heart J.,* **66:**443, 1963.

42. Nixon, P. G. F., Wooler, G. H., and Radigon, L. R.: The Opening Snap in Mitral Incompetence, *Brit. Heart J.,* **22:**396, 1960.

43. Nixon, P. G. F., and Woller, G. H.: Left Ventricular Filling Pressure Gradient in Mitral Incompetency, *Brit. Heart J.,* **25:**382, 1963.

44. Rivero-Carvallo, J. M.: El diagnostico de la estenosis tricuspidea, *Arch. Inst. cardiol. México,* **20:**1, 1950.

45. Kelly, J. J., Jr.: Diagnostic Value of Phonocardiography in Mitral Stenosis, *Am. Heart J.,* **19:**682, 1955.

46. Messer, A. L., Counihan, T. B., Rappaport, M. B., and Sprague, H. B.: Effect of Cycle Length on Time of Occurrence of First Heart Sound and Opening Snap in Mitral Stenosis, *Circulation,* **4:**576, 1951.

47. Margolies, A., and Wolferth, C. C.: Opening Snap ("claquement d'overture de la mitrale") in Mitral Stenosis, Its Characteristics, Mechanism of Production and Diagnostic Importance, *Am. Heart J.,* **7:**443, 1932.

48. Leatham, A., and Gray, I.: Auscultatory and Phonocardiographic Signs of Atrial Septal Defect, *Brit. Heart J.,* **18:**193, 1956.

49. Aygen, M. M., and Braunwald, E.: The Splitting of the Second Heart Sound in Normal Subjects and in Patients with Congenital Heart Disease, *Circulation,* **25:**328, 1962.

50. Van Der Hauwaert, L., and Nadas, A.: Auscultatory Findings in Patients with a Small Ventricular Septal Defect, *Circulation,* **23:**886, 1961.

51. Craige, E.: Phonocardiography in Interventricular Septal Defects, *Am. Heart J.,* **60:**51, 1960.

52. Leatham, A., and Segal, B.: Auscultatory and Phonocardiographic Signs of Ventricular Septal Defect with Left-to-Right Shunt, *Circulation,* **25:**318, 1962.

53. Feruglio, B. A., and Gunton, R. W.: Intracardiac Phonocardiography in Ventricular Septal Defect, *Am. J. Cardiol.,* **5:**191, 1960.

54. Burchell, H. B.: Variations in the Clinical and Pathological Picture of Patent Ductus Arteriosus, *M. Clin. North America,* **32:**911, 1948.

55. Myers, G. S., Scannell, J. G., Wyman, S. M., and Hurst, J. W.: Atypical Patent Ductus Arteriosus with Absence of the Usual Aortic-Pulmonary Pressure Gradient and of the Characteristic Murmur, *Am. Heart J.,* **41:**819, 1951.

56. Spencer, M. P., Johnston, F. R., and Meredith, J. H.: The Origin and Interpretation of Murmurs in Coarctation of the Aorta, *Am. Heart J.,* **56:**722, 1958.

57. Still, G. F.: Common Disorders and Diseases of Childhood, H. Frowde, Hodder, and Stoughton, London, 1909, p. 434.

58. Wells, B.: The Graphic Configuration of Innocent Systolic Murmurs, *Brit. Heart J.,* **19:**129, 1957.

59. Barlow, J., and Shillingford, J.: The Use of Amyl

Nitrite in Differentiating Mitral and Aortic Systolic Murmurs, *Brit. Heart J.,* **20**:162, 1958.

60. January, L. E., Fisher, J. M., and Ehrenhaft, J. L.: Mitral Insufficiency Resulting from Rupture of Normal Chordae Tendinae, *Circulation,* **26**:1329, 1962.

61. Shapiro, H. A., and Weiss, R.: Mitral Insufficiency Due to Ruptured Chordae Tendinae Simulating Aortic Stenosis, *New England J. Med.,* **261**:272, 1959.

62. Phillips, J. H., Burch, G. E., and De Pasquale, N. P.: The Syndrome of Papillary Muscle Dysfunction, *Ann. Int. Med.,* **59**:508, 1963.

63. Bishop, L., and Logue, B.: External Rupture of Heart Causing Systolic Murmur and Thrill, *J.A.M.A.,* **144**:757, 1950.

64. Johnston, F. D., and Kline, E. M.: An Acoustical Study of the Stethoscope, *A.M.A. Arch. Int. Med.,* **65**:328, 1940.

65. Rappaport, M. B., and Sprague, H. B.: Physiologic and Physical Laws That Govern Auscultation and the Clinical Application, *Am. Heart J.,* **21**:257, 1941.

66. Rappaport, M. B., and Sprague, H. B.: The Effects of Improper Fitting of Stethoscope to Ears on Auscultatory Efficiency, *Am. Heart J.,* **43**:713, 1952.

67. Geckler, G. D., Likoff, W., Mason, D., Riesz, R. R., and Wirth, C. H.: Cardiospectrograms, *Am. Heart J.,* **48**:189, 1954.

EXAMINATION
OF THE RETINAL FUNDI

Joseph A. Wilber, M.D.

Sir George Pickering, Regius Professor of Medicine at Oxford, when making ward rounds would use the house man's ophthalmoscope to examine the patient's eyes, and he would comment that one could always tell a good doctor by the strength of the batteries in his ophthalmoscope. Professor Pickering, an eminent observer and investigator, obviously thought it was important to be able to see the retinal fundi as clearly as possible. It is important, because it is the only opportunity the doctor has of seeing the living blood vessels and nerves of his patient, and of observing the flow of blood to tissues.

If the optic fundus is involved, three broad categories of disease may be detected with the ophthalmoscope: (1) systemic diseases that affect small blood vessels, either arterioles or venules (e.g., hypertension or diabetes); (2) diseases that interfere with retinal blood flow (embolic disease, leukemia, or atherosclerosis of the central retinal artery); and (3) diseases causing generalized anoxemia, including anoxemia of the retina (severe anemia, carbon monoxide poisoning). It is important to realize, however, that the optic fundus frequently looks perfectly normal when the patient

has serious vascular disease elsewhere. In particular, the fundus is frequently normal when there is severe atherosclerosis of the coronary, cerebral, or other arteries of the body. Conversely, minor changes in the retinal blood vessels are difficult even for experts to evaluate. Too much emphasis should not be placed on slight degrees of narrowing or tortuosity, or questionable changes in light reflexes that may well fall within the range of normal. White or yellow glistening spots in the retina, called *drusen bodies,* are occasionally seen and frequently mistaken for exudates. They are not associated with any known disease and occur in healthy persons.

TECHNIQUE

Correct use of the ophthalmoscope is simple and can be learned rapidly. With a cooperative patient in a darkened room, a satisfactory view of the fundus can often be obtained without dilating the pupil. However, for the wide-range view necessary to assess generalized vascular changes, dilatation is of prime importance. Sympathomimetic agents (such as one drop of 10 per cent Neo-synephrine in each eye, 30 min before the examination) are quicker, safer, and shorter-acting than mydriatics, such as homatropine. Precipitation of acute glaucoma with these agents is extremely rare, even in the elderly.

A few points should be emphasized. The patient must keep his eye still, and to do this he must be able to fixate on a distant object straight ahead with the opposite eye. Therefore, the examiner must not obstruct the view of this eye. To examine the right eye the examiner must hold the ophthalmoscope in his right hand, be on the right side of the patient, and look with his right eye into the patient's right eye. Similarly, when the left eye is examined, the examiner uses his left hand and left eye, and is on the patient's left side.

Before the fundus is examined the examiner must check the transparency of the cornea, aqueous, lens, and vitreous. This inspection is best made with the examiner at a distance, using an 8-D lens about 8 in. from the eye.

To examine the fundus, the ophthalmoscope is brought directly in front of and *as close as possible* to the patient's eye. The patient is told to look directly forward, but not into the light. First the optic disk is examined; then each of the four major branches of the retinal artery and vein is followed out to the periphery as far as possible. Lastly, the macular region is brought directly into view by asking the patient to look directly into the light. Macular inspection usually requires full dilatation of the pupil.

THE HISTOLOGY OF THE RETINAL BLOOD VESSELS

When we look at the optic fundus through an ophthalmoscope, we are using the patient's eye as a lens which magnifies structures about fourteen times. We are looking at moving streams of blood encased in walls so thin that they are practically transparent, and held in place by transparent layers of nerve fibers.

Normally, we cannot see the blood vessel walls except indirectly as a white line or "light reflex" formed by reflection of light from the ophthalmoscope off the convex surface of the blood column. This light reflex is important, as it tells us the state of health and thickness of the wall of the vessel. Since the arteriolar wall is thicker than that of the venule, the light streak on the arteriole is normally wider and brighter than that on the accompanying venule. Thickening of these blood vessel walls, with concomitant loss of transparency and widening of the light reflex, is one of the major signs of retinal vascular disease.

Certain peculiarities of the retinal blood vessels are important to the understanding of some of the common pathologic changes observed. The central retinal artery is a branch of the ophthalmic artery which enters the optic nerve at some distance behind the eyeball and courses through the nerve in close association with its corresponding vein. It is a typical small artery with three well-defined layers —an endothelium with an internal elastic membrane, a muscularis, and an adventitia. But when the artery pierces the cribriform plate of the sclera and enters the eye, it changes drastically. The thickness of the wall suddenly diminishes; the internal elastic membrane thins and disappears by the first or second bifurcation within or close by the disk margin. The muscular coat of the artery abruptly thins, also, at the cribiform plate. By the first or second bifurcation, it is found only as widely separated muscle fibers. Vasomotor nerves have not been demonstrated in human retinas. There is some question of neural control of tone in the retinal vessels. There is no doubt, however, that humoral factors affect retinal arteriolar tone.

Thus the arterial vessel we see leaving the disk margin and coursing out over the retina is basically an *arteriole* consisting of an endothelial layer with a thin basement membrane, a few scattered muscle fibers, and an adventitia.

The retinal venules which are visible have even thinner walls than the arterioles. Their adventitia lie directly on the basement membrane of their endothelium. They are wider than the arterioles, the ratio of the diameter of an arteriole to its accompanying venule being about 2:3. Because of the difference in oxygenation of the blood, the veins are dark red, in contrast to the arterioles. Unlike the blood vessels in other organs in the body, the arterial and venous vessels in the retina lie close together; they take parallel courses, and their branches frequently cross one another. The importance of this is that where there is an arteriovenous crossing, both vessels share the same adventitia, and the basement membrane of the vein lies directly on the basement membrane of the arteriole. This arrangement may explain why any disease of the arteriole often directly affects the vein and, in fact, may be most obvious by its effect on the AV crossing. Seitz has postulated that each arterial pulse wave indents the vein at this site and causes, even under physiologic conditions, considerable stress on the venous wall. This stress in systemic hypertension would be much greater and is a potent argument for the recent concept that AV crossing changes are indicative of long-standing blood pressure elevation.

THE PATHOLOGY OF THE OPTIC FUNDUS

Like many other specialized tissues of the body, the optic fundus can react only in a limited number of ways to a variety of noxious stimuli or diseases. Thus we often see a similar retinal picture in a diversity of systemic disorders. Rather than describe the combinations of these nonspecific changes that occur in specific diseases, let us consider individually some of the common ophthalmoscopic findings and correlate them with the pathophysiology as presently known. Illustrations of these abnormalities are shown in Plates 4 and 5.

Vascular Sclerosis

Because of its vagueness the term *arteriosclerotic retinopathy* should be discarded. Rather, let us consider vascular sclerosis under the headings of *arteriolar sclerosis* and *atherosclerosis*.

Arteriolar Sclerosis. In the author's opinion, most evidence points to the concept that this is the specific lesion of "high blood pressure" and probably is a direct result of the mechanical effect of the elevated pressure. It occurs in all types of hypertension and histologically is characterized by intimal hyalinization and proliferation, progressing to medial hypertrophy and adventitial fibrosis. It is rarely seen in the absence of hypertension of several years' duration, and it indicates similar small–blood vessel changes throughout the entire body. Some investigators believe it may occur as an aging phenomenon in the absence of hypertension. (Since we do not really know what the normal blood pressure should be with increasing age, and since blood pressure variation may be of large magnitude from minute to minute, it is difficult to say when hypertension is absent or has never been present.)

As the arteriolar wall thickens, it becomes less translucent and the light reflex seen with the ophthalmoscope becomes wider and extends further toward the periphery, including the small branches. The normal bright red color of the arterial blood column changes to orange ("copper-wire vessels") as the wall thickens, and less commonly a "silver-wire" effect is produced when the wall becomes completely opaque.

It should be emphasized that normal retinal vessels do not rule out hypertension. The pressure in blood vessels can be doubled with only one-sixth decrease in vascular caliber. Such a change would not be visible with the ophthalmoscope.

This same process of sclerosis of the arteriolar walls produces characteristic changes in the retinal veins where they *cross* the arterioles. At these crossing points the arteriole and venule *share the same adventitia,* and disease of the arteriole wall obscures, compresses, and indents the visible venous blood column. Various classifications have been devised to grade this continuous process of the arteriolar sclerosis with concomitant venous crossing changes, but since each author has his own classification it is clinically better to describe what is seen in each individual.

Although the sclerosis of the arteriolar wall in hypertensive disease may be uniformly distributed in the retinal vessels, producing a generalized vascular narrowing with more acutely branching angles and loss of visibility of small twig branches, in severe hypertensive disease one more commonly sees gross irregularity of arteriolar caliber in the same blood vessel. These irregular narrowings and constrictions have been attributed to "vasospasm," but clinical evidence for this is scant. Since the irregular caliber of retinal arterioles in hypertensive disease rarely is reversible (though the papilledema and hemorrhages and exudates will disappear with chronic lowering of the blood pressure), it seems that most of the localized narrowings are due to focal organic sclerosis. In acute forms of hypertension, such as acute glomerulonephritis and toxemia of pregnancy, sharply localized, symmetric, "waistlike" constrictions are seen that vary in number and may disappear when the hypertension is relieved.

Atherosclerosis. Atherosclerosis is a spotty disease of large blood vessels and is *rarely visible* with the ophthalmoscope. Since the visible retinal vessels are mainly "arteriolar" in nature, atheromas in vessels this size rarely occur. The central retinal artery within the optic nerve does develop atheroma, however, and occlusion of it causes sudden complete loss of vision, with mild or marked pallor

of the entire retina, attenuation of all the retinal vessels, and a "cherry-red" spot at the macula. Hemorrhages and exudates are infrequent with central retinal artery occlusion.

Central vein occlusion and venous occlusions at AV crossings near the disk may be due to atherosclerotic disease since they may represent invisible atheroma of the associated arterial vessels with invasion or thrombosis of the vein. Central venous occlusion is characterized by sudden loss of vision, but there are also marked retinal edema, papilledema, and massive diffuse hemorrhages.

Rarely, atheromatous plaques may break off the basilar or carotid artery walls and be seen as shiny, yellow, irregular patches lodged at a retinal bifurcation ("Hollenhorst bodies," see Plate 7. The transient, migrating white "gaps" in the blood columns of retinal vessels have been photographed by Pickering. He suggests that they may be platelet-leucocyte-thrombin aggregations fragmnted from partial occlusions centrally. Retinal infarcts may be produced on occasion; they may simulate retinal detachment.

Hemorrhages

Retinal hemorrhages occur in a wide variety of diseases. They are not specific for hypertension and are also seen in a variety of disorders including leukemias, severe anemia of any cause, embolic disease, macroglobulinemias, diabetes, subarachnoid hemorrhage, any disease causing vascular stasis, septicemia, carcinomatosis, and various collagen diseases such as polyarteritis.

The shape of the hemorrhage depends on its location on or in the various layers of the retina. Hemorrhages in the nerve-fiber layer are linear or flame-shaped, because of the orientation of these fibers. Round hemorrhages are located deeper in the nerve cell or plexiform layers and are round because of the orientation of the elements in these layers. Large irregular pools of blood called *preretinal hemorrhages* occur when the hemorrhage is very superficial and is lying between the limiting membrane of the vitreous and the retina. Such hemorrhages occur in diabetic patients in particular and may leak into the vitreous, with sudden loss of vision and subsequent fibrosis which is called *retinitis proliferans.*

Capillary Aneurysms

Small round "red spots," located principally between the disk and macular region, that are unusually persistent and unchanging in appearance, are clinically called "capillary aneurysms." They are frequently seen in diabetes of many years' duration. By injection techniques, Cogan and coworkers have shown that they are saccular dilatations coming off

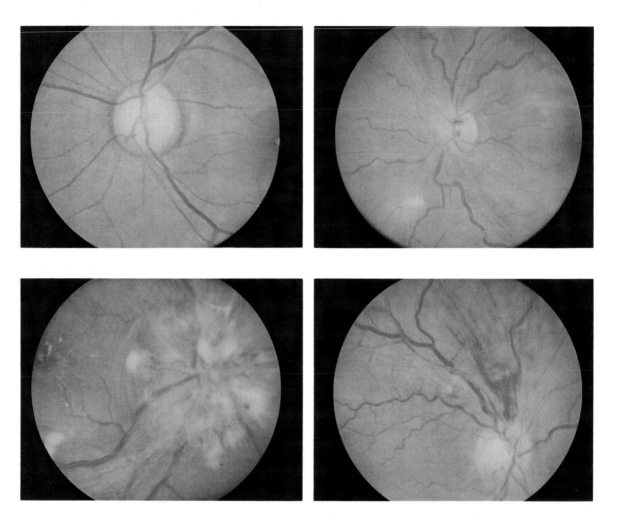

Plate 4. *Upper left.* The retina of a 49-year-old Negro female with asymptomatic "essential hypertension" of at least 10 years' duration showing generalized arteriolar narrowing and straightening, increased light reflex, irregular caliber, loss of small arteriolar branches, and early AV crossing changes. *Upper right.* The retina of a 42-year-old Negro female with "essential hypertension" with blood pressure levels averaging 260/130. She was asymptomatic except for headaches. Note the severe vascular sclerosis seen as marked irregularity of arteriolar caliber, "sheathing," and nearly complete loss of transparency of the arterioles. A "cotton wool" exudate is seen at 7 o'clock. The nasal disk margin is blurred, which may occur normally. *Lower left.* The retina of a 38-year-old Negro male with "malignant hypertension" with bilateral papilledema and azotemia. There was no visual disturbance. Note the massive edema, hemorrhages, and exudates, completely obscuring the disk and burying the blood vessels. The veins are congested and the arterioles show diffuse thickening ("copper wire"). There are hard exudates (edema residues) forming in the nerve bundle grooves in the macular region at 10 o'clock. *Lower right.* The retina of a 50-year-old Negro female with severe hypertension of 25 years' duration. *Arteriolar* sclerosis is shown by the marked narrowing, irregular caliber, increased light reflex, and AV crossing changes. *Atherosclerosis* is suggested by the large fan-shaped superficial hemorrhage, due to occlusion of a branch of the superior temporal vein as it enters the disk region.

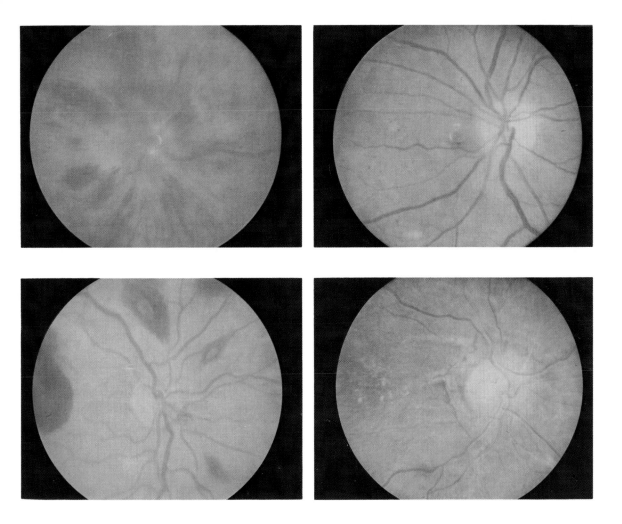

Plate 5. *Upper left.* The retina of a 74-year-old white male with normal blood pressure who complained of sudden loss of vision in one eye. This shows the typical picture of central retinal vein occlusion, probably due to *atherosclerosis* of its adjacent artery behind the disk. Diffuse edema (loss of retinal detail), massive hemorrhages, and papilledema are present. *Upper right.* The retina of a 68-year-old white male with hypertension and mild diabetes mellitus. Note the very small red dots, or capillary aneurysms, scattered between the disk and the macular region. There is also a faint "cotton wool" exudate at 7 o'clock. *Lower left.* The retina of a 24-year-old white female with acute myeloblastic leukemia and severe anemia. The blood pressure was normal. Note the scattered hemorrhages, some with whitish centers (Roth spots), and the portion of the large *preretinal* hemorrhage at 9 o'clock. The blood vessels are pale but otherwise normal. *Lower right.* The retina of a 36-year-old white female with *pseudoxanthoma elasticum.* Severe hypertension, marked visual disturbance, and renal insufficiency were present. Note the characteristic brownish "angioid streaks" around the disk and extending toward the macula. Also seen are marked retinal arteriolarsclerotic changes, sheathing, irregular caliber, occluded vessels, and hard exudates with a "smudge" hemorrhage at 7 o'clock.

one side of a capillary, terminal arteriole, or venule, and are not derived preferentially from the venous side. Microscopically they tend to be oriented, bulging toward an avascular zone in the retina, and probably can occur in any type of disease associated with localized areas of retinal vascular occlusion. Though numerous and common in diabetes, they are occasionally seen in other diseases such as hypertension, or the "aortic arch syndrome."

Exudates

Exudates are not specific for hypertension. They occur in a wide variety of disorders that involve vascular stasis and increased permeability of the capillary wall. Generally speaking, any disease that can cause retinal hemorrhages may also cause exudates.

Clinically, three types of exudates are recognized: (1) "cotton-wool," (2) "hard," and (3) "macular star." All three types occur in severe hypertension.

1. Cotton-wool exudates. These are superficial white lesions with a hazy, frayed border. They are located in the nerve-fiber layer and histologically are composed of eosinophilic globules with dark-staining central zones called *cytoid bodies*. Their exact composition and origin are unknown. They may be thought of as retinal ischemic areas and have been shown to be located in areas supplied by a single end-arteriole. They may appear suddenly, persist several weeks, and gradually fade away without leaving any residual defect. Fluorescent dye studies suggest that they represent areas of transient increased vascular permeability and may resolve without permanent vascular occlusion. Scattered cotton-wool exudates are an important clue to severe, premalignant hypertension.

2. Hard exudates. These are smaller, more dense, shinier, and more persistent than cotton-wool exudates. They may be white or yellowish. Histologically, they are located in the deeper layers of the retina and probably represent collections of old edema fluid containing lipids and protein. They, too, may be absorbed without residual effect. They are considered residua of retinal edema.

3. Macular star exudates. These are not pathologically a different type of exudate but merely a radial arrangement of hard exudates in the macular region, indicating that a massive retinal edema occurred some time in the past. Since edema fluid tends to collect at the posterior pole of the eye (in the macular region), when this fluid coalesces to form hard exudates it lines up in the grooves of the nerve bundles leading to the macula, forming a partial starlike arrangement. Macular stars occur in all types of severe hypertensive disease as well as in other conditions with retinal edema. The terms "nephritic" or "albuminuric" retinopathy should be discarded, since in this author's opinion retinopathy due to severe renal disease never occurs in the absence of hypertension or severe anemia, which by themselves may account for the retinal findings.

Papilledema

Papilledema (swelling of the nerve head) should be distinguished if possible from papillitis (inflammation of the nerve head). Often this is not easy, even for experts.

Papilledema is usually *bilateral* and in its early stage entails no *impairment in vision*. The physiologic cupping of the disk disappears first, followed by blurring of the disk margin, distortion of the retinal veins as they cross the disk margin, vascular engorgement, generalized haziness of the retinal background, and, finally, diffuse hemorrhages and exudates on and around the disk region. Papilledema occurs with increased intracranial pressure from any cause, but the more severe forms are usually seen with *"malignant hypertension"* in which increased intracranial pressure (for reasons unknown) may not be present. In hypertensive disease with papilledema, together with the arteriolar sclerotic changes previously described, scattered hemorrhages and exudates are seen widely distributed toward the periphery. In brain tumor or other forms of intracranial disease, the papilledema is usually less severe, and the retinal vessels out from the disk are normal (in the absence of coincident chronic hypertension). It should be noted that papilledema may occur in patients with advanced pulmonary insufficiency with marked respiratory acidosis. With treatment, papilledema frequently subsides without damage to vision or any visible residual effect.

Papillitis is usually *unilateral* and is always associated with *severe visual impairment*, even in the early stages. The disk is swollen and grayish white, and, as in papilledema, though less commonly, the veins may be engorged and hemorrhages and exudates may occur. Causes include syphilis, multiple sclerosis, and encephalitis, but more often papillitis is idiopathic. It frequently progresses to optic atrophy.

Pseudopapilledema is not rare and may lead to unnecessary extensive neurologic diagnostic procedures. It is distinguished by usually being unilateral, and is an irregular, asymmetric blurring of the disk margins with normal-appearing vessels. Hemorrhages never occur.

Angioid Streaks

Dark brown or black pigmented "cracks" radiating out from the disk, or forming concentric partial rings near the disk, are a rare finding called *angioid streaks.* Pathologically, they are linear defects in the lamina vitrea (Bruch's membrane) separating the retina from the dark brown choroid. They are frequently associated with a rare hereditary disease of elastic tissue, pseudo-xanthoma elasticum. This is a widespread disease of elastic tissue throughout the body, and the streaks frequently extend into the macular region, causing blindness. Renal damage, hypertension, and gastrointestinal hemorrhage also occur, because of the generalized elastic defect.

Angioid streaks have been reported also in osteitis deformans (Paget's disease of the bone), sickle-cell disease, and high myopia.

SUGGESTED READING

Ashton, N., Pears, M. A., and Pickering, G. W.: Neuroretinopathy Following Hemorrhage, *Brit. J. Ophth.,* **45**:385, 1961.

Carr. R. E., and Henkind, P.: Retinal Findings Associated with Serum Hyperviscosity, *Am. J. Ophth.,* **56**:23, 1963.

Cogan, D. G., Toussaint, D., and Kuwabara, T.: Retinal Vascular Patterns, IV, *Arch. Ophth.,* **66**:366, 1961.

Hogan, M. J.: "Ophthalmic Pathology," W. B. Saunders Company, Philadelphia, 1962.

Klein, B. A.: Retina and Optic Nerve: Annual Review, *Arch. Ophth.,* **67**:622, 1962.

Kuwabara, T., Carroll, J., and Cogan, D. G.: Retinal Vascular Patterns, III, *Arch. Ophth.,* **65**:708, 1961.

Pickering, G. W.: "High Blood Pressure," Grune & Stratton, Inc., New York, 1955.

Scheie, H. G.: Evaluation of Ophthalmoscopic Changes of Hypertension and Arteriolar Sclerosis, *Arch. Ophth.,* **49**:117, 1953.

Toussaint, D., Knirvabara, T., and Cogan, D. G.: Retinal Vascular Patterns. II, *Arch. Ophth.,* **65**:575, 1961.

Wagener, H. P.: Retinal Arterial and Arteriolar Lesions Associated with Systemic Vascular Hypertension: A View of Some Recent Opinions, *Amer. J. M. Sc.,* **241**:240, 1961.

Wagener, H. P., and Keith, N. M.: Diffuse Arteriolar Disease with Hypertension and Associated Retinal Lesions, *Medicine,* **18**:317, 1939.

Section B: Routine Diagnostic Procedures

6 ELECTROCARDIOGRAPHY AND VECTORCARDIOGRAPHY

E. Harvey Estes, M.D.

INTRODUCTION

In the 60 years of its existence, electrocardiography has become established as an atraumatic, relatively inexpensive, and extremely useful technique for gaining information about the heart. Once the tool of the cardiologist, it is now commonly used by the general internist, the general practitioner, the surgeon, and others. In spite of its age and utility, the art is still on a somewhat insecure theoretical base.

The surface electrocardiogram is related to the electrical activity of myriads of single-fiber units, each having an action potential of a characteristic amplitude, configuration, and duration, and each having a particular spatial structural relationship to other units. The electrical activity of these individual units is programmed by a conduction system, which determines the sequence of activation by virtue of a higher conduction velocity. The surface electrocardiogram is assumed to be a complex mathematic summation of this activity, but in spite of the fundamental nature of this relationship, it is not possible to predict the configuration of the surface electrocardiogram from a knowledge of the configuration of the action potentials of individual units, nor is it possible to predict the details of the surface electrocardiogram from the sequence of activation.

It is hoped that knowledge of those factors affecting the transmembrane action potential of single cardiac fibers, more precise knowledge of the sequence of activation, and further clarification of the characteristics of transmission to the surface of the body will eventually place electrocardiography on a more rational foundation; but for the moment most of the information which we use in the interpretation of the electrocardiogram is derived from empirical observation. The various theories of electrocardiography have arisen retrospectively and represent attempts to formulate a framework which will bind the individual bits of empirical data into a meaningful whole, thus making them easier to recall and to use. These theories have to a degree achieved their goal; yet we should not forget their humble origin and tentative nature. Each new observation constitutes a "test" of the theory. It may fit the theory, in which case the theory is bolstered. On the other hand, it may not fit, in which case the theory must be altered, stretched, or discarded.

It is the feeling of the author that the "spatial vector" approach to the electrocardiogram most completely incorporates the empirical data into a meaningful whole, that it is an easier system to learn and to teach, and that it simplifies the transition from the electrocardiogram to the closely related vectorcardiogram. The method assumes that the electrical activity from all fiber units undergoing excitation at a given moment of time can be represented by a single resultant electrical force, with a finite direction and magnitude, and that this force is transmitted equally well in all directions. This force can be recorded on a surface lead, and the magnitude and direction of the recorded deflection are dependent on the distance of the lead from the point of origin of the force, and the relationship between the direction of the resultant force and the axis of the surface lead. If the resultant force is perpendicular to the axis of a given surface lead, no deflection is seen on the surface lead. If the resultant force is directed toward the positive end of the axis of the surface lead, a positive deflection is obtained; if the force is directed toward the negative end, a negative deflection is obtained.

These broad principles can be applied to an entire P, QRS, or T deflection to obtain the direction of the mean P, QRS, and T vectors, and can also be applied to a given portion of a complex, such as the initial or terminal 0.04 sec of QRS, to obtain a vector for that part of the complex. The reader is referred to other sources[1] for a more complete discussion of these techniques.

The vectorcardiogram is a plot of the pathway of instantaneous vectors, usually during one cardiac cycle. It is inscribed by plotting on an oscilloscope the voltage obtained from one surface lead against the voltage obtained from a second surface lead perpendicular to the first lead. By plotting two perpendicular leads lying in the frontal plane, a frontal-plane vectorcardiogram is obtained. In a similar manner, horizontal and sagittal vectorcardiograms can be obtained.

There has been much discussion regarding the choice of leads to be used in recording the vectorcardiogram. Several recent lead systems, based on torso model studies, seem to offer advantages of a closer approach to the ideal of three mutually perpendicular (orthogonal) leads which can be paired to form frontal, horizontal, and sagittal vectorcardiograms. These systems (Frank,[2] Schmitt SVEC III,[3] and McFee[4] systems) seem to offer the additional advantage of being more interchangeable than previous systems (tetrahedron,[5] rectangular,[6] and cube[7]). For this reason the author has chosen

one of the orthogonal systems (Frank), and the examples and discussion refer to this system.

Information derived from standard scalar electrocardiograms can be used to plot a rough approximation of the vectorcardiogram, and a rough prediction of the configuration of a given surface lead can be made from the vectorcardiogram. This relationship is only approximate, since it is not possible to reconstruct accurately the phase relationships between two scalar leads recorded at different points in time, and since assumptions are made regarding the axis of standard and unipolar leads which are only approximately correct. Nevertheless, the relationship is useful and enables one to apply knowledge derived from one system to the other with a fair degree of confidence.

The newer vectorcardiogram will probably never displace the scalar electrocardiogram. The vectorcardiogram, being a plot of voltage against voltage, does not permit an appreciation of time. Time is usually introduced by interruption of the tracing, but this is effective only when the beam is in motion. The P and T waves produce very small loops on the usual vectocardiogram, and these loops must be amplified considerably more than the QRS loop for interpretation. These electrical events are currently more easily evaluated on scalar leads. The vectorcardiogram, on the other hand, is a more precise tool for the appreciation of details of the QRS complex. Phase relationships are also appreciated by the vectorcardiogram. A difference in the time of onset of two scalar complexes may produce a totally different direction of rotation of a QRS loop and yet not be appreciated on sequentially recorded scalar leads (Fig. 6-1). Thus the two techniques are complementary, each offering advantages over the other.

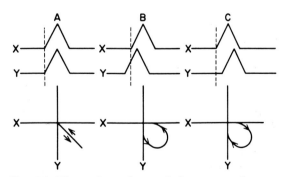

Fig. 6-1. Phase relationships and the vectorcardiogram. In *A*, the complexes occur simultaneously, and the resultant vectorcardiogram (below) is a straight line. In *B*, complex Y begins earlier than complex X and a counterclockwise loop is recorded. A slight time displacement in the other direction, as in *C*, produces an opposite (clockwise) rotation of the loop.

THE APPROACH TO
THE ELECTROCARDIOGRAM

There are two parts to the interpretation of an electrocardiogram and/or vectorcardiogram: (1) one must make certain routine measurements and observations, and evaluate whether or not they fit into the accepted range of normal; (2) one must fit these observations into the situation of the individual patient and determine whether they support the clinical impression, deny the clinical impression, or suggest hitherto unconsidered diagnostic possibilities. The experienced electrocardiographer performs these two parts of interpretation without consciously separating them, but it is useful for the beginner to consider each separately. The first is quickly learned and indeed can be carried out with extreme speed and precision by a digital computer. The second is a much more complex and difficult problem. Although this, too, can conceivably be programmed for a computer, the number of variables and modifying factors which must be considered in evaluating the problem of each patient would make this an extremely tedious procedure. The first part of the interpretation is that which is usually carried out in the electrocardiographic laboratory. These observations, plus a few facts, such as age, height, weight, blood pressure, history of digitalis ingestion, chest pain, etc., enable the ECG reader to make a reasonable guess as to how these observations fit into the clinical picture, but in most instances it is the patient's physician who must carry out the second phase of interpretation.

As implied above, certain routine measurements are carried out before seriously attempting any interpretation of the findings. An old rule of roentgenologic interpretation is applicable: If an abnormality is obvious at first glance, disregard it and survey the rest of the picture first. It is easy to become so much engrossed with the rhythm disturbance that an obvious QRS or T abnormality is ignored.

The "routine" measurements and observations are as follows: atrial and ventricular rate and rhythm, P-R interval, QRS interval, Q-T interval, mean frontal P, QRS, and T vectors, spatial orientation of these vectors; relationship between QRS and T vectors, the direction of the initial QRS vector, the relationship between this vector and the mean QRS vector, and the presence and orientation of S-T segment forces.

The atrial and ventricular rates are usually determined, in the presence of a normal rhythm, by dividing the P-P and R-R intervals, in seconds, into 60 sec, which gives the heart rate in cycles per minute. If irregular, the extremes can be counted, or an average value over a number of cycles can be calculated. A quick method of arriving at an approximation of rate is to divide the number of large squares between complexes into 300, the number of large squares representing 1 min of time at normal paper speed. Usually atrial and ventricular rates are equal, but habit of measuring both rates independently prevents the overlooking of AV dissociation, variable AV block, etc.

The normal P-R interval varies with heart rate and the age of the patient. In the normal adult with a slow heart rate, the P-R interval rarely exceeds 0.20 sec; thus, for practical purposes, this figure may be considered the upper limit of normal. In children, or in adults with very slow rates, standard tables may be consulted.

The Q-T interval also varies with heart rate. There are two methods of comparing a given Q-T interval with the normal range: (1) Correct the observed Q-T interval by means of a formula such as that of Bazett:

$$Q - Tc = \sqrt{\dfrac{Q - T \quad \text{sec}}{R - R \text{ interval} \quad \text{sec}}}$$

then compare the corrected interval with the range of normal (0.35 to 0.44 sec in the adult). (2) Compare the observed value directly with a table of normal values for the observed heart rate as seen in Fig. 6-2.

The mean frontal P, QRS, and T-vector axes are next calculated by inspection of standard and unipolar limb leads, as described by Grant,[1] and their directions are compared with the expected direction. The mean P-wave axis is generally directed in the left lower quadrant, at about +60°, the range being from 0 to +75°. The direction of the frontal-plane QRS axis varies tremendously with age. In the newborn infant,[8] the axis is in the right lower quadrant at +135°. The axis moves to the left with advancing months and years. It moves into the left lower quadrant at about 2 years, and is at +60 to +90° in the young adult. Horizontal direction of the mean QRS axis is seen with increasing frequency in older age groups, but only rarely does it move more leftward than −15°.

The axis of the T vector in the frontal plane is determined by inspection in the same manner as the QRS axis. In the newborn infant,[8] the frontal-plane T axis is more leftward than QRS, at 0 to +60°. In the adult, the frontal-plane position of the T axis is usually within 50° of the QRS axis, but it is also related to the direction of the QRS axis. If the QRS axis is vertical or semivertical (+75 to +90°), the normal T axis is to the left of the QRS axis. If the QRS axis is horizontal or semihorizontal (−15 to +30°), the normal T axis is to the right of the QRS axis. Thus a frontal QRS-vector direction of 0° and a T-vector direction of −10° is abnormal, though the angle between the QRS and T vectors is well within 50°.

An appreciation of the spatial direction of mean QRS and mean T-vector axes is gained from the precordial lead transition of QRS and T waves. In the infant,[8] the axis of the QRS vector lies anterior to the frontal plane and presents as a predominant upright QRS complex in the right precordial leads. At about age 2 to age 5, the QRS vector moves posterior to the frontal plane, and the QRS in the right precordial leads assumes the more usual adult configuration—a QRS complex which is more negative than positive in the right precordial leads.

The axis of the T vector is posterior in orientation in the newborn infant;[8] thus the T wave is usually inverted in the right precordial leads. This pattern persists until adolescence or early adulthood, when the T axis moves anterior to the frontal plane. The T waves become flat in V_1 and V_2, then still later become upright in these leads. In the usual adult ECG, the T waves are upright in all precordial leads. A persistence of the juvenile pattern of T-wave inversion in right precordial leads is occasionally seen into adulthood, especially in young women.

The spatial relationship between QRS and T axes changes from an anterior QRS axis with a posterior T axis (the infant relationship) to that of a posterior QRS axis with an anterior T axis (the adult relationship). An exaggeration of this trend, in which the T-vector axis moves anteriorly, to the extent that the T waves in V_5 and V_6 become flat or inverted, is occasionally seen but is probably related to heart disease (usually ischemic).

THE ATRIAL ELECTROCARDIOGRAM
(P and Ta waves)

The atrium is usually considered as a thin-walled, hollow mass of homogeneous cardiac muscle, in which activation is initiated by the spontaneous rhythmicity of a well-defined group of specialized cells (the sinoatrial node). Activation is considered as spreading uniformly outward from this site, first to the right atrium, then to the left, without the benefit of a specialized conduction pathway.

Almost all these classic views have been seriously challenged. Specialized cells indeed exist in the area of the junction of the venae cavae and atrium, but they probaby exist in a band, or ring, which merges with other fibers of an intermediate character that extend down to the AV ring and to the AV nodal area. This vague strip has been thought by some to serve a role similar to that of the conduction pathway in the ventricles. It is likely that neural and other influences are able to shift impulse formation from one site to another within the area

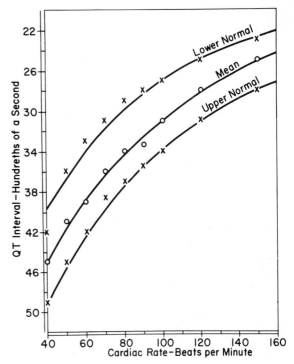

Fig. 6-2. The Q-T interval at various cardiac rates. The actual values for lower normal are from Lepeschkin, and the values for mean and upper normal are from Ashman.

of the sinoatrial band. It is also likely that several distinct groups of atrial fibers exist, and that each group responds in a somewhat different way to influences such as vagal and sympathetic stimulation. These phenomena may explain the remarkable variability of the P wave from time to time in the same patient, such as the commonly observed increase in P-wave amplitude with a rapid heart rate. Changes in configuration are also seen, but less regularly than the amplitude change.

The atrial complex is most useful in judging the site of impulse formation, and in the clarification of the nature of various arrhythmias. It does, however, have other value. It often adds to the precision of electrocardiographic interpretation. Right ventricular hypertrophy (RVH), as diagnosed from the QRS complex and T waves, may have many causes. The additional presence of left atrial enlargement would allow the electrocardiographer to conclude that mitral stenosis is the most likely cause of the RVH.

A number of methods have been proposed for the diagnosis of atrial enlargement. The classic "P pulmonale" (tall P wave in leads II and III, with a tall, peaked configuration) and "P mitrale" (notched P wave in leads I and II, with a broad, prolonged configuration) have been unreliable as sole criteria of right and left atrial enlargement. The more recently proposed Macruz[9] index, which measures the ratio of P duration to P-R segment duration (less than 1.0 in right atrial enlargement, greater than 1.6 in left atrial enlargement), has also proved more unreliable than expected from earlier reports. The most reliable criterion of atrial enlargement has proved to be the configuration and size of the P wave in V_1.

In left atrial enlargement the P wave in V_1 is diphasic, with a large terminal negative portion. Morris[10] has proposed the following criteria for the diagnosis of left atrial enlargement from the P wave in V_1. The P wave is divided into two portions, an initial (usually positive) deflection and a terminal (usually negative) deflection. The duration (in seconds) and magnitude (in millimeters at normal standardization) of the terminal force is measured and the algebraic product is determined. A value more negative than −0.03 mm-sec is considered abnormal and indicative of left atrial enlargement. These criteria correctly categorized 92 per cent of a group of 200 patients (100 normal, 100 with valvular heart disease expected to cause left atrial enlargement).

P-wave abnormalities meeting the above criteria for left atrial enlargement are frequently seen in disease of the left ventricle, such as hypertensive vascular disease, idiopathic myocardial hypertrophy, and muscular subaortic stenosis. The cause of such abnormalities is unknown. Morris has observed that the P wave in V_1 may be abnormal in the face of normal left atrial pressure and atrial size by x-ray examination. The size of the terminal negative portion of the P wave in V_1 may also change from day to day in the same patient. Congestive failure due to left ventricular disease is often accompanied by very large terminal P-wave forces, which rapidly decrease in size (but usually remain abnormal) over a period of several days.

Right atrial enlargement is characterized by a large upright P wave in V_1, with no terminal negative component. Although this configuration is highly specific (i.e., if the configuration is present, right atrial enlargement is very likely to be present), it is not a very sensitive criterion. In many cases in which right atrial enlargement is expected, the P wave is normal in V_1. The same may be said of the more convential criteria of a large peaked P wave of 2.5 mm or higher amplitude in leads II and III, with a mean P axis of greater than +60°.

Repolarization in a given atrial area probably begins immediately after depolarization in the same area. The atrial repolarization wave (Ta) thus begins after the first portion of the P wave and continues through the P-R interval. It is generally not identified unless it is larger than usual, or unless the P wave occurs independently of QRS, as in complete AV block. When seen, the Ta wave is in an opposite direction from the P wave. Since the mean P vector is usually at about +30 to +60°, the vectoral direction of the Ta wave is usually at about −120 to −150°. When the P wave is large, the Ta wave is also generally large and may be seen to extend beyond the QRS complex and to distort the initial portion of the S-T segment. It may be mistaken for the S-T segment depression of subendocardial injury, since it has a similar vectoral direction. The configuration of the atrial repolarization wave (smooth curve with upward concavity, Fig. 6-3), the recognition of similar deviation of the baseline before QRS is written, and the recognition of a large P wave usually enable a correct interpretation. A frequent clinical setting in which this problem arises is that of chronic pulmonary disease, in which a rapid heart rate is common and in which large, tall P waves are seen in leads II and III.

The atrium is also occasionally involved in myocardial infarction and in trauma, both accidental and surgical. Atrial injury is usually suspected because of the presence of atrial irritability in a suitable clinical setting, and because of the presence of a deviation of the P-R segment in a direction other than that expected with atrial repolarization.

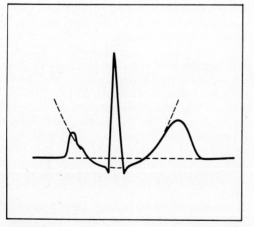

Fig. 6-3. Atrial repolarization as a cause of S-T segment deviation. Note that the P-R and S-T segments can be connected by a smooth curve, and that the direction of the deviation is opposite in direction to the P wave.

THE VENTRICULAR ELECTROCARDIOGRAM (QRS and T waves)

Activation and Form of the Electrocardiogram and Vectorcardiogram

The ventricular myocardium is depolarized in a more or less predictable sequence, programmed by the ventricular conduction system (the AV node, the common bundle, the left and right bundle branches, and the Purkinje network). The electrical activity of the specialized conduction tissue cannot be detected on the surface electrocardiogram, but it can be identified by local leads in close proximity to these structures. There is general agreement that ventricular depolarization begins on the left side of the interventricular septum, near the central portion. This is followed in as little as 1 to 2 msec by depolarization on the right side of the septum, and by depolarization near the tip of the right ventricle (Fig. 6-4A). The mean vector for the first 5 to 10 msec of ventricular depolarization has a direction which is anterior, to the right, and either inferior or superior. The most consistent feature is its anterior direction, probably representing the consistency of earlier left septal depolarization and the anterior position of the right ventricle. These first vectoral forces are responsible for the initial "Q" loop of the vectorcardiogram, which is consistently anterior when viewed in the horizontal plane.

The orientation of these early forces in the supero-inferior direction is much less consistent and is related to the direction of the body of the QRS loop. In subjects in whom the mean QRS is horizontal, the initial forces are usually inferiorly directed, producing a counterclockwise QRS loop in the frontal plane. With a vertical mean QRS, the initial forces are usually superiorly directed, and the frontal QRS loop is thus written in a clockwise direction. Disturbance of this expected relationship is occasionally an alerting feature, suggesting previous myocardial infarction.

The scalar electrocardiogram also reflects these early forces. The anterior direction produces a constant R wave in the early precordial leads (see Figs. 6-5 and 6-6). The variable supero-inferior direction is reflected in the occurrence of "normal" Q waves in all standard limb leads from time to time in normal subjects. The relationship between early forces and mean QRS direction is again useful. Q waves in leads II and III, reflecting a superior orientation of early forces, are not unusual with a vertical mean QRS vector, but they would be unusual enough to demand explanation with a horizontal mean QRS vector. Similarly, inferiorly directed early forces producing a Q wave in leads I and AVL are usual with a horizontal QRS vector but unusual with a vertical QRS vector. These *normal* Q waves are usually of short duration, less than 0.02 sec, but may occasionally reach 0.04 sec and become confused with *abnormal* Q waves associated with myocardial infarction. This is especially frequent in association with a commonly encountered nonpathologic conduction variant, called the $S_1S_2S_3$ type of conduction disturbance, which will be discussed below.

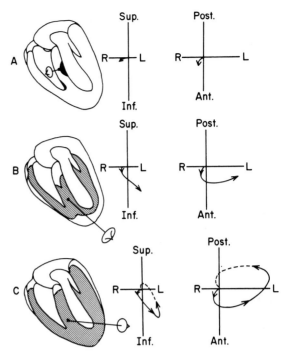

Fig. 6-4. Ventricular activation and the vectorcardiogram. *A, B,* and *C* represent depolarization at three stages: early, mid, and late. To the right of each is a representation of the resultant electrical force at this stage as seen in the frontal- and horizontal-plane vectorcardiograms.

The size of normal initial forces is extremely variable, but they are generally more prominent in young subjects and become more attenuated in older age groups. In the horizontal plane vectorcardiogram, for example, in an older man large anterior forces are highly suggestive of an old posterior myocardial infarct, yet they are not abnormal in a young man, especially when there is an $S_1S_2S_3$ type of conduction disturbance (see Figs. 6-6 and 6-17).

The depolarization of the interventricular septum occurs as a double envelopment, from both left and right sides toward the center and toward the base. At the same time, depolarization of the free walls is proceeding from endocardium to epicardium. The resultant vectoral forces are represented by the outward, or efferent, limb of the QRS loop, and have an orientation to the left, inferiorly and slightly anteriorly (Fig. 6-4B). Associated with the breakthrough of depolarization on the epicardial surface of the right ventricle, there is increasing dominance of vectoral forces directed from endocardium to epicardium in the left ventricular free wall. These forces are more posteriorly oriented, and the afferent limb of the QRS loop has a pos-

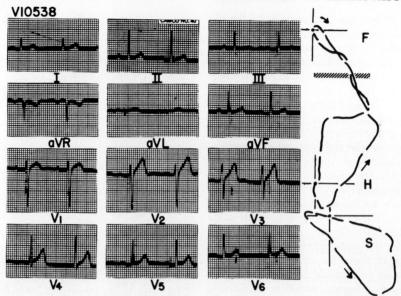

Fig. 6-5. Normal electrocardiogram and vectorcardiogram. A normal 28-year-old male. The initial forces are almost directly anterior and do not produce Q waves in leads I, II, or III. In this and subsequent examples, tracings of the QRS loop of the vectorcardiogram are seen to the right, each plane being identified as *F* (frontal), *H* (horizontal), and *S* (left sagittal). The interruptions are spaced at 0.01-sec intervals. The shaded bar on each figure indicates the distance equivalent to 1 mv.

terior orientation, though it is generally still oriented to the left and inferiorly (Fig. 6-4*C*). These forces account for the initial positive, then negative configuration of the precordial leads.

The last area of the ventricles to be depolarized is the posterobasal region, and the vectoral forces resulting from depolarization of this area are gen-

erally directed to the right, superiorly and posteriorly.

Some normal persons demonstrate an exaggeration in the size of these terminal forces. This normal conduction variant is termed the $S_1S_2S_3$ type of conduction disturbance (Fig. 6-6). It is also seen in mild right ventricular hypertrophy, but it is

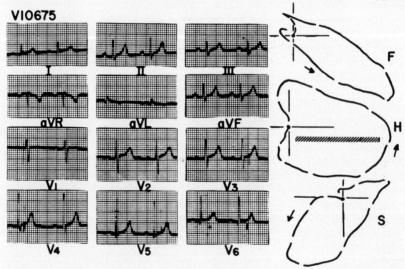

Fig. 6-6. Normal $S_1S_2S_3$ type of conduction. A normal 31-year-old male. Note that the terminal QRS loop is prominent and is posterior and superior in position. In this example, there is no S in lead I, since the terminal force is directly superior. Note the prominence of the initial anterior forces in the horizontal plane, and compare with the prominent anterior forces in Fig. 6-17.

not diagnostic of any etiologic form of heart disease. QRS loops of the $S_1S_2S_3$ type have smaller maximum vectors than other normal loops and tend to be counterclockwise in direction.

Ventricular Hypertrophy

One of the most frequent reasons for obtaining an electrocardiogram is to determine whether or not ventricular hypertrophy is present, or to determine the relative degree of left and right ventricular hypertrophy.

The identification of hypertrophy from the electrocardiogram is not simple. Those ECG parameters which we use for this purpose are probably not specifically altered by the presence of hypertrophy. For example, there is no correlation between heart weight and QRS amplitude in hearts less than 400 to 450 Gm in total weight.[11] The amplitude begins to correlate with heart weight only when the heart becomes definitely enlarged. The available evidence indicates that the electrical activity of the individual myocardial unit is not altered by hypertrophy,[12] so it seems likely that the observed effects are related to (1) an altered sequence of depolarization and repolarization (altered endocardial-epicardial sequence), (2) an altered relationship between the depolarization and repolarization of one ventricle with respect to the other ventricle (altered phase relationships between large areas), (3) an alteration in the anatomic relationship of the heart to the recording electrodes (proximity or rotational effect), or (4) a combination of these effects. The problem is compounded by the frequent coincident occurrence of hypertrophy with emphysema and/or pleural or pericardial fluid. These considerations do not help in the interpretation of an individual ECG, but they do help us understand the frequent false-negative and occasional false-positive electrocardiographic diagnoses of left or right ventricular hypertrophy.

Left Ventricular Hypertrophy

There are certain differences between the progression of the ECG and VCG abnormalities in hypertrophy associated with a pressure-type overload (systolic overload) and that associated with a volume-type overload (diastolic overload). As has been emphasized by Cabrera and coworkers,[13] these differences are of considerable diagnostic importance, especially in the child or young adult. In the adult, these differentiating features are less specific but nevertheless useful.

In pressure overload, the QRS loop becomes larger and is displaced posteriorly and to the left (see Fig. 6-7). There is also a change in the initial forces, as well as in the configuration of the loop. The initial forces, which are normally to the right

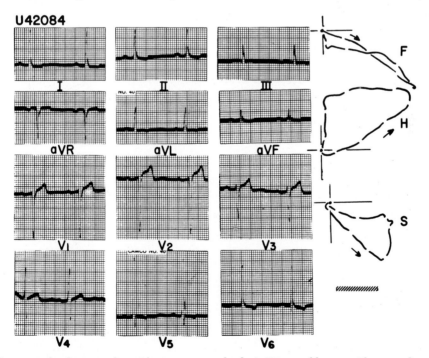

Fig. 6-7. Left ventricular hypertrophy with pressure overload. A 32-year-old man with severe hypertensive cardiovascular disease. The early forces move to the left, and the Q wave is diminutive in leads I and V_6. Note that the ST-T wave changes of left ventricular strain are present.

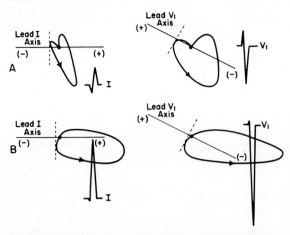

Fig. 6-8. Influence of position of initial force on size of Q and R waves. *A.* A normal frontal-plane QRS loop (on the left) and left sagittal loop (on the right), showing the projection of initial forces on lead I and lead V_1 axes. In the frontal plane, the initial force projects on the negative side of the axis of lead I, producing a Q wave proportional to the distance from the origin of the loop to the dotted line. In the sagittal plane, the initial force projects on the positive side of the V_1 axis, thus producing an R wave proportional to the distance from the origin to the dotted line. *B.* A left ventricular hypertrophy loop, showing how a change in orientation of initial forces produces a smaller Q wave in lead I and a smaller R wave in V_1.

and anteriorly, are shifted inferiorly. These forces may be larger than normal initial forces when measured on the VCG, yet because of the directional change, the projection of these forces on lead I and the right precordial leads is reduced, as seen in Fig. 6-8. The Q wave becomes smaller in lead I, and the R wave becomes smaller in V_1 and V_2 (see Fig. 6-8). With more advanced degrees of left ventricular hypertrophy, the initial forces shift into the left lower quadrant, so that there is no Q wave in lead I. There are also a prolongation of conduction time and a change in the configuration of the body of the QRS loop, so that it assumes a figure-of-eight configuration in the horizontal plane, similar to that seen in left bundle branch block (Fig. 6-9).

These changes are reflected in the scalar electrocardiogram in the following ways. There is an increase in QRS amplitude, which is most readily appreciated in the precordial leads. The R wave becomes taller in leads V_5 and V_6, and the S wave becomes deeper in V_1, V_2, and V_3. The Q wave tends to become smaller in leads I and V_6, and the R wave tends to become smaller in V_1, reflecting the change in initial forces mentioned above. The mean QRS vector moves to the left and posteriorly, and the QRS duration becomes somewhat prolonged. With advanced, long-standing hypertrophy, and usually after congestive heart failure

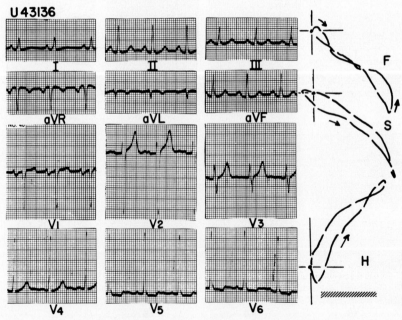

Fig. 6-9. Severe left ventricular hypertrophy. A 24-year-old man with rheumatic heart disease, severe aortic insufficiency, and mild aortic stenosis. Note that the horizontal loop (below) shows a figure-of-eight configuration very similar to that seen in left bundle branch block (Fig. 6-13).

has supervened, the configurational change in the body of the loop mentioned above becomes apparent and is reflected in the scalar electrocardiogram by a further delay in the QRS duration and a prolonged intrinsicoid deflection time as measured in leads V_5 and V_6.

The S-T segment of the electrocardiogram becomes altered, probably as a result of disturbances in the pathway of conduction and the duration of the depolarized state, rather than as a result of a current of injury. The vectoral direction of the S-T segment shift is opposite to that of the mean QRS vector and is often accompanied by a similar shift in the direction of the mean T vector. This shift of the S-T segment is called left ventricular strain, a term which is ill chosen physiologically but which is well established in usage.

Volume (or diastolic) overload eventually results in the same changes as does pressure overload, but there are differences along the way which are worthy of note. First, the shift in direction of the initial forces of the QRS loop is not so striking, and the initial forces may become larger in their normal direction. This at times results in an accentuation of the normal Q waves in leads I, V_5, and V_6 of the scalar electrocardiogram (see Fig. 6-10). Next,

the ST-T wave changes are much delayed, and the T waves may become somewhat larger while maintaining a normal direction. In such cases the normally upright precordial T waves become larger and somewhat peaked.

The establishment of a hard set of criteria for the ECG diagnosis of hypertrophy is difficult, since any criteria which aim at a high degree of sensitivity will erroneously diagnose hypertrophy in a large proportion of normal persons, particularly in the younger age group. The following criteria for the ECG diagnosis of left ventricular hypertrophy have been useful, but it should be realized that sensitivity has been sacrificed to attain increased specificity.

The ECG findings of left ventricular hypertrophy are given a point "score." The point score is totaled for each electrocardiogram and is used for weighing the certainty of the diagnosis. The scoring system is as follows:

1. Amplitude criteria: presence of one or more of the following = 3 points.
   Largest R or S wave in limb leads $\geq$ 20 mm.
   Largest S wave in V_1, V_2, V_3 $\geq$ 25 mm.
   Largest R wave in V_4, V_5, V_6 $\geq$ 25 mm.

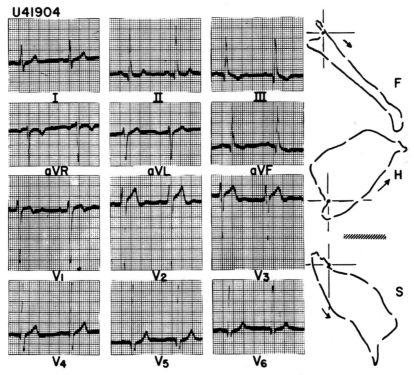

Fig. 6-10. Left ventricular hypertrophy with volume overload. A 22-year-old man with rheumatic heart disease and aortic insufficiency. The QRS amplitude is large in the electrocardiogram (S wave, 30 mm in V_2) and in the vectorcardiogram. Note that the initial forces remain prominent in the loop and in the ECG (Q in V_5, V_6). Also note that the T vector is in a normal direction.

2. S-T segment criteria:

Any S-T segment shift with a vectoral direction opposite to mean QRS *in the absence of digitalis* = 3 points.

If digitalis *has* been administered, ST-T segment typical of "left ventricular strain" (sloping contour, S-T and T vectors opposite to mean QRS vector) = 1 point.

3. Axis criteria:

Left axis deviation $\geqq -15°$ = 2 points.

4. Duration criteria:

QRS duration $\geqq 0.09$ sec = 1 point.

Intrinsicoid deflection in V_5 or $V_6 \geqq 0.04$ sec = 1 point.

The maximum possible score is 10 points, which is only rarely attained. A score of 5 or more points is interpreted as indicating left ventricular hypertrophy. A score of 4 points is interpreted as probably indicative of left ventricular hypertrophy. In use, most "points" are scored on amplitude criteria, but the use of the scoring system does not permit a definite ECG interpretation with this as a sole criterion.

It should be emphasized that this is a score,

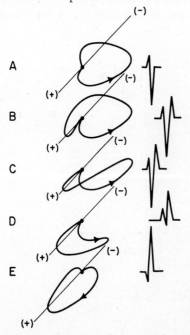

Fig. 6-11. Horizontal QRS loop and lead V_1 with right bundle branch block and increasing right ventricular hypertrophy. *A.* A normal horizontal QRS loop, showing the axis of V_1 and the resulting V_1 complex to the right. *B.* A horizontal-plane QRS loop in right bundle branch block, with the axis of V_1 and the resulting V_1 complex. *C, D,* and *E.* Increasing degrees of right ventricular hypertrophy. Note that with each step the loop becomes abnormal at an earlier point in the loop. In *E,* the loop is abnormal from its outset.

which is a part of the first phase of interpretation, as mentioned in a previous section. A physician would be foolish to disregard the presence of high QRS amplitude in the ECG of a patient with aortic stenosis, for example, even though it does not reach a diagnostic point score. Phase 2 interpretation would include the fact that many patients with distinct left ventricular hypertrophy have normal ECGs, and in this setting high amplitude alone would have both diagnostic meaning and therapeutic implications.

Right Ventricular Hypertrophy

As in left ventricular hypertrophy, there are differences in the evolution of pressure and volume overload of the right ventricle. As with left ventricular hypertrophy, these differences are more specific in the younger age groups.

Pressure overload produces a change in the rotation and configuration of the QRS loop, so that it becomes clockwise and "open" as viewed in the frontal plane. It also becomes directed to the right and anteriorly. The scalar counterparts of these changes in the loop are as follows: the mean QRS axis moves to the right, so that lead I becomes more negative than positive. The clockwise rotation produces a small Q wave in lead III and an R-S configuration in lead I. The broad open character of the loop is reflected in the diphasic character of the limb leads. The anterior shift is reflected in a predominantly upright QRS in leads V_1 and V_2.

Volume overload is more likely to cause incomplete or complete right bundle branch block, in which the initial forces are in a relatively normal position but the terminal forces are directed rightward and anteriorly, producing an S wave in leads I and V_6, and a terminal R' deflection in V_1 and V_2.

The following empirical rules, as set forth by Milnor,[14] are useful in the diagnosis of right ventricular hypertrophy in the adult, when the QRS duration is less than 0.12 sec.

1. Right axis deviation of more than +110°.

2. An R or R' wave in V_1 of 5 mm or greater, with an R/S ratio in V_1 of 1.0 or greater.

These rules are applicable to tracings with an R' in V_1, as long as the QRS duration is less than 0.12 sec.

The vectorcardiogram has been particularly helpful in assessing the degree of right ventricular hypertrophy in those tracings with R' waves in V_1 and V_2. The degree of right ventricular hypertrophy is roughly correlated with the point in time at which the forces forming the loop begin to deviate from their normal or expected position (see Fig. 6-11). In complete or incomplete right bundle branch block in the absence of right ventricular hypertrophy, as occasionally occurs in otherwise normal persons, the abnormal forces occur very late, as the loop approaches the point of origin. In more severe grades of right ventricular hypertrophy the loop becomes abnormal quite early in its course, turning anteriorly as viewed in the horizontal plane, so that the terminal loop is written in a clockwise instead of counterclockwise direction. The duration of the QRS loop (whether complete or incomplete right bundle branch block) seems to be less helpful than the configuration in deciding whether or not right ventricular hypertrophy is present. With more severe grades of right ventricular hypertrophy, the loop becomes abnormal from the outset, the initial forces being directed posteriorly, and the entire loop being written in a clockwise direction in the frontal plane (see Fig. 6-12).

The scalar leads are less useful than the vectorcardiogram in the assessment of the degree of RVH in cases of incomplete or complete right bundle branch block probably because phase relationships play an important role in production of the loop abnormalities and these are not readily appreciated from sequentially recorded scalar leads. However, with marked RVH as described above, in which the QRS loop is abnormal from its outset, the abnormality can be readily identified from scalar leads. The QRS is tall and upright in V_1 and is preceded by a small Q wave. This picture is unusual in volume overload, unless right ventricular hypertension approaching systemic levels has supervened.

There is a third form of an abnormal QRS loop which can be seen in right ventricular hypertrophy. Occasionally an exaggerated form of the $S_1S_2S_3$

type of conduction disturbance is the only manifestation. In the vectorcardiogram, this differs from the $S_1S_2S_3$ configuration, seen in a large number of "normal" individuals, in several respects. The loop tends to be clockwise and more "open" in the frontal plane. The terminal forces in the horizontal plane are larger than usual and may be larger than the forces forming the body of the QRS loop. A posteriorly directed T loop, the VCG counterpart of "right ventricular strain," is occasionally seen. The ECG features of this group are as implied in the term "$S_1S_2S_3$ type of conduction disturbance." There are deep S waves in leads I, II, and III, with a biphasic character to the QRS complexes in all limb leads and in the left precordial leads. This configuration is not diagnostic of any cause of RVH, but in the younger age groups it is more often seen with tetralogy of Fallot, and in the adult it is more often seen with mitral stenosis, the obesity cardiopulmonary syndrome (Pickwickian syndrome), and chronic lung disease.

It is necessary to emphasize that occasional patients with well-developed right ventricular enlargement manifest none of the ECG changes of right ventricular hypertrophy, again emphasizing the fallibility of the method and the need for an intelligent "phase-2" interpretation.

Ventricular Conduction Disturbances

A discussion of conduction disturbances, if extended, could well include most of electrocardiographic interpretation. As implied in a previous section, it is likely that a large part of the changes of

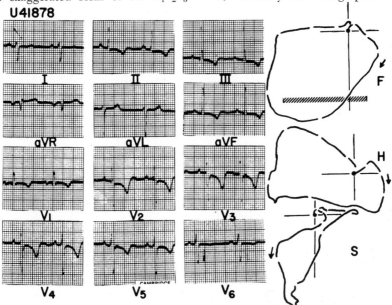

Fig. 6-12. Severe right ventricular hypertrophy. A 39-year-old man with an atrial septal defect and pulmonary hypertension. Note that the horizontal loop shows an initial posterior QRS, followed by a clockwise, anterior QRS.

ventricular hypertrophy are related to altered conduction. Myocardial infarction also manifests itself as a conduction disturbance. This section will include those conduction disturbances which are not specifically covered in other paragraphs.

A brief classification of conduction disturbances is as follows:

I. Classic bundle branch blocks
   A. Left bundle branch block
      1. Complete
      2. Incomplete
   B. Right bundle branch block
      1. Complete
      2. Incomplete
II. Peripheral or parietal blocks
   A. Peri-infarction block
   B. Parietal block (must be further classified as to cause, if known)

The classic bundle branch blocks are usually assumed to be related to a specific lesion in one of the major (left or right) divisions of the bundle of His. In an extensive study, Lenègre[15] found such lesions in a high percentage of cases of left bundle branch block (75 per cent of cases) and right bundle branch block (96 per cent of cases), but hypertrophy of the respective ventricle was also frequently seen. Incomplete left bundle branch block was associated with a similar high incidence of lesions of the left bundle branch, but in incomplete right bundle branch block, only 25 per cent of cases were found to have lesions of the right conduction system. Right ventricular enlargement was found in 93 per cent of the cases of incomplete

right bundle branch block. Thus an impressive number of specific conduction system lesions was found, but the possibility remains, on the basis of these same studies, that ventricular hypertrophy is also in some manner related to this electrocardiographic picture, especially in incomplete right bundle branch block.

Left Bundle Branch Block

In left bundle branch block, the QRS duration is prolonged beyond 0.12 sec. As viewed in the QRS loop (see Fig. 6-13), the slowing is in the midportion and in the returning (afferent) limb. The vectorcardiographic configuration is very characteristic. The early forces are anteriorly directed, but, in contrast to the normal, they consistently move toward the left in the frontal plane, thus producing no Q wave in scalar leads I and V_6. The body of the frontal-plane QRS loop is generally to the left of its normal position in the left inferior quadrant, but marked left axis deviation is not usually found, either in the vectorcardiogram or in the scalar electrocardiogram. The terminal forces are also to the left.

The horizontal loop moves anteriorly, then sharply reverses its direction and moves posteriorly. This posterior movement is followed by a rightward and anterior movement, which is considerably slowed, forming the characteristic figure-of-eight loop of this conduction disturbance. The scalar counterparts of this disturbance are easily correlated with the loop. There is a small but consistent R wave in the right precordial leads, followed by a deep, prolonged S wave, with considerable slurring. In the left precordial leads, there is usually

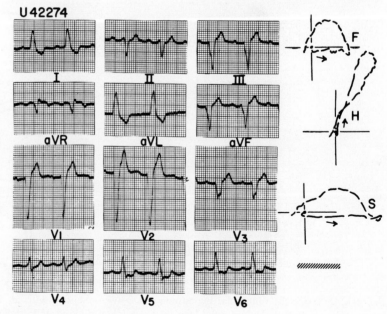

Fig. 6-13. Left bundle branch block. A 67-year-old man with a history of diabetes mellitus and an episode of precordial pain and diaphoresis about 2 weeks before this record. The record shows left bundle branch block, the only unusual feature being the presence of striking left axis deviation. Note the small but definite anterior QRS forces in the horizontal and sagittal QRS loops, and the small R wave in V_1 and V_2

no Q or S wave, but a broad, upright, slurred R wave.

The mechanism of production of these loop and scalar lead abnormalities is not completely clear. One would expect, for example, that with a block of the left bundle branch, the earliest forces would be written from right to left, and from anterior to posterior. As seen above, the right-to-left direction fits the observations, but the expected posterior direction of earliest forces is *not* seen. This is presumed to be a result of early depolarization of some portion of the right ventricle, probably the anterior paraseptal region. The abrupt posterior movement of the efferent limb of the QRS loop is felt to represent septal depolarization from the right ventricular to the left ventricular surface. The anatomic position of the ventricles is such that this would fit the observed direction. The last portion of the loop is felt to be formed by forces arising from the free wall of the left ventricle.

The significance of left bundle branch block in a given person rests on other historical and physical data, but statistically, a high percentage of patients (probably 95 per cent) with this condition are found to have serious heart disease such as valvular disease, hypertension, or coronary artery disease. The presence of a myocardial infarct with left bundle branch block is difficult to detect but is occasionally suggested by marked left axis deviation, by the absence of the expected early anterior forces (no initial R wave in right precordial leads), or by the presence of large rightward and inferior initial forces (a Q wave in leads I and AVL).

Secondary T-wave abnormalities are expected to occur in uncomplicated left bundle branch block. By using the ventricular gradient concept, it is occasionally possible to recognize T-wave abnormality in the presence of left bundle branch block; the combination suggests that the left bundle branch block is complicated by an additional ischemic process. In uncomplicated left bundle branch block the mean ST vector should parallel the mean T vector. Occasionally myocardial infarction complicating left bundle branch block can be recognized when the mean ST vector is not found in the expected position in relationship to the mean T vector.

Incomplete left bundle branch block is less well defined in usage, yet it is frequently encountered. Occasionally one has the opportunity to follow the vectorcardiographic course of left ventricular hypertrophy as it gradually evolves into a picture identical with that of left bundle branch block, yet without the expected slowing of the midforces and the afferent limb. In the scalar leads, this same evolution is manifest as a gradual prolongation of QRS duration to 0.10 or 0.11 sec, with a delay in the intrinsicoid deflection time in V_5 or V_6. This is felt to be incompelte left bundle branch block. As implied, it usually develops as a result of left ventricular hypertrophy (97 per cent of Lenègre's 37 cases) (see Fig. 6-9).

Right Bundle Branch Block

As stated in the previous discussion, right bundle branch block is seen in right ventricular hypertrophy, especially of the volume-overload variety. Although this is true, a view from another perspective is indicated. In the younger person, right ventricular hypertrophy is commonly associated with right bundle branch block, either complete or incomplete. In the older age group (40 years and up), coronary artery disease becomes the most likely cause. The QRS duration also has a relationship to the underlying etiologic factor. Those tracings with a QRS duration of over 0.12 sec are more likely to be related to coronary artery disease than those of 0.12 sec or under.

Some observers feel that complete right bundle block is present when the QRS duration exceeds 0.11 sec. Others feel that a QRS duration of over 0.09 sec indicates complete right bundle branch block. In evaluating right ventricular hypertrophy, this is largely an academic point, since the vectorcardiographic configurational changes are the same in incomplete and complete block. As stated above, a very long QRS duration has a higher statistical chance of being related to degenerative heart disease. It is common for complete right bundle branch block to occur following surgical closure of ventricular septal defect.

The common feature of vectorcardiographic loops with right bundle branch block is a terminal force which is directed to the right and anteriorly (see Fig. 6-14). The initial and midforces are in a more or less normal position in the uncomplicated example, but they may be deviated anteriorly in right ventricular hypertrophy. Leftward deviation of the midforces (producing left axis deviation in the frontal plane) generally indicates the coincident presence of left ventricular disease, usually of the degenerative variety.

In uncomplicated right bundle branch block, the initial forces are normal, the midforces are normal, and only the terminal forces are abnormal. These are written slowly and are directed anteriorly and to the right, characteristically forming an R′ configuration in V_1 and V_2 and a broad S wave in V_5 and V_6. The rightward terminal force direction as viewed in the frontal plane produces an S wave in leads I and II, and a terminally positive or isoelectric complex in lead III. Leftward terminal forces, producing a deep broad S wave in lead III

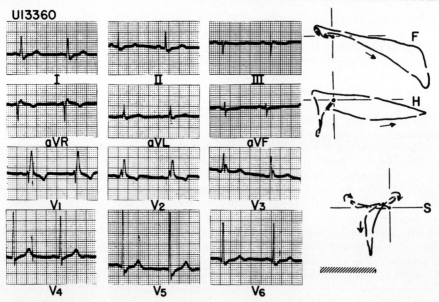

Fig. 6-14. Right bundle branch block. A 68-year-old man, known to have moderate hypertension (170/90), but with no cardiovascular complaints. Note that the horizontal-plane loop becomes abnormal very late in its course. The frontal-plane QRS loop is unusual in that the initial forces are superior in spite of a horizontal QRS loop. There was no history in this patient of previous chest pain.

are more likely to be associated with left ventricular disease.

Peripheral or Parietal Blocks

In 1950, First, Bayley, and Bedford [16] described a form of conduction disturbance, peri-infarction block, which occurred with myocardial infarction and which could be confused with the classic bundle branch blocks. The characteristics were as follows: (1) an initial QRS deformity of an infarct, (2) a QRS duration of 0.11 sec or greater, and (3) terminal forces opposite in direction to the initial forces (directed toward the infarct). This abnormality was felt to be due to a disturbance in the usual outward spread of depolarization in the region of the infarct, rather than to a lesion in the central conduction system.

In 1956, Grant [17] pointed out that left axis deviation of greater than −30° was associated, in a large percentage of cases, with diffuse myocardial fibrosis or myocardial infarction. In later publications,[1] he concluded that if left axis deviation was accompanied by a wide angle (greater than 110°) between initial and terminal forces, myocardial infarction was the most common cause. He recognized that other forms of heart disease, such as severe left ventricular hypertrophy, could cause left axis deviation of this type, but he felt that in view of the frequency of myocardial infarction in association with this abnormality, this was most often a form of parietal block related to infarction (a form

of peri-infarction block). As experience has grown, an increasing number of other causes has been recognized for left axis deviation, with and without a wide initial-terminal angle. Among them are idiopathic myocardial hypertrophy, scleroderma heart disease, cardiac amyloidosis, progressive muscular dystrophy, etc. In view of the varieties of heart disease with this ECG abnormality but with different origins, it is felt that the term *peri-infarction block* should not be used to describe this entity but should be restricted to the abnormality reported by First, Bayley, and Bedford as described above. The term *parietal block*, with a proposed causative factor, seems more appropriate (such as "parietal block due to coronary artery disease," "parietal block due to scleroderma heart disease," etc.). In most cases, the cause is suggested by ancillary historical or physical examination data, rather than by the electrocardiogram.

Myocardial Infarction

The most consistent and most striking electrical alteration produced by a myocardial infarction is a change in the initial forces so that they move away from the area of the infarct. Current electrocardiographic theory associates the initial forces with depolarization of the midseptal area; thus it becomes very difficult to explain observed alteration of these forces in the absence of septal involvement by the infarct. The usual "window" theory postulates that the lack of forces from an infarcted area allows normal forces from the opposite wall to dominate, deviating the resultant electrical activity away from the infarcted area. This fails to account for the fact that the abnormality is manifest before depolarization reaches the free wall of the left ventricle. This explanation would better explain abnormalities of the mid- and terminal forces; yet these forces, when altered, tend to move toward the infarct (peri-infarction block).

The explanation may lie in an alteration of the conduction system by the infarction, producing a different sequence of ventricular depolarization from that at its outset. Robb[18] has suggested that the conduction system does not derive its blood supply from the muscle through which it passes, but that it carries its own blood supply. It is possible that an occlusion of an anterior descending artery producing an anterior infarct might, at the same time, produce a lesion in a specific portion of the conduction system which derives its blood supply from this vessel, thus accounting for the consistent ECG picture and the early alteration in the QRS forces.

In addition to the initial QRS abnormalities of an infarct, terminal QRS abnormalities are also frequently seen, as has been discussed under "Peripheral and Parietal Blocks." S-T segment and T-wave alterations are also seen. They are felt to be related to the areas of injury and ischemia surrounding the area of dead tissue. The vectoral direction of the S-T segment shift is toward the area of infarction; the T-vector direction is away from this area. These force abnormalities have an expected sequence of appearance and disappearance, which allows a rough approximation of the age of an infarct. These expected sequences are summarized in the following table.

It may be seen that a given ECG, showing QRS and S-T segment abnormalities, but no T-wave reversal is likely to be a hyperacute infarct, less than 24 hr old. An ECG showing initial QRS and T-wave changes but no S-T segment shift is likely to be more than 6 weeks old, etc. It is emphasized that these are average sequences, and that a given case might deviate strikingly from the expected pattern.

The direction of the abnormal forces in an infarct is related to the position of the infarct, which may be in any area of the left ventricle. Right ventricular and atrial infarcts occasionally occur as a part of a left ventricular infarct, but they are very unusual as isolated entities. Thus the variety of locations of infarcts, and the resultant ECG or VCG patterns, is almost endless. The location of the infarct is determined by plotting the direction of the abnormal forces and determining the area of the left ventricle which fits the force abnormality. Several locations occur with relative frequency; they will be briefly discussed in order to emphasize the relationship between area of infarct and the abnormality and between the vectorcardiogram and electrocardiogram. The reader is referred to other sources for a more complete discussion.[19]

Anteroseptal infarcts are so named because they involve the anterior wall and the anterior portion of the interventricular septum. As viewed in the QRS loop (see Fig. 6-15), the initial forces move posteriorly from the outset, and the usual anterior "Q" loop is not seen in the horizontal and sagittal plane. The ECG is characterized by an absence of the usual R wave in V_1, V_2, and V_3.

Anterolateral infarcts are characterized by initial forces which move to the right and posteriorly, away from the anterior free wall of the left ventricle. In the horizontal plane the QRS loop usually moves anteriorly, then to the right and posteriorly, forming a clockwise initial loop (see Fig. 6-16). In the electrocardiogram, the rightward direction of the initial forces is seen as a Q wave in leads I and AVL. In the precordial leads the R wave may be present in V_1 and V_2, but disappears in the more lateral V leads, so that a broad Q wave with a Q-S or Q-R complex is seen in V_4, V_5, or V_6.

"Posterior" infarcts are usually posteroinferior in location, and the initial forces are displaced superiorly and anteriorly (see Fig. 6-17). The superior projection is seen as a clockwise rotation with a large superior "Q" loop in the frontal-plane vectorcardiogram, and the anterior projection is seen as an exaggeration in the size of the anterior "Q" loop in the horizontal and sagittal planes. In the electrocardiogram, these abnormalities present as a large Q wave in leads II, III, and AVF and as an unusually broad R wave in the right precordial leads.

Lesser degrees of coronary artery disease may produce one of several other ECG pictures, ranging from a widening of the QRS-T angle due to myocardial ischemia to S-T segment deviation due to subendocardial ischemia and injury. A wide QRS-T angle may develop in an asymptomatic person and remain for years without other developments, but it may also develop in the setting of symptoms of coronary artery disease. The most frequently encountered direction of the T vector is

Table 6-1. APPEARANCE AND DISAPPEARANCE OF THE ELECTROCARDIOGRAPHIC ABNORMALITIES ASSOCIATED WITH MYOCARDIAL INFARCTION

Abnormality	Appears	Disappears
Initial QRS	Immediately	Years to never
S-T segment	Immediately	3–6 weeks
T wave	In 6–24 hr	Months to years

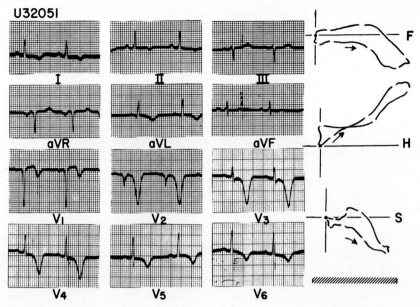

Fig. 6-15. Anteroseptal myocardial infarct. A 49-year-old man with a classical history of chest pain 1 month prior to this record. Note the immediate posterior movement of the early forces in the hoorizontal- and sagittal-plane loops, and the QS complexes in V_1 and V_2.

inferior and anterior, producing flat or inverted T waves in leads AVL, I, V_5, and V_6.

Subendocardial injury usually appears in a dramatic clinical setting, e.g., with anginal pain, shock, pulmonary embolism, or similar castrophic events.

The mechanism by which these changes are produced is obscure, but under such circumstances small petechial hemorrhages are often seen in the subendocardial layers of both ventricles and in the tips of the papillary muscles. The changes are usu-

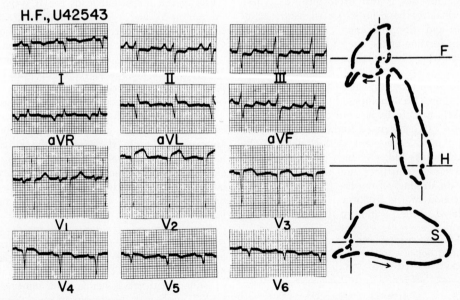

Fig. 6-16. Anterolateral myocardial infarct. A 48-year-old man with a history consistent with a myocardial infarct about 4 months prioor to this record. The QRS loop is so distorted that the mean axis is rightward in the frontal plane. Note the counterclockwise direction oof the horizontal loop, and the loss of R waves from V_2 through V_6.

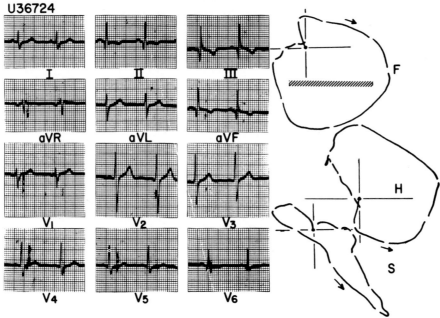

U36724

Fig. 6-17. Posteroinferior myocardial infarct. A 46-year-old man with a history of an infarct 1 year previously. Note the superioor direction of initial forces in the frontal and sagittal planes, foroming a Q in leads II, III, and AVF. These forces are also seen to be anterior in the horizontal and sagittal loops.

ally transient, disappearing in a few hours. The direction of the S-T segment vector is rightward, superior, and anterior, so that S-T segment depression is seen in leads I, II, III, and in V_5 and V_6. Morphologically the junction between the QRS and S-T segment ("J" point) is depressed and the depression is relatively uniform over the S-T segment, in contrast to the sloping and sagging S-T segment contours of left ventricular strain and digitalis effect.

The persistence over a period of days of the electrocardiographic picture of subendocardial injury developing in a setting such as those described above is characteristic of subendocardial infarction, which usually involves the whole inner shell of the left ventricle. The lack of changes in the initial QRS forces is a remarkable feature of such infarcts; it may be explained by postulating, as previously, a separate blood supply to the conduction tissue.

Miscellaneous

Pericarditis is characterized by the appearance of S-T segment shift with a vectoral direction toward the left, inferior, and anterior. This is felt to be related to the presence of a thin shell of myocardial injury in the subepicardial layers. In the ECG this is manifest as an elevated S-T segment in limb leads I, II, and III, and in V_5 and V_6. This S-T segment shift is characteristically short-lived, disappearing over a period of 2 or 3 days and being

followed by a shift in the vectoral direction of the T wave away from the left side—usually toward the right shoulder. There are no QRS changes, except for the occasionally encountered diminution in amplitude secondary to pericardial fluid.

Pulmonary embolism changes many parts of the electrocardiogram. The cardiac rate rises, and arrhythmias (especially atrial fibrillation) occasionally appear. The QRS loop is altered so that it becomes broad, clockwise, and displaced to the right. Subendocardial injury is produced, with its characteristic S-T segment shift, and the T vector is displaced posteriorly and to the left. The QRS-loop alterations may produce Q waves in leads III and AVF, where none existed previously, and right axis deviation. The T-vector shift may produce T-wave inversion in leads V_1 to V_3. None of these findings can be considered diagnostic, but as a "constellation" they are very helpful in confirming a clinical impression of pulmonary embolism.

Drugs are among the more frequent causes of electrocardiographic abnormalities. Digitalis produces an S-T segment deviation with a vectoral direction to the right, superior and anterior, similar to that produced by subendocardial injury. This change is accompanied by a shortened Q-T interval and a diminution in the size of the T wave. Quinidine produces a prolonged Q-T interval, and if the level is in the toxic range, a prolongation of the QRS interval.

REFERENCES

1. Grant, R. P.: "Clinical Electrocardiography: The Spatial Vector Approach," McGraw-Hill Book Company, New York, 1957.
2. Frank, E.: An Accurate, Clinically Practical System for Spatial Vectorcardiography, *Circulation,* 13:737, 1956.
3. Schmitt, O. H., and Simonson, E.: The Present Status of Vectorcardiography, *A.M.A. Arch. Int. Med.,* 96:574, 1955.
4. McFee, R., and Parungao, A.: An Orthogonal Lead System for Clinical Electrocardiography, *Am. Heart J.,* 62:93, 1961.
5. Wilson, F. N., Johnson, F. D., and Kossman, C. E.: The Substitution of a Tetrahedron for the Einthoven Triangle, *Am. Heart J.,* 62:93, 1961.
6. Duchosal, P. W., and Sulzer, R.: "La vectorcardiographie," S. Karger, Basle, 1949.
7. Grishman, A., and Sherlis, L.: "Spatial Vectorcardiography," W. B. Saunders Company, Philadelphia, 1952.
8. Craige, E., and Harned, H. S.: Phonocardiographic and Electrocardiographic Studies in Normal Newborn Infants, *Am. Heart J.,* 65:180, 1963.
9. Macruz, R., Perlof, J. K., and Case, R. B.: A Method for the Electrocardiographic Recognition of Atrial Enlargement, *Circulation,* 17:882, 1958.
10. Morris, J. J., Estes, E. H., Jr., Whalen, R. E., Thompson, H. K., and McIntosh, H. D.: P Wave Analysis in Valvular Heart Disease, *Circulation,* 29:242, 1964.
11. Carter, W. A., and Estes, E. H., Jr.: Electrocardiographic Manifestations of Ventricular Hypertrophy; A Computer Study in 319 Cases, *Am. Heart J.,* 68:173, 1964.
12. Uhley, H. N.: Study of the Transmembrane Action Potential, Electrogram, Electrocardiogram and Vectorcardiogram in Rats with Left Ventricular Hypertrophy, *Am. J .Cardiol.,* 7:211, 1961.
13. Cabrera, E. C., and Monroy, J. R.: Systolic and Diastolic Overloading of the Heart. II. Electrocardiographic Data, *Am. Heart J.,* 43:669, 1952.
14. Milnor, W. R.: Electrocardiogram and Vectorcardiogram in Right Ventricular Hypertrophy and Right Bundle Branch Block, *Circulation,* 16:348, 1957.
15. Lenègre, J.: Contribution à l'étude des blocs de branche comportant notamment les confrontations électriques et histologiques, *Arch. mal. coeur,* Suppl. 1, 1957.
16. First, E. R., Bayley, R. H., and Bedford, D. R.: Peri-infarction Block: Electrocardiographic Abnormality Occasionally Resembling Bundle Branch Block and Local Ventricular Blocks of Other Types, *Circulation,* 2:31, 1950.
17. Grant, R. P.: Left Axis Deviation, *Circulation,* 14:233, 1956.
18. Robb, J. S.: The Conducting Tissue and Cardiac Electrophysiology, *Ann. New York Acad. Sc.,* 65:818, 1957.
19. Hugenholtz, P. G., Forkner, C. E., and Levine, H. D.: A Clinical Appraisal of the Vectorcardiogram in Myocardial Infarction. II. The Frank System, *Circulation,* 24:828-850, 1961.

7 RADIOLOGIC EXAMINATION OF THE HEART

*H. Stephen Weens, M.D., and
Brit B. Gay, Jr., M.D.*

Since the discovery of the roentgen rays, radiologic procedures have made many important contributions to the study of the normal and abnormal heart. The earliest methods developed, fluoroscopy and roentgenography, still remain essential in the general evaluation of cardiac disease. Subsequently, more specialized radiologic methods were introduced which further clarified certain anatomic and physiologic changes of the cardiovascular system. With recent efforts to keep somatic and gonadal radiation exposure at a necessary minimum, our concepts of the relative merits of individual x-ray methods have changed to some extent. The procedures which are considered important or essential can be selected only with sound clinical judgment.

The following are the more commonly used principal radiologic methods:

1. *Teleoroentgenography.* Roentgenograms taken at sufficient distance depict the cardiac contours in great detail and provide adequate information about heart size and configuration, as well as anatomic changes of individual heart chambers. If the esophagus is opacified with contrast medium, displacement of this organ by adjacent structures, such as the left atrium or the aorta, may be readily recorded.

Teleoroentgenograms should be obtained in the upright position, with the exposure of the film at the end of normal inspiration. A distance of 72 in., or 150 to 200 cm, is usually selected, to reduce magnification of the heart by the divergent x-ray beam. At these distances, magnification of the heart is small (5 to 10 per cent) and may be disregarded. The radiation exposure of the thorax is less than that expected with cardiac fluoroscopy, and gonadal radiation exposure is insignificant.

2. *Fluoroscopy.* The fluoroscopic examination of the heart should be carried out with the fluoroscopic image intensifier. The greater brightness levels of this fluoroscope permit better perception of detail in the presence of reduced radiation ex-

posture. As already emphasized, roentgenograms appear entirely satisfactory for the evaluation of cardiac size and configuration.

Fluoroscopy possesses, however, certain advantages which make it an essential procedure in the study of certain phases of heart disease. The amplitude of the heart borders and the pulsation of the aorta and pulmonary artery may be readily observed. Cardiac calcifications are recognized with greater ease on account of their characteristic motion. With the fluoroscope, motility of other thoracic structures, such as the mediastinum and diaphragm, is readily studied, and detection of small pleural fluid collections is facilitated.

3. *Cineradiography.* A permanent record of all fluoroscopic observations may be obtained with cineradiographic equipment. A movie record depicting only a limited number of cardiac cycles may provide very complete information with regard to all cardiac activities in various projections. One of the most important uses for cineradiography appears to be, however, its application to angiocardiography.

4. *Angiocardiography.* Conventional radiographic and fluoroscopic examinations have distinct limitations, as they permit only the contours of the cardiac surface to be evaluated. The introduction of angiocardiography has brought about one of the greatest advances in cardiac diagnosis as it renders the cardiac chambers, heart valves, large vessels, and coronary vessels directly visible in the living organism.

In spite of considerable progress in the development of safer contrast media, angiocardiography is not entirely without risk and cannot be regarded as a routine procedure. It has to be carefully selected and devised for solution of specific radiologic problems.

Though the injection of contrast medium by the intravenous route (intravenous angiocardiography) has provided significant information about many anatomic and physiologic features of the heart and large vessels, it has been largely replaced by selective angiocardiography. In this method the contrast medium is directly injected into the individual heart chambers or large vessels through a catheter. The advantages of the selective method are that the bolus of contrast medium can be injected as close as feasible to the area of interest, and that the segment of the heart under special investigation is not obscured by other opacified cardiac and vascular structures.

For successful selective angiocardiography, meticulous attention to detail is required. An adequate bolus of contrast medium cannot be administered unless a proper injection speed is attained. For these reasons injection pressure, concentration and viscosity of contrast medium, and catheter dimensions have to be taken into proper consideration.

Another prerequisite for successful angiocardiography is a suitable system which records x-ray images in rapid sequence in order to depict the full range of cardiac activities. Large-size films obtained with rapid biplane film changers provide without question a maximum of anatomic detail. The disadvantage of large-film angiocardiography is, however, the cumbersome apparatus, as well as the film expense.

In many institutions single or biplane angiocardiography with cineradiographic apparatus has yielded entirely acceptable information. The apparatus is less complicated, and a greater number of x-ray images is readily obtained. Frequently the demonstration of intracardiac shunts is accomplished with less difficulty than with large-size film angiocardiography.

Though angiocardiography in practically all instances is carried out with the aid of iodinated water-soluble compounds, carbon dioxide has found limited applications as a contrast medium in the demonstration of the right atrium, particularly in the study of pericardial effusion. Special precautions have to be taken to retain the gas in the right atrium until it is absorbed in the bloodstream.

5. *Tomography.* The principal application of cardiac tomography is in the analysis of various types of cardiac calcifications. With this method, the extent and position of the calcifications can be determined with reasonable accuracy. This has been found to be of particular value in the preoperative study of valvular and pericardial diseases.

CARDIAC MENSURATION

Since the introduction of roentgen methods into the diagnosis of heart disease, considerable effort has been spent to determine heart size under normal and pathologic conditions. Generally, those methods which attempt to establish a relationship between the transverse diameter of the heart with the transverse diameter of the chest (cardiothoracic ratio) are found to be of limited value, as body build is not taken into proper consideration.

Mensuration techniques which correlate the cardiac dimensions with individual weight and height or body surface provide more meaningful information. In the presence of borderline values, heart size alone should not be a determining factor in the establishment of heart disease, as there is an overlap of normal and pathologic values. Nevertheless, if cardiac size is properly appraised in relation to the type of heart disease under study, important information as to the degree and prognosis of heart disease may be obtained.

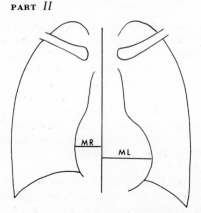

Fig. 7-1. Measurement of transverse diameter of heart. The transverse diameter equals the sum of the midright (*MR*) and midleft (*ML*) measurements.

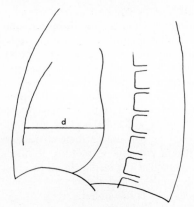

Fig. 7-3. The measurement of cardiac depth (*d*) as determined in the lateral projection.

The following methods have been found to be of practical value in the determination of heart size:

1. Correlation of the transverse diameter of the heart with height and weight. The transverse diameter of the heart is determined from teleoroentgenograms by drawing a line midway between the medial ends of the clavicles. Perpendicular lines from the midline to the most lateral portions of both heart borders are termed the midright (MR) and midleft (ML) diameters (Fig. 7-1). The total transverse diameter of the heart is the sum of these two measurements, and may be correlated with normal values in tables established by Ungerleider and Clark for various heights and weights. The transverse diameter of the heart in normal persons will rarely exceed 10 per cent of the predicted values.*

2. The frontal area of the heart. The frontal area

of the heart as determined by planimetry may be correlated with height and weight. As the upper and lower margins of the heart area would have to be arbitrary, the frontal area of the heart may be calculated from the formula $A = \pi/4 \times l \times b$. The letter l represents the longitudinal diameter of the heart measured from the junction of the right atrium and superior vena cava to the apex of the heart (Fig. 7-2). The letter b represents the diameter of the heart represented by a perpendicular to the long diameter of the heart extending from the right cardiophrenic angle to the left upper heart border. Measurements of the heart area may be evaluated with the aid of nomograms correlating cardiac area with height and weight.

3. Heart-volume determinations. Most methods of heart-volume determination are based on formulas originally proposed by Rohrer and Kahlstorf. A practical method of heart-volume determination from teleoroentgenograms has been established by Jonsell, utilizing the long (*l*) and broad (*b*) diameters of the heart in the frontal plane as well as the cardiac depth in the sagittal plane (*d*) (Fig. 7-3).

Amundsen, introducing slight modifications of the formula employed by Jonsell and others, has evaluated the merits of the relative heart volume (relative heart volume = heart volume per square meter of body surface) under normal and pathologic conditions. The formula employed in his calculations was $V = K \times l \times b \times d$. The value for K was fixed at 0.4, taking into consideration the ellipsoid shape of the heart and certain magnification corrections on teleoroentgenographic measurements.

On the basis of his studies, three groups of individuals could be established (Table 7-1).

The group with hearts that are not enlarged will include normal persons, but also patients who have

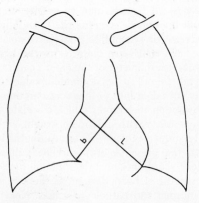

Fig. 7-2. The broad (*b*) and long (*l*) diameters of the heart.

* These tables may be obtained from the Picker X-Ray Corporation, White Plains, N.Y.

Table 7-1. RELATIVE HEART VOLUMES

Heart size	Male, ml/m²	Female, ml/m²
Not enlarged	<500	<400
Borderline	500–540	450–490
Enlarged	>540	>490

hypertension without coronary artery disease and some milder pathologic cardiac states. The immediate likelihood of congestive heart failure is small in these individuals, and prognosis is generally good. If congestive heart failure is present, it will usually be found in association with myocardial infarction, mitral stenosis, corpulmonale, or, rarely, constrictive pericarditis.

In the group with definitely enlarged hearts, all hearts are considered to be diseased. These patients usually exhibit signs of congestive failure or are very likely to develop it. Exceptions to these rules are patients with aortic insufficiency, certain types of mitral valvular disease, myocardial aneurysm, and pericardial effusion.

THE NORMAL CARDIAC CONTOUR

Posteroanterior Projection (PA). In this projection the patient's chest faces the x-ray cassette or fluoroscopic screen.

From the diaphragm upward the right cardiac border is formed by the right atrium and superior vena cava, the junction of which may be indicated by a distinct angle (Fig. 7-4A and B). Only in the presence of marked elongation or dilatation does the aorta participate in the formation of the right upper cardiac and mediastinal border. On deep inspiration a small triangular shadow, cast by the inferior vena cava, is frequently visible in the region of the angle between the right side of the diaphragm and the right atrium.

On fluoroscopy the right border of the heart shows a slight inward motion synchronous with the more pronounced inward motion of the left lower heart border. As atrial and ventricular pulsations are superimposed in this region, the motion of the right border of the heart is difficult to analyze.

The left border of the heart consists usually of three well-defined segments. The most superior segment consists of the aortic knob, which represents that portion of the aortic arch observed in an end-on projection. Below the aortic arch the pulmonary artery and/or its main descending branch form a well-defined segment of the left border of the heart. The tip of the left auricle may extend to the left border of the heart at the inferior aspect of the pulmonary artery segment. The left ventricular wall forms the lowest segment of the left cardiac margin. The motion of the left ventricle is inward on systole, opposite to the outward pulsation of the pulmonary artery segment and aortic knob. This change of the direction of cardiac amplitude creates at the junction of the pulmonary artery segment and the ventricular segment a point of opposite pulsation which may serve as an important anatomic landmark. The left cardiophrenic angle is often occupied by a small triangular shadow, representing the epicardial fat pad of the heart.

Right Anterior Oblique Projection (RAO). In this projection the patient's right axilla faces the x-ray cassette or fluoroscopic screen.

The posterior border of the heart is formed from below upward by the inferior vena cava in continuity with the right atrium (Fig. 7-5A and B). At a slightly higher position the shadow of the left atrium is visible; it overlaps the posterior border of the right atrium. The space between the atria and the spine (retrocardiac space) appears clear and is occupied by mediastinal structures such as the esophagus. In the upright position the esophagus pursues a fairly straight course or one that curves gently backwards along the posterior surface of the heart in this projection. As the esophagus lies adjacent to the posterior wall of the left atrium, dilatation of this chamber readily dislodges this structure from its normal position.

Anteriorly, the heart border is formed above the

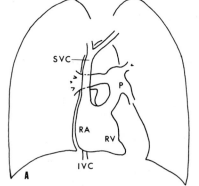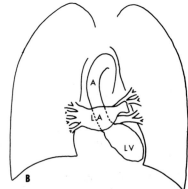

Fig. 7-4A and B. Posteroanterior projection (PA) of the normal heart. The cardiac contours are shown in relation to the heart chambers and large vessels. SVC, superior vena cava; IVC, inferior vena cava; RA, right atrium; RV, right ventricle; P, pulmonary artery; LA, left atrium; LV, left ventricle; A, aorta.

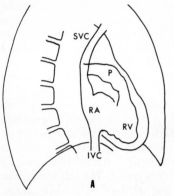

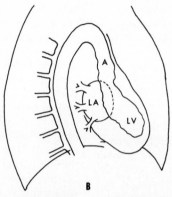

Fig. 7-5A and B. Right anterior oblique projection (*RAO*). For explanation of symbols, see Fig. 7-4A and B.

diaphragm by the right ventricle, though in slighter degrees of rotation the left ventricle may also participate in the formation of the lower anterior cardiac segment. More superiorly, the outflow tract of the right ventricle in continuity with the pulmonary artery makes up the anterior heart border in this projection.

Left Anterior Oblique Projection (LAO). In this projection the left axilla of the patient faces the x-ray cassette or fluoroscopic screen.

Superiorly the aortic arch and, to some extent, also the arch of the pulmonary artery form the upper portion of the cardiac shadow (Fig. 7-6A and B).

The posterior portion of the heart is formed from below upward by the left ventricle and left atrium; often at the junction of left atrium and ventricle an indentation is visible, the so-called atrioventricular groove. Along the posterosuperior aspect of the left atrial shadow the air-filled left main bronchus is distinctly visible in this projection.

The anterior border of the heart in the left anterior oblique projection is formed from below upward by the right ventricle and right atrium, above which the overlapping outlines of the pulmonary artery and ascending aorta blend with the superior mediastinum.

Left Lateral Projection. In this projection the chest wall of the patient's left side faces the x-ray cassette or fluoroscopic screen (Fig. 7-7A and B).

Anteriorly the heart border is formed by the superimposed right atrium and right ventricle, though that segment of the anterior cardiac margin below the vascular pedicle of the heart is largely atrial in character. The posterior cardiac surface consists of the posterior wall of the left ventricle below and the left atrium above. Between the left side of the diaphragm and the left ventricle a clear space is often visible, the so-called posteroinferior recess, in which the shadow of the inferior vena cava may be seen. Enlargement and displacement of the ventricle may obliterate this recess.

CARDIAC ENLARGEMENT

One of the most important radiologic signs of cardiac abnormality is a change of the cardiac configuration or an enlargement of the heart shadow. Cardiac enlargement may be generalized or may affect predominantly individual heart chambers. For a systematic analysis of cardiac diseases, it is most helpful to recognize those radiologic patterns which may be attributed to enlargement of individual atria or ventricles. Admittedly, criteria established in the past for enlargement of heart chambers have certain limitations, as angiocardiographic or surgical observations have shown. Nevertheless, they serve in many instances as useful guides to roentgen diagnosis of heart disease. The physician should realize, however, that in conventional radiologic examina-

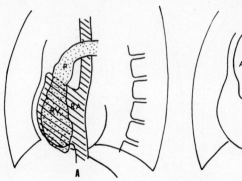

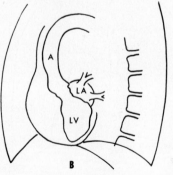

Fig. 7-6A and B. Left anterior oblique projection (*LAO*). For explanation of symbols, see Fig. 7-4A and B.

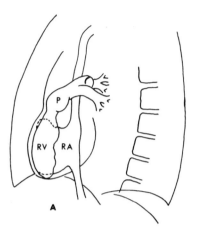
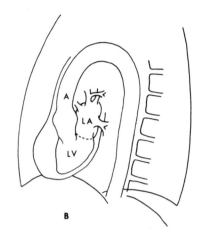

Fig. 7-7A and B. Left lateral projection of heart. For explanation of symbols, see Fig. 4-A and B.

tions the diagnosis of heart-chamber enlargement is largely inferred from changes in the configuration of the cardiac surface. If more precise radiologic volume determinations of the heart chambers are desired, angiocardiographic studies have to be performed. Further difficulties are introduced by the fact that in the presence of ventricular enlargement, cardiac rotation may take place, which in itself will contribute to changes of cardiac configuration.

LEFT VENTRICULAR ENLARGEMENT

Minor degrees of left ventricular hypertrophy do not produce significant changes in the cardiac configuration. With increasing enlargement of the left ventricle, particularly its outflow tract, the border of the left side of the heart becomes progressively rounded and more convex and the distance from the point of opposite pulsation to the cardiac apex becomes increased. The lower left border of the heart may extend more to the left side, and the cardiac apex appears depressed, extending below the level of the diaphragm (Fig. 7-8A). With progressive left ventricular enlargement, posterior bulging of the left ventricle may be demonstrated in the left anterior oblique and lateral projections (Fig.

7-8B). Normally, on rotation into the left anterior oblique position, the posterior aspect of the left ventricle will clear the spine at angles of 60° or less. In the presence of marked left ventricular enlargement, the left ventricle may overlap the spine even in full left lateral position. The posteroinferior recess of the heart may likewise be obliterated by the enlarged left ventricle. It is noteworthy, however, that obliteration of the posteroinferior recess of the heart in the lateral view may also be caused by other conditions, such as downward extension of a markedly enlarged left atrium and distension of the pericardial sac as the result of fluid formation.

RIGHT VENTRICULAR ENLARGEMENT

Anterior bulging of the region of the right ventricular outflow tract in the oblique projections and lateral views is considered evidence of right ventricular enlargement (Fig. 7-9A). On the frontal projection little change in the cardiac configuration may develop, but prominence of the pulmonary artery segment of the border of the left side of the heart serves as a valuable indirect sign of right ventricular changes (Fig. 7-9B). It is rare to find right ventricular enlargement not accompanied by these changes in the pulmonary artery. The promi-

Fig. 7-8. A. Left ventricular enlargement (PA). The left ventricle bulges downward and to the left. B. Left ventricular enlargement (LAO). The enlarged left ventricle does not clear the spine and extends downward.

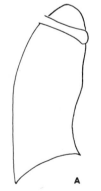
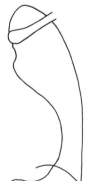
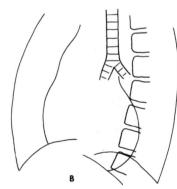

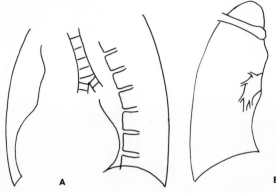
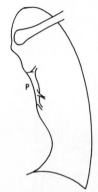

Fig. 7-9. *A*. Right ventricular enlargement (*LAO*). Anterior bulging of the heart into the retrosternal space. *B*. Right ventricular enlargement (*PA*). Prominence of pulmonary artery segment (*P*) and dilatation of main branches of pulmonary arteries as indirect signs of right ventricular enlargement.

nence of the pulmonary artery segment along the left border of the heart is usually accentuated by rotation of the heart to the left in the presence of right ventricular enlargement. In patients with mitral stenosis, anterior bulging of the right ventricle in the oblique and lateral projections may be attributed to some extent to the forward displacement of the right ventricular chamber by the enlarged left atrium.

ENLARGEMENT OF THE LEFT ATRIUM

The left atrium occupies the posterior aspect of the cardiac mass and does not ordinarily participate in the formation of the left or right borders of the heart. Enlargement of the left atrium is characteristically indicated by a posterior bulge of the dorsal heart surface. This posterior expansion of the heart at the level of the left atrium may be demonstrated to advantage in the lateral and right anterior oblique position by posterior displacement of the opacified esophagus. One should keep in mind, however, that opacification of the esophagus is not always necessary to demonstrate this phenomenon. Attempts should be made to delineate the posterior surface of the heart in the same way as the right and left borders of the heart. With more marked degrees of left atrial enlargement this chamber may extend beyond the right border of the heart, lead-

ing to the development of a double contour (Fig. 7-10A and B). As the left atrium distends it may form a separate arc between the pulmonary artery segment and left ventricle. Occasionally the dilated left atrium may assume gigantic proportions, extending actually to the chest walls.

In mitral stenosis prominence of the pulmonary artery segment is caused not only by pulmonary artery dilatation, but also by displacement of this vessel by the dilated left atrium. Rotation of the heart to the left further contributes to these changes in cardiac configuration.

As enlargement of the left atrium dislodges the esophagus posteriorly, displacement of this organ may be demonstrated in both the right anterior oblique and lateral views (Fig. 7-11A and B). In the frontal projection the esophagus may be found to be displaced to the right side at the level of the atrium, although in a few cases deviation of the esophagus to the left side will be observed, usually in association with tortuosity of the aorta.

As the left atrium is situated just below the tracheobronchial angle, dilatation of this chamber may cause a widening of the tracheal bifurcation. Elevation of the left main bronchus is best observed in the posteroanterior and left anterior oblique projections (Figs. 7-10A and B, 7-12A and B). In young persons, in addition to elevation of the left main bronchus, deformity of the left main bronchus may take place; it is indicated by a shal-

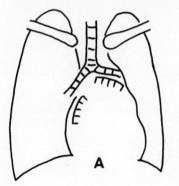
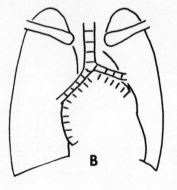

Fig. 7-10. *A*. Moderate and marked dilatation of the left atrium in the posteroanterior projection. The left main bronchus is markedly elevated. In *B* the enlarged left atrium extends beyond the border of the right side of the heart.

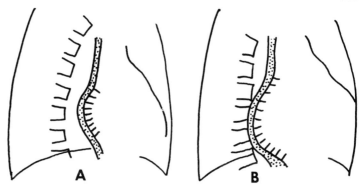

Fig. 7-11. Moderate and marked degrees of left atrial enlargement as seen in the right anterior oblique projection. The left atrium displaces the opacified esophagus posteriorly.

low indentation of the left bronchus along its inferior aspect.

ENLARGEMENT OF THE RIGHT ATRIUM

Enlargement of the right atrium manifests itself by displacement and bulging of the right border of the heart to the right side (Fig. 7-13A). In the left anterior oblique projections, distension of the atrium is indicated by anterior bulging of the cardiac silhouette in the supradiaphragmatic portion (Fig. 7-13B). The roentgen diagnosis of enlargement of the right atrium is, however, subject to many errors, as this chamber may be readily displaced by other cardiac structures. A more precise determination of right atrial enlargement is often impossible without contrast visualization.

CARDIAC CALCIFICATIONS

Radiologic methods play an all-important role in the recognition of cardiac and pericardial calcifications. Though some of these calcifications may be of little clinical importance, others are most significant in the diagnosis and classification of heart disease. Experience has shown that fluoroscopy with image intensification, tomography, and cineradiography are superior methods for the detection of these calcifications.

Coronary Artery Calcifications

The calcifications observed on radiologic examination consist of small flecks of plaques, often arranged in two parallel lines or in tubular form (Fig. 7-14). Calcification of the left coronary artery occurs about three times as often as that of the right artery, and the circumflex branch of the left coronary artery is most frequently involved. In a large series of patients above the age of 55, Jorgens found an incidence of coronary artery calcification in over 30 per cent of patients, as determined by cineradiographic studies. Though coronary artery calcifications may exist in the absence of any clinical and electrocardiographic abnormalities, the presence of ischemic heart disease and myocardial infarction is more common in this group of patients. The movement of the coronary artery calcification occurs in synchronism with the movements of the cardiac surfaces, which should aid in the differentiation of coronary artery calcification from other types of calcification.

Left Atrial Calcification

Calcification may develop in the wall of the left atrium or in an organized thrombus and occurs nearly always in association with severe mitral valvular disease of long duration. The endocardial calcification is most commonly found along the poste-

Fig. 7-12. Left atrial enlargement in the left anterior oblique projection. Elevation and inferior indentation of the left main bronchus by the dilated atrium.

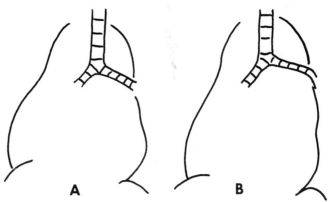

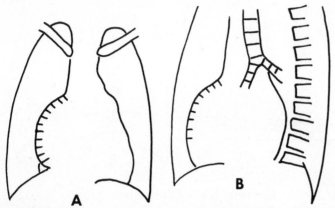

Fig. 7-13. Right atrial enlargement. In the posteroanterior projection, a marked bulging of the right border of the heart into the right lung field is noted. In the left anterior oblique projection the heart extends anteriorly into the retrosternal space.

rior aspect of the atrial wall above the posterior mitral leaflet. Radiologically, these calcifications appear as curvilinear densities confined to the wall of the left atrium, as demonstrated in the standard projections (Fig. 7-15).

If the calcification has a laminated character, a calcified mural thrombus should be suspected, though it is not always possible to differentiate between thrombus and endocardial calcification. In some cases, calcified atrial thrombi have shown a striking dancing motion on fluoroscopy.

Calcification in Cardiac Tumors

In very few instances, cardiac tumors have exhibited striking calcification on fluoroscopic and roentgenographic examination. These calcifications appear to occur most commonly in myxomas and are then found within the confines of the atrial chambers, usually on the left side. The motion of the calcification will be synchronous with the heart action (Fig. 7-16A and B). Differentiation of a calcified myxoma from a calcified thrombus appears, however, difficult or impossible.

Pericardial Calcification

In nearly one-half of patients with constrictive pericarditis, pericardial calcifications can be demonstrated radiologically, a finding which may be de-

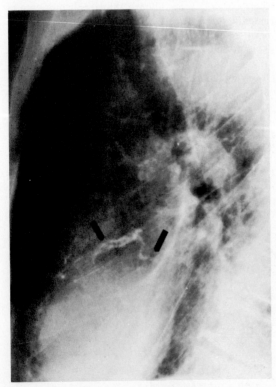

Fig. 7-14. Calcification of coronary arteries (anterior descending branch and circumflex branch of left coronary artery).

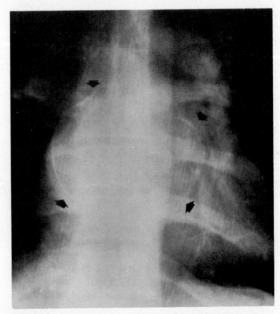

Fig. 7-15. Extensive curvilinear calcifications of the dilated left atrium.

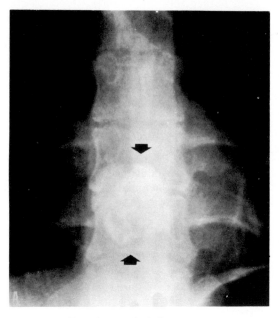
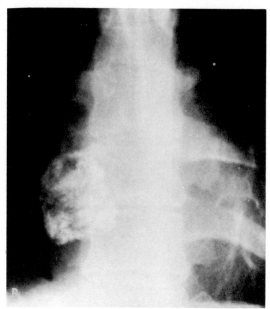

Fig. 7-16. Calcified myxoma of the right atrium in atrial systole and atrial diastole.

cisive in the establishment of a clinical diagnosis (Fig. 7-17A and B). It is noteworthy, however, that pericardial calcifications are also sometimes found in persons without any clinical evidence of constrictive pericarditis. Most commonly, pericardial calcifications are found along the diaphragmatic aspect of the ventricles, from which location they may extend to the region of the atria and atrioventricular groove. Occasionally, the differentiation from

calcific myocardial calcification is difficult. Myocardial calcifications are usually deeper within the outline of the heart and anatomically confined to one ventricle or cardiac septum.

Myocardial Calcifications

Myocardial calcifications are usually secondary to arteriosclerotic heart disease and may occur following myocardial infarction or in conjunction with

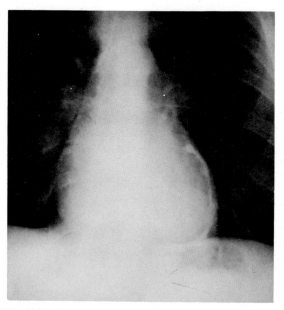
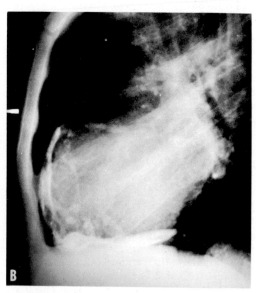

Fig. 7-17. Constrictive pericarditis with extensive pericardial calcification as demonstrated in posteroanterior and lateral views.

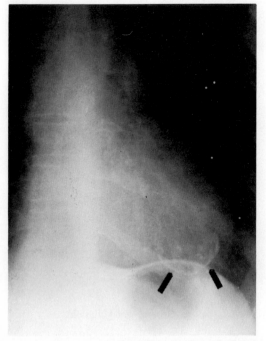

Fig. 7-18. Myocardial calcification in the region of the apex of the left ventricle. History of myocardial infarct.

ventricular aneurysm. Calcifications appear most commonly in the region of the apex of the left ventricle and are usually associated with abnormal pulsations of the adjacent heart border (Fig. 7-18).

Valvular Calcifications

With rare exception valvular calcifications are found in the mitral and aortic valves. Most authors accept that calcification of the leaflets of the mitral valve is nearly always caused by rheumatic infection whereas calcification of the mitral annulus is most often degenerative in character. There appears to be more controversy concerning the cause of aortic valvular calcification. Evidence has been presented that both inflammatory as well as degenerative processes may play an important role in the aortic valvular changes (Fig. 7-19). In some instances, congenital defects of the aortic valve, such as bicuspid aortic stenosis, predispose to calcification of the aortic valve.

On fluoroscopy, heart valves display an unusual degree of motility synchronous with the cardiac cycle, far exceeding the surface activity of the heart.

It is important to differentiate calcification of the mitral leaflet from that of the mitral annulus (Fig. 7-20A and B). Calcification found in the mitral annulus is usually smooth, dense, and homogeneous. The calcified structure has a diameter much larger

than that of the mitral orifice and usually assumes a J- or U-shaped pattern. If a nearly complete ring-like calcification is observed, involvement of the membranous septum has to be postulated, a condition frequently associated with conduction defects. On the other hand, calcification in the leaflets of the mitral valve is more irregular, patchy, and nodular in character (Fig. 7-23B). If the calcification is extensive, it may resemble a small string of beads.

The position of the heart valves may be of considerable aid in separating calcification of the aortic valve from that of the mitral valve. On the postero-anterior projection, the aortic valve occupies a more cranial position, close to the spine; the mitral valve appears lower and somewhat more laterally to the left (Fig. 7-21A). In the left anterior oblique projection the aortic valve is found in the middle third of the cardiac shadow, whereas the mitral valve assumes a more dorsal position, close to or within the posterior third of the cardiac mass (Fig. 7-21B).

It is noteworthy that the position of the heart valves is subject to considerable variations which may be attributed to displacement of the valvular planes by enlargement of individual heart chambers.

THE LUNGS IN HEART DISEASE

Perhaps the most important contribution of the roentgenologic examination of the chest in a cardiac patient is the demonstration of physiologic alterations in the pulmonary circulation. The vascular

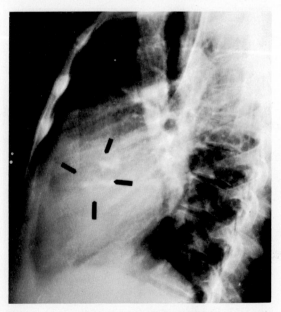

Fig. 7-19. Calcification in calcific aortic stenosis. The patient had a bicuspid aortic valve.

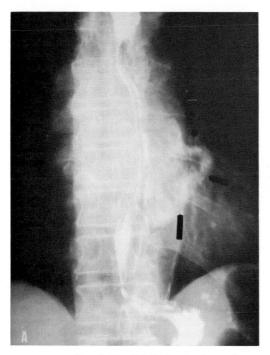
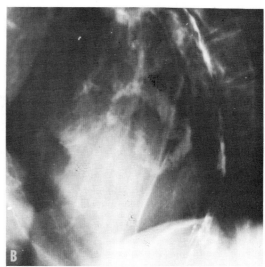

Fig. 7-20. Calcified mitral annulus in anteroposterior and lateral projections.

shadows in the frontal roentgenogram of the chest are produced by the pulmonary arteries and veins as they extend into the various pulmonary segments. The major "comma" shadow in each hilus is produced by the descending branch of the pulmonary artery, from which arise the smaller segmental branches to the lower and middle lobes (Fig. 7-22B). On the right side, the descending pulmonary artery branch measures normally in the adult between 9 to 16 mm in greatest transverse diameter on a conventional roentgenogram of the chest. The segmental arteries at the lung bases average 2 to 4 mm in size. The ratio of the size of the central to the peripheral arterial shadows varies between 3:1 and 5:1. The pulmonary veins in the lower lobe of the right lung can be traced to the right border of the heart. These venous shadows are more horizontal in position and are medial to the major arterial trunks. The upper lobe pulmonary venous shadows, however, are lateral to the major arterial branches in the superior part of the hilar shadow. This difference in position of the vascular shadows aids in differentiating arterial from venous trunks. The inferior two-thirds of the hilar shadow on the chest roentgenogram is produced by the arterial trunks; the upper one-third of the hilar shadow is produced by the major superior pulmonary veins.

The greatest amount of information can be obtained when the pulmonary vascular shadows are interpreted in terms of physiologic alterations in the pulmonary circulation. The major changes in the pulmonary circulation are related to pulmonary

Fig. 7-21. A. Diagram of the position of the heart valves in the posteroanterior projection. B. Diagram indicating position of the aortic and mitral valves in the left anterior oblique projection.

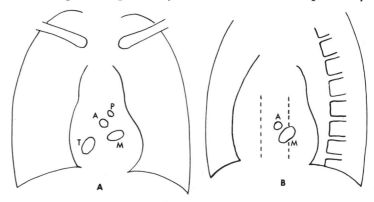

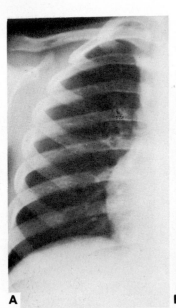 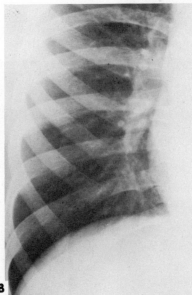 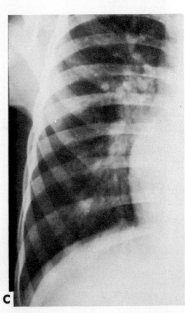

Fig. 7-22. *A.* Roentgenologic pattern of decreased pulmonary blood flow. Pulmonary arterial and venous shadows are small generally. Patient has tetralogy of Fallot. *B.* Normal pulmonary blood-flow pattern in patient with co-arctation of the aorta. *C.* Roentgenologic pattern of increased pulmonary blood flow associated with large ventricular septal defect. Note the enlargement of pulmonary arteries and veins centrally and peripherally.

arterial and venous pressure, pulmonary blood flow, and pulmonary edema.

PULMONARY VENOUS HYPERTENSION

The first roentgenologic change which occurs following an increase of the pulmonary venous pressure above the maximum mean normal of 10 mm Hg is dilatation of the pulmonary venous shadows, which can be seen as enlarged vascular trunks in the superior lateral aspect of the hilus and horizontal vascular shadows along the margin of the right side of the heart inferiorly and behind the heart shadow in the lower field of the left lung. In the more chronic forms of pulmonary venous hypertension (as in mitral stenosis, chronic left ventricular failure, left atrial tumor, and cor triatriatum), with mean pressures near 18 mm Hg, a different roentgenologic pattern is seen. The superior pulmonary veins become prominently dilated; the inferior pulmonary veins are normal or constricted (Fig. 23A and B). This asymmetry between the superior and inferior pulmonary venous shadows results in the "antler pattern" of the hilar shadows so frequently seen in mitral stenosis. This pattern has been explained on the basis of vasoconstriction in the lower lobes with redirection of blood flow into the upper lobes. The mechanism of this change has been discussed by Simon. The venous dilatation in the

upper lobes is the result of the effect of increased pressure and increased regional blood flow. As the pulmonary venous pressure exceeds the oncotic pressure of the blood, edema fluid accumulates in the tissues of the lungs.

Pulmonary edema is of two types: (1) alveolar and (2) interstitial. Alveolar edema occurs most often in an acute left-sided heart failure and is characterized roentgenographically by bilateral confluent lung densities in the central lung fields (butterfly wing pattern of consolidation). Interstitial edema results from more chronic elevation of pulmonary venous pressure or from incipient left ventricular failure. The edema fluid accumulates in the interstitial tissues of the lung and results in several roentgenologic changes. Edema fluid in the perivascular tissues of the lung produces haziness and clouding of the vascular shadows, which lose their sharp definitions. The background density of the lung is increased, giving the lung a "cloudy" appearance. When the fluid collects in the interlobular septums of the lung, septal lines can be seen roentgenographically. These lines, originally described by Kerley, appear as sharply demarcated linear densities in the lung base perpendicular to the pleura (Fig. 7-24), or they may be more centrally located, in which case they are longer and may be seen coursing in any direction. These septal lines can be produced by any process which thickens the

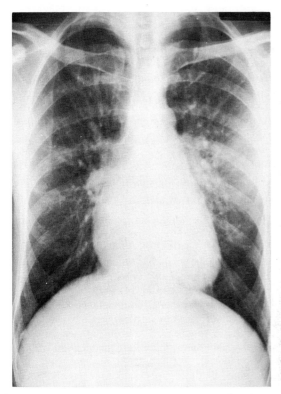 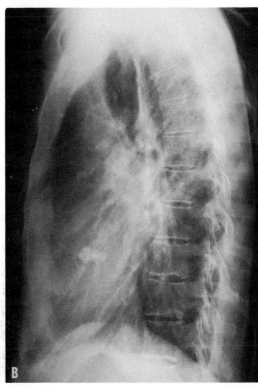

Fig. 7-23. *A.* Patient with mitral stenosis and pulmonary venous hypertension. Note the enlarged superior pulmonary veins in association with constriction of the lower lobe vascular shadows. *B.* Lateral roentgenogram of the same patient showing the enlarged left atrium and calcification of the mitral valve.

interstitial septal tissue planes (e.g., fibrosis, tumor infiltrate, edema fluid, or inflammatory infiltrate). Any cause of pulmonary edema may produce septal lines roentgenologically.

In more chronic forms of heart failure, pleural fluid may accumulate in small amounts, blunting the costophrenic sulci or thickening the shadows of the interlobar fissures. Sometimes this pleural change may be seen only in the lateral roentgenogram of the chest. Accumulation of edema fluid beneath the visceral pleura may simulate the roentgenographic appearance of free pleural fluid in the lateral costophrenic sulci.

PULMONARY ARTERIAL HYPERTENSION

When the pulmonary arterial pressure is increased, certain characteristic roentgenologic changes are produced in the pulmonary vascular pattern of the lungs. The causes of pulmonary arterial hypertension are many and are considered in more detail in Chap. 48, Pulmonary Hypertension. Elevated pulmonary artery pressure most commonly follows pulmonary venous hypertension and is referred to as secondary or postcapillary pulmonary arterial hypertension. In the group of patients with this condition, the lungs roentgenographically will show the changes of pulmonary venous hypertension discussed above, in addition to the changes in the pulmonary arterial pattern described below.

Precapillary pulmonary arterial hypertension produces alterations in the pulmonary vascular pattern when the pulmonary artery pressure reaches the range of 50/25 mm Hg. Slight elevations of pressure below this level may not produce abnormal clinical or roentgenologic signs. The characteristic roentgenologic change in the pulmonary arterial pattern is marked enlargement or dilatation of the main pulmonary artery and the central right and left main pulmonary artery branches down to the origin of the segmental arteries (Fig. 7-25). The segmental arterial branches to the lung are normal or constricted so that the ratio of the size of the central pulmonary artery branches to the peripheral ones is greater than 7:1. In acquired pulmonary hypertension the pulsations of the pulmonary arteries as seen with image amplification are usually normal. When pulmonary valvular insufficiency is present, the pulsations of the central pulmonary

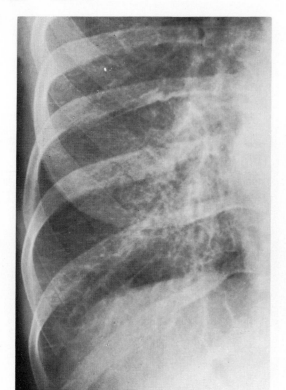

Fig. 7-24. Pulmonary venous hypertension in a patient with mitral stenosis. Note the multiple transverse septal lines perpendicular to the pleura and the haziness of vascular markings due to interstitial edema.

arteries become increased. Congenital pulmonary hypertension (as in Eisenmenger's complex) is usually associated with increased pulsations in the pulmonary arteries similar to the pulsations seen with the large left-to-right shunts. The pulmonary veins remain normal in precapillary pulmonary arterial hypertension; septal lines are not present in cases of precapillary pulmonary hypertension.

INCREASED PULMONARY BLOOD FLOW

Normally the cardiac output of the right side of the heart is equal to that of the left side, so that the systemic and pulmonary blood flows are equal. When a left-to-right shunt or a complex admixture lesion is present, the pulmonary blood flow will exceed the systemic blood flow. Roentgenologic evidence of this excess will be present when the pulmonary blood flow is one and one-half to two times greater than the systemic flow, and the greater the difference between the two circulations, the more marked will be the roentgenologic change.

With increased pulmonary blood flow there occurs enlargement of the shadows of the pulmonary

arteries and veins throughout both lungs (Fig. 7-22C). The central arteries enlarge proportionately to the peripheral segmental arteries, so that the ratio of the size of the central to the peripheral arteries remains normal (less than 6:1). Roentgenoscopy with image amplification is helpful in those cases where the roentgenographic signs are borderline. An increase in the intrinsic pulsations of the pulmonary arteries occurs when the pulmonary blood flow is excessive; the greater the flow, the more marked the visible pulsation of the pulmonary artery branches.

DECREASED PULMONARY BLOOD FLOW

Since the size of the pulmonary vessels is closely related to pulmonary blood flow, one would expect that when a right-to-left shunt is present, as with tetralogy of Fallot, and the systemic blood flow exceeds the pulmonary blood flow, the pulmonary vascular shadows would be smaller than normal. Both the pulmonary arterial and venous shadows appear small; because of decreased blood flow the lungs have a more radiolucent appearance (Fig. 7-22A). The main pulmonary artery segment along the left border of the heart is concave usually, and the hilar shadows are small and poorly defined.

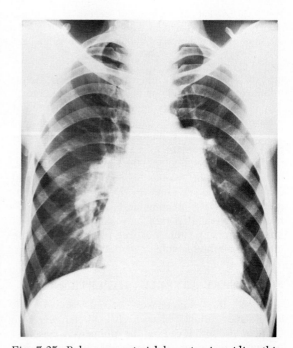

Fig. 7-25. Pulmonary arterial hypertension, idiopathic. The roentgenologic signs include marked enlargement of the main pulmonary artery segment, dilatation of the central hilar pulmonary artery branches, and constriction of the segmental pulmonary arteries. The pulmonary veins are not enlarged.

Intrinsic pulsations in the central and peripheral pulmonary arteries are not visible with roentgenoscopic image amplification.

COLLATERAL OR BRONCHIAL CIRCULATION TO THE LUNGS

When pulmonary atresia is present, blood supply to the lungs and pulmonary arterial bed must come from some other source. There may be enlargement of the bronchial arteries which arise from the aorta, or anomalous arteries from the aorta may join the smaller branches of the pulmonary arteries in the lungs. Through these collateral routes poorly oxygenated blood finds its way from the aorta into the lung hilus and, through numerous anastomoses with the pulmonary arteries, eventually reaches the capillary bed of the lung to become oxygenated. The roentgenologic pattern of the lung is fairly characteristic of this anatomic and physiologic change associated with pulmonary atresia. The pulmonary veins are very small and poorly defined. The arterial branches in the lung are very small and show an irregular reticular pattern; the number of these small vessels, however, is usually increased. When there is atresia of a main right or left pulmonary artery, the hilar shadow is abnormal. No continuous vascular structure can be seen, as normally, between the mediastinum and the hilar shadow. The hilus is situated away from the mediastinum as an island of irregular vascular shadows (Fig. 7-26).

SUGGESTED READING

Abrams, H. L.: Radiologic Apsects of Increased Pulmonary Artery Pressure and Flow, *Stanford M. Bull.*, **14**:97–111, 1956.

Amundsen, P.: The Diagnostic Value of Conventional Radiological Examination of the Heart in Adults, *Acta radiol., Suppl.* 181, 1959.

Campbell, M., and Gardner, F.: Radiological Features of Enlarged Bronchial Arteries, *Brit. Heart J.*, **12**:183–200, 1950.

Dotter, C. T., and Steinberg, I.: Angiocardiography, *Ann. Roentgenol.*, **20**:1–304, 1952.

Gay, B. B., Jr., and Franch, R. H.: Pulsation in the Pulmonary Arteries as Observed with Roentgenoscopic Image Amplification: Observations in Patients Having Increased Pulmonary Blood Flow, *Am. J. Roentgenol.*, **85**:1025–1036, 1961.

Grainger, R. G.: Interstitial Edema and Its Radiological Diagnosis: A Sign of Pulmonary Venous and Capillary Hypertension, *Brit. J. Radiol.*, **31**:201–217, 1958.

Jonsell, S.: A Method for Determination of the Heart Size by Teleoroentgenography, *Acta radiol.*, **20**: 325–340, 1939.

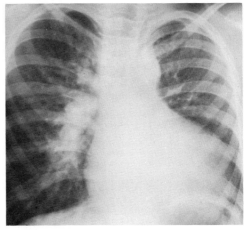

Fig. 7-26. Patient with truncus arteriosus where the right pulmonary artery arises from the trunk and the left lung is supplied by the bronchial circulation, there being no left pulmonary artery as such. The right lung shows the pattern of increased pulmonary blood flow; the left lung shows the pattern of decreased pulmonary blood flow, and the irregular pattern associated with bronchial collateral circulation.

Jorgens, J., Blank, N., and Wilcox, W. A.: The Cineflurographic Detection and Recording of Calcifications within the Heart, *Radiology*, **74**:550–554, 1960.

Kjellberg, S. E., et al.: "Diagnosis of Congenital Heart Disease," 2d ed., Edition, The Year Book Medical Publishers, Inc., Chicago, 1959.

Lavender, M. B., and Doppman, S.: The Hilum in Pulmonary Venous Hypertension, *Brit. J. Radiol.*, **35**: 303–313, 1962.

Lehman, J. S., and Curry, J. L.: A Correlation of Roentgen and Surgical Findings in Two Hundred Cases of Rheumatic Mitral Valvular Disease, *Am. J. Roentgenol.*, **71**:599–610, 1954.

Logue, R. B., Rogers, J. V., Jr., and Gay, B. B., Jr.: Subtle Roentgenographic Signs of Left Heart Failure, *Am. Heart J.*, **65**:464–473, 1963.

Schwedel, J. B.: "Clinical Roentgenology of the Heart," Paul B. Hoeber, Inc., New York, 1946.

Shapiro, J. H., et al.: "Calcifications of the Heart," Charles C Thomas, Publisher, Springfield, Ill., 1963.

Simon, M.: Pulmonary Veins in Mitral Stenosis, *J. Fac. Radiologists*, **9**:25–32, 1958.

Sosman, M. C.: The Technique for Locating and Identifying Pericardial and Intracardiac Calcification, *Am. J. Roentgenol.*, **50**:461–468, 1943.

Steiner, R. E.: Radiological Appearances of Pulmonary Vessels in Pulmonary Hypertension, *Brit. J. Radiol.*, **31**:188–200, 1958.

Ungerleider, H. E., and Clark, C. P.: A Study of the Transverse Diameter of Heart Silhouette, with Prediction Table Based on Teleoroentgenogram, *Am. Heart J.*, **17**:92–102, 1939.

Ungerleider, H. E., and Gubner, R.: Evaluation of Heart Size Measurements, *Am. Heart J.*, 24:494–510, 1942.

Windholz, F., and Grayson, C.: The Roentgen Demon-

stration of Calcification in the Interventricular Septum in Cases of Heart Block, *Am. J. Roentgenol.*, 58:411–421, 1947.

Section C: Special Laboratory Procedures

8 CARDIAC CATHETERIZATION

Robert H. Franch, M.D.

In 1905 Fritz Bleichroeder, medical director of a small hospital for women in Berlin, had a ureteral catheter placed in his axillary vein from the arm and in his inferior vena cava from the thigh.[1,2] In 1929 Werner Forssman (born 1904), a resident surgeon at Eberswalde, catheterized his right atrium from a left antecubital vein cutdown, utilizing self-fluoroscopy with a mirror.[3] The position of the catheter tip was verified by an x-ray film (Fig. 8-1). The extensive use of the catheter by Cournand in the early 1940s in the study of human cardiovascular physiology[4-7] led his group and those of Dexter,[8-12] McMichael,[12a] and Bing[13] to explore the use of this technique for the study of heart dis-

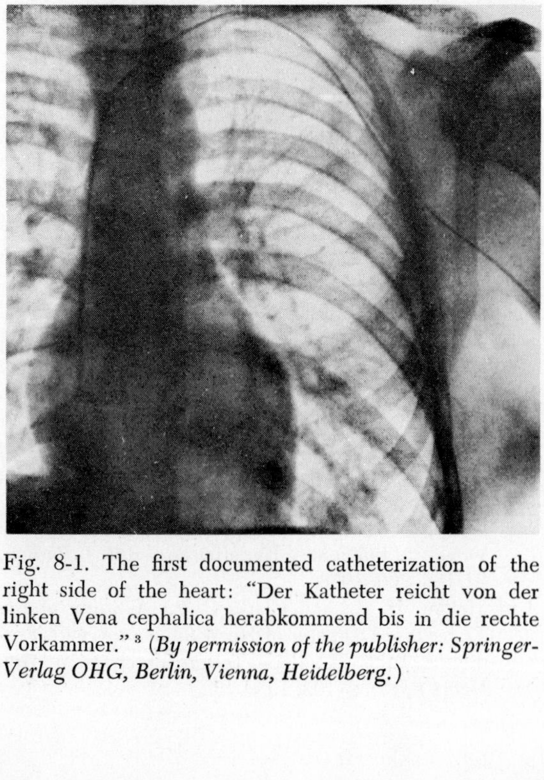

Fig. 8-1. The first documented catheterization of the right side of the heart: "Der Katheter reicht von der linken Vena cephalica herabkommend bis in die rechte Vorkammer." [3] (*By permission of the publisher: Springer-Verlag OHG, Berlin, Vienna, Heidelberg.*)

ease.[14,15] At Emory University in 1945 Brannon, Weens, and Warren[16] described the hemodynamics of atrial septal defect in four patients. From this point on, steady, imaginative, bold advances have occurred, with progressive refinement of laboratory techniques, including indicator-dilution methods, selective angiography, and catheterization of the left side of the heart.[17-21]

GENERAL ASPECTS OF CARDIAC CATHETERIZATION

The physician who is to do the catheterization should examine the patient completely, review the history, films, and electrocardiogram, and have a clinical diagnosis and a planned approach formulated before beginning the procedure. The catheterization may then be intelligently modified as various data become available during the procedure.

The patient should be in the hospital the afternoon prior to study. A relaxed meeting with the patient and his family serves to lessen long-standing apprehension and to correct any misunderstanding. Since catheterization is frequently the first major step on the road to cardiac surgery, a tolerable experience now fosters an improved attitude in the patient and his family toward future events. This visit may also be used to familiarize the patient with the bicycle ergometer, nose clips, and breathing valves. Breakfast is withheld for a morning procedure; for an afternoon procedure breakfast consists of toast and coffee or juice, and lunch is withheld. The cyanotic infant with a high hematocrit is permitted fluids up to 2 hr before catheterization. In our experience, prophylactic antibiotics are not necessary.

General anesthesia is neither necessary nor desirable. It is particularly to be avoided in small infants. A combination of 6.25 mg Phenergan (promethazine), 6.25 mg Thorazine (chlorpromazine), and 25 mg Demerol (meperidine hydrochloride) per cubic centimeter of mixture provides excellent sedation.[22,23] The intramuscular dose is 0.5 to 2.0 ml, depending on the age and weight of the child, and is given 1 hr before the procedure. The mixture is not given intravenously, nor do we repeat it after the initial loading dose. If additional sedation is required, small doses of intravenous Demerol may be used. In the neonatal period or in the small infant, Demerol alone, 1 mg per lb, is adequate, especially if combined with a glucose pacifier. In the adult, Seconal (secobarbital sodium) gr 1½ is used; Demerol is added if arterial catheterization or transthoracic puncture is planned.

The sedated infant or small child is gently strapped to a thin plywood or plastic frame covered with foam rubber and a plastic cover. There may be a brief arousal to the needle prick or to the sensation of burning of the subcutaneous 1 per cent Xylocaine (lidocaine). Demerol tends to release endogenous histamine; if nasal itching occurs, it should be controlled by gentle rubbing. Vomiting is unusual, but occasionally, in the adult, vagal slowing of the pulse, nausea, and perspiration are noted. Intravenous atropine is antidotal. No data should be obtained until pulse, respiration, and blood pressure are completely stable. Adults and adolescents may be more fearful than children. Loose talk should be avoided in the catheterization room. During the procedure the cardiac rhythm is continuously monitored, using the electrocardiogram.

It is desirable that the laboratory be involved almost daily in diagnostic work. General efficiency is increased, costly equipment and space are utilized, and, most important, all personnel become confident and knowledgeable with experience. Certainly the most important ingredient in the laboratory is the thoroughly experienced technical-professional team. The procedure must move briskly. The primary object is to make complete and accurate diagnosis at one sitting, with least possible risk and discomfort to the patient. The availability of angiocardiographic techniques in the same room is absolutely necessary if this is to be accomplished.

TECHNIQUE

Catheterization of the Right Side of the Heart. In the infant, the saphenous vein or the superficial femoral vein distal to its junction with a deep femoral vein is used.[24] If the common femoral vein is needed, a purse-string repair is done to avoid the temporary coldness, blueness, and edema of the leg that follow complete interruption of this vein. Occasionally the pelvic brim may arrest the catheter tip, or rarely the catheter tip may enter the hemiazygous vein and pass into the right atrium via a left superior vena cava. From the saphenous approach, the pulmonary artery may be slightly more difficult to enter, especially if there is a narrowed and/or hypertrophied right ventricular outflow tract. A patent foramen ovale is easily crossed as the catheter tip tends to curve gently from the inferior vena cava toward the atrial septum; a patent ductus arteriosus is frequently entered as the tip of the catheter points to the "roof" of the junction of the main and left pulmonary artery. The external jugular vein or the axillary vein may also be used. In the newborn infant, a relatively large catheter may be passed via the umbilical vein or artery for catheterization of the heart and for selective angiocardiography.[25]

Flow-guided catheterization permits a small silastic catheter to be carried into the pulmonary artery by the blood stream without fluoroscopic guidance.[26] Its use remains limited.

In the older child and adult, the right arm is preferred; the basilic or median cubital vein is utilized. From the left arm, the catheter tip may enter a persistent left superior vena cava, exiting via the coronary sinus into the right atrium in an awkward position for entering the right ventricle. Catheterization of a persistent left superior vena cava may disclose anomalous pulmonary venous drainage (Fig. 8-2) or, rarely, communication between the left atrium and the coronary sinus. If the superficial veins are small, the venae comitantes of the brachial artery may be used. A deep inspiration will often enable the catheter tip to pass the subclavian vein–brachiocephalic vein junction. The catheter tip frequently forms a loop against the tricuspid ring and passes directly into the pulmonary artery from the right ventricle in a quick motion. Often a loop is formed against the lateral wall of the right atrium, which is rotated tip headward through the tricuspid valve into the right ventricle and pulmonary artery. It is not good practice to form a loop in the ventricle. A deep inspiration while advancing the catheter facilitates the seating of the catheter tip in the pulmonary artery wedge position (Fig. 8-3).[27,28]

Direct puncture of the exposed artery at the venous cutdown site with a short beveled No. 22 needle is a useful procedure in the infant. Arterial pressure may then be recorded continuously, the recording being unaffected by the slow drip needed to keep the needle open.[18] In adults and older children, an inlying needle is easily introduced percutaneously into the radial artery. Arterial saturation is ideally checked by simultaneous pulmonary vein and peripheral arterial sampling in order to exclude a pulmonary cause for desaturation.

Catheterization of the Left Side of the Heart. In general, transbronchial[29-33] and posterior transthoracic puncture of the left atrium[34-38] as an avenue to the left side of the heart has been supplanted by transseptal left heart catheterization, retrograde

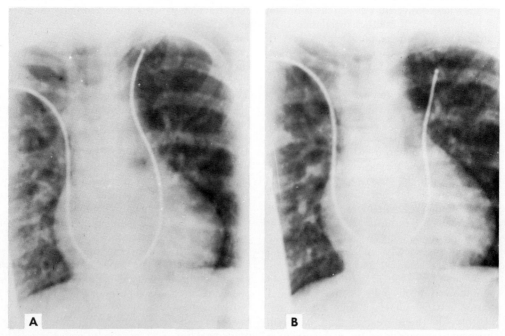

Fig. 8-2. *A.* The catheter tip passes from the right superior vena cava to the right atrium, thence to the coronary sinus, thence to the left superior vena cava. *B.* The catheter tip passes from the left superior vena cava to an anomalous left upper lobe pulmonary vein.

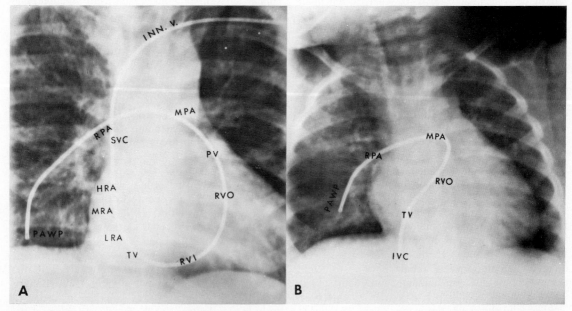

Fig. 8-3. Sites of pressure recording and/or blood sampling during catheterization of the right side of the heart. *A.* Catheter introduced from the left basilic vein into the right pulmonary artery. *B.* Catheter introduced from the saphenous vein into the right pulmonary artery. *Inn. V.*, innominate vein (brachiocephalic vein); *SVC, IVC,* superior and inferior venae cavae; *HRA, MRA, LRA,* high, mid-, and low right atria; *RVI, RVO,* right ventricular inflow and outflow tracts; *TV, PV,* tricuspid and pulmonary valves; *MPA, RPA:* main and right pulmonary arteries; *PAWP:* pulmonary artery wedge position.

aortic catheterization of the left ventricle, and percutaneous left ventricular puncture.[56] Suprasternal puncture of the left atrium and aortic arch and pulmonary artery[40,41] have not proved popular in this country.

In retrograde aortic catheterization, the catheter may be introduced percutaneously[42] over a spring guide wire previously introduced by puncture of the brachial, axillary, subclavian,[43] or femoral artery.[44-50] The open technique usually utilizes the brachial artery or ulnar artery.[51-53] The arteriotomy is closed by either a purse-string suture in the adventitia[54] or one or two interrupted sutures.[55] A dilute solution of heparin should be injected distally at the time of arteriotomy and again just before closure. The normal aortic valve is easily crossed in order to gain access to the left ventricle for pressure, sampling, indicator-dilution, or opaque-media studies (Fig. 8-4). In acquired aortic stenosis, the left ventricle is entered in approximately two-thirds of the cases;[56] in congenital aortic stenosis, in 89 per cent of the cases.[57-59]

Transseptal catheterization is widely used.[60-71] From the right femoral vein, percutaneously[68,72] or via a saphenous vein cutdown, a long needle with a curved tip is advanced through a thin-walled catheter in a posteromedial direction so as to puncture the lower third of the atrial septum or preferably higher, beneath the ledge of the limbus fossa ovalis.[73] The left atrial pressure is checked, and a

blood sample is obtained. The catheter tip is advanced with the needle until it is free in the left atrium (Fig. 8-5). The needle is withdrawn and the footward-curved catheter tip may be advanced across the mitral valve into the left ventricle (Fig. 8-5). Left ventricular angiography may be performed.[74,75] Left ventricular pressure is measured; a pullback pressure across the mitral valve is obtained. Recently puncture of the atrial septum by the catheter alone has been advocated. The left atrium is difficult to enter if there is deformity of the thoracic or lumbar spine or if there is a very large right atrium.[76]

A brief, direct percutaneous puncture through the palpable apex of the left ventricle for left ventricular pressure measurement is surprisingly free of complications.[77-80] Left ventricular angiography performed through the needle[81,82] adds to the length of time the rigid needle is in the left ventricular cavity.[83,84] There is also the risk of intramyocardial injection of contrast material.[85-87] A coil spring guidewire has been advanced into the left ventricle through an 18-gauge needle. The needle is then replaced by a Teflon tubing, which is advanced over the guidewire into the ventricular cavity. This catheter may be advanced antegrade across the aortic valve and occasionally retrograde through the mitral valve into the left atrium.[77,88,89] Children should have light anesthesia during this procedure.[90]

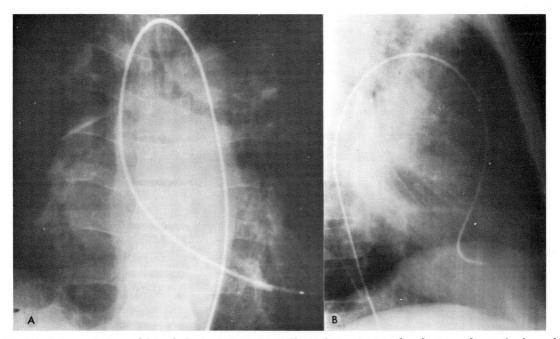

Fig. 8-4. Anteroposterior and lateral chest roentgenogram. The catheter tip, introduced retrograde via the femoral artery, passes up the thoracic aorta, around the aortic arch and across the aortic valve to the apex of the left ventricle.

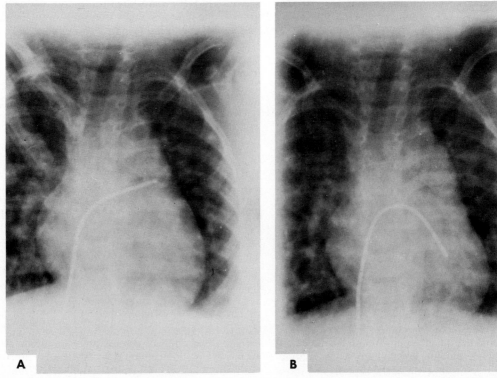

Fig. 8-5. Transseptal catheterization of the left side of the heart. *A.* The catheter tip, introduced from the saphenous vein, passes from the right atrium through the atrial septum to the left atrium. *B.* The catheter tip is manipulated across the mitral valve into the left ventricle.

EQUIPMENT

Catheters. Catheters in a wide range of sizes and lengths should be available. All catheters are autoclaved or gas-sterilized. Cold sterilization is less desirable; bloodstream infection has been reported when this sterilization technique was used.[91] Foreign-protein reactions, or "catheter fever," are prevented by continuous flushing of the catheters with tap water for 24 hr and with 3 per cent hydrogen peroxide or an 8 per cent ammonium hydroxide solution to clear the catheter of foreign protein. For the infant, a No. 5 French thin-walled catheter with an end hole and two side holes has wide use. One should avoid the use of stiff catheters because of the risk of perforation. The use of limp catheters should be avoided because of the likelihood of knotting. Also, both stiff and limp catheters are difficult to manipulate. The ideal catheter is soft enough to permit bending as required, yet it should hold its shape and have enough body to permit the curve of the tip to be advanced intact.

In the adult, image intensification fluoroscopy and adequate pressure transducers have made the use of a 100-cm No. 6 French thin-walled catheter feasible. For pulmonary artery wedge pressure measurements in adults, an end-hole catheter is optimal. A special side-hole catheter presenting a tapered, blind, easily looped tip may be used for passage through angulated channels. An electrode catheter permits[92,93] identification of the P waves of the intracardiac electrocardiogram during cardiac dysrhythmia.[94] Intracardiac phonocardiograms are obtained by a catheter with a barium titanate crystal inside its tip.[95]

Fluoroscopy. Conventional fluoroscopy should no longer be used. Image intensification fluoroscopy provides markedly increased visibility at one-tenth the radiation exposure to the operator and the patient. The room need not be darkened, and television monitoring is available.

Recording Systems. The three major components of a modern physiologic recording system are the transducer, amplifier, and recorder.[96,97]

The unbonded strain-gauge or wire-resistance manometer that has sufficient sensitivity to drive a recording galvanometer is sensitive, durable, stable, and comparatively inexpensive. Its high-resonant frequency makes it the extracardiac transducer of choice in recording from the fluid-filled catheter.[98]

The transducer measures the relative pressure between two systems, one limb of which is open to air or ambient pressure. The tubing should transmit the pressure pulse wave without energy loss. Examples of other transducers include:

1. A conductor moving in a magnetic field (flowmeter)

2. Thermistors and thermocouples (body-temperature studies)

3. Photoelectric devices using transmitted or reflected light (densitometers, reflection oximeters)

Electronic amplification of the transducer signal is obtained by one of three kinds of amplifiers: carrier, direct-coupled, or chopper. Each has desirable and undesirable characteristics in regard to stability, gain, signal-to-noise ratio, and frequency response. Problems common to all are those of stability and noise suppression. Amplifiers that are sensitive, accurate, and linear are available; generally amplifiers are not a limiting factor in physiologic recording.

Recorders may be divided into direct-writer or optical recorders. The direct writer has a writing arm and provides an immediate record. Optical recorders provide records on film. Several variables may be recorded from the same base line (cross-over tracings). The mirror galvanometer uses a light-beam writing arm. The cathode-ray oscilloscope uses an electron beam. Information may also be stored on electromagnetic tape in analogue or digital form for future computer use or for scanning by other playback devices.

A pressure recording system is said to be adequate if the tenth harmonic of the fundamental frequency of a wave can be recorded with uniform sensitivity. Thus a system with a uniform response from 0 to 40 cps would be adequate for heart rates up to 240 beats per minute. The limiting factor in all manometer systems is the cardiac catheter itself, whose accelerating and decelerating movements in the beating heart superimpose artifacts on the pressure tracing.[99] Distortion of the catheter-obtained phasic pressure tracings is avoided by use of a catheter-tip micromanometer, whose small mass is not greatly affected by acceleration and deceleration.[100,101]

Oxygen Analysis. The total oxygen content of the blood may be determined by the classical Van Slyke manometric technique[102] or, more rapidly, by gas chromatography.[103-107] Direct oximetry of unhemolized, undiluted blood by flow through cuvettes connected directly to the catheter utilizes either transmission[108-113] or reflection methods[114-118] in order to determine blood-oxygen saturation, rapidly and accurately, during catheterization. Small samples of blood from a syringe may also be analyzed in these cuvettes, or after hemolysis, by a precision spectrophotometer.[119-121] In the transmission technique, the oxygen saturation is proportional to the ratio of the optical density of blood at 605 μ to the optical density of blood at 805 μ; in the dual-beam reflection oximeter, the oxygen saturation of heparinized whole blood is proportional to the intensity of light scattered at 805 μ divided by the intensity scattered at 660 μ. A fiberoptic reflection oximeter catheter permits intracardiac oxygen-saturation measurements without withdrawal of blood.[122-124] In the future, direct measurements of oxygen tension may be made routinely from the tip of the catheter.[125]

Analysis of expired air for oxygen and carbon dioxide may be made by extraction techniques,[126] paramagnetic analyzers,[127] or a closed-circuit method.

DATA OBTAINED AT CATHETERIZATION

One must be familiar with the limitations of cardiac catheterization in order to avoid mistakes in diagnosis.[128,129] There may be technical errors in obtaining the data, or properly recorded data may be misinterpreted or may not be specific.

Pressure Measurements

Caution is advisable in interpreting pressure curves that may be distorted by artifact. High-fidelity phasic pressure curves are not obtainable from the pulmonary artery. The undamped curve gives falsely high systolic and falsely low diastolic readings, and the overdamped curve has a smooth shape with disappearance of the incisura. The mean pulmonary artery pressure is reliable for clinical purposes. Wide abrupt swings in pressure, premature beats, and intermittent abutting of the catheter tip against the ventricular wall make the ventricular pressure curve subject to even greater alteration. The shape of the ventricular pressure trace is thus rarely of primary diagnostic importance. A significant abrupt fall in pressure in early diastole (early diastolic dip) followed by a sudden rise to a high end-diastolic pressure plateau does not differentiate among constrictive pericarditis, myocardial failure, and/or fibrosis and endocardial fibroelastosis. It is not inevitably true that in isolated pulmonic stenosis the configuration of the right ventricular pressure curve is peaked or triangular,[130-132] but, is trapezoidal in shape, if a large ventricular septal defect is associated with pulmonic stenosis. End-diastolic pressure in the ventricle may be a relatively insensitive index of end-diastolic volume, since diastolic pressure is also dependent on the physical properties of the ventricular muscle.[133]

A satisfactory pulmonary artery wedge pressure provides a good estimate of pulmonary venous and

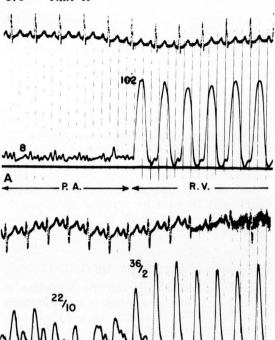

Fig. 8-6. Pullback pressure record in: *A.* Valvular pulmonic stenosis; the phasic pulmonary artery pressure pulse is completely distorted. The rise in right ventricular systolic pressure is abrupt; there is no evidence of an intermediate pressure zone. *B.* "Relative" valvular pulmonic stenosis in a young girl with a large left-to-right shunt. The systolic pressure differential disappeared after successful closure of the atrial septal defect.

left atrial mean pressure.[134] In infants and children, the wedge pressure may be significantly higher than left atrial mean pressure;[135] and in adults, it may be up to one-third higher than a simultaneously recorded left atrial mean pressure.[136] Incomplete wedging, or wedging of the catheter tip into the wall of a sharply angulated tortuous pulmonary artery, is a common cause of an unsatisfactory pulmonary artery wedge pressure tracing.[137,138]

The pressure curves in the atria are more easily recorded. The pressure changes are of less amplitude; catheter motion is less. The catheter should lie free in the mid-atrium. If it lies near the atrioventricular valve or in the atrial appendage, an abnormally shaped curve with a high c or a wave is recorded.[128,139,140] If it enters the coronary sinus, an atrial, or, if the catheter tip is wedged, a ventricular pressure curve is recorded. The direct analysis of the left atrial pressure pulse has not proved completely satisfactory in quantitating the degree of mitral regurgitation.[141-145]

One of the most useful contributions of pressure recording is that it permits measurement of either the peak or the mean pressure differential across a stenotic semilunar (Figs. 8-6, 8-7) or atrioventricular valve (Fig. 8-8) or a segmentally narrowed blood vessel[146] (Fig. 8-9). If possible, simultaneous pressure recordings across a valve should be obtained, especially if there is atrial fibrillation. If the pulmonary artery wedge pressure is used as an estimate of left-atrial mean pressure, the error in assessing mitral stenosis is small, provided the gradient across the mitral valve is large.[147]

Blood-oxygen Measurements

An increased oxygen step-up in the right side of the heart must be closely correlated with the clinical findings. Normally there is significant variability in the oxygen content of blood withdrawn from the right atrium because of laminar flow from the coronary sinus, superior vena cava, and inferior vena

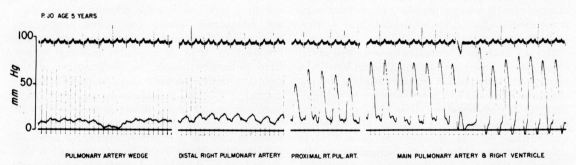

Fig. 8-7. Pressure record in multiple congenital stenosis of the right and left pulmonary artery branches, illustrating a systolic pressure differential between the distal, proximal, and main pulmonary artery. There are systolic hypertension and a wide pulse pressure in the proximal right and main pulmonary arteries, related to a reduction in the capacity of the pulmonary artery compression chamber.

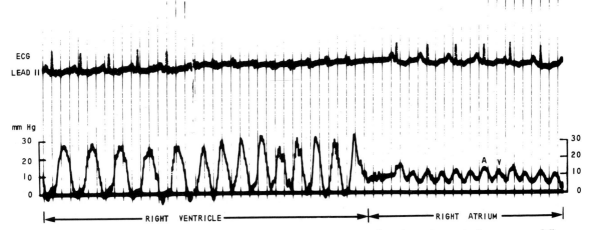

Fig. 8-8. Pullback pressure tracing in rheumatic tricuspid stenosis. Note that the atrioventricular pressure differential persists throughout ventricular diastole. Right atrial A and V waves are prominent.

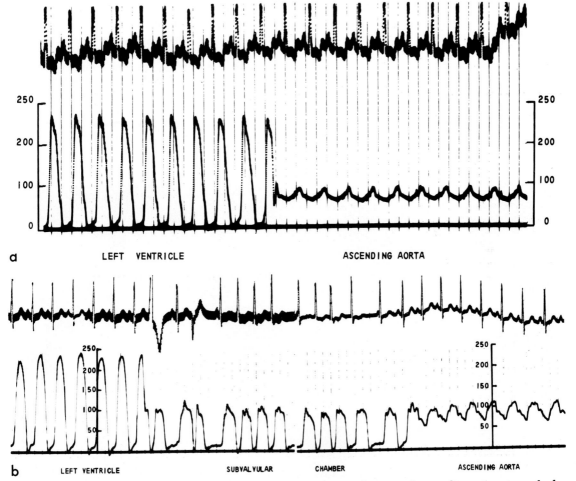

Fig. 8-9. Withdrawal pressure record in A. *Valvular aortic stenosis:* Left ventricular systolic pressure is much elevated. The pressure transition at the valve is abrupt. Coarse systolic vibrations are superimposed on the slowly ascending limb of the aortic pressure pulse. B. *Subvalvular aortic stenosis:* The locus of peak systolic pressure change is in the left ventricular outflow tract. No peak systolic pressure differential is present across the aortic valve.

cava. Therefore mixed venous blood is best obtained from the pulmonary artery. Serial sampling should be done as quickly as possible; there should be minimal change in the steady state during sampling. Contamination with pulmonary venous blood may occur if the catheter tip is placed too far peripherally in the pulmonary artery, where it may migrate into a partially wedged position. Oxygenated blood from a ventricular septal defect may stream across the pulmonary valve so that the oxygen step-up occurs only in the pulmonary artery. Oxygenated blood from a patent ductus may reflux back into the right ventricle from the pulmonary artery if there is pulmonary regurgitation. Therefore, precise localization of a left-to-right shunt in certain cases and detection of multiple sites of shunting are limited if only the oxygen sampling technique is used.[148]

In the normal circulation on random sampling, early studies[10] showed least oxygen difference between right ventricular and pulmonary artery blood (0.5 vol per cent maximally) and the largest oxygen difference between the venae cavae and right atrium (1.9 vol per cent maximally); the right atrial–right ventricular oxygen-content difference was 0.9 vol per cent maximally. An oxygen step-up in excess of the maximal differences was evidence for a left-to-right shunt. By these criteria, false-positive results are rare but false-negative results occur in patients with small shunts. Recent studies show that sensitivity in detecting left-to-right shunts is improved if numerous serial blood samples are withdrawn in rapid succession for photometric analysis. If two sets of interrupted samples are taken from the superior vena cava, right atrium, right ventricle, and pulmonary artery, then a 9 per cent saturation increase indicates an atrial shunt; 5 per cent, a ventricular shunt; and 3 per cent, a pulmonary artery shunt.[18] Sensitivity can be further improved if blood samples are obtained in multiple pairs in a rapid serial sweep without saline flushing between samples; then a 3 per cent atrial step-up or a 3 per cent ventricular oxygen step-up or a 2 per cent pulmonary artery oxygen step-up is 95 per cent likely to be due to a left-to-right shunt.[149] Increment criteria based on the *t* distribution have been recently proposed.[150,151]

The normal range of difference in saturation between chambers is approximately the same in adults and in children. If differences in oxygen content are used to detect a shunt, a decrease in oxygen capacity (anemia) may cause a false-negative result by lowering the oxygen-content differences due to shunting to within the range of normal variation.[18] Left-to-right shunts less than 20 per cent of pulmonary flow are not detectable by the conventional blood-oxygen saturation methods. Selective angiography and/or use of the hydrogen electrode provide maximal sensitivity and reliability in the detection of small shunts.

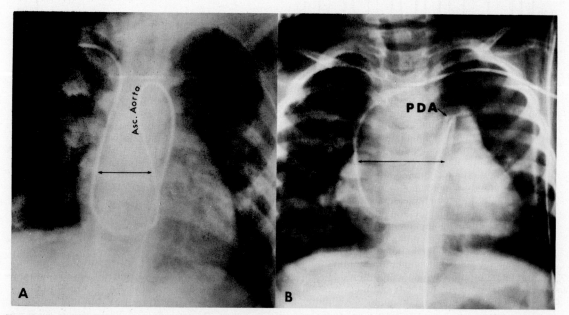

Fig. 8-10. Anteroposterior roentgenograms to demonstrate the difference in width of the catheter loop when *A.* The catheter tip passes in a hairpin loop (arrow) from the right ventricle to the ascending aorta via a ventricular septal defect. *B.* The catheter tip passes in a wide U loop (arrow) from the right ventricle to the pulmonary artery, thence to the descending thoracic aorta via a patent ductus arteriosus.

Catheter Position

Localization of a right-to-left shunt by simple catheterization of the right side of the heart alone is difficult unless the shunt is bidirectional or unless the catheter passes through a defect. The catheter position then becomes useful in identifying the anatomic location of the defect. In ventricular septal defect in the anteroposterior view, the catheter enters the ascending aorta from the right ventricle in a hairpin loop (Fig. 8-10) and enters the pulmonary artery from the right ventricle in a wider U loop; in the lateral projection, the catheter is anterior if it is in the pulmonary artery, and in the middle of the heart shadow if it is in the aortic root. In patent ductus arteriosus, the tip first passes from the pulmonary artery to the descending aorta (Fig. 8-10); in aortopulmonary septal defect, the tip passes directly up the ascending aorta from the pulmonary artery. When the catheter tip enters a pulmonary vein within the heart shadow, angiocardiography or indicator-dilution studies are necessary to ascertain whether the pulmonary vein drains into the left or the right atrium.

In the occasional patient with pulmonary stenosis and right ventricular systolic pressure greater than left ventricular systolic pressure,[152,153] a ventricular septal defect is detected solely by being catheterized. A shunt is not apparent, since the ventricular septal defect tends to close with systole or to be obstructed by the septal leaflet of the tricuspid valve. These patients with concealed ventricular septal defect are frequently operated on for isolated valvular or infundibular stenosis.[132] If the ventricular septal defect is unsuspected at surgery, a left-to-right shunt may become apparent in the postoperative period. If the tricuspid valve is congenitally displaced into the right ventricle, the pressure transition from right ventricle to right atrium may occur while the catheter tip is far to the left of the spine. Simultaneous intracardiac electrocardiography is confirmatory (Fig. 8-11).[154,155]

Flow and Shunt Calculations by Dilution Methods

Fick Method. *Cardiac Output.* Adolph Fick, in 1870, in a brief note before the Society of Physiology and Medicine of Wurzburg, expounded a theory for the measurement of blood flow that he never used in the laboratory: "The total uptake or release of a substance by an organ is the product of the blood flow to the organ and of the arteriovenous concentration of the substance."[156,157] The Fick principle was applied by Grehant and Quinquaud in 1886, utilizing venous catheterization of dogs.[158] The work of Forssman led Klein, in 1930,

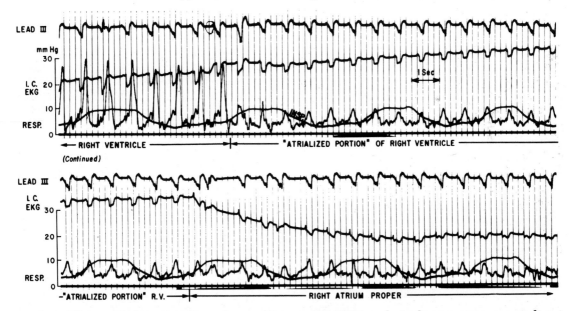

Fig. 8-11. The use of the intracavitary electrocardiogram (IC ECG) and simultaneous pressure recording in the diagnosis of Ebstein's disease. Lead III of the standard electrocardiogram shows a short P-R interval and a prolonged QRS complex associated with WPW syndrome. The IC ECG of the "atrialized portion" of the right ventricle resembles the IC ECG of the right ventricle, but the pressure pulse of the atrialized portion of the right ventricle is the same as that of the right atrium proper. This finding suggests displacement of the tricuspid valve into the right ventricle. The IC ECG in the right atrium proper shows characteristic peaked biphasic P waves and reduction in voltage of the QRS.

to obtain mixed venous blood from the right side of the heart of man for the calculation of cardiac output.[159] Cournand and coworkers in the early 1940s applied cardiac catheterization and the Fick method to a systematic study of cardiovascular physiology in man; the achievements of Forssman, Cournand, and Richards were recognized by the award of the Nobel prize in medicine and physiology in 1956.

Accurate measurement of pulmonary blood flow by the Fick technique requires a stable respiratory rate, heart rate, oxygen consumption, and respiratory exchange ratio.[160-163] Under conditions of exercise, 5 to 7 min are usually required until a steady state is obtained.

The cardiac output may be calculated given the following values:

Total oxygen consumption:	300 ml per min (collection and analysis of expired air or via a closed-circuit technique)
Arterial blood–oxygen content:	19 ml per 100 ml blood (arterial puncture)
Mixed venous blood–O_2 content:	14 ml per 100 ml blood (pulmonary artery catheterization sample)
Body-surface area:	2 m²

Cardiac output, cc/min =

$$\frac{\text{oxygen consumption (ml/min)} \times 100}{\substack{\text{arterial } O_2 \text{ content (ml/100 ml blood)} - \\ \text{mixed venous blood–}O_2 \text{ content (ml/100 ml blood)}}}$$

Cardiac output, ml/min = $\dfrac{300 \times 100}{19 \times 14}$

Cardiac output, ml/min = $\dfrac{30,000}{5}$ (arteriovenous difference)

Cardiac output, ml/min = 6,000
Cardiac output, L/min = 6.0

Cardiac output may be related to the body-surface area as the cardiac index:

Cardiac index (C.I.) = $\dfrac{\text{cardiac output (L/min)}}{\text{body-surface area (m}^2)}$[164]

C.I. = 6/2
C.I. = 3 L/min/m²

The arteriovenous oxygen difference may be a better standard relating to the normality of blood-flow values than the cardiac index.[165]

As the arterial-venous oxygen difference narrows, small errors in the collection or analysis of blood samples make large variations in the cardiac output possible. Theoretically, then, the Fick method is

more accurate in low–cardiac output states; the indicator-dilution technique may be more accurate in high-output states. In 19 normal subjects at supine rest with an average of three samples of blood from the pulmonary artery separated by a mean interval of 37 min, the mean of the maximal variation in oxygen saturation was 3.3 per cent, with a range of 0 to 10 per cent. Thus, repeated measurement of the cardiac output by the Fick technique in a given person may vary to a maximum of ±17 per cent, presuming oxygen consumption and arterial oxygen saturation remain constant.[149]

Shunt Calculations. Shunt calculations utilizing the Fick principle tend to be approximations. The nearness of the pulmonary artery to the site of shunt makes complete mixing of venous and shunted blood unlikely. Extremely narrow arteriovenous oxygen differences may occur, yielding very high pulmonary flow values. Too, samples are usually not collected simultaneously from the pulmonary artery, systemic artery, and proximal to the site of shunt. The calculation of shunts, however, is useful; it provides a quantitative index that is combined with clinical findings in order to assess operability.

Numerous formulas have been developed, particularly those of Cournand, Dexter, and Bing.[166,9,13,167]

1. Calculation of left-to-right shunt:

Total oxygen consumption (VO_2)	240 ml/min
Pulmonary artery blood–O_2 content (PAO_2)	17 ml/100 ml blood
Mixed venous blood–O_2 content (MVO_2)	15 ml/100 ml blood
Arterial blood–oxygen content (SAO_2) (assumed to equal pulmonary venous oxygen content)	19 ml/100 ml blood

Pulmonary flow (Q_p) = $\dfrac{VO_2}{SAO_2 - PAO_2}$

$$= \frac{240}{19 - 17} = 12 \text{ L/min}$$

Systemic flow (Q_s) = $\dfrac{VO_2}{SAO_2 - MVO_2}$

$$= \frac{240}{19 - 15} = 6 \text{ L/min}$$

a. Pulmonary flow/systemic flow ratio
$$= Q_p/Q_s = 12/6 = 2$$

b. Left-to-right shunt (overall shunt)
$$= Q_p - Q_s = 12 \text{ L} - 6 \text{ L} = 6 \text{ L/min}$$

c. Percentage of left-to-right shunt, expressed as the percentage of pulmonary flow that originates from the pulmonary veins:

$$\% \text{ L-R shunt} = \frac{Q_p - Q_s}{Q_p} = \frac{12 - 6}{12} = 50\%$$

or if one substitutes for Q_s and Q_p in the above formula, and reduces to a common denominator, the percentage of left-to-right shunt is obtained from a formula requiring only the oxygen content:

$$\% \text{ L-R shunt} = \frac{Q_p - Q_s}{Q_p} = \frac{PAO_2 - MVO_2}{SAO_2 - MVO_2}$$

$$= \frac{17 - 15}{19 - 15} = 50\% \text{ L-R shunt}$$

2. Calculation of right-to-left shunt:

$$VO_2 = 240 \text{ ml/min}$$
$$MVO_2 = 13 \text{ ml/100 ml blood}$$
$$SAO_2 = 17 \text{ ml/100 ml blood}$$

Pulmonary vein blood-oxygen content is as follows:

$$PVO_2 = 19 \text{ ml/100 ml blood}$$

(Assumed to be 98 per cent of oxygen capacity,[168,169] + 0.3 ml of dissolved oxygen.)

$$Q_p = \frac{VO_2}{PVO_2 - MVO_2} = \frac{240}{19 - 13} = 4 \text{ L/min}$$

$$Q_s = \frac{VO_2}{SAO_2 - MVO_2} = \frac{240}{17 - 13} = 6 \text{ L/min}$$

a. Pulmonary/systemic flow ratio = $Q_p/Q_s = 0.7$
b. Right-to-left shunt (overall shunt)
$$= Q_s - Q_p = 6 \text{ L} - 4 \text{ L} = 2 \text{ L}$$

c. $\% \text{ R-L shunt} = \dfrac{Q_s - Q_p}{Q_s} = \dfrac{6 - 4}{6} = 33\%$

or, substituting for Q_s and Q_p,

$$\% \text{ R-L shunt} = \frac{Q_s - Q_p}{Q_s} = \frac{PVO_2 - SAO_2}{PVO_2 - MVO_2}$$

$$= \frac{19 - 17}{19 - 13} = \frac{2}{6} = 33\%$$

3. Calculation of bidirectional shunt:

$$VO_2 = 240 \text{ ml/min}$$
$$PAO_2 = 15 \text{ ml/100 ml blood}$$
$$MVO_2 = 13 \text{ ml/100 ml blood}$$
$$SAO_2 = 18 \text{ ml/100 ml blood}$$
$$PVO_2 = 19 \text{ ml/100 ml blood}$$

$$Q_p = \frac{VO_2}{PVO_2 - PAO_2} = \frac{240}{19 - 15} = 6 \text{ L/min}$$

$$Q_s = \frac{VO_2}{SAO_2 - MVO_2} = \frac{240}{18 - 13} = 4.8 \text{ L/min}$$

$$Q_{ep}* = \frac{VO_2}{PVO_2 - MVO_2} = \frac{240}{19 - 13} = 4.0 \text{ L/min}$$

* Effective pulmonary flow is that portion of mixed venous blood that reaches the pulmonary capillaries.

Left-to-right shunt = $Q_p - Q_{ep} = 6 - 4 = 2$ L/min
Right-to-left shunt = $Q_s - Q_{ep} = 4.8 - 4.0$
$$= 0.8 \text{ L/min}$$

Indicator-dilution Technique (Injection Method). *Cardiac Output.* The cardiac output, or the mean volume rate of flow, may be determined by using a modification of the standard concentration equation used for the determination of a static fluid volume such as the blood volume:

V (vol of fluid, ml)

$$= \frac{I \text{ (indicator added to fluid, mg)}}{C \text{ (concentration of indicator}}$$
$$\text{in each ml of fluid, mg/ml)}$$

For determination of a moving-fluid volume (cardiac output):[170,171]

$V = \dfrac{I}{C \times t}$ (time required for all the indicator-fluid

mixture to pass the sampling site once)

If the indicator particles are injected into the circulation as a bolus and measured in the initial passage at a downstream site, they distribute themselves in a time concentration plot of grossly predictable form called an indicator-dilution curve. The descending limb of the indicator-dilution curve is distorted by indicator-blood mixture that has begun a second circulation. To exclude recirculating indicator, the concentration is plotted logarithmically against time.[172-175] The early portion of the disappearance slope is linearly extrapolated on semilogarithmic paper to obtain a primary curve, on the premise that if indicator-blood mixing is complete, the washout of indicator is an exponential function of time (Fig. 8-12).[176] Each artery is presumed to get a homogeneous, completely mixed quantity of indicator. A cuvette densitometer is used to obtain conveniently a continuous arterial time-concentration curve.[177] Thus

Cardiac output (L/min)

$$= \frac{I \times 60 \text{ sec}}{C \text{ (mean concentration of indicator}}$$
$$\text{in one circulatory passage, mg/L) } \times t$$
$$\text{(passage time, sec}$$

The mean transit time is the average time interval required for all the indicator particles to go from the injection site to the sampling site in the primary curve; the mean transit time divides the primary curve into two equal portions. The cardiac output multiplied by the mean transit time measures the blood volume between the site of injection and the site of sampling. In a central injection, it includes the volume of all arteries equidistant from the ascending aorta to the arterial sampling site.[178] In a peripheral venous injection, the volume meas-

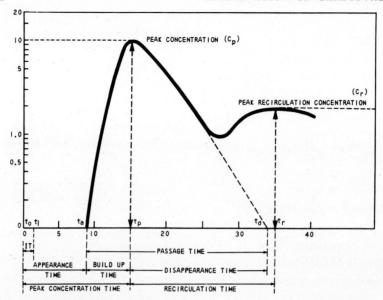

Fig. 8-12. Time and concentration components of a normal indicator-dilution curve that has been replotted semi-logarithmically, with extrapolation of the declining slope of concentration to eliminate the effect of recirculated indicator. The logarithm of the concentration on the ordinate is plotted against time on the abscissa.

t_o, time of onset of injection of the indicator slug; t_i, time from t_o to the end of injection; t_a, time from t_o to the first detectable appearance of indicator at the sampling site; t_p, time from t_o to the peak (maximal) concentration of the indicator; t_d, time when the declining concentration of indicator reaches a minimally detectable value; t_r, time from t_o to the time of the secondary concentration peak due to systemic recirculation of indicator. *IT*, the injection time. (*After Wood and Swan.*[176])

urement includes all veins that have equivalent circulation times.

The central or pulmonary blood volume is determined by pulmonary artery injection with left atrial sampling, or by injecting both the pulmonary artery and the left atrium and sampling the brachial artery to determine mean pulmonary artery–left atrial transit time.[179,180] The latter method avoids the possibility of poor mixing in the left atrium. By either technique the pulmonary blood volume is 10 per cent of the total circulating blood volume. With pulmonary artery injection and peripheral arterial sampling, the central blood volume is approximately 20 to 25 per cent of the total blood volume.

The indicator used is one that is easily and accurately detected because of its chemical, electrical, optical, or thermal properties.[181] It should be stable, nontoxic, and sterile for intravenous use; there should be no loss from the circulation in the first passage. The volume of injectate needed should be small and measurable with precision, and repeated doses should be possible without staining;[182] its quantitative detection should not be influenced by changes in oxyhemoglobin concentration.[183,184]

In the absence of shunt, the indicator-dilution curve shows an uninterrupted buildup slope, a sharp concentration peak, a steep disappearance slope (short disappearance time), and a prominent recirculation peak (Fig. 8-13A). Two major types of distortion are produced by central shunting.[185-187] In a left-to-right shunt, there are decreased peak concentration of dye, a gentle disappearance slope (prolonged disappearance time), and absence of the recirculation peak (Fig. 8-13B). These alterations are produced by the recirculation of indicator particles through the lungs, resulting in a slow release of indicator to the peripheral circulation. The typical curve produced by a venoarterial, or right-to-left, shunt shows deformity of the buildup slope by an abnormal early-appearing hump, or reflection, representing indicator that has been shunted from right to left (Fig. 8-13C).

The distortion in contour of the indicator-dilution curve in valvular regurgitation is similar to that occurring with left-to-right shunts.

The shape of the curve is also affected by changes in volume between the injection and the sampling sites and by changes in cardiac output. When an injection site is moved progressively to the periphery, there is an increased appearance time, decreased concentration peak, and all time components are lengthened except the recirculation time. With exercise and increased cardiac output, all time components are decreased and the peak concentration is decreased. In congestive heart failure with low cardiac output, all time components are prolonged and there is a small and poorly defined concentration peak.

The output is falsely high if some indicator is lost. If some indicator is counted twice, i.e., if undetected recirculation occurs, the cardiac output is falsely low. Curves that have an abnormal gradual downslope or a very high recirculation takeoff should be suspect. Evidence for nonuniform arterial distribution of dye has been presented.[188] In general, however, values for cardiac output obtained with the indicator-dilution technique compare closely with those obtained by the Fick method.[189-192]

Many investigators have attempted to define mathematically the factors that alter the shape of the indicator-dilution curve.[193-195] Efforts have been made to predict all or part of the curve from certain other curve components. The forward-triangle method compares favorably with the Hamil-

ton analysis. In this technique, the initial portion of the indicator-dilution curve is considered to be a triangle.[196] The area of this triangle multiplied by a constant gives the area of the primary dilution curve. Thus:

$$\text{Cardiac output} = \frac{60 \times I \times K}{\frac{1}{2}\,C_p \times BT}$$

where K = 0.35 (peripheral) or 0.37 (central), depending on the site of injection

C_p = peak concentration of indicator particles at sampling site, mg/L

BT = buildup time, sec, which equals time of peak concentration PCT minus time of first appearance of dye particles AT

The method of Dow gives similar results.[197]

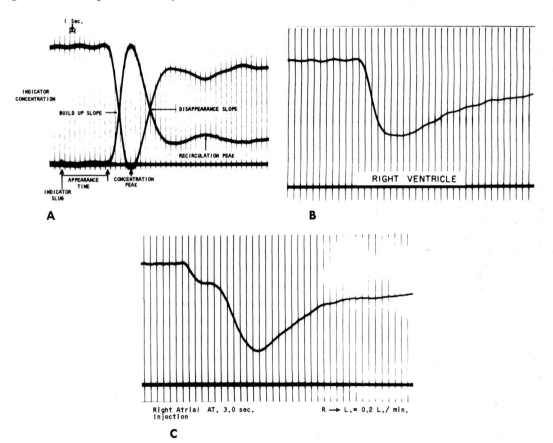

A

B

C

Fig. 8-13. *A.* Simultaneously recorded, oppositely inscribed indicator-dilution curves from the femoral arteries of a normal subject. The polarity of the recorded curve depends on local convention. Note the uninterrupted buildup slope, the steep disappearance slope, and the prominent recirculation peak characteristic of the normal indicator-dilution curve. *B.* Peripheral indicator-dilution curve following injection of indicator into the right ventricle of a patient with a left-to-right shunt. The peak concentration of indicator is decreased, the disappearance slope is gentle (prolonged disappearance time), and the recirculation peak is absent. *C.* Peripheral indicator-dilution curve following right atrial injection in a patient with a right-to-left shunt. The buildup slope is deformed by an early-appearing hump representing shunted indicator.

Quantification of Shunts. The forward-triangle method of indicator-dilution curve analysis is also used to quantitate shunts. The values obtained correlate well with those from the Fick method. In a left-to-right shunt, the pulmonary blood flow is calculated by using the forward triangle from a systemic artery curve following the injection of indicator into the *distal* pulmonary artery. If the forward-triangle area of a venous dilution curve, simultaneously obtained from the *proximal* pulmonary artery, is used, the fraction of pulmonary flow due to shunted blood may be found.[198,199]

The estimation of a right-to-left shunt[200] by indicator-dilution techniques is based on the supposition that the area under the early-appearing hump of the dilution curve is proportional to the volume of shunt flow.[201] This area plus the area of the remainder of the curve is then a measure of the total systemic flow. The ratio of shunt area to total area gives the percentage of right-to-left shunt (Fig. 8-14). This technique detects and quantitates a right-to-left shunt of 5 per cent of systemic flow. Injection is made upstream from the site of right-to-left shunt, and sampling is from a peripheral artery.

Despite continuing effort,[202] there is at present no satisfactory method of quantitating accurately the volume of valvular regurgitation by indicator-dilution techniques.[144,203-208]

Detection and Localization of Shunts. The configuration of the peripheral dye-dilution curve is not usually altered by a left-to-right shunt of less than 20 per cent of pulmonary flow. The search for increased sensitivity in the detection of small left-to-right shunts has led to much ingenious methodology.[209] The use of tricarbocyanine green dye with peak absorption at an isobestic point for both reduced hemoglobin and oxyhemoglobin, and thus relative insensitivity to fluctuation in oxygen saturation, has made venous dye-dilution curves possible for the right side of the heart.[183,184] Following an injection into a distal lobar pulmonary artery catheter, a shunt as small as 5 per cent of pulmonary flow may be detected by a second proximal catheter, sampling from the main pulmonary artery.[210,223] In a left-to-right shunt, the venous return curve from the main pulmonary artery sampling site shows an early appearance peak. For localization, the sampling site is moved retrograde until early dye is no longer detected. Only a single catheter is required if a radioactive gas, ethyl or methyl iodide, is introduced into the left side of the heart by a single inhalation.[211-213] In a left-to-right

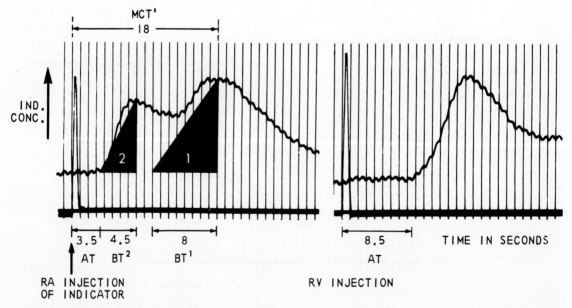

Fig. 8-14. The use of buildup triangles for the calculation of right-to-left shunt in a patient with reversal of flow through an atrial septal defect. There is early appearance of indicator following right atrial injection. Note the normal appearance time following right ventricular injection of indicator. Triangles 1 and 2 represent the areas of the buildup triangles of the primary and secondary curves, respectively. BT' is theoretically derived (BT^1 = 0.44 MCT^1). AT, appearance time; BT^1 and BT^2, buildup times of primary and secondary curves; MCT^1, maximal concentration time. The peak concentration of the primary and secondary curves is measured directly from the record. The quotient (area of triangle 2 divided by the area of triangles 1 plus 2) times 100 equals the right-to-left shunt in percentage of systemic flow. In this example, 30 per cent of the systemic flow was shunted from the venous side.

shunt, appearance at the pulmonary artery catheter and in sites distal to the shunt significantly precedes the appearance of gas proximal to the left-to-right shunt. After nitrous oxide is breathed, the content of gas is elevated in right heart blood samplings obtained at or downstream from the site of left-to-right shunt.[214,215] Simultaneous sampling from the pulmonary artery and the peripheral artery during a 30-sec inhalation of the inert radioactive gas krypton (Kr^{85}) may also be used to detect small left-to-right shunts. In normal persons, the venous-to-arterial ratio of radioactivity is less than 15 per cent and in shunts is nearly always greater than 20 per cent.[216-218] Recording isotope dilution curves directly by precordial counting[219,220] is not adequate for detection of small left-to-right shunts. Shunts of less than 10 per cent of pulmonary flow can be detected and quantitated if helium or nitrogen is inhaled briefly and if the transient reduction in blood-oxygen saturation is monitored simultaneously and continuously in a peripheral artery and in the right side of the heart.[221]

Localization of a shunt requires comparisons of injections made proximal to or at the site of the shunt with those made distal to the site of shunt.[222,223,199] The accurate localization of shunts may occasionally be subject to error related to streaming of indicator forward or backward from the chamber of injection.[224]

The catheter tip may enter the root of a great vessel whose identity cannot be ascertained by the position of the catheter or by determinations of pressure or oxygen saturation. The appearance time of injected dye may be used to identify the vessel as either the pulmonary artery or the aorta.[225] An injection made into an anomalous pulmonary vein would resemble a curve from an injection made in the venae cavae.[226] In pulmonary atresia the heart ejects via a single great vessel, the aorta, and thus the contours of dilution curves following injection into the right ventricle and the aorta are similar.[227] In tricuspid atresia the blood flow to both ventricles comes by a common path across the mitral valve; thus dilution curves following injection into the right atrium and left atrium are similar.[228]

Peripheral dye-dilution curves following central injection are highly successful in detecting small right-to-left shunt (5 per cent of the systemic flow). The detection of the early appearance of cyanide[229] or of fluorescein at the histamine-prepared ear under Wood's light following an injection of 2 ml of the 20 per cent solution, and detection of the decrease in arm-facial paresthesia time following ether injection[230] were among the first circulatory measurements in venoarterial shunts. Since then, numerous dyes have been used as indicators, as well as concentrated saline solution detected by conductivity cell,[231] P^{32}-tagged red blood cells, cold saline solution or blood,[232-234] and radioactive Renografin. Radioactive krypton (Kr^{85}) in solution injected centrally is detected in high concentration in arterial blood in a right-to-left shunt. Normally 95 per cent of the gas is cleared in one passage through the lungs, and the arterial concentration is low. Kr^{85} may be detected early in expired air following injection into the left side of the heart proximal to the site of a left-to-right shunt.[216-218]

The *hydrogen electrode* utilizes the principle of potentiometry in measuring the direct voltage between a silver and platinum electrode.[235-239] Unlike the polarographic technique, this method requires no membrane. Hydrogen gas (dissolved in blood) yields, reversibly, two hydrogen ions plus two electrons on contact with a platinum surface. The potential developed (300 to 400 mv) is easily recorded. The hydrogen electrode is sensitive to other redox substances, such as ascorbic acid [240] or isoproterenol. The platinum electrode is easily mounted on a catheter tip[241] or a needle obturator. The patient inhales hydrogen gas from a conductive bag. It is dissolved in the alveolar capillary blood and enters the left side of the heart. If a left-to-right shunt is present, the hydrogen gas will be detected within 4 sec of the time of inhalation at the site of shunt (Fig. 8-15) or downstream from it.[242] The site of shunt can be detected by varying the position of the platinum electrode–tipped catheter.[243,244] Rapid circulation as a cause of early-appearing hydrogen can be excluded by a simultaneous recording from a peripheral artery electrode.

An intravenous injection of hydrogen dissolved in saline solution or blood is completely cleared in one passage through the lung. Hydrogen detected early in the aorta or its branches is due to right-to-left shunt.[245] The site of shunt can be detected by varying the site of central injection.

The hydrogen-electrode system is extremely sensitive[246,247] and is easy to use. Inhalations may be repeated numerous times. Hydrogen gas is explosive at a concentration of 5 per cent or greater, and the intracardiac electrode has a low resistance to stray current flow, but these potential disadvantages do not militate against the value of its daily use.

Ventricular Volume Measurements (Thermodilution)

The thermodilution technique was introduced by Fegler in 1953 in order to measure volume flow rate.[248-250] The indicator may be either warmer[251] or colder than circulating blood, but usually cold blood or saline solution is injected.[252] The detector is a thermistor-tipped conventional cardiac catheter.

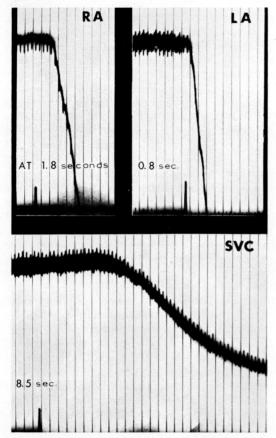

Fig. 8-15. Use of the platinum electrode catheter in the detection and localization of left-to-right shunts. Note the abnormal early appearance of inhaled hydrogen gas at the right atrial level in a patient with atrial septal defect. A normal venous circulation curve is noted in the superior vena cava.

The apparatus is simple and relatively inexpensive, and repeated measurements may be made without withdrawal of blood. The excellent response time of the thermistor makes the temperature record suitable for the calculation of ventricular end-diastolic volume.[253]

A bead thermistor–tipped catheter is placed beyond the aortic or pulmonary artery semilunar valve. A slug of ice-cold saline solution or cold blood is injected by a second catheter into the ventricle, during diastole. As the cold solution is ejected from the heart, the thermistor temperature drops and then progressively rises in a beat-to-beat, steplike disappearance slope as the cold solution is washed out of the ventricle (Fig. 8-16). Recirculation does not occur. Cardiac output may be calculated by the modified Stewart-Hamilton method.

The end-diastolic volume measurement is that of a static volume; the end-diastolic volume equals

"the amount of cold injected" divided by the temperature or concentration of the "cold-" blood mixture at the first systole following the injection of cold saline solution.[254,253] The formula, using the ratio of any two successive washout steps[254] and the stroke volume, is especially reliable for high end-diastolic volumes. Other indicators, including dye,[255,254] concentrated saline solution,[254] and radioactive isotopes,[256] may be used for the measurement of ventricular volume. The optical density changes associated with the washout of opaque media from the ventricle may be quantitated by analysis of the cinecardiogram.[199]

The following assumptions are made in this determination:[257]

1. That complete mixing of blood and indicator occurs in the ventricle.

2. That there is a constant end-diastolic, end-systolic, and stroke volume during the few seconds of the determination.

3. That the concentration recorded in the aorta during diastole is equal to the concentration in the ventricle during the immediately preceding systole.

Left ventricular volumes have been measured by angiocardiography using opaque media.[258-265] The left ventricle shadow is treated as an ellipsoid, and its end-systolic and end-diastolic surface area is measured on the film in two planes, with correction for magnification. Right ventricular volume is not directly determinable by x-ray techniques because of the shape of the right ventricle.[266] By radiologic techniques the percentage emptying of the ventricle is 50 to 70 per cent, and by the washout technique the percentage emptying is 30 to 40 per cent.[269] Close agreement between the two methods awaits refinement in both techniques. By both techniques, the stroke volume agrees well with indicator-dilution and Fick determinations.[267-269] The volume of one ventricle or of both may be derived from washout curves obtained by precordial counting of the passage of radioactive gamma–emitting tracer through the heart and lungs.[256,270-272]

The direct measurement of end-diastolic volume is extremely important in the study of ventricular function and may be useful in helping to define early heart failure.

Resistance

Vascular resistance is impedance to blood flow in systemic, pulmonary, or regional vascular beds. It is estimated by analogy to Ohm's law:

$$\text{Resistance} = \frac{\text{pressure, volts}}{\text{flow, amp}}$$

$$= \frac{\text{mean pressure differential across the vascular bed}}{\text{blood flow}}$$

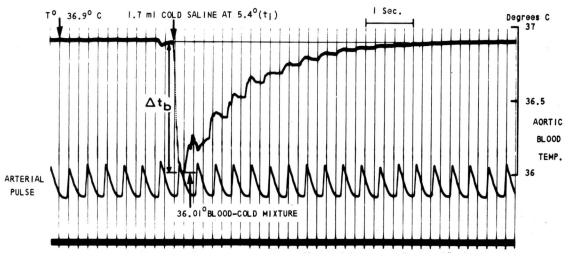

Fig. 8-16. Thermodilution curve recorded from the aorta following the injection of cold normal saline solution into the left ventricle during diastole. A 95 per cent response to an instantaneous temperature change occurs in 0.2 sec.

$$\text{End-diastolic volume} = \frac{\text{amount of cold shared by the injectate and the blood}}{\Delta t_b \text{ (change in the aortic blood temperature during the first systole after injection)}}$$

$$\text{End-diastolic volume} = \frac{(36.9 - 5.4) \times (1.7 \text{ ml})}{(36.9 - 36.01)} - \frac{53.55}{0.89} = 60 \text{ ml}$$

One converts to the metric centimeter-gram-second (cgs) scale as follows:

1. Pressure = density of fluid (mass per unit volume) $\times$ gravity acceleration factor $\times$ height of fluid column

1 mm Hg pressure

$$= 13.6 \frac{\text{Gm}}{\text{cm}^3} \times 980 \frac{\text{cm}}{\text{sec}^2} \times 0.1 \text{ cm}$$

$$= 1{,}332 \frac{\text{Gm-cm-cm}}{\text{cm}^3 \text{ sec}^2} = 1{,}332 \left(\frac{\text{Gm-cm}}{\text{sec}^2}\right) \frac{1}{\text{cm}^2}$$

By definition, 1 dyne = 1 $\dfrac{\text{Gm-cm}}{\text{sec}^2}$

Therefore 1 mm Hg pressure = $1{,}332 \left(\dfrac{\text{dynes}}{\text{cm}^2}\right)$

2. Blood flow is the cardiac output in milliliters per second. In cgs units, then:

$$\text{Resistance} = \frac{\text{mean pressure differential, mm Hg,}}{\text{blood flow (cardiac output in ml/sec)}} \times 1{,}332 \text{ dynes/cm}^2$$

$$R = \frac{\text{mean pressure differential}}{\text{flow in ml/sec}} \times 1{,}332 \text{ dynes-sec-cm}^{-5}$$

Conversion into cgs units does not add to the intrinsic significance of the measurements. Resistance may be expressed simply as:

$$R \text{ in units} = \frac{\text{pressure difference}}{\text{cardiac output}}$$

but preferably in order to obtain data that are comparable in infants, children, and adults, the pressure drop is related to the flow index, thus:

$$R = \frac{\text{pressure difference}}{\text{cardiac index}}$$

Generally, 1 resistance unit = 80 dynes-sec-cm^{-5} or 80 dynes per cm^2 per ml/sec of blood flow.

Another technique is to relate all resistances to the standard adult surface area of 1.7 m^2.

In a physiologic sense the term *resistance* avoids specific definition. A change in resistance usually means a change in cross-sectional area of the vascular bed but does not indicate the mechanism behind the change.[273] Passive widening of the vessels by increases in intravascular pressure as well as the opening of previously closed channels may produce changes in resistance similar to those of active vasomotion. The ideal state of constant flow must be present before a change in pulmonary artery pressure can be interpreted as due to vasomotion.

Calculation of Valve Areas

The equation for resistance (Poiseuille's law) applies to the pressure differential or decay due to friction or impedance in a long multiple-tube system at relatively steady velocity and flow. In contrast the equation for calculation of valve areas (Torricelli's orifice equation) uses a standard hydrokinetic formula for a rounded-edge orifice or a short tube. When flow occurs across a narrow orifice, the pressure differential or decay is related to the conversion of pressure into high-velocity flow. The Gorlin formula derivation for calculation of valve area is from two standard formulas:[274]

Formula I.

$$F = AVC_c$$

where F = volume rate of flow during the time the valvular orifice is open, ml/sec of diastole or systole

    A = area of fixed orifice, cm²

    V = velocity flow, cm/sec

    C_c = coefficient of orifice contraction compensating for the physical phenomenon of reduction of the orifice stream to an area less than the area of the actual orifice

Formula II.

$$V^2 = C_v^2 \; 2gh \quad \text{or} \quad V = C_v \; \sqrt{2gh}$$

where g = gravity acceleration (980 cm/sec/sec)

    V = as above

    h = pressure head or differential across the orifice, cm water

    C_v = coefficient of velocity (allowing for some loss in conversion of pressure energy to velocity)

Combining I and II:

$$A = \frac{F}{C_c \times C_v \; \sqrt{2gh}} \qquad A = \frac{F}{C \times 44.5 \; \sqrt{P_1 - P_2}}$$

where C = discharge coefficient (an empirical constant obtained by comparing calculated with measured valve areas at postmortem,[274,275] which combined C_c, C_v, conversion factor, mm Hg to cm H₂O, other unknown factors)

$$44.5 = \sqrt{2g} = \sqrt{1,960}$$

$h = P_1 - P_2$

    = pressure differential across the orifice, mm Hg

The duration of ventricular filling or emptying is measured in seconds from the arterial pressure tracing, or from simultaneous pressure records obtained on the immediate upstream and downstream sides of the valve. The systolic or diastolic time per beat multiplied by the heart rate gives the number of seconds in each minute during which either filling or emptying occurs across the valve. Thus, the volume rate of flow in milliliters per second of systole or diastole is the mean volume rate of flow (cardiac output, ml/min) divided by the filling or emptying time in seconds per each minute.

A sample calculation of mitral valve area is as follows:

Cardiac output (*CO*)   = 5,000 ml/min
Diastolic filling period
   (*Dfp*) beat   = 0.38 sec/beat
Pulse rate   = 90 beats/min
Dfp/min   = 34 sec/min
Left atrial mean
   pressure (*LAP*)   = 30 mm Hg
Left ventricular mean
   diastolic pressure (*LVDP*) = 5 mm Hg
C   = 0.7 (empirical constant for the mitral valve)

$$\text{Mitral valve flow } (MVF) = \frac{CO}{Dfp/\text{min}}$$

$$= \frac{5,000 \text{ ml/min}}{34 \text{ sec/min}} = 147 \text{ ml/sec of diastole}$$

Mitral valve orifice area (*MVA*) =

$$\frac{MVF}{0.7 \times 44.5 \; \sqrt{LAP - LVDP}} = \frac{147}{31 \; \sqrt{25}} = 0.9 \text{ cm}^2$$

The calculation for the aortic valve area is as follows:

AVA, cm²

$$= \frac{F}{C \times 44.5 \; \sqrt{P_1 - P_2}}$$

$$= \frac{\text{aortic valve flow, ml/systolic sound}}{1 \times 44.5 \; \sqrt{LVS - ASP}}$$

where LVS = left ventricular systolic mean pressure, mm HG

    ASP = aortic systolic mean pressure, mm Hg

Similarly, valve areas may be calculated for the tricuspid and pulmonary valves. The approximations and systematic errors in the formulas do not detract from their usefulness in providing objectivity in the classification of patients with valvular disease. If flow is normal, reducing the orifice diameter to less than half or the cross-sectional area to one-fourth is required to offer significant obstruction. Calculation of valve orifices is not possible in the presence of valvular regurgitation, since the amount of regurgitant flow cannot be accurately measured. Any such calculation would overestimate the severity of the stenosis.

INDICATIONS FOR CARDIAC CATHETERIZATION

Cardiac catheterization is performed (1) to confirm the presence of a clinically suspected lesion and simultaneously to exclude associated hidden lesions; (2) to evaluate the severity of a known cardiac lesion; (3) to establish a diagnosis when the specific lesion is not certain but heart disease is known to be present;[276] (4) to establish or disprove the presence of a cardiac lesion when it is not known whether heart disease is present; and (5) to evaluate the completeness and long-term effect of surgical repair. There is no absolute contraindication to cardiac catheterization. Increased risk is expected in the severely cyanotic infant, in the infant with markedly elevated pulmonary venous pressure, and in those subjects with severe semilunar valve stenosis. The techniques used, the number of selective angiocardiograms and catheterizations on the left side of the heart that are performed, the proportion of sick infants studied, and the experience of the catheterization unit are factors that determine the overall risk.

COMPLICATIONS OF CARDIAC CATHETERIZATION

The experienced operator can carry out catheterization of the right side of the heart without difficulty in practically all cases.[277] Reported complications, however, have included knotting, looping, kinking, or partially breaking the catheter so that it cannot be withdrawn freely; excessive blood loss, pyrogen reaction, perforation of the atrium, ventricle, or coronary vein,[278,279,295,296] hypoxia due to reduction in effective orifice area of a severely stenotic pulmonary valve by the catheter,[280] venous spasm, air embolism, pulmonary infarction from flushing a small clot while in the pulmonary artery wedge position or in a lobar pulmonary artery, localized phlebitis and thrombosis, and cutdown infection. Prolonged ventricular or atrial arrhythmia may occur. Nonspecific elevation of the level of serum glutamic oxaloacetic transaminase has been noted after catheterization and angiocardiography.[281] Small currents due to improper grounding may easily pass into the heart via an electrode catheter or a saline solution–filled conventional catheter, causing ventricular fibrillation.[282] All electronic and x-ray equipment should have an ample common ground.[283] The catheterization room should have as standard equipment an external defibrillator and a bag and mask for supplying oxygen. Personnel should be competent in external cardiac massage.[284,285]

Catheterization of the left side of the heart entails a moderate increase in the opportunity for complications.[286,287] If arterial catheterization is used, complete or partial thrombosis may occur at the cannulation site with or without propagation of the clot. Recurrent neurovascular pain may rarely persist after brachial artery catheterization, and claudication occasionally follows femoral artery catheterization. Bleeding may occur at the percutaneous puncture site or retroperitoneally if perforation of the artery occurs at a tortuous abdominal or pelvic site.[288,289] Intravascular breakage of a spring guide wire has occurred.[290] Direct left ventricular puncture may be complicated by hemopericardium, cardiac tamponade, pneumothorax, pleural effusion, and pulmonary atelectasis. The transseptal approach may result in inadvertent puncture of the aorta or the free wall of the atrium, with resultant hemopericardium and cardiac tamponade.[291,76] A persistent puncture defect of the atrial septum with left-to-right shunt has been noted;[292] a broken tip of the transseptal needle has embolized to the liver;[293] a left atrial mural thrombus has formed.[294]

REFERENCES

1. Bleichroeder, F.: Intra arterielle Therapie, *Berlin klin. Wchnschr.*, 49:1503, 1912.
2. Benatt, A. J.: Cardiac Catheterization: A Historical Note, *Lancet*, 1:746, 1949.
3. Forssman, W.: Die Sondierung des rechten Herzens, *Berlin klin. Wchnschr.*, 8:2085, 1929.
4. Cournand, A., and Ranges, H. A.: Catheterization of the Right Auricle in Man, *Proc. Soc. Exper. Biol. & Med.*, 46:462, 1941.
5. Cournand, A., Bloomfield, R. A., and Lauson, H. D.: Double Lumen Catheter for Intravenous and Intracardiac Blood Sampling and Pressure Tracing, *Proc. Soc. Exper. Biol. & Med.*, 60:73, 1945.
6. Cournand, A., Riley, R. L., Breed, E. S., Baldwin, E. deF., and Richards, D. W., Jr.: Measurement of Cardiac Output in Man Using the Technique of Catheterization of the Right Auricle or Ventricle, *J. Clin. Invest.*, 24:106, 1945.
7. Richards, D. W., Jr., Cournand, A., Darling, R. C., Gillespie, W. H., and Baldwin, E. DeF.: Pressure of Blood in the Right Auricle, in Animals and in Man, under Normal Conditions and in Right Heart Failure, *Am. J. Physiol.*, 136:115, 1942.
8. Dexter, L., Burwell, C. S., Haynes, F. W., and Seibel, R. E.: Oxygen Content of Pulmonary "Capillary" Blood in Unanesthetized Human Beings, *J. Clin. Invest.*, 25:913, 1946.
9. Dexter, L., Haynes, F. W., Burwell, C. S., Eppinger, E. C., Seibel, R. E., and Evans, J. M.: Studies of Congenital Heart Disease. I. Technique of Venous Catheterization as a Diagnostic Procedure, *J. Clin. Invest.*, 26:547, 1947.
10. Dexter, L., Haynes, F. W., Burwell, C. S., Eppinger, E. C., Sagerson, R. P., and Evans, J. M.: Studies of Congenital Heart Disease. II. Pressure and Oxygen Content of Blood in Right Auricle, Right Ventricle, and Pulmonary Artery in Control Patients, with Observations on Oxygen Saturation and Source of Pulmonary "Capillary" Blood, *J. Clin. Invest.*, 26:554, 1947.
11. Dexter, L., Haynes, F. W., Burwell, C. S., Eppinger, E. C., Sosman, M. C., and Evans, J. M.:

Studies of Congenital Heart Disease. III. Venous Catheterization as a Diagnostic Aid in Patent Ducts Arteriosus, Tetralogy of Fallot, Ventricular Septal Defect, and Auricular Septal Defect, *J. Clin. Invest.*, **26**:561, 1947.

12. Dexter, L.: Venous Catheterization of the Heart. II. Results, Interpretation and Value, *Radiology*, **48**:451, 1947.

12*a*. McMichael, J., and Sharpey-Schafer, E.: Cardiac Output in Man by a Direct Fick Method, *Brit. Heart J.*, **6**:33, 1944.

13. Bing, R. J., Vandam, L. D., and Gray, F. D., Jr.: Physiological Studies in Congenital Heart Disease. I. Procedures, *Bull. Johns Hopkins Hosp.*, **80**:107, 1947.

14. Baldwin, E. deF., Moore, L. V., and Noble, R. P.: The Demonstration of Ventricular Septal Defect by means of Right Heart Catheterization, *Am. Heart J.*, **32**:152, 1946.

15. Bloomfield, R. A., Lauson, H. D., Cournand, A., Breed, E. S., and Richards, D. W., Jr.: Recording of Right Heart Pressures in Normal Subjects and in Patients with Chronic Pulmonary Disease and Various Types of Cardiocirculatory Disease, *J. Clin. Invest.*, **25**:639, 1946.

16. Brannon, E. S., Weens, H. S., and Warren, J. V.: Atrial Septal Defect: Study of Hemodynamics by the Technique of Right Heart Catheterization, *Am. J. M. Sc.*, **210**:480, 1945.

17. Holling, H. E., and Zak, G. A.: Cardiac Catheterization in the Diagnosis of Congenital Heart Disease, *Brit. Heart J.*, **12**:153, 1950.

18. Rudolph, A. M., and Cayler, G. G.: Cardiac Catheterization in Infants and Children, *Pediat. Clin. North America*, **5**:907, 1958.

19. Selzer, A., Willet, F. M., McCaughey, D. J., and Feichtmeir, T. V.: Uses of Cardiac Catheterization in Acquired Heart Disease, *New England J. Med.*, **257**:66, 121, 1957.

20. Selzer, A., Poppes, R. W., Lau, F. Y. K., Morgan, J. J., and Anderson, W. L.: Present Status of Diagnostic Cardiac Catheterization, *New England J. Med.*, **268**:589, 654, 1963.

21. Richards, D. W.: Right Heart Catheterization: Its Contributions to Physiology and Medicine, *Science*, **125**:1181, 1957.

22. Smith, C., Rowe, R. D., and Vlad, P.: Sedation of Children for Cardiac Catheterization with an Ataractic Mixture, *Canad. Anaesth. Soc. J.*, **5**:35, 1958.

23. Moffitt, E. A., Dawson, B., and O'Neill, N. C.: Anesthesia for Pediatric Cardiac Catheterization and Angiography, *Anesth. & Analg.*, **40**:483, 1961.

24. Hohn, A. R., and Vlad, P.: A Guide for Introducing Catheterization Cannulating Small Vessels, *Pediatrics*, **24**:636, 1959.

25. Sapin, S. O., Linde, L. M., and Emmanouilides, G. C.: Umbilical Angiocardiography, *Pediatrics*, **31**:946, 1963.

26. Dotter, C. T., and Straube, K. R.: Flow Guided Cardiac Catheterization, *Am. J. Roentgenol.*, **88**:27–30, 1962.

27. Hellems, H. K., Haynes, F. W., and Dexter, L.: Pulmonary "Capillary" Pressure in Man, *J. Appl. Physiol.*, **2**:24, 1949.

28. Lagerlof, H., and Weiko, L.: Studies on the Circulation of Blood in Man. VI. The Pulmonary Capillary Venous Pressure Pulse in Man, *Scandinav. J. Clin. & Lab. Invest.*, **1**:147, 1949.

29. Facquet, J., Lemoin, J. M., Alhomme, P., and Lefeboie, J.: La mesure de la pression auriculaire gauche par voie transbronchique, *Arch. mal. coeur*, **48**:741, 1952.

30. Allison, P. R., and Linden, R. J.: Bronchoscopic Measurement of Left Auricular Pressure, *Circulation*, **7**:669–673, 1953.

31. Crymes, T. P., Fish, R. G., Smith, D. E., and Takaro, T.: Complications of Transbronchial Left Atrial Puncture, *Am. Heart J.*, **58**:46, 1959.

32. Morrow, A. G., Braunwald, E., Haller, J. A., and Sharp, E. H.: Left Heart Catheterization by Transbronchial Route: Technic and Applications in Physiologic and Diagnostic Investigations, *Circulation*, **16**:1033–1039, 1957.

33. Morrow, A. G., Braunwald, E., and Tanenbaum, H. L.: Transbronchial Left Heart Catheterization: Modified Technique and Its Physiologic Evaluation, *S. Forum*, **8**:390–392, 1958.

34. Bjork, V. O., Malmstrom, G., and Uggla, L. G.: Left Auricular Pressure Measurements in Man, *Ann. Surg.*, **138**:718–725, 1953.

35. Bjork, V. O.: Direct Pressure Measurement in the Left Atrium, the Left Ventricle, and the Aorta, *Acta chir. scandiav.*, **107**:466, 1954.

36. Bjork, V. O., Blakemore, W. S., and Malmstrom, G.: Left Ventricular Pressure Measurement in Man: New Method, *Am. Heart J.*, **48**:197–203, 1954.

37. Fisher, D. L.: Use of Pressure, Recordings Obtained at Transthoracic Left Heart Catheterization in Diagnosis of Valvular Heart Disease, *J. Thoracic Surg.*, **30**:379–396, 1955.

38. Musser, B. G., and Goldberg, H.: Left Heart Catheterization: Evaluation of Its Clinical Application in 450 Cases, *J. Thoracic Surg.*, **34**:414–420, 1957.

39. Brock, R., Milstein, B. B., and Ross, D. N.: Percutaneous Left Ventricular Puncture in the Assessment of Aortic Stenosis, *Thorax*, **11**:163, 1956.

40. Radner, S.: Suprasternal Puncture of Left Atrium for Flow Studies, *Acta med. scandinav.*, **148**:57–60, 1954.

41. Radner, S.: Extended Suprasternal Puncture Technique, *Acta med. scandinav.*, **151**:223, 1955.

42. Seldinger, S. I.: Catheter Replacement of the Needle in Percutaneous Arteriography, *Acta radiol.*, **39**:368, 1953.

43. Amplatz, K., and Harner, H.: A New Subclavian

Artery Catheterization Technic, *Radiology*, **78**:963, 1962.

44. Prioton, J. B., Thévenet, A., Pelissier, M., Puech, P., Latour, H., and Pourquier, J.: Cardiographie ventriculaire gauche par catheterisme retrograde percutane femorale; Technique et premiers resultats, *Presse méd.*, **65**:1948–1951, 1957.

45. Odman, P., and Philipsson, J.: Aortic Valvular Diseases Studied by Percutaneous Thoracic Aortography, *Acta radiol.*, Suppl. 172, 1958.

46. Odman, P.: The Radiopaque Polythene Catheter, *Acta radiol.*, **52**, fasc. 1, 1959.

47. Dotter, C. T., and Gensini, G. G.: Percutaneous Retrograde Catheterization of the Left Ventricle and Systemic Arteries of Man, *Radiology*, **75**:171–184, 1960.

48. Dotter, C. T.: Left Ventricular and Systemic Arterial Catheterization; Simple, Percutaneous Method Using Spring Guide, *Am. J. Roentgenol.*, **83**:969–984, 1960.

49. Lurie, P. R., Armer, R. M., and Klatte, E. C.: Percutaneous Guide Wire Catheterization in Diagnosis and Therapy, *Am. J. Dis. Child.*, **106**:189, 1963.

50. Littmann, D., Starobin, O. E., Hall, J. H., Matthews, R. J., and Williams, J. A.: New Method of Left Ventricular Catheterization, *Circulation*, **21**:1150–1155, 1960.

51. Limon Lason, R., Rubio Alvarez, V., and Bouchard, F.: El cateterismo intracardiaco: Cateterizacion de las cavidades izquierdas en el hombre. Registro simultaneo de presion y electrocardiograma intracavitarios, *Arch. Inst. cardiol. México*, **20**:147, 1950.

52. Green, E. W., Ziegler, R. F., and Kavanagh-Gray, D.: Clinical Use of Retrograde Left Ventricular Catheterization in Congenital Heart Disease, *Circulation*, **20**:704, 1959.

53. Zimmerman, H. A., Scott, R. W., and Becker, N. D.: Catheterization of Left Side of Heart in Man, *Circulation*, **1**:357, 1950.

54. Husson, G. S., and Blackman, M. S.: Arteriotomy for Catheterization of the Left Side of the Heart in Children, *New England J. Med.*, **268**:545, 1963.

55. Vengsarkar, A. S., and Swan, H. J. C.: Arteriotomy for Cardiac Catheterization and Angiocardiography in Infants and Children, *Proc. Staff Meet. Mayo Clin.*, **37**:619, 1962.

56. Gray, I. R., and Joshepura, C. S.: Retrograde Left Ventricular Catheterization and Cardioangiography in Aortic Stenosis, *Brit. Heart J.*, **26**:199, 1964.

57. Vlad, P., Hohn, A., and Lambert, E. C.: Retrograde Arterial Catheterization of the Left Heart: Experience with 500 Infants and Children, *Circulation*, **29**:787, 1964.

58. Lambert, E. C., and Vlad, P.: Retrograde Arterial Catheterization of Left Heart: Experience with 117 Infants and Children, *Circulation*, **20**:724, 1959 (Abstract).

59. Honick, G. L., Cayler, G. G., Richardson, W. R., and Taybi, H.: New Type of Catheter Tip for Retrograde Catheterization of the Left Ventricle in Congenital Aortic Stenosis, *New England J. Med.*, **266**:1101, 1962.

60. Ross, J., Jr.: Catheterization of the Left Heart through the Interatrial Septum: A New Technique and Its Experimental Evaluation, *S. Forum*, **9**:297, 1959.

61. Ross, J., Jr.: Transseptal Left Heart Catheterization: A New Method of Left Atrial Puncture, *Ann. Surg.*, **149**:395, 1959.

62. Ross, J., Jr., Braunwald, E., and Morrow, A. G.: Transseptal Left Atrial Puncture: New Technique for Measurement of Left Atrial Pressure in Man, *Am. J. Cardiol.*, **3**:653, 1959.

63. Ross, J., Jr., Braunwald, E., and Morrow, A. G.: Transseptal Left Heart Catheterization: A New Diagnostic Method, *Progr. Cardiovasc. Dis.*, **2**:315, 1960.

64. Ross, J., Jr., Braunwald, E., and Morrow, A. G.: Left Heart Catheterization by the Transseptal Route, *Circulation*, **22**:927, 1960.

65. Brockenbrough, E. C., and Braunwald, E.: A New Technique for Left Ventricular Angiocardiography and Transseptal Left Heart Catheterization, *Am. J. Cardiol.*, **6**:1062, 1960.

66. Peckham, G. B., Chrysohou, A., Aldridge, H. E., and Wigle, E. D.: Combined Percutaneous Retrograde Aortic and Transseptal Left Heart Catheterization, *Brit. Heart J.*, **26**:460, 1964.

67. Brockenbrough, E. C., Braunwald, E., and Ross, J., Jr.: Transseptal Left Heart Catheterization: Review of 450 Studies and Description of Improved Technique, *Circulation*, **25**:15, 1962.

68. Cope, C.: Technique for Transseptal Catheterization of the Left Atrium: Preliminary Report, *J. Thoracic Surg.*, **37**:482, 1959.

69. Cope, C.: Newer Techniques of Transseptal Left Heart Catheterization, *Circulation*, **27**:758, 1963.

70. McGaff, C. J., Roveti, G. C., Glassman, E., and Ross, R. S.: An Experience with Transseptal Left Heart Catheterization, *Am. Heart J.*, **61**:161, 1961.

71. Miller, B. L., and Medd, W. E.: Transseptal Left Heart Catheterization, *Brit. Heart J.*, **26**:33, 1964.

72. Endys, J., and Steinhart, L.: Transseptal Catheterization and Cardioangiography of the Left Heart by a Percutaneous Route through the Femoral Vein, *Cardiologia*, **41**:47, 1962.

73. Bloomfield, D. A., and Sinclair-Smith, B. C.: The Limbic Ledge. A Landmark for Transseptal Left Heart Catheterization, *Circulation*, **31**:103, 1965.

74. Beuren, A. J., and Apitz, J.: Left Ventricular Angiocardiography by Transseptal Puncture of the Left Atrium, *Circulation*, **28**:209, 1963.

75. Braunwald, E., Brockenbrough, E. C., Talbert, J. L., Folse, J. R., and Rockoff, S. D.: Selective Left Heart Angiocardiography by the Transseptal Route, *Am. J. Med.*, **33**:213, 1962.

76. Russell, R. O., Carroll, J. F., and Hood, W. G., Jr.: Cardiac Tamponade: A Complication of the Transseptal Technique of Left Heart Catheterization Resulting in a Fatality, *Am. J. Cardiol.*, **13**:558, 1964.

77. Fleming, H. A., Hancock, E. W., Milstein, B. B., and Ross, D. N.: Percutaneous Left Ventricular Puncture with Catheterization of Aorta, *Thorax*, **13**:97, 1958.

78. Yu, P. N., Lovejoy, F. W., Schreiner, B. F., Leahy, R. H., Stanfield, C. A., and Walther, H.: Direct Left Ventricular Puncture in the Evaluation of Aortic and Mitral Stenosis, *Am. Heart J.*, **55**:926, 1958.

79. Hamer, N. A. J., and Dow, J. W.: Selection of Techniques for Measurements of Left Heart Pressures, *Brit. Heart J.*, **23**:317, 1961.

80. Morrow, A. G., Braunwald, E., and Ross, J., Jr.: Left Heart Catheterization: An Appraisal of Techniques and Their Applications in Cardiovascular Diagnosis, *A.M.A. Arch. Int. Med.*, **105**:645, 1960.

81. Nuvoli, I.: Arteriografia dell'aorta toracica mediante puntura dell'aorta ascendente o del ventricolo, *Policlinico* (*sez. prat.*), **43**:227, 1936.

82. Ponsdomenech, E. R., and Nunez, V. B.: Heart Puncture in Man for Diodrast Visualization of the Ventricular Chambers and Great Arteries, *Am. Heart J.*, **41**:643, 1951.

83. Uricchio, J. F., Lehman, J. S., Lemmon, W. M., Boyer, R. A., and Likoff, W.: Cardiac Ventriculography in Selection of Patients for Mitral Valve Surgery, *Am. J. Cardiol.*, **3**:22, 1959.

84. Lehman, J. S., Musser, B. G., and Lykens, H. D.: Cardiac Ventriculography: Direct Transthoracic Needle Puncture Opacification of Left (or Right) Ventricle, *Am. J. Roentgenol.*, **77**:207, 1957.

85. Bjork, V. O., Cullhed, I., Hallen, A., Lodin, H., and Maless, E.: Sequelae of Left Ventricular Puncture with Angiocardiography, *Circulation*, **24**:204, 1961.

86. Lehman, J. S.: Cardiac Ventriculography: Practical Considerations, *Progr. Cardiovasc. Dis.*, **2**:52, 1959.

87. Greenberg, B. E., and Knox, F. H.: Faulty Contrast Medium Injection in Percutaneous Ventricular Puncture, *Radiology*, **75**:85, 1960.

88. Grajo, M. Z., and Lurie, P. R.: Evaluation of Method of Direct Left Heart Puncture, *J. Lab. & Clin. Med.*, **53**:140, 1959.

89. Amplatz, K., Levy, M., and Lillehei, C. W.: Transthoracic Left Heart Catheterization and Angiocardiography for Combined Assessment of Mitral and Aortic Valves, *Radiology*, **78**:638, 1962.

90. Lurie, P. R., Armer, R. M., and Klatte, E. C.: An Apical Technique for Catheterization of the Left Side of the Heart Applied to Infants and Children, *New England J. Med.*, **264**:1182, 1961.

91. Shickman, M. D., Guze, L. B., and Pearce, M. L.: Bacterimia Following Cardiac Catheterization, *New England J. Med.*, **260**:1164, 1959.

92. Watson, H.: Electrode Catheter and the Diagnostic Application of Intracardiac Electrography in Small Children, *Circulation*, **24**:284, 1964.

93. Bertrand, C. A., Zohman, L. R., and Williams, M. H., Jr.: Intracardiac Electrocardiography in Man, *Am. J. Med.*, **26**:534, 1959.

94. Vogel, J. H. K., Tabari, K., Averill, K. H., and Blount, S. G.: A Simple Technique for Identifying P Waves in Complex Arrhythmias, *Am. Heart J.*, **67**:158, 1964.

95. Lewis, D. H., Deitz, G. W., Wallace, J. D., and Brown, J. R., Jr.: Present Status of Intracardiac Phonocardiography, *Circulation*, **18**:991, 1958.

96. Fry, D. L.: Physiologic Recording by Modern Instruments with Particular Reference to Pressure Recording, *Physiol. Rev.*, **40**:753, 1960.

97. Wood, E. H.: Special Instrumentation Problems Encountered in Physiological Research Concerning the Heart and Circulation in Man, *Science*, **112**:707, 1950.

98. Wood, E. H., and Sutterer, W.: Improved Resistance Wire Strain Gauge Manometers Adaptable for Biologic Measurements, *J. Lab. & Clin. Med.*, **45**:153, 1955.

99. Fry, D. L., Noble, F. W., and Malles, A. J.: An Evaluation of Modern Pressure Recording Systems, *Circulation Res.*, **5**:40, 1957.

100. Allard, E. M.: Sound and Pressure Signals Obtained from a Single Intracardiac Transducer, *IRE Tr. Biomed. Elec.*, BME-9:74, 1962.

101. Shaw, D. B.: The Pressure Wave Form in the Pulmonary Artery, *Brit. Heart J.*, **25**:347, 1963.

102. Van Slyke, D. D., and Neill, J. M.: The Determination of Gases in Blood and Other Solutions by Vacuum Extraction and Manometric Measurements, *J. Biol. Chem.*, **61**:523, 1924.

103. Chambliss, K. W., and Nouse, D. C.: Blood Oxygen Determinations by Gas Chromatography, *Clin. Chem.*, **8**:654–659, 1962.

104. Lukas, D. S., and Ayers, S. M.: Determination of Blood Oxygen Content by Gas Chromatography, *J. Appl. Physiol.*, **16**:371–374, 1961.

105. Ramsey, I. H.: Analysis of Gas in Biological Fluids by Gas Chromatography, *Science*, **129**, 900, 1959, (abstract).

106. Wilson, R. H., Jay, B., Doty, V., Pingree, H., and Higgins, E.: Analysis of Blood Gases with Gas Absorption Chromatographic Technique, *J. Appl. Physiol.*, **16**:374, 1961.

107. Wilson, R. H., Jay, B., and Holland, R. H.: Gas Chromatography: A Simple, Rapid, Reliable Method for Blood Gas Analyses, *J. Thoracic & Cardiovasc. Surg.*, **42**:575, 1961.

108. Comroe, J. H., and Wood, E. H.: Measurement of Oxygen Saturation by Filter Photometers (Oximeters), in J. H. Comroe (ed.), "Methods in Medical Research," The Year Book Medical Publishers, Inc., Chicago, 1950, vol. 2.

109. Gordy, E., and Drabkin, D. L.: A Simplified Spectrophotometric Technique Applicable to Standard Equipment for Determining Oxygen Saturation, *Am. J. M. Sc.*, **221**:231, 1951.

110. Harned, H. S., Lurie, P. R., Croethers, C. H., and Whittemore, R.: Use of the Whole Blood Oximeter during Cardiac Catheterization, *J. Lab. & Clin. Med.*, **40**:445, 1952.

111. Wood, E. H., Geraci, J. E., and Groom, D. L.: Photoelectric Determination of Blood Oxygen Saturation in Man, *Fed. Proc.*, **7**:137, 1948.

112. Wood, E. H., Lambert, E., and Burchell, H. B.: Application of Strain Gauge Manometer, Modified Ear Oximeter and Whole Blood Cuvette Oximeter to Technique of Cardiac Catheterization, *J. Clin. Invest.*, **28**:819, 1949.

113. Wood, E. H.: The Oximeter, in Otto Glasser, "Medical Physics," 2d ed., The Year Book Medical Publishers, Inc., Chicago, 1950.

114. Zijlstra, W. G.: "A Manual of Reflection Oximetry," Van Gorcum's Medical Library, N.R. 152, Assen, Netherlands, 1958.

115. Zijlstra, W. G., and Mook, G. A.: "Medical Reflection Photometry," Royal Van Gorcum Ltd., Assen, Netherlands, 1962.

116. Rodrigo, F. A.: Determination of the Oxygen Saturation of Blood in Vitro by Using Reflected Light, *Am. Heart J.*, **45**:809, 1953.

117. Ware, P. F., Polanyi, M. L., Hehir, R. M., Stapleton, J. F., Sanders, J. I., and Kocot, S. L.: A New Reflection Oximeter, *J. Thoracic & Cardiovas. Surg.*, **42**:580, 1961.

118. Brinkman, R., and Zijlstra, W. G.: Determination and Continuous Registration of the Percentage Oxygen Saturation in Clinical Conditions, *Arch. chir. neerl.*, **1**: 177, 1949.

119. Hickam, J. B., and Frazer R.: Spectrophotometric Determination of Blood Oxygen, *J. Biol. Chem.*, **180**:457, 1949.

120. Holling, H. E., MacDonald, I., O'Halloran, J. A., and Venner, A.: Reliability of a Spectrophotometric Method of Estimating Blood Oxygen, *J. Appl. Physiol.*, **8**:249, 1955.

121. Jonxis, J. H. P., and Boeve, J. H. W.: A Spectrophotometric Determination of Oxygen Saturation in Small Amounts of Blood, *Acta med. scandinav.*, **155**:157, 1956.

122. Enson, Y., Briscoe, W. A., Polanyi, M. L., and Cournand, A.: In Vivo Studies with an Intravascular and Intracardiac Reflection Oximeter, *J. Appl. Physiol.*, **17**:552, 1962.

123. Enson, Y., Jameson, A. G., and Cournand, A.: Intracardiac Oximetry in Congenital Heart Disease, *Circulation*, **29**:499, 1964.

124. Gamble, W. J., Hugenholtz, P. G., Monroe, R. G., Polanyi, M., and Nadas, A. S.: The Use of Fiberoptics in Clinical Cardiac Catheterization. I. Intracardiac Oximetry, *Circulation*, **31**:328, **1965.**

125. Bargeron, L., Clark, L. C., and Lyons, C.: Use of an Electrode for Continuously Recording Intracardiac pO_2 Changes in Cardiac Catheterizations, *Circulation*, **24**:881, 1961.

126. Scholander, P. F.: Analyser for Accurate Estimation of Respiratory Gases in One-half Cubic Centimeter Samples, *J. Biol. Chem.*, **167**:235, 1947.

127. Pauling, L., Wood, R. E., and Sturtevant, J. H.: Oxygen Meter, *Science*, **103**:338, 1946.

128. Fowler, N. O., Mannix, E. P., Jr., and Noble, W.: Difficulties in Interpretation of Right Heart Catheterization Data, *Am. Heart J.*, **53**:343, 1957.

129. Milnor, W. R.: Evaluation of Diagnostic Tests in Cardiovascular Disease, *Mod. Concepts Cardiovas. Dis.*, **31**, no. 2, 1962.

130. Harris, P.: Some Variations in the Shape of the Pressure Curve in the Human Right Ventricle, *Brit. Heart J.*, **17**:173, 1955.

131. Bouchard, F., and Cornu, C.: Etude des couches de pressions ventriculaire droite et arterielle pulmonaire dans les retrecessements pulmonaires, *Arch. mal. coeur*, **47**:417, 1954.

132. Hoffman, J. I. E., Rudolph, A. M., Nades, A. S., and Paul, M. H.: Physiologic Differentiation of Pulmonic Stenosis with and without an Intact Ventricular Septum, *Circulation*, **12**:385, 1960.

133. Braunwald, E., and Ross, J., Jr.: The Ventricular End Diastolic Pressure: Appraisal of Its Value in the Recognition of Ventricular Failure in Man, *Am. J. Med.*, **34**:147, 1963.

134. Connolly, P. C., Kirklin, J. W., and Wood, E. H.: Relationship between Pulmonary Artery Wedge Pressure and Left Atrial Pressure in Man, *Circulation Res.*, **2**:434, 1954.

135. Nadas, A. S.: "Pediatric Cardiology," W. B. Saunders Company, Philadelphia, 1963.

136. Luchsinger, P. C., Seipp, H. W., Jr., and Patel, D. J.: Relationship of Pulmonary Artery Wedge Pressure to Left Atrial Pressure in Man, *Circulation Res.*, **11**:315, 1962.

137. Bell, L. A. L., Haynes, W. F., Jr., Shimomura, S., and Dallas, D. P.: Influence of Catheter Tip Position on Pulmonary Wedge Pressures, *Circulation Res.*, **10**:215, 1962.

138. Wiggers, G. J.: Editorial: Pulmonary Wedged Catheter Pressures, *Circulation Res.*, **1**:371, 1953.

139. Miller, D. E., Tucker, D. H., and Jacoby, W. J., Jr.: The Giant "A" Wave of the Left Atrial Appendage, *Circulation*, **28**:1110, 1963.

140. Johansson, B. W., and Ohlsson, W. M.: Falsely High Pressure Curve from the Right Atrial Appendage, *Brit. Heart J.*, **23**:281, 1961.

141. Owen, S. G., and Wood, P.: A New Method of Determining the Degree or Absence of Mitral Obstruction, *Brit. Heart J.*, **17**:41, 1955.

142. Morrow, A. G., Braunwald, E., Haller, J. A., and Sharp, E. H.: Left Atrial Pressure Pulse in Mitral Valve Disease, *Circulation*, **16**:399, 1957.

143. Hancock, E. W.: Assessment of Mitral Valve Disease by Left Heart Catheterization, *Brit. Heart J.*, **21**:389, 1959.

144. Marshall, H. W., Woodward, E., Jr., and Wood,

E. H.: Hemodynamic Methods for Differentiation of Mitral Stenosis and Regurgitation, *Am. J. Cardiol.*, 2:24, 1958.

145. Shillingford, J. P.: The Estimation of Severity of Mitral Incompetence, *Progr. Cardiovas. Dis.*, 5:248, 1962.

146. Franch, R. H., and Gay, B. B.: Congenital Stenosis of the Pulmonary Artery Branches, *Am. J. Med.*, 35:512, 1963.

147. Hamer, N. A. J., and Dow, J. W.: The Indications for Measurement of Left Heart Pressures in Mitral and Aortic Valvular Disease, *Am. Heart J.*, 62:344, 1961.

148. Bowers, D., Burchell, H. B., and Wood, E. H.: Difficulty in the Precise Localization by Cardiac Catheterization of Left to Right Shunts Near the Pulmonary Valve, *Proc. Staff Meet. Mayo Clin.*, 30:261, 1955.

149. Barratt-Boyes, B. G., and Wood, E. H.: The Oxygen Saturation of Blood in the Venae Cavae, Right Heart Chambers and Pulmonary Vessels of Healthy Subjects, *J. Lab. & Clin. Med.*, 50:93, 1957.

150. Grayzel, J., and Jameson, G. A.: Optimum Criteria for the Diagnosis of Ventricular Septal Defect from Measurements of Blood Oxygen Saturation, *Circulation*, 27:64, 1963.

151. Grayzel, J., and Jameson, A. G.: Optimum Criteria for the Diagnosis of Patent Ductus Arteriosus from Measurements of Blood Oxygen Saturation, *Am. Heart J.*, 67:23, 1964.

152. Neufeld, H. N., McGoon, D. C., Dushane, J. W., and Edwards, J. E.: Tetralogy of Fallot with Anomalous Tricuspid Valve Simulating Pulmonary Stenosis with Intact Septum, *Circulation*, 22:1083, 1960.

153. Hoffman, J. I. E., Rudolph, A. M., Nadas, A. S., and Gross, R. E.: Pulmonic Stenosis, Ventricular Septal Defect, and Right Ventricular Pressure above Systemic Level, *Circulation*, 22:405, 1960.

154. Hernandez, F. A., Rochkind, R., and Cooper, H. R.: Intracavitary Electrocardiogram in the Diagnosis of Ebstein's Anomaly, *Am. J. Cardiol.*, 1:181, 1958.

155. Yim, B. J. B., and Yu, P. N.: Value of an Electrode Catheter in Diagnosis of Ebstein's Disease, *Circulation*, 17:543, 1958.

156. Fick, A.: Ueber die messung des blutquantums in der herzventrikeln, Reprinted and trans. by H. E. Hoff and H. J. Scott, *New England J. Med.*, 239:120, 1948.

157. Fick, A. Ueber die messung den blutquantums in der herzventrikeln, *Sitzungsb. Phys. med. Ges. Würzburg*, 1870, 36.

158. Grehant, H., and Qurnquad, C. E.: Recherches expérimentales sur la mésure du volume de sang qui traverse les poumons en un temps donné, *Compt. rend. Soc. Biol.*, 30:159, 1886.

159. Klein, O.: Zur Bestimmung der zirkulatorischen Minutenvolumens beim Menschen nach dem

Fickschen Prinzip, *München. med. Wchnschr.*, 77:1311, 1930.

160. Visscher, M. B., and Johnson, J. A.: The Fick Principle: Analysis of Potential Errors in Its Conventional Application, *J. Appl. Physiol.*, 5:635, 1953.

161. Warren, J. V., Stead, E. A., Jr., and Brannon, E. S.: Cardiac Output in Man: A Study of Some of the Errors in the Method of Right Heart Catheterization, *Am. J. Physiol.*, 145:458, 1946.

162. Wood, E. H., Bowers, D. G., Shepherd, J. T., and Fox, I. J.: Oxygen Content of "Mixed" Venous Blood in Man during Various Phases of the Respiratory and Cardiac Cycles in Relation to Possible Errors in Measurement of Cardiac Output by Conventional Application of the Fick Method, *J. Appl. Physiol.*, 7:621, 1955.

163. Thomasson, B.: Cardiac Output in Normal Subjects under Standard Basal Conditions: Repeatability of Measurements by the Fick Method, *Scandinav. J. Clin. & Lab. Invest.*, 9:365, 1957.

164. Dubois, D., and Dubois, E. F.: Clinical Calorimetry: A Formula to Estimate the Approximate Surface Area if Height and Weight Be Known, *Arch. Int. Med.*, 17:863, 1916.

165. Reeves, J. T., Groves, R. F., Filley, G. F., and Blount, S. G., Jr.: Cardiac Output of Normal Resting Man, *J. Appl. Physiol.*, 16:276, 1961.

166. Cournand, A., Baldwin, J. S., and Himmelstein, A.: "Cardiac Catheterization in Congenital Heart Disease," The Commonwealth Fund, New York, 1949.

167. Bing, R. J., Vandam, L. D., and Gray, F. D., Jr.: Physiologic Studies in Congenital Heart Disease. II. Results of Preoperative Studies in Patients with Tetralogy of Fallot, *Bull. Johns Hopkins Hosp.*, 80:121, 1947.

168. Sendroy, J., Jr.: Manometric Determination of Hemoglobin by the Oxygen Capacity Method, *J. Biol. Chem.*, 91:307, 1931.

169. Roughton, F. J. W., Darling, R. C., and Root, W. S.: Factors Affecting the Determination of Oxygen Capacity Content and Pressure in Human Arterial Blood, *Am. J. Physiol.*, 142:708, 1944.

170. Stewart, G. N.: Researches on the Circulation Time and on the Influences Which Affect It. IV. The Output of the Heart, *J. Physiol.*, 22:159, 1897.

171. Stewart, G. N.: The Pulmonary Circulation Time: Quantity of Blood in Lungs and Output of Heart, *Am. J. Physiol.*, 58:20, 1921.

172. Hamilton, W. F., Moore, J. W., Kinsman, J. M., and Spurling, R. C.: Simultaneous Determination of the Greater and Lesser Circulation Times, of the Mean Velocity of Blood Flow through the Heart and Lungs, of the Cardiac Output and an Approximation of the Amount of Blood Actively Circulating in the Heart and Lungs, *Am. J. Physiol.*, 85:377, 1928a.

173. Hamilton, W. F., Moore, J. W., Kinsman, J. M., and Spurling, R. G.: Simultaneous Determination of the Pulmonary and Systemic Circulation Times

in Man and of a Figure Related to the Cardiac Output, *Am. J. Physiol.*, **84**:338, 1928.

174. Hamilton, W. F., Moore, J. W., Kinsman, J. M., and Spurling, R. G.: Studies on the Circulation. IV. Further Analysis of the Injection Method, and of Changes in Hemodynamics under Physiological and Pathological Conditions, *Am. J. Physiol.*, **99**:534, 1932.

175. Kinsman, J. M., Moore, J. W., and Hamilton, W. F.: Studies on the Circulation. I. Injection Method: Physical and Mathematical Consideration, *Am. J. Physiol.*, **89**:322, 1929.

176. Wood, E. H., and Swan, H. J. C.: Definition of Terms and Symbols for Description of Circulatory Indicator-dilution Curves, *J. Appl. Physiol.*, **6**:797, 1954.

177. Gilford, S. R., Gregg, D. E., Shadle, O. W., Ferguson, T. B., and Marzetta, L. A.: An Improved Cuvette Densitometer for Cardiac Output Determination by the Dye-dilution Method, *Rev. Scient. Instruments*, **24**:696, 1953.

178. McIntosh, H. D., Gleason, W. L., Miller, D. E., and Bacos, J. M.: Major Pitfall in the Interpretation of "Central Blood Volume," *Circulation Res.*, **9**:1223, 1961.

179. Milnor, W. R., Vose, A. D., and McGaff, C. J.: Pulmonary Vascular Volume, Resistance, and Compliance in Man, *Circulation*, **22**:130, 1960.

180. Dock, D. S., Kraus, W. S., McGuire, L. B., Hyland, J. W., Haynes, E. W., and Dexter, L.: Pulmonary Blood Volume in Man, *J. Clin. Invest.*, **40**:317, 1961.

181. Fox, I. J.: Indicators and Detectors for Circulatory Dilution Studies and Their Application to Organ or Regional Blood-flow Determination, *Circulation Res.*, **10**:447, 1962.

182. Taylor, S. H., and Shillingford, J. P.: Clinical Application of Coomassie Blue, *Brit. Heart. J.*, **21**:497, 1959.

183. Fox, I. J., Brooker, L. G. S., Heseltine, D. W., Essex, H. E., and Wood, E. H.: A Tricarbocyanine Dye for Continuous Recording of Dilution Curves in Whole Blood Independent of Variation in Blood Oxygen Saturation, *Proc. Staff Meet. Mayo Clin.*, **32**:478, 1957.

184. Fox, I. J., and Wood, E. H.: Indocyanine Green: Physical and Physiologic Properties, *Proc. Staff Meet. Mayo Clin.*, **35**:732, 1960.

185. Prinzmetal, M., Corday, E., Spritzler, R. J., and Flieg, W.: Radiocardiography and Its Clinical Applications, *J.A.M.A.*, **139**:617, 1949.

186. Hetzel, P. S., Swan, H. J. C., and Wood, E. H.: The Applications of Indicator-dilution Curves in Cardiac Catheterization, in H. A. Zimmerman, "Intravascular Catheterization," Charles C Thomas, Publisher, Springfield, Ill., 1959, p. 539.

187. Wiederhelm, C. A., Bruce, R. A., Hamilton, C., and Parker, R.: Diagnosis of Central Shunts from Abnormalities of Peripheral Dye Dilution Curves, *Am. Heart J.*, **54**:205, 1957.

188. Sleeper, J. C., Thompson, H. K., Jr., McIntosh, H. D., and Elston, R. C.: Reproducibility of Results Obtained with Indicator-Dilution Technique for Estimating Cardiac Output in Man, *Circulation Res.*, **11**:712, 1962.

189. Hamilton, W. F., Riley, R. S., Attyah, A. M., Cournand, A., Fowell, D. M., Himmelstein, A., Noble, R. P., Remington, J. W., Richards, D. W., Jr., Wheeler, N. C., and Witham, A. C.: Comparison of the Fick and Dye Injection Methods of Measuring the Cardiac Output in Man, *Am. J. Physiol.*, **153**:309, 1948.

190. Moore, J. W., Kinsman, J. M., Hamilton, W. F., and Spurling, R. G.: Studies on the Circulation. II. Cardiac Output Determinations: Comparison of the Injection Method with the Direct Fick Procedure, *Am. J. Physiol.*, **89**:331, 1929.

191. Doyle, J. T., Wilson, J. S., Lepine, C., and Warren, J. V.: An Evaluation of the Measurement of the Cardiac Output and of the So-called Pulmonary Blood Volume by the Dye-Dilution Method, *J. Lab. & Clin. Med.*, **41**:29, 1953.

192. Dow, P.: Estimations of Cardiac Output and Central Blood Volume by Dye-Dilution, *Physiol. Rev.*, **38**:77, 1956.

193. Emanuel, R. W., Lacy, W. W., and Newman, E. V.: Relative Effects of Heart Chambers, Lungs, and Mitral Insufficiency on the Shape of Indicator Dilution Curves, *Circulation Res.*, **7**:141, 1959.

194. Lacy, W. W., Emanuel, R. W., and Newman, E. V.: Effect of the Sampling System on the Shape of Indicator Dilution Curves, *Circulation Res.*, **5**:568, 1957.

195. Marshall, R. J.: Factors Modifying the Contours of Indicator-dilution Curves, *Circulation Res.*, **10**:123, 1962.

196. Hetzel, P. S., Swan, W. J. C., Ramirez de Arellano, A. A., and Wood, E. H.: Estimation of Cardiac Output from First Part of Arterial Dye-Dilution Curves, *J. Appl. Physiol.*, **13**:92, 1958.

197. Dow, P.: Dimensional Relationships in Dye-Dilution Curves from Humans and Dogs with an Empirical Formula for Certain Troublesome Curves, *J. Appl. Physiol.*, **7**:399, 1955.

198. Ramirez de Arellano, A. A., Hetzel, P. S., and Wood, E. H.: Measurement of Pulmonary Blood Flow Using the Indicator-dilution Technique in Patients with a Central Arteriovenous Shunt, *Circulation Res.*, **4**:400, 1956.

199. Wood, E. H.: Diagnostic Applications of Indicator-dilution Techniques in Congenital Heart Disease, *Circulation Res.*, **10**:531, 1962.

200. Prinzmetal, M.: Calculation of Venous-Arterial Shunt in Congenital Heart Disease, *J. Clin. Invest.*, **20**:705, 1941.

201. Swan, H. J. C., Zapata-Diaz, J., and Wood, E. H.: Dye-Dilution Curves in Cyanotic Congenital Heart Disease, *Circulation*, **8**:70, 1953.

202. Warner, H. R.: An Analysis of the Role of Indi-

cator Technics in Quantitation of Valvular Regurgitation, *Circulation Res.*, **10**:519, 1962.

203. Newcombe, C. P., Sinclair, J. D., Donald, D. F., and Wood, E. H.: The Detection and Assessment of Mitral Regurgitation by Left Atrial Indicator Dilution Curves, *Circulation Res.*, **19**:1196, 1961.

204. Braunwald, E., and Morrow, A. E.: A Method for the Detection and Estimation of Aortic Regurgitant Flow in Man, *Circulation*, **17**:505, 1958.

205. Korner, P. I., and Shillingford, J. P.: Further Observations on the Estimation of Valvular Incompetence from Indicator-Dilution Curves, *Clin. Sc.*, **15**:417, 1956.

206. Warner, H. R., and Toronto, A. F.: Quantitation of Backflow in Patients with Aortic Insufficiency Using an Indicator Technique, *Circulation Res.*, **6**:29, 1958.

207. Warner, H. R., and Toronto, A. F.: Effect of Heart Rate on Aortic Insufficiency as Measured by a Dye-dilution Technique, *Circulation Res.*, **9**:413, 1961.

208. Levinson, G. E., Stern, S. W., Carleton, R. A., and Abelman, W. H.: Measurement of Mitral Regurgitation in Man from Simultaneous Atrial and Arterial Dilution Curves of the Ventricular Injection, *Circulation*, **24**:720, 1961.

209. Wood, E. H.: Speculations Concerning Present and Future Developments in Indicator-Dilution Techniques, *Circulation Res.*, **10**:569, 1962.

210. Hyman, A. L., DeGraff, A. C., Jr., and Quiroz, A. C.: Double Catheter Dye Technique for Detection of Left to Right Shunts, *S. Forum*, **10**:450, 1959.

211. Case, R. B., Horley, H. W., Keating, R., Keating, P., Sachs, H. L., and Loeffler, E. E.: Detection of Circulatory Shunts by Use of Radioactive Gas, *Proc. Soc. Exper. Biol. & Med.*, **97**:4, 1958.

212. Case, R. B., Hurley, H. W., and Keating, P.: Detection and Measurement of Circulatory Shunts by Use of a Radioactive Gas, *Progr. Cardiovas. Dis.*, **2**:186, 1959.

213. Amplatz, K., and Marvin, J. F.: A Simple and Accurate Test for Left to Right Cardiac Shunts, *Radiology*, **72**:585, 1959.

214. Sanders, R. J., Cooper, T., and Morrow, A. G.: An Evaluation of the Nitrous Oxide Method for the Quantification of Left-to-Right Shunts, *Circulation*, **19**:898, 1959.

215. Morrow, A. G., Sanders, R. J., and Braunwald, E.: The Nitrous Oxide Test: An Improved Method for the Detection of Left to Right Shunts, *Circulation*, **17**:284, 1958.

216. Long, R. T. L., Braunwald, E., and Morrow, A. G.: The Intracardiac Injection of Radioactive Krypton: the Clinical Applications of New Methods for the Characterization of Circulatory Shunts, *Circulation*, **21**:1126, 1960.

217. Sanders, R. J.: Use of Radioactive Gas (Kr⁸⁵) in Diagnosis of Cardiac Shunts, *Proc. Soc. Exper. Biol. & Med.*, **97**:1, 1958.

218. Sanders, R. J., and Morrow, A. G.: The Identification and Quantification of Left to Right Circulatory Shunts: A New Diagnostic Method Utilizing the Inhalation of Radioactive Gas (Kr⁸⁵) *Am. J. Med.*, **26**:508, 1959.

219. Cornell, P. W., Braunwald, E., and Morrow, A. G.: External Precordial Scanning: Preliminary Report of a Simplified Method for the Detection of Left to Right Shunts, *M. Ann. District of Columbia*, **29**:67, 1960.

220. Cornell, W. P., Braunwald, E., and Morrow, A. G.: Precordial Scanning: Applications in the Detection of Left to Right Circulatory Shunts, *Circulation*, **23**:21, 1961.

221. Wood, R. C., Marshall, H. W., and Wood, E. H.: Detection and Quantitation of Intracardiac Left to Right Shunts by an Oximetric Inert Gas Technique, *Circulation*, **27**:351, 1963.

222. Wood, E. H., Swan, H. J. C., Fox, I. J., Kirklin, J. W., Helmholtz, H. F., Jr., Brooker, L. G. S., Heseltine, D. W., Essex, H. F., Burchell, H. B., Wright, L. J., Penido, J. R. F., Weil, M. H., Birkhead, N. C., Toscano-Barboza, E., and Woodward, E., Jr.: Symposium on Diagnostic Applications of Indicator-dilution Techniques, *Proc. Staff Meet. Mayo Clin.*, **32**:463, 1957.

223. Wood, E. H., Swan, H. J. C., and Marshall, H. W.: Technical and Diagnostic Applications of Dilution Curves Recorded Simultaneously from the Right Side of the Heart and from the Arterial Circulation, *Proc. Staff Meet. Mayo Clin.*, **33**:536, 1958.

224. Franch, R. H.: The Clinical Usefulness of the Dye-dilution Curve, *South. Med. J.*, **53**:821, 1960.

225. Penindo, J. R. F., and Swan, H. J. C.: Identification of Central Great Vessels by Indicator-dilution Curves, *Proc. Staff Meet. Mayo Clin.*, **32**:500, 1957.

226. Swan, H. J. C., and Wood, E. H.: Anomalous Connection of the Pulmonary and Systemic Veins, *Proc. Staff Meet. Mayo Clin.*, **32**:496, 1957.

227. Weil, M. H., and Swan, H. J. C.: Demonstration of Ejection Pathways from the Right Ventricle, *Proc. Staff Meet. Mayo Clin.*, **32**:502, 1957.

228. Berkhead, N. C., and Wood, E. H.: The Diagnosis of Tricuspid Atresia, *Proc. Staff Meet. Mayo Clin.*, **32**:506, 1957.

229. McGuire, J., and Goldman, F.: Apparent Increased Velocity of Blood Flow in Cases of Congenital Heart Disease with Septal Defects Having Right to Left Shunt, *Am. Heart J.*, **14**:230, 1937.

230. Benenson, W., and Hitzig, W. M.: Diagnosis of Venous-arterial Shunt by Either Circulation Time Method, *Proc. Soc. Exper. Biol. & Med.*, **38**:256, 1938.

231. Booth, R. W., Ryan, J. W., and Goodwin, R. S.: A Saline Conductivity Method for Detection of Cardiac Shunts by Indicator-dilution Technique, *Circulation Res.*, **6**:142, 1958.

232. Cooper, T., Braunwald, E., Riggle, G. C., and Morrow, A. G.: Thermal Dilution Curves in the Study of Circulatory Shunts: Instrumentation and Clinical Applications, *Am. J. Cardiol.,* 6:1065, 1960.

233. Paul, R. E., Oppenheimer, M. J., Lynch, P. R., and Stauffer, A. M.: Regurgitation of Radiopaque Contrast Material through Normal Mitral Valves in Cinefluoroscopic Studies of Dogs, *J. Appl. Physiol.,* 12:98, 1958.

234. Paul, M. H., Rudolph, A. M., and Rappaport, M. D.: Temperature Dilution Curves for the Detection of Cardiac Shunts (Abstract), *Circulation,* 18:765, 1958.

235. Clark, L. C., Jr.: Intravascular Polarographic and Potentiometric Electrodes for the Study of Circulation, *Tr. Am. Soc. Artificial Int. Organs,* 6:348, 1960.

236. Arcasoy, M. M.: Guntheroth, W. G., and Mullins, G. L.: Simplified Intravascular Hydrogen Electrode Method, *Am. J. Dis. Child.,* 104:349, 1962.

237. Hyman, A. L., Hyman, E. S., Quiroz, A. C., and Gantt, J. R.: Hydrogen Platinum Electrode System in the Detection of Intravascular Shunts, *S. Forum,* 11:450, 1960.

238. Hyman, A. L., Hyman, E. S., Quiroz, A. C., and Gantt, J. R.: Hydrogen Platinum Electrode System in Detection of Intravascular Shunts, *Am. Heart J.,* 61:53, 1961.

239. Vogel, J. H. K., Grover, R. F., and Blount, S. G., Jr.: The Platinum Electrode, *Am. Heart J.,* 65:841, 1963.

240. Pfaff, W. W., Frommer, P., and Morrow, A. G.: Ascorbic Acid Dilution Curves in Cardiovascular Diagnosis, *S. Forum,* 11:147, 1960.

241. Levy, L., Fowler, R., Kirkley, D., Albert, H., and Martinez, J. L.: Multiple Hydrogen-electrode Catheter for Determination of Cardiac Shunts, *New England J. Med.,* 264:1356, 1961.

242. Hugenholtz, P. G., Schwark, T., Monroe, R. G., Gamble, W. J., Hauck, A. J., and Nadas, A. S.: The Clinical Usefulness of Hydrogen Gas as an Indicator of Left to Right Shunts, *Circulation,* 28:542, 1963.

243. Clark, L. C., Jr., and Bargeron, L. M., Jr.: Left to Right Shunt Detection by an Intravascular Electrode with Hydrogen as an Indicator, *Science,* 130:709, 1959.

244. Clark, L. C., Jr., and Bargeron, L. M., Jr.: Detection and Direct Recording of Left to Right Shunts with the Hydrogen Electrode Catheter, *Surgery,* 46:797, 1959.

245. Clark, L. C., Jr., Bargeron, L. M., Jr., Lyons, C., Bradley, M. N., and McArthur, K. T.: Detection of Right to Left Shunts with an Arterial Potentiometric Electrode, *Circulation,* 22:949, 1960.

246. Hyman, A. L., Myers, W., Hyatt, K., DeGraff, A. C., Jr., and Quiroz, A. C.: A Comparative Study of the Detection of Cardiovascular Shunts by Oxygen Analysis and Indicator Dilution Methods, *Ann. Int. Med.,* 56:535, 1962.

247. Vogel, J. H. K., Averell, K. H., Tabou, K., and Blount, S. G.: Detection of Intracardiac Shunts with the Platinum Electrode, Using a Simplified Percutaneous Approach, *Am. Heart J.,* 67:610, 1964.

248. Fegler, G.: Measurement of Cardiac Output in Anaesthetized Animals by a Thermo-dilution Method, *Quart. J. Exper. Physiol.,* 39:153, 1954.

249. Fegler, G.: The Reliability of the Thermo-dilution Method for Determination of the Cardiac Output and the Blood Flow in Central Veins, *Quart. J. Exper. Physiol.,* 42:254, 1957.

250. Goodyer, A. V. N., Huvos, A., Eckhardt, W. F., and Ostberg, R. H.: Thermal Dilution Curves in the Intact Animal, *Circulation Res.,* 7:432, 1959.

251. Khalil, H. H.: Determination of Cardiac Output in Man by a New Method Based on Thermodilution, *Lancet,* 1:1352, 1963.

252. Hosie, K. F.: Thermal-dilution Techniques, *Circulation Res.,* 10:491, 1962.

253. Luthy, F.: Die Haemodynamik des suffizienten und insuffizienten rechten Herzens, Bibliotheca Cardiologica, fasc. 11, Karger Edit., Basel, 1962.

254. Holt, J. P.: Estimation of the Residual Volume of the Ventricle of the Dog's Heart by Two Indicator-dilution Techniques, *Circulation Res.,* 4:187, 1956.

255. Bing, R. J., Heimbecker, R., and Falholt, W.: An Estimation of the Residual Volume of Blood in the Right Ventricle of Normal and Diseased Human Hearts in Vivo, *Am. Heart J.,* 42:483, 1951.

256. Folse, R., and Braunwald, E.: Determination of Fraction of Left Ventricular Volume Ejected per Beat and Clinical Observations with a Precordial Dilution Technique, *Circulation,* 25:674, 1962.

257. Swan, H. J. C., and Beck, W.: Ventricular Non-mixing as a Source of Error in the Estimation of Ventricular Volume by the Indicator Dilution Technic, *Circulation Res.,* 8:989, 1960.

258. Liljestrand, G., Lysholm, E., Nylin, G., and Zachrison, C. G.: The Normal Heart Volume in Man, *Am. Heart J.,* 4:406, 1939.

259. Arvedsson, H.: Angiocardiographic Determination of Left Ventricular Volume, *Acta radiol.,* 56:321, 1961.

260. Axen, O., and Lind, J.: Recording in Angiocardiography with Synchronous Serial Photography at Right-angled Planes, *Cardiologia,* 16:60, 1950.

261. Bjork, G.: On the Relationship between the Heart Volume and Various Physical Factors, *Acta radiol.,* 25:373, 1944.

262. Chapman, C. B., Baker, O., Reynolds, J., and Bonte, F.: Use of Biplane Cine-fluorography for Measurement of Ventricular Volume, *Circulation,* 18:1105, 1958.

263. Dodge, H. T., Sandler, H., Ballew, D. H., and Lord, J. D., Jr.: Use of Biplane Angiocardiography for the Measurement of Left Ventricular Volume in Man, *Am. Heart J.,* 60:762, 1962.

264. Gribbe, P., Hirvonen, L., Lind, J., and Wegelius, C.: Cineangiocardiographic Recordings of the Cyclic Changes in Volume of the Left Ventricle, *Cardiologia*, **34**:348, 1959.

265. Kahlstorf, A.: Ueber eine orthographische Herzvolumen bestimmung, *Fortschr. Geb. Röntgenstrahlen*, **45**:123, 1932.

266. Reedy, T., and Chapman, C. B.: Measurement of Right Ventricular Volume by Cineangiofluorography, *Am. Heart J.*, **66**:221, 1963.

267. Dodge, H. T., Hay, R. E., and Sandler, H.: An Angiocardiographic Method for Directly Determining Left Ventricular Stroke Volume in Man, *Circulation Res.*, **11**:739, 1962.

268. Gribbe, P.: Comparison of the Angiocardiographic and the Direct Fick Methods in Determining Cardiac Output, *Cardiologia*, **36**:20, 1960.

269. Hallerman, F. J., Rastelli, G. C., and Swan, H. J. C.: Comparison of Left Ventricular Volumes by Dye Dilution and Angiographic Methods in the Dog, *Am. J. Physiol.*, **204**:446, 1963.

270. Donato, L., Giuntini, C., Lewis, M. L., Durand, J., Rochester, D. F., Harvey, R. M., and Cournand, A.: Quantitative Radiocardiography, *Circulation*, **26**:174, 1962.

271. Donato, L.: Selective Radiocardiography, *Progr. in Cardiovas. Dis.*, **5**:1, 1962.

272. Cournand, A., Donato, L., Durand, J., Rochester, D. F., Parker, J. O., Harvey, R. M., and Lewis, M. L.: Separate Performance of Both Ventricles in Man during the Early Phase of Exercise, as Analyzed by the Method of Selective Radiocardiography, *Tr. A. Am. Physicians*, **73**:283, 1960.

273. Rudolph, A. M., and Nadas, A. S.: The Pulmonary Circulation and Congenital Heart Disease, *New England J. Med.*, **267**:968; 1022, 1962.

274. Gorlin, R., and Gorlin, S. G.: Hydraulic Formula for Calculation of the Area of the Stenotic Mitral Valve, Other Cardiac Valves, and Central Circulating Shunts, *Am. Heart J.*, **41**:1, 1951.

275. Richter, H. S.: Mitral Valve Area: Measurement Soon after Catheterization: Report of a Case, *Circulation*, **28**:451, 1963.

276. Kelly, E. R., Morrow, A. G., and Braunwald, E.: Catheterization of the Left Side of the Heart, *New England J. Med.*, **262**:162, 1960.

277. Cournand, A., Bing, R. J., Dexter, L., Dotter, C., Katz, L. N., Warren, J. V., and Wood, E.: Report of Committee of Cardiac Catheterization and Angiocardiography of the American Heart Association, *Circulation*, **7**:769, 1953.

278. Stern, T. N., Tacket, H. S., and Zachary, E. G.: Penetration into Pericardial Cavity during Cardiac Catheterization, *Am. Heart J.*, **44**,448, 1952.

279. Read, J. L., Bond, E. G., Porter, R. R.: The Hazard of Unrecognized Catheterization of the Coronary Sinus, *A.M.A. Arch. Int. Med.*, **96**:176, 1955.

280. Paul, M. H., and Rudolph, A. M.: Pulmonary Valve Obstruction during Catheterization, *Circulation*, **18**:53, 1958.

281. Adrouny, Z. A., Stephenson, M. J., Straube, K. R., Dotter, C. T., and Griswold, H. E.: Effect of Cardiac Catheterization and Angiocardiography on the Serum Glutamic Oxaloacetic Transaminase, *Circulation*, **27**:565, 1963.

282. Burchell, H. B.: Electrocution Hazards in the Hospital or Laboratory, *Circulation*, **27**:1015, 1963.

283. Weinberg, D. I., Artley, J. L., Whalen, R. E., and McIntosh, H. D.: Electric Shock Hazards in Cardiac Catheterization, *Circulation Res.*, **11**:1004, 1962.

284. Dawson, B., Moffitt, E. A., Glover, W. J., and Swan, H. J. C.: Closed Chest Resuscitation in a Cardiac Catheterization Laboratory, *Circulation*, **25**:976, 1962.

285. Kouwenhoven, W. B., Jude, J. R., and Knickerbocker, G. G.: Closed-chest Cardiac Massage, *J.A.M.A.*, **173**:1064, 1960.

286. Laurence, G. H.: Risk of Catheterization of the Left Side of the Heart, *New England J. Med.*, **255**:180, 1956.

287. Venables, A. W., and Hiller, H. G.: Complications of Cardiac Investigation, *Brit. Heart J.*, **25**:334, 1963.

288. Lang, E. K.: A Survey of the Complications of Percutaneous Retrograde Arteriography, Seldinger Technique, *Radiology*, **81**:257, 1963.

289. Lang, E. K.: Hazards of Percutaneous Arteriography, *J. Urol.*, **90**:604, 1963.

290. Cope, C.: Intravascular Breakage of Seldinger Spring Guide Wires, *J.A.M.A.*, **180**:1061, 1962.

291. Androuny, Z. A., Southerland, D. W., Greswold, H. E., and Ritzmann, L. W.: Complications with Transseptal Left Heart Catheterization, *Am. Heart J.*, **65**:327, 1963.

292. Ross, J. R., Jr., Braunwald, E., Mason, T., Braunwald, N. S., and Morrow, A. G.: Interatrial Communication and Left Atrial Hypertension: A Cause of Continuous Murmur, *Circulation*, **28**:853, 1963.

293. Susmano, A., and Carleton, R. A.: Transseptal Catheterization of the Left Atrium: Report of an Unusual Complication, *New England J. Med.*, **270**:897, 1964.

294. Pinkerson, A. L., Kelser, G. A., Jr., Adkins, P. C.: Left Atrial Mural Thrombus Secondary to Transseptal Left Heart Catheterization, *New England J. Med.*, **268**:367, 1963.

295. McMichael, J., and Mounsey, J. P. D.: Complication Following Coronary Sinus and Cardiac Vein Catheterization in Man, *Brit. Heart J.*, **13**:397, 1951.

296. Smith, W. W., Albert, R. E., and Rader, B.: Myocardial Damage following Inadvertent Deep Cannulation of the Coronary Sinus during Right Heart Catheterization, *Am. Heart J.*, **42**:661, 1951.

9 SELECTIVE ANGIOCARDIOGRAPHY, NEGATIVE-CONTRAST ROENTGENOGRAPHY, AND RADIOISOTOPE PHOTOSCANNING

Robert H. Franch, M.D., and
Wade H. Shuford, M.D.

SELECTIVE ANGIOCARDIOGRAPHY

In 1947 contrast media was injected through a rubber catheter placed in the right ventricle.[1] For the first time, opaque media could be delivered to a specific intracardiac site so that overlapping shadows might be avoided. The right atrium no longer needed to obscure the right ventricular outflow tract in the lateral projection. Other investigators carried this technique to an advanced state of development,[2-7] and in the past 10 years, selective angiocardiography has assumed a major role in the diagnostic laboratory.

A catheter with a large lumen facilitates rapid delivery of a single bolus of the contrast agent.[8] A closed-end catheter with laterally directed openings reduces recoil.[9] A power injector increases the flow rate of contrast substance five times over a hand injection.[10] The injection is usually made at a random time. Contrast media in smaller volume may be delivered at a specific time in the cardiac cycle by an injection triggered by the R wave of the electrocardiogram or a variable delay after the R wave. In the past 10 years, contrast agents have been developed which have high opacity, lower viscosity, and less toxicity.[11,12] The present opaque media contain an organic iodide with a stabilizer and a buffer. All media are uniformly hypertonic (greater than 1,500 mOsm-liter); excretion is by the kidney tubules. Tachycardia and a modest decrease in systemic blood pressure occur for 2 min after injection. The cardiovascular response also includes a sustained use in cardiac output and a sharp increase in muscle blood flow.[13]

A single or biplane roll or cut-film changer provides 2 to 12 frames per minute. These studies have the advantage of excellent detail; disadvantages are the high film costs, necessity for meticulous attention to the mechanism of the film-changing device, and in practice, inability to monitor the injection. A second technique, cineangiocardiography, was made generally available by the development of intensification and amplification fluoroscopy, whereby the conventional fluoroscopic light image is converted into an equivalent electron image.[14-17] The electron image is focused by electrostatic lenses on a small fluorescent screen in order to increase electron concentration.[18-21] The electrons are also accelerated with high voltage, increasing their energy as they strike the fluorescent screen.[22] Thus the electron image is reconverted into a light image of much-increased brightness, permitting movie, television, or television tape recording and, of course, fluoroscopy with the cone cells of the retina.[23]

This technique provides for monitoring at the time of injection and inexpensive, trouble-free filming by a motor-driven 16- or 35-mm movie camera. Though the detail of the individual cineframe is only one-third the total resolution of the conventional x-ray, the motion of itself increases visual perception and makes details apparent that are not appreciated on the static-image x-ray. Variations in cineangiocardiographic optical density may be quantitated by applying the indicator-dilution principle: using one film strip, cinedensograms could be obtained from the atria, ventricles, and great vessels.

A successful procedure is the product of an adequate catheter, properly placed, proper positioning of the patient, a rapid injection, and detailed attention to radiologic technique.[10]

In congenital heart disease, a right ventricular injection is used in order to study the level of obstruction to right ventricular outflow[24] (Figs. 9-1 to 9-3), to identify whether communication of the right ventricle with the aorta or left ventricle is present (Figs. 9-4 to 9-6), and to study the pulmonary artery tree (Fig. 9-7). If the catheter tip cannot be advanced across a patent foramen ovale or atrial septal defect (Fig. 9-8) into the left atrium, a pulmonary artery injection may be used to fill the left side of the heart with opaque media in order to visualize left-to-right shunts from the left atrium, left ventricle, or aorta. A pulmonary artery injection is also useful for detecting the site of partial (Figs. 9-1–9-23) or total anomalous venous drainage of the pulmonary veins. An aortic injection or, in infants, a left brachial artery countercurrent injection[25-27] demonstrates an aortopulmonary window, aortic valve atresia (Fig. 9-10), patent ductus arteriosus (Fig. 9-11), and coarctation of the aorta (Fig. 9-12). A left ventricular injection determines the level of obstruction to left ventricular outflow[28] (Figs. 9-13, 9-14) and detects mitral regurgitation.[29-34] The oblique projections, especially the right anterior oblique, are best for demonstrating the mitral valve.[35,36]

In valvular or acquired heart disease, left ventricular injection is used to detect and grossly to quantitate mitral regurgitation[37] (Fig. 9-15). A normal mitral valve may leak during diastole because of momentary reversal of the pressure gradient if there is extreme bradycardia or asystole or if there are premature ventricular beats with a long diastolic pause (see references 233 and 234 in Chap. 8). In mitral stenosis a domelike filling defect is frequently noted in diastole in the left ventricular cavity, presumably because of fusion of the valve leaflets[38] (Fig. 9-16). During left ventricular injection a Valsalva maneuver may increase opacity by decreasing the volume rate of flow.[39]

Injections made above the aortic valve serve to detect diseases of the aorta (Figs. 9-17 to 9-19) and to show aortic regurgitation (Fig. 9-20). The catheter tip should be above the maximum upward deflection of the valve cusps so that artifactual aortic insufficiency is not produced. If possible, a side-hole catheter should be used. In an aortic injection, size and mobility of a stenotic aortic valve may be visualized by negative-contrast washout of the opacified aorta with nonopaque ventricular blood. (Selective coronary arteriography is discussed in Chap. 10.)

The *complications* of selective angiocardiography are as follows. Major reactions from contrast media, such as respiratory arrest, convulsions, shock, and renal toxicity, are extremely rare. Sensitivity testing of opaque media is done only in those who have specific, allergic history. Warmth and a flush are universally experienced. Occasionally there are vomiting and headache; urticaria may occur. In desperately ill, cyanotic infants with a high hemoglobin concentration, the hypertonicity of the contrast media may cause osmotic red-cell agglutination.[40-43] Some prophylaxis may be offered by use of a plasma expander, such as Dextran,[44] or by use of parenteral fluids.[45]

Pressure injection of a large volume of opaque media into the wedged coronary sinus, wedged pulmonary artery,[46] and wedged pulmonary vein positions should be avoided (Fig. 9-21). If the catheter tip passes into the coronary sinus and thence into the great cardiac vein, the anteroposterior projection may resemble that of a catheter tip positioned in the right ventricular outflow tract, the main pulmonary artery, or the left pulmonary artery hidden behind an enlarged heart shadow.[47,48] The record obtained from a wedged coronary vein position simulates that of a ventricular tracing (see reference 279 in Chap. 8) (Fig. 9-22). Clues to coronary sinus catheterizations are (1) the acute angle that the catheter shaft makes as it enters the coronary sinus, especially in the right anterior oblique position (see position 13 in Chap. 8); (2) the marked desaturation of coronary sinus blood; (3) the inability to withdraw blood through the catheter in the coronary vein wedge position; (4) the posterior position of the catheter.

Perforation of the atria, ventricles, or large veins[49] with the catheter tip either before or during the injection is possible (Fig. 9-23).[50,51] One should be careful of inadvertently advancing the tip of the catheter while turning or positioning the patient. The catheter tip should lie free in the cardiac cavity, well away from the endocardium; otherwise some opaque media will be delivered into the subendocardial muscle. The opaque media is quickly dissipated from the intramural site, and intramyocardial hematoma does not result, apparently because of the efficient sinusoidal drainage system. Usually no sequelae are noted unless perforation with intrapericardial bleeding is an accompanying complication.[52] The danger of injecting opaque media into a false passage may occur when retrograde arterial catheterization and angiography are done in cases of dissecting aneurysm of the aorta.[53]

Ventricular fibrillation is a potential danger, especially if the catheter tip abuts against the ventricular endocardium. In the elderly, a hypotensive reaction, apparently of reflex origin, is occasionally noted. Generally, selective angiocardiography is well tolerated and complications are minimal in experienced hands.

NEGATIVE-CONTRAST ROENTGENOGRAPHY

Animal studies have shown that the high solubility of carbon dioxide in the serum at body temperature permits its safe use for negative-contrast visualization of intracardiac structures.[54] In the human being, its major use is to distinguish the large cardiac silhouette of myocardial dilatation from that of pericardial thickening or effusion.[55-57] The patient is placed in the left lateral decubitus position (right side up) and a 6-ft anteroposterior scout roentgenogram is obtained. Air is removed from a 100-ml syringe and its connections by flushing with carbon dioxide gas. The syringe is filled with 50 to 100 ml of pure carbon dioxide, which[58] is injected as rapidly as possible via an 18-gauge needle in the left antecubital vein.[59] Films are obtained in 4, 8, and 15 sec. The patient remains in position, with the right side of the chest up, for 10 min to permit complete absorption of carbon dioxide.

The gas entering the right atrium from the

superior vena cava rises, to layer out along the right atrial border. Thus the right atrial wall and the overlying pericardium and pleura are sandwiched as an opaque band between the radiolucent air-filled lung and the carbon dioxide–containing right atrium (Fig. 9-24). The normal right atrial opaque band is 5 mm or less in width. In a large pericardial effusion, the band may increase to 20 mm in width.[59]

An effusion in the pleural space overlying the right atrial border may mimic pericardial effusion or thickening. A false-negative result occurs if pericardial fluid shifts from the right atrial border to the dependent portion of the pericardial sac while the patient is in position with the left side of the chest down.[60] Venous angiography with the right side of the chest down avoids this problem (Fig. 9-25).

RADIOISOTOPE PHOTOSCANNING

Automatic radioisotope photoscanning of the heart and great vessels is dependent on the addition of a gamma-emitting isotope to the blood, usually I_{131} human serum albumin.[61] I_{131} sodium iodipamide (Cholografin sodium) may be preferable, since it has a shorter effective half-life, rapid liver clearance, and less total-body radiation.[62,63]

The size and shape of the radioactive blood pool within the heart and the aorta are detected by a scintillation crystal, then amplified and photo-recorded.[64,65] While the patient is on the scanning table, a special recumbent anteroposterior chest roentgenogram is taken by a technique that minimizes distortion of the heart image.

In a normal heart and aorta, the photoscan of the blood pool matches the size of the heart and aorta on the roentgenogram. In the dilated heart, the blood pool is large but it equals the roentgenographic image in size. As in the normal person, the photoscan shows the liver and heart blood pools to be fused. In a pericardial effusion (250 ml or greater) the heart blood pool is of normal size, but it is smaller than (less than 80 per cent the diameter of) the roentgenographic image and the heart blood pool is separated from the liver and lung blood pools (Fig. 9-26).[62] A lipoma within the pericardium has given a false-positive result.[64] Image-intensification fluoroscopy detects epicardial fat in 75 per cent of patients as a line of negative contrast; the presence of such a "fat line" well inside the cardiac silhouette is indicative of pericardial effusion.[66]

The blood pool in a giant left atrium, a ventricular aneurysm, or an aortic aneurysm is detectable. A neoplasm or thrombus may encroach on the blood pool. The vascular origin of mediastinal masses may be established.

Asplenia and a bilaterally symmetric liver may be detected by photoscan in cases of dextrocardia and in situs inversus with levocardia that have complicated cardiac malformations.[67] In the future, pulmonary[68] and myocardial infarction may be pinpointed by gamma-ray emission.

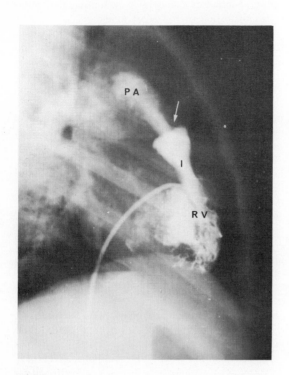

Fig. 9-1. Valvular pulmonary stenosis (lateral view). Right ventricular injection of opaque medium. Contrast material exits through central orifice of pulmonary valve in form of a jet (arrow). *RV*, right ventricle; *I*, infundibulum of right ventricle; *PA*, pulmonary artery.

Fig. 9-2. Valvular pulmonary stenosis (lateral view). Right ventricular injection of opaque medium reveals bulging of fused cusps (arrow) into dilated pulmonary artery and narrowing of infundibulum of right ventricle. *PA*, pulmonary artery; *I*, infundibulum.

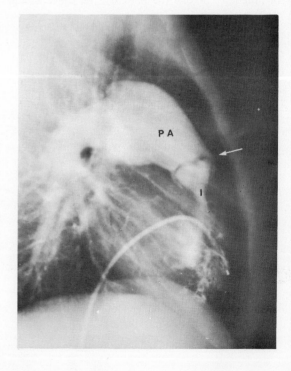

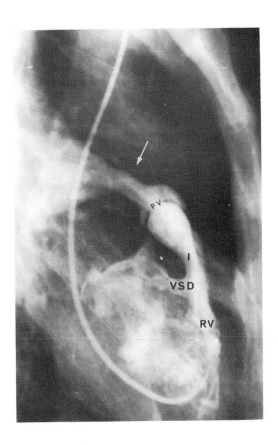

Fig. 9-3. Pulmonary stenosis and ventricular septal defect (lateral view). Selective right ventricular angiocardiogram. Thickened pulmonary valve cusps bulge into base of pulmonary artery, which shows marked supravalvular stenosis (arrow). *RV*, right ventricle; *VSD*, ventricular septal defect; *I*, infundibulum of right ventricle; *PV*, pulmonary valve.

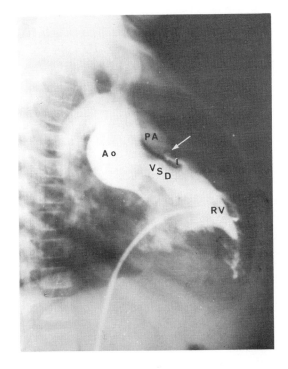

Fig. 9-4. Severe tetralogy of Fallot (lateral view). Right ventricular injection of contrast material. Infundibulum is constricted into a narrow tube, and arrow indicates stenosis of the pulmonary valve. Aorta is large and overriding, and receives blood from both ventricles. Nonopaque blood from the left ventricle passes to the aorta below the ventricular septal defect. *Ao*, aorta; *PA*, pulmonary artery; *VSD*, ventricular septal defect; *RV*, right ventricle; *I*, infundibulum.

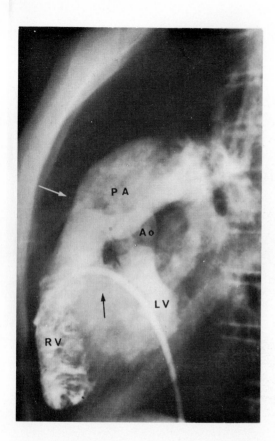

Fig. 9-5. Ventricular septal defect and pulmonary hypertension (lateral view). Right ventricular injection reveals normal outflow and moderate-sized VSD (bottom arrow) in membranous portion of ventricular septum. Contrast material passes into the aorta, which is slightly small. Observe large size of main pulmonary artery and normal pulmonary valve (top arrow). *PA*, pulmonary artery; *Ao*, aorta; *RV*, right ventricle; *LV*, left ventricle.

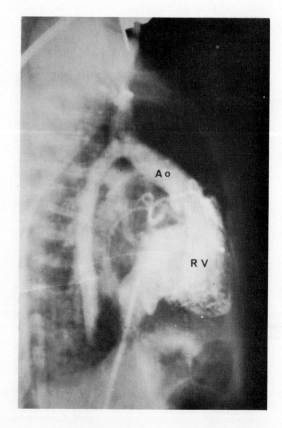

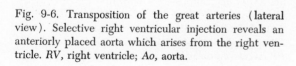

Fig. 9-6. Transposition of the great arteries (lateral view). Selective right ventricular injection reveals an anteriorly placed aorta which arises from the right ventricle. *RV*, right ventricle; *Ao*, aorta.

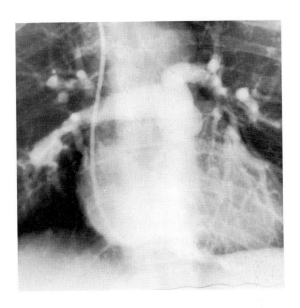

Fig. 9-7. Peripheral pulmonary artery stenoses (frontal view). Right ventricular injection of opaque material. There are multiple stenoses of the peripheral segmental arteries to both lungs, with no involvement of the main pulmonary arteries.

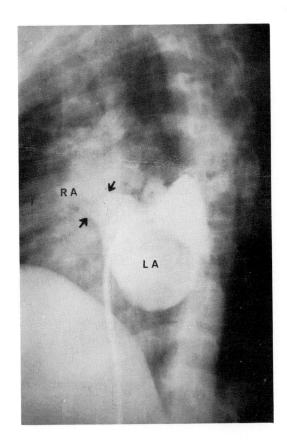

Fig. 9-8. Atrial septal defect (left anterior oblique position). Trip of the catheter is in the left atrial appendage. The left atrium is injected, and the secundum septal defect lies between the arrows, with a moderate shunt to the right atrium. *RA*, right atrium; *LA*, left atrium.

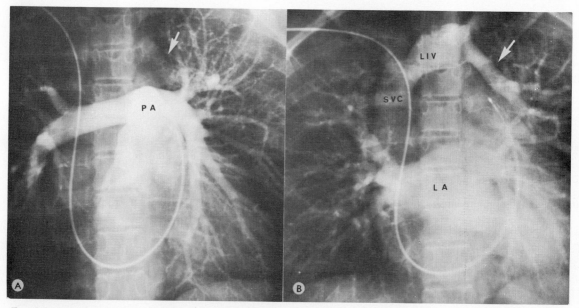

Fig. 9-9. Partial anomalous drainage of pulmonary veins (frontal view). *A.* The catheter has been introduced into the right atrium and ventricle and positioned in the main pulmonary artery, where selective injection is performed. *B.* Pulmonary venous phase. A large pulmonary vein (arrow) drains the upper lobe of the left lung, with anomalous venous return to the left innominate vein. *PA,* pulmonary artery; *LIV,* left innominate vein (brachiocephalic vein); *SVC,* superior vena cava; *LA,* left atrium.

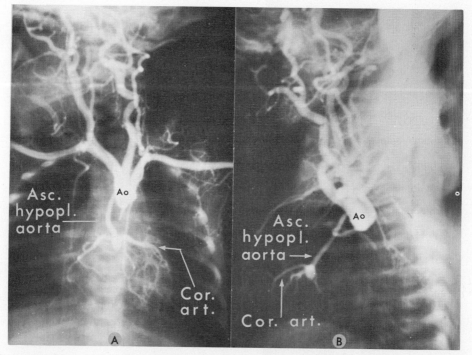

Fig. 9-10. Aortic valvular atresia (frontal and lateral views). Contrast media injected through cannula in left brachial artery. Excellent opacification of aortic arch, hypoplastic ascending aorta, and coronary arteries.

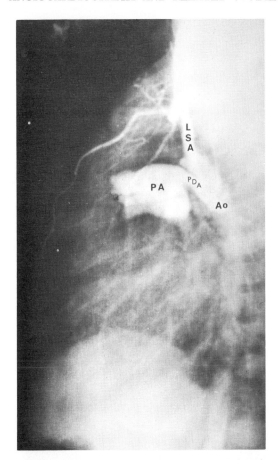

Fig. 9-11. Patent ductus arteriosus (lateral view). Countercurrent injection of opaque media through cannula in left brachial artery. Contrast material fills the left subclavian artery and aorta and flows into dilated pulmonary artery through large ductus arteriosus. *PA*, pulmonary artery; *PDA*, patent ductus arteriosus; *LSA*, left subclavian artery; *Ao*, aorta.

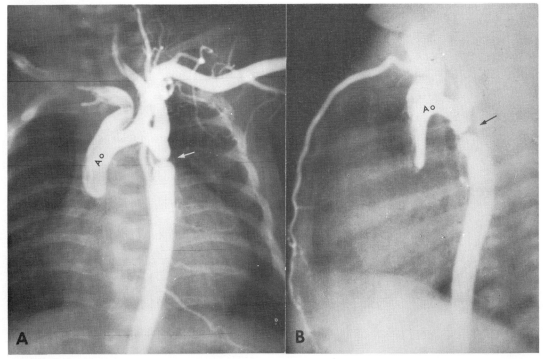

Fig. 9-12. Coarctation of the aorta (frontal and lateral views). Injection of opaque material through cannula in left brachial artery. There is a localized, diaphragm-like constriction of the aorta beyond the left subclavian artery, with dilatation of the aorta below the constricted segment (arrow).

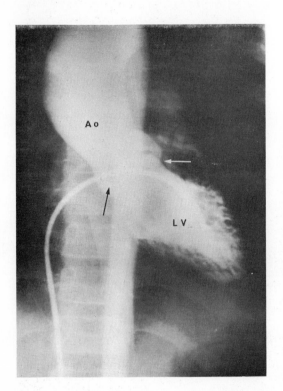

Fig. 9-13. Valvular aortic stenosis (frontal view). Catheter passed from right atrium to left atrium by transseptal puncture and advanced into left ventricle. Selective left ventricular injection reveals dome-shaped defect of aortic valve with bulging of leaflets into dilated ascending aorta (arrows). *Ao*, aorta; *LV*, left ventricle.

Fig. 9-14. Supravalvular aortic stenosis (frontal view). Left ventricular injection of contrast media reveals marked tubular narrowing of entire ascending aorta and constriction of the innominate (brachiocephalic and left carotid arteries near their origins. Arrow points to level of the aortic valve.

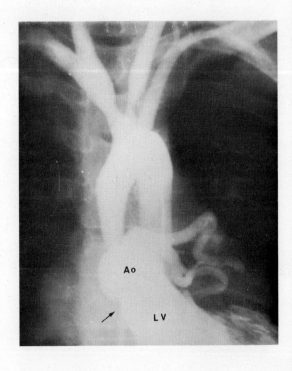

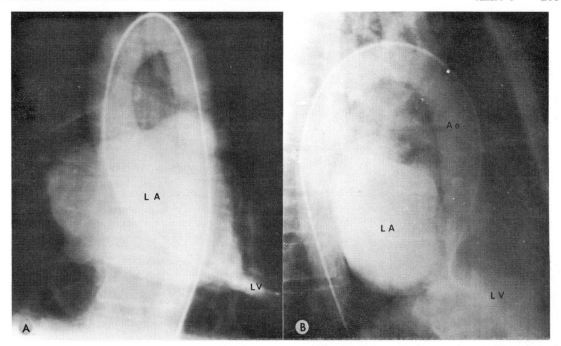

Fig. 9-15. Mitral insufficiency (frontal and lateral views). Left ventricular injection of contrast material. Densely opacified left atrium indicates a severe degree of mitral insufficiency. *Ao,* aorta; *LV,* left ventricle; *LA,* left atrium.

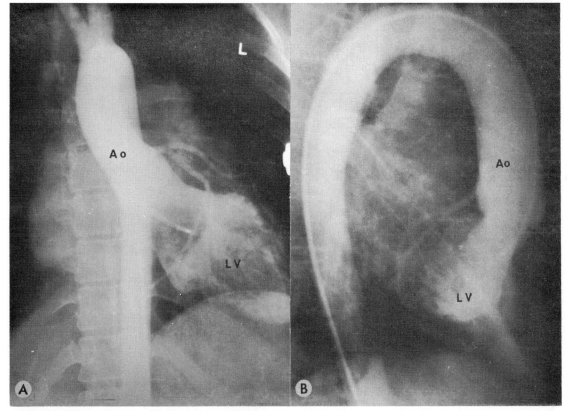

Fig. 9-16. Selective left ventricular angiocardiography in mitral stenosis (frontal and lateral views). The femoral artery has been catheterized and the catheter passed through the aortic valve into the left ventricle. Absence of left atrial opacification is good evidence against significant mitral insufficiency. *Ao,* aorta; *LV,* left ventricle.

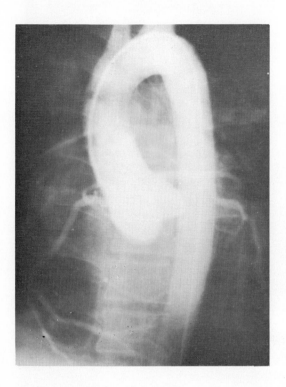

Fig. 9-17. Normal aortogram (frontal view). Injection of opaque material through catheter lying just above the aortic valve. Root of aorta well outlined, with no spill of contrast material into left ventricle, excluding significant aortic insufficiency.

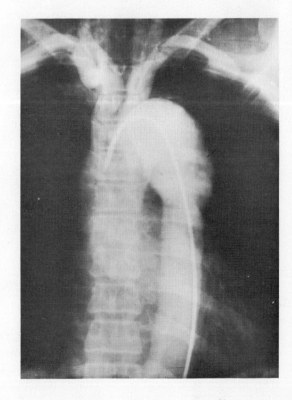

Fig. 9-18. Aneurysm of aorta (frontal view). Catheter tip in ascending aorta following percutaneous catheterization of the femoral artery. Syphilitic sacular aneurysm beginning just beyond left subclavian artery is well outlined. In this area traumatic aneurysms may also be found.

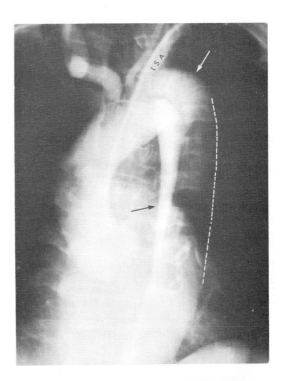

Fig. 9-19. Dissecting aneurysm of the aorta (frontal view). Thoracic aortogram with tip of catheter in normal ascending aorta. Top arrow outlines large hematoma of aortic wall beginning just beyond the left subclavian artery. Lower arrow indicates compressed true channel of the aorta. *LSA*, left subclavian artery.

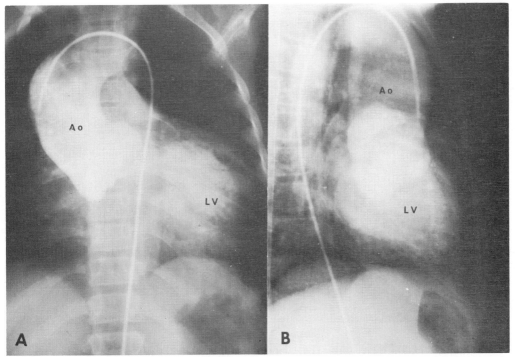

Fig. 9-20. Aortic insufficiency (frontal and lateral views). Following injection of opaque media into the ascending aorta, there is opacification of the left ventricle, indicating a moderate degree of aortic valve incompetence. Note widening of the ascending aorta. *Ao*, aorta; *LV*, left ventricle.

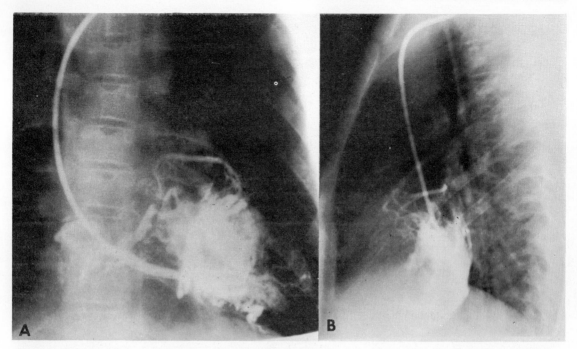

Fig. 9-21. During catheterization of the right side of the heart the coronary sinus was catheterized and the catheter tip advanced into a large coronary vein. Observe the posterior direction of the catheter. Injection of opaque material resulted in rupture of the coronary vein and myocardial and pericardial extravasation.

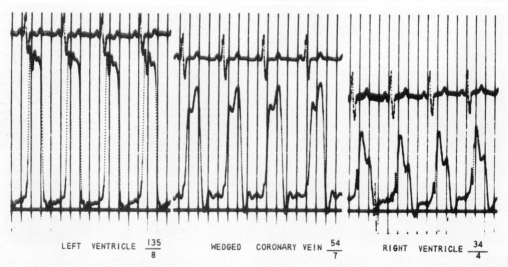

LEFT VENTRICLE $\frac{135}{8}$ WEDGED CORONARY VEIN $\frac{54}{7}$ RIGHT VENTRICLE $\frac{34}{4}$

Fig. 9-22. The pressure pulse in the wedged coronary vein position may be similar in configuration and amplitude to the ventricular pressure curve.

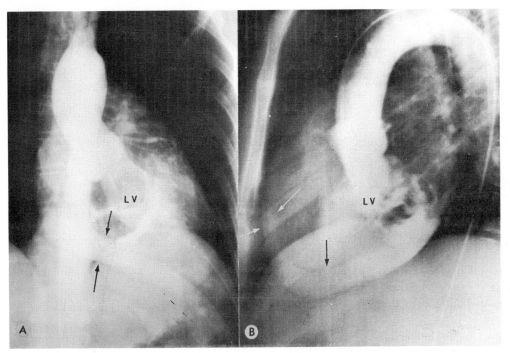

Fig. 9-23. Myocardial rupture following selective left ventricular angiocardiography (frontal and lateral views). Following pressure injection through open-end catheter, contrast media is irregularly deposited beneath endocardium and in wall of left ventricle, with rupture into the pericardial space. Arrows indicate opaque material in pericardial sac. Patient made satisfactory recovery.

Fig. 9-24. Pericardial effusion (frontal view, left lateral decubitus position). Carbon dioxide angiocardiogram. Following intravenous injection of 100 ml of CO_2, the right atrium is outlined by nonopaque contrast media. Distance between right border of the heart (arrow) and right atrium of 18 mm is indicative of pericardial effusion. *RA*, right atrium.

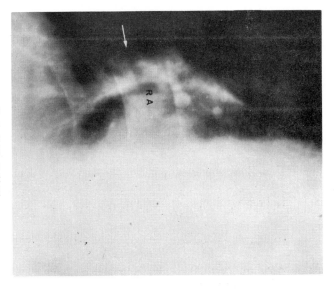

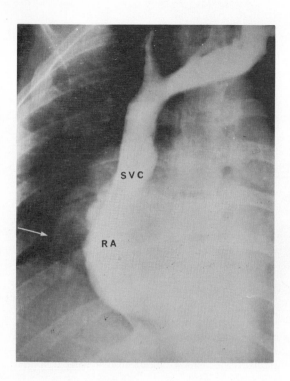

Fig. 9-25. Pericardial effusion (frontal view, supine position). Venous angiocardiogram. Distance between right border of the heart (arrow) and opacified right atrium of 20 mm is indicative of large pericardial effusion. *RA*, right atrium; *SVC*, superior vena cava.

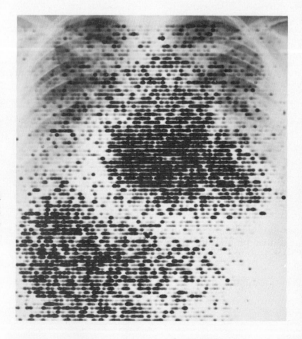

Fig. 9-26. Radioactive Cholografin scan in pericardial effusion, showing difference between outline of the total cardiac shadow and that of the heart blood pool. Note the separation between the liver and heart blood pools.

REFERENCES

1. Chavez, I., Dorbecker, N., and Celis, A.: Direct Intracardiac Angiocardiography: Its Diagnostic Value. *Am. Heart J.*, **33**:560, 1947.
2. Keith, J. D., and Munn, J. D.: Angiocardiography in Infants and Children: New Technique, *Pediatrics*, **6**:20, 1950.
3. Jonsson, G., Broder, B., and Karnell, J.: Selective Angiocardiography, *Acta Radiol.*, **32**:486, 1949.
4. Jonsson, G.: Selective Visualization in Angiocardiography, *J. Fac. Radiologists*, **3**:125, 1951.
5. Rowe, G. C., Huston, J. H., Tuchman, H., Maxwell, G. M., Weinstein, A. B., and Crumpton, C. W.: The Physiological Effect of Contrast Media Used for Angiocardiography, *Circulation*, **13**:896, 1956.
6. Rowe, R. D., Vlad, P., and Keith, J. D.: Selective Angiocardiography in Infants and Children, *Radiology*, **66**:344, 1956.
7. Sones, F. Mason, Jr.: "Cinecardioangiography. Clinical Cardiopulmonary Physiology," 2d ed., Grune & Stratton, Inc., 1960, p. 130.
8. Dow, J., and Taylor, D. G.: Angiocardiographic Technique in Intracardiac Shunts, *Brit. J. Radiol.*, **35**:241, 1962.
9. Rodriguez-Alvarez, A., and Martinez de Rodriguez, G.: Studies in Angiocardiography: The Problems Involved in the Rapid, Selective, and Safe Injections of Radiopaque Materials; Development of a Special Catheter for Selective Angiocardiography, *Am. Heart J.*, **53**:841, 1957.
10. Klatte, E. C., Campbell, J. A., and Lurie, P. R.: Technical Factors in Selective Cinecardioangiography, *Radiology*, **73**:539, 1959.
11. Wallingford, V. H.: General Aspects of Contrast Media Research, *Ann. New York Acad. Sc.*, **78**:709, 1959.
12. Lehman, J. S., and Debbas, J. N.: Evaluation of Cardiovascular Contrast Media, *Radiology*, **76**:548, 1961.
13. Brown, R., Rahimtoola, S. H., Davis, G. D., Swan, H. J. C.: The Effect of Angiocardiographic Contrast Medium on Circulatory Dynamics in Man, *Circulation*, **31**:234, 1965.
14. Abrams, H. L.: Approach to Biplane Cineangiocardiography. 1. Background and Objectives, *Radiology*, **72**:735; 741, 1959.
15. Abrams, H. L.: Approach to Biplane Cineangiocardiography. 4. Technical Data. *Stanford M. Bull.*, **19**:82–88, 1961.
16. Abrams, H. L.: Present Status of Biplane Cineangiocardiography, *J.A.M.A.*, **184**:91, 1963.
17. Campbell, J. A., Klatte, E. C., and Shalkowski, R. A.: Factors Influencing Image Quality in Cineroentgenography, *Am. J. Roentgenol.*, **83**:345, 1960.
18. Coltman, J. W.: Fluoroscopic Image Brightening by Electronic Means, *Radiology*, **51**:359, 1948.
19. Coltman, J. W.: Scintillation Limit in Fluoroscopy, *Radiology*, **63**:867, 1954.
20. Moon, R. J.: Amplifying and Intensifying Fluoroscopic Image by Means of Scanning X-ray Tube, *Science*, **112**:389, 1950.
21. Morgan, R. H.: Screen Intensification: Review of Past and Present Research with Analysis of Future Development, *Am. J. Roentgenol.*, **75**:69, 1956.
22. Sturm, R. E., and Morgan, R. H.: Screen Intensification Systems and Their Limitations, *Am. J. Roentgenol.*, **62**:617, 1949.
23. Potsaid, M. S.: Kineradiography, *New England J. Med.*, **264**:178, 1961.
24. Coelho, E., de Parva, E., Nunes, A., and Tavares, V.: Angiocardiographic Studies of Valvular Malformations in Pulmonary Stenosis: Relationship to Physiologic Alterations, *Am. J. Cardiol.*, **10**:634, 1962.
25. Castellanos, A., and Pereiras, R.: Retrograde or Countercurrent Aortography, *Amer. J. Roentgenol.*, **63**:559, 1950.
26. Abrams, H. L.: Retrograde Brachial Arteriography, *Circulation*, **14**:593, 1956.
27. Keith, J. D., and Forsyth, C.: Aortography in Infants, *Circulation*, **2**:907, 1950.
28. Bjork, V. O., Cullhed, I., and Lodin, H.: Aortic Stenosis: Correlations between Pressure Gradient and Left Ventricular Angiocardiography, *Circulation*, **23**:509, 1961.
29. Amplatz, K., Ernst, R., Lester, R. G., Lillehei, C. W., and Lillie, A.: Retrograde Left Cardioangiography as Test of Valvular Competence, *Radiology*, **72**:268, 1959.
30. Paulin, S., and Vainauskas, E.: Selective Transseptal Angiocardiography, *Acta radiol.*, **57**:3, 1962.
31. Ross, D. N.: Left Heart Angiography, *Brit. J. Radiol.*, **35**:525, 1962.
32. Starobin, O. E., Littmann, D., Sanders, C. A., and Turner, J. D.: Retrograde Catheterization of the Left Ventricle and Angiography in the Diagnosis of Mitral-valve Disease, *New England J. Med.*, **265**:462, 1961.
33. Khalaf, J. D., Chapman, C. B., and Ernst, R.: The Cinefluorographic Approach to the Diagnosis of Mitral Regurgitation, *Progr. Cardiovas. Dis.*, **5**:230, 1962.
34. Dow, J.: Left Angiocardiography in Congenital Heart Disease, *Brit. J. Radiol.*, **35**:530, 1962.
35. Kjellberg, S. R., Nordenstrom, B., Rudhe, U., et al.: Cardioangiographic Studies of the Mitral and Aortic Valves, *Acta radiol.*, Suppl. 204, 1961.
36. Ross, R. S., and Creley, J. M.: Contrast Radiography in Mitral Regurgitation, *Progr. Cardiovas. Dis.*, **5**:195, 1962.
37. Bjork, V. O., Lodin, H., and Malers, E.: The Evaluation of the Degree of Mitral Insufficiency by Selective Left Ventricular Angiocardiography, *Am. Heart J.*, **60**:691, 1960.
38. Bjork, V. O., and Lodin, H.: Evaluation of Mitral Stenosis with Selective Left Ventricular Angiocardiography, *J. Thoracic & Cardiovas. Surg.*, **40**:17, 1960.
39. Nordenstrom, B.: Methods of Altering Circulatory

Dynamics to Improve Roentgen Examination of the Cardiovascular System, Chamberlain Lecture, 1961, *Am. J. Roentgenol.*, 89:233, 1963.

40. Mudd, J. G., Wong, J. C., Wyatt, J. P., and Hanlon, C. R.: An Experimental Study of Toxic Factors in Angiocardiography, *S. Forum*, 6:262, 1955.

41. Read, R. C.: Cause of Death in Cardioangiography, *J. Thoracic & Cardiovas. Surg.*, 38:685, 1959.

42. Read, R. C., et al.: Vascular Effects of Hypertonic Solutions, *Circulation Res.*, 8:538, 1960.

43. Giammona, S. T., Lurie, P. R., and Segar, W. E.: Hypertonicity Following Selective Angiocardiography, *Circulation*, 28:1096, 1963.

44. Bernstein, E. F., Evans, R. L., Blum, J. A., and Avant, R. F.: Further Experimental and Early Clinical Observations Concerning Protective Action of Low Molecular Weight Dextran on Intravenous Hypaque Toxicity, *Radiology*, 76:260, 1961.

45. Garber, G. L., and Read, R. C.: Protective Effect of Hypervolemia in Cardioangiography, *J.A.M.A.*, 180:116, 1962.

46. Bell, A. L. L., Jr., Shimomura, S., Guthrie, W. J., Hempel, H. F., Fitzpatrick, H. F., and Begg, C. F.: Wedge Pulmonary Arteriography, *Radiology*, 73:566, 1959.

47. McMichael, J., and Mounsey, J. P. D.: Complication Following Coronary Sinus and Cardiac Vein Catheterization in Man, *Brit. Heart J.*, 13:397, 1951.

48. Smith, W. W., Albert, R. E., and Rader, B.: Myocardial Damage Following Inadvertent Deep Cannulation of the Coronary Sinus during Right Heart Catheterization, *Am. Heart J.*, 42:661, 1951.

49. Koehler, P. R., and Isard, H. J.: An Unusual Complication of Inferior Venacavography, *Circulation*, 26:935, 1962.

50. Cheng, T. O.: Myocardial Infarction Following Transmural Extravasation of Contrast Medium during Left Ventricular Cineangiography, *Circulation*, 28:105, 1963.

51. Keates, P. G., and Wagner, G. R.: Perforation of Heart during Cardiac Catheterization and Selective Angiocardiography, *Circulation*, 28:585, 1963.

52. Hilbish, T. F., and Herdt, J. R. L.: Complications of Selective Angiocardiography, *Radiology*, 75:197, 1960.

53. Hart, W. L., Berman, E. J., and LaCom, R. H.: Hazard of Retrograde Aortography in Dissecting Aneurysm, *Circulation*, 27:1140, 1963.

54. Oppenheimer, M. J., Durant, T. M., Stauffer, H. M., Stewart, G. H., Lynch, T. R., and Barrera, F.: In-vivo Visualization of Intracardiac Structures with Gaseous Carbon Dioxide: Cardiovascular-Respiratory Effects and Associated Changes in Blood Chemistry, *Am. J. Physiol.*, 186:325, 1956.

55. Durant, T. M., Stauffer, H. M., Oppenheimer, M. J., and Paul, R. E.: The Safety of Intravascular Carbon Dioxide and Its Use for Roentgenologic Visualization of Intracardiac Structures, *Ann. Int. Med.*, 44:191, 1951.

56. Scatliff, J. H., Kummer, D. J., and Janzen, A. H.: The Diagnosis of Pericardial Effusion with Intracardiac Carbon Dioxide, *Radiology*, 73:871, 1959.

57. Phillips, J. H., Jr., Burch, G. E., and Hellinger, R.: Use of Intra-Cardiac Carbon Dioxide in Diagnosis of Pericardial Disease, *Am. Heart J.*, 61:748, 1961.

58. Burch, G. E., and Phillips, J. H.: A Miniature Tank for Supply of Carbon Dioxide for Carboangiocardiography, *J.A.M.A.*, 183:154, 1963.

59. Burch, G. E., and Phillips, J. H., Jr.: Methods in Diagnostic Differentiation of Myocardial Dilatation from Pericardial Effusion, *Am. Heart J.*, 64:266, 1962.

60. Weens, H. S.: Personal communication.

61. Rejali, A. M., MacIntyre, W. J., and Friedell, H. L.: Radioisotope Method of Visualization of Blood Pools, *Am. J. Roentgenol.*, 79:129–137, 1958.

62. Charkes, N. D., and Sklaroff, D. M.: Radioisotope Photoscanning as a Diagnostic Aid in Cardiovascular Disease, *J.A.M.A.*, 186:134, 1963.

63. MacIntyre, W. J., Crespo, G. G., and Christie, J. H.: Use of Radioiodinated (I 131) Iodipamide for Cardiovascular Scanning, *Am. J. Roentgenol.*, 89:315, 1963.

64. Wagner, H. N., Jr., McAfee, J. G., and Mozley, J. M.: Diagnosis of Pericardial Effusion by Radioisotope Scanning, *Arch. Int. Med.*, 108:679, 1961.

65. Bonte, F. J., et al.: Radioisotope Scanning in Detection of Pericardial Effusions, *South. M. J.*, 55:577, 1962.

66. Jorgens, J., Kundel, R., and Lieber, A.: The Cinefluorographic Approach to the Diagnosis of Pericardial Effusion, *Am. J. Roentgenol.*, 87:911, 1962.

67. Shah, K. D., Neill, C. A., Wagner, H. N., Jr., and Taussig, H.: Radioisotope Scanning of the Liver and Spleen in Dextrocardia and in Situs Inversus with Levocardia, *Circulation*, 29:231, 1964.

68. Wagner, H. N., Jr., Sabiston, D. C., Jr., McAfee, J. G., Tow, D., and Stern, H. S.: Diagnosis of Massive Pulmonary Embolism in Man by Radioisotope Scanning, *New England J. Med.*, 271:377, 1964.

10 OTHER DIAGNOSTIC PROCEDURES

Robert H. Franch, M.D.

CIRCULATION (APPEARANCE) TIME

Clinically the circulation time is the earliest subjective appearance of an intravascular indicator material at a sampling site, usually the tongue or the lung. The circulation time between any two points is directly proportional to the vascular volume between the two points and is inversely proportional to volume rate of flow.[1] If the volume of the vascular bed rises secondary to a flow increase, the circulation time may be unchanged.

A wide range of indicators has been used, and new ones are being added.[2,3] Indicators may utilize color, vasodilator effect, radioactivity,[4,5] effect on respiration, neuromuscular stimulation, smell, or taste as end points.

The test is usually performed in a supine resting steady state with the arm abducted at the midchest level.[3] The largest vein is punctured with a 19-gauge needle. If a subjective end point is used, the patient is previously instructed to say "now" on *first* experiencing the appropriate sensation. After removing the tourniquet and observing that respiration is normal, a rapid injection of indicator is made. It is convenient to have the stopwatch already running; this permits both hands to be free for the injection. The injection is begun as the stopwatch hand passes a given point. The test may be repeated with a different agent, or a nonindicator blank, e.g., saline solution, may be injected to assess the patient's reliability. Injection time is usually 1 to 2 sec. Three milliliters of a 20 per cent magnesium sulfate solution produces a sensation of warmth in the tongue and pharynx in 7 to 17 sec. Decholin, 3 to 5 ml, in 20 per cent concentration produces a bitter taste in 10 to 16 sec. A mixture of 0.3 ml of ether mixed with 0.6 ml of normal saline solution is detected in 4 to 8 sec by smell or cough during passage through the lungs.[6]

The arrival of indicator is noted only when it reaches a detectable or threshold concentration. The circulation time is shorter with 20 per cent Decholin than with 10 per cent Decholin.[7] This difference tends to be accentuated in patients with heart failure.[7] Circulation time with magnesium sulfate is about 3 sec longer than with Evans blue detected by an ear oximeter.[8] The latter technique is especially useful in patients who lack sensory discrimination.

Normal variations in circulation time when a single indicator is used depend on whether the arm is raised during injection, on age, sex, and central blood volume.[8] The appearance time in the adult male is longer than in the adult female or in teenagers of both sexes.[4,8,9] The circulation time tends to be longer in subjects over 40.[8] The prolonged arm-to-tongue time in left ventricular failure (greater than 20 sec) is related to the increase in pulmonary, left atrial, and left ventricular blood volume. The circulation time is usually normal in dyspnea due to pulmonary disease. In high-output failure, the circulation time may be normal or shortened in the presence of congestive heart failure. Circulation time is prolonged in pericardial disease if the venous pressure is elevated; it may be normal or abnormal in early heart failure. Serial circulation times are useful in documenting the course of heart failure. In the future, all circulation times may well be objective measurements, recorded as part of a time-concentration curve that gives, in addition, flow and volume data.

VENOUS PRESSURE

Venous pressure is usually measured to obtain an index of mean right atrial pressure. Frey in 1902 used an indirect method to measure venous pressure: A bar capable of moving in a vertical plane rested on the skin and was weighted until the vein collapsed. From the surface area exposed and the amount of weight, the venous pressure could be calculated.[10] Other investigators used a transparent air chamber over the vein and measured the air pressure necessary to produce a venous collapse.[11-13] An indirect method was proposed which required no apparatus: the distance above heart level at which the superficial veins of the hand were noted to collapse was represented as the venous pressure.[14]

In 1910 Moritz and D. von Tabora measured venous pressure directly by needling a superficial vein.[15] The arm is abducted to 60° and the antecubital fossa is supported either at a level 10 cm up from the dorsal spine of the supine patient or at midchest. Puncture is made with an 18-gauge needle so that there is brisk retrograde blood flow. A 10-ml flushing syringe and heparine-saline filled manometer tube are connected to the needle by a three-way stopcock. The manometer is then turned in to monitor the venous pressure now represented by the height of the saline column above the selected reference level. Readings should be repeated until they are constant. The normal venous pressure range is 2 to 12 ml of water. (A pressure of 1 mm Hg = 1.36 ml of water.) Accurate measurement of venous pressure as an index of right atrial mean pressure presumes:

1. That the venous channel extends uncompressed and unkinked into the right atrium.

2. That the intrathoracic and intraabdominal pressure vary within normal limits.

3. That the needle lies free in the vein lumen. Respiratory variations in the fluid level and a rise with venous obstruction above the needle confirm an unobstructed system. The patient with right ventricular failure should show a rise of several centimeters of water with abdominal compression.[16,17]

4. That the zero reference level and the technique of measurement be constant in serial observations. The normal value for venous pressure depends on the reference level—the further toward the back, the higher the venous pressure. In supine adults a distance of 10 cm (in children, 5 cm)

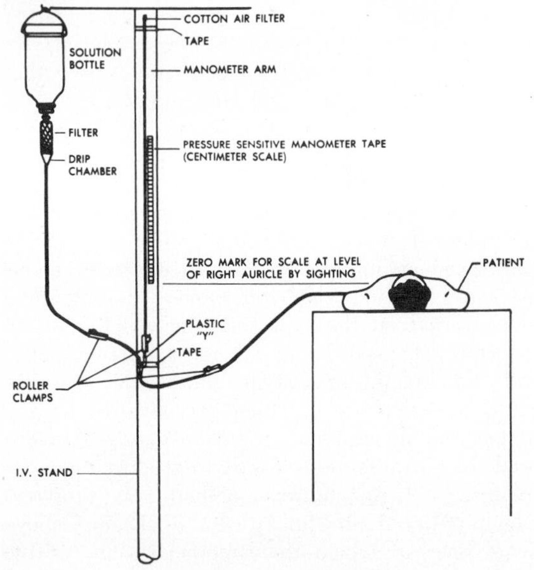

Fig. 10-1. A technique for intermittent monitoring of central venous pressure via a small plastic catheter in the superior vena cava or the right atrium. (*By permission of Fenwal Laboratories.*)

(see reference 135 in Chap. 8) up from the back places the zero level at the entrance of the venae cavae into the right atrium.[18,19] A caliper may be used for measuring the anteroposterior diameter of the chest at the level of the fourth left intercostal space at the sternum, and the standard level of reference is taken to be one-half this diameter.[20] If the patient shifts to a semisitting position, a plane parallel to the floor passing through the zero reference point is taken as the reference level.[20,21] A careful observer will establish normal values for his particular reference point and technique.

Recently, the direct measurement of venous pressure in right ventricular failure has given way to indirect estimation by the inspection of the jugular venous system. For training purposes, however, it is desirable to apply the direct techniques as a proficiency check. Continuous or intermittent monitoring of venous pressure during and after open-heart surgery (Fig. 10-1) is useful as an index of blood volume. The course of localized venous obstruction, e.g., superior vena cava syndrome, may be documented.

ARTERIAL PULSE

The rapid displacement of blood (45 ml in 0.1 sec) from the left ventricle into the aorta (a fixed-capacity, high-pressure reservoir) produces a forward movement of blood with distension of the elastic aortic arch through an increase in lateral pressure.[22] The pressure change is transmitted as a wave over the entire aorta and its many branches, so that arteries as far away as the dorsalis pedis are expanding before ventricular systole has terminated.[22]

The arterial pulse is divided into the systolic phase (during which pressure rises, plateaus, and falls) and the diastolic phase (during which pressure falls). The two phases are separated by an incisura, which is related to closure of the aortic semilunar valve. At the beginning of systole the initial part of the curve is steep. The pressure rises rapidly because of[23] (1) the viscoelastic resistance of the aorta to rapid stretch, and (2) the inertial resistance of the nearly stationary column of blood in the upper aorta. The first part of ejection expands only the upper part of the aorta and produces a pressure rise that is much greater than if the whole of the aorta were distended by the same volume. By mid-systole the whole aorta is expanded, and a given amount of ejected blood does not produce so great a rise as occurred in early systole; thus pressure rises slowly or may plateau.

As the pressure pulse moves to the periphery, there is a change in temporal relationships, contour, and amplitude.[24,25] The distance between the R wave of the electrocardiogram and the onset of the pulse wave is increased. The incisura, which is sharp and short in the aortic pressure pulse, is lost during transmission to the extremities, as is the anacrotic wave. The dicrotic depression is drawn out and deep in the brachial-radial system, approaches diastolic pressure in the dorsalis pedis, but is practically nonexistent in the femoral pressure pulse. A tidal wave following the primary peak, but preceding the dicrotic notch, is usually present in the brachial-radial system, but not in the femoral-dorsalis pedis system. In the periphery, there is an increase in pulse pressure, a decrease in dicrotic pressure, a decrease in diastolic and mean pressure, and a slight tendency for systolic pressure to increase.[24]

The mechanism of the change in form and amplitude of the pressure pulse skeleton as it moves to the periphery is not completely understood. Classically, the pressure wave is said to rebound from the periphery, producing a standing-wave system that adds or subtracts from different portions of the pressure pulse.[22,26-28] In addition, there is damping of the pressure wave in the elastic compression chamber. Too, the pressure pulse can be resolved into a series of sinusoidal waves of different frequencies.[29] The amplitude and phase relationship of the various frequency components determine the size and shape of the pulse wave.[30] The arterial system functions as a damped, resonant transmission line which will transmit different frequencies with varying degrees of attenuation.[31] As the pulse wave passes through the system, the attenuation of certain frequency components will result in a reshaping of the wave.

The pressure pulse is transmitted slowly in a distensible tube and quickly in a rigid tube. The pulse-wave velocity is 3 to 4 m per sec in the distensible aorta but 7 to 14 m per sec in the muscular arteries of the limbs.[32,33] The velocity of blood flow is approximately ½ to 1 m per sec. The pulse-wave velocity is a highly variable measurement. It is affected by age, blood pressure, vessel disease, and other physiologic variables.[23] In general, pulse-wave velocity increases with age and with decreased distensibility. The pulse-wave velocity might be used to measure the relative distensibility of a vessel if the exact volume of the aorta in diastole were known.[23]

It would be useful if the ventricular stroke volume could be estimated from the pulse pressure.[34-37] For this calculation, the capacitance ($\Delta V/\Delta P$) of the aorta should be determined for each individual. Capacitance varies significantly in different aortas; nor is it linear over a high-to-low pressure range. A surprisingly close correlation with stroke volume determined by the Fick method has been found in one study;[38] however, widespread assessment of the pulse-contour method has not yet been made.

The externally recorded arterial pulse measures the expansion and elongation of the arterial wall induced by the transmitted central pressure wave. The external arterial pulse may be recorded by (1) a funnel-shaped or cup pickup connected to a piezoelectric crystal or strain-gauge transducer;[39-41] (2) photoelectric recording of digital transparency changes;[42] (3) electrical resistance recording of a mercury-filled rubber tube encircling the limb,[43] or measurement of electrical impedance between two skin areas;[44-46] and (4) by amplification of the pressure changes in an air-filled cuff surrounding the limb or the neck.[47-50]

The pressure with which the volume-sensing elements are applied against the artery influences the size and contour of the recorded pulse without significantly altering intraarterial pressure. In general, the extraarterial pulse increases in amplitude, without contour distortion, with increasing counterpressure of the pickup unit up to about diastolic pressure (Marey's principle).[46]

If a rubber cuff, 23 × 4 cm, inflated to 3 mm Hg pressure is held in place about the neck by a leather band and is connected to an air-filled transducer and photographic recording system with a frequency response flat to 60 cycles, the normal carotid pulse is as follows:[49]

There are two major peaks during systole, either of which may be greater. The first peak, called the percussion wave, always rises rapidly, occurring 0.1 to 0.12 sec after onset. The second peak, called the tidal wave or end-systolic shoulder, occurs 0.20 to 0.24 sec after the onset of systole. The pulse between the two peaks may rise, fall, or remain a plateau. The upstroke time is measured to the higher peak.[49,51] The normal brachial pulse upstroke time is shorter than the carotid, since the first peak is always higher than the second in the brachial pulse. Coarse systolic upstroke vibrations are lost in the brachial tracing. The incisura is sharp in the carotid but attenuated in the brachial artery.[52]

The externally recorded carotid pulse serves as a suitable time reference for phonocardiography (0.02 to 0.04 sec transmission delay) (Fig. 10-2) and trains the finger to appreciate the pulse contour. There is close agreement, in curve contour, duration of left ventricular ejection, and upstroke time between the direct aortic or carotid pressure pulse and the indirect carotid pulse tracing.[41,22]

VENOUS PULSE

Lancisi in 1728 described "systolic fluctuation" of the jugular vein in a patient with tricuspid regurgitation proved at autopsy.[54] In 1863 Chauveau and Marey developed a mechanical-graphic recording technique that was utilized by Friedreich in 1866 to obtain jugular venous pulse tracings from patients.[55] Potain in 1867 recorded simultaneous tracings with the apex beat and recognized the presystolic timing and atrial origin of the *a* wave.[56] MacKenzie in 1893 recognized, named, and provided a hemodynamic explanation for the *a*, *c*, and *v* waves. In the pre- and early-electrocardiographic era, he applied venous poly-

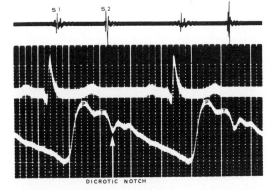

Fig. 10-2. Indirect recording of the normal carotid pulse with simultaneous electrocardiogram and phonocardiogram. Vertical time lines, 0.04 sec. *P*, percussion wave; *T*, tidal wave. (*After Myers,*[53] *with permission of the publisher.*)

graph tracings to the bedside study of arrhythmias.[57,58]

The Marey tambour had much inertia and a low fundamental frequency.[59] Though the Frank segment capsule ingeniously used a beam of light for a writing pen, the limitations of its rubber membrane remained.[60] The development of a crystal microphone, utilizing the piezoelectric effect, provided a voltage output proportional to the pressure changes that occurred in the air-filled tubing connected to the venous cup.[61,62] When combined with a satisfactory amplifier recorder system, a flat frequency response from ⅓ to 40 cps was available.

By virtue of its proximity to the heart, the internal jugular vein reflects rather closely the pressure changes that occur in the right atrium. The venous pulse is usually recorded over the base of the right internal jugular vein at a dilatation called the *jugular bulb*. The pressure-volume changes in an overlying cup airtight with the skin are relayed to a transducer recorder system. The subject is positioned so that maximum pulse amplitude is present in the deep vein. The head may be turned slightly to the right to relax the right sternocleidomastoid muscle. The sensing cup, usually held by hand, may require several trial placements; its rim may be used to displace gently the carotid artery. A normal resting heart rate is desirable, since the venous pulse is primarily a diastolic phenomenon. Respiration is best stopped in the neutral or end-expiratory phase. Occasionally the pulse may be optimally recorded at a higher position in the right side of the neck or from the left internal jugular vein.

In the normal jugular pulse (Fig. 10-3), (1) the *a* wave is a presystolic pressure wave due to atrial contraction; it disappears when atrial fibrillation

is present. The descending limb of the *a* wave, or the venous systolic collapse, has its nadir at X. It is related to atrial relaxation and to the movement of the tricuspid valve plane toward the ventricular apex during systole. The X descent is interrupted by the *c* wave. (2) The *c* wave is largely related to the transmission of the carotid artery pulsation to the jugular vein or of the aortic root pulsation to the superior vena cava. Other factors include bulging of the tricuspid valve into the atrium during isovolumetric contraction and a momentary pressure rise when atrial inflow temporarily exceeds the volume change of the right atrium. The *c* wave is not regularly conspicuous in the right atrial pressure tracing. (3) The *v* wave is a diastolic "volume" wave due to progressive filling of the right atrium. Its apex signals the opening of the tricuspid valve. The descending limb of the *v* wave, or the venous diastolic collapse, has its nadir at Y. (4) **The *h* wave** is a shoulder or a slight promontory rising immediately before the *a* wave and visible only at slow heart rates. It marks the pause following the end of ventricular filling and is the reference point about which the venous pulse fluctuates.

Measurements of the transmission delay from the right atrium to the right jugular bulb have ranged from insignificant[63] to as much as 0.2 sec.[64] One may take 0.02 sec as a mean value. The jugular phlebogram does not present quantitative pressure information. The distance from *a* to *c* may give a rough approximation of the P-R interval; the distance, *c* to *v*, of ventricular systole; the distance, *v* to *y*, a rough estimate of the duration of the rapid-filling phase; and from *y* to the beginning of *a* or to *h*, if present, an estimate of the reduced filling phase. The *c* wave tends to occur 0.1 sec before the radial upstroke and is simultaneous with the beginning of the carotid upstroke. In making measurements, the peak of the venous waves is difficult to determine within 0.04 sec.

The phlebogram is of usefulness as a timing reference for phonocardiography, but primarily it serves to train the eye in the recognition of deviations of the jugular pulse from the normal pattern.

PHONOCARDIOGRAM

The phonocardiogram is discussed in Chap. 5, under "Auscultation of the Heart."

APEX CARDIOGRAM

The kinetocardiogram (KCG) or the apex cardiogram (ACG) is a graphic record of ultra-low-frequency precordial chest-wall movements (0.1 to 20 cps). A flexible metal bellows, 7 mm in diameter

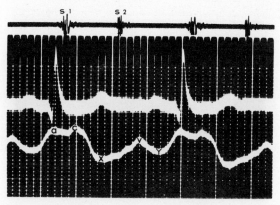

Fig. 10-3. Indirect recording of the normal jugular venous pulse, with simultaneous electrocardiogram and phonocardiogram. Vertical time lines, 0.04 sec. (*After Myers,*[53] *with permission of the publisher.*)

at the skin contact point, is connected via rubber tubing to a pressure-sensitive transducer. Displacement movements of the precordium are sensed and recorded (kinetocardiogram).[65–68] Another technique of sensing displacement uses a sound microphone, placed over the apex, in tandem with a crystal microphone connected to an amplifier recorder system, thus providing simultaneous phonocardiogram and apex cardiogram.[69] The record is made in end expiration. A precordial electrocardiographic lead via the aluminum microphone bell confirms a left ventricular complex at the recording site. The records are reproducible, but careful positioning over the center of the apex beat is required. Using this method, the components of the ultra-low-frequency precordial movements may be related to the cardiac cycle as follows (Fig. 10-4): the *a* wave coincides with the fourth heart sound and with the *a* wave of the atrial pressure curve. It reflects the transmission of atrial contraction to the ventricle. In patients with complete heart block, the *a* wave follows the *p* wave of the electrocardiogram. The point E represents the opening of the aortic valve; thus from the end of A to point E represents isovolumetric contraction. The point O represents the opening of the mitral valve. The time span from E to O represents the systolic wave of the ACG. The time span from E to S-2 on the phonocardiogram is a measure of left ventricular ejection. The total height or amplitude of the ACG is represented by the vertical distance E to O. The isovolumetric relaxation period is not well defined. The rapid ventricular filling wave (RFW) is represented by the rise toward the base line from point O. It tends to disappear in mitral stenosis[70] and to reappear after valvulotomy; it tends to be exaggerated in mitral insufficiency. The slow ventricular filling wave duration varies with heart rate. The *a* wave is increased in patients who have a high left ventricular end-diastolic pressure, left ventricular hypertrophy, or loss of ventricular distensibility. A large *a* wave has been recorded during angina, with return to the pre-pain amplitude 5 min after administration of nitroglycerin. In some patients with hypertension, the *a* wave may be taller than the E wave. The *a* wave tends to increase with exercise in patients with ischemic heart disease, but not in normal persons.[71,72] The E to O configuration may be double-peaked in subaortic hypertrophic stenosis and may be bisferiens in aortic stenosis and aortic insufficiency combined.

This technique requires experience. A satisfactory instrument should record a sustained plateau if it is present to palpation. The ACG is an important objective aid to those interested in evaluating the apical impulse at the bedside.

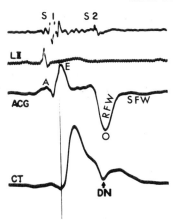

Fig. 10-4. Simultaneous recording of the phonocardiogram, electrocardiogram (lead II), apex cardiogram (*ACG*), and carotid pulse (*CT*). A, coincides with atrial systole; E, represents opening of the aortic valve; O, the opening of the mitral valve; RFW and SFW, the rapid and slow ventricular filling waves; DN, the dicrotic notch. (*After Benchimol and Dimond, with permission of the authors and publisher.*[69])

BALLISTOCARDIOGRAM

The ballistocardiogram (BCG) records the movements of the body or of a table top on which the body lies; motion is produced by alternate speeding and slowing of masses of blood and soft tissue as a result of cardiac contraction. The BCG pattern is determined, in addition, by the mechanical characteristics of the body-table system.

Generally there are four types of ballistocardiographs in use (Fig. 10-5):[73]

1. The ultra-low-frequency instrument has a natural frequency of vibration less than 0.5 cps.[74,75] The ultra-low-frequency system is said to measure the true displacement caused by the heartbeat. The bed follows the movement of the body freely so that distortion due to elastic forces is minimized.

2. The low-frequency, critically damped instrument has a small elastic force applied to the table to yield a natural frequency of vibration of 1 cps or slightly greater.[76–80] Critical damping seeks to prevent the overshoot or undershoot that distorts the BCG wave.

3. The high-frequency BCG table works against a strong spring; the patient-table system has a natural frequency of vibration above 10 cps.[81,36,82] The high-frequency BCG tends to reflect the force of the heartbeat.

4. The direct body ballistocardiograph of Dock utilizes the movements of a bar placed across a patient's shins for its record.[83] The patient lies on a rigid table and moves against the elasticity of his own tissues. The curve obtained resembles the record of the high-frequency table.

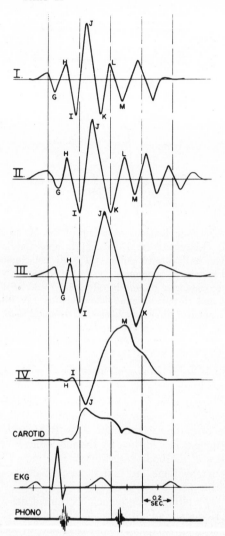

above 40 years of age, and 90 per cent of tracings in the eighth decade are abnormal.[85] If the amplitude of motion were proportional only to the force of the heartbeat, an easily obtainable index of the force of myocardial contraction would be available. As yet, however, the contribution of the motion of blood in the vessels cannot be clearly separated. The study of the dynamics of ventricular ejection or "the initial ventricular impulse" may be a promising field for ballistocardiography. The measurement of cardiac output by the BCG is grossly unreliable, especially in the presence of cardiac disease.

Occlusion of an arteriovenous fistula causes decreased amplitude in BCG complexes. Administration of nitroglycerin causes increased amplitude of the complexes. Inspiration, for unknown reasons, tends to cause larger BCG complexes.

BCG tracings are read and graded by a pattern method, and time measurements are made. The BCG may be abnormal because of alteration in the wave pattern, increased respiratory variation, or abnormal amplitude. The potential of the BCG is in the evaluation of the mechanical function of the heart as a pump, but at present it is not an important diagnostic tool.

ELECTROKYMOGRAM

The electrokymogram is a record of the movement of a small section or a single border of the heart or of a great vessel.[86,87] The electrokymograph consists of a photoelectric cell or photomultiplier tube that receives light from a small fluorescent screen activated by x-rays that pass through a slitlike, lead window that lies on the patient's chest. As the heart border moves across the window, more

Fig. 10-5. The relationship of displacement records from different ballistocardiographic systems to the carotid pulse, electrocardiogram, and phonocardiogram. The initial solid vertical line marks the Q wave of the electrocardiogram. Compare the difference in timing and relationship of waves in: I. High-frequency ballistocardiogram. II. Direct body ballistocardiogram. III. Low-frequency ballistocardiogram. IV. Ultra-low-frequency ballistocardiogram. (*By permission of the authors and publisher.*[73])

In addition to the displacement BCG that records body headward and footward movement during the heart cycle, the velocity of body movements (velocity BCG) and a record of the force causing body movements during the heart cycle (acceleration BCG)[84] may be obtained.

The clinical and physiologic significance of the BCG, especially in the older normal age groups, is poorly understood. Abnormal BCGs are common

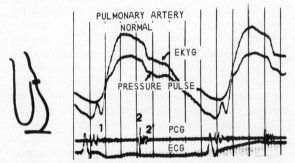

Fig. 10-6. Normal pulmonary artery electrokymogram (EKYG) recorded simultaneously with pulmonary pressure pulse, phonocardiogram (PCG), and electrocardiogram (ECG). Note the general agreement in contour of the EKYG and the pressure pulse; EKYG time lag is 0.01 sec. 2 and 2', aortic and pulmonary components of the second sound. (*With permission of the authors and publisher.*[86])

or less emitted light from the fluoroscope stimulates the photoelectric cell. The output of the cell is filtered, amplified, and recorded to provide a record of the phasic motion of the heart border plotted against time. Excellent border electrokymograms, resembling their pressure curves closely, are obtained from the pulmonary artery (Fig. 10-6) and the aorta. The reference tracings include the electrocardiogram, the phonocardiogram, and the apex cardiogram. The electrokymograph filter introduces a 0.01-sec time lag between the electrocardiogram and the electrokymogram. The attractiveness of the method lies in the painless ease with which cyclic changes in the great vessels and heart chambers may be recorded with the hope of using these changes as an index of flow. Studies have also been made of the paradoxical motion of the ventricle after myocardial infarction and of early diastolic filling in patients with constrictive pericarditis. A cooperative patient is needed. Small children may be difficult subjects. Uniform sensitivity of the detecting phototube and uniform frequency response have not been completely obtained.

LUNG FUNCTION AND HEART DISEASE

Arterial blood-oxygen saturation is decreased by one or a combination of factors: (1) uneven relation between pulmonary ventilation and perfusion, (2) alveolar hypoventilation, (3) decreased diffusion of oxygen, (4) anatomic shunts. A fall in arterial oxygen saturation during exercise is a sign of advanced pulmonary disease, if shunt is excluded. In pulmonary insufficiency, the CO_2 tension of arterial blood rises; respiratory acidosis occurs when renal compensation becomes inadequate. Determination of arterial blood pH and CO_2 tension is necessary to separate respiratory acidosis and metabolic alkalosis.

In heart failure accompanied by dyspnea the vital capacity is usually decreased,[88] as is the total lung capacity. The timed vital capacity is normal or only slightly decreased. The residual volume may be normal or increased in relation to total lung capacity. In failure of the left side of the heart the arterial oxygen tension is normal or slightly decreased, falling further with pulmonary edema.[89] The arterial pH may be normal or elevated, depending on whether respiratory alkalosis is present.

The isotope oxygen-15 with a half-life of 2 min may be piped from a cyclotron to be inhaled by the subject as radioactive carbon dioxide.[90] The latter is removed from the alveoli rapidly in direct proportion to the regional pulmonary blood flow. If counting is performed over the chest, the clearance of CO_2 is decreased from the upper part of the chest in the upright normal human being (de-

creased upper lobe blood flow compared to lower lobe blood flow). This difference tends to be less with exercise or with high-flow left-to-right shunts. The difference between upper and lower zone is abolished if the patient is supine. In moderate mitral stenosis, there is equal clearance from the upper and lower lobes in the upright position, but if mitral stenosis is severe, CO_2 clearance is increased from the upper zone (upper lobe flow is increased).[91]

EXAMINATION OF THE BLOOD, URINE, AND EXTRAVASCULAR FLUIDS

A white blood cell count, a blood smear, and a hemoglobin or hematocrit are basic screening tests. The red blood cells of infants and children with secondary polycythemia may become microcytic and hypochromic for lack of large iron stores;[92] the hemoglobin concentration in relation to the hematocrit (reduced mean corpuscular hemoglobin concentration) and the blood smear form the laboratory basis for beginning iron therapy. Cyanotic infants who show numerous nucleated red blood cells and Howell-Jolly bodies in a peripheral smear may have absence of the spleen and serious associated cardiac anomalies.[93,94] In secondary polycythemia of advanced degree, complex thrombotic and hemorrhagic manifestations may occur. Poor clot retraction reflects relative deficiency of fibrinogen (low plasma volume with a high red-cell mass).[95] Production of platelets and other clotting elements may be decreased.

Phase reactants are sensitive indicators of inflamation and tissue damage. Critical clinical judgment must be applied to decide whether their presence is of major or minor significance. The erythrocyte sedimentation rate (ESR) is also elevated in pregnancy and in dysproteinemias. In the patient with rheumatic fever followed serially, an erythrocyte sedimentation rate of greater than 20 mm per hr (Westergren), or greater than 15 mm (Wintrobe), corrected, may be indicative of rheumatic activity. The ESR is occasionally normal in acute rheumatic fever with heart failure (see reference 135 in Chap. 8). The C-reactive protein (CRP) is absent from the blood of normal individuals; hence there is no normal range. It is increased in patients with acute rheumatic fever, including those with heart failure. It is useful in following the course of rheumatic activity; it may be normal in isolated manifestations of rheumatic fever such as chorea or erythema marginatum (see reference 135 in Chap. 8).

Serum enzymes provide useful confirmation of tissue damage, but as yet no specific enzymes for myocardial necrosis have been found.

Antistreptolysin-O titers of 400 Todd units or

greater occur 4 to 6 weeks following a β-hemolytic streptococcus infection and may return to control levels in 4 months. An evaluation of paired serums is important in cases with lower titers. Serums for this determination may be stored at −20°C. A throat swab on a 5 per cent sheep blood agar plate is used to culture β-hemolytic streptococcus. A group-specific antiserum against an acid extract of the bacteria may be used to exclude the 10 to 15 per cent of β-hemolytic streptococcus isolated from nose and throat that are other than group A.

In preparation for obtaining a blood culture, the skin is cleaned with 70 per cent alcohol before and after being painted with a 2.5 per cent tincture of iodine solution. The quantity of blood added should be approximately 10 per cent of the volume of culture medium in the container.[96] Media suitable for both anaerobic and aerobic and microaerophilic bacterial growth are necessary. An antagonist to sulfa or penicillin should be added. Incubation is for 21 days and up to 42 days if brucellosis is suspected.

In failure of the right side of the heart the elevated right atrial pressure rise is transmitted to the hepatic veins and the venous vasculature of the liver becomes distended. There is parenchymal-cell hypoxia,[97] the pressure dynamics of bile secretion may be altered, and estimated hepatic blood flow is decreased. Bromsulfalein removal is slowed, the serum-bilirubin level may rise, especially if there is associated hemolysis or pulmonary infarction, protein synthesis is disturbed, particularly in constrictive pericarditis, and the serum-transaminase level may be much elevated, in the absence of shock or myocardial or pulmonary infarction.[98,99]

In heart failure, renal plasma flow is decreased and glomerular filtration rate is reduced; a smaller reduction in tubular function provides increased reabsorption of water and electrolytes. With normal protein breakdown, an increase in blood–urea nitrogen concentration occurs when the glomerular filtration rate is reduced to 35 per cent of normal. At present the 24-hr endogenous-creatinine clearance is the best test for the clinical evaluation of renal function. Only serial renal function tests in the patient with heart failure separate anatomic from functional or reversible renal impairment.

The measurement of serum electrolytes is of importance in the management of patients with congestive heart failure.[100] Hypokalemia, hypernatremia, hypochloremia, hypomagnesemia, and alkalosis are serum alterations observed in primary aldosteronism.[101]

The urine is best examined fresh, well-concentrated, and at an acid pH. In heart failure, the day volume of urine may be one-third to one-half the night volume.[102] Mild-to-moderate proteinuria, less than 1 Gm per liter is usually present;[103] urine urobilinogen is increased.[97] White blood cells may be found in the urine sediment, but red cells are uncommon in simple congestive heart failure.[104] The urinary sediment in endocarditis may occasionally mimic that of advanced renal disease.[105] In the carcinoid syndrome, a urinary excess of 5-hydroxyindole acetic acid, a metabolic product of serotonin, is easily and simply detected.[106]

Serous effusion into the body cavities may occur in congestive heart failure, cardiac tamponade, localized venous obstruction, cirrhosis, renal failure, cancer, and hypoproteinemia. A transudate has a low protein content, low specific gravity, and low osmolarity. There is absence of fibrinogen; clotting does not occur. Malignant cells should be sought by the cell block or the Papanicolau method. The fat content of any milky serous effusion should be determined. Pericardial fluid may be inoculated into day-old suckling mice and into tissue culture systems in an attempt to isolate Coxsackie virus.

REFERENCES

1. Burton, A. C.: "A Ciba Foundation Symposium; Peripheral Circulation in Man," Little, Brown and Company, Boston, 1954, p. 7.
2. Hitzig, W. M.: The Value of Circulation Times, *Mod. Concepts Cardiovas. Dis.,* 16(No. 8): 1947.
3. Morris, L. E., and Blumgart, H. L.: Velocity of Blood Flow in Health and Disease, *Circulation,* 15:448, 1957.
4. Blumgart, H. L., and Yens, O. C.: Studies on the Velocity of Blood Flow. I. The Method Utilized, *J. Clin. Invest.,* 4:1, 1927.
5. Blumgart, H. L.: The Velocity of Blood Flow in Health and Disease, *Medicine,* 10:1, 1931.
6. King, H., and Hawtof, D. B.: Accidental Intraarterial Injection of Ether, *J.A.M.A.,* 184:241, 1963.
7. Pearce, M. L., Lewis, A. E., and Kaplan, M. R.: The Factors Influencing the Circulation Time, *Circulation,* 5:583, 1952.
8. Dees, T. M., Rumsfeld, J. A., Miller, W. F., and Chapman, C. B.: Clinical Measurement of Circulation Time: A Comparison of Magnesium Sulphate and Evans Blue Dye in Normal Subjects, *J. Appl. Physiol.,* 10:451, 1957.
9. Carter, S. A., Swan, H. J. C., and Wood, E. H.: Time and Concentration Components of Indicator-dilution Curves Recorded Following Central Injections of Dye in Normal Human Subjects, *Circulation,* 19:430, 1959.
10. Frey, A. Ueber die Bedeutung der Venendruckmessung bei der diatetisch-physikalischen Behandlung der Kreislaufstörungen, *Deutsches Archiv. Für Klinische Medicin,* 73:511, 1902.
11. von Basch, S.: Ehrfahrungen uber den Venen-

druck des Menschen, *Arch. Biol. Nauk..*, 1904–1905, 11 (Suppl.), 117.

12. Hooker, D. R., and Eyster, J. A. E.: An Instrument for the Determination of Venous Pressure in Man, *Johns Hopkins Hosp. Bull.*, **19**:274, 1908.

13. Hooker, D. R.: The Influence of Age upon the Venous Blood Pressure in Man, *Am. J. Physiol.*, **40**:43, 1916.

14. Gaertner, G.: Die Messung des Drucks in rechten Vorhof, *München. med. Wchnschr.*, 1903, 1, 2038.

15. Moritz, F., and von Tabora, D.: Uber eine Methode beim Menschen den Druck in oberflachlichen Venen exakt zu Bestimmen, *Deutsches Arch. Klin. Med.*, **98**:475, 1910.

16. Rondot, E.: Le réflux hepato-jugulaire, Gaz. hebd. sc. méd. Bordeaux, **19**:567, 1898.

17. Hitzig, W. M.: Venous Pressure Curves in Normal and Abnormal Circulatory States; Normal Venous Pressure Curves and Negative "Hepato-jugular Reflux Phenomenon," *J. Mt. Sinai Hosp.*, **12**:309, 1945.

18. Lyons, R. H., Kennedy, J. A., and Burwell, C. S.: Measurement of Venous Pressure by Direct Method, *Am. Heart J.*, **16**:675, 1938.

19. Hussey, H. H., and Jeghers, H.: Practical Considerations of Venous Pressure, *New England J. Med.*, **237**:776, 1947.

20. Burch, G. E.: "A Primer of Venous Pressure," Lea & Febiger, Philadelphia, 1950, p. 85.

21. Winsor, T., and Burch, G. E.: Phlebostatic Axis and Phlebostatic Level: Reference Levels for Venous Pressure Measurements in Man, *Proc. Soc. Exper. Biol. & Med.*, **58**:165, 1945.

22. Wiggers, C. J.: "Circulatory Dynamics: Physiologic Studies," Modern Medical Monographs, Grune & Stratton, Inc., New York, 1952.

23. Hamilton, W. F.: The Arterial Pulse, in A. A. Luisada (ed.), "Cardiology: An Encyclopedia of the Cardiovascular System," McGraw-Hill Book Company, New York, 1959, pp. 2–132.

24. Kroeker, E. J., and Wood, E. H.: Comparison of Simultaneously Recorded Central and Peripheral Arterial Pressure Pulses during Rest, Exercise, and Tilted Position in Man, *Circulation Res.*, **3**:623, 1955.

25. Salans, A. H., Katz, L. N., Graham, G. R., Gordon, A., Elisberg. E. I., and Gerber, A.: A Study of the Central and Peripheral Arterial Pressure Pulse in Man: Correlation with Simultaneously Recorded Electrokymograms, *Circulation*, **4**:510, 1951.

26. Alexander, R. S.: The Genesis of the Aortic Standing Wave, *Circulation Res.*, **1**:145, 1953.

27. Hamilton. W. F., and Dow, P.: An Experimental Study of the Standing Waves in the Pulse Propagated through the Aorta, *Am. J. Physiol.*, **125**:48, 1939.

28. Hamilton, W. F.: The Patterns of the Arterial Pulse, *Am. J. Physiol.*, **141**:235, 1944.

29. Henley, E. J., Lukas, D. S., Staffin, H. K., and

Staffin, R.: Application of Signal Analysis Methods to Arterial and Aortic Pressure Curves, *J. Appl. Physiol.*, **18**:1025, 1963.

30. Warner, H. R.: A Study of the Mechanism of Pressure Wave Distortion by Arterial Walls Using an Electrical Analog, *Circulation Res.*, **5**:79, 1957.

31. Peterson, L. H., and Gerst, P. H.: Significance of Reflected Waves within the Arterial System, *Fed. Proc.*, **15**:144, 1956.

32. Sands, J.: Studies in Pulse Wave Velocity. III. Pulse Velocity in Pathological Conditions, *Am. J. Physiol.*, **71**:519, 1925.

33. Bazett, H. C., Cotton, F. S., Laplace, L. B., and Scott, J. C.: Calculation of Cardiac Output and Effective Peripheral Resistance from Blood Pressure Measurements, with an Appendix on the Size of the Aorta in Man, *Am. J. Physiol.*, **113**:312, 1935.

34. Erlanger, J., and Hooker, D. R.: An Experimental Study of Blood Pressure and of Pulse Pressure in Man, *Johns Hopkins Hosp. Rep.*, **12**:145, 1904.

35. Remington, J. W., Noback, C. R., Hamilton, W. F., and Gold, J. J.: Volume Elasticity Characteristics of the Human Aorta and Prediction of the Stroke Volume from the Pressure Pulse, *Am. J. Physiol.* **153**:298, 1948.

36. Starr, I., Schnabel, T. G., Jr., Askovitz, S. I., and Schild, A.: Studies Made by Simulating Systole at Necropsy. IV. On the Relation between Pulse Pressure and Cardiac Stroke Volume, Leading to a Clinical Method of Estimating Cardiac Output from Blood Pressure and Age, *Circulation*, **9**:648, 1954.

37. Brotmacher, M. D.: Evaluation of Derivation of Cardiac Output from Blood Pressure Measurements, *Circulation Res.*, **5**:589, 1957.

38. Warner, H. R., Swan, H. J. C., Connolly, D.C., Tompkins, R. G., and Wood, E. H.: Quantitation of Beat-to-Beat Changes in Stroke Volume from the Aortic Pulse Contour in Man, *J. Appl. Physiol.*, **5**:495. 1953.

39. Smith, J. E.: A Technique for Recording Carotid Artery Pulsations, with Special Reference to Aortic Stenosis, *Am. Heart J.*, **49**:428, 1955.

40. Smith, J. E., Hsu, I., Evans, J. M., and Lederer, L. G.: Aortic Stenosis: A Study with Particular Reference to an Indirect Carotid Pulse Recording in Diagnosis, *Am. Heart J.*, **58**:527, 1959.

41. Weissler, A. M., Peeler, R. G., and Rochell, W. H., Jr.: Relationships between Left Ventricular Ejection Time, Stroke Volume, and Heart Rate in Normal Individuals and Patients with Cardiovascular Disease, *Am. Heart J.*, **62**:367, 1961.

42. Simonson, E., Koff, S., Keys, A., and Minckler, J.: Contour of the Toe Pulse: Reactive Hyperemia and Pulse Transmission Velocity with Group and Repeat Variability Effect of Age, Exercise and Disease, *Am. Heart J.*, **50**:260, 1955.

43. Whitney, R. J.: The Measurement of Volume

Changes in Human Limbs, *J. Physiol.*, **121**:1, 1953.

44. Nyboer, J.: Electrical Impedance Plethysmography, *Circulation*, **2**:811, 1950.

45. Van den Berg, J. W., and Alberts, A. J.: Limitations of Electrical Impedance Plethysmography, *Circulation Res.*, **2**:233, 1954.

46. Dontas, A. S., and Cottas, C. S.: Arterial Volume and Pressure Pulse Contours in the Young Human Subject, *Am. Heart J.*, **61**:676, 1961.

47. Daoud, G., Reppert, E. H., Jr., and Butterworth, J. S.: Basal Systolic Murmurs and the Carotid Pulse Curve in the Diagnosis of Calcareous Aortic Stenosis, *Ann. Int. Med.*, **50**:323, 1959.

48. Duchosal, P. W., Ferrero, C., Leupin, A., and Urdaneta, E.: Advance in the Clinical Evaluation of Aortic Stenosis by Arterial Pulse Recordings of the Neck, *Am. Heart J.*, **51**:861, 1956.

49. Robinson, B.: The Carotid Pulse, Diagnosis of Aortic Stenosis: External Recordings, *Brit. Heart J.*, **25**:51, 1963.

50. Dontas, A. S.: Comparison of Simultaneously Recorded Intra-arterial and Extra-arterial Pressure Pulses in Man, *Am. Heart J.*, **59**:576, 1960.

51. Epstein, E. J., and Coalshed, N.: Assessment of Aortic Stenosis from the External Carotid Pulse Wave, *Brit. Heart J.*, **26**:84, 1964.

52. Hancock, E. W., and Abelmann, W. H.: A Clinical Study of the Brachial Arterial Pulse Form with Special Reference to the Diagnosis of Aortic Valvular Disease, *Circulation*, **16**:572, 1957.

53. Myers, G. B.: "The Interpretation of the Unipolar Electrocardiogram," The C. V. Mosby Company, St. Louis, 1956, p. 12.

54. Lancisi, G. M.: "De motu cordis et aneurysmatibus," Rome, 1728.

55. Friedreich, N.: Über den Venenpuls, *Deutsches Arch. klin. Med.*, **1**:241, 1866.

56. Potain, P. C. E.: Des mouvements et des bruits qui se passant dans les veines jugulaires, *Mém. Soc. méd. hôp. Paris*, **3**, 1867.

57. MacKenzie, J.: "A Study of the Pulse, Arterial, Venous and Hepatic, and of the Movements of the Heart," The MacMillan Company, New York, 1902.

58. MacKenzie, J.: The Ink Polygraph, *Brit. M. J.*, **1**:1411, 1908.

59. Marey, E. J.: "La circulation du sang á'létat physiologique et dans les maladies," G. Masson, Paris, 1881.

60. Frank, O.: Segment Capsule Theory, *Ztschr. Biol.*, **50**:281, 1908.

61. Miller, A., and White, P.: Crystal Microphone for Pulse Wave Recording, *Am. Heart J.*, **21**:504, 1941.

62. Rappaport, M. B., and Sprague, H. B.: Physiologic and Physical Laws That Govern Auscultation and Their Clinical Application: The Acoustic Stethoscope and the Electrically Amplifying Stethoscope and Stethograph, *Am. Heart J.*, **21**:257, 1941.

63. Hartman, H.: The Jugular Venous Tracing, *Am. Heart J.*, **59**:698, 1960.

64. Kuo, P. T., Schnabel, T. G., Jr., Blakemore, W. S., and Whereat, A. F.: Diastolic Gallop Sounds: The Mechanism of Production, *J. Clin. Invest.*, **36**:1035, 1957.

65. Eddleman, E. E., Jr., Hefner, L., Reeves, T. J., and Harrison, T. R.: Movements and Forces of the Human Heart, *A.M.A. Arch. Int. Med.*, **99**:401, 1957.

66. Eddleman, E. E., Jr., and Harrison, T. R.: The Kinetocardiogram in Patients with Ischemic Heart Disease, *Progr. Cardiovas. Dis.*, **6**:189, 1963.

67. Harrison, T. R.: Movements of the Heart and Velocity of Pressure Change during the First Part of Systole, *Johns Hopkins Hosp. Bull.*, **104**:290, 1959.

68. Harrison, T. R.: Movements of the Heart, *Arch. Int. Med.*, **109**:64, 1962.

69. Benchimol, A., and Dimond, E. G.: The Normal and Abnormal Apex-cardiogram: Its Physiologic Valuation and Its Relation to Intracardiac Events, *Am. J. Cardiol.*, **12**:368, 1963.

70. Legler, J. F., Benchimol, A., and Dimond, E. G.: The Apex-cardiogram in the Study of the 2-OS Interval, *Brit. Heart J.*, **25**:246, 1963.

71. Benchimol, A., and Dimond, E. G. The Apex-cardiogram in Normal Older Subjects and in Patients with Arteriosclerotic Heart Disease: Effect of Exercise on the "A" Wave, *Am. Heart J.*, **65**:789, 1963.

72. Benchimol, A., and Dimond, E. G.: The Apex Cardiogram in Ischaemic Heart Disease, *Brit. Heart J.*, **24**:581, 1962.

73. Scarborough, W. R., and Talbot, S. A.: Proposals for Ballistocardiographic Nomenclature and Conventions: Revised and Extended, *Circulation*, **14**:435, 1956.

74. Scarborough, W. R.: The Nature of Records from Ultra-low Frequency BCG Systems and Their Relations to Circulatory Events, *Am. J. Cardiol.*, **5**:613, 1958.

75. Von Wittein, W.: Ballistocardiography with Elimination of the Influence of the Vibration Properties of the Body, *Am. Heart J.*, **46**:705, 1953.

76. Nickerson, J. L.: The Design of the Ballistocardiograph, *Am. J. Physiol.*, **142**:1, 1944.

77. Nickerson, J. L., Warren, J. V., and Brannon, E. S.: Cardiac Output in Man: Studies with Low Frequency, Critically Damped Ballistocardiograph and Method of Right Atrial Catheterization, *J. Clin. Invest.*, **26**:1, 1947.

78. Nickerson, J. L.: Some Observations on the Ballistocardiographic Pattern with Special Reference to the H and K Waves, *J. Clin. Invest.*, **28**:369, 1949.

79. Nickerson, J. L., and Mathers, J. A. L.: A Study of the Physical Properties of the Ballistocardiograph, *Am. Heart J.*, **47**:1, 1954.

80. Burger, H. C., Noordergraaf, A., and Verhagen, A. M. W.: Physical Basis of the Low Frequency Ballistocardiograph, *Am. Heart J.*, **46**:71, 1953.

81. Starr, I. A., Rawson, J., Schroder, H. A., and Joseph, N. R.: Studies on the Estimation of Cardiac Output in Man, and of Abnormalities in Cardiac Function, from the Heart's Recoil and the Blood's impacts: The Ballistocardiogram, *Am. J. Physiol.*, **127**:1, 1939.

82. Braunstein, J. R., Delker, C. F., and Gowdy, R. C.: Design of a Two-dimensional Ballistocardiograph, *J. Clin. Invest.*, **29**:1219, 1950.

83. Dock, W., and Taubman, F.: Some Techniques for Recording the Ballistocardiogram, *Am. J. Med.*, **7**:751, 1949.

84. Elliot, R. V., Packard, R. G., and Kyrazis, D. T.: Acceleration Ballistocardiography: Design, Construction and Application of a New Instrument, *Circulation*, **9**:2, 1954.

85. Scarborough, W. R.: Current Status of Ballistocardiography, *Progr. Cardiovas. Dis.*, **2**:263, 1959.

86. Kjellberg, S. R., Mannheimer, E., Rudhe, U., and Jonsson, B.: "Diagnosis of Congenital Heart Disease, 2d ed., The Year Book Medical Publishers, Inc., Chicago, 1959.

87. Rushmer, R. F.: "Cardiovascular Dynamics," 2d ed., W. B. Saunders Company, Philadelphia, 1961, p. 381.

88. Fowler, N. O.: The Lung in Congestive Heart Failure, *Heart Bull.*, **9**:5, 1960.

89. Cosby, R. S., Stowell, E. C., Jr., Hartwig, W. R., and Mayo, M.: Pulmonary Function in Left Ventricular Failure, Including Cardiac Asthma, *Circulation*, **15**:492, 1957.

90. Dyson, N. A., Hugh-Jones, P., Newberry, G. R., and West, J. B.: The Preparation and Use of Oxygen-15, with Particular Reference to Its Value in the Study of Pulmonary Malfunction, in "Proceedings Second U.N. International Conference on Peaceful Uses of Atomic Energy; Isotopes in Medicine," 1958, vol. 26, p. 103.

91. Dollery, C. T., West, J. B., Goodwin, J. F., Hugh-Jones, P., and Wilckins, D. E. L.: Regional Pulmonary Blood Flow in Mitral and Congenital Heart Disease, in Ciba Foundation Study Group, No. 8, "Problems of Pulmonary Circulation," Little, Brown and Company, Boston, 1961, p. 17.

92. Rudolph, A. M., Nadas, A. S., and Borges, W. H.: Hematologic Adjustments to Cyanotic Congenital Heart Disease, *Pediatrics*, **11**:454, 1953.

93. Willi, H., and Gasser, C.: The Clinical Diagnosis of the Triad Spleen Agenesis, Defects of the Heart and Vessels and Situs Inversus, *Études néonatales*, **4**:25, 1955.

94. Bush, J. A., and Dinger, L. E.: Congenital Absence of the Spleen with Congenital Heart Disease: Report of a Case with Antemortem Diagnosis on the Basis of Hematologic Morphology, *Pediatrics*, **15**:93, 1955.

95. Hartmann, R. C.: A Hemorrhagic Disorder Occurring in Patients with Cyanotic Congenital Heart Disease, *Bull. Johns Hopkins Hosp.*, **91**:49, 1952.

96. Goldberg, J., and Shaffer, J. G.: Serology and Bacteriology, in A. A. Luisada (ed.), "Cardiology: An Encyclopedia of the Cardiovascular System," McGraw-Hill Book Company, New York, 1959, vol. 2, pp. 4–286.

97. Sherlock, S.: "Diseases of the Liver and Bilary System," Charles C Thomas, Publisher, Springfield, Ill., 1955, p. 401.

98. Richman, S. M., Delman, A. J., and Grob, D.: Alteration in Indices of Liver Function in Congestive Heart Failure, with Particular Reference to Serum Enzymes, *Am. J. Med.*, **30**:211, 1961.

99. Logan, R. G., Mowry, F. M., and Judge, R. D.: Cardiac Failure Simulating Viral Hepatitis: Three Cases with Serum Transaminase Levels above 1000, *Ann. Int. Med.*, **56**:784, 1962.

100. Laragh, J. H., and Bradley, S. E.: Diuretic Therapy in Cardiac Failure, *Mod. Concepts Cardiovas. Dis.*, **39**:619, 1960.

101. Conn, J. W.: Aldosteronism in Man: Some Clinical and Climatological Aspects, *J.A.M.A.*, **183**:871, 1963.

102. Goldman, R.: Studies in Diurnal Variation of Water and Electrolyte Excretion: Nocturnal Diuresis of Water and Sodium in Congestive Cardiac Failure and Cirrhosis of the Liver, *J. Clin. Invest.*, **29**:187, 1950.

103. Race, G. A., Scheifley, C. H., and Edwards, J. E.: Albuminuria in Congestive Heart Failure, *Circulation*, **13**:329, 1956.

104. Sternheimer, R.: Urinalysis in Cardiovascular Disease, in A. A. Luisada (ed.), "Cardiology: An Encyclopedia of the Cardiovascular System," McGraw-Hill Book Company, New York, 1959, vol. 2 (suppl.), p. 442.

105. Schreiner, G. E.: Some Observations on Telescoped Urinary Sediments, *Ann. Int. Med.*, **42**:826, 1955.

106. Sjoerdsma, A., Weissbach, H., and Udenfriend, S.: A Simple Test for Diagnosis of Metastatic Carcinoid (Argentaffinoma), *J.A.M.A.*, **159**:397, 1955.

SUGGESTED READING

Bramwell, C.: The Arterial Pulse in Health and Disease, *Lancet*, **2**:239, 301, 366, 1937.

Braunwald, E., Fishman, A. P., and Cournand, A.: Time Relationship of Dynamic Events in the Cardiac Chambers, Pulmonary Artery and Aorta in Man, *Circulation Res.*, **4**:100, 1956.

Comroe, J. H., Forster, R. E., Dubois, A. B., Briscoe, W. A., and Carlsen, E.: "The Lung: Clinical Physiology and Pulmonary Function Tests," The Year Book Medical Publishers, Inc., Chicago, 1962.

Fowler, N. O.: "Physical Diagnosis of Heart Disease," The Macmillan Company, New York, 1962.

"Handbook of Physiology," sec. 2, "Circulation," vols. 1, 2, section editor, W. F. Hamilton, American Physiological Society, Washington, D. C., 1962–1963.

Keith, J. D., Rowe, R. D., and Vlad, P.: "Heart Disease in Infancy and Childhood," The MacMillan Company, New York, 1958.

"Medical Electronics in Cardiovascular Disease," C. K. Friedberg and E. Donoso, (eds.), Grune & Stratton, Inc., New York, 1963.

Page, L. B., and Culver, P. J.: "A Syllabus of Laboratory Examinations in Clinical Diagnosis," Harvard University Press, Cambridge, Mass., 1960.

Proceedings of the Staff Meetings of the Mayo Clinic: 1. Symposium on Diagnostic Applications of Indicator Dilution Techniques, **32:**463–551, 1957. 2. Symposium on Diagnostic Applications of Indicator Dilution Curves Recorded from the Right and Left Sides of the Heart, **33:**535–609, 1958. 3. Symposium on Indocyanine Green and Its Clinical Applications, **35:**729–744, 1960.

Relman, A. S., and Levinsky, N. G.: Clinical Examination of Renal Function, in M. B. Strauss and L. G. Welt, (eds.), "Diseases of the kidney," Little, Brown and Company, Boston, 1963.

Symposium on Use of Indicator-dilution Technique in the Study of the Circulation, *Circulation Res.* **10,** no. 3, part 2, 1962.

Wood, E. H., Sutterer, W. F., and Cronin, L.: "Oximetry in Glasser, Otto: Medical Physics," The Year Book Medical Publishers, Inc., Chicago, 1960, vol. 3, p. 416.

Ziegler, R. F.: Clinical Cardiac Catheterization in Infants and Children, *Pediat. Clin. North America,* **1:**93, 1954.

Zimmerman, H. A. (ed.): "Intra-vascular catheterization." Charles C Thomas, Publisher, Springfield, Ill., 1959.

Section A: Heart Failure

11 ALTERED PHYSIOLOGY OF THE CARDIOVASCULAR SYSTEM IN HEART FAILURE

Robert C. Schlant, M.D.

INTRODUCTION

One of the more important current problems is communication between individuals, and one of the major factors in this problem is a lack of agreement on definitions of terms. Fortunately, in clinical medicine, there is an increasing appreciation of the need for precise physiologic definitions. Nevertheless, at times there is still a considerable difference between the physiologic and clinical uses of similar terms. This situation is particularly common in considerations of patients with "heart failure." The following definitions and classification are presented with the realization that future research will allow a much more precise analysis and classification of different types of heart failure based on differences in their molecular biology.

Circulatory failure refers to an inadequacy of the cardiovascular system in performing its basic function of providing nutrition to the tissue cells and removing metabolic products from the cells. It may be caused primarily by either cardiac or peripheral (noncardiac) conditions.

The term *heart failure* or *cardiac failure* refers to the condition in which the heart is no longer able to pump an adequate supply of blood in relation to the venous return and in relation to the metabolic needs of the tissues of the body at that particular moment. The actual amount of blood pumped by the heart per minute (the cardiac output) may be normal, increased, or decreased. In most patients with heart failure, the cardiac output is decreased. Even in patients in whom the cardiac output is elevated or normal, *heart failure* is present if there is a discrepancy between the *needs* of the body and the *supply* of blood pumped by the heart. These patients with high-output failure[1,2] have a cardiac output which may be normal or higher than normal but which is lower than the metabolic needs of the body at that particular time. The expression *high-output failure* should not be used to refer to conditions associated with an elevated cardiac output,

including circulatory congestion or overloading (see below), unless there is evidence that the heart is failing to pump an adequate amount of blood to meet the metabolic needs of the body in relation to the venous return of the heart.[3]

The expression *congestive heart failure* refers to that state in which abnormal circulatory congestion exists as a result of heart failure. When this is present for any length of time, there is usually increased transudation of fluid from the capillaries into the interstitial spaces. In the pulmonary circulation, if the rate of transudation exceeds the rate of lymphatic drainage, there may initially be only interstitial edema on x-ray examination and only later may audible rales be detected on physical examination. In the systemic venous system, the venous congestion itself may be visible and may result in the development of peripheral edema or of hepatomegaly. In most instances, congestive heart failure develops chronically and is associated with the retention of sodium and water by the kidneys. It may also develop acutely following a myocardial infarction of the left ventricle. In this situation there may be an acute shift of blood from the systemic circulation to the pulmonary circulation before sodium or water retention occurs. It should be emphasized that the term *congestive heart failure* should not be used unless the congestion is of cardiac origin. When the cause of the congestion is not clear, it is preferable to describe the symptoms or signs, which are nonspecific, and to avoid improperly diagnosing of heart failure.

In patients in whom there is evidence that the pumping ability of the left side of the heart is primarily impaired, the failure is said to be *left-sided failure;* conversely, if the pumping ability of the right side of the heart is primarily impaired, the failure is said to be *right-sided*. Since both sides of the heart are in a circuit, it is apparent that one side cannot pump significantly more blood than the other for any length of time in the absence of abnormal shunts or communications. Accordingly, even though the pumping ability of one side may be primarily impaired, the output of the other side is secondarily decreased. In either left-sided or right-sided failure, the cardiac output may be decreased, normal, or increased. In most situations, left-sided failure is evidenced by symptoms and signs of elevated pressure and congestion in the pulmonary veins and capillaries, whereas right-sided failure is apparent from signs and symptoms of elevated pressures and congestion in the systemic veins and capillaries. Although reasonably pure forms of left-sided and right-sided failure occur, it should be emphasized that the most common cause of right-sided failure is left-sided failure and that often both ventricles fail nearly simultaneously.

Heart failure is said to be *latent* when it is not apparent at rest but is apparent only under certain circumstances, such as exercise, fever, or emotion. Failure may be *compensated* as a result of normal compensatory mechanisms [i.e., increased sympathetic adrenergic stimulation of the heart, fluid retention, hypertrophy, etc. (see below)] or by the improvement of myocardial function by the administration of digitalis glycosides or by diuresis if the fluid retention is excessive.

Heart failure may be caused by *atrial failure*, by *ventricular failure*, or by both. Heart (atrial or ventricular) failure may be classified (see the classification below) into three main categories: (1) myocardial (muscular) failure, (2) failure related to mechanical abnormalities, and (3) failure related to cardiac arrhythmias. It should be emphasized that patients may have heart failure from more than one of the causes listed in this classification and also that the causes of failure in a given patient may change during the course of his disease.

CLASSIFICATION OF CIRCULATORY FAILURE AND CIRCULATORY OVERLOAD

I. Circulatory failure
  A. Heart (cardiac) failure
    1. Myocardial (muscular) failure
      a. Primary
        (1) Primary diseases of muscle
        (2) Metabolic
        (3) Inadequate muscle mass
      b. Secondary
        (1) Dysdynamic (physicochemical) failure
        (2) Metabolic
        (3) Inflammatory
    2. Mechanical abnormalities
      a. Increased resistance to forward blood flow (pressure load)
      b. Valvular regurgitation; shunts (volume or flow load)
      c. Pericardial tamponade, constriction
      d. Endocardial or myocardial restriction
      e. Ventricular aneurysm
    3. Arrhythmia
      a. Standstill
      b. Fibrillation
      c. Extreme tachycardia or bradycardia

  B. Peripheral (noncardiac) failure
    1. Decreased return of blood to heart
    2. Increased capacity of vascular bed
    3. Peripheral vascular abnormalities or disease
II. Circulatory overload
  A. Increase in blood volume
  B. Increase in venous return and/or decrease in peripheral vascular resistance

The expression *myocardial failure* is used to refer to heart failure primarily produced by an inadequacy of the myocardial contractile or muscular mechanisms. Myocardial failure is said to be "primary" when it is caused by (1) primary disease of muscle, such as muscular dystrophy, (2) metabolic deficiencies of the myocardium, such as hyperthyroidism, hypothyroidism, or beriberi, or (3) inadequate quantity of myocardium, such as might result from myocardial infarction, hypoplasia, or replacement by fibrosis, tumor, or other masses. Myocardial failure is said to be "secondary" when it is caused by (1) largely unknown physicochemical factors producing *dysdynamic* (impaired force or power) *myocardial failure*. (This is the most common form of myocardial failure and is frequent in hypertension, aortic valve disease, and mitral regurgitation. The term implies that there has been a change in the contractility of the myocardium, with the result that the muscle no longer responds with an adequate contraction in response to the amount of end-diastolic stretch of the fibers. This type of myocardial failure undoubtedly is produced by different mechanisms in different patients and diseases. Some of the factors currently thought to be important are discussed below.); (2) metabolic factors such as ischemia, chronic shock, or depression by drugs or toxins; or (3) myocardial inflammation.

Heart failure, i.e., an inability of the heart to pump an adequate amount of blood to the body relative to the needs of the body, may be produced by *mechanical abnormalities* without physiologic "failure" of the myocardium, although secondary dysdynamic myocardial failure may eventually develop. As with other forms of heart failure, either the right or the left side of the heart may be primarily involved and the primary burden may be on either the atria or the ventricle. At times more than one chamber is involved. The more common mechanical causes of heart failure are (1) increased resistance to the ejection of blood from a cardiac chamber (obstruction at the arteriolar, arterial, supravalvular, valvular, or subvalvular level), (2) organic or "functional" valvular regurgitation, or abnormal shunting of blood between cardiac chambers and/or great vessels, (3) pericardial tamponade or constriction, (4) endocardial or myocardial restriction, and (5) ventricular aneurysm.

Heart failure may also be caused by *cardiac arrhythmias,* such as standstill, fibrillation, or extreme tachycardia or bradycardia. In most instances *atrial failure* which is caused by an arrhythmia does not by itself produce significant heart failure unless there is an additional, usually ventricular, cause of heart failure.

Peripheral (noncardiac) circulatory failure may be caused by (1) decreased return of blood to the heart (as by obstruction to venous return or by decreased blood volume secondary to hemorrhage, dehydration, altered capillary permeability, etc.); (2) increased capacity or decreased "tone" of the peripheral vascular bed; or (3) peripheral vascular abnormalities or disease.

Circulatory overload or *congestion* may have noncardiac causes, although secondary heart failure may eventually occur in many of these conditions. Circulatory overload may be divided into two categories: (1) those conditions in which the primary defect appears to be an increase in blood volume (the accumulation of excess amounts of salt and water due to salt-retaining steroids, excess blood or fluid administration, acute glomerulonephritis, oliguria, or anuria); and (2) those conditions in which the primary defect appears to be an increased venous return and/or decreased peripheral resistance (arteriovenous fistula, beriberi, possibly cirrhosis or severe anemia, etc.). In many of these conditions, the cardiac output is elevated; however, the term *heart failure* should not be applied so long as the output is adequate to meet the demands of the body. When *secondary heart failure* does develop, the absolute level of cardiac output may remain elevated (so-called "high-output failure" [1,2]) or may decrease to normal or low levels. Generally digitalis glycosides produce little or no change in hemodynamics in patients with noncardiac circulatory overload or congestion unless there is secondary myocardial failure (usually "dysdynamic") or arrhythmia. Eichna[3] has emphasized the differences between myocardial failure and noncardiac circulatory congestion. He used the latter term in referring to three types of congestion: (1) mechanical obstruction in or about the heart (mitral or tricuspid stenosis, pericardial tamponade); (2) circulatory overloading due to the accumulation of excessive amounts of salt and water (salt-retaining steroids, anuria, oliguria, acute glomerulonephritis); and (3) circulatory congestion in the hyperkinetic or high-output circulatory states (arteriovenous fistula, beriberi, severe anemia, etc.). In the classification of heart failure presented in this chapter, conditions producing congestion secondary to mechanical obstruction have been included under "heart failure" (rather than under "noncardiac circulatory congestion"), since in most instances there is some decrease in cardiac output occurs by the time the obstruction produces significant congestion.

The expressions *forward failure* and *backward failure* have been used at times with somewhat different meanings. In oversimplified terms, "forward failure" has been used to imply that most of the patient's symptoms resulted from a low cardiac output with resultant easy fatigability, weakness, or even shock, whereas "backward failure" has been used to imply that most of the patients' symptoms resulted from elevation of venous pressure behind the failing ventricle. This elevation of venous pressure was usually thought to be caused by obstruction to ventricular filling (mitral or tricuspid stenosis) or by the inability of the ventricle to empty itself properly. The two expressions have also been used in reference to concepts of the pathogenesis of the retention of salt and water. Thus, according to some, in "forward failure," the decreased cardiac output at one time was postulated to produce tissue edema by an increase in capillary permeability secondary to tissue hypoxia. Later, when this theory became untenable, it was postulated that the decreased cardiac output altered renal plasma flow and glomerular filtration, thereby contributing to the retention of salt and water and producing a secondary increase in blood volume, elevation of venous pressure, and edema formation. It was further postulated that in backward failure most of the patient's symptoms and signs of congestion resulted from an elevation of venous pressure upstream from the ventricle. The cardiac output might be reduced or might be returned to normal by the increased venous pressure behind the ventricle and the resultant increase in diastolic filling of the ventricle. When right ventricular failure developed, systemic venous and capillary pressures became elevated and edema developed, producing a decrease in effective circulating blood volume. An increase in tubular reabsorption of salt and water was thought to occur as a result of renal vasoconstriction secondary to the change in effective blood volume or as a result of an elevation of renal venous pressure. More recent studies have demonstrated that both the forward-failure and the backward-failure theories were usually oversimplifications of the pathogenesis of salt and water retention and edema formation in heart failure (see Chap. 12, p. 239). Accordingly, even though the expressions are no longer completely applicable in this regard, they may still be useful to describe the clinical symptoms. Thus, when the symptoms are predominantly related to venous congestion, backward failure, which is usually, but not always, chronic, may be said to exist. If the symptoms are predominantly related to a marked decrease in cardiac output, forward cardiac failure, which is usually acute, may be said to exist.

Since the basic fundamental of heart failure is an inability of the heart to supply the demands of the body, it is apparent that the term is applicable whenever the demands are not met as a result of cardiac limitations. This implies that any heart would eventually fail if the demands were increased sufficiently. This may in fact occur during very extreme exertion in subjects with apparently normal hearts. In most individuals, however, the exercise is probably stopped prior to heart failure by the subjective sensation of fatigue and by the limitations of the respiratory system. In some elderly individuals there may be involutional changes of the myocardium, which are usually associated with decreased elasticity of the skeleton of the heart and with mild fibrotic changes of the valves. The chemical basis of these aging changes and of the associated pigmentation of the heart is not known. This condition, known as *presbycardia*, or *senile heart disease*,[4-6] probably only rarely produces heart failure by itself; however, it does decrease the adaptive capacity or reserves of the heart. Accordingly, patients with this condition more readily develop heart failure in the presence of other forms of heart disease or, occasionally, even from the increased demands of fever, moderate anemia, mild hyperthyroidism, excess fluid administration, etc.

Dysdynamic (i.e., with impaired force or power) *myocardial failure* is the most common type of secondary myocardial failure. In most instances there is an apparent form of heart disease (hypertension, coronary artery disease, valvular heart disease, etc.) which has either increased the work load on the ventricle or impaired blood flow to the myocardium. The exact physicochemical changes responsible for dysdynamic myocardial failure are uncertain. The important factor of chamber dilatation and its effects on ventricular function are discussed below, as are some of the other physicochemical changes which may contribute to "myocardial" failure. Although dysdynamic myocardial failure may involve either atria or ventricles, the discussion below is mainly concerned with the more common type of myocardial failure involving the ventricles, particularly the left ventricle.

Atrial failure refers to the condition in which the atrium fails to provide adequate filling and distension of the ventricle in relation to the venous return to the atrium. In most instances atrial failure results from failure of the atrial *pumping* mechanism, although rarely the *reservoir* function of the atrium may also be involved. The studies of Sarnoff and Mitchell[7-9] have emphasized the important role of the atria, particularly when the usual cardiac reserve and compensatory mechanisms are limited by heart disease. Atrial failure may be due to most of the causes of heart failure presented in the classification above. The more common forms of atrial failure are "dysdynamic" failure of the atrial myocardium, which is usually secondary to ventricular failure; atrial failure due to mechanical abnormalities (e.g., mitral or tricuspid valvular disease); and atrial failure produced by arrhythmia (e.g., atrial fibrillation). The detrimental effects of atrial fibrillation or flutter on hemodynamics have been documented by numerous clinical studies.[10-18] Atrial failure due to arrhythmia may be seen in patients with compensated heart disease who develop congestive heart failure with the onset of atrial fibrillation or flutter. In these patients the restoration of normal sinus rhythm often results in a marked improvement in their hemodynamics. This worsening of congestive failure by atrial fibrillation may occur even when the ventricular response rate is controlled by digitalis. Presumably, it is caused by the loss of the normal "booster-pump" function of the atrium.

MECHANISMS OF DYSDYNAMIC MYOCARDIAL FAILURE

The precise anatomic, biochemical, and physiologic changes responsible for dysdynamic "failure" of the myocardium are not known. It is particularly difficult to tell whether some of the changes which have been described are primary *causes* of the "failure" or whether they are merely secondary *consequences* of failure. It is probable that dysdynamic myocardial failure results from different combinations of mechanisms in different conditions.

The available evidence indicates that in the usual secondary dysdynamic myocardial failure there is no defect in the liberation or conservation of energy by the myocardium. Instead there is a failure of energy utilization, i.e., the *conversion* of this readily available chemical energy into effective physical work.[19-25] This is in contrast to thyroid heart disease (Chap. 54), beriberi, or thiamine deficiency (Chap. 61), and acute hypoxia, in which there is evidence of defective liberation or conservation of energy by the myocardium. In heart failure, evidence has been reported of osmiophilic degeneration of sarcosomes;[26] a decrease in ATPase activity;[27] an uncoupling of oxidative phosphorylation in mitochondria;[28] a decrease in myocardial norepinephrine;[29] a decreased contractility of actomyosin bands;[30] and abnormal polymerization of myosin.[31] Buckley and Tsuboi[32] found no difference between the nucleotides and nucleosides of failing and nonfailing hearts. Nebel and Bing[33] have reviewed the differences in contractile proteins of normal and failing human hearts.

The studies of Huxley and Peachey[34] and of Sonnenblick, Spotnitz, and Spiro[34] suggest that physical "overstretch" of the sarcomeral units may be an important defect in ventricular myocardial failure. Against this appealing theory are the observations of Linzbach,[35] who was unable to demonstrate significant increase in the distance between the Z bands of the myocardial fibers of patients with heart failure. He emphasized the detrimental rearrangements of the surviving muscle fibers found in hearts with eccentric dilatation and hypertrophy. He referred to the regional irreversible "overstretch" as *irreversible plastic dilatation*. Linzbach pointed out that a dilated, hypertrophied ventricle has the normal adult ratio of one capillary to one myocardial fiber. He concluded that the limitation of coronary flow in ventricular hypertrophy was caused by the limited size of the coronary ostiums and an inadequate growth of the coronary arteries and that the essence of myocardial failure was the discrepancy between the amount of energy available and the increased amount of energy necessary to expel a stroke volume from a ventricle with structural dilatation. The areas of focal necrosis and scarring frequently found in hypertrophied hearts were accepted by Linzbach as evidence of myocardial hypoxia.

HEMODYNAMIC CHARACTERISTICS OF DYSDYNAMIC MYOCARDIAL FAILURE OF THE VENTRICLE

In ventricular myocardial failure the ventricle fails to contract with a sufficient force to eject a stroke volume appropriate for the filling load upon the ventricle. It is perhaps best described in terms of the normalcy of the ventricular function curve (ventricular work vs. ventricular end-diastolic fiber length). Although there were some early investigations of the law of the heart related the performance of ventricular muscle to end-diastolic pressure or volume, subsequent investigations indicated that end-diastolic fiber length is a more significant determinant of contractility. It is possible, however, that the main determinant of ventricular function is the end-diastolic tension *within the muscle fibers*, rather than end-diastolic fiber length or end-diastolic pressure within the ventricular cavity. These variables are usually, but not always, related to each other. Since pressure is the easiest of the variables to measure, it is most commonly measured in clinical studies. In most patients with ventricular myocardial failure there is an abnormal

elevation of both end-diastolic pressure and end-diastolic volume in relation to the force of contraction and the stroke volume achieved by the ventricle. On the other hand, patients are occasionally encountered who have pulmonary congestion secondary to elevations of the left ventricular mean diastolic and end-diastolic pressures, but in whom the amount of *total* work the ventricle performs at rest and exercise may be normal or even supernormal. If the ventricular function curve (relating end-diastolic fiber length to total ventricular work) in these patients is normal, ventricular "failure" is physiologically not present, despite the presence of pulmonary congestion. This is especially likely to occur in patients with concentric ventricular hypertrophy secondary to aortic stenosis or hypertension. In these patients some of the elevation of ventricular diastolic pressure may at times be related to an increased *impedance*, or resistance to filling, of the thick, hypertrophied ventricle. Conversely, occasional patients with ventricular failure may have marked ventricular dilatation, decreased rate and force of contraction, and decreased stroke volume but normal end-diastolic ventricular pressures at rest. The possible errors in equating an elevation of ventricular end-diastolic pressure with *ventricular failure* have been discussed by Braunwald and Ross.[36]

The failing ventricle, which is operating on a decreased ventricular function curve, is characterized by a decreased force of contraction and a decreased accomplishment of work for a given amount of diastolic load. In most situations there is an inadequate systolic emptying of the ventricle and an increased end-systolic volume, which reflects the basic inability of the heart to empty itself. There is also a decrease in net, or effective, stroke volume relative to the needs of the body and relative to the elevations of end-diastolic ventricular pressure and volume and in end-diastolic myocardial fiber length and tension. The *total* volume of stroke output is usually decreased but may be normal or even elevated, particularly with valvular regurgitation. Atrial pressure is elevated secondary to the changes in ventricular diastolic pressure and to changes in the pressure-volume characteristics or impedance of the ventricle during diastolic filling. Buckley and Zeig[37] found relatively irreversible changes in the resistance, or *impedance*, to diastolic filling in experimental ventricular failure.

The decreased myocardial contractility in ventricular failure is evidenced by a *slower rate of rise of pressure* within the ventricle during contraction and a slower rate of decrease in pressure during ventricular relaxation. The mean rate of left ventricular ejection is also usually decreased in congestive heart failure.[38,39] The decreased rate of myocardial fiber shortening and ejection is in part secondary to the greater tension or force required by the myocardial fibers to develop and maintain pressure within, and to eject blood from, a dilated ventricle;[39–47] (see below, "Effects of Dilatation on Ventricular Function.") The peak systolic pressure within the failing ventricle is often somewhat lower than it would be if the failure were not present, but it is usually within normal limits until the failure is extremely severe. *Pulsus alternans* may be present in ventricular failure, particularly if the failure is caused by aortic stenosis. It is probably caused by alternation of the end-diastolic length of the myocardial fibers.[48,49] Mitral or tricuspid regurgitation frequently develops secondary to marked ventricular dilatation and may further increase the volume load on a failing ventricle.[50] The atrial pressure tracing may have a large regurgitant or *v* wave if functional regurgitation across the AV valve is produced by ventricular dilatation.[51] This type of "functional" regurgitation across an AV valve is predominantly the result of inability of the papillary muscles and chordae tendinae to anchor the valve leaflets properly, whereas actual dilatation of the AV valve ring is less important. The pressures in the left atrium, pulmonary artery, and right ventricle may become elevated secondary to left ventricular failure. This may eventually result in right ventricular failure.

In response to exercise, patients with dysdynamic ventricular myocardial failure, as in many other forms of heart failure, have an exaggeration of their hemodynamic abnormalities. In most instances of ventricular myocardial failure, the cardiac output fails to increase normally and may even decrease despite an elevation of end-diastolic pressure. If the failure is severe, exercise may be associated with a further *increase* in both end-diastolic and end-systolic volumes of the ventricle. This response contrasts with the decrease in these volumes found in normal persons during exercise. The *rate of increase of pressure in the ventricle* and the mean rate of ventricular ejection,[38,39] which are indices of the rate of myocardial fiber shortening and of myocardial contractility, fail to increase during exercise in patients with ventricular failure as they do in normal subjects. In normal individuals the stroke volume during exercise may or may not increase (see Chap. 2), although it often does increase about 10 to 20 per cent during moderate exertion in young persons and even more in athletes. In dysdynamic myocardial failure, the stroke volume often *decreases* during exertion. In some patients this is caused by an increase in the "functional" mitral or tricuspid regurgitation.[50,51]

CARDIOVASCULAR RESERVE MECHANISMS IN HEART FAILURE

The adjustments of the body to heart failure may be divided into acute, subacute, and chronic, depending on how long it takes the adjustment to become effective. Most of the acute and subacute reserve mechanisms persist in the chronic stage unless the failure becomes compensated by the chronic adjustments.

Acute Adjustments

The acute adjustments to heart failure are similar to the homeostatic mechanisms utilized by the body in response to circulatory failure from any cause, whether acute blood loss or acute myocardial infarction. Many of these mechanisms and reflex pathways are the same as the normal cardiac *reserve mechanisms* utilized by normal subjects during exercise or during periods of increased stress. In human beings, it is usually impossible to separate the different mechanisms of adjustment to acute heart failure. This separation is particularly difficult since each mechanism of adjustment affects and modifies the others.

The most important acute adjustment is a reflex increase in autonomic *sympathetic* excitation to most of the arteries and veins of the body and to the heart. This is associated with an inhibition of cardiac *parasympathetic* activity. The increased sympathetic ("adrenergic") stimulation of the peripheral arteries contributes to the maintenance of arterial pressure despite a decrease in stroke volume. As a result of the vasomotor regulation of peripheral arteries and arterioles, blood flow to the more essential organs—brain and heart—is maintained at the expense of blood flow to other areas, such as skin, kidneys, splanchnic organs, and skeletal muscles. The sympathetic stimulation of the veins contributes to the increase in venous tone present in congestive heart failure.[52–54] This increase in venous tone increases venous pressure above what it would otherwise be even though the pressure may be within normal limits. This "increased" venous pressure helps to maintain venous return, ventricular filling, and diastolic stretch of the ventricular fibers. The increased sympathetic and decreased parasympathetic impulses to the heart usually increase the heart rate and increase myocardial contractility. Occasionally, patients with untreated, severe congestive failure do not have a significant increase in pulse rate; the explanation for this is unknown. As a result of increased myocardial contractility from sympathetic stimulation, the myocardium contracts more forcefully and more rapidly than it otherwise would for the same diastolic load or end-diastolic myocardial fiber tension, fiber length, or pressure. The associated increased rate of ventricular relaxation following contraction contributes to increased ventricular filling. The increased contractility produced by sympathetic myocardial stimulation is reflected in a "shift to the left" of the atrial and ventricular function curves. The increased sympathetic activity may also result in the release of epinephrine or norepinephrine from the adrenal medulla. These compounds further enhance myocardial contractility.

Chidsey, Harrison, and Braunwald [55] have shown that patients in congestive failure have a greater than normal release of norepinephrine into the coronary sinus blood during exercise. Chidsey et al.[29] reported that the myocardial concentration of norepinephrine was lower in patients with chronic congestive heart failure than in subjects without heart failure. The low levels in congestive failure were often similar to the low levels produced by reserpine. Gaffney and Braunwald [56] have emphasized the importance of the sympathetic adrenergic system in helping to maintain ventricular function in congestive heart failure and have pointed out that congestive heart failure is occasionally made worse by drugs, such as reserpine or guanethidine, which interfere with the myocardial sympathetic-adrenergic system. Braunwald et al.[57] have subsequently postulated a possible role of the heart as an endocrine organ, capable of releasing significant quantities of norepinephrine.

The reflex mechanisms initiating the autonomic sympathetic activity in acute heart failure are extremely complex and they require some discussion here. Reflexogenic areas have been described in most of the chambers of the heart and great vessels, in addition to the brain and brain stem. The relative importance of the various reflex areas in acute ventricular failure in the human being is uncertain. The stretch receptors in the carotid sinus and aorta seem to be of major importance. It should be noted that the activity of the carotid sinus stretch receptors is affected not only by the pressure within the sinus but also by the rate of change of the pressure and by the "tone" of the wall of the carotid sinus. The carotid sinus may also be of major importance in the regulation of renal hemodynamics and the retention of salt and water during ventricular failure.[58,59]

The law of the heart is an additional mechanism brought into play following acute heart failure. If the ventricle fails to eject a normal quantity of blood during one beat, the blood entering the ventricle during the subsequent diastole usually produces ventricular dilatation with a greater ventricular end-diastolic volume, pressure, fiber

length, and tension within the myocardial fibers. Unless the ventricle is operating on the "descending limb" of its function curve, these changes will result in a greater amount of work and a greater stroke volume with the subsequent ventricular contraction.

In response to acute heart failure and a decrease in stroke volume, the available blood flow is redistributed by the integrative autonomic response mentioned above and by local regulatory mechanisms. In addition, the tissues of the body which receive less blood than required may utilize anaerobic metabolism[60,61] and/or may extract more oxygen from each unit of blood reaching the tissues. This "venous oxygen reserve" is potentially less useful to the myocardium, which even normally extracts about 70 to 75 per cent of the oxygen coming to it.[62,63]

Subacute Adjustments

The subacute adjustments to acute heart failure are principally those mechanisms which cause the retention of salt and water by the kidneys. Renal retention of salt and/or water may result from increased tubular reabsorption in association with decreased renal blood flow and decreased glomerular filtration. At times other mechanisms may also be important: increased renal venous pressure, sympathetic impulses to the kidney or the release of hormones (aldosterone, antidiuretic hormone) from other organs (see Chap. 12). Largely as a result of excess salt and water retention by the kidney, blood volume is increased in congestive heart failure.[64,65] In general, the mean pressures within the vascular tree are elevated by increases in blood volume and in vasomotor tone caused by sympathetic activity. The increase in venous pressure tends to increase venous return to the heart and to increase ventricular diastolic filling and stretch. The generalized increase in the pressure within the vascular system tends to increase the transudation of fluid out of the capillaries into the interstitial spaces, elevating interstitial pressure. This increase in interstitial pressure may also contribute to an increase in venous pressure and venous return. The localization of edema produced by "excess" fluid and salt retained by the body in its interstitial spaces is largely dependent on hydrostatic factors such as the position of the patient.

In some patients with congestive heart failure due to ventricular failure from various causes, Rader et al.[66] have demonstrated that diuresis produced by the administration of mercurial diuretics in the absence of digitalis may result in the relief of subjective symptoms and removal of the characteristic signs of circulatory congestion. In a significant number of the patients, they found an improvement towards normal in cardiac output and arteriovenous oxygen difference associated with a reduction in the elevated intracardiac pressures. The results in these patients suggested that the reduction in intracardiac pressures produced by diuresis allowed a "reascent along the descending limb of the pressure-output curve with resultant increase in cardiac output as the diastolic intracardiac pressures fall." (See below, "Effects of Dilatation on Ventricular Function.") These studies also demonstrate that the "compensatory mechanisms" of the body may "overcompensate," to the detriment of the organism.

Chronic Adjustment

The principal chronic hemodynamic adjustment to heart failure is hypertrophy of the ventricular myocardium. The stimulus is presumably a chronic increase in the systolic force or tension developed by the myocardial fibers. According to Linzbach,[35] there may also be an absolute increase in the *number* of muscle fibers, nuclei, and capillaries, in addition to hypertrophy of the individual muscle fibers. He postulated that the increase in number of muscle fibers was the result of longitudinal cleavage between points of anastomosis of the myocardial syncytium.

In an individual patient, compensation may be achieved by acute, subacute, and/or chronic adjustments. If a ventricle becomes fully compensated by hypertrophy, the acute and subacute adjustments may no longer be present. This type of compensation may occur spontaneously without therapy with digitalis or diuretics.

Patients with acute myocardial infarction usually have a decreased minute output and stroke output; arterial blood pressure is usually not markedly diminished.[67-71] Occasionally, patients with acute myocardial infarction fail to have the usual increase in systemic arteriolar resistance. In these patients, the arterial hypotension is related to the lack of peripheral arteriolar vasoconstriction, in addition to the obvious loss of pumping ability by the left ventricle.

EFFECTS OF DILATATION ON VENTRICULAR FUNCTION

The effects of ventricular dilatation on the mechanics and energetics (and ultimately the physicochemical reactions) of myocardial contraction are very important factors contributing to *ventricular failure*. Burch,[41] Burton,[42] and Gorlin,[44] in particular, have emphasized the importance of dilatation in the mechanics of ventricular contraction.

On first thought it would seem that ventricular dilatation is advantageous. With a greater end-diastolic ventricular volume and fiber length, each ventricular fiber would have to shorten less to eject a given volume of blood and each fiber would be able to perform more work by virtue of the law of the heart. In many situations, however, these seeming advantages are negated by several hemodynamic consequences of dilatation. The more important of these is the need for the myocardial fibers in the wall of a dilated ventricle to develop a greater *contractile tension* in order to produce a given *pressure* within the ventricle. Ventricular myocardial tension has been calculated by employing the law of Laplace, which applies to a distensible membrane which has a spherical or cylindrical shape, and by assuming that the ventricle has a spherical cavity. Figure 11-1 illustrates three definitions of contractile tension in the ventricular myocardium as used by different authors. Badeer[72] has recently recommended that calculations of myocardial tension be expressed in terms of force per unit of cross-section area (formula shown on right of Fig. 11-1). By all three formulas, however, it is apparent that as the radius increases, more tension must be developed by each fiber to produce or maintain a given intraventricular pressure. This basic relationship expressed by the law of Laplace gives the dilated ventricle an additional disadvantage during ejection. The tangential wall tension or force is constantly changing during ejection as a result of the change in average radius of the ventricular cavity. In a normal ventricle during ejection the change in average radius of the ventricle is relatively large. During ejection the effect of the decrease in radius on wall tension is normally greater than the effect of the increasing pressure in the ventricle. As a result, the myocardial fiber tension or force may actually *decrease* soon after the beginning of ejection and is usually less at the moment of peak systolic pressure than at the beginning of ejection. On the other hand, if the ventricle is significantly dilated, the relative and absolute decrease in average radius will be less during the ejection of an equal volume. In a markedly dilated ventricle during the ejection of blood and the continued increase in ventricular pressure, the average tension in the myocardial fibers continues to increase up to the peak systolic pressure. In a sense, this is a type of "afterload" encountered by the dilated ventricle during ejection. A further disadvantage of dilatation is that the increased force, or tension, in the myocardial fibers required to develop a given pressure inside a dilated ventricle results in a decrease in the *rate* of myocardial fiber shortening.[40,43,46,47] The obvious effect of this is to decrease the ability of the ventricle to eject blood.

The oxygen requirement of a dilated ventricle is increased since myocardial oxygen requirement

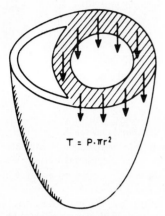

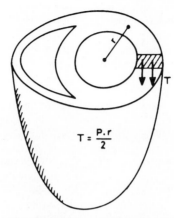

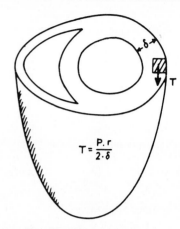

T = Force across the total cross-sectional area of muscle.

T = Force per unit length of circumference and the entire thickness of wall.

T = Force per unit cross-sectional area of muscle.

Fig. 11-1. Three definitions of contractile force in the myocardium and the formulas based on the law of Laplace used to calculate each. Abbreviations: *T*, contractile tangential tension or force in the wall of the ventricle; *P*, transmural pressure across the wall of the ventricle; *r*, average radius of the ventricle assuming it to be spherical; and δ, ventricular wall thickness. (*From H. S. Badeer, Contractile Tension in the Myocardium, Am. Heart J.,* **66**:433, 1963. *Reprinted with the permission of the author and The C. V. Mosby Company.*)

is directly related to total myocardial fiber tension, which is a function of both the intraventricular pressure and the mean radius of the ventricle.[39,44,45,63] Measurements of myocardial oxygen consumption in patients with chronic congestive failure with ventricular dilatation and hypertrophy reveal the oxygen consumption to be normal per 100 Gm of heart.[19,24,25,39,62,73,74] The *total* amount of oxygen consumed by the hypertrophied heart, however, is increased at rest and is much more increased during exercise. Levine and Wagman[45] found that the left ventricle in left ventricular failure consumed an average of 16 per cent of the total amount of oxygen consumed by the body, as compared to 5 per cent in normal subjects. They reported one patient with severe aortic valve disease in whom the left ventricle accounted for 27 per cent of the total amount of oxygen consumed by the body.

In normal subjects the calculated left ventricular mechanical efficiency at rest is about 25 to 35 per cent.[24,39,75] In normal persons the calculated efficiency increases during exercise,[45,62,63] possibly because of the greater *rate* of fiber shortening and/or because of the normal *decrease* in end-diastolic and end-systolic diameters during exercise. Patients with dilated, "failing" ventricles have a basic defect in the ability of their fibers to shorten. During exercise, these patients are often unable to increase their stroke volume significantly despite an *increase* in end-diastolic volume and fiber length. During exercise, patients with severe left ventricular failure may also increase end-systolic volumes and diameters. In these patients, the myocardial

oxygen consumption often increases markedly during exercise. The result of these changes is an inability of the dilated ventricle to increase its calculated mechanical efficiency in a normal fashion during exercise.[39,34,62,63,74]

Most patients with left ventricular failure have a normal volume of coronary blood flow (per 100 Gm of myocardium) at rest despite the elevated myocardial oxygen requirements.[39,63] As a result, there is an elevated extraction of oxygen from each unit of coronary flow and a resultant fall in coronary venous oxygen content and in myocardial oxygen tension. During exercise, many patients with congestive heart failure have an elevated coronary blood flow associated with coronary vasodilatation; however, the exaggerated oxygen requirements of the dilated, failing ventricle usually result in a further lowering of coronary venous oxygen content.[39,63] Some patients with very severe left ventricular failure and low cardiac output (cardiac index below 3 liters per min per m²) have a lower than normal coronary blood flow at rest and consequent marked lowering of the coronary venous oxygen content. In these patients, Messer et al.[63] have suggested that the chronic reduction of cardiac output in congestive heart failure may initiate reflex coronary vasoconstriction which is not completely overridden by the local metabolic factors at rest.

PULMONARY EDEMA

Transudation of fluid out of the pulmonary capillaries occurs when the pressure in the capillaries, which is normally 7 to 12 mm Hg at rest in the supine position, exceeds the plasma oncotic pressure, which is normally 25 to 30 mm Hg.[76-83] Thus, any condition with a sustained increase in pulmonary capillary pressure may produce pulmonary edema if the important rate of lymphatic drainage is exceeded by the rate of capillary transudation. If the serum oncotic pressure is low because of a low concentration of serum proteins, transudation of fluid across the pulmonary capillaries occurs at even lower pressure.[84] There is little evidence that an alteration of pulmonary capillary permeability by anoxia or central nervous system influences is ordinarily an important factor in the production of pulmonary edema. The major factor of importance is an elevation of pulmonary capillary pressure.[78] It should be noted, however, that the pulmonary capillaries have a significant "reserve" compared to systemic capillaries, since the pulmonary capillary pressure can increase about 15 to 20 mm Hg before significant transudation occurs.

An important consideration in the pulmonary circulation is the normal increased hydrostatic pressure in both the arteries and veins in the dependent areas of the lungs. This increased pressure accounts for the initial appearance of pulmonary edema in the lower lobes in many patients with congestive failure. In normal persons in the upright position relatively little pulmonary blood flow goes to the upper areas of the lungs; however, in severe left ventricular failure, as in severe mitral stenosis, the relative blood flow to the upper lobes may equal or even exceed that to the lower lobes.

It is as yet uncertain whether this change in distribution of pulmonary blood flow is caused by local vasoconstriction produced by alveolar hypoxia, by reflexes from the left atrium or pulmonary veins, or by a reactive hypertrophy and increased vascular tone of small arteries secondary to the elevation of pulmonary arterial pressure. Patients with marked elevation of left atrial pressure for long periods of time may often withstand elevations of pulmonary capillary pressure reasonably well, whereas the same level of pulmonary capillary pressure might produce severe fulminating pulmonary edema in 5 to 10 min in a patient whose pulmonary circulation was not accustomed to the high pressure levels. The explanation for this difference may be that patients with chronic transudation of fluid from pulmonary capillaries often develop capacious lymphatic channels which are capable of removing large quantities of fluid from the pulmonary interstitial spaces. The pericapillary thickening associated with chronic pulmonary capillary hypertension may also tend to decrease the rate of fluid transudation. Since pulmonary lymphatic drainage empties into systemic veins, any elevation of central systemic venous pressure tends to decrease pulmonary lymphatic drainage. The importance of pulmonary lymphatic vessels in pulmonary edema has been studied by Uhley et al.[85,86] It is possible that the occurrence of localized pulmonary edema in areas of acute infection or of previous infection[87] may be partially related to alterations in lymphatic drainage. It is also possible that the relative rareness of pulmonary rales in infants with left ventricular failure is in part related to the presence of a pulmonary lymphatic system unscarred by respiratory tract infection. Vasoconstriction of the pulmonary *veins* may be an important factor in the pulmonary edema produced by certain endotoxins.[88] The pulmonary edema of high altitude is apparently associated with marked pulmonary artery hypertension and pulmonary arteriolar vasoconstriction but normal pulmonary artery wedge ("pulmonary capillary") pressure.[89] The mechanism of pulmonary edema in this syndrome is uncertain.

PULMONARY FUNCTION IN CONGESTIVE HEART FAILURE

As a result of pulmonary congestion caused by mechanical obstruction at the mitral valve or by left ventricular failure, the ventilatory functions of the lungs may be impaired [90-95] and the patient may experience dyspnea. The amount of space in the thorax available for ventilation may be decreased by hydrothorax, by an increase in the amount of blood in the pulmonary blood vessels, or by the increased amount of fluid in the pulmonary interstitial tissues, in the walls of the bronchi and bronchioles, and in the alveoli. The increased amount of fluid and congestion in the lungs increases the stiffness (decreases the *compliance*) of the lungs and thereby increases the work of breathing and the oxygen cost of this work. The presence of fluid in the alveolar spaces may also decrease pulmonary compliance by altering the normal alveolar surface-tension characteristics. Pericapillary thickening and interstitial edema may interfere with alveolar-capillary diffusion of oxygen. The respiratory muscles, which have an increased work load because of the decreased pulmonary compliance, may have their blood supply limited by the decreased cardiac output and may suffer from relative ischemia. This ischemia at times produces chest pain which may be difficult to distinguish from pain of myocardial origin. Many patients with pulmonary congestion have a compensatory hyperventilation which results in respiratory alkalosis. Since pulmonary congestion alters many pulmonary function tests, it is often difficult by such tests to distinguish between dyspnea due to cardiac causes and dyspnea due to pulmonary causes. In clear-cut instances, however, such a separation is often possible.

REFERENCES

1. Youmans, W. B.: Mechanism of High Output Circulatory Failure, *Ann. Int. Med.*, **41**:747, 1954.
2. Youmans, W. B.: High Output Circulatory Failure as a Distinct Syndrome, *Mod. Concepts Cardiovas. Dis.*, **26**:389, 1957.
3. Eichna, L. W.: The George E. Brown Memorial Lecture: Circulatory Congestion and Heart Failure, *Circulation*, **22**:864, 1960.
4. Dock, W.: Presbycardia or Aging of the Myocardium, *New York J. Med.*, **45**:983, 1945.
5. Morgan, H. J.: Senescence and Heart Disease, *Tr. A. Am. Physicians*, **44**:54, 1951.
6. Morgan, H. J.: Senile Heart Disease (Presbycardia). *Tr. Am. Clin. & Climatol. A.*, **65**:64, 1954.
7. Linden, R. J., and Mitchell, J. H.: Relation between Left Ventricular Diastolic Pressure and Myocardial Segment Length, and Observations on the Contribution of Atrial Systole, *Circulation Res.*, **8**:1092, 1960.
8. Mitchell, J. H., Gilmore, J. P., and Sarnoff, S. J.: The Transport Function of the Atrium: Factors Influencing the Relation between Mean Left Atrial Pressure and Left Ventricular End-diastolic Pressure, *Am. J. Cardiol.*, **9**:237, 1962.
9. Skinner, N. S., Jr., Mitchell, J. H., Wallace, A. G., and Sarnoff, S. J.: Hemodynamic Consequences of Atrial Fibrillation at Constant Ventricular Rates, *Am. J. Med.*, **36**:342, 1964.
10. Phillips, E., and Levine, S. A.: Auricular Fibrillation without Other Evidence of Heart Disease: A Cause of Reversible Heart Failure, *Am. J. Med.*, **7**:478, 1949.
11. Kory, R. C., and Meneely, G. R.: Cardiac Output in Auricular Fibrillation with Observations on the Effects of Conversion to Normal Sinus Rhythm, *J. Clin. Invest.*, **30**:653, 1951.
12. Hecht, H. H., Osher, W. J., and Samuels, A. J.: Cardiovascular Adjustments in Subjects with Organic Heart Disease before and after Conversion of Atrial Fibrillation to Normal Sinus Rhythm, *J. Clin. Invest.*, **30**:647, 1951.
13. Hansen, W. R., McClendon, R. L., and Kinsman, J. M.: Auricular Fibrillation: Hemodynamic Studies before and after Conversion with Quinidine, *Am. Heart J.*, **44**:499, 1952.
14. Harvey, R. M., Ferrer, M. I., Richards, D. W., and Cournand, A.: Cardiocirculatory Performance in Atrial Flutter, *Circulation*, **12**:507, 1955.
15. Hecht, H. H., and Lange, R. L.: The Hemodynamic Consequences of Atrial Fibrillation, *Mod. Concepts Cardiovas. Dis.*, **25**:351, 1956.
16. Broch, O. J., and Müller, O.: Haemodynamic Studies during Auricular Fibrillation and after Restoration of Sinus Rhythm, *Brit. Heart J.*, **19**:222, 1957.
17. Dodge, H. T., Kirkham, F. T., Jr., and King, C. V.: Ventricular Dynamics in Atrial Fibrillation, *Circulation*, **15**:335, 1957.
18. Brill, I. C., Rosenbaum, E. E., and Flanery, J. R.: Congestive Failure Due to Auricular Fibrillation in an Otherwise Normal Heart, *J.A.M.A.*, **173**:784, 1960.
19. Wollenberger, A.: Energy Metabolism of the Failing Heart and the Metabolic Action of Cardiac Glycosides, *Pharm. Rev.*, p. 311, 1949.
20. Olson, R. E., and Schwartz, W. B.: Myocardial Metabolism in Congestive Heart Failure, *Medicine*, **30**:21, 1951.
21. Olson, R. E.: Molecular Events in Cardiac Failure, *Am. J. Med.*, **20**:159, 1956.
22. Olson, R. E., and Piatnek, D. A.: Conservation of Energy in Cardiac Muscle, *Ann. New York Acad. Sc.*, **72**:466, 1959.
23. Olson, R. E.: Abnormalities in Myocardial Metabolism, *Circulation Res.*, **14** and **15** (Supp. II): 109, 1964.
24. Blain, J. M., Schafer, H., Siegel, M. S., and Bing, R. J.: Studies on Myocardial Metabolism. VI. Myocardial Metabolism in Congestive Failure, *Am. J. Med.*, **20**:820, 1956.
25. Danforth, W. H., Ballard, F. B., Kako, K., Choudhury, J. D., and Bing, R. J.: Metabolism of the Heart in Failure, *Circulation*, **21**:112, 1960.
26. Kisch, B.: A New Concept of Cardiac Failure, *Am. J. Cardiol.*, **5**:383, 1960.
27. Alpert, N. R., and Gordon, M. S.: Myofibrillar ATPase in Congestive Heart Failure, *Amer. J. Physiol.*, **202**:940, 1962.
28. Schwartz, A., and Lee, K. S.: Study of Heart Mitochondria and Glycolytic Metabolism in Experimentally Induced Cardiac Failure, *Circulation Res.*, **10**:321, 1962.
29. Chidsey, C. A., Braunwald, E., Morrow, A. G., and Mason, D. T.: Myocardial Norepinephrine Concentration in Man: Effects of Reserpine and of Congestive Heart Failure, *New England J. Med.*, **269**: 653, 1963.
30. Kako, K., and Bing, R. J.: Contractility of Actomysin Bands Prepared from Normal and Failing Hearts, *J. Clin. Invest.*, **37**:465, 1958.
31. Olson, R. E., Ellenbogen, E., and Iyengar, R.: Cardiac Myosin and Congestive Heart Failure in the Dog, *Circulation*, **24**:471, 1961.
32. Buckley, N. M., and Tsuboi, K. K.: Cardiac Nucleotides and Derivatives in Acute and Chronic Ventricular Failure of the Dog Heart, *Circulation Res.*, **9**:618, 1961.
33. Nebel, M. L., and Bing, R. J.: Contractile Proteins of Normal and Failing Human Heart, *Arch. Int. Med.*, **111**:190, 1963.
34. Huxley, A. F., and Peachey, L. D.: Maximum Length for Contraction in Striated Muscle, *J. Physiol.*, **146**:55P, 1959.
34a. Sonnenblick, E. H., Spotnitz, H. M., and Spiro, D.: Role of the Sarcomere in Ventricular Function

and the Mechanism of Heart Failure, in J. R. Evans (guest ed.), Symposium: Structure and Function of Heart Muscle, *Circulation Res.*, **15** (Supp. II): 70, 1964.

35. Linzbach, A. J.: Heart Failure from Point of View of Quantitative Anatomy, *Am. J. Cardiol.*, **5**:370, 1960.

36. Braunwald, E., and Ross, J. Jr.: The Ventricular End-diastolic Pressure: Appraisal of Its Value in the Recognition of Ventricular Failure in Man (Editorial), *Am. J. Med.*, **34**:147, 1963.

37. Buckley, N. M., and Zeig, N. J.: Acute Unilateral Ventricular Failure in the Isolated Dog Heart, *Am. J. Physiol.*, **197**:247, 1959.

38. Levine, H. J., Neill, W. A., Wagman, R. J., Krasnow, N., and Gorlin, R.: The Effect of Exercise on Mean Left Ventricular Ejection Rate in Man, *J. Clin. Invest.*, **41**:1050, 1962.

39. Levine, H. J., Messer, J. N., Neill, W. A., and Gorlin, R.: The Effect of Exercise on Cardiac Performance in Human Subjects with Congestive Heart Failure, *Am. Heart J.*, **66**:731, 1963.

40. Hill, A. V.: The Heat of Shortening and the Dynamic Constants of Muscle, *Proc. Roy. Soc. London, ser. B.*, **126**:136, 1938.

41. Burch, G. E., Ray, C. T., and Cronvich, J. A.: Certain Mechanical Peculiarities of the Human Cardiac Pump in Normal and Diseased States, *Circulation*, **5**:504, 1952.

42. Burton, A. C.: The Importance of the Size and Shape of the Heart, *Am. Heart J.*, **54**:801, 1957.

43. Abbott, B. C., and Mommaerts, W. F. H. M.: A Study of Inotropic Mechanisms in the Papillary Muscle Preparation, *J. Gen. Physiol.*, **42**:533, 1959.

44. Gorlin, R.: Recent Conceptual Advances in Congestive Heart Failure, *J.A.M.A.*, **179**:441, 1962.

45. Levine, H. J., and Wagman, R. J.: Energetics of the Human Heart, *Am. J. Cardiol.*, **9**:372, 1962.

46. Sonnenblick, E. H.: Force-Velocity Relations in Mammalian Heart Muscle, *Am. J. Physiol.*, **202**:931, 1962.

47. Fry, D. L., Griggs, D. M. Jr., and Greenfield, J. C. Jr.: Myocardial Mechanics: Tension-Velocity-Length Relationships of Heart Muscle, *Circulation Res.* **14**:73, 1964.

48. Gleason, W. L., and Braunwald, E.: Studies on Starling's Law of the Heart. VI. Relationships between Left Ventricular End-diastolic Volume and Stroke Volume in Man, with Observations on the Mechanics of Pulsus Alternans, *Circulation*, **25**:841, 1962.

49. Mitchell, J. H., Sarnoff, S. J., and Sonnenblick, E. H.: The Dynamics of Pulsus Alternans: Alternating End-diastolic Fiber Length as a Causative Factor, *J. Clin. Invest.*, **42**:55, 1963.

50. McMichael, J., and Shillingford, J. P.: The Role of Valvular Incompetence in Heart Failure, *Brit. M. J.*, **1**:537, 1957.

51. Korner, P., and Shillingford, J.: The Right Atrial Pulse in Congestive Heart Failure, *Brit. Heart J.*, **16**:447, 1954.

52. Burch, G. E.: Evidence for Increased Venous Tone in Chronic Congestive Heart Failure, *A.M.A. Arch. Int. Med.*, **98**:750, 1956.

53. Wood, J. E., Litter, J., and Wilkins, R. W.: Peripheral Venoconstriction in Human Congestive Heart Failure, *Circulation*, **13**:524, 1956.

54. Wood, J. E.: The Mechanism of the Increased Venous Pressure with Exercise in Congestive Heart Failure, *J. Clin. Invest.*, **41**:2020, 1962.

55. Chidsey, C. A., Harrison, D. C., and Braunwald, E.: Augmentation of the Plasma Nor-epinephrine Response to Exercise in Patients with Congestive Heart Failure, *New England J. Med.*, **267**:650, 1962.

56. Gaffney, T. E., and Braunwald, E.: Importance of the Adrenergic Nervous System in the Support of Circulatory Function in Patients with Congestive Heart Failure, *Am. J. Med.*, **34**:320, 1963.

57. Braunwald, E., Harrison, D. C., and Chidsey, C. A.: The Heart as an Endocrine Organ, *Am. J. Med.*, **36**:1, 1964.

58. Barger, A. C.: The Kidney in Congestive Heart Failure, *Circulation*, **21**:124, 1960.

59. Gilmore, J. P.: Contribution of Baroreceptors to the Control of Renal Function, *Circulation Res.*, **14**:301, 1964.

60. Huckabee, W. E., and Judson, W. E.: The Role of Anerobic Metabolism in the Performance of Mild Muscular Work. I. Relationship to Oxygen Consumption and Cardiac Output and the Effect of Congestive Heart Failure, *J. Clin. Invest.*, **37**:1577, 1958.

61. Huckabee, W. E.: The Role of Anaerobic Metabolism in the Performance of Mild Muscular Work. II. The Effect of Asymptomatic Heart Disease, *J. Clin. Invest.*, **37**:1593, 1958.

62. Gorlin, R.: Measurement of Coronary Flow in Health and Disease, in A. M. Jones (ed.), "Modern Trends in Cardiology," Butterworth & Co. (Publishers), Ltd., London, 1960, p. 191.

63. Messer, J. V., and Neill, W. A.: The Oxygen Supply of the Human Heart, *Am. J. Cardiol.*, **9**:384, 1962.

64. Gunton, R. W., and Paul, W.: Blood Volume in Congestive Heart Failure, *J. Clin. Invest.*, **34**:879, 1955.

65. Samet, P., Fritts, H. W., Jr., Fishman, A. P., and Cournand, A.: The Blood Volume in Heart Disease, *Medicine*, **36**:211, 1957.

66. Rader, B., Smith, W. W., Berger, A. R., and Eichna, L. W.: Comparison of the Hemodynamic Effects of Mercurial Diuretics and Digitalis in Congestive Heart Failure, *Circulation*, **29**:328, 1964.

67. Freis, E. D., Schapner, H. W., Johnson, R. L., and Schreiner, G. E.: Hemodynamic Alterations in Acute Myocardial Infarction. I. Cardiac Output, Mean Arterial Pressure, Total Peripheral Resistance, "Central" and Total Blood Volumes, Venous Pres-

sure and Average Circulation Time, *J. Clin. Invest.,* 31:131, 1952.

68. Smith, W. W., Winkler, N. S., and Fox, A. G.: Hemodynamic Studies of Patients with Myocardial Infarction, *Circulation,* 9:352, 1954.

69. Gilbert, R. P., Goldberg, M., and Griffin, J.: Circulatory Changes in Acute Myocardial Infarction, *Circulation,* 9:847, 1954.

70. Gammill, J. F., Applegarth, J. J., Reed, C. E., Fernald, J. D., and Antenucci, A. J.: Hemodynamic Changes Following Acute Myocardial Infarction Using the Dye Injection Method for Cardiac Output Determination, *Ann. Int. Med.,* 43:100, 1955.

71. Broch, O. J., Humerfelt, S., Haarstad, J., and Myhre, J. R.: Hemodynamic Studies in Acute Myocardial Infarction, *Am. Heart J.,* 57:522, 1959.

72. Badeer, H. S.: Contractile Tension in the Myocardium, *Am. Heart J.,* 66:432, 1963.

73. Bing, R. J.: The Coronary Circulation in Health and Disease as Studied by Coronary Sinus Catheterization, *Bull. New York Acad. Med.,* 27:407, 1951.

74. Lombardo, T. A., Rose, L., Taeschler, M., Tuluy, S., and Bing, R. J.: The Effect of Exercise on Coronary Blood Flow, Myocardial Oxygen Consumption and Cardiac Efficiency in Man, *Circulation,* 7:71, 1953.

75. Bing, R. J., and Michal, G.: Myocardial Efficiency, *Ann. New York Acad. Sc.,* 72:555, 1959.

76. Lewis, B. M., Houssay, H. E. J., Haynes, F. W., and Dexter, L.: The Dynamics of Both Right and Left Ventricles at Rest and During Exercise in Patients with Heart Failure, *Circulation Res.,* 1:312, 1953.

77. Luisada, A. A., and Cardi, L.: Acute Pulmonary Edema: Pathology, Physiology and Clinical Management, *Circulation,* 13:113, 1956.

78. Visscher, M. B., Haddy, F. J., and Stephens, G.: The Physiology and Pharmacology of Lung Edema, *Pharmacol. Rev.,* 8:389, 1956.

79. Wasserman, S.: "Acute Cardiac Pulmonary Edema," Charles C Thomas, Publisher, Springfield, Ill., 1959.

80. Fejfar, Z., Fejfarová, M., Bergmann, K., and Brod, J.: Haemodynamic Changes during Acute Pulmonary Edema, *Cardiologia,* 34:233, 1959.

81. Luisada, A. A.: Pathogenesis of Paroxysmal Pulmonary Edema, in A. A. Luisada (ed.), "Cardiology. An Encyclopedia of the Cardiovascular System," McGraw-Hill Book Company, New York, 1959, vol. 4, p. 18-79.

82. Sarnoff, S. J.: Some Physiologic Considerations in the Genesis of Acute Pulmonary Edema, in A. Wright and I. Veith (eds.), "Pulmonary Circulation," Grune & Stratton, Inc., New York, 1959, p. 273.

83. Finlayson, J. K., Luria, M. N., Stanfield, C. A., and Yu, P. N.: Hemodynamic Studies in Acute Pulmonary Edema, *Ann. Int. Med.,* 54:244, 1961.

84. Guyton, A. C., and Lindsey, A. W.: Effect of Elevated Left Atrial Pressure and Decreased Plasma Protein Concentration on the Development of Pulmonary Edema, *Circulation Res.,* 7:649, 1959.

85. Uhley, H. N., Leeds, S. E., Sampson, J. J., and Friedman, M.: Some Observations on the Role of the Lymphatics in Experimental Acute Pulmonary Edema, *Circulation Res.,* 9:688, 1961.

86. Uhley, H. N., Leeds, S. E., Sampson, J. J., and Friedman, M.: Role of Pulmonary Lymphatics in Chronic Pulmonary Edema, *Circulation Res.,* 11:966, 1962.

87. Robin, E. D., and Thomas, E. D.: Some Relations between Pulmonary Edema and Pulmonary Inflammation (Pneumonia), *Arch. Int. Med.,* 93:713, 1954.

88. Kuida, H., Hinshaw, L. B., Gilbert, R. P., and Visscher, M.: Effect of Gram-negative Endotoxin on Pulmonary Circulation, *Am. J. Physiol.,* 192:335, 1958.

89. Hultgren, H. N., Lopez, C. E., Lundberg, E., and Miller, H.: Physiologic Studies of Pulmonary Edema at High Altitude, *Circulation,* 29:393, 1964.

90. Richards, D. W., Jr.: The Nature of Cardiac and of Pulmonary Dyspnea, *Circulation,* 7:15, 1953.

91. Brown, C. C., Jr., Fry, D. L., and Ebert, R. V.: Mechanics of Pulmonary Ventilation in Patients with Heart Disease, *Am. J. Med.,* 17:438, 1954.

92. Saxton, G. A., Jr., and Bliss, H. A.: Physiological Factors in the Differential Diagnosis of Chronic Cardiac and Pulmonary Disease, *M. Clin. North America,* 42:165, 1958.

93. McIlroy, M. B.: Dyspnea and the Work of Breathing in Diseases of the Heart and Lungs. *Progr. Cardiovas. Dis.,* 1:284, 1958/59.

94. Donald, K. W.: Disturbances in Pulmonary Function in Mitral Stenosis and Left Heart Failure, *Progr. Cardiovas. Dis.,* 1:298, 1958/59.

95. Butler, J.: Pulmonary Function in Heart Disease, in A. M. Jones (ed.), "Modern Trends in Cardiology," Butterworth & Co., Publishers, Ltd., London, 1961, p. 18.

SUGGESTED READING*

Altschule, M. D.: "Acute Pulmonary Edema," Grune & Stratton, Inc., New York, 1954.

Altschule, M. D.: "Physiology in Diseases of the Heart and Lungs," 2d ed., Harvard University Press, Cambridge, Mass., 1954.

Badeer, H. S.: Biological Significance of Cardiac Hypertrophy, *Am. J. Cardiol.,* 14:133, 1964.

Badeer, H. S.: The Stimulus to Hypertrophy of the Myocardium, *Circulation,* 30:128, 1964.

Barger, A. C., Ross, R. S., and Price, H. L.: Reduced Sodium Excretion in Dogs with Mild Valvular Lesions of the Heart, and in Dogs with Congestive Failure, *Am. J. Physiol.,* 180:249, 1955.

Barger, A. C., Muldowney, F. P., and Leibowitz, M. R.: Role of the Kidney in the Pathogenesis of Congestive Heart Failure, *Circulation,* 20:273, 1959.

Bing, R. J., Wu, C., and Gudbjarnason, S.: Mechanism

* See also References and Suggested Reading in Chap. 15.

of Heart Failure, in J. R. Evans (guest ed.), Symposium: Structure and Function of Heart Muscle, *Circulation Res.*, **15** (Supp. II): 64, 1964.

Bishop, J. M., Donald, K. W., and Wade, O. L.: Circulatory Dynamics at Rest and on Exercise in the Hyperkinetic States, *Clin. Sc.*, **14**:329, 1955.

Blacket, R. B., and Palmer, A. J.: Hemodynamic Studies in High Output Beriberi, *Brit. Heart J.*, **22**:483, 1960.

Bondurant, S., Hickam, J. B., and Isley, J. K.: Pulmonary and Circulatory Effects of Acute Pulmonary Vascular Engagement in Normal Subjects, *J. Clin. Invest.*, **36**:59, 1957.

Büchner, F.: "Die Koronarinsuffizienz," Dresden, Steinkopff, 1939.

Burch, G. E., and Ray, C. T.: A Consideration of the Mechanism of Congestive Heart Failure, *Am. Heart J.*, **41**:918, 1951.

Case, R. B., Berglund, E., and Sarnoff, S. J.: Ventricular Function. II. Quantitative Relationship between Coronary Flow and Ventricular Function with Observations of Unilateral Failure, *Circulation Res.*, **2**:319, 1954.

Chapman, C. B., and Fraser, R. S.: Studies on the Effect of Exercise on Cardiovascular Function. III. Cardiovascular Response to Exercise in Patients with Healed Myocardial Infarction, *Circulation*, **9**:347, 1954.

Clements, J. A.: Pulmonary Edema and Permeability of Alveolar Membranes, *Arch. Environmental Health*, **2**:280, 1961.

Cournand, A.: A Discussion of the Concept of Cardiac Failure in the Light of Recent Physiologic Studies in Man, *Ann. Int. Med.*, **37**:649, 1952.

Daley, R., Goodwin, J. F., and Steiner, R. E.: "Clinical Disorders of the Pulmonary Circulation," Boston: Little, Brown and Company, 1960.

Davis, J. O., and Smith, J. R.: Pathogenesis of Peripheral Cardiac Edema, *Am. J. Med.*, **3**:704, 1947.

Davis, J. O.: Mechanisms of Salt and Water Retention in Congestive Heart Failure: The Importance of Aldosterone, *Am. J. Med.*, **29**:486, 1960.

Davis, J. O.: Adrenocortical and Renal Hormonal Function in Experimental Cardiac Failure, *Circulation*, **25**:1002, 1962.

Dumont, A. E., Clauss, R. H., Reed, G. E., and Tice, D. A.: Lymph Drainage in Patients with Congestive Heart Failure: Comparison with Findings in Hepatic Cirrhosis, *New England J. Med.*, **269**:949, 1963.

Eddleman, E. E., Jr.: Chronic Congestive Heart Failure, in B. L. Gordon (ed.), "Clinical Cardiopulmonary Physiology," 2d ed., Grune & Stratton, Inc., New York, 1960, p. 355.

Dock, D. S., Kraus, W. L., McGuire, L. B., Hyland, J. W., Haynes, F. W., and Dexter, L.: The Pulmonary Blood Volume in Man, *J. Clin. Invest.*, **40**:317, 1961.

Donald, K. W.: Exercise Studies in Heart Disease, *Mod. Concepts Cardiovas. Dis.*, **28**:529, 1959.

Donald, K. W.: Hemodynamics in Chronic Congestive Heart Failure, *J. Chronic Dis.*, **9**:476, 1959.

Eichna, L. W., Farber, S. J., Berger, A. R., Earle, D. P., Rader, B., Pellegrino, E., Albert, R. E., Alexander, J. D., Taube, H., and Youngwirth, S.: The Interrelationship of the Cardiovascular, Renal and Electrolyte Effects of Intravenous Digoxin in Congestive Heart Failure, *J. Clin. Invest.*, **30**:1250, 1951.

Eichna, L. W., Farber, S. J., Berger, A. R., Earle, D. P., Rader, B., Pellegrino, E., Albert, R. E., Alexander, J. D., Taube, H., and Yonngwirth, S.: Cardiovascular Dynamics, Blood Volumes, Renal Functions and Electrolyte Excretions in the Same Patients during Congestive Heart Failure and after Recovery of Cardiac Compensation, *Circulation*, **7**:674, 1953.

Eichna, L. W., Farber, S. J., Berger, A. R., Rader, B., Smith, W. W., and Albert, R. E.: Non-cardiac Circulatory Congestion Simulating Congestive Heart Failure, *T. A. Am. Physicians*, **67**:72, 1954.

Evans, J. R. (ed.): Symposium: Structure and Function of Heart Muscle, *Circulation Res.*, **14** and **15** (Supp. II): 1-224, 1964.

Farber, S. J., Becker, W. H., and Eichna, L. W.: Electrolyte and Water Excretions and Renal Hemodynamics during Induced Congestion of the Superior and Inferior Vena Cava of Man, *J. Clin. Invest.*, **32**:1145, 1953.

Fejfar, Z., and Brod, J.: The Mechanism of General Haemodynamic Changes in Heart Failure, *Acta med. scandinav.*, **148**:247, 1954.

Ferrer, M. I., Harvey, R. M., Cournand, A., and Richards, D. W.: Cardiocirculatory Studies in Pulsus Alternans of the Systemic and Pulmonary Circulations, *Circulation*, **14**:163, 1956.

Ferrer, M. I., and Harvey, R. M.: Decompensated Pulmonary Heart Disease, with a Note on the Effect of Digitalis, in W. R. Adams and I. Veith (eds.), "Pulmonary Circulation," Grune & Stratton, Inc., New York, 1959, p. 171.

Grimm, A. F., Kubota, R., and Whitehorn, W. V.: Properties of Myocardium in Cardiomegaly, *Circulation Res.*, **12**:118, 1963.

Guyton, A. C.: Cardiac Output and Venous Return in Heart Failure, in A. A. Luisada (ed.), "Cardiology. An Encyclopedia of the Cardiovascular System," McGraw-Hill Book Company, New York, 1959, vol. 4, p. 18-8.

Hamilton, W. F.: The Physiology of Congestive Failure of the Circulation, *Minnesota Med.*, **37**:36, 1954.

Harris, P., and Heath, D.: "The Human Pulmonary Circulation: Its Form and Function in Health and Disease," The Williams & Wilkins Company, Baltimore, 1962.

Harrison, T. R.: "Failure of the Circulation," 2d ed., The Williams & Wilkins Company, Baltimore, 1939.

Harvey, R. M., Ferrer, M. I., Cathcart, R. T., Richards, D. W., Jr., and Cournand, A.: Some Effects of Digoxin upon the Heart and Circulation in Man:

Digoxin in Left Ventricular Failure, *Am. J. Med.*, 7:439, 1949.

Harvey, R. M., Ferrer, M. I., Cathcart, R. T., and Alexander, J. K.: Some Effects of Digoxin on the Heart and Circulation in Man, *Circulation*, 4:366, 1951.

Hickman, J. B., and Cagill, W. H.: Effects of Exercise on Cardiac Output and Pulmonary Arterial Pressure in Normal Persons and in Patients with Cardiovascular Disease and Pulmonary Emphysema, *J. Clin. Invest.*, 27:10, 1948.

Holland, W. C., and Klein, R. L.: "Chemistry of Heart Failure," Charles C Thomas, Publisher, Springfield, Ill., 1960.

Humerfelt, S., Müller, O., and Sorstein, O.: The Circulation in Hyperthyroidism: A Cardiac Catheterization Study before and after Treatment, *Am. Heart J.*, 56:87, 1958.

Iseri, L. T., Evans, J. R., and Evans, M.: Pathogenesis of Congestive Heart Failure: Correlation between Anaerobic Metabolism and Plasma Volume Changes Following Exercise, *Ann. Int. Med.*, 59:788, 1963.

Johnson, R. D., and Conn, J. W.: Aldosterone, Antidiuretic Hormone and Congestive Heart Failure, *Mod. Concepts Cardiovas. Dis.*, 27:431, 1958.

Judson, W. E., Hollander, W., Hatcher, J. D., and Halperin, M. H.: The Effects of Exercise on Cardiovascular and Renal Function in Cardiac Patients with and without Heart Failure, *J. Clin. Invest.*, 34:1546, 1955.

Kabins, S. A., Fridman, J., Neustadt, J., Espinosa, G., and Katz, L. N.: Mechanisms Leading to Lung Edema in Pulmonary Embolization, *Am. J. Physiol.*, 198:543, 1960.

Katz, L. N.: The Mechanism of Cardiac Failure, *Circulation*, 10:663, 1954.

Katz, L. N.: Analysis of the Several Factors Regulating the Performance of the Heart, *Physiol. Rev.*, 35:91, 1955.

Katz, L. N., Feinberg, H., and Shaffer, A. B.: Hemodynamic Aspects of Congestive Heart Failure, *Circulation*, 21:95, 1960.

Katz, L. N.: The Lewis A. Conner Memorial Lecture: The Performance of the Heart, *Circulation*, 21:483, 1960.

Katz, L. N.: Recent Concepts of the Performance of the Heart, *Circulation*, 28:117, 1963.

Kisch, B., Cavusoglu, M., and Marangoni, B.: Electron Microscopic Changes in the Human Heart in Cardiac Failure, *Exper. Med. & Surg.*, 17:85, 1959.

Krasnow, N., and Gorlin, R.: Myocardial Lactate Metabolism in Coronary Insufficiency, *Ann. Int. Med.*, 59:781, 1963.

LaDue, J. S.: Cardiac Failure and Function Tests, in W. A. Sodeman (ed.), "Pathologic Physiology: Mechanisms of Disease," W. B. Saunders Company, Philadelphia, 1961, p. 551.

Laragh, J. H.: Hormones and the Pathogenesis of Congestive Heart Failure: Vasopressin, Aldosterone, and Angiotensin II: Further Evidence for Renal-Adrenal Interactions from Studies in Hypertension and in Cirrhosis, *Circulation*, 25:1015, 1962.

Levine, H. J., and Britman, N. A.: Force-Velocity Relations in the Intact Dog Heart, *J. Clin. Invest.*, 43:1383, 1964.

Lindsey, A. W., Banahan, B. F., Cannon, R. N., and Guyton, A. C.: Pulmonary Blood Volume of the Dog and Its Changes in Acute Heart Failure, *Am. J. Physiol.*, 190:45, 1957.

Lindsey, A. W., and Guyton, A. C.: Continuous Recording of Pulmonary Blood Volume and Pulmonary Pressure and Volume Changes, *Am. J. Physiol.*, 197:959, 1959.

Luethy, E.: "Die Haemodynamik des suffizienten und insuffizienten rechten Herzens Biblioteca Cardiologica, Fasc. II, S. Karger, Basel, 1962.

McMichael, J.: Heart Failure of Pulmonary Origin, *Edinburgh M. J.*, 55:65, 1948.

McMichael, J.: Cardiac Venous Congestion: Its Causes and Consequences, *Am. J. Med.*, 6:651, 1949.

McMichael, J.: Changing Views on Heart Failure, *Ann. Int. Med.*, 51:635, 1959.

Meerson, F. Z.: Compensatory Hyperfunction of the Heart and Cardiac Insufficiency, *Circulation Res.*, 10:250, 1962.

Merrill, A. J.: Edema and Decreased Renal Blood Flow in Patients with Chronic Congestive Heart Failure: Evidence of "Forward Failure" as the Primary Cause of Edema, *J. Clin. Invest.*, 25:389, 1946.

Merrill, A. J.: Mechanisms of Salt and Water Retention in Heart Failure, *Am. J. Med.*, 6:357, 1949.

Miller, A. J., Pick, R., and Katz, L. N.: Ventricular Endomyocardial Pathology Produced by Chronic Cardiac Lymphatic Obstruction in the Dog, *Circulation Res.*, 8:941, 1960.

Moyer, J. H., and Fuchs, M. (eds.): "Edema: Mechanism and Management," W. B. Saunders Company, Philadelphia, 1960.

Muldowney, F. P., Veith, F. J., Olesen, K. H., Haxhe, J. J., Boyden, C. M., and Moore, F. D.: Body Composition in the Dog. II. The Effect of Progressive Congestive Heart Failure, *J. Surg. Res.*, 2:254, 1962.

Müller, O., and Rorvik, K.: Haemodynamic Consequences of Coronary Heart Disease, *Brit. Heart J.*, 20:302, 1958.

Norman, T. D.: The Pathogenesis of Cardiac Hypertrophy, *Progr. Cardiovas. Dis.*, 4:439, 1962.

Ogden, D. A., Spritz, N., and Rubin, A. L.: Fluid and Electrolyte Distribution in Congestive Heart Failure, *Progr. Cardiovas. Dis.*, 3:580, 1961.

Orgain, E. S., and Stead, E. A. Jr.: Clinical Progress: Congestive Heart Failure, *Circulation*, 16:291, 1957.

Paine, R., and Smith, J. R.: The Mechanism of Heart Failure, *Am. J. Med.*, 6:84, 1949.

Richards, D. W., Jr.: The Dynamics of Congestive Heart Failure, *Am. J. Med.*, 6:772, 1949.

Samet, P., and Bernstein, W. H.: Cardiac Catheterization in Heart Failure, in A. A. Luisada (ed.), "Cardiology. An Encyclopedia of the Cardiovascular System," McGraw-Hill Book Company, New York, 1959, vol. 4, p. 18-87.

Sarnoff, S. J., and Sarnoff, L. C.: Neurohaemodynamics of Acute Pulmonary Edema. I. Autonomic Influence on Pulmonary Vascular Pressures and the Acute Pulmonary Edema State, *Dis. Chest*, **22**:685, 1952.

Sarnoff, S. J., Berglund, E., and Sarnoff, L. C.: Neurohemodynamics of Pulmonary Edema. III. Estimated Changes in Pulmonary Blood Volume Accompanying Systemic Vasoconstriction and Vasodilation, *J. Appl. Physiol.*, **5**:367, 1953.

Sarnoff, S. J., and Berglund, E.: Neurohemodynamics of Pulmonary Edema. IV. Effect of Systemic Vasoconstriction and Subsequent Vasodilation on Flow and Pressures in Systemic and Pulmonary Vascular Beds, *Am. J. Physiol.*, **170**:588, 1952.

Sarnoff, S. J., Braunwald, E., Welch, G. H., Jr., Case, R. B., Stainsby, W. N., and Macruz, R.: Hemodynamic Determinants of the Oxygen Consumption of the Heart with Special Reference to the Tension-Time Index, *Am. J. Physiol.*, **192**:148, 1958.

Selzer, A.: Hemodynamic Sequelae of Sustained Elevation of Left Atrial Pressure, *Circulation*, **20**:243, 1959.

Selzer, A., and McCaughey, D. J.: Hemodynamic Patterns in Chronic Cardiac Failure, *Am. J. Med.*, **28**:337, 1960.

Sensenbach, W., Madison, L., and Eisenberg, S.: Cerebral Hemodynamic and Metabolic Studies in Patients with Congestive Heart Failure, *Circulation*, **21**:697, 1960.

Sharpey-Schafer, E. P.: Circulatory Dynamics and the Left Heart, in A. M. Jones (ed.), "Modern Trends in Cardiology," Butterworth & Co. (Publishers), London, 1961, p. 9.

Singer, D., Saltzman, P. W., Rivera-Estrada, C., Pick, R., and Katz, L. N.: Hemodynamic Alterations Following Miliary Pulmonary Embolization in Relation to the Pathogenesis of the Consequent Diffuse Edema, *Am. J. Physiol.*, **191**:437, 1957.

Smith, R. C., Burchell, H. B., and Edwards, J. E.: Pathology of the Pulmonary Vascular Tree: IV. Structural Changes in the Pulmonary Vessels in Chronic Left ventricular failure, *Circulation*, **10**:801, 1954.

Sobol, B. J., Kessler, R. H., Rader, B., and Eichna, L. W.: Cardiac, Hemodynamic and Renal Function in Congestive Heart Failure during Peripheral Vasodilatation: Relationship to Starling's Law of the Heart in Man, *J. Clin. Invest.*, **38**:557, 1959.

Soloff, L. A.: On the Lack of Meaning of Heart Failure, *Am. Heart J.*, **66**:276, 1963.

Stead, E. A., Jr.: The Role of the Cardiac Output in the Mechanisms of Congestive Heart Failure, *Am. J. Med.*, **6**:232, 1949.

Starr, I.: Our Changing Viewpoint about Congestive Failure, *Ann. Int. Med.*, **30**:1, 1949.

Symposium on Congestive Heart Failure, *Circulation*, **21**:95-128, 218-255, 424-447, 1960.

Visscher, M. B.: The Energy Transformation by the Heart and the Mechanism of Experimental Cardiac Failure, in American Association for the Advancement of Science, "Blood, Heart and Circulation," Publ. No. 13, Lancaster, Pennsylvania, 1940, p. 176.

Werkö, L., and Lagerlöff, H.: Studies on the Circulation in Man; Cardiac Output and Blood Pressure in the Right Auricle, Right Ventricle, and Pulmonary Artery in Patients with Hypertensive Cardiovascular Disease, *Acta med. scandinav.*, **133**:427, 1949.

Werkö, L.: The Kidney in Heart Disease, in A. M. Jones (ed.), "Modern Trends in Cardiology," Butterworth and Co., London, 1961, p. 53.

Wood, P.: "Diseases of the Heart and Circulation," 2d ed., J. B. Lippincott Co., Philadelphia, 1956.

12 HORMONAL FACTORS IN THE EDEMA OF HEART FAILURE

Elbert P. Tuttle, Jr., M.D.

For many years there has been an implied hope in much cardiovascular-renal research that a unitary explanation might be found for the retention and abnormal distribution of water and salt in the body in congestive heart failure. It is much more likely, from the complexity of the circulatory controls outlined in the chapter on hypertension, that many mechanisms must be involved.

Efforts to evaluate the role of individual control components in water and salt retention in man have been made difficult by several circumstances. Studies in diseased states have failed to recognize that as a negative feedback mechanism in a control system succeeds in reducing the "error signal," its functional state approaches normal. The deviation of control functions from normal in a sensitive system may be imperceptible except in their net cumulative effect, and experimental studies in intact man are met by compensating feedback responses.

The fact that the untreated cardiac patient with edema does not at the time examined have a reduced cardiac output, reduced renal blood flow, excessive aldosterone secretion, or evidence of antidiuretic activity need not be surprising. It does not prove that these factors did not play a role in bringing about the edematous state. It may be simply an indication of the success of the control mechanisms in restoring to normal the critical force or function which stimulated the sensing transducers in the circulatory system and led to salt retention.

The humoral agents which have been examined in greatest detail for a role in the retention of water and salt in heart failure are renin, angiotensin, aldosterone, vasopressin, estrogen, and norepinephrine. Pure renin has not been available for study, but it has been shown that none of the other agents, administered alone to normal man, can produce a picture of the edema of congestive heart failure. Infusions of angiotensin for 2 to 8 hr in normal persons on normal sodium diets cause sodium retention.[1] Infusions in hypertensive patients pro-

duce a large diuresis of water and sodium.[2] Data from our laboratory[3] indicate that with prolonged infusions of angiotensin for 24 to 48 hr in normal man, a response somewhat similar to that of the hypertensive patient is seen (Fig. 12-1). A diuresis of water and salt occurs though renal plasma flow and glomerular filtration rate are still below control levels. This breakthrough minimizes the cumulative retention of water and sodium.

Aldosterone has been studied by August, Nelson, and Thorn.[4] Injection of high doses produces a weight gain of 2 to 4 kg, but is followed by increasing urinary sodium output and the achievement of stable weight in a new balance state before edema is manifest. Patients with aldosterone tumors

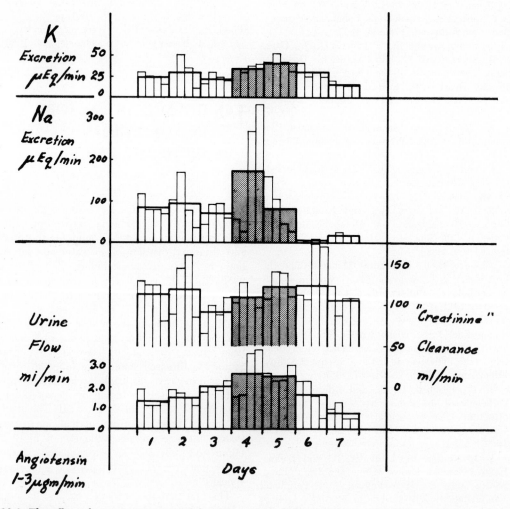

Fig. 12-1. The effect of angiotensin on renal function and electrolyte excretion. (Small bars represent 6-hr excretion periods. Large bars represent mean excretion for 24 hr. Angiotensin was infused throughout the shaded periods.) Patient at bed rest on moderate sodium intake responds to a prolonged infusion of angiotensin with initial retention of sodium. At 12 to 24 hr after beginning angiotensin infusion, there is a diuresis of sodium and water of a magnitude which creates a net negative sodium balance for the first 24-hr period.

rarely develop heart failure or edema.[5] This over-riding of the pharmacologic effect of aldosterone is the result of the engagement of negative feedback mechanisms, some of which have been indicated. Expansion of blood volume, elevation of blood pressure, suppression of renin and endogenous aldosterone secretion must contribute to the reduced fraction of the filtered sodium which is reabsorbed.

Vasopressin, the antidiuretic hormone, when administered to normal man with large water intake leads only to mild edema because of the large negative sodium balance which ensues.[6] This permits the major portion of the retained water to enter cells and may lead to the convulsions of water intoxication before congestive heart failure is seen. The control mechanisms involved here again seem to be those of elevated blood pressure, increased renal perfusion, suppression of renin and aldosterone release, and probably redistribution of renal blood flow.

It has been postulated that failure of the congested liver to detoxify estrogen might be partially responsible for the abnormal retention of water and sodium seen in congestive heart failure. It was beautifully shown by Preedy and Aitken[7] that in normal man exogenous estrogen in large doses was incapable of producing edema. In patients with heart failure, however, edema was increased by the administration of estrogen.[8]

Norepinephrine is reported to cause retention of sodium during the first 3 hr of infusion in normal man.[9] Within 6 hr of the onset of a constant infusion in man, a diuresis of sodium begins, and a net negative sodium balance is seen within the first 24 hr.[1,2,10] Patients with pheochromocytomas rarely have edema. They are often, in fact, depleted of sodium and water, and following extirpation of a pheochromocytoma, expansion of the circulating blood volume or substitution pressor therapy is usually required.[11]

It would seem from this analysis that excessive secretion of no single hormone can produce the syndrome of cardiac edema. Moreover, not even the reduction of glomerular filtration or the reduction of renal perfusion pressure can be called on for explanation. Many patients with severe reduction of glomerular filtration rate never get edema, and patients with coarctation of the aorta above the renal arteries develop heart failure late, if at all.

The syndrome of passive congestive heart failure must be interpreted, then, as the consequence of an integrated response to the inability of the heart to do the work demanded of it within the normal range of operation of the circulatory control mechanisms. Either the effector organs or their controls must operate outside their usual range.

When water and salt retention have occurred and cardiac and blood volume are elevated, then other control and effector organs may return to their normal operating range.

There is evidence from animal experiments and from studies in man that each of these hormones may play a role in the creation and/or preservation of the edematous state in congestive heart failure. It is not necessary that the rate of secretion of a hormone be found to be absolutely elevated above the normal range to reach this conclusion. The mere fact that the hormone is being secreted at a normal rate, when the usually accepted determinants of its secretion would long since have dictated its suppression, is abnormal. The secretion of a normal amount of aldosterone at a time when the total body sodium store is 20 per cent above normal is indication that it is collaborating in the preservation of the edematous state. Only in severe states of "decompensation," meaning a state of metabolic imbalance tending to rapid *accumulation* of edema, or during pharmacologic blockade of some of the physiologic responses, would one expect to find elevated levels of the salt- and water-retaining hormones. This does not imply, however, that blockade of, or suppression of, any one of these humors would not lead to a diuresis.

A pressor substance considered to be renin was obtained from the renal blood of patients in congestive heart failure by A. J. Merrill and colleagues in 1946.[12] Precise measurement of renin in blood has remained difficult, as has the assay of its product, angiotensin, but Davis et al. have shown that the renin content of the kidneys of dogs with experimental congestive heart failure is increased and the blood of these animals contains a humoral agent which stimulates aldosterone secretion.[13] The lack of a pressor response in heart failure patients is not surprising in view of the relative resistance to the pressor effects of angiotensin in animals with experimental congestive heart failure.[13] The likelihood is good at present that human kidneys secrete more than normal amounts of renin and generate more than normal amounts of angiotensin in congestive heart failure, but definitive proof of this has not yet been produced.

Aldosterone has been widely thought to contribute to the edema of congestive heart failure. As pointed out by Laragh,[14] many of the physiologic responses of the patient with heart failure suggest excessive aldosterone activity: increased renal tubular reabsorption of sodium and wastage of potassium when diuretics are administered; low Na/K ratio of body secretions; diuresis with spirolactones. Measurements of aldosterone secretion in congestive heart failure in man have occasionally, but not consistently, shown elevation.[14-16] The significance of this needs to be examined in the light of Ayers's demonstration that the metabolism of aldosterone is reduced to one-half to one-third the normal turnover rate when the liver is experimentally congested by high inferior caval pressures.[17] In any case, it has been shown by Duncan, Liddle, and Bartter that depletion of sodium toward normal by resins and low-sodium diet resulted in increased aldosterone excretion in four out of five patients.[18] Blockade of the renal effects of aldosterone by the spironolactones frequently produces a diuresis of sodium and water.[19] It may fail to do so, even if aldosterone secretion is high, when reduced filtration rate and avid proximal reabsorption of water and salt preclude an adequate presentation of sodium to the distal tubular exchange sites.

The secretion of hypertonic urine in the presence of marked hypotonicity of the body fluids has raised the possibility that vasopressin might be secreted in excessive amounts or detoxified at a slow rate in congestive heart failure.[20] Assays of the urine have indeed shown increased amounts of antidiuretic material in patients with heart failure.[21] Specific measurements of vasopressin have not been made. The discovery of intrathoracic stretch receptors in low-pressure vascular compartments by Henry, Gauer, and Reeves[22] that appear to modulate diuresis offers a possible pathway, particularly in cor pulmonale and constrictive pericarditis, by which vasopressin secretion might be stimulated.

The demonstration by Berliner and Davidson[23] that reduction of renal perfusion pressure could cause a fall in free-water clearance and the demonstration by Schedl and Bartter[24] that the failure to secrete a dilute urine could be relieved by the administration of an osmotic diuretic, mannitol, offer alternative explanations of the antidiuresis. Avid proximal tubular reabsorption of sodium and water was thought to explain the impairment of free-water clearance.

If the mechanism is only a renal one, it is difficult to understand why simple restriction of water intake cannot be used to correct the hyponatremia. Intense thirst usually prevents successful use of this tactic, and gives evidence that the water retention involves at least some central nervous support.

In the present state of our knowledge it seems most likely that at times all three of these mechanisms are involved in the impaired capacity to excrete free water. Under these circumstances the tonicity of body fluids is dependent on the solute-to-water ratio of the daily intake. In cardiac patients, because of restriction of dietary sodium, this is usually low.

Although exogenous estrogen does not produce edema in normal man, Preedy and Aitken[8] showed that in congestive heart failure with hepatic congestion marked sodium and water retention can be induced by this hormone. This was presumed to be the consequence of impaired hepatic inactivation of estrogen. If impaired inactivation does not suppress synthesis of estrogen in man, this might be an added stimulus to sodium retention. The appearance of cardiac edema in man as well as woman would suggest that this is not a major determinant of the edema of heart failure, but the occasional occurrence of spider hemangiomas with cardiac cirrhosis would indicate the definite possibility of a contributory role.

The final hormone to be considered is norepinephrine, though this is perhaps better considered a neurohumor or transmitter of the sympathetic nerve impulse. Studies by Barger et al.[25] have shown in experimental heart failure in the dog that sympathetic blockade of the renal blood vessels by phenoxybenzamine hydrochloride will produce a diuresis of sodium and water. Selective pharmacologic blockade of renal sympathetic nerves in man has not been reported. It is clear from studies on the explanted, denervated kidney in the dog that sympathetic innervation is not essential to the production of edema, but species differences in the neurogenic control of the circulation and in the responses to changes in perfusion are so great between man and the dog that caution must be exercised in drawing conclusions from the information currently available. It is plausible to consider that the fall in renal blood flow in heart failure, even in the absence of a reduced cardiac output or blood pressure, may in part be due to sympathetic constriction of renal vessels.

It has recently been shown by Davis[26] that the retention of water and sodium with the production of edema and ascites cannot be induced in the dog with a single denervated, explanted kidney exposed to high levels of salt-retaining hormone unless an added circulatory lesion, such as constriction of the inferior vena cava above the hepatic vein, is present. This suggests that an added hormone from outside the kidney must be called forth by the lesion, such as, for instance, increased secretion of vasopressin, or that intrarenal redistribution of blood flow from the transient reduction of cardiac output increases sodium reabsorption.

In summary, no single hormone accounts for the edema of congestive heart failure. Though edema be present, no hormone must be presumed to be present in amounts above those found in normal persons. During periods of severe decompensation, or under conditions of vigorous diuretic therapy, renin, angiotensin, aldosterone, vasopressin, and norepinephrine, released in an integrated response, may together or in varying combinations contribute to the retention of sodium and water, but conditions of renal perfusion are of equal importance.

REFERENCES

1. Laragh, J. H., Angers, M., Kelly, W. G., and Lieberman, S.: Hypotensive Agents and Pressor Substances: Effect of Epinephrine, Norepinephrine, Angiotensin II and Others on the Secretory Rate of Aldosterone in Man, *J.A.M.A.*, **174**:234, 1960.
2. Peart, W. S., and Brown, J. J.: Effect of Angiotensin (Hypertensin or Angiotonin) on Urine Flow and Electrolyte Excretion in Hypertensive Patients, *Lancet*, **1**:28, 1961.
3. Tuttle, E. P., Jr.: Saluresis and Potassium Retention Induced by Pressor Amines (Abstract), *Clin. Res.*, **8**:89, 1960.
4. August, J. T., Nelson, D. H., and Thorn, G. W.: Response of Normal Subjects to Large Amounts of Aldosterone, *J. Clin. Invest.*, **37**:1549, 1958.
5. Conn, J. W., Aldosteronism in Man, *J.A.M.A.*, **183**:871, 1963.
6. Leaf, A., Bartter, F. C., Santos, R. F., and Wrong, O.: Evidence in Man That Urinary Electrolyte Loss Induced by Pitressin Is a Function of Water Retention, *J. Clin. Invest.*, **32**:868, 1953.
7. Preedy, J. R. K., and Aitken, E. H.: The Effect of Estrogen on Water and Electrolyte Metabolism. I. The Normal, *J. Clin. Invest.*, **35**:423, 1956.
8. Preedy, J. R. K., and Aitken, E. H.: The Effect of Estrogen on Water and Electrolyte Metabolism. III. Cardiac and Renal Disease, *J. Clin. Invest.*, **35**:443, 1956.
9. Nickel, J. F., Smythe, C. M., Papper, E. M., and Bradley, S. E.: A Study of the Mode of Action of the Adrenal Medullary Hormones on Sodium, Potassium and Water Excretion in Man, *J. Clin. Invest.*, **33**:1687, 1954.
10. Biron, P., Koiw, E., Nowaczynski, W., Brouillet, J., and Genest, J.: The Effects of Intravenous Infusions of Valine-5 Angiotensin II and Other Pressor Agents on Urinary Electrolytes and Corticosteroids, Including Aldosterone, *J. Clin. Invest.*, **40**:338, 1961.
11. Brunjes, S., Johns, V. J., and Crane, M. G.: Pheochromocytoma: Postoperative Shock and Blood Volume, *New England J. Med.*, **262**:393, 1962.
12. Merrill, A. F., Morrison, J. L., and Brannon, E. S.: Concentration of Renin in Renal Venous Blood in Patients with Chronic Heart Failure, *Am. J. Med.*, **1**:468, 1946.
13. Davis, J. O., Hartroft, P. M., Titus, E. O., Carpenter, C. J., Ayers, C. R., and Spiegel, H. E.: The Role of Renin-Angiotensin System in the Control of Aldosterone Secretion, *J. Clin. Invest.*, **41**:378, 1962.
14. Laragh, J. H.: Hormones and the Pathogenesis of Congestive Heart Failure: Vasopressin, Aldosterone and Angiotensin II, *Circulation*, **25**:1015, 1962.
15. Cox, J. R., Davies-Jones, G. A. B., and Leonard, P. J.: Sodium Content and Urinary Aldosterone Excretion in Patients with Congestive Heart Failure before and after Treatment and Comparison with Normal Subjects Undergoing Salt Restriction, *Clin. Sc.*, **26**:177, 1964.
16. Wolff, H. P., Koczorek, K. R., Buchborn, E., and Rieker, G.: Endocrine Factors (in Symposium: Congestive Heart Failure), *J. Chron. Dis.*, **9**:554, 1959.
17. Ayers, C. R., Davis, J. O., Lieberman, F., Carpenter, C. C. J., and Berman, M.: The Effects of Chronic Hepatic Venous Congestion on the Metabolism of *d,l*-aldosterone and *d*-aldosterone, *J. Clin. Invest.*, **41**:884, 1962.
18. Duncan, L. E., Liddle, G. W., and Bartter, F. C.: The Effect of Changes in Body Sodium on Extracellular Fluid Volume and Aldosterone and Sodium Excretion by Normal and Edematous Men, *J. Clin. Invest.*, **35**:1299, 1956.
19. Liddle, G. W.: Sodium Diuresis Induced by Steroidal Antagonists of Aldosterone, *Science*, **126**:1016, 1957.
20. Leaf, A., and Mamby, A. R.: An Antidiuretic Mechanism Not Regulated by Extracellular Fluid Tonicity, *J. Clin. Invest.*, **31**:60, 1952.
21. Bercu, B. A., Rokaw, S. N., and Massie, E.: Antidiuretic Action of the Urine of Patients in Cardiac Failure, *Circulation*, **2**:409, 1950.
22. Henry, J. P., Gauer, O. H., and Reeves, J. L.: Evidence of the Atrial Location of Receptors Influencing Urine Flow, *Circulation Res.*, **4**:91, 1956.
23. Berliner, R. W., and Davidson, D. G.: Production of Hypertonic Urine in the Absence of Pituitary Antidiuretic Hormone, *J. Clin. Invest.*, **36**:1416, 1957.
24. Schedl, H. P., and Bartter, F. C.: An Explanation for and Experimental Correction of the Abnormal Water Diuresis in Cirrhosis, *J. Clin. Invest.*, **39**:248, 1960.
25. Barger, A. C., Muldewney, F. P., and Liebowitz, M. R.: Role of the Kidney in the Pathogenesis of Congestive Heart Failure, *Circulation*, **20**:273, 1959.
26. Davis, J. O., Holman, J. E., Carpenter, C. C. J., Urquhart, J., and Higgins, J. T., Jr.: An Extraadrenal Factor Essential for Chronic Renal Sodium Retention in Presence of Increased Sodium-Retaining Hormone. *Circulation Res.*, **14**:17, 1964.

13 DISTURBANCE OF INORGANIC METABOLISM IN HEART FAILURE

William C. Waters, III, M.D.

OUTLINE OF WATER AND ELECTROLYTE PHYSIOLOGY OF THE NEPHRON

Deficits and excesses of sodium, potassium, and water are averted in health by means of delicate control mechanisms which involve the pituitary, the adrenal, and the kidney. It is perhaps simplest to consider these devices from the point of view of the nephron, the "final common pathway" through which selective excretion or reabsorption of these substances is accomplished.

Approximately one-fifth of the minute cardiac output is diverted into the renal circulation. This blood (approximately 1 liter per min) is filtered at the glomerulus, and one-tenth of this volume (approximately 100 ml per min) enters the nephron as the *glomerular filtrate*. At this point, in the proximal renal tubule, the filtrate is approximately isotonic with plasma and the active processes concerned with reabsorption begin. Best available evidence indicates that sodium is actively pumped from the tubular lumen, to be followed by the passive migration of an equivalent quantity of anion; simultaneously osmotic forces impel water to move from the tubular lumen into the interstitium of the kidney and thence to the peritubular blood.[1,2] This process thus accounts for the isotonic reabsorption of some 85 per cent of the glomerular filtrate. The influences which control the degree of reabsorption are poorly understood, but much information indicates that a greater percentage of reabsorption takes place when glomerular filtration rate is depressed, as for example in renal artery constriction, extracellular fluid volume depletion, or congestive heart failure.[3–6] Hormonal influences have been suggested, but proof is lacking. In this proximal segment, potassium is virtually completely reabsorbed.[7]

The tubular fluid subsequently passes through the loop of Henle and then to the distal tubule and finally into the collecting duct. During its passage through these structures, a series of operations takes place in which an osmotic *countercurrent gradient*[8,9] is established within the interstitial portion of the kidney, so that as tubular fluid passes down the final segment of the nephron it is exposed to progressively greater forces tending to abstract water from the interior of the tubule.[2] Passive movement of water can then take place, providing the tubular wall is rendered water-permeable through the presence of *antidiuretic hormone* (ADH) from the posterior pituitary gland.[2] Thus, in hydropenic states, high concentrations of ADH are available, water is removed from the filtrate, and a concentrated urine results; when the fluid bathing the hypophyseal osmoreceptors is diluted, ADH is withheld, water remains within the tubule, and a dilute urine is produced.

In the *distal tubule* and *collecting duct*, sodium reabsorption—still an active process—is matched by passive chloride reabsorption, or by exchange for potassium and hydrogen.[10] In this distal site, the potent mineralocorticoid *aldosterone* is operative, high concentrations tending to accelerate sodium reabsorption (resulting in hydrogen and potassium loss).[11] It now appears that factors which result in a shrinkage of intravascular volume activate juxtaglomerular cells to produce renin, which results in production of angiotensin II, which in turn stimulates the adrenal cortex to elaborate aldosterone.[12] The resultant sodium retention tends to return extracellular fluid volume toward normal.

PATHOPHYSIOLOGY OF THE NEPHRON IN CONGESTIVE HEART FAILURE: CLINICAL CONSEQUENCES

When these delicately balanced mechanisms are subjected to the changes produced by congestive heart failure, the role of these systems in preserving homeostasis may be so altered that they may contribute to, rather than offset, the pathologic process. Indeed, most of the familiar objective findings of congestive heart failure are the direct result of altered fluid and electrolyte handling deriving from physiologic disturbance in the nephron.

Disturbances of Sodium Metabolism

With a fall in effective cardiac output, a commensurate reduction in renal plasma flow occurs. However, since the filtration fraction is often elevated, glomerular filtration rate may be relatively well preserved.[13,14] Because of this phenomenon, the "forward-failure" theory has been regarded as an inadequate explanation for the positive salt and water balance of congestive failure.[15,16] Nonetheless, methods for measuring glomerular filtration rate are sufficiently inaccurate that even minor alterations in proximal tubular flow may be important. For example, if proximal sodium and water reabsorption rate remains fixed while a 2 per cent fall in glomerular filtration rate occurs, an enormous daily addition of fluid to the body will occur.* At any rate, very substantial evidence indicates that the most quantitatively important site for salt and water retention in congestive heart failure lies within the proximal tubule, and distal mechanisms may be regarded as only "fine tuning" devices for further adjustment of fluid excretion.

In far-advanced heart failure, or in moderate heart failure under vigorous therapy with diuretics and salt restriction, detectable or even very striking increases in aldosterone production have been noted.[17-19] Influences of this hormone produce a further retention of sodium, largely in the distal tubule, and an augmented excretion of potassium. As a result, it is common to find urinary sodium concentrations of less than 1 mEq per 24 hr even when intake of sodium is normal. In such patients, daily weight gain can be predicted from the sodium content of the diet (e.g., 8 Gm daily = 136 mEq daily = 1 L of extracellular fluid = 2.2 lb weight gain daily).

It is these exaggerations of physiologic mechanisms that diuretic therapy is designed to oppose. Aminophylline (theophylline), for example, operates by increasing cardiac output and renal plasma flow and also opposes sodium reabsorption in the proximal tubule; mercurials inhibit proximal reabsorptive processes; and the thiazides both antagonize proximal retention and inhibit distal sodium removal by interfering with the enzyme carbonic anhydrase. The spirolactones oppose the action of aldosterone.[20] It is also through the agency of diuretics that many of the clinical disturbances of body electrolyte composition in congestive heart failure occur (see below).

Disturbances of Potassium Metabolism

As in the normal nephron, potassium is filtered at the glomerulus, virtually completely reabsorbed in the proximal tubule, and excreted in the distal tubule and collecting duct in exchange for sodium.[10] The rate of excretion at the distal site will therefore be dependent on three factors: (1) the degree of aldosterone activity; (2) the rate of sodium delivery to the distal exchange site; and (3) the presence or absence of carbonic anhydrase inhibition by diuretics. As might be predicted, potassium deficiency is common and potassium excess is occasionally noted in patients under therapy for congestive heart failure.

1. Potassium depletion. Like other chronically ill individuals, patients with congestive heart failure are subject to episodes of anorexia, vomiting, and diarrhea, with consequent increased potassium loss and decreased intake. In addition, these patients may exhibit a continuously accelerated potassium excretion rate resulting from secondary hyperaldosteronism. Even more important, however, is the effect of diuretics in augmenting distal tubular sodium delivery; indeed the major reason for the kaliopenic effects of the thiazide diuretics is this tendency to flood the distal exchange site.[20] It can be predicted, in fact, that potassium depletion of some degree will result if thiazide-induced diuresis of more than 4 or 5 lb occurs within 1 or 2 days unless supplementary potassium is given, and severe degrees of potassium depletion with weakness or paralysis have been reported. Even more treacherous, of course, is the augmentation of digitalis effect produced by hypokalemia; the "postdiuretic redigitalization phenomenon" with digitalis intoxication and arrhythmia is well known.

2. Potassium intolerance. Because of the high rate of proximal tubular sodium removal (and, hence, low distal sodium delivery) characteristic of patients with moderate to severe heart failure, maximum potassium excretion can approach a "ceiling." Since the body has no provision for storing "excess" potassium, extracellular potassium concentration may rise, and cardiotoxicity may result. It is not widely appreciated that potassium intoxication occurs outside the setting of renal failure, but the author has personally seen nine patients with severe heart failure and no overt renal disease who first announced their state of potassium intoxication by development of complete heart block or sinus arrest. In all instances where therapy was effective in correcting hyperkalemia, a return to normal sinus rhythm ensued. All these patients were receiving supplementary potassium salts (3 to 4 Gm daily). Some had stopped taking diuretic agents, but others had continued them; it is significant that where diuretics were being employed, they were ineffective in producing further loss of weight. It appears clear that, although patients with congestive heart failure in an active stage of diuresis require supplementary potassium, such supplements must be used with caution when heart failure is severe or when refractoriness to diuretic agents appears. It should here be noted that the degree of cardiotoxicity, as mirrored by the electrocardiogram, correlates extremely well with the serum-potassium level, not with total body potassium or tissue potassium, as has been suggested. Indeed, many of the measures designed to combat hyperkalemia result in increased cellular uptake of potassium but with reversion of the electrocardiogram to normal.

* Two per cent × 85 per cent × 100 ml/min = 1.7 ml additional fluid retained per minute = 1.5 L/24 hr.

Table 13-1. THERAPY OF HYPERKALEMIC CARDIOTOXICITY IN CONGESTIVE HEART FAILURE

Method	Dose (adult)	Onset of effect	Duration of effect
Calcium (gluconate)*	10–20 ml 10% solution	1 min	10 min–2 hr
Artificial hyperventilation (positive pressure device)		1–2 min	Only while in use
Intravenous sodium bicarbonate	45 mEq I.V. or 90 mEq/500 ml 10% glucose in water	4–5 min	1–24 hr
Hypertonic glucose and insulin	50 ml 50% solution c. 10 units regular insulin	15 min–1 hr	1–24 hr
Na-K cycle exchange resins	20 Gm orally q 6 h	6–18 hr	Indefinite
Peritoneal or extracorporeal dialysis		1–3 hr	Indefinite

* Intravenous calcium salts probably should not be used in a patient receiving digitalis.

Where the potassium intolerance of congestive heart failure has resulted in hyperkalemia, the measures employed in immediate therapy are similar to those used in acute renal failure (Table 13-1).

Disturbances of Water Metabolism

One of the most familiar and often perplexing therapeutic problems in congestive heart failure is reduction of the serum-sodium concentration. Hyponatremia, often loosely called "the low-salt syndrome," may occur as the result of several entirely different circumstances. It is certainly true that sodium depletion not infrequently occurs as a consequence of continued administration of diuretics and enforcement of sodium restriction beyond a desirable level of reduction in extracellular fluid volume. Patients treated thus complain of thirst, show a narrowing of the pulse pressure (frequently with postural hypotension), have diminished skin turgor, anorexia, and a rise in blood–urea nitrogen and serum-creatinine levels. Generally, addition of small quantities of salt to the diet and temporary interruption of diuretic therapy are all that is required.

On the other hand, the larger group of hyponatremic cardiac patients exhibit low serum-sodium concentrations at a time when edema is present, their chest x-rays reveal evidence of pulmonary congestion, and they are obviously in a state of both sodium and water overload.[21] Mechanisms responsible for this paradoxic state of dilutional hyponatremia are not entirely clear, but several studies have demonstrated that water accumulation, rather than salt loss, is the defect involved.[21,22] Some patients excrete substances with antidiuretic potency, and increased ADH activity undoubtedly plays a role. On the other hand, avid proximal tubular sodium reabsorption—with dimin-

ished urine flow to the distal tubular site where free water is generated ("Berliner effect")[23]—is likely to be a feature of the disturbed physiologic function in at least some patients. Administration of sodium to such patients in an effort to correct serum-electrolyte concentrations regularly results in worsening of the clinical state and may even produce pulmonary edema.[21,22] Most such individuals are not symptomatic from the disturbed electrolyte concentrations but suffer only the effects of heart failure. On the other hand, an occasional patient will exhibit a rapid or profound drop in serum osmolarity and develop "hyponatremic encephalopathy," with stupor, irritability, or even seizures; in such cases cautious administrations of small amounts of hypertonic saline solution, together with water restriction, can be life-saving.

By far the largest proportion of such patients are best managed by regarding the hyponatremia as a symptom, not only of metabolic distress but of further impairment of cardiac function. Several studies have shown that underlying the development of hyponatremia may be such factors as unrecognized pulmonary emboli, unsuspected bronchopulmonary infection, or inadequate digitalization.[22] On the other hand, some patients with congestive heart failure exhibit findings of water intoxication only when presented with an excessive water load, as in phenolsulfonphthalein tests or with too rapid administration of intravenous solutions. The postoperative period is especially treacherous in this respect, and severe degrees of hyponatremia have repeatedly been observed following mitral commissurotomy even though "normal" amounts of water had been administered.[24] In all such cases of dilutional hyponatremia, rational therapy will include water restriction, sometimes to as little as 100 to 300 ml daily. Insensible loss and obligatory urinary losses will effect a slow improvement. Furthermore, the finding of a low serum-sodium concentration is by no means a contraindication to further diuretic therapy. In fact, since the composition of urine during diuresis is almost always hypotonic, a rise in serum-solute concentration can often be effected by employing mercurials or, when circulatory dynamics will permit, osmotic diuretics such as mannitol. Recent evidence has indicated that some hypotonic states will respond to short (1-week) courses of corticosteroids, presumably as a result of the effects of these agents on the water permeability of the distal renal tubule.[25] In addition, of course, the cardiac patient is subject to many other causes of low serum-sodium concentration. A differential diagnosis for this condition is presented in Table 13-2.

Disturbances of Acid-Base Balance

The only common alterations of acid-base balance in congestive heart failure represent the effects of diuretic agents.[20] Carbonic anhydrase inhibitors, such as Diamox (acetazoleamide), produce a mild metabolic acidosis which is of no clinical significance in therapeutic doses and even may favorably prepare the patient for mercurial action. Mercurials, on the other hand, tend to produce a hypochloremic alkalosis which, when established, inhibits the efficacy of subsequent mercurial injections.[26] Although the potassium-depleting effect and carbonic anhydrase inhibition of the thiazide group produce a mild metabolic alkalosis, the acid-base disturbance is rarely of

clinical consequence. When renal disease complicates congestive failure, chronic metabolic acidosis may constitute a therapeutic problem, since administration of sodium bicarbonate may result in sodium retention. In such instances, sodium bicarbonate therapy may be advantageously combined with vigorous sodium chloride restriction. In rare instances unsupervised administration of ammonium chloride may precipitate severe metabolic acidosis which may be accompanied by a moderate degree of azotemia. In general, however, disturbance in the regulation of plasma bicarbonate is not an important feature of cardiac failure.

In summary, the disturbances of inorganic metabolism in congestive heart failure are most simply viewed as an exaggeration of normal physiologic processes taking place in the nephron. Avid proximal sodium and water reabsorption, coupled with, in many cases, accelerated aldosterone activity, results in expansion of extracellular fluid volume. When sodium reabsorption is blocked and access to dietary sodium prohibited, the tubular effort to conserve volume proceeds without regard for tonicity, and dilutional hyponatremia ensues. Diuretic agents, when effective, may result in potassium depletion; when they are not effective, potassium intoxication may result from injudicious use of potassium supplements.

Abnormalities of blood chemistry in congestive heart failure are in themselves not therapeutic objectives but clues to a clinical disturbance; recognition of the clinical problem and understanding of the pathogenesis of the electrolyte aberration

Table 13-2. CLASSIFICATION OF TYPES OF HYPONATREMIA

Mechanism	Serum Na	Urine Na	BUN*	Body weight	Skin turgor
Cardiac Hyponatremia					
Salt depletion: diuretics, salt restriction	Low	Low	High	Reduced	Reduced
Water retention: postoperative state, bronchopulmonary infection, pulmonary emboli, "escape from digitalization," recurrent myocardial infarctions, excessive water loading, progressive congestive failure	Low	Low	Normal	Increased	Edema
Noncardiac Hyponatremia					
Other edema states: hepatic cirrhosis, nephrotic syndrome	Low	Low	Normal	Increased	Edema
"Pseudohyponatremia": hyperglycemia, hyperlipemia	Low	Normal	Normal	Normal	Normal
Gastrointestinal salt losses	Low	Low	High	Reduced	Reduced
Adrenal insufficiency	Low	High	High	Reduced	Reduced
Renal salt wasting	Low	High	High	Reduced	Reduced
Inappropriate ADH syndrome	Low	High	Low	Increased	Normal

* BUN, blood urea nitrogen.

remain the most important prerequisites to appropriate therapy.

REFERENCES

1. Ussing, H. H.: Transport of Ions across Cellular Membranes, *Physiol. Rev.*, **29:**127, 1949.
2. Berliner, R. W., Levinsky, N. G., Davidson, D. G., and Eden, M.: Dilution and Concentration of the Urine and the Action of Antidiuretic Hormone, *Am. J. Med.*, **24:**730, 1958.
3. Post, R. S.: Decrease of Cardiac Output by Acute Pericardial Effusion and Its Effect on Renal Hemodynamics and Electrolyte Excretion, *Am. J. Physiol.*, **165:**278, 1951.
4. Thompson, D. D., and Pitts, R. F.: Effects of Alterations of Renal Arterial Pressure on Sodium and Water Excretion, *Am. J. Physiol.*, **168:**490, 1952.
5. Levitt, N. F., Turner, L. B., and Sweet, A. Y.: The Effect of Experimental Venous Obstruction on Salt and Water Distribution and Excretion in Man, *J. Clin. Invest.*, **31:** 885, 1952.
6. Farber, S. J., Becher, W. H., and Eidma, I. W.; Electrolyte and Water Excretion and Renal Hemodynamics during Induced Congestion of the Superior and Inferior Vena Cava of Man, *J. Clin. Invest.*, **32:**1145, 1953.
7. Berliner, R. W., Kennedy, T. J., Jr., and Hilton, J. G.: Renal Mechanism for the Excretion of Potassium, *Am. J. Physiol.*, **162:**348, 1950.
8. Kuhn, W., and Ruffel, K.: Herstellung konzentrieter Losungen aus verdunnten durch blosse Membranwirkung: Ein Modellversuch zur Funktion der Niere, *Ztschr. physiol. Chem.*, **276:**145, 1942.
9. Gottschalk, C. W.: Micropuncture Studies of tubular Function in the Mammalian Kidney, *Physiologist*, **4:**35, 1961.
10. Berliner, R. W., Kennedy, T. J., Jr., and Orloff, J.: Factors Affecting the Transport of Potassium and Hydrogen Ions by the Renal Tubules, *Arch Internat. pharmacodyn.*, **97:**299, 1954.
11. Bartter, F. C.: The Role of Aldosterone in Normal Homeostasis and in Certain Disease States, *Metabolism*, **4:**369, 1956.
12. Carpenter, C. C. J., Davis, J. O., and Ayers, C. R.: Relation of Renin, Angiotensin II, and Experimental Renal Hypertension to Aldosterone Secretion, *J. Clin. Invest.*, **40:**2026, 1961.
13. Barger, A. C.: The Pathogenesis of Sodium Retention in Congestive Heart Failure, *Metabolism*, **5:**480, 1956.
14. Werko, L., Varnauskas, W., Eliasch, H., Ek, J., Bueht, H., Thomasson, B., and Bergstrom, J.: Studies on the Renal Function in Mitral Valvular Disease. 1. Effect of Exercise, *Circulation*, **9:**687, 1954.
15. Briggs, A. P., Fowell, D. M., Hamilton, W. F., Remington, J. W., Wholler, N. C., and Winslow, J. W.: Renal and Circulatory Factors in the Edema Formation of Congestive Heart Failure, *J. Clin. Invest.*, **27:**810, 1948.
16. Heller, B. I., and Jacobson, W. E.: Renal Hemodynamics in Heart Disease, *Am. Heart J.*, **39:**188, 1950.
17. Duncan, L. E., Jr., Liddle, G. W., and Bartter, F. C.: The Effect of Changes in Body Sodium on Extracellular Fluid Volume and Aldosterone and Sodium Excretion by Normal and Edematous Man, *J. Clin. Invest.*, **35:**1299, 1956.
18. Singer, B., and Wenes, J.: Excretion of Sodium-retaining Substances in Patients with Congestive Heart Failure, *Am. Heart J.*, **45:**795, 1953.
19. Luetscher, A. J., Jr., Neher, R., and Weltstein, A.: Isolation of Crystalline Aldosterone from the Urine of a Nephrotic Patient, *Experimentation*, **10:**456, 1954.
20. Pitts, R. F.: Some Reflections on Mechanisms of Action of Diuretics, *Am. J. Med.*, **24:**745, 1958.
21. Orloff, J., Walser, M., Kennedy, T. J., and Bartter, F. C.: Hyponatremia. *Circulation*, **19:**284, 1959.
22. Weston, R. E., Grossman, J., Borun, E. R., and Hanenson, I. B.: The Pathogenesis and Treatment of Hyponatremia in Congestive Heart Failure, *Am. J. Med.*, **25:**558, 1958.
23. Berliner, R. W., and Davidson, D. G.: Production of Hypertonic Urine in the Absence of Pituitary Antidiuretic Hormone, *J. Clin. Invest.*, **36:**1416, 1957.
24. Wilson, G. M., Edelman, I. S., Brooks, L., Myrden, J. A., Harken, D. E., and Moore, F. D.: Metabolic Changes Associated with Mitral Valvuloplasty, *Circulation*, **9:**199, 1954.
25. Orloff, J., and Berliner, R. W.: Renal Pharmacology, *Ann. Rev. Pharm.*, **1:**287, 1961.
26. Schwartz, W. B., and Wallace, W. M.: Electrolyte Equilibrium during Osmotic Diuresis, *J. Clin. Invest.*, **30:**1089, 1951.

14 ETIOLOGY AND CLINICAL RECOGNITION OF HEART FAILURE

R. Bruce Logue, M.D., and
J. Willis Hurst, M.D.

ETIOLOGY OF HEART FAILURE

It is not sufficient merely to establish the presence of heart failure—the *cause* must be found. The cause may be elusive and unknown, but it must be sought. There is a marked difference between not knowing the cause of a type of heart failure and disregarding its cause. Not only must the cause of the basic heart disease be established, but the factors that might precipitate or aggravate heart failure must also be identified.

The diagnostic clues that enable one to identify specific types of heart disease are discussed in detail throughout the book and will not be repeated here. The *age* of the patient is extremely important in establishing the general type of heart disease responsible for heart failure. Accordingly, this statistical information has been consolidated here for convenience. Heart failure during the early years of life is usually due to congenital heart disease but may, on occasion, be due to myocarditis or ectopic tachycardia.[1–3] Between birth and 1 week of age, aortic atresia is the most frequent cause of congestive heart failure. Between 1 week and 1 month of age, coarctation of the aorta and transposition of the great vessels are the most common causes of failure and are followed in frequency by endomyocardial disease, ventricular septal defect, and patent ductus arteriosus. Between 3 and 6 months of age, endomyocardial disease is the most frequent cause of failure, followed in frequency by ventricular septal defect, patent ductus arteriosus, total anomalous pulmonary venous return, coarctation of the aorta, and transposition of the great vessels. Note that transposition of the great vessels, a condition usually associated with cyanosis, is a common cause of heart failure during the early months of life. Therefore, heart failure in this age group associated with definite, persistent cyanosis suggests the diagnosis of transposition of the great vessels. From birth to 6 months of age, paroxysmal atrial tachycardia may precipitate acute, catastrophic heart failure in the absence of other evidence of heart disease.

When heart failure develops in infants between 6 and 12 months of age, it is wise to search for ventricular septal defect and endomyocardial disease. Between 5 and 15 years of age, the cause of failure is likely to be acute rheumatic myocarditis, acute glomerulonephritis, or less commonly congenital heart disease (ventricular septal defect, atrial septal defect of the ostium primum type, or patent ductus arteriosus). Note that uncomplicated tetralogy of Fallot is not a common cause of heart failure. Atrial septal defect, of the secundum type, and congenital and acquired valve disease rarely produce heart failure during early life. In young adults, however, congestive heart failure is frequently due to rheumatic mitral and aortic valve disease. Young women more often have mitral valve disease, especially mitral stenosis, which is the most common cause of heart failure. In young adults, acute rheumatic carditis should be considered when the valve disease seems to be an inadequate cause for heart failure. Young adults also have nonrheumatic myocardial disease, and congenital heart disease may occasionally produce heart failure at this age. The congenital abnormalities which are likely to be responsible include ventricular septal defect, atrial septal defect, and patent ductus arteriosus.

After the age of 40, heart failure is usually due to one of the following causes: coronary atherosclerosis with myocardial infarction, diastolic hypertension (usually above 110 mm Hg), valvular heart disease, pulmonary disease, or diffuse myocardial disease. At times, heart failure may be due to a combination of congenital heart disease and acquired disease. It is not unusual, in such cases, for the congenital disease to be misdiagnosed, since the clinical picture is likely to be altered considerably by the acquired disease.

After age 50, the most commonly overlooked cause of congestive heart failure[4] due to valve disease is calcific aortic stenosis, due either to congenital bicuspid valves or to rheumatic heart disease. This is particularly true if the patient is male.

The following discussion deals mainly with congestive heart failure as found in adults. Congestive heart failure in children is discussed in Chap. 20.

FACTORS THAT PRECIPITATE AND AGGRAVATE HEART FAILURE

Although congestive heart failure may occur in the natural history of organic heart disease, it is prudent to look for certain additional factors which may either *precipitate or aggravate heart failure*. The patient with organic heart disease who is active and asymptomatic does not usually develop heart failure within a few minutes, hours, or days unless some new factor has been added. Common causes of acute changes in cardiac compensation are myocardial infarction, ectopic cardiac rhythms, and pulmonary emboli. Extraordinary effort and excessive intravenous fluids may also acutely precipitate heart failure in patients who have heart disease. It is wise to search for additional cardiac and extracardiac factors when heart failure develops more gradually, for example, over a period of a few days to several weeks. These factors may include myocardial infarction, ectopic cardiac rhythm, pulmonary emboli, pulmonary infection, renal disease including infection, acute rheumatic fever in the child, bacterial endocarditis, prostatic obstruction in the elderly male, cerebral vascular accident, thyrotoxicosis, anemia, liver disease, pregnancy, corticosteroid or estrogen administration, increased work load, and emotional stress. These same factors may also be responsible for poorly controlled or even refractory heart failure in some patients.

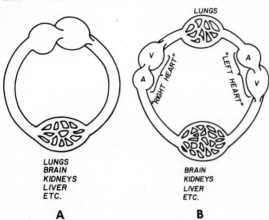

Fig. 14-1A. Schema of a theoretical one-pump circulatory system. The pump is composed of one atrium and one ventricle. The lungs, brain, kidneys, liver, etc., are downstream from the pump. All diseases of the pump would affect the organs and the peripheral circulation in the same way. When it fails to pump out the blood that comes to it, the pump becomes larger. The pressure in the circulation gradually approaches that of a stagnant circulation. Inadequate perfusion of the organs would produce dysfunction of the organs. The dysfunction of the kidneys would lead to retention of salt and water which, along with venous constriction, would produce engorgment of the organs and increase in venous pressure. The lungs would be ineffective in this system. *B.* The two-pump system. The two-pump system is composed of the left atrium and ventricle and the right atrium and ventricle. (The two atria act as reservoirs and booster pumps for the ventricles.) The lungs are uniquely located between the two pumps. Diseases affecting the left side of the heart can produce different symptoms compared with diseases of the right side. Acute disease of the left side of the heart is associated with an abrupt fall in output while the right side of the heart continues to pump normally. The lungs suffer and edema develops. After a short time the outputs of the two ventricles become equal again. At the same time, the perfusion of the kidneys, brain, liver, etc., is altered. If the inadequacy continues, the kidneys will retain salt and water. Poor function of the right ventricle will not flood the lungs with excess blood. The left ventricle ejects only the blood delivered to it by the right ventricle plus the amount in the lungs. This amount of blood is not sufficient to raise the venous pressure and produce engorgment of the organs. The increased blood volume and systemic venous constriction produce the increased peripheral venous pressure and organ engorgment. The lungs in such a system have the vital advantage of being able to gather oxygen and eliminate carbon dioxide efficiently, but they have the disadvantage of being vulnerable to pulmonary edema. (*Adapted from G. E. Burch and C. T. Ray, Am. Heart J.,* 41:918–946, 1951, *with permission of the authors and publisher.*)

SYMPTOMS AND CLINICAL SYNDROMES ASSOCIATED WITH HEART FAILURE

Failure of the circulation occurs whenever the circulatory system is unable to meet the metabolic needs of the body. *Peripheral circulatory failure* (shock) occurs when the amount of blood is not sufficient to fill the vascular bed adequately, whether or not the heart is normal. *Heart failure* occurs when the diseased heart is unable to pump an adequate amount of blood to meet the particular metabolic demands of the body at the moment.[5–8]

In order to understand the signs and symptoms of heart failure, it is necessary to consider certain aspects of the physiologic derangement associated with the disorder known as heart failure.

Viewed simply, the heart is a pump that receives blood from the veins and ejects blood into the arteries. The uniqueness of the human circulation is best emphasized by contrasting and comparing a theoretical one-pump circulatory system with a two-pump system (Fig. 14-1A and *B*).[9,10]

In a theoretical *one-pump* circulatory system (Fig. 14-1A), the heart would pump blood through the arteries to all the veins and the veins would return the blood to the heart. In this system the imaginary heart is composed of two parts: a ventricle, which is the major pump for the system, and an atrium, which functions as a reservoir and as a booster pump for the ventricle. Note that all organs, including the lungs, are located in the peripheral part of the vascular circuit. Since only a portion of the blood would pass through the lungs with each passage, only that portion of the blood flow passing through the lungs would be normally oxygenated. This blood would then mix with the blood returning from the other organs to return to the heart and eventually to become the arterial blood for all organs.

In such a one-pump system, failure of the pump would cause similar changes in the circulation irrespective of the cause of the heart failure. If the ventricle were unable to empty itself completely, its end-systolic and end-diastolic volumes would increase very slightly. This amount of blood would be transferred from the systemic (mainly venous) circulation to the heart without a significant change in venous pressure. The change in ventricular and end-diastolic fiber length produced by this transfer might compensate the ventricle for a while. If the ventricle were to fail more markedly, the output of the ventricle and the arterial pressure would decrease, but the venous pressure would not increase significantly unless there were an increase either in blood volume or in venous vasoconstriction. If the pump stops completely, the arterial and venous pressures equilibrate at the static, or stagnant, pressure of the system.

In this system, the basic consequence of failure of the pump from whatever cause is an inadequate perfusion of all organs, and there is no significant change in venous pressure (i.e., no congestion or damming up of blood) produced by the failure per se. The venous pressure increases significantly only if there is an increase in blood volume or if there is reflex venous vasoconstriction.

The human heart is, fortunately, made up of two pumps: the right atrium and ventricle (referred to as the right side of the heart) and the left atrium and ventricle (referred to as the left side of the heart). The atria serve as reservoirs and booster pumps for the more powerful ventricles. This more efficient system retains certain characteristics of the one-pump system but has some unique features. In this system, the lungs are located between the two pumps while all other organs are located downstream from the pumping system. Since certain diseases damage mainly the left side of the heart and others damage mainly the right side of the heart, it is *possible for the lungs to be affected differently, depending on which side of the heart is damaged.*

When the left ventricle cannot eject blood normally following a sudden insult, such as occurs with acute myocardial infarction, the lungs suffer, since they still receive blood from the right side of the heart.

For a short period of time, the right ventricle may pump more blood to the lungs than the left side of the heart pumps to the body. The result of this inequality is an increase in pulmonary blood volume. This increase may be produced acutely without a change in total blood volume by a redistribution of blood to the lungs from the peripheral venous system without a significant change in venous pressure. Eventually, however, the output of the two ventricles must equilibrate. This may occur as the result of an increase in left ventricular output secondary to the increased pulmonary venous pressure and greater filling of the left ventricle or as the result of a decrease in right ventricular output.

The engorgement of lungs due to failure of the left side of the heart is clinically termed left-sided *backward failure.* Unless the output of the left ventricle is restored to normal by greater filling, there is also *forward failure,* since the peripheral organs do not receive an adequate supply of blood. As the result of this forward failure, many complex feedback mechanisms are brought into action. Three of the more important of these are selective alterations in peripheral vascular tone and altered renal function produced by reflexes from stretch receptors in the carotid sinus ond other areas, retention of sodium and water produced by the altered renal hemodynamics, and changes in the renin-angiotensin-aldosterone system.

When the right ventricle fails acutely and is unable to pump a normal amount of blood to the lungs, a somewhat different syndrome is produced. In this situation it is not possible for the left ventricle to pump more blood than the right ventricle for any significant length of time, since the amount of blood in the lungs (400 to 800 ml) and in the left side of the heart would rapidly be depleted. Even if a large proportion of this blood were redistributed behind the right ventricle in the venous system, it would not by itself produce a significant increase in venous pressure. In this situation venous pressure increases predominantly as the consequence of an increased blood volume secondary to renal retention of sodium and water and of an increase in systemic venous vasoconstriction.[11-14] Both these responses are, at least in part, the result of inadequate flow from the left side of the heart (forward failure).

In most situations, the clinical syndrome of congestive heart failure is the result both of mechanisms referred to as forward failure and of mechanisms referred to as backward failure. The major consequences of forward failure are produced by an inadequate output of the left ventricle and by an abnormal arterial pressure pulse. These may produce important alterations in renal function and in peripheral arterial and venous tone. Backward failure is responsible for the accumulation of blood behind the involved ventricle. Pure backward failure of the left ventricle may produce severe pulmonary congestion; pure backward failure of the right ventricle rarely, if ever, produces significant systemic venous congestion.

This discussion of forward failure and of backward failure is not intended to overemphasize these concepts. It is realized that these terms are oversimplifications of very complex reactions and that many persons have abandoned the use of these expressions. Nevertheless, it is felt that these concepts still have some value in a discussion of the basic mechanisms of heart failure.

Although both backward and forward failure is usually present in a given patient, it is valuable to divide the clinical syndromes of heart failure into "left-sided heart failure" and "right-sided heart failure." This is possible because the lungs are "trapped" between the two pumps. Accordingly, diseases of the left side of the heart are more likely to produce pulmonary congestion, whereas poor function of the right side of the heart is more likely to produce peripheral edema and increased venous engorgement and pressure. Since the left side of the heart is more often affected by disease than the right side, and since left-sided heart failure produces an increase in pressures in the pulmonary circuit—and, in time, produces an increase in both pulmonary and total blood volume—the most common cause of "right-sided heart failure" is "left-sided heart failure" of long duration. Accordingly, it is possible for a patient to have both left- and right-sided heart failure. Despite the overlap of symptoms and signs in such patients, considerable useful clinical information may be gained from a careful evaluation of the patient's symptoms and from examination of the heart, arteries, veins, and other organs. The ultimate goal is the therapy of the patient. This is best accomplished by the physician's thinking in terms of the altered physiologic function in an individual patient. Often, when the cause of the basic heart disease is known, it is possible to predict and to look for signs of heart failure which are characteristic of that lesion. Conversely, when the basic heart disease is not known, or is poorly understood, it is possible to gain insight regarding the cause of the disease by carefully identifying the particular signs and symptoms of heart failure.

As a rule, the diagnosis of congestive heart failure in a patient is made from the presence of a group of signs and symptoms. Clues to the existence of heart failure are usually found in the patient's history, physical examination, and chest x-ray. Special tests, such as venous pressure, circulation time, and vital capacity are usually not necessary; and the electrocardiogram gives absolutely no information regarding the presence or absence of heart failure.

Symptoms Due to Failure of the Left Side of the Heart

Most types of heart disease affect primarily and initially the left side of the heart. The output from the left atrium may be blocked by mitral stenosis, or the left ventricle may function abnormally as a result of coronary artery disease, myocardial disease, systemic hypertension, or disease of the aortic or mitral valves. The patient with "left-sided heart failure" complains of "breathlessness" or "shortness of breath." The medical term for this unpleasant subjective sensation is *dyspnea*.[15–18] In many situations it occurs when emptying of the left ventricle becomes impaired. As a result of this impairment, the left ventricular residual volume increases and the left ventricular diastolic pressure increases. In turn, there is an elevation of left atrial, pulmonary venous, and pulmonary capillary pressures. When the pulmonary capillary pressure is below the level of the oncotic pressure of plasma proteins (25 to 30 mm Hg), there is minimal

exudation of fluid from the pulmonary capillaries and there are no physical signs such as rales. When the hydrostatic pressure in the pulmonary capillary bed exceeds the oncotic pressure of plasma proteins, however, transudation into surrounding tissue occurs. This produces *interstitial pulmonary edema* and, when advanced in degree, *alveolar pulmonary edema*. The increased turgidity and decreased compliance of the congested lung increases the work of breathing and is in part responsible for the subjective symptom of dyspnea. Dyspnea may also be related to an inadequate blood flow to the respiratory muscles. This latter mechanism may be in part responsible for the dyspnea associated with cardiac lesions which are not associated with pulmonary congestion, e.g., pulmonary stenosis.

Dyspnea on Effort.[19,20] Dyspnea on effort is a common and relatively early symptom of left ventricular failure. This is not surprising since one of the characteristics of heart failure is the inability of the heart to increase its output normally in response to exercise. Dyspnea on effort may be obscured in the following circumstances:

1. When the patients decrease their physical activities. Patients may not be completely aware that this has occurred. Patients with congenital disease or slowly progressive acquired disease may gradually adjust to less physical activity and may not recognize an abnormality of breathing. Such patients may recognize dyspnea only in retrospect after corrective surgery.

2. Sedentary persons whose activity is so limited for other reasons that respiratory symptoms do not develop.

3. Chronically ill or bedridden patients.

4. Patients who are phlegmatic or who are stoical may not appreciate the symptom of dyspnea as early as anxious patients. This variable factor makes it difficult to correlate the symptoms of dyspnea with the degree of heart failure.

5. Patients with cerebral disease with obtunded consciousness may be completely unaware of symptoms.

The symptom of dyspnea on effort is not specific for congestive heart failure. Chronic lung disease, obesity, and poor physical fitness can produce this complaint. The latter two conditions are usually obvious, but the effect of chronic lung disease is not so easily eliminated, especially when heart disease and lung disease coexist. When there has been a rather definite change in exercise tolerance over a short period of time, heart failure rather than lung disease should be suspected. As a rule, the dyspnea associated with chronic lung disease develops more gradually and the patient learns to live within certain limits in order to avoid the unpleasant symptoms. On the other hand, when pulmonary infection, increased bronchospasm, or pneumothorax becomes superimposed on the basic lung disease, abrupt changes in effort tolerance may develop and the dyspnea may closely mimic congestive heart failure.

Patients with diabetic acidosis or renal acidosis may breathe deeply and rapidly and may appear to have respiratory distress; however, these patients rarely complain of dyspnea.

During the late stage of pregnancy the patient may "huff and puff"—even noisily—and may complain in a detached manner of difficulty with breathing. She is rarely concerned or distressed about it.

The dyspnea of anxiety is quite different from the dyspnea of heart failure. The patient with anxiety has deep, sighing respirations and a feeling that the "breath does not go down." [4] Hyperventilation, fatigue, and other symptoms of anxiety are often present.

Patients with severe anemia may become dyspneic with effort. It is surprising how a phlegmatic patient at times may experience neither dyspnea nor fatigue despite a hematocrit of 10 per cent.

Orthopnea. Patients who have more advanced degrees of pulmonary congestion due to failure of the left side of the heart sleep more comfortably with the upper part of their body elevated. They experience dyspnea in the recumbent position and have less dyspnea in the upright position. This is because of (1) decreased venous return in the upright position, (2) decreased hydrostatic pressure in the upper portion of the lungs in the upright position, (3) increase in vital capacity in the upright position. At times the patient may go to sleep lying flat but later awaken because of breathlessness, which requires him to sit upright.

At times, patients with mitral stenosis may lose the symptom of orthopnea as their disease progresses.[21] This phenomenon has been attributed to the development of relative tricuspid regurgitation, which may indeed be present; it may also be due to the development of pulmonary arteriosclerosis and increased pulmonary arteriolar resistance, which tends to "protect" the pulmonary capillaries. In exceptional cases of mitral stenosis, the pulmonary arteriolar resistance may develop so rapidly and to such a marked degree that orthopnea and paroxysmal nocturnal dyspnea do not occur. In such patients fatigue and evidence of right-sided heart failure may dominate the clinical picture, although dyspnea on exertion is still experienced. In these patients the marked elevations of left atrial pressure, which are ordinarily associated with effort and excitement in patients with mitral stenosis, may not occur. Orthopnea may also decrease in patients who have left ventricular failure

due to other causes. This decrease may be due to the development of tricuspid regurgitation although other factors may be present.

The symptom of orthopnea is not specific for left-sided heart failure. The patient with chronic lung disease, such as pulmonary emphysema, may choose to sleep with his head and trunk elevated: the abdominal organs crowd the lung space in the recumbent position, the bronchi may become smaller when the patient lies down, and the work of breathing may be greater in the recumbent position. In such patients, other clues usually indicate that lung disease is present but it may be difficult to exclude associated left heart disease. Clues which are useful in separating the symptoms of heart disease from lung disease are discussed in Chap. 4.

Cardiac Asthma.[22-27] Wheezing due to bronchospasm, termed *cardiac asthma,* may be the dominant complaint of patients with left-sided heart failure. Individuals with interstitial pulmonary edema vary in their susceptibility to bronchospasm. Patients with left-sided heart failure who have a tendency to bronchospasm from other causes, such as chronic bronchitis or allergy, are more likely to wheeze than those without such a condition; however, wheezing due to heart failure may occur without associated lung disease. In the absence of pulmonary disease, the presence of asthma should be considered a symptom of left-sided heart failure. Cardiac asthma usually occurs on effort or paroxysmally during the night. The patient may or may not be aware of wheezing, and occasionally he may complain only of restlessness and cough. Patients who complain of a "rattling sensation" in the chest, as contrasted to wheezing, usually have more advanced alveolar pulmonary edema rather than the more common and milder interstitial edema.

Patients with bronchial asthma, with or without chronic lung disease, may also experience increasing wheezing and coughing with effort. As a rule, the long history of these symptoms will aid in identifying the nature of the problem. The clinical distinction between these two causes of wheezing becomes more difficult when chronic lung disease is associated with left-sided heart disease. Additional clues found on physical examination and x-ray of the chest may aid in identifying the relative contribution of the lung disease and the heart disease to the clinical picture. Occasionally, the response of the patient to therapy for heart failure may be necessary to clarify the problem.

Paroxysmal Nocturnal Dyspnea.[28,29] Patients with left-sided heart failure are said to have paroxysmal nocturnal dyspnea when they suddenly awaken with dyspnea a few hours after retiring.

They often sit on the side of the bed or get up for a drink of water. Occasionally they go to the window for "a breath of fresh air." The symptoms may subside on return to bed and may not recur during the remainder of the night. When the patient is examined by a physician some hours later, there may be no rales or venous distension; and there may or may not be a ventricular diastolic gallop rhythm. The chest x-ray at this time may reveal evidence of interstitial pulmonary edema, which may be an earlier manifestation of left-sided heart failure than orthopnea or even paroxysmal nocturnal dyspnea.

Paroxysmal nocturnal dyspnea is one of the most specific symptoms of left-sided heart failure. The symptom complex must occur as described above, since many patients who are initially thought to have paroxysmal nocturnal dyspnea do not have these symptoms as described if they are carefully questioned. Even this symptom complex is not specific for left-sided heart failure. Patients with advanced pulmonary emphysema and chronic bronchitis may have "paroxysmal nocturnal dyspnea" because of increased wheezing associated with the recumbent position and perhaps because of the accumulation of bronchial secretions when lying flat. Pulmonary emboli may of course occur at night and produce paroxysmal nocturnal dyspnea, but it is unlikely that a patient would have repeated pulmonary emboli for several nights in succession. Anxious patients may awaken from sleep, with or without recalling a nightmare, and sit on the side of the bed and have an episode of extreme hyperventilation. They may go to the window searching for air and finally return to bed. Such an episode is rarely as "paroxysmal"as the type related to heart failure, and it is just as likely to occur soon after the patient drops off to sleep as it is to awaken the patient a few hours later. The collateral evidence of anxiety noted at the time of the episode or obtained by history, and the absence of signs of heart disease serve to identify this rather common problem. The diagnostic difficulty arises in the anxious patient with known heart disease.

Cough, Insomnia, and Cheyne-Stokes Respirations. The complaint of cough may be the dominant symptom of left-sided heart failure, rather than dyspnea on exertion, paroxysmal nocturnal dyspnea, or orthopnea.[30] Cough due to congested bronchial mucosa is usually dry, nonproductive, and nocturnal. Cough due to heart failure may appear on first assuming the recumbent position or may be troublesome throughout the night. Its cardiac origin is frequently overlooked, particularly when the cough first appears after a respiratory infection. It is common in children with congenital heart disease due to left-to-right shunts. The re-

current attacks of coughing, which are frequent in patients with mitral stenosis, are occasionally misdiagnosed as "winter bronchitis." Cough due to heart failure may be present with or without rales; the cardiac origin of the cough may occasionally be revealed by the pattern of interstitial edema in the chest x-ray. In some patients, a therapeutic trial of digitalis and diuresis may be needed to differentiate cough due to bronchial infection or disease from cough due to left-sided heart failure. The prompt subsidence of cough after several days of therapy favors a cardiac origin.

Patients with left-sided heart failure may complain of restlessness and inability to sleep. In some, the insomnia is due to Cheyne-Stokes breathing, which may be the dominant symptom of heart failure. This type of breathing tends to occur soon after the patient goes to sleep. The patient may awaken during the rapid, deep-breathing phase which follows a period of apnea. Cheyne-Stokes respiration is more likely to occur in association with central nervous system disease. In patients in whom Cheyne-Stokes breathing is caused by heart disease, it appears to be due to a prolonged lung-to-brain circulation time which disturbs the feedback mechanism regulating respiration.[31] Cheyne-Stokes respiration rarely occurs in children and is seldom observed in patients with cor pulmonale. The breathing abnormality is increased by opiates and sedatives and may be prevented or relieved by aminophylline.

Acute Pulmonary Edema.[32-34] The sudden onset of alveolar pulmonary edema is catastrophic; its prompt and proper management is life-saving. To the patient, it is terrifying and he is filled with the fear of impending death, as he literally drowns in his own secretions. He may also complain of faintness and dizziness. Acute pulmonary edema may occur in patients with known symptomatic heart disease, but often it is the presenting symptom complex in a patient whose heart disease has not previously been recognized. It is an expression of disease of the left side of the heart: acute myocardial infarction with or without associated chest pain, tight mitral stenosis, advanced aortic stenosis or insufficiency, or malignant hypertension. In the newborn infant it may occur with ectopic tachycardia.

Acute fulminating alveolar pulmonary edema is uncommon with predominant mitral regurgitation unless this disease is aggravated by uncontrolled arrhythmia. In patients with tight mitral stenosis, severe acute alveolar pulmonary edema is less common when there is marked pulmonary arteriolar disease. Acute alveolar pulmonary edema rarely occurs secondary to left-to-right shunts or diffuse myocardial disease, although pulmonary edema of the interstitial type is common in these conditions. Acute alveolar pulmonary edema does not occur with cor pulmonale, pulmonary stenosis, tetralogy of Fallot, or constrictive pericarditis. The patient with chronic heart failure due to coronary artery disease may develop acute pulmonary edema as the result of further acute myocardial infarction, which may be painless; the onset of ectopic tachycardia; or pulmonary embolism. Ectopic tachycardia or pulmonary embolism may also precipitate acute pulmonary edema in a person with a normal heart.

The circumstances in which an episode of acute pulmonary edema may occur are varied. A middle-aged man with acute myocardial infarction may be awakened from sleep or may develop the symptoms during the course of a normal day's activities; a young woman with tight mitral stenosis may develop pulmonary edema for the first time during sexual intercourse on her wedding night. The patient with pulmonary edema may sit or stand in the upright position. Frequently, he is anxious, pale, or even drenched with sweat. The skin may be cyanotic, cold, and clammy. The respiratory rate is rapid; the depth of respiration may be deep or shallow. Infants often have a respiratory rate of 100 beats per minute; adults commonly have rates of 30 to 40 beats per minute. The alae nasi may be dilated, and the accessory muscles of respiration may be prominent. Retraction of the intercostal spaces and supraclavicular areas is frequently present. There may be coughing, prolonged expiratory wheezing, and rattling sensations in the trachea. The sputum may be profuse, frothy, watery, or even blood-tinged. The pulse rate is rapid. The systolic and diastolic blood pressures may be elevated to high levels; however, if there is profound pulmonary edema, the systemic blood pressure may drop to shock levels. The venous pressure is elevated and the neck veins are distended when the trunk of the patient is at an angle of 45° or greater. The venous hypertension is partly the result of systemic venous constriction. Bubbling rales, wheezing, and rhonchi may be heard throughout the lungs and may obscure the auscultatory findings of underlying valvular heart disease or ventricular diastolic gallop rhythm. The chest x-ray may show the characteristic pattern of alveolar pulmonary edema upon examination. The symptoms of acute pulmonary edema may subside after an interval of 15 min to several hours. Pulmonary edema of various types may occur in the absence of primary heart disease; with acute glomerulonephritis, after inhalation of noxious gas, in acute heroin poisoning,[35] with viral pneumonia, with drowning, or at high altitudes[36] (Figs. 14-13 and 14-14).

Acute pulmonary edema is unmistakable in its classic form. When the sputum is not frothy and pink-tinged, acute pulmonary edema may resemble acute bronchial asthma, although the evidence of heart failure can usually be found. On the other hand, when the patient is too sick to give a history and the heart is not audible because of chest wheezing, it may be difficult to distinguish pulmonary edema from acute bronchial asthma. In such a case, it is wise to avoid administering morphine, which is ordinarily used for pulmonary edema, or epinephrine—which is often used for bronchial asthma—until the situation is clarified. Aminophylline and oxygen are useful in both pulmonary edema and acute asthma; their administration may bring enough relief to enable one to complete the evaluation of the patient.

Symptoms Due to Failure of the Right Side of the Heart

Failure of the right side of the heart is associated with systemic venous hypertension, edema, hepatomegaly, and ascites. Symptoms may originate in the gastrointestinal tract because of congestion; *anorexia, nausea, vomiting, and abdominal distension* are common symptoms of heart failure and at times may be difficult to differentiate from over-digitalization. Congestion of the liver may also produce upper abdominal pain, which may be aggravated by effort. *The liver is commonly tender.* Occasionally an erroneous diagnosis of primary liver disease may be made if the observer misses the obvious *abnormal neck vein distension and pulsations.* This diagnostic error is also likely since liver-function tests may be abnormal because of heart failure; the retention of Bromsulphalein to levels of 35 per cent or more, hypoalbuminemia, positive cephalin flocculation test, elevation of serum-transaminase and alkaline-phosphate levels, and hyperbilirubinemia may all occur. Indeed, levels of bilirubin of 12 mg per 100 ml with serum-transaminase levels greater than 1,000 units per ml have been reported. As a rule, however, the serum-bilirubin level is seldom above 2 mg per 100 ml as a result of heart failure.[39] Higher levels than this increase the likelihood of associated pulmonary infarction or liver disease. Congestive *splenomegaly* is occasionally noted in right-sided heart failure.[37] Ascites and an *increase in girth* constitute a late sign of the right-sided heart failure. *Constipation* may be troublesome and is explained in part by inactivity.

Although pulmonary edema due to acute left ventricular failure may occur without weight gain, patients with chronic heart failure may gain weight because of abnormal retention of salt and water by the kidneys, and the cause of the weight gain may not be appreciated. Ten pounds or more of *weight gain* may occur in a patient with chronic heart failure without the development of pitting edema of the feet and ankles. Because of this fact, peripheral edema is a late sign and a poor sign of heart failure. During the period of retention of fluid, the patient may have *decreased urinary frequency and volume* during the day, but *increased frequency and volume (nocturia)* at night; the patient drinks water during the day and passes his urine during the night.[8] At the end of the day, he may note *swelling of the feet and ankles which subsides at night with recumbency.* There are many noncardiac causes of edema: varicose veins, obesity, phlebitis, pregnancy, liver disease, renal disease, cyclical edema, lymphedema, steroid administration, and retroperitoneal tumor. The distinction of heart failure from renal disease may be difficult, since patients with either condition may have oliguria, nocturia, facial edema, albuminuria, elevated blood–urea nitrogen level, decreased creatine clearance, or occasional microscopic hematuria. In the elderly male with heart failure these findings may be wrongly attributed to prostatism.

The location of *edema* is determined by local factors; the most important factor determining the localization of edema due to heart failure is increased hydrostatic pressure.[38] This may be increased by gravity (the erect position favors collection of the fluid in the feet, ankles, and lower portion of the legs, whereas the recumbent position favors the accumulation of the fluid in the sacral region) or by localized obstruction. (Venous obstruction from phlebitis or varicose veins leads to unilateral edema of the extremities.) *Ascites* is another type of localized accumulation of extracellular fluid.[39] Ascites is not rare in constrictive pericarditis, in which liver damage is often moderate. Ascites is more likely to occur in patients with heart failure who have primary liver disease than in patients with heart failure who do not have primary liver disease.

Additional Symptoms Associated with Heart Failure

As a result of the impaired cerebral blood flow associated with a marked decrease in cardiac output, patients with heart failure may have dizziness, somnolence, restlessness, and confusion. These may be the initial or most prominent symptoms of heart failure, and their cause may be overlooked when other cardiac complaints are not present. The occurrence of these central nervous system symptoms is particularly likely in elderly patients with cerebral atherosclerosis or with obstructive lesions in the carotid or basilar vertebral system.

Inadequate blood flow to the muscles with exercise may be manifested by *weakness.*[8] In some patients with advanced heart failure in whom congestion of lungs or viscera is well controlled by therapy, the major symptom may be weakness. At times this symptom may be aggravated by electrolyte depletion.

PHYSICAL FINDINGS ASSOCIATED WITH HEART FAILURE

Many signs indicative of heart failure may be found on physical examination. These diagnostic clues are commonly overlooked, misinterpreted, or disregarded. Some of these signs may be the only evidence of heart failure in patients who are examined before the development of the signs of congestion or edema, or the symptoms of severe heart failure. (See Chap. 20 for discussion of congestive heart failure in children.)

Since most of the symptoms of heart failure may be caused by noncardiac disorders, it is prudent to search for evidence of heart disease on physical examination. In particular, we wish to emphasize signs of heart failure which are often neglected, and certain clues to the diagnosis of other conditions which may aggravate or precipitate heart failure.

Evidence of Heart Disease[40–44]

It is folly to diagnose heart failure in a patient unless there is some evidence of heart disease. It is also folly to diagnose heart failure just because heart disease is present. The causation of the heart disease, which must be known for proper treatment, may often be identified on physical examination; the diastolic blood pressure may be persistently elevated to moderate levels; abnormal murmurs may originate in the heart or peripheral vessels; a myocardial aneurysm may be palpated; and pulmonary emphysema may be suspected. Congenital heart disease, valvular heart disease, and heart disease due to hypertension are usually suspected by physical examination. There are, of course, exceptions to the general rule, and additional information may be needed in order to define the abnormalities with precision. Ischemic heart disease, which is usually due to coronary atherosclerosis, is frequently recognized by the symptoms of angina pectoris or myocardial infarction. In this disease the physical examination is not so important as the history, although certain diagnostic signs may occasionally be detected. In addition, the electrocardiogram assumes a semidiagnostic role in the recognition of myocardial infarction.

One of the more important aspects of the physical examination is the determination of *heart size. Definite cardiac enlargement is reliable evidence of heart disease, and hearts of normal size are rarely associated with heart failure.* This statement although true and helpful must be qualified in order to minimize errors. It does not imply that mild heart disease (such as slight aortic regurgitation) or severe heart disease (such as angina pectoris or myocardial infarction) may not be present when the heart size is normal. The statement does indicate that *if* there is definite evidence of cardiac enlargement, some form of cardiac abnormality *is* present.

In years past, the term *cardiac enlargement* referred to the size of the heart as determined by percussion. This, in effect, was no more than the estimation of the frontal projection of the cardiac silhouette on the anterior surface of the chest. Today, the term *cardiac enlargement* refers to hypertrophy or dilatation of the individual cardiac chambers as well as to the overall size of the heart. Percussion, of course, is not so valuable as inspection and palpation in determining chamber enlargement. For example, the left border of cardiac dullness may be well within the midclavicular line in a patient with tight mitral stenosis, but there may be a sustained and abnormal lift of the sternum which indicates right ventricular hypertrophy. The normal range of the heart size is great. Accordingly, a patient whose heart size was previously near the lower limits of normal may develop definite cardiac enlargement and the heart may still *seem* to be within normal limits of size. This problem may sometimes be resolved if the physician's skill of cardiac inspection and palpation is developed, since he may be able to detect that the apex impulse is abnormal—even though it is located inside the midclavicular line. The usual evidence of right ventricular hypertrophy may be obscured by emphysema. In such cases the right ventricular hypertrophy may be detected by palpating beneath the anterior portion of the thoracic cage. Emphysema may also obscure evidence of left ventricular hypertrophy.

In addition to evidence of *heart disease,* one may obtain evidence of *heart failure* from physical examination of the patient. Heart failure may be associated with moist rales which may be heard at the lung bases or over the entire lung field. Rales due to heart failure are often attributed to poor ventilation. It is not generally appreciated that the rales of heart failure may be heard only on the dependent side, and that they may shift to the opposite side immediately when the patient turns. Heart failure may, of course, be present without rales. On the other hand, rales may also be due to noncardiac disease. Bronchial wheezing is often caused by heart failure and is frequently misinterpreted as being produced by bronchial asthma. Hydrothorax may develop in patients with heart failure.[45,46] It may occur on either side but is more frequently located predominantly or solely on the right side.

The finding of hydrothorax on the left side with little fluid on the right side suggests the diagnosis of pulmonary infarction. Edema, a late sign of heart failure, occurs in the dependent parts of the body, usually the feet and ankles. In the bedridden patient it may be localized to the presacral area. Unilateral edema suggests local disease, especially venous insufficiency. The liver may become large and tender and may seem to pulsate in some patients with heart failure. Ascites may be due to heart failure. There are numerous other causes of a large liver and of ascites, both of which are late signs of heart failure.

Proper examination of the *heart, arteries, and veins* for evidence of heart failure is often neglected (Fig. 14-2). (The details of these physical signs are discussed in Chap. 5; they are briefly described here for emphasis.)

A *ventricular gallop* sound (protodiastolic gallop or third heart sound gallop) is the hallmark of ventricular failure.[47,48] This low-pitched sound is heard best when the bell of the stethoscope is applied with light pressure. This sound occurs in early diastole at the end of rapid ventricular filling. A left ventricular gallop sound is best heard at the apex, and a right ventricular gallop sound is best heard over the right ventricle. The normal third sound of the child or adolescent is identical to the abnormal gallop sound. Therefore, the finding of a ventricular gallop (S_3) does not indicate heart failure in the child or in the young adult. The normal adult rarely has a ventricular gallop. In patients with mitral regurgitation, a ventricular gallop does not always indicate ventricular failure. Young adults who are pregnant or who have thyrotoxicosis or anemia may also develop a third heart sound which is not necessarily an indication of heart failure. Obviously, a patient with tricuspid stenosis cannot have a right ventricular gallop, nor can a patient with tight mitral stenosis have a left ventricular gallop. In years past, the term "gallop rhythm" was applied to the heart sounds when a third sound was heard in a patient with tachycardia. It is now clear that this extra sound has the same significance regardless of the heart rate. It is still true that the abnormal ventricular gallop sound may be intensified when the heart rate increases. The ventricular gallop sound becomes a reliable sign of early myocardial failure when its development is observed in a patient with heart disease. For example, a ventricular gallop at the apex, which is heard for the first time the day after a myocardial infarction, represents a definite sign of left ventricular myocardial failure. As a rule therapy for heart failure should be started if a ventricular gallop sound is noted in a patient with heart disease.

An *atrial gallop* sound (presystolic gallop, fourth heart sound gallop) is not a reliable sign of heart

SIGNS OF HEART FAILURE

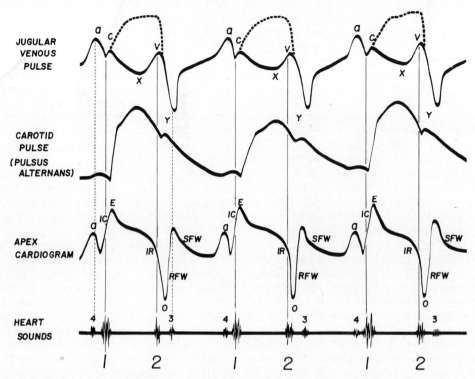

Fig. 14-2. Physical signs of heart failure. The diagram depicts the signs of heart failure which are found on examination of the heart itself, the arteries, and the veins. These signs are often ignored. The heart sounds at the bottom are reference points for the examination of the heart, arteries, and veins. One should listen to the heart sounds and simultaneously examine the arteries, veins, and precordial pulsations.

The *jugular venous pulsation* (solid line) in heart failure shows a reasonably normal wave form but at a higher level than normal. The A *wave*, occurring before the first sound, is a little large, and the Y *descent* a bit deep. The dotted line indicates a large V wave of tricuspid regurgitation which often accompanies right-sided heart failure.

The *carotid pulse* tracing shows pulsus alternans.

The *apex cardiogram* (piezoelectric crystal) in heart failure has a prominent A wave suggesting high left ventricular diastolic pressure, a prolonged E (indicating left ventricular disease), an obvious O, and a prominent change in slope or even an outward wave which occurs at the end of the rapid-filling wave (RFW) and the beginning of the slow-filling wave (SFW). The left ventricular "gallop" sound (S_3) occurs at the end of the RFW, and the left atrial "gallop" sound (S_4) occurs during the A wave of the apex cardiogram. These waves are often palpable in patients with clear left ventricular disease. A definite anterior lift of the right ventricle is also a sign of heart failure.

The phonocardiogram at the bottom shows a fourth heart sound (atrial gallop) and a third heart sound (left ventricular gallop). Although the atrial gallop is not so specific for heart failure as the ventricular gallop, at times this finding is a valuable sign of heart failure.

failure and may occur in patients with a long P-R interval, in patients with hypertension or coronary disease, and in some patients for unknown reasons.[49,50] Recent observations, however, indicate that an atrial gallop sound may at times assume more significance than was formerly appreciated. Specifically, an atrial gallop developing after myocardial infarction may herald early heart failure. At times subaudible ventricular or atrial gallop sounds may be seen or felt.[51,52] In order to identify the precordial "movements" associated with audible atrial or ventricular gallop sounds, it is necessary to listen to the heart, to identify the first and second sounds, and to determine whether the abnormal movement occurs just before the first sound (atrial gallop) or shortly after the second heart sound (ventricular gallop).

In a patient with disease of the left side of the heart, a sustained lift of the sternum due to right ventricular enlargement suggests heart failure, since it is unlikely that left ventricular enlargement alone will displace the right ventricle anteriorly.

In such cases the right ventricle is large secondary to the elevation of pressure in the pulmonary circuit produced by the left-sided heart failure. In other patients a large right ventricle may force the left ventricle posteriorly and may replace the normal left ventricular apical impulse with a large right ventricular impulse. This finding does not indicate heart failure.

Pulsus alternans in the peripheral arterial system indicates heart failure due to disease of the left ventricle. It may be associated with alternation of other cardiac events which depend on left ventricular contraction. For example, the intensity of the heart sounds may be faint one cycle and louder the next cycle. Heart murmurs, especially the murmur of aortic stenosis, may alternate in intensity from cycle to cycle. Most patients with pulsus alternans have a left ventricular gallop sound produced by left ventricular failure.

The effect of the Valsalva (Weber) maneuver on blood pressure can be used as a test for heart failure. The test consists of having the patient blow into a simple tube connected to a manometer. The forced expiration should be maintained at a level of 40 to 50 mm Hg for 15 sec. When this test is being performed in a patient with heart failure, the response is abnormal in that there is persistent elevation of systolic and diastolic systemic pressure, giving the arterial pressure tracing a "square" wave effect. After the maneuver has been discontinued, the normal arterial pressure overshoot and the reflex bradycardia do not occur.[53] This abnormal response is identified best by obtaining an arterial tracing, but certain aspects of the response can be determined at the bedside by simply obtaining the systolic pressure and noting the heart rate. The absence of a pressure overshoot associated with bradycardia supports a diagnosis of heart failure. The test, unfortunately, does not identify minor degrees of heart failure, and when failure is severe, other signs are usually present.

Abnormalities of the *neck veins* are frequently overlooked during physical examination. Signs of heart failure which may be detected from examination of the neck veins include the following: pulsations of the deep jugular veins when the trunk of the body is elevated 45°, a prominent early V wave, prominent sustained A and V waves with a rapid and deep Y descent, and an abnormal hepatojugular reflux test.

Heart failure may be *precipitated* or *aggravated* by certain conditions. Many of these conditions may be recognized or suspected on physical examination: uncontrolled heart rhythm, enlargement of the prostate and bladder, or evidence of thrombophlebitis, hydrothorax, hyperthyroidism, hypothyroidism, anemia, or infection.

RADIOGRAPHIC SIGNS OF HEART FAILURE[54-64]

An early hemodynamic change of left-sided heart failure is pulmonary venous hypertension, which may occur without auscultatory abnormalities. In some patients evidence of very early left-sided heart failure may be detected in the chest x-ray before it can be detected with the stethoscope. When the pulmonary venous pressure becomes raised over the normal value (about 5 to 13 mm Hg) and approaches and exceeds the oncotic pressure of plasma protein (25 to 30 mm Hg), there may be exudation of fluid from the capillary into the interstitial tissue. This engorgement may lead to stiffening of the lung and decreased compliance. The concentration of plasma proteins, the efficiency of lymphatic drainage, and the character of the alveolar membrane and the interstitial tissue determine the level of oncotic pressure at which exudation occurs. When most physicians think of pulmonary edema, they think in terms of the alveolar variety, which represents a more advanced state than the more common interstitial type. The latter variety of pulmonary edema is often overlooked or ascribed to technically poor films.

When excess exudation of fluid into the tissues immediately surrounding the pulmonary capillary membrane occurs, interstitial edema is said to be present. This stage of pulmonary edema can often be detected by x-ray examination before it becomes clinically apparent; in a recent series of 114 patients at Emory University Hospital who had radiologic diagnosis of interstitial edema, heart failure was previously unrecognized by the clinician in 24 per cent.[65] The transverse diameter of the heart was less than half the transverse diameter of the chest (cardiothoracic ratio) in 28 per cent of the patients. The heart size is often normal when acute heart failure is secondary to acute myocardial infarction, mitral stenosis, and acute renal failure.

Since the radiographic evidence of heart failure is important and since it is often overlooked, this aspect of heart failure will be emphasized.

When pulmonary venous hypertension occurs, dilatation of the pulmonary veins ensues; there is constriction of the arteries and veins to the lower lobes so that dilatation is particularly noted in the superior pulmonary veins, often giving rise to the "antler" appearance. The pulmonary veins to the upper lobes lie lateral to the major arterial branches, and they cross the main right and left branches of the pulmonary artery at right angles (Figs. 14-3 and 14-4).

Shortly after the pulmonary venous pressure becomes elevated in left-sided heart failure, the *pulmonary artery pressure* becomes elevated. On x-ray

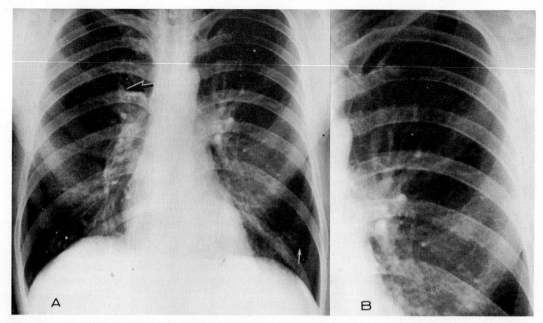

Fig. 14-3. T. S., a 41-year-old man with mild mitral stenosis, was initially diagnosed as having bronchiectasis as the cause of his hemoptysis. A. Note the distension of superior pulmonary veins (large arrow) and costophrenic septal lines (small arrow). B, The antler-like appearance of the superior pulmonary veins.

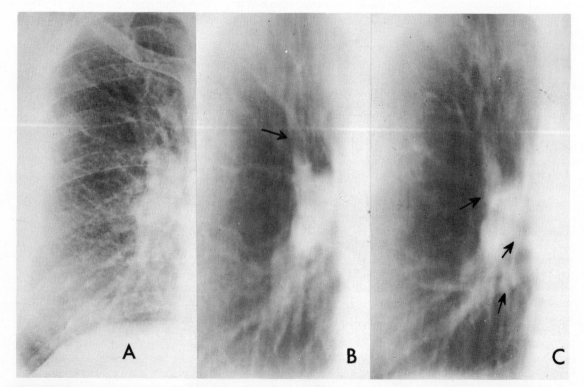

Fig. 14-4. B. D., a 73-year-old man, had arteriosclerotic heart disease and several old myocardial infarctions. A. The chest film shows early changes of interstitial pulmonary edema, with dilatation of pulmonary veins and pulmonary clouding. Tomograms B and C emphasize the dilated pulmonary veins.

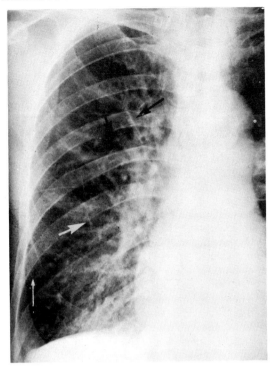

examination this may be noted as a dilatation of the central right and left pulmonary artery shadows. The right descending pulmonary artery, which forms the major vascular structure in the right hilum, normally measures 9 to 16 mm in greatest diameter. When it measures 17 mm or more, it is a reasonably reliable sign of elevation of the pulmonary artrey pressure if pulmonary blood flow is not increased (Fig. 14-3). At times both the major arteries and the veins are obscured by the pulmonary clouding of interstitial edema.

Pulmonary clouding with increased interstitial density of the central lung markings is frequent early in the course of interstitial edema. This x-ray finding is often attributed by the unsophisticated radiologist to "poor technique." The arteries and veins are surrounded by connective tissue containing lymphatic vessels. The accumulation of edema fluid in the perivascular tissues and in the pulmonary lymphatic vessels causes haziness and a loss of sharp outline of the arteries and veins (Figs. 14-4–14-8, 14-10, 14-12).

The accumulation of fluid in the subpleural fibrous planes and lymphatic vessels and in the interlobar fissures and lymphatic vessels causes a *thickening*, which may be visible on the radiograph (Figs. 14-5, 14-7, 14-11). As the interstitial edema clears, the septa may no longer be apparent.

The secondary lobules of the lung are separated

Fig. 14-5. H. P., a 57-year-old man, suffered an acute myocardial infarction. Note "A" lines (large arrows) and "B" lines (small arrow), pulmonary clouding, and hilar engorgement.

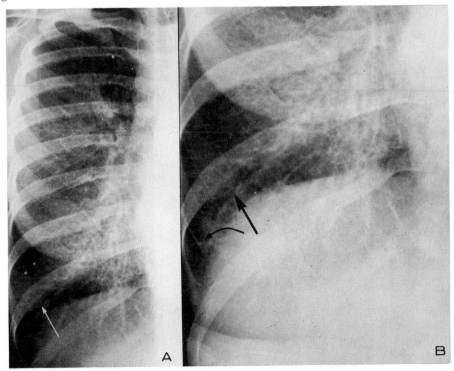

Fig. 14-6. A. O., a 43-year-old man, has mitral stenosis. Note costophrenic septal lines, dilated superior pulmonary veins, and increased interstitial density (clouding) of the lungs.

by fine septums containing lymphatic vessels and the vein draining the lobule. At the periphery of the lungs these septa lie perpendicular to the pleural surface and are continuous with the subpleural fibrous and lymphatic tissue. These septa near the periphery of the lung are normally microscopic in size and therefore they are not seen in the chest x-ray. When they are thickened by edema fluid, however, they are apparent as sharp linear lines. They are more common in the lower portion of the lungs because the hydrostatic pressure is greatest in this location. These thickened septa and lymphatic vessels are usually horizontal, and they may extend to the pleural surface. Occasionally they are vertical and project perpendicular to the pleural surface over the diaphragms. These peripheral markings were termed "B" lines by Kerley (Figs. 14-3, 14-5, 14-6). Similar longer lines extending peripherally from the hilum have been termed "A" lines (Figs. 14-5 and 14-6). Both types of septal lines may result from any condition which thickens the fibrous septa: inflammation such as that produced by viral infection, hemochromatosis, infiltration by tumor, or fibrosis. They are not specific for left-sided heart failure. When they are due to heart failure, however, the pulmonary capillary pressure and the pulmonary artery diastolic pressure usually exceed 18 mm Hg.

Subpleural fluid may also accumulate in the area of the costophrenic sulci and simulate free pleural fluid (Fig. 14-11). When localized in the basal subpleural space, it may simulate elevation of the diaphragm.

Free pleural fluid may occur with blunting or obstruction of the costophrenic angles. This occurs more frequently on the right side; at times it may be best seen in a film taken in the lateral projection (Fig. 14-7).

Any or all of the above findings may be present in any patient with heart failure, and at times there may be, in addition, localized areas of *alveolar edema*. When these areas are large or confluent, they may simulate pneumonia, tumor, or infarction (Fig. 14-8). Clinically, the differentiation may be made by the rapid clearing after several days of digitalis and diuretic therapy.

Accumulation of fluid in the interlobar spaces may also simulate tumor. Such a "pseudotumor" or "phantom tumor" is illustrated in Fig. 14-9.

The superior vena cava and azygos veins often become dilated when there is right-sided failure in association with increases in blood volume and in systemic vasoconstriction.

Advanced pulmonary alveolar edema is recognized without difficulty. Fluid fills the alveolar spaces in the central area of the chest, giving a "butterfly" appearance to the chest film. [The heart makes the body of the butterfly and the alveolar edema makes the wings (Fig. 14-12).] Pulmonary edema may occur from noncardiac causes (Figs. 14-13, 14-14).

LABORATORY EVIDENCE OF HEART FAILURE

There is absolutely *no electrocardiographic finding* which indicates the presence or absence of con-

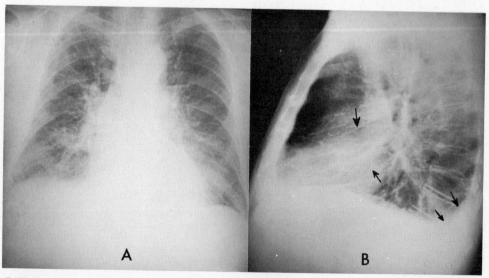

Fig. 14-7. T. G., a 74-year-old man, has arteriosclerotic heart diseases with old myocardial infarctions. A. Typical changes of interstitial pulmonary edema. In the lateral film (*B*) fluid is seen in the posterior costophrenic sulcus, which cannot be seen well in the posteroanterior view. There is also thickening of the interlobar fissures, which is usually more apparent in the lateral views.

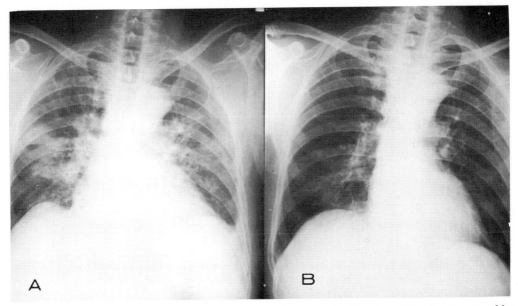

Fig. 14-8. L. S., a 64-year-old man, has arteriosclerotic heart disease with old myocardial infarction, in addition to aortic regurgitation. *A.* Alveolar edema of lobular type which may be mistaken for pneumonia, pulmonary infarction, or pulmonary neoplasm. *B.* Clearing obtained after 4 days of treatment for congestive heart failure.

gestive heart failure. Accordingly, there is no electrocardiographic change which indicates when treatment is required. An electrocardiogram should be obtained for the following reasons:

1. When correlated with other findings, it may give information regarding the cause of the condi-

tion. For example, unsuspected myocardial infarction may be detected or mitral stenosis may be suggested by the presence of right axis deviation of the QRS and atrial fibrillation, or by abnormal "m-shaped" P waves.

2. It serves as a base line to evaluate further

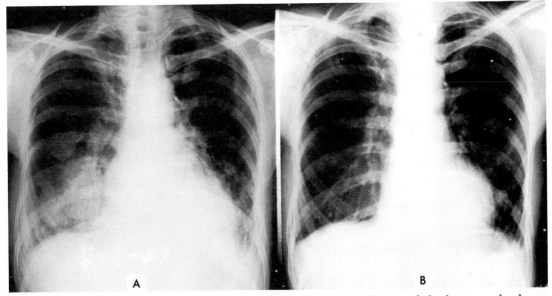

Fig. 14-9. R. R., a 76-year-old man, has arteriosclerotic heart disease with old myocardial infarction and pulmonary emphysema. *A.* Changes of interstitial pulmonary edema and the "pseudotumor" due to loculated interlobar pleural effusion. *B.* Considerable clearing, obtained after 4 days of treatment for congestive heart failure.

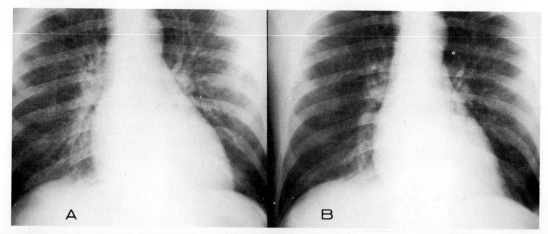

Fig. 14-10. W. O., 48 years old, with old and acute myocardial infarction. At this time the pulse rate was 84; there were no ventricular gallop, pulmonary rales, or edema. The neck veins were slightly distended at 30°. There were no symptoms. *A*. Note changes of pulmonary edema. *B*. A degree of clearing, 24 hr after digitalization and diuresis.

changes regarding overdigitalization, electrolyte disturbance, acute myocardial infarction, unrecognized arrhythmias, or changes in atrioventricular or intraventricular conduction.

For practical purposes, congestive heart failure may be recognized *without resort to laboratory procedures*. The techniques of measuring *venous pressure*,[66] circulation time,[67] and vital capacity are discussed in Chap. 10. Ordinarily, the height of the venous pressure may be adequately determined by inspection of the neck veins. It should be noted, however, that heart failure may be present with a normal peripheral venous pressure and that elevation of the systemic venous pressure is often preceded by changes of interstitial pulmonary edema on chest x-ray.

Since the *circulatory* time is in part a reflection of the volume of the pulmonary vascular bed and

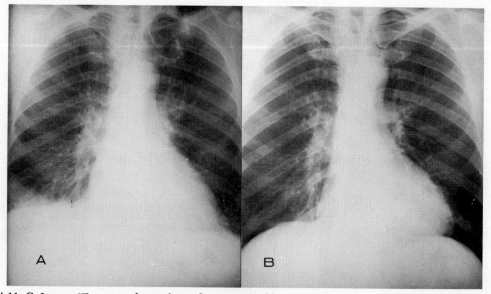

Fig. 14-11. C. L., age 57; arteriosclerotic heart disease with old myocardial infarctions. Transient paroxysmal nocturnal dyspnea developed the night prior to the initial film (*A*). There were no rales, cough, wheezing, ventricular gallop, venous distension, hepatomegaly, or edema. The pulse rate was 80. *B*. Clearing of the interstitial edema and subpleural fluid in the costophrenic sulci, 4 days after digitalization and diuresis.

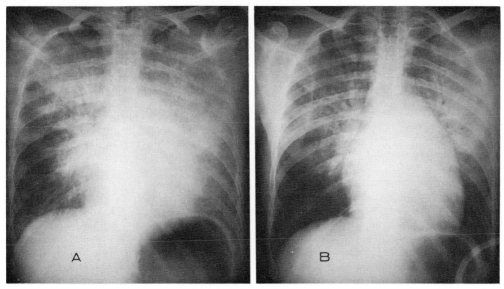

Fig. 14-12. Roentgenogram of a 24-year-old man with tight mitral stenosis. *A.* Intraalveolar pulmonary edema. *B.* Partial clearing, 24 hr later, of the intraalveolar edema on the right side, but persistent interstitial edema on the left side.

of the volume of the heart in addition to the cardiac output, patients with acute heart failure induced by myocardial infarction may occasionally have normal circulation time. The circulation time may also not be significantly prolonged with mild degrees of heart failure due to other causes. This measurement does have value in the identification of patients with high-output heart failure, in whom the circulation time is shorter than expected. The value of measurements of *vital capacity* in assessing the presence of heart failure is greatest when managing patients with heart disease during pregnancy.

Normally the vital capacity increases or remains the same during pregnancy, whereas it decreases with the onset of congestive heart failure.

As with clinical evidence of heart failure, there is no single finding at *cardiac catheterization* which indicates heart failure. The patient with heart failure may have findings at cardiac catheterization of one of the following: an elevated end-diastolic

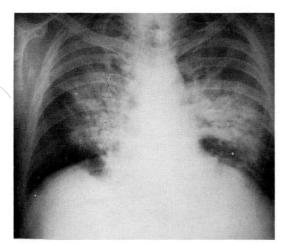

Fig. 14-13. S., a 53-year-old man, developed toxic nephritis as a result of carbon tetrachloride ingestion. The chest film illustrates alveolar pulmonary edema.

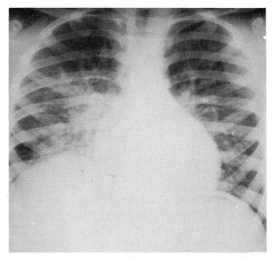

Fig. 14-14. L., a 10-year-old boy, was admitted following drowning and resuscitation. The chest film shows confluent intraalveolar pulmonary edema on the right and interstitial edema on the left. (*Courtesy, Dr. Howard Lee and Dr. Frank Morgan.*)

pressure in the involved ventricle or atrium; a lower resting cardiac output as compared to that prior to the onset of failure; an inability to increase cardiac output in response to exercise; or an abnormally high arteriovenous oxygen difference at rest or during exercise. One does not subject a patient to cardiac catheterization to determine the presence or absence of heart failure; rather, this procedure is used to determine the cause or the severity of the underlying heart disease.

The total *blood volume* may be normal or increased in the patient with heart failure.[68–70] Occasionally the total volume may be normal whereas the pulmonary blood volume may be increased.

Dysfunction of the liver, kidney, or brain may develop as a result of altered cardiac output and diminished organ perfusion, or as a result of increased venous pressure. This causes no permanent structural changes in the kidney and brain; however, permanent changes due to chronic passive congestion may be produced in the liver. Urinalysis may reveal moderate albuminuria. The specific gravity of the urine may be high during the phases of salt and water retention and low during periods of diuresis. The blood–urea nitrogen level may be moderately elevated, usually no higher than 50 mg per 100 ml, secondary to heart failure (prerenal azotemia).

Hepatic dysfunction, often with structural damage to the liver, may result in moderate retention of Bromsulphalein, abnormal cephalin flocculation test, slight elevation of serum-bilirubin level, and serum–glutamic oxaloacetic transaminase level.[71–74]

The erythrocyte sedimentation rate may be retarded during congestive heart failure. This occurs because the fibrinogen level is decreased secondary to impaired liver function.[75]

THE CONSTELLATION

There is no single diagnostic sign of heart failure. The diagnosis is based on a constellation of symptoms, physical signs, and laboratory findings in a patient with heart disease. For generations symptoms such as dyspnea and signs such as rales and edema have been emphasized. These findings are well known to all men of medicine. We have chosen not to emphasize such findings but rather have strongly emphasized those signs of heart failure which are less generally recognized but which may be found on examination of the heart, arteries, or veins or which may be detected by careful examination of the chest x-ray.

REFERENCES

1. Keith, J. D.: Congestive Heart Failure, *Pediatrics*, 18:491, 1956.

2. McCue, C. M., and Young, R. B.: Cardiac Failure in Infancy, *J. Pediat.*, **58**:330, 1961.

3. Hubbard, J. P.: Paroxysmal Tachycardia and Its Treatment in Young Infants, *Am. J. Dis. Child.*, **61**:687, 1941.

4. Logue, R. B., and Hurst, J. W.: Errors in the Recognition and Treatment of Heart Disease, *Circulation*, **10**:920, 1954.

5. Warren, J. V., and Stead, E. A., Jr.: Fluid Dynamics in Chronic Congestive Heart Failure, *A.M.A. Arch. Int. Med.*, **73**:138, 1944.

6. Stead, E. A., Jr., and Warren, J. V.: Cardiac Output in Man: Analysis of the Mechanisms Varying the Cardiac Output Based on Recent Clinical Studies, *A.M.A. Arch. Int. Med.*, **80**:237, 1947.

7. Stead, E. A., Jr., Warren, J. V., and Brannon, E. S.: Cardiac Output in Congestive Heart Failure, *Am. Heart J.*, **35**:529, 1948.

8. Stead, E. A., Jr., and Hickam, J.: Heart Failure. *Disease-a-Month*, January, 1955.

9. Burch, G. E. and Ray, C. T.: A Consideration of the Mechanism of Congestive Heart Failure, *Am. Heart J.*, **41**:918, 1951.

10. Burch, G. E., Ray, C. T., and Cronvich, J. A.: Certain Mechanical Peculiarities of Human Cardiac Pump in Normal and Disease States, *Circulation*, **5**:504, 1952.

11. Warren, J. V., and Stead, E. A., Jr.: Fluid Dynamics in Chronic Congestive Heart Failure: Interpretations of Mechanism Producing Edema, Increased Plasma Volume and Elevated Venous Pressure in Certain Patients with Prolonged Congestive Heart Failure, *A.M.A. Arch. Int. Med.*, **73**:138, 1944.

12. Burch, G. E.: Evidence for Increased Venous Tone in Chronic Congestive Heart Failure, *A.M.A. Arch. Int. Med.*, **98**:750, 1956.

13. Merrill, A. J.: Edema and Decreased Renal Blood Flow in Patients with Chronic Congestive Heart Failure: Evidence of "Forward Failure" as Primary Cause of Edema, *J. Clin. Invest.*, **25**:389, 1946.

14. Merrill, A. J.: Mechanisms of Salt and Water Retention in Heart Failure, *Am. J. Med.*, **6**:357, 1949.

15. Harrison, T. R.: Cardiac Dyspnea, *West. J. Surg.*, **52**:407, 1944.

16. Stead, E. A.: Edema and Dyspnoea of Heart Failure, *Bull. New York Acad. Sc.*, **28**:159, 1952.

17. Richards, D. W.: The Nature of Cardiac and of Pulmonary Dyspnea (The Lewis A. Conner Memorial Lecture); *Circulation*, **7**:15, 1953.

18. Comroe, J. H., Jr.: Dyspnea. *Mod. Concepts Cardiovas. Dis.*, **25**:347, 1956.

19. Harrison, T. R., Harrison, W. G., Jr., Calhoun, J. A., and March, J. P.: Congestive Heart Failure. XVII. The Mechanism of Dyspnea on Exertion, *A.M.A. Arch. Int. Med.*, **50**:690, 1932.

20. Christie, R. V.: Dyspnoea: A Review, *Quart. J. Med.*, **7**:421, 1938.

21. Wood, P.: An Appreciation of Mitral Stenosis. Part I. Clinical Features. Part II. Investigations

and Results, *Brit. M. J.*, 1:1051–1063; 1113–1124, 1954.

22. Palmer, R. S., and White, P. D.: The Clinical Significance of Cardiac Asthma: Review of Two Hundred and Fifty Cases, *J.A.M.A.*, 92:431, 1929.

23. Weiss, S., and Robb, G. P.: Cardiac Asthma (Paroxysmal Cardiac Dyspnea) and the Syndrome of Left Ventricular Failure, *J.A.M.A.*, 100:1841, 1933.

24. Heyer, H. E., Abnormalities of the Respiratory Pattern in Patients with Cardiac Dyspnea, *Am. Heart J.*, 32:457, 1946.

25. Heyer, H. E.: Significance and Management of the Obstructive Factor in Cardiac Asthma and Cardiac Dyspnea, *Am. Pract.*, 1:121, 1946.

26. Plotz, M.: Bronchial Spasm in Cardiac Asthma, *Ann. Int. Med.*, 26:521, 1947.

27. Swineford, O., Jr.: Cardiac Asthma, *Postgrad. Med.*, 24:577, 1958.

28. Altschule, M. D.: "Physiology in Diseases of the Heart and Lung," 2d ed., Harvard University Press, Cambridge, Mass., 1954.

29. Perera, G. A., and Berliner, R. W.: The Relation of Postural Hemodilution to Paroxysmal Dyspnea, *J. Clin. Invest.*, 22:25, 1943.

30. Currens, J. H., and White, P. D.: Cough as a Symptom of Cardiovascular Disease, *Ann. Int. Med.*, 30:528, 1949.

31. Lange, R. L., and Hecht, H. H.: The Mechanism of Cheyne-Stokes Respiration, *J. Clin. Invest.*, 41:42, 1962.

32. Drinker, C. K.: "Pulmonary Oedema and Inflammation," Harvard University Press, Cambridge, Mass., 1945.

33. Hilden, T.: On the Pathogenesis of Acute Pulmonary Edema, *Acta med. scandinav.* (Suppl. 234), 136:162, 1949.

34. Sharp, J. T., Griffith, G. T., Bunnell, I. L., and Green, D. G.: Ventilatory Mechanics in Pulmonary Oedema in Man, *J. Clin. Invest.*, 37:111, 1958.

35. Silber, R., and Clerkin, E. P.: Pulmonary Edema in Acute Heroin Poisoning: Report of Four Cases, *Am. J. Med.*, 27:187, 1959.

36. Hultgren, H. N., Lopez, C. E., Lundberg, E., and Miller, H.: Physiologic Studies of Pulmonary Edema at High Altitude, *Circulation*, 29:393, 1964.

37. Fowler, N. O.: Splenomegaly in Congestive Heart Failure, *Ann. Int. Med.*, 27:733, 1947.

38. Stead, E. A., Jr.: Edema of Heart Failure, *Bull. New York Acad. Med.*, 24:607, 1948.

39. Hyatt, R. E., and Smith, J. R.: Mechanism of Ascites: A Physiologic Appraisal, *Am. J. Med.*, 16:434, 1954.

40. White, P. D.: "Heart Disease," 7th ed., The Macmillan Company, New York, 1951.

41. Hochstein, E.: Detection of the Early Signs of Heart Disease in General Practice, *New York J. Med.*, 53:2227, 1953.

42. White, P. D.: "Clues in the Diagnosis and Treatment of Heart Disease," Charles C Thomas, Publisher, Springfield, Ill., 1955.

43. Levine, S. A.: "Clinical Heart Disease," 5th ed., W. B. Saunders Company, Philadelphia, 1958.

44. Levine, S. A.: Some Prevalent Errors in the Practice of Cardiology, *Am. J. Cardiol.*, 7:132, 1961.

45. Bedford, D. E., and Lovibond, J. L.: Hydrothorax in Heart Failure, *Brit. Heart J.*, 3:93, 1941.

46. Race, G. A., Scheifly, C. H., and Edwards, J. E.: Hydrothorax in Congestive Heart Failure, *Am. J. Med.*, 22:83, 1957.

47. Dock, W., Grandell, F., and Taubman, F.: The Physiologic Third Heart Sound: Its Mechanism and Relation to Protodiastolic Gallop, *Am. Heart J.*, 50:449, 1955.

48. Warren, J. V., Leonard, J. J., and Weissler, A. M.: Gallop Rhythm, *Ann. Int. Med.*, 48:580, 1958.

49. Leonard, J. J., Weissler, A. M., and Warren, J. V.: Observations on the Mechanism of Atrial Gallop Rhythm, *Circulation*, 17:1007, 1958.

50. Crevasse, L., Wheat, M. W., Wilson, J. R., Leeds, R. F., and Taylor, W. J.: The Mechanism of the Generation of the Third and Fourth Heart Sounds, *Circulation*, 25:635, 1962.

51. Dressler, W.: Pulsations of the Chest Wall as Diagnostic signs, *Mod. Concepts Cardiovas. Dis.*, 26:421, 1957.

52. Benchimol, A., and Dimond, E. G.: The Normal and Abnormal Apexcardiogram: Its Physiological Variation and Its Relation to Intracardiac Events, *Am. J. Cardiol.*, 12:368, 1963.

53. Sharpey-Schafer, E. P.: Effects of Valsalva's Manoeuvre on the Normal and Failing Circulation, *Brit. M. J.*, 1:693, 1955.

54. Kerley, P.: Radiology in Heart Disease, *Brit. M. J.*, 2:594, 1933.

55. Hodson, C. J.: Pulmonary Oedema and the "Batswing" Shadow, *J. Fac. Radiologists* (*London*), 1:176, 1950.

56. Kerley, P.: "A Textbook of X-ray Diagnosis," 2d ed., ed. by Shanks and Kerley, H. K. Lewis, London, 1951, vol. 2, p. 404.

57. Carmichael, J. H. E., Julian, D. J., Jones, P. G., and Wren, E. M.: Radiological Signs in Pulmonary Hypertension: The Significance of Lines B of Kerley, *Brit. J. Radiol.*, 27:393, 1954.

58. Steinbach, H. L., Keats, T. K., and Sheline, G. E.: The Roentgen Appearance of the Pulmonary Veins in Heart Disease, *Radiology*, 65:158, 1955.

59. Keats, T. E., Kreis, A., and Simpson, E.: The Roentgen Manifestations of Pulmonary Hypertension in Congenital Heart Disease, *Radiology*, 66:693, 1956.

60. Short, D. S.: Radiology of the Lung in Left Heart Failure, *Brit. Heart J.*, 18:233, 1956.

61. Grainger, R. G.: Interstitial Pulmonary Oedema and Its Radiological Diagnosis: A Sign of Pulmonary Venous and Capillary Hypertension, *Brit. J. Radiol.*, 31:201, 1958.

62. Simon, M.: The Pulmonary Vessels in Incipient Left Ventricular Decompensation: Radiologic Observations, *Circulation*, 24:185, 1961.

63. Harley, H. R. S.: The Radiological Changes in Pulmonary Venous Hypertension, with Special Reference to the Root Shadows and Lobular Pattern, *Brit. Heart J.*, 23:75, 1961.

64. Soter, C. S., Berkmen, Y., Hadzidakis, A., Gur, H., Zannis, A., and Gilmore, J. H.: Roentgenologic Diagnosis of Incipient Left Heart Failure, *J.A.M.A.*, 175:1136, 1961.

65. Logue, R. B., Rogers, J. V., Jr., and Gay, B. B., Jr.: Subtle Roentgenographic Signs of Left Heart Failure, *Am. Heart J.*, 65:464, 1963.

66. Wood, P. H.: Right and Left Ventricular Failure: A Study of Circulation Time and Venous Blood Pressure, *Lancet*, 2:15, 1936.

67. Knott, D. H., and Barlow, G.: The Comparison of Fluorescein and Decholin Circulation Times, *Am. J. M. Sc.*, 247:304, 1964.

68. Samet, P., Fritts, H. W., Jr., Fishman, A. P., and Cournand, A.: The Blood Volume in Heart Disease, *Medicine*, 36:211, 1957.

69. Gunton, R. W., and Paul, W.: Blood Volume in Congestive Heart Failure, *J. Clin. Invest.*, 34:879, 1955.

70. Warren, J. V., and Stead, E. A., Jr.: Fluid Dynamics in Chronic Congestive Heart Failure: An Interpretation of the Mechanisms Producing the Edema, Increased Plasma Volume and Elevated Venous Pressure in Certain Patients with Prolonged Congestive Failure, *A.M.A. Arch. Int. Med.*, 73:138, 1944.

71. Sherlock, S.: The Liver in Heart Failure: Relations of Anatomical, Functional, and Circulatory Changes, *Brit. Heart J.*, 13:273, 1951.

72. Zak, E. R.: Liver Function in Cardiac Failure, *Acta med. scandinav.*, 134:428, 1949.

73. Blumberg, N., and Schloss, E. M.: The Effect of Circulatory Factors on the Bromsulphalein Test in Liver Disease, *Am. J. M. Sc.*, 213:470, 1947.

74. Evans, J. M., Zimmerman, H. J., Wilmer, J. G., Thomas, L. J., and Ethridge, C. B.: Altered Liver Function of Chronic Congestive Heart Failure, *Am. J. Med.*, 13:705, 1952.

75. Sanghvi, L. M., and Bohra, B. M.: The Retardation of Erythrocyte Sedimentation in Congestive Heart Failure, *Brit. Heart J.*, 24:180, 1962.

SUGGESTED READING

Altschule, M. D., Zamcheck, N., and Iglauer, A.: The Lung Volume and Its Subdivisions in the Upright and Recumbent Positions in Patients with Congestive Failure: Pulmonary Factors in the Genesis of Orthopnea, *J. Clin. Invest.*, 22:805, 1943.

Burchell, H. B.: Unusual Causes of Heart Failure, *Circulation*, 21:436, 1960.

Burroughs, R. W., and Bruce, R. A.: Significance of Abnormal Phase II Response to Valsalva Maneuver in Cardiac Patients, *Circulation*, 14:72, 1956.

Burwell, C. S.: The Pathological Physiology of the Early Manifestations of Left Ventricular Failure, *Ann. Int. Med.*, 16:104, 1942.

Chinard, F. P.: Starling's Hypothesis in the Formation of Edema, *Bull. New York Acad. Med.* 38:375, 1962.

Cosby, R. S., Stowell, E. C., Jr., Hartwig, W. R., and Mayo, M.: Pulmonary Function in Left Ventricular Failure, Including Cardiac Asthma, *Circulation*, 15:492, 1957.

Cournand, A.: Discussion of the Concept of Cardiac Failure in the Light of Recent Physiologic Studies in Man, *Ann. Int. Med.*, 37:649, 1952.

Ebert, R. V.: The Lung in Congestive Heart Failure, *Arch. Int. Med.*, 107:450, 1961.

Eichna, L. W.: Circulatory Congestion and Heart Failure, *Circulation*, 22:864, 1960.

Epstein, B. S., and Young, D.: A Correlation between Roentgenographic Changes in the Lungs in Left Ventricular Failure and the Circulation Rates, *Am. J. Roentgenol.*, 50:316, 1943.

Finlayson, J. K., Luria, M. N., Stanfield, C. A., and Yu, P. N.: Hemodynamic Studies in Acute Pulmonary Edema, *Ann. Int. Med.*, 54:244, 1961.

Davis, J. O.: Mechanisms of Salt and Water Retention in Congestive Heart Failure: The Importance of Aldosterone, *Am. J. Med.*, 29:486, 1960.

Dock, W.: Congestive Heart Failure: Adaptation of the Body to Inadequate Cardiac Output, *J.A.M.A.*, 140:1135, 1949.

Goodyear, A. V. N.: Renal Function and Renal Impairment in Congestive Heart Failure, *Progr. Cardiovas. Dis.*, 3:483, 1961.

Gorlin, R.: Recent Conceptual Advances in Congestive Heart Failure, *J.A.M.A.*, 179:441, 1962.

Gorlin, R., Knowles, J. H., and Storey, C. F.: The Valsalva Maneuver as a Test of Cardiac Function, *Am. J. Med.*, 22:197, 1957.

Hecht, H. H.: Clinical Progress: Heart Failure and Lung Disease, *Circulation*, 14:265, 1956.

Hope, J.: "A Treatise on the Diseases of the Heart and Great Vessels," William Kidd, London, 1832.

Lewis, T., Ryffel, J. H., Wolf, C. G. L., Cotton, R., and Barcroft, J.: Observations Relating to Dyspnea in Cardiac and Renal Patients, *Heart*, 5:45, 1913.

Mackenzie, J.: The Nature and Significance of Heart Symptoms, *Brit. M. J.* 1:505, 1922.

Merrill, A. J., and Cargill, W. H.: The Effect of Exercise on the Renal Plasma Flow and Filtration Rate of Normal and Cardiac Subjects, *J. Clin. Invest.*, 27:272, 1948.

Nadas, A. S., and Hauck, A. J.: Pediatric Aspects of Congestive Heart Failure, *Circulation*, 21:424, 1960.

Peabody, F. W.: Cardiac Dyspnea, *The Harvey Lectures*, series 12, 1916–1917, p. 248.

Sarnoff, S. J., Berglund, E., and Sarnoff, L. C.: Neurohemodynamics of Pulmonary Edema: Estimated Changes in Pulmonary Blood Volume Accompanying Systemic Vasoconstriction and Vasodilatation, *J. Appl. Physiol.*, 5:367, 1953.

Sarnoff, S. J., and Sarnoff, L. C.: Neurohemodynamics of Pulmonary Edema. I. Autonomic Influence on Pulmonary Vascular Pressures and the Acute Pulmonary Edema State, *Dis. Chest*, **22**:685, 1952.

Scharpey-Schafer, E. P.: The Peripheral Circulation in Circulatory Failure, *Brit. M. Bull.*, **8**:331, 1952.

Seminar on Congestive Heart Failure, *Circulation*, **21**: 95, 218, 424, 1960.

Stewart, P. B.: The Rate of Formation and Lymphatic Removal of Fluid in Pleural Effusions, J. Clin. Invest. 42:258, 1963.

Thompson, D. P.: Salt and Water Excretion in Heart Failure, *Progr. Cardiovas. Dis.*, **3**:520, 1961.

Walther, R. J., Griffin, J., and Moschos, C. B.: Recognition and Treatment of Congestive Heart Failure in Infants, *GP*, **26**:94, 1962.

White, P. D.: Weakness and Failure of the Left Ventricle without Failure of the Right Ventricle, *J.A.M.A.*, **100**:1993, 1933.

Youmans, W. B.: High Output Circulatory Failure as a Distinct Syndrome, *Mod. Concepts Cardiovas. Dis.*, **26**:389, 1957.

15 TREATMENT OF HEART FAILURE

R. Bruce Logue, M.D., and
J. Willis Hurst, M.D.

The treatment of congestive heart failure is designed (1) to reduce the work load of the heart; (2) to increase myocardial contractility and, in most instances, cardiac output; (3) to decrease visceral congestion; and (4) to remove precipitating and aggravating factors leading to decompensation and to modify the underlying heart disease. (Although these four facets of therapy are discussed separately, in practice they are instituted in combination.)

REDUCTION OF WORK LOAD

The work load of the heart may be *decreased by physical and emotional rest*.[1] The objective of therapy is to decrease the work load within the limits of practicability for an individual patient.[2] The majority of patients with heart failure must continue to earn a living; therefore, the physician must review the patient's workday in order to advise him intelligently regarding his activity. Many patients with mild heart failure require little or no change in their activities. Others may need adjustments in hours of work and manner of work, as well as curtailment of nonessential activities. For example, the business man may benefit from having someone else drive him to work. His load of business should be decreased as much as possible. He might break his routine by an hour's rest in the middle of the day. The housewife may need domestic help, or her housework may be reorganized to require the smallest expenditure of energy and to allow appropriate periods of rest. Shopping trips, which can be quite tiring, may need to be restricted. Some patients are not seen by a physician until they are symptomatic at rest. The activity of these patients should be greatly restricted until effective therapy has been established, diuresis has occurred, and symptoms have been relieved. The patient should be encouraged to sit in a comfortable chair, and while in bed, he should be placed in the "head up–legs down" position which aids in the relief of dyspnea.[3] The decreased venous return achieved by this position may improve cardiac efficiency, and edema fluid may accumulate in the subcutaneous portion of the dependent parts rather than in the lungs. The harmful effects of bed and chair rest must be avoided. Especial attention to the avoidance of venous stasis is essential, since pulmonary emboli are so common in this setting. After the patient has improved, he may gradually assume more activity and should then be returned to work. At this point, adjustments in his workday and other restrictions may be needed. Unfortunately, the natural course of disease is such that patients may eventually be unable to work, and their activity becomes more and more restricted until they must be confined to a bed or chair in order to avoid symptoms.

When congestive heart failure occurs during pregnancy, its treatment may require more prolonged rest, or, occasionally, complete inactivity until the pregnancy is terminated (see Chap. 62). The treatment of failure due to acute rheumatic myocarditis may require long periods of rest in a chair or bed until the acute activity subsides (see Chap. 25). Patients with certain types of idiopathic diffuse myocardial disease may benefit from rest for prolonged periods of up to a year.[4]

Prolonged bed rest induces poor muscle tone, poor cardiovascular reactivity, venous stasis with a predisposition to thromboembolism, mental depression, and anxiety on resuming activity. Therefore, critical judgment is needed in assessing the need for long periods of rest, and brief periods of mobilization and change in posture are desirable throughout the course of treatment.[5]

Emotional rest is more difficult to achieve. An outsider cannot judge the degree of emotional turmoil and its effect on a patient as accurately as he can judge the effect of physical activity. When a patient has hungry children to feed, it may be more detrimental for the patient not to work at all than to perform light work. In some patients, rest may not be possible until an important document is read or difficult decisions have been made. There is no facet of medicine which requires more insight than the analysis of emotional factors as they relate to cardiac work. Slight sedation at night and during the day may be needed, but should not be routinely prescribed.

INCREASED MYOCARDIAL CONTRACTILITY AND CARDIAC OUTPUT

Myocardial contractility and cardiac output can be improved by *digitalis* (see p. 000 for a complete discussion of the pharmacologic action of digitalis). The major actions of digitalis are to increase myocardial contractility and to slow the ventricular rate when atrial fibrillation is present. We agree with Brenner that "The simple, safe (and old) rule is that digitalis is needed in all patients with heart failure, right and left-sided, low output and high output, with atrial fibrillation, normal rhythm, or heart block." [1] This statement is true even though compensation may be restored with rest, sodium restriction, or diuretics. There are quantitative differences in response to digitalis therapy; for example, patients with heart failure due to acute rheumatic myocarditis respond less well than do patients with failure due to hypertensive heart disease. Excellent response to digitalis therapy for heart failure may be noted in patients with the following: mitral stenosis with atrial fibrillation, valvular aortic stenosis or regurgitation, rheumatic mitral regurgitation, coronary disease, or congenital heart disease with left-to-right shunts. Less satisfactory response may be noted in patients with the following conditions: mitral stenosis with sinus rhythm; diffuse myocardial disease; chronic cor pulmonale; acute myocarditis; constrictive pericarditis; primary pulmonary hypertension; Eisenmenger syndrome or congestive heart failure asociated with thyrotoxicosis, beriberi, anemia, acute glomerulonephritis and peripheral AV fistula. The absolute contraindication to the use of digitalis in a patient with heart failure is digitalis intoxication. (The problem is to make the diagnosis of subtle forms of digitalis intoxication.) Following the use of digitalis, some patients with functional hypertrophic subaortic stenosis have had an increase in symptoms related to this unique disorder.[6] If atrioventricular block is not produced by digitalis intoxication, it is not a contraindication to the use of digitalis, although caution may be needed to avoid producing higher grades of AV block, SA block, or inducing Stokes-Adams attacks.

Certain investigators have suggested that digitalis should be administered to patients with well-compensated heart disease in an effort to delay the appearance time of congestive failure.[7] More experience is needed to determine whether digitalis therapy in such patients is of prophylactic value, as Christian earlier suggested.[8] There is, however, no evidence that digitalis in subtoxic doses is injurious to the normal or compensated heart.

Digitalis is useful in the reversion of ectopic rhythms, especially atrial and nodal tachycardia; and in the control of the ventricular rate in other arrhythmias, such as atrial fibrillation and flutter. In these conditions an uncontrolled ventricular rate may produce or aggravate heart failure.[9,10]

The early recognition of heart failure has been stressed in preceding sections of this book. We now wish to stress the early treatment of heart failure. Thus, digitalis is indicated for slight dyspnea on effort due to heart failure, a nonproductive nocturnal cough, the development of a ventricular gallop sound or rhythm, or the presence of pulmonary congestion due to left-sided heart failure, detected either on physical examination or by x-ray of the chest. Pulsus alternans and abnormal neck vein pulsations are often overlooked as signs of heart failure. The late signs of heart failure, such as orthopnea and peripheral edema, are less often overlooked.

The authors believe that digitalization should be promptly instituted for early signs of left-sided heart failure due to acute myocardial infarction. Since a hemodynamic effect can be obtained with an average dose that is significantly smaller than the dose producing toxic effects, it is desirable to err on the side of underdigitalization. It should be emphasized that in the setting of myocardial infarction, heart failure may be present when any of the following signs is present, either alone or in combination: ventricular or atrial gallop, pulmonary rales, or x-ray evidence of interstitial pulmonary edema. Symptoms such as dyspnea, wheezing, cough, and orthopnea are late signs of left-sided heart failure. Persistent shock, which is often associated with myocardial infarction, may improve with digitalization. When digitalis is used cautiously for heart failure due to myocardial infarction, we have not seen treacherous arrhythmias produced, nor have we noted any evidence of increased incidence of myocardial rupture or aneurysm formation.

The following general principles regarding the administration of digitalis deserve emphasis:

1. Be certain that digitalis has not been given within the prior week or two. It is important to determine the presence of renal failure, since this may predispose to toxic effects during maintenance therapy.

2. The route and rapidity of digitalization are determined by the circumstances. For example, the patient with uncontrolled atrial fibrillation and severe dyspnea deserves prompt treatment by intravenous route; the patient with slight dyspnea on exertion or ventricular diastolic gallop rhythm may be digitalized slowly by oral administration.

3. Beneficial hemodynamic response can be obtained without following the time-honored advice to administer the drug until minor toxic symptoms develop; all too often when the latter method has been employed, the patient has subsequently refused to take this needed drug.

4. The physician must individualize the dosage, always working with an average dose schedule and observing for toxic effects. On rare occasions a patient cannot tolerate any digitalis whatever; other patients may tolerate large amounts without toxicity. The elderly person is generally more susceptible to the toxic effects.

5. The use of the pulse rate to determine the need for digitalis has certain limitations. Heart failure may occur—in fact, it often occurs—with a normal pulse rate. Occasionally, severe failure with marked sinus bradycardia may be evidence of early digitalis intoxication. On the other hand, when heart failure is due to or aggravated by pulmonary embolism, thyrotoxicosis, or myocarditis, the heart rate may be rapid. When digitalis is given to slow the rate of such patients, especially when the rhythm is sinus tachycardia, toxic effects of the drug may develop before slowing is satisfactory.

6. Numerous preparations of digitalis glycosides are available.[11] It is wise to become familiar with the use of no more than two or three preparations. The majority of situations can be handled by digoxin (Lanoxin), digitoxin, and digitalis leaf. The authors use digoxin for parenteral and oral digitalization and rarely use ouabain, acetyl strophanthidin, or lanatoside C (Cedilanid). Attempts to become familiar with the innumerable preparations on the market add to insecurity and confusion.

7. All digitalis preparations have toxic effects, and it is usually worthless to shift from one to another in the hope of finding a better-tolerated product.

8. Potassium loss sensitizes the myocardium to the toxic effects of digitalis. Accordingly, it is essential to assess potassium depletion in evaluating the dosage of digitalis.[12]

9. The electrocardiogram does not indicate the need for digitalis and does not indicate when optimum dosage is reached. The ST-T changes characteristic of "digitalis effect" do not correlate with either optimum or toxic effects. On the other hand, various toxic effects of digitalis may be detectable only in the electrocardiogram; e.g., AV dissociation.

10. The majority of patients with congestive heart failure require permanent digitalis therapy. A common error is the omission of the drug when compensation has been restored over a period of time; all too often the symptoms promptly recur. On the other hand, digitalis may be omitted after surgical correction of remedial lesions, after normal metabolism is restored in thyrotoxicosis, and after renal function improves with acute renal failure, etc. In many instances of acute left-sided heart failure associated with acute myocardial infarction, the drug may be omitted after an interval of several months if the exercise tolerance is good, the heart size is normal, and there is no evidence of heart failure.

Digoxin may be given orally for *routine digitalization* when there is no urgency. The maximum effect is reached in about 6 hr, and the duration of action is 3 to 6 days. The total oral dose is usually 2.0 to 3.0 mg given over a period of 48 hr. The dose may be divided into any convenient schedule, such as 0.5 mg three times daily, or 1.0 mg initially followed by 0.25 mg at intervals of 4 to 6 hr. When congestive failure is moderately severe, it is desirable to accomplish digitalization in a shorter period of time. As always, the dosage must be individualized, and an occasional patient may develop toxic symptoms on these schedules. It is better to err on the side of underdigitalization than to arouse the patient's antagonism to the continued use of the drug. It is important to check the patient during the early days of digitalization. More patients tolerate a maintenance dose of 0.25 mg digoxin daily, with satisfactory hemodynamic effect and freedom from toxicity, than are able to tolerate doses of 0.5 mg. However, many patients require 0.5 mg daily and a few require 0.75 mg daily for optimal effects. Patients with atrial fibrillation or flutter should receive the daily requirement of digoxin in divided doses to lessen the rare possibility of "nocturnal escape" with acceleration of the ventricular rate.

Digoxin may be used for *rapid digitalization.* The effects of intravenous digoxin begin within 5 to 10 min and reaches a peak in 4 to 6 hr (recent observations by Weissler[13]). The rapid action lessens the need for such preparations as ouabain or acetyl strophanthidin, which in our experience, are only rarely needed. In the patient who has received no prior digitalis preparation, an initial dose of 1.0 mg may be given slowly intravenously. Additional increments of 0.25 mg may be given orally, in the muscle, or intravenously in 4 to 6 hr for two to three doses, depending on the need.

The maintenance dose may be started the following day. Since 50 to 60 per cent of digoxin is absorbed from the gastrointestinal tract, the parenteral dosage is one-half to two-thirds of the oral dose. The digitalization of infants and children is discussed in Chap. 20.

Digitoxin is completely absorbed from the gastrointestinal tract. The oral digitalizing dose in the adult varies from 1.2 to 1.6 mg, given in divided doses over a period of 24 to 48 hr. The onset of action occurs in about 4 hr; the maximum effect is reached in 6 to 8 hr, and the duration of action is 14 to 21 days. A convenient schedule is 0.6 mg initially, followed by 0.2 every 6 hr for three doses, or until satisfactory response is achieved. The maintenance dose is usually in the range of 0.1 to 0.15 mg. Although 0.2 mg is occasionally necessary, this dosage is generally excessive. The oral and parenteral dosages of digitoxin are identical. When digitoxin is given intravenously, it has an onset of effect in 30 min to 2 hr, and a peak effect in about 8 hr.

Digitalis leaf, which is administered only orally, has an onset of action in 4 to 6 hr; it reaches a maximum effect in 6 to 8 hr and has a duration of effect for 14 to 21 days. The oral dose for the average adult varies from 1.0 to 2.0 Gm, given in divided doses over a period of 3 to 4 days; the average maintenance dose is 0.1 Gm daily.

Lanatoside C can be used intravenously when a rapid effect is desired. The effect begins within 5 min and reaches a peak action in about 20 min. The peak action is maintained for about 2 hr and is then dissipated over a period of 3 to 5 days. Lanatoside C is not used for maintenance therapy. In our experience, intravenous digoxin has an effect that begins almost as quickly without the variables inherent in switching to another preparation for maintenance therapy. On the other hand, the short period required to attain the peak effect of lanatoside C can be used to advantage under certain circumstances. The dose of lanatoside C varies from 1.2 to 2.0 mg given in divided doses. In most situations, an initial dose of 0.8 mg is administered and is followed by increments of 0.4 mg at 2-hr intervals.

When it is difficult to ascertain whether or not the patient has been on digitalis, the following approach is recommended: Carefully survey the patient's symptoms and electrocardiogram for possible evidence of digitalis toxicity. If none is present, one may give 0.25 to 0.5 mg digoxin orally and observe hemodynamic effect and response. If no toxicity occurs, additional increments may be given after 4 to 6 hr. The patient must be seen and an electrocardiographic "rhythm strip" obtained before each additional dose.

In urgent situations in which the state of digitalization is unknown and in which there is electrocardiographic evidence of possible digitalis intoxication, such as frequent ventricular premature beats, one can cautiously administer 0.25 mg digoxin intravenously. If this produces an increased frequency of premature beats, further administration of the drug is omitted. On the other hand, if the response is satisfactory and there is no increase in ventricular beats, additional doses may be given, with proper assessment before each increment. Since the peak effect of digoxin occurs at 4 to 6 hr, it is necessary to observe the rhythm for this period of time. Lanatoside C, 0.2 mg intravenously, can also be used for this purpose. Close observation for 2 hr is mandatory when this drug is used. Lown has successfully used acetyl strophanthidin for this purpose,[14] but this drug is not recommended for general use. Unfortunately, there is no sure way of determining the state of digitalization in such patients. One should have lidocaine, or procainamide hydrochloride (Pronestyl) available for intravenous use to counteract toxicity, such as evidenced by increased frequency of ventricular premature beats or ventricular tachycardia. In addition, the use of potassium therapy in digitalis intoxication must be understood. The physician who gives additional digitalis to a patient who might have digitalis intoxication must be prepared to institute external cardiac massage and to maintain pulmonary ventilation. Equipment for defibrillation and cardiac pacing should be available (see Chap. 16). If these measures are not available, it is far better to manage the congestive failure by means other than digitalis until the problem has been resolved with the passage of time.

Another situation posing a problem is the patient on known digitalis preparation who has omitted the drug for an unknown number of days. The need for partial redigitalization presents itself. Depending on the urgency, one may give a small amount of digoxin intravenously as described above or may begin with an increased maintenance dose.

Digitalis, like all drugs, has *toxic effects*. Since the days of Withering, physicians have been aware that anorexia, nausea, vomiting, diarrhea, and yellow vision may be due to overdigitalization. Abdominal pain and toxic psychosis with delirium have been rarely noted. Gazes reported mesenteric venous occlusion secondary to digitalis toxicity.[15] Gynecomastia may be associated with digitalis administration in the absence of cardiovascular evidence of toxicity. Rarely, the chronically overdigitalized patient may be erroneously suspected of having carcinoma because of anorexia and weight loss. An occasional patient may be troubled by increased vigor of cardiac contraction, but this alone does not indicate a harmful effect. Trigeminal neuralgia due to digitalis toxicity has been reported, but its occurrence is probably coincidental. The visual disturbances include scotomas, bluish vision, and the conventional yellow vision.

The cardiac effects of digitalis intoxication cannot be overemphasized. In this situation the electrocardiogram may furnish the sole evidence of toxicity. Chlorothiazide diuretics produce potassium depletion, and the use of these drugs has resulted in widespread digitalis intoxication. Reserpine and guanethidine sulfate (Ismelin) less often predispose to toxicity. Calcium preparations given intravenously induce ventricular arrhythmias in patients receiving digitalis. Many common manifestations of overdigitalization may be readily recognized by physical examination: frequent premature beats, bigeminy, the irregularity due to Wenckebach's phenomena, marked bradycardia, or a striking increase in rate which may be regular or irregular. On the other hand, more subtle signs of toxic effects should be suspected in the following situations: when the rate increases slightly rather than slows with therapy (AV dissociation may be present), when atrial fibrillation is replaced by a regular rate (atrial tachycardia with block, atrial flutter, ventricular tachycardia, nodal tachycardia may be present), or when response to therapy is unsatisfactory. In each instance, the electrocardiogram is essential for identification of the disturbance. Digitalis may produce virtually all cardiac arrhythmias, including frequent ventricular premature contractions, often with coupling of multifocal origin, interference dissociation, paroxysmal atrial tachycardia with AV block, nonparoxysmal nodal tachycardia, varying degrees of AV block, commonly Wenckebach's phenomenon, and rarely complete heart block; atrial fibrillation, atrial flutter, ventricular tachycardia, occasionally bidirectional type, and ventricular fibrillation. These arrhythmias are usually recognized by a "rhythm strip," which should be taken using a lead axis which shows the P waves of maximum amplitude. Cautious carotid sinus massage may be helpful in selected instances. At times, cardiac arrhythmias due to digitalis may be so complex that expert electrocardiographers argue the mechanism. A given tracing may suggest a variety of mechanisms, including AV dissociation with interference, atrial tachycardia, aberrant conduction simulating ventricular tachycardia, etc. Such tracings frequently depict an acceleration of the nodal pacemakers which periodically competes with the atrial pacemakers. An argument regarding the mechanism of an arrhythmia in itself is sufficient grounds to suspect digitalis intoxication.

Mild digitalis toxicity producing symptoms such as anorexia, nausea, vomiting, diarrhea, infrequent ventricular ectopic beats, and Wenckebach's phenomenon can be managed by omission of digitalis for several days. Certain arrhythmias deserve additional measures. Frequent *ventricular ectopic beats*, especially those occurring near the peak of the T wave, bigeminy, or multifocal ventricular premature beats are managed by discontinuance of the drug and by the oral administration of 1 Gm potassium chloride every 4 hr (Fig. 15-1). One gram of potassium chloride contains 13 mEq of potassium. If oral medication is not feasible because of nausea, vomiting, or intolerance to the drug, one may give 40 to 60 mEq potassium chloride in 500 ml of 5 per cent glucose in water intravenously over a period of 2 to 4 hr. Urinary output of more than 20 ml per hour or a serum-potassium level of less than 6 mEq per liter should be confirmed before giving large amounts of potassium, in order to avoid potassium intoxication. If the situation warrants, one may give procaine amide hydrochloride intravenously in a dose of 250 to 500 mg diluted in 100 ml of 5 per cent glucose in water, over a period of 5 to 15 min. A maintenance dose of 200 to 500 mg every 4 to 6 hr may be used.

Although paroxysmal atrial tachycardia with varying AV block may occur in the absence of digitalis administration, the majority of instances are due to toxicity to digitalis (Fig. 15-2). The clinical setting may be one in which the dose of digitalis has been increased or its excretion impaired, or in which the dose of digitalis is unchanged but potassium loss has occurred. The latter may be due to diuretics, particularly the thiazide derivatives, vomiting, diarrhea, gastrointestinal suction, glucose administration without potassium supplementation, corticosteroid administration, or potassium-losing nephropathy. The serum-potassium level may be unchanged and cannot be used to indicate the need for potassium. It may be that the decreased potassium content of red cells furnishes a more accurate estimate of potassium depletion. The management consists of omission of digitalis and the intravenous administration of 40 to 60 mEq potassium chloride in 500 ml of 5 per cent glucose in water, over a period of 4 hr. Adequate renal function should be present before intravenous potassium salts are given. Electrocardiographic monitoring during potassium therapy is desirable. Resuscitative measures should be available in the event that a catastrophe occurs. The rhythm may also be reverted using electrical cardioversion (direct current). Patients with AV node disease due either to intrinsic disease or to digitalis may have unusual arrhythmias after electrical cardioversion.[16] Because of this, the

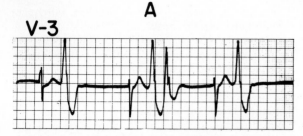

A

V-3

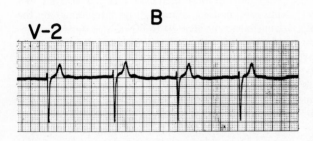

B

V-2

Fig. 15-1. *A*. Digitalis intoxication. Atrial fibrillation is present with an extremely slow ventricular rate, suggesting depressed conduction in the AV node. Ventricular ectopic contractions occur after each normal beat and in rapid succession after the second normal beat. *B*. Digitalis has been omitted and potassium chloride has been given. The ventricular ectopic beats have vanished, but atrial fibrillation with a slow ventricular rate continues.

patient with digitalis intoxication is not considered to be an ideal candidate for this form of therapy. Despite this danger, it may be needed if potassium therapy fails. At times, procainamide or quinidine may be effective in the reversion of this arrhythmia. When there is atrial tachycardia with varying AV block (2:1 and 3:1) and the ventricular rate is not rapid, oral potassium salts may be used (Fig. 15-2).

Interference dissociation due to digitalis will usually respond to omission of the drug and oral administration of potassium salts (Fig. 15-3). Intravenous potassium is rarely needed unless oral therapy is not feasible. Procainamide hydrochloride, lidocaine, or quinidine may be effective, but their mechanisms of action are not so physiologic as potassium supplements.

Atrial tachycardia with high-grade AV *block*

(3:1 and 4:1) or complete heart block due to digitalis should *not* be treated with potassium, quinidine, or procaine amide hydrochloride, since all these drugs may accentuate impaired conduction and suppress needed ectopic pacemakers. In this situation, these drugs may induce ventricular fibrillation. Digitalis must be omitted, and the rhythm should be continuously or intermittently monitored. If AV block increases or if episodes of ventricular standstill occur, electronic cardiac pacing is indicated. This may be accomplished by right ventricular catheter pacing or by external pacing if the equipment for internal pacing is not available. If no electronic equipment is available, isoproterenol (Isuprel) may be used. This drug should be used with caution, since there is a hazard of inducing ventricular tachycardia or fibrillation. It may be administered sublingually, 5 to 20

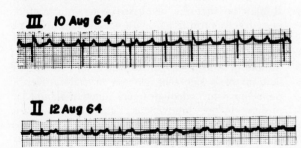

III 10 Aug 64

II 12 Aug 64

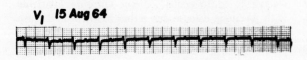

V₁ 15 Aug 64

Fig. 15-2. Upper, atrial tachycardia with varying AV block (2:1, 3:1, and 4:1) secondary to digitalis intoxication; middle, Wenckebach's phenomenon, recorded 2 days after digitalis was discontinued and oral potassium chloride was begun; lower, 3 days later, first-degree heart block.

mg every 2 to 4 hr, or 30 mg or more of proterenol (sustained-action isoproterenol) orally every 4 to 6 hr; or in the form of a slow intravenous drip of 1 mg of isoproterenol in 500 ml of 5 per cent glucose distilled water.

Ventricular tachycardia due to digitalis intoxication is treated with intravenous potassium chloride as described earlier for paroxysmal atrial tachycardia with block. If reversion does not occur in a short period of time, electrical therapy using direct current should be used. In urgent situations, controlled electrical therapy can be used initially and should be followed by potassium therapy. Intravenous procainamide, 1 gm in 200 ml of 5 per cent glucose in water, administered over a period of 30 to 45 min with appropriate monitoring, may be used if a d-c cardioverter is not available. Intravenous quinidine sulfate, 0.6 Gm in 200 ml of 5 per cent glucose in water, administered over a period of 30 to 45 min with appropriate electrocardiographic monitoring, may also be used if equipment for electrical reversion is not available.

Ventricular fibrillation is treated by emergency measures, including external massage and pulmonary ventilation. If spontaneous reversion does not occur, electrical defibrillation must be used and potassium repletion undertaken (see Chap. 69).

Chelating agents, such as sodium ethylenediaminetetraacetate (EDTA), which bind calcium have been used in the treatment of cardiac arrhythmias, but the toxic effects of these agents are so great that they are not recommended.

The *prevention* of digitalis intoxication by care in dosage and by observation of the side effects of diuresis is important. With increasing heart or renal failure, the excretion of digitalis may be impaired and toxicity may develop on a previously well-tolerated regimen. A reduction of the maintenance dosage may be needed in this setting. Currently, the major cause of digitalis intoxication is potassium depletion induced by chlorothiazide derivatives. Accordingly, potassium chloride should be administered along with the diuretics. Patients with renal failure who are receiving chlorothiazide may not require supplemental potassium. Added potassium may not be needed when an aldosterone antagonist is given in conjunction with chlorothiazide or similar drugs.

METHODS OF DECREASING VISCERAL CONGESTION

Patients with congestive heart failure may experience diuresis, weight loss, and decreased visceral congestion when placed at rest (decrease in demand) and when digitalized (improvement

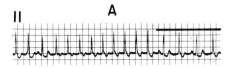

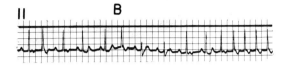

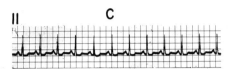

Fig. 15-3. Interference dissociation due to digitalis intoxication. *A.* P waves are difficult to identify, but there appears to be a short run of nodal tachycardia. The dark horizontal line seen at the end of *A* and throughout *B* indicates the duration of carotid sinus pressure (applied continuously—see text). P waves are clearly seen during the early part of *B.* Nodal tachycardia returns at the end of *B. C.* Digitalis has been omitted and potassium chloride has been given. The rhythm is normal sinus rhythm. The ST-T abnormalities are characteristic of digitalis effect but are not in themselves evidence of toxicity.

in cardiac function). Since these measures are not always successful and since permanent inactivity is obviously a poor solution to the problem, it is fortunate that the *diet* can be altered and that *diuretics* can be employed with enormous benefit to the patient.

Diet.[1] Many individuals eat more sodium than they need, but the excess is excreted in the urine when the kidneys and other organs are functioning normally. Most of this excess is in the form of sodium chloride, and a normal diet contains about 10 Gm daily. Heart failure causes the kidneys to function abnormally and leads to sodium and water retention, weight gain, visceral congestion, and increased venous pressure. The amount of sodium and water retained by the body as a result of heart failure can be altered by decreasing the amount of salt ingested in the diet.[17] Sodium and water retention may also be prevented by certain diuretic drugs. The low-sodium diet and diuretics may be used simultaneously with other measures for heart failure. The object is to make the total treatment as effective, simple, pleasant, and safe as possible. Accordingly, the therapy for heart failure is individualized.

The usual patient with heart failure does not require rigid restriction of sodium. The newly developed oral diuretics (despite their complicating difficulties) have decreased the need for unpleasant diets and salt substitutes. Even so, it is wise for the patient with the slightest heart failure to avoid obviously salty foods and to restrict the use of salt after the food is served. This will decrease the salt intake to about 5 Gm daily. The patient should try to accustom his palate to less salt. In practice it is generally more acceptable to the patient when the diet is altered as little as possible, even though more oral medication may be needed. When failure is not controlled by slight restriction of salt intake and reasonable diuretic therapy, more stringent restriction of salt intake is indicated. Under these circumstances, a diet containing only 2 to 3 Gm sodium chloride daily may be indicated. This can be attained by omitting certain naturally salty foods, salt during cooking, and at the table. A strict low-salt diet containing 0.5 Gm salt is used only after the preceding has failed. This diet is not palatable and is deficient in many badly needed foodstuffs such as protein. Such a diet may be used for short periods of time but it is the exceptional patient who tolerates the diet for a long period, because his appetite fails, his tissues waste away, and he becomes increasingly unhappy.

As a rule, water need not be restricted except at

Table 15-1. ORAL DIURETIC PREPARATIONS

Preparation	Daily dosage range, mg	Duration of action, hr
Thiazides:		
Polythiazide (Renese)	1–4	24–48
Trichlormethiazide (Naqua)	2–4	+24
Methyclothiazide (Enduron)	2.5–10	+24
Bendroflumethiazide (Naturetin)	5–20	+18
Benzthiazide (Exna)	25–200	12–18
Hydro Chlorothiazide (Esidrix, HydroDiuril, Oretic)	25–200	12–18
Chlorothiazide (Diuril)	500 mg–1 Gm	6–12
Related sulfonamide compounds:		
Chlorthalidone (Hygroton)	50–200; usually every other day	48–72
Quinethazone (Hydromox)	50–200	18–24

SOURCE: Reprinted with permission of the Journal of the American Medical Association.[20]

the stage of heart failure characterized by dilutional hyponatremia.

The diet may be important aside from the consideration of sodium balance. The obese patient should lose weight. This is another way to reduce the demand the body places on the heart. When appetite is poor and the diet is not palatable, vitamin B complex should be given.

Diuretics. The pharmacologic aspects of the diuretic agents are discussed in Chap. 68. The practical use of the drugs is considered below.

Diuretics are eventually needed in most patients with heart failure. They are used to remove and prevent the accumulation of body fluid and sodium in an effort to relieve or forestall symptoms due to visceral congestion. Pitting edema is a late sign of heart failure. An accurate record of the daily weight affords the best method of determining the amount of fluid accumulation and the need for diuretics. A gain of 3 to 4 lb of weight in a period of a few days indicates the need for additional diuretic administration. It must be remembered, however, that with anorexia, poor food intake, and resultant tissue wasting, the weight may remain unchanged or even decrease in the presence of persistent edema and congestion. Thus, the weight alone is only one factor in judging the need for diuretic therapy.

Chlorothiazide Derivatives. The advantages of these drugs are that they are extremely effective orally, that there is lessened need for sodium restriction with its associated unpalatable diet, that more even control of congestive heart failure can be obtained, and that there is a greater margin of safety in patients with intrinsic renal disease. Furthermore, the drug may be effective in the treatment of coexisting hypertension. The enormous advantage is counterbalanced by the major disadvantages of potassium depletion, the accentuation of hyperglycemia in the diabetic patient, and the depression of uric acid excretion, which may lead to clinical gout in some patients.

Numerous preparations are available, but it is desirable to become familiar with the use of a single preparation (Table 15-1).[20] Chlorothiazide (Diuril) may be administered as a single daily dose of 500 mg upon awakening, or it may be repeated at lunch time. Depending on the need, the daily dose (0.5 to 1 Gm) may be given twice a week, every other day; and if absolutely necessary, daily. Diuretics produce a greater diuresis of sodium and water per unit dose if taken at bedtime, but the inconvenience of nocturia may counterbalance the intensification of the desired effect. Potassium depletion occurs more often when the diuretic is given daily. Most patients receiving thiazide diuretics need supplements of 50 to 100 mEq potassium daily. Many preparations containing a mixture of potassium salts may be ineffective in restoring or maintaining potassium balance, and it is essential to give potassium in the form of chloride.[20a] Orange juice does not furnish adequate potassium. Unfortunately potassium chloride may not be tolerated by the patient and often produces gastric irritation. Enteric coated potassium chloride is frequently not absorbed and circumferential, stenosing, or ulcerative lesions of the small bowel may occur, rarely, due to potassium administration alone (especially when used as enteric coated tablets) or in combination with thiazide drugs.[20b,20c] Accordingly, it is best to administer liquid potassium chloride in some vehicle such as tomato juice.

Mercurial Diuretics. Serious electrolyte depletion is less likely than with chlorothiazide drugs, although hypochloremic alkalosis may still occur. They are occasionally effective when chlorothiazides fail to produce a response. The disadvantages are that they must be given intramuscularly or intravenously, which makes self-administration difficult; and they produce more nephrotoxicity, although this is not a serious drawback when the kidneys are not diseased. The presence of albuminuria and mildly elevated level of blood urea nitrogen per se are not absolute contraindications to their use. Meralluride sodium with theophylline (Mercuhydrin) or mercaptomerin sodium (Thiomerin), 1 to 2 ml, is commonly given intramuscularly; however, they may be given intravenously with reasonable safety (mercaptomerin sodium may be given subcutaneously). The toxicity when given by this route has been overemphasized. The administration of these preparations intramuscularly often produces pain; and when severe congestive heart failure is present, there may be impaired absorption from the muscle. In the presence of renal disease, it is unwise to repeat the mercurials when diuresis fails to occur. When frequent injections are given, chloride supplementation is often needed and potentiates response (ammonium chloride or potassium chloride, 1 Gm three times daily). Diuresis begins in 1 to 2 hr after intramuscular injection. The diuretic effect reaches a peak in about 8 hr and continues for 24 hr. The frequency of administration of mercurial diuretics varies from once a week to several times weekly, depending on the clinical status, the dietary intake of sodium, and associated diuretic therapy. It is unwise to repeat mercurial injections at daily intervals when diuresis is continuing from the initial dose, since a satisfactory response may persist for several days. Toxic effects are discussed in Chap. 68.

The simplicity of using the oral diuretics has dampened the enthusiasm formerly held for the mercurial diuretics. This is unfortunate, and we wish to emphasize that the diuresis associated with the intermittent use of mercurial diuretics is less likely to produce the frightening potassium loss so often seen with the daily use of thiazide diuretics. This advantage is especially desirable when patients are unable to tolerate potassium supplements. Also, the therapeutic response may be easier to identify following a mercurial diuretic. This feature is useful when one is attempting to separate dyspnea due to heart failure from that due to pulmonary disease. In addition, the mercurials act more promptly and therefore are useful when diuresis is needed quickly.[21] Patients with gout may have these symptoms aggravated by mercurial diuretics but not to the extent noted after thiazide drugs. Diabetic patients tolerate mercurial diuretics better than thiazide derivatives.

The normal serum contains more sodium than chloride. The urine, following a mercurial diuretic, contains more chloride than sodium, and in addition, there is increased loss of potassium. This produces a greater fall in concentration of serum chloride than of sodium. The serum-potassium level may or may not be decreased. Hypochloremic alkalosis is therefore to be expected in patients receiving mercurial diuretics. The responsiveness of the mercurials is decreased when this electrolyte disorder occurs.[22] The potassium and chloride deficit must be corrected. Mercurial diuretics should be omitted, and 4 to 6 Gm ammonium chloride should be administered daily for 3 to 4 days prior to the next mercurial injection. Beware of using ammonium chloride in patients with severe liver disease or renal acidosis. Appropriate amounts of potassium replacement, given as potassium chloride, are also indicated. The responsiveness to mercurial diuretics may also be restored by creating a state of systemic acidosis by one of several methods. Ten grams of L-lysine mono-hydrochloride may be given by mouth, in milk or juice, three times daily for several days prior to and on the day of the mercurial injection. This drug produces systemic acidosis and causes chloruresis. The responsiveness to mercurial diuretics can be restored by producing systemic acidosis even when the plasma-chloride level is not raised. Carbonic anhydrase inhibitors, such as acetazoleamide (Diamox), may be used to restore the effect of mercurial diuretics by reversing hypochloremic alkalosis. Acetazoleamide is given orally (250 to 375 mg daily) for several days prior to mercurial injection. The drug should not be given 24 hr before mecurial injection because this drug seems to interfere with the action of the mercurial diuretic on the tubule.

Other Diuretics. Aldosterone antagonists and corticosteroids are not used in the management of the usual cases of heart failure; they are discussed further on in this chapter, under "Refractory Heart Failure." Osmotic diuretics, such as mannitol and urea, are rarely used in the treatment of heart failure. Ammonium chloride has some diuretic effect on its own, but its major value is in potentiating the effect of mercurial diuretics. Xanthines are weak diuretics. The major use of theophylline ethylenediamine (aminophylline) is to increase cardiac output after a mercurial injection. Resins which bind sodium in the gastrointestinal tract are now seldom employed. Ethacrynic acid is an extremely potent diuretic that blocks sodium and chloride excretion in both proximal and distal tubules. It may be useful in refractory edema, when electrolyte disturbances are present, and in the presence of azotemia. The dose is 50 mg four times daily for 1 to 3 days. It must be used with great caution since severe depletion of electrolytes may occur, and metabolic alkalosis with reduced blood volume is not uncommon.[22a,b,c]

ELECTROLYTE DISTURBANCES[23,24]

Disturbances of inorganic metabolism occur in untreated heart falure. This primary disturbance of electrolytes can be altered greatly by modern therapy. The alteration of electrolytes may be beneficial, but many harmful effects may be observed. They are discussed in Chap. 13.

Hyponatremia, or low serum-sodium concentration, is a recurrent problem—often of ominous significance—which deserves reemphasis. As shown by Edelman, the serum-sodium level may be low as a result of excess body water or reduced body content of either sodium or potassium. The ratio of body content of sodium and potassium to body water determines the serum-sodium concentration.

Hyponatremia in congestive heart failure is almost always associated with excess body water, and therefore is often called "dilutional hyponatremia." The body stores of sodium are almost always increased but, because of low-salt diets and diuretics, not so much as the total body water is increased. In addition, potassium depletion may occasionally be present. These factors combine to reduce the measured concentration of sodium in the blood.

On very rare occasions, with maximum measures to produce sodium excretion, the total body stores of sodium may be reduced below normal; but if detectable edema is present, then excess body water is also present. The absolute levels of body water and sodium content are of little significance in heart failure. What is important is their values relative to each other and relative to the function of the heart.

It can be stated as a general rule that whenever hyponatremia is present, it is desirable to try and reduce body water content relative to cation (Na + K) content. This reduction should be sought by restriction of water intake and by diuretics (which always produce loss of more water than sodium), as long as clinical considerations indicate that reduction of cardiac filling pressure is desirable. Potassium supplements should also be given if not previously supplied. Sodium should not be used lest the load on the heart be further increased.

Occasionally diuretics may be used in a patient to the point that the reduction of venous filling pressure reduces cardiac output. This may occur even with a venous pressure above normal and with some edema present, as in some cases of constrictive pericarditis and cor pulmonale. Patients at this stage complain less of dyspnea and more of an extreme degree of muscular weakness, lassitude, and inability to get up from bed. This point is best detected by observing a drop in arterial blood pressure when the patient stands up. Under these circumstances, if the serum-sodium concentration is low, cautious administration of sodium may be desirable.

TREATMENT OF ACUTE PULMONARY EDEMA

Sudden flooding of the lungs in alveolar pulmonary edema is life-threatening and requires prompt measures. The physician should be prepared to act in a decisive and confident manner. Steps in management, many of which are carried out simultaneously, are as follows:

1. The majority of patients are more comfortable in the upright *position* and assume it spontaneously.[3] When shock is present, this position may be modified.

2. The single most important medication is morphine sulfate. From 10 to 15 mg should be given slowly by vein, with close scrutiny for respiratory depression. Morphine antagonists such as nalorphine hydrochloride (Nalline) should be available. Hypotension may be induced by morphine and nalorphine hydrochloride, but this does not limit their use; indeed, with advanced pulmonary edema, shock may be present prior to treatment.

3. Oxygen is given by mask or nasal catheter.[25] The proper administration of oxygen by positive pressure may be helpful; however, one must be careful not to produce a decrease in cardiac output by excessive impairment of venous return or to produce abdominal distension. An oxygen tent is ineffective and impractical.

4. Tourniquets applied sufficiently tight to occlude venous return may be applied to three extremities and rotated every 15 min.[26-29] Equipment designed to inflate and deflate blood pressure cuffs automatically is available.[30] One may use stethoscope tubing or any rubber tube or binder available. Tourniquets usually suffice and, in fact, may be superior to phlebotomy, but if response is not adequate, the withdrawal of 500 ml blood may turn the tide.

5. Aminophylline may be given intravenously, 10 ml (0.24 Gm), if response to other measures is not prompt, but it should be used with caution in shock.

6. In the undigitalized patient, 1.0 mg digoxin may be given by vein, followed by additional increments as indicated. This drug is usually secondary in importance to morphine, oxygen, and tourniquets unless there is an ectopic tachycardia which is responsive to this drug. Such rhythm as supraventricular tachycardia, atrial flutter, and atrial fibrillation with uncontrolled ventricular rate, may respond dramatically to rapid digitalization.

7. When supraventricular ectopic tachycardia and ventricular tachycardia do not respond to the usual therapy, the rhythm may be reverted by electrical means using d-c synchronized equipment (Fig. 15-4).[16] It may be used at the bedside with the patient under the influence of morphine. In urgent cases it may be used from the outset.

8. One milliliter of a mercurial diuretic such as meralluride sodium with theophylline or mercaptomerin sodium may be given intramuscularly or intravenously. Little immediate benefit is expected from diuretic agents, but it is wise to administer these drugs early in anticipation of a diuresis several hours later.[20] Mercurial diuretics are contraindicated when the pulmonary edema is secondary to acute renal failure.

9. Some normotensive patients develop paroxysmal hypertension early in an attack, presumably because of fear and apprehension and an increased liberation of catecholamines, but the blood pressure returns to normal when the symptoms are controlled. Acute pulmonary edema, related to systemic hypertension, may respond to small doses of ganglionic blocking drugs, such as 1 to 3 mg mecamylamine (Ansolysen) diluted in 50 ml glucose in water and given slowly by vein.[30] The smallest amount which produces a satisfactory blood pressure response is used. This drug should not be used when acute myocardial infarction is suspected.

10. In our hands, agents such as alcohol that reduce surface tension of alveolar fluid have been of limited value in the treatment of pulmonary

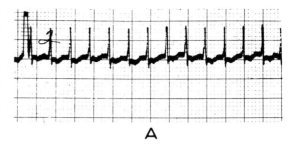

A

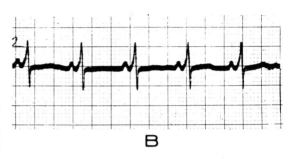

B

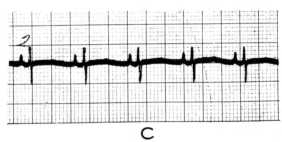

C

Fig. 15-4. A. Supraventricular tachycardia in a newborn infant with a normal heart. The heart rate is almost 300 beats per minute. The child had acute, severe, life-threatening heart failure. B. The rhythm was reverted to normal (sinus bradycardia for newborn), utilizing a d-c synchronized cardioverter. Fifty watt-seconds was required for reversion. Wolff-Parkinson-White syndrome is present. C. Normal sinus rhythm. The P waves are slightly pointed. The QRS conduction is normal. (*Case material furnished by Dr. Thomas L. Ross, Jr., of Macon, Georgia.*)

edema and they are therefore not recommended.

After the emergency has been controlled, one should seek the exact cause and the precipitating factors, keeping in mind that there are three etiologic categories of pulmonary edema: cardiac, cardiac plus extracardiac factors, and noncardiac. The therapy may vary in the three groups, e.g., morphine may be contraindicated in patients with pulmonary edema associated with increased intracranial pressure and in patients with pulmonary disease, such as extensive viral pneumonitis.

OTHER MEASURES USEFUL IN THE ROUTINE MANAGEMENT OF CONGESTIVE HEART FAILURE

The proper position of the patient in the bed, the use of a large comfortable chair, and the dangers of bed rest have been discussed earlier in this chapter.

Since heat and humidity increase cardiac work, an air-conditioned room is desirable in hot climates.[31] Oxygen is generally not required in the management of chronic heart failure; it is useful in severe failure and pulmonary edema. The nasal tube is satisfactory if care is taken so that the patient does not swallow oxygen. A tent is less efficient but offers the additional advantage of a cool environment. The use of hyperbaric oxygen with its attendant side effects remains experimental. Opiates, such as morphine, are not advised for the usual patient with chronic heart failure. On the other hand, such a drug may give rest and comfort to the exhausted patient who has been unable to sleep. Morphine is also useful in preventing initial or recurrent pulmonary edema. The side effects include nausea, vomiting, bladder retention, abdominal distension, constipation, respiratory depression, hypotension, and a modest antidiuretic effect.

Phenobarbital or meprobamate may be administered several times daily in an effort to decrease nervous tension and to thereby decrease cardiac work. A short-acting barbiturate may be used at night for sleep if necessary. Mental depression is not uncommon in patients with congestive heart failure, and occasionally drug therapy, such as imipramine hydrochloride (Tofranil), 25 mg three to four times daily, is helpful. Opiates and sedatives may accentuate insomnia due to Cheyne-Stokes respirations and at times are contraindicated in cor pulmonale due to chronic lung disease.

The oral xanthines are relatively ineffective, but suppositories containing aminophylline or intravenous aminophylline (10 ml: 0.24 Gm) may prevent or relieve Cheyne-Stokes respirations and wheezing.

Corticosteroid administration is useful in the management of heart failure secondary to acute rheumatic myocarditis or to myocarditis secondary to hypersensitivity states.

Thoracentesis may be desirable in patients in whom pleural fluid impairs ventilation. Diuresis may follow this procedure. Abdominal paracentesis is generally not advisable, since severe electrolyte depletion may occur. The removal of edema fluid from the legs with needles (Southey tubes) is not wise and is seldom necessary.[32]

REVERSIBLE FACTORS ASSOCIATED WITH HEART FAILURE

Certain cardiac and vascular abnormalities can be corrected, and cardiac function may be restored to the point that heart failure no longer develops. Also, the removal of aggravating and precipitating factors in patients with heart disease may reduce the cardiac work load so that improvement occurs, although the basic heart disease remains.

Heart failure due to peripheral AV fistula, patent ductus arteriosus, coarctation of the aorta, constrictive pericarditis, or atrial and ventricular septal defects may be eliminated when these abnormalities are surgically corrected. Generally, surgical correction of acquired or congenital valvular disease (see Chaps. 21 and 26) is not curative but ameliorative. The correction of a ventricular septal defect or ventricular aneurysm caused by a myocardial infarction may at times decrease the heart failure but is obviously not curative (see Chap. 26). Reversible hypertensive heart disease is represented by pheochromocytoma, aldosteronism, and some instances of Cushing's disease and of unilateral renal disease.

Pulmonary emboli are so common in patients with congestive heart failure that they seem to be part of the clinical syndrome. Furthermore, pulmonary emboli often precipitate and aggravate congestive heart failure. Long-term anticoagulant therapy has been used in an effort to decrease the thromboemboli complications in patients with congestive heart failure. Several groups of investigators have reported favorable results with Dicumarol.[33,34] Despite the studies which indicate the beneficial effect of long-term anticoagulant therapy in patients with heart failure, the procedure has not been generally adopted as a routine prophylactic measure in the management of such patients, perhaps because of the difficulties of controlling prothrombin levels as a result of hepatic congestion. Anticoagulants are clearly indicated when the pulmonary emboli are obvious, but it must be recalled that only 10 per cent of pulmonary emboli produce the clinical picture of pulmonary infarct and that the majority of emboli go unrecognized. Anticoagulants, especially heparin, are indicated in patients with cor pulmonale who have high hematocrit levels and in whom a vigorous diuresis is expected.

Cossio investigated the value of ligating the inferior vena cava in patients with chronic congestive heart failure.[35] This procedure does seem to decrease the number of microemboli; and in addition it has a long-term tourniquet effect. The procedure has not been adopted as a routine measure and is reserved for situations where the diagnosis is definite. It is obvious that we have not as yet solved the serious problem of thromboembolism in patients with heart failure.

When heart failure is due solely to thyrotoxicosis, cure may follow control of metabolism; on the other hand, in the overwhelming majority of patients, the hypermetabolism is an aggravating factor in the presence of underlying heart disease, and its control results in improvement but not in cure (see Chap. 61).

In the infant, heart failure may be due to paroxysmal supraventricular tachycardia alone, and correction of the arrhythmia may be life-saving (Fig. 15-4).[36] Ectopic tachycardia in the patient with heart disease frequently precipitates or aggravates heart failure; accordingly, the control of arrhythmia may be paramount in management.[16]

With the exception of sickle-cell disease, in which multiple factors are involved (Chap. 54), anemia rarely produces heart failure unless the hemoglobin level is below 5 Gm per 100 ml. Anemia may be an aggravating factor in patients with heart disease, and specific therapy of the anemia is indicated. If the anemia is sufficiently severe to warrant transfusion, small amounts of packed red blood cells, rather than whole blood, should be used. Erythrocytosis predisposes to thromboembolism, particularly after vigorous diuresis. Periodic phlebotomy in patients with cor pulmonale of 300 to 400 ml from patients with hematocrits of 50 to 60 or higher can be tried but is usually of limited value.

An obstructing prostate may be an aggravating factor in the male. Prostatic swelling may be aggravated by heart failure, and, in turn, it may impair renal function and aggravate the heart failure.

Viral pneumonitis may be catastrophic to cardiac patients. Other pulmonary or urinary tract infections may accentuate or precipitate heart failure; they should be treated by specific measures when possible. Pulmonary infection is an extremely common precipitating factor in children.

REFRACTORY HEART FAILURE

Many patients who do not respond to conventional therapy outside the hospital environment may do so when hospitalized; this is because of better control of dietary sodium and of activity, assessment of the need for and administration of additional digitalis and diuretics, or, conversely, the determination that electrolyte depletion or digitalis intoxication has followed excessive medication, and to the relief of anxiety. A careful search for the factors known to aggravate heart failure may be rewarding. The correction of arrhythmias may be especially rewarding. Atrial fibrillation is a common arrhythmia, and the loss of the atrial booster pumps

may compromise the cardiac output by 20 per cent. The reversion of this rhythm to normal, using small amounts of quinidine sulfate and d-c synchronized electrical therapy, may be of considerable benefit to patients with heart failure. Even when normal rhythm cannot be maintained with quinidine sulfate, the period of normal rhythm may benefit the patient considerably so that when the arrhythmia returns the patient may remain improved.[16] Congestive heart failure may be associated with a heart rate of 30 to 40 beats per minute because of complete heart block. The insertion of a catheter pacemaker or a permanently implanted cardiac pacemaker in order to increase the heart rate to 65 to 70 beats per minute may produce marked improvement. Cardiac arrhythmias due to digitalis intoxication must be corrected.

Electrolyte abnormalities, including hypochloremic alkalosis and potassium deficits, must be corrected. Refractoriness to mercurial diuretics should be corrected by creating systemic acidosis with ammonium chloride, acetazoleamide, or L-lysine monohydrochloride.

The reabsorption of sodium can be blocked in the proximal tubule of the nephron by mercurial diuretics and by thiazide derivatives. The distal tubular reabsorption of sodium can be blocked by administering an antagonist to aldosterone.[37] Spironolactone (Aldactone-A), 25 mg four times daily, may be given orally. The effect of the drug is not immediate and may be delayed for 5 to 7 days. This drug promotes sodium excretion and potassium reabsorption. The drug should be used in combination with thiazide diuretics, rather than alone. When this is done, it is usually not necessary to give supplemental potassium, since spironolactone reduces the amount of potassium loss associated with thiazide diuretics.

In order to be certain that the mercurial diuretic reaches the kidney in adequate concentration, the drug may be given intravenously. To optimize the hemodynamic conditions for diuresis, the patient should remain at bed rest for 2 or 3 hr after the injection. (Patients with heart failure, unlike normal subjects, may have a higher cardiac output at rest than when walking about.[3]) Aminophylline (0.25 Gm) may be given intravenously an hour after the mercurial injection in order to increase the cardiac output so that renal blood flow containing the diuretics may be enhanced.[40] Even though mercurial diuretics, thiazide drugs, and aldosterone antagonists reach the renal tubule, they may fail in blocking the renal tubular reabsorption of sodium and water, under the hemodynamic conditions of severe heart failure.

A constant drip of epinephrine has been used in

a small number of infants who had refractory heart failure due to large left-to-right shunts.[38] Dopamine (3,4-dihydroxyphenylamine) has a positive inotropic effect, increases cardiac output, decreases peripheral resistance, and promotes sodium excretion.[39] Unfortunately, its long-term use is not practical.

A short course (1 week) of adrenal corticosteroids has, on occasion, been followed by a diuresis in patients with refractory heart failure.[41] The mechanism of this effect is obscure. These drugs may affect favorably the water permeability of the distal renal tubule, exert a positive inotropic action on the heart, or modify the distribution of body fluids. The long-term benefit of such an approach is minimal.

Rarely, the euthyroid patient with refractory heart failure may benefit from the production of hypothyroidism by the administration of radioactive iodine.

Hyperbaric oxygen therapy for refractory heart failure is experimental at the time of this writing.

When intractable heart failure develops and dilutional hyponatremia is evident, the patient may not tolerate a no-sodium diet or restriction of fluid intake. The former leads to nausea, vomiting, weakness, drowsiness, and even coma; and the latter leads to overpowering thirst. Merrill has suggested that fasting for 5 to 7 days may be of benefit to some patients.[42] This intriguing idea needs to be investigated further. The administration of hypertonic saline solution is almost never indicated.

Another approach suggested for dilutional hyponatremia has been hemodialysis; however, this experimental approach should currently be confined to those patients with remedial lesions.

After all the avenues of treatment have been explored, a state of absolute refractory failure may develop. At this point, further unwarranted attempts at tightening the control may make life more miserable. At this state the wise physician's foremost concern is the comfort of his patient. ✳

PROGNOSIS

The prognosis of heart failure cannot be stated in a meaningful way. One patient may die with his first episode of acute fulminating pulmonary edema; another patient with chronic heart failure may live for 20 years. For example, the patient with heart failure due to aortic stenosis or aortic insufficiency seldom lives more than 2 years after decompensation occurs. By contrast, the patient with mitral stenosis may live many years even though the course is punctuated by recurrent bouts of heart failure. Patients with coronary disease may have recurrent heart failure incidental to myocardial

necrosis but may remain compensated between attacks. Even with chronic heart failure, patients may live for many years.

Today, more is known about sodium balance in heart failure, and therefore the diet can be modified and diuretics given. Many aggravating factors can be removed, and the basic heart disease itself can often be altered. Fortunately, congestive heart failure can be managed far better today than it was 10 years ago.

REFERENCES

1. Brenner, O.: The Management of Heart Failure in A. M. Jones (ed.), "Cardiology," Hoeber Medical Division, Harper & Row, Publishers, Incorporated, New York, 1961, p. 84.
2. Rusk, H. A., and Gertler, M. M.: Rehabilitation in Congestive Heart Failure, *Circulation*, **21**:444, 1960.
3. Stead, E. A., and Hickam, J.: Heart Failure, *Disease-a-Month*, January, 1955.
4. Burch, G. E., Walsh, J. J., and Black, W. C.: Value of Prolonged Bedrest in Management of Cardiomegaly, *J.A.M.A.*, **183**:81, 1963.
5. Levine, S. A.: Some Harmful Effects of Recumbency in the Treatment of Heart Disease, *J.A.M.A.*, **126**:80, 1944.
6. Braunwald, E., Brockenbrough, E. C., and Frye, R. L.: Studies on Digitalis. V. Comparison of the Effects of Ouabain on Left Ventricular Dynamics in Valvular Aortic Stenosis and Hypertrophic Subaortic Stenosis, *Circulation*, **26**:166, 1962.
7. Selzer, A.: Clinical Use of Digitalis: Science or Empiricism? *Circulation*, **28**:1031, 1963.
8. Christian, H. A.: The Use of Digitalis Other Than in the Treatment of Cardiac Decompensation, *J.A.M.A.*, **100**:789, 1933.
9. Skinner, N. S., Jr., Mitchell, J. H., Wallace, A. G., and Sarnoff, S. J.: Hemodynamic Consequences of Atrial Fibrillation at Constant Ventricular Rates, *Am. J. Med.*, **36**:342, 1964.
10. Burchell, H. B.: A Clinical Appraisal of Atrial Transport Function, *Lancet*, **1**:775, 1964.
11. Kay, C. F.: The Clinical Use of Digitalis Preparations, *Circulation*, **12**:116–123, 291–304, 1955.
12. Lown, B.: Digitalis and Potassium, *Advances Int. Med.*, **8**:125, 1956.
13. Weissler, A. Personal communication.
14. Lown, B., Crocker, A. T., and Levine, S. A.: A Digitalis Tolerance Test, *Proc. New England Cardiovas. Soc.*, **11**:17, 1953.
15. Gazes, P. C., Holmes, C. R., Moseley, V., and Pratt-Thomas, H. R.: Acute Hemorrhage and Necrosis of the Intestines Associated with Digitalization, *Circulation*, **23**:358, 1961.
16. Hurst, J. W., Paulk, E. A., Jr., Proctor, H. D., and Schlant, R. C.: The Management of Patients with Atrial Fibrillation, *Am. J. Med.*, **37**:728, 1964.

17. Schroeder, H. A.: The Importance of Restriction of Salt as Compared to Water, *Am. Heart J.,* **22:** 141, 1941.

18. Ray, C. T., and Bresler, E. H.: Diuretic Drugs in Congestive Heart Failure, *M. Clin. North America,* **41:**433, 1957.

19. Schreiner, G. E., and Bloomer, H. A.: Effect of Chlorothiazide on the Edema of Cirrhosis, Nephrosis, Congestive Heart Failure, and Chronic Renal Insufficiency, *New England J. Med.,* **257:**1012, 1957.

20. Council on Drugs: Thiazides and Related Oral Diuretics, *J.A.M.A.,* **188:**162, 1964.

20a. Kassirer, J. P., Berkman, P. M., Lawrenz, D. R., and Schwartz, W. B.: The Critical Role of Chloride in the Correction of Hypokalemic Alkalosis in Man, *Am. J. Med.,* **38:**172, 1965.

20b. Baker, D. R., Schroder, W. H., and Hitchcock, C. R.: Small Bowel Ulceration Apparently Associated with Thiazide and Potassium Therapy, *J.A.M.A.,* **190:**586, 1964.

20c. Lawrason, F. D., Alpert, E., Mohr, F. L., and McMahon, F. G.: Ulcerative Obstructive Lesions of the Small Intestine, *J.A.M.A.,* **191:**641, 1965.

21. Alsever, J. B., and Levine, S. A.: The Immediate Effect of Mercurial Diuretics on the Vital Capacity of the Lungs, *Am. Heart J.,* **15:**201, 1938.

22. Weston, R. E., Escher, D. J. W., Grossmann, J., and Leiter, L.: Mechanisms Contributing to Unresponsiveness to Mercurial Diuretics in Congestive Cardiac Failure, *J. Clin. Invest.,* **31:**901, 1952.

22a. Cannon, P. J., Heinemann, H. O., Stason, W. B., and Laragh, J. H.: Ethacrynic Acid. Effectiveness and Mode of Diuretic Action in Man, *Circulation,* **31:**5, 1965.

22b. Beyer, K. H., Baer, J. E., Michaelson, J. K., and Russo, H. F.: Renotropic Characteristics of Ethacrynic Acid: A Phenoxyacetic Saluretic-Diuretic Agent, *J. Pharmacol. & Exper. Therap.,* **147:**1, 1965.

22c. Maher, J. F., and Schreiner, G. E.: Studies on Ethacrynic Acid in Patients with Refractory Edema, *Ann. Int. Med.,* **62:**15, 1965.

23. Seldin, D. S.: Management of Congestive Heart Failure: Management Designed to Avoid Serious Disturbance of Electrolyte and Water Balance, *A.M.A. Arch. Int. Med.,* **95:**385, 1955.

24. Friedberg, C. K.: Fluid and Electrolyte Disturbances in Heart Failure and Their Treatment, *Circulation,* **16:**437, 1957.

25. Daly, W. J., and Behnke, R. H.: Hemodynamic Consequences of Oxygen Breathing in Left Ventricular Failure, *Circulation,* **27:**252, 1963.

26. Weiss, S., and Robb, G. P.: The Treatment of Cardiac Asthma (Paroxysmal Cardiac Dyspnea), *M. Clin. North America,* **16:**961, 1933.

27. Ebert, R. V., and Stead, E. A., Jr.: The Effect of the Application of Tourniquets on the Hemodynamics of the Circulation, *J. Clin. Invest.,* **19:**561, 1940.

28. Kountz, W. B., Smith, J. R., and Wright, S. T.: Observations on the Effect of Tourniquets on Acute Cardiac Crises, Normal Subjects, and Chronic Heart Failure, *Am. Heart J.,* **23:**624, 1942.

29. Hellerstein, H. K., Rand, H. J., and Brinza, J.: Automatic Rotating Cuff Apparatus, *J. Lab. & Clin. Med.,* **46:**615, 1955.

30. Kelley, R. T., Fries, E. D., and Higgins, T. F.: The Effects of Hexamethonium on Certain Manifestations of Congestive Heart Failure, *Circulation,* **7:**169, 1953.

31. Burch, G. E., and Hyman, J.: Influence of a Hot and Humid Environment upon Cardiac Output and Work in Normal Man and in Patients with Chronic Congestive Heart Failure at Rest, *Am. Heart J.,* **53:**665, 1957.

32. Vere, D. W., and King, C. E.: The Reaction to Subcutaneous Drainage in Anasarca, *Lancet,* **1:** 779, 1960.

33. Anderson, G. M., and Hull, E.: The Effect of Dicoumerol upon the Mortality and Incidence of Thromboembolic Complications in Congestive Heart Failure, *Am. Heart J.,* **39:**697, 1950.

34. Levinson, D. C., and Griffith, G. C.: Evaluation of Anticoagulant Therapy in Congestive Heart Failure, *Circulation,* **4:**416, 1951.

35. Cossio, P.: Ligation of the Inferior Vena Cava in the Treatment of Heart Failure, *Am. Heart J.,* **43:** 97, 1952.

36. Young, D.: Treatment of Paroxysmal Supraventricular Tachycardia in Infancy, *Am. Heart J.,* **67:** 565, 1964.

37. Liddle, G. W.: Aldosterone Antagonists, *A.M.A. Arch. Int. Med.,* **102:**998, 1958.

38. Rudolph, A. M., Mesel, E., and Levy, J. M.: Epinephrine in the Treatment of Cardiac Failure Due to Shunts, *Circulation,* **28:**3, 1963.

39. McDonald, R. H., Jr., Goldberg, L. I., McNay, J. L., and Tuttle, E. P., Jr.: Effects of Dopamine in Man: Augmentation of Sodium Excretion, Glomerular Filtration Rate, and Renal Plasma Flow, *J. Clin. Invest.,* **43:**1116, 1964.

40. David, J. O., and Shock, N. W.: The Effect of Theophylline Ethylene Diamine on Renal Function in Control Subjects and in Patients with Congestive Heart Failure, *J. Clin. Invest.,* **28:**1459, 1949.

41. Mickerson, J. N., and Swale, J.: Diuretic Effect of Steroid Therapy in Obstinate Heart Failure, *Brit. M. J.,* **1:**876, 1959.

42. Merrill, A. J.: Intractable Heart Failure—Management with 5 to 7 Days of Fasting: A Preliminary Trial, *Am. Heart J.,* **67:**433, 1964.

SUGGESTED READING

Baum, G. L., Dick, M. M., Blum, A., Kaupe, A., and Carballo, J.: Factors Involved in Digitalis Sensitivity in Chronic Pulmonary Insufficiency, *Am. Heart J.,* **57:**460, 1959.

Black, A. B., and Litchfield, J. A.: Uraemia Complicating Low Salt Treatment of Heart Failure, *Quart. J. Med.,* 20:149, 1951.

Blumgart, H. L.: The Management of Congestive Heart Failure, *Circulation,* 7:127, 1953.

Blumgart, H. L., and Zoll, P. M.: The Clinical Management of Congestive Heart Failure, *Circulation,* 21:218, 1960.

Brenner, O.: Electrolyte Disturbances in Heart Failure, in E. J. Ross (ed.), "Clinical Effects of Electrolyte Disturbances," J. B. Lippincott Co., Philadelphia, 1954.

Burack, W. R., Pryce, J., and Goodwin, J. F.: A Reversible Nephrotic Syndrome Associated with Congestive Cardiac Failure, *Circulation,* 18:562, 1958.

Cort, J. H., and Matthews, H. L.: Potassium Deficiencies in Congestive Heart Failure, *Lancet,* 1:1202, 1954.

Davies, C. E.: The Effect of Treatment on Renal Circulation in Heart Failure, *Lancet,* 2:195, 1951.

DeGraff, A. C., and Lyon, A. F.: Diuretic Therapy. Part I, *Am. Heart J.,* 67:840, 1964.

DeGraff, A. C., and Lyon, A. F.: Diuretic Therapy. Part II. Pharmacology of Mercurial Diuretics, *Am. Heart J.,* 68:131, 1964.

DeGraff, A. C., and Lyon, A. F.: Diuretic Therapy. Part III. Clinical Use of Mercurial Diuretics, *Am. Heart J.,* 68:278, 1964.

Edelman, I. S.: Pathogenesis of Hyponatremia: Physiological and Therapeutic Implication, *Metabolism,* 5:500, 1956.

Elkington, J. R.: Hyponatraemia: Clinical State or Biochemical Sign, *Circulation,* 14:1027, 1956.

Ferrer, M. I., Conroy, R. J., and Harvey, R. M.: Some Effects of Digoxin upon the Heart and Circulation in Man: Digoxin in Combined (Right and Left) Ventricular Failure, *Circulation,* 21:372, 1960.

Friend, D. C.: Current Concepts in Therapy: Cardiac Glycosides, *New England J. Med.,* 266:88–89, 187–189, 300–302, 402–404, 1962.

Horan, L. G., and Flowers, N. C.: Trial by Digitalis, *Am. Heart J.,* 67:567, 1964.

Hurst, J. W., and Schlant, R. C. (eds.): Treatment of Cardiac Arrhythmias, *Mod. Treatment,* 1:665, 1964.

Kay, C. F.: Current Status of Therapy for Congestive Heart Failure: Special Report to A.M.A. Council on Drugs, *J.A.M.A.,* 164:659, 1957.

Levine, H. J.: The Treatment of Congestive Heart Failure, *M. Clin. North America,* 46:1261, 1962.

Love, W. D.: Digitalis Dosage—Individualized or Confused? *Am. Heart J.,* 63:575, 1962.

Lown, B., and Levine, S. A.: "Current Concepts in Digitalis Therapy," Little, Brown and Company, Boston, 1954.

Lown, B., Black, H., and Moore, F. D.: Digitalis, Electrolytes and the Surgical Patient, *Am. J. Cardiol.,* 6:309, 1960.

Lown, B., Marcus, F., and Levine, H.: Digitalis and Atrial Tachycardia with Block: A Year's Experience, *New England J. Med.,* 260:301, 1959.

Lyon, A. F., and DeGraff, A. C.: Diuretic Therapy. Part IV. Pharmacology of Thiazide Diuretics, *Am. Heart J.,* 38:421, 1964.

Lyon, A. F., and DeGraff, A. C.: Diuretic Therapy. Part V. Clinical Use of Thiazide Diuretics, *Am. Heart J.,* 68:569, 1964.

Lyon, A. F., and DeGraff, A. C.: Diuretic Therapy. Part VI. Metabolic Complications of Thiazide Therapy and Their Correction, *Am. Heart J.,* 68:710, 1964.

Morse, W. H., and Bing, R. J.: Congestive Heart Failure: Its Physiopathology and Treatment, with Special Reference to Intractable Heart Failure, *Postgrad. Med.,* 30:293, 1961.

Orgain, E. S., and Stead, E. A., Jr.: Clinical Progress: Congestive Heart Failure, *Circulation,* 16:291, 1957.

Schroeder, H. A.: Renal Failure Associated with Low Extracellular Sodium Chloride, *J.A.M.A.,* 141:117, 1949.

Sharp, J. T., Bunnell, I. L., Griffith, G. T., and Greene, D. G.: The Effects of Therapy on Pulmonary Mechanics in Human Pulmonary Edema, *J. Clin. Invest.,* 40:665, 1961.

Singer, M. M., and DeGraff, A. C.: Diuretic Therapy. Part VII. Spironolactone, *Am. Heart J.,* 68:835, 1964.

Stead, E. A.: Edema and Dyspnoea of Heart Failure, *Bull. New York Acad. Sc.,* 28:159, 1952.

Symposium on Congestive Heart Failure, *Circulation,* 21:95–128, 218–255, 424–447, 1960.

Wasserman, S.: "Acute Cardiac Pulmonary Edema: Its Pathogenesis and Treatment," Charles C Thomas, Publisher, Springfield, Ill., 1959.

Welt, L. G.: Edema of Hyponatraemia, *A.M.A. Arch. Int. Med.,* 89:931, 1952.

Section B: Disturbances of Rhythm and Conduction, Syncope, Shock, and Sudden Death

16 CARDIAC ARRHYTHMIAS AND CONDUCTION DISTURBANCES *

INTRODUCTION

J. Willis Hurst, M.D.

Abnormalities of the heart beat may not be recognized by the patient. Some patients with these disorders complain of palpitation, which is an unpleasant awareness of the heart beat. This complaint is virtually unrelated to the seriousness of the underlying disorder but is greatly influenced by the

* Dr. Eliot Corday and Dr. Tzu-Wang Lang furnished all the illustrations and legends used in this chapter.

We wish to thank the W. B. Saunders Company for permission to reprint a number of the illustrations originally used in the book *Disturbances of Heart Rate, Rhythm and Conduction,* by E. Corday, M.D., and D. W. Irving, M.D. (Philadelphia, 1961).

We also thank the publishers of *Annals of Internal Medicine,* the *American Journal of Cardiology,* and the *American Journal of Medicine* for permission to use the illustrations originally printed in those journals and so identified in the legends of this chapter.

The articles marked with an asterisk (*) were reprinted with permission of the authors, editors, and publisher, Paul B. Hoeber, Inc., medical division of Harper & Row, Publishers, New York, from *Treatment of Cardiac Arrhythmias,* in *Modern Treatment,* vol. 1, No. 3, pp. 665–776, 1964. The material has been modified slightly and brought up to date.

The articles marked with a dagger (†) and Tables 16-1, 16-2, and 16-3 were reprinted with permission of the authors and publisher from the article The Management of Patients with Atrial Fibrillation, by J. Willis Hurst, M.D., E. Alan Paulk, M.D., Herbert D. Proctor, M.D., and Robert C. Schlant, M.D., *American Journal of Medicine,* vol. 37, No. 5, pp. 728–741, 1964. The material has been modified slightly and brought up to date.

emotional status of the patient. Cardiac arrhythmias and conduction disturbances may or may not impair the function of the heart and circulation. The final effect produced by these disorders is determined by the specific nature of the arrhythmia and by the integrity of the circulatory system, including the heart and peripheral arteries. For example, atrial fibrillation with a ventricular rate of 145 heart beats per minute may create very little hemodynamic change in the normal resting individual; the same arrhythmia with the same heart rate may precipitate pulmonary edema in a patient with tight mitral stenosis, or angina pectoris in a patient with coronary atherosclerosis. Certain arrhythmias may be relatively unimportant but may be the forerunner of potentially lethal disorders. For example, ventricular ectopic beats occurring after myocardial infarction may be followed by ventricular tachycardia or ventricular fibrillation. Sudden death may occur without warning of any sort as a result of ventricular fibrillation or cardiac standstill.

Disorders of the heart beat are common. They may occur in patients who have no other evidence of heart disease and may, of course, occur in patients who have clear evidence of heart disease.

The ability to recognize and treat cardiac arrhythmias and conduction disturbances has changed considerably during the last several years because of the advances in the electronic field which led to the development of monitoring devices, electrical defibrillators, and cardiac pacemakers.

HEMODYNAMIC CONSEQUENCES OF CARDIAC ARRHYTHMIAS

Eliot Corday, M.D., and
Tzu-Wang Lang, M.D.

Cardiac arrhythmias may precipitate or aggravate congestive heart failure in certain clinical situations (Chap. 14). In addition, the circulation to the brain, heart, kidneys, gastrointestinal tract, muscles, and skin may be profoundly altered by cardiac arrhythmias. This aspect of cardiac arrhythmias has not been generally appreciated until recently and, therefore, is emphasized in the following discussion.

The normal resting subject will have little disturbance of circulatory hemodynamics unless the heart rate drops below 40 beats per minute or exceeds 160 beats per minute.[1] Under these circumstances, numerous reserve mechanisms are utilized to maintain normal blood pressure and cardiac output (see Chap. 2). (Fig. 16-1). On the other hand patients with disease of the heart or blood vessels may not have the reserve capacity which enables them to tolerate these extremes of heart rate. At excessively rapid or slow heart rates the cardiac output, systemic blood pressure, and blood flow to the vital organs may become so reduced that ischemia of the brain, myocardium, liver, kidney, gastrointestinal tract, and musculocutaneous system may develop[2-5] (Fig. 16-1).

Ischemia of these "target" organs can occur when the heart rate is no slower than 50 beats per minute or no faster than 120 beats per minute if there is

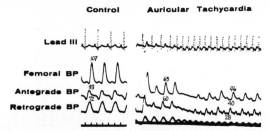

Fig. 16-2. Simultaneous recording of the electrocardiogram, femoral blood pressure, and antegrade and retrograde coronary blood pressures, before and following the induction of a paroxysm of atrial tachycardia. Note the marked drop in femoral and coronary blood pressures subsequent to the induction of atrial tachycardia. (*From Fig. 4, E. Corday, H. Gold, L. B. DeVera, J. H. Williams, and J. Fields: Effect of the Cardiac Arrhythmias on the Coronary Circulation, Ann. Int. Med.,* **50:**540, 1959.)

associated heart disease or peripheral arterial disease.

Cerebral Circulation. Recent experimental studies using electromagnetic flowmeter and computer techniques indicate that the cerebral blood flow may be reduced by an average of 8 per cent during frequent premature atrial systoles and by 12 per cent during premature ventricular systoles.[2] Occasional premature systoles have little effect on the cerebral circulation. When they occur very frequently, symptoms may occur because the cerebral blood flow may be diminished as much as 25 per cent. During atrial tachycardia, fibrillation, or flutter with rapid ventricular rates, the average reduction in cerebral blood flow is 23 per cent. However, if the ventricular rate is extremely rapid, it may decrease as much as 40 per cent. Normal subjects may tolerate a reduction in cerebral blood flow due to cardiac arrhythmias without having symptoms of ischemia; patients with cerebral vascular disease may develop signs and symptoms of cerebral vascular insufficiency.[6] The common symptoms are dizziness, weakness, syncope, convulsions, visual disturbances such as blurring, and hemianopsia, regional paresis, or paralysis.[7] The patient might even be unaware of the irregular or rapid heart action, but complain of the peripheral cerebral manifestations. If the collateral circulation is not compromised, and if the drop in cardiac output or pressure is profound, the symptoms might be those of generalized cerebrovascular ischemia, i.e., confusion, psychosis, and weakness.[2,8] Patients with transient focal or generalized neurologic signs and symptoms which cannot otherwise be explained should be monitored electrocardiographically over a period of hours to determine whether the episode might be due to transient arrhythmias.

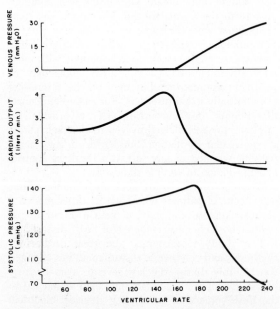

Fig. 16-1 The effect of increasing ventricular rate on systolic blood pressure, cardiac output, and venous pressure. The cardiac output gradually increases when the heart rate speeds up to 170 beats per minute, and then as the rate increases it gradually diminishes. As the rate speeds up, the systolic pressure gradually increases, and because peripheral vasoconstriction occurs, the pressure is sustained until the rate is about 190 to 210 beats per minute. Because of low cardiac output and despite vasoconstriction, which is not sufficient to maintain pressure above this rate, the systolic pressure begins to diminish. The venous pressure remains normal until around 180 beats per minute.

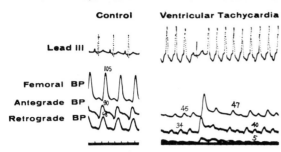

Fig. 16-3. The effect of ventricular tachycardia on the systemic and coronary blood pressures. Note that both the antegrade and retrograde coronary blood pressures drop markedly during a paroxysm of ventricular tachycardia. (*From Fig. 7, E. Corday, H. Gold, L. B. DeVera, J. H. Williams, and J. Fields: Effect of the Cardiac Arrhythmias on the Coronary Circulation, Ann Int. Med., 50;542, 1959.*)

Coronary Circulation. Coronary arterial blood flow diminishes when the systemic pressure drops during rapid supraventricular or ventricular arrhythmias (Figs. 16-2 and 16-3). The coronary blood flow falls an average of 35 per cent during rapid supraventricular tachycardia and 40 per cent during uncontrolled atrial fibrillation.[5,9,10] The heart may have time to fill when atrial flutter is associated with a slow ventricular rate, (thus coronary blood flow may be near normal), but with more rapid ventricular rates the coronary blood flow falls an average of 22 per cent. During ventricular tachycardia the average reduction in coronary blood flow is 60 per cent, and during ventricular fibrillation the coronary flow is imperceptible. Irregular rhythms, such as premature atrial systoles and premature ventricular systoles, cause a reduction in the coronary

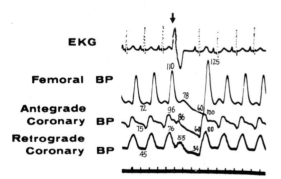

Fig. 16-4. Simultaneous recordings of the electrocardiogram, femoral blood pressure, and antegrade and retrograde coronary blood pressures which demonstrate the marked drop in systolic and diastolic blood pressures associated with premature ventricular systole. (*From Fig. 2, E. Corday, H. Gold, L. B. DeVera, J. H. Williams, and J. Fields: Effect of the Cardiac Arrhythmias on the Coronary Circulation, Ann. Int. Med., 50:539, 1959.*)

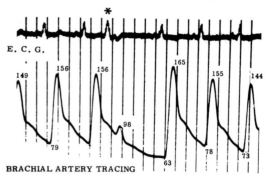

Fig. 16-5. Electrocardiogram and brachial artery tracing in a patient with severe coronary artery disease, which demonstrate the marked drop in systemic pressure with a single premature ventricular systole. Note that the T wave inverts after the QRS that follows premature systole. (*From Fig. 3, E. Corday, H. Gold, L. B. DeVera, J. H. Williams, and J. Fields: Effect of the Cardiac Arrhythmias on the Coronary Circulation, Ann. Int. Med., 50:539, 1959.*)

flow of 5 to 12 per cent, respectively, but very frequent premature ventricular systoles may reduce the flow by as much as 25 per cent.[5] Premature ventricular systoles cause the systemic pressure to drop momentarily because insufficient blood is ejected (Fig. 16-4). In the patient with coronary artery narrowing, this lowered coronary perfusion pressure is apt to cause transient T-wave inversion for one or two beats after the premature systoles (Fig. 16-5). Depression of the S-T segment and/or T-wave inversion are common during rapid tachycardia (Fig. 16-6). These electrocardiographic changes which may persist for 3 or 4 days after conversion, have been called the post-tachycardia T-wave syndrome. The patient with a normal coro-

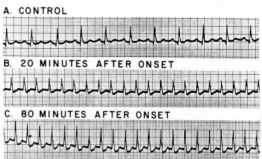

Fig. 16-6. Electrocardiogram of patient during a paroxysm of supraventricular tachycardia. Note that 20 min after the onset of the paroxysm there is an S-T segment depression, and the tracing recorded 80 min after the onset shows more marked S-T segment depression and diphasic T waves. In this patient, these findings were considered indicative of coronary insufficiency.

nary circulation will not be disturbed by the drop in coronary perfusion pressure and flow during transient arrhythmias. However, a patient with coronary atherosclerosis may develop heart failure or angina pectoris when the heart rate is as low as 140 beats per minute.

Renal Circulation. Renal blood flow may be reduced by 8 to 10 per cent during frequent atrial or ventricular premature systoles. The blood flow may be reduced by 18 per cent during paroxysmal atrial tachycardia, 20 per cent during rapid atrial fibrillation, and 60 per cent during ventricular tachycardia.[4] Progressive vasoconstriction of the renal circulation occurs during rapid arrhythmias and persists for several hours after the rhythm has returned to normal.[3] Ischemia of the kidney secondary to cardiac arrhythmias may produce azotemia, proteinuria, and oliguria. Lower-nephron nephrosis has been reported to follow ventricular tachycardia.[11]

Mesenteric Circulation. Vasoconstriction of the mesenteric circulation occurs soon after the onset of cardiac arrhythmias. It is a natural protective process which attempts to maintain systemic pressure and perfusion pressure of the brain, liver, and myocardium.[4,12] Rapid supraventricular tachycardia reduces the blood flow as much as 34 per cent. Mesenteric angiospasm terminates as soon as the arrhythmia is corrected. This is in contrast to the renal vasoconstriction, which persists when the arrhythmia terminates. Mesenteric angiospasm may result in the syndrome of acute mesenteric vascular insufficiency, in which ischemia of the gastrointestinal tract causes abdominal distension, para-

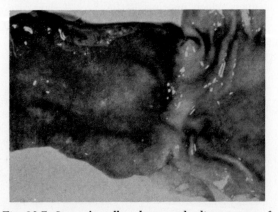

Fig. 16-7. Stomach wall, pylorus, and adjacent area of duodenum after an episode of ventricular tachycardia following a myocardial infarction, showing marked hemorrhagic necrosis of the duodenum (*From E. Corday, D. W. Irving, H. Gold, H. Bernstein, and R. B. T. Skelton: Mesenteric Vascular Insufficiency: Intestinal Ischemia Induced by Remote Circulatory Disturbances, Am. J. Med., 33:369, 1962.*)

lytic ileus, pain, peptic ulceration, or diarrhea with or without bleeding. Hemorrhagic necrosis and gangrene of the duodenum and bowel may occur as a complication of rapid tachycardia (Fig. 16-7).[4,12,13]

Musculocutaneous Circulation. As the cardiac output or systemic pressure falls during a cardiac arrhythmia, angiospasm of the musculocutaneous system occurs in an attempt to maintain systemic pressure. This results in purplish cyanosis of the extremities and cold, clammy skin. Gangrene of the fingers and toes has been reported following ventricular tachycardia.[14]

MONITORING CARDIAC RHYTHM TO EXPLAIN OBSCURE HEMODYNAMIC EVENTS [15]

Eliot Corday, M.D., and Tzu-Wang Lang, M.D.

Fewer than 50 per cent of patients recognize an irregularity or rapid beating of the heart. Thus, many patients are unaware that they are experiencing a cardiac arrhythmia and note only the peripheral manifestations due to ischemia of the "target" organs. The clinician must be constantly aware that recurrent ischemic symptoms may be produced by a transient arrhythmia. To be sure that an arrhythmia is the causative factor, a monitoring apparatus (such as the Holter AVSEP manufactured by Avionics) should be used. This instrument records the electrocardiogram on magnetic tape over a period of 10 hr while the patient conducts normal activities (Fig. 16-8). The magnetic tape may be rapidly analyzed by computers which measure R-R intervals (Figs. 16-9 and 16-10). Thus, 10 hr of electrocardiogram may be analyzed in 10 min. This technique vividly demonstrates an arrhythmia, and indicates when it occurred. Segments of the tape recording can be reproduced on regular electrocardiographic paper. The patient should keep a diary of symptoms which occur during the period of monitoring in order to correlate the symptoms with the electrocardiographic findings. We have found this apparatus of great help in establishing whether arrhythmias are the cause of syncope, transient aphasia, hemiparesis, acute dyspnea, or angina pectoris.

CLASSIFICATION

Disorders of the heart beat may be classified into two broad categories: (1) disorders of pacemaker formation and function; (2) disorders of cardiac conduction (Figs. 16-11 and 16-12).

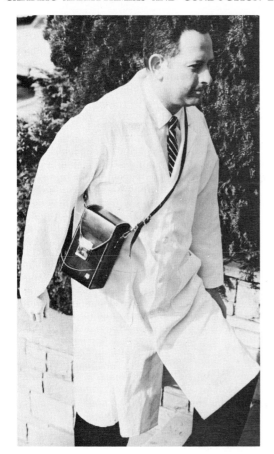

Fig. 16-8. Subject wearing the Holter monitor as he climbs steps. The Electrocardiogram may be recorded on electromagnetic tape over a 10-hr period while the patient performs normal duties.

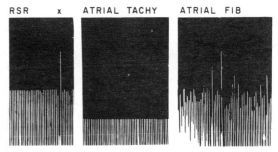

Fig. 16-10. Cathode-ray oscilloscope (Holter apparatus, Fig. 10-9), illustrating changing R-R intervals in patients who were not aware of cardiac arrhythmia. First segment, a premature ventricular systole with a short R-R interval followed by a long R-R interval due to the compensatory pause. Middle segment, shortened R-R intervals due to a paroxysm of atrial tachycardia. Third segment, irregular R-R intervals due to atrial fibrillation. (*Reprinted with permission of the publisher.*[15])

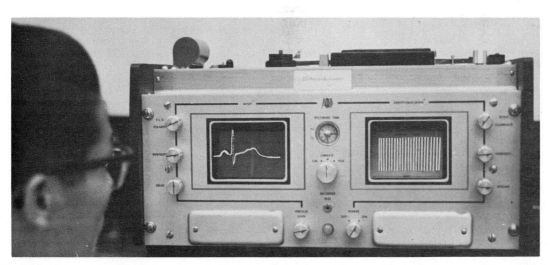

Fig. 16-9. Holter apparatus for scanning the tape-recorded electrocardiogram. The cathode-ray oscilloscope on the left superimposes one electrocardiographic complex on top of the next. The cathode-ray oscilloscope on the right demonstrates the R-R interval of each beat. With this scanning apparatus, 10 hr of electrocardiogram can be studied in a 10-min period. Any pertinent segment of electrocardiogram can be written out on the standard paper. (*Reprinted with permission of the publisher.*[15])

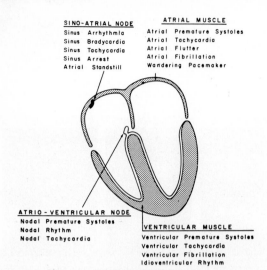

Fig. 16-11. Abnormalities in formation of the excitatory impulse may occur in the sinoatrial node, atrial muscle, atrioventricular node, or ventricular muscle. (*From Fig. 21, E. Corday and D. W. Irving: "Disturbances of Heart Rate, Rhythm and Conduction," W. B. Saunders Company, Philadelphia, 1961.*)

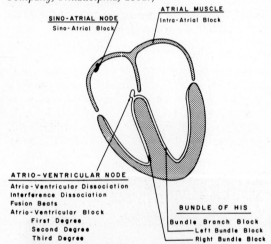

Fig. 16-12. Possible defects in conduction of the excitatory impulse. Disorders in conduction may occur in the sinoatrial node, atrial muscle, atrioventricular node, or bundle of His. (*From Fig. 22, E. Corday and D. W. Irving: "Disturbances of Heart Rate, Rhythm and Conduction," W. B. Saunders Company, Philadelphia, 1961.*)

DISORDERS OF PACEMAKER FORMATION AND FUNCTION

A NOTE ON CARDIAC AUTOMATICITY* [16]

*Robert C. Schlant, M.D., and
J. Willis Hurst, M.D.*

A characteristic property of cardiac tissue is automaticity, or the ability to beat rhythmically with-

out external stimuli. The specialized cardiac cells with the most rapid inherent rhythm are called "pacemaker" cells. In man this pacemaker activity is normally confined to the sinoatrial (SA) node and the atrioventricular (AV) node. (The anatomy of the conduction system is discussed in Chap. 29.) Although the other parts of the conducting network may also normally be capable of generating impulses, it is not definite that in man all cardiac tissue normally has this capability, even though in disease states ectopic beats may originate from either atrial or ventricular foci.

Under normal conditions, the cardiac pacemaker with the highest inherent rate, the SA node, will dominate the heart rate and will depolarize the slower pacemaker before they can generate beats. On the other hand, if the SA node fails to start an impulse or if its rate is markedly slowed, the AV node, which has the second highest inherent rate, will usually take over the function of cardiac pacemaker. The exact mechanism by which the SA and AV nodes generate impulses and function as pacemakers is not known, but it may be that these cells are more permeable than other cardiac tissue to sodium in the resting state, so that at the end of each cycle they become gradually depolarized to the level at which rapid depolarization and impulse formation occur.

Although the SA node possesses inherent automaticity, its rate of impulse formation is normally controlled by vagal and sympathetic impulses. When an increase in the rate of the SA node impulse formation occurs, it is not definitely known whether the impulses continue to originate from the same cells in the SA node or whether the decrease in vagal inhibition shifts the pacemaker activity to a slightly higher area of the SA node possessing a more rapid inherent rate.

After originating in the SA node the normal excitatory impulse spreads through both atria in a wavelike fashion, with the auricles being the last portions depolarized. There is conflicting evidence as to whether, in man, the atrial excitation spreads over a specialized atrial conducting system[17]—as in the ventricles—or whether it spreads predominantly through the ordinary atrial myocardial cells.

The mechanisms of the origin and propagation of the activation impulse in the atria which results in atrial flutter and fibrillation have been the subject of numerous investigations for more than half a century. Despite these studies, however, there is still not universal agreement on the mechanisms of these arrhythmias.[18] Three major theories are currently used to explain atrial flutter and fibrillation. The first, largely popularized by Lewis and associates,[19-21] is the concept of circus movement. By this theory, a primary activation wave called a mother wave follows a circular, unidirectional path

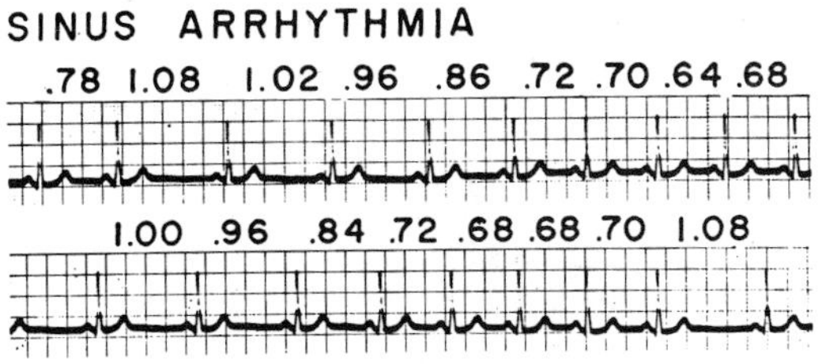

SINUS ARRHYTHMIA

.78 1.08 1.02 .96 .86 .72 .70 .64 .68

1.00 .96 .84 .72 .68 .68 .70 1.08

Fig. 16-13. Electrocardiogram of a patient with sinus arrhythmia. The figures mounted above the electrocardiogram indicate the R-R interval. The heart speeds up during inspiration and slows during expiration.

around the ostiums of the two venae cavae, and from this wave are given off irregular daughter waves, which then proceed erratically to depolarize the atria. The second theory, largely supported by the work of Rothberger,[22,23] Prinzmetal,[24] and Scherf,[25] postulates that an ectopic focus, or more than one, in the atria initiates impulses at an extremely rapid rate and takes over the function of the normal SA node. A third theory, proposed by Katz and Pick,[26] explains these arrhythmias by the mechanism of multiple reentry. According to this last theory, which in some regards is a compromise between the other two, a sinus or an atrial ectopic impulse occurring in a vulnerable period of the heart's cycle initiates either atrial flutter or fibrillation, which is perpetuated by the development of multiple reentries and multiple simultaneous circulating waves, each with its "gap" and its "head" trying to reach and swallow its "tail." This is in lieu of a primary circulating wave, as proposed by Lewis. At the present time, it is not possible to

state which of these concepts is more nearly correct: the ultimate explanation must await future research.

SINUS ARRHYTHMIAS[*][16]

Robert C. Schlant, M.D., and
J. Willis Hurst, M.D.

A normal sinus rhythm is usually slightly irregular because of the moment-to-moment normal homeostatic variations in vagal tone. When the irregularity is such that the difference between the longest and shortest cycle is 0.12 sec or more, "sinus arrhythmia" is said to be present. The most common variety of sinus arrhythmia is "phasic sinus arrhythmia" or "respiratory arrhythmia," in which there is a cyclic speeding of the heart rate during inspiration with a slowing during expiration (Figs. 16-13 and 16-14). It is thought that the respiratory variations in reflex stimulation of the lungs and great vessels produce a varying degree of vagal tone, inhibiting the SA node. At times the sinus arrhythmia may be nonphasic and not related to the respiratory cycle, although occasionally deep breathing may make nonphasic sinus arrhythmia become phasic with respiration. The phasic type of sinus arrhythmia is common in normal persons, particularly in children, adolescents, and young adults. It tends to become less marked with aging and also becomes less marked as the heart rate increases. The less common nonphasic type of sinus arrhythmia is more likely to be encountered in older individuals with or without heart disease. Neither form of sinus arrhythmia is responsible for symptoms,

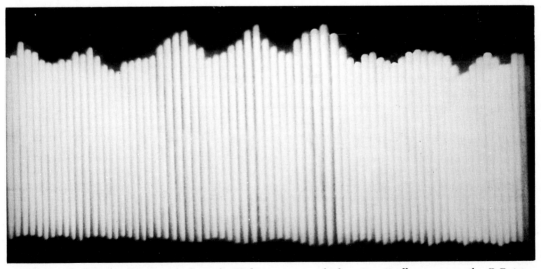

Fig. 16-14. Arrhythmiagraphic tracing from the Holter scanner, which automatically measures the R-R interval, showing the phasic variation of the R-R interval sinus arrhythmia.

and neither form is thought to be produced by disease; consequently, no treatment is indicated.

SINUS TACHYCARDIA* 16

Robert C. Schlant, M.D., and
J. Willis Hurst, M.D.

When the SA node causes the heart to beat at a rate faster than 100 beats per minute in adults, the rhythm is referred to as "sinus tachycardia." The rate in sinus tachycardia is seldom faster than 140 to 165 beats per minute in adults or 200 beats per minute in children. The more common causes of sinus tachycardia are excitement, nervousness, exercise, fever, anoxia, hypotension, hyperthyroidism, and drugs such as epinephrine, isoproterenol (Isuprel), or atropine sulfate. In the occasional instances of sinus tachycardia at rates between 160 and 180 beats per minute in adults, the differentiation between sinus tachycardia and atrial tachycardia may be difficult. If the heart rate is almost perfectly regular and unchanging over minutes or even several hours, the rhythm is more likely to be atrial tachycardia; if even a slight variation in heart rate can be detected, the rhythm is more likely to be sinus tachycardia. It should be noted that the variation in rate in rapid sinus tachycardia is often so slight that it can be reliably detected only by electrocardiography. At times, carotid sinus massage may help to differentiate between these rhythms. With atrial tachycardia, carotid sinus massage will either produce no effect or cause an abrupt cessation of the tachycardia. In sinus tachycardia, carotid sinus massage may produce a temporary slowing of the rate followed by a gradual speeding up of the rate (Fig. 16-15). Often the changes in rate of sinus tachycardia produced by carotid sinus massage are so slight that they can be detected only by electrocardiography. On the electrocardiogram the P waves during sinus tachycardia are more likely to resemble those during slower normal sinus rhythm, although their amplitude is usually increased. Paroxysmal atrial tachycardia, on the other hand, is often associated with a more marked change in configuration of the P waves. Since sinus

SINUS TACHYCARDIA

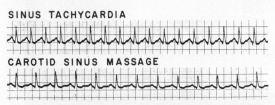

Fig. 16-15. Electrocardiogram of a patient with sinus tachycardia (upper strip) which the P wave joins the T wave. During carotid sinus massage the rate slows down and the P wave separates from the T wave.

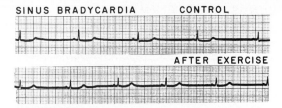

Fig. 16-16. Electrocardiogram of patient with sinus bradycardia before and after exercise. Note that the rhythm accelerates following exercise. In contrast, the rate does not significantly increase following exercise in patients with complete heart block. This feature is used in bedside, diagnosis in differentiating between sinus bradycardia and heart block.

tachycardia usually is a manifestation of a circulatory compensatory mechanism, treatment must be directed against the underlying or precipitating condition rather than against the sinus tachycardia per se.

SINUS BRADYCARDIA* 16

Robert C. Schlant, M.D., and
J. Willis Hurst, M.D.

A sinus rhythm at a rate less than 60 beats per minute is referred to as "sinus bradycardia" in the adult (Fig. 16-16). This rhythm usually varies slightly with respiration; its rate is seldom less than 45 beats per minute. Sinus bradycardia is probably produced by a high degree of vagal tone (Fig. 16-17). It is not uncommon in normal young adults, particularly athletes accustomed to prolonged exertion, although it may be encountered in patients with myxedema or in older patients with arteriosclerosis. In an otherwise normal individual, sinus bradycardia produces no symptoms and no interference with cardiac function. Indeed, it probably reflects that the person has a more efficient heart than normal.

ATRIAL ECTOPIC BEATS* 16

Robert C. Schlant, M.D., and
J. Willis Hurst, M.D.

When an impulse arises in the atria outside the SA node, the ensuing impulse is referred to as an "ectopic atrial beat." Such beats are not uncommon in apparently normal persons, particularly when the individuals are under emotional stress or have indulged excessively in smoking or in drinking alcoholic beverages or coffee. They may also be initiated by digitalis and by atrial stretching or ischemia. In most instances atrial ectopic beats may be recognized by hearing a premature beat and

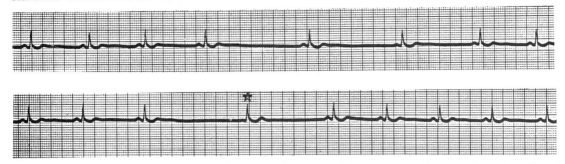

Fig. 16-17. Upper strip, electrocardiogram of a patient during a Valsalva maneuver. Because of vagotonia there is slowing of the sinus rate so that the P-P interval becomes prolonged. Second strip, on repetition of the Valsalva maneuver, a prolonged sinus arrest resulted in a nodal escape (indicated by star) in which the QRST appears normal but is not preceded by a P wave.

noting that the following compensatory pause is not complete; however, it should be noted that at times atrial ectopic beats may be followed by a full compensatory pause and that ventricular ectopic beats at times are not followed by a full compensatory pause. The differentiation between atrial and ventricular ectopic beats is also helped by the tendency of the heart sounds to be more nearly "normal" with an atrial than with a ventricular ectopic beat. When atrial ectopic beats occur very frequently, it may not be possible by auscultation to differentiate this condition from atrial fibrillation. Indeed, the presence of frequent atrial ectopic beats often precedes the development of atrial fibrillation. It is always best to confirm the exact arrhythmia present by electrocardiography, since the clinical differentiation between these and other arrhythmias is so often difficult or impossible (Fig. 16-18).

Atrial or nodal ectopic beats usually produce no symptoms, although they may be responsible for a sensation of a pause of the heart rhythm or an awareness of a forceful heartbeat or palpitation, particularly in a person with increased heart consciousness. In such patients reassurance regarding the significance of the ectopic beats and the avoidance of possibly precipitating habits or drugs may relieve the ectopic beats and the palpitations. Often a trial of phenobarbital, 15 to 30 mg three or four times a day, will decrease the symptoms. Some patients who are not relieved by these measures may require a therapeutic trial of quinidine sulfate, 200 to 400 mg every 4 to 6 hr orally, to control the atrial ectopic beats. When quinidine sulfate is employed for this purpose, it is important after 2 to 3 months to discontinue the medication to determine whether the ectopic beats recur. The patient should also be reassured that the occurrence of the ectopic beats themselves is relatively unimportant. In patients receiving digitalis, the development of atrial ectopic beats occasionally is evidence of digi-

talis intoxication and may precede the development of paroxysmal atrial tachycardia with block. When frequent atrial ectopic beats occur following acute myocardial infarction, particularly of the posterior or inferior variety, and paticularly when the SA rate is slow or relatively slow, the administration of atropine sulfate, 1.0 mg intravenously or intramuscularly every 6 to 8 hr, may block vagal impulses which are slowing the SA rate. The speeding of the SA node impulse formation produced by atropine may be associated with abolishment of the ectopic beats. In other instances, correction of hypotension of congestive heart failure will often abolish ectopic atrial beats.

Nodal Premature Beats. A cardiac impulse which arises prematurely in the AV node is referred to as an atrioventricular (AV) nodal premature beat. It is characterized by the premature QRST contour which is usually identical to the form during sinus rhythm but which may be occasionally deformed by ventricular aberration of the right bundle branch type, and by retrograde P waves which may occur before, during, or after the QRS complex. If the retrograde P wave occurs before the QRS complex, the P-R interval is characteristically less than 0.12 sec. The relationship between the onset of the retrograde P wave and the onset of the QRS complex is thought to be related to the location of the pacemaker within the atrioventricular junc-

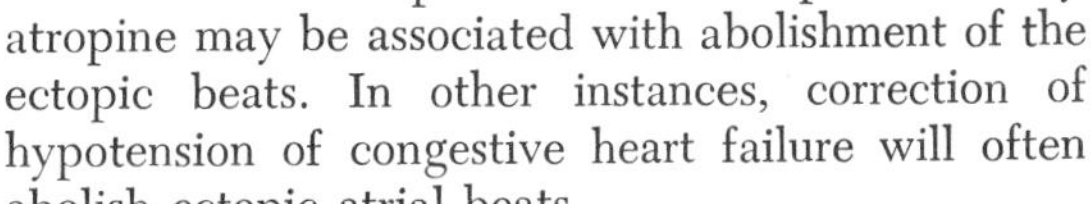

Fig. 16-18. Frequent premature atrial systoles characterized by an inverted P wave, and QRS complexes of normal configuration and a P-R interval greater than 0.12 sec. The alteration in the shape of the P wave signifies that the premature atrial systole arises in an ectopic focus. Some cardiologists designate this particular type of atrial premature beat as a coronary sinus ectopic beat.

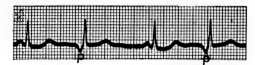

Fig. 16-19. Electrocardiogram of a patient with nodal premature systoles. Note that the P wave is inverted and precedes the QRS complex by less than 0.12 sec; the QRS is of normal configuration. This suggests that the ectopic focus is in the upper part of the AV node.

tional tissues. Accordingly, AV nodal beats may be classified into upper AV nodal beats, middle AV nodal beats, and lower AV nodal beats (Figs. 16-19 to 16-21). The term "coronary sinus beat" is sometimes used in reference to beats which are thought to originate near the orifice or the coronary sinus and which are characterized by retrograde P waves with a P-R interval of greater than 0.12 sec. The compensatory pause following an AV nodal premature beat may be complete if there is no retrograde conduction of the premature nodal impulse to the atria or if the retrograde impulse arrives at the SA node after the sinus impulse has been initiated, whereas the compensatory pause is incomplete if the retrograde impulse arrives in time to discharge the cells of the SA node.

Atrioventricular nodal premature beats are relatively common in patients both with and without heart disease. In general, they have the same clinical significance as atral ectopic beats and are treated similarly. At times nodal premature beats occur prior to the development of AV nodal tachycardia because of digitalis intoxication.

NODAL ESCAPE AND NODAL RHYTHM* 16

Robert C. Schlant, M.D., and
J. Willis Hurst, M.D.

Following an acute posterior myocardial infarction or associated with such procedures as bronchoscopy, abdominal surgery, or carotid sinus massage, it is frequently noted that the site of origin of the atrial impulse electrocardiographically appears to migrate in the atrium downward toward

PREM. NODAL SYSTOLE

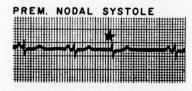

Fig. 16-20. Premature nodal systole arising in the midportion of the AV node. The characteristic features are that a P wave cannot be recognized, and the QRS complex is of normal configuration. (*From Fig. 33.*¹)

NODAL PREMATURE SYSTOLES

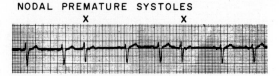

Fig. 16-21. Electrocardiogram demonstrating two nodal premature systoles. The QRS is of normal configuration but is premature and an inverted P wave follows the QRS complex. This suggests that the ecopic focus is in the lower part of the AV node. A compensatory pause follows each premature nodal systole.

the AV node, apparently as a result of intense reflex vagal stimulation. When the SA node is markedly inhibited and the pacemaker function of the heart is not taken over by a focus lower in the atrium, the AV node will usually take over the pacemaker function of the heart. If this occurs for a single beat, the resultant delayed impulse originating in the AV node is referred to as a "nodal escape beat" (Fig. 16-17). If there is a persistent failure of the SA node to form impulses or if the impulses are not transmitted to the AV node, the AV node may take over the pacemaker function entirely, producing an "atrioventricular nodal rhythm" (Fig. 16-22). Usually this rhythm has a rate between 40 and 70 beats per minute. While nodal rhythm is usually regular, it may vary slightly with exercise or emotional stress. When nodal rhythm results from vagal inhibition of the SA node, it may be treated with atropine sulfate, 1.0 mg intravenously or intramuscularly every 6 to 8 hours, to allow the SA node to regain its normal pacemaker function. When nodal rhythm is associated with myocardial infarction, the correction of hypotension or congestive failure may restore the normal dominance of the SA node. It should also be kept in mind that nodal rhythm may result from digitalis intoxication, in which case administration of digitalis must be discontinued.

The excellent studies of James[27-29] on the anatomy of the coronary arteries and the relation of atrial arrhythmias and AV block to occlusive coronary artery disease offer much promise for better understanding and treatment of these arrhythmias (Chaps. 28 and 29). His studies indicate that the SA node receives its blood supply from the right coronary artery in approximately 60 per cent of human beings and from the left circumflex or the left main coronary artery in the remaining 40 per cent. From the knowledge of the blood supply to the SA and AV nodes and to the different areas of ventricular myocardium, it is often possible to predict with good accuracy the location of an occlusion in a specific coronary artery from the electrocardiographic localization of the myocardial injury and

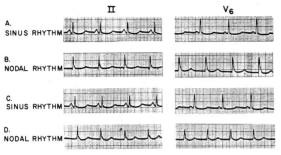

Fig. 16-22. Electrocardiogram of patient during sinus rhythm (A) and (C) and minodal rhythm (B) and (D)—standard lead II and lead V₆. In strips B and D there is a P wave buried in the QRS complex. This signifies that the activation of the atria and that of the ventricles occur at the same time.

from the presence of or absence of abnormal function of the SA or AV node.[29]

PAROXYSMAL ATRIAL AND NODAL TACHYCARDIA IN ADULTS[*][16]

Edward R. Dorney, M.D.

Paroxysmal atrial and paroxysmal nodal tachycardias are rapid, regular supraventricular rhythms which are for the most part indistinguishable on clinical or routine electrocardiographic examination (Figs. 16-23–16-27). For this reason, it is fortunate that they respond in a similar manner to all forms of treatment and for therapeutic purposes may be considered to be the same disorder.

Diagnosis. The diagnosis may be suspected clini-

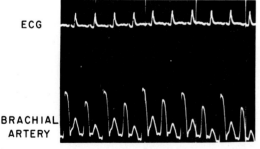

Fig. 16-23. Brachial artery pressure tracing during a paroxysm of atrial tachycardia, demonstrating that there is a regular variation in the pulse pressure because alternate ventricular contractions are more forceful. This phenomenon is called "mechanical alternans." It can be detected by the sphygmomanometer, which demonstrates two different levels of the systolic pressure. Alternate beats will be heard at a higher level. This phenomenon is not uncommon with paroxysmal atrial tachycardia.

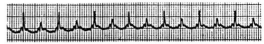

Fig. 16-24. Electrocardiogram demonstrating electrical alternans in a patient with supraventricular tachycardia. Alternate ventricular complexes are lower than the preceding ones. Electrical alternans is not directly related to mechanical alternans.

cally on the basis of a regular tachycardia with a rate between 140 and 220, usually about 180, beats per minute in a patient who has a 1:1 correlation between the neck vein pulsations and the apical rate and in whom the first heart sound remains constant. Nodal tachycardia at times produces a sharp pulsation in the neck veins which was not present prior to this arrhythmia, and thus may be distinguished from the atrial variety. If, in addition, the patient is able to give a history of sudden onset of the present attack, or better still if he can state that previous attacks of rapid heart action have begun and terminated suddenly, the diagnosis becomes almost certain. Confirmation can be obtained by the response of the arrhythmia to carotid sinus pressure (Figs. 16-28 and 16-29). In paroxysmal atrial or nodal tachycardia, the response will be either immediate termination of the arrhythmia or no effect whatsoever. This maneuver is also valuable in differentiating atrial or nodal tachycardia from atrial flutter, in which the ventricular rate will slow momentarily and then rapidly return to its former rate, or from sinus tachycardia, in which the rate will slow gradually and then gradually return to its former speed when pressure on the carotid sinus is released. The diagnosis can also be confirmed by electrocardiography (Figs. 16-28 and 16-29). Here, too, carotid sinus pressure is valuable in slowing the ventricular response of flutter so that the characteristic sawtooth base line may be identified. Nodal tachycardia may sometimes be distinguished on the routine electrocardio-

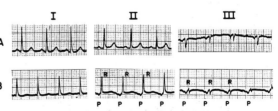

Fig. 16-25. Electrocardiogram of a patient during sinus rhythm (A) and nodal tachycardia (B). In nodal tachycardia, arising high in the node, the P wave precedes the QRS complex and the P-R interval is less than 0.12 sec. It is inverted, suggesting that the activation of the atria is in a retrograde direction. The QRS complexes are of normal amplitude and shape.

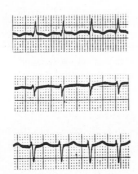

Fig. 16-26. Electrocardiogram of patient with midnodal tachycardia. The P wave cannot be identified because it is buried in the QRS complex. The QRS complex was identical to that found in the patient's control tracing. Upper tracing is lead I, the middle tracing, lead II, and the lower tracing, lead III.

gram by the finding of an inverted P wave in leads 2, 3, and AVF; but more often, the use of an esophageal lead is needed (Fig. 16-30).

Treatment. Although paroxysmal atrial or nodal

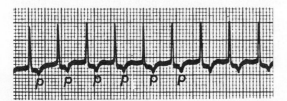

Fig. 16-27. Nodal tachycardia. The P wave is inverted and follows the QRS complex, because of retrograde activation of the atria, demonstrating that the ectopic focus is low in the AV node. (*From Fig.* 110.[1]) E. Corday and D. W. Irving: "Disturbances in Heart Rate, Rhythm and Conduction," W. B. Saunders Company, Philadelphia, 1961.

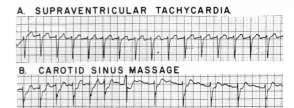

Fig. 16-28. Electrocardiogram demonstrating the effect of carotid sinus pressure in a patient with supraventricular tachycardia. In the upper tracing the P waves cannot be identified, but the slight variation in the shape of the T wave suggests that there is a P wave superimposed upon it. Immediately following carotid sinus massage the rhythm converts to regular sinus rhythm, thereby proving that the rhythm was paroxysmal atrial tachycardia rather than sinus tachycardia.

tachycardia may be seen in patients with acute and chronic rheumatic heart disease, coronary artery disease, digitalis intoxication, the Wolff-Parkinson-White syndrome, and many other cardiac abnormalities, it most often occurs in adults with normal hearts, and for this reason, is usually well tolerated. Symptoms are due mainly to anxiety secondary to the racing heart, but chest pain, dyspnea, synscope, and congestive heart failure have occurred, particularly in those patients with underlying heart disease. Since the arrhythmia is well tolerated in normal hearts for periods up to several days, and since the majority of these patients have normal hearts, it is important that the aggressiveness of treatment be dictated by the individual situation. The treatment should not be more dangerous than the disease.

The patient should first be reassured that his problem is not life-threatening and at the same time should be given sedation in the form of

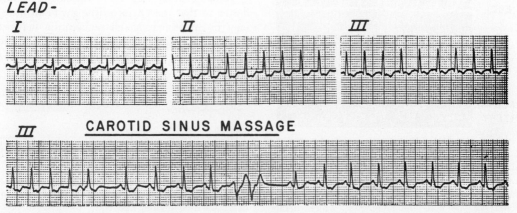

Fig. 16-29. Electrocardiogram showing the termination of a paroxysm of supraventricular tachycardia by carotid sinus massage. The upper strips, leads I, II, and III, demonstrate supraventricular tachycardia. Carotid sinus massage converted the rhythm to normal in the lower strip. This response proves that the tachycardia was not of sinus origin. This tracing is shown to demonstrate that certain arrhythmias can occur at the time of reversion. In this case, note ventricular ectopic beats.

phenobarbital (Sodium Luminal), 130 mg by intramuscular injection, or secobarbital (Seconal) or pentobarbital sodium (Nembutal), 100 to 200 mg by mouth. It is important that these patients not be given narcotics for sedation, since paroxysms tend to recur and addiction may become a real problem.

If, after sedation and reassurance, the tachycardia has not spontaneously reverted, various mechanical and pharmacologic maneuvers to enhance vagal tone should be employed. The Valsalva maneuver is accomplished by having the patient inhale deeply, hold his breath, and then strain down hard while he counts slowly to 10. This is a most effective treatment for paroxysmal atrial tachycardia when properly performed. When unsuccessful, the usual mistake has been failure to sustain the straining for a full 10 sec. Whether or not the Valsalva maneuver terminates this particular attack, it is important to instruct the patient that this maneuver, coughing, gagging, or even self-induced vomiting may be successful in future episodes.

Following an unsuccessful Valsalva maneuver, the next logical step is enhancement of vagal tone through the carotid sinus reflex (Figs. 16-28 and 16-29). This reflex, and that of the aortic arch, are the normal regulators of the blood pressure and heart rate. Carotid sinus stimulation is a safe procedure if carried out carefully and in a proper manner. It should not be attempted in patients who have a history of carotid or basilar artery insufficiency or in patients who have had previous cerebrovascular accidents. With the patient in a supine position and the examiner at the patient's right side, the examiner's right hand is placed on the patient's neck so that the index finger is just behind the angle of the right mandible and the middle finger is just below the horizontal ramus of this bone. Firm pressure with a massaging motion is then applied posteriorly and medially to compress the carotid sinus between the examiner's fingers and the cervical vertebrae. Pressure should never be applied for more than 3 to 5 sec at any given time. During the procedure, the physician should monitor the patient's heartbeat with a stethoscope applied to the chest or with a direct-writing electrocardiograph. Pressure should be withdrawn immediately when there is any change in the cardiac rhythm. This maneuver should be carried out several times, first on the right and then on the left side. Never massage both carotid vessels at the same time. The vagal stimulus may be augmented by having the patient perform a Valsalva maneuver during the carotid compression.

If these maneuvers, repeated several times, have been unrewarding, then the use of a pressor amine to enhance vagal effect is indicated. This treatment

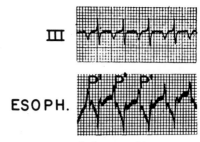

Fig. 16-30. Esophageal electrocardiogram in a patient with atrial tachycardia. The P waves cannot be seen in standard leads but can be readily recognized in the esophageal lead.

should be limited, however, to those patients with otherwise normal cardiovascular systems. Treatment consists of 5 mg of phenylephrine hydrochloride (Neo-synephrine) diluted in 100 ml of 5 per cent dextrose in water given as a rapid intravenous infusion; constant monitoring of the blood pressure is essential. The infusion should be continued until a systolic pressure of 180 mm Hg is reached. Levels higher than this are seldom necessary. In a home situation where an infusion is not practical, Neo-synephrine may be given intravenously by syringe in the following manner. Dilute 2 mg Neo-synephrine to make 10 ml. Give 2.5 ml of this mixture rapidly by vein and record the blood pressure and pulse every minute for 5 min. If the tachycardia does not cease or if a systolic pressure of 160 to 180 mm Hg is not reached, then give 5 ml (1 mg) rapidly. In most cases this will result in conversion of the tachycardia. Metaraminol (Aramine) and levarterenol norepinephrine, Levophed) have both been used for the same purpose, but since they are no more effective than Neo-synephrine in this particular arrhythmia, and since they also have a greater tendency to produce ventricular arrhythmias and skin sloughs, I see no need to employ them.[30]

Neostigmine (Prostigmine), 0.5 to 1.0 mg given intramuscularly, will produce considerable parasympathomimetic action and will terminate paroxysmal atrial tachycardia, particularly if carotid sinus pressure or the Valsalva maneuver is carried out 15 to 30 min after the injection. Prostigmin may also be used to augment digitalis and has been used alone as initial therapy.[31]

Methacholine bromide (Mecholyl) and acetylcholine have both been used to terminate paroxysmal atrial tachycardia. These drugs frequently produce unpleasant and dangerous side effects and are not so effective as the safer drugs already outlined; I see no need for their use.

If these procedures are not successful, or in patients with frequently repetitive tachycardia who will need prophylactic medication, or in those with significant heart disease, the use of digitalis or a synchronized d-c converter is indicated. The mode of action of digitalis in this particular arrhythmia is not clear. It may act directly by depressing the ectopic focus or by increasing the refractory period of the atrial fibers, or indirectly by increasing vagal tone or sensitizing the carotid sinus reflex. Most probably, it acts by a combination of all these factors.[32] The reason for choosing digoxin is that this particular drug is available in intravenous and oral preparations. It acts rapidly and is excreted quickly. Onset of action, when given intravenously, is 15 to 30 min, with a maximum reached in 2 to 3 hr. It is excreted within 3 to 4 days, and toxic symptoms, when produced, usually last about 24 hr. If continuation of digitalis is desired, maintenance doses may be started orally without redigitalization. In the previously undigitalized patient with a normal heart, 1 mg digoxin may be given slowly intravenously over an interval of 5 to 10 min. In older patients, in those with known heart disease, or in those with recent myocardial infarction, 0.5 mg intravenously is a more prudent initial dose. Many times, conversion of the tachycardia occurs shortly after administration of the drug.[33] If not, carotid sinus pressure augmented by a Valsalva maneuver, if necessary, should be repeated at about 15-min intervals for a period of 2 to 3 hr. If, after this period of time has elapsed, the rhythm is unchanged, digitalization should be completed by the oral route and the patient given sedation and allowed to rest overnight. In practice, it is only a rare case that is this resistant.

If digitalization, reinforced by the various maneuvers and drugs to increase vagal tone, is not successful, the use of selectively *synchronized d-c countershock* is indicated. I feel that this is a more reliable and safer procedure than the administration of quinidine, but if such equipment is not available, then quinidine sulfate, given by mouth, is the next drug employed. Quinidine is particularly toxic and tricky when given intravenously, and there is rarely any need for this mode of administration in paroxysmal atrial tachycardia.

Quinidine acts by depressing ectopic foci and prolonging the refractory period of the atria musculature.[34] It should not be used in patients with known sensitivity. Patients who are to have rhythm conversion with quinidine should be admitted to the hospital. Starting early in the morning, a dose of 400 mg quinidine sulfate is given by mouth every 2 hr for a total of five doses.[35] A control electrocardiogram should be taken before therapy is started. Blood pressure and pulse should be checked before each dose and the cardiac rhythm monitored by electrocardiogram before each of the last three doses. If the QRS complex increases by more than 50 per cent of its control value, if frequent prema-

ture ventricular contractions or dissociated rhythm should appear, or if the rhythm reverts to normal sinus, the medication should be immediately discontinued. Other side effects such as nausea, diarrhea, and tinnitus are only relative contraindications to continuation of therapy. If nausea occurs, it may be controlled by 10 to 25 mg chlorpromazine (Thorazine) given by mouth. Diphenoxylate hydrochloride (Lomotil), 5 mg, and paregoric, 5 to 10 ml, have been effective in checking the diarrhea caused by quinidine.

In the very rare cases where therapy has progressed to this point and the rhythm has not reverted, the patient should be reevaluated for the presence of a persistent inciting mechanism such as thyrotoxicosis. If this is eliminated, procaine amide hydrochloride (Pronestyl) may be given intravenously. This drug, while having much the same pharmacologic action as quinidine, is not so toxic nor so potent by either the oral or the intravenous route.[36] Pronestyl may be used as a continuous intravenous drip of 1 Gm in 100 ml of 5 per cent dextrose in water or may be given directly by syringe (1 Gm diluted with 5 per cent dextrose in water to make 50 ml), 100 mg every 3 to 4 min. Occasionally, it may be necessary to increase the rate of administration of Pronestyl to 100 mg per min, but this should be reserved for resistant cases. The drug should be discontinued immediately upon conversion of the rhythm or the appearance of toxic symptoms, particularly ventricular tachycardia or fibrillation, widening of the QRS complex, or hypotension. Continuous electrocardiographic and blood pressure determinations should be performed during its use. Cardiotoxic manifestations of Pronestyl or quinidine sulfate may be treated with 40 ml of 1 *m* sodium lactate and sympathomimetic drugs given rapidly intravenously and repeated as necessary.[37, 38] Electronic pacemaking equipment should be readily available.

Prophylactic and Maintenance Measures. Tobacco, alcohol, excitement, and fatigue all can precipitate attacks of paroxysmal atrial or nodal tachycardia. A careful history should be taken to ascertain, if possible, the exciting cause in the particular patient. Patients having one or two widely separated attacks of paroxysmal atrial tachycardia do not need preventive medication. If the paroxsms are frequent, occurring every few days, or if they are particularly resistant to treatment or disturbing to the patient because of anxiety, pain, or production of congestive heart failure, then prophylaxis should be attempted.

A simple and very effective form of prophylaxis is full digitalization with daily maintenance doses of the drug.[32] This may not only prevent recurrence of the attacks but, in many instances, will also enable the patient to stop his own attacks quickly by use of the Valsalva or other maneuvers, as described above. If digitalization is unsuccessful, the patient should be started on quinidine sulfate, 200 mg, taken with meals and at bedtime. This dose may be increased to 400 mg taken at the same intervals if necessary.

Occasionally, the problem of maintenance quinidine during the night hours may be met by substituting quinidine gluconate (Quinaglute), 300 mg each night for the bedtime dose. Some patients may be maintained entirely on Quinaglute, 300 to 600 mg given in the morning and evening. Quinaglute is not used as the first choice for quinidine prophylaxis, principally because of its cost to the patient.

For those patients in whom the side effects of quinidine are intolerable, Pronestyl may be used as a substitute medication. Usually, at least 500 mg of the drug taken orally four times a day is the basic minimum dose.

In particularly resistant cases, or when the quinidine or Pronestyl in therapeutic doses cannot be tolerated by the patient, reserpine (Serpasil), 0.25 mg taken by mouth three times a day, or guanethedine, 25 mg taken by mouth every day,[39] may be helpful. These drugs are said to act through their ability to reduce the catecholamine content of the myocardium.

Other drugs, such as hydroxyzine pamoate (Vistaril), 25 mg taken three to four times a day, have been effective as preventive therapy in some instances.

When various combinations of quinidine sulfate, Pronestyl, Vistaril, Serpasil, and digitalis have failed to prevent frequently recurring attacks, destruction or depression of thyroid function by the use of radioactive iodine has produced striking results.[32] This treatment is not relegated only to those cases associated with hyperthyroidism but has been equally useful in euthyroid patients. It is not suggested that this mode of therapy be employed unless all others have failed or are contraindicated by the side effects of the drugs. Myxedema is often produced and introduces many new problems, including the need for maintenance with exogenous thyroid hormone. When needed, the hormone may be started at daily doses of 8 mg and gradually increased so that the metabolic state may be brought as close to normal as possible without reinstituting the tachycardia. Recent trials with the dextrorotatory form of triiodothyronine, used to lower blood-cholesterol level, seem to indicate that this drug may be able to alter some of the metabolic deficiencies of myxedema in doses smaller than would be necessary for myocardial stimulation.

In tachycardias occurring with the Wolff-Parkinson-White syndrome, quinidine sulfate has proved more satisfactory as a prophylatic medication than digitalis.

PAROXYSMAL ATRIAL TACHYCARDIA IN CHILDREN[*] [16]

Edward R. Dorney, M.D.

Paroxysmal atrial tachycardia in children presents a somewhat different problem. The arrhythmia is seen throughout childhood but is more common in the first 2 years. It is relatively well tolerated in older children, but in the group under 3 months of age congestive failure is common. In most cases, the heart rate is 200 beats per minute or over. The arrhythmia is usually not recognized until the appearance of cyanosis, rapid respirations, and large liver signal congestive heart failure. Death may result if prompt treatment is not carried out. In young children carotid sinus massage is seldom successful, perhaps because of the difficulty in carrying out the maneuver. Nevertheless, it should be tried. The drug of choice for treatment of paroxysmal atrial tachycardia in children is digoxin (Lanoxin). It should be given by mouth if congestive failure has not yet appeared. It may be used intravenously if necessary.[40] In children under 2 years of age, the oral dose is calculated at 0.035 mg per lb (0.07 mg per kg) of body weight. One-half the calculated dose is given initially, followed by one-quarter the calculated dose given at 4-hr intervals until the total dose has been given. The maintenance dose is calculated at one-quarter the total digitalizing dose and is given each day. For children over the age of 2 years, the dose is reduced to 0.025 mg per lb (0.05 mg per kg) of body weight, with one-quarter the digitalizing dose as the maintenance amount. Above the age of 10 years, depending on the size and weight of the child, the digitalizing dose averages 2.5 mg given orally in divided doses over a space of 24 to 36 hr. The maintenance dose is about 0.25 mg each day. For small infants and children, pediatric elixir of digoxin is the most convenient to use; it is quick-acting and rapidly excreted. If intravenous administration is necessary, it is a good rule of thumb to calculate the total oral digitalizing dose of Lanoxin and use one-half this amount. For example, if the calculated total oral dose is 0.6 mg, the total intravenous dose will be 0.3 mg. The first injection, then, would contain 0.15 mg; the second injection, given after 2 hr, would be 0.075 mg; and the third, 2 hr later, 0.075 mg. Since it is known that this is probably a suboptimal dose, an additional dose of 0.075 mg could be given if needed.[41] In infants, maintenance digitalization should be carried out until the age of 2 years. Periodic changes in the maintenance dose will be necessary as the child's weight increases. In older children, the frequency and severity of attacks determine the need for preventive therapy, as in adults.

To date there has been little experience with the use of the selectively synchronized d-c converter in infants under 2 years of age, but congestive heart failure or refractory tachycardia certainly would represent a definite indication for its use.

PAROXYSMAL ATRIAL TACHYCARDIA WITH BLOCK[*][16]

Edward R. Dorney, M.D.

When second-degree AV block is present with paroxysmal atrial tachycardia, the problems of diagnosis and treatment are greatly compounded. Although the arrhythmia may be seen as a complication of rheumatic or arteriosclerotic heart disease, it is most important to recognize the possible association with digitalis intoxication (Chap. 15). This cannot be stressed too strongly, for what would constitute adequate treatment of the arrhythmia in the former case may result in death in the latter. The arrhythmia may be precipitated by excessive ingestion of digitalis or by potassium depletion secondary to vomiting, diarrhea, or strenuous diuresis, particularly with thiazide compounds.

Diagnosis. From a clinical standpoint, paroxysmal atrial tachycardia with block may be difficult to recognize, since the atrial rate varies between 140 and 250 beats per minute, and with a 2:1 or 3:1 block, the ventricular rate may be as slow as 50 or as fast as 125 beats per minute. The rhythm may be entirely irregular, with a shifting 1:1, 2:1, 3:1 conduction. Atrial tachycardia with block should be suspected in the digitalized patient who notes a change in heart rhythm or complains of palpitation. Nausea, visual difficulties, and other signs of digitalis intoxication may not be present. Often previously unsuspected paroxysmal atrial tachycardia with block is discovered through an electrocardiogram taken as a control measure in an asymptomatic digitalized patient.

Electrocardiographic diagnosis also presents problems. The nonconducted P waves may be buried in the preceding T wave and may be difficult to identify, or the atrial rate may be such that the rhythm resembles atrial flutter. In the case of the buried P waves, any of the following procedures may make the P waves more easily seen: carotid sinus pressure alone or accompanied by an esophageal lead, a high lead V_1, a standard lead I with the right-arm electrode on the V_1 position and the left-arm electrode on the V_2 position. Electrocardiographic differentiation from atrial flutter is made by noting the presence of the characteristic undulating base line in at least one lead in atrial flutter but an isoelectric base line in paroxysmal atrial tachycardia with block. This differentiation is usually made in standard leads 2 and 3, AVF, or in chest lead V_1. The atrial rate in untreated flutter is almost always 300, plus or minus 20, while in paroxysmal atrial tachycardia with block it is seldom greater than 250 beats per minute. Carotid sinus pressure applied during electrocardiography may be quite helpful by increasing the block and spreading the QRS complexes far enough apart so that the base-line characteristics may be studied. Even with these criteria and with electrocardiographic help, differentiation is not always certain.

Treatment. Since paroxysmal atrial tachycardia with block in the absence of digitalis intoxication is usually seen in the presence of severe heart disease, the first step in treatment is to gain control of the ventricular rate by increasing the block at the AV node. This is done to prevent or lessen congestive heart failure and is best accomplished by digitalization.[42] The speed of digitalization depends on the gravity of the situation. If the ventricular response is not more than 100 or if the patient is tolerating the rate well, then digoxin, 0.5 mg given orally every 4 hr for five doses, will usually suffice. If more is needed to increase the block and slow the ventricular rate, it may be given by continuing the same dosage schedule. A daily maintenance dose of 0.25 mg by mouth is usually sufficient once the rate is slowed, but the dose must be adjusted for the individual patient.

If, for example, the paroxysmal atrial tachycardia is occurring at a rate of 130 beats per minute and shows a variable 1:1 or 2:1 response so that the ventricular rate varies from 65 to 130, and if the heart is in failure at this time, more rapid digitalization is necessary. In this situation, 0.5 mg digoxin should be given intravenously and repeated at 2-hr intervals until the rate is controlled. In addition, simultaneous use of opiates, diuretics, and tourniquets would be indicated for rapid control of congestive heart failure.

In paroxysmal atrial tachycardia with block not due to digitalis intoxication, the selectively synchronized d-c converter could be used as initial therapy or could be employed to revert the rhythm after the ventricular rate had been controlled through the use of digitalis.

If a synchronized d-c converter is not available, a trial of quinidine sulfate by mouth as outlined in the section on paroxysmal atrial and nodal tachycardia would be indicated, with prophylactic therapy to follow if the rhythm is reverted. This rhythm may be quite refractory to treatment, however, and many times the physician is forced to accept the paroxysmal atrial tachycardia and be satisfied with control of the ventricular rate with digitalis.

When paroxysmal atrial tachycardia with block appears in the patient who is receiving digitalis, the treatment is quite different. In this case, it must be assumed that the digitalis is responsible for the arrhythmia, and administration of the drug should be immediately discontinued. As stated previously, it is not necessary that either recent increase in the maintenance dose or an excessive maintenance dose be involved. Any situation which may result in depletion of body potassium may induce intoxication of the digitalized patient. The more common inciting causes are the thiazide diuretics, diarrhea, and vomiting. As indicators of whether paroxysmal atrial tachycardia with block is due to digitalis, the serum electrolytes are often misleading, since intoxication may occur with normal levels of serum potassium. When the diagnosis of digitalis intoxication has been reached, the following three factors are important in dictating the treatment: (1) the type of digitalis preparation used, (2) the condition of the patient, and (3) the mode of precipitation of the intoxication.

For patients who have been taking excessive maintenance doses of short-acting preparations, who are tolerating the arrhythmia well, and who have no reason for potassium depletion, discontinuing the drug will usually result in a cure in 36 to 48 hr.

If in the same circumstances, the longer-acting preparations such as digitalis leaf or digitoxin are responsible for the toxic reaction, 4 to 6 Gm potassium chloride by mouth in divided doses should be given each day in chilled tomato juice. It is well to remember that before potassium is administered to any patient, the physician must first ascertain that adequate renal function is present to prevent development of toxic levels.[43] Repeated monitoring of renal function and blood levels of potassium should be carried out in any patient being given potassium for prolonged periods, particularly if congestive failure or renal disease is present. In either case, if the arrhythmia has been precipitated by sudden or gradual potassium depletion, the cause of the loss should be eliminated and the potassium replaced as described above. In patients with a tendency to potassium depletion following diuresis, it is advisable to avoid thiazide diuretics in favor of the injectable mercurials, which have less tendency to cause potassium depletion.

In patients with more severe digitalis intoxication who are tolerating the arrhythmia poorly, intravenous administration of potassium is indicated. This is accomplished by the use of 40 to 60 mEq potassium in 500 ml of 5 per cent dextrose and water, given intravenously as an infusion at a rate of 20 to 40 mEq per hr. This may be repeated until a total of 120 mEq is given or the rhythm is corrected. Potassium therapy should be carried out under continuous electrocardiographic control. The toxic effects of potassium are similar to those described for quinidine and Pronestyl given in a similar fashion.

It should be recognized that potassium is not a panacea for digitalis intoxication; it is not a direct antagonist to the effects of digitalis; and its mode of action in paroxysmal atrial tachycardia with block is poorly understood. The treatment itself can be dangerous. It should not be used unless necessary.[43,44]

In the past few years there have been many reports of the use of chelating agents in the treatment of paroxysmal atrial tachycardia with block secondary to digitalis intoxication.[45] Our own experience with this material is not great, and our results have been poor in the few cases when it was tried. It is thought that these compounds act through their ability to bind calcium and thereby decrease the effectiveness of the digitalis bodies.

The value of the selectively synchronized d-c converter in paroxysmal atrial tachycardia with block due to digitalis intoxication is not clear at this time. If severe congestive heart failure is present and immediate termination of the arrhythmia is desirable, it would be worth trying. The converter was successful in the single instance with which I have had experience, but I suspect the abnormal rhythm will return promptly in most cases if pharmacologic treatment with potassium is not carried out immediately following conversion.

ATRIAL FLUTTER* [16]

Edward R. Dorney, M.D.

Atrial flutter is an arrhythmia which usually is first noted as a rapid, regular tachycardia with a ventricular rate of 150 beats per minute, plus or minus 10. It is not a common arrhythmia, and unlike paroxysmal atrial tachycardia is almost always seen in association with significant heart disease and only rarely in normal hearts. It can occur at any age, but the majority of patients are over the age of 40 and have coronary artery disease.

Clinically, the rhythm must be differentiated from paroxysmal atrial tachycardia, which it very closely resembles. It is said that the diagnosis may be made at the bedside by the simple observation that the neck veins are pulsating at a rate twice that of the cardiac apex. In my experience, this particular sign is not especially helpful and can rarely be recognized even when the true character of the arrhythmia is already known (Fig. 16-31).

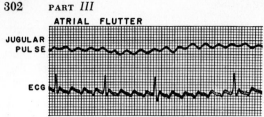

Fig. 16-31. Jugular venous pulse and electrocardiogram recorded during atrial flutter. Note the rapid, regular venous pulsation with each atrial systole. (*From Fig. 88, E. Corday and D. W. Irving: "Disturbances in Heart Rate, Rhythm and Conduction, W. B. Saunders Company, Philadelphia, 1961.*)

A better clinical impression may be had by the ventricular response to carotid sinus massage. In the case of flutter, the apical rate responds with a sudden cessation of beat and then a jerky return to its former rapid, regular rate as soon as the carotid stimulation is removed. The final identification of the arrhythmia is made by the presence of the characteristic sawtooth undulations of the base line in

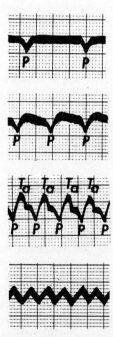

Fig. 16-32. The true configuration of the atrial electrocardiogram in atrial flutter. As the atrial rate increases, the Ta wave develops. The faster the rate, the larger the Ta wave. The isoelectric interval between the end of the Ta wave and the next P wave becomes shorter and shorter until finally the electrocardiographic configuration appears to have a sawtooth pattern. (*From Fig. 82, E. Corday and D. W. Irving: "Disturbances in Heart Rate, Rhythm and Conduction," W. B. Saunders Company, Philadelphia, 1961.*)

one or more leads of the electrocardiogram (Fig. 16-32). For this observation, standard leads 2 and 3, the augmented foot lead (AVF), or the chest leads V_1 and V_2 are the most useful. When the atrial flutter has not been treated, the atrial rate is usually 300 beats per minute, and since the usual degree of AV block is 2:1, the ventricular rate is usually 150 beats per minute. The AV block may be greater than 2:1 and may be variable. Accordingly, the ventricular rate may be irregular and as slow as 60 to 75 beats per minute (Figs. 16-33 and 16-34).

Probably because it is usually seen in the presence of severe cardiac disease and in the older age groups, atrial flutter is frequently associated with symptoms. These take the form of congestive heart failure, chest pain, and various cerebrovascular disturbances. For this reason prompt treatment is indicated.

Treatment. The treatment of choice in atrial flutter is reversion of the rhythm with a synchronized d-c converter. If the converter is unsuccessful or if this equipment is not available or cannot be applied because of refusal by the patient or mechanical difficulties with the chest wall, then drug therapy should be employed.

Since the basic defect is an excessively rapid atrial pacemaker resulting in a rapid and many times ineffective ventricular response, the first aim of treatment is to increase the block at the AV node so that fewer impulses reach the ventricle and a more efficient rate can be established. This is best accomplished by the use of digitalis. An initial dose of 0.5 mg digoxin may be given intravenously and repeated at 2- to 3-hr intervals until the ventricular rate is controlled. There is no formula for precalculating the dose of digitalis required in any given case of flutter. The physician must give as much as is needed to gain the desired effect. As always when digitalis is pushed, electrocardiograms should be obtained frequently in order to permit prompt

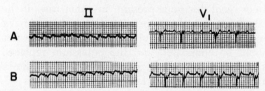

Fig. 16-33. Electrocardiogram of a patient with atrial flutter. Top, variable ventricular response—2:1 and 3:1. Lower, *regular* ratio, i.e., two atrial complexes to each QRS complex. There is a sawtooth appearance in the base line of lead 2 *but* a distinct P wave with isoelectric interval in lead V_1. This illustrates the difficulty encountered in utilizing the "isoelectric period" between P waves to separate atrial tachycardia with block from atrial flutter.

identification of signs of digitalis intoxication, such as ventricular ectopic beats or paroxysmal atrial tachycardia with block. For unknown reasons, however, patients with atrial flutter are particularly tolerant of both the cardiac and gastrointestinal effects of digitalis preparations, so that the large doses needed to gain sufficient block may often be used over short periods of time without toxic manifestations. Occasionally during this stage of treatment, atrial flutter will revert to sinus rhythms.

When the ventricular rate has been controlled and if reversion of the rhythm has not occurred, the next step would be to continue the digoxin, 0.5 mg by mouth every 4 hr, until toxic symptoms result or until the rhythm converts to a sinus mechanism. Reversion to sinus rhythm will occur in about 40 to 60 per cent of the patients when digitalis is used in this manner. In the remainder, the rhythm will remain as atrial flutter with a slow ventricular response or will change to atrial fibrillation. If atrial fibrillation should appear during the digitalis administration, treatment should be continued as outlined until reversion to sinus rhythm occurs or until toxic symptoms appear.

When it has been demonstrated that atrial flutter cannot be terminated by digitalis or that the rhythm has converted to a fixed atrial fibrillation with a controlled ventricular rate, a decision must be made as to the advisibility of further attempts at reversion of this rhythm to normal sinus rhythm. If a d-c converter is available, it should again be tried at this point. If a converter is not available, quinidine sulfate therapy as outlined in the section on paroxysmal atrial tachycardia may be employed. The dangers of quinidine therapy should be weighed against the possible benefits of reversion of the rhythm to normal sinus rhythm in the individual patient. It must be remembered that either atrial fibrillation or atrial flutter can be well tolerated for many years as long as a slow ventricular response is maintained through the use of digitalis, even though some decrease in cardiac output is most probably present. Either inability to gain adequate control of the ventricular rate or persistence of congestive heart failure despite a slow ventricular rate is indication for quinidine therapy. The possibility of embolization from a fibrillating or fluttering atrium is only a relative indication except in mitral valve disease. Actual embolization, either pulmonary or peripheral, is a positive indication for reversion to a normal sinus rhythm.

Embolization at the time of reversion has not proved to be a problem, so anticoagulation is not done routinely before reversion. If there has been previous pulmonary or peripheral embolization, however, anticoagulants should be employed for several weeks prior to the reversion to allow firm fixation of previously formed thrombi while new thrombus formation is prevented.

Atrial flutter with rapid ventricular response has been reported in very young children and, just as with paroxysmal atrial tachycardia, may result in congestive heart failure and death if not controlled. The treatment of choice is reversion of the rhythm with a d-c converter; if this is not available, digitalis should be administered in the same manner as described for paroxysmal atrial tachycardia in children. As mentioned previously, the dose necessary to control the arrhythmia may be much greater than the calculated dose for the age and weight. Digitalis

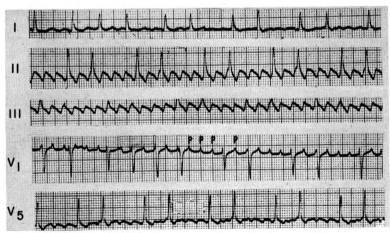

Fig. 16-34. Electrocardiogram which demonstrates the typical sawtooth waves of atrial flutter in leads II and III but shows distinct P waves followed by isoelectric intervals in V_1. Many electrocardiographers would call the rhythm in lead V_1 atrial tachycardia with block, but if all the leads were recorded at the same time, typical sawtooth deflections and P waves with isoelectric intervals would occur simultaneously. Considerable confusion in terms exists regarding whether this rhythm is atrial flutter or atrial tachycardia with block.

should be maintained for about 6 to 12 months after reversion as a prophylactic measure.

The indications for prophylactic therapy after reversion of atrial flutter are much the same as for paroxysmal atrial tachycardia. When atrial flutter recurs frequently, when it results in congestive failure, or when significant heart disease is present, a maintenance dose of quinidine sulfate, 300 to 500 mg orally every 6 hr, should be given for an indefinite period.

ATRIAL FIBRILLATION

DIAGNOSIS OF ATRIAL FIBRILLATION

Eliot Corday, M.D., and
Tzu-Wang Lang, M.D.

Atrial fibrillation is a common arrhythmia and has been the subject of much study for many years.

There are two theories of the *mechanism* of atrial fibrillation, the unifocal theory of Rothberger[22,23] and the circus theory of Lewis (Figs 16-35 and 16-36).[19,20] Recent experimental evidence favors the unifocal theory, according to which the rate of stimulation from an ectopic focus exceeds the rate at which the atria can respond and recover. Then a chaotic atrial rhythm results. Normal ventricular conduction occurs, but the AV node is activated

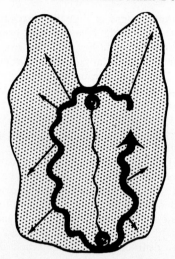

Fig. 16-36. Diagram of the hypothetical circus movement during atrial fibrillation as conceived by Lewis. Note that the wave of excitation follows an irregular circus pathway around the superior and inferior venae cavae, giving off daughter waves which excite the remaining portions of the atria.

irregularly. The fact that atrial fibrillation is often preceded by premature atrial systoles, atrial tachycardia, or flutter would favor the unifocal theory (Fig. 16-37). The circus movement theory, for which there has been no satisfactory experimental evidence to date, would suggest that the wave of excitation follows an irregular circus pathway around the vena cava and gives off daughter waves which cause an irregular contraction of the atria.

High-speed cinematography reveals that there are two types of contraction waves in the atrium: large waves called "L" waves which occur irregularly in frequency and in force; and, superimposed on the L waves, micro "M" waves which cause a constant, irregular wrinkling of the atrial surface.[46] The electrical impulses which have been recorded during atrial fibrillation also suggest the presence of these large L waves at a rate of 400 to 800 beats per minute and minute M waves at a frequency of around 40,000 beats per minute. Occasionally, there is a forceful contraction which propels the blood into the ventricle. Usually it is so irregular and weak that it does not force the blood into the ventricles, or, because of its irregular timing, it contracts when the AV valves are closed.

Usually the patient with atrial fibrillation and a slow ventricular rate is not aware of the irregular rhythm; however, if the rate is rapid, he might notice an irregular thumping or pounding in the chest or head or complain of "momentary stoppage of the heart." If the ventricular rate is extremely rapid, the cardiac output and systemic pressure usu-

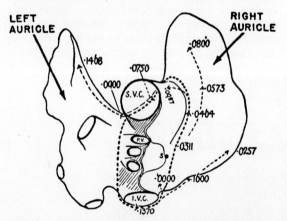

LEFT AURICLE   RIGHT AURICLE

Fig. 16-35. Reproduction of Lewis's results. From these determinations he assumed that the course of the flutter wave was in a circular direction around the superior and inferior venae cavae in what he called a "circus movement." According to his circus movement theory, the impulse traveled up the right atrium and down the left. He did not make any determinations on the long downward path over the left atrium. *From Sir Thomas Lewis: "The Mechanism and Graphic Registration of the Heart Beat,"* 3d *ed., courtesy of Shaw and Sons, Ltd., London,* 1925.

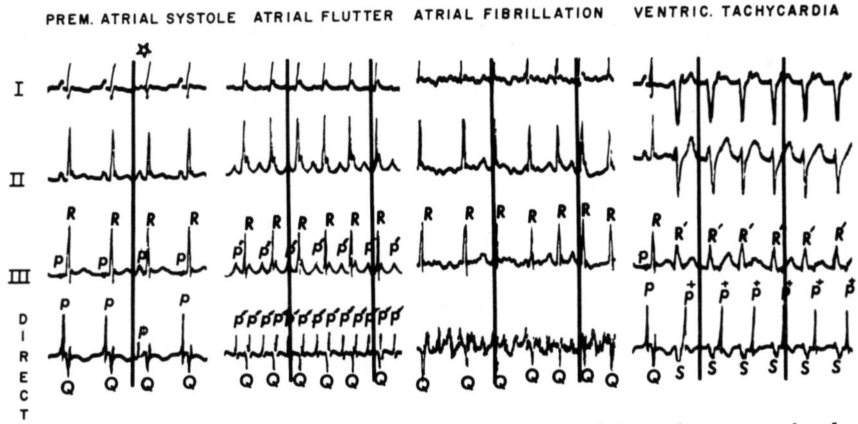

PREM. ATRIAL SYSTOLE   ATRIAL FLUTTER   ATRIAL FIBRILLATION   VENTRIC. TACHYCARDIA

Fig. 16-37. Standard limb leads and a lead recorded from the surface of the right atrium of a dog. Stroking the atrium with an applicator produced premature atrial systoles, atrial flutter, and fibrillation. In the direct lead, the P wave during regular sinus rhythm is larger than the QRS wave, whereas the direct P wave of the premature systole is of much lower amplitude. During the paroxysm of atrial flutter, the direct P waves are of lower amplitude than those of sinus rhythm but identical to those of the premature atrial systoles. In atrial fibrillation, the direct atrial lead reveals a constantly moving pattern with no particular form. During ventricular tachycardia, the QRS is followed by a retrograde P wave. This illustration shows that the P waves in leads II and III and directly from the atrium are identical during premature atrial systoles and atrial flutter and are produced by stimulation of the same ectopic focus, suggesting the unitarian nature of these atrial arrhythmias. (*From Fig. 80, E. Corday and D. W. Irving: "Disturbances in Heart Rate, Rhythm and Conduction," W. B. Saunders Company, Philadelphia, 1961.*)

ally decrease, and the patient might complain of angina because of the lowered coronary perfusion pressure, or complain of weakness, dyspnea, and cough due to the heart failure.[47] Because of the reduction in cerebral perfusion pressure, syncope or dizziness may occur; and if cerebral artery narrowing is present, the rapid ventricular rate might result in focal neurologic symptoms such as hemiparesis, aphasia, hemianopsia, etc.[2,6-8] If the patient has no underlying heart disease, few cardiac symptoms will be evident.[48] Where heart disease, such as coronary atherosclerosis or valvular disease, is present, heart failure and coronary insufficiency may quickly supervene.[22,24,34] Hemianopsia, hemiparesis, or hemiplegia may be due to emboli.[2,5,48] Emboli to the kidney cause flank pain and, later, hematuria. Splenic emboli refer pain, which varies with respiration, to the lower left part of the chest or to the left upper quadrant of the abdomen. Emboli to the gastrointestinal tract will cause abdominal pain, abdominal rigidity, distension, ileus, and often bloody diarrhea. Peripheral emboli to the arms or legs will induce pain, pallor, inability to use the limb, and gangrene.

The *characteristic feature* of atrial fibrillation is an apical rate usually between 60 and 180 beats per minute, grossly irregular in intensity and rhythm. The radial pulse is usually lower than the apical rate because some systolic contractions are feeble. The discrepancy between the radial pulse and apex beat is called the pulse deficit. During atrial fibril-

lation the cervical veins pulsate irregularly. Often a large cervical venous pulse wave will become evident. Because rheumatic heart disease is commonly found with this condition, an apical diastolic rumble may be evident; but because the atrial systolic contraction is often inadequate, the typical presystolic murmur may be heard only during an occasional beat of the heart. The second sound may not be heard with each beat because the ventricle fails to propel sufficient blood to open the aortic and pulmonic valves.

THE ELECTROCARDIOGRAM IN ATRIAL FIBRILLATION

Eliot Corday, M.D., and
Tzu-Wang Lang, M.D.

The characteristic feature of atrial fibrillation is that the base line is constantly moving (Fig. 16-38). No P waves can be regularly identified. There are irregularly occurring L waves of various shapes, but occasionally they have the uniform appearance of flutter waves except that they are slightly irregular in frequency (Fig. 16-39). The QRS complexes are usually of the same shape as in normal sinus rhythm, but they occur at irregular intervals. However, when the ventricular rate is rapid and almost regular, the QRS complex may become abnormal because of aberrant conduction and the rhythm may resemble ventricular tachycardia. Very rarely carotid sinus massage may convert atrial fibrillation.

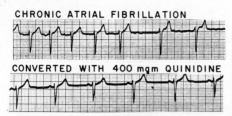

Fig. 16-38. Electrocardiogram demonstrating typical characteristics of atrial fibrillation. Top, the R-R interval varies considerably because of atrial fibrillation, later converted with 400 mg of quinidine. Note that the base line during atrial fibrillation is grossly irregular compared to that of normal sinus rhythm. No P waves, such as are seen on the lower strip during sinus rhythm, can be identified during the atrial fibrillation. The QRS complexes are of similar configuration in both.

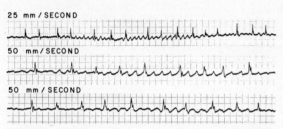

Fig. 16-39. Electrocardiogram showing the undulating base line of atrial fibrillation recorded at a paper speed of 25 and 50 mm per sec. Note that at times there is a sawtooth deflection almost resembling that of atrial flutter, but when these deflections are measured out they do not occur regularly as in atrial flutter. Many authorities would call this "flutter fibrillation," but such an interpretation is not possible; it is either flutter or fibrillation.

MANAGEMENT OF PATENTS WITH ATRIAL FIBRILLATION† [49]

J. Willis Hurst, M.D.,
E. Alan Paulk, Jr., M.D.,
H. D. Proctor, M.D., and
Robert C. Schlant, M.D.

The recent development of new therapeutic tools in the management of cardiac arrhythmias has stimulated us to reconsider the problems related to atrial fibrillation and its management. Our present views regarding this arrhythmia are based on our past experience, the medical literature, and our recent experiences with 230 carefully evaluated patients.

It would be unreasonable, naive, and short-sighted to think that this document represents the final word in the management of this arrhythmia. We anticipate that our views will change in the months and years ahead.

Clinical Situations in Which Atrial Fibrillation Is frequent. Atrial fibrillation may develop and persist for the remainder of the patient's life (*chronic* atrial fibrillation). At times, atrial fibrillation may occur in paroxysms, which may last from a few minutes to a few days. Some patients have recurrent paroxysmal episodes prior to the development of chronic atrial fibrillation. In other patients the episodes of atrial fibrillation occur as isolated episodes and are not recurrent or followed by the development of chronic atrial fibrillation.

Chronic atrial fibrillation is most frequently associated with rheumatic heart disease (particularly mitral valve disease), ischemic heart disease, hypertensive heart disease, and diffuse myocardial disease.[50-52] It occasionally occurs in patients with constrictive pericarditis or hyperthyroidism, and in adult patients with atrial septal defect who have developed severe pulmonary vascular disease and heart failure. It is not common in congenital heart disease,[40,53] although it may occasionally be noted in children with atrial septal defect, tricuspid atresia, or Ebstein's disease. In most of the conditions associated with chronic atrial fibrillation, either there is ischemia of the atrial musculature or of the sinoatrial node[29] or there is dilatation and hypertrophy of the atria. At times, it occurs secondary to neural-humoral or metabolic abnormalities.[54,55] The left atrium appears to be predominantly involved in most clinical conditions associated with chronic atrial fibrillation. In contrast, in disease associated with chronic dilatation and hypertrophy of only the right atrium, e.g., chronic cor pulmonale or pulmonary stenosis, atrial fibrillation is less common. In some patients chronic atrial fibrillation may occur with no demonstrable heart disease and may be associated with only minimal limitation of function.[47,56-59] On the other hand, several reports[57,60,61] have clearly shown that cardiac enlargement and congestive heart failure occasionally may be produced by atrial fibrillation in patients who have no demonstrable organic heart disease. In addition to the above conditions, atrial fibrillation may rarely occur as a familial finding.[58,62,63] This condition appears to be more common in males. In most instances of familial atrial fibrillation, there are usually no symptoms of congestive heart failure although exercise tolerance is diminished and palpitations may be troublesome.

Paroxysmal atrial fibrillation is probably quite frequent. It is likely that many persons have brief, transient episodes of atrial fibrillation which do not cause the patient to be seen by a physician, either because they are of such short duration or because they do not produce sufficient symptoms. To determine the exact incidence of such episodes would require long-term monitoring of many individuals.

Paroxysmal atrial fibrillation which comes to the attention of a physician is particularly likely to occur in healthy, young adults under increased emotional tension, particularly associated with lack of sleep and excess alcohol. In some patients, excess smoking, excess coffee, or other stimulants may be responsible. Paroxysmal atrial fibrillation may also be produced by thyrotoxicosis, digitalis toxicity, and pulmonary embolism. This arrhythmia may also occur following the administration of catecholamines, such as epinephrine. Paroxysms of atrial fibrillation often occur in patients with rheumatic mitral valve disease prior to the establishment of chronic atrial fibrillation.

Isolated episodes of atrial fibrillation may occur in most of the above conditions. They are particularly likely to occur in otherwise normal individuals. Head injuries, thoracic surgery, acute pericarditis, acute rheumatic fever, and febrile disease, such as lobar pneumonia, are occasionally associated with isolated atrial fibrillation. It is relatively common following an acute myocardial infarction which is produced by occlusion of the coronary artery supplying the sinoatrial node[55].

Two of the authors, Paulk and Proctor, have recently completed the evaluation of 230 patients with atrial fibrillation. These patients have been seen in a special atrial fibrillation clinic established at Grady Memorial Hospital in order to reappraise atrial fibrillation and its related problems, including management. Efforts were made to have the physicians on the medical service of this large municipal hospital refer patients without any selection other than the presence of this arrhythmia. Although not all patients with atrial fibrillation seen at the hospital were evaluated in this clinic, an attempt was made to see as many of them as possible. The preselection of patients by the referring physicians in such a study is obvious although a strong attempt was made to minimize this bias as much as possible. Patients were classified by the criteria of the New York Heart Association.[64] The findings in this study serve as partial basis for much of this discussion.

The ages and diagnoses of these 230 patients are listed in Table 16-1. Except for four patients whose heart rhythm spontaneously reverted shortly after they were first seen, all the patients had atrial fibrillation of more than 4 weeks' duration. The design of the study limited the opportunity for patients with paroxysmal or isolated atrial fibrillation to be seen in this clinic. The nature of the patient population available for study tended to exclude "normal fibrillators" and to increase the incidence of organic heart disease in the group.

There were 79 patients in this series who had coronary artery atherosclerosis and 27 who had

Table 16-1. AGE OF PATIENT AND CAUSE OF HEART DISEASE ASSOCIATED WITH ATRIAL FIBRILLATION IN 230 PATIENTS*

Clinical classification	To-tal No.	Age Mean	Median	Range
Atherosclerotic coronary disease	79	68.8	69	43–84
Hypertensive heart disease	25	71.8	63	30–78
Hypertensive and atherosclerotic coronary disease	27	69.2	70	53–84
Rheumatic heart disease	46	66.1	38	14–78
Diffuse myocardial disease	13	58.9	56	28–78
Hyperthyroidism	10	66.7	66	57–75
Cor pulmonale	9	67.2	69	51–82
Syphilitic heart disease	8	67.6	64.5	65–73
Atrial septal defect	4	74	74.5	63–75
Hypothyroidism	1	66	66	66
Unclassified†	8	64.1	61	49–79
Total	230			

* Classification according to the New York Heart Association.

† Four patients with chronic alcoholism; one patient with malignancy in pericardium; one patient with history of carcinoma of breast; one patient with no associated disease; one patient with moderately severe obesity.

both coronary artery atherosclerosis and hypertensive heart disease. Of the total of 106 patients with coronary artery atherosclerosis 54 had angina pectoris, 12 had evidence of previous myocardial infarction, and 40 had both.

There were 46 patients with rheumatic heart disease. Of these, 5 had aortic valve disease, 27 had mitral valve disease, and 14 had combined aortic and mitral valve disease. Of the 5 patients with aortic valve disease, 4 had predominant stenosis and 1 had predominant regurgitation. Of the 27 patients with mitral valve disease, 11 had predominant stenosis, 8 had predominant regurgitation, and 8 had combined stenosis and regurgitation. Of the 14 patients with combined mitral and aortic valve disease, 8 had combined mitral regurgitation and aortic regurgitation, 2 had combined mitral stenosis and aortic regurgitation, 2 had mitral regurgitation and aortic stenosis, and 2 had mitral regurgitation in addition to combined aortic stenosis and regurgitation.

Ten of the 230 patients were found to have evidence of hyperthyroidism. All these patients were seen in the first 100 cases. We believe that the decreased incidence of this condition in the patients seen subsequently is the result of increased awareness of this diagnostic possibility on the part of the referring physicians. At this time in our study there are a number of patients with atrial fibrillation due to hyperthyroidism who are undergoing therapy for hypermetabolism which developed prior to their referral and who are not included in the present figures.

Disadvantages of Atrial Fibrillation. The three major disadvantages of atrial fibrillation are as follows: (1) clinical problems associated with a decrease in cardiac reserve, (2) the occurrence of pulmonary or peripheral emboli, and (3) the presence of bothersome palpitations which persist despite adequate therapy with digitalis.

Decreased Cardiac Reserve. Measurements of cardiac output before and after reversion of atrial fibrillation have been reported by several groups of investigators.[65-73] The reversion of atrial fibrillation to normal sinus rhythm increases the resting cardiac output by 20 to 40 per cent in most, but not in all, patients who have heart failure associated with the arrhythmia. In those patients who do not have heart failure during atrial fibrillation, there is usually no increase in the resting cardiac output after reversion. After reversion to normal sinus rhythm, however, many of these patients are able to increase their cardiac output during exercise much more substantially than before reversion of the atrial fibrillation.

The two major factors affecting cardiac output in atrial fibrillation are atrial failure and the rapid, irregular ventricular rate.

Atrial Failure. Medical giants, including William Harvey, have emphasized the contribution of atrial contraction to cardiac function.[74] This contribution was relatively ignored in the daily practice of medicine until the last few years. The atria have two main functions in the human circulation. The more important function is as a booster pump which increases ventricular filling and end-diastolic fiber length.[74-78] This pumping action not only increases the end-diastolic volume of the corresponding ventricle, but also causes the ventricle to contract with greater force, by virtue of Starling's law of the heart. When atrial fibrillation is present, the atria "fail" in their pumping function, although they may still maintain their second function as reservoirs for ventricular filling.[78]

The loss of the atrial booster pump associated with atrial fibrillation is usually well tolerated by the normal human heart if the ventricular rate is not excessively rapid. In patients with heart disease, however, the presence of "atrial failure" with the development of atrial fibrillation may cause failure of the overall function of the heart.

Braunwald[79] observed that following the reversion of atrial fibrillation there may be no immediate effective atrial contraction despite the presence of P waves on the electrocardiogram. This interesting phenomenon seems to occur more frequently following the reversion of patients whose atrial fibrillation was of long duration.

Uncontrolled Ventricular Rate. The rapid, irregular ventricular rate occasionally associated with atrial fibrillation decreases the cardiac reserve. In some patients it is impossible to control the ventricular rate despite the administration of adequate amounts of digitalis. This clinical situation is most often encountered in patients with other complications, e.g., atelectasis, pulmonary emboli, anemia, infection, bacterial endocarditis, hyperthyroidism, or even digitalis toxicity. Even after these conditions have been ruled out, however, there remain some patients in whom it is impossible to achieve an adequate slowing of the ventricular rate—both at rest and in response to exercise—without producing serious digitalis toxicity, which is usually manifest by ventricular ectopic beats or even bigeminy. These patients frequently are dramatically improved by reversion of their atrial fibrillation.

The clinical consequences of the decreased cardiac reserve associated with the development of atrial fibrillation are congestive heart failure, angina pectoris, and syncope. In the normal individual, these disorders rarely occur as the consequence of atrial fibrillation. In patients with underlying heart disease, however, atrial fibrillation may precipitate or aggravate congestive heart failure. In other patients with heart disease, especially coronary atherosclerosis, the clinical manifestations of decreased cardiac reserve may be angina pectoris or even myocardial infarction. In patients with underlying heart disease and peripheral vascular disease, atrial fibrillation may predispose to the development of ischemia of various organs, e.g., of the brain, abdomen, or extremities.

In some patients without organic heart disease, atrial fibrillation may produce cardiac enlargement and congestive heart failure.[57,60,61] Phillips and Levine[57] demonstrated frank or latent heart failure in 14 of 84 patients with atrial fibrillation who had no apparent organic heart disease. After the heart beats of these patients were converted to normal sinus rhythm, their circulatory dynamics, heart size, and compensation changed toward normal. In their study, heart failure usually developed within weeks or months after the onset of atrial fibrillation; if this arrhythmia was tolerated without difficulty for a year, subsequent heart failure was unusual.

In the present series, there were 149 patients in whom reversion was accomplished once or more than once. In 57 (38 per cent) of these patients, reversion was thought to have produced a significant improvement in symptoms and signs of heart failure or in angina pectoris (Table 16-2). Occasionally, reversion was associated with a change in status from bedridden with complete disability to a return to gainful employment with only moderate symptoms. Similar benefits have been reported in the literature.[69–71,80–85] Interestingly, several patients who had a marked improvement in symptoms following reversion were considerably less disabled by the recurrence of atrial fibrillation after several weeks of normal sinus rhythm. In the majority of the 12 patients who had an improvement in angina pectoris following the reversion of atrial fibrillation, the angina pectoris completely disappeared.

Emboli. Approximately 30 per cent of all persons with chronic atrial fibrillation experience at least one serious embolic phenomenon during the course of the fibrillation.[85] Emboli had been said to be responsible for about 10 to 20 per cent of all deaths in rheumatic heart disease.[80,86,87] Atrial fibrillation is present in about 90 per cent of patients with mitral stenosis who have peripheral emboli.[86,88,89] In one series of 257 patients with atrial fibrillation who died, 42 per cent had an embolus, or more than one.[40] Although sudden death may occur in any patient with heart disease, it has been estimated that 2.5 to 4 per cent of patients with atrial fibrillation die suddenly and unexpectedly.[31,60,82,84,90–92] It is probable that patients with a history of an embolus have a significantly greater chance of having another embolus, with or without

reversion, than patients with atrial fibrillation who have never had an embolus.

In the 230 patients with atrial fibrillation evaluated in the present series, 48 (30.9 per cent) had a history of previous pulmonary embolus and 17 (7.4 per cent) had a history of previous systemic embolus. It is obvious that many emboli do not produce recognizable symptoms. It is also clear that many pulmonary emboli come from the veins of the legs, rather than from the fibrillating atria, and that peripheral emboli may originate from the left ventricle. In the present series the incidence of a history of pulmonary embolus was significantly greater in patients with underlying mitral valve disease than in patients with arteriosclerotic, hypertensive, or diffuse myocardial disease, whereas a history of peripheral embolus was slightly more common in patients with coronary atherosclerotic heart disease. It should be noted, however, that in this series more patients with rheumatic heart disease had severe congestive heart failure than did patients in the other diagnostic categories.

Palpitation. The occurrence of severe, bothersome palpitations which persist despite adequate control of the ventricular rate with digitalis occasionally is the major indication for reversion of atrial fibrillation. In the present series, however, this symptom by itself was never the sole indication for reversion.

General Principles Governing the Management of Patients with Atrial Fibrillation. The discovery of atrial fibrillation in a patient should be a mental

Table 16-2. PATIENTS SHOWING MARKED IMPROVEMENT IN SYMPTOMS
FOLLOWING REVERSION OF ATRIAL FIBRILLATION

Etiology of heart disease	No. of patients with reverted rhythms	Congestive failure*		Angina pectoris†	
		Present before reversion	Significantly improved	Present before reversion	Significantly improved
Atherosclerotic coronary disease	49	27	8	19	8
Hypertensive and atherosclerotic coronary disease	20	9	4	7	4
Hypertensive heart disease	15	11	6		
Rheumatic heart disease	40	38	18		
Syphilitic heart disease	3	2	1		
Diffuse myocardial disease	10	10	5		
Thyrotoxicosis	2	1	1		
Miscellaneous	6				
Atrial septal defect	4	4	2	—	—
Total	149	102	45	26	12

* Congestive failure: marked improvement signifies great subjective and objective change in the clinical status of the patient. It is not dependent on the long-term status of the rhythm.

† Angina pectoris: the majority of these patients (9 of 12) had complete disappearance of angina. The other three were markedly improved. This was dependent on the maintenance of sinus rhythm by the patient.

stimulus to the physician to search for the cause of the underlying disease and to institute measures to control the ventricular rate. Many times, the basic disease responsible for the arrhythmia is apparent at the outset; in other patients the diagnosis is apparent only after the rate is slowed or is reverted to regular rhythm or after special diagnostic procedures are performed. In many patients with tight mitral stenosis and atrial fibrillation, the condition is not recognized initially. The diastolic rumble may not be heard when the ventricular response is rapid. It is not unusual for digitalis to be administered and repeated auscultation for evidence of mitral stenosis to be omitted after the ventricular rate is controlled. Although it is uncommon, the diastolic rumble may be inaudible or faint even when the ventricular rate is controlled. Although there may be other clues to the diagnosis of mitral stenosis in this group of patients, the clues may be overlooked and the diagnosis may be missed until the rhythm is returned to normal. This situation illustrates the necessity of re-evaluating all patients with atrial fibrillation after the ventricular rate has slowed and again after the restoration of normal sinus rhythm, if this is accomplished. Hyperthyroidism should be considered in every patient with atrial fibrillation even when another cause of heart disease is present and assumed to be responsible for the arrhythmia. This is especially true when the ventricular rate is difficult to control with digitalis.

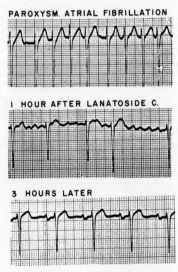

PAROXYSM. ATRIAL FIBRILLATION

I HOUR AFTER LANATOSIDE C.

3 HOURS LATER

Fig. 16-40. The upper tracing shows atrial fibrillation. An hour after the administration of lanatoside C, the ventricular rate slowed because the glycoside increased the degree of block in the atrioventricular node. Three hours after administration of the drug rhythm converted to sinus rhythm.

In most patients with untreated atrial fibrillation, the ventricular rate is 130 to 160 beats per minute. A cardinal rule of therapy in patients with atrial fibrillation is to slow the ventricular rate (Fig. 16-40). This is usually accomplished by the administration of digitalis. The clinical status of the patient determines the necessary speed of digitalization. A peripheral pulse rate of 70 to 80 beats per minute does *not* indicate that adequate digitalis has been administered. The resting apical beat of 70 to 80 beats per minute does *not* indicate that adequate digitalis has been administered. It is necessary to administer digitalis until the ventricular rate, determined by auscultation or by the electrocardiogram, is controlled in the range of 60 to 80 beats per minute at rest and 90 to 110 after slight exercise or after the sick patient has coughed several times. Should the ventricular rate increase following an initial period of slowing, it is necessary to obtain an electrocardiogram to make certain that multiple ventricular ectopic beats, the forerunner of ventricular tachycardia and ventricular fibrillation, are not responsible. Whenever the ventricular rate becomes regular during digitalization, it is also necessary to obtain an electrocardiogram. The regular rhythm may be due to the restoration of normal sinus rhythm or sinus tachycardia or it may be due to the development of digitalis toxicity with paroxysmal atrial tachycardia with atrioventricular block, AV nodal tachycardia, or ventricular tachycardia. An extra dividend of obtaining an electrocardiogram after the restoration of normal sinus rhythm is the ability to analyze the P waves, which may reveal a diagnostic clue to the diagnosis of mitral stenosis.

Digitalis not only slows the ventricular rate in most patients with atrial fibrillation, but may also be responsible for the reversion to normal sinus rhythm (Fig. 16-40). This is particularly likely in patients without demonstrable heart disease in whom the atrial fibrillation is of short duration. It may also occur in patients with mild heart disease. In patients who develop atrial fibrillation following myocardial infarction, the atrial fibrillation frequently reverts to normal sinus rhythm while the patient is being maintained on digitalis. Even in severe valvular heart disease the rhythm may rarely revert from atrial fibrillation to normal sinus rhythm with digitalization.

Special problems are presented by patients with atrial fibrillation in whom the ventricular rate is slow, i.e., 40 to 60 beats per minute, before receiving digitalis. These patients are usually in the older age group. It is likely that they have vascular or other disease of the atrioventricular node. The urgency of digitalization is obviously not so great in these patients as in those with a rapid ventricular response. When these patients have congestive heart failure, however, digitalization is indicated. On the other hand, if there is no evidence of heart failure and if the ventricular rate does not become excessive with moderate exercise, digitalis is probably not indicated, but it should be administered when the need arises. Patients in this group appear to have a high incidence of undesirable rhythm disturbances associated with reversion of their atrial fibrillation. These rhythm disturbances include sinoatrial standstill, with the supraventricular impulse originating in an ectopic atrial focus or from the atrioventricular node; sinoatrial block; slow AV nodal rhythm; and frequent relapse to atrial fibrillation. At times it is difficult to determine whether these disturbances following reversion are related to the basic disease process, to digitalis, or to quinidine.

We suspect that near-intoxication with digitalis is frequently needed to control adequately the ventricular rate in some patients with atrial fibrillation. Support for this view is found in the observation that patients with known digitalis intoxication have an increased incidence of abnormal atrial or nodal rhythm disturbances following reversion of atrial fibrillation. In addition, we have observed patients whose ventricular rate with atrial fibrillation was apparently well controlled without any evidence of digitalis toxicity, who had evidence suggestive of digitalis toxicity (atrial, nodal, or ventricular rhythm disturbances, particularly AV dissociation and bigeminy) following reversion of atrial fibrillation. Accordingly, it has seemed prudent to omit digitalis for 1 or 2 days prior to attempted reversion.

It is particularly necessary to keep a careful record of all the peripheral arterial pulses in patients with atrial fibrillation in order to detect the occurrence of arterial embolism during atrial fibrillation or subsequent to reversion.

Some authorities have recommended long-term anticoagulant therapy for patients with atrial fibrillation and a history of embolic phenomena, particularly systemic emboli.[93,96] Although there are still no completely adequate, well-controlled studies to support the hope that this therapy does decrease the incidence of emboli, it is prudent on the basis of current knowledge to administer long-term anticoagulant therapy to patients with a definite history of arterial embolus unless there is a definite contraindication.

Since the development of techniques (d-c defibrillation) which allow one to revert the rhythm in practically all patients with atrial fibrillation (95.8 per cent in our experience), it is mandatory to consider reversion in the management of all patients with this rhythm. In the treatment of an individual patient it is necessary to balance the dangers of reversion against the problems and dangers of allowing the abnormal rhythm to continue. The indications and contraindications listed below are merely general guide lines to therapy and are not to be considered dogma.

Patients in Whom Rerversion of Atrial Fibrillation is Indicated.

1. Young or middle-aged patients, with or without heart disease or heart failure.

2. Patients with hyperthyroidism in whom atrial fibrillation persists after the hyperthyroidism has been controlled.

3. Patients with congestive heart failure in whom ordinary methods of therapy have not controlled the decompensation.

4. Certain patients with angina pectoris which is not easily controlled by ordinary methods of treatment, whether or not congestive heart failure is present.

5. Patients with peripheral or pulmonary emboli thought to orginate from the atria.

6. Patients with atrial fibrillation in whom the ventricular rate cannot be adequately controlled with digitalis.

7. Patients in whom palpitation is very bothersome.

Patients in Whom Reversion of Atrial Fibrillation is Contraindicated.

1. Patients who are unable to tolerate prophylactic agents, such as quinidine, because of idiosyncrasy, hypersensitivity, or cinchonism.

2. Patients whose rhythm has been reverted many times without significant improvement but who have repeatedly relapsed to atrial fibrillation despite adequate prophylactic quinidine.

3. Patients with complete heart block.

Patients in Whom Reversion of Atrial Fibrillation is Relatively Contraindicated.

1. Asymptomatic elderly patients with atrial fibrillation which is easily controlled with digitalis may not need reversion.

2. Patients with intraventricular or bundle branch block conduction defects should have their atrial fibrillation reverted by electrical means rather than by pharmacologic methods.

3. Patients with extremely slow ventricular rates without digitalis. The frequency of disease of the SA and AV nodes is high in this group; and treacherous arrhythmias, including sinoatrial block, slow AV nodal rhythm, and sinoatrial standstill, may occur at the time of reversion.

4. Patients with atrial fibrillation precipitated by digitalis toxicity or patients with atrial fibrillation with other evidence of digitalis toxicity must be carefully evaluated prior to electrical reversion since more serious arrhythmias may be produced by

reversion. Certain of these patients may need potassium.

5. Patients in whom mitral valve surgery is planned in the near-future. These patients should have their atrial fibrillation reverted after recovery from surgery.

In years past, contraindications to the reversion of atrial fibrillation included long duration of the atrial fibrillation, marked cardiac failure, peripheral emboli, and severe angina pectoris. It is interesting to note how many of these former contraindications are now considered to be indications for reversion.

The value of anticoagulation in preventing embolization at the time of reversion is unknown. Some reports have indicated that all patients received anticoagulation prior to reversion;[70,102] other studies have indicated that anticoagulation was used only in patients with a history of an embolic phenomenon or in women with asymptomatic mitral valve disease and atrial fibrillation of recent onset.[91,92,121,122] Since the risk of embolization associated with the reversion of atrial fibrillation is estimated to be only 1.0 to 1.5 per cent,[91,92] it is obvious that a very large and well-controlled study would be required to demonstrate the efficacy of anticoagulation. In our own group of 186 reversions in 149 patients, we did not employ anticoagulant therapy. It seems prudent, however, to administer anticoagulant therapy for 3 to 4 weeks prior to reversion and for 1 week after the reversion of patients with atrial fibrillation who have a definite history of embolic phenomena.

Techniques of Reversion. The drugs used for the reversion of atrial fibrillation include quinidine sulfate (Fig. 16-38), procainamide hydrochloride (Pronestyl), and, for certain patients, potassium chloride. Reversion of atrial fibrillation may also be effected by electrical means (Figs. 16-41 and 16-42). The majority of patients with atrial fibrillation should be placed on digitalis prior to reversion (Fig. 16-40). Occasionally, normal sinus rhythm may result from the use of this drug alone. Certain drugs, such as quinidine sulfate, are usu-

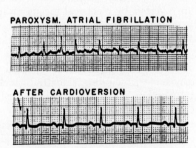

Fig. 16-41. Electrocardiogram of patient with paroxysmal atrial fibrillation which was converted by programmed electrical d-c capacitor discharge.

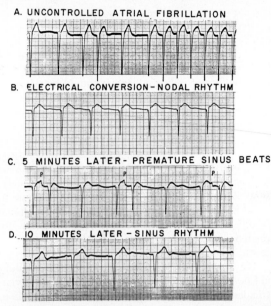

Fig. 16-42. Electrocardiogram of patient with uncontrolled atrial fibrillation (*A*) which was converted by programmed d-c capacitor discharge. Note that initially after the electric shock, nodal rhythm (*B*) resulted (P waves cannot be identified before the QRS complexes). Five minutes later (*C*), premature sinus beats occur, but the basic rhythm is that of nodal rhythm. Ten minutes later (*D*) the sinus node has taken over the pacemaking function.

ally necessary to prevent the recurrence of atrial fibrillation.

Reversion with Quinidine. In years past, many different schedules have been recommended for the reversion of atrial fibrillation with quinidine.[60,69,81,82,84,85,91,92,97–103] As will be pointed out later, larger dosage schedules of this drug are seldom justified at this time. Two-tenths of a gram of quinidine sulfate every 6 hr for several days will produce reversion in a small percentage of patients (14 per cent in our experience), and 0.4 Gm every 6 hr is safely tolerated by most patients. If equipment for electrical defibrillation is not available and if the smaller dosages have not been successful in reverting the rhythm, it is possible to administer 0.2 Gm every 2 hr for five doses. If this schedule fails to produce reversion, one must seriously consider that the risk of a larger dosage schedule may be greater than the risk of simply controlling the ventricular rate with digitalis. If compelling reasons for reversion are present, quinidine sulfate, 0.4 Gm every 2 hr for five doses, may be given. It is wise to begin the dosage regimen in the early morning in order that the patient can be observed more carefully during the day. Electrocardiograms should be obtained frequently whenever quinidine is administered for reversion of atrial fibrillation in order to detect early evidence of myocardial toxicity.

Complications. Quinidine toxicity may occur in patients given quinidine for any reason, including its use for prophylactic purposes after the reversion of atrial fibrillation by quinidine or by electrical means. The most common untoward effect of quinidine is cinchonism, which may be manifested by anorexia, nausea, vomiting, abdominal cramps of varying severity, diarrhea, tinnitus, and weakness. Quinidine idiosyncrasy may rarely produce peripheral vascular collapse, coma, or convulsions within 30 min or a few hours after a small initial oral dose. Some of these reactions are probably produced by ventricular tachycardia or ventricular fibrillation. True idiosyncrasy is an absolute contraindication to the use of quinidine at any future time. Quinidine hypersensitivity may be manifested by thrombocytopenic purpura,[104–107] which occurs in 0.1 to 0.2 per cent of patients[105–108] and may be lethal.[109,110] Other possible hypersensitivity reactions include drug fever, skin rashes, leukopenia, splenomegaly, hemolytic anemia,[113] nonthrombocytopenic purpura, and toxic amblyopia.[114] The cardiovascular toxicity of quinidine includes cardiac arrhythmias, conduction disturbances, hypotension, and sudden death. Unfortunately, these toxic reactions may occur without preceding cinchonism or widening of the QRS on the electrocardiogram. Syncope is a frequently unrecognized manifestation of myocardial toxicity. It is probable that many episodes of sudden death and of death attributed to central nervous system depression or to respiratory failure are primarily due to the myocardial toxicity. The incidence of myocardial toxicity has been indicated to be relatively low in many series.[81,84,85,91,92,97,100,115] However, in a recent review of quinidine therapy in 274 unselected patients, there were 12 episodes of sudden loss of consciousness, with respiratory and circulatory depression requiring resuscitative measures.[102] In most of these 12 patients, the episodes were produced by cardiac arrhythmias. Another report described 8 patients with quinidine synscope, which was thought to be produced by paroxysmal ventricular fibrillation.[116] These 8 cases were in a group of patients estimated to be between 200 and 300 in number.

There is no satisfactory method to prevent some of the untoward reactions to quinidine. All patients receiving quinidine should be observed closely for any evidence of toxicity, in particular, a change in rhythm or syncope. Frequent electrocardiograms should be obtained whenever patients receive more than minimal doses of quinidine.

The catastrophic reactions may also occur following small doses of quinidine, although they are rare. The incidence of serious myocardial toxicity is usually related to the dosage and blood level of quinidine. Sokolow and Ball[100,117] reported that episodes of serious myocardial toxicity did not occur with serum quinidine levels below 3 mg per liter and occurred in only 1.6 per cent of patients with levels less than 6 mg per liter. They found the incidence of toxicity increased markedly with higher serum concentrations. We suspect that the incidence of serious toxicity from quinidine is much higher than their studies indicate when this drug is administered by others with less experience and without the extremely careful observation and monitoring which their patients received. In addition, in patients with very severe heart disease, the incidence of myocardial toxicity to quinidine appears to be higher than their report indicates.

If it is desirable or necessary to attempt reversion with quinidine sulfate, this drug may be administered in divided doses not exceeding a total of 2.0 to 3.0 Gm per day. By restricting the dosage to no more than 3.0 Gm per day, one may accomplish most of the reversions which will occur and avoid most of the episodes of serious myocardial toxicity.[91,92,100,117]

Our own observations in patients receiving quinidine sulfate, 0.2 Gm every 6 hr, revealed that the prevalence of toxicity was surprisingly high. In these 186 patients, many of whom have severe organic heart disease, the effects of this small dose of quinidine have been observed over a period of months. Minor symptoms of cinchonism have been relatively frequent, and 34 patients were noted to have moderate to severe symptoms of cinchonism or other toxic manifestations of quinidine. In 26 patients, discontinuance of the drug was mandatory because of these effects. The commonest cause of stopping the drug was intractable diarrhea, but it was also stopped because of unexplained syncope (3 cases), onset of seizure (1 case), hemolytic anemia (1 case), electrocardiographic changes (4 cases), and unexplained fever (1 case). There were 4 cases of unexplained sudden death in patients receiving quinidine; however, there were also instances of sudden unexplained death in patients, not included in our series of 230 patients, who were still undergoing diagnostic evaluation before receiving quinidine. Two deaths in our series which were attributable to quinidine are discussed further on, under Complications [of electrical reversion].

In different large series, the incidence of reversion of atrial fibrillation with quinidine has varied from about 50 to 90 per cent. Holzman and Brown[98] reviewed 1,082 cases in the literature and found an overall conversion rate of 71 per cent with quinidine. Sokolow and Ball[100] accomplished reversion with quinidine in 74 per cent of 214 attempts in 177 patients. Eighty per cent of these reversions occurred while the patients were on a daily dose of 3.0 Gm or less of quinidine.

In most of the reported studies of the reversion of atrial fibrillation with quinidine sulfate, the incidence of reversion has varied with the cause of the heart disease. Thus, Sokolow[84] reported successful conversion with quinidine in 80 per cent of a miscellaneous group of patients with mitral stenosis. Goldman[91] reported over 90 per cent conversion in patients in whom atrial fibrillation persisted after control of thyrotoxicosis. In patients with coronary artery disease or hypertensive heart disease, he reported success in 87 per cent of patients. In patients with predominant mitral stenosis the incidence of successful conversion with quinidine is reported to be 50 to 55 per cent; in patients with predominant mitral regurgitation, the expected conversion rate was only 20 to 25 per cent.[91,101] McMillan and Welfare,[97] however, found no difference in the incidence of conversion in patients with mitral stenosis as compared to patients with other types of heart disease.

Procaine amide hydrochloride has not achieved the therapeutic eminence of quinidine in the management of atrial arrhythmias. It can be tried when patients do not tolerate quinidine.[123]

Embolization associated with reversion is a feared complication. Goldman[91] has estimated that emboli occur in 1.5 per cent of patients whose atrial fibrillation is reverted to normal sinus rhythm. Sokolow and Perloff[92] concluded that the incidence of embolism with reversion was probably less than 1 per cent.

Atrial fibrillation related to digitalis toxicity, which is often precipitated by the potassium loss produced by thiazide diuretics, should be treated with potassium chloride.

Technique of Electrical Reversion. The technique of electrical reversion we have used is similar to the technique which has been described by others.[121,122,124,125] Except for minor variations, the same technique has been employed in all our electrical reversions.

Prior to electrical reversion, the patients are given quinidine sulfate, 0.2 Gm every 6 hr, for 2 days. This is administered for the following reasons: (1) to test the patient's tolerance or sensitivity to this drug, which must be continued after reversion, (2) to achieve a level of quinidine in the blood and heart in order to lessen the likelihood of relapse immediately following electrical reversion, and (3) to revert the small percentage (10 to 15 per cent in our experience) of patients who

require only this small amount to revert atrial fibrillation to normal sinus rhythm.

The strength of all peripheral pulses is carefully noted before reversion and periodically after reversion in order to detect peripheral arterial embolism.

We do not administer barbiturates or narcotics prior to reversion, since they may mask subtle symptoms and signs after reversion. Reversion is performed in the patient's room whenever possible in order to allay his anxiety. If this is not possible, reversion is performed in the ward treatment room.

An anesthetic drug is administered during electrical reversion to produce transient narcosis or amnesia. This is preferred for the following reasons: (1) It is often necessary to administer more than one shock to the patient and stronger shocks may be particularly uncomfortable for the patient. (2) The use of small intravenous doses of thiopentothal sodium, 75 to 250 mg, produces rapid, adequate, and transient amnesia and the patient is not sedated following the procedure. (3) The presence of an anesthesiologist helps to assure that the patient will be well ventilated and that the heart will be maximally oxygenated.

Electrocardiographic recording of the electrical activity of the heart is recorded before and after the procedure. In addition, the patient's electrocardiogram is continuously monitored and displayed on an oscilloscope. During the actual reversion, a continuous record is obtained of the electrocardiogram before, during, and following the electrical shock. This is recorded on a standard electrocardiographic machine connected by a cable to the defibrillator.

Prior to administering the electrical shock to the patient, the operator test-fires the instrument several times to check the accuracy of the synchronization of the electrical shock. We routinely use the minimal setting on the synchronizer, which places the electrical shock about 20 msec after the R or S wave.

We prefer to use large electrodes which are applied to the front and back of the patient. The advantages of these electrodes are greater safety for the operator, greater ease in positioning the patient, and the ability to accomplish reversion with less electrical energy.[125] The electrodes are liberally covered with electrode jelly and placed posteriorly just below the left scapula and anteriorly over the heart just to the left of the sternum. The initial shock administered is 75-watt-sec unless the patient is very thick-chested. If repeated shocks are required, the strength of subsequent shocks is increased by increments of 100 watt-sec up to a maximum of 400 watt-sec.

If the cardiac rhythm is regular after the shock

has been administered, an electrocardiogram is used to distinguish between atrial fibrillation and sinus rhythm with atrial or nodal ectopic beats. Lead V_1 is especially valuable for this purpose. Occasionally we have seen apparent atrial fibrillation persist for 5 to 10 sec after the shock and then revert to normal sinus rhythm. The explanation for this phenomenon is not apparent. In two of our patients complete cardiac asystole followed the electrical shock. In these patients immediate resuscitation was initiated and normal sinus rhythm commenced in less than 1 min.

Intramuscular quinidine gluconate, 200 mg, is administered immediately following successful reversion. For several hours after reversion is accomplished, the patient is watched very closely to observe the adequacy of ventilation, to monitor the electrocardiogram, and to measure the blood pressure. The patients are carefully evaluated for evidence of arterial embolization during this period and during their entire follow-up period.

Special precautions are used to ensure that no one is in contact with the patient when the electrical shock is administered. Electrodes used to monitor the electrocardiograms should not be applied near the sites used for the defibrillation electrodes, since this might allow an electrical arc to jump to the monitor electrode and burn the skin.

Complications.[125a] Many of the patients have minor irritation and erythema at the major electrode sites, but most burns have been prevented by adequate amounts of electrode jelly.

Immediately following the reversion of atrial fibrillation and the restoration of normal sinus rhythm, there may be conduction disturbances or atrial, nodal, or ventricular ectopic beats (Fig. 16-42). In most patients in whom these have occurred, one of the following factors was thought to be responsible: (1) poor ventilation and oxygenation of the patient; (2) digitalis toxicity (It appears that the amount of digitalis necessary to control the ventricular rate during atrial fibrillation may produce evidence of toxicity during normal sinus rhythm. In most instances, these disturbances disappear when digitalis is withheld. If the patient reverts to atrial fibrillation in the intervening period, successful electrical reversion is usually obtained.); (3) hyperexcitability of the myocardium may be induced by the electrical current, particularly when high-energy shocks are necessary. In those instances thought to represent this phenomenon, the arrhythmia or conduction disturbance usually subsides in 5 to 10 min, and the rhythm either persists in normal sinus rhythm or soon reverts to atrial fibrillation. If the rhythm relapses to atrial fibrillation, repeated shocks at the same or higher settings are not

given to patients in this particular group, since the shocks are likely to induce ventricular tachycardia or ventricular fibrillation.

Although there were no deaths attributable to electrical shock in this series of patients, there were two patients who did die following reversion. In one patient, who had preexisting severe CO_2 narcosis, death 18 hr after reversion was thought to be due to respiratory depression. The second death, which occurred 24 hr after electrical reversion, was attributed to quinidine intoxication.

Embolus. There were two embolic episodes associated with 186 reversions (5 spontaneous, 23 quinidine, and 158 electrical) of atrial fibrillation of 149 patients. No embolic episodes occurred in the 5 patients whose rhythm was reverted spontaneously or in the 23 patients whose rhythm was reverted while they were receiving maintenance quinidine in preparation for electrical reversion. Following 158 episodes of electrical reversion in 121 patients, there were two embolic phenomena. One patient had an embolus to his left superficial femoral artery 8 days after successful electrical reversion. This was removed by embolectomy and the patient recovered satisfactorily. A second patient had an embolus to her right common iliac artery 3 days after transiently successful electrical reversion. The patient was treated surgically with an arterial bypass but died of surgical complications 6 weeks later. This incidence of embolic phenomena associated with the reversion of atrial fibrillation is comparable to that previously reported.[91,92,100,121,122,125]

Success. Electrical reversion of atrial fibrillation was successful in 151 (95.8 per cent of 158 attempts in 121 patients. In 25 patients, more than one electrical reversion of atrial fibrillation was performed. In most of these patients, the relapse to atrial fibrillation occurred a day or two following the initial reversion and the procedure was repeated within another day or two.

Frequency of Relapse after Conversion of Atrial Fibrillation. The important problem of relapse following the reversion of atrial fibrillation with quinidine has been considered by numerous investigators.[60,81,84,91,92,97,126] In general, it is agreed that the vast majority, or about 85 per cent, of patients in whom chronic atrial fibrillation has been reverted to normal sinus rhythm will relapse to atrial fibrillation if the patients are not maintained on an adequate maintenance schedule of quinidine.[42,43] About 80 to 90 per cent of all patients whose rhythm has been converted can be maintained in normal sinus rhythm on 0.4 Gm four times daily. Patients who require a higher dosage of quinidine for reversion tend to require a higher maintenance dosage. Thus, patients who revert readily on 2.0 Gm

Table 16-3. FOLLOW-UP STUDY OF 149 PATIENTS WHOSE HEART BEAT WAS REVERTED TO SINUS RHYTHM AND PERCENTAGE OF REVERSION IN 193 EPISODES OF ATRIAL FIBRILLATION

Etiology of heart disease	Total No. of patients	Episodes of atrial fibrillation treated by reversion				No. of patients reverting to atrial fibrillation		No. of patients remaining in normal sinus rhythm†	
		Successful*		Failed		−1 mo	+1 mo	No.	%
		No.	%	No.	%				
Atherosclerotic coronary disease	49	60	94	4	6	11	1	36	74
Hypertensive heart disease	15	23	96	1	4	3	2	9	60
Hypertensive and atherosclerotic coronary disease	20	26	93	2	7	4	1	14	70
Rheumatic heart disease	40	50	100			8	5	25	63
Diffuse myocardial disease	10	10	100			4		6	60
Hyperthyroidism	2	2	100					2	100
Syphilitic heart disease	3	3	100			1		2	67
Intraatrial septal defect	4	4	100			2		2	50
Miscellaneous	6	8	100					6	100
Totals	149	186	96	7	4	33	9	102	68

* Success is defined as the presence of normal sinus rhythm for at least 6 hr following reversion which occurred either spontaneously (5 patients), on prophylactic quinidine sulfate (23 patients), or with electrical defibrillation (158 episodes in 121 patients).

† The follow-up periods in these patients range from a minimum of 3 months to a maximum of 12 months.

or less of quinidine frequently can be maintained on 0.2 Gm four times a day, whereas patients who require 4 to 5 Gms quinidine in 1 day for conversion may need 0.6 Gm four times a day for several weeks following conversion before one should attempt to reduce the dosage to 0.4 Gm four times a day.[91]

In our series of 230 patients there were 149 patients whose heart beat was reverted to normal sinus rhythm (Table 16-3). The reversion occurred spontaneously in 5 patients and occurred in 23 patients while they were receiving 0.2 Gm of quinidine sulfate every 6 hr prior to contemplated electrical reversion. There were 121 patients whose rhythm was reverted once or more than once electrically. There were 117 who were successfully maintained on quinidine. In this group of 117 patients, there were 102 patients (87 per cent who were maintained in normal sinus rhythm for the current follow-up period of at least 3 months and up to 12 months. Fifteen patients relapsed, usually in less than 3 months, despite prophylactic quinidine sulfate. There were 38 patients who were not maintained on prophylactic quinidine. In 26 of these 38 patients, quinidine had to be stopped because of toxic symptoms. In 20 of these patients the heart beat promptly reverted to atrial fibrillation, and no further attempts at reversion have been made in these

patients. Six patients have maintained normal sinus rhythm despite not receiving prophylactic quinidine sulfate. Twelve patients accidentally stopped or did not receive quinidine prophylaxis. In 6 of these patients the rhythm was subsequently reverted electrically to normal sinus rhythm. Of these, 5 patients have remained in normal sinus rhythm on quinidine prophylaxis; 1 patient reverted to atrial fibrillation. The remaining 6 patients, who did not receive quinidine prophylaxis and who developed atrial fibrillation, still have this arrhythmia.

The following conclusions can be drawn from the previous discussion:

1. Quinidine sulfate in small dosage will cause toxic symptoms in a small percentage of patients. It is likely that the incidence of toxicity with both small and large dosage is higher than has previously been suspected. The problem of quinidine toxicity exists whether the drug is used prior to and after electrical reversion or whether it is used to accomplish reversion and is administered prophylactically following reversion. When larger amounts of quinidine are used for the purpose of reversion, the incidence of serious toxicity increases, especially when there is severe heart disease. Large dosage schedules of quinidine sulfate for reversion can no longer be justified when a defibrillator is available for the reversion of atrial fibrillation.

2. A major advantage of electrical defibrillation is that certain vital medical personnel are assembled at the time of reversion. If a catastrophe occurs, prompt resuscitation is possible and it is even possible for the defibrillator to be used again in the treatment of the new, undesirable rhythm. On the other hand, if an undesirable arrhythmia, such as ventricular fibrillation, develops during reversion with quinidine sulfate, it may not be recognized promptly. In addition, the treatment of a heart poisoned with quinidine may be difficult.

Clinical Sketches Depicting the Problems and Management of Atrial Fibrillation. The following case histories have been selected to illustrate in a more specific and vivid manner some of the general principles concerning the problems of atrial fibrillation and its management.

No. 1. A 26-year-old male developed atrial fibrillation following a sleepless night, liberal alcoholic ingestion, and excessive smoking. There was no evidence of heart disease or heart failure. He was aware of cardiac irregularity. The ventricular rate was 140 beats per minute and blood pressure was normal. Treatment consisted of bed rest, mild sedation, and oral administration of 1.5 mg digoxin in divided doses. His heart beat reverted to normal sinus rhythm after several hours.

Comment. Young persons with no evidence of heart disease usually tolerate atrial fibrillation without significant clinical difficulty. Normal sinus rhythm can be established in the majority of such patients by simple measures. Digoxin is administered in order to control the ventricular rate; however, reversion to normal rhythm frequently occurs

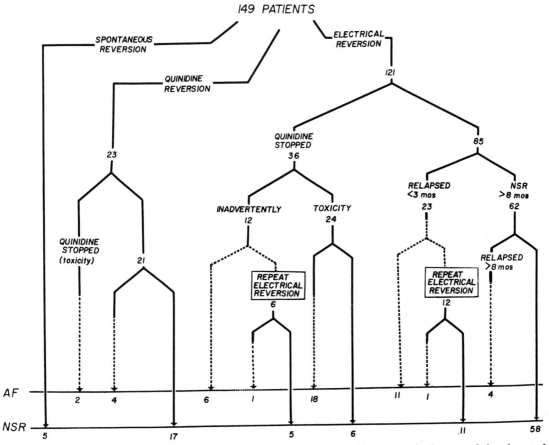

(*Table 16-4.*)
149 PATIENTS

* The current status of the 149 patients is shown by the two horizontal lines at the bottom of the chart indicating atrial fibrillation (*AF*) and normal sinus rhythm (*NSR*). In the group of 121 patients whose rhythm was reverted by electrical means, there were 19 patients who relapsed, usually within a day or two, after their initial electrical reversion and whose rhythm was promptly reverted a second time by electrical means. All patients now in NSR are receiving prophylactic quinidine sulfate except those who cannot tolerate this drug. Electrical reversion, either initial or repeat, is planned for some of those patients who are now in atrial fibrillation and who can tolerate prophylaxis.

as an extra dividend, possibly because of improved hemodynamics. As a rule, the oral use of digoxin is adequate; however, the intravenous administration of digoxin 0.75 mg may be used in the patient complaining of weakness, intolerable palpitations, or other evidence of circulatory insufficiency. If the rhythm does not revert spontaneously after a day or so, quinidine sulfate in a dose of 0.2 Gm every 6 hr for 24 to 48 hr is indicated. If reversion does not occur on this regimen, doses of 0.4 Gm every 6 hr may be given for 48 hr. If this fails to accomplish reversion, electrical (d-c) reversion is warranted.

Atrial fibrillation occurring in the above clinical setting does not usually require prophylactic medication.

No. 2. A 49-year-old female had a history of two or three episodes of atrial fibrillation each year for approximately 8 years; however, during the year prior to admission, she had an increased incidence of these paroxysms (five or six in the past 6 months) and the duration of each episode increased. There was no evidence of heart disease, cardiac enlargement, or thyrotoxicosis. The electrocardiogram between episodes remained normal except for frequent premature atrial contractions. The episodes of atrial fibrillation usually reverted spontaneously in 1 to 12 hr. Because of these prolonged and frequent episodes, the patient sought medical attention. Oral digoxin, 1.5 mg in divided doses over 24 hr, slowed the ventricular rate, and the patient's heart beat reverted to normal sinus rhythm. Prophylactic quinidine sulfate (0.2 Gm every 6 hr) subsequently eliminated the atrial ectopic beats and has prevented recurrent episodes.

Comment. If this amount of prophylactic quinidine is not sufficient, an increase in dosage to 0.4 Gm every 8 hr would be justified. In some patients maintenance digoxin and prophylactic quinidine sulfate may be used simultaneously to prevent paroxysms of this arrhythmia. Digitalis is used primarily for control of ventricular rate should atrial fibrillation occur. Electrical reversion has little place in the management of atrial fibrillation in this clinical setting. If frequent paroxysms cannot be prevented by moderate amounts of quinidine sulfate and if the patient tolerates atrial fibrillation without serious cardiovascular consequences, it is prudent to maintain the patient on adequate digitalis in order to control the ventricular rate.

No. 3. A 40-year-old normal asymptomatic male had a documented history of atrial fibrillation for 5 years. He was placed on maintenance digoxin shortly after the onset of the arrhythmia. Heart size was normal. The ventricular rate was 80 to 85 beats per minute at rest and accelerated to 135 to 140 per minute following moderate exercise. The digitalis was increased for bet-

ter control of the ventricular response. The patient was then placed on quinidine sulfate, 0.2 Gm every 6 hr, to test tolerance to the drug. At times, this dosage may also produce reversion. Reversion in this patient occurred during the following night. For the past 3 months, he has been maintained on this same dosage of quinidine.

Comment. This case illustrates that many patients with atrial fibrillation are not adequately digitalized. The ventricular rate following exercise should be sufficiently controlled as a guide to proper maintenance dosage of digitalis. Our studies indicate that in about 15 per cent of patients with atrial fibrillation due to various forms of heart disease reversion of rhythm is accomplished on 0.2 Gm quinidine sulfate every 6 hr. This is more likely when atrial fibrillation is associated with less severe forms of heart disease.

What would be the proper management had reversion not occurred in this patient? At the present time, it is acceptable to administer quinidine sulfate 0.4 Gm every 6 hr orally for 2 to 3 days. If this does not revert the rhythm, d-c defibrillation should be employed. If the equipment for defibrillation is not available, it is wiser to discontinue quinidine and to control the ventricular rate with digitalis; higher doses of quinidine, with its associated toxicity, are not indicated in an asymptomatic case of this sort.

No. 4. A 33-year-old female had presented symptoms of hyperthyroidism for 1 year and irregular heart action for 1 month. The heart was slightly enlarged, and there was atrial fibrillation with a ventricular response of 130 to 135 beats per minute. The patient was receiving digitalis and reserpine. After receiving antithyroid medication for several weeks, her heart beat spontaneously reverted to normal sinus rhythm as the hypermetabolic state subsided.

Comment. It is often difficult to control the ventricular rate with digitalis when atrial fibrillation is associated with hyperthyroidism. This difficulty may be the first clue to the diagnosis of thyrotoxicosis. In this clinical situation, reserpine is of great value in controlling the ventricular rate. In many patients with atrial fibrillation and hyperthyroidism, spontaneous reversion to normal sinus rhythm occurs during treatment of the metabolic condition. If atrial fibrillation persists for several weeks after the patient becomes euthyroid, reversion may be attempted with small or moderate doses of quinidine sulfate (0.2 to 0.4 Gm every 6 hr). If this is unsuccessful in producing reversion, d-c defibrillation should be performed.

Radioactive iodine may be used in euthyroid patients when the ventricular rate is not controlled with digitalis. The need for this therapy is, however, quite rare (Fig. 16-43).

No. 5. A 72-year-old male had had known atrial fibrillation for the past 20 years, for which he had been taking digitalis. No symptoms, other than very mild exertional dyspnea, were referable to the cardiovascular system. His heart was not enlarged, and his ventricular rate was adequately controlled at rest and during exercise.

Comment. This elderly man with chronic atrial fibrillation of many years' duration had no definite symptoms of congestive failure or history of embolic episodes. There is no need to attempt reversion in this type of patient.

No. 6. A 31-year-old female with mitral stenosis had few symptoms until the development of atrial fibrillation on the night of admission to the hospital, when she was awakened with extreme shortness of breath. She was admitted to the hospital with acute pulmonary edema and hypotension. Routine measures, including elevation of the trunk of the body, tourniquets to the extremities, oxygen, intravenous morphine sulfate, and digoxin produced partial improvement, but her state remained precarious. At this point, the patient underwent d-c defibrillation (75 watt-sec) while under the influence of morphine, and her heart beat reverted to normal sinus rhythm. The blood pressure returned to normal, and the patient was continued on digoxin and quinidine sulfate. After thorough evaluation, sufficient evidence was found to indicate mitral commissurotomy, which was performed several weeks later.

Comment. Tight mitral stenosis is a common form of valvular heart disease and is frequently associated with atrial fibrillation. Patients with this lesion tolerate atrial fibrillation poorly when the ventricular rate is rapid. The onset of atrial fibrillation in patients with mitral stenosis may precipitate acute pulmonary edema, as in this patient, or lesser degrees of pulmonary congestion, such as dyspnea on effort or orthopnea. The severity of the pulmonary congestion and its response to routine measures determine the immediate mode of therapy. Often pulmonary congestion is not severe and responds promptly to routine measures. After the acute pulmonary edema has cleared, the patient should be maintained on a dosage of digitalis adequate to control the ventricular response and other measures should be taken to help prevent recurrence of congestive failure.

These patients should all be carefully evaluated for mitral valve surgery. If surgery is indicated and is accepted by the patient, reversion of the heart rhythm should be postponed until after the operation. (If atrial fibrillation is reverted to normal sinus rhythm in such patients, experience has shown that

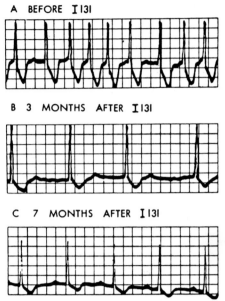

Fig. 16-43. Patient with uncontrolled atrial fibrillation. *A.* The ventricular rate could not be slowed with digitalis. *B.* Three months after the administration of radioactive iodine, the ventricular rate was slowed, but atrial fibrillation continued. *C.* Seven months after radioiodine administration, when the patient was hypometabolic, the rhythm spontaneously converted to regular sinus rhythm. This patient, with giant left atria due to mitral stenosis and insufficiency, had had chronic atrial fibrillation for 30 years. (*From Fig.* 6, *E. Corday, H. L. Jaffe, and D. W. Irving: Hypometabolic Treatment of Heart Disease, Am. J. Cardiol.,* **6:** 952, 1960.)

it will recur before, at the time of, or shortly after surgery despite quinidine prophylaxis). After recovery from surgery (1 to 2 weeks), the patient should be given 0.2 Gm quinidine sulfate every 6 hr. If reversion of the rhythm does not occur on this regimen, it is carried out with d-c defibrillation and the patient is placed on maintenance quinidine, 0.2 Gm every 6 hr. If reversion is not accomplished or if atrial fibrillation recurs after a short time, the patient should be brought back for at least two additional attempts. If sinus rhythm is only transient in these cases, the prophylactic quinidine may be increased to 0.4 Gm every 6 hr. In those patients in whom mitral surgery is not indicated after careful evaluation, or in patients who refuse surgery, early reversion, as described above, should be attempted.

In this patient, who is in the child-bearing age, pregnancy may be the *precipitating* cause of pulmonary congestion. It is mandatory to determine whether or not pregnancy is present, since electrical reversion and quinidine therapy may be contraindicated, although data on this point are not available.

No. 7. A 20-year-old female with aortic and mitral regurgitation secondary to rheumatic fever remained well compensated on digoxin and diuretics. She had only moderate cardiomegaly until the onset of atrial fibrillation. Following this, she gradually developed uncontrolled congestive failure and marked cardiomegaly. After her ventricular rate had been controlled with digoxin, the patient was started on 0.2 Gm quinidine sulfate every 6 hr. When reversion was not accomplished in 48 hr, the patient's heart beat was electrically reverted to normal sinus rhythm during thiopental sodium narcosis. Her cardiac compensation rapidly returned, and she was able to resume her normal activities. She was continued on digoxin and on prophylactic quinidine, 0.2 Gm every 6 hr. Four months later, she again reverted to atrial fibrillation and to her previous state of cardiac decompensation. Electrical reversion was again successful, and the patient was continued on the original maintenance dosage of quinidine sulfate.

Comment. This patient was controlled satisfactorily with drugs only as long as she remained in normal sinus rhythm. Corrective surgery in her situation would require the insertion of two artificial valves and would be associated with greater mortality than is justified in her particular case at the present time. Reversion of atrial fibrillation is indicated, since it is such a great liability to this patient. Electrical reversion with d-c defibrillation is relatively innocuous and may be performed on repeated occasions, whereas repeated reversions with quinidine would be dangerous.

No. 8. A 28-year-old manual laborer, who probably has had idiopathic myocardial disease for 3 years, was well compensated on no medication until he developed atrial fibrillation 1 month prior to admission to the hospital. He had moderate cardiomegaly, pulmonary edema, and atrial fibrillation with a ventricular rate of 160 to 170 beats per minute. Routine measures improved most of his symptoms; however, his ventricular rate could not be adequately controlled despite 4 mg digoxin in the first 36 hr and 0.75 mg daily. Maintenance quinidine sulfate (0.2 Gm every 6 hr) was begun, and reversion to normal sinus rhythm was accomplished with d-c defibrillation. The ventricular rate immediately decreased from 140 to 150 to 88 beats per minute. Cardiac compensation rapidly returned, and the patient was placed on maintenance digoxin and quinidine.

Comment. This patient illustrates the occasional inability of digitalis to control the ventricular rate in atrial fibrillation. At times, pulmonary emboli may contribute to the onset of this condition and to inability to control the ventricular rate. Regard-

less of the exact cause of the atrial fibrillation, it could not be controlled with safe doses of digitalis, whereas electrical reversion produced an improvement in the patient's cardiac status.

No. 9. A 52-year-old female, who had had stenosis and regurgitation of both the mitral and aortic valves, had severe congestive failure with massive edema, ascites, and pulmonary congestion. She was totally disabled and required frequent hospital admissions of 1 to 2 months' duration for more stringent cardiac care. Her heart was markedly enlarged and demonstrated atrial fibrillation with a ventrcular rate of 50 beats per minute. She was placed on 0.2 Gm quinidine sulfate every 6 hr for 2 days, and her heart beat was then reverted to normal sinus rhythm with synchronized electrical countershock (400 watt-sec). Diuresis began promptly, and the patient lost 32 lb during the next 12 days. There was remarkable improvement in all her symptoms. Atrial fibrillation returned in 13 days; a repeated attempt at electrical reversion was unsuccessful. Despite the recurrence of atrial fibrillation, however, the remarkable clinical improvement has persisted for 1 year.

Comment. This case illustrates the remarkable clinical improvement which may follow restoration of normal sinus rhythm. In addition, it illustrates a type of response which requires emphasis. Although the duration of sinus rhythm following electrical reversion was only 13 days, the resumption of atrial fibrillation was not associated with the recurrence of either subjective symptoms or objective signs of congestive failure of the severity present before her reversion. The exact mechanism of this phenomenon is unknown but is currently under investigation.

No. 10. Six months prior to admission to the hospital, a 14-year-old student developed rheumatic fever, with severe carditis, mitral regurgitation, uncontrolled congestive heart failure, massive cardiomegaly, and atrial fibrillation. In addition to the usual measures, including adequate digitalis and diuretics, a course of corticosteroids was administered without apparent benefit. The atrial fibrillation was not reverted by quinidine in moderate dosage, but electrical reversion was successful. The restoration of normal sinus rhythm produced a dramatic improvement in the signs and symptoms of congestive heart failure, which persisted until maintenance quinidine was discontinued 3½ months later. Subsequently, the patient's rhythm has been reverted on two occasions. For the past 4 months, he has remained in normal sinus rhythm with excellent cardiac compensation. He has continued to take digitalis and prophylactic quinidine.

Comment. This case is distinctive because the patient had two conditions which have sometimes been said to be contraindications to the reversion of atrial fibrillation: acute rheumatic carditis and severe mitral regurgitation. The success in this case illustrates that rigidity of thought regarding contraindications based on previous experience with quinidine in similar situations is not justified. One difficulty in assessing mitral regurgitation, a condition sometimes considered a contraindication to reversion, is determining the relative degree of organic valve dysfunction and of functional valve dysfunction.

No. 11. A 60-year-old night watchman who was admitted to the hospital because of an acute inferior myocardial infarction developed atrial fibrillation a few days after admission. The ventricular rate was easily controlled with digitalis, and no attempt was made at reversion of the heart rhythm during the hospital admission. Following discharge from the hospital, the patient developed incapacitating angina pectoris without evidence of heart failure. Eight weeks after his infarction, the patient was readmitted to the hospital and his heart rhythm was electrically reverted after 2 days of quinidine sulfate (0.2 Gm every 6 hr). He was discharged on maintenance quinidine, 0.2 Gm every 6 hr, completely free of angina pectoris. He has returned to work and has remained free from angina for the past year.

Comment. This case illustrates the development of atrial fibrillation associated with myocardial infarction. When this occurs, the first obligation is to control the ventricular rate with digitalis. If the circulation is not compromised and if the arrhythmia persists, the patient should be considered for electrical reversion of the rhythm several weeks later. On the other hand, if the atrial fibrillation is associated with circulatory failure, such as shock, pulmonary congestion, or angina decubitus, earlier electrical reversion should be considered; it may be needed as an emergency procedure. This patient also illustrates the dramatic improvement in angina that sometimes occurs with the resumption of normal rhythm.

No. 12. A 60-year-old female had syphilitic heart disease and congestive heart failure which was well controlled for several years until the onset of atrial fibrillation. At that time, the congestive heart failure became much worse and the patient was admitted to the hospital. She had marked cardiomegaly and atrial fibrillation with moderately rapid ventricular rate. The electrocardiogram showed the pattern of left bundle branch block with a QRS duration of 0.14 sec. She was treated with an increased amount of digitalis and with diuretics and sodium restriction. Some improvement was noted, but she remained in atrial fibrillation. Because of the widened QRS, she was not treated with quinidine. Several months later, when electrical defibrillation became available, she was readmitted to the hospital and started on quinidine sulfate, 0.2 Gm every 6 hr, in preparation for electrical reversion. The pa-

tient's heart rhythm reverted after 36 hr on this regimen, before electrical reversion could be performed. There was much improvement in the congestive heart failure, and she has been maintained on digitalis and quinidine.

Comment. This patient illustrates the therapeutic problem encountered in the reversion of rhythm in patients with prolonged intraventricular conduction. Although there is probably some increased risk in the administration of quinidine to such patients, one may be justified in using small doses of quinidine as long as there is no evidence of quinidine toxicity, particularly widening of the QRS duration by more than 25 per cent of the control value. If this patient's heart rhythm had not reverted to sinus rhythm on small doses of quinidine, it would have been reverted with electrical defibrillation, which is safer than large doses of quinidine.

No. 13. A 78-year-old male with calcific aortic stenosis had a history of slowly progressive congestive heart failure. Several months prior to admission the patient developed atrial fibrillation associated with increased congestive heart failure and the onset of claudication of the calves. He had moderate cardiomegaly and atrial fibrillation with a rapid ventricular response. There were no palpable pulses below weak femorals. He was treated for congestive heart failure, but the ventricular response could not be controlled with digitalis. The patient was placed on 0.2 Gm quinidine sulfate for 2 days and his heart beat was then electrically reverted. With establishment of normal sinus rhythm there was marked improvement in his congestive failure and the claudication disappeared. The patient has continued to be free of congestive heart failure and claudication, and since discharge from the hospital has been maintained on digitalis and quinidine.

Comment. In this patient there was marked clinical improvement in both congestive heart failure and peripheral vascular insufficiency following reversion of atrial fibrillation. It was impossible to control the ventricular rate adequately during atrial fibrillation. It is likely that many patients with peripheral vascular disease (cerebral, abdominal, renal, or in the extremities) will be significantly improved by the reversion of atrial fibrillation to normal sinus rhythm.

No. 14. This 55-year-old female with combined mitral stenosis and regurgitation had evidence of moderate congestive failure for several years which was well controlled by digitalis and diuretics. During the preceding 2 years, she had one definite cerebral embolus and probably had several other systemic emboli. She was placed on anticoagulant therapy, but it was not possible to maintain her safely in a therapeutic range of anticoagulation. Her heart was moderately enlarged, and there was atrial fibrillation with a ventricular rate of 54 beats per minute even though her digitalis dosage had been decreased for 1 month. She was placed on quinidine sulfate, 0.2 Gm every 6 hr for 2 days, and electrical reversion was attempted. After her second shock (200 watt-sec), she developed multifocal ectopic ventricular beats, which persisted for several minutes. She relapsed to atrial fibrillation, but no further shocks were administered.

Comment. In this patient, reversion of atrial fibrillation was attempted because of multiple emboli which were thought to originate from the left atrium. There are inadequate data from which to decide the value of anticoagulant therapy prior to the reversion of patients with a history of emboli. At the present time, we do not continue with attempts at electrical reversion of atrial fibrillation when the electrical shocks are followed by multiple ectopic beats.

No. 15. A 61-year-old male, who had had frequent anginal attacks following the onset of atrial fibrillation 1½ months previously, was admitted to the hospital for elective reversion of atrial fibrillation. He was given quinidine sulfate, 0.2 Gm every 6 hr for 2 days, and then underwent electrical reversion. Following the first shock, the patient developed asystole, requiring resuscitation and external massage. After 1½ minutes, normal sinus rhythm resumed and the patient was unaware of any difficulty. He has remained in sinus rhythm and has been free from angina pectoris during the past 8 months, while receiving only maintenance quinidine.

Comment. Whenever a major change occurs in cardiac rhythm, asystole or ventricular fibrillation may intervene. These are no more likely with synchronized d-c defibrillation than with drugs. This case illustrates the advantage of having an anesthesiologist present during electrical reversion. The technique of electrical reversion schedules the attendance of an anesthesiologist. If this catastrophic event occurred secondary to the administration of quinidine, it is unlikely that such prompt assistance would be available.

VENTRICULAR ECTOPIC BEATS* [16]

*Robert C. Schlant, M.D., and
J. Willis Hurst, M.D.*

When a cardiac impulse arises spontaneously from either ventricle and is not the result of an impulse received from the atria, it is referred to as a ventricular ectopic beat. When the beat occurs earlier than the next expected excitation of ventricles from the atria, it is referred to as a premature ventricular beat or contraction. When a premature ventricular beat occurs, the ventricle is usually refractory to the normal impulse coming down from the atria at about the same time. Consequently,

there is a pause until the next normal impulse causes the ventricles to beat. This pause is completely compensatory when the duration of the two beats, including the premature beat, is equal to two normal heart cycles. Less frequently, the pause is not fully compensatory. Occasionally, with a slow heart rate, a ventricular ectopic beat may occur between two normally occurring ventricular beats without delaying or interrupting the subsequent ventricular beat. Such an impulse is referred to as an interpolated ventricular ectopic beat. The configuration of the QRS complex associated with a ventricular ectopic contraction, as seen in the electrocardiogram, is reasonably distinctive. The QRS complex is quite different from normal QRS complexes and is broad in duration and slurred in shape. A premature atrial contraction with aberrant conduction may resemble a ventricular ectopic beat.

Ventricular ectopic beats either may have no clinical significance or may be of the greatest significance, depending on the circumstances in which they occur. In some apparently normal persons they may occur for many years without producing any symptoms and without any apparent relation to cardiac disease. They may be produced by any form of heart disease and are frequently caused by digitalis intoxication, particularly following diuresis. They may also be produced by epinephrine (Adrenalin), isoproterenol (Isuprel), caffeine, amphetamine compounds, and even sympathomimetic vasoconstrictor compounds found in nose drops, nasal sprays, or inhalers. Ventricular ectopic beats frequently occur in congestive heart failure and disappear when the failure is corrected with digitalis, even though digitalis may produce them at other times. In the presence of left bundle branch block, the occurrence of a ventricular ectopic beat without the conduction defect may assist in the diagnosis of acute myocardial infarction. Occasionally, there are significant changes in the T wave of the beat following a premature ventricular beat—the so-called "postextrasystolic T-wave changes"—which are statistically indicative of the presence of heart disease, either symptomatic or occult.[127,128]

Ventricular ectopic beats may produce symptoms either by causing a sensation of the heart's stopping during the compensatory pause or by causing discomfort, palpitation, or pain in the chest or neck when the subsequent, more forceful, ventricular beat occurs. When these symptoms occur in a normal person, reassurance regarding their significance should be given, and an attempt should be made to eliminate substances such as tobacco, coffee, tea, or other stimulants, which commonly precipitate such symptoms. If the symptoms continue to bother the patient excessively, he may be given a trial of phenobarbital, 15 to 30 mg three to

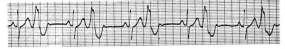

Fig. 16-44. Electrocardiogram of a patient demonstrating a bigeminal rhythm. A premature ventricular systole follows each regular sinus beat. The prolonged pause after each premature ventricular systole is called a compensatory pause. This is typical of premature ventricular systoles.

four times a day for a few months. If this regimen fails and the patient is still bothered excessively by symptoms, he may be given a trial of quinidine sulfate, 200 to 400 mg every 6 to 8 hr, or procaine amide hydrochloride (Pronestyl), 250 mg orally every 6 to 8 hr. After a trial of any of these drugs, the medication should be discontinued after 2 to 3 months to determine whether the ectopic beats persist or recur and to determine whether the patient can learn to live with the ectopic beats rather than having to take pills indefinitely.

When premature ventricular ectopic beats occur alternately with a normal sinus beat, the cardiac rhythm will be bigeminal, while if premature ventricular ectopic beats occur regularly after every pair of normal beats, the resulting rhythm will be trigeminal. When ventricular ectopic beats appear to arise from different areas of the ventricles, they are referred to as multifocal ventricular ectopic beats (Figs. 16-44 through 16-50).

Ventricular ectopic beats are particularly dangerous and likely to lead to the development of ventricular tachycardia in the following circumstances: when they occur during the vulnerable period of the preceding beat, usually at or just prior to the peak of the T wave; when several or more occur each minute; when they produce bigeminy or trigeminy; when several occur in a row; or when they are multifocal. When any of these situations occurs as a result of digitalis, and particularly following diuresis, digitalis should be discontinued and potassium administered either orally or intravenously, as described by Dorney in this book. On the other hand, premature ventricular beats occurring during congestive failure often disappear when the failure is corrected. When these situations occur following a myocardial infarction and do not disappear after treatment of shock or congestive failure, quinidine sulfate, 0.2 to 0.4 Gm

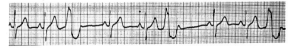

Fig. 16-45. Electrocardiogram of a patient demonstrating trigeminal rhythm. After two succeeding regular sinus beats there is a premature ventricular systole.

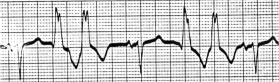

Fig. 16-46. Another instance of trigeminy, but this time it is due to two succeeding ventricular premature systoles followed by a regular sinus beat.

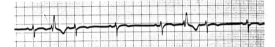

Fig. 16-47. Interpolated premature ventricular systoles. The premature ventricular systole falls immediately between two normal sinus beats. The premature systole does not interfere with the normal sinus cadence. There is no compensatory pause following the premature ventricular systole. This is truly an extra beat.

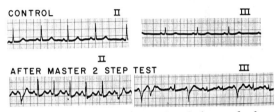

Fig. 16-48. Electrocardiogram taken before and after Master two-step test which demonstrates the occurrence of frequent premature ventricular systoles immediately after exercise. In addition to premature ventricular systoles, S-T segment depressions occur, which also signify ischemia of the myocardium.

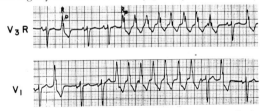

Fig. 16-49. Electrocardiogram of a patient with frequent premature ventricular systoles and paroxysms of ventricular tachycardia. The shapes of the QRS complexes of the premature ventricular systoles and during ventricular tachycardia are identical, suggesting that both arrhythmias arise from the same ectopic focus. A retrograde P wave occurs in the downslope of the QRS after each ectopic ventricular complex.

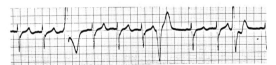

Fig. 16-50. Premature ventricular systoles arising from several different foci, each characterized by a different shape.

every 4 to 6 hr, should be administered to depress the excitability of the ectopic ventricular focus. If quinidine relieves the ectopic beats and the patient progresses well, it is best to continue quinidine in the minimum dose necessary to depress the ectopic beats for about 1 week, at which time one should gradually discontinue quinidine if this is possible without the recurrence of the ectopic beats. Since ventricular ectopic beats may serve as the forerunner of ventricular tachycardia or ventricular fibrillation, and since it was formerly thought that most patients dying of myocardial infarction die of these arrhythmias, some physicians formerly recommended the routine administration of quinidine following myocardial infarction. This practice is not recommended, since quinidine is a general myocardial depressant; it is particularly contraindicated following a posterior or inferior infarction, when AV block is particularly likely to occur. In addition, the studies of Hellerstein and Turell indicate that ventricular standstill, rather than ventricular fibrilaltion, is the most common terminal rhythm in patients dying of myocardial infarction.[129] Accordingly, quinidine is not administered routinely following a myocardial infarction, but only if specific indications are present. Recent studies of this subject are discussed in Chap. 35.

VENTRICULAR TACHYCARDIA

Eliot Corday, M.D., and
Tzu-Wang Lang, M.D.

General Features. Paroxysmal ventricular tachycardia, although relatively uncommon, is a serious arrhythmia. Its hemodynamic effects may be benign, but at the other extreme it frequently causes serious hemodynamic disturbances.[2,4,5,12,48,130] It is considered a very dangerous arrhythmia because it

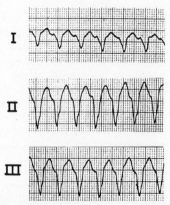

Fig. 16-51. Electrocardiogram of patient with ventricular tachycardia. The QRS complexes are widened and distorted in shape, and there is a slight variation in the interval between the ventricular complexes.

may subsequently convert to ventricular fibrillation, which is usually fatal.

Etiology. Herrmann has demonstrated that 71 per cent of paroxysms of ventricular tachycardia occur in patients with ischemic heart disease; 12 per cent, in those with rheumatic valvular disease; 3 per cent, in those with thyrotoxicosis; and 3 per cent, in those with congenital heart disease.[131] It occurs in patients with diffuse myocardial disease. Ventricular tachycardia is relatively common in digitalis toxicity[131-133] and electrolyte disturbances[134-136] and also occurs in diphtheria and streptococcal infections. It rarely occurs in patients with normal hearts,[137] although Strauss,[138] Lundy and McLellan,[139] Armbrust and Levine,[140] and Herrmann[131] have reported this in 10 to 13 per cent of their series. Then it was usually associated with excessive use of tobacco, severe emotional disturbances,[141,142] or electrolyte derangements resulting from severe diarrhea. It is also known to occur from cerebral electric shock therapy. It has recently been demonstrated that many episodes of Stokes-Adams syndrome in patients with heart block are actually due to ventricular tachycardia, which is an escape rhythm. Anesthesia with chloroform or cyclopropane may induce ventricular tachycardia, particularly if epinephrine has been administered.[143-145]

Mechanism. When an ectopic pacemaker in the ventricle produces stimuli faster than that of the sinus pacemaker, the ectopic focus is apt to take over the pacemaking function. This may also occur as an escape rhythm when the sinus pacemaker is depressed by either drugs or excessive vagotonia. An occasional ectopic stimulus will result in premature ventricular systoles; however, if six or more premature systoles occur in succession it is considered to constitute a paroxysm of ventricular tachycardia. Occasionally two or more pacemakers in the ventricle take on the pacemaking function and this results in a multidirectional ventricular tachycardia.[133,146] The reentry phenomenon has also been described as a mechanism for paroxysmal ventricular tachycardia.[147,148] Ventricular tachycardia is usually slightly irregular (Fig. 16-51). It may be extremely rapid or only slightly faster than that of the regular sinus rhythm. The cardiac impulse at times is conducted through the AV node to the atria in a retrograde fashion, and under such circumstances atrial excitation will follow ventricular depolarization and contraction. In this situation the AV valves are closed at the time the atria contract. This causes the atria to regurgitate their contents into the venous circulation, and therefore large cannon waves can be seen in the neck veins (Chap. 5).

Hemodynamics. The rhythm might be benign, in that it causes no hemodynamic effect, but in other instances it may be malignant and have severe hemodynamic consequences.[2,4,5,12,48,130] For instance, the patients may have a rate of 160 beats per minute and the cardiac output and systemic pressure will be normal, but in other instances a rate of 100 beats per minute will produce a catastrophic drop in systemic pressure, cardiac output, and coronary flow. It has been theorized that the reason for the marked variation in hemodynamics might lie in the different location of the ectopic focus. If the focus is near the base of the heart, the blood will first be propelled toward the apex and then be shuttled back into the outflow track. It has been theorized that the outflow track may be constricted by the time the blood is shuttled back into it and that this will throttle the cardiac output. The benign type originates near the apex and the hemodynamics are little disturbed except for the rapid rate when the heart will not have time to fill. This could explain the difference between the benign and malignant types of ventricular tachycardia. Vasoconstriction of the mesenteric, renal, and musculoskeletal circulations occurs as soon as the cardiac output is diminished or systemic pressure drops.[4,12,13,15] This may result in ischemia of the organs supplied by these circulations and may result in peptic ulceration, hemorrhagic duodenitis, hemorrhagic necrosis of the bowel, distension, or paralytic ileus.[23,28,33] It may result in azotemia and diminished urinary output, and tubular necrosis has been described.[11,149] The cerebral circulation and the coronary circulation may be markedly reduced if hypotension supervenes during a paroxysm (Fig. 16-5). This may result in myocardial and cerebrovascular ischemia, with the focal damage in the myocardium or brain.[2,3,5,28] When a paroxysm of tachycardia causes ischemia of the liver, the serum–glutamic oxaloacetic transaminase (SGOT) and serum–glutamic pyruvic transaminase (SGPT) levels may become abnormally elevated.[1,150]

Symptoms and Signs. The benign type may produce very few signs and symptoms except if the rate is very rapid, but in the malignant type vascular collapse results and produces the symptoms and signs of shock, including pallor, cold and clammy skin, and dyspnea. Syncopal attacks are common.[151] The rate is usually 150 to 160 beats per minute, there being a slight irregularity which might confuse the diagnosis with that of atrial fibrillation or frequent premature ventricular systoles. The patient may complain of substernal pain, dyspnea, dizziness, and confusion. Focal neurologic signs may develop if cerebral arterial narrowing is present. The patient may not be aware that he is having a rapid arrhythmia and may seek medical advice because of neurologic symptoms. The diagnosis of ventricular tachycardia should always be considered in a patient who complains of sudden dizziness, weakness, dyspnea, or precordial distress and who has a history of previous arrhythmias.

There might be a slight variation in the intensity of the first sound, although the rhythm may seem regular. The jugular pulse might reveal distinct *a* waves which are regular or slightly irregular, depending on whether or not there is retrograde atrial conduction. The ventricular rate associated with ventricular tachycardia does not change with carotid sinus massage. This distinguishes it from atrial tachycardia or atrial flutter. The rhythm usually lasts for a few minutes to several hours but has lasted as long as 32 days.[152]

The Electrocardiogram. The electrocardiogram of ventricular tachycardia is characterized by a widened, slurred, QRS complex, and the rhythm may be slightly irregular (Fig. 16-51). It is usually 150 to 200 beats or more per minute, but it may occur at rates around 100 beats. The QRS complexes of ventricular tachycardia resemble those of premature ventricular systoles which often precede the paroxysm (Fig. 16-52).[153] When the QRS complexes of a paroxysm of ventricular tachycardia have the same configuration as premature systoles, it suggests that they both arise from the same ectopic focus and emphasizes the unitarian nature of these ventricular rhythms. When the QRS complexes are multidirectional and alternate with each other periodically, the prognosis is very ominous because this pattern often precedes ventricular fibrillation (Fig. 16-53).[133,146] Because of retrograde atrial excitation, the P waves might be visible immediately following the QRS complexes. If AV dissociation is present, P waves occur at a slower rate than the QRS complexes. If ventricular tachycardia supervenes on chronic atrial fibrillation, the irregular atrial deflections will distort the baseline QRS complexes.[154]

It is very difficult to differentiate ventricular tachycardia from supraventricular tachycardia with aberrant ventricular conduction except with the aid of an esophageal electrocardiogram (Fig. 16-54).[131,155,156] The differential characteristic of ventricular tachycardia is that there is a slight variation in the pulse rate of ventricular tachycardia. In addition, in patients with supraventricular tachycardia with aberrant ventricular conduction, carotid sinus massage may convert the arrhythmia, whereas ventricular tachycardia is rarely converted by this maneuver.

Treatment. Ventricular tachycardia must be considered a grave emergency because it is apt to convert to fatal ventricular fibrillation at any time.

Sedation. Relief of anxiety in any rhythm disturbance is most important because anxiety perpetuates the arrhythmia. Therefore, the patient

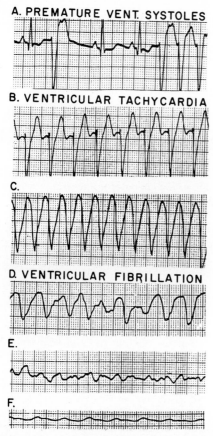

Fig. 16-52. Electrocardiogram of patient with frequent premature ventricular systoles (*A*), then paroxysmal ventricular tachycardia (*B*), followed by terminal ventricular fibrillation (*C*), (*D*), (*E*), (*F*). Note that during ventricular fibrillation, the QRS complexes are initially of large amplitude but gradually become more distorted and of lower voltage. Some authorities would call strip (*C*) ventricular flutter, which they consider an intermediate rhythm between ventricular tachycardia and ventricular fibrillation.

should first receive a barbiturate by mouth or by injection. Morphine, which also has an antiarrhythmic action, is most effective in relieving anxiety.

Electric Countershock. Synchronized capacitor

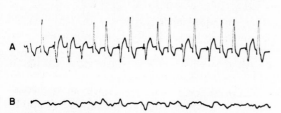

Fig. 16-53. A. Multidirectional ventricular tachycardia demonstrates ventricular complexes of various configurations arising from many foci. Ventricular fibrillation occurs in strip *B*.

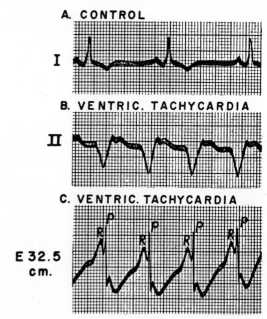

Fig. 16-54. Esophageal lead (*C*) recorded during an episode of ventricular tachycardia. The P waves which follow the normal QRS deflections can be identified only by the esophageal leads. (*From Fig. 118, E. Corday and D. W. Irving: "Disturbances of Heart Rate, Rhythm and Conduction," W. B. Saunders Company, Philadelphia, 1961.*)

discharge when available is the treatment of choice for this serious arrhythmia (Fig. 16-55).[121,122,157-159] Usually the rhythm instantly converts to sinus rhythm after an initial shock of 100 to 300 watt-sec. However, it is important to administer antiarrhythmic medications such as quinidine or procaine amide before the depolarization in order to prevent the recurrence of ventricular tachycardia.[84]

Quinidine. Quinidine restores normal rhythm when administered orally, intramuscularly, or intra-

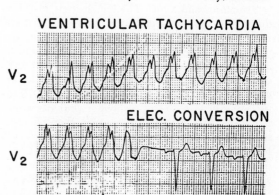

Fig. 16-55. Paroxysm of ventricular tachycardia converted to normal sinus rhythm by d-c electrical capacitor discharge.

venously.[115,262-264] If the patient cannot take the oral form and treatment with quinidine is imperative, it may be administered intramuscularly or intravenously. The oral administration of quinidine sulfate is safest, and the average dose ranges between 0.2 and 0.4 Gm every 2 hr for a total of five doses. Quinidine depresses ventricular conduction, and if this effect becomes too profound, ventricular fibrillation may supervene.[160,161] It is important to monitor such effects with an electrocardiogram before each subsequent dose. Widening of the QRS more than 25 per cent is an indication that further quinidine should not be administered. Once the arrhythmia is converted, a maintenance dose of 0.2 to 0.4 Gm four times a day should be prescribed. For the intramuscular route quinidine gluconate 0.4 to 0.8 Gm may be used. Intravenous quinidine must be given over a long period of time as 0.5 to 1 Gm diluted in 50 to 100 ml saline solution injected slowly at a maximal rate of 2 ml per minute.[162] The electrocardiograph should be monitored when this is given intravenously.

Procaineamide. This is also an effective agent for the treatment of ventricular tachycardia.[163,164] It is a safer drug for parenteral administration than quinidine. The oral dose is 0.5 to 1 Gm every 2 to 3 hr. If the oral treatment cannot be used, it may be given intramuscularly or intravenously. The intramuscular dose is 0.5 to 1 Gm repeated every 1 to 2 hr until the arrhythmia is corrected. In resistant cases as much as 4 Gm has been administered intravenously, diluted in 200 ml of 5 per cent dextrose in water given over a period of 36 min.[270] During such an infusion, widening of the QRS interval may precede ventricular fibrillation; therefore, electrocardiographic monitoring should be used whenever procaine amide hydrochloride is given by parenteral route or in large dosage.

Vasopressor Drugs. The restoration of systemic pressure often converts ventricular tachycardia.[165,166] The most effective vasopressor drugs are norepinephrine (Levophed) and metaraminol (Aramine). The blood pressure must be carefully controlled when these drugs are dripped intravenously because extremely high pressure levels might induce ventricular fibrillation. From 40 to 60 per cent of paroxysms of ventricular tachycardia convert spontaneously when the systemic pressure is restored.

Rhythmol. This is a new antiarrhythmic drug which has been effective in converting ventricular tachycardia but has not been approved for general use.[167,168] It may be administered intramuscularly in a single dose of 200 mg.

Diphenylhydantoin (Dilantin).[169,170] This drug appears to be effective in converting ventricular tachycardia in the experimental animal, particularly when this condition is due to digitalis toxicity and aconitine. In the human being 100 mg intramuscularly converted the rhythm in 15 to 20 mins in our cases.

Atropine. Atropine has been used to terminate attacks. A dosage of 1 to 2 mg, intravenously or intramuscularly, has been used.[171,172]

Magnesium. Magnesium sulfate has been used to terminate arrhythmias. From 15 to 20 ml of a 20 per cent solution may be administered intravenously.[146,173-175]

Treatment of Recurrent Ventricular Tachycardia. As in all other arrhythmias, tobacco, alcohol, and coffee should be stopped for a trial period to determine if they are causative factors. The most effective drugs to prevent recurrent paroxysms are procaine amide, 250 mg, four times a day, or quinidine sulfate, 0.2 Gm four times a day. Diphenylhydantoin, 100 mg four times daily has recently been used to prevent recurrences.[169,170] Where all other measures have failed, the induction of hypometabolism has proved to be effective.[176,177]

Prognosis. Because ventricular fibrillation may supervene following the onset of ventricular tachycardia, the latter is considered to be a serious arrhythmia. Vascular collapse may occur in ventricular tachycardia and result in renal failure, azotemia, and proteinuria. The drop in blood pressure may cause cerebral ischemia and result in hemiparesis, visual disturbances, and aphasia. Ischemia of the gastrointestinal tract because of intense mesenteric angiospasm may result in peptic ulceration and hemorrhagic necrosis of the bowel. Because the blood supply of the myocardium may drop appreciably during a paroxysm, cardiac decompensation and necrosis of the myocardium may result. The prognosis, therefore, is very serious if shock or cardiac decompensation supervenes. The longer the duration of the paroxysm, the more serious the prognosis because of the secondary ischemia to other organs. Patients who have severe heart disease may die of ventricular tachycardia within a few hours.

VENTRICULAR FIBRILLATION

Eliot Corday, M.D., and
Tzu-Wang Lang, M.D.

Ventricular fibrillation is the most serious of all arrhythmias; unless the patient is treated with a defibrillator, death usually ensues. The rhythm is characterized by an irregular, uncoordinated twitching movement of the ventricles. The circulation completely fails, and death of the vital organs follows.[181-186]

Etiology. It usually occurs when the heart has

been severely damaged, or as a result of certain toxic drugs, but it may occur in patients with completely normal hearts.[187-189] The most common cause is ischemia of the myocardium due to coronary insufficiency or acute coronary occlusion. It often is the cause of death on the operating table, when it may be caused by ischemia of the heart due to asphyxia or irritability of the heart due to such drugs as chloroform or cyclopropane, particularly when used in conjunction with epinephrine.[1,190] High voltages of electricity, particularly if the patient is standing in water so that he may be grounded, may result in fatal ventricular fibrillation. Drugs, such as digitalis,[191] quinidine,[160] and procaine amide, when used in toxic doses, may result in ventricular fibrillation. Ventricular fibrillation may supervene in extreme sinus bradycardia or follow an extremely slow ventricular rate associated with heart block. Hypoxemia such as occurs in pulmonary edema, obstructed airway in anesthesia, or strangulation may result in ventricular fibrillation. A severe blow to the chest, bullet wounds to the heart, and cardiac catheterization[192-194] may also result in ventricular fibrillation. In debilitating conditions such as cancer, toxic infections, renal or hepatic failure, ventricular fibrillation may be the terminal event. Unexplained "mechanisms death," for which no anatomic cause can be found at autopsy, may be due to ventricular fibrillation.[195]

Mechanism. Although ventricular fibrillation was first described by Hoffa and Ludwig in 1850,[196] only recent rapid cinematographic studies have demonstrated that there is an irregular contraction of the heart, which gradually becomes more incoordinated and ineffectual. Finally, the myocardial contractions seem to be so ineffective that the heart is merely a quivering mass of muscle.[197,198] After a period of 5 min there is no movement except for feeble contraction waves which pass across the heart in various directions. The cardiac output falls completely, as does the coronary and cerebral blood flow.

Ventricular fibrillation is often preceded by ventricular tachycardia which emanates from a single ectopic focus or from several ectopic foci. When the rate of excitation exceeds that to which the ventricle may rhythmically respond, the chaotic arrhythmia of ventricular fibrillation results.

Signs and Symptoms. Usually the onset is rapid. The patient will suddenly lose consciousness and appear pale, and he may have a few gasping respirations. The condition is characterized by absent pulse, blood pressure, and cardiac sounds. It must always be suspected during general surgery when there is a sudden desaturation of arterial blood, with disappearance of pulse or blood pressure.[190] If the chest is then opened, one may observe the characteristic twitching of the myocardium, which is similar to the appearance of a wriggling bag of worms.

Electrocardiogram. Immediately prior to the onset of fibrillation there may be many premature ventricular systoles, of multifocal origin, or ventricular tachycardia of unifocal or multifocal origin.[199] Suddenly irregular deflections of large magnitude will be noted. Actually, just preceding the onset of fibrillation, the QRS interval may become widened and irregular in amplitude at a rate of 175 to 250 beats per minute. Then it is impossible to differentiate between the waves of depolarization and repolarization because the QRS complexes and waves fuse (Fig. 16-56). The waves become more irregular and coarse, and they vary in amplitude and configuration. Gradually, the voltages become less and the base line merely undulates irregularly (Fig. 16-52).

Treatment. A defibrillating shock usually results in immediate return to normal sinus rhythm. The object of the sudden depolarization of the heart is to produce one strong simultaneous depolarization of all the fibrillating muscle fibers, which is followed by a period of complete relaxation of the myocardium. It is hoped that then a preexisting pacemaker in the atrium or ventricle may recapture the rhythmic functioning. Closed-chest cardiac massage is effective in maintaining the circulation during ventricular fibrillation until a defibrillator may be used (see Chap. 69). Therefore should ventricular fibrillation occur, immediate closed-chest cardiac massage with mouth-to-mouth respiration should be performed to maintain the circulation and oxygenation. However, this must be followed by electrical defibrillation. Resuscitative measures must be instituted almost immediately, since it has been determined that permanent damage to the brain may result if cardiac arrest persists for longer than a 4-min interval.[200,201] During open resuscitation adequate ventilation must be provided with positive-pressure breathing or a pressure rebreathing bag and an airway, or resuscitative measures will fail. The application of 440 volts of alter-

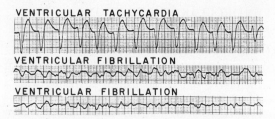

Fig. 16-56. Ventricular tachycardia converting to ventricular fibrillation. During ventricular fibrillation the electrical complexes are irregular and coarse, and they vary in amplitude and configuration.

nating current across the heart for 0.25 sec may be used for external defibrillation.[202,203] More recently direct current (100 to 400 watt-sec) has been used externally to defibrillate the ventricles and is preferred to alternating current.[159] If the heart cannot be defibrillated promptly, closed-chest cardiac resuscitation must be reinstituted in order to provide oxygen to the myocardium and brain. This must be done before an electrical defibrillation is attempted again.

The cardiac surgeon may purposely induce ventricular fibrillation to stop contractions of the heart in order to accomplish cardiac surgery. The heart-lung pump is used to perfuse the peripheral organs and myocardium until the surgery is completed, following which the heart is defibrillated.

Various drugs, such as quinidine, procaine amide, and Dilantin, may be used to prevent a recurrence of ventricular fibrillation. Ventricular fibrillation due to digitalis intoxication should be treated with electrical defibrillation and potassium chloride. Drugs such as quinidine gluconate, 600 mg intramuscularly, or procaine amide (Pronestyl), 500 mg intravenously, may be given. We have found diphenylhydantoin (Dilantin), 6 to 15 mg per kg body weight, administered intravenously, to be effective in preventing recurrences of fatal digitalis-induced ventricular fibrillation.[169,170] This usually is sufficient to prevent the heart from returning into ventricular fibrillation following the electrical depolarization. Anesthetic agents should be withdrawn, and the patient should be well oxygenated with a positive-pressure apparatus and a good airway. Lidocaine hydrochloride (Xylocaine) is very effective in preventing return of ventricular fibrillation in dogs.[204,205]

Prognosis. When ventricular fibrillation occurs away from the hospital and if resuscitative procedures are not instituted, death almost always occurs. If ventricular fibrillation occurs in the hospital where resuscitative equipment is available and it is recognized immediately after the onset, patients can usually be defibrillated and many of them survive. If a period of longer than 4 min has elapsed before resuscitative procedures are attempted, the brain becomes irreparably damaged. The prognosis of patients with ventricular fibrillation is very grave. The best prognosis is found in the patient who develops ventricular fibrillation during cardiac surgery, when it can be recognized as soon as it occurs and resuscitative measures can be performed immediately. Day has demonstrated that if coronary patients are monitored constantly by electronic techniques for the first 12 days following a coronary occlusion, many of them may be resuscitated immediately and will survive ventricular fibrillation.[206]

VENTRICULAR STANDSTILL

See Chap. 69.

DISORDERS OF CARDIAC CONDUCTION

ATRIOVENTRICULAR
CONDUCTION * 16

Robert C. Schlant, M.D., and
J. Willis Hurst, M.D.

The phenomenon of conduction of the excitatory impulse from the atria through the atrioventricular (AV) node and bundle to the ventricles is one of the more intriguing in all medicine or biology. It has been, and still is, the subject of innumerable investigations.[29,207-217] Of particular interest to physicians is a consideration of the actual mechanism of this conduction—a conduction associated with what is seemingly an abnormally long delay in impulse transmissions. Is it actually helpful that this strange little bundle of tissue delays the excitation of the ventricles? How many impulses per minute can the AV node transmit, and how many does it prefer to transmit? How does abnormality of the AV node or of its blood supply alter this conduction? What is the clinical significance of altered AV conduction, and how can it be managed? These are some of the questions which will be considered and partially answered in the following discussion, much of which is based on the excellent investigations by James[211,212] of the anatomy of the heart and its blood vessels and conducting system (see Chaps. 28 and 29).

ANATOMIC AND PHYSIOLOGIC
CONSIDERATIONS* 16

Robert C. Schlant, M.D., and
J. Willis Hurst, M.D.

In the average adult, the AV node is about 1 by 3 by 6 mm in size and is located somewhat posteriorly more or less in the center of the heart in the lower portion of the interatrial septum near its junction with the membranous portion of the interventricular septum and the attachments of the mitral and tricuspid valves. It is somewhat oblong and flattened, with a slight concavity toward the base of the mitral valve and a slight convexity toward the attachment of the tricuspid valve.

As discussed and illustrated in Chap. 29, the AV node receives two groups of fibers on its posterior and superior aspects from the interatrial septum. One group passes down the center of the interatrial septum and divides just above the AV node; most of the fibers pass directly into the node, and a smaller tract bypasses the AV node and courses toward the right atrial endocardium. The second group of fibers apparently comes primarily from the eustachian ridge. This group also divides into two tracts: one enters the posterosuperior portion of the AV node, and the other bypasses the node and extends down the right atrial endocardium to the base of the tricuspid valve. The bypass tracts from the septum and from the eustachian ridge join and then divide into fibers terminating in most cases either at the inferior margin of the AV node or at the base of the tricuspid valve. Since some of these right atrial endocardial bypass tracts lack Purkinje fibers, and since it is not certain that rapid conduction occurs in other types of myocardial fibers, one cannot assume that these tracts regularly carry excitation impulses around the main body of the AV node—either to the lower margin of the node or to the bundle of His.

The AV node itself is composed of profusely ramifying and interlacing atriated fibers and has relatively little collagen matrix. The profuse arborization and apparent labyrinth of short circuitous pathways within most of the substance of the node suggest that during its passage through the AV node the impulse is divided and rejoined many times, with multiple electrical cancellations taking place, thus producing the normal AV node transmission delay.[211] Some investigators,[217] however, believe that most of the delay occurs at the atrionodal junction, rather than within the node itself.

The blood supply to the AV node and to the initial portion of the bundle of His is by means of the ramus septi fibroso, which usually is located in the center of the AV node, though its presence and location are less certain than those of the sinus node artery. According to the studies of James,[29,211] the blood vessel supplying the AV node and the nearby area originates from the right coronary artery in 90 per cent of human beings. In the remaining 10 per cent, and more commonly in men, he found this area to be supplied by a branch of the left circumflex artery. These facts probably explain why posterior wall myocardial infarctions, which are usually produced by occlusion of the right coronary artery, are particularly apt to be associated with disturbances of the AV node conduction and with sudden death. In addition, the presence[218] of an area of vagal neuroreceptors in the region of the ostium of the coronary sinus, only a few millimeters from the AV node and probably having the same blood supply, may explain why ischemia of this area is so commonly associated with evidence of intense vagal discharge, manifested by bradycardia, nausea, vomiting, sweating, sialorrhea, tracheal burning or spasm, and even syncope. Clin-

ically, it is necessary to consider the state of increased vagotonia commonly present in posterior myocardial infarction whenever drugs must be used which may have either a vagomimetic or a direct depressant effect on AV conduction. In fact, it may be often desirable to use a vagolytic agent such as atropine when increased vagotonia might be present or might develop.

It has become apparent that disease of the AV node may either accelerate[207] or slow AV conduction. The anatomic considerations just described make it possible to explain both these phenomena. The presence of fibers bypassing the AV node makes it possible for the circumferential pathway to be a potential mechanism of the "accelerated" AV conduction occasionally produced by ischemia or disease of the AV node. An alternate explanation for accelerated conduction is that ischemia of the AV node may, under certain conditions, eliminate some of the normal intranodal pathways and associated cancellation effects, thereby actually decreasing the delay in the node itself.[211] The accelerated conduction encountered in the Wolff-Parkinson-White syndrome, in congenital heart disease, particularly Ebstein's syndrome, and in coronary artery disease may be explained by the above two mechanisms, although one cannot completely exclude the occurrence of accelerated conduction through a bundle of Kent, even though to date no Purkinje fibers have been demonstrated in such bundles.

Accelerated conduction per se requires no treatment, except when it is associated with paroxysms of atrial tachycardia, as in the Wolff-Parkinson-White syndrome (p. 340).

More commonly encountered clinically is an abnormal prolongation of the AV conduction time. This is usually produced by severe interference with the normal conduction mechanisms and pathways by such agents as ischemia, infarction, trauma, drugs, or foreign masses in the node.

Physiologically, the normal prolongation of the AV conduction time allows the atria adequate time to contract and thus to contribute more to ventricular filling. The contribution by atrial systole probably accounts for about 20 per cent of ventricular filling at rest, but when tachycardia or some condition associated with increased sympathetic stimulation of the atria is present, systole is probably even more important. If there were no delay at the AV node, ventricular contraction would occur so soon after atrial conduction that much of the additional ventricular filling produced by atrial conduction would be lost because the AV valves would close before the end of atrial ejection.

The AV node will not transmit an unlimited number of impulses per minute. In addition, the rate at which the ventricles can contract is limited by the effective refractory period of the ventricular musculature. These two mechanisms probably explain why even in untreated atrial fibrillation, the ventricular rate is usually less than 160 beats per minute, even though hundreds of impulses presumably reach the AV node each minute. Indeed, if the ventricles were to respond to all the atrial impulses presumably reaching the AV node, atrial fibrillation would be uniformly fatal, since there appears to be a ventricular rate above which the ventricles literally do not have time to fill adequately during diastole, whether or not the atria are contracting normally. This rate, above which cardiac output will decrease, is probably about 170 to 180 beats per minute for a normal human heart with normal sinus rhythm, but is considerably lower when disease is present. This is particularly true in the presence of significant mitral stenosis, in which the shortening of diastole by tachycardia usually produces both a decrease in the flow across the stenotic mitral valve and a marked elevation of left atrial pressure, which may in turn produce acute pulmonary edema.

FIRST-DEGREE HEART BLOCK * 16

Robert C. Schlant, M.D., and
J. Willis Hurst, M.D.

The definition of first-degree heart block, like the definition of overweight, is rather arbitrary, since the condition varies widely both in itself and under the influence of age, heart rate, disease, or pharmacologic agents. The usually stated upper limit of P-R interval is 0.20 sec in adults. For infants and children, tables of normal limits should be consulted to determine the upper limit of the "normal" P-R interval. When the P-R interval is longer than normal, first-degree heart block is said to be present (Fig. 16-57A and B).

The P-R interval represents the electrocardiographic interval between the beginning of detectable excitation of the atrial myocardium and the beginning of detectable electrical excitation of the ventricular myocardium. It is measured to the beginning of detectable ventricular excitation, whether the latter begins with an R wave or a Q wave.

It should be noted that occasional persons will have P-R intervals longer than 0.20 sec in the absence of apparent disease or disability. Although many diseases, such as acute rheumatic fever, diphtheria, coronary artery disease, congenital heart disease (particularly atrial septal defect), or viral diseases such as mumps, may prolong the AV conduction time, these diseases cannot be reliably diagnosed solely on the findings of first-degree heart

block. Among the commonly used drugs, digitalis, quinidine, procainamide hydrochloride, and potassium may produce prolongation of the AV conduction. Increased levels of adrenal corticosteroids tend to shorten the P-R interval while low levels of these hormones may be associated with longer P-R intervals than normal.[219] In reality, prolongation of the P-R interval in most patients serves merely as a small diagnostic clue which must be evaluated in the light of the entire clinical picture.

In many instances, it is possible to deduce the presence of a prolonged P-R interval from physical examination. Usually, the intensity of the first heart sound will be diminished when there is first-degree heart block; however, when the P-R interval is markedly prolonged, above about 0.28 sec, the intensity may, paradoxically, become more accentuated.

First-degree heart block is not responsible for symptoms and produces no significant alteration of cardiac function. Accordingly, treatment is usually not indicated. Slight prolongation of the P-R in-

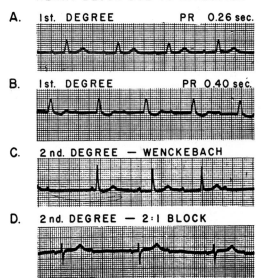

HEART BLOCK DUE TO INFECTION

Fig. 16-57. Electrocardiogram of patient with various degrees of heart block, following an acute infection. A. The P-R interval is 0.26 sec; B. it is increased to 0.40 sec. As the AV conduction becomes more seriously involved, second-degree heart block results, in C and D. In C the P-R interval lengthens progressively untily it is maximally prolonged, AV conduction fails, and a dropped beat results. In D every second atrial complex is blocked at the AV node and 2:1 heart block results. (*From Fig. 130B, E. Corday and D. W. Irving: "Disturbances of Heart Rate, Rhythm and Conduction," W. B. Saunders Company, Philadelphia, 1961.*)

terval, when due to digitalis, is not a contraindication for continuing digitalis; however, progressive and marked prolongation of the P-R interval may serve as a warning that higher degrees of AV block might develop.

SECOND-DEGREE
HEART BLOCK * 16

Robert C. Schlant, M.D., and
J. Willis Hurst, M.D.

Types of Second-degree Heart Block. Second-degree heart block may be arbitrarily divided into two types. In the first type, the Wenckebach phenomenon, there is a progressive lengthening of the P-R interval for several beats until one P wave representing atrial excitation occurs which is not followed by ventricular excitation (Figs. 16-57C and 16-58). The subsequent atrial impulse is then conducted with a shorter P-R interval, and the entire sequence is repeated. In most instances, the P-R interval is at least moderately prolonged for all beats of the sequence. Common causes of the Wenckebach type of second-degree heart block are rheumatic fever, coronary artery disease, digitalis, diphtheria, and viral infections. At the bedside, it may be recognized by the occurrence of a dropped beat without the occurrence of a preceding premature beat and by the intensity of the first heart sound, which either may be constantly faint or may decrease in intensity over several heartbeats. Such a progressive change in intensity of the first heart sound is thought to be related to the progressive lengthening of the P-R interval.

In the second type of second-degree heart block, there is a failure of AV conduction so that only every second, third, or fourth impulse from the atria is conducted to the ventricles. For example, if there is 2:1 block, and the atrial rate is 80 beats per minute, the ventricular rate will be 40 beats per minute (Fig. 16-57D). In this type of second-

degree heart block, the ventricular rhythm may be either regular or irregular depending on whether the block is constant or variable. Occasionally, if the block is variable, it may cause palpitation, though more commonly it is not associated with any symptoms. This type of second-degree heart block is caused by the same conditions which produce the Wenckebach phenomenon. At the bedside this type of heart block may be detected by simultaneous inspection of the neck and auscultation of the heart. This may reveal several venous A waves, representing atrial contraction, occurring for each ventricular contraction. Occasionally, it may be possible to hear atrial heart sounds, thought to be caused by the movements of the AV valves produced by the atrial contractions.

Treatment. Both these forms of second-degree heart block probably interfere mildly with cardiac function. When second-degree heart block seems related to drugs such as digitalis or quinidine, these drugs should be withheld until the block disappears (Chap. 15). Although administration of potassium is usually indicated for paroxysmal tachycardia with 2:1 and 3:1 block due to digitalis and/or potassium loss, potassium is usually not indicated for AV block due to digitalis when atrial tachycardia is not present. In fact, potassium may be contraindicated. When second-degree heart block occurs following myocardial infarction, the right coronary artery, which supplies the inferior or posterior aspect of the heart and AV node in 90 per cent of individuals, is likely to be involved.[212] Occasionally, the block may be relieved by correction of hypotension or pulmonary congestion. Pain associated with the block may be relieved by various medications. Meperidine hydrochloride (Demerol), 50 to 100 mg intramuscularly, is probably preferable for the relief of pain in patients with AV block or posterior infarction because of its atropine-like action. If morphine is used for the relief of pain, atropine sulfate, 0.4 mg intramuscularly, should be given for each 15 mg of morphine sulfate to block the vagomimetic effect of morphine, which might contribute to the block. Since patients with second-degree heart block due to myocardial infarction may suddenly develop complete heart block or complete arrest, the cardiac electrical activity of these patients should be monitored continuously and an external pacemaker should be used to pace the heart if complete block with standstill or marked slowing occurs. If external pacing of the heart is required even once, a special bipolar electrode pacemaker catheter should be placed in the right ventricle to take over the pacing activity. In these patients this right ventricular electrode catheter should be left in place for several days even though the block may disappear.

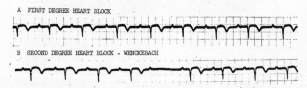

A FIRST DEGREE HEART BLOCK

B SECOND DEGREE HEART BLOCK - WENCKEBACH

Fig. 16-58. Patient with first-degree and second-degree heart block. In *A*, the P-R interval is prolonged to 0.30 sec; in *B* successive P-R intervals gradually prolonged, and following the fifth atrial complex, failure of atrioventricular conduction results in a dropped beat. After the sixth P wave the P-R interval again is shortened, but then progressively increases. This is known as the Wenckebach phenomenon.

SINUS RHYTHM

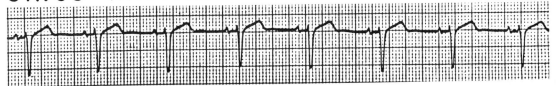

COMPLETE HEART BLOCK

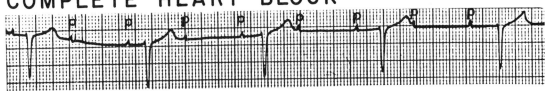

Fig. 16-59. Electrocardiogram of patient during regular sinus rhythm (*A*) and later during complete heart block (*B*). The atria and ventricles are beating at their own independent rhythms during heart block, and the P waves and QRS complexes are completely disassociated. There may be a tendency for the atrial and ventricular impulses to synchronize, even though the impulse is not conducted.

COMPLETE (THIRD-DEGREE) HEART-BLOCK * 16

Robert C. Schlant, M.D., and J. Willis Hurst, M.D.

Electrocardiographic Characteristics. Complete heart block is generally said to exist when the AV node fails to conduct any impulses from the atria to the ventricles. Electrocardiographically, there is usually no relation between the atrial and the ventricular complexes, although on occasion there may be a tendency for their rates to synchronize, even though the impulse is apparently not conducted (Fig. 16-59).

The form of the ventricular QRS complex may be normal (Fig. 16-59) if the ventricular focus is in the lower portion of the AV node or in the upper portion of the ventricular septum, but the QRS form becomes more bizarre the further the idioventricular focus is from the AV node (Fig. 16-60).

Causes. Complete heart block may be congenital[220] or may be produced by drugs or by any disease affecting the AV conduction system. The most frequent cause is ischemia or infarction produced by coronary artery atherosclerosis,[221,222] particularly in the right coronary artery. Complete heart block due to coronary atherosclerosis either occurs acutely following a posterior infarction, in which case it is usually transient[222] and seldom lasts longer than 3 to 4 weeks, or occurs without apparent relation to an acute infarction, in which case it may be either transient or permanent. We have encountered a number of adult patients with complete heart block who were labeled as having coronary atherosclerosis. This, of course, is the common practice today. Since at autopsy the major coronary arteries of some of these patients revealed minimal atherosclerosis, we assumed that the disease was in the small vessels of the AV node. We have the impression that not all these cases are related to atherosclerosis of the small vessels and wonder if other unknown causes may be responsible. To restate, we are not convinced that atherosclerosis is the *only* vascular disease responsible for complete heart block, although it undoubtedly is the cause in most cases.

Drugs, including digitalis, procaine amide hydrochloride, and quinidine, may produce complete heart block, as may infection, particularly diphtheria and myocarditis of various sorts.[223] In acute rheumatic fever, complete heart block occurs rarely; first- or second-degree block is more common. The presence of masses, such as primary or metastatic tumors, sarcoidosis, abscesses related to endo-

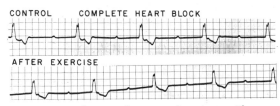

Fig. 16-60. Electrocardiogram of patient with complete heart block which demonstrates that the ventricular rate does not speed up after exercise. This is characteristic of the patient with complete heart block. In comparison, sinus bradycardia speeds up following exercise. The bizarre forms of the QRS complex indicate that the idioventricular focus is probably below the lower part of the AV node or the upper part of the interventricular septum.

carditis, tubercles, or gummas may produce complete heart block. In calcific aortic stenosis or calcified mitral annulus, there may be deposition of calcium salts in the AV node which may produce complete heart block, although in many of these patients there is also significant coronary artery atherosclerosis. Complete heart block may occur as an isolated congenital heart defect,[220] although ventricular septal defect is perhaps the most common congenital defect associated with complete heart block. In recent years, the surgical correction of ventricular septal defect, with the production of complete heart block by the surgical procedure, has introduced a new cause. Hyperkalemia secondary to hypoaldosteronism has been reported as a cause of syncopal attacks in a patient with complete heart block. In some apparently normal persons, complete heart block may be produced by increased vagal tone such as is induced by carotid sinus pressure; in many other patients, particularly those with coronary atherosclerosis, increased vagal tone often seems to be an additional factor in producing complete heart block.

Characteristics Detectable on Physical Examination. Complete heart block should be suspected when physical examination yields the following clues: (1) *A waves in the neck unrelated to the pulse or heart sounds* (Fig. 16-61), (2) *cannon waves* which may be produced if the atria contract when the AV valves are closed (Fig. 16-61), (3) a regular ventricular rate which is usually slow (30 to 50 beats per minute) and which does not usually increase significantly with physical activity (Fig. 16-60), (4) a marked variation in the intensity of the first heart sound related to the changing position of the AV valves at the onset of ventricular contraction, (5) and detection of heart sounds related to atrial contraction. The systolic pressure and pulse pressure may be elevated because of an increase in stroke output associated with the slow ventricular rate.

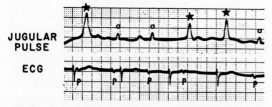

Fig. 16-61. Large cannon waves (★) occur during complete heart block when the P wave falls during ventricular systole between the QRS and the T wave. The atria contract but cannot empty against a closed AV valve. (*From Fig. 194, E. Corday and D. W. Irving: "Disturbances in Heart Rate, Rhythm and Conduction," W. B. Saunders Company, Philadelphia, 1961.*)

Treatment. In our experience, most patients with complete heart block can be classified in five groups on the basis of the clinical manifestations of the disorder. The management of these patients will be discussed using this classification, even though an individual patient may not fit exactly into one group or may change from one group to another.

1. Asymptomatic heart block. The first group is composed of patients with chronic complete heart block who are active and essentially asymptomatic. Some patients may note slightly decreased exercise tolerance resulting from the relatively slow and fixed ventricular rate, but they are rarely incapacitated. The complete heart block in this group of patients may be first detected by routine physical examination or electrocardiography. In these patients, when the block is essentially asymptomatic, no treatment is indicated. This group makes up a small percentage of patients with complete heart block.

2. Heart block associated with cerebral symptoms. For patients in the second group, complete heart block is associated with several episodes of syncope or convulsions per year. The term Morgagni-Stokes-Adams syndrome has been used in reference to attacks of such cerebral symptoms occurring in patients who exhibit some degree of heart block. Although most patients with Morgagni-Stokes-Adams attacks exhibit some degree of AV block between attacks, we have observed patients with paroxysmal complete heart block in whom the AV conduction was entirely normal between episodes. Schwartz and Schwartz have reported similar patients. During a true Morgagni-Stokes-Adams attack, the electrocardiogram reveals either ventricular standstill, ventricular fibrillation, ventricular tachycardia, or a slowing of the idioventricular impulses below a critical rate (Figs. 16-62 and 16-63). It is important to document the cardiac mechanism responsible for the episode of syncope whenever possible, since, for example, the treatment for ventricular tachycardia associated with AV block may be quite different from the treatment of ventricular tachycardia interrupting normal sinus rhythm. When such episodes occur two to three times a year, it is difficult not only to obtain electrocardiographic proof of the mechanism responsible for the attack but also to be sure that any prescribed treatment is beneficial. Since cerebral episodes due to ventricular standstill or slowing seem to be more common than those due to ventricular fibrillation or tachycardia, patients with cerebral symptoms should be given a trial of isoproterenol hydrochloride (Isuprel), 5 to 20 mg sublingually every 2 to 6 hr, or ephedrine sulfate, 25 mg orally every 4 to 6

hr. It is important to start with small doses and to monitor the electrocardiographic effects for several hours when patients are started on these medications. Usually one should not try to maintain a rate above 50 to 60 beats per minute with these drugs, since there is a real danger of producing excessive ventricular tachycardia or fibrillation. Isuprel may also be given as a long-acting preparation, 30 mg orally every 4 to 6 hr.[224] Epinephrine in oil, 1 ml of a 1:500 solution every 12 to 24 hr, was formerly used more than it is currently employed. Occasionally, the occurrence of Morgagni-Stokes-Adams syndrome may be decreased by the use of chlorothiazide in amounts adequate to lower the serum-potassium level to between 3.5 and 3.9 mEq per liter.[225] The usual initial dose is 0.5 to 1.0 Gm daily. Presumably the decrease in intracellular and extracellular potassium alters the resting potential of the membrane of myocardial cells. In some patients, chlorothiazide may decrease the incidence of Morgagni-Stokes-Adams attacks even without altering AV conduction; in a few patients it has reportedly caused even complete heart block to disappear.[225] Of course, potassium supplement should not be given when chlorothiazide is administered for the treatment of AV block. Corticosteroids have also been used in the treatment of chronic complete heart block.[226] The exact dose of any medication employed varies greatly from patient to patient. Even in one patient, it may need to be varied markedly in short periods of time. In the future, as more experience is gained, even those patients with infrequent episodes of Morgagni-Stokes-Adams attacks may have myocardial electrodes and a battery pacemaker implanted to take over the pacing of the ventricles.

The above group of patients makes up a large percentage of patients with complete heart block.

3. Heart block associated with congestive heart failure. A third group is composed of patients whose complete heart block is associated with chronic severe congestive heart failure. If the failure does not readily and easily respond to treatment with sublingual Isuprel, oral ephedrine, or oral chlorothiazide, in the doses given above, in addition to the cautious administration of digitalis, a bipolar electrode catheter should be placed in the right ventricle[227-232] and connected to an external pacemaker to take over the pacing of the ventricles. The ventricular rate can thereby be increased to approximately 70 beats each minute. If the increase in heart rate can be accomplished and if it is associated with an increase in cardiac output and a decrease in heart failure,[233] the patient should be considered as a candidate for the implantation of a permanent cardiac pacemaker.[234] This is accomplished by connecting the bipolar

electrode catheter to a battery-operated pacemaker in order to transport the patient to the operating room. Myocardial electrodes are then sutured in place and a subcutaneous pacemaker is implanted.[235-241] Once the latter has been accomplished, the external pacemaker can be turned off

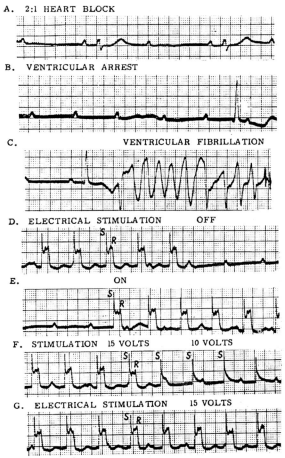

Fig. 16-62. Electrocardiogram of patient with 2:1 heart block (*A*). Ventricular arrest occurred in *B*, followed by ventricular fibrillation in *C*. Patient was defibrillated, and an external electric pacemaker was applied (*D*). Following each stimulus (*S*) there was a ventricular response. When the electric stimulator was turned off (*E*), there was no ventricular response, but when it was turned on again a ventricular response recurred. In *F* when the stimulus was reduced from 15 to 10 volts, the ventricular stimulus was not followed by a ventricular complex; but when the stimulus was again increased to 15 volts (*G*), it was followed by ventricular complexes. This demonstrates that sufficient electrical voltage must be used to cause excitation of the ventricle. (*From Fig. 163, E. Corday and D. W. Irving: "Disturbances in Heart Rate, Rhythm and Conduction," W. B. Saunders Company, Philadelphia, 1961.*)

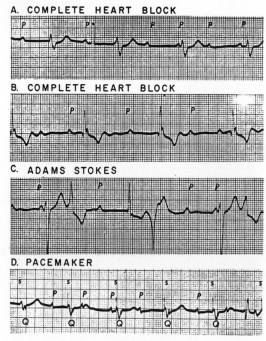

Fig. 16-63. Patient with complete heart block. During strip *C* frequent premature ventricular systoles of multifocal origin occurred and produced the Adams-Stokes syndrome. An external pacemaker was attached to the patient's chest (*D*), and a ventricular QRS deflection followed each stimulus indicated by S.

and the implanted pacemaker turned on. This can be done without the loss of a single heartbeat.

This group makes up a small percentage of patients with complete heart block.

4. Heart block associated with myocardial infarction. The treatment of complete heart block associated with fresh inferior or posterior myocardial infarction by using the bipolar catheter pacemaker is now being investigated. Nine of our cases have been published as part of a larger study by Bruce et al.[241a] Forty-one of our patients with acute infarction and complete heart block have now been studied by Dr. E. Alan Paulk, in the Department of Medicine, Emory University School of Medicine, at Grady Memorial Hospital.[241b] Thirty-five of this series of patients had, in addition to complete heart block, episodes of ventricular standstill or fibrillation. All forty-one patients were treated by placing a bipolar electrode catheter into the right ventricle in order to pace the heart at a rate of 70 times a minute with an external battery operated pacemaker. The value of the procedure is still being studied but there is no doubt that this technique prevented the death from cardiac arrhythmia of some of these patients. The mortality rate is high in patients with complete heart block

due to acute myocardial infarction. In addition, it is often difficult to be certain whether or not syncope has occurred. Accordingly we are now trying the bipolar electrode catheter pacemaker initially in such patients rather than waiting for documented evidence of ventricular standstill or fibrillation. If death can be prevented during the acute stage of the infarction, the high-grade AV block usually disappears. After the heart has been paced with the catheter electrode for several days, one may attempt to *wean* the patient from the catheter pacing by slowly turning down the external pacemaker and observing whether the complete block persists and, if it does, the rate of the idioventricular beat. We shall use the word *wean* again; therefore, a clear definition of the term is in order. We use the word here to explain the process of discontinuing controlled electrical pacing of the heart in anticipation that the normal pacemakers of the heart will take over. During the weaning period, certain drugs may be tried. Occasionally, atropine sulfate, 1 mg intravenously or intramuscularly every 6 to 8 hr, may cause complete heart block to disappear, presumably by blocking vagomimetic impulses which are contributing to the block. Occasionally, corticosteroids are of benefit in the treatment of complete heart block following an acute myocardial infarction.[242] Presumably, corticosteroids decrease the amount of inflammatory edema in the AV node and perhaps increase the cardiac responsiveness to catecholamines and to sympathetic stimuli and sympathomimetic drugs. During the weaning stage, short periods of asystole may appear, or the complete heart block may persist with an extremely slow ventricular rate. During this weaning period, an intravenous infusion of either Isuprel or epinephrine may be useful. Generally, if the patient is normotensive or hypertensive, Isuprel is preferred, since it has no peripheral vasopressor action. In patients who have very recently suffered disorders of AV conduction, epinephrine, which is a less potent stimulator of the sinoatrial pacemaker than is Isuprel, may be more suitable, since AV conduction might return with an excessively rapid ventricular rate. It is usually best to adjust the rate of infusion until the idioventricular rate is about 50 beats per minute. Useful dilutions are 4 ml of a 1:1,000 solution of epinephrine (4 mg) in 1 liter of 5 per cent dextrose in water, or 1 mg (5 ampules of 0.2 mg each) of Isuprel in 250 ml of 5 per cent dextrose in water. The initial rate of administration of these solutions is 4 mg per min (15 drops or 1 ml per min). At times, when treating patients with intravenous epinephrine or Isuprel, it may be necessary to administer levarterenol concurrently to help maintain the blood pressure. The rate of administration of levarterenol (norepinephrine or Levophed, 4 to 8 mg in 1 liter of 5 per cent dextrose in water) must be adjusted individually to the blood pressure response; the physician should keep in mind that levarterenol may also increase the rate of an idioventricular focus.[243] While the patient is being weaned from electrical pacing and the above medications are being employed, *the pacemaker catheter should at all times be in the right ventricle, either pacing the ventricle or set with a cardiac monitor to take over pacing if it should be necessary.* Although it is unusual for heart block following acute infarction to persist more than a few weeks, the catheter should be left in the right ventricle ready to pace for several days after the complete block disappears. Very rarely, the complete block will persist despite all measures. When it is impossible to wean the patient away from a catheter pacemaker without inducing episodes of standstill, it may be necessary to continue to pace the heart by the right ventricular pacemaker catheter for several weeks and then to operate and implant myocardial electrodes and a subcutaneous pacemaker.

This group makes up a large percentage of patients with complete heart block.

5. Heart block associated with change in frequency of syncopal attacks. The fifth group of patients is composed of those with complete heart block who have a significant change in the frequency of syncopal attacks. The patient may have had no attacks for several months and then begin to have "clusters" of attacks, several per week or even several per day. The development of such clusters of attacks may be caused by a recent myocardial infarction, but, as a rule, infarction is not evident. These patients should all be promptly hospitalized. If the cardiac mechanism responsible for the attacks can be documented, this should be done; however, a bipolar electrode pacemaker catheter should be placed in the right ventricle as soon as possible and its frequency set high enough to take over from the idioventricular focus. This program should be used whether the cardiac mechanism is not known, is documented as ventricular standstill or marked slowing, or is shown to be ventricular fibrillation. Although there is no really satisfactory treatment for attacks of ventricular fibrillation that interrupt complete heart block, at times pacing the ventricles at 60 to 70 beats per minute by the right ventricular bipolar electrode catheter will prevent the development of this arrhythmia. A d-c defibrillator should be constantly available in case the patient develops persistent ventricular fibrillation. Once the pacemaker catheter has taken over, it is best to let it

pace the ventricles for several days, during which one may, if desired, administer chlorothiazide as described above. If, after several days, there is no evidence of fresh myocardial infarction, the bipolar electrode catheter should be connected to a battery pacemaker and the patient sent to the operating room for implantation of myocardial electrodes and a subcutaneous pacemaker. This precaution is desirable because most of these patients tend to have repeated episodes despite the most meticulous drug therapy.

This group makes up a large percentage of patients with complete heart block.

Treatment with Drugs Alone. In situations in which artificial pacing equipment is not available so that electrical therapy as described above cannot be used, drugs such as atropine, Isuprel, epinephrine, chlorothiazide, or corticosteroids, in the doses described above must be relied on. Although drugs are far less efficient than electrical therapy in preventing ventricular fibrillation or tachycardia following AV block, Isuprel, epinephrine, or ephedrine sulfate, in the doses described above, is occasionally successful.[243,244]

Warnings. When episodes of ventricular tachycardia or fibrillation interrupt AV block, quinidine and Pronestyl are usually *contraindicated.* This situation is entirely different from the interruption of normal sinus rhythm by ventricular tachycardia, a disorder for which Pronestyl and quinidine may be quite useful.

Atrial tachycardia with 2:1 AV block is frequently due to digitalis intoxication and potassium loss. Multiple ventricular ectopic beats and ventricular tachycardia also may be due to digitalis intoxication and potassium loss. These arrhythmias are remedied by discontinuing digitalis and restoring potassium. Complete heart block also may result from digitalis intoxication; it should be treated by discontinuing digitalis and using an electrical pacer if necessary until the drug has been eliminated. Potassium medication in such cases may be detrimental.

AV DISSOCIATION [* 16]

*Robert C. Schlant, M.D., and
J. Willis Hurst, M.D.*

Of the complex cardiac arrhythmias, those described by the term *AV dissociation* are perhaps the most difficult to recognize and to understand (Fig. 16-64). Much of this confusion has arisen from a diversity in terms employed by different authors. Jacobs, Donoso, and Friedberg[244a] have applied the term only to those arrhythmias which meet the following criteria:

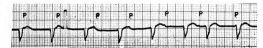

Fig. 16-64. Electrocardiogram of a patient with heart block demonstrating interference dissociation. Note that the first six ventricular QRS complexes occur at a faster rate than the P waves. The sixth atrial deflection is followed by a QRS complex, because this wave of excitation is conducted through to the ventricle. The regular cadence of the QRS is interrupted and this is called "interference dissociation."

(1) the atria and ventricles are controlled by independent pacemakers; (2) retrograde VA block is present, since without such block two independent pacemakers cannot exist; (3) the capacity for forward conduction is intact, although occasionally incomplete AV block may be present, and (4) the ventricular rate is less than 150 beats per min when the ventricles are governed by an idioventricular pacemaker.

In their series, the most common cause was digitalis intoxication, particularly associated with the administration of diuretics or with cerebral vascular accident. Less common causes were acute rheumatic fever, quinidine overdosage, cardiac catheterization, coronary artery disease, and pulmonary embolization. When AV dissociation occurs without AV block development, it may require no specific treatment because of its transient nature; however, when it results from the administration of a drug, the drug should be discontinued. When it has resulted from digitalis, the administration of potassium may speed the restoration of normal sinus rhythm. When the AV dissociation seems to result from vagal hypersensitivity, atropine, 1 mg intravenously, may restore normal sinus rhythm, even though in other circumstances it may aggravate or even produce AV dissociation.

BUNDLE BRANCH BLOCK

Eliot Corday, M.D., and
Tzu-Wang Lang, M.D.

When conduction of the excitatory impulse is delayed through a portion of the bundle of His, the right or left bundle, one ventricle will be activated and contract before the other; this condition is described as bundle branch block[245] (see Chap. 6). The QRS complex is widened above 0.1 sec.

Etiology. Ischemia of the myocardium (as in coronary atherosclerosis), acute myocardial infarction,[246,247] hypertension, and rheumatic disease are the most common causes of bundle branch block. It may be found in congenital heart disease, as in interventricular or interatrial septal defect. It is found in fibrosis and other degenerative changes in the conduction bundles.[248,249] Aortic valvular disease with calcific stenosis may impinge upon the left bundle and cause left bundle branch block.[1] Conduction disturbances of the bundle are known to occur because of tumors of the myocardium[250-252] diphtheria,[253-255] rheumatic fever,[256,257] bacterial endocarditis,[258] syphilitic aortitis[259-261] and other acute infections.[262-265] Toxic substances such as digitalis, quinidine, procaine amide, and potassium[266] might also induce conduction disturbances of the bundle. Bundle branch block may result from cardiac surgery and then might be transient or permanent.[267] Ischemia of the bundle of His due to rapid ventricular rate as in supraventricular tachycardias might also produce delayed ventricular conduction.[249,268,269] Some patients with normal hearts are born with a congenital disturbance of the conduction system.[270,271]

Mechanism. In bundle branch block conduction down the intact bundle produces a normal excitation process of that side, but because of a conduction delay in the bundle of the opposite side, excitation and ventricular contraction will be delayed on the side of the disturbed bundle. In order for the ventricles to be excited on the side of the bundle block, the impulse must bypass through the muscle from the normal side into the affected side. This requires a transmission through muscle tissue which is relatively slow; thus the excitation of the remaining portion of the ventricle is delayed. Then abnormal conduction through the muscle mass will cause a distortion of the QRS complex, the delay causing a widening of the QRS above 0.1 sec. A partial delay of 0.1 to 0.12 sec is called "incomplete" bundle branch block.[272] If the duration of the QRS is greater than 0.12 sec it is called "complete" bundle branch block. The block may be permanent or may last for from only a few beats to several hours. It often alternates with periods of normal conduction. When the block occurs in paroxysms, it is referred to as recurrent or paroxysmal bundle branch block.[249,268,269] If the block occurs periodically in a ratio of 2:1 or 3:1 with normal conduction it is termed "partial" or "periodic" bundle branch block.[274,275] A delay in the conduction of the terminal bundle of the Purkinje network is called "arborization" block.

Fluoroscopic studies of patients with bundle branch block indicate that the two ventricles do not contract at the same time.

Signs and Symptoms. Usually there are no symptoms of bundle branch block. However, prolongation or splitting of the first and second sounds may occur. In complete right bundle branch block there is a persistent splitting of the second sound, which becomes more noticeable with inspiration.

This is because of asynchronous contraction of the ventricles.[276,277] In complete left bundle branch block, paradoxic splitting of the second sound is heard during expiration[277] (see Chap. 5).

Electrocardiogram. There is a prolongation of the QRS complex above 0.1 sec. The P wave and the P-R interval are usually normal; however, bundle branch block also often occurs with atrial fibrillation. The characteristic pattern of standard leads of typical left complete bundle branch block are (1) notching or slurring of the QRS complex; (2) widening of the QRS complexes to 0.12 sec or longer; (3) the ventricular deflection of the greatest duration is upward in lead I and downward in lead III; (4) large T waves in leads I and III which are opposite in direction to the deflections of major duration (Fig. 16-65).

The precordial leads of complete left bundle branch block demonstrate a delay in the intrinsicoid deflection over the left precordium; i.e., the latest peak of the R wave, which is inscribed as the wave of depolarization passes toward and beneath the exploring electrode, occurs later in the left precordial leads. The absence of the Q wave in the left precordial leads is due to the disappearance of the vector which normally represents early activation of the septum from left to right.[278] An initial R wave may be present in the left precordial leads because the activation of the septum is now abnormal from right to left, toward the exploring electrode. The R wave is usually notched because of slow activation of the left septal mass. The right precordial leads usually demonstrate a decrease in the amplitude of the R wave because the septum is now activated from right to left. This is followed by a deep S wave, because of the vector force moving slowly away from the exploring electrode through the left ventricle. Many variations in the pattern of left bundle branch block may occur because of associated enlargement of cardiac chambers, location of myocardial damage, and the geographic position of the heart. The electrocardiographic features of myocardial infarction may mask or distort those of bundle branch block. When these variations occur, the condition is termed "atypical" bundle branch block.

In typical complete right bundle branch block, the electrocardiographic patterns are essentially the reverse of those for left complete bundle branch block (Fig. 16-66): (1) the QRS complexes are notched or slurred. The QRS complexes are widened to 0.12 sec or more. (3) The widest deflection is upward in lead III and downward in lead I. (4) As in left bundle branch block, the T wave is inscribed in the opposite direction to the QRS complex.

The precordial leads are very helpful in the

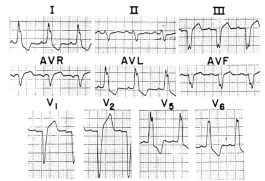

Fig. 16-65. Electrocardiogram of a patient with typical complete left bundle branch block. The QRS complex is slurred and widened to 0.12 sec. In lead I and the left precordial leads, the ventricular deflections of greatest duration are upward and the T waves are inverted. The intrinsicoid deflection is of maximum duration in the left precordial leads. In lead III and the right precordial leads, the ventricular deflections of widest duration are downward and the T waves are opposite in direction to the major deflection.

diagnosis of right bundle branch block. In leads V_1 and V_2, prominent R waves, which are often wide and notched, are frequently seen. The right precordial leads show an intitial R wave, because of the early normal activation of the left aspect of the septum. This is followed by a deep S wave, because of the normal activation passing through the left ventricle and causing forces which are moving away from the right precordial electrodes and which are strong enough to produce negativity. The second R wave, which is of greater magnitude and duration, represents the abnormal delayed

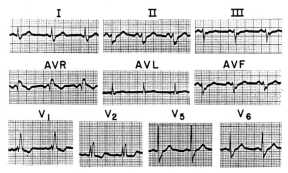

Fig. 16-66. Electrocardiogram from a patient demonstrating typical complete right bundle branch block. The duration of the QRS complex is 0.12 sec. The ventricular deflections of widest duration are downward in lead I and upward in lead III. The intrinsicoid deflection is of maximum duration in the right precordial leads. The T waves are opposite in direction to the deflection of greatest duration.

activation of the right ventricular mass. The left precordial leads in right bundle branch block show a Q wave because the initial activation of the septum still takes place in the normal direction, i.e., from left to right. Following this, the left ventricle is activated normally and produces a tall R wave. As the activation travels away from the electrode to the right side, a widened, slurred S is inscribed. Typically the T waves are oppositely directed to the ventricular deflection of maximum duration, inverted in the right but upright in the left precordial leads. The intrinsicoid deflection is more delayed over the right precordial leads than over the left because of the late activation of the right ventricular mass.

The pattern of right bundle branch block in the standard leads may be distorted by associated myocardial disease, right ventricular hypertrophy, or changes in the position of the heart. The electrocardiographic pattern is then called atypical.

The electrocardiographic patterns of *incomplete bundle branch block* are similar to those of complete bundle branch block except that the QRS interval is of shorter duration, usually between 0.10 to 0.11 sec.[273,276]

In *atypical left or right bundle branch block,* the QRS reflections are similar to those described above, but the T wave is in the same direction as the principal deflection of the QRS.

In *periodic left or right bundle branch block,* normal QRS complexes alternate with bundle blocked complexes in a ratio of 2:1, 3:1, 4:3, etc.[274,275]

The QRS complexes in arborization block tend to be low in amplitude and are frequently splintered.

Treatment. Bundle branch block is usually asymptomatic and requires no treatment. However, if it is due to digitalis, quinidine, or procaine amide, the drugs should be withdrawn.

Prognosis. Prognosis is usually that of the underlying disease, and if there is no disease present, the life span is usually normal.[279,280] The block may be permanent or transient.[267,281,282] The permanent type usually carries a more significant prognosis because of the underlying cardiac disease. The prognosis is usually worse in left bundle branch block.[279,280]

WOLFF-PARKINSON-WHITE SYNDROME

Eliot Corday, M.D., and
Tzu-Wang Lang, M.D.

Wolff-Parkinson-White syndrome is a disorder of activation of the heart due to accelerated conduction between the atria and ventricles and an abnormal excitation of the ventricles. It is characterized by a P-R interval of less than 0.12 sec and a widened, distorted QRS complex. Persons with Wolff-Parkinson-White syndrome often develop paroxysmal supraventricular tachycardia.[283,284] Because of its characteristic rapid atrioventricular excitation, it has also been called preexcitation syndrome.

Etiology. Wolff-Parkinson-White syndrome often occurs in infants,[285-289] but it may be found in any age group.[289,290] There appears to be a congenital form because it has been found in twins[291] and often in several members of a family.[292,293] However, the hearts of such persons have appeared completely normal on autopsy.[292-294] The syndrome may first occur following a myocardial infarction in which the AV node has been damaged. This has provided support to the theory of accelerated conduction through some fibers of the AV node when that AV node is damaged.[1,295]

Mechanism. There are three theories of the mechanism of the preexcitation syndrome: according to the bundle of Kent[296-298] theory, there is a special rapid-conduction pathway between the atria and ventricles which may cause preexcitation of part of the ventricle;[296-302] according to the second theory, a disturbance, either functional or organic, of the AV node causes an unusually rapid excitation through some fibers of the AV node, which quickly activate part of the ventricle, but the rest of the ventricular fibers are activated at their normal time;[1,295] according to the third theory, the preexcitation is due to vagotonia which affects the conduction through the AV node.[303]

The excitations of the atria and then of the ventricles allow just sufficient time for the atria to empty before ventricular systole.

Supraventricular tachycardia occurs very often in patients with Wolff-Parkinson-White syndrome, and ventricular tachycardias occur occasionally. Sudden death has been attributed to the sudden onset of a ventricular arrhythmia.[299,304-306]

Signs and Symptoms. There are no characteristic symptoms of the Wolff-Parkinson-White syndrome, and the patient will not be aware of the syndrome until it is first observed in an electrocardiogram. Often the first inclination that the condition exists is the sudden onset of tachycardia which causes the patient to seek medical advice and have an electrocardiogram.

Electrocardiogram. The characterizing features of Wolff-Parkinson-White syndrome (Fig. 16-67) are: (1) the P-R interval is short, less than 0.12 sec, (2) the QRS complex is wide, 0.11 to 0.14 sec, (3) the upslope of the R wave is slowed, giving it the characteristic delta wave appearance, (4) depression of the S-T segment and inversion of the

T waves may occur. Occasionally the administration of atropine, procaine amide, or quinidine[302] or exercise might cause the abnormal electrocardiogram to revert to normal. In some instances Wolff-Parkinson-White complexes might be interspersed with normal sinus rhythm. Also a "concertina" effect might be noted, with the P-R interval progressively narrowing beat by beat as the QRS widens, and then the P-R interval lengthening again as the QRS shortens.[1]

Treatment. The patient does not require treatment except when the rapid tachycardia occurs, and then the treatment is that of the tachycardia per se. Occasionally the administration of atropine will correct the arrhythmia, but the methods used for treatment of supraventricular tachycardias, such as digitalis, quinidine, procaine amide, radioiodine, and cardioversion, are usually successful.

Prognosis. Prognosis of Wolff-Parkinson-White is usually normal;[287] however, sudden death is known to occur in younger persons from this condition, possibly because of cardiac arrhythmias.[299,306] If the syndrome follows a myocardial infarction, the prognosis is that of the causative condition. If it is found during examination for aircraft pilot training, most examiners reject the candidate because of the high incidence of associated arrhythmias.[1]

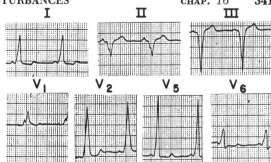

Fig. 16-67. Electrocardiogram of a patient with typical features of the Wolff-Parkinson-White syndrome. The P-R interval is short, measuring 0.09 sec; the QRS complex is widened to more than 0.12 sec. In the left precordial leads, the slurred upstroke of the R waves (delta wave), S-T segment depression, and diphasic T waves are demonstrated. The slurred downslope of the S wave in lead II corresponds to the slurred upstroke of the R wave in other leads.

REFERENCES

1. Corday, E., and Irving, D. W.: "Disturbances of Heart Rate, Rhythm and Conduction," W. B. Saunders Company, Philadelphia, 1961.

2. Corday, E., and Irving, D. W.: Effect of Cardiac Arrhythmias on the Cerebral Circulation, *Am. J. Cardiol.*, 6:803, 1960.

3. Corday, E., and Williams, J. H.: Effect of Shock and of Vasopressor Drugs on the Regional Circulation of the Brain, Heart, Kidney and Liver, *Am. J. Med.*, 29:228, 1960.

4. Irving, D. W., and Corday, E.: Effect of the Cardiac Arrhythmias on the Renal and Mesenteric Circulations, *Am. J. Cardiol.*, 8:32, 1961.

5. Corday, E., Gold, H., De Vera, L. B., Williams, J. H., and Fields, J.: Effect of the Cardiac Arrhythmias on the Coronary Circulation, *Ann. Int. Med.*, 50:535, 1959.

6. Corday, E., Rothenberg, S. F., and Putnam, T. J.: Cerebral Vascular Insufficiency: An Explanation of Some Types of Localized Cerebral Encephalopathy, *Arch. Neurol. & Psychiat.*, 69:551, 1953.

7. Corday, E., Rothenberg, S. F., and Weiner, S. M.: Cerebral Vascular Insufficiency: An Explanation of the Transient Stroke, *A.M.A. Arch. Int. Med.*, 98:683, 1956.

8. Corday, E., and Rothenberg, S. F.: Primary Cerebral Angiospasm, in J. S. Myers (ed.), "Monograph of Cerebral Hypoxia," Charles C Thomas, Publisher, Springfield, Ill., 1961.

9. De Vera, L. B., Gold, H., and Corday, E.: Simultaneous Comparison of Antegrade and Collateral Coronary Blood Flows, *Circulation Res.*, 6:26, 1958.

10. Corday, E., Williams, J. H., De Vera, L. B., and Gold, H.: Effect of Systemic Blood Pressure and Vasopressor Drugs on Coronary Blood Flow and the Electrocardiogram, *Am. J. Cardiol.*, 3:626, 1959.

11. Galbraith, B. T.: Lower Nephron Nephrosis Associated with Prolonged Shock from Ventricular Tachycardia, *Am. Heart J.*, 42:766, 1951.

12. Corday, E., Irving, D. W., Gold, H., Bernstein, H., and Skelton, R. B. T.: Mesenteric Vascular Insufficiency: Intestinal Ischemia Induced by Remote Circulatory Disturbances, *Am. J. Med.*, 33:365, 1962.

13. Sedlacek, R. A., and Bean, W. B.: Abdominal "Angina": The Syndrome of Intermittent Ischemia of Mesenteric Arteries, *Ann. Int. Med.*, 46:148, 1957.

14. Greenbaum, D.: Gangrene of the Extremities Following Cardiac Infarction and Noradrenalin Therapy, *Lancet*, 1:1102, 1958.

15. Corday, E., Bazika, V., Lang, T., Pappelbaum, S., Gold, H., and Bernstein, H.: Detection of Phantom Arrhythmias and Evanescent Electrocardiographic Abnormalities. *J.A.M.A.*, 193:417, 1965.

16. Hurst, J. W., and Schlant, R. C. (eds.): Treatment of Cardiac Arrhythmias, *Mod. Treatment*, 1:665, 1964.

17. James, T. N.: The Connecting Pathways between the Sinus Node and A-V Node and between the Right and Left Atrium in the Human Heart, *Am. Heart J.*, 66:498, 1963.

18. Katz, L. N., and Pick, A.: Current Status of Theories of Mechanisms of Atrial Tachycardias, Flutter, and Fibrillation, *Progr. Cardiovas. Dis.*, 2:650, 1960.

19. Lewis, T., Feil, H. S., and Stroud, W. D.: Observations upon Flutter and Fibrillation. II. The Nature of Auricular Flutter, *Heart,* 7:191, 1920.

20. Lewis, T., Drury, A. N., and Iliescu, C. C.: A Demonstration of Circus Movement in Clinical Fibrillation of the Auricles, *Heart,* 8:361, 1921.

21. Lewis, T.: "The Mechanism and Graphic Registration of the Heart Beat," Shaw, London, 1925.

22. Rothberger, C. J.: Neue Theorien über Flimmern und Flattern, *Klin. Wchnschr.,* 1:82, 1922.

23. Rotherberger, C. J.: Normale und pathologische Physiologie der Rhythmik und Koordination des Herzens, *Ergebn. Physiol.,* 32:472, 1931.

24. Prinzmetal, M., Corday, E., Brill, I. C., Oblath, R. W., and Kruger, H. E.: "The Auricular Arrhythmias, Charles C Thomas, Publisher, Springfield, Ill., 1952.

25. Scherf, D., Schaffer, A. I., and Blumenfeld, S.: Mechanism of Flutter and Fibrillation, *A.M.A. Arch. Int. Med.,* 91:333, 1953.

26. Katz, L. N., and Pick, A.: The Mechanism of Auricular Flutter and Auricular Fibrillation, *Circulation,* 7:601, 1953.

27. James, T. N.: "Anatomy of the Coronary Arteries," Hoeber Medical Division, Harper & Row, Publishers, Incorporated, 1961.

28. James, T. N.: Myocardial Infarction and Atrial Arrhythmias, *Circulation,* 24:761, 1961.

29. James, T. N.: Arrhythmias and Conduction Disturbances in Acute Myocardial Infarction, *Am. Heart J.,* 64:416, 1962.

30. Dorney, E. R.: Complications of Pressor Amine Therapy, *South. M. J.,* 53:875, 1960.

31. Wadman, S., and Pelner, L.: The Action of Prostigmine in Supraventricular Tachycardia, *Ann. Int. Med.,* 29:53, 1948.

32. Orgain, E. S.: Current Status of Treatment of Paroxysmal Atrial Tachycardia, *Progr. Cardiovas. Dis.,* 2:663, 1959.

33. Barrow, J. G.: Treatment of Paroxysmal Supraventricular Tachycardia with Lanatoside C, *Ann. Int. Med.,* 32:116, 1950.

34. Sokolow, M., and Perloff, D. B.: The Clinical Pharmacology and Use of Quinidine in Heart Disease, *Progr. Cardiovas. Dis.,* 3:316, 1960–1961.

35. Sokolow, M., and Ball, R. E.: Factors Influencing Conversion of Chronic Atrial Fibrilation with Special Reference to Serum Quinidine Concentration, *Circulation,* 14:568, 1956.

36. Kayden, H. J., Brodie, B. B., and Steele, J. M.: Procaine Amide: A Review, *Circulation,* 15:118, 1957.

37. Gottsegen, G., and Östär, E.: Drug to Reduce Quinidine Cardiotoxicity, *Am. Heart J.,* 65:102, 1963.

38. Wasserman, F., Brodsky, L., Dick, M. M., Kathe, J. M., and Rodensky, P. L.: Successful Treatment of Quinidine and Procaine Amide Intoxication, *New England J. Med.,* 259:797, 1958.

39. Jackson, G. L.: Paroxysmal Atrial Tachycardia: Its Possible Management by Decrease in Myocardial Norepinephrine Content, *New England J. Med.,* 269:518, 1963.

40. Nadas, A. S.: "Pediatric Cardiology," W. B. Saunders Company, Philadelphia, 1963.

41. Rodensky, P. L., and Wasserman, F.: Observations on Digitalis Intoxication, *Arch. Int. Med.,* 108:61, 1961.

42. Morgan, W. L., and Breneman, G. M.: Atrial Tachycardia with Block Treated with Digitalis, *Circulation,* 25:787, 1962.

43. Lown, B., and Levine, S. A.: "Current Concepts in Digitalis Therapy," Little, Brown and Company, Boston, 1954.

44. Zimmerman, H. B., Gentsh, K. W., and Gale, A. H.: Potassium Potentiation of Digitalis, *Dis. Chest,* 43:377, 1963.

45. Surawicz, B.: Use of Chelating Agent, EDTA, in Digitalis Intoxication and Cardiac Arrhythmias, *Progr. Cardiovas. Dis.,* 2:432, 1959.

46. Prinzmetal, M., Corday, E., Brill, I. C., Oblath, R. W., and Kruger, H. E.: "The Auricular Arrhythmias," Charles C Thomas, Publisher, Springfield, Ill., 1952.

47. Corday, E., Williams, J. H., De Vera, L., and Gold, H.: Hemodynamics of Coronary Circulation in Cardiac Arrhythmias, *Mod. Concepts Cardiovas. Dis.,* 27:493, 1958.

48. Phillips, E., and Levine, S. A.: Auricular Fibrillation without Other Evidence of Heart Disease, *Am. J. Med.,* 7:478, 1949.

49. Hurst, J. W., Paulk, E. A., Jr., Proctor, H. D., and Schlant, R. C.: The Management of Patients with Atrial Fibrillation, *Am. J. Med.* 37 (No. 5): 728, 1964.

50. White, P. D., and Jones, T. D.: Heart Disease and Disorders in New England, *Am. Heart J.,* 3:302, 1928.

51. Cookson, H.: The Aetiology and Prognosis of Auricular Fibrillation, *Quart. J. Med.,* 23:309, 1930.

52. McEachern, D., and Baker, B. M., Jr.: Auricular Fibrillation: Its Etiology, Age Incidence and Production by Digitalis Therapy, *Am. J. M. Sc.,* 183:35, 1932.

53. Wood, P.: "Diseases of the Heart and Circulation," 2d ed., J. B. Lippincott Company, Philadelphia, 1956.

54. Cohen, M. G., and Pastor, B. H.: Delayed Cardiac Arrhythmias Following Non-cardiac Thoracic Surgery, *Dis. Chest,* 32:435, 1957.

55. Dodd, R. B., Sims, W. A., and Bone, D. J.: Cardiac Arrhythmias Observed during Anesthesia and Surgery, *Surgery,* 51:400–447, 1962.

56. Orgain, E. S., Wolff, L., and White, P. D.: Uncomplicated Auricular Fibrillation and Auricular Flutter: Frequent Occurrence and Good Prognosis in Patients without Other Evidence of Cardiac Disease, *A.M.A. Arch. Int. Med.,* 57:493, 1936.

57. Evans, W., and Swann, P.: Lone Auricular Fibrillation, *Brit. Heart J.,* 16:189, 1954.

58. Hanson, H. H., and Rutledge, D. I.: Auricular Fibrillation in Normal Hearts, *New England J. Med.*, 240:947, 1949.

59. Evans, W., and Swann, P.: Lone Auricular Fibrillation, *Brit. Heart J.*, 16:189, 1954.

60. Parkinson, J., and Campbell, M.: The Quinidine Treatment of Auricular Fibrillation, *Quart. J. Med.*, 22:281, 1929.

61. Brill, I. C.: Auricular Fibrillation with Congestive Failure and No Other Evidence of Organic Heart Disease, *Am. Heart J.*, 13:175, 1937.

62. Wolff, L.: Familial Auricular Fibrillation, *New England J. Med.*, 229:396, 1943.

63. Gould, W. L.: Auricular Fibrillation: Report on a Study of a Familial Tendency, 1920–1956, *A.M.A. Arch. Int. Med.*, 100:916, 1957.

64. New York Heart Association: "Diseases of the Heart and Blood Vessels: Nomenclature and Criteria for Diagnosis," 6th ed., Little, Brown and Company, Boston, 1964.

65. Kerkhof, A. C., and Baumann, H.: Minute Volume Determinations in Mitral Stenosis during Auricular Fibrillation and When Restored to Normal Rhythm, *Proc. Soc. Exper. Biol. & Med.*, 31:168, 1933.

66. Hecht, H. H., Osher, W. J., and Samuels, A. J.: Cardiovascular Adjustments in Subjects with Organic Heart Disease before and after Conversion of Atrial Fibrillation to Normal Sinus Rhythm, *J. Clin. Invest.*, 30:647, 1951.

67. Kory, R. C., and Meneely, G. R.: Cardiac Output in Auricular Fibrillation with Observations on the Effects of Conversion to Normal Sinus Rhythm, *J. Clin. Invest.*, 30:653, 1951.

68. Wetherbee, D. G., Brown, M. G., and Holzman, D.: Ventricular Rate Response Following Exercise during Auricular Fibrillation and after Conversion to Normal Sinus Rhythm, *Am. J. M. Sc.*, 223:667, 1952.

69. Storstein, O., and Tveten, H.: Quinidine Treatment of Established Auricular Fibrillation, *Acta med. Scandinav.*, 153:57, 1955.

70. Maurice, P., Rulliere, R., Acar, J., and Lenegre, J.: Étude clinique de 90 cas de fibrillation auriculaire idiopathique, *Bull. et mém. Soc. méd. hôp. Paris*, 72:607, 1956.

71. Broch, O. J., and Muller, O.: Haemodynamic Studies during Auricular Fibrillation and after Restoration of Sinus Rhythm, *Brit. Heart J.*, 19:222, 1957.

72. Gilbert, R., Eich, R. H., Smulyan, H., Keighley, J., and Auchincloss, J. H., Jr.: Effect on Circulation of Conversion of Atrial Fibrillation to Sinus Rhythm, *Circulation*, 27:1079, 1963.

73. Morris, J. J., Jr., Entman, M. L., Thompson, H. K., Jr., North, W. C., and McIntosh, H. D.: Cardiac Output in Atrial Fibrillation and Sinus Rhythm, *Circulation*, 28:772, 1963.

74. Burchell, H. B.: A Clinical Appraisal of Atrial Transport System, *Lancet*, 1:775, 1964.

75. Sarnoff, S. J., and Mitchell, J. H.: The Regulation of the Performance of the Heart, *Am. J. Med.*, 30:747, 1961.

76. Braunwald, E., and Frahm, C. J.: Studies on Starling's Law of the Heart. IV. Observations on the Hemodynamic Functions of the Left Atrium in Man, *Circulation*, 24:633, 1961.

77. Mitchell, J. H., Gilmore, J. P., and Sarnoff, S. J.: The Transport Function of the Atrium: Factors Influencing the Relation between Mean Left Atrial Pressure and Left Ventricular and Diastolic Pressure, *Am. J. Cardiol.*, 9:237, 1962.

78. Grant, C., Bunnell, I. L., and Greene, D. G.: The Reservoir Function of the Left Atrium during Ventricular Systole, *Am. J. Med.*, 37:36, 1964.

79. Braunwald, E.: Personal communication.

80. Lewis, T.: The Value of Quinidine in Cases of Auricular Fibrillation and Methods of Studying the Clinical Reaction, *Am. J. M. Sc.*, 163:781, 1922.

81. Fahr, G.: Treatment of Cardiac Irregularities, *J.A.M.A.*, 111:2268, 1938.

82. Askey, J. M.: Quinidine in the Treatment of Auricular Fibrillation in Association with Congestive Failure, *Ann. Int. Med.*, 24:371, 1946.

83. Sokolow, M., and Edgar, A. L.: Blood Quinidine Concentration as a Guide in the Treatment of Cardiac Arrhythmias, *Circulation*, 1:576, 1950.

84. Sokolow, M.: The Present Status of Therapy of the Cardiac Arrhythmias with Quinidine, *Am. Heart J.*, 42:771, 1951.

85. Goldman, M. J.: Quinidine Treatment of Auricular Fibrillation, *Am. J. M. Sc.*, 222:382, 1951.

86. Laws, C. L., and Levine, S. A.: Clinical Notes on Rheumatic Heart Disease with Special Reference to the Cause of Death, *Am. J. M. Sc.*, 186:833, 1933.

87. Weiss, S., and Davis, D.: Rheumatic Heart Disease. III. Embolic Manifestations, *Am. Heart J.*, 9:45, 1933–1934.

88. Daley, R., Mattingly, T. W., Holt, C. L., Bland, E. F., and White, P. D.: Systemic Arterial Embolism in Rheumatic Heart Disease, *Am. Heart J.*, 42:566, 1951.

89. Hall, H.: Beitrag zur Behandlung der Vorhofsflimmerns: Zusammenfassung, *Acta med. scandinav.*, 108, Suppl. 123, p. 162, 1941.

90. DeGraff, A. C., and Lingg, C.: The Course of Rheumatic Heart Disease in Adults. III. The Influence of Auricular Fibrillation on the Course of Rheumatic Heart Disease, *Am. Heart J.*, 10:630, 1934–1935.

91. Goldman, M. J.: The Management of Chronic Atrial Fibrillation: Indications for and Methods of Conversion to Sinus Rhythm, *Progr. Cardiovas. Dis.*, 2:465, 1960.

92. Sokolow, M., and Perloff, D. B.: The Clinical Pharmacology and Use of Quinidine in Heart Disease, *Progr. Cardiovas. Dis.*, 3:316, 1961.

93. Wright, I. S., and Foley, W. T.: Use of Anti-

coagulants in the Treatment of Heart Disease, *Am. J. Med.,* 3:718, 1947.

94. Askey, J. M.: "Systemic Arterial Embolism: Pathogenesis and Prophylaxis," Grune & Stratton, Inc., New York, 1957, p. 102.

95. Askey, J. M., and Bernstein, S.: The Management of Rheumatic Heart Disease in Relation to Systemic Arterial Embolism, *Progr. Cardiovas. Dis.,* 3:220, 1961.

96. Freeman, I., and Wexler, J.: Anticoagulants for Treatment of Atrial Fibrillation, *J.A.M.A.,* 184:1007, 1963.

97. McMillan, R. L., and Welfare, C. R.: Chronic Auricular Fibrillation: Its Treatment with Quinidine Sulfate, *J.A.M.A.,* 135:1132, 1947.

98. Holzman, D., and Brown, M. G.: The Use of Quinidine in Established Auricular Fibrillation and Flutter, *Am. J. M. Sc.,* 222:644, 1951.

99. Weisman, S. A.: Review and Evaluation of Quinidine Therapy for Auricular Fibrillation, *J.A.M.A.,* 152:496, 1953.

100. Sokolow, M., and Ball, R. E.: Factors Influencing Conversion of Chronic Atrial Fibrillation with Special Reference to Serum Quinidine Concentration, *Circulation,* 14:568, 1956.

101. Sokolow, M.: Some Quantitative Aspects of Treatment with Quinidine, *Ann. Int. Med.,* 45:582, 1956.

102. Rokseth, R., and Storstein, O.: Quinidine Therapy of Chronic Auricular Fibrillation: The Occurrence and Mechanism of Syncope, *Arch. Int. Med.,* 111:184, 1963.

103. Freeman, I., and Wexler, J.: Quinidine in Chronic Atrial Fibrillation, *Am. J. M. Sc.,* 239:181, 1960.

104. Nudelman, P. L., Leff, I. L., and Howe, C. D.: Thrombopenic Purpura Following Quinidine, *J.A.M.A.,* 137:1219, 1948.

105. Bolton, F. G., and Damashek, W.: Thrombocytopenic Purpura Due to Quinidine. I. Clinical Studies, *Blood,* 11:527, 1956.

106. Bolton, F. G.: Thrombocytopenic Purpura Due to Quinidine. II. Serologic Mechanisms, *Blood,* 11:547, 1956.

107. Shulman, N. R.: Immunoreactions Involving Platelets. IV. Studies on the Pathogenesis of Thrombocytopenia in Drug Purpura Using Test Doses of Quinidine in Sensitized Individuals: Their Implications in Idiopathic Thrombocytopenic Purpura, *J. Exper. Med.,* 107:711, 1958.

108. Hunt, J. C., Anderson, M. W., and Hanlon, D. G.: Hemorrhagic Diathesis Related to Quinidine Therapy, *Proc. Staff Meet. Mayo Clinic,* 33:87, 1958.

109. Bourne, S., and O'Sullivan, D. J.: Fetal Thrombocytopenic Purpura Due to Quinidine, *Brit. M. J.,* 1:1046, 1957.

110. Bishop, R. C., Spencer, H. H., and Bethell, F. H.: Quinidine Purpura: Report of Six Cases, *Ann. Int. Med.,* 50:1227, 1959.

111. Sprague, H. B., and Tensey, W. A.: Fever as a Sign of Quinidine Toxicity: Report of Sensitivity in Two Brothers with Thyroid Disease, *New England J. Med.,* 249:796, 1953.

112. Dreyfuss, F., Ehrenfeld, E. N., and Smir, N.: Fever Due to Quinidine, *Acta med. orient.,* 15:241, 1956.

113. Freedman, A. L., Barr, P. S., and Brody, E. A.: Hemolytic Anemia Due to Quinidine: Observations on Its Mechanism, *Am. J. Med.,* 20:806, 1956.

114. Monninger, R., and Platt, D.: Toxic Amblyopia Due to Quinidine, *Am. J. Ophthalmol.,* 43:107, 1957.

115. Goldman, M. J.: Quinidine Therapy of Auricular Fibrillation, *Am. Heart J.,* 40:93, 1950.

116. Selzer, A., and Wray, H. W.: Quinidine Syncope: Paroxysmal Ventricular Fibrillation Occurring during Treatment of Chronic Atrial Arrhythmias, *Circulation,* 30:17, 1964.

117. Sokolow, M., and Ball, R. E.: Interrelationships between Dose, Serum Concentration and Toxicity in the Treatment of Atrial Fibrillation with Quinidine, *Circulation,* 14:1003, 1956.

118. Young, E. H., Rosenblum, M., and McMillan, R. L.: Quinidine for Chronic Auricular Fibrillation in the Patient over 60, *Geriatrics,* 8:19, 1953.

119. Bedard, O.: Quinidine in the Treatment of Auricular Fibrillation, *Am. J. M. Sc.,* 227:530, 1954.

120. Beckwith, J. R., Ibarra, J. A., and Wood, J. E., Jr.: The Problem of Established Atrial Fibrillation, *Am. J. M. Sc.,* 231:519, 1956.

121. Lown, B., Perlroth, M. G., Kaidbey, S., Abe, T., and Harken, D. E.: "Cardioversion" of Atrial Fibrillation: A Report on the Treatment of 65 Episodes in 50 Patients, *New England J. Med.,* 269:325, 1963.

122. Lown, B.: "Cardioversion" of Arrhythmias (I and II), *Mod. Concepts Cardiovas. Dis.,* 33:863, 869, 1964.

123. Goldman, M. J.: Combined Quinidine and Procaine Amide Treatment of Chronic Atrial Fibrillation, *Am. Heart J.,* 54:742, 1957.

124. Lown, B., Kleiger, R., and Wolff, G.: The Technique of Cardioversion, *Am. Heart J.,* 67:282, 1964.

125. Morris, J. J., Jr., Kong, Y., North, W. C., and McIntosh, H. D.: Experience with "Cardioversion" of Atrial Fibrillation and Flutter, *Am. J. Cardiol.,* 14:94, 1964.

125a. Paulk, E. A., and Hurst, J. W.: Clinical Problems of Cardioversion, *Am. Heart J.* (in press).

126. Harris, K. E.: A Series of Cases of Auricular Fibrillation Treated with Quinidine Sulfate, with Special Reference to Duration of Restored Normal Mechanism, *Heart,* 14:283, 1929.

127. Levine, H. D., Lown, B., and Streeper, R. B.: The Clinical Significance of Postextrasystolic T-wave Changes, *Circulation,* 6:538, 1952.

128. Mann, R. H., and Burchell, H. B.: The Significance of T-wave Inversion in Sinus Beats follow-

ing Ventricular Extrasystoles, *Am. Heart J.,* 47:504, 1954.

129. Hellerstein, H. K., and Turell, D. J.: Mode of Death in Coronary Artery Disease: Electrocardiographic and Clinical-Pathologic Correlation, *Circulation,* 18:735, 1958.

130. Wegria, R., Frank, C. W., Wang, H. H., and Kanter, D. M.: The Effect of Auricular and Ventricular Tachycardias on Cardiac Output, Coronary Blood Flow, and Arterial Blood Pressure, *Fed. Proc.,* 12:151, 1953.

131. Herrmann, G. R., Park, H. M., and Hejtmancik, M. R.: Paroxysmal Ventricular Tachycardia: A Clinical and Electrocardiographic Study, *Am. Heart J.,* 57:166, 1959.

132. Fremont, R. E., and King, H.: Digitoxin Causing Ventricular Tachycardia with Peripheral Vascular Collapse: Report of an Unusual Case, *J.A.M.A.,* 143:1052, 1950.

133. Zimdahl, W. T., and Townsend, C. D.: Bidirectional Tachycardia Due to Digitalis Poisoning, *Am. Heart J.,* 47:304, 1954.

134. Lown, B.: "Atrial Arrhythmias, Digitalis and Potassium," Appleton-Century-Crofts, Inc., New York, 1958.

135. Sampson, J. J.: The Relation of Potassium to Digitalis Effectiveness and Toxicity, *California Med.,* 98:249, 1963.

136. Levine, H. D., Merrill, J. P., and Somervilles, W.: Advanced Disturbances of the Cardiac Mechanism in Potassium Intoxication in Man, *Circulation,* 3:889, 1951.

137. Dimond, E. G., and Hayes, W. L.: Benign Paroxysmal Ventricular Tachycardia: Report of a Case, *Ann. Int. Med.,* 53:1255, 1960.

138. Strauss, M. B.: Paroxysmal Ventricular Tachycardia, *Am. J. M. Sc.,* 179:337, 1930.

139. Lundy, C. J., and McLellan, L. L.: Paroxysmal Ventricular Tachycardia, *Ann. Int. Med.,* 7:812, 1934.

140. Armbrust, C. A., Jr., and Levine, S. A.: Paroxysmal Ventricular Tachycardia: A Study of 107 Cases, *Circulation,* 1:28, 1950.

141. Ring, A., and Blankfein, J.: Paroxysmal Ventricular Tachycardia in an Apparently Normal Heart, *Ann. Int. Med.,* 42:680, 1955.

142. Froment, R., Gallavardin, L., and Cahen, P.: Paroxysmal Ventricular Tachycardia: A Clinical Classification, *Brit. Heart J.,* 15:172, 1953.

143. Hoff, H. E., and Nahum, L. H.: The Role of Adrenaline in the Production of Ventricular Rhythms and Their Suppression by Acetyl-β-methylcholine Chloride. *J. Pharmacol. & Exper. Therap.,* 52:235, 1934.

144. Hoff, H. E., and Nahum, L. H.: The Nature of Ventricular Fibrillation Following Electric Shock and Its Prevention by Acetyl-β-methylcholine Chloride, *Am. J. Physiol.,* 110:675, 1935.

145. Nahum, L. H., and Hoff, H. E.: The Experimental Production of Ventricular Fibrillation and Its Pre-

vention by β-methyl-acetyl Choline Chloride, *Am. J. Physiol.,* 109:78, 1934.

146. Hellman, E., and Lind, A.: Bidirectional Tachycardia, *Am. Heart J.,* 51:140, 1956.

147. Langendorf, R. Pick, A., and Winternitz, M.: Mechanisms of Intermittent Ventricular Bigeminy. I. Appearance of Ectopic Beats Dependent upon Length of the Ventricular Cycle, the "Rule of Bigeminy," *Circulation,* 11:422, 1955.

148. Langendorf, R., and Pick, A.: Mechanisms of Intermittent Ventricular Bigeminy. II. Parasystole and Parasystole or Re-entry with Conduction Disturbance, *Circulation,* 11:431, 1955.

149. Sheehan, H. L.: Symmetrical Cortical Necrosis of Kidneys, *Brit. M. J.,* 2:1327, 1950.

150. Chinsky, M., Wolff, R. J., and Sherry, S.: Serum Transaminase Activity: A Comparison of the Pyruvic and Oxaloacetic Transaminase, *Am. J. M. Sc.,* 233:400, 1957.

151. Berte, S. J., and Smith, A. T.: Adams-Stokes Syndrome Due to Ventricular Fibrillation and Tachycardia, *New England J. Med.,* 248:282, 1953.

152. Elliot, A. R., and Fenn, G. K.: Long Continued Ventricular Tachycardia: Report of an Unusual Case, *Am. Heart J.,* 9:806, 1933–1934.

153. Dressler, W., and Rossler, H.: The Occurrence in Paroxysmal Ventricular Tachycardia of Ventricular Complexes Transitional in Shape to Sino-auricular Beats, *Am. Heart J.,* 44:485, 1952.

154. Gouaux, J. L., and Ashman, R.: Auricular Fibrillation with Aberration Simulating Ventricular Paroxysmal Tachycardia, *Am. Heart J.,* 34:366, 1947.

155. Pick, A., and Langendorf, R.: Differentiation of Supraventricular and Ventricular Tachycardias, *Progr. Cardiovas Dis.,* 2:291, 1960.

156. Langendorf, R.: Differential Diagnosis of Ventricular Paroxysmal Tachycardia, *Exper. Med. & Surg.,* 8:228, 1950.

157. Lown, B., Neuman, J., Amarasingham, R., and Berkovits, B. V.: Comparison of Alternating Current with Direct Current Electroshock Across the Closed Chest, *Am. J. Cardiol.,* 10:223, 1962.

158. Lown, B., Amarasingham, R., Neuman, J., and Berkovits, B. V.: The Use of Synchronized Direct Current Countershock in the Treatment of Cardiac Arrhythmias, *Tr. Am. Soc. Clin. Invest.,* Apr. 30, 1962.

159. Lown, B., Amarasingham, R., and Neuman, J.: New Method for Terminating Cardiac Arrhythmias: Use of Synchronized Capacitor Discharge, *J.A.M.A.,* 182:548, 1962.

160. Acierno, L. J., and Gubner, R.: Utility and Limitations of Intravenous Quinidine in Arrhythmias, *Am. Heart J.,* 41:733, 1951.

161. Binder, M. J., and Rosove, L.: Paroxysmal Ventricular Tachycardia and Fibrillation Due to Quinidine, *Am. J. Med.,* 12:491, 1952.

162. Marriott, H. J. L.: Rational Approach to Quini-

dine Therapy, *Mod. Concepts Cardiovas. Dis.*, 31:745, 1962.

163. Lucas, B. G. B., and Short, D. S.: Procaine Amide in the Control of Cardiac Arrhythmias, *Brit. Heart J.*, 14:470, 1952.

164. Kayden, H. J., Steele, J. M., Mark, L. C., and Brodie, B. B.: The Use of Procaine Amide in Cardiac Arrhythmias, *Circulation*, 4:13, 1951.

165. Fernandez, Barbieri F., Corday, E., Lang, T. W.: Tratamiento de Arritmias con Drogas Vasopresoras, *Arch. Inst. Cardiol. Mex.*, 34:395, 1964.

166. Gold, H., and Corday, E.: Vasopressor Therapy in the Cardiac Arrhythmias, *New England J. Med.*, 260:1151, 1959.

167. Brest, A. N., Staughin, J., Singer, A., and Likoff, W.: Preliminary Observations on a New Antiarrhythmic Agent (RO-2-5803), *Am. J. Cardiol.*, 5:811, 1960.

168. Green, R. S., Geiss, P. G., Sumen, A., and Schuster, J.: Preliminary Evaluation of RO-2-5803, an Antiarrhythmic Agent, *Am. J. Cardiol.*, 5:806, 1960.

169. Lang, T. W., Bernstein, H., Barbieri, F. F., and Corday, E.: Diphenylhydantoin in the Treatment of Cardiac Arrhythmias. I. Treatment of Digitalis Toxic Arrhythmias (In press).

170. Bernstein, H., Lang, T. W., Gold, H., and Corday, E.: Diphenylhydantoin in the Treatment of Cardiac Arrhythmias. II. Treatment of Drug Resistant Cardiac Arrhythmias (In press).

171. Salley, S. M.: Unusual Atropine Effect on Ventricular Tachycardia, *Am. J. M. Sc.*, 183:256, 1932.

172. Wilburne, M., Surtshin, A., Rodbard, S., and Katz, L. N.: Inhibition of Paroxysmal Ventricular Tachycardia by Atropine, *Am. Heart J.*, 34:860, 1947.

173. Zwillinger, L.: Über die Magnesiumwirking auf das Herz, *Klin. Wchnschr.*, 14:1429, 1935.

174. Boyd, L. J., and Scherf, D.: Magnesium Sulfate in Paroxysmal Tachycardia, *Am. J. M. Sc.*, 206:43, 1943.

175. Szekely, P., and Wynne, N. A.: Effects of Magnesium on Cardiac Arrhythmias Caused by Digitalis, *Clin. Sc.*, 10:241, 1951.

176. Corday, E., Gold, H., and Jaffe, H. L.: Radioiodine Treatment of Paroxysmal Supraventricular Tachycardia in the Euthyroid Patient, *Circulation*, 17:900, 1958.

177. Corday, E., Jaffe, H. L., and Irving, D. W.: Hypometabolic Treatment of Heart Disease, *Am. J. Cardiol.*, 6:952, 1960.

178. Prevost, J. L., and Battelli, F.: On Some Effects of Electrical Discharges on the Heart of Mammals, *Compt. rend. Acad. sc.*, 129:1267, 1899.

179. Hooker, D. R.: On the Recovery of the Heart in Electric Shock, *Am. J. Physiol.*, 91:305, 1930.

180. Hooker, D. R., Kouwenhoven, W. B., and Langworthy, O. R.: The Effect of Alternating Electric Currents on the Heart, *Am. J. Physiol.*, 103:444, 1933.

181. Beck, C. S., Pritchard, W. H., and Feil, S. H.: Ventricular Fibrillation of Long Duration Abolished by Electric Shock, *J.A.M.A.*, 135:985, 1947.

182. Zoll, P. M., Linenthal, A. J., Gibson, W., Paul, W. H., and Norman, L. R.: Termination of Ventricular Fibrillation in Man by Externally Applied Electric Countershock, *New England J. Med.*, 254:727, 1956.

183. Kouwenhoven, W. B., Milnor, W. R., Knickerbocker, G. G., and Chestnut, W. R.: Closed Chest Defibrillation of the Heart, Surgery, 42:550, 1957.

184. Peleska, B.: Transthoracic and Direct Defibrillation, *Rozhl. chir.*, 26:731, 1957.

185. Hellerstein, H., and Hornstein, T. R.: Treatment of Ventricular Tachycardia and Ventricular Fibrillation, *Mod. Treatment*, 1:725–760, 1964.

186. Bellet, S.: "Clinical Disorders of the Heart Beat," 2d ed., Lea & Febiger, Philadelphia, 1963.

187. Moe, T.: A Case of Morgagni-Adams-Stokes Attacks Caused by Transient Recurrent Ventricular Fibrillation without Apparent Organic Disease, *Acta med. scandinav.*, 130:416, 1948.

188. Stern, T. N.: Paroxysmal Ventricular Fibrillation in the Absence of Other Disease, *Ann. Int. Med.*, 47:552, 1957.

189. Storstein, O.: Stokes-Adams Attacks Caused by Ventricular Fibrillation in a Man with Otherwise Normal Heart, *Acta med. scandinav.*, 133:437, 1949.

190. Harris, A. S.: Terminal Electrocardiographic Patterns in Experimental Anoxia, Coronary Occlusion and Hemorrhagic Shock, *Am. Heart J.*, 35:895, 1948.

191. Enselberg, C. D., Croce, J. P., Jr., and Lown, B.: Ventricular Fibrillation Due to Digitalis Preparations, *Circulation*, 3:647, 1951.

192. Michel, J., Johnson, A. D., Bridges, W. C., Lehmann, J. H., Gray, F., Field, L., and Green, D. M.: Arrhythmias during Intracardiac Catheterization, *Circulation*, 2:240, 1950.

193. Fowler, N. O., Westcott, R. N., and Scott, R. C.: Disturbances in Cardiac Mechanism of Several Hours' Duration Complicating Cardiac Venous Catheterization, *Am. Heart J.*, 42:652, 1951.

194. Weinberg, D. I., Artley, J. L., Whalen, R. E., and McIntosh, H. D.: Electric Shock Hazards in Cardiac Catheterization, *Circulation Res.*, 11:1004, 1962.

195. Stroud, M. W., and Feil, H. S.: The Terminal Electrocardiogram, *Am. Heart J.*, 35:910, 1948.

196. Hoffa, M., and Ludwig, C.: Einige neue Versuche über Herzbewegung, *Ztschr. f. rat. Med.*, 9:107, 1850.

197. Wiggers, C. J.: The Mechanism and Nature of Ventricular Fibrillation, *Am. Heart J.*, 20:399, 1940.

198. Schwartz, S. P., and Jezer, A.: Transient Ventricular Fibrillation: The Clinical and Electro-

cardiographic Manifestations of the Syncopal Seizures in a Patient with Auriculoventricular Dissociation, *Arch. Int. Med.,* **50**:450, 1932.

199. Schwartz, S. P., Orloff, J., and Fox, C.: Transient Ventricular Fibrillation. I. The Prefibrillary Period During Established Auriculoventricular Dissociation with a Note on the Phonocardiogram Obtained at Such Times, *Am. Heart J.,* **37**:21, 1949.

200. Cole, S. L., and Corday, E.: Four-minute Limit for Cardiac Resuscitation, *J.A.M.A.,* **161**:1456, 1956.

201. Leeds, S. E.: Cardiac Resuscitation, *J.A.M.A.,* **152**:1409, 1953.

202. Jude, J. R., Kouwenhoven, W. B., and Knickerbocker, G. G.: Cardiac Arrest, *J.A.M.A.,* **178**:1063, 1961.

203. Zoll, P. M., Linenthal, A. J., and Zarsky, L. R. N.: Ventricular Fibrillation: Treatment and Prevention by External Electric Currents, *New England J. Med.,* **262**:105, 1960.

204. Carden, M. L., and Steinhaus, J. E.: Lidocaine in Cardiac Resuscitation from Ventricular Fibrillation, *Circulation Res.,* **4**:680, 1956.

205. Von Dougen, K.: The Action of Xylocaine on Fibrillation of the Heart, *Arch. internat. pharmacodyn.,* **96**:45, 1953.

206. Day, H.: Summary of Current Therapy: An Intensive Coronary Care Area, *Dis. Chest,* **44**:423, 1963.

207. Borduas, J. L., Rakita, L., Kennamer, R., and Prinzmetal, M.: Studies on the Mechanisms of Ventricular Activity. XIV. Clinical and Experimental Studies on Accelerated Auriculoventricular Conduction, *Circulation,* **11**:69, 1955.

208. Grant, R. P.: The Mechanism of A-V Arrhythmias with an Electrical Analogue of the Human A-V Node, *Am. J. Med.,* **20**:334, 1956.

209. Hoffman, B. F.: Physiology of Atrioventricular Transmission, *Circulation,* **24**:506, 1961.

210. Hoffman, B. F., Moore, N., Stuckey, J. H., and Cranefield, P. F.: Functional Properties of the Atrioventricular Conduction System, *Circulation Res.,* **13**:308, 1963.

211. James, T. N.: Morphology of the Human Atrioventricular Node, with Remarks Pertinent to Its Electrophysiology, *Am. Heart J.,* **62**:756, 1961.

212. Scherf, D., and Cohen, J.: The Atrioventricular Node and Selected Cardiac Arrhythmias, Grune & Stratton, Inc., New York, 1964.

213. Lev, M., and Unger, P. N.: The Pathology of the Conduction System in Acquired Heart Disease. I. Severe Atrioventricular Block, *A.M.A. Arch. Path.,* **60**:502, 1955.

214. Moe, G. K., Preston, J. B., and Burlington, H.: Physiologic Evidence for a Dual A-V Transmission System, *Circulation Res.,* **4**:357, 1956.

215. James, T. N., and Reynolds, E. W., Jr.: Pathology of the Cardiac Conduction System in a Case of Diphtheria Associated with Atrial Arrhythmia and Heart Block, *Circulation,* **28**:283, 1963.

216. Rosenblueth, A.: Two Processes for Auriculo-Ventricular and Ventriculo-Auricular Propagation of Impulses in the Heart, *Am. J. Physiol.,* **194**:495, 1958.

217. Scher, A. M., Rodriguez, M. I., Likane, J., and Young, A. C.: The Mechanism of Atrioventricular Conduction, *Circulation Res.,* **7**:54, 1959.

218. Juhasz-Nagy, A., and Sventivanyi, M.: Localization of the Receptors of the Coronary Chemoreflex in the Dog, *Arch. internat. pharmacodyn.,* **131**:39, 1961.

219. Lown, B., Arons, W. L., Ganong, W. F., Vazifdar, J. E., and Levine, S. A.: Adrenal Steroids and Auriculoventricular Conduction, *Am. Heart J.,* **50**:70, 1955.

220. Paul, M. H., Rudolph, A. M., and Nadas, A. S.: Congenital Complete Atrioventricular Block: Problems of Clinical Assessment, *Circulation,* **18**:183, 1959.

221. Penton, G., Miller, H., and Levine, S. A.: Some Clinical Features of Complete Heart Block, *Circulation,* **13**:801, 1956.

222. Rowe, J. C., and White, P. D.: Complete Heart Block: A Follow-up Study, *Ann. Int. Med.,* **49**:260, 1958.

223. Lev, M.: The Pathology of Complete Heart Block, *Progr. Cardiovas. Dis.,* **6**:317, 1964.

224. Dack, S., and Robbin, S. R.: Treatment of Heart Block and Adams-Stokes Syndrome with Sustained-action Isoproterenol, *J.A.M.A.,* **176**:505, 1961.

225. Tobian, L.: Prevention of Stokes-Adams Seizures with Chlorothiazide, *New England J. Med.,* **265**:623, 1961.

226. Friedberg, C. K., Kahn, M., Scheuer, J., Bleifer, S., and Dack, S.: Adams-Stokes Syndrome Associated with Chronic Heart Block: Treatment with Corticosteroids, *J.A.M.A.,* **172**:1146, 1960.

227. DeSanctis, R. W.: Short-term Use of Intravenous Electrode in Heart Block, *J.A.M.A.,* **184**:544, 1963.

228. Furman, S., and Robinson, G.: Stimulation of the Ventricular Endocardial Surface in Control of Complete Heart Block, *Ann. Surg.,* **150**:841, 1959.

229. Goetz, R. H.: Bi-polar Catheter Electrode as Temporary Pacemaker in Stokes-Adams Syndrome, *Surg. Gynec. & Obst.,* **116**:712, 1963.

230. Parsonnet, V., Zucker, I. R., Gilbert, L., and Asa, M. M.: An Intracardiac Bipolar Electrode for Interim Treatment of Complete Heart Block, *Am. J. Cardiol.,* **10**:261, 1962.

231. Samet, P., Jacobs, W., and Bernstein, W. H.: Electrode Catheter Pacemaker in the Treatment of Complete Heart Block in the Presence of Acute Myocardial Infarction: Report of Four Cases, *Am. J. Cardiol.,* **11**:379, 1963.

232. Schwedel, J. B., Furman, S., and Escher, D. J. W.: Use of Intracardiac Pacemaker in Treatment of Stokes-Adams Seizures, *Progr. Cardiovas. Dis.,* **3**:170, 1960.

233. Benchimol, A., Li, Y.-B., Voth, R. B., and Roland, A. S.: Effect of Heart Rate, Exercise, and Nitroglycerin on the Cardiac Dynamics in Complete Heart Block, *Circulation*, **28**:510, 1963.

234. Müller, O. F., and Bellet, S.: Treatment of Intractable Heart Failure in the Presence of Complete Atrioventricular Heart Block by the Use of the Internal Cardiac Pacemaker: Report of Two Cases, *New England J. Med.*, **265**:768, 1961.

235. Nathan, D. A., Center, S., Wu, C., and Keller, W.: An Implantable Synchronous Pacemaker for the Long Term Correction of Complete Heart Block, *Am. J. Cardiol.*, **11**:362, 1963.

236. Chardack, W. M., Gage, A. A., Schimert, G., Thomson, N. B., Sanford, C. E., and Greatbatch, W.: Two Years' Clinical Experience with Implantable Pacemaker for Complete Heart Block, *Dis. Chest*, **43**:225, 1963.

237. Dressler, W., Jonas, S., and Kantrowitz, A.: Observations in Patients with Implanted Cardiac Pacemaker. I. Clinical Experience, *Am. Heart J.*, **66**:325, 1963.

238. Elmquist, R., Landegren, J., Pettersson, S. O., Senning, A., and William-Olsson, G.: Artificial Pacemaker for Treatment of Adams-Stokes Syndrome and slow Heart Rate, *Am. Heart J.* **65**:731, 1963.

239. Landegren, J., and Biörck, G.: The Clinical Assessment and Treatment of Complete Heart Block and Adams-Stokes Attacks, *Medicine*, **42**:171, 1963.

240. Weirich, W. L., Paneth, M., Gott, V. L., and Lillehei, C. W.: Control of Complete Heart Block by Use of an Artificial Pacemaker and a Myocardial Electrode, *Circulation Res.*, **6**:410, 1958.

241. Zoll, P. M., and Linenthal, A. J.: External and Internal Electric Cardiac Pacemakers, *Circulation*, **28**:455, 1963.

241a. Bruce, R. A., Blackmon, J. K., Cobb, L. A., and Dodge, H. T.: Treatment of Asystole of Heart Block during Acute Myocardial Infarction with Electrode Catheter Pacing, *Am. Heart. J.*, **69**:460, 1965.

241b. Paulk, E. A. and Hurst, J. W.: Unpublished data.

242. Perry, E. L., and Jaeck, J. L.: Use of Corticosteroids in Stokes-Adams Syndrome, *Ann. Int. Med.*, **53**:589, 1960.

243. Zoll, P. M., Linenthal, A. J., Gibson, W., Paul, M. H., and Norman, L. R.: Intravenous Drug Therapy of Stokes-Adams Disease: Effects of Sympathomimetic Amines on Ventricular Rhythmicity and Atrioventricular Conduction, *Circulation*, **17**:325, 1958.

244. Linenthal, A. J., and Zoll, P. M.: Prevention of Ventricular Tachycardia and Fibrillation by Intravenous Isoproterenol and Epinephrine, *Circulation*, **27**:5, 1963.

244a. Jacobs, D. R., Donoso, E., and Friedberg, C. K.:

A-V Dissociation: A Relatively Frequent Arrhythmia, *Medicine*, **40**:101, 1961.

245. Wilson, F. N., Johnston, R. F. D., Hill, I. G. W., Macleod, A. G., and Barker, P S.: The Significance of Electrocardiograms Characterized by an Abnormally Long QRS Interval and by Broad S Deflection in Lead I, *Am. Heart J.*, **9**:459, 1934.

246. Pick, A.: Recent Posterior Wall Infarction in the Presence of Left Bundle Branch Block, with Pseudo-ventricular Tachycardia and Pseudo-preexcitation, *Dis. Chest*, **37**:693, 1960.

247. Somerville, W., and Wood, P.: Cardiac Infarction with Bundle Branch Block, *Brit. Heart J.*, **11**:305, 1949.

248. Lenègre, J., Chevalier, H., and Jacquot, R.: Étude histologique de sept cas de bloc de la branch droite, *Arch. mal. coeur*, **44**:481, 1951.

249. Papp, C., and Smith, K. S.: The Changing Electrocardiogram in Wilson Block, *Circulation*, **11**:53, 1955.

250. Willius, F. A., and Amberg, S.: Two Cases of Secondary Tumor of the Heart in Children, in One of Which the Diagnosis Was Made During Life, *M. Clin. North America*, **13**:1307, 1930.

251. Lloyd, P. C.: Heart Block Due to Primary Lymphangioendothelioma of A-V Node, *Bull. Johns Hopkins Hosp.*, **44**:149, 1929.

252. Amsterdam, H. J., Grayzel, D. M., and Louria, A. L.: Hemangioendothelioblastoma of the Heart, *Am. Heart J.*, **37**:291, 1949.

253. Burkhardt, E. A., Eggleston, C., and Smith, L. W.: Electrocardiographic Changes and Peripheral Nerve Palsies in Toxic Diphtheria, *Am. J. M. Sc.*, **195**:301, 1938.

254. Begg, N. D.: Diphtheritic Myocarditis: Electrocardiographic Study, *Lancet*, **1**:857, 1937.

255. Benchimon, A. B., and Dias Carneiro, R.: Diphtheritic Myocarditis, *Arq. brasil. med.*, **42**:85, 1952.

256. Levander-Lindgren, M.: "Electrocardiographic Structures in Scarlet Fever," Affarstryek, Stockholm, 1952.

257. Shookhoff, C., and Taran, L. M.: Electrocardiographic Studies in Infectious Diseases. II. Scarlet Fever, *Am. J. Dis. Child.*, **42**:554, 1931.

258. Kerr, S.: "Subacute Bacterial Endocarditis," Charles C Thomas, Publisher, Springfield, Ill., 1955.

259. Leonard, J. C., and Smith, W. G.: Syphilitic Aortic Incompetence with Specific Reference to Prognosis and Effect of Treatment, *Lancet*, **1**:234, 1957.

260. Major, R. H.: Stokes-Adams Disease Due to Gumma of the Heart, *A.M.A. Arch. Int. Med.*, **31**:857, 1923.

261. Weinstein, A., Kampmeier, R. H., and Harwood, T. R.: Complete Heart Block Due to Syphilis, *A.M.A. Arch. Int. Med.*, **100**:90, 1957.

262. Ross, L. J.: Electrocardiographic Findings in Measles, *Am. J. Dis. Child.*, **83**:282, 1952.

263. Master, A. M., Romanoff, A., and Jaffe, H.: Electrocardiographic Changes in Pneumonia, *Am. Heart J.*, **6**:696, 1930.

264. Thomson, K. J., Rutstein, D. D., Tlomach, D. M., and Walker, W.: Electrocardiographic Studies during and after Pneumococcus Pneumonia, *Am. Heart J.*, **31**:565, 1946.

265. DeGraff, A. C., Travell, J. G., and Yager, J. A.: An Electrocardiographic Study of the Heart in Lobar Pneumonia, *J. Clin. Invest.*, **10**:633, 1931.

266. Mirrill, J. P., Levine, H. D., Somerville, W., and Smith, S.: Clinical Recognition and Treatment of Acute Potassium Intoxication, *Ann. Int. Med.*, **33**:797, 1950.

267. Kittle, C. F., Santos, E. M., and Dimond, E. G.: Persistent Right Bundle Branch Block Due to Pulmonic Valvotomy and Infundibulectomy, *Am. Surgeon*, **22**:80, 1956.

268. Sandberg, L.: Studies on Electrocardiographic Changes during Exercise Tests, *Acta med. scandinav.* (Suppl.) **169**:365, 1961.

269. Sandberg, A. A., Wener, J., Master, A. M., and Scherlis, L.: Intermittent and Transient Bundle Branch Block: A Clinical and Electrocardiographic Study, *Ann. Int. Med.*, **35**:1085, 1951.

270. Sanabria, T.: Étude anatomo-pathologique du bloc de branche, *Acta cardiol.*, **8**:145, 1953.

271. Deforest, R. E.: Four Cases of "Benign" Left Bundle Branch Block in the Same Family, *Am. Heart J.*, **51**:398, 1956.

272. Barker, J. M. and Valencia, F.: The Precordial Electrocardiogram in Incomplete Right Bundle Branch Block, *Am. Heart J.*, **38**:376, 1946.

273. Sodi-Pallares, D., Estandia, G. A., Soberón, J., and Rodríguez, M. I.: The Left Intraventricular Potential of the Human Heart. II. Criteria for Diagnosis of Incomplete Bundle Branch Block, *Am. Heart J.*, **40**:655, 1950.

274. Shearn, M. A., and Rytand, D. A.: Intermittent Bundle-branch Block: Observations with Special Reference to the Critical Heart Rate, *Arch. Int. Med.*, **91**:448, 1953.

275. Vesell, H., and Frieldfeld, L.: Critical Rates in Ventricular Conduction. IV. Duration of Unstable Bundle Branch Block, *Am. Heart J.*, **44**:830, 1952.

276. Contro, S., and Luisada, A. A.: Modifications of the Heart Sounds in Bundle Branch Block, *J. Mt. Sinai Hosp.*, **19**:70, 1952.

277. Wolferth, C. C., and Margolies, A.: Asynchronism in Contraction of the Ventricles in the So-called Type of Bundle-branch Block, *Am. Heart J.*, **10**:425, 1935.

278. Sodeman, W. A., Johnston, F. D., and Wilson, F. N.: The Q1 Deflection of the Electrocardiogram in Bundle Branch Block and Axis Deviation, *Am. Heart J.*, **28**:271, 1944.

279. Perera, G. A., Levine, S. A., and Erlanger, H.: Prognosis of Right Bundle Branch Block, *Brit. Heart J.*, **4**:35, 1942.

280. Vazifdar, J. P., and Levine, S. A.: Benign Bundle Branch Block, *Arch. Int. Med.*, **89**:568, 1952.

281. Kurtz, C. M.: Transient Complete Bundle-branch Block, *Am. Heart J.*, **11**:212, 1936.

282. Packard, J. M., and Graybiel, A.: Bundle Branch Block as a Temporary Phenomenon in Thyrotoxicosis: Report of a Case, *Am. Heart J.*, **39**:144, 1950.

283. Wolff, L.: Anomalous Atrioventricular Excitation (Wolff-Parkinson-White) Syndrome, *Circulation*, **19**:14, 1959.

284. Wolff, L.: Wolff-Parkinson-White Syndrome: Historical and Clinical Features, *Progr. Cardiovas. Dis.*, **2**:677, 1960.

285. Averill, K. H., Fosmoe, R. J., and Lamb, L. E.: Electrocardiographic Findings in 67,375 Asymptomatic Subjects. IV. Wolff-Parkinson-White Syndrome, *Am. J. Cardiol.*, **6**:108, 1960.

286. Engle, M. A.: Wolff-Parkinson-White Syndrome in Infants and Children, *Am. J. Dis. Child.*, **84**:692, 1952.

287. Sondergaard, G.: The Wolff-Parkinson-White Syndrome in Infants, *Acta med. scandinav.*, **145**:386, 1953.

288. Schiebler, G. L., Adams, P., and Anderson, R. C.: Wolff-Parkinson-White Syndrome, *Pediatrics*, **29**:585, 1959.

289. Heftmancik, M. R., and Herrmann, G. R.: Electrocardiographic Syndrome of Short P-R Interval and Broad QRS Complexes: Clinical Study of 80 Cases, *Abst. 30th Scient. Sess. Am. Heart Assoc.*, 1957, p. 892.

290. Lyle, A. M.: Latent Wolff-Parkinson-White Syndrome, *Am. Heart J.*, **46**:49, 1953.

291. Averill, J. H.: Wolff-Parkinson-White Syndrome Occurring in Brothers, *Am. Heart J.*, **51**:943, 1956.

292. Harnischfeger, W. W.: Hereditary Occurrence of Pre-excitation (W-P-W) Syndrome) with Reentry Mechanism and Concealed Conduction, *Circulation*, **19**:28, 1959.

293. Willis, W. H., and Shepard, C. C.: The Familial Incidence of Certain Unusual Diseases, *North New York M. J.*, **10**:19, 1953.

294. Öhnell, R. F.: "Pre-excitation: A Cardiac Abnormality," P. A. Norstedt & Söner, Stockholm, 1944.

295. Borduas, J. L., Rakita, L., Kennamer, R., and Prinzmetal, M.: Studies on the Mechanism of Ventricular Activity. XIV. Clinical and Experimental Studies of Accelerated Aurico-ventricular Conduction, *Circulation*, **11**:69, 1955.

296. Kent, A. F. S.: Research on the Structure and Function of the Mammalian Heart, *J. Physiol.*, **14**:233, 1893.

297. Kent, A. F. S.: Observations on the Auriculoventricular Junction of the Mammalian Heart, *Quart. J. Exper. Physiol.*, **7**:193, 1914.

298. Wood, F. C., Wolferth, C. C., and Geckeler, G. D.: Histologic Demonstration of Accessory Muscular Connections between Auricle and Ven-

tricle in a Case of Short P-R Interval and Prolonged QRS Complex, *Am. Heart J.*, 25:454, 1943.

299. Holzmann, M., and Scherf, D.: Über Elektro-
kardiogramme mit verkurzter Vorhof-Kammer-
Distanz und positiven P-Zacken, *Ztschr. klin.
Med.*, 121:404, 1932.

300. Wolferth, C. C., and Wood, F. C.: Further Observations on the Mechanism of the Production
of a Short P-R Interval in Association with Prolongation of QRS Complex, *Am. Heart J.*, 22:450,
1941.

301. Butterworth, J. S., and Poindexter, C. A.: Short
P-R Interval Associated with a Prolonged QRS
Complex, *A.M.A. Arch. Int. Med.*, 59:431, 1942.

302. Roberts, G. H., and Abramson, D. I.: Ventricular
Complexes of Bundle Branch Block Type Associated with Short P-R Intervals, *Ann. Int. Med.*,
9:983, 1936.

303. Wilson, F. N.: A Case in Which the Vagus Influenced the Form of the Ventricular Complex of
the Electrocardiogram, *A.M.A. Arch. Int. Med.*,
16:1008, 1915.

304. Dunn, J. J., Sarrell, W., and Franklin, R. B.: The
Wolff-Parkinson-White Syndrome Associated with
Paroxysmal Ventricular Tachycardia, *Am. Heart
J.*, 47:462, 1954.

305. Levine, S. A., and Beeson, P. B.: The Wolff-
Parkinson-White Syndrome with Paroxysms of
Ventricular Tachycardia, *Am. Heart J.*, 22:401,
1941.

306. Silverman, J. L., and Werner, M.: Fatal Paroxysmal Tachycardia in a Newborn Infant with the
Wolff-Parkinson-White Syndrome, *J. Pediat.*, 37:
765, 1950.

17 SYNCOPE, SHOCK, AND SUDDEN DEATH

*Arnold M. Weissler, M.D., and
James V. Warren, M.D.*

SYNCOPE

Definition and Pathogenesis of Syncope

The terms *syncope* and *fainting* refer to a dramatic clinical syndrome characterized by sudden
and transient loss or impairment of consciousness
associated with inability to maintain postural tone.
It should be recognized that these terms refer
to symptom pictures which can be induced by a
variety of mechanisms. Despite the frequency with
which syncope is encountered, knowledge of its
mechanisms and of the varied circumstances which
may induce fainting was sparse until recent years.
The loss or impairment of consciousness reflects

an alteration in cerebral function which is fundamental to the development of syncope. Such
changes in cerebral function may be produced by
circulatory, metabolic, or neuropsychologic mechanisms, or by a combination of these factors. In the
following discussion, we will focus attention on
syncope of circulatory origin. Such disease states
as the cerebral dysrhythmias, vertigo, cataplexy,
and hysteria will be stressed only to elucidate the
differentiation of their mechanisms from that of
syncope of circulatory origin.

The loss of consciousness accompanying a
sudden episode of syncope of circulatory origin
reflects an impairment in cerebral cellular metabolism usually resulting from an inadequacy of
blood flow to the brain. The circulation and metabolism of the brain have certain unique characteristics, the understanding of which lends insight
into the various mechanisms of fainting.[1] The brain
maintains a remarkably stable rate of oxygen utilization, in the range of 3.5 ml oxygen per 100 Gm
per min and corresponding to an average oxygen
consumption of 50 ml per min for the adult brain.[2]
This level of oxygen consumption remains constant
over a wide spectrum of cerebral and cardiovascular performance. The brain is unique in its
lack of storage capacity for readily available
energy substrate and in its reliance predominantly
on glucose to subserve its energy needs.[3] Thus,
adequate cerebral function is highly dependent on
the omnipresent maintenance of an adequate cerebral blood flow. In the normal adult, in the
recumbent position, cerebral blood flow is 55 ml
per 100 Gm of brain per min, corresponding
to a total cerebral blood flow of 700 to 750 ml
per min. The critical dependence of the level of
consciousness on the adequacy of blood flow to
the brain is emphasized in the observation that
with sudden complete interruption of cerebral
arterial inflow, consciousness is lost within 10 sec.[4]

Among the major determinants of cerebral blood
flow are the cardiac output, the perfusion pressure
at the level of the brain, and the resistance of the
cerebral vascular bed.[1,5] The low resistance in the
cerebral vascular bed relative to the total peripheral resistance provides the brain with a significant
component of the cardiac output (15 per cent in the
normal resting individual). With a fall in cardiac
output, cerebral vascular resistance decreases relative to total vascular resistance, allowing the maintenance of adequate cerebral blood flow. The delivery of this blood is dependent on the maintenance of an adequate perfusion pressure to the
brain. This perfusion pressure is essentially the
mean arterial pressure minus venous pressure at
the level of the brain. The anatomic position of
the brain above the level of the heart in the stand-

ing posture adds a circulatory stress relative to the maintenance of perfusion which is not present in other vital vascular beds.[6,7] The fall in jugular venous pressure accompanying a change from recumbent to upright posture assists in maintaining adequacy of perfusion pressure, while the decrease in intracranial pressure due to the shifts in cerebrospinal fluid aids in maintaining patency of the cerebral capillary bed.

Probably of greatest significance in the regulation and adaptation of the cerebral vascular bed is the intrinsic adjustment of the cerebral vessels to changes in perfusion pressure and cardiac output.[8] Although there is sympathetic and parasympathetic innervation to the cerebral vessels in man, alterations in autonomic tone appear to exert little effect in regulating the blood flow to the brain. On the other hand, local factors, particularly the tension of carbon dioxide in the cerebral bed, play a dominant role in cerebral vascular adaptation to peripheral circulatory changes. In view of the constancy of cerebral metabolism, a fall in cerebral blood flow is attended by a rise in cerebral capillary CO_2 tension, while oxygen tension diminishes. Both these changes induce potent vasodilator effects on the cerebral vascular bed, which serve to lower cerebral vascular resistance and reequilibrate cerebral flow to cerebral demand.

Syncope may then be conveniently classified according to the alteration in physiologic mechanism involved. Although a combination of mechanisms is often present, the primary factors form the basis for the present classification:[*]

1. Syncope due to decrease of cerebral perfusion pressure
   a. Vasodepressor syncope
   b. Orthostatic hypotension
   c. Cerebral-occlusive syncope
   d. Carotid sinus syncope—vasodepressor type
   e. Cough syncope
   f. Postmicturition syncope
2. Syncope due to inadequacy of cardiac output—cardiac syncope
   a. Syncope in cardiac disease
   b. Cardiac arrhythmias and Morgagni-Adams-Stokes attacks
   c. Reflex asystole
3. Syncope due to metabolic causes
   a. Hypoxia
   b. Hypoglycemia
   c. Hyperventilation syndrome
4. Syncope due to neuropsychologic factors
   a. Carotid sinus syncope—cerebral type
   b. Hysterical syncope

[*] In this classification, the term *syncope* refers to either loss or impairment of consciousness.

    c. Cerebral dysrhythmias
    d. Syncopal migraine
    e. Vertigo

Syncope Due to Decrease of Cerebral Perfusion Pressure

Vasodepressor Syncope

Vasodepressor syncope, or the common faint, is the most frequently encountered clinical form of syncope. This form of fainting may occur as a response to sudden emotional stress or in a setting of real, threatened, or fantasied injury. The reaction is not infrequently brought on by venepuncture or the sight of blood, and is also observed after sudden painful experiences such as may occur during surgical manipulation or following severe tissue injury. It is particularly likely to occur in certain environmental settings, such as in a hot and crowded room, especially if the individual is fatigued, hungry, or ill or has experienced recent blood loss. The common faint is usually encountered when the patient is in the upright or sitting posture but may rarely occur while the patient is recumbent. Clinically, vasodepressor syncope is characterized by a fall in blood pressure associated with impairment or loss of consciousness and accompanied by a marked degree of autonomic overactivity, as evidenced by pallor, sweating, nausea, mydriasis, hyperventilation, and bradycardia. So dramatic is the clinical picture of the common faint that it has often stimulated authors to eloquent description. Weiss's portrayal is particularly vivid:

In the severe type with rapid onset the patient collapses instantly without warning. The body lies crumpled and motionless. The face and the body surface are ghastly pale. The pupils usually are dilated, and the conjunctival reflexes are absent. Respiration usually is either shallow and slow, or deep and sighing. The heart sounds are slow or normal in rate, barely audible. The radial pulse may be imperceptible or weak, but the carotid and femoral pulsations usually are easily palpable. There may be rather slow, clonic movements localized over the facial muscles or over the upper part of the body; in rare instances they may be generalized. There is no other condition including the deepest coma which so closely resembles death. No wonder that a simple benign syncope is often described as "an attack in which the patient almost died."

Less dramatic than the sudden collapse but of equal importance in recognizing the clinical syndrome are the premonitory symptoms of the fainting reaction. These more gradually occurring changes may appear minutes before the loss of consciousness and postural tone. One often observes first the occurrence of pallor accompanied by beads of perspiration. The subject soon experiences an upper-gastric discomfort which is frequently likened to nausea but often distinguished as a separate sensation. There are associated yawning and sighing, leading to frank hyperventilation. Close observation reveals the presence of pupillary dilatation, and the individual reports the occurrence of visual blurring just prior to loss of hearing. Although the sudden nature of the fainting episode, with precipitous fall in arterial pressure, is commonly emphasized, one observes in laboratory-induced syncope a relentless and more gradual fall in systolic and diastolic pressure prior to collapse. During this period, which is referred to as "presyncope," the patient has difficulty in concentrating; he gradually becomes unaware of his surroundings and in his discomfort almost prefers the anticipated unconsciousness to the generalized distress in this presyncopal phase. Although bradycardia is regularly present at the time of unconsciousness, this premonitory phase of the fainting reaction is most often associated with a relatively rapid heart rate.[9] With continuing hypotension, progressive slowing of the pulse appears and may be marked at the moment that the individual loses consciousness. When the subject of a syncopal reaction is allowed to rest with his head down, consciousness is rapidly regained, while the relative bradycardia persists. Of additional importance in the overall clinical picture of vasodepressor syncope are the postsyncopal findings, which are characterized by a persistence of pallor, nausea, weakness and sweating, oliguria, and a proneness for recurrence of the reaction if the individual is returned to the upright posture.

The hemodynamic mechanisms responsible for vasodepressor syncope have interested authors for over a century.[10] Although it was first felt that fainting may represent a severe depression of cardiac output, scrutiny of changes in cardiac output, as measured by the indicator-dilution and Fick oxygen techniques, has demonstrated little tendency for cardiac output to fall beyond that which occurs with assumption of the head-up posture.[11-13] Though it has been observed that cardiac output tends to diminish in the advanced stages of syncope[14] and in the unusual circumstance in which syncope is observed in the recumbent position,[15] the development of the entire reaction in the absence of diminished cardiac output in subjects studied in the upright posture would mitigate against the explanation that the fall in cardiac output is the primary event. It is rather the marked fall in total peripheral resistance in vasodepressor syncope that must be the essential element responsible for the fall in arterial pressure and the diminished perfusion pressure to the brain. The peripheral hemodynamic factors responsible for the marked fall in

arterial pressure were first suggested in observations made by John Hunter in 1793, when he wrote,[16] "I bled a lady but she fainted and while she continued in the fit the colour of the blood that came from the vein was a fine scarlet." This description of arterialization of venous blood was the first observation reflecting on the greatly increased blood flow to the forearm during fainting, a finding which has been confirmed repeatedly in studies employing modern plethysmographic techniques.[17-20] From such studies, it is apparent that vascular resistance in the skeletal muscle bed is markedly reduced. Resistance is reduced, as well, in other major vascular areas, such as the mesenteric,[21] the renal,[22,23] and indeed the cerebral beds.[24,25] In contrast to skeletal muscle, blood flow in the skin,[17,26] mesenteric,[21] renal,[22,23] and indeed the cerebral beds.[24,25] In contrast to skeletal muscle, blood flow in the skin,[17,26] mesenteric,[21] renal,[22,23] and cerebral vascular beds[24,25] is reduced during syncope. Of particular importance is the fact that the fall in total peripheral resistance is not compensated by a rise in cardiac output, as usually occurs in normal individuals in the presence of widespread vascular dilatation. Why the heart fails to respond to this stimulus is not entirely clear. While vagal inhibition[27] may be a contributory factor, it has been observed repeatedly that vasodepressor syncope may occur even when vagal activity is blocked by atropine.[13,28] Recent observations have demonstrated that cardiac responses to both a fall in peripheral vascular resistance and to pharmacologic stimulation may be markedly diminished when the normal individual assumes the upright posture.[29-32] This failure of the heart to respond appears to be related to postural shifts in blood volume in which the central venous volume is diminished. The decrease in the central venous reservoir is sufficient to diminish the rate of ventricular filling, which cannot be maintained adequately to sustain cardiac responses in the face of known stimulation. The absence of cardiac response in the face of a marked increase in flow to skeletal muscle with an overall profound fall in peripheral resistance results in the fall in arterial pressure, and hence in the decreased perfusion to the brain.

The onset of unconsciousness in syncope is associated with the sudden appearance in the electroencephalogram of large-amplitude slow-wave activity.[9,33,34] This dramatic change in the electroencephalogram occurs only after severe diminution in mean arterial pressure (average pressure, 25 mm Hg at heart level) and is accompanied by a fall in cerebral blood flow to 50 to 70 per cent of normal.[9,14,24,25]

It is of interest to note that if one considers the average distance from the heart to the brain of 45 cm and the specific gravity of blood (1.058), an adequate pressure head of at least 31 mm Hg at heart level is required to maintain cerebral perfusion in the upright posture. Considering the average decrease of 7 mm Hg in venous pressure at the level of the brain when the upright posture is assumed, the arterial pressure at which fainting occurs in the upright tilt under laboratory conditions coincides well with that predicted on the basis of physical factors alone.

Accompanying the common faint there is usually a moderate-to-severe degree of hyperventilation, most probably the result of the associated anxiety as well as of the cerebral hypoxia. Associated with hyperventilation there is a fall in arterial carbon dioxide content.[13] The recognized effect of hypocapnia in lowering cerebral blood flow[35] and arterial pressure and in increasing forearm blood flow[36] may well serve to accentuate the circulatory embarrassment in syncope.

A particularly intriguing aspect of the fainting reaction is the postsyncopal oliguria. It would appear from studies of Brun, Knudsen, and Raaschou[23] that this antidiuresis is related to excessive secretion of antidiuretic hormone. The possible role of the posterior pituitary substance in inducing some of the other alterations in syncope, viz., pallor and nausea, has been stressed by some investigators.[37]

The underlying precipitating event in vasodepressor syncope has been the subject of considerable speculation. Vasodepressor syncope most frequently occurs in the normal person in the upright posture and under circumstances that he finds distasteful. Social behavior or other situational factors force him to stand his ground, and thus a state occurs in which the body reactions for flight or fight are in part mobilized, yet in part suppressed. Extensive peripheral muscle dilatation occurs, unaccompanied by a supporting cardiac response. The incomplete circulatory response results in a fall in arterial pressure and syncope. The emotional factors involved in the above interpretation were proposed initially by Darwin[38] and have been elaborated in recent years by Engel and Romano.[39] A possible neurogenic network connecting the emotional and the cardiovascular changes in the syncopal response were suggested in the studies of Uvnas,[40] who described a central vasomotor outflow pathway responsible for generalized dilatation and a fall in arterial pressure in animals.

Although vasodepressor syncope is most often observed in individuals with a normal circulation, the syncopal reaction is not at all uncommon in patients with cardiovascular disease. The mechanism of the fainting reaction under these circumstances is similar to that in the normal person, viz., a fall in arterial pressure consequent upon a sudden decrease in peripheral vascular resistance, occurring in a setting where the heart fails to compensate by an increase in output. The fall in peripheral resistance in these disease states may be induced by emotion or exercise. Syncope of this type may be observed in patients with aortic stenosis, less commonly in aortic regurgitation, in various forms of congenital heart disease, and in primary pulmonary hypertension.[41-45] Under these circumstances the cardiac lesion offers an additional impediment to cardiac responses. Syncope is often noted in patients with acute or chronic anemia, and in individuals who have received surgical or pharmacologic sympathectomy.[14,46-50] Under these circumstances, the lowered blood volume or the diminished vascular responsiveness in the upright posture creates a hemodynamic setting predisposing to the fainting reaction. Occasionally, vasodepressor syncope occurs immediately following acute myocardial infarction,[51] or during a severe attack of angina pectoris.[52] In addition to vasodepressor syncope, fainting due to cardiac arrhythmia must always be considered under these circumstances. Typical vasodepressor syncope is not uncommon in the course of pregnancy. It is notable that this form of syncope may actually be precipitated by lying down and relieved by standing.[20,53] Syncope has also been noted to occur following strenuous exercise,[54] after the intake of vasodilating drugs such as nitrite and nitroglycerin,[26] and in patients receiving various tranquilizing agents.[55] Fainting is particularly likely to occur in the course of acute febrile infections and following prolonged recumbency in chronic illness. Normal persons maintained at bed rest for several days have a propensity for fainting, particularly when arising abruptly from the recumbent position.[56] A problem of importance in aviation medicine is the vasodepressor syncope occurring during acceleration, particularly when centrifugal force is applied in the head-to-foot position.

The therapy of vasodepressor syncope consists of placing the patient in the recumbent position with the head lower than the rest of the body.

Orthostatic Hypotension

When the normal individual assumes the upright posture, the attendant gravitational stresses on the circulation are compensated by several mechanisms, viz., reflex arteriolar and venous constriction, acceleration of heart rate, and mechanical factors including the venous valvular system, the mechanical pumping of the leg muscles, and the decreased intrathoracic pressure. In addition, there is an increase in plasma catecholamine levels with standing.[57] Chronic orthostatic hypotension is a disorder in which the autonomic and humoral factors compensating for the upright posture are inadequate or absent. Assumption of the upright posture in such patients is associated with a prompt fall in arterial pressure. Hypotension is progressive over a period of seconds to minutes, depending on the degree of loss in the adaptive responses, until the point where perfusion pressure to the brain is inadequate to maintain consciousness. When the recumbent posture is resumed, there is rapid increase in blood pressure and consciousness is regained. The failure of reflex hemodynamic adaptation in the upright posture in chronic orthostatic hypotension is a reflection of an overall deficiency in autonomic function. Thus, during the presyncopal period in these patients there is little or no change of pulse rate, as well as absence of the pallor, sweating, pupillary dilatation, and upper-gastric distress seen in vasodepressor syncope. In addition, these patients demonstrate other defects in autonomic function between episodes of fainting, including impotence, bladder and bowel disturbances, and absence or loss of sweating. Urinary excretion of catecholamines may be diminished, and plasma catechol levels fail to rise during head-up tilt.[57-59] It is of interest that when individuals with chronic orthostatic hypotension are observed under laboratory conditions, the role of mechanical factors alone in maintaining arterial pressure in the upright posture is reflected in the transient elevations in arterial pressure induced by leg motion, deep inspiration, and infusions of blood-volume expanders.

Orthostatic hypotension with syncope is seen under a variety of clinical situations, including diseases involving the autonomic nervous system, such as tabes dorsalis, syringomyelia, diabetic neuropathy, and subacute combined sclerosis.[60-62] A similar, but perhaps not identical, picture is seen with prolonged recumbency during protracted illness, following surgical sympathectomy or pharmacologic blockade of the autonomic ganglions, and with pharmacologic suppression of sympathetic nerve activity.[14,47-50] There is, in addition, an idiopathic form of chronic orthostatic hypotension in which no etiolgic factor has yet been elucidated.[63]

Orthostatic hypotension associated with prolonged bed rest can be lessened by early ambulation. When it is medically permissible, the chronically ill patient should spend some time in a chair each day. Orthostatic hypotension of the idiopathic variety or that associated with a known abnormality of the autonomic nervous system is difficult to manage. The treatment depends on the specific cause, when known, and is tempered always by the associated medical problems. Therapy ranges from the use of elastic stockings and pressure suits to high salt intake and corticosteroids. Hypotensive agents, such as ganglionic blocking drugs, rauwolfia deriv-

atives, chlorothiazide drugs, monoamine oxidase inhibitors, and certain tranquilizers, should be avoided in such patients.

Cerebral-occlusive Syncope

With partial or complete occlusion of the major arteries of the neck, the maintenance of perfusion to the brain becomes a more direct function of the level of arterial pressure. The greater the degree of cerebral vascular involvement, the more likely it is that syncope will become a part of the clinical picture.[64,65] Thus, with extensive involvement of the carotidovertebral arterial inflow in patients with pulseless disease (aortic arch syndrome), syncope occurs with a high degree of frequency.[66] With lesser degrees of cerebral vascular inflow occlusion, transient lowering of arterial pressure, e.g., immediately following the assumption of the upright posture, may be followed by vague symptoms suggesting impaired or marginal cerebral blood flow. Such postural symptoms as lightheadedness, dizziness, weakness, and visual disturbances are not uncommon in elderly individuals and particularly in patients with hypertensive disease. Associated with such symptoms there may be signs of focal neurologic deficit, such as hemiparesis, unilateral sensory signs and symptoms, altered speech, and cranial nerve dysfunction. In patients with major occlusive disease of the carotidovertebrobasilar arterial system, manual compression of either carotid artery may provoke syncope associated with focal neurologic signs.[67] One must, therefore, be extremely cautious in using carotid sinus massage in patients with suspected occlusive cerebral vascular disease. Fainting induced in this manner may be erroneously interpreted as carotid sinus syncope. Frequently recurring transient losses or impairment of consciousness in patients with cerebral vascular disease should be recognized as an ominous sign, often heralding a major cerebral vascular accident. Impairment or loss of consciousness in relation to changing positions of the head, particularly hyperextension and lateral rotation, has been described in occlusion of the vertebral arteries. Such symptoms have been observed in patients with lesions of the upper cervical spine, such as the Klippel-Feil deformity,[68] and in cervical osteoarthritis.[69,70]

Carotid Sinus Syncope—Vasodepressor Type[72-73]

Massage or compression of the carotid sinus in normal persons is often attended by transient slowing of the heart rate and mild hypotension. In a rare group of patients, such stimulation of the carotid sinus is followed by a profound fall in blood pressure or marked slowing in heart rate or a combination of these findings. In these individuals, the disorder is referred to as "carotid sinus syncope" or "hyperirritable carotid sinus syndrome." This syndrome is observed most commonly in elderly patients, the majority of whom have organic heart disease (coronary atherosclerosis with disease of the SA node or AV node or aortic stenosis) and diffuse atherosclerosis. Hyperirritability of the carotid sinus has also been observed in patients with disease processes localized to the carotid sinus area, such as neoplasm and inflammatory masses in the neck. The administration of digitalis appears to accentuate such hyperirritability. In patients with hyperirritable carotid sinus reflex, symptoms of light-headedness and impaired consciousness may be initiated by relatively minor stimulation of the carotid sinus by head motion, shaving, or, classically, a tight collar. Carotid sinus syncope of the vasodepressor type is that form of the syndrome in which fainting or impaired consciousness occurs in the absence of change in heart rate. Presyncopal signs such as nausea, sweating, and pallor are usually not observed under these circumstances, in which the fall in perfusion pressure to the brain is precipitous. Syncope due to hyperirritable carotid sinus in other individuals is associated primarily with slowing of the heart rate because of marked sinus bradycardia, sinoatrial block, or high-degree atrioventricular block. In such circumstances syncope is related more to the prolonged asystole than to the marked fall in peripheral vascular resistance. Such episodes of carotid sinus syncope due to slowing of the heart rate are referred to as the *cardioinhibitory type* of carotid sinus syncope. A third form of carotid sinus syncope, referred to as the *cerebral type,* in which loss of consciousness is unassociated with fall in arterial pressure or bradycardia, will be discussed in a later section.

Tumors of the carotid sinus are rare. The common disorders associated with a hypersensitive carotid sinus reflex are coronary atherosclerosis, with impaired circulation to the SA and AV nodes, and cerebral atherosclerosis. Although results are not reproducible, the use of atropine and related drugs and sympathomimetic amines, such as arterenol (norepinephrine), may be effective in preventing attacks. External stimulation of the carotid sinus, such as produced by turning the head, wearing a tight collar, or performing a Valsalva maneuver, should be avoided. The presence of associated occlusive disease of the carotid or vertebrobasilar arterial system predisposes to attacks and enjoins caution in performing carotid sinus massage in the elderly.

Cough Syncope[74]

Although at one time fainting during paroxysms of cough was considered rare, it is now recognized as a relatively common cause of fainting. In cough syncope (also called "laryngeal vertigo" and "tussive syncope"), loss of consciousness occurs following a paroxysm of vigorous coughing. It is commonly observed in robust men and children, rarely in women. This syndrome is particularly frequent among individuals with chronic bronchitis and "hacking cough." The impairment in cerebral blood flow is related to the marked increase in intrathoracic pressure during the coughing episode. Several factors may be implicated in the mechanism of cough syncope, including a sharp decrease in cardiac output, peripheral vasodilatation following cough, a marked increase in cerebrospinal fluid pressure with resultant compression of the intracranial capillary and venous beds, an increase in cerebral vascular resistance induced by the hypocapnia of coughing, and a "concussive" effect caused by the sudden rise in intracranial pressure transmitted from the thorax and abdomen via the cerebrospinal fluid.[75-77] The latter mechanism has been involved to explain those episodes of laboratory-induced cough syncope in which no change in the electroencephalogram suggesting cerebral anoxia has been observed.

Omission of smoking is mandatory in the treatment of this disease. Therapy of associated bronchitis should be carried out.

Syncope related to more prolonged increases in intrathoracic pressure may be observed during a sustained Valsalva maneuver. With prolonged exhalation against a closed glottis, there is progressive fall in arterial pressure and cardiac output, which may be of sufficient degree to impair cerebral circulation. The "fainting lark," a trick indulged in by school children and consisting of sudden manual compression of the chest of the victim made sensitive following a period of hyperventilation, is most probably caused by this mechanism. Some instances of drowning may be induced by this mechanism. Syncope following a similar schoolboy prank in which the individual squats and hyperventilates and quickly stands and performs a Valsalva maneuver has a similar mechanism.

Postmicturition Syncope

Micturition syncope[78] or, more properly, postmicturition syncope is often seen in adult men with nocturia. During or immediately following voiding there is sudden loss of consciousness, often without premonitory symptoms. Many such persons give the history of drinking large quantities of alcoholic beverage before retiring. A similar type of syncope may be observed following drainage of a distended bladder or after removal of large quantities of ascitic fluid. It has been suggested by some investigators that the loss of consciousness in these circumstances is related to a sudden reflex decrease in peripheral vascular resistance stimulated by the precipitous fall in intraabdominal volume. Others have felt the loss of consciousness in postmicturition syncope to be related to typical vasodepressor syncope accentuated by such factors as the Valsalva maneuver and the widespread peripheral vasodilatation associated with a warm bed and recent alcohol consumption.

Syncope Due to Inadequacy of Cardiac Output —Cardiac Syncope

Syncope in Cardiac Disease

The term *cardiac syncope* refers to fainting related primarily to a sudden and marked decrease in cardiac output. Although syncope of cardiac origin is often accompanied by heart disease, fainting due to a marked and precipitous fall in cardiac output does not necessarily denote the presence of underlying disease in the heart.

It has been noted previously that vasodepressor syncope may accompany various forms of heart disease in which the cardiac output response to a sudden fall in peripheral resistance is impaired. Typical vasodepressor syncope may occur in the course of such diseases as aortic stenosis, aortic insufficiency, various congenital abnormalities of the heart, primary pulmonary hypertension, and ischemic heart disease.[41–45,51,52] In these disease states, a sudden fall in peripheral vascular resistance is unattended by an increase in cardiac output, with a consequent fall in arterial pressure and diminished perfusion to the brain. The fall in peripheral vascular resistance is most commonly induced by exercise under these circumstances, in contrast to the peripheral vascular dilatation mediated by emotion in the typical vasodepressor faint. The term *effort syncope* is often applied in these cases. Although additional reflex mechanisms have often been implicated as a cause for cardiac syncope, laboratory studies to date have not yielded definitive data supporting such mechanisms.

A dramatic form of cardiac syncope is that associated with mechanical obstruction of the mitral orifice in patients with a ball-valve type of thrombus or a myxomatous tumor of the left atrium.[79,80] Obstruction of the mitral valve in these circumstances is associated with a sudden loss of consciousness and often occurs with changing position. There may be associated signs of mitral stenosis and peripheral embolic phenomena.

Cardiac Arrhythmias and Morgagni-Adams-Stokes Attacks

A major mechanism in many episodes of syncope of cardiac origin consists of alterations in cardiac rhythm. These alterations in cardiac rhythm may be associated with either rapid or slow heart rate, with regular or irregular rhythm, and may have as their basis, block in the conduction or initiation of depolarization.

Loss or impairment of consciousness associated with alterations in cardiac rhythm is related to a precipitous fall in cardiac output accompanying the rhythm change. In paroxysmal atrial and ventricular tachycardia and in paroxysmal atrial fibrillation, syncope may occur at the onset or termination of the cardiac arrhythmia. At these times, when the cardiac pacemaker shifts its locus, there is often a period of asystole, with cessation of the heart beat. A sudden run of ventricular extrasystoles or transient ventricular fibrillation with a sharp diminution in cardiac output may also occur at these times. Often the patient becomes aware of rapid heart action before he loses consciousness; this suggests an alternate explanation for the syncope. With onset of an extremely rapid tachycardia (i.e., heart rates above 200 beats per minute) there may be an associated marked drop in cardiac output. Such a fall in cardiac output is attended by reflex vasoconstriction. Until the time that the reflex phenomena restore arterial pressure and aid ventricular filling, the fall in cardiac output may be sufficient to impair cerebral blood flow and account for the alterations in consciousness. Such a mechanism is likely to occur in the cardiac patient or when the individual is standing. In the course of atrial arrhythmias, a sudden decrease in the degree of AV block may induce a similar hemodynamic change. One need not therefore invoke a cardiac arrest mechanism to explain loss of consciousness in cardiac arrhythmias in all cases. In many circumstances, however, transient syncope in the course of cardiac arrhythmias remains unexplained. With the more frequent use of cardiac monitoring devices in such patients, the mechanism of syncope may be clarified.

Syncope occurring in patients with heart block is termed "Morgagni-Adams-Stokes syndrome." Several mechanisms are responsible for fainting in such patients, including (1) failure of the idioventricular pacemaker, with delay or lack of new pacemaker formation, (2) asystole in the transition from normal sinus rhythm to partial or complete heart block or when the level of heart block increases, and (3) the superimposition of ectopic ventricular arrhythmia, such as ventricular tachycardia or ventricular fibrillation.

Syncope associated with the cardiac arrhythmias and heart block is characterized by the suddenness of its onset and the lack of premonitory symptoms of cerebral hypoxia and autonomic discharge. The fainting episode may occur either in the erect or the upright posture. It is notable that with cardiac arrest, loss of consciousness ensues more rapidly when the individual is standing (4 to 8 sec) than when he is recumbent (12 to 15 sec). With prolonged periods of asystole, convulsions usually ensue. (For therapy, see Chap. 16).

Reflex Asystole

Suppression of atrial pacemaker activity and of atrioventricular conduction by the vagus plays an important role in several forms of syncope. Thus, in the course of vasodepressor syncope, sinus bradycardia and various levels of incomplete heart block are often noted. Although the vagal mechanism may not be the primary cause of fainting under these circumstances, the slowing of the heart rate to critically low levels is certainly a contributing factor. Vagal influences may also play an important role in the course of atrial arrhythmias when sudden slowing or acceleration in ventricular rate due to varying atrioventricular block may occur. Similarly, alterations in vagal tone may account for episodes of syncope in patients with heart block, when changes from incomplete to complete block are responsible for the fainting reaction. The role of the vagus in the vasodepressor type of carotid sinus syncope has been emphasized previously. In the cardioinhibitory type of carotid sinus syncope, suppression of atrial pacemaker activity and of AV node conduction by the vagus is a primary cause of syncope.

In rare instances, syncope may occur in individuals without evidence of heart disease as a result of reflex cardiac asystole. The term *vagovagal syncope* is applied to such syncope of reflex origin, in which the entire reflex arc is located within the vagal system.[81] Syncope associated with distension of an esophageal diverticulum and in the course of pathologic lesions in the larynx and mediastinum has been explained on this basis. A similar mechanism for cardiac standstill arising from vagal reflex activity has been attributed to syncope following distension of the viscera, fainting associated with irritation of the pleura or peritoneum, the cardiac asystole associated with esophagoscopy or bronchoscopy, and the syncope associated with glossopharyngeal neuralgia and cardiospasm. Recurrent syncope of this type is often relieved or prevented by administration of anticholinergic agents, such as atropine sulfate, in adequate dosage.

Syncope Due to Metabolic Causes

Hypoxia

Fainting due to hypoxia may be related primarily to the lack of oxygen or, as is often encountered, may be due to vasodepressor syncope initiated during a period of oxygen lack.[19] The effect of hypoxia alone is best observed in persons studied in altitude chambers.[82] Though there is considerable individual variation, the onset of the hypoxic symptoms under these circumstances depends primarily on the level of altitude and, in addition, on the rate of ascent. With exposure to altitudes of 10,000 ft or greater, the point in the oxyhemoglobin dissociation curves is reached at which an abrupt decrease in oxygen saturation occurs with further fall in oxygen tension. Oxygen saturation falls rapidly from approximately 90 per cent saturation at 10,000 ft to 80 per cent at 15,000 ft and 63 per cent at 20,000 ft. At the latter altitudes there is an insidious progressive mental deterioration associated with visual disturbances, headache, and breathlessness. At the time of impairment of consciousness one may note cyanosis; with severe oxygen deprivation, convulsive movements are seen. With cardiovascular disease, pulmonary insufficiency, and anemia, symptoms of hypoxia occur at lower levels of altitude. The impairment of consciousness due to hypoxia is accompanied by sinus tachycardia and maintenance of arterial blood pressure. The environmental setting in which impaired consciousness due to hypoxia occurs usually leaves little difficulty in differentiating it from other forms of syncope.

Hypoglycemia

Severe hypoglycemia is associated with weakness, sweating, a sensation of hunger, confusion, and altered consciousness. The symptoms are unrelated to posture and respond promptly to food ingestion or intravenous glucose administration. Altered consciousness associated with overdosage of insulin, islet-cell adenomas of the pancreas, certain retroperitoneal tumors, in patients with reactive hypoglycemia, and in the presence of advanced adrenal, pituitary, or hepatic disease may be explained on this basis. Impaired consciousness associated with hypoglycemia is associated with a sinus rhythm and is rarely accompanied by hypotension; in contrast to syncope of circulatory origin, it is gradual in onset.

Hyperventilation Syndrome[83]

In normal persons anxiety is regularly accompanied by varying degrees of hyperventilation. In the hyperventilation syndrome, anxiety is associated with an inordinate degree of hyperventilation. The symptoms of hypocapnia dominate the clinical picture under these circumstances and may actually replace the anxiety as the major discomfort. Early during the episode, the patient complains of smothering, a tightness in the chest, and a feeling of suffocation. Later, there appear confusion, a sense of unreality, bewilderment, and in time a feeling of panic. Symptoms of palpitation, precordial oppression, and dyspnea may suggest an acute cardiac or pulmonary catastrophe. Associated with the above, there are sensations of "numbness" or coldness of the extremities and the circumoral areas. The symptoms may last as long as 30 min, and in the most severe episodes frank tetany with carpopedal spasm may be noted. Of particular note in differentiating hyperventilation attacks from other forms of syncope is the fact that the episodes may occur in the sitting or recumbent posture; there is often slight hypotension, but not a profound drop in blood pressure, and the heart rate is rapid. The episode is terminated usually after the patient is calmed and the hyperventilation is stopped. One may aid the resolution of symptoms of hypercapnia by having the patient rebreathe in a paper or plastic bag. It is notable that although consciousness is impaired, actual loss of consciousness usually does not occur. Typical vasodepressor syncope may be superimposed on the hyperventilation attack, making the delineation of the syndrome more difficult.

The pathogenesis of the hyperventilation syndrome is incompletely understood. While an underlying emotional disorder is almost invariably present, the factors leading to hyperventilation in these patients are not clearly defined. Much of the clinical findings in the hyperventilation syndrome can be explained by the effects of hypocapnia, namely the lowering of cerebral blood flow, and the alkalosis. The reproduction of a typical episode by voluntary hyperventilation in patients with the syndrome is a helpful diagnostic maneuver, and in addition, aids in educating the patient regarding the prevention and control of attacks.

Syncope Due to Neuropsychologic Factors

Carotid Sinus Syncope—Cerebral Type

In addition to carotid sinus syncope of the vasodepressor and cardioinhibitory types, Weiss and coworkers have described an additional form of syncope following carotid sinus massage in which loss of consciousness is unassociated with change in blood pressure or pulse.[71–73] In this type of carotid sinus syncope symptoms may occur in any position and the loss of consciousness may be preceded or accompanied by focal neurologic manifestations. It has been suggested by Weiss and coworkers that inhibition of the center for regulation of consciousness by a reflex mechanism or by secondary focal circulatory disturbance may account for these episodes of syncope. In view of recent reports of the occurrence of syncope during carotid sinus manipulation in patients with carotidovertebral artery insufficiency, some question has arisen as to whether some of these episodes are related primarily to cerebral ischemia.[67,84] The possibility of hysterical syncope must also be raised in some instances in which a diagnosis of the cerebral type of hypersensitive carotid sinus is made. However, there are a sufficient number of carefully observed episodes of syncope of this type to suggest that it is a clinical entity among the carotid sinus syndromes.

Hysterical Syncope[85]

Hysterical fainting is of particular importance because it may mimic altered consciousness of an organic origin. Hysterical episodes most frequently occur in young females, often with severe emotional illness. The episode usually occurs in the presence of an audience. The patient slumps gently and gracefully to the floor or in a convenient chair or sofa, typically without injury or awkwardness. The patient may be motionless at the time of the episode or may show symbolic and resistive movements. The episode is of varying duration and may last for as long as an hour or more. Although the patient is unresponsive to verbal stimulation, there is often evidence that he has not lost consciousness, and there are no abnormalities in pulse, blood pressure, or skin color. A distinctive characteristic in the hysterical faint is the calm emotional detachment with which the patient describes symptoms and the fact that there is no sharp reversal in their progress when the recumbent posture is assumed.

Cerebral Dysrhythmias

The differentiation of the various forms of syncope of circulatory origin from the transitory loss of consciousness during a generalized seizure is often easy on the basis of history alone. One form of epilepsy, viz., the akinetic form of petit mal epilepsy, does offer particular difficulty in differentiation. Epilepsy as a cause of sudden loss of consciousness is suggested in the dramatic nature of the onset often preceded by an aura, the lack of change in skin color, the lack of hypotension or rhythm change other than that of sinus tachycardia, tonic convulsive movements with upturning of the eyes, the prolonged period of unconsciousness, the urinary incontinence, and the postictal drowsiness, headache, and confusion. Although any of the above findings may occur in individual episodes of syncope of circulatory origin, the frequent combination of these events in epilepsy allows differentiation of the cause of the event. The finding of an abnormal electroencephalographic picture suggesting epilepsy between episodes of unconsciousness is most helpful in this differentiation.[34]

Syncopal Migraine

Symptoms suggesting syncope are rarely if ever encountered in ordinary types of migraine headache. Recent observations have suggested one type of migraine associated with loss of consciousness.[86] In rare instances in which the basal arterial system is involved, instead of the more usually affected carotid system, the premonitory aura of migraine terminates in a period of unconsciousness of several minutes' duration. When the patient awakens there is severe headache, typically in the occipital area. This form of migraine usually afflicts adolescent girls. The period of unconsciousness is associated with no other apparent circulatory change.

Vertigo

Though recurrent episodes of vertigo may first be described by the patient as a loss or impairment of consciousness, careful direction of the history will often reveal the true nature of this symptom. In vertigo there is a keen sense of movement, either of the environment or of the patient himself. Falling may be abrupt; it is due not to weakness of postural muscles but to a loss of balance. Nausea, pallor, and cold perspiration may suggest vasodepressor syncope, but the lack of true loss or impairment of consciousness, the increased distress with head movement and the associated nystagmoid movements of the eyes, together with the finding of a normal blood pressure and pulse, will help differentiate the syndrome.

Treatment of Syncope

The alterations in the physiologic mechanism responsible for the syncope must be identified when possible, and treatment must be aimed at its correction. The therapy of syncope related to the cardiovascular system is mentioned in this portion of the text but is covered in detail elsewhere in the book. Obviously, as all physicians know, the patient who has "fainted" should be placed in the recumbent position with the lower extremities higher than the head until the clinical situation can be appraised properly.

SHOCK

Clinical Picture of Shock

Through the years there have been numerous attempts to classify shock and give the term specific meaning. All these efforts have met with difficulty, and there is still no unanimity of opinion. It would appear advisable, therefore, to limit the term *shock* to a simple descriptive meaning. The classic clinical picture is that of a patient who lies somewhat restlessly in bed, whose level of consciousness is blunted, but who is usually not comatose. The skin is pale, moist, and often slightly cyanotic. The extremities are cool. The pulse is feeble and often rapid. The veins are usually collapsed, except in special circumstances. The arterial blood pressure is low or unobtainable by the conventional means. The urinary output is scanty or absent. Unless successfully treated, it may progress to a situation in which shock persists despite usually effective therapeutic measures. This is the state of "irreversible shock."

Pathophysiology of Shock

The study, classification, and treatment of shock would be much simpler if a simple physiologic deficit could be ascribed to all cases. Unfortunately this is not possible at present. A recent attempt at definition is that "shock is a default in the transport mechanisms of the body, generally affecting vital cells." [117] So-called irreversible shock would represent an absolute and nonremediable form of transport damage. Even with the breadth of this definition, there are still some problems in interpretation. It would be desirable to have a more specific definition. In terms of early shock many, but not all, forms would come under the category of acute and severe impairment of the total circulation. Most shock occurring in the course of cardiovascular disease would be of this type. In those patients who have bacterial infections, shock may occur without initial circulatory impairment of the usual sort. In so-called irreversible shock, cellular damage affecting transport may be more important than the circulatory factor in producing the clinical picture and its resistance to therapy. Since circulation is a closed vascular loop, measurement of cardiac output would be an indicator of the deficiency in the circulatory function. Such deficiency could be caused by a variety of factors. It could be brought about by the loss of blood or plasma, such as one sees in bleeding due to injury or in internal bleeding or due to crushing injuries of the extremities. It may be due to interference with the flow of blood by massive pulmonary embolus or by the impairment of cardiac function caused by pericardial tamponade. It may be caused in the heart itself, as in massive myocardial infarction. Thus, cardiovascular diseases may initiate the shock picture in a variety of ways.

Once shock has been established, from whatever cause, cardiovascular factors are thought to be of great importance in its prolongation and in its eventual outcome. Marked vasoconstriction is a concomitant of most types of shock. It may at times be protective and may serve as a mechanism of sustaining arterial blood pressure in the face of diminished cardiac output. However, there is increasing evidence that vasoconstriction at times may be deleterious, leading to ischemia and cellular damage of vital organs. Recent studies on various forms of shock have indicated the importance of the heart as a determinant of the final outcome, regardless of the initial cause of the shock state. If the heart becomes seriously damaged, the outcome may well prove fatal. The kidneys also are importantly involved in the determination of a fatal outcome.

Discussion of the cause, mechanisms, and treatment of all types of shock is far beyond the scope of this volume. Attention in greater detail will be paid to "cardiogenic shock" as it occurs in the course of heart disease, particularly acute myocardial infarction.

Cardiogenic Shock and Its Treatment

While it is generally accepted that the essential hemodynamic factor in the circulatory collapse in cardiogenic shock is related to the impairment of cardiac output,[87-89] there is considerable evidence, as suggested by Fishberg and Boyer, that peripheral circulatory mechanisms play an additional significant role.[90,91] Of note in this regard is the finding that the level of the cardiac output in the patient with cardiogenic shock need not be any lower than that seen in patients with severe cardiac disease or following myocardial infarction in the absence of peripheral circulatory failure. A diminution in total blood volume cannot be implicated as a primary factor in the hypotension under most circumstances of cardiogenic shock.[87,88,92,93] It would appear, therefore, that inadequacy in the peripheral circulatory response to a fall in cardiac output might supervene under these circumstances. This inadequacy might be due either to suppression of the usual peripheral circulatory constrictor mechanisms, or to a disorganization in the peripheral circulatory response akin to that seen in the more acute forms of circulatory embarrassment discussed previously under "Vasodepressor Syncope."

As in most cases when complete understanding of the mechanism of disease is absent, the therapy of cardiogenic shock has remained largely empirical. When a potent remediable etiologic factor can be identified, dramatic recovery often follows when the responsible mechanism is reversed. This is particularly evident on reversion of cardiac arrhythmias with extremely rapid ventricular rate or when pericardiocentesis relieves pericardial tamponade. In the usual case of cardiogenic shock, as is seen accompanying an acute myocardial infarction, such dramatic events are rare and a more general approach to therapy is instituted.

It is important to recognize at the outset that in the early course of an acute myocardial infarction, the patient may exhibit many of the peripheral manifestations of the shock syndrome, including peripheral vasoconstriction, with pallor and sweating, and hypotension. With attention focused on the relief of pain, administration of oxygen, and maintaining the patient in the supine position, there is gradual reversal of this picture and recovery without the need of potent circulatory stimulants.[94,95] In many regards, the picture of shock under these circumstances is comparable to that of a prolonged episode of vasodepressor syncope. In this phase of cardiogenic hypotension, one must be careful not to administer excessive doses of narcotics which might precipitate further circulatory embarrassment.[96]

The persistence of hypotension and signs of peripheral circulatory failure for more than 30 min is the major indication for introducing vasopressor therapy. There is little doubt, on clinical grounds, that the addition of vasopressor agents in the therapy of postmyocardial infarction shock has contributed significantly to the diminution in the mortality from this process.[95,97] It is evident, in addition, that the potency of these agents makes vasopressor therapy a double-edged sword. This reflects both our incomplete understanding of the specific peripheral circulatory phenomena that need to be reversed in order to achieve adequate circulatory balance, and the fact that the pressor agents induce a significant increase in left ventricular work because of their action in enhancing peripheral resistance and left ventricular work load. Thus, although coronary perfusion may be increased by the pressor agents following an acute myocardial infarction,[98] the increased work load may outbalance the improvement in coronary perfusion and result in enhancement of circulatory deterioration, heart failure, or arrhythmia. In addition to such hemodynamic considerations, the agents themselves promote myocardial irritability[99] and may induce subendocardial hemorrhage. Any specific recommendations for therapy with the vasopressor agents should be tempered by the above considerations.

In general, with the administration of vasopressors in shock one attempts to reestablish a balance in circulatory equilibrium, in which blood pressure is maintained at levels approaching normotension for the individual, and in which there is evidence of improved cerebral and renal perfusion, at a time when cardiac rhythm is stable and signs of pulmonary congestion are minimal. With establishment of such an equilibrium, the physician hopes to allow the normal homeostatic mechanisms and myocardial repair processes to supervene. Beyond these principles, much remains controversial in the treatment of cardiogenic shock. Some investigators have claimed superiority of agents which enhance ventricular inotropy in addition to their potent peripheral constrictor effect.[100,101] It would appear that in modern-day treatment the vasopressor agents with at least some positive inotropic influence on the heart, such as norepinephrine and metaraminol or mephentermine, are the preferred agents. The pressor amines with almost pure peripheral constriction activity, such as phenylephrine and methoxamine, are also widely employed.

In recent years the potent pressor, polypeptide angiotensin amide, has proved effective as a vasopressor agent, even when the infusion of norepinephrine has failed to elevate arterial pressure.[102] There is recent evidence that this agent exerts a positive inotropic effect as well.[103] It has the distinct advantage over norepinephrine in that it does not induce tissue sloughing on subcutaneous infiltration and exhibits no tachyphylaxis.[104] The exact place of angiotensin in the therapy of coronary shock remains to be established.

The precise contribution of autonomic stimulation to the development of the peripheral circulatory failure in cardiogenic shock is unknown. Evidence in hypovolemic shock would suggest that sympathetic stimulation exerts a strongly negative influence and promotes the circulatory embarrassment and tissue deterioration in this form of circulatory collapse.[105] There is some evidence that sympathetic block might actually be of benefit in the course of coronary shock as well.[106,107] Further experimental and clinical data are required, however, before an acceptable approach to coronary shock on the basis of autonomic or sympathetic blockade could be recommended.

The use of transfusions and infusions to enhance blood volume is no longer in vogue in the treatment of coronary shock. Similarly, the use of steroids is not recommended for this form of circulatory collapse.

A modern and extremely useful therapeutic measure in the treatment of coronary shock complicated by heart block or ventricular arrhythmia consists of the electrical pacing and cardioversion techniques. Ventricular pacing of the heart employing a catheter pacemaker appears to be a most effective approach in situations where complete heart block or high-degree atrioventricular block develops in the course of an acute myocardial infarction.[108] In our hands, transient atrial or ventricular pacing has proved effective in establishing regularity of the ventricular response where multiple ventricular or atrial contractions appear. The increase in ventricular rate and the regularization of the ventricular response under these circumstances serve to enhance cardiac output and contribute significantly to the improvement in the circulatory status of the patient. Where atrial or ventricular arrhythmia with rapid ventricular re-

sponse supervenes, electrical conversion is often rewarding in reversing the state of circulatory embarrassment.[109,110] The use of cardioversion and pacing when ventricular fibrillation or cardiac asystole develops has been discussed in Chap. 16.

Another recent approach to the patient with cardiogenic shock involves the use of extracorporeal circulatory assist techniques.[111,112] The contribution of such measures in the treatment of circulatory collapse following myocardial infarction will best be evaluated in future clinical observations.

An additional clinical consideration is the use of anticoagulant therapy in cardiogenic shock. In view of the altered coagulation observed in shock,[113,114] and the impaired peripheral perfusion and clumping of red cells,[115,116] there appears to be good physiologic rationale for the administration of anticoagulants to patients with sustained cardiogenic shock.[117]

SUDDEN DEATH

Sudden death is a dramatic event. It has recently engaged the increased attention of physicians because of the possibility of resuscitation in those instances where structural changes are minimal. Sudden death, in the absence of trauma, is said to occur when death takes place in a matter of seconds. The terminal event in such situations is usually of cardiovascular origin. It is probably most frequently the result of sudden stoppage of effective heart action by asystole or arrhythmia. Almost all types of cardiovascular disease may at times produce sudden catastrophes of this sort. Recent studies indicate that sudden death occurs in patients with coronary atherosclerosis as an initial catastrophe more often than was formerly appreciated. Sudden death may also occur secondary to the rupture of an aortic aneurysm or to pulmonary embolism. In general, episodes of cerebral vascular disease with bleeding into the brain, although they may produce death in minutes, do not truly produce "sudden death" in the terms of this discussion. As noted earlier, syncope may be a prolonged event, but when it becomes prolonged enough to have a fatal outcome it is then classified as a cause of sudden death.

Two major mechanisms appear to be operative in producing sudden death in heart disease. In some instances actual cardiac standstill or asystole appears to take place; in others, ventricular fibrillation with ineffective contraction is found. Information regarding the relative frequency of these two mechanisms is not entirely satisfactory[118] but would indicate that there is about even distribution of the two types. Monitoring and telemetering equipment now being placed in use will eventually lead to a more accurate appraisal of the problem as it occurs in a hospital. It is obviously difficult to know what takes place in those events occurring in the circumstances of daily life.

There is no general agreement regarding the time limits of cessation of the circulation for effective resuscitation. It would appear that the sooner resuscitation is instituted, the more likely one is to have success. Many factors are apparently involved. Outer limits of 4 min seem to apply generally, although successful resuscitation has occurred after even longer periods of inadequate circulation.[119] In some instances, body functions may be resumed but the higher levels of brain function do not return. Fortunately, this is not a common problem, but, again because of inadequacy of present information, its frequency cannot be stated with accuracy.

In the past, efforts at resuscitation were limited to use of intracardiac epinephrine or artificial respiration. In the 1950s open-chest cardiac massage was introduced.[120] It requires surgical opening of the chest and manual massage of the heart. Although these methods were occasionally successful, they were predominantly restricted to the operating room and were not generally employed. The more recent introduction of closed chest cardiac massage has greatly increased the potential of resuscitation.[121] Early reports in the literature have indicated moderate degrees of success.[122,123] There have at the same time been complications such as fractured ribs, and at times more serious complications such as a rupture of the liver.[122] The exact benefits of so-called coronary care units and resuscitative efforts are yet to be determined.[123–125] Nevertheless, there is adequate information to indicate that successful resuscitations can take place, and there is every reason to pursue these attempts enthusiastically in those patients whose general clinical condition indicates that survival is possible.

REFERENCES

1. Lassen, N. A.: Cerebral Blood Flow and Oxygen Consumption in Man, *Physiol. Rev.*, 39:183, 1959.
2. Kety, S. S., and Schmidt, C. F.: The Nitrous Oxide Method for the Quantitative Determination of Cerebral Blood Flow in Man: Theory, Procedure and Normal Values, *J. Clin. Invest.*, 27:476, 1948.
3. Himwich, H. E.: "Brain Metabolism and Cerebral Disorders," The Williams & Wilkins Company, Baltimore, 1951.
4. Kabat, H., Rossen, R., and Anderson, J. P.: Acute Arrest of Cerebral Circulation in Man, *A.M.A. Arch. Neurol. & Psychiat.*, 50:519, 1943.
5. Patterson, J. L., Jr.: Circulation through the Brain, in T. C. Ruch and J. R. Fulton, "Medical

Physiology and Biophysics" 18th ed., W. B. Saunders Company, Philadelphia, 1960, p. 741.
6. Scheinberg, P., and Stead, E. A., Jr.: The Cerebral Blood Flow in Male Subjects as Measured by the Nitrous Oxide Technique: Normal Values for Blood Flow, Oxygen Utilization, Glucose Utilization and Peripheral Resistance with Observations on the Effect of Tilting and Anxiety, *J. Clin. Invest.*, 28:1163, 1949.
7. Patterson, J. L., Jr., and Warren, J. V.: Mechanisms of Adjustment in the Cerebral Circulation upon Assumption of the Upright Position, *J. Clin. Invest.*, 31:653, 1952.
8. Schmidt, C. F.: "The Cerebral Circulation in Health and Disease," Charles C Thomas, Publisher, Springfield, Ill., 1950.
9. Karp, H. R., Weissler, A. M., and Heyman, A.: Vasodepressor Syncope: EEG and Circulatory Changes, *Arch. Neurol.*, 5:94, 1961.
10. Weissler, A. M., and Warren, J. V.: Vasodepressor Syncope, *Am. Heart J.*, 57:786, 1959.
11. Barcroft, H., Edholm, O. G., McMichael, J., and Sharpey-Schafer, E. P.: Posthemorrhagic Fainting, Study by Cardiac Output and Forearm Flow, *Lancet*, 1:489, 1944.
12. Warren, J. V., Brannon, E. S., Stead, E. A., Jr., and Merrill, A. J.: The Effect of Venesection and the Pooling of Blood in the Extremities on the Arterial Pressure and Cardiac Output in Normal Subjects, with Observations on Acute Circulatory Collapse in Three Instances, *J. Clin. Invest.*, 24:337, 1945.
13. Weissler, A. M., Warren, J. V., Estes, E. H., Jr., McIntosh, H. D., and Leonard, J. J.: Vasodepressor Syncope, Factors Influencing Cardiac Output, *Circulation*, 15:875, 1957.
14. Finnerty, F. A., Jr., Guillaudeu, R. L., and Fazekas, J. F.: Cardiac and Cerebral Hemodynamics in Drug-induced Postural Collapse, *Circulation Res.*, 5:34, 1957.
15. Greene, M. A., Boltax, A. J., and Ulberg, R. J.: Cardiovascular Dynamics of Vasovagal Reactions in Man, *Circulation Res.*, 9:12, 1961.
16. Hunter, J.: "Works of John Hunter," J. F. Palmer, London, 1837, vol. 3.
17. Barcroft, H., and Edholm, O. G.: On the Vasodilatation in Human Skeletal Muscle during Posthemorrhagic Fainting, *J. Physiol.*, 104:161, 1945.
18. Greenfield, A. D. M.: An Emotional Faint, *Lancet*, 1:1302, 1951.
19. Anderson, D. P., Allen, W. J., Barcroft, H., Edholm, O. G., and Manning, G. W.: Circulatory Changes during Fainting and Coma Caused by Oxygen Lack, *J. Physiol.*, 104:426, 1946.
20. Brigden, W., Howarth, S., and Sharpey-Schafer, E. P.: Postural Changes in the Peripheral Blood Flow of Normal Subjects, with Observations on Vasovagal Fainting Reactions as a Result of Tilt-

ing, the Lordotic Posture, Pregnancy and Spinal Anaesthesia, *Clin. Sc.*, 9:79, 1950.

21. Bearn, A. G., Billing, B., Edholm, O. G., and Sherlock, S.: Hepatic Blood Flow and Carbohydrate Changes in Man during Fainting, *J. Physiol.*, 115:442, 1951.

22. DeWardener, H. E., and McSwiney, R. R.: Renal Haemodynamics in Vasovagal Fainting Due to Hemorrhage, *Clin. Sc.*, 10:209, 1951.

23. Brun, C., Knudson, E. O. E., and Raaschou, F.: Kidney Function and Circulatory Collapse, Postsyncopal Oliguria, *J. Clin. Invest.*, 25:568, 1946.

24. Finnerty, F. A., Jr., Witkin, L., and Fazekas, J. F.: Cerebral Hemodynamics during Cerebral Ischemia Induced by Acute Hypotension, *J. Clin. Invest.*, 33:1227, 1954.

25. McHenry, L. C., Fazekas, J. F., and Sullivan, J. F.: Cerebral Hemodynamics of Syncope, *Am. J. M. Sc.*, 241:173, 1961.

26. Weiss, S., Wilkins, R. W., and Haynes, F. W.: The Nature of Circulatory Collapse Induced by Sodium Nitrite, *J. Clin. Invest.*, 16:73, 1937.

27. Dermksian, G., and Lamb, L. E.: Syncope in Population of Healthy Young Adults, *J.A.M.A.*, 168:1200, 1958.

28. Lewis, T.: Vasovagal Syncope and the Carotid Sinus Mechanism, *Brit. M. J.*, 1:873, 1932.

29. Weissler, A. M., Leonard, J. J., and Warren, J. V.: Effect of Posture and Atropine on the Cardiac Output, *J. Clin. Invest.*, 36:1656, 1957.

30. Weissler, A. M., Leonard, J. J., and Warren, J. V.: The Hemodynamic Effects of Isoproterenol in Man: With Observations on the Role of the Central Blood Volume, *J. Lab. & Clin. Med.*, 53:921, 1959.

31. Bevegard, S.: Studies on the Regulation of the Circulation in Man, *Acta physiol. scandinav.*, 57: Suppl. 200, 1962.

32. Weissler, A. M., Roehll, W. H., Jr., and Peeler, R. G.: Effect of Posture on the Cardiac Response to Increased Peripheral Demand, *J. Lab & Clin. Med.*, 59:1000, 1962.

33. Engel, G. L., Romano, J., and McLin, T.: Vasodepressor and Carotid Sinus Syncope: Clinical, Electroencephalographic and Electrocardiographic Observations, *A.M.A. Arch. Int. Med.*, 74:100, 1944.

34. Gastaut, H., and Fischer-Williams, M.: Electroencephalographic Study of Syncope, *Lancet*, 2: 1018, 1957.

35. Kety, S. S., and Schmidt, C. F.: The Effects of Active and Passive Hyperventilation on Cerebral Blood Flow, Cerebral Oxygen Consumption, Cardiac Output and Blood Pressure of Normal Young Men, *J. Clin. Invest.*, 25:107, 1946.

36. Burnum, J. F., Hickam, J. B., and McIntosh, H. D.: The Effect of Hypocapnia on Arterial Blood Pressure, *Circulation*, 9:89, 1954.

37. Stead, E. A., Jr., Kunkel, P., and Weiss, S.: Effect

of Pitressin in Circulatory Collapse Induced by Sodium Nitrite, *J. Clin. Invest.*, 18:673, 1939.

38. Darwin, C.: "Expression of the Emotions," Murray, London, 1872. (Philosophical Library, New York, 1955).

39. Engel, G. L., and Romano, J.: Studies of Syncope. IV: Biological Interpretations of Vasodepressor Syncope, *Psychosom. Med.*, 9:288, 1947.

40. Uvnas, B.: Sympathetic Vasodilator Outflow, *Physiol. Rev.*, 34:608, 1954.

41. Marvin, H. M., and Sullivan, A. G.: Clinical Observations upon Syncope and Sudden Death in Relation to Aortic Stenosis, *Am. Heart J.*, 10:705, 1935.

42. Hammarsten, J. F.: Syncope in Aortic Stenosis, *A.M.A. Arch. Int. Med.*, 87: 274: 1951.

43. Mitchell, A. M., Sackett, C. H., Hunzicker, W. J., and Levine, S. A.: The Clinical Features of Aortic Stenosis, *Am. Heart J.*, 48:684, 1954.

44. Tyler, H. R., and Clark, D. B.: Loss of Consciousness and Convulsions with Congenital Heart Disease, *A.M.A. Arch. Neurol. & Psychiat.*, 79:506, 1958.

45. Dressler, W.: Effort Syncope as an Early Manifestation of Primary Pulmonary Hypertension, *Am. J. M. Sc.*, 223:131, 1952.

46. Ebert, R. V., Stead, E. A., Jr., and Gibson, J. G.: Response of Normal Subjects to Acute Blood Loss, *A.M.A. Arch. Int. Med.*, 68:578, 1941.

47. Gambill, E. E., Hines, E. A., Jr., and Adson, A. W.: The Circulation in Man in Certain Postures before and after Extensive Sympathectomy for Essential Hypertension, *Am. Heart J.*, 27:360, 1944.

48. Grimson, K. S., Orgain, E. S., Rowe, C. R., and Sieber, H. A.: Caution with Regard to Use of Hexamethonium and "Apresoline," *J.A.M.A.*, 149: 215, 1952.

49. Freis, E. D., Stanton, J. R., Finnerty, F. A., Jr., Schnaper, H. W., Johnson, R. L., Rath, C. E., and Wilkins, R. W.: The Collapse Produced by Venous Congestion of the Extremities or by Venesection Following Certain Hypotensive Agents, *J. Clin. Invest.*, 30:435, 1951.

50. O'Donnell, T. V.: Studies in Postural Hypotension Following Ganglion Blocking Drugs, *Clin. Sc.*, 18:237, 1959.

51. Cookson, H.: Fainting and Fits in Cardiac Infarction, *Brit. Heart J.*, 4:163, 1952.

52. Golden, A.: Syncope Associated with Exertional Dyspnea and Angina Pectoris, *Am. Heart J.*, 28:689, 1944.

53. Howard, B. K., Goodson, J. H., and Mengert, W. F.: Supine Hypotensive Syndrome in Late Pregnancy, *Obst. & Gynec.*, 1:371, 1953.

54. Eichna, L. W., Horvath, S. M., and Bean, W. B.: Post Exertional Orthostatic Hypotension, *Am. J. M. Sc.*, 213:641, 1947.

55. Hollister, L. E.: Medical Progress: Complications

from the Use of Tranquilizing Drugs, *New England J. Med.*, **257**:170, 1957.

56. Deitrick, J. E., Whedon, O. G. D., and Shorr, E.: Effects of Immobilization on Various Metabolic and Physiologic Functions of Normal Men, *Am. J. Med.*, **4**:3, 1948.

57. Hickler, R. B.: Plasma Catechol Amine and Electroencephalographic Responses to Acute Postural Change, *Am. J. Med.*, **26**:410, 1959.

58. Luft, R., and Von Euler, U. S.: Two Cases of Postural Hypotension Showing a Deficiency in Release of Norepinephrine and Epinephrine, *J. Clin. Invest.*, **32**:1065, 1953.

59. Benestad, A. M., and Boe, J.: Idiopathic Orthostatic Hypotension, *Acta med. scandinav.*, **150**:1, 1954.

60. Bradbury, S., and Eggleston, C.: Postural Hypotension, *Am. Heart J.*, **1**:73, 1925.

61. Rundles, R. W.: Diabetic Neuropathy, *Medicine*, **24**:111, 1945.

62. Young, R. H.: Association of Postural Hypotension with Sympathetic Nervous System Dysfunction: Case Report with a Review of Neurological Features Associated with Postural Hypotension, *Ann. Int. Med.*, **15**:910, 1941.

63. Stead, E. A., Jr., and Ebert, R. V.: Postural Hypotension, a Disease of the Sympathetic Nervous System, *A.M.A. Arch. Int. Med.*, **67**:546, 1941.

64. Denny-Brown, D.: Recurrent Cerebrovascular Episodes, *A.M.A. Arch. Neurol.*, **2**:194, 1960.

65. Meyer, J. S.: Occlusive Cerebrovascular Disease, *Am. J. Med.*, **30**:577, 1961.

66. Currier, R. D., DeJong, R. N., and Bole, G. G.: Pulseless Disease: Central Nervous System Manifestations, *Neurology*, **4**:818, 1954.

67. Webster, J. E., and Gurdjian, F. S.: Observations upon Response to Digital Carotid Artery Compression in Hemiplegic or Hemiparetic Patients, *Neurology*, **7**:757, 1957.

68. Illingworth, R. S.: Attacks of Unconsciousness in Association with Fused Cervical Vertebrae, *Arch. Dis. Childhood*, **31**:8, 1956.

69. Tatlow, W. F. T., and Banner, N. G.: Syndrome of Vertebral Artery Compression, *Neurology*, **7**:331, 1957.

70. Hardin, C. A., Williamson, W. P., and Steegman, A. T.: Vertebral Artery Insufficiency Produced by Cervical Osteoarthritic Spurs, *Neurology*, **10**:855, 1960.

71. Weiss, S., and Baker, J. P.: The Carotid Sinus Reflex in Health and Disease: Its Role in the Causation of Fainting and Convulsions, *Medicine*, **12**:297, 1933.

72. Ferris, E. B., Capps, R. B., and Weiss, S.: Carotid Sinus Syncope and Its Bearing on the Mechanism of the Unconscious State and Convulsions, *Medicine*, **14**:377, 1935.

73. Weiss, S., Capps, R. B., Ferris, E. B., and Munro, D.: Syncope and Convulsions Due to a Hyperactive Carotid Sinus Reflex: Diagnosis and Treatment, *A.M.A. Arch. Int. Med.*, **58**:407, 1936.

74. Derbes, V. J., and Kerr, A., Jr.: "Cough Syncope," Charles C Thomas, Publisher, Springfield, Ill., 1955.

75. McIntosh, H. D., Estes, E. H., and Warren, J. V.: The Mechanisms of Cough Syncope, *Am. Heart J.*, **52**:70, 1956.

76. Sharpey-Schafer, E. P.: The Mechanism of Syncope after Coughing, *Brit. M. J.*, **2**:860, 1953.

77. Kerr, A., Jr., and Eich, R. H.: Cerebral Concussion as a Cause of Cough Syncope, *Arch. Int. Med.*, **108**:138, 1961.

78. Lyle, C. B., Jr., Monroe, J. T., Jr., Flinn, D. E., and Lamb, L. E.: Micturition Syncope: Report of 24 Cases, *New England J. Med.*, **265**:982, 1961.

79. Schwartz, S. P., and Billon, S.: The Clinical Signs of Occluding Thrombi of the Left Auricle, *Am. Heart J.*, **7**:84, 1931.

80. Harvey, J. K.: Myxoma of the Left Auricle, *Ann. Int. Med.*, **47**:1067, 1957.

81. Weiss, S., and Ferris, E. B.: Adams-Stokes Syndrome with Transient Complete Heart Block of Vagovagal Reflex Origin, *A.M.A. Arch. Int. Med.*, **54**:931, 1934.

82. Schwichtenberg, A. H., Luft, U. C., and Stratton, K. L.: Altitude Physiology: Air Travel in the Jet Age, in "Clinical Cardiopulmonary Physiology," 2d ed., Grune & Stratton, Inc., New York, 1960, p. 936.

83. Engel, G. L., Ferris, E. B., and Logan, M.: Hyperventilation Analysis of Clinical Symptomatology, *Ann. Int. Med.*, **27**:683, 1947.

84. Gurdjian, E. S., Webster, J. E., Hardy, W. G., and Lindner, D. W.: Nonexistence of the So-called Cerebral Form of Carotid Sinus Syncope, *Neurology*, **8**:818, 1958.

85. Romano, J., and Engel, G. F.: Studies of Syncope. III. The Differentiation between Vasodepressor and Hysterical Fainting, *Psychosom. Med.*, **7**:3, 1945.

86. Bickerstaff, E. R.: Impairment of Consciousness in Migraine, *Lancet*, **2**:1057 1961.

87. Freis, E. D., Schnaper, H. W., Johnson, R. L., and Schreiner, G. E.: Hemodynamic Alterations in Acute Myocardial Infarction, *J. Clin. Invest.*, **31**:131, 1952.

88. Smith, W. W., Wikler, N. S., and Fox, A. C.: Hemodynamic Studies of Patients with Myocardial Infarction, *Circulation*, **9**:352, 1954.

89. Gilbert, R. P., Goldberg, M. A., and Griffin, J.: Circulatory Changes in Acute Myocardial Infarction, *Circulation*, **9**:847, 1954.

90. Fishberg, A. M., Hitzig, W. M., and King, F. H.: Circulatory Dynamics in Myocardial Infarction, *A.M.A. Arch. Int. Med.*, **54**:977, 1934.

91. Boyer, N. H.: Medical Progress: Cardiogenic Shock, *New England J. Med.*, **230**:226, 256, 1944.

92. Agress, C. M., Rosenburg, M., Schneiderman, A., and Brotman, E. J.: Blood Volume Studies in Shock Resulting from Myocardial Infarction. I.

Studies with Evans Blue Dye, *J. Clin. Invest.*, 29: 1267, 1950.

93. Agress, C. M., Rosenburg, M. J., Binder, M. J., Schneiderman, A., and Clark, W. G.: Blood Volume Changes in Protracted Shock Resulting from Experimental Myocardial Infarction, *Am. J. Physiol.*, 166:603, 1951.

94. Blumgart, H. L.: Treatment of Acute Myocardial Infarction with Particular Reference to Shock, *J.A.M.A.*, 154:107, 1954.

95. Agress, C. M.: Therapy of Cardiogenic Shock, *Progr. in Cardiovas. Dis.*, 6:236, 1963.

96. Altschule, M. D.: Hazards in Treatment of Cardiac Decompensation, *New England J. Med.*, 248:493, 1953.

97. Binder, M. J., Ryan, J. A., Marcus, S., Mugler, F., Strange, D., and Agress, C. M.: Evaluation of Therapy in Shock Following Acute Myocardial Infarction, *Am. J. Med.*, 18:622, 1955.

98. Sarnoff, S. J., Case, R. B., Berglund, E., and Sarnoff, L. C.: Ventricular Function: Circulatory Effects of Aramine, *Circulation*, 10:84, 1954.

99. Littler, T. R., and McKendrick, C. S.: L-Noradrenaline in Myocardial Infarction, *Lancet*, 2:825, 1957.

100. Gazes, P. C., Goldberg, L. I., and Darby, T. D.: Heart Force Effects of Sympathomimetic Amine as Basis for Their Use in Shock Accompanying Myocardial Infarction, *Circulation*, 8:883, 1953.

101. West, J. W., Faulk, A. T., and Guzman, S. V.: Comparative Study of Effects of Levarterenol and Methoxamine in Shock Associated with Acute Myocardial Ischemia in Dogs, *Circulation Res.*, 10:712, 1962.

102. del Greco, F., and Johnson, D. C.: Clinical Experience with Angiotensin II in the Treatment of Shock, *J.A.M.A.*, 178:994, 1961.

103. Koch-Weser, J.: Myocardial Actions of Angiotensin, *Circulation Res.*, 14:337, 1964.

104. Derrick, J. R., Anderson, J. R., and Roland, B. J.: Adjunctive Use of a Biologic Pressor Agent, Angiotensin, in Management of Shock, *Circulation*, 25:263, 1962.

105. Nickerson, M.: Sympathetic Blockade in Therapy of Shock, *Am. J. Cardiol.*, 12:619, 1963.

106. Agress, C. M.: Management of Coronary Shock, *Am. J. Cardiol.*, 1:231, 1958.

107. Manning, G. W., et al.: Use of Cardiac Sympathetic Denervation to Reduce Mortality Due to Ventricular Arrhythmias: Report to Royal College of Physicians and Surgeons of Canada, 1962.

108. Humphries, J. O.: Treatment of Heart Block with Artificial Pacemakers, *Mod. Concepts Cardiovas. Dis.*, 33:857, 1964.

109. Alexander, S., Kleiger, R., and Lown, B.: Use of External Countershock in the Treatment of Ventricular Tachycardia, *J.A.M.A.*, 177:916, 1961.

110. Lown, B., Amarasingham, R., and Neuman, J.: New Method for Terminating Cardiac Arrhythmias, *J.A.M.A.*, 182:548, 1962.

111. Stuckey, J. H., Newman, M. M., Dennis, C., Berg, E. H., Goodman, S. E., Fries, C. C., Karlson, K. E., Blumenfeld, M., Weitzner, S. W., Binder, L. S., and Winston, A.: The Use of the Heart-Lung Machine in Selected Cases of Acute Myocardial Infarction, *S. Forum*, 8:342, 1957.

112. Corday, E., Dennis, C., LaDue, J. S., Master, A. M., and Zimmerman, H. A.: Emergency Management of Complications of Acute Coronary Occlusion, *Dis. Chest*, 42:6, 1962.

113. Matthes, K.: Myocardial Shock, in "CIBA Foundation Symposium on Shock," Little, Brown and Company, Boston, 1962, pp. 253–266.

114. Crowell, J. W., and Read, W. L.: In Vivo Coagulation—A Probable Cause of Irreversible Shock, *Am. J. Physiol.*, 183:565, 1955.

115. Zweifach, B. W.: Tissue Mediators in the Genesis of Experimental Shock, *J.A.M.A.*, 81:866, 1962.

116. Knisely, M. H., Eliot, T. S., and Block, E. H.: Sludged Blood in Traumatic Shock, *A.M.A. Arch. Surg.*, 51:220, 1945.

117. Rhoads, J.: Recent Progress and Present Problems in the Field of Shock (Summation of Conference), *Fed. Proc.*, 20:235, 1961.

118. Stroud, M. W., and Feil, H. S.: The Terminal Electrocardiogram: Twenty-three Case Reports and a Review of the Literature, *Am. Heart J.*, 35:910, 1948.

119. Cole, S. L., and Corday, E.: Four Minute Limit for Cardiac Resuscitation, *J.A.M.A.*, 161:1454, 1956.

120. Beck, C. S., and Leighninger, D. S.: Death after Clean Bill of Health, *J.A.M.A.*, 174:133, 1960.

121. Kouwenhoven, W. B., Jude, J. R., and Knickerbocker, G. G.: Closed-Chest Cardiac Massage, *J.A.M.A.*, 173:1064, 1960.

122. Himmelhock, S. R., et al.: Closed-chest Cardiac Resuscitation, *New England J. Med.*, 270:118, 1964.

123. Day, H. W.: An Intensive Coronary Care Area, *Dis. Chest*, 44:423, 1963.

124. Wilburne, M., and Fields, J.: Cardiac Resuscitation in Coronary Artery Disease, *J.A.M.A.*, 184:453, 1963.

125. Lockward, H. J., Lundberg, A. F., Jr., and Odoroff, M. E.: Effect of Intensive Care on Mortality Rate of Patients with Myocardial Infarcts, *Pub. Health Rep.*, 78:655, 1963.

PART IV

Common Diseases of the Heart and Pericardium

Section A: Congenital Heart Disease

18 PATHOLOGY OF CONGENITAL HEART DISEASE

Robert S. Eliot, M.D., and
Jesse E. Edwards, M.D.

The pathology of congenital heart disease is most useful to the clinician when it is presented within the framework of clinical patterns. The clinician has certain readily available tools with which he can establish a broad functional category; i.e., the working diagnosis. From this, special studies may be intelligently planned from which a specific anatomic anomaly may be identified. The tools at the clinician's disposal are (1) presence or absence of cyanosis (in this presentation, the term *cyanosis* will refer to incomplete oxygen saturation of the systemic arterial blood, whether or not visible bluing of the skin and mucous membranes occurs), (2) the radiologic appearance of the pulmonary arterial vessels, whether of increased, normal, or decreased prominence, and (3) the presence or absence of electrocardiographic evidence of hypertrophy of one or both of the ventricles.

With these considerations as a background, the following classification, modified from Kanjuh and Edwards,[1] will be used:

CLASSIFICATION OF CONGENITAL HEART DISEASE

I. Increased prominence of the pulmonary arterial vessels
  A. Without cyanosis
  B. With cyanosis
    1. Delayed
    2. From birth
II. Decreased or normal prominence of the pulmonary arterial vessels with cyanosis
  A. With right ventricular hypertrophy
  B. Without right ventricular hypertrophy
III. Normal pulmonary vessels without cyanosis and with right ventricular hypertrophy
IV. Normal pulmonary vessels without cyanosis and with left ventricular hypertrophy
V. Prominent pulmonary arterial and venous vessels with right ventricular hypertrophy and without cyanosis (pulmonary venous obstruction)

Several anatomic entities usually conform to any one functional class. In the following, these will be considered, but for more detailed coverage of the various anatomic entities, the reader is referred to two publications in which one of us (J. E. E.) was involved in authorship.[2,3]

Material on incidence, age and sex distribution, and coexistence of one malformation with another is covered comprehensively elsewhere.[4]

INCREASED PROMINENCE OF THE PULMONARY ARTERIAL VESSELS WITHOUT CYANOSIS

Under this heading are the anomalies which are associated with a left-to-right shunt. The shunt may be either into a right-sided cardiac chamber or into the pulmonary trunk. The specific anomalies will be considered according to the anatomic site into which the left-to-right shunt occurs.

Left-to-right Shunt into the Right Atrium

The common anomaly which allows a left-to-right shunt into the right atrium is the atrial septal defect, of which there are several anatomic varieties. Of these, the most prevalent is the defect at the fossa ovalis. This anomaly is not specifically associated with any other, although there is some association with rheumatic mitral stenosis, a combination called the *Lutembacher syndrome*. In the latter, it is probable that the atrial septal defect does not predispose to the occurrence of rheumatic mitral valvular disease. Rather, it is conceivable that the mitral valvular disease is primary and that the atrial septal defect develops from a valvular competent patent foramen ovale as a consequence of left atrial dilatation incident to the mitral stenosis.

Classically, atrial septal defect is not associated with pulmonary hypertension, except as a late complication. The right-sided chambers and the pulmonary arterial vessels are enlarged, as anatomic expressions of the large volume of the shunt that usually pertains (Fig. 18-1a).

Another form of atrial septal defect is that which occurs in the lowermost part of the atrial septum and which is associated with some maldevelopment of the atrioventricular valves and the ventricular septum. Together, these anomalies form the complex known as *persistent common atrioventricular canal.* Two major forms of this malformation are identifiable, the partial and the complete. In the partial form, the atrial septal defect is associated with a cleft in the anterior leaflet of the mitral valve, while the tricuspid valve is not cleft. The basal aspect of the ventricular septum is deficient, but since the mitral valve is adherent to the posterior edge of the deficiency, no interventricular communication occurs, although this arrangement may cause subaortic stenosis.

In the complete variety of persistent common atrioventricular canal, there is a greater tendency for association with mongolism than in the partial variety. In the complete form, both the anterior mitral and septal tricuspid leaflets are cleft, so that there is, in effect, one atrioventricular valve which is common to both sides of the heart. Beneath the common atrioventricular valve, spaces usually occur which allow interventricular communication. The latter circumstance introduces functional factors like those in ventricular septal defect.

A third form of atrial septal defect is that which occurs superior to the fossa ovalis. This defect is in close proximity to the superior vena cava, which may straddle it. As part of a developmental complex, this defect is associated with anomalous connection of some or all of the right pulmonary veins, either to the superior vena cava or to the right atrium.

A fourth variety of atrial septal defect is that which occurs in the posteroinferior angle of the septum and is associated with termination of a persistent left superior vena cava in the left atrium. This variety, as well as the third type of atrial septal defect mentioned, may be associated with an element of a right-to-left shunt in association with the major left-to-right shunt.

There are other anomalies in acyanotic patients which allow fully saturated blood to enter the left atrium. These include (1) a peculiar form of ventricular septal defect which allows a left ventricular–right atrial communication, (2) rupture of an aortic sinus aneurysm into the right atrium, (3) communication of a coronary artery either with the coronary sinus or with the right atrium, and (4) anomalous communication of some of the pulmonary veins with the right atrium or with a systemic vein.

It is also to be mentioned that a ventricular septal defect associated with tricuspid insufficiency will cause fully oxygenated blood to enter the right atrium.

Left-to-right Shunt into the Right Ventricle

The common anomaly which allows abnormal delivery of fully saturated blood into the right ventricle is the ventricular septal defect. Though any portion of the ventricular septum may show a defect, the common location is in relation to the membranous septum. Such defects, commonly called *membranous ventricular septal defects,* usually involve not only the membranous portion but also some of that muscular part of the septum which lies anterior and inferior to the membranous portion.

Though ventricular septal defects are usually solitary, there are examples of multiple defects. The latter represent retention of the normally occurring intertrabecular spaces in the ventricular septum of the embryo. In the mature heart these defects are tortuous channels in the muscular part

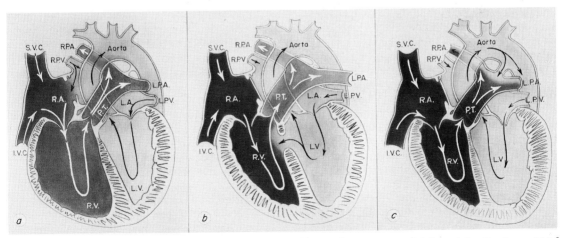

Fig. 18-1. Diagrammatic portrayal of central circulation in common varieties of left-to-right shunt. *a.* Atrial septal defect. *b.* Ventricular septal defect. *c.* Classical patent ductus arteriosus. (*With permission of the author and the publisher.*[1])

of the septum. Lying in the contractile part of the septum, such channels may change in size with different phases of the cardiac cycle. Also, as the septum grows, such channels may become obliterated postnatally, if still present at birth.

The functional disturbance caused by a ventricular septal defect is dependent primarily on its size and on the nature of the pulmonary vascular bed rather than on the position of the defect.[5] Two functional types of ventricular septal defects may be recognized, the small and the large. The dividing line is usually compared with the size of the aortic valvular orifice. Those defects which are smaller than this orifice are classified as *small;* those as large as the aortic orifice or larger are designated as *large.*

In cases with small ventricular septal defect the pulmonary arterial and right ventricular pressures are either normal or at least below aortic and left ventricular pressures, respectively. The shunt is in a left-to-right direction and is usually of lesser magnitude than in comparable cases with large defects. Small ventricular septal defect, the so-called *maladie de Roger,* has, as its chief complication, bacterial endocarditis.

When a ventricular septal defect is large, there is, invariably, equalization of pulmonary arterial and right ventricular systolic pressures, on one hand, with the aortic and left ventricular pressures, on the other (Fig. 18-1*b*). The pulmonary hypertension in this situation is to be considered an integral part of the functional derangement, not a complication. In infancy, and in most cases through childhood, the resistance offered to pulmonary blood flow is less than the resistance offered to systemic flow. During this period in life the shunt is usually entirely in a left-to-right direction. This places a strain on the left ventricle, to which the shunted blood returns, and death in infancy from left ventricular failure is common. It is perhaps the exceptional patient, in terms of the total number of patients born with ventricular septal defect, regardless of the absolute number of cases that exist beyond infancy, who survives for more than 6 months after birth.

Among most patients with ventricular septal defect the great vessels are normally oriented. Uncommonly, *corrected transposition of the great vessels* is associated. In corrected transposition, although the great vessels are transposed, the route for the flow of blood is normal. The venous connections with the heart and the atria are normal. The venous ventricle, although exhibiting a mirror-image structure of a normal left ventricle, lies between the venous atrium and the pulmonary trunk. Likewise, the arterial ventricle, which shows a mirror-image structure of a right ventricle, lies be-

tween the arterial atrium and the transposed aorta.

There are other conditions which cause a left-to-right shunt into the right ventricle. In *ventricular septal defect associated with aortic valvular insufficiency* some of the "arterialized" blood reaching the right ventricle originates above the incompetent aortic valve. *Rupture of an aneurysm of the right aortic sinus* leads into the outflow tract of the right ventricle. Such aneurysms may be associated with a subjacent ventricular septal defect. *Anomalous communication of a coronary artery with the right ventricle* is yet another cause of abnormal delivery of fully oxygenated blood into the right ventricle.

Left-to-right Shunt into the Pulmonary Arterial System

The classic condition responsible for a shunt of fully saturated blood into the pulmonary arterial system is *patent ductus arteriosus* (Fig. 18-1*c*). As with ventricular septal defect, the functional state is dependent on the resistance offered to flow through the abnormal opening. Those cases in which the ductus is narrow or long and narrow, states offering high levels of resistance to flow, yield a picture of *classical patent ductus arteriosus* in which the pulmonary pressure is not elevated and in which the characteristic "machinery" murmur occurs. Patients with this condition usually live to adult life and are faced with the potential complications either of left ventricular failure or of bacterial endarteritis. When the ductus offers little resistance to flow it is usually short and *wide.* In such cases, as with large ventricular septal defect, there is pulmonary hypertension with equalization of systemic and pulmonary arterial pressures. The hazards of the large left-to-right shunt in this condition are like those in large ventricular septal defect.

Considerably less common than patent ductus arteriosus, but having a functional pattern fundamentally similar to that of wide patent ductus arteriosus, is the *aorticopulmonary septal defect.* The synonym "aorticopulmonary window" is descriptive of the anomaly, which is a window-like communication between the left side of the ascending aorta and the right side of the pulmonary trunk. Although the possibility of aorticopulmonary septal defect is to be entertained in the differential diagnosis of patent ductus arteriosus, the two conditions may, uncommonly, coexist.[6]

Uncommon causes of "arterialization" of pulmonary arterial blood are anomalies of the coronary arterial system. These anomalies take two forms. In one form the two usual coronary arteries arise from the aorta, while an *accessory coronary artery* arises from the pulmonary trunk. Through communications between the normal and abnormal coronary arteries, systemic arterial blood may be carried into the pulmonary trunk.

The second type of coronary arterial anomaly is that in which, of the two coronary arteries, one arises from the aorta while the other *arises from the pulmonary trunk.* In the postnatal period, numerous collateral connections develop between the two arteries. As the pulmonary arterial pressure is lower than the aortic pressure, a state is reached in which aortic blood flows from the normal coronary artery into the abnormal one and finally into the pulmonary trunk.

INCREASED PROMINENCE OF THE PULMONARY ARTERIAL VESSELS WITH DELAYED CYANOSIS

The septal defects, including patent ductus arteriosus, which were considered in the foregoing section usually are not associated with cyanosis during infancy. In each of these defects, cyanosis may appear at a later date. In atrial septal defect, this complication is not usual before adult life is reached; in ventricular septal defect or patent ductus arteriosus, cyanosis may appear during childhood but more commonly appears during adolescence or early adult life. In each type of septal defect, cyanosis is an ultimate sign of complicating occlusive pulmonary vascular disease.

When a large ventricular septal defect or wide patent ductus arteriosus is present, there is equalization of pulmonary and systemic arterial pressures from birth. The direction of the shunt through the defect depends on the state of the small pulmonary arterial vessels (Fig. 18-2*a* and *b*). In the early years of life these changes are such as to allow a left-to-right shunt. With time, and as a consequence of the pulmonary hypertension (and possibly increased flow), occlusive lesions develop in the pulmonary vascular bed. These lesions, which reduce the capacity of the pulmonary vascular bed, may become so extensive as to tip the balance in favor of a reduced left-to-right shunt and, ultimately, a right-to-left shunt through the defect.

In atrial septal defect, the relationship between occlusive pulmonary vascular disease, on one hand, and cyanosis, on the other, is not so direct. In this condition, although a large left-to-right shunt may exist for many years, no pulmonary hypertension is present until occlusive pulmonary vascular disease develops. When this occurs the pulmonary arterial pressure rises and the right ventricular wall hypertrophies.

The direction of flow through an atrial septal defect depends on the distensibility of the right ventricle relative to the distensibility of the left ventricle. With the right ventricular hypertrophy that accompanies pulmonary hypertension, the right ventricle offers more resistance to filling. This effects a reduction in the left-to-right shunt, and ultimately, the right ventricle may offer such levels of resistance to filling as to tip the balance in favor of a right-to-left shunt through the atrial septal defect (Fig. 18-2*c*).

INCREASED PROMINENCE OF THE PULMONARY ARTERIAL VESSELS WITH CYANOSIS FROM BIRTH

Included under this heading are those anomalies which fulfill the following criteria: (1) there is a common mixing chamber or vessel, and (2) pul-

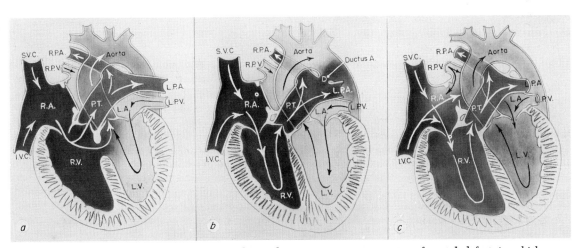

Fig. 18-2. Diagrammatic portrayal of central circulation in common varieties of septal defect in which cyanosis may be acquired. *a.* Large ventricular septal defect. *b.* Wide patent ductus arteriosus. *c.* Atrial septal defect. (*With permission of the author and publisher.*[1])

monary stenosis is absent. Cyanosis is primarily dependent on the presence of a common mixing chamber which establishes the basis for obligatory bidirectional shunts. Pulmonary blood flow is usually greater than systemic flow in most of the conditions in this category, and pulmonary hypertension is universally present, except when the mixing occurs at the atrial level. The pulmonary hypertension may lead to occlusive pulmonary vascular disease and cause a reduction in the volume of left-to-right shunt and accentuation of the degree of cyanosis.

The anomalies which pertain to this category will be considered according to the anatomic site of the mixing chamber or vessel. In *total anomalous pulmonary venous connection,* none of the pulmonary veins joins the left atrium. Instead, these veins join either the right atrium or one (usually) or several of the systemic veins. Mixing of systemic and pulmonary venous blood occurs in the right atrium. Systemic blood flow depends on flow into the left atrium from the right atrium across an interatrial communication. Common systemic venous sites for anomalous termination of the pulmonary veins are the left innominate vein, the coronary sinus, and the superior vena cava and intraabdominal visceral veins, particularly the portal vein or the ductus venosus.

Pulmonary venous obstruction may be an added element of the functional derangement in total anomalous pulmonary venous connection. This is most apt to occur when the pulmonary veins terminate in an abdominal vein, but it is also seen in some cases of intrathoracic termination of the pulmonary veins. Pulmonary venous obstruction tends to influence survival adversely. Patients with this condition tend to succumb in infancy, and in those patients with total anomalous pulmonary venous connection but without pulmonary venous obstruction, survival to adult life is uncommon.

Cor Triloculare Biatriatum without Pulmonary Stenosis

This condition is characterized by a common ventricle which supplies both the systemic and pulmonary arterial circulations, while two atria are present. In those cases of cor triloculare biatriatum which conform to the functional category in which there is increased prominence of the pulmonary vessels, no pulmonary stenosis is present and the great vessels are transposed, the ascending aorta lying anterior to the pulmonary trunk. When two atrioventricular valves are present, mixing in the single ventricle is not complete, as the stream of blood from the left atrium tends to be directed toward the aorta, while the right atrial blood tends

to be directed toward the pulmonary trunk. Under these circumstances, the clinical picture may resemble that of ventricular septal defect. When either the mitral or tricuspid valve is atretic, more uniform mixing occurs than when each of these valves is patent.

Origin of Both Great Vessels from the Right Ventricle without Pulmonary Stenosis

An interesting anomaly is that in which the heart possesses the usual four chambers but in which both great arterial vessels arise from the right ventricle. The only outlet for the left ventricle is a ventricular septal defect, usually of the large variety. The origin of the pulmonary trunk from the right ventricle is in a normal position, while the aortic origin lies to the right of the pulmonary origin. Above the heart, the positions of the two great arteries, as viewed in a frontal plane, cannot be distinguished from normal. Viewed from the side, the proximal segment of the aorta is abnormally anterior and fails to make the curvature posteroinferiorly toward the left ventricle.

Two major forms of origin of both great vessels from the right ventricle have been defined,[7] according to the position of the ventricular septal defect. In the first form, the defect lies relatively low, being separated from both the semilunar valves by muscular tissue of the ventricular septum. In the second type, which is synonymous with the *Taussig-Bing heart,* the ventricular septal defect lies immediately subjacent to the pulmonary trunk. On the basis of preferential flow of streams through the ventricular portion of the heart, greater degrees of right-to-left shunt, and consequently greater degrees of cyanosis, are seen in the second type than in the first.

Complete Transposition of Great Vessels

A common condition, and one that is usually lethal during infancy, is complete transposition of the great vessels. The venous connections with the heart are normal, and as the aorta arises from the right ventricle and the pulmonary trunk from the left, intense cyanosis is the rule. Survival depends on the presence of communications between the two sides of the heart. A ventricular septal defect is present in about one-half the cases.[8] An interatrial communication is present in all cases and takes the form either of valvular competent patent foramen ovale or of a small true atrial septal defect (Fig. 18-3a). Patency of the ductus arteriosus is common. A favorable combination of coexisting malformations in complete transposition is pulmonary or subpulmonary stenosis distal to a ventricular septal defect in association with either a patent ductus or an interatrial communication.

DECREASED OR NORMAL PROMINENCE OF THE PULMONARY ARTERIAL VESSELS WITH CYANOSIS AND RIGHT VENTRICULAR HYPERTROPHY

The cyanotic patient with normal or decreased prominence of the pulmonary arterial vessels is often seen among subjects with congenital heart disease. In such patients, both pulmonary stenosis and right ventricular hypertrophy are common.

In an exceptional case of cyanosis without increased prominence of the pulmonary arterial vessels, right ventricular hypertrophy is absent. Such cases, which form a group represented by a small number of malformations, will be considered further on in this chapter. Here we are concerned with those conditions which, in the presence of cyanosis and of normal or decreased pulmonary arterial prominence, display right ventricular hypertension and hypertrophy.

In this category each condition is characterized by the right-to-left shunt, which is responsible for the cyanosis and which usually occurs at the ventricular level. In only two of the conditions which pertain to this group, viz., pulmonary stenosis and pulmonary atresia, each with intact ventricular septum, does the right-to-left shunt occur at the atrial level. The latter two conditions will be considered after those in which the right-to-left shunt is at the ventricular level.

Tetralogy of Fallot

This is the most common condition which obeys the definition of cyanosis associated with right ventricular hypertrophy and normal or decreased prominence of the pulmonary arterial vessels. Anatomically, this condition is characterized by a biventricular origin of the aorta above a large ventricular septal defect and obstruction to pulmonary blood flow (Fig. 18-3*b*). The latter usually results from narrowness of the right ventricular infundibulum. The pulmonary valve is usually bicuspid and may also be stenotic. The right-to-left shunt occurs between the right ventricle and the aorta. Its magnitude depends on the degree of obstruction to pulmonary blood flow. Although in most cases of the tetralogy of Fallot only a right-to-left shunt occurs, there are examples with fundamentally the same anatomic features, but in which the degree of pulmonary stenosis is mild. In these cases, a bidirectional or only a left-to-right shunt occurs. Clinically the patients are said to have "pink tetralogies" or "acyanotic tetralogies."

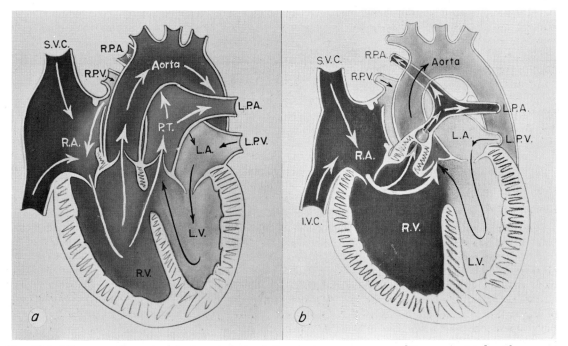

Fig. 18-3. Diagrammatic portrayal of central circulation in two common conditions associated with cyanosis from birth and right-to-left shunt at ventricular level. *a.* Complete transposition of great vessels. A ventricular septal defect and interatrial communication are commonly observed. *b.* Tetralogy of Fallot with pulmonary stenosis. (*With permission of the author and publisher.*[1])

When, in the tetralogy, the obstruction to pulmonary flow takes the form of atresia, either of the right ventricular infundibulum or of the pulmonary valve, the condition may be called *pseudo-truncus arteriosus*. In such cases the pulmonary trunk and its branches are present. Flow of blood to the lungs is mainly through enlarged bronchial arteries and, at times, also through a patent ductus arteriosus.

A right aortic arch is found in about 20 per cent of all patients with the tetralogy of Fallot, with a greater tendency for this associated malformation to occur among patients with the tetralogy who have pulmonary atresia rather than pulmonary stenosis. Usually the aortic malformation does not interfere with the function of the trachea or of the esophagus, as the branches of the arch are in mirror image of the normal and there is no retroesophageal aortic segment. Less commonly, the left subclavian artery arises as the fourth branch of the aorta. In this form, as the left subclavian artery passes behind the esophagus and receives the systemic end of the ductus arteriosus, it may be responsible for a vascular ring. A double aortic arch is rarely associated with the tetralogy of Fallot. Also uncommon is the situation in which there is a right aortic arch but no connection is present between the aorta and the left subclavian artery. The latter vessel is joined to the origin of the left pulmonary artery by the ductus arteriosus.

Among the complications of the tetralogy of Fallot are (1) hypoxic fainting spells, (2) cerebral abscess, and (3) bacterial endocarditis.

Origin of Both Great Vessels from the Right Ventricle with Pulmonary Stenosis

Anatomically, except for the presence of infundibular stenosis, this condition is like origin of both great vessels from the right ventricle without pulmonary stenosis. The presence of infundibular stenosis favors a right-to-left shunt, and the clinical picture resembles closely that of the tetralogy of Fallot. Angiocardiographic studies may be helpful in establishing the diagnosis.

Common Ventricle with Pulmonary Stenosis

When a common ventricle is associated with pulmonary stenosis, the great vessels either may be transposed or may occupy normal positions. The obstruction to pulmonary blood flow usually is on the basis of a narrow subpulmonary infundibular chamber. Clinically, resemblance to the tetralogy of Fallot is great. The features of the two conditions are especially likely to coincide when, in common ventricle with pulmonary stenosis, the great vessels are normally related. Both atrioventricular valves may be patent or one may be atretic. When the tricuspid valve is atretic, there is a tendency

for the electrocardiogram to show signs of left ventricular hypertrophy. When mitral atresia is present, the anticipated signs of pulmonary venous obstruction may be absent, in view of the low volumes of pulmonary blood flow incident to the pulmonary stenosis (or atresia).

Congenital Heart Disease Associated with Asplenia

Asplenia is usually part of a developmental complex in which multiple and major cardiovascular anomalies occur. These anomalies almost invariably include severe obstruction to pulmonary blood flow. Either a ventricular septal defect or a common ventricle is present. The atrial portion of the heart is commonly normal, and usually bilateral superior venae cavae are present. Total anomalous pulmonary venous connection occurs frequently. A right-sided stomach is common. As the lobes of the liver are of about equal size, a hint of this complex may be obtained from roentgenograms that include the upper abdomen. A horizontal rather than an oblique course of the lower edge of the liver in a cyanotic subject is to be considered almost pathognomonic. Heinz bodies and multiple Howell-Jolly bodies in the erythrocytes in smears of the peripheral blood add to the likelihood of this complicated developmental aberration.

Persistent Truncus Arteriosus with Pulmonary Stenosis

In most examples of persistent truncus arteriosus there is no obstruction to pulmonary blood flow and the cases are in the category of cyanosis from birth associated with increased prominence of the pulmonary arterial vessels. Uncommonly, there may be stenosis of the pulmonary arterial branches, or, indeed, there may be no pulmonary arteries. The latter arrangement is designated as persistent truncus arteriosus, type IV, in the classification of Collett and Edwards.[9] In the latter type, pulmonary blood flow depends on bronchial arteries, which may be enlarged enough to distort the esophagus. The type IV variety of persistent truncus arteriosus may be impossible to distinguish from pseudo-truncus arteriosus even by angiocardiography if in the latter, the pulmonary arteries are not visualized. Patients with persistent truncus arteriosus, type IV, in general have a better outlook than those with pseudo-truncus arteriosus. The former have occasionally been reported to live to adult life; the latter usually succumb in infancy.

Pulmonary Stenosis with Intact Ventricular Septum and Transatrial Right-to-left Shunt

Varying in manifestation, from severe cyanosis in infancy, to survival to adult life with mild cyanosis, is pulmonary stenosis with intact ventricular septum and transatrial right-to-left shunt.

The primary anomaly is in the pulmonary valve. The valvular tissue fails to form the usual semilunar cusps. Instead, the valve is represented by a dome-shaped structure resembling a truncated cone.

Poststenotic dilatation of the pulmonary trunk is common. As the right ventricular pressure is elevated, there is right ventricular hypertrophy. The latter frequently is of major proportion, and the thickness of the right ventricle may exceed that of the left. The hypertrophied wall of the right ventricle may encroach upon the chamber, and in the infundibular region, this process may be responsible for secondary subpulmonary stenosis.

The right-to-left shunt takes place across the atrial septum, usually through a valvular competent foramen ovale (Fig. 18-4a), less often through a true atrial septal defect.

The complications of the condition include cardiac failure, cerebral abscess, and right-sided bacterial endocarditis.

Pulmonary Atresia with Intact Ventricular Septum

Having a more consistently poor prognosis than pulmonary stenosis with intact ventricular septum and transatrial right-to-left shunt is pulmonary atresia with intact ventricular septum. In this condition the pulmonary valve is represented by a fibrous membrane. There is no normal outlet for the right ventricle. Two basic forms are recognized. In one, the right ventricle is small or tiny; in the other, the right ventricle is of normal size or even larger than normal. The latter form probably is dependent on coexistent tricuspid insufficiency. The major outlet for blood from the right side of the heart is across the atrial septum. Mixing occurs in the left atrium, and the entire cardiac output passes into the aorta. Blood supply to the lungs is usually by way of a patent ductus arteriosus, but since the ductus arteriosus has a tendency to close in the postnatal period, the commonly poor prognosis in this condition is attributed to an inadequate pulmonary blood flow.

When the right ventricle is small or tiny, the tricuspid valve is small but probably functions competently. In such cases, the right ventricular pressure may reach excessively high levels and trapped blood in the right ventricle may be forced through myocardial sinusoids into the epicardium, where sinusoidal vessels may join the coronary arterial ramifications.

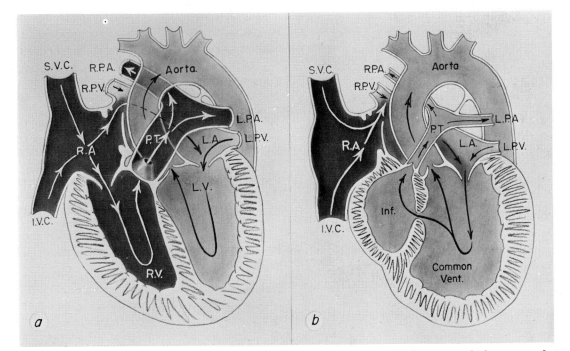

Fig. 18-4. Diagrammatic portrayal of central circulation in two common conditions in which cyanosis from birth is on the basis of a transatrial right-to-left shunt. *a.* Pulmonary valvular stenosis with intact ventricular septum and right-to-left transatrial shunt. *b.* Tricuspid atresia with subpulmonary stenosis. (*With permission of the author and publisher.*[1])

DECREASED OR NORMAL PROMINENCE OF THE PULMONARY ARTERIAL VESSELS WITH CYANOSIS BUT WITHOUT RIGHT VENTRICULAR HYPERTROPHY

Any of the following small number of conditions may be present when there is cyanotic congenital heart disease without signs of right ventricular hypertrophy.

Tricuspid Atresia

In tricuspid atresia there is no tricuspid orifice or valvular tissue in this area. All the blood returning from the systemic circulation is shunted from the right atrium across the atrial septum into the left atrium and, ultimately, into the ventricular portion of the heart. With pulmonary stenosis being present, the major part of the left ventricular output is into the aorta (Fig. 18-4*b*). The left ventricle, which functions as a common ventricle, is enlarged and probably accounts for the electrocardiographic signs of left ventricular hypertrophy. Most commonly, the great vessels are normally related; less commonly the vessels are transposed.

Ebstein's Malformation of the Tricuspid Valve

In this condition the tricuspid valve is abnormal in several ways. The annular attachment of the septal and posterior leaflets is usually lower than normal, the leaflets being attached to the right ventricular wall. In addition, valvular tissue may show multiple adhesions to the right ventricular wall, so that, in some areas, only histologic examination may identify valvular tissue, as such. Anatomically, the derangement causes the inflow portion of the right ventricle to function as a receiving chamber, along with the right atrium. The pumping part of the right ventricle is consequently diminished in size. Thinning of the right ventricular wall, both proximal and distal to the tricuspid valve, is common. In some instances the outflow portion of the thin right ventricle may be so prominent as to yield a shadow along the left cardiac border in roentgenograms. In most instances the atrial septum shows either a defect or a valvular competent patent foramen ovale, and under these circumstances, it is usual that a right-to-left shunt occurs from the right atrium into the left. Survival in this condition varies. Some patients succumb in infancy. Others live to adult life. Treacherous cardiac arrhythmias, congestive cardiac failure, and cerebral abscess are the major complications.

Communication of Superior Vena Cava or Inferior Vena Cava with the Left Atrium

Under rare circumstances, either a persistent left superior vena cava or the inferior vena cava enters the left atrium, carrying unsaturated blood into the systemic side of the circulation. This accounts for cyanosis, and as the right ventricular portion of the heart is normal, no evidence of right ventricular hypertrophy is found in the clinical examination. An atrial septal defect may be associated.

Pulmonary Arteriovenous Fistula

Although not a malformation of the heart, pulmonary arteriovenous fistula is frequently confused with congenital heart disease because the patient is cyanotic. The heart is of normal size. The shunt of pulmonary arterial blood (systemic venous) into the pulmonary veins without passing through pulmonary parenchyma is the basis for the desaturation of the systemic arterial blood. A special form of pulmonary arteriovenous fistula is that in which a pulmonary artery makes direct communication with the left atrium.[10]

NORMAL PULMONARY VESSELS WITHOUT CYANOSIS AND WITH RIGHT VENTRICULAR HYPERTROPHY

A relatively uncommon state is that in which right ventricular hypertrophy is unattended by cyanosis. Two conditions are most commonly encountered in this functional state: (1) pulmonary valvular stenosis with intact ventricular septum and without a right-to-left shunt at the atrial level; (2) stenosis of the peripheral pulmonary arteries.

Pulmonary Stenosis with Intact Ventricular Septum and without Transatrial Shunt

The anomaly in this condition is identical with the pulmonary valve in examples of pulmonary stenosis with intact ventricular septum and transatrial right-to-left shunt. The only difference is that no right-to-left shunt occurs at the atrial level. In some instances this is because of closure of the foramen ovale. In other instances, although the foramen ovale is potentially capable of carrying a shunt, none occurs. The basis for this may be that the right ventricle, although hypertrophied, may still offer less resistance to filling than the left ventricle. The cardiac output frequently is normal, as, with a buildup of right ventricular pressure, blood flows at high velocity through the stenotic pulmonary valve.

Peripheral Pulmonary Arterial Stenosis

Stenosis occurring either in the major pulmonary arteries or in their peripheral branches may be responsible for right ventricular hypertrophy in a manner similar to that which results from pulmonary valvular stenosis. The obstruction may be localized to the bifurcation of the pulmonary trunk, it may occupy multiple zones in peripheral

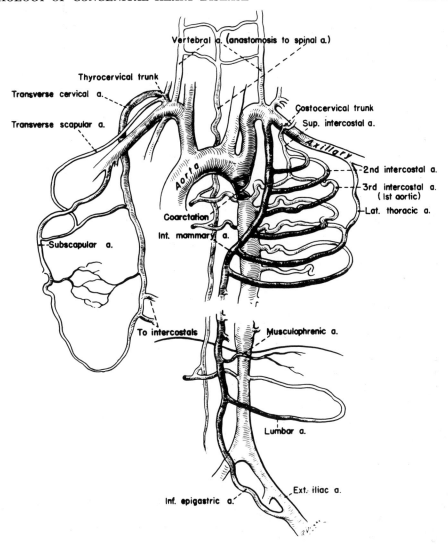

Fig. 18-5. Diagrammatic portrayal of collateral circulation in coarctation of the aorta. (*With permission of the author and publisher.*[17])

branches, or it may be a combination of these two conditions. There may be associated pulmonary valvular stenosis (either with intact ventricular septum or as part of the tetralogy of Fallot). As the pressure is built up in the pulmonary artery proximal to the zone of obstruction, flow occurring through the stenotic points in the pulmonary arterial system may be responsible for a continuous murmur.

NORMAL PULMONARY VESSELS WITHOUT CYANOSIS AND WITH LEFT VENTRICULAR HYPERTROPHY

Another group of conditions is characterized by obstruction to left ventricular outflow in the absence of a shunt and in the absence of significant pulmonary venous obstruction. The major condition in this category is coarctation of the aorta. Other conditions involve the region of the aortic valve.

Coarctation of the Aorta

The characteristic lesion in coarctation of the aorta is the deformity of the media of the aorta at the origin of its descending portions. The deformity involves the anterior, superior, and posterior walls and is represented by a curtain-like infolding of the wall which causes the lumen to be narrowed and eccentric.[17] The outlook for the patient varies according to the position of the coarctation with respect to the ductus arteriosus. When the coarctation lies peripheral to the ductus arteriosus, survival to adult life is common. When the coarctation lies proximal to the ductus arteriosus, there may be signs of left ventricular failure in infancy and death may occur suddenly during that period. In coarctation of the aorta, survival depends on the development of a collateral system between the aortic segment proximal to the coarctation and that segment distal to the coarctation. The major sources for collaterals are branches of the subclavian arteries, with the internal mammary, scapular, and intercostal arteries playing prominent roles (Fig. 18-5).

A bicuspid aortic valve is commonly associated with coarctation of the aorta, being present in about 85 per cent of the cases of coarctation, and may on occasion result in aortic insufficiency. Subaortic stenosis may be a coexistent lesion. The major complications in coarctation of the aorta[11] include congestive cardiac failure, dissecting aneurysm of the aorta, bacterial endocarditis of the bicuspid aortic valve, aortic valvular insufficiency, and rupture of an aneurysm of the circle of Willis. Thrombosis at the anterior spinal artery is an uncommon complication. Rupture of the aorta without dissection and rupture of an aneurysm of an intercostal artery are rare complications.

Stenosis in the Region of the Aortic Valve

Congenital obstruction in the region of the aortic valve may involve the aortic valve itself, the aorta in a supravalvular position, or the left ventricle in a subaortic position. *Aortic valvular stenosis* is usually characterized by a dome-shaped deformity of the valve which, in some respects, is similar to the pulmonary valve in congenital pulmonary stenosis. In most instances, instead of a true dome stenosis, there is a modified dome stenosis in which the valve possesses one commissure.[12]

Supravalvular aortic stenosis may involve an hourglass-shaped deformity of the ascending aorta above the valve. In other instances there may be a localized, fibrous, diaphragm-like stenosis of the ascending aorta, and in still other instances, there may be tubular narrowing of the ascending aorta. With the latter state, there may be associated tubular narrowing of the pulmonary trunk. The basic malformation of the aorta in this condition, is represented, structurally, by a mosaic distribution of the elements of the aortic media. A familial tendency occurs in this condition.

Subaortic stenosis may result from one of several anatomic situations. Two classic varieties of subaortic stenosis are usually considered, membranous and muscular. The membranous type of subaortic stenosis is characterized by a fibrous collar encircling the left ventricular outflow tract a short distance below the aortic valve. The anterior leaflet

of the mitral valve is involved in receiving attachment to this membrane. The muscular type of subaortic stenosis has a familial tendency and is characterized by a deformity of the muscular portion of the ventricular septum concentrated in the subaortic area.

Other forms of subaortic stenosis result from primary malformations of the mitral valve, including accessory tissue of the mitral valve; a cleft in the anterior leaflet of the mitral valve with insertion of chordae from the mitral valve to the ventricular septum, thereby binding the anterior leaflet of the mitral valve against the ventricular septum and causing obstruction to the outflow tract during ventricular systole; the malformation of the mitral valve which forms part of the complex known as persistent common atrioventricular canal, in which a basic deficiency of the ventricular septum causes the outflow tract of the left ventricle to be narrowed.

Functional hypertrophic muscular stenosis is discussed in Chaps. 5 and 25.

PROMINENT PULMONARY ARTERIAL AND VENOUS VESSELS WITH RIGHT VENTRICULAR HYPERTROPHY AND WITHOUT CYANOSIS (PULMONARY VENOUS OBSTRUCTION)

In a number of conditions, there is coexistence of right ventricular hypertrophy, prominence of the pulmonary arterial vessels, and a ground-glass haziness in the thoracic roentgenograms suggesting pulmonary venous obstruction. In some instances, in addition, there are Kerley lines in the lungs. Two major groups may be recognized among malformations responsible for pulmonary venous obstruction, those secondary to elevation of left ventricular diastolic pressure, and those related to primary obstruction in the pulmonary veins, in the left atrium or at the mitral valve.[13]

Elevation of Left Ventricular Diastolic Pressure

Elevation of left ventricular diastolic pressure may occur as the result of failure of the left ventricle, or hypertrophy of the left ventricle incident to an obstructive lesion, or a combination of the two. Among the conditions responsible for this functional derangement are *coarctation of the aorta* and *obstructive lesions of or in relation to the aortic valve*. Other conditions include primary lesions of the left ventricle, such as *glycogen-storage disease* and *endocardial sclerosis of the left ventricle*.

Obstructive Lesions in the Pulmonary Veins, in the Left Atrium or at the Mitral Valve

A series of malformations involves this portion of the cardiovascular system. Obstruction of the pulmonary veins may take one of the following forms: (1) *stenosis of the individual pulmonary veins,* in which the pulmonary veins join the left atrium at normal sites, but at the junction of each vein with the left atrium, there is a fibrotic lesion in the intima, causing the venous lumen to be narrowed; (2) *atresia of the common pulmonary vein,*[14] in which the four pulmonary veins converge to join a common receiving venous chamber, which, however, fails to make junction with the heart. The only avenue for pulmonary venous flow is through collateral vessels. Signs of pulmonary venous obstruction are severe. When the pulmonary veins converge to form a venous recess which, in turn, joins the left atrium through a stenotic opening, the condition *cor triatriatum* is said to be present.

In examples of total anomalous pulmonary venous connection, particularly to veins of the abdomen, an element of pulmonary venous obstruction is frequently observed. In this condition, however, cyanosis is an integral part of the functional derangement.

Congenital mitral stenosis as an isolated entity is rare. Grossly, the leaflets and chordae bear close resemblance to the alterations seen in rheumatic mitral stenosis. A complex of malformations has recently been reported,[15] in which (1) there is a stenosing ring in the left atrium just above the mitral valve, (2) the mitral valve itself is deformed, having a structure that has been compared to a parachute, (3) subaortic stenosis forms a third obstructive lesion, and (4) coarctation of the aorta completes the complex (Fig. 18-6).

Congenital mitral insufficiency may be seen as an integral part of several complex situations. It may occur in endocardial sclerosis (fibroelastosis) of the left ventricle. It may also be observed in instances of *anomalous origin of the left coronary artery from the pulmonary trunk* where, in association with endocardial sclerosis of the left ventricle, there may be infarction of the posterior papillary muscle of the left ventricle. Mitral insufficiency may occur as an isolated entity in which there is an isolated cleft in the anterior leaflet of the valve. In an additional situation, mitral insufficiency may occur as part of *corrected transposition of the great vessels.* In this condition, it is common that the ventricular septal defect is also present.[16]

REFERENCES

1. Kanjuh, V. I., and Edwards, J. E.: A Review of Congenital Anomalies of the Heart and Great Vessels According to Functional Categories, *Pediat. Clin. North America,* **11:**55, 1964.
2. Edwards, J. E.: Congenital Malformations of the

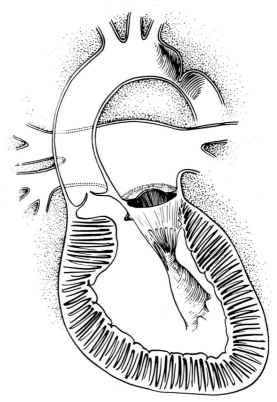

Fig. 18-6. Diagrammatic portrayal of the four obstructive anomalies in the complex described by Shone and associates.[15] Note (1) stenosing ring of left atrium, (2) parachute deformity of mitral valve, (3) subaortic stenosis of mitral valve, (4) coarctation of aorta. (*With permission of the author and publisher.*)

Heart and Great Vessels, in Gould's "Pathology of the Heart," 2d ed., Charles C Thomas, Publisher, Springfield, Ill., 1960, pp. 260–496.
3. Edwards, J. E., Dry, T. J., Parker, R. L., Burchell, H. B., Wood, E. H., and Bulbulian, A. H.: "An Atlas of Congenital Anomalies of the Heart and Great Vessels," Charles C Thomas, Publisher, Springfield, Ill., 1954, p. 202.
4. Fontana, R. S., and Edwards, J. E.: "Congenital Cardiac Disease: A Review of 357 Cases Studied Pathologically," W. B. Saunders Company, Philadelphia, 1962, p. 291.
5. Edwards, J. E.: Functional Pathology of the Pulmonary Vascular Tree in Congenital Cardiac Disease, *Circulation,* **15:**164, 1957.
6. Neufeld, H. N., Lester, R. G., Adams, P., Jr., Anderson, R. C., Lillehei, C. W., and Edwards, J. E.: Aorticopulmonary Septal Defect, *Am. J. Cardiol.,* **9:**12, 1962.
7. Neufeld, H. N., Lucas, R. V., Jr., Lester, R. G., Adams, P., Jr., Anderson, R. C., and Edwards, J. E.: Origin of Both Great Vessels from the Right

Ventricle without Pulmonary Stenosis, *Brit. Heart J.,* 24:393, 1962.

8. Levy, M. J., Lillehei, C. W., Elliott, L. P., Carey, L. S., Adams, P., Jr., and Edwards, J. E.: Accessory Valvular Tissue Causing Subpulmonary Stenosis in Corrected Transposition of Great Vessels, *Circulation,* 27:494, 1963.

9. Collett, R. W., and Edwards, J. E.: Persistent Truncus Arteriosus: A Classification According to Anatomic Types, *Surg. Clin. North America,* 29: 1245, 1949.

10. Lucas, R. V., Jr., Lund, G. W., and Edwards, J. E.: Direct Communication of a Pulmonary Artery with the Left Atrium: An Unusual Variant of Pulmonary Arteriovenous Fistula, *Circulation,* 24:1409, 1961.

11. Reifenstein, G. H., Levine, S. A., and Gross, R. E.: Coarctation of the Aorta, *Am. Heart J.,* 33:146, 1947.

12. Edwards, J. E.: Pathologic Aspects of Cardiac Valvular Insufficiencies, *A.M.A. Arch. Surg.,* 77:634, 1958.

13. Lucas, R. V., Jr., Anderson, R. C., Amplatz, K., Adams, P., Jr., and Edwards, J. E.: Congenital Causes of Pulmonary Venous Obstruction, *Ped. Clin. North America,* 10:781, 1963.

14. Lucas, R. V., Jr., Woolfrey, B. F., Anderson, R. C., Lester, R. G., and Edwards, J. E.: Atresia of the Common Pulmonary Vein, *Pediatrics,* 29:729, 1962.

15. Shone, J. D., Sellers, R. D., Anderson, R. C., Adams, P., Lillehei, C. W., and Edwards, J. E.: The Developmental Complex of "Parachute Mitral Valve," Supravalvular Ring of Left Atrium, Subaortic Stenosis and Coarctation of the Aorta, *Am. J. Cardiol.,* 11:714, 1963.

16. Edwards, J. E.: Differential Diagnosis of Mitral Stenosis: Clinicopathologic Review of Simulating Conditions, *Lab. Invest.,* 3:89, 1954.

17. Edwards, J. E., Clagett, O. T., Drake, R. L., and Christensen, N. A.: The Collateral Circulation in Coarctation of the Aorta, *Proc. Staff Meet. Mayo Clin.,* 23:333, 1948.

19 ALTERED CARDIAC FUNCTION IN CONGENITAL HEART DISEASE

Robert C. Schlant, M.D.

INTRODUCTION

The obvious complexity and variability of congenital heart defects make it impossible to discuss in detail the hemodynamics of all lesions. In this chapter, in which the hemodynamic alterations of only a few selected defects are discussed, an attempt is made to emphasize general principles applicable to the hemodynamics of individual patients. The hemodynamics of valvular stenosis and regurgitation are discussed in more detail in Chap. 24, Altered Cardiovascular Function in Rheumatic Heart Disease.

FETAL CIRCULATION AND CHANGES ASSOCIATED WITH BIRTH

Prior to birth the fetus must obtain its nutritional requirements, including oxygen, by the placental circulation. Consequently, while there is need for a high blood flow to the placenta, there is no need to pass all the blood through the lungs. The fetal circulation accomplishes its function with the aid of three vascular channels which normally disappear after birth. (1) The *foramen ovale* in the interatrial septum allows blood to pass from the right atrium to the left atrium in utero, but the *septum primum,* which serves as the valve of the foramen ovale, prevents the right-to-left shunting of blood after birth when the left atrial pressure rises. (2) The *ductus arteriosus* connects the pulmonary artery to the aorta and enables blood reaching the pulmonary artery to bypass the pulmonary circulation. (3) The *ductus venosus* shunts blood returning from the placenta in the umbilical cord through the liver to the inferior vena cava.

These structures allow more than half the output of both ventricles to go to the placenta for oxygen and carbon dioxide exchange. It has been estimated that only 10 to 15 per cent passes through the lungs and that about a third goes to the body of the fetus. Fetal arterial blood has an oxygen saturation of only 50 to 60 per cent and an O_2 tension of 30 mm Hg, as compared to 94 to 100 per cent and 95 mm Hg in the adult. The low arterial oxygen saturation is a result of two factors: (1) the gradient for the diffusion of oxygen in the placenta limiting the oxygen saturation of blood returning to the fetus in the umbilical vein to 80 per cent, and (2) the subsequent mixture of this blood in the heart with the unsaturated blood returning from the body of the fetus.

During delivery of the fetus, the umbilical cord is compressed and the placenta begins to separate. In addition, the newborn baby is suddenly exposed to a cold, strange environment. Both the asphyxia and the cold environment are strong respiratory stimuli, and the baby usually begins to breathe soon after birth. Within seconds after the expansion of the lungs, pulmonary blood flow increases tremendously. This occurs as the consequence of many events occurring at that time. One of the most important of these is the marked decrease in resistance to blood flow through the lungs. This decrease is due not only to the result of gaseous expansion of the lungs with a decrease in the kinking and compression of the pulmonary blood vessels, but also due to a marked decrease in vasoconstriction of the pulmonary vessels. In addition, with compression or tying of the umbilical cord, systemic resistance is markedly increased and the return of blood from the placenta ceases. As a result of these events, the pressure in the inferior vena cava and right atrium falls while the pressure in the left atrium increases and the foramen ovale is thereby functionally closed by the septum primum. After birth, the ductus arteriosus usually constricts, although it may remain partially patent for several days or weeks. The major stimulus for closure of the ductus is thought to be an increase in arterial pO_2 acting upon the specialized smooth-muscle cells in the ductus, although some constriction can also be produced by sympathetic amines released by partial asphyxia. Patency of the ductus for several days is relatively easy to detect by auscultation in calves, sheep, or foals, but patency in human infants is more difficult to detect, although it can often be demonstrated by special techniques. In the first few days after birth, most of the flow through a patent ductus is probably from aorta to pulmonary artery, although it may at times be bidirectional or even reversed, particularly if there is respiratory distress or crying.

Subsequent to the above events, there occurs a marked involution of the fetal pulmonary vasculature and right ventricular hypertrophy. Prior to birth the systemic and pulmonary circuits are in communication by the ductus arteriosus. Consequently, the systolic pressures in both ventricles, aorta, and pulmonary artery are all about equal, although the right ventricular and pulmonary artery systolic pressure is probably a few millimeters higher than that in the aorta. In association with the fall in pulmonary vascular resistance at birth and the closure of the ductus arteriosus, the pulmonary artery pressure falls, at first rather abruptly to a mean pressure of about 20 to 30 mm Hg and thereafter more slowly until it reaches normal childhood values in a few weeks. Subsequently, the main pulmonary artery, which at birth histologically resembles the aorta, and the pulmonary arteries and arterioles, which at birth are thick-walled and muscular, regress to have much thinner walls. At birth the wall of the right ventricle is about equal in thickness to that of the left ventricle. As a result of the decrease in pressure load following birth, the right ventricle regresses and by a few months achieves the normal childhood thickness. Interestingly, the electrocardiographic evidence of right ventricular predominance seems to persist for sev-

eral months or even years after the development of anatomic left ventricular predominance.

OBSTRUCTIVE CONGENITAL EFFECTS

Congenital heart disease due to obstructive or stenotic and regurgitant lesions of the heart valves is generally similar in altered physiology to acquired valvular heart disease (see Chap. 24). There are, however, several important characteristic congenital obstructive lesions which must be considered separately.

Coarctation of the Aorta

Coarctation of the aorta, by obstructing the flow of blood in the aorta, increases the resistance to aortic flow. The most common site is at a point distal to the origin of the left subclavian artery. When the coarctation is located below the ductus arteriosus, it is referred to as a *postductal coarctation;* when it is located above the ductus arteriosus, it is referred to as a *preductal coarctation.* The ductus arteriosus may either remain open or may close in each type, although it is more likely to remain open in preductal coarctation.

Prior to birth, in both types of coarctation increased pressure work is performed by both ventricles. In patients with the preductal, or "infantile," coarctation, the ductus usually remains patent in early life and usually there is a shunting of blood from aorta to pulmonary artery unless the ductus is very large and pulmonary vascular disease develops. In patients with the postductal, or "adult," coarctation, the ductus is usually closed, particularly after 1 year of age, and the major burden is a pressure load on the left ventricle. The resistance to blood flow in most blood vessels is increased relatively little until the cross-sectional area is decreased by about 60 to 70 per cent; however, the resistance increases strikingly if the cross-sectional area is further decreased. In most coarctations which produce hemodynamic alterations there is a significant narrowing of the aortic lumen, which is often only 1 to 2 mm in diameter. In addition to the increased resistance to left ventricular output, the coarctation produces other important hemodynamic changes. In most instances the systolic, and usually the diastolic, arterial pressure above the coarctation is elevated above normal levels, whereas the pressure pulse in the femoral artery below the coarctation has a systolic pressure which is lower than that in the upper extremities and a diastolic pressure which is usually above the normal range (Fig. 19-1). These pressure changes are, in part, caused by the damping effect of the coarctation. Also as a result of the damping

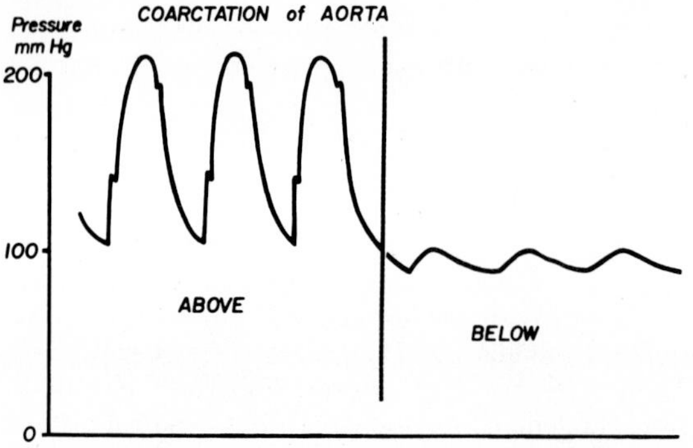

Fig. 19-1. Characteristic tracings above and below a coarctation of the aorta. The arterial pressure pulse below the coarctation is damped by the coarctation and is characterized by a slow rate of rise of pressure and a delayed peak pressure.

effect on the transmission of the pulse wave, the onset of the femoral pulse wave is delayed about 0.03 sec beyond that of the radial pulse wave, and the femoral pulse wave has a prolongation of the buildup time, i.e., the systolic upstroke time, or the time from the onset to the peak of the pulse wave, is prolonged from a normal of about 0.15 to about 0.23 sec.

The mechanism of the hypertension in the upper limbs has been the subject of numerous investigations. It appears to involve mechanical factors (the increased resistance to aortic flow produced by the coarctation and a decreased capacity and distensibility of the vessels into which the left ventricle ejects its contents during systole) and possibly humoral factors [the release of vasopressor substances (renin?) by the kidney as a consequence of a decrease in either renal blood flow and/or renal pulse pressure]. Once the pressure is increased by other mechanisms, it is also probable that the hypertension is maintained in part by an increase in capability of the blood vessels to respond to increased intraluminal pressure, secondary to increased tone and muscular hypertrophy. At present there is little good evidence of a significant neurogenic mechanism in the production of the hypertension above the coarctation. Surgical removal of the coarctation results in marked improvement of the circulatory dynamics with long-lasting correction of the hypertension in most cases. A bicuspid aortic valve has been reported to occur in as many as 80 per cent of patients with coarctation of the aorta. The major importance of the bicuspid valve lies in its liability to bacterial endocarditis, although on occasion it may produce significant obstruction to left ventricular outflow, and less commonly, it may cause significant regurgitation.

Aortic Stenosis

Aortic stenosis may be supravalvular, valvular, or subvalvular. Occasionally more than one type of obstruction is present. *Supravalvular aortic stenosis* is usually produced by a congenital fibrous band or constriction resembling a coarctation just above the aortic valve. The diagnosis is best established by left ventricular angiography, although it may be possible to record pressures in the supravalvular "chamber." Typically the systolic pressure in this chamber should be the same as that in the left ventricle but significantly higher than in the aorta above the obstruction. The diastolic pressure in the chamber is essentially the same as in the aorta. The arterial systolic pressure in the subclavian artery which originates from the brachiocephalic artery is higher than in the other subclavian artery, i.e., the right subclavian and brachial artery systolic pressures are higher than the left unless there is dextrocardia. (See Chap. 20 for additional clinical characteristics.) The hemodynamics of *congenital valvular aortic stenosis* are similar to those of acquired aortic stenosis, which is discussed in Chap. 24. *Subvalvular* aortic stenosis may be caused either by a fibrous band or ring or by hypertrophic subaortic muscular stenosis.

Hypertrophic Subaortic Muscular Stenosis

Hypertrophic subaortic muscular stenosis may be familial and/or congenital, or it may be acquired. It sometimes appears to develop secondary to a condition leading to left ventricular hypertrophy such as valvular aortic stenosis, hypertension, coarctation of the aorta, patent ductus arteriosus, or ventricular septal defect. Two hemodynamic characteristics of hypertrophic subaortic muscular stenosis frequently aid in establishing its presence. The peripheral arterial pressure pulse (Fig. 19-2) often has a characteristic bisferiens form, with an initial rapid upstroke (the "percussion wave") followed by a descent of the pulse wave, attributed to the ("muscle-bound") muscular obstruction to left ventricular output becoming apparent and/or a rapid deceleration of ejection. Reflected waves from the peripheral arterial tree may also contribute to the dip in pressure. This downward wave is followed by a slow rise in the pressure pulse wave (the "tidal wave") to a delayed second peak. The left ventricular pressure pulse may show a notch on the ascending portion shortly before the peak systolic pressure, at about the moment of maximum ejection. Pressure tracings taken during withdrawal of the catheter from left ventricle to aorta may reveal an outflow-tract chamber with diastolic pressure corresponding to that in the left ventricle and systolic pressure corresponding to aortic pressures but lower than that in the main left ventricular chamber (Fig. 19-2). An additional feature of hypertrophic muscular subaortic stenosis is the fact that the arterial pressure pulse of the beat following a premature beat is smaller than the ordinary beat. Normally, this succeeding pulse is larger than the ordinary beat. It is thought that the longer period of diastolic filling following the premature beat allows greater end-diastolic fiber stretch and increases the contractile force of the entire ventricular musculature, including the area producing the muscular obstruction. Hypertrophic subaortic muscular stenosis at times appears to be absent, in which case its presence may be demonstrated by

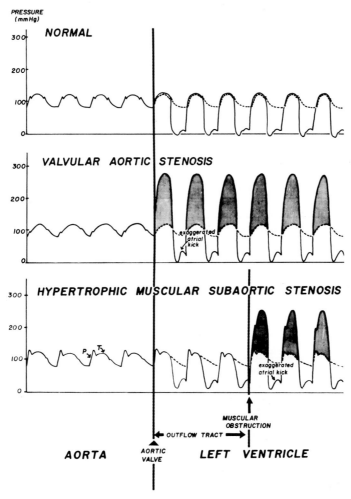

Fig. 19-2. Characteristic pressure tracings in the aorta and left ventricle in aortic stenosis. Upper, normal pressure tracing, characterized by the absence of a significant systolic pressure tracing between the left ventricle and aorta. The central aorta pressure tracing is characterized by an anacrotic notch on the ascending limb of the pressure pulse and by an incisura. The middle panel illustrates the findings in valvular aortic stenosis. The systolic pressure gradient between left ventricle and aorta is indicated by the shaded areas. The left ventricular pressure tracing shows the exaggerated "atrial kick" produced by the powerful atrial contraction. The aortic pressure tracing shows a parvus et tardus wave form with a prominent anacrotic notch, a slow rise of pressure to a low and delayed peak, and a prolongation of the total period of ejection indicated by the delay in the incisura, which is less distinct than normal. Lower panel, the findings in hypertrophic muscular subaortic stenosis. The systolic pressure gradient between the main left ventricular chamber and the outflow-tract "chamber" is indicated by the shaded area. The pressure tracing in the left ventricular tracing often has a notch on the ascending limb shortly before the peak pressure. The aortic pressure tracing is characterized by an initial rapid rise of pressure indicated by "P" ("percussion wave"), followed by a decrease in pressure, and a secondary rise in pressure indicated by "T" ("tidal wave"). The second pressure peak and the damped incisura are both delayed.

the administration of isoproterenol or levarterenol (norepinephrine). Digitalis, nitroglycerin, exercise, and the Valsalva maneuver may also increase the pressure gradient of the muscular subvalvular obstruction. The increased obstruction produced by these pharmacologic agents or activities appears to be the result of either an increase in myocardial contractility, particularly of the obstructing area, or a decrease in heart size.

Coarctation (Stenosis) of the Pulmonary Artery

Coarctation also occurs in the pulmonary arterial system, where it may involve the main pulmonary artery, the main branches of the pulmonary artery, or many smaller branches of the pulmonary artery. The diagnosis is established by demonstrating a systolic pressure difference while withdrawing a cardiac catheter from a free position in a small pulmonary artery distal to the main pulmonary artery and right ventricle. Angiography is helpful in demonstrating the extent of the coarctations, if they are multiple. The hemodynamic consequences are basically similar to that of valvular pulmonic stenosis. Coarctation (or "stenosis") of the pulmonary artery may be associated with coarctation of the aorta. It may also be associated with patent ductus arteriosus, particularly if the mother had rubella during pregnancy.

Pulmonic Stenosis

General

Pulmonic stenosis with intact septum may be caused by either valvular or infundibular stenosis, or both. Infundibular, or outflow-tract, obstruction may be caused either by a fibrous band or ring or by muscular hypertrophy (see below). As a result of pulmonic stenosis, which may vary from mild to severe, there is a pressure difference during systole between the main right ventricular cavity and the pulmonary artery. The effective valve area usually must be decreased by 60 per cent before there is hemodynamically significant obstruction to flow. The peak systolic pressure difference may reach 240 mm Hg; rarely it may be higher. A proper appreciation of the degree of obstruction requires knowledge not only of the mean pressure gradient but also of the amount of flow across the valve, since a relatively mild degree of stenosis may have a significant pressure gradient if the pulmonary flow is very high, and conversely severe stenosis may be associated with a relatively small gradient if the flow is very low as a result of right ventricular failure (see the Gorlin and Gorlin formula, Chap. 8). In most instances, patients at rest with pressure gradients less than 50 mm Hg have mild

stenosis, those with gradients between 50 and 100 mm Hg have moderate stenosis, and those with gradients over 100 mm Hg have severe stenosis.

When the stenosis is severe, the right ventricle may fail and there may be a decreased cardiac output even at rest, associated with elevation of both the right ventricular end-diastolic pressure and the right atrial mean pressure. The elevated right atrial pressure may produce signs of systemic venous congestion. At times, it may cause the foramen ovale to open and allow some shunting of blood from right atrium to left atrium. Arterial unsaturation and cyanosis may result from this shunt, although in severe pulmonic stenosis, cyanosis may also result from a decreased cardiac output with a stasis type of cyanosis resulting from the low flow to the peripheral tissues. In the latter situation, the arterial saturation is normal.

Valvular Pulmonic Stenosis

In patients with severe valvular stenosis, the pulmonary artery pressure is usually lower than normal and has a pulse wave which is less distinct than normal. Just distal to the stenotic valve, there may be negative systolic waves referred to as *Venturi waves*, which are ascribed to the conversion of pressure energy into velocity energy as the blood passes through the small valve orifice and/or to the sucking action of this stream on the column of fluid in the cardiac catheter facing downstream. As the catheter is withdrawn to the right ventricle in valvular pulmonic stenosis, there is an abrupt change to a high ventricular pressure (Fig. 19-3). The right ventricular pressure pulse typically has a rapid rate of increase in pressure to a delayed but sharp peak pressure and a rapid fall in pressure. The pressure during diastole is usually within normal limits until ventricular failure develops, but even before failure develops there is a prominent elevation of the end-diastolic pressure produced by atrial systole—the "atrial kick." The right atrial pressure similarly shows a prominent or even giant *a* wave, but the mean atrial pressure is usually not significantly elevated unless ventricular failure develops. Similar prominent right atrial *a* waves are present in other conditions in which right atrial contraction encounters increased resistance, i.e., tricuspid stenosis or right ventricular hypertrophy secondary to pulmonary hypertension from various causes. The amplitude of such *a* waves is less when there is a septal defect, particularly at the atrial level.

In most patients with significant valvular stenosis, the resting cardiac output is within normal limits although during exercise the cardiac output does not usually increase normally. Since a *doubling* of flow across a stenotic valve requires a *four*fold

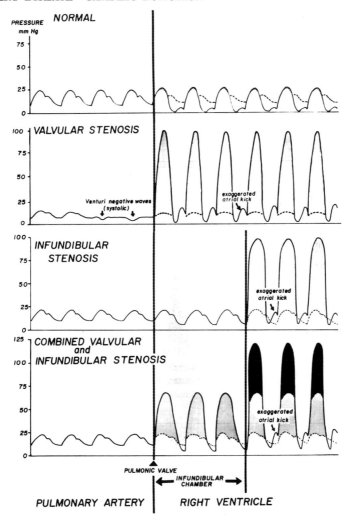

Fig. 19-3. Characteristic pressure tracings during withdrawal of catheter from pulmonary artery to right ventricle. Upper tracing, normal pressure tracings with no significant pressure difference between right ventricle and pulmonary artery during systole. Second tracing, the characteristic findings in pure valvular pulmonic stenosis—a systolic pressure difference between right ventricle and pulmonary artery indicated by the shaded areas, a sharp rise of pressure in the right ventricle, an exaggerated "atrial kick" in the right ventricular tracings, a prolonged systolic ejection period of the right ventricle, negative systolic waves ("Venturi waves") in the pulmonary artery just above the pulmonary valve, and damped, low-amplitude pressure pulses in the pulmonary arterial system. Third tracing, the findings in infundibular pulmonic stenosis, characterized by an "infundibular chamber," which has a systolic pressure lower than in the main right ventricular cavity but equal to the systolic pressure in the pulmonary artery. During diastole the pressure in the infundibular chamber is equal to that in the main right ventricular chamber. The right ventricular pressure tracing has an exaggerated atrial kick, and the rate of increase in pressure in the main right ventricular cavity during systole is less than in valvular stenosis. The systolic pressure difference between the main right ventricular chamber and the infundibular chamber is indicated by the shaded areas. Lower tracings, the findings in combined valvular and infundibular stenosis. The systolic pressure difference between the main right ventricular chamber and the infundibular chamber is indicated by cross hatching; the pressure difference between the infundibular chamber and the pulmonary artery is indicated by the shaded areas.

increase of pressure and since the peak pressure in either ventricle rarely exceeds 320 mm Hg, flow through a severely stenotic valve is limited. An inability of coronary blood flow to increase suffi-ciently may also contribute to the limited response to exercise. Coronary blood flow may be limited by several mechanisms: the degree of ventricular hypertrophy in relation to the amount of coronary capillary circulation, the fixed size of the coronary ostia, the relative shortening of diastole especially with tachycardia, the very high pressures in the right ventricular wall decreasing the coronary flow during systole, and a decreased pressure gradient across the coronary bed produced by elevation of right atrial pressure.

Infundibular Pulmonic Stenosis

Obstruction to the infundibulum, or outflow tract, of the right ventricle is usually caused by (1) a fibrous band or ring or (2) infundibular hypertrophic muscular stenosis. At times the two types of obstruction are both present.

Hypertrophic Infundibular Muscular Stenosis. Hypertrophic subvalvular muscular stenosis may occur as a congenital lesion, alone or in combination with other defects, or it may develop secondary to other lesions. It may occur in the outflow tract of either the right ventricle (hypertrophic infundibular muscular stenosis) or the left ventricle (hypertrophic subaortic muscular stenosis). In the right ventricle, it may occur alone or together with valvular pulmonic stenosis, often in association with ventricular septal defect. In some instances of medium to large-sized ventricular defects, muscular obstruction to right ventricular outflow develops after birth and may then protect the pulmonary vasculature from increased flow and the high right ventricular pressure. The continuous recording of pressure while withdrawing a cardiac catheter from the pulmonary artery will frequently reveal whether pulmonic stenosis is valvular, infundibular, or both (Fig. 19-3). Pressure tracings will not usually distinguish between muscular infundibular obstruction and infundibular obstruction produced by a fibrous band, or an obstruction produced by both. If the evidence on the pressure tracings of infundibular obstruction becomes apparent or becomes more marked during the administration of an inotrophic drug such as isoproterenol or levarterenol (norepinephrine), it is likely that there is a muscular element in the infundibular obstruction. Although angiography is invaluable in the evaluation of infundibular stenosis, pressure tracings should also be obtained whenever possible. The outflow tract of either ventricle may be hypertrophied as a result of many conditions, and it is very difficult to distinguish radiographically between hypertrophy producing obstruction and that producing no significant outflow-tract obstruction.

If the pulmonic stenosis is of the "pure" infundibular type, it may be possible to identify an "infundibular chamber" by cardiac catheterization, although the catheter tip frequently flips through the area. Typically, as the catheter is withdrawn from the pulmonary artery across the pulmonary valve into the infundibular chamber, systolic pressure stays the same but the diastolic pressure decreases to right ventricular level (Fig. 19-3). When the catheter is further withdrawn to the main right ventricular cavity, the systolic pressure is significantly higher than in the infundibular chamber or pulmonary artery. If both infundibular and valvular pulmonic stenosis are present, the pressure tracings will be similar except that the systolic pressure in the infundibular chamber will be at a level between that in the main right ventricle and the pulmonary artery.

Tricuspid Atresia

Tricuspid atresia signifies an absence of the usual inflow orifice to the right ventricle. Therefore, the only outlet for blood returning to the right atrium is through an interatrial communication, which is usually a patent foramen ovale. In the left atrium, the systemic venous blood mixes with oxygenated blood returning from the pulmonary veins. Consequently, there is always arterial unsaturation, the extent of which is inversely proportional to pulmonary blood flow. In most cases there is an associated interventricular septal defect through which blood passes to the right ventricle and the lungs. At times, pulmonary circulation is maintained by a patent ductus arteriosus. There may be a transposition of the aorta and pulmonary artery or even a truncus arteriosus. Occasionally, pulmonic valvular or infundibular stenosis is present. In most cases of tricuspid atresia, the right ventricle is diminutive. Cardiac catheterization demonstrates an elevation of right atrial pressure, often with a prominent a wave, particularly if the interatrial communication is not large. The catheter cannot be passed into the right ventricle but passes into the left atrium, which may have a slightly lower pressure than the right atrium. The arterial saturation is low, but if pulmonary flow is high enough in relation to systemic flow, clinical cyanosis may be absent. Angiography is generally preferable to determine the associated defects present.

Ebstein's Malformation

Ebstein's malformation results in obstruction to right ventricular filling because of malposition of the septal and posterior cusps of the tricuspid valve with a decrease in size of the right ventricle, part of which is incorporated into the right atrium. The deformed tricuspid valve also frequently allows tricuspid regurgitation. As a consequence of the obstruction to right ventricular filling, there is usually a large right-to-left shunt through either the foramen ovale or the atrial septal defect, with arterial hypoxemia and cyanosis. The right atrial mean pressure may be normal or elevated. The right atrial pressure pulse usually has a prominent a wave, and if there is tricuspid regurgitation, it may have a prominent V, or regurgitant, wave. There is no significant diastolic pressure gradient across the tricuspid valve, and the right ventricular and pulmonary artery pressures are normal.

VALVULAR REGURGITATION

The basic hemodynamic changes brought about by valvular regurgitation are similar to those of acquired valvular regurgitation (see Chap. 24).

ABNORMAL COMMUNICATIONS BETWEEN CHAMBERS OR VESSELS

General

Abnormal communications between chambers or vessels comprise one of the largest groups of congenital heart defects. The important factors of the direction and magnitude of shunts are basically determined by the relative resistances of the possible outlets available to the blood. This basic concept will be found as a common denominator in the following discussion of individual defects.

The diagnosis of intracardiac shunting of blood is often based on changes in oxygen content or saturation of blood samples obtained during catheterization of the right side of the heart. Since normal subjects usually have more oxygen in blood in the inferior vena cava than in blood in the superior vena cava and since there is incomplete mixing of blood in the right atrium and in the right ventricle, it is important to know the extent of changes in oxygen content or saturation which may be encountered in the absence of a shunt. Table 19-1 gives these values reported by two groups of investigators. In patients with left-to-right shunts of a small magnitude, inadequate to produce a significant difference between cardiac chambers, special diagnostic methods may enable one to establish the presence of the shunt (see Chap. 8). It also should be noted that at times there may be streaming of the shunted blood, causing it to be detected in the downstream chamber. In addition, occasionally valvular regurgitation may cause shunted blood to be detected in the chamber upstream to the shunt.

Atrial Septal Defect

Atrial septal defect may be either the "secundum" type or the "primum" type, a form of endocardial cushion defect. In the latter type, there is often associated tricuspid and/or mitral regurgitation in addition to a possible communication between left ventricle and either right ventricle or right atrium. In this section only the hemodynamics of the *secundum* type of atrial septal defect will

Table 19-1. NORMAL VARIATIONS IN VENOUS OXYGEN CONTENT AND SATURATION

Site	Maximum variations in oxygen content of successive samples, vol %* Within chambers	Between chambers‡	Oxygen saturation† Mean	Range (95% band)
Pulmonary artery:				
Right and/or left	0.4			
Main		+0.5	78	73–83
Right ventricle:				
Below pulmonary valve	0.8			
Mid-ventricle	1.0	+0.9	79	71–87
Right atrium:§				
Lower	1.5			
Mid	2.3		80	74–86
Upper		+1.9 (sup.) −1.5 (inf.)		
Vena cava:				
Superior	0.6		77	67–87
Inferior	0.8		83	77–89

* L. Dexter et al.[1]

† B. G. Barratt-Boyes and E. H. Wood.[2]

‡ + = maximum increase over the more proximal chamber; − = maximal decrease over the more proximal chamber.

§ Occasionally sampling near coronary sinus will give an abnormally low oxygen content out of line with other atrial samples.

be discussed. In this type of atrial septal defect the mean left atrial pressure may be slightly higher, usually less than 3 mm Hg, than that in the right atrium if the cross-sectional area of the defect is not over 2 cm². If the total cross-sectional area of the defect(s) is larger, however, there is essentially no resistance to blood flow across the defect and hence no significant pressure difference between the two atria. Thus, both atria may be considered functionally to be a common atrial chamber from which blood will flow to areas of least resistance. Since the right atrial system is more distensible than the left, since the tricuspid valve is normally somewhat more capacious than the mitral valve, and since the thinner-walled right ventricular chamber will more readily accommodate a larger volume of blood at the same filling pressure than the left ventricle (i.e., the right ventricle has greater distensibility), most of the blood from the functional common pressure chamber will go to the right ventricle, producing a left-to-right shunt of blood. Actually, in about 70 per cent of cases, a very small amount of blood passes from right atrium to left atrium, but this is so slight that it usually does not lower arterial saturation below normal; in fact, this right-to-left shunt often may be detected only by special indicator-dilution techniques. In atrial septal defect there is probably little or no left-to-right shunting of blood immediately after birth before the right ventricle has had opportunity to involute and lose its normal fetal hypertrophy and before the left ventricle hypertrophies. In most instances of atrial septal defect the right ventricle accommodates the large, "torrential" left-to-right shunt with moderate dilatation but with no elevation of end-diastolic pressure and only slight elevation of systolic pressure. There is a preferential shunting of the blood returning to the left atrium in the right pulmonary veins, caused by their proximity to the atrial septal defect. Because of the massive flow across the tricuspid valve, there is usually a diastolic flow murmur, which at times has been misinterpreted as being produced by mitral stenosis. The large flow across the normal pulmonary valve not only produces the usual systolic murmur heard with atrial septal defect but may produce a systolic gradient across the pulmonic valve, because of a "relative" or "functional" stenosis. The peak systolic pressure difference across the pulmonic valve is usually less than 10 mm Hg, although occasionally it may be 10 to 20 mm Hg and very rarely it has been reported to be 50 to 60 mm Hg in the absence of pulmonic stenosis.

Patients with atrial septal defect may tolerate the tremendous volume load on the right ventricle and pulmonary circuit quite well for many years. In a minority of patients, pulmonary vascular disease develops and alters the situation considerably. Normally the pulmonary arterial system in atrial septal defect undergoes regression following birth. In some patients, presumably as a consequence of the tremendous volume of blood flow through the lungs and possibly aggravated by the slight increase in pulmonary artery pressure, the pulmonary arterial system develops pulmonary vascular disease and an increased vascular resistance. This rarely occurs before the age of 20. It has even been suggested that some of the very rare cases in which severe pulmonary vascular disease occurs earlier are instances of coincidental primary pulmonary hypertension. Once pulmonary vascular disease begins, a vicious cycle seems to be set up in some patients in which the right ventricular and pulmonary artery pressures are elevated secondary to the increased pulmonary vascular resistance. This results in greater right ventricular hypertrophy and in some patients seems to result in even greater pulmonary vascular disease, perhaps as a consequence of the additional trauma of elevated pressure in addition to high flow. In patients who develop pulmonary vascular disease with high vascular resistance, the left-to-right shunt decreases largely because of the increased thickness and decreased distensibility of the right ventricle. In some patients the process continues until there is no significant left-to-right shunting of blood. Eventually, the shunt may be from right atrium to left atrium if the right ventricle has even less distensibility than the left. If there is a significant right-to-left shunt, arterial unsaturation and cyanosis may develop.

The key role in the physiology of atrial septal defect played by the pulmonary vasculature should be emphasized. It should be noted that in most patients with atrial septal defect, who have a large pulmonary blood flow and a normal or only slightly elevated pulmonary artery pressure, there is actually a decrease in calculated pulmonary vascular resistance. This is thought to be due to both utilization of all pulmonary vascular channels (normally some channels are thought to be only partially or intermittently utilized to any large degree) and probably to some degree of dilatation of the pulmonary vasculature. It is unknown why some patients with atrial septal defect develop pulmonary vascular disease while other patients with the same apparent hemodynamics do not suffer the same disability.

Endocardial Cushion Defect

Patients with endocardial cushion defects have extremely variable hemodynamics as well as clinical patterns. If the communication is mainly at the ventricular level, the right ventricular and pulmonary artery pressures will be elevated and the pulmonary flow will be increased unless the pulmonary vascular resistance is severely elevated. These patients are often hemodynamically similar to patients with large ventricular septal defects. Some patients with the main communication at the atrial level have normal pressures in the right side of the heart and a large pulmonary blood flow, as in the secundum type of atrial septal defect. At times, there may be direct shunting of blood from left ventricle to right atrium, detected by angiography. There may also be defects in the tricuspid or mitral valve, or both, which may result in severe regurgitation through the respective valve(s).

Ventricular Septal Defect

The physiology of ventricular septal defect is largely dependent on the area of the defect and the reaction of the pulmonary vasculature. Generally, one may divide patients with isolated ventricular septal defect into three groups, depending on the size of the defect. In the first group of patients, the defect is less than 0.5 cm² and consequently the defect itself offers a large resistance to flow from the left ventricle to the right ventricle. The magnitude of the shunt is determined mainly by the size of the defect. In such patients there is usually no elevation of right ventricular or pulmonary artery pressures and the left-to-right shunt may be so small that it is not detected by oxygen analysis of blood samples from the right side of the heart and pulmonary artery but can be detected only by special indicator (hydrogen, krypton, nitrous oxide, dye) techniques. Usually, this type of defect imposes little burden on the heart except for the danger of bacterial endocarditis; however, it is possible that it is a contributing factor to congestive failure in patients with other forms of heart disease such as coronary artery disease or systemic hypertension. It is also probable that many of the 25 per cent of all ventricular septal defects which spontaneously close after birth are these relatively small defects.

In the second group of patients the ventricular septal defect is 0.5 to 1.0 cm² in effective cross-sectional area. In this situation there are three main areas of resistance to the left-to-right shunting of blood: (1) the orifice of the defect itself, which offers some resistance to the passage of blood from left to right ventricle; (2) the right ventricle which does not regress normally after birth and is therefore less distensible than normal; (3) the pulmonary vasculature, which in this situation with moderate increase in flow (about 1.5 to 3.0 times systemic) and moderate increase in systolic pressure in the right ventricle and pulmonary artery, develops some degree of pulmonary vascular disease, which either may stay moderate and relatively unchanged or may, for unexplained reasons, become progressively severe with a marked elevation of pulmonary vascular resistance. As the pulmonary vascular resistance becomes elevated, the right ventricle will usually become thicker and less distensible and its systolic pressure rises. Consequently, the pressure difference across the defect may be less, and the left-to-right shunt actually decreases or it may even reverse.

In the third group of patients with ventricular septal defect, the effective area of the defect is 1.0 cm² or larger. As a result of this large defect, which

offers virtually no resistance to the flow of blood, the two ventricles are essentially in free communication at all times. Consequently, the systolic pressure in both ventricles, the aorta, and pulmonary artery is essentially the same at all times, in utero and after birth. In this situation, very similar to that which exists with a common ventricle, there are two outlets, i.e., the pulmonary valve and the aortic valve, through which blood in the functional single pumping chamber may pass when the ventricles contract. The relative proportion of blood going to the two circulations is directly governed by the relative resistance of the two circulations. Any condition or drug affecting either of these resistances will therefore affect the distribution of blood flow from the common pressure ventricles. At birth the pulmonary vasculature in infants with a large (over 1.0 cm²) ventricular septal defect has the normal high resistance. In the neonatal period the normal decrease in pulmonary vascular resistance commences. As a consequence, more and more blood will be shunted from the left to the right ventricle and into the lungs. As this happens both ventricles are required to increase their volume load of work. In some instances the left ventricle "fails" and develops an elevated diastolic pressure. As a result the pressure becomes elevated in the left atrium and in the pulmonary capillaries. At the same time, if the pulmonary vessels involute excessively, the pulmonary capillaries will be "unprotected" from the high pressure in the pulmonary arteries. The consequence of these events is an elevation of pulmonary capillary pressure, pulmonary edema, and possible death. Edwards[3] has suggested that this syndrome is produced by pulmonary arteriolar "failure," i.e., failure to maintain a degree of resistance adequate to protect the pulmonar capillaries from the high pulmonary artery pressure and failure to protect against left ventricular failure by limiting the volume of the shunt.

As a result of the partial involution of the pulmonary vasculature and the resultant marked increase in pulmonary blood flow, clinical pulmonary congestion frequently occurs at about 3 to 12 months of age. In most instances, however, the pulmonary vasculature eventually responds to the combined high-pressure and high-flow stimulus by the apparent "redevelopment" of high pulmonary vascular resistance, which results in a decreased pulmonary blood flow, a lessened left-to-right shunt across the interventricular septum, and decreased volume load on both ventricles. Indeed it is necessary for the survival of patients with a large ventricular septal defect to have an increased resistance to outflow from the right ventricle. The high pulmonary vascular resistance is caused both by hypertrophy and vascular disease of the pulmonary arteries and arterioles and by increased vasomotor tone and vasoconstriction of these vessels. Unfortunately, however, the pulmonary vascular disease in some patients appears to become progressively severe during the subsequent years, and eventually the pulmonary vascular resistance ·may equal or exceed systemic resistance. When the pulmonary vascular disease is very severe, there may be little or no vasoconstrictive element to the pulmonary vascular resistance, which is then relatively "fixed." When the two resistances are equal, the pulmonary and systemic· net flows are equal, with either no shunting of blood or bidirectional shunting with an equal small amount of blood shunted in each direction. When the pulmonary resistance is even higher than systemic, the right-to-left shunt predominates and may be sufficient to produce detectable cyanosis—the "Eisenmenger complex." Although the expressions "Eisenmenger's syndrome" and "Eisenmenger physiology" have been rather loosely applied to any condition with a left-to-right shunt which subsequently develops pulmonary vascular disease and a predominant right-to-left shunt, there is no advantage to this usage, which often generates more confusion than clarity.

At times, patients with medium or large-sized ventricular septal defect develop right ventricular hypertrophic infundibular muscular stenosis. This obstruction, not present at birth, may also serve to protect the pulmonary vasculature from the high pressure and flow to which it otherwise would be exposed (see reading lists, pp. 397 and 398).

Patent Ductus Arteriosus

Patients with patent ductus arteriosus may be divided into those in whom the vascular resistance through the ductus itself is small, moderate, or large. Since the resistance of the ductus is related not only to its cross-sectional area but also to its length, it is more difficult to define the anatomic size of the ductus in the different groups. In patients with a small internal-diameter ductus with a high resistance, the flow across the ductus will be relatively small, the extra volume work on the left ventricle is tolerated well, and the pulmonary pressure and resistances are not elevated and usually do not become elevated. Patients with only moderate resistance in the ductus have some increase in pulmonary artery pressure and resistance and usually have a moderately greater volume of shunting across the ductus. The hemodynamics of this group of patients is similar to that of patients with intermediate-size (0.5 to 1.0 cm^2) ventricular septal defects except that the latter group of patients also have a volume load on the right ventricle corresponding to the shunt. In patent ductus, the vol-

ume load is on the left ventricle, which may "fail" and develop an elevated end-diastolic pressure which is reflected in the left atrium and pulmonary capillaries.

The right ventricle is burdened mainly by a pressure load in the pulmonary circuit caused by pulmonary vasoconstriction and pulmonary vascular disease. Eventually, some of these patients develop more severe pulmonary vascular disease and increased pulmonary artery and right ventricular systolic pressures. If the pulmonary vascular resistance becomes high enough, the shunt through the ductus may reverse; in this situation, unsaturated arterial blood and possibly cyanosis are present in the lower portion of the body.

In patients with a large patent ductus which offers minimal resistance to blood flow, the aorta and pulmonary artery are in essentially free communication and the pressure in the pulmonary artery will be equal or close to that in the aorta. As in patients with a large ventricular defect, these patients may develop pulmonary congestion. This results from left ventricular failure with increased pressure in the left atrium and pulmonary capillaries and the failure of the pulmonary vasculature to "protect" the pulmonary capillaries from the high pulmonary artery pressure and flow. In this regard these patients are hemodynamically similar to patients with large ventricular septal defects.

In early life patients with a large patent ductus may also go through a period of pulmonary congestion; however, in most patients, adequate therapy can maintain them while giving time for (1) the left ventricle to compensate with dilatation and hypertrophy to carry the volume load, and (2) the pulmonary vasculature to respond to the high pressure by developing and maintaining adequate vasomotor tone and resistance to "protect" the pulmonary capillaries. It is likely that the high pressure in the pulmonary circuit induces a "reactive" type of muscular hypertrophy, probably giving the arteries and arterioles greater ability to have and to maintain greater vasoconstriction. If the hypertrophy itself has decreased the cross-sectional area of a given vessel, any additional narrowing will be proportionately even more effective in increasing the resistance of the vessel. The role of reflexes in the development and maintenance of "functional" pulmonary vasoconstriction is uncertain.

In patients with extreme degrees of pulmonary vascular disease, the structural changes in the vessels themselves account for most of the vascular resistance, which can no longer be decreased with pulmonary vasodilators such as oxygen administration or acetylcholine infusion. When this stage is reached, the pulmonary resistance may equal or exceed the resistance of systemic circulation and there may be shunting of unsaturated blood from pulmonary artery to aorta. This often causes the arterial saturation to be higher in the arms, especially the right, than the legs.

Patients with a patent ductus arteriosus and a large shunt from the aorta to the pulmonary artery have exaggerated systemic arterial pressure pulse waves compatible with a rapid runoff from the aorta, i.e., a rapid rise of the pulse wave to a systolic peak which may be higher than normal, followed by a rapid fall in pressure to a dicrotic notch and to a diastolic pressure lower than normal. With the development of high pulmonary vascular resistance and decreased shunting of blood to the lungs, the arterial pulse may lose these characteristics.

The hemodynamics of patients with an *aorticopulmonary septal defect* or "window" are basically the same as the hemodynamics in patients with a large patent ductus arteriosus or, except for the absence of volume load upon the right ventricle, patients with a large ventricular septal defect.

Partial Anomalous Pulmonary Venous Connection

Partial anomalous pulmonary venous connection with or without associated atrial septal defect is hemodynamically similar to an uncomplicated atrial septal defect. When it occurs without an associated atrial septal defect, however, the magnitude of pulmonary blood flow rarely reaches the very high values found in atrial septal defect. Arterial unsaturation and cyanosis are rare unless there are an associated atrial septal defect and the development of pulmonary hypertension.

Total Anomalous Pulmonary Venous Connection

Total anomalous pulmonary venous connection is compatible with life only if there is a communication between the right and left sides of the heart. This usually is a patent foramen ovale or atrial septal defect. In this type of anomaly all the blood from both pulmonary and systemic circulations returns to the right atrium. In most situations the pulmonary resistance is low and most of the blood from the right atrium flows to the right ventricle and pulmonary circuit. Consequently, there is a large volume of fully saturated blood returning to the right atrium, where it mixes with the unsaturated blood returning from the systemic circulation. Since systemic arterial blood comes from this mixture of blood in the right atrium (via the defect in the atrial septum), the systemic arterial saturation remains high as long as the pulmonary blood flow

remains high. If the pulmonary resistance increases and pulmonary blood flow decreases or if the oxygen content of blood returning from the systemic circulation is decreased by exercise, the systemic arterial saturation will fall. The amount of pulmonary blood flow may be expressed as follows:

$$Qp = \frac{\dot{V}_{O_2}}{Cpv - Cpa}$$

where Qp = pulmonary blood flow, liters per min
        $\dot{V}_{O_2}$ = oxygen consumption, ml per min
      Cpv = oxygen content of pulmonary venous blood, ml per liter
      Cpa = oxygen content of pulmonary arterial blood, ml per liter

If the equation is rewritten

$$Cpa = Cpv - \frac{\dot{V}_{O_2}}{Qp}$$

it is apparent that pulmonary arterial oxygen content *decreases* with increased oxygen utilization but *increases* with pulmonary blood flow. If complete mixing in the right atrium is assumed (even though strictly not true), the blood going to the left atrium and to the systemic circulation will be the same as that going to the pulmonary artery, and these same relationships will be true for *systemic* arterial oxygen content and saturation. This same basic relationship exists whenever there is venoarterial or "right-to-left" shunting of blood.

Complete Transposition of the Great Vessels

In complete transposition of the great vessels, the aorta originates from the right ventricle and the pulmonary artery originates from the left ventricle; the systemic veins drain into the right atrium, and the pulmonary veins into the left atrium. For survival there must be communication between the two circulations. Almost all patients have an atrial septal defect or patent foramen ovale, about two-thirds have a patent ductus arteriosus and about one-half have a ventricular septal defect. The hemodynamics are dependent on the combination of defects present, but the basic finding at cardiac catheterization is a greater oxygen content in blood obtained from the pulmonary artery, which originates from the left ventricle, than in blood in the aorta, which originates from the right ventricle. The right ventricular systolic pressure is essentially the same as systemic arterial pressure. There must be evidence of shunts at various levels. Usually, the atrial shunt is from left to right; if a patent ductus arteriosus is present the shunt is usually from aorta to pulmonary artery. The ventricular shunting is commonly bidirectional, although the magnitude of the shunt and the pressure in the left ventricle and pulmonary artery depend on the size of the ventricular defect and the relative resistance in the pulmonary and systemic circulations, as in uncomplicated ventricular septal defects. Angiography is of great value in establishing the anatomic type of transposition present.

"Corrected" Transposition of the Great Vessels

In corrected transposition of the great vessels, the aorta originates from the left-sided ventricle and the pulmonary artery originates from the right-sided ventricle; however, the aorta is anterior to the pulmonary artery. Rhythm disturbances, incompetence of the left atrioventricular valve, or a ventricular septal defect may be present, but otherwise there may be no functional disturbance in these patients.

SEPTAL DEFECTS ASSOCIATED WITH VALVULAR OBSTRUCTION

Atrial Septal Defect Associated with Mitral Stenosis

Atrial septal defect associated with mitral stenosis, referred to as the "Lutembacher syndrome," has varying hemodynamic patterns, depending mainly on the size of the stenotic mitral valve orifice, the size of the atrial septal defect, and the severity of the pulmonary vascular disease. If the mitral stenosis is severe, there necessarily must be an elevation of left atrial pressure to provide an adequate gradient across the mitral valve to force enough blood into the left ventricle to sustain life. If the atrial septal defect is large and there is pressure equalization in both atria, there will be a large flow into the right ventricle and pulmonary artery. Pulmonary hypertension occurs earlier and more frequently than in uncomplicated atrial septal defect. If the mitral stenosis is severe and the atrial defect is large, the elevated pressure in the functional common atrium is associated with significant elevation of systemic venous pressure. Occasionally patients with acquired or congenital mitral valve disease may have an interatrial communication because of incompetence of the foramen ovale secondary to dilatation of the left atrium[4] (see reading list, p. 401).

Atrial Septal Defect Associated with Pulmonic Stenosis

Atrial septal defect associated with pulmonic stenosis, referred to as the "trilogy of Fallot," presents a wide spectrum of hemodynamic alterations mainly depending on the severity of the pulmonic stenosis. If the stenosis is mild, the right ventricular pressure is moderately elevated and the shunt may be predominantly left to right, although seldom does it have the "torrential" volume found in uncomplicated atrial septal defect. When the ventricle "fails" or becomes so hypertrophied that its filling characteristics are markedly altered, the shunting of blood at the atrial level may reverse and become predominantly right to left. If the stenosis is very severe from birth, the right atrial pressure will be greater than that in the left atrium from birth, causing a right-to-left shunt with arterial hypoxia and cyanosis. There is some evidence that the atrial septal defect (or foramen ovale) thus acts as a safety valve to prevent overloading of the right ventricle. In addition, the presence of the interatrial communication tends to prevent excessive elevation of right atrial pressure and may thus prevent a decrease in the pressure gradient between the coronary arteries and the coronary sinus. The prominent *a* wave of atrial contraction seen in pulmonic stenosis are much less prominent in the presence of an atrial (or ventricular) septal defect. The right ventricular systolic pressure may be lower than, equal to, or greater than the systolic pressure in the aorta.

Ventricular Septal Defect and Pulmonic Stenosis

Ventricular septal defect and pulmonic stenosis are the essential features of the "tetralogy of Fallot." The other features are right ventricular hypertrophy and an overriding aorta. It is probable that the altered relationship of the aortic root to the ventricular septal defect plays no important role in the altered hemodynamics of this condition. Since the ventricular septal defect is usually large, both ventricles and the systemic arteries have essentially the same systolic pressures. The basic hemodynamic factor determining how well these patients tolerate their disease is the ratio between the resistance to flow into the aorta and the resistance to flow across the stenotic right ventricular infundibulum and/or stenotic pulmonic valve. If the latter resistances are not large, the pulmonary flow may be twice the systemic flow and the arterial saturation may be normal (so-called "acyanotic tetralogy of Fallot"). On the other hand, if the resistance to pulmonary flow is severe, the pulmonary flow may be markedly decreased and there may be arterial unsaturation and cyanosis even at rest. When the pulmonary stenosis is very severe, much or even most of the pulmonary blood flow may be by way of collateral blood flow by large bronchial arteries, particularly after childhood.

The mechanism by which "squatting" relieves breathlessness and faintness after exercise in patients with pulmonary stenosis and ventricular septal defect is unknown. It is known that the arterial saturation returns to its resting value more rapidly if the patient squats after exercise. It is probable that squatting also produces an increase in systemic arterial blood pressure and in systemic cardiac output in normal subjects. Presumably squatting produces these same changes in patients with pulmonic stenosis and ventricular septal defect. In patients with this combination of lesions, as in patients with a large ventricular septal defect, the relative amount of blood passing to the lungs and to the aorta depends on the relative resistances of the two circuits (including the resistance of the pulmonic stenosis for the pulmonic circuit). It is possible that the increase in arterial saturation produced by squatting in these patients is in part related to an increase in peripheral resistances. The studies of Sharpey-Shafer[5] and O'Donnell and McIlroy[6] suggest that one of the major mechanisms responsible for producing this increase in peripheral resistance may be the removal of the distending force of gravity upon the systemic arterial bed rather than the more traditional viewpoint that the increased arterial resistance was produced by kinking of the femoral arteries. It was formerly suggested that squatting improved arterial saturation by obstructing the return of markedly unsaturated blood from the legs, which would then be gradually returned to the heart and circulation. Actually, there is evidence that squatting increases venous return to the heart and shifts blood from the legs to the heart and lungs. It is probable that the arterial saturation increases as the result of (1) a relative and perhaps absolute increase in pulmonary blood flow which increases the return of fully saturated blood to the left ventricle, and (2) a decrease in shunting of unsaturated blood from the right ventricle to the aorta. These changes apparently are associated with an increased venous return to the heart, an increase in peripheral resistance, and an increase in left ventricular and probably right ventricular pressure.

Hypercyanotic episodes in patients with pulmonic stenosis and ventricular septal defect are of uncertain origin. It is possible that some episodes are caused by periods of unusual hyperactivity of fibers in the right ventricular outflow tract producing, or exaggerating, previously present functional hypertrophic infundibular muscular stenosis.

As a result of arterial unsaturation, patients with pulmonic stenosis and ventricular septal defect may develop marked polycythemia. This may be severe enough to increase the viscosity of blood and thereby impede flow, particularly in small vessels. In addition, polycythemia may increase the tendency to thrombosis, particularly in the cerebral and pulmonary vessels.

The mechanism of the systemic arterial hypertension occasionally encountered in patients with pulmonic stenosis and ventricular septal defect is unknown. In some patients it probably is initiated by an increased production of renin.

Pulmonic stenosis with both ventricular and atrial septal defect is referred to as "pentalogy of Fallot." The presence of the additional defect at the atrial level does not significantly modify the basic hemodynamics.

Ventricular Septal Defect Associated with Aortic Stenosis

Ventricular septal defect and aortic stenosis, when present in the same patient, produce more severe alterations than either one alone, since the high pressure in the left ventricle necessary to force blood out the stenotic aortic valve also increases the left-to-right shunt through the ventricular septal defect. If the ventricular septal defect is large with equalization of pressures in the two ventricles, the right ventricular and the pulmonary artery systolic pressure will be higher than that in the systemic arteries. As in other large ventricular septal defects, the magnitude and direction of shunting depends on the relative resistance to the outflow of blood from the right and left ventricles. In addition to the high pressure load, both ventricles and pulmonary circulation sustain a high volume load. This combination usually leads to early severe pulmonary vascular disease and ventricular failure. At times, these two defects are associated with a coarctation of the aorta and a patent ductus distal to the coarctation. In this combination, there is usually a very high pulmonary blood flow, and most of the blood supply to the lower body is through the ductus, while the upper part of the body is perfused from the left ventricle through the stenotic aortic valve.

REFERENCES

1. Dexter, L., Haynes, F. W., Burwell, C. S., Eppinger, E. C., Sagerson, R. P., and Evans, J. M.: Studies of Congenital Heart Disease. II. The Pressure and Oxygen Content of Blood in the Right Auricle, Right Ventricle, and Pulmonary Artery in Control Patients, with Observations on the Oxygen Saturation and Source of Pulmonary "Capillary" Blood, *J. Clin. Invest.*, **26**:554, 1947.

2. Barratt-Boyes, B. G., and Wood, E. H.: The Oxygen Saturation of Blood in the Venae Cavae, Right-heart Chambers, and Pulmonary Vessels of Healthy Subjects, *J. Lab. & Clin. Med.*, **50**:93, 1957.

3. Edwards, J. E.: Functional Pathology of the Pulmonary Vascular Tree in Congenital Heart Disease, *Circulation*, **15**:164, 1957.

4. Marshall, R. J., and Warden, H. E.: Mitral Valve

Disease Complicated by Left-to-right Shunt at Atrial Level, *Circulation,* 29:432, 1964.

5. Sharpey-Shafer, E. P.: Effects of Squatting on the Normal and Failing Circulation, *Brit. M. J.,* 1:1072, 1956.

6. O'Donnell, T. V., and McIlroy, M. B.: The Circulatory Effects of Squatting, *Am. Heart J.,* 64:347, 1962.

SUGGESTED READING[*]

General

Allan, G. A.: A Schema of the Circulation with Experiments to Determine the Additional Load in the Apparatus Produced by Conditions Representing Valvular Lesions, *Heart,* 12:181, 1925.

Barratt-Boyes, B. G., and Wood, E. H.: Cardiac Output and Related Measurements and Pressure Valves in the Right Heart and Associated Vessels, Together with an Analysis of the Hemodynamic Response to Inhalation of High Oxygen Mixtures in Healthy Subjects, *J. Lab. & Clin. Med.,* 51:72, 1958.

Bass, A. D., and Moe, G. K. (eds.): "Symposium on Congenital Heart Disease," American Association for the Advancement of Science, publ. no. 63, Washington, D.C., 1960.

Campbell, M. (chairman): Symposium on Congenital Heart Disease, *Brit. Heart J.,* 20:261, 1958.

Cournand, A., Baldwin, J. S., and Himmelstein, A.: "Cardiac Catheterization in Congenital Heart Disease: A Clinical and Physiological Study in Infants and Children," The Commonwealth Fund, New York, 1949.

Dexter, L., Haynes, F. W., Burwell, C. S., Eppinger, E. C., Seibel, R. E., and Evans, J. M.: Studies of Congenital Heart Disease. I. Technique of Venous Catheterization as a Diagnostic Procedure, *J. Clin. Invest.,* 26:547, 1947.

Holling, H. E., and Zak, G. A.: Cardiac Catheterization in the Diagnosis of Congenital Heart Disease, *Brit. Heart J.,* 12:153, 1960.

Keith, J. D., Rowe, R. D., and Vlad, P.: "Heart Disease in Infancy and Childhood," The Macmillan Company, New York, 1958.

Kjellberg, S. R., Mannheimer, E., Rudhe, U., and Jonsson, B.: "Diagnosis of Congenital Heart Disease," 2d ed, The Year Book Medical Publishers, Inc., Chicago, 1959.

Lagerlöf, H., and Werkö, L.: Studies on the Circulation in Man. II. Normal Values for Cardiac Output and Pressure in the Right Auricle, Right Ventricle and Pulmonary Artery, *Acta physiol. scandinav.,* 16: 75, 1949.

McCord, M. C., Komesu, S., and Blount, S. G., Jr.: The Characteristics of the Right Atrial Pressure Wave Associated with Right Ventricular Hypertrophy, *Am. Heart J.,* 45:706, 1953.

Marshall, H. W., Helmholz, H. F., Jr., and Wood, E. H.: Physiologic Consequences of Congenital Heart Disease, in W. F. Hamilton and P. Dow (eds.), "Handbook of Physiology, sec 2, "Circulation," vol. 1, American Physiological Society, Washington, D.C., 1962, p. 417.

Nadas, A. S. (ed.): Symposium on Pediatric Cardiology, *Pediat. Clin. North America,* 5:835–1159, 1958.

Nadas, A. S.: "Pediatric Cardiology," 2d ed, W. B. Saunders Company, Philadelphia, 1963.

Praagh, R. van, Praagh, S. van, Vlad, P., and Keith, J. D.: Anatomic Types of Congenital Dextrocardia: Diagnostic and Embryologic Implications, *Am. J. Cardiol.,* 13:510, 1964.

Taussig, H. B.: "Congenital Malformations of the Heart," 2d ed., vols. 1 and 2, The Commonwealth Fund, New York, 1960.

Wood, P.: "Diseases of the Heart and Circulation," 2d ed., J. B. Lippincott Company, Philadelphia, 1956.

Wood, P., McDonald, L., and Emanuel, R.: The Clinical Picture Correlated with Physiological Observations in the Diagnosis of Congenital Heart Disease, *Pediat. Clin. North America,* 5:981–1010, 1958.

Wright, J. L., and Wood, E. H.: Value of Central and Peripheral Intra-arterial Pressures and Pulse Contours in Cardiovascular Diagnosis, *Minnesota Med.,* 41:215, 1958.

Zimmerman, H. A. (ed.): "Intravascular Catheterization," Charles C. Thomas, Publisher, Springfield, Ill., 1959.

Fetal and Neonatal Circulation

Adams, F. H., and Lind, J.: Fetal and Neonatal Circulation: Observations in Humans, in A. D. Bass and G. K. Moe (eds.), "Symposium on Congenital Heart Disease," American Association for the Advancement of Science, publ. no. 63, Washington, D.C., 1960, p. 51.

Ardran, G. M., Dawes, G. S., Pritchard, M. M., Reynolds, S. R., and Wyatt, D. G. J.: The Effect of Ventilation on the Foetal Lungs upon the Pulmonary Circulation, *J. Physiol.,* 118:12, 1952.

Assali, N. S., Sehgal, N., Marable, S.: Pulmonary and Ductus Arteriosus Circulation in the Fetal Lamb before and after Birth, *Am. J. Physiol.,* 202:536, 1962.

Barclay, A. E., Franklin, K. J., and Prichard, M. M. L.: "The Foetal Circulation and Cardiovascular System and Changes That They Undergo at Birth," Charles C Thomas, Publisher, Springfield, Ill., 1944.

Cook, C. D., Drinker, P. A., Jacobson, H. N., Levinson, H., and Strang, L. B.: Factors Determining the Increase in Pulmonary Blood Flow on Ventilation of the Foetal Lamb Lung, *J. Physiol.,* 166: 9P, 1963.

[*] See also references from Chapters 11 and 24 on heart failure and valvular disease, respectively.

Dawes, G. S.: Changes in the Circulation at Birth and the Effects of Asphyxia, in D. Gairdner (ed.), "Recent Advances in Pediatrics," Churchill, London, 1958, p. 1.

Dawes, G. S.: Fetal and Neonatal Circulation in Relation to Congenital Heart Disease, in A. D. Bass and G. D. Moe (eds.), "Symposium on Congenital Heart Disease," American Association for the Advancement of Science, publ. no. 63, Washington, D.C., 1960, pp. 39–49.

Dawes, G. S.: Changes in the Circulation at Birth, *Brit. M. Bull.,* **17**:149, 1961.

Dawes, G. S., and Mott, J. C.: Vascular Tone of the Foetal Lung, *J. Physiol.,* **164**:465, 1962.

Lind, J., and Wegelius, C.: Human Foetal Circulation: Changes in the Cardiovascular System at Birth and Disturbances in the Post-natal Closure of the Foramen Ovale and Ductus Arteriosus, *Cold Spring Harbor Symp. Quant. Biol.,* **19**:109, 1954.

Rowe, R. D., and James, L. S.: The Normal Pulmonary Arterial Pressure during the First Year of Life, *J. Pediat.,* **51**:1, 1957.

Rudolph, A. M., Auld, A. M., Golinko, R. J., and Paul, M. H.: Pulmonary Vascular Adjustments in the Neonatal Period, *Pediatrics,* **28**:28, 1961.

Young, M.: The Fetal and Neonatal Circulation, in W. F. Hamilton and P. Dow (eds.), "Handbook of Physiology, sec. 2: "Circulation," vol. 2, American Physiological Society, Washington, D.C., 1963, p. 1619.

Pulmonary Vasculature in Congenital Heart Disease

Auld, P. A. M., Gibbons, J. E., and McGregor, M.: Vasomotor Tone in the Pulmonary Vascular Bed in Patients with Left-to-right Shunts, *Brit. Heart J.,* **25**:257, 1963.

Auld, P. A. M., Johnson, A. L., Gibbons, J. E., and McGregor, M.: Changes in Pulmonary Vascular Resistance in Infants and Children with Left-to-Right Intracardiac Shunt, *Circulation,* **27**:257, 1963.

Bayliss, W. M.: On the Local Reactions of the Arterial Wall to Changes in Internal Pressure, *J. Physiol.,* **28**:220, 1902.

Burchell, H. B.: Studies in Pulmonary Hypertension in Congenital Heart Disease, *Brit. Heart J.,* **21**:255, 1959.

Civin, W. H., and Edwards, J. E.: The Postnatal Structural Changes in the Intrapulmonary Arteries and Arterioles, *A.M.A. Arch. Path.,* **51**:192, 1951.

Downing, S. E., Vidone, R. A., Brandt, H. M., and Liebow, A. A.: The Pathogenesis of Vascular Lesions in Experimental Hyperkinetic Pulmonary Hypertension, *Am. J. Path.,* **43**:739, 1963.

Folkow, B.: Intravascular Pressure as a Factor Regulating the Tone of Small Vessels, *Acta physiol. scandinav.,* **17**:289, 1949.

Friedberg, C. K.: Pulmonary Hypertension with Special Reference to Its Occurrence in Congenital Heart Disease, *Progr. Cardiovas. Dis.,* **1**:356, 1958–59.

Goodwin, J. F.: Congenital Heart Disease, in R. Daley, J. F. Goodwin, and R. E. Steiner (eds.), "Clinical Disorders of the Pulmonary Circulation," Little, Brown and Company, Boston, 1960, p. 229.

Heath, D., and Edwards, J. E.: The Pathology of Hypertensive Pulmonary Vascular Disease: A Description of Six Grades of Structural Changes in the Pulmonary Arteries with Special Reference to Congenital Cardiac Septal Defects, *Circulation,* **18**:533, 1958.

Heath, D., Helmholz, H. F., Jr., Burchell, H. B., DuShane, J. W., Kirklin, J. W., and Edwards, J. E.: Relation between Structural Changes in the Small Pulmonary Arteries and the Immediate Reversibility of Pulmonary Hypertension Following Closure of Ventricular and Atrial Septal Defects, *Circulation,* **18**:1167, 1958.

Heath, D., and Whitaker, W.: Hypertensive Pulmonary Vascular Disease, *Circulation,* **14**:323, 1956.

Heath, D., Wood, E. H., DuShane, J. W., and Edwards, J. E.: The Structure of the Pulmonary Trunk at Different Ages and in Cases of Pulmonary Hypertension and Pulmonary Stenosis, *J. Path. & Bact.,* **77**:443, 1959.

Muller, W. H., Jr., Dammann, J. F., Jr., and Head, W. H., Jr.: Changes in the Pulmonary Vessels Produced by Experimental Pulmonary Hypertension, *Surgery,* **34**:363, 1953.

Rudolph, A. M., and Nadas, A. S.: The Pulmonary Circulation and Congenital Heart Disease: Considerations of the Role of the Pulmonary Circulation in Certain Systemic-pulmonary Communications, *New England J. Med.,* **267**:968, 1022, 1962.

Shepherd, J. T., Semler, H. J., Helmholz, H. F., Jr., and Wood, E. H.: Effects of Infusion of Acetylcholine on Pulmonary Vascular Resistance in Patients with Pulmonary Hypertension and Congenital Heart Disease, *Circulation,* **20**:381, 1959.

Shepherd, J. T., and Wood, E. H.: The Role of Vessel Tone in Pulmonary Hypertension, *Circulation,* **19**:641, 1959.

Swan, H. J. C., Zapata-Diaz, J., Burchell, H. B., and Wood, E. H.: Pulmonary Hypertension in Congenital Heart Disease, *Am. J. Med.,* **16**:12, 1954.

Swan, H. J. C., Burchell, H. B., and Wood, E. H.: Effect of Oxygen on Pulmonary Vascular Resistance in Patients with Pulmonary Hypertension Associated with Atrial Septal Defect, *Circulation,* **20**:66, 1959.

Wagenvoort, C. A., Heath, D., and Edwards, J. E.: "The Pathology of the Pulmonary Vasculature," Charles C Thomas, Publisher, Springfield, Ill., 1963.

Wood, P.: The Vasoconstrictive Factor in Pulmonary Hypertension, in W. R. Adams and I. Veith (eds.), "Pulmonary Circulation: An International Symposium," Grune & Stratton, Inc., New York, 1959, p. 294.

Coarctation of the Aorta

Beard, E. F., Wood, E. H., and Clagett, O. T.: Studies of Hemodynamics in Coarctation of the Aorta Using Dye Dilution and Direct Intra-arterial Pressure Recording Methods, *J. Lab. & Clin. Med.*, 38:858, 1951.

Bing, R. J., Hendelsman, J. C., Campbell, J. A., Griswold, H. E., and Blalock, A.: The Surgical Treatment and Physio-pathology of Coarctation of the Aorta, *Ann. Surg.*, 128:803, 1948.

Gross, R. E.: Hypertension from Coarctation of the Aorta, *Am. J. Surg.*, 107:14, 1964.

Gupta, T. C., and Wiggers, C. J.: Basic Hemodynamic Changes Produced by Aortic Coarctation of Different Degrees, *Circulation*, 3:17, 1951.

Katz, L. N., Ralli, E. P., and Cheer, S. N.: The Cardiodynamic Changes in the Aorta and Left Ventricle Due to Stenosis of the Aorta, *J. Clin. Invest.*, 5:205, 1928.

March, H. W., Hultgren, H. N., and Gerbode, F.: Immediate and Remote Effects of Resection on the Hypertension in Coarctation of the Aorta, *Brit. Heart J.*, 22:361, 1960.

Newcombe, C. P., Ongley, P. A., Edwards, J. E., and Wood, E. H.: Clinical, Pathologic and Hemodynamic Considerations in Coarctation of the Aorta Associated with Ventricular Septal Defect, *Circulation*, 24:1356, 1961.

Rathi, L., and Keith, J. D.: Post-Operative Blood Pressures in Coarctation of the Aorta, *Brit. Heart J.*, 26:671, 1964.

Scott, H. W., Jr., Collins, H. A., Langa, A. M., and Olson, N. S.: Additional Observations Concerning the Physiology of Hypertension Associated with Experimental Coarctation of the Aorta, *Surgery*, 36:445, 1954.

Werkö, L., Ek, J., Bucht, H., and Karnell, J.: Cardiac Output, Blood Pressures and Renal Dynamics in Coarctation of the Aorta, *Scandinav. J. Clin. & Lab. Invest.*, 8:193, 1956.

Wright, J. L., Burchell, H. B., Wood, E. H., Hines, E. A., Jr., and Clagett, O. T.: Hemodynamic and Clinical Appraisal of Coarctation Four to Seven Years after Resection and End-to-End Anastomosis of the Aorta, *Circulation*, 14:806, 1956.

Supravalvular Aortic Stenosis

Beuren, A. J., Schulze, C., Eberle, P., Harmjanz, D., and Apitz, J.: The Syndrome of Supravalvular Aortic Stenosis, Peripheral Pulmonary Stenosis, Mental Retardation and Similar Facial Appearance, *Am. J. Cardiol.*, 13:471, 1964.

Denie, J. J., and Verheught, A. P.: Supravalvular Aortic Stenosis, *Circulation*, 18:902, 1958.

Morrow, A. G., Waldhausen, J. A., Peters, R. L., Bloodwell, R. D., and Braunwald, E.: Supravalvular Aortic Stenosis: Clinical, Hemodynamic and Pathologic Observations, *Circulation*, 20:1003, 1959.

Williams, J. C. P., Barratt-Boyes, B. G., and Lowe, J. B.: Supravalvular Aortic Stenosis, *Circulation*, 24:1311, 1961.

Valvular Aortic Stenosis*

Braunwald, E., Goldblatt, A., Aygen, M. M., Rockoff, S. D., and Morrow, A. G.: Congenital Aortic Stenosis. I. Clinical and Hemodynamic Findings in 100 Patients, *Circulation*, 27:426, 1963.

Braunwald, E., and Morrow, A. G.: Obstruction to Left Ventricular Outflow: Current Criteria for the Selection of Patients for Operation, *Am. J. Cardiol.*, 12:53, 1963.

Buteler, B. S.: The Relation of Systolic Upstroke Time and Pulse in Aortic Stenosis, *Brit. Heart J.*, 24:657, 1962.

Dexter, L., Harken, D. E., Cobb, L. A., Jr., Novack, P., Schlant, R. C., Phinney, A. O., Jr., and Haynes, F. W.: Aortic Stenosis, *A.M.A. Arch. Int. Med.*, 101:254, 1958.

Dow, P.: The Development of the Anacrotic and Tardus Pulse of Aortic Stenosis, *Am. J. Physiol.*, 131:432, 1940.

Epstein, E. J., and Coulshed, N.: Assessment of Aortic Stenosis from the External Carotid Pulse Wave, *Brit. Heart J.*, 26:84, 1964.

Feil, H. S., and Katz, L. N.: The Transformation of the Central into the Peripheral Pulse in Patients with Aortic Stenosis, *Am. Heart J.*, 2:12, 1926.

Gorlin, R., McMillan, I. K. R., Medd, W. E., Matthews, M. B., and Daley, R.: Dynamics of the Circulation in Aortic Valvular Disease, *Am. J. Med.*, 18:855, 1955.

Hastreiter, A. R., Oshima, M., Miller, R. A., Lev, M., and Paul, M. H.: Congenital Aortic Stenosis Syndrome in Infancy, *Circulation*, 28:1084, 1963.

Jones, R. C., Walker, W. J., Jahnke, E. J., and Winn, D. F., Jr.: Congenital Aortic Stenosis: Correlation of Clinical Severity with Hemodynamic and Surgical Findings in Forty-three Cases, *Ann. Int. Med.*, 58:486, 1963.

Nadas, A. S., Hauwaert, L. van der, Hauck, A. J., and Gross, R. E.: Combined Aortic and Pulmonic Stenosis, *Circulation*, 25:346, 1962.

Peckham, G. B., Keith, J. D., and Evans, J. R.: Congenital Aortic Stenosis: Some Observations on the Natural History and Clinical Assessment, *Canad. M. A. J.*, 91:639, 1964.

Sissman, N. J., Neill, C. A., Spencer, F. C., and Taussig, H. S.: Congenital Aortic Stenosis, *Circulation*, 19:458, 1959.

Tjong, O. S., and Verheught, A. P. M.: Peripheral and Central Arterial Pressure Pulse in the Estimation of the Severity of Aortic Stenosis, *Am. Heart J.*, 62:180, 1961.

Wood, P.: Aortic Stenosis, *Am. J. Cardiol.*, 1:553, 1958.

* See also references in Chapter 24 on rheumatic heart disease.

Hypertrophic Subaortic Muscular Stenosis

Boiteau, G. M., and Allenstein, B. J.: Hypertrophic Subaortic Stenosis: Clinical and Hemodynamic Studies with Special Reference to Pulse Contour Measurement, *Am. J. Cardiol.*, 8:614, 1961.

Brachfeld, N., and Gorlin, R.: Subaortic Stenosis: A Revised Concept of the 'Disease, *Medicine*, 38:415, 1959.

Braunwald, E., Morrow, A. G., Cornell, W. P., Aygen, M. M., and Hilbish, T. F.: Idiopathic Hypertrophic Subaortic Stenosis: Clinical, Hemodynamic and Angiographic Manifestations, *Am. J. Med.*, 29:924, 1960.

Braunwald, E., Brockenbrough, E. C., and Morrow, A. G.: Hypertrophic Subaortic Stenosis—A broadened Concept, *Circulation*, 26:161, 1962.

Braunwald, E., and Ebert, P. A.: Hemodynamic Alterations in Idiopathic Hypertrophic Subaortic Stenosis Induced by Sympathomimetic Drugs, *Am. J. Cardiol.*, 10:489, 1962.

Braunwald, E., Brockenbrough, E. C., and Frye, R. L.: Studies on Digitalis. V. Comparison of the Effects of Ouabain on Left Ventricular Dynamics in Valvular Aortic Stenosis and Hypertrophic Subaortic Stenosis, *Circulation*, 26:166, 1962.

Braunwald, E., Oldham, H. N., Jr., Ross, J., Jr., Linhart, J. W., Mason, D. T., and Fort, L., III: The Circulatory Response of Patients with Idiopathic Hypertrophic Subaortic Stenosis to Nitroglycerin and to the Valsalva Maneuver, *Circulation*, 29:422, 1964.

Braunwald, E., Lambrew, C. T., Rockoff, S. D., Ross, J., Jr., and Morrow, A. G.: Idiopathic Hypertrophic Subaortic Stenosis: I. A Description of the Disease Based upon an Analysis of 64 Patients, *Circulation*, 30 (supp. IV): 3, 1964.

Brockenbrough, E. C., Braunwald, E., and Morrow, A. G.: A Hemodynamic Technic for the Detection of Hypertrophic Subaortic Stenosis, *Circulation*, 23:189, 1961.

Calvin, J. L., Perloff, J. K., Conrad, P. W., and Hufnagel, C. A.: Idiopathic Hypertrophic Subaortic Stenosis, *Am. Heart J.*, 63:477, 1962.

Cohen, J., Effat, H., Goodwin, J. F., Oakley, C. M., and Steiner, R. E.: Hypertrophic Obstructive Cardiomyopathy, *Brit. Heart J.*, 26:16, 1964.

Hancock, E. W.: Differentiation of Valvular, Subvalvular, and Supravalvular Aortic Stenosis, *Guy's Hosp. Rep.*, 110:1, 1961.
Stenosis, *Brit. Heart J.*, 21:581, 1959.

Hancock, E. W.: The Diagnosis of Subvalvular Aortic Stenosis, *Brit. Heart J.*, 21:581, 1959.

Harrison, D. C., Braunwald, E., Glick, G., Mason, D. T., Chidsey, C. A., and Ross, J., Jr.: Effects of Beta Adrenergic Blockade on the Circulation, with Particular Reference to Observations in Patients with Hypertrophic Subaortic Stenosis, *Circulation*, 29:84, 1964.

Hernandez, R. R., Greenfield, J. C., and McCall, B. W.: Pressure-flow Studies in Hypertrophic Subaortic Stenosis, *J. Clin. Invest.*, 43:401, 1964.

Krasnow, N., Rolett, E., Hood, W. B., Jr., Yurchak, P. M., and Gorlin, R.: Reversible Obstruction of Ventricular Outflow Tract, *Am. J. Cardiol.*, 11:1, 1963.

Lauer, R. M., DuShane, J. W., and Edwards, J. E.: Obstruction of Left Ventricular Outlet in Association with Ventricular Septal Defect, *Circulation*, 22:110, 1960.

Manchester, G. H.: Muscular Subaortic Stenosis, *New England J. Med.*, 269:300, 1963.

Marcus, F. I., Westura, E. E., and Summa, J.: The Hemodynamic Effect of the Valsalva Maneuver in Muscular Stenosis, *Am. Heart J.*, 67:324, 1964.

Neufeld, H. N., Ongley, P. A., and Edwards, J. E.: Combined Congenital Subaortic Stenosis and Infundibular Pulmonary Stenosis, *Brit. Heart J.*, 22:686, 1960. Symposium: Left Ventricular Outflow Tract Obstruction, *Circulation*, 31:585–621, 1965.

Wigle, E. D.: The Arterial Pressure Pulse in Muscular Subaortic Stenosis, *Brit. Heart J.*, 25:97, 1963.

Pulmonary Artery Stenosis or Coarctation

Agustsson, M. H., Arcilla, R. A., Gasul, B. M., Bicoff, J. P., Nassif, S. I., and Lendrum, B. L.: The Diagnosis of Bilateral Stenosis of the Primary Pulmonary Artery Branches Based on Characteristic Pulmonary Trunk Pressure Curves, *Circulation*, 26:421, 1962.

Arvidsson, H., Carlsson, E., Hartmann, A., Jr., Tsifutis, A., and Crawford, C.: Supravalvular Stenosis of the Pulmonary Arteries, *Acta radiol.*, 56:466, 1961.

Baum, D., Khoury, G. H., Ongley, P. A., Swan, H. J. C., and Kincaid, O. W.: Congenital Stenosis of the Pulmonary Artery Branches, *Circulation*, 29:680, 1964

d'Cruz, I. A., Agustsson, M. H., Bicoff, J. P., Weinberg, M., Jr., and Arcilla, R. A.: Stenotic Lesions of the Pulmonary Arteries: Clinical and Hemodynamic Findings in 84 Cases, *Am. J. Cardiol.*, 13:441, 1964.

DeLaney, T. B., and Nadas, A. S.: Peripheral Pulmonic Stenosis, *Am. J. Cardiol.*, 13:451, 1964.

Franch, R. H., and Gay, B. B., Jr.: Congenital Stenosis of the Pulmonary Artery Branches. A Classification, with Post-mortem Findings in Two Cases, *Am. J. Med.*, 35:512, 1963.

Gyllensward, A., Lodin, H., Lundberg, A., and Möller, T.: Congenital Multiple, Peripheral Stenoses of the Pulmonary Artery, *Pediatrics*, 19:399, 1957.

Luan, L. L., D'Silva, J. L., Gasul, B. M., and Dillon, R. F.: Stenosis of the Right Main Pulmonary Artery: Clinical, Angiocardiographic, and Catheterization Findings in Ten Patients, *Circulation*, 21:1116, 1960.

Shafter, H. A., and Bliss, H. A.: Pulmonary Artery Stenosis, *Am. J. Med.*, 26:517, 1959.

Valvular Pulmonic Stenosis

Barritt, D. W.: Simple Pulmonary Stenosis, *Brit. Heart J.*, **16**:381, 1954.

Bassingthwaighte, J. B., Parkin, T. W., DuShane, J. W., Wood, E. H., and Burchell, H. B.: The Electrocardiographic and Hemodynamic Findings in Pulmonary Stenosis with Intact Ventricular Septum, *Circulation*, **28**:893, 1963.

Campbell, M.: Relationship of Pressure and Valve Area in Pulmonary Stenosis, *Brit. Heart J.*, **22**:101, 1960.

Dow, J. W., Levine, H. D., Elin, M., Haynes, F. W., Hellems, H. K., Whittenberger, J. W., Ferris, B. G., Goodale, W. T., Harvey, W. P., Eppinger, E. C., and Dexter, L.: Studies of Congenital Heart Disease: IV. Uncomplicated Pulmonic Stenosis, *Circulation*, **1**:267, 1950.

Joos, H. A., Yu, P. N., Lovejoy, F. W., Jr., Nye, R. E., Jr., and Simpson, J. H.: Clinical and Hemodynamic Studies of Congenital Pulmonic Stenosis with Intact Ventricular Septum, *Am. J. Med.*, **17**:6, 1934.

Kirklin, J. W., Connolly, D. C., Ellis, F. H., Burchell, H. B., Edwards, J. E., and Wood, E. H.: Problems in the Diagnosis and Surgical Treatment of Pulmonic Stenosis with Intact Ventricular Septum, *Circulation*, **8**:849, 1953.

Rashkind, W. J.: Pressure Pulse Waves in the Right Ventricle: Alteration in Patients with Pulmonic Stenosis and Pulmonary Hypertension, *Am. Heart J.*, **59**:36, 1960.

Silverman, B. K., Nadas, A. S., Whittenborg, M. H., Goodale, W. T., and Gross, R. F.: Pulmonary Stenosis with Intact Ventricular Septum: Correlation of Clinical and Physiologic Data with Review of Operative Results, *Am. J. Med.*, **20**:53, 1956.

Watson, H., and Lowe, K. G.: Ventricular Pressure Flow Relationships in Isolated Valvular Stenosis, *Brit. Heart J.*, **24**:431, 1962.

Hypertrophic Infundibular Stenosis

Blount, S. G., Vigoda, P. S., and Swan, H.: Isolated Infundibular Stenosis, *Am. Heart J.*, **57**:684, 1959.

Johnson, A. M.: Functional Infundibular Stenosis: Its Differentiation from Structural Stenosis and Its Importance in Atrial Septal Defect, *Guy's Hosp. Rep.*, **108**:373, 1959.

Rodbard, S., and Schaffer, A. B.: Muscular Contraction in the Infundibular Region as a Mechanism of Pulmonic Stenosis in Man, *Am. Heart J.*, **51**:885, 1956.

Ebstein's Malformation

Blount, S. G., Jr., McCord, M. C., and Gelb, I. J.: Ebstein's Anomaly, *Circulation*, **15**:210, 1957.

Brown, J. W., Heath, D., and Whitaker, W.: Ebstein's Disease, *Am. J. Med.*, **20**:322, 1956.

Gøtzsche, H., and Falholt, W.: Ebstein's Anomaly of the Tricuspid Valve: A Review of the Literature and Report of Six New Cases, *Am. Heart J.*, **47**:587, 1954.

Kilby, R. A., DuShane, J. W., Wood, E. H., and Burchell, H. B.: Ebstein's Malformation: A Clinical and Laboratory Study, *Medicine*, **35**:161, 1956.

Livesay, W. R.: Clinical and Physiologic Studies in Ebstein's Malformation, *Am. Heart J.*, **57**:701, 1959.

Mayer, F. E., Nadas, A. S., and Ongley, P. A.: Ebstein's Anomaly: Presentation of Ten Cases. *Circulation*, **16**:1057, 1957.

Sinha, K. P., Uricchio, F. J., and Goldberg, H.: Ebstein's Syndrome, *Brit. Heart J.*, **22**:94 1960.

Atrial Septal Defect

Beck, W., Swan, H. J. C., Burchell, H. B., and Kirklin, J. W.: Pulmonary Vascular Resistance after Repair of Atrial Septal Defects in Patients with Pulmonary Hypertension, *Circulation*, **22**:938, 1960.

Bedford, D. E., and Sellors, T. H.: Atrial Septal Defect, in A. M. Jones (ed.), "Modern Trends in Cardiology," Hoeber Medical Division, Harper & Row, Publishers, Incorporated, New York, 1961, p. 138.

Campbell, M., Neill, C., and Suzman, S.: The Prognosis of Atrial Septal Defect, *Brit. M. J.*, **1**:1375, 1957.

Dexter, L.: Atrial Septal Defect, *Brit. Heart J.*, **18**:209, 1956.

Dexter, L.: Pulmonary Hypertension Developing in Atrial Septal Defect, in W. R. Adams and R. Veith (eds.) "Pulmonary Circulation: An International Symposium," Grune & Stratton, Inc., New York, 1959, p. 227.

Dow, J. W., and Dexter, L.: Circulatory Dynamics in Atrial Septal Defects, *J. Clin. Invest.*, **29**:809, 1950.

Hull, E.: The Cause and Effects of Flow through Defects in the Atrial Septum, *Am. Heart J.*, **38**:350, 1949.

Little, R. C., Opdyke, D. F., and Hawley, J. G.: Dynamics of Experimental Atrial Septal Defects, *Am. J. Physiol.*, **158**:241, 1949.

McDonald, L., Emanuel, R., and Towers, M.: Aspects of Pulmonary Blood Flow in Atrial Septal Defect, *Brit. Heart J.*, **21**:279, 1959.

Novack, P., Segan, B., Kasparian, H., and Likoff, W.: Atrial Septal Defect in Patients over 40, *Geriatrics*, **18**:421, 1963.

Rowe, G. G., Castillo, C. A., Maxwell, G. M., Clifford, J. E., and Crumpton, C. W.: Atrial Septal Defect and the Mechanism of Shunt, *Am. Heart J.*, **61**:369, 1961.

Soulié, P., Carlotti, J., Joly, F., Acar, J., and Forman, J.: Les communications inter-auriculaires; à propos de 81 cas, *Semaine hôp. Paris*, **35**:669/SP 81–708/SP 120, 1959.

Swan, H. J. C., Burchell, H. B., and Wood, E. H.: The Presence of Venoarterial Shunts in Patients with Interatrial Communications, *Circulation*, **10**:705, 1954.

Swan, H. J. C., Burchell, H. B., and Wood, E. H.: Effect of Oxygen on Pulmonary Vascular Resistance in Patients with Pulmonary Hypertension Associated with Atrial Septal Defect, *Circulation*, **20**:66, 1959.

Weidman, W. H., Swan, H. J. C., DuShane, J. W., and Wood, E. H.: A Hemodynamic Study of Atrial Septal Defect and Associated Anomalies Involving the Atrial Septum, *J. Lab. & Clin. Med.*, **50**:165, 1957.

Zimmerman, H. B. (ed.): Symposium on Atrial Septal Defect, *Am. J. Cardiol.*, **2**:664, 1958.

Endocardial Cushion Defect, Atrioventricular Canal, Ostium Primum Defect

Blount, S. G., Jr., Balchum, O. J., and Gensini, G.: The Persistent Ostium Primum Atrial Septal Defect, *Circulation*, **13**:499, 1956.

Braunwald, E., and Morrow, A. G.: Left Ventriculo–Right Atrial Communication: Diagnosis by Clinical, Hemodynamic and Angiographic Methods, *Am. J. Med.*, **28**:913, 1960.

Campbell, M., and Missen, G. A. K.: Endocardial Cushion Defects: Common Atrio-Ventricular Canal and Ostium Primum, *Brit. Heart J.*, **19**:403, 1957.

Kiely, B., Adams, P., Jr., Anderson, R. C., and Lester, R. G.: The Ostium Primum Syndrome, *A.MA. J. Dis. Child.*, **96**:381, 1958.

Levy, M. J., Cuello, L., Tuna, N., and Lillehei, C. W.: Atrioventricularis Communis. Clinical Aspects and Surgical Treatment, *Am. J. Cardiol.*, **14**:587, 1964.

Omeri, M. A., Bishop, M., Oakley, C., Bentall, H. H., and Cleland, W. P.: The Mitral Valve in Endocardial Cushion Defects, *Brit. Heart J.*, **27**:161, 1965.

Symposium on Persistent Atrioventricular Canal, *Am. J. Cardiol.*, **6**:565, 618, 1960.

Wakai, C. S., Swan, H. J. C., and Wood, E. H.: Hemodynamic Data and Findings of Diagnostic Value in Nine Proved Cases of Persistent Common Atrioventricular Canal, *Proc. Staff Meet. Mayo Clin.*, **31**:500, 1956.

Ventricular Septal Defect

Agustsson, M. H., Arcilla, R. A., Bicoff, J. P., Moncada, R., and Gasul, B. M.: Spontaneous Functional Closure of Ventricular Septal Defects in Fourteen Children Demonstrated by Serial Cardiac Catheterizations and Angiocardiography, *Pediatrics*, **31**:958, 1963.

Arcilla, R. A., Agustsson, M. H., Bicoff, J. P., Lynfield, J., Weinberg, M., Jr., Fell, E. H., and Gasul, B. M.: Further Observations on the Natural History of Isolated Ventricular Septal Defects in Infancy and Childhood: Serial Cardiac Catheterization Studies in 75 Patients, *Circulation*, **28**:560, 1963.

Ash, R.: Natural History of Ventricular Septal Defects in Childhood Lesions with Predominant Arteriovenous Shunts, *J. Pediat.*, **64**:45, 1964.

Bloomfield, D. K.: The Natural History of Ventricular Septal Defect in Patients Surviving Infancy. *Circulation*, **29**:914, 1964.

Blount, S. G., Mueller, H., and McCord, M. C.: Ventricular Septal Defect: Clinical and Hemodynamic Patterns, *Am. J. Med.*, **18**:871, 1955.

Blount, S. G., Jr., and Woodward, G. M.: Considerations Involved in the Selection for Surgery of Patients with Ventricular Septal Defects, *Am. J. Cardiol.*, **5**:223, 1960.

Brown, J. W., Heath, D., and Whitaker, W.: Eisenmenger's Complex, *Brit. Heart J.*, **17**:273, 1955.

Dammann, J., F., Jr., Thompson, W. M., Jr., Sosa, O., and Christlieb, I.: Anatomy, Physiology and Natural History of Simple Ventricular Septal Defects. *Am. J. Cardiol.*, **5**:136, 1960.

Eisenmenger, V.: Die angeborenen Defecte der Kammerscheidewand der Herzens, *Ztschr. klin. Med.*, **32** (Suppl.): 1, 1897.

Evans, J. R., Rowe, R. D., and Keith, J. D.: Spontaneous Closure of Ventricular Septal Defects, *Circulation*, **22**:1044, 1960.

Fyler, D. C., Rudolph, A. M., Wittenborg, M. H., and Nadas, A. S.: Ventricular Septal Defect in Infants and Children: A Correlation of Clinical, Physiologic, and Autopsy Data, *Circulation*, **18**:833, 1958.

Grant, R. P., Downey, F. M., and MacMahon, H.: The Architecture of the Right Ventricular Outflow Tract in the Normal Heart and in the Presence of Ventricular Septal Defects, *Circulation*, **24**:223, 1961.

Howitt, G., and Wade, E. G.: Repeat Catheterization in Ventricular Septal Defect and Pulmonary Hypertension, *Brit. Heart J.*, **24**:649, 1962.

Imperial, E. S., Nogueira, C., Kay, E. B., and Zimmerman, H. A.: Isolated Ventricular Septal Defects: An Anatomic-Hemodynamic Correlation, *Am. J. Cardiol.*, **5**:176, 1960.

Kohout, F. W., Silbero, E. N., Schlicter, J. G., and Katz, L. N.: Dynamics of the Eisenmenger Complex, II. *Am. Heart J.*, **50**:337, 1955.

Keck, E. W. O., Ongley, P. A., Kincaid, O. W., and Swan, H. J. C.: Ventricular Septal Defect with Aortic Insufficiency: A Clinical and Hemodynamic Study of 18 Proved Cases, *Circulation*, **27**:203, 1963.

Lucas, R. V., Jr., Adams, P., Jr., Anderson, R. C., Meyne, N. G., Lillehei, C. W., and Varco, R. L.: The Natural History of Isolated Ventricular Septal Defect: A Serial Physiologic Study, *Circulation*, **24**:1372, 1961.

Lynfield, J., Gasul, B. M., Arcilla, R., and Luan, L. L.: The Natural History of Ventricular Septal Defects in Infancy and Childhood: Based on Serial Cardiac Catheterization Studies, *Am. J. Med.*, **30**:357, 1961.

Marshall, H. W., Swan, H. J. C., Burchell, H. B., and Wood, E. H.: Effect of Breathing Oxygen on Pulmonary Artery Pressure and Pulmonary Vascular

Resistance in Patients with Ventricular Septal Defect, *Circulation*, 23:241, 1961.

Morgan, B. C., Griffiths, S. P., and Blumenthal, S.: Ventricular Septal Defect. I. Congestive Heart Failure in Infancy, *Pediatrics*, 25:54, 1960.

Morgan, J., Pitman, R., Goodwin, J. F., Steiner, R. E., and Hollman, A.: Anomalies of the Aorta and Pulmonary Arteries Complicating Ventricular Septal Defect, *Brit. Heart J.*, 24:279, 1962.

Nadas, A. S., Scott, L. P., Hauck, A. J., and Rudolph, A. M.: Spontaneous Functional Closing of Ventricular Septal Defects, *New England J. Med.*, 264:309, 1961.

Savard, M., Swan, H. J. C., Kirklin, J. W., and Wood, E. H.: Hemodynamic Alterations Associated with Ventricular Septal Defect, in A. D. Bass and G. K. Moe (eds.), "Symposium on Congenital Heart Disease," American Association for the Advancement of Science, Washington, D.C., 1960, publ. No. 63, p. 141.

Selzer, A., and Laquer, G. L.: The Eisenmenger Complex and Its Relation to the Uncomplicated Defect of the Ventricular Septum: Review of Thirty-five Autopsied Cases of Eisenmenger Complex, Including Two New Cases, *A.M.A. Arch. Int. Med.*, 87:218, 1951.

Wagenvoort, C. A., Neufeld, H. N., DuShane, J. W., and Edwards, J. E.: The Pulmonary Arterial Tree in Ventricular Septal Defect: A Quantitative Study of Anatomic Features in Fetuses, Infants, and Children, *Circulation*, 23:740, 1961.

Weidman, W. H., DuShane, J. W., and Kincaid, O. W.: Observations Concerning Progressive Pulmonary Vascular Obstruction in Children with Ventricular Septal Defects, *Am. Heart J.*, 65:148, 1963.

Wood, P.: The Eisenmenger Syndrome or Pulmonary Hypertension with Reversed Central Shunt, *Brit. M. J.*, 2:701, 755, 1958.

Zacharioudakis, S. C., Tearplan, K., and Lambert, E. C.: Ventricular Septal Defects in the Infant Age Group, *Circulation*, 16:374, 1957.

Patent Ductus Arteriosus

Adams, F. H., and Lind, J.: Physiologic Studies on the Cardiovascular Status of Normal Infants (with Special Reference to the Ductus Arteriosus), *Pediatrics*, 19:431, 1957.

Burchell, H. B.: Variations in the Clinical and Pathologic Picture of Patent Ductus Arteriosus, *M. Clin. North America*, 32:911, 1948.

Cooley, J. C., Kirklin, J. W., Clagett, O. T., DuShane, J. D., Burchell, H. B., and Wood, E. H.: Coarctation of the Aorta Associated with Patent Ductus Arteriosus, *Circulation*, 13:843, 1956.

Dailey, F. H., Genovese, P. D., and Behnke, R. H.: Patent Ductus Arteriosus with Reversal of Flow in Adults, *Ann. Int. Med.*, 56:865, 1962.

Eldridge, F. L., and Hultgren, H. N.: The Physiologic Closure of the Ductus Arteriosus in the Newborn Infant, *J. Clin. Invest.*, 34:987, 1955.

Eliasch, H., Eriksson, K., and Werkö, L.: Patent Ductus Arteriosus in the Adult, *Acta med. scandinav.*, 155:135, 1956.

Gonzales-Cerna, J. L., and Lillehei, C. W.: Patent Ductus Arteriosus with Pulmonary Hypertension Simulating Ventricular Septal Defects: Diagnostic Criteria in Ten Surgically Proven Cases, *Circulation*, 18:871, 1958.

Hultgren, H., Selzer, A., Purdey, A., Holman, E., and Gerbode, F.: The Syndrome of Patent Ductus Arteriosus with Pulmonary Hypertension, *Circulation*, 8:15, 1953.

Lukas, D. S., Araujo, J., and Steinberg, I.: Syndrome of Patent Ductus Arteriosus with Reversal of Flow, *Am. J. Med.*, 17:298, 1954.

Rudolph, A. M., Mayer, F. E., Nadas, A. S., and Gross, R. E.: Patent Ductus Arteriosus: A Clinical and Hemodynamic Study of 23 Patients in the First Year of Life, *Pediatrics*, 22:892, 1958.

Taylor, B. E., Pollock, A. A., Burchell, H. B., Clagett, O. T., and Wood, E. H.: Studies of the Pulmonary and Systemic Arterial Pressure in Cases of Patent Ductus Arteriosus with Special Reference to Effects of Surgical Closure, *J. Clin. Invest.*, 29:745, 1950.

Aorticopulmonary Septal Defect

Morrow, A. G., Greenfield, L. J., and Braunwald, E.: Congenital Aorticopulmonary Septal Defect. Clinical and Hemodynamic Findings, Surgical Technic, and Results of Operative Correction, *Circulation*, 25:463, 1962.

Neufeld, H. N., Lester, R. G., Adams, P., Jr., Anderson, R. C., Lillehei, C. W., and Edwards, J. E.: Aorticopulmonary Septal Defect, *Am. J. Cardiol.*, 9:12, 1962.

Anomalous Pulmonary Venous Drainage

Burchell, H. B.: Total Anomalous Pulmonary Venous Drainage: Clinical and Physiologic Patterns, *Proc. Staff Meet. Mayo Clin.*, 31:161, 1956.

Burroughs, J. T., and Edwards, J. E.: Total Anomalous Pulmonary Venous Connection, *Am. Heart J.*, 59:913, 1960.

Gott, V. L., Lester, R. G., Lillehei, C. W., and Varco, R. L.: Total Anomalous Pulmonary Return: An Analysis of Thirty Cases, *Circulation*, 13:543, 1956.

Hickie, J. B., Gimlette, T. M. D., and Bacon, A. P. C.: Anomalous Pulmonary Venous Drainage, *Brit. Heart J.*, 18:365, 1953.

Keith, J. D., Rowe, R. D., Vlad, P., and O'Hanley, J. N.: Complete Anomalous Pulmonary Venous Drainage, *Am. J. Med.*, 16:23, 1954.

Morrow, A. G., Anderson, R. P., and Braunwald, E.: Total Anomalous Pulmonary Venous Connection Associated with Incomplete Persistent A-V Canal or Common Atrium (Clinical, Hemodynamic, and Operative Findings), *J. Cardiovas. Surg.*, 4:795, 1963.

Sepulveda, G., Lukas, D. S., and Steinberg, I.: Anomalous Drainage of Pulmonary Veins: Clinical, Physiologic, and Angiocardiographic Features, *Am. J. Med.*, 18:883, 1955.

Swan, H. J. C., Toscano-Barboza, E., and Wood, E. H.: Hemodynamic Findings in Total Anomalous Pulmonary Venous Drainage, *Proc. Staff Meet. Mayo Clin.*, 31:177, 1956.

Swan, H. J. C., Kirklin, J. W., Becu, L. M., and Wood, E. H.: Anomalous Connection of Right Pulmonary Veins to Superior Vena Cava with Interatrial Communications: Hemodynamic Data in Eight Cases. *Circulation*, 16:54, 1957.

Transposition of the Great Vessels

Anderson, R. C., Lillehei, C. W., and Lester, R. G.: Corrected Transposition of the Great Vessels of the Heart, *Pediatrics*, 20:626, 1957.

Beck, W., Schrire, V., Vogelpoel, L., Nellen, M., and Swanepoel, A.: Corrected Transposition of the Great Vessels, *Brit. Heart J.*, 23:497, 1961.

Berry, W. B., Robert, W. C., Morrow, A. G., and Braunwald, E.: Corrected Transposition of the Aorta and Pulmonary Trunk: Clinical, Hemodynamic and Pathologic Findings, *Am. J. Med.*, 36:35, 1964.

Boesen, I.: Complete Transposition of the Great Vessels: Importance of Septal Defects and Patent Ductus Arteriosus: Analysis of 132 Patients Dying before Age 4, *Circulation*, 28:885, 1963.

Chiechi, M. A.: Incomplete Transposition of the Great Vessels with Biventricular Origin of the Pulmonary Artery (Taussig-Bing Complex): Report of Four Cases and Review of the Literature, *Am. J. Med.*, 22:234, 1957.

Elliott, L. P., Carey, L. S., Adams, P., Jr., and Edwards, J. E.: Left Ventricular–Right Atrial Communication in Complete Transposition of the Great Vessels, *Am. Heart J.*, 66:29, 1963.

Goodman, A. H., and Kuzman, W. J.: Functionally Corrected Transposition of the Great Vessels without Significant Associated Defects, *Am. Heart J.*, 61:811, 1961.

Honey, M.: The Diagnosis of Corrected Transposition of the Great Vessels, *Brit. Heart J.*, 25:313, 1963.

Keith, J. D., Neill, C. A., Vlad, P., Rowe, R. D., and Chute, A. L.: Transposition of the Great Vessels, *Circulation*, 7:830, 1953.

Noonan, J. A., Nadas, A. S., Rudolph, A. M., and Harris, G. B. C.: Transposition of the Great Arteries: A Correlation of Clinical, Physiologic and Autopsy Data, *New England J. Med.*, 263:637, 684, 1960.

Schiebler, G. L., Edwards, J. E., Burchell, H. B., DuShane, J. W., Ongley, P. A., and Wood, E. H.: Congenital Corrected Transposition of the Great Vessels: A Study of 33 Cases, *Pediatrics*, 27:851, 1961.

Shaher, R. M.: The Syndromes of Corrected Transposition of the Great Vessels, *Brit. Heart J.*, 25:431, 1963.

Shaher, R. M.: Complete and Inverted Transposition of the Great Vessels, *Brit. Heart J.*, 26:51, 1964.

Shaher, R. M.: The Hemodynamics of Complete Transposition of the Great Vessels, *Brit. Heart J.*, 26:343, 1964.

Atrial Septal Defect with Mitral Stenosis

Angelino, P. F., Garbagni, R., and Tartara, D.: Le syndrome de Lutembacher: Observations cliniques et hémodynamiques avant et après intervention, *Arch. mal. coeur*, 54:511, 1961.

Espino-Vela, J.: Rheumatic Heart Disease Associated with Atrial Septal Defect: Clinical and Pathologic Study of 12 Cases of Lutembacher's Syndrome, *Am. Heart J.*, 57:185, 1959.

Lutembacher, R.: De le stenose mitrale avec communication interauriculaire, *Arch. mal. coeur*, 9:237, 1916.

Sambhi, M. P., and Zimmerman, H. A.: Pathologic Physiology of Lutembacher Syndrome, *Am. J. Cardiol.*, 2:681, 1958.

Atrial Septal Defect with Pulmonary Stenosis

Broadbent, J. C., Wood, E. H., and Burchell, H. B.: Left-to-right Intracardiac Shunts in the Presence of Pulmonary Stenosis, *Proc. Staff Meet. Mayo Clin.*, 28:101, 1953.

Callahan, J. A., Brandenburg, R. O., and Swan, H. J. C.: Pulmonary Stenosis and Interatrial Communication with Cyanosis: Hemodynamic and Clinical Study of 10 Patients. *Am. J. Med.*, 19:189, 1955.

Magidson, O., Cosby, R. S., Dimitroff, S. P., Levinson, D. C., and Griffith, G. C.: Pulmonary Stenosis with Left to Right Shunt, *Am. J. Med.*, 17:311, 1954.

Moffitt, G. R., Zinsser, H. F., Kuo, P. T., Johnson, J., and Schnabel, T. G.: Pulmonary Stenosis with Left to Right Intracardiac Shunts, *Am. J. Med.*, 16:521, 1954.

Rudolph, A. M., Nadas, A. S., and Goodale, W. T.: Intracardiac Left-to-right Shunt with Pulmonic Stenosis, *Am. Heart J.*, 48:808, 1954.

Selzer, A., Carnes, W. H., Noble, C. A., Higgins, W. H., and Holmes, R. O.: The Syndrome of Pulmonary Stenosis with Patent Foramen Ovale, *Am. J. Med.*, 6:3, 1949.

Swan, H., Marchioro, T., Kinard, S., and Blount, S. G.: Trilogy of Fallot: Experience with Twenty-two Surgical Cases, *A.M.A. Arch. Surg.*, 81:291, 1960.

Ventricular Septal Defect with Pulmonary Stenosis

Bing, R. J., Vandam, L. D., and Gray, F. D., Jr.: Physiological Studies in Congenital Heart Disease. II. Results of Preoperative Studies in Patients with Tetralogy of Fallot, *Bull. Johns Hopkins Hosp.*, 80:121, 1947.

Brotmacher, L., and Campbell, M.: Ventricular Septal Defect with Pulmonary Stenosis, *Brit. Heart J.*, 20:379, 1958.

Brotmacher, L.: Haemodynamic Effects of Squatting

during Recovery from Exertion, *Brit. Heart J.,* 19:567, 1957.

Fallot, A.: Contribution à l'anatomie pathologique de la maladie bleue (cyanose cardiaque), *Marseille-méd.,* 25:77, 138, 207, 270, 341, 403, 1888.

Lurie, P. R.: Postural Effects in Tetralogy of Fallot, *Am. J. Med.,* 15:297, 1953.

McCord, M. D., Van Elk, J., and Blount, S. G., Jr.: Tetralogy of Fallot: Clinical and Hemodynamic Spectrum of Combined Pulmonary Stenosis and Ventricular Septal Defect, *Circulation,* 16:736, 1957.

Ross, R. S., Taussig, H. B., and Evans, M. H.: Late Hemodynamic Complications of Anastomotic Surgery for Treatment of the Tetralogy of Fallot, *Circulation,* 18:553, 1958.

Wood, P.: Attacks of Deeper Cyanosis and Loss of Consciousness (Syncope) in Fallot's Tetralogy (in Symposium on Congenital Heart Disease), *Brit. Heart J.,* 20:282, 1958.

Wood, P., Magidson, O., and Wilson, P. A. O.: Ventricular Septal Defect, with a Note on Acyanotic Fallot's Tetralogy, *Brit. Heart J.,* 16:387, 1954.

20 CLINICAL RECOGNITION AND MEDICAL MANAGEMENT OF CONGENITAL HEART DISEASE

F. Kathryn Edwards, M.D., and Dorothy Brinsfield, M.D.

Definition. Congenital heart disease may be defined as a gross structural malformation of the heart or great vessels which is present at birth. In general, these conditions are the result of abnormal embryonic development, or the persistence beyond the time of normal involution of a fetal structure such as the ductus arteriosus.

Incidence. The exact incidence of congenital heart disease in live-born infants is not known. The most complete recent figures are shown in Table 20-1.

Using the incidence of MacMahon,[1] it is estimated that over 13,000 infants, with congenital heart disease were born in the United States in 1961. Were it not for the high mortality rate in the first year of life, a large population of individuals with congenital heart defects would soon accumulate. Certainly in the pediatric age group, congenital heart disease is a common problem. Nadas[5] estimated that there are ten times as many new patients with congenital heart disease admitted to

Table 20-1. INCIDENCE OF CONGENITAL HEART DISEASE IN LIVE-BORN INFANTS

Author	No. per 1,000 live-born
MacMahon et al.[1]	3.2
Richards et al.[2]	7.6
Mustacchi[3]	5.9
Carlgren[4]	6.4

the Boston Children's Medical Center as new patients with rheumatic fever. Keith[6] states that congenital heart disease is the leading cause of death at the Toronto Hospital for Sick Children. The fact that these reports are from dissimilar groups results in the variability of the data on the incidence of specific lesions. Table 20-2 shows the percentage incidence of the various congenital cardiac lesions in Abbott's[7] series of 1,000 autopsied cases, Wood's[8] clinical series which excludes infants, Keith's[6] series in children from birth to 14 years of age, and Nadas's[5] series of 3,786 cases diagnosed at catheterization, operation, or postmortem examination. It certainly appears that ventricular septal defects are most common and make up about 15 to 20 per cent of the cases. Atrial septal defect, patent ductus arteriosus, coarctation of the aorta, tetralogy of Fallot, pulmonary stenosis, aortic stenosis, and transposition of the great vessels make up all but a small percentage of the remainder.

Of 356 patients with congenital heart disease in the Toronto Heart Registry, 49 per cent were males and 51 per cent were females.[6] Certain defects, however, are more common in one sex than the other. Patent ductus arteriosus and atrial septal defect are more common in females. Aortic stenosis, coarctation of the aorta, and transposition of the great vessels are more common in males.

Two or more cases of congenital heart disease in a family have been noted by most observers. The incidence among siblings of patients with congenital heart disease has been reported as 18 per 1,000; the incidence in the general population on the same series was only 3.2 per 1,000 live births.[9,1] Although this is six times the rate of the general population, it is still relatively low and parents should be encouraged to have other children if they desire.

The Infant with Congenital Heart Disease

Over half the infants born with congenital heart disease die before 1 year of age if proper diagnosis is not made and treatment instituted.[1] The difficulties in clinical recognition of heart disease in the young infant are related to: (1) the unfamiliar manifestations of heart disease in the infant in comparison to the older individual, and (2) inade-

Table 20-2. PERCENTAGE INCIDENCE OF VARIOUS CONGENITAL CARDIAC LESIONS

Lesion	Abbott[7]	Wood[8]	Keith[6]	Nadas[5]
Pulmonic stenosis with ventricular septal defect	11.5	12.3	11	14.55
Patent ductus arteriosus	10.5	15.0	17	12.31
Coarctation of aorta	8.5	9.0	6	4.99
Ventricular septal defect	6.2	11.0	25	19.97
Transposition of the great vessels	4.9	1.0	8	3.96
Pulmonic stenosis without ventricular septal defect	3.5	17.0	7	11.97
Atrial septal defect	3.3	19.5	7	10.04
Dextrocardia	2.9	0.5		
Aortic stenosis	2.3	3.0	4	5.73
Persistent truncus arteriosus	2.1	Rare	1	
Tricuspid atresia	1.6	1.5	3	1.24
Aortopulmonary fenestration	1.0	0.3		
Anomalous pulmonary venous drainage	0.4	Rare	2	
Miscellaneous	41.3	9.9	10	15.24

quate physical examination of the infant's cardiovascular system. With present advances in medical and surgical treatment, over half these infants may be helped and many may be cured.

Cyanosis is one of the more frequent first signs of cardiac disease in the infant, but it may also be an early sign of pulmonary disease, central nervous system disease, or methemoglobinemia. The "respiratory distress syndrome" of the newborn baby occurs most frequently in the premature infant, the infant of a diabetic mother, or the infant delivered by Cesarean section, and the cyanosis is almost invariably preceded by tachypnea and retraction of the chest wall. Early in this syndrome, the heart is not enlarged and there are usually no murmurs. Later, there may be a striking anterior lift of the sternum, hepatomegaly, rales, a systolic murmur, and cardiomegaly.[10] Chest x-ray may show the characteristic granular appearance of the lungs or areas of atelectasis.[11] Transient right-to-left shunting of blood may occur at the foramen ovale and ductus in newborns with severe respiratory distress. With improvement in respiration, left-to-right shunting may occur through the ductus prior to its functional closure.[10a] The infant with cyanosis secondary to central nervous system disease will have other neurologic manifestations. Flaccidity, spasticity, or convulsions may be present, or the periodic breathing and peripheral vasomotor instability found in the normal newborn infant may be accentuated. In methemoglobinemia, blood exposed to air will retain a brownish color instead of becoming a normal bright red.

The cyanosis of congenital heart disease is due to shunting of venous blood into the arterial system or to heart failure. The cyanosis due to heart failure will improve or disappear with the administration of oxygen; that due to the shunting of venous blood into the arterial system will remain even though high concentrations of oxygen are administered.

There are 5 T's and 2 AT's that should be considered in the differential diagnosis of the cyanotic infant with venoarterial shunting. *T*ransposition of the great vessels, *t*etralogy of Fallot, *t*ricuspid atresia, *t*otal anomalous pulmonary venous return, and persistent *t*runcus make up the 5 T's and aortic *at*resia and pulmonary *at*resia with normal aortic root, the 2 AT's. Except in tetralogy of Fallot, the cyanosis is grayish blue or has an underlying pallor.

The normal newborn infant has a hemoglobin concentration of 17 to 22 Gm per 100 ml.[12] It will usually drop to 10.5 to 11.5 Gm per 100 ml at 3 months and then slowly rises to 12 to 13 Gm per 100 ml by 2 years. If the hemoglobin level is higher than these normal values after the newborn period, arterial unsaturation is probably present.

Even with severe cyanosis, clubbing will not appear before approximately 3 months of age and is first detected as a fullness at the base of the thumb nail.

Tachypnea may be due to pulmonary congestion or to low arterial oxygen saturation. In the paroxysms of hypoxia, as seen in tetralogy of Fallot, there are increased rate and depth of respiration without obstruction to the movement of air and with no retraction of the chest wall. If the tachypnea is secondary to left-sided heart failure, there is usually lower costal retraction. The infant's respirations are not nearly so deep but may be as rapid as 150 per minute.

Effort intolerance in the infant is usually manifested as a feeding problem. The infant may take a small amount of feeding and then, because of respiratory distress, he may aspirate, cough, or even vomit. After a short rest, he will be hungry again, only to repeat the same episode.

Failure to gain weight or grow properly is usually an indication of a large left-to-right shunt or congestive heart failure. The ordinary stenotic lesions without congestive failure do not interfere with growth.

Profuse sweating with exertion or excessive sweating in ordinary temperatures are common in infants with left-sided heart failure or with large left-to-right shunts.[13]

It is impossible to examine adequately the cardiovascular system of an infant who is not quiet. The infant should be placed in a stable position where sudden motion can be avoided. The young infant may often be quieted with a pacifier or bottle. The infant from 3 months to 1 year can be quieted by holding his attention with a colorful, moving, or shiny object. The child from 1 year to 3 years often is examined better while he sits on his mother's lap.

It is sometimes difficult to palpate the radial or dorsalis pedis pulse in the newborn infant. The femoral pulsations, however, are usually easily felt in the inguinal region and can be compared to the brachial pulsations. When there is a large aortic runoff, the pulse can be felt by simply holding the infant's palm or fingers.

Blood pressure determinations in the infant require some patience but are extremely rewarding in the diagnosis of coarctation of the aorta or patent ductus arteriosus. If the cuff is too small, pressure measurements are obtained which are extremely high and do not compare with intraarterial pressure recordings. A deliberately large cuff has been shown to give blood pressure readings by auscultation that are most nearly the same as intraarterial pressures. The first muffling of the sound compares well with intraarterial diastolic pressure.[14] Auscultation can be accomplished by using a simple seal with a stethoscope over the flat surface just distal and somewhat medial to the antecubital fold. Since most stethoscopes have too large a bell, it is often necessary to remove the larger piece in order to obtain blood pressure determinations by auscultation in the infant. Blood pressure in the legs is best determined with the infant lying on his abdomen. The "flush" technique of blood pressure recording, which has been widely used in pediatrics, will record essentially a systolic pressure in the infant and a mean pressure in the older child. This method fails to reveal the wide pulse pressure of aortic runoff, the "alternans" that is often seen in left ventricular failure, or the "paradox" of cardiac tamponade. Even in coarctation of the aorta, the mean blood pressure in the arms is often the same as in the legs.

The liver is palpable 2 cm below the costal mar-

gin in the normal infant up to age 2 years. The liver in the infant enlarges rapidly with right-sided heart failure, has a somewhat firmer edge than normal, and may be tender. A rapid decrease in size may occur in response to treatment.

A downward systolic pulsation of the liver may be felt in most infants who have cardiomegaly. To evaluate intrinsic pulsations, such as the presystolic pulsations seen in tricuspid atresia, it is best to note whether there is an anterior pulsation of the liver in the midclavicular line with very gentle pressure over the liver.

In those conditions with a large left-to-right shunt or persistent chronic congestive heart failure, the precordium may have an anterior bulge and there may be asymmetric fullness over the precordium. The lower costal margins are often pulled in at the area of attachment of the diaphragm. Cardiac size is best determined in the infant by palpation with the fingertips in the intercostal spaces. The total cardiac size should be evaluated, and some estimate of ventricular hypertrophy or dilatation should be made. In the normal infant, the apical impulse can usually be felt in the fourth or fifth intercostal space at the left midclavicular line. The precordial impulse or the impulse at the left parasternum is normally very slight. Thrills are best palpated with the palm of the hand. However, they are localized in the infant more easily with the fingertips.

The normal heart sounds of the newborn infant have been well described.[15–17] A systolic ejection sound is frequently heard in the first few days of life. The normal splitting of the second heart sound is usually not appreciated until the infant is beyond 24 hr of age even though two semilunar valves may be present. Murmurs due to stenotic lesions are usually audible at birth; those due to shunt lesions usually do not appear until after the third day of life. Even in ventricular septal defects, the murmurs may not be characteristic until later. The murmur of an atrial septal defect is not present in the infant. Although a heart murmur makes one suspicious of underlying heart disease, murmurs in the newborn period are often unassociated with heart disease.[15] Also, many severe congenital cardiac lesions in the newborn period do not cause murmurs. Certainly, severe congenital heart disease cannot be excluded simply by the absence of a heart murmur.

Since the infant's breath sounds are extremely loud, the cardiac sounds may be obscured. Slowly applied, firm pressure over the infant's abdomen will usually stop respirations long enough to allow auscultation of four or five cardiac cycles. In the very young infant the examiner may touch the end of the baby's nose for an instant and this will also interrupt respiration temporarily.

The accuracy of diagnosis in congenital heart disease is greatly enhanced with the addition of chest x-rays and the electrocardiogram. Poor technical quality of either of these examinations makes interpretation impossible. The electrocardiogram from the infant should be obtained using electrodes 1.5 cm in diameter. The standard linear electrocardiogram should include a precordial lead to the right of V_1 (V_3 or V_4 on the right side of the chest). The use of the electrodes of adult size or failure to remove excess electrode paste will give an electrocardiogram with abnormal voltage and configuration (Fig. 20-1).

No estimation of heart size can be obtained from a chest roentgenogram which is obtained in expiration. If an x-ray is to be technically suitable for the evaluation of heart size, the right leaf of the diaphragm should be at the level of the ninth rib. If the film is taken with the patient rotated, the cardiac silhouette cannot be evaluated properly. It has been pointed out that the vascular markings cannot be estimated in the x-ray unless the thoracic intervertebral spcaes are just faintly visible through the heart shadow.[18] More darkness or lightness in the film technique makes estimation of the pulmonary blood flow extremely difficult. In the first 2 to 3 days of life, pulmonary resistance is still somewhat elevated and there is usually very little flow across a defect. As pulmonary resistance decreases, the flow across a defect increases, and pulmonary plethors may develop by the seventh to tenth day of life.

Congestive Failure in the Infant. Keith,[19] in an analysis of 1,580 patients with congenital heart disease, noted that 20 per cent developed congestive

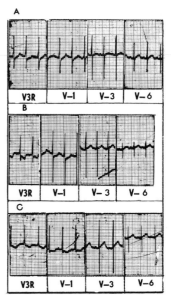

Fig. 20-1. Precordial leads of the electrocardiogram from an infant: *A,* taken with too much electrode paste. *B,* taken with an adult electrode. *C,* taken with an electrode 1.5 cm in diameter with proper amount of electrode paste. Note that complexes differ in voltage and configuration.

heart failure during childhood, 90 per cent having the onset in the first year of life. The clinical picture of congestive heart failure in infants differs somewhat from that seen in adults in that it is often unrecognized, more fulminating in its course, and associated with respiratory tract infection. The percentage incidence of signs of congestive failure

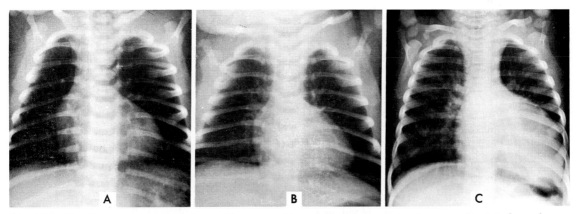

Fig. 20-2. Roentgenograms of an infant with transposition of the great vessels. *A* was made at 2 days of age; pulmonary blood flow appeared normal. *B* was made at 10 days of age and shows definite pulmonary plethora. *C,* taken at 1 year of age, shows cardiomegaly and pulmonary plethora. Progressive cardiomegaly, the narrow cardiac base, "egg-on-side" contour, and pulmonary plethora are characteristic roentgenologic findings in transposition of the great vessels.

Table 20-3. PERCENTAGE FREQUENCY OF SIGNS
OF CONGESTIVE FAILURE IN INFANTS

Sign	Hauck[20]	McCue[21]
Tachypnea	91	100
Tachycardia	88	66
Cardiomegaly	*	90
Hepatomegaly	88	85
Rales	35	62
Edema	19	23

* Not recorded.

in infants is recorded in Table 20-3. Certainly, the most common single finding is tachypnea. Cardiomegaly is present in most types of congestive heart failure; the rare exceptions are total anomalous pulmonary venous return below the diaphragm, congenital mitral stenosis, a few cases of supraventricular tachycardia, aortic atresia, and acute myocarditis.

The infant with left-sided heart failure often presents with prolongation of expiration and lower costal retraction with inspiratory and expiratory wheezes and rales. It may be difficult to distinguish this condition from pneumonia or bronchiolitis. Indeed, in many infants, pulmonary infection may precipitate failure. Episodes of paroxysmal pulmonary edema are uncommon in infants but may be seen with large left-to-right shunts or conditions which cause left atrial blockade, such as sever mitral stenosis or total anomalous pulmonary venous return below the diaphragm. There may be a short period of tachypnea and lower costal retraction with rapid progression to respiratory and cardiac arrest. If peripheral edema is present, it is usually noted around the eyes or on the dorsum of the feet.

The most common congenital cardiac defects causing heart failure in children are transposition of the great vessels, endomyocardial diseases, ventricular septal defect, coarctation of the aorta, aortic atresia, endocardial cushion defects, and patent ductus arteriosus; these make up 75 per cent of McCue's[21] series and 69 per cent of Keith's[19] series. Interestingly, both series show that aortic atresia is the most frequent cause of congestive failure between birth and 1 week of age. Coarctation of the aorta and transposition of the great vessels are the leading causes of congestive failure between 1 week and 1 month of age. Transposition of the great vessels followed by endomyocardial disease, coarctation, and ventricular septal defect are the most common causes of failure between 1 and 3 months of age. In the 3 to 6 months age group, endomyocardial disease is the most frequent cause of failure, followed by transposition of the great vessels, ventricular septal defect, total anomalous pulmonary venous return, and coarctation of the aorta. In our experience, these incidence figures by age have been extremely useful and far more reliable than "playing the horses."

The principles of medical treatment of congestive heart failure in infants are the same as in adults.[22,23] A semierect position can be maintained in an infant seat. Oxygen is best administered in a tent with proper moisture. The temperature inside the tent should be maintained at 70°F. Since respiratory tract infections are so commonly associated with congestive failure, any acutely ill child should receive antibiotics. If tachypnea is severe or vomiting is present, feedings should be omitted for 12 hr. When feedings are reinstituted, glucose water should be tried before milk, because of the danger of aspiration. Morphine sulfate, in a dosage of $\frac{1}{2}$ to 1 mg per 5 kg body weight, may be used for immediate sedation; however, long-term sedation is best maintained with phenobarbital, 6 mg per kg per day divided into three doses. Intramuscular meralluride should be used in severe failure.[24] Long-term diuretic therapy can be accomplished with chlorothiazide suspension in a single oral dose of 25 mg per kg per day. To avoid hypokalemia, the diet should include mashed bananas or orange juice, or an oral liquid potassium chloride supplement may be given. Low-sodium milks are available, if needed, but care should be taken to avoid hyponatremia. Intravenous aminophylline is not recommended in infants because of the severe toxic manifestations.[25] In the acutely ill infant, digitalization should be rapid, by the parenteral route.*

The prognosis in the infant who develops congestive failure is very poor.[19] If the failure cannot be controlled medically, it is imperative that a definitive diagnosis be made in order to determine the need for surgery.

Classification of Congenital Heart Disease

Abbott[7] originally divided the types of congenital heart disease into major groups: (1) those with cyanosis at rest, (2) those without cyanosis or with cyanosis occurring late, (3) those with no cyanosis.

* This may be accomplished parenterally with Lanoxin (digoxin) 0.02 to 0.03 mg per lb body weight in children less than 2 years old or 0.01 to 0.02 mg per lb body weight in children more than 2 years of age. One-half this total digitalizing dose is often given immediately, followed by one-fourth the total dose 6 and 12 hr later. In premature infants a total digitalizing dose of 0.01 to 0.02 mg per lb body weight is recommended. With parenteral digitalization repeated evaluation for signs of toxicity, including electrocardiographic signs, is essential.

Since the presence or absence of cyanosis is dependent on the relative resistance in the two circulations (pulmonary and systemic) and whether or not there is a possible means of communication between the two circulations, there is considerable overlap in that classification. For this reason, other classifications have been suggested which are based on the anatomic defects as well as the hemodynamics. Using the general classification of Nadas,[5] this text is arranged as follows:

1. Communications between systemic and pulmonary circulation without cyanosis (left-to-right shunt)
2. Valvular and vascular lesions with right-to-left shunt or no shunt
3. The transpositions

COMMUNICATIONS BETWEEN SYSTEMIC AND PULMONARY CIRCULATION WITHOUT CYANOSIS (LEFT–TO–RIGHT SHUNTS)

Intracardiac Shunts

Atrial Septal Defects. Four types of openings may be present in the atrial septum. *Probe patency of the foramen ovale* is normal and will not be discussed here. *Secundum atrial septal defects* may be single or multiple. *Sinus venosus atrial septal defects* frequently have one or two anomalous pulmonary veins from the right lung emptying into the superior vena cava. *Ostium primum atrial septal defects* are the partial form of endocardial cushion defect and are discussed in that section.

Clinical Picture. The majority of patients with ostium secundum defects and sinus venosus defects are asymptomatic, although an asthenic build is common. A heart murmur is usually first detected on routine preschool examination. There may be a history of frequent respiratory tract infections. Mild exertional dyspnea is occasionally experienced by adults, but congestive failure is rare before the third decade.[8] On rare occasions, congestive failure may occur in infancy or early childhood.[26a] Atrial fibrillation, usually having its onset in the fourth decade, occurs in 10 to 20 per cent of the adults and may lead to rapid progression of congestive failure.[8] Approximately 10 per cent of the patients with ostium secundum defects or sinus venosus defects develop pulmonary vascular obstruction and present the features of Eisenmenger's syndrome.[27,28] The average life expectancy of a patient with an atrial septal defect is 40 years. However, cases have been reported in the seventh decade.

Physical examination shows a hyperdynamic right ventricle with a systolic lift at the left parasternum. The left ventricular impulse is often not palpable. There is no systolic thrill in uncomplicated cases, but a systolic pulsation of the pulmonary artery may be felt in the second left intercostal space. On auscultation, there is a grade II to III pulmonic ejection systolic murmur, followed by a widely split second heart sound that does not vary with respiration. A middiastolic rumble is heard at the lower left sternal border or apex.[29,30] At the apex the first heart sound often is accentuated, is split, and has a loud tricuspid component.[31] In the absence of congestive failure, the jugular venous pressure is normal and there is no hepatomegaly.

The electrocardiogram shows the pattern of incomplete right bundle branch block with evidence of right ventricular hypertrophy (Fig. 20-3). The P-R interval is prolonged in 20 per cent of the patients, and the mean QRS axis is between 0 and +180° in 96 per cent of the cases.[32,33] The roentgenographic findings include mild to moderate cardiomegaly, enlargement of the pulmonary artery, and increased pulmonary blood flow. The right atrium and right ventricle are enlarged. On fluoroscopy the intrinsic pulsations of the pulmonary artery are more prominent than in any other left-to-right shunt lesion. The aorta is usually small and inconspicuous (Fig. 20-4). The sinus venosus defect with partial anomalous pulmonary veins may be suspected if the hilar markings of the right lung are more prominent than those of the left (Fig. 20-55) and if there is no shadow of the superior vena cava, which is usually shifted somewhat to the left.[34,35] At cardiac catheterization the catheter may be passed into the left atrium or into the anomalous pulmonary veins. The phasic and mean pressures in both atria are similar.[8] Oxygen studies reveal a left-to-right shunt at the atrial level. The systolic pressure of the right ventricle and pulmonary artery is usually less than 50 mm Hg. Secondary to the large

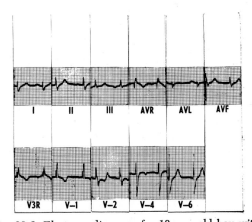

Fig. 20-3. Electrocardiogram of a 10-year-old boy with an uncomplicated secundum atrial septal defect shows a right ventricular conduction delay, right ventricular hypertrophy, and a prolonged P-R interval.

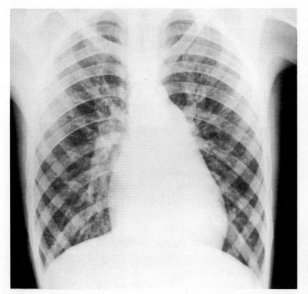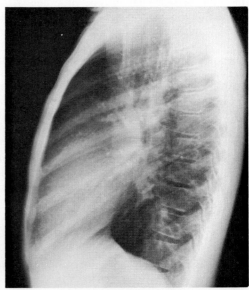

Fig. 20-4. Posteroanterior roentgenogram (left) from the same patient as in Fig. 20-3 (secundum atrial septal defect) shows moderate cardiomegaly, pulmonary plethora, and a prominent pulmonary artery with a small aorta. The lateral projection (right) shows right ventricular hypertrophy and no left atrial enlargement.

flow, a systolic gradient of 10 to 20 mm Hg may be recorded across the normal pulmonary valve. The pulmonary resistance is usually low, and the pulmonary to systemic flow ratio is quite large. Selective left atrial angiocardiography will demonstrate the defect.

One of the most difficult problems in differential diagnosis of atrial septal defects is recognition of the innocent pulmonary systolic ejection murmur of children between the ages of 3 and 12 years. The absence of the wide, fixed splitting of the second heart sound, the absence of the middiastolic rumble, the normal cardiac size, pulmonary blood flow, and pulmonary pulsations indicate that the murmur is of benign origin. Extremely mild degrees of valvular pulmonic stenosis may produce an electrocardiogram similar to that in atrial septal defect. The murmur, however, is much more harsh and is preceded by a systolic ejection sound.

The medical management includes proper antibiotic therapy for respiratory tract infections, which may precipitate congestive heart failure. If atrial fibrillation occurs, attempts should be made to convert the rhythm back to normal, since congestive failure is severe and progressive with atrial fibrillation. If fibrillation has a rapid ventricular response, digitalis should be given to slow the ventricular rate. Although bacterial endocarditis is uncommon in atrial septal defects, prophylactic antibiotics should be given as with other forms of congenital heart disease. If congestive failure develops, its treatment should be instituted prior to surgery.

With the present low operative mortality in atrial septal defects, surgery is probably indicated in all uncomplicated cases with a significant left-to-right shunt.

Ventricular Septal Defects. In uncomplicated ventricular septal defects, the magnitude of the left-to-right shunt is dependent on the size of the defect and the difference between systemic and pulmonary resistance. If the defect is less than 1 cm in diameter (or less than half the diameter of the aorta), the small to moderate shunt is always from the left to the right ventricle and is limited by the size of the opening. If the defect is larger than 1 cm in diameter (or greater than half the diameter of the aorta),[36] pressures in the two ventricles are virtually equal. The shunt size is determined by the relative peripheral resistance in the pulmonary and systemic circuits. If pulmonary resistance is low, the left-to-right shunt may be quite large, but if pulmonary resistance is equal to or greater than the systemic resistance there may be a bidirectional or even a right-to-left shunt, as found in Eisenmenger's syndrome.

Clinical Picture. The majority of patients with a *small* ventricular septal defect are asymptomatic, although a murmur may have been heard since the patient was a few days old. If the left-to-right shunt is moderate in size, mild exercise intolerance and repeated respiratory infections may occur. Congestive failure is rare unless there is an added insult to the cardiovascular system. The jugular venous pulse and arterial pulses are normal, and cyanosis is absent. The precordium may be normal except for a thrill over the lower left parasternum and xiphoid area. Some of these patients have a prominent apical impulse. The second heart sound is frequently widely split and varies normally with respiration, and a third heart sound is commonly heard at the apex.[37] The harsh murmur originally described by Roger[38] is usually grade III to VI, pansystolic, and heard best in the third, fourth, and fifth left intercostal spaces. A middiastolic flow rumble is found in 60 per cent of the patients with moderate shunts but is unusual with small shunts. The classic murmurs may not be present in patients with very small ventricular septal defects or a defect undergoing spontaneous closure. In such instances the short, harsh systolic murmur at the lower left sternal border may be decrescendo or ejection in type.[39,40]

The electrocardiogram commonly shows a normal mean QRS axis and P-R interval. In moderate-size shunts there may be a prominent q and increased voltage of the R and T waves in the left precordial leads.[41,42] Radiologic findings may be normal in a patient with a small ventricular septal defect. In defects of moderate size, there is usually slight cardiomegaly, with left atrial enlargement and prominence of the main pulmonary artery. The pulmonary vasculature appears engorged, and moderate pulsations are seen at fluoroscopy. At cardiac catheterization, a left-to-right shunt is found at the ventricular level. Right ventricular and pulmonary artery systolic pressures are within normal range or slightly elevated. Pulmonary resistance is low, and pulmonary blood flow is usually no greater than two times the systemic. The catheter may pass from the right ventricle through the defect into the left ventricle or ascending aorta. Left ventricular angiocardiography may be used to demonstrate the exact location of the defect.

Patients with *large* ventricular septal defects invariably are symptomatic during the first year of life. These infants are poorly developed and nourished and may present severe congestive failure in the first few months of life. Cyanosis is usually not present except with episodes of congestive failure or pneumonia. There is often some deformity of the left side of the chest, with a vigorous left parasternal lift as well as a prominent apical impulse. A thrill at the lower left sternal border is present in only 50 per cent o fthese patients, and a basal ejection systolic murmur and ejection click may be superimposed on the holosystolic murmur of the defect.[37,42] The arterial pulse may be normal or small. Hepatomegaly, elevated jugular venous pressure, and other evidence of heart failure are often seen. Pulmonary rales and expiratory wheezes are heard on auscultation. The electrocardiographic findings

are extremely variable. However, ventricular septal defects with a large left-to-right shunt and equal ventricular pressures will produce evidence of combined ventricular hypertrophy. There are usually high-voltage R waves in V_1 and V_2, normal T waves rather than peaked and tall in V_6,[42] and large complexes in the midprecordial leads (Katz-Wachtel sign).[43] Wide-peaked P waves are often seen. There is a pattern of incomplete right bundle branch block in 25 per cent of the cases, and the P-R interval is prolonged in 10 per cent.[5] In our experience, the mean QRS axis may fall between -30 and $+120°$ (Fig. 20-5). Chest roentgenograms reveal moderate to severe cardiomegaly, a large pulmonary artery segment, and left atrial enlargement. The aortic knob appears small, and pulmonary arteries are engorged with increased pulsation (Fig. 20-6). Evidence of pulmonary edema, particularly well seen in the right upper lobe, is common in the infant. Cardiac catheterization reveals approximately equal systolic pressures in both ventricles, aorta, and pulmonary artery. Pulmonary flow is usually twice the systemic, and pulmonary resistance is near normal. Left atrial and left ventricular end-diastolic pressures are elevated when heart failure is present. Right ventricular angiocardiography may be needed to exclude forms of incomplete transposition (see "Double-outlet Right Ventricle, further on in this chapter).

An unusual form of ventricular septal defect may occur in which there is a *left ventricular–right atrial shunt*. Since the tricuspid valve is lower than the mitral valve, a defect in the uppermost portion of the ventricular septum results in a shunt from left ventricle to right atrium through a defect in the medial leaflet of the tricuspid valve or through an opening just above the tricuspid valve. These patients usually present clinical, radiologic, and electrocardiographic findings virtually indistinguishable

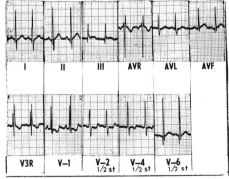

Fig. 20-5. Electrocardiogram of an infant with a large ventricular septal defect shows a normal mean QRS axis and biventricular hypertrophy with prominent voltage in the midprecordial leads.

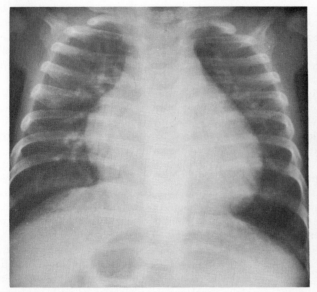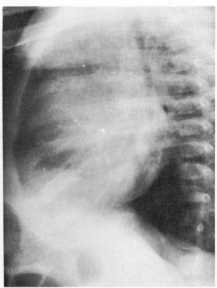

Fig. 20-6. Roentgenograms of an infant with a large ventricular septal defect show moderate cardiomegaly, a large pulmonary artery segment, and pulmonary plethora. The left atrium is enlarged on the lateral view (right).

from those of a small to moderate size ventricular septal defect. This defect may be suspected if an enlarged right atrium is found on the roentgenogram[44] or first-degree block is seen on the electro-

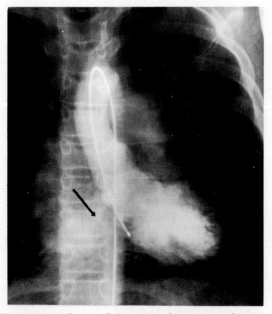

Fig. 20-7. Selective left ventricular angiocardiogram from a patient with a left ventricular–right atrial shunt. Note the opacification of the right atrium directly from the left ventricle (arrow). The clinical findings were those of a ventricular septal defect, small to moderate in size, except that the roentgenogram suggested right atrial enlargement.

cardiogram in a patient with findings of a small ventricular septal defect. At cardiac catheterization, a left-to-right shunt at the atrial level is demonstrated although the catheter cannot be advanced across the atrial septum.[45,46] Left ventricular angiocardiography will demonstrate the left ventricular–right atrial shunt and any associated defects of the ventricular septum or tricuspid valve[45,47] (Fig. 20-7).

The differentiation of ventricular septal defects from other shunt lesions is included in the discussions of atrial septal defects, patent ductus arteriosus, endocardial cushion defects, aortopulmonary shunts, and incomplete transposition.

In early infancy, aortic stenosis may simulate ventricular septal defects. The harsh ejection systolic murmur may be located along the lower left sternal border, and a sustained apical impulse may be present. In infants, the systolic murmur is only rarely accompanied by a thrill until it migrates to the more typical position at the base of the heart.[6] A systolic ejection sound may be present at the apex if the aortic stenosis is valvular. Idiopathic hypertrophic muscular subaortic stenosis may be confused with ventricular septal defect in the older patient.

The findings in severe mitral insufficiency differ from those of a ventricular septal defect in that the systolic murmur and thrill are invariably maximum at the apex rather than at the lower left sternal border and the murmur radiates into the left axilla. Pulmonary pulsations are normal, but pulmonary venous engorgement may be striking.

The natural history of ventricular septal defect is

unknown. With few exceptions, the course and prognosis of an individual case of ventricular septal defect cannot be predicted. Asymptomatic patients with small ventricular septal defects probably have a normal life expectancy but have a higher risk of contracting bacterial endocarditis than those with larger ventricular septal defects.[48] Indisputable data exist that ventricular septal defects may close spontaneously during the first 3 years of life or even up to 6 years of age.[48-50] In contrast, a small percentage of patients with ventricular septal defects may die during the first few years of life from intractable heart failure.[51,52] Of the infants with large left-to-right shunts who survive the first 2 years of life, the majority will show a marked reduction in symptoms and some improvement in their hemodynamic status.[53] Some of these patients undoubtedly develop hypertrophy of the crista supraventricularis, with transformation of the condition into an acyanotic or cyanotic type of tetralogy.[54] Of the remainder who show temporary improvement in childhood, a small number develop irreversible pulmonary arteriolar obstruction in their teens, with classic findings of Eisenmenger's syndrome and early death in the third decade.[55] The progression of pulmonary vascular disease is usually relatively slow, but on rare occasions, progression may be rapid during childhood.[56] On occasion, pulmonary vascular disease or abnormal pulmonary vascular response is thought to be present from birth.[57]

The prevention or treatment of bacterial endocarditis is part of the medical management of ventricular septal defects of any size. In the small infant with a large left-to-right shunt, congestive failure may be severe but surgery should be considered only when adequate control of congestive failure is impossible. Vigorous therapy of respiratory infections is required.

The detection of other cardiac anomalies associated with ventricular septal defects is imperative if surgery is contemplated. The most common associated defects are patent ductus arteriosus, ostium secundum atrial defects, pulmonic stenosis, aortic insufficiency, coarctation of the aorta, and corrected transposition of the great arteries.

When a small patent ductus arteriosus or an ostium secundum atrial defect accompanies a ventricular septal defect, the murmurs of the second defect may be obscured by the loud, holosystolic, and diastolic murmurs of the ventricular septal defects. Cardiac catheterization and angiocardiography may be the only means of detecting the second anomaly.

Ventricular septal defect with mild pulmonic stenosis is characterized by a ventricular shunt that is predominantly left to right.[58,59] The pulmonic stenosis is usually infundibular in type and may be congenital or acquired.[54] The clinical features of these combined defects are similar to those of a small ventricular septal defect with a few exceptions. The pulmonary component of the second heart sound is diminished, and although the pulmonary blood flow appears increased radiologically, pulmonary artery pulsations are often equivocal. Mild left atrial enlargement may be noted. The electrocardiogram shows more evidence of right ventricular hypertrophy than expected from an asymptomatic patient with a ventricular septal defect. Cardiac catheterization, in addition to the left-to-right shunt at the ventricular level, reveals systemic pressure in the right ventricle with a gradient in the infundibular area. The systolic pressure in the pulmonary artery is rarely below 40 mm Hg.[5] Right ventricular angiocardiography will demonstrate narrowing of the infundibulum.

High *ventricular septal defects* may have associated *aortic insufficiency* because of unsupported or deformed aortic valve cusps. The murmur of aortic regurgitation may be present at birth or may appear suddenly at any age. The prolapsed right coronary cusp herniates through the ventricular septal defect, causing obstruction to the left-to-right shunt or even obstruction to the right ventricular outflow.[60] The auscultatory findings are those of a ventricular septal defect plus a high-pitched diastolic, descrescendo murmur along the left sternal border. A wide pulse pressure and peripheral signs of aortic insufficiency may dominate the clinical findings. Congestive failure and angina herald a rapid downhill course with a poor prognosis. The electrocardiogram usually shows dominant left ventricular hypertrophy. Roentgenograms may show marked cardiomegaly.[61] Retrograde aortography is essential to differentiate these combined defects from a ruptured sinus of Valsalva.[62]

Endocardial Cushion Defects. Failure of the embryonic atrioventricular endocardial cushions to fuse properly in the midline results in a spectrum of anomalies referred to as endocardial cushion defects.[63] Although these defects are closely allied embryologically, the clinical picture is quite varied. In the *partial* form of endocardial cushion defect (*ostium primum defect*), there is an opening between the atria which has a crescent superior margin; the inferior margin is formed by the two atrioventricular valves. If there is no deformity of the atrioventricular valves, the clinical picture is indistinguishable from that of secundum atrial septal defect. Usually, however, the aortic leaflet of the mitral valve is cleft and thickened and has abnormal chordae tendineae, which result in varying degrees of insufficiency of the mitral valve.[30] If the septal leaflet of the tricuspid valve is cleft, it may be insufficient. The severity of the symptoms depends on the degree of abnormal function of the atrioventricular valves. Symptoms may not occur until the third decade. Usually, however, there are frequent respiratory tract infections, poor growth and development, exertional fatigue, and congestive failure in early childhood. Prominence of the left side of the chest and lower costal retraction are common. The liver may be enlarged and the jugular venous pressure elevated. If there is significant regurgitation at the atrioventricular valves, there are a systolic pulsation of the liver and a prominent systolic pulsation of the neck veins. Total heart size is moderately to greatly enlarged, with a sustained left parasternal and apical impulse. A thrill is frequently felt at the apex. The pulmonary valve closure may be palpable in the second left intercostal space, and there may be a systolic pulsation in the same area. On auscultation in the second left intercostal space, there is a grade II to III ejection systolic murmur followed by a second heart sound that is widely split, does not vary with respiration, and has a loud pulmonic component. At the apex, there are a low-pitched middiastolic rumble and a loud, high-frequency holosystolic murmur of mitral insufficiency.[64,65]

In the *complete* form of endocardial cushion defect (*atrioventricularis communis*), there is complete failure of fusion of the embryonic endocardial cushions, resulting in a large atrial septal defect, a single atrioventricular valve ring with deformity of the leaflets, and a large ventricular septal defect functionally resulting in a two-chambered heart. This defect has been found to occur in 36 per cent of persons who have Down's syndrome (mongolism), and it is estimated that about half of all diagnosed cases of atrioventricularis communis have associated monogolism.[6,65,66] Symptoms usually occur in early infancy. There are severe congestive failure, poor growth and development, repeated respiratory tract infections, and chronic cough.

There may be bouts of paroxysmal pulmonary edema or ectopic rhythm; cyanosis is usually not visible except with pulmonary infections or congestive failure. There are usually asymmetry of the chest and lower costal retraction. There may be rales, elevated jugular venous pressure, hepatomegaly, tachypnea, and pulsus alternans. There is biventricular enlargement of the heart. A systolic thrill may be present along the left sternal border. On auscultation, the murmurs are indistinguishable from those produced by a large ventricular septal defect. The prognosis is poor, and only a few infants survive the first 2 years of life.[6] Those who do survive have obstruction to pulmonary blood flow; they may live to adolescence or young adult life.[67]

The linear electrocardiogram characteristically shows biventricular hypertrophy in the precordial leads, with a prominent R' in the right precordial leads. The P-R interval is frequently prolonged, and the P waves may be tall, bifid, and broad. The QRS complexes have large voltage in all leads. The mean QRS axis is between 0 and −180° in 87 per cent of the cases[33] (Fig. 20-8). The vectorcardiogram shows a superiorly oriented counterclockwise loop in the frontal plane.[68,69] These electrocardiographic findings are highly suggestive of endocardial cushion defects. However, they are not specific for this condition.[70] The roentgenologic examination shows marked cardiac enlargement involving both ventricles and both atria. Pulmonary flow is increased, and there is often a fullness at the base of the enlarged pulmonary artery.[6] Pulmonary edema may be present (Fig. 20-9).

At catheterization of the right side of the heart the catheter may pass from right to left atrium at a low level and may, in the complete form, pass directly from the right atrium to the left ventricle. In the complete form, a loop of the catheter may be formed which will traverse all four cardiac chambers. Right ventricular and pulmonary arterial systolic pressures are elevated and may be the same as the systemic. Oxygen saturations will demonstrate the left-to-right shunt, which may be present in the low right atrium as well as in the right ventricle. Phasic and mean pressures from both atria are similar. In the complete form of endocardial cushion defect, there is frequently slight systemic arterial unsaturation. Selective right ventricular angiocardiography may show dilatation of the infundibulum.[6] Selective left ventricular angiocardiograms will often demonstrate the insufficiency of the atrioventricular valve, the left-to-right shunt, and an abnormal outline along the septal surface of the left ventricle.[71]

If there is no involvement of the atrioventricular valves in the partial form of endocardial cushion defect, the differential diagnosis is one of distin-

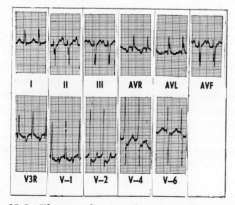

Fig. 20-8. Electrocardiogram from an infant with a complete endocardial cushion defect shows left axis deviation (−60°), first-degree heart block with large-notched P waves, and biventricular hypertrophy.

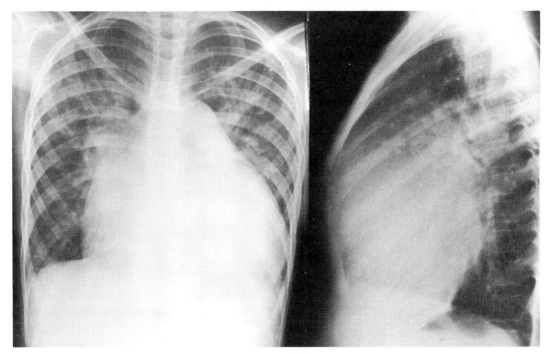

Fig. 20-9. Roentgenograms from an adolescent with the partial form of endocardial cushion defect (ostium primum defect). Kerley lines may be seen at the base of the right lung in the posteroanterior projection (left). There are marked cardiomegaly with enlargement of all chambers and pulmonary plethora. Marked right ventricular enlargement is present in the lateral projection (right).

guishing this defect from secundum atrial septal defect. The low passage of the cardiac catheter from right atrium to left atrium may suggest an ostium primum defect, and left atrial selective angiocardiograms may show that the defect is very low. It may, however, be impossible to distinguish these two except by direct visualization. If mitral insufficiency is present, ostium primum defects may be confused with rheumatic mitral insufficiency. The widely split, fixed second heart sound, the typical electrocardiographic findings, and the pulmonary plethora with increased pulsations on fluoroscopy should make the diagnosis of ostium primum defect. The complete form of endocardial cushion defect must be differentiated from the combined secundum atrial septal defect and ventricular septal defect. In the combined lesion, the mean QRS axis is normal or slightly to the right. However, cardiac catheterization and selective angiocardiography may be necessary for a definitive diagnosis. On rare occasions, direct observation of the defect at surgery is necessary to distinguish these two conditions. A large ventricular septal defect in early infancy may be very similar clinically and electrocardiographically to an atrioventricularis communis. Cardiac catheterization and angiocardiography may be necessary to distinguish these two conditions, also.

There are *transitional* forms of endocardial cushion defects between these extremes. Also, there are other congenital cardiac lesions which are embryologically related to endocardial cushion defects. *Isolated ventricular septal defects of the atrioventricular canal type* have been reported.[72] In this condition, the electrocardiogram is the same as in other forms of endocardial cushion defects and there may be some deformity of one or both of the atrioventricular valves. These cases clinically present as large ventricular septal defects. *Congenital mitral insufficiency* is an uncommon isolated lesion and is usually the result of a cleft in the aortic leaflet of the mitral valve. There may or may not be a hemodynamically insignificant atrial septal defect of the primum type associated with this lesion. The murmur of mitral insufficiency is usually present at birth, or shortly thereafter, and the clinical picture is that of isolated rheumatic mitral insufficiency. The electrocardiogram is not typical of an endocardial cushion defect in the majority of the cases reported.[73-75] *Left ventricular–right atrial shunts* are probably embryologically related to endocardial cushion defects. Clinically, this condition simulates ventricular septal defect and is discussed under that subject.

The medical treatment for endocardial cushion defects should include prompt and vigorous treatment for intercurrent respiratory tract infections. Congestive heart failure should be treated in the usual manner. The course in the complete form of this condition is rapidly downhill once congestive failure occurs. Therefore, surgery should be strongly considered even though the risk is high.[76,76a] In the incomplete forms, surgery may be delayed if symptoms can be controlled. Because of the deformity of the atrioventricular valve leaflets and the location of the conducting system, there may be residual mitral insufficiency and severe conduction disturbances after surgery.[76,77] Prophylactic antibiotics should be given for the prevention of bacterial endocarditis even if the patient has had surgery.

Extracardiac Shunts

Patent Ductus Arteriosus. Patent ductus arteriosus results from the persistence of the normal embryonic channel which connects the left pulmonary artery to the descending aorta just distal to the left subclavian artery.

Clinical Picture. Children with uncomplicated patent ductus arteriosus are asymptomatic and have normal growth and development. Underdevelopment, seen occasionally, is probably due to a large ductus with altered cardiac function or is secondary to some associated congenital anomaly such as the rubella syndrome.[78] The diagnosis is most often made when a continuous murmur is found in a well child on routine physical examination. Occasionally, repeated respiratory infections may occur. The peripheral arterial pulses are bounding, and a conspicuous Corrigan pulse may be present. The jugular venous pressure is normal. The total cardiac size is usually normal, but the apical impulse may be slightly prominent. A systolic thrill may be palpable in the second left intercostal space and in the suprasternal notch. The most significant single finding is a harsh, "machinery," continuous murmur which is maximum in the second left intercostal space radiating toward the left clavicle. The systolic component may radiate down the left sternal border. The murmur is heard throughout the cardiac cycle or may wane in the latter part of diastole. The maximum intensity is in late systole and frequently obscures the second heart sound. A systolic ejection sound, a third heart sound, and a mid-diastolic rumble may be heard at the apex.[79] The systolic component of the peripheral arterial pressure is usually slightly higher and the diastolic component slightly lower than normal, giving a pulse pressure of 45 mm Hg or more in 75 to 90 per cent of cases.[6]

The asymptomatic patient with a small left-to-right shunt probably has a normal life expectancy provided bacterial endarteritis can be avoided. If bacterial endarteritis occurs, the lesion is usually found on the pulmonary artery side of the ductus and results in septic embolization to the lung.[8]

The electrocardiogram is frequently within normal limits. If the left-to-right shunt is of moderate size, there are usually a normal mean QRS axis, somewhat broadened and notched P waves, and left ventricular hypertrophy. The characteristic pattern seen in the left precordial leads is a prominent q, followed by a tall R and tall peaked T waves.[80] On roentgenographic examination the heart and lungs are normal in one-third of the cases. Depending on the size of the shunt, there may be slight to moderate cardiomegaly. The aortic knob is prominent and has increased pulsations on fluoroscopy. The pulmonary artery and pulmonary vascular markings are prominent. Left atrial and left ventricular enlargement may be present. Cardiac catheterization is rarely indicated for the diagnosis and management of a typical patent ductus arteriosus. When catheterization of the right side of the heart is performed, however, the catheter may pass from the pulmonary artery, through the ductus arteriosus, into the descending aorta. A left-to-right shunt is present at the pulmonary artery level. Arterial saturation is normal. The pulmonary arterial and right ventricular pressures are normal or slightly elevated. Aortography will show opacification of the ductus and pulmonary artery.

The two major complications that may develop in the patient with a moderate to large patent ductus arteriosus are congestive failure and pulmonary hypertension. The incidence of either of these complications is not known. However, if congestive failure does not appear during infancy, it is unlikely to occur before the third decade. A small percentage of patients with left-to-right shunts during childhood develop pulmonary hypertension with a reversal of flow through the ductus in later life[81] and have the clinical features of Eisenmenger's syndrome, with cyanosis and clubbing in the lower trunk and extremities. On rare occasions calcification or aneurysm of the ductus may occur.[79,82]

The classic case of patent ductus arteriosus is easily diagnosed clinically. However, other causes of *continuous murmurs* may be a source of confusion. The *venous hum,* so frequently heard in normal children,[16] is maximum over the base of the neck on the right. It varies with rotation of the patient's head or with gentle compression over the ipsilateral veins, increases in intensity on inspiration, is louder in diastole, and usually disappears when the patient is in the recumbent position. *Pulmonary arteriovenous fistulas* may cause continuous murmurs over the peripheral lung fields and mild to moderate cyanosis with a normal heart size. Other signs suggesting hereditary telangiectasia, the Rendu-Osler-Weber disease, should arouse suspicion, and the fistulous mass may be visible on roentgenogram.[83] The continuous murmur of a *ruptured sinus of Valsalva* is sudden in onset and is similar to that of a *coronary arteriovenous fistula* in that it is found almost invariably lower on the precordium than is the murmur of a patent ductus.[84,85] Multiple *coarctations of the pulmonary arteries* or *bronchial collateral vessels* off the descending aorta may cause continuous murmurs which are louder on the back and over the peripheral lung fields.[86] In *persistent truncus arteriosus*, the continuous murmur is more widely distributed; there are arterial unsaturation and, usually, severe congestive heart failure. Clinically and hemodynamically, *aortopulmonary fistulas* and patent ductus arteriosus are frequently indistinguishable except at cardiac catheterization and aortography.[87,88] A continuous venous hum can occasionally be heard in *transposition of the pulmonary veins*.[6]

Medical treatment for the patient with patent ductus arteriosus is directed towards the prevention or treatment of bacterial endarteritis and routine measures for the control of congestive failure until the optimal time for surgical correction.

Symptomatic Patent Ductus of Infancy. Patent ductus arteriosus may cause cardiomegaly and severe congestive failure during the first few weeks or months of life.[89,90] The murmur is often primarily systolic but may extend into the first part of diastole, depending on the pressure relationship between the aorta and the pulmonary artery.[91] In about half these infants, the murmur may be heard maximally in the third and fourth left intercostal spaces but retains the late systolic accentuation of the typical ductus murmur.[92] There is a hyperdynamic precordium, with signs of biventricular enlargement. An apical middiastolic rumble is present. The peripheral pulses are bounding and "physiologic coarctation" may be noted.[86] Cyanosis may be present with severe congestive failure, and episodes of pulmonary edema may occur. Although the second heart sound is covered by the murmur, paradoxical splitting may be shown by phonocardiography.[93] The electrocardiogram demonstrates a normal mean QRS axis, broad-notched P waves, and evidence of biventricular hypertrophy (Fig. 20-10). Radiologically there is a marked increase in pulmonary blood flow and, as in other large left-to-right shunts in infancy, there may be pulmonary edema, particularly well seen in the right upper lobe. The left atrium is enlarged, and there is moderate cardiomegaly (Fig. 20-11). Since this is a surgically correctable lesion, any infant with congestive failure in whom a patent ductus cannot be excluded clinically, should have cardiac catheterization or aortography[94] (see Chaps. 8 and 9, pp. 172, 173, and 201).

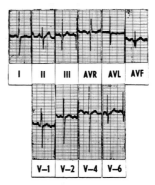

Fig. 20-10. Electrocardiogram from an infant with symptomatic patent ductus arteriosus shows broad and notched P waves in lead I, a normal mean QRS axis, and probable biventricular hypertrophy.

Occasionally, infants are born with severe pulmonary vascular disease and retain a patent ductus arteriosus. There may be associated hypoplasia of the arch of the aorta or preductal coarctation. These infants have severe right ventricular hypertrophy from birth, and eventually cyanosis of the lower trunk and extremities will appear. Maternal rubella, occurring in the first 2 months of gestation, may cause congenital cataracts, mental retardation, deafness, microcephaly, and congenital heart disease in the infant.[95,96] After the rubella epidemic in the spring of 1964, 26 infants with congenital rubella syndrome were followed at Grady Memorial Hospital by the Department of Pediatrics of Emory University School of Medicine. Many of these infants had low birth weights, neonatal jaundice, hepatosplenomegaly, thrombocytopenia, and a variety of anomalies of the eye (cataracts, microphthalmia, retinal dystrophy, glaucoma, and coloboma of the optic nerve). Three of these infants died in the neonatal period. Such infants may show other evidences of their disease in the neonatal period and have rubella virus in their stool, nasopharynx, and tissues for several months. The virus has been shown to be transmitted from these infants to susceptible persons.[97] The most frequent cardiac lesion is patent ductus arteriosus which occurred in 21 of these patients and was noted in 22 out of 31 of Rowe's cases.[97a] Other forms of heart disease have been noted, including coarctations of the pulmonary arteries, atrial septal defects, ventricular septal defects, valvular pulmonic stenosis, tetralogy of Fallot, coarctation of the aorta, aortic stenosis, transposition of the great vessels, and tricuspid atresia.[97a,98]

Aortopulmonary Septal Defects. Aortopulmonary septal defect is an uncommon anomaly in which there is an opening between the aorta and the pulmonary artery just above the aortic valve. The

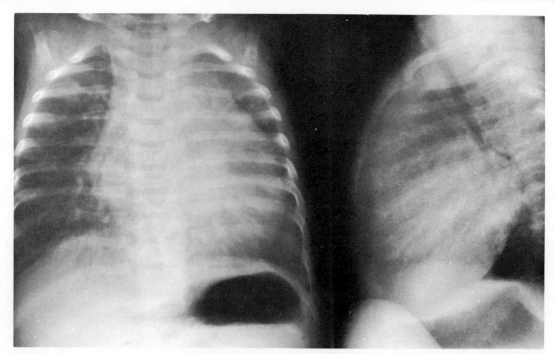

Fig. 20-11. Posteroanterior roentgenogram (left) from an infant with a large patent ductus shows marked cardio-megaly with increased pulmonary blood flow and suggests pulmonary edema, particularly in the area of the right upper lobe. The lateral projection (right) shows left atrial enlargement.

clinical picture depends on the size of the defect and the resistance in the pulmonary vascular bed. If the defect is small and the pulmonary resistance is near normal, the clinical picture is similar to that of a patent ductus arteriosus except that the continuous murmur is usually somewhat lower and more medial.[5] In the majority of the patients, the defect is large and the pulmonary pressure and resistance are elevated. The clinical picture, in this situation, is similar to that of a large ventricular septal defect with pulmonary hypertension. There may be a systolic murmur and thrill along the left sternal border.

The electrocardiographic findings may be similar to those of a large patent ductus or a large ventricular septal defect with biventricular hypertrophy. The roentgenologic picture is indistinguishable from that of a ventricular septal defect with pulmonary hypertension. At cardiac catheterization, there is evidence of a left-to-right shunt at the pulmonary artery level. The pulmonary artery pressure is elevated, and the catheter may cross the defect into the ascending aorta.[88] Retrograde aortography will demonstrate the opening between the ascending aorta and the pulmonary artery.[87,99] The prognosis and medical treatment are the same as for a large patent ductus arteriosus. The risk at surgery is somewhat greater than with simple patent ductus since the pulmonary resistance is often

higher and cardiopulmonary bypass is usually necessary for the closure of the defect.

Persistent Truncus Arteriosus. When the embryonic bulbar ridges fail to develop, there is persistence of the fetal common trunk, or persistent truncus arteriosus. Since the ridges contribute to the development of the ventricular septum, a defect or complete absence of the ventricular septum is invariably present. The pulmonary arteries arise as a single trunk from the dorsal wall or independently from either side of the truncus. The clinical picture is primarily that of a large left-to-right shunt associated with a mild degree of cyanosis. Failure to thrive and congestive failure are observed from the first few months of life. There is usually a prominent parasternal lift and apical impulse with progressive cardiomegaly. After the first month of life, 70 per cent of these patients have a systolic murmur, occasionally accompanied by a thrill, in the third and fourth left intercostal spaces similar to the murmur of a large ventricular septal defect.[6,8] Continuous murmurs may be heard over the lung fields if pulmonary resistance is near normal. The second heart sound is single and accentuated.[86] Increased venous pressure, hepatomegaly, and rales over the lung fields are frequently found with other evidence of congestive heart failure. A wide pulse pressure and vigorous pulses usually suggest an aortic runoff. The majority of these infants do not survive past 6 months of age. If hypoplastic pulmonary arteries arising from the truncus are present or if pulmonary vascular disease develops, life expectancy is prolonged. On rare occasions, such patients may reach the third or fourth decade. When the pulmonary flow is obstructed, the clinical picture is that of Eisenmenger's syndrome or may simulate tetralogy of Fallot. The electrocardiographic findings are not characteristic. The mean QRS axis is frequently within normal range, and biventricular hypertrophy is probably the most common finding in the precordial leads[100] (Fig. 20-12). The roentgenograms reveal moderate or severe cardiomegaly without a characteristic contour. The pulmonary arteries appear engorged and pulsate vigorously at fluoroscopy. If the left pulmonary artery is noted to be high near the level of the aortic arch, persistent truncus should be suspected.[101] The "aorta" may be enlarged and have increased pulsations, and a right arch is present in 25 per cent of the cases.[5] At cardiac catheterization, the catheter may be advanced into the truncus and out each pulmonary artery. Arterial unsaturation is found in all cases and may be severe if pulmonary resistance is elevated. If there is no obstruction to pulmonary blood flow, the unsaturation may be mild. Similar oxygen saturations and systolic pressures are found in the aortic arch and pulmonary arteries. Selective angiocardiography from the proximal truncus may demonstrate the truncus, origin of the pulmonary arteries, and the frequently associated insufficiency of the truncal valve.[101,101a] Medical management is primarily directed towards the treatment of congestive failure, the prevention of bacterial endocarditis, and the complications of right-to-left shunts. The differential diagnosis should include large ventricular septal defects of infancy, tricuspid atresia with transposition of the great vessels, severe forms of tetralogy of Fallot, and aortopulmonary septal defects. These conditions are discussed elsewhere.

VALVULAR AND VASCULAR LESIONS WITH RIGHT–TO–LEFT SHUNT OR NO SHUNT

Aortic Arch Anomalies. A *right aortic arch* may occur as a mirror image of the normal structure without associated anomalies. However, right aortic arches have been noted to be associated with other vascular anomalies within the thorax such as bilateral ductus arteriosus, contralateral absence of the pulmonary arteries, and large bronchial arteries. Also, it has been estimated that if a right aortic arch is present, there is a 40 per cent chance of having intracardiac anomalies.[102] A right aortic arch may occur in approximately 25 per cent of the

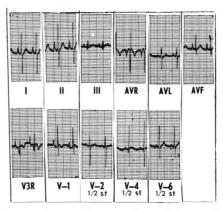

Fig. 20-12. Electrocardiogram obtained from a 2-week-old infant who had persistent truncus arteriosus shows a normal mean QRS axis, giant P waves, and biventricular hypertrophy.

cases of tetralogy of Fallot and persistent truncus arteriosus, and in 5 per cent of the cases of tricuspid atresia. If remnants of both the right and left aortic arches (*double aortic arch*) remain, there may be complete encircling of the trachea and esophagus,[103] with symptoms of recurrent respiratory tract infections, a brassy cough, and difficulty in feeding in the first few months of life. These infants are more comfortable when the neck is hyperextended. The vascular anomaly may be demonstrated by its impingement on the barium-filled esophagus or compression of the trachea (Fig. 20-13). The vessels are outlined by angiocardiography (Fig. 20-14). If obstructive symptoms are severe, surgery is indicated.[104]

If a portion of the right arch persists, the right subclavian may arise from the descending aorta (*aberrant right subclavian artery*). The aberrant right subclavian artery passes posterior to the esophagus, and occasionally there is a large arterial diverticulum known as *Kommerell's diverticulum*. The aberrant right subclavian artery usually causes no symptoms but may be found on roentgenography in approximately 1 per cent of individuals.[102]

Coarctation of the Aorta. A constriction of varying length may occur anywhere along the aorta[105,106] but, in 95 per cent of the cases it is a localized constriction just distal to the left subclavian artery near the site of the ligamentum arteriosum.

Clinical Picture. Coarctation of the aorta is twice as common in males as females but is commonly seen in ovarian agenesis (*Turner's syndrome*) in the female.[107] Symptoms are uncommon in children and young adults, but attention is directed to the cardiovascular system when a heart murmur or hypertension in the upper extremities is noted at routine physical examination. Growth and develop-

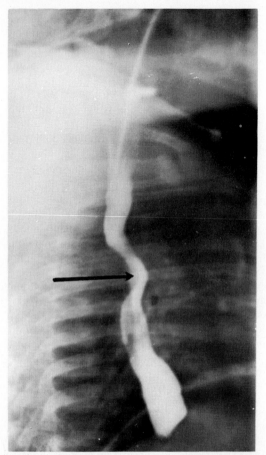

Fig. 20-13. Barium esophagram obtained on a 2-month-old infant who had respiratory stridor and recurrent pneumonia shows anterior displacement of the esophagus (arrow) by the posterior segment of the double aortic arch.

ment are usually normal, and excessive development of the muscles of the arms and shoulders may be noted. Complaints of leg pain with exercise, epistaxis, headaches, or, rarely, dyspnea on exertion may be elicited on questioning. The arterial pulsations in the suprasternal notch and carotids are forceful. Visible and palpable collateral vessels on the back do not usually appear before adolescence. The blood pressure in the arms is elevated, and the systolic pressure in the legs is 20 to 30 mm Hg less than in the arms. If the pulse pressure is greatly diminished, it may be impossible to obtain blood pressures in the legs by auscultation. There is a delay in the upstroke of the femoral pulse. On rare occasions, pulsations in the left arm may be diminished if the coarctation involves the aorta near the origin of the left subclavian artery. If an aberrant right subclavian artery is present, the pressures

in the right arm and legs are lower than the pressure in the left arm. The total heart size is usually normal, but the apical impulse is forceful and sustained. A thrill may be palpable in the suprasternal notch but is uncommon over the precordium. A grade II ejection systolic murmur is heard along the left sternal border in 80 per cent of the cases. A middiastolic rumble is heard at the apex in 10 to 50 per cent of the cases.[5,8] A systolic aortic ejection sound is frequently present at the apex. The systolic ejection murmur is well heard in the neck and is maximal on the left back between the scapula and spine. Collateral vessels may cause a continuous murmur over the back.

Complications of coarctation are uncommon between the ages of 2 to 20 years. A bicuspid aortic valve is estimated to occur in 10 to 70 per cent of the cases of coarctation and may give rise to a murmur of aortic insufficiency or aortic stenosis.[7,108] Rarely, dilatation of the aorta may produce aortic insufficiency in the absence of a bicuspid valve. Bacterial endocarditis may occur at the site of coarctation or on the bicuspid aortic valve. Cerebrovascular accidents due to rupture of intracranial arteries have been noted in about 10 per cent of the cases coming to autopsy in the third decade.[7,109] Hypertensive encephalopathy has been noted in both children and adults. Retinal hemorrhages and exudates are uncommon. Aneurysmal dilatation of the aorta may occur in the proximal aorta or just distal to the coarctation. Rupture is more likely to occur in the ascending aorta, with dissection into the pericardium, and is found in 20 per cent of the autopsy cases. Rupture may occur in late pregnancy.[110] If congestive failure does not develop in the first year of life, it is unlikely to occur until the third decade. The average life expectancy in coarctation of the aorta is 35 years.[111–113]

The electrocardiogram is normal in half the cases,[8] and in the remainder, there is left ventricular hypertrophy by voltage in the precordial leads with a normal mean QRS axis. Evidence of severe left ventricular hypertrophy with T-wave changes suggests associated aortic stenosis.[5,8] Young children with no associated anomaly may have some residual right ventricular hypertrophy on the electrocardiogram. Roentgenograms show the shadow of the dilated left subclavian artery high on the left mediastinal border. The total heart size and pulmonary flow are usually normal, but the left ventricle is prominent. Rib notching, secondary to dilatation of intercostal arteries, may be seen after the age of 6 on the lower aspect of the ribs (Fig. 20-15). The barium-filled esophagus will often show the E sign, which is due to the dilated aorta

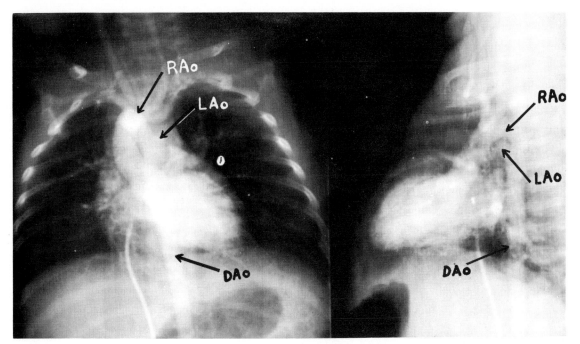

Fig. 20-14. Angiocardiogram in same patient as in Fig. 20-13 outlines the left side of the heart and aorta. The persistent right aortic arch (*RAo*) lies posterior to the esophagus. A segment of the left arch (*LAo*) is also opacified. Note that the descending aorta (*DAo*) crosses the midline to descend on the left in the anteroposterior view.

proximal to the coarctation, the coarctation itself, and the poststenotic dilatation beyond the coarctation (Fig. 20-16).

Cardiac catheterization is rarely indicated in coarctation of the aorta but is useful in excluding associated anomalies. Aortography best demonstrates the area of coarctation. The arterial pressure pulse proximal to the coarctation will have a rapid upstroke, an elevation of systolic pressure, and an increased pulse pressure. Distal to the coarctation, the upstroke time is delayed, the systolic pressure is lower, and the pulse volume is decreased. The mean pressure distal to the coarctation is usually near normal.

Medical treatment should include the prevention and treatment of bacterial endocarditis. Routine prophylaxis for bacterial endocarditis should be continued postoperatively because of the high incidence of associated bicuspid aortic valve. The optimal time for surgery is between the ages of 8 to 20 years.[112,114] Mild hypertension may remain for a few weeks postoperatively. A syndrome of necrotizing arteritis of the bowel may occur between the third and tenth postoperative days and may lead to bowel necrosis. Symptoms of progressive hypertension and abdominal pain with leuko-

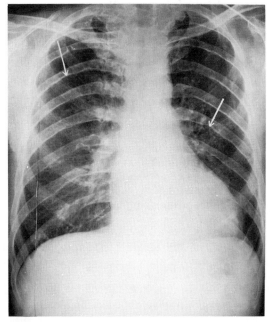

Fig. 20-15. Posteroanterior roentgenogram of a young adult with coarctation of the aorta shows notching along the lower aspects of the ribs (arrow).

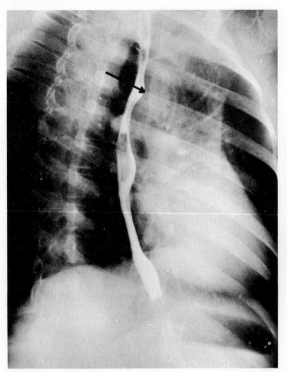

Fig. 20-16. Barium esophagram in a case of coarctation of the aorta. The arrow marks the area of coarctation. Above and below the area of coarctation, the aorta is dilated, producing the "E sign."

cytosis are indications for antihypertensive drug therapy. If necrosis has not developed, symptoms usually subside promptly with treatment.[115]

Symptomatic Coarctation of Infancy. It has been estimated that 55 per cent of the patients with coarctation discovered in childhood will have symptoms in the first year of life, usually between 1 week and 3 months of age.[6,116] Congestive failure with poor weight gain, tachypnea, cough, and feeding difficulties is rapidly progressive. Severe congestive heart failure and death may occur with no associated lesions. However, many of these infants have associated cardiac defects such as patent ductus arteriosus, aortic stenosis, mitral stenosis, ventricular septal defect, transposition of the great vessels, single ventricle, and endocardial fibroelastosis of the left side of the heart.[117,118] The diagnosis of coarctation can be made in over 90 per cent of the cases by proper blood pressure determinations.[6] The liver may be greatly enlarged, and the jugular venous pressure may be elevated. Significant murmurs are uncommon in the absence of other anomalies. The heart is moderately to greatly enlarged, and there is usually a sustained left parasternal impulse. A systolic ejection click and third heart sound are frequently heard at the apex. If a

patent ductus is present, the shunt will be from the aorta to the pulmonary artery unless there is severe pulmonary vascular disease (Eisenmenger's syndrome).

The electrocardiogram usually has a normal mean QRS axis. Right ventricular hypertrophy is present on the precordial leads until the age of 6 months (Fig. 20-17). If right ventricular hypertrophy alone is present after the age of 6 months, associated defects are probably present.[5] Roentgenographic studies show moderate to gross cardiac enlargement with biventricular and left atrial enlargement. Pulmonary blood flow is normal in the absence of associated defects, but pulmonary edema may be very prominent (Fig. 20-18). *Catheterization of the right side of the heart,* useful in excluding associated anomalies, shows a moderate increase in pulmonary arterial and right ventricular pressure and elevation of pulmonary capillary pressure. Retrograde aortography will show the site of coarctation and the collateral vessels (see p. 201).

Medical treatment of congestive failure should be vigorous. In the absence of associated anomalies, these infants usually improve in the first 12 to 24 hr after treatment is instituted. If improvement does not occur, diagnostic studies are indicated and emergency surgery may be necessary.[117] Those infants who respond to medical treatment usually improve over the next few months, although they may be retarded in their growth. They usually become asymptomatic after 2 years of age, and surgery may then be delayed until the optimal age.

Congenital Aortic Stenosis. Congenital obstruction to the outflow of the left ventricle may occur above, below, or at the aortic valve, but in 75 per cent of the cases, the obstruction is valvular.[5]

Clinical Picture. Valvular aortic stenosis is four times as common in males as in females. A heart

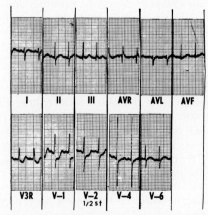

Fig. 20-17. Electrocardiogram obtained from a 1-month-old infant with symptomatic coarctation of the aorta shows a normal mean QRS axis with right ventricular hypertrophy.

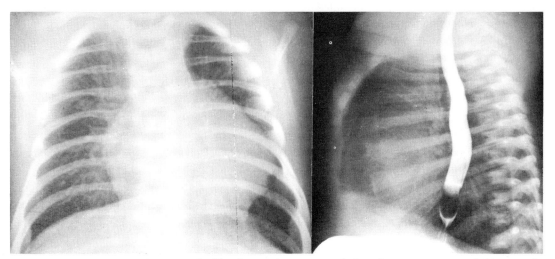

Fig. 20-18. Roentgenograms of a 1-month-old infant with congestive failure due to coarctation of the aorta show moderate cardiomegaly and pulmonary edema.

murmur is usually present at birth, but symptoms do not appear before adolescence unless the obstruction is severe. Exertional dyspnea and angina usually signify moderately severe stenosis, and exertional syncope often indicates severe obstruction.[119] Sudden death may occur at any age but is preceded by symptoms or electrocardiographic changes in most instances.[5] Growth and development are normal, and there is no cyanosis. The pulse volume may be decreased, and the pulse is anacrotic. Total heart size is not increased but the apical impulse is sustained. In over 80 per cent of the cases, a systolic thrill is palpable in the second right intercostal space and over the carotids.[120] The absence of a left ventricular sustained impulse and a systolic thrill usually indicates that the obstruction is mild.[119] A systolic ejection sound is frequently heard at the apex, and if the stenosis is severe, there may be paradoxical splitting of the second heart sound.[93] A third heart sound is audible at the apex in many cases. An early, high-pitched, blowing diastolic murmur of aortic insufficiency is heard in 10 to 20 per cent of the cases.[119,121] The classic finding on auscultation is a grade III to VI harsh, ejection systolic murmur in the second right intercostal space, radiating into the neck, down the left sternal border, and towards the apex. If the peak intensity of the murmur is in the latter part of systole or if a left atrial fourth heart sound is heard at the apex after adolescence, the degree of stenosis is likely to be severe.[119,122]

The electrocardiogram may be normal or may have evidence of left ventricular hypertrophy with T-wave and S-T segment changes.[123] The magnitude of the maximum QRS vectors correlates well with the degree of left ventricular hyperten-

sion.[124,124a] On roentgenographic examination, the total heart size is usually normal but the left ventricle may be prominent. There is poststenotic dilatation of the ascending aorta (Fig. 20-19), and calcification of the aortic valve may occur after adolescence. Cardiac catheterization is indicated if symptoms appear or if there are changes in the S-T segment or T waves of the electrocardiogram.[123] Catheterization of the right side of the heart is indicated, primarily to exclude associated lesions. The combination of aortic and pulmonic stenosis is

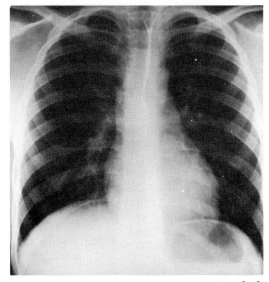

Fig. 20-19. Posteroanterior roentgenogram in valvular aortic stenosis in an adolescent boy shows a prominent ascending aorta and aortic knob. The total heart size and pulmonary blood flow are normal.

common enough that it should be excluded prior to surgery.[125] Catheterization of the left side of the heart will demonstrate a systolic gradient between the left ventricle and the aorta. Selective left ventricular angiocardiography demonstrates the site of obstruction and shows the poststenotic dilatation of the aorta (see p. 202). Medical treatment of aortic stenosis should include the prophylaxis for bacterial endocarditis, and it should be continued after surgery since the valve remains deformed. At the present time, surgery is recommended for those individuals who have a calculated valve area of 0.5 cm² or less.[121]

A *discrete fibrous subvalvular ring*, located approximately 5 mm below the aortic leaflets, is the second most common type of left ventricular outflow obstruction. Symptoms, physical signs, and electrocardiographic signs are usually more pronounced and occur at an earlier age than in isolated valvular stenosis. A systolic ejection sound is only rarely heard, and a diastolic murmur of aortic insufficiency is found in 55 to 100 per cent of the patients.[119,121] Poststenotic dilatation of the ascending aorta usually is not present. Pressure recordings from the left ventricle to the aorta may show a drop in systolic pressure, with a continuation of the low diastolic pressure of the left ventricle before the valve is crossed. Left ventricular angiocardiography may demonstrate the discrete sub-

valvular ring. Medical treatment is the same as for valvular aortic stenosis.

Idiopathic hypertrophic muscular subaortic stenosis usually does not cause a murmur until adolescence. The disease may be familial and appears to occur equally in males and females.[126–128] Angina, exertional dyspnea, palpitations, and syncope are frequent. The apical impulse is bifid, and a systolic thrill may be palpable at the apex.[129] The peripheral pulses are brisk, with a percussion and tidal wave.[130] The murmur is loudest at the lower left sternal border and apex and rarely transmits to the neck. Although the murmur is ejection, it is frequently mistaken for the murmur of ventricular septal defect or mitral insufficiency. A middiastolic rumble is frequently heard at the apex, but the murmur of aortic insufficiency has been reported only twice.[128] Sympathomimetic drugs with a positive inotropic effect and digitalis increase the degree of obstruction.[131,132] Unlike that in other forms of aortic stenosis, the arterial systolic pressure, following a premature ventricular contraction, is usually less than the preceding pressure.[133] The electrocardiogram may show prominent q waves in lead I, II, III, AVL, AVF, V_5 and V_6 in association with tall R waves in AVR, V, and V_2.[133a] Ventricular extrasystoles are more common in this form of aortic stenosis, and the heart is usually larger on physical and roentgenographic examination. Post-

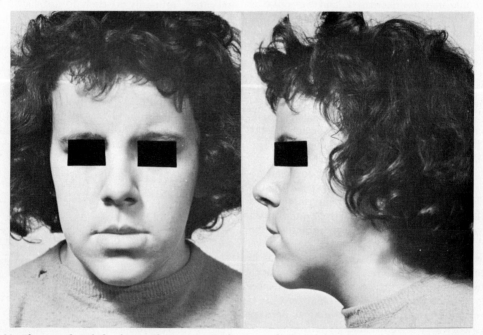

Fig. 20-20. Photographs of the facies of a patient with supravalvular aortic stenosis show a long upper lip, full cheeks with prominent chin, up-turned nose, and full, pouting lower lip. Strabismus, seen in some cases, was not present in this patient.

stenotic dilatation of the aorta and a systolic ejection sound are uncommon. At catheterization of the left side of the heart, a notch is noted on the upstroke of the left ventricular pressure pulse, and pullback pressure recordings may suggest an infundibular type of stenosis.[129] No specific medical treatment is presently available for this condition. Certain drugs, such as digitalis, nitroglycerin, or isoproterenol, may precipitate or accentuate symptoms.[129a] If vasopressor drugs are indicated, those without a positive inotropic effect should be used. Drugs which have a negative inotropic effect on the myocardium or beta adrenergic blocking drugs may prove to be of value in medical management of these patients.

Supravalvular aortic stenosis, another uncommon form of obstruction to the left ventricular outflow tract, has been noted to be familial in approximately one-third of the cases. An unusual facies, characterized by strabismus, fullness of the lower lip and cheeks, and prominence of the chin and nose, has been described (Fig. 20-20).[134,135] Mental and physical retardation are common in this group. A difference of 20 mm Hg, or more, in the systolic pressure of the arms has been recorded in approximately one-half the patients.[134–138] The systolic ejection murmur is maximal in the suprasternal notch or over the right side of the neck. A systolic ejection sound is not heard,[139] but a murmur of aortic insufficiency has been noted in approximately a quarter of the cases. Since the free edges of the aortic leaflets may be attached to the area of constriction and cause obstruction to coronary blood flow, angina is common and the electrocardiogram may show severe S-T segment and T-wave changes. Roentgenograms usually show moderate cardiac enlargement, no poststenotic dilatation of the ascending aorta, and a small aortic knob (Fig. 20-21). Left ventricular angiocardiography will demonstrate the site of obstruction and may show asymmetric filling of dilated coronary arteries and narrowing of the vessels arising from the aortic arch (see p. 202). Pulmonary stenosis, especially peripheral coarctation, is commonly associated with supravalvular aortic stenosis.[140] The documented report of the association of idiopathic hypercalcemia of infancy with the syndrome of supravalvular aortic stenosis and unusual facies suggest that excessive vitamin D or a defect in vitamin D metabolism may be the etiologic basis of the entire syndrome.[140a] Surgical treatment has been recommended for this condition, but the frequent association of anomalies of the aortic valve leaflets makes the postoperative prognosis uncertain.[140b]

Symptomatic Valvular Aortic Stenosis in Infancy. Although the majority of cases of congenital aortic stenosis are asymptomatic in the first decade, oc-

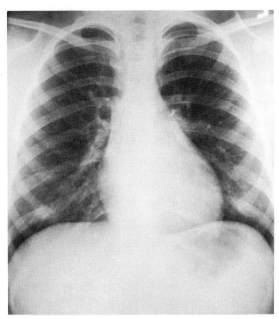

Fig. 20-21. Posteroanterior roentgenogram of the same patient seen in Fig. 20-20 (supravalvular aortic stenosis) shows slight cardiomegaly with no poststenotic dilatation of the aorta. The aortic knob is not visible.

casionally severe congestive failure develops in the first few months of life. There may be marked cardiomegaly, tachypnea, lower costal retraction, cyanosis, and pulmonary edema. The ejection systolic murmur often is heard best at the apex or along the lower left sternal border, and it may be unaccompanied by a thrill.[6,141] Secondary endocardial fibroelastosis of the left ventricle is common. The electrocardiogram frequently shows signs of severe left ventricular hypertrophy with S-T segment and T-wave changes.[5] The diagnosis is confirmed by catheterization of the left side of the heart and selective left ventricular angiocardiography. Surgery in the symptomatic infant is imperative. Because the annulus is frequently small and endocardial fibroelastosis is common, the ultimate prognosis is guarded.

Bicuspid Aortic Valve. A bicuspid aortic valve may occur in completely asymptomatic persons but is often associated with coarctation of the aorta and valvular aortic stenosis.[108] This anomaly should be suspected if bacterial endocarditis occurs in a patient who has no known heart disease. Bicuspid aortic valve may be the underlying and predisposing cause of calcific aortic stenosis or aortic insufficiency in adults.[108,142]

Aortic Atresia. Aortic atresia, or severe aortic stenosis with hypoplasia of the ascending aorta and left ventricle, is an uncommon anomaly. It occurs more often in males than in females and usually re-

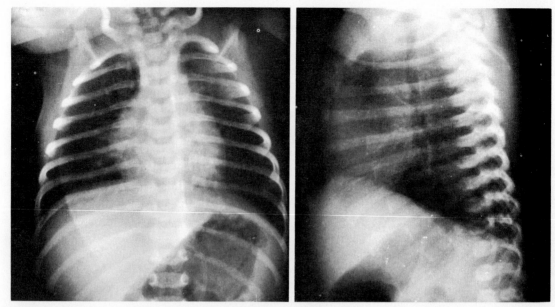

Fig. 20-22. Posteroanterior (left) and lateral (right) roentgenograms of a 2-day-old infant with aortic atresia with hypoplasia of the left side of the heart and ascending aorta show only slight cardiomegaly and pulmonary plethora. The infant had clinical evidence of congestive failure, and there was marked right ventricular hypertrophy on the electrocardiogram.

sults in death in the first week of life. Infants with this complex anomaly may be thought to be normal at birth, but they develop severe congestive failure with cyanosis during the first 24 to 48 hr of life.[143,144] The peripheral pulses are difficult to palpate, especially in the right arm. If the foramen ovale is closed and there is a small opening in the mitral and aortic valve, a color differential, with pinkness of the right upper quadrant and cyanosis of the remainder of the body, may be noted.[145] The heart is moderately to grossly enlarged, and there is a forceful sternal and left parasternal lift. The second heart sound is loud and single, and murmurs are usually absent.

The electrocardiogram shows tall, spiked P waves, marked right ventricular hypertrophy, and S-T segment changes. Roentgenograms usually show cardiac enlargement with pulmonary plethora, but on rare occasions the heart is not greatly enlarged (Fig. 20-22).[21] Retrograde aortography will demonstrate the hypoplasia of the aorta (see Chap. 9, p. 200, Fig. 9-10). Treatment is directed toward control of congestive failure, but the prognosis is invariably poor and no patients have lived past 4 months of age.[143]

Mitral Atresia. Mitral atresia is a rare congenital anomaly in which there are complete closure of the mitral valve, an opening between the atria, hypoplasia of the left ventricle, and a ventricular septal defect. The aorta frequently overrides both ventricles.[143,146] Generalized cyanosis and congestive fail-

ure frequently develop in the first 2 weeks of life. The peripheral pulses are weak. The heart is greatly enlarged, and there is a prominent sternal and left parasternal impulse. A loud systolic murmur is usually audible along the left sternal border, and the second heart sound is split, with an accentuated second component.

The electrocardiogram shows tall, notched, and broad P waves and marked right ventricular hypertrophy (Fig. 20-23). Radiologic examination shows cardiomegaly, primarily due to enlargement of the right ventricle and both atria, pulmonary plethora, and edema (Fig. 20-24). Medical management should include the treatment of intercurrent infections and congestive failure. Response is poor, most infants dying in the first few months of life.

Atresia of the Aortic Arch. Interruption of the aortic arch most commonly occurs between the left common carotid and the site of insertion of the ductus.[147] Arterial unsaturation is present in the lower trunk and extremities, but differential cyanosis is rarely noted clinically.[143] There may be a systolic murmur along the left sternal border. Congestive failure occurs early, and average life expectancy is less than 1 month.[147] Diagnosis can be made by venous angiocardiography or retrograde aortography.

Congenital Mitral Stenosis. Congenital mitral stenosis is another rare anomaly, frequently involving underdevelopment of the left ventricle and endocardial fibroelastosis of the left atrium.[148] In-

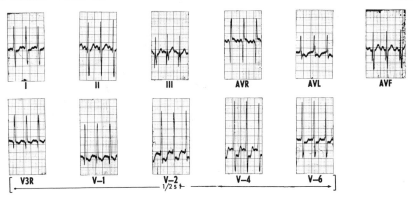

Fig. 20-23. Electrocardiogram of a 2-month-old infant with congenital mitral atresia shows prominent, notched P waves and marked right ventricular hypertrophy.

tracardiac and extracardiac anomalies are frequent.[149] The most common associated anomalies are coarctation of the aorta and defects in the atrial and ventricular septums. Patients with isolated mitral stenosis may present in early infancy or childhood with poor growth and development, paroxysmal edema, syncope, recurrent respiratory tract infections, and congestive heart failure. A heart murmur is frequently present from birth, and the heart may be slightly to moderately enlarged, with a prominent left parasternal impulse. A diastolic thrill is found at the apex, and a diastolic murmur with presystolic accentuation and an opening snap may be present.[150] The first heart sound at the apex is loud; the second heart sound is physiologically split, with accentuation of the pulmonary component. A systolic ejection murmur of grade II intensity is commonly heard along the left sternal border.

The electrocardiogram shows tall, bifid, and broad P waves and right ventricular hypertrophy. The roentgenogram shows slight to moderate cardiomegaly with left atrial and right ventricular enlargement. The pulmonary veins are engorged, and pulmonary edema may be present (Fig. 20-25). The findings at cardiac catheterization are essentially the same as those found in acquired mitral stenosis. Left atrial angiocardiography demonstrates delayed emptying of the left atrium, shows the stenotic valve, and outlines the left ventricular chamber (Fig. 20-26). Treatment for congestive failure may be indicated. It is probably wise to consider

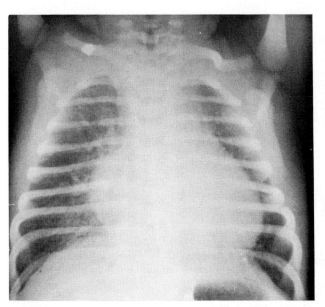
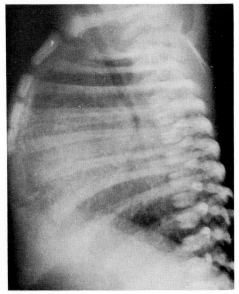

Fig. 20-24. Posteroanterior (left) and lateral (right) roentgenograms of a 10-day-old infant with congenital mitral atresia shows marked cardiomegaly involving the right ventricle, right atrium, and left atrium. Severe pulmonary edema is also present.

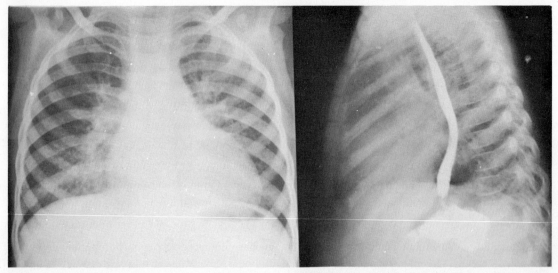

Fig. 20-25. Posteroanterior roentgenogram (left) of a 3-year-old boy with congenital mitral stenosis shows cardiomegaly and pulmonary edema. The lateral (right) roentgenogram shows left atrial and right ventricular enlargement.

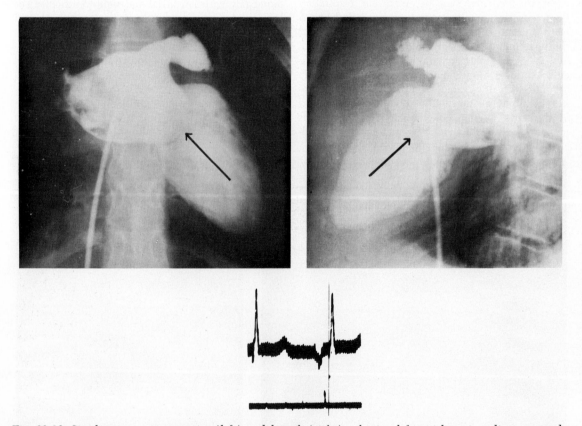

Fig. 20-26. Simultaneous anteroposterior (left) and lateral (right) selective left atrial angiocardiograms made during atrial systole (timer mark below) show that the mitral valve (arrows) does not open normally. The left atrium is large, and the contrast material remained in the atrium longer than usual after a pressure injection. Diagnosis is congenital mitral stenosis (same case as in Fig. 20-25).

surgery before severe vascular disease develops. Since the valve is grossly abnormal, the surgical results are not curative and the mortality is high.[151] Prophylaxis should be given to avoid bacterial endocarditis. The differential diagnosis in congenital mitral stenosis should include the acquired and congenital forms of left atrial blockade.

Cor Triatriatum. Cor triatriatum is a congenital lesion in which the pulmonary veins enter a third atrial-like chamber from which a small outlet communicates with the normal left atrium. There is obstruction to pulmonary venous return, and the findings are similar to those of congenital mitral stenosis except that a presystolic apical murmur and opening snap are not heard. Without surgical treatment, 75 per cent of the patients will die before 1 year of age.[6] However, survival beyond the fourth decade may occur.[152] The diagnosis should be suspected if pulmonary capillary pressure is higher than left atrial pressure at cardiac catheterization. Selective pulmonary arterial angiocardiography may demonstrate the triatrial chamber. The differential diagnosis should include the acquired and congenital forms of left atrial blockade. Medical management includes the treatment of intercurrent infection, congestive failure, and bacterial endocarditis. If symptoms appear, surgical removal of the obstructing diaphragm is indicated.[153]

Endocardial Fibroelastosis. *Secondary endocardial fibroelastosis* may occur in association with other forms of congenital heart disease. The most frequent causes of secondary endocardial fibroelastosis of the left ventricle are severe aortic stenosis, aortic atresia, and coarctation of the aorta.[154] Secondary endocardial fibroelastosis may occur on the right side of the heart with severe pulmonary stenosis or pulmonary atresia. *Primary endocardial fibroelastosis* is one of the more frequent causes of congestive heart failure in infants.[19] The cause is not known, but the condition has been shown to follow acute viral myocarditis, glycogen storage disease of the heart, anomalous origin of a coronary artery, and other types of endomyocardial injury. Symptoms are related to heart failure.

Clinical Picture. Primary endocardial fibroelastosis is about equally common in males and females and has been reported rarely in siblings.[154] Growth and development are usually normal until the onset of congestive failure. Cough, tachypnea, poor feeding, and low-grade fever are early symptoms and are often misinterpreted as indicating respiratory tract infection. Cyanosis, if present, is due to congestive failure. Symptoms usually appear before 6 months of age, and few infants survive past 1 year of age. [21,154,155] Death is usually due to congestive heart failure, with or without associated respiratory infection. There may be sudden death from embolization of mural thrombi or arrhythmias. Sudden episodes of crying, probably due to angina-like pain, may occur.[154,156] Tachypnea, retraction of the chest wall, expiratory wheezes, and left lower lobe atelectasis are frequent. The jugular venous pressure may be elevated and the liver enlarged. There are usually no murmurs, or there may be a soft systolic murmur along the left sternal border. However, if the mitral and aortic valves are involved, there may be murmurs of aortic stenosis, mitral stenosis, or mitral insufficiency. A third heart sound, pulsus alternans, and an accentuation of the normal respiratory effect on the pulse may be present.

The electrocardiogram shows left ventricular hypertrophy with T-wave changes over the left precordium. The mean QRS axis is usually normal.[157] The P waves may be prominent, broad, and notched. Low-voltage and conduction disturbances are rare, which helps to exclude acute idiopathic myocarditis.[5] Rarely, there is contraction of the left ventricle with resulting right ventricular hypertrophy.[156] Radiologically, there are gross cardiomegaly, predominantly involving the left ventricle and left atrium, normal pulmonary blood flow, and pulmonary edema (Fig. 20-27). The heart may appear relatively quiet at fluoroscopy. Atelectasis of the left lower lobe is frequently present, because of obstruction of the bronchus by the enlarged heart. Cardiac catheterization is rarely indicated in endocardial fibroelastosis since the clinical picture is

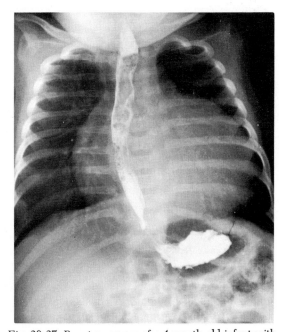

Fig. 20-27. Roentgenogram of a 4-month-old infant with primary endocardial fibroelastosis shows marked cardiomegaly and normal pulmonary blood flow.

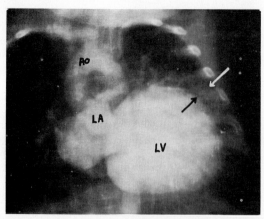

Fig. 20-28. Venous angiocardiogram of the same case as in Fig. 20-27 (endocardial fibroelastosis) shows contrast material in the left atrium (*LA*), left ventricle (*LV*), and aorta (*Ao*). The left ventricular cavity is dilated, and the left ventricular wall is moderately thick (between arrows).

characteristic. If congestive failure is present, the pulmonary "capillary" and arterial as well as right ventricular pressures, may be elevated.[158] Angiocardiography shows little change in heart size with cardiac contraction and prolonged retention of contrast medium.[159] The muscle mass of the left ventricle appears moderately thick, and the cavity is dilated (Fig. 20-28).

The differential diagnosis should include those conditions causing congestive failure without cyanosis or murmurs. Coarctation of the aorta can be excluded by physical examination, since a difference in blood pressure in the upper and lower extremities will be noted in all except the moribund patient. Rarely, infants with severe aortic stenosis and congestive failure have no murmur,[141] and catheterization of the left side of the heart may be necessary to exclude this condition. Pericarditis with effusion and other forms of endomyocardial disease of infancy must be excluded.

Treatment. The treatment for primary endocardial fibroelastosis is supportive. Respiratory tract infections should be treated with proper antibiotic therapy. Vigorous treatment of congestive failure is recommended, and early response is frequently very gratifying. An occasional patient with this clinical syndrome may recover.[5] In general, however, there are recurrent bouts of congestive heart failure, and few infants with this disease survive past 1 year of age.

Eisenmenger's Syndrome. When in the presence of a large communication between the two circulations, the pulmonary resistance is equal to or greater than the systemic, the clinical picture is more or less similar regardless of the shunt site.[28,79,160] This condition is known as Eisenmenger's syndrome.

Clinical Picture. The syndrome developes most frequently in those conditions in which increased pulmonary flow is associated with elevated pressure.[161] As secondary changes in the pulmonary vascular bed lead to increasing pulmonary resistance, the shunt becomes bidirectional or reversed.[161,162] This is estimated to occur in 8 to 10 per cent of the cases of congenital heart disease.[5,8] Symptoms may be slight until after adolescence, and effort dyspnea seems to be due to arterial unsaturation.[160] Angina and syncope with exertion occur in 10 per cent of adults. Mild cyanosis, clubbing, and polycythemia are present; if the central shunt is a patent ductus, the cyanosis and clubbing are differential, involving the lower trunk and legs only. Hemoptysis occurs in one-third of those over 20 years of age and was the cause of death in one-fourth of Wood's series.[28,160] Anesthesia, thoracotomy, and angiocardiography are poorly tolerated. Sudden death, probably due to arrhythmia, or right-sided heart failure with a rapid downhill course, is frequent after the third decade, and few patients survive the fourth decade. The jugular venous pulse and liver are usually normal. The total heart size is normal. The left ventricular impulse is impalpable, but a tapping impulse of right ventricular hypertrophy is felt at the left parasternum. If pulmonary insufficiency is present, the left parasternal impulse may be hyperdynamic. A systolic pulsation of the pulmonary artery, followed by a palpable impulse of valve closure, can be felt in the second left intercostal space. On auscultation, there is a pulmonary systolic ejection sound, a pulmonary ejection systolic murmur of soft to moderate intensity, a loud pulmonary valve closure sound, and a high-frequency diastolic murmur of pulmonic insufficiency. The second heart sound is split and fixed if the central shunt is an atrial septal defect, is split and varies physiologically if the shunt is a patent ductus, and is closely or inaudibly split and fixed if the shunt is a ventricular or aortopulmonary septal defect.[160] A right ventricular third heart sound and right atrial fourth heart sound may be present.

The electrocardiogram shows right ventricular hypertrophy (Fig. 20-29). The roentgenogram shows dilated hilar vessels, clear peripheral lung fields, and marked enlargement of the main pulmonary artery (Fig. 20-30). Right ventricular enlargement is present. Catheterization of the right side of the heart will show a marked increase in pulmonary vascular resistance. Right-sided heart pressures are essentially the same as systemic if the shunt is at the ventricular or pulmonary arterial level, but may be lower than systemic with an

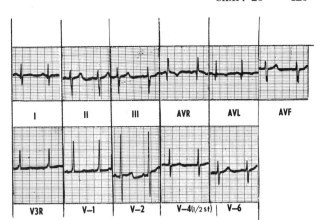

Fig. 20-29. Electrocardiogram of a cyanotic adolescent with a large ventricular septal defect and severe pulmonary vascular disease showing marked right ventricular hypertrophy.

atrial shunt. The site of the central shunt may be demonstrated by dye dilution or angiocardiography. Systemic arterial saturation will be decreased distal to the shunt. No specific medical treatment is available for Eisenmenger's syndrome. Heart failure, complications of right-to-left shunt, and bacterial endocarditis are treated in the usual manner. Surgical intervention is usually lethal.

Pulmonary Stenosis with Intact Ventricular Septum. Obstruction to the outflow of the right ventricle may occur at the pulmonary valve, the infundibulum of the right ventricle, or in the pulmonary arteries. Unlike tetralogy of Fallot, there is no ventricular septal defect, and the aortic arch is normal.

Clinical Picture. Valvular pulmonic stenosis, four times as common as the other forms of right ventricular obstruction, may be familial.[163,164] At least a quarter of the patients are asymptomatic although a murmur is present from birth. If the obstruction is severe, dyspnea on exertion, right-sided heart failure, syncope, and sudden death may occur.[165,166] Squatting is rare, but cyanosis may be present if there is an opening in the atrial septum. Growth and development are normal in the absence of congestive heart failure. Hypertelorism

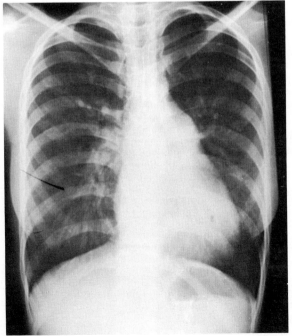
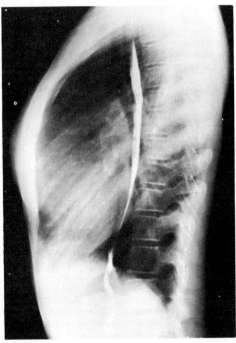

Fig. 20-30. Roentgenograms of same patient as in Fig. 20-29 (ventricular septal defect with pulmonary vascular disease) show an enlarged main pulmonary artery and hilar vessels with clear peripheral lung fields in the postero-anterior view (left). There are right ventricular enlargement and no left atrial enlargement on the lateral view (right).

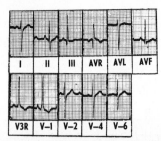

Fig. 20-31. The electrocardiogram of a 2-year-old boy with moderately severe valvular pulmonic stenosis shows prominent P waves and right ventricular hypertrophy.

and a "moon facies" have been noted in patients with severe obstruction.[8] If the obstruction is not severe, the liver is not enlarged but a presystolic pulsation in the jugular veins may be noted. The heart is not enlarged, but a left parasternal sustained impulse is felt. A systolic thrill is palpable in the second left intercostal space and may be felt in the suprasternal notch and over the left side of the neck. On auscultation in the second left intercostal space, a systolic ejection sound, which increases in intensity on expiration,[167] is followed by a grade III to V ejection systolic murmur which may extend beyond aortic closure. The second heart sound may be widely split with decreased intensity of the pulmonic component.[168,169] The obstruction has been shown to be severe if the ejection sound is absent or early in onset and unvarying with respiration, if the systolic murmur has its peak in late systole, and if the second heart sound is fixed and split more than 0.08 sec with a very soft or inaudible pulmonic component.[169a] A giant *a* wave in the venous pulse, a presystolic pulsation of the liver, a right atrial fourth heart sound, and cardiomegaly with a prominent left parasternal impulse are also present in severe stenosis.

In mild pulmonic stenosis, the electrocardiogram may be normal. Right ventricular hypertrophy and tall, spiked P waves are seen with moderately severe pulmonic stenosis (Fig. 20-31). The height of the R in V_1 has fair correlation with the right ventricular systolic pressure.[170,171] Better correlation is found when the R-wave amplitude in V_1 is compared to the calculated right ventricular work.[172] The mean QRS axis is usually anterior and to the right in severe stenosis, and the frontal QRS loop is clockwise.[173] Progression of T-wave inversion from V_1 to V_5 in a short period of time is indicative of critical obstruction.[174] On roentgenologic examination poststenotic dilatation of the main pulmonary artery is usually present after the first few months of life, even in mild obstruction. Cardiomegaly, primarily due to right ventricular and right atrial enlargement, is present in severe obstruction, and the apex is not elevated (Fig. 20-32). Pulmo-

nary blood flow is normal in the absence of a right-to-left atrial shunt; the left pulmonary artery pulsation is greater than that of the right on fluoroscopy. At catheterization of the right side of the heart, an abrupt systolic gradient is present at the pulmonary valve. The ventricular pressure pulse may have symmetrically pointed systolic waves, and right ventricular systole may be prolonged. The pulse form is poor in the pulmonary artery, but the mean pressure is near normal. The *a* wave is prominent in the right atrial pulse, and there may be right-to-left shunting across a patent foramen.[175] If the obstruction is severe, passage of the catheter into the pulmonary artery is technically difficult and may obstruct cardiac output severely.[176] The relatively immobile, cone-shaped pulmonary valve and the systolic jet into the dilated main pulmonary artery may be visualized at right ventricular angiocardiography (Fig. 20-33). In severe valvular pulmonic stenosis, there may be hypertrophy of the crista supraventricularis, with narrowing of the infundibulum. Regression of this infundibular obstruction occurs in the majority of these patients within 18 months after valvulotomy.[177,178] The medical management should include the prevention of bacterial endocarditis. Congestive failure is treated in the usual manner. Surgery is indicated if symptoms or signs of severe obstruction occur or if right ventricular systolic pressure is greater than 60 mm Hg with a normal cardiac output.

Isolated infundibular pulmonary stenosis is found in fewer than 10 per cent of the cases of right ventricular obstruction. Characteristically, the sys-

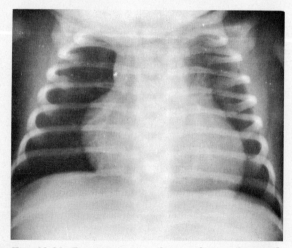

Fig. 20-32. Roentgenogram of a newborn infant with severe valvular pulmonic stenosis and a patent foramen ovalue shows cardiomegaly, decreased pulmonary blood flow, and right atrial enlargement. Poststenotic dilatation of the pulmonary artery is not usually present on chest films until after the age of 1 year.

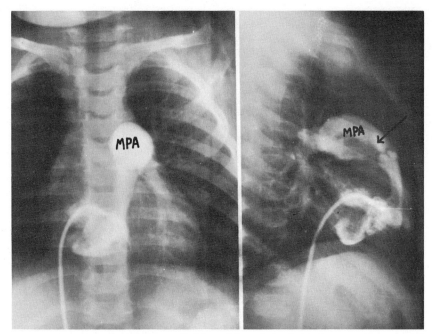

Fig. 20-33. These simultaneous anteroposterior (left) and lateral (right) selective right ventricular angiocardiograms of the same case as in Fig. 20-31 (valvular pulmonic stenosis) are made during ventricular systole and show the dilated main pulmonary artery *MPA*. The jet (arrow) is shown above the cone-shaped pulmonary valve.

tolic thrill and ejection murmur are lower down the left sternal border. No ejection sound is heard, the pulmonic component of the second heart sound is clearly audible, and there is no poststenotic dilatation of the pulmonary artery.[175] At cardiac catheterization the pressure pulse indicates infundibular obstruction and has a sloping plateau with a late systolic peak.[179] Right ventricular angiocardiography will demonstrate the obstruction. Since ventricular septal defects are commonly associated with infundibular obstruction, every attempt should be made to exclude this defect prior to surgery.

Supravalvular pulmonic stenosis and *multiple peripheral coarctations* of the pulmonary arteries are rare anomalies, which may be familial.[180,181] Most of the patients are relatively asymptomatic, but a few of them experience exertional dyspnea, hemoptysis, and transient cyanosis, and some even die early.[5,181] The physical findings are similar to those of valvular pulmonic stenosis with a few exceptions. The systolic ejection murmur is usually heard as well over the lungs as it is over the second left intercostal space, and frequently the murmur is continuous.[182] There is no systolic ejection sound, and the second heart sound is well split, with a normal or loud pulmonary component. The electrocardiographic (Fig. 20-34) and roentgenographic findings are similar to those of valvular stenosis. Occasionally, the hilar vessels appear narrow in contrast to the dilated peripheral pulmonary arteries.[180] At cardiac catheterization a systolic gradient is noted at the site of the coarctation, and the pressure pulse from the main pulmonary artery resembles that of the right ventricle if the obstruction is severe.[183] Right ventricular or pulmonary artery angiocardiography will demonstrate the areas of coarctation and poststenotic dilatation (Fig. 20-35). Medical treatment for coarctations of the pulmonary arteries and isolated infundibular stenosis is the same as for valvular pulmonic stenosis.

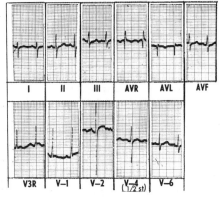

Fig. 20-34. Electrocardiogram of a child with multiple peripheral coarctations of the pulmonary arteries shows right ventricular hypertrophy.

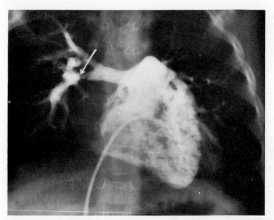

Fig. 20-35. Selective right ventricular angiocardiogram from the same case as in Fig. 20-34 shows an area of peripheral coarctation of a pulmonary artery (arrow) with poststenotic dilatation.

Unilateral or bilateral peripheral pulmonic stenoses may be associated with other cardiac anomalies, such as valvular pulmonic stenosis, tetralogy of Fallot, patent ductus arteriosus, ventricular and atrial septal defects, truncus arteriosus, and tricuspid atresia.[5,97]

Pulmonary Atresia with Intact Ventricular Septum. If the pulmonary valve is completely closed by fusion of its leaflets, the right ventricular chamber is small and thick-walled, and frequently there is endocardial fibroelastosis of the chambers of the right side of the heart.[184] In 20 per cent of the cases the right ventricle is large and there may be tricuspid valve insufficiency. For survival, there must be an opening between the atria and a patent ductus arteriosus or bronchial collateral vessels. Cyanosis and dyspnea on exertion appear soon after birth, and hypoxic attacks may be severe. Progressive hepatic enlargement with presystolic pulsation, a giant a wave in the jugular veins, and moderate to gross cardiac enlargement with a prominent sternal and left parasternal impulse distinguish this condition from tetralogy of Fallot. On auscultation, the second heart sound is single and a right atrial fourth heart sound is heard. Murmurs are usually absent, but on occasion, the murmur of a patent ductus or bronchial collaterals may be present. In cases with tricuspid incompetence, there may be a loud systolic murmur and thrill at the lower left sternal border.[5,6,184] The prognosis is poor; only those infants with a large patent ductus survive the first few weeks of life.

The electrocardiogram, which is the most characteristic part of the clinical features, has a clockwise frontal QRS loop with a mean axis between +30 and +130°.[5,6] Initially, the precordial leads show dominant left ventricular hypertrophy, but,

in contrast to tricuspid atresia, serial tracings in the first few days of life show increasing evidence of right ventricular enlargement (Fig. 20-36).[6] The P waves are tall and spiked. In those cases with a large right ventricle, the electrocardiogram is indistinguishable from that in severe valvular pulmonic stenosis. The roentgenogram is not characteristic but usually shows progressive cardiac enlargement, marked pulmonary ischemia, and a concave pulmonary artery segment. At cardiac catheterization, the findings are similar to those of severe valvular pulmonic stenosis with an open foramen ovale except that the pulmonary artery cannot be entered from the right ventricle. At venous angiocardiography the sequence of contrast through the heart is similar to that in tricuspid atresia. Selective right ventricular injection shows occlusion of the pulmonary artery and may demonstrate sinusoids communicating with the coronary vessels.[184,184a] Medical management is the same as for severe valvular pulmonic stenosis. Surgical opening of the diaphragm occluding the pulmonary artery should be attempted.

Tetralogy of Fallot. Tetralogy of Fallot, which is the combination of pulmonary stenosis with a ventricular septal defect, dextroposition of the aorta, and right ventricular hypertrophy, is physiologically explained as pulmonary stenosis with a right-to-left shunt at the ventricular level. Approximately three-fourths of cyanotic patients over 2 years of age will be found to have this defect.[5]

Clinical Picture. Cyanosis, a prominent feature in tetralogy of Fallot, usually appears between birth and 6 months of age. Dyspnea with exertion, retarded growth and development, clubbing, and polycythemia are common. Squatting, which occurs between 1½ and 10 years of age, is almost pathognomonic of tetralogy. Hypoxic attacks, a major

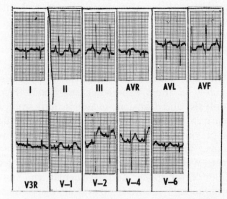

Fig. 20-36. Electrocardiogram of a 2-day-old infant with pulmonary atresia and intact ventricular septum shows tall, spiked P waves and right ventricular hypertrophy. Tracing made the previous day did not show definite evidence of right ventricular hypertrophy.

problem in infants between 2 months and 2 years of age,[86] may be precipitated by infection or exertion, are more common in the summer than in the winter, and occur most often in the mornings. Characteristically, there is irritability or crying, with increasing cyanosis and tachypnea. Attacks may occur as frequently as several times a day, may last from a few minutes to several hours, and may progress to syncope, convulsions, and death. The systemic blood pressure usually remains normal, but arterial oxygen saturation is greatly decreased. The systolic murmur, which may have been quite loud prior to the attack, is decreased during the episode. Since congestive heart failure is not a part of the usual picture of tetralogy of Fallot, the jugular venous pressure, heart and liver size are normal. If congestive failure does occur, a diligent search should be made for complications or associated diseases which, in our experience, are most likely to be anemia, acute glomerulonephritis, systemic hypertension, rheumatic fever, or bacterial endocarditis. The apex may be difficult to palpate, but a faint tapping impulse is felt at the left parasternum. A systolic thrill is present in the third left intercostal space in 50 per cent of the patients.[8] On auscultation along the mid-left sternal border, there is usually a grade III to V ejection systolic murmur which stops before a loud single second heart sound. If severe stenosis is present, the systolic murmur is almost inaudible and the continuous murmur of a patent ductus or dilated bronchial collaterals may

be present. A systolic ejection sound is frequently heard at the left sternal border and apex.[79] The course and prognosis in tetralogy of Fallot vary with the degree of pulmonary stenosis and the complications which may occur secondary to the right-to-left shunt. Prior to the advent of surgery, approximately one-third of these individuals died in infancy. However, there are occasional reports of survival to the sixth or seventh decade.[185]

The mean QRS axis of the electrocardiogram is usually to the right, between +60 and −120°, and there is right ventricular hypertrophy, characterized by a tall R wave in the right precordial leads and a deep S wave in the left precordial leads.[100] The P waves are prominent in 10 per cent of the cases.[8] On the anteroposterior roentgenogram, the total heart size is normal but the right ventricle is moderately enlarged on the lateral projection. The aorta is large and has a right arch in 25 per cent of the cases. The pulmonary blood flow is decreased, the pulmonary segment is concave, and the apex is somewhat elevated, giving the *coeur en sabot* contour (Fig. 20-37). Catheterization of the right side of the heart shows a normal right atrial pressure, a plateau at the peak of the right ventricular pressure pulse, and the same systolic pressure in the right ventricle, left ventricle, and aorta. On rare occasions, the pressure in the right ventricle may be higher than that in the left ventricle and aorta.[186] The pulmonary artery mean pressure is usually near normal. The cardiac catheter may cross the ven-

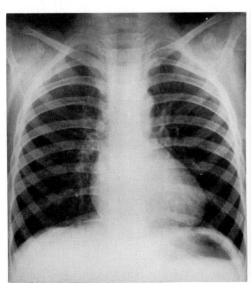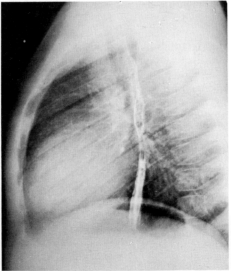

Fig. 20-37. Posteroanterior roentgenogram (left) of a 3-year-old girl with tetralogy of Fallot shows the total heart size within normal limits, a prominent aorta which descends on the left, a concave pulmonary artery segment, and decreased pulmonary blood flow. There is an increased number of small vessels in the lung fields, suggesting increased collateral circulation. The lateral view (right) shows moderate right ventricular enlargement and no left atrial enlargement.

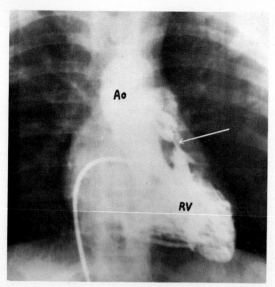

Fig. 20-38. Anteroposterior view of the selective right ventricular (*RV*) angiocardiogram in a child with tetralogy of Fallot shows premature opacification of the large aorta (*Ao*) and infundibular pulmonic stenosis (arrow).

tricular septal defect and enter the ascending aorta more easily than it enters the pulmonary artery. Pressure recordings from the pulmonary artery to the right ventricle usually demonstrate an infundibular chamber. Selective right ventricular angiocardiography is extremely valuable in the evaluation of a patient for surgery. The pulmonary obstruction, ventricular septal defect, and early opacification of the aorta are easily visualized (Fig. 20-38).

The differential diagnosis in tetralogy of Fallot should include those conditions with cyanosis, pulmonary ischemia, and right ventricular hypertrophy. The complete and incomplete forms of transposition with pulmonary stenosis usually show biventricular hypertrophy by electrocardiography, but cardiac catheterization and angiocardiography may be necessary to distinguish these conditions.[187–190] Endocardial cushion defects with pulmonary stenosis will have a mean electrical axis between −90 and ±180° (Fig. 20-39).[67] Severe valvular pulmonic stenosis with intact ventricular septum may be confused with tetralogy of Fallot. In such cases the heart is usually larger and has a more hyperdynamic left parasternal impulse; a presystolic jugular venous pulsation and hepatomegaly are usually present. Persistent truncus arteriosus with obstruction to pulmonary blood flow shows definite biventricular hypertrophy on the electrocardiogram.[191]

Complications of Cyanotic Congenital Heart Disease. Secondary to the polycythemia and often

precipitated by dehydration, spontaneous thrombosis may occur at any location. The most serious type is *central nervous system thrombosis,* which is most apt to occur in the child under 2 years of age who is deeply cyanotic and has a relative iron-deficiency anemia.[192] Evidence of minor occlusive vascular disease has been reported in 10 per cent of patients with congenital heart disease at autopsy.[193] The thrombi may be arterial or venous. Venous thrombosis is usually more insidious in onset, with irritability and anorexia occurring before localizing signs appear. The cerebrospinal fluid may be bloody, and the intracranial pressure may be slightly to moderately increased. Focal signs and seizures may also be present.[194] Treatment of this complication should be directed toward the maintenance of fluid and electrolyte balance. Intravenous hypertonic urea may be indicated if cerebral edema and increased intracranial pressure are present. Anticoagulant therapy is not generally recommended.[194]

It has been estimated that the incidence of *brain abscess* in cyanotic congenital heart disease is 2 to 4 per cent.[195] In cyanotic congenital heart disease, venous blood bypasses the normal filtering action of the lung to enter the systemic circulation so that arterial bacteremia may occur in the absence of bacterial endocarditis. Abscess formation is thought to occur in the central nervous system in areas of previous vascular damage.[193,194,196] There is usually a history of a preceding infection, headache, fever, leukocytosis, and signs of increased intracranial pressure. There may be convulsions and hemiparesis.[194,197] The cerebrospinal fluid may show mild leukocytosis with some elevation of the

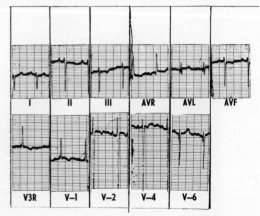

Fig. 20-39. Electrocardiogram of an adolescent who had Down's syndrome with the complete form of endocardial cushion defect and pulmonary stenosis. Although there is right ventricular hypertrophy, note that the mean QRS axis is approximately −150°. This would be an unusual finding in tetralogy of Fallot.

protein level, but organisms are rarely cultured from the spinal fluid. The electroencephalogram is of value in localizing the site of the abscess, but contrast x-ray studies are usually needed. Treatment should include surgical drainage with antibiotic therapy.[194,197]

Multiple pulmonary arterial thrombi may occur in cyanotic heart disease with pulmonary ischemia.[198] The extensiveness of the thrombosis seems to be directly related to the age of the patient.[199] These lesions do not occur if pulmonary blood flow is adequate, and they may subside following surgical procedures that increase pulmonary blood flow.[200]

A relative *anemia* is especially common in the cyanotic infant and may cause an accentuation of symptoms.[201] Patients with severe arterial unsaturation probably function best with a hematocrit in the range of 55 to 70 per cent.[5] If iron deficiency is present, therapy with intramuscular or oral iron is indicated. If the hematocrit is higher than 75 per cent, blood viscosity is increased and phlebotomy may be indicated.[201] Phlebotomy should be undertaken with great caution, since it may precipitate severe hypoxic episodes.

A variety of blood *coagulation defects*, including thrombocytopenia, low fibrinogen and prothrombin, and poor clot retraction, have been noted in association with cyanotic heart disease.[187,202,203] Coagulation studies should be obtained on all cyanotic patients before surgery is considered. Most of these hematologic abnormalities can be temporarily corrected by repeated removal of small amounts of blood.

Hemoptysis may occur secondary to rupture of extensive bronchial collateral vessels, from previous spontaneous thrombi or coagulation defects. Hemoptysis occurs more frequently in persons who have severe pulmonary vascular disease (Eisenmenger's syndrome).

Gout has been found in adults with cyanotic congenital heart disease but is uncommon in children.[204]

The medical treatment in tetralogy of Fallot is directed primarily to the prevention and treatment of complications. The hypoxic episodes of infants should be treated by placing the infant in the knee-chest position. Oxygen therapy may be helpful. Morphine sulfate is almost specific for these episodes and should be given in a dosage of ½ to 1 mg per 5 kg body weight.[86] Early and vigorous treatment should be given for intercurrent infections, and prophylactic antibiotics are recommended for the prevention of bacterial endocarditis.

Associated Anomalies. A secundum atrial septal defect may be associated with tetralogy of Fallot (*pentalogy of Fallot*). In this condition, there is usually a left-to-right or bidirectional shunt at the

atrial level, but cardiac catheterization is necessary to demonstrate the associated defect. On rare occasions, a *unilateral atresia* of one pulmonary artery, usually the left, is present in tetralogy of Fallot. There is often compensatory dilatation of the contralateral pulmonary artery, and a continuous murmur may be audible over the lung with the pulmonary atresia.[205] *Absence of the pulmonary valve* will cause aneurysmal dilatation of the pulmonary artery and a diastolic murmur of pulmonary insufficiency over the precordium.[206] *Anomalies of the aortic arch and coarctations of the peripheral pulmonary arteries* may also occur in tetralogy of Fallot; angiocardiography is necessary to demonstrate these associated defects. Those patients with a right aortic arch frequently have anomalous origin of the brachiocephalic vessels.[102,207] If complete atresia of the pulmonary artery with a right-to-left shunt at the ventricular level (*severe tetralogy of Fallot*) occurs, bronchial collateral vessels or a patent ductus are necessary for survival. Symptoms occur early and are very severe. The systolic ejection murmur is absent; the heart is usually larger and has a more sustained left parasternal impulse. The electrocardiogram is the same as in typical tetralogy of Fallot (Fig. 20-40); however, pulmonary blood flow is greatly decreased and the heart is moderately enlarged (Fig. 20-41).

Tricuspid Atresia. Tricuspid atresia is a complex anomaly of the heart in which there is complete closure of the tricuspid valve, an opening in the atrial septum, underdevelopment of the right ventricle, and a large but usually normally formed mitral valve and left ventricle. In most cases, there are a small ventricular septal defect and hypoplasia of the pulmonary artery, with some degree of infundibular stenosis.

Clinical Picture. Although the degree of cyanosis is directly dependent on the pulmonary blood flow, most infants are cyanotic soon after birth. Clubbing,

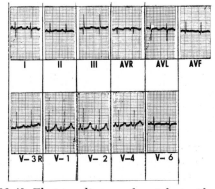

Fig. 20-40. Electrocardiogram of an infant with severe tetralogy of Fallot showing right ventricular hypertrophy.

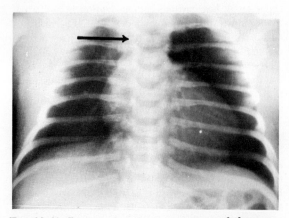

Fig. 20-41. Posteroanterior roentgenogram of the same case as in Fig. 20-40 (tetralogy of Fallot) shows that the heart is moderately enlarged and the pulmonary blood flow is greatly decreased. A right aortic arch (arrow) is present in this case.

polycythemia, and exertional dyspnea occur early, and hypoxic episodes are frequent. Taussig[86] states that squatting occurs in these children with a frequency equal to that seen in tetralogy of Fallot. However, only 1 of the 8 patients in Keith's series[6] who were of walking age squatted. There is a prominent presystolic pulsation in the jugular veins and liver, and the liver may be slightly to moderately enlarged. The heart is not enlarged. The impulse at the left parasternum may be similar to that found in tetralogy of Fallot, but the apical impulse is more easily felt and sustained. The second heart sound is single. Murmurs depend on the associated defects. If the ductus is patent, a soft systolic or continuous murmur may be heard. If the pulmonic stenosis is not too severe, there may be an ejection systolic murmur and thrill along the left sternal border. In approximately 10 per cent of the cases, there is complete atresia of the main pulmonary artery and the blood supply to the lungs is from a patent ductus or bronchial collaterals off the descending aorta. Cyanosis is severe, and murmurs may be absent. The prognosis in these patients is extremely poor; the average life expectancy is 3 months. Approximately one-fourth of the patients with tricuspid atresia have associated transposition of the great vessels, with the aorta arising anteriorly from the underdeveloped right ventricle.[6] A ventricular septal defect is always present, and the pulmonary artery is usually normal or large. Cyanosis is only slight, but congestive failure and progressive cardiomegaly occur very early. There is a loud holosystolic murmur with a thrill at the lower left sternal border, a middiastolic rumble at the apex, and a split second heart sound at the base. The prognosis in all cases of tricuspid atresia is

poor. Approximately one-half the infants will die by 6 months of age, and two-thirds will not survive beyond the first year of life. Only 1 in 10 patients will survive to 10 years of age.[6] Hypoxia is the usual cause of death. Those patients with transposition of the great vessels usually die of congestive failure in the first few months of life.

Precordial leads of the electrocardiogram will show either an absence of the normal right ventricular dominance of infancy or true left ventricular hypertrophy. The mean QRS axis is between +30 and −90°, and the frontal plane QRS loop is counterclockwise (Fig. 20-42).[5] The P waves of the electrocardiogram are large and peaked in over half the cases. The height of the P wave is thought to be inversely related to the size of the interatrial communication.[5] In about one third of the cases the P wave is prolonged, with a bifid contour. In those cases with associated transposition of the great vessels, the electrocardiogram is usually the same (Fig. 20-43), but on rare occasions, the mean QRS axis is within normal range.

On the anteroposterior roentgenogram in tricuspid atresia, the cardiac silhouette is characterized by a straight right-heart border which does not extend beyond the spine or occasionally, the dilated superior vena cava causes a fullness at the base on the right. The total heart size is not greatly enlarged (CT ratio of 60 per cent or less), and progressive enlargement in childhood does not occur. A right aortic arch occurs in 5 per cent of the patients. The lungs are ischemic, the pulmonary artery segment is concave, and the vascular pedicle is narrow. In the lateral view, there may be left atrial enlargement, which is a valuable point of difference from tetralogy of Fallot. Since the right ventricular muscle mass is underdeveloped, the cardiac border may not extend beyond the shadow of the aorta in the left anterior oblique view (Fig.

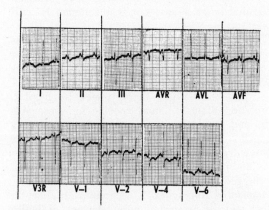

Fig. 20-42. Electrocardiogram of a 3-week-old infant with tricuspid atresia shows a mean QRS axis of −30° and left ventricular hypertrophy.

20-44). In about 10 per cent of the cases of tricuspid atresia, the chest x-ray is indistinguishable from that of tetralogy of Fallot. If transposition of the great vessels is associated with tricuspid atresia, the roentgenogram is the same as that in complete transposition of the great vessels (Fig. 20-45).

At *cardiac catheterization,* the right ventricle cannot be entered directly from the right atrium but the left atrium is easily entered. There is a prominent a wave in the right atrial pressure pulse. If there is no more than 5 mm Hg difference in the mean pressures of the two atria and the phasic patterns are similar, the atrial opening is probably adequate for good mixing.[5,86] There is always a right-to-left shunt at the atrial level, and the oxygen saturations are similar in the left atrium, left ventricle, and great arteries. Systemic arterial saturation is always decreased. On venous angiocardiography, the course of the contrast medium through the heart is invariably from right atrium to left atrium and then to the left ventricle. The left ventricle always opacifies before the right ventricle, and frequently the right ventricle is never seen. A triangular, nonopaque area may be seen on the anteroposterior projection; it has been called the "right ventricular window" (Fig. 20-46).[208] Although the sequence of opacification should make one highly suspicious of tricuspid atresia, it is not diagnostic, since other conditions with hypoplasia of the right ventricle can have the same sequence. Selective left ventricular angiocardiography, with

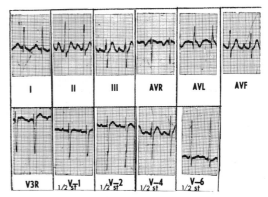

Fig. 20-43. Electrocardiogram of a 3-year-old boy with tricuspid atresia and transposition of the great vessels shows a prolonged P-R interval, large, notched P waves, a mean QRS axis of +30°, and left ventricular hypertrophy.

lateral views, will demonstrate the great vessels and the ventricular septal defect.

The differential diagnosis involves basically the exclusion of other cyanotic conditions with left ventricular hypertrophy. *Pulmonary atresia* with an intact ventricular septum may have hypoplasia of the right ventricle. However, the electrocardiogram has a normal mean QRS axis and the frontal QRS loop is clockwise. In some of the more complex forms of *transposition of the great vessels,* there may be a rudimentary right ventricle. The electro-

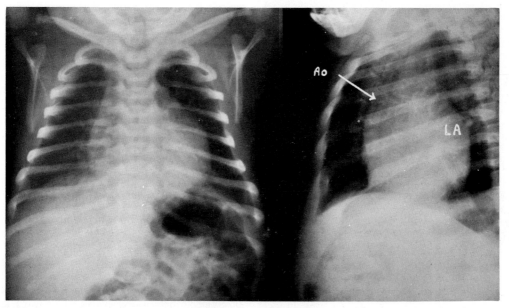

Fig. 20-44. Posteroanterior roentgenogram (left) of an infant with tricuspid atresia shows moderate cardiomegaly and pulmonary ischemia. In the left anterior oblique view (right) the cardiac border does not extend beyond the shadow of the aorta (*Ao*). The left atrium (*LA*) causes posterior displacement of the air-filled esophagus.

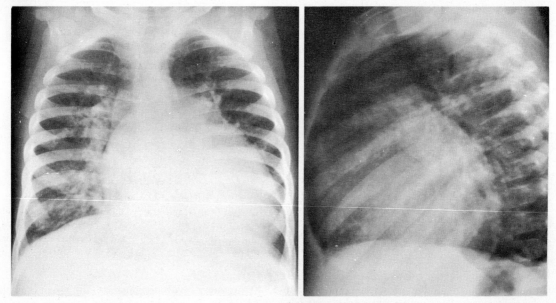

Fig. 20-45. Posteroanterior roentgenogram (left) of the same patient as in Fig. 20-43 (transposition of the great vessels and tricuspid atresia) shows marked cardiomegaly, narrow cardiac base, and pulmonary plethora. The lateral view (right) suggests left atrial enlargement. These findings are the same as in uncomplicated transposition of the great vessels.

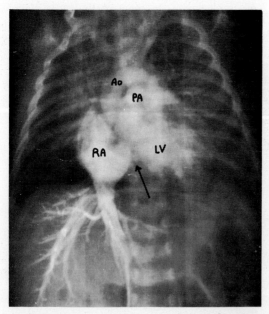

Fig. 20-46. Anteroposterior venous angiocardiogram in a case of tricuspid atresia shows an area of nonopacification (arrow) called the "right ventricular window." In this view contrast material may be seen in right atrium (*RA*), left ventricle (*LV*), aorta (*Ao*), and pulmonary artery (*PA*).

cardiogram may show dominant left ventricular hypertrophy, but the mean QRS axis is usually vertical (Fig. 20-47). It may be impossible to tell these complex variations of transposition of the great vessels from transposition of the great vessels with associated tricuspid atresia except by special studies. *Persistent truncus* may have mild cyanosis, and in about 5 per cent of the cases the mean QRS axis is to the left. However, biventricular hypertrophy is usually seen on the precordial leads. The pulmonary blood flow is usually increased, and the peripheral pulses may be bounding. Severe tetralogy of Fallot may be indistinguishable by history, physical examination, and chest x-ray from tricuspid atresia. The electrocardiogram, in contrast, shows right ventricular hypertrophy.

Early and vigorous treatment of intercurrent infections is recommended. Medical care of the complications of cyanosis and congestive failure and the prophylaxis of bacterial endocarditis are discussed elsewhere. Early surgical intervention is indicated if hypoxic episodes occur.

Ebstein's Anomaly. In Ebstein's anomaly the anterior leaflet of the tricuspid valve is attached normally to the annulus fibrosus while the septal and posterior leaflets are displaced downward and attached to the ventricular wall near its apex. The upper part of the right ventricle is thin-walled and continuous with the right atrium, and the functional right ventricle is made up of the apical and infundibular portion of the right ventricle. Tricuspid regurgitation and pulmonary stenosis are frequently present. The foramen ovale is usually patent, and there may be a right-to-left shunt at this level. This anomaly has been found on the left in corrected transposition of the great vessels.[209]

Clinical Picture. In about one-half the patients, difficulty is first noted in infancy;[5] however, on occasion, symptoms are very mild even in adult life. There may be exertional fatigue, mild cyanosis, paroxysms of arrhythmia, and right-sided heart failure.[8] A prominent systolic pulsation in the jugular venous pulse and a systolic thrill and murmur of tricuspid insufficiency may be present.[210] The most striking finding on palpation of the precordium is the extremely poor cardiac impulse in the face of marked cardiomegaly. The liver may be enlarged and have a systolic pulsation. On auscultation, there is a diastolic sound along the lower left sternal border which is superficial and has characteristics much like a pericardial rub. The four heart sounds, usually audible over the precordium, are made up of a loud first sound, a widely split second sound with decreased intensity to the pulmonary component, and an atrial sound.[5] The prognosis in Ebstein's anomaly is quite variable.[5,211] However, death may be sudden because of arrhythmias or congestive heart failure.

The electrocardiogram shows giant P waves, a prolonged P-R interval, and complete or incomplete right bundle branch block. Occasionally, there is a short P-R interval with the pattern of Wolff-Parkinson-White syndrome. The voltage of the P wave may be as great as that of the QRS in the right precordial leads. Arrhythmias are common. Roentgenographic studies may show marked cardiomegaly, which is predominantly due to right atrial enlargement. Pulmonary blood flow is decreased if a right-to-left shunt is present and normal if there is no shunt. Cardiac pulsations are feeble at fluoroscopy.

Cardiac catheterization and angiocardiography carry a higher risk than usual, because of the frequency of rhythm disturbances.[8,210] These studies are probably not indicated in cases which can be clearly recognized clinically. However, cardiac catheterization can be carried out when the condition is not clinically obvious provided the higher risk is accepted. At catheterization, a patent foramen is usually found, and occasionally a right-to-left shunt at the atrial level. Prominent systolic pulsations may be present in the right atrial pressure pulse; this may be helpful in differentiating this anomaly from aplasia of the myocardium of the

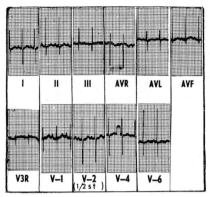

Fig. 20-47. Electrocardiogram of an infant with transposition of the great vessels and both atrioventricular valves emptying into the left ventricle shows a normal mean QRS axis and left ventricular hypertrophy. A ventricular septal defect and rudimentary right ventricle were also present.

right ventricle (Uhl's anomaly), which usually has a prominent presystolic *a* wave and an electrocardiogram which shows a lack of normal right ventricular activity.[212,212a] Right ventricular pressure curves are noted only as the catheter approaches the apex or outflow of the right ventricle.[213] Intracardiac electrocardiograms show a right ventricular type of complex, while the pressure recorded is that of the right atrium.[214-216]

Medical treatment includes the management of right-sided heart failure, rhythm disturbances, and complications of cyanosis, as well as prevention of bacterial endocarditis. Surgical bypass of the right side of the heart, reconstruction of the tricuspid valve or prosthetic replacement, has been recommended in selected cases.[216,217,217a]

THE TRANSPOSITIONS

Transposition of the Arteries

Complete Transposition of the Great Vessels. In complete transposition of the great vessels, the aorta arises anteriorly from the right ventricle and the pulmonary artery arises posteriorly from the left ventricle. Life is possible only if there are openings to allow shunting between the two circulations.

Clinical Picture. Cyanosis is present at birth or in the immediate newborn period in over 80 per cent of the cases.[187] Congestive heart failure does not usually occur until after 2 weeks of age, but this defect is the most frequent cause of congestive failure in the first 2 months of life.[6] It is four times more common in males than in females, and the average weight at birth is greater than 7 lb.[5] If a large ventricular septal defect and near-normal pulmonary resistance are present, the cyanosis is mild to moderate but congestive failure is severe. There are usually a holosystolic murmur along the left sternal border and a middiastolic murmur at the apex. The second heart sound is split and can usually be heard equally well in the right and left second intercostal spaces. The majority of infants die before 6 months of age from severe congestive heart failure, but these patients may survive for a few years if pulmonary vascular obstruction develops. If the only shunts present are a patent foramen and/or a small ductus, cyanosis is the most prominent feature and death from hypoxia usually occurs in the first 3 months of life. Murmurs may be absent, but both components of the second heart sound are usually audible. If a large ventricular septal defect and pulmonary stenosis are found in association with transposition of the great vessels, there may be deep cyanosis but only occasionally are there signs of congestive failure before adolescence. There is usually a loud ejection systolic murmur followed by a single second heart sound along the left sternal border. Clinically, transposition of the great vessels with pulmonary stenosis may be indistinguishable from tetralogy of Fallot, except that squatting is not common and the electrocardiogram shows biventricular hypertrophy. Anoxic episodes, congestive heart failure, and the complications of cyanotic heart disease are frequent findings in transposition of the great vessels. If pulmonary vascular resistance is equal to, or greater than, systemic resistance, there may be flow through a patent ductus from the pulmonary artery to the descending aorta. This reversed shunt presents an unusual clinical picture of cyanosis in the upper trunk and extremities and normal color in the lower trunk and legs.

The electrocardiogram, in cases of transposition

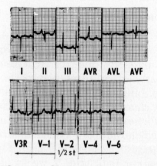

Fig. 20-48. Electrocardiogram of a week-old infant with complete transposition of the great vessels and an intact ventricular septum shows prominent P waves and right ventricular hypertrophy. Frequently the only abnormality noted in the electrocardiogram in the newborn period is the persistence of the upright T wave in the right precordial leads after 48 hr of age.

of the great vessels in which the shunts are small, usually shows a mean QRS axis to the right and right ventricular hypertrophy. In the immediate newborn period the only indication of right ventricular hypertrophy may be positive T waves in the right precordial leads (Fig. 20-48). If a large shunt is present, the electrocardiogram usually shows biventricular hypertrophy and, occasionally, even dominant left ventricular hypertrophy.[218] Rarely, the electrocardiogram is similar to that seen in tricuspid atresia. The radiologic findings in transposition of the great vessels characteristically show progressive cardiac enlargement, pulmonary plethora, a narrow cardiac base, and the "egg-on-side" contour (Fig. 20-2).[219] In those cases with pulmonary stenosis, the x-ray findings may be indistinguishable from those in tetralogy of Fallot.

Cardiac catheterization always shows some arterialization of the blood in the right atrium or right ventricle and a lower oxygen saturation in the aorta than in the pulmonary artery. Angiocardiography demonstrates the aorta arising anteriorly from the right ventricle, with its valve more superior than normal, and the pulmonary artery arising posteriorly from the left ventricle (Fig. 20-49). The remainder of the findings depends on the associated defects.

Medical management of transposition of the great vessels is directed toward the treatment of congestive heart failure and the associated respiratory tract infections, as well as the prevention of bacterial endocarditis and the complications of cyanosis. Survival past 6 months of age is unusual. Those patients who survive past 1 year of age usually have an associated ventricular septal defect with obstruction to pulmonary blood flow. It appears that if surgical treatment is to be of any real value in salvaging these infants, it must be early.

Incomplete Transposition of the Great Vessels. *Transposition of the Aorta with Overriding Pulmonary Artery.* In one variant of this condition, called the *Taussig-Bing syndrome,*[220] the aorta arises from the right ventricle and is slightly posterior to the pulmonary artery, which arises anteriorly from both ventricles. In a second, more common form of incomplete transposition of the great vessels, the aorta arises from the right ventricle anterior to the pulmonary artery, which overrides both ventricles.[221] A ventricular septal defect is present in both variants, and unless there is secondary pulmonary vascular disease, there are a holosystolic murmur along the left sternal border and a middiastolic rumble at the apex. Cyanosis is present at birth.

The electrocardiogram usually shows biventricular hypertrophy but may have dominant right ventricular hypertrophy (Fig. 20-50). The chest x-ray of the Taussig-Bing variant is very similar to that

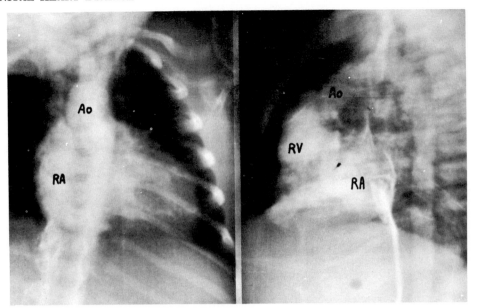

Fig. 20-49. Simultaneous anteroposterior (left) and lateral (right) venous angiocardiogram of the same case as in Fig. 20-2 with complete transposition of the great vessels shows the aorta arising anteriorly from the right ventricle. Contrast material is shown in the right atrium (*RA*), right ventricle (*RV*), and aorta (*Ao*).

seen in a large ventricular septal defect, in that the pulmonary artery is usually visible and somewhat enlarged, pulmonary blood flow is increased, and biventricular and left atrial enlargement are present (Fig. 20-51). In the more common variant, the chest x-ray is similar to that seen in complete transposition of the great arteries. Although an occasional infant survives to childhood, death usually occurs in infancy. The medical management of incomplete forms of transposition of the great vessels is the same as for complete transposition.

Double-outlet Right Ventricle. In this unusual malformation the aorta and pulmonary artery both arise from the right ventricle. The aorta is usually slightly posterior and receives its blood supply from the left ventricle through the ventricular septal defect. These cases may look clinically like a ventricular septal defect, or, if pulmonary stenosis is present, they may resemble tetralogy of Fallot.[189,222-224] The most reliable clinical clue to this diagnosis is that the electrocardiogram is similar to that seen in endocardial cushion defects.[5,188] Selective left ventricular angiocardiography will show that the only outlet from the left ventricle is the ventricular septal defect. Right ventricular angiocardiography with lateral view will show the aorta and pulmonary artery in the same plane and the aortic valve more superior than normal.[224] Medical treatment is the same as for complete transposition.

Corrected Transposition of the Great Vessels. In corrected transposition of the great vessels, the aorta arises anterior to the pulmonary artery. Since there is inversion of the ventricles, the pulmonary artery arises from a functional venous ventricle which anatomically resembles the left ventricle; the aorta arises, anteriorly and somewhat to the left, from a functional arterial ventricle which anatomically resembles the right ventricle. The atrioventricular valves remain with the anatomic ventricular chamber with which they are usually associated. The flow of blood through the heart is normal unless there are associated defects. A variety of congenital defects occurs with this condition. Most commonly, these are deformed atrioventricular valves, rhythm

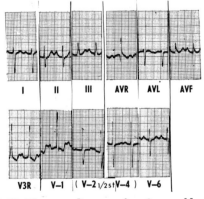

Fig. 20-50. Electrocardiogram of an 8-year-old girl with incomplete transposition of the great vessels, Taussig-Bing syndrome, shows a prolonged P-R interval, prominent P waves, and right ventricular hypertrophy.

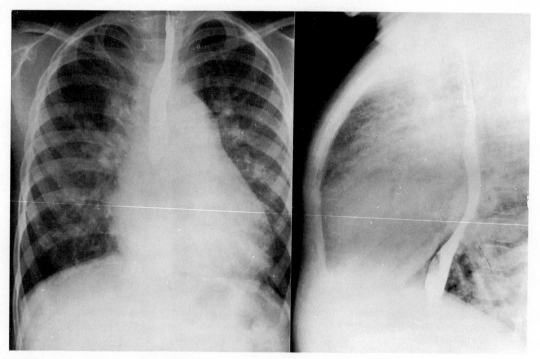

Fig. 20-51. Roentgenograms of a child with Taussig-Bing syndrome (same case as in Fig. 20-50) are similar to those found in a large ventricular septal defect. There are a prominent pulmonary artery, pulmonary plethora, and cardiomegally in the posteroanterior view (left). Left atrial and right ventricular enlargement are shown in the lateral view (right).

disturbances, ventricular septal defect, and pulmonary stenosis.[5,190,225,226] The roentgenologic findings, highly suggestive of the diagnosis, are a full area at the left cardiac base and the absence of a normally placed aortic knob.[190,226,227] At cardiac catheterization it is difficult to direct the catheter into the great vessels.[228] Other findings will depend on the associated defects. Rhythm disturbances are frequently encountered at cardiac catheterization, probably because of the inversion of the conducting system.[229] The electrocardiogram of corrected transposition, with or without associated intracardiac defects, characteristically reveals abnormal initial QRS forces which are directed to the left, superiorly and anteriorly. This is reflected by the presence of a Q wave in V_3R and V, and the absence of a Q wave in V_6.[229a] Angiocardiography will outline the anatomic features of the chambers and their relationship to the great vessels.[226] Medical treatment is indicated only if there are associated anomalies.

Transposition of the Pulmonary Veins

Complete Transposition of the Pulmonary Veins. In total anomalous pulmonary venous return, both the pulmonary and systemic venous blood enter the right atrium. There is always an opening in the

atrial septum, either a patent foramen ovale or a true atrial septal defect.

Clinical Picture. If the pulmonary venous connection is to a vessel within the thoracic cavity or directly to the right atrium, there is usually no anatomic obstruction to the flow of blood into the right atrium.[230,231] On the rare occasions in which these is obstruction, the clinical findings are similar to those in total anomalous pulmonary venous return below the diaphragm.[232,233] Most patients with anomalous pulmonary venous return above the diaphragm have severe tachypnea and congestive heart failure in the first 6 months of life. Cyanosis is present, but minimal, and clubbing is only slight. The jugular venous pressure is elevated and has a prominent presystolic pulsation. There are hepatomegaly and often a presystolic pulsation of the liver. The heart is greatly enlarged, with a prominent left parasternal lift and a poorly defined apical impulse. On auscultation there is usually a grade II to III ejection systolic murmur at the second left intercostal space. At the lower left sternal border and towards the apex, there are four distinct heart sounds. The second sound over the second left intercostal space is usually widely split but varies physiologically with respiration and has accentuation of the pulmonic component. A middiastolic rumble is usually heard at the lower left sternal border. A continuous murmur, which is increased on inspiration, may be audible over the large venous channel.[6] If severe congestive heart failure develops in the first 6 months of life, the prognosis is extremely poor and few infants survive past 1 year of age. Children who develop failure at an older age may be incapacitated with exertional fatigue, dyspnea, and mild cyanosis, but they tolerate their lesion well.[234]

The electrocardiogram shows right ventricular hypertrophy with a qR pattern in the right precordial leads and enlarged P waves (Fig. 20-52). The roentgenograms of the chest show increased pulmonary blood flow with a prominent pulmonary artery, right atrium, and right ventricle. When there is a persistent left superior vena cava, a "snow-man" or "figure-of-eight" contour may be seen after the age of 1 year (Fig. 20-53).[235] When the anomalous venous return is to the coronary sinus, a box-shaped heart may be visualized on the anteroposterior projection (Fig. 20-54).[236] Cardiac catheterization will show an increase in oxygen content of the blood at the site of the anomalous venous connection. The cardiac catheter may enter the anomalous venous trunk. Oxygen saturations are similar in all cardiac chambers and great arteries. The right atrial, right ventricular, and pulmonary artery pressures are usually elevated.[237] Angiocardiography, with injection into the pulmonary artery, may show the anomalous venous connection. If the anomalous trunk can be entered with a cardiac catheter, injection here will outline its course and connection.[238]

Total anomalous pulmonary venous drainage below the diaphragm or *total anomalous pulmonary venous return with obstruction* to the venous channel will cause marked pulmonary edema, hepatomegaly, and severe tachypnea in the neonatal

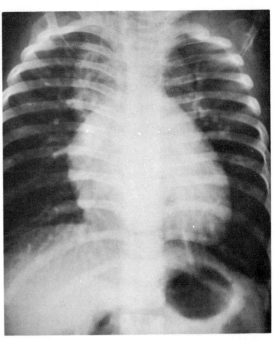

Fig. 20-53. Roentgenogram of a child with total anomalous pulmonary venous return to a persistent left superior vena cava shows fullness above the cardiac shadow, giving the "snow-man" or "figure-of-eight" contour. Cardiomegaly and pulmonary plethora are also shown.

period. Retraction of the chest wall is prominent, and cyanosis is present. The prognosis is very poor, most infants dying of congestive failure in the newborn period. The electrocardiogram shows progressive right ventricular and right atrial hypertrophy.[233] Chest roentgenogram shows severe pulmonary edema with a granular appearance to the lung fields and a total heart size which is near normal.[6,239]

Medical treatment for total anomalous pulmonary venous return is essentially the treatment of congestive failure, respiratory tract infection, and complications of cyanosis. If symptoms are present, surgery is indicated. All infants who develop failure before 1 year of age should be offered surgical treatment, since response to medical therapy is extremely poor.

Partial Anomalous Pulmonary Venous Return. In partial anomalous pulmonary venous return, one or more of the pulmonary veins enters the right side of the heart. The connection may be below the diaphragm or in the thoracic cavity. There may be associated hypogenesis and sequestration of part of the lung from which the anomalous vessel arises.[240,241] Partial anomalous venous return from the right lung is often associated with a sinus venosus defect; the findings in this condition are de-

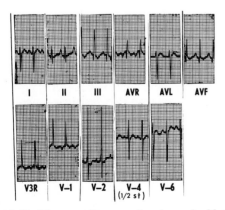

Fig. 20-52. Electrocardiogram of a 4-month-old infant with total anomalous pulmonary venous return to the coronary sinus shows prominent peaked P waves and right ventricular hypertrophy.

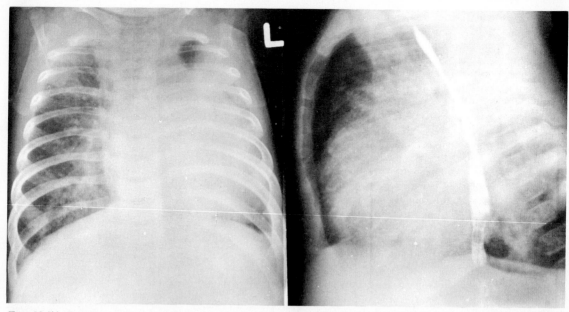

Fig. 20-54. Posteroanterior roentgenogram (left) of an infant (same case as Fig. 20-52) with total anomalous pulmonary venous return to the coronary sinus suggests a box-shaped contour. Pulmonary plethora and cardiomegaly are also shown. In the lateral view (right) the right ventricle is prominent and there is no left atrial enlargement,

scribed with atrial septal defects. If less than 50 per cent of the pulmonary venous blood enters the right atrium and if there are no major intracardiac anomalies, there are no symptoms and the electrocardiogram is within normal limits. On chest x-ray the anomalous veins may cause an abnormal shadow

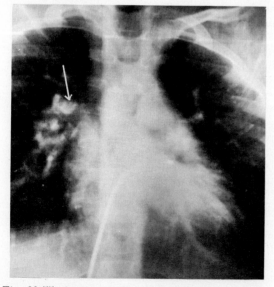

Fig. 20-55. Anteroposterior angiocardiogram of a case with atrial septal defect and partial anomalous pulmonary venous return. The anomalous veins from the right lung are shown (arrow).

in the lungs (Fig. 20-55), and the right atrium may be slightly enlarged.[240] The fact that the cardiac catheter passes into a pulmonary vein from the right side of the heart does not prove that the connection is anomalous, for the catheter may have passed to the left atrium through a patent foramen ovale. An anomalous connection can be proved with dye-dilution studies. The circulation time obtained when dye is injected into the pulmonary artery of the lung having the anomalous venous drainage will be longer than that obtained when the injection is made into the pulmonary artery which has normal venous connections.[242] Usually no medical treatment is indicated for partial anomalous pulmonary venous return.

Transposition of Systemic Veins and Anomalies of the Venae Cavae

Incomplete. As an isolated defect, a persistent left superior vena cava,[243,6,86] a right superior vena cava,[8] or the inferior vena cava[244,5] may drain directly to the left atrium. Although mild central cyanosis is present, symptoms are uncommon. Wood[8] noted that the second heart sound was single and attributed this to slight delay in aortic closure and an early pulmonic closure. If a persistent left superior vena cava is present, there may be fullness at the left upper mediastinal border on the roentgenogram. The electrocardiogram is within normal limits or shows slight left ventricular hypertrophy. Cardiac catheterization and angiocardiography are necessary to establish the diagnosis. No medical treatment is indicated since these patients are asymptomatic, but surgical correction has been accomplished.[243]

Complete. Rarely, all of the systemic venous return is to the left atrium.[86] In this condition there is hypoplasia of the right side of the heart, with severe symptoms and death in the neonatal period. Few physiologic data are available in this condition.

Anomalies. A *persistent left superior vena cava,* draining superiorly into the brachiocephalic vein and inferiorly into the coronary sinus, is a common finding at autopsy; it may cause technical difficulty when cardiac catheterization is attempted from the left arm. The condition is hemodynamically insignificant unless open-heart surgery is anticipated. A persistent left superior vena cava is found most commonly in patients who have intracardiac anomalies.[245,246] It may be suspected on the roentgenogram because of a fullness of the left mediastinum.

A failure of the distal inferior vena cava to fuse normally with the hepatic portion results in an *anomalous inferior vena cava with azygous continuation.* Although it may occur as an isolated and hemodynamically insignificant condition, it is usually associated with severe cyanotic congenital heart disease and is often a part of the dextroversion complexes.[246,247] If the drainage is to the azygous system, there is fullness of the right mediastinal silhouette; if the drainage is to the hemiazygous system, there may be fullness at the left mediastinal area.[246] There may be multiple splenic masses within the abdomen, but there were no instances of absent spleen in the series reported by Anderson.[246] The diagnosis can be made by venous angiocardiography with injection into a leg vein. The outline of the inferior vena cava will show the typical "candy cane" of the anomalous venous pathway.

Transposition of the Heart

There is a great deal of confusion in the classification of dextrocardia and levocardia. For simplification in this text the terms will be defined as follows:

Levocardia. The heart and abdominal viscera are normally placed in the body.

Levoversion. The heart is located in the left hemithorax with its apex to the left, but there is partial or complete heterotaxia of the other viscera.

Dextrocardia. The heart is on the right, a mirror image of the normal, and the abdominal viscera are also mirror images of the normal (situs inversus totalis).

Dextroversion. The heart is in the right hemithorax with its apex to the right, but there is partial or complete heterotaxia of the other viscera.

In dextrocardia (situs inversus totalis), the incidence of congenital heart disease is probably no greater than that seen when the heart and viscera are normally placed (levocardia).[248] The triad of sinusitis, bronchiectasis, and dextrocardia (Kartagener's syndrome) is reported to occur frequently when there is situs inversus totalis. The electrocardiogram in dextrocardia will show inverted P_1, QRS_1, and T_1, upright P_{AVR}, and inverted P_{AVL} Physical and radiologic examinations reveal the mirror-image position of all viscera.

In dextroversion and levoversion, congenital malformations of the heart, especially the cyanotic varieties, are extremely common. The anomalies most frequently found are transpositions of the great arteries and of the systemic and pulmonary veins; incomplete forms of transposition of the arteries, including corrected transposition; single ventricle or atrium; complete endocardial cushion defects; pulmonary stenosis; and tricuspid atresia.[5,6,86,190,227,248-250] Anomalous inferior vena cava with azygous drainage, commonly found in the cardioversions,[246] may make cardiac catheterization from a leg vein confusing and technically difficult. Although tetralogy of Fallot may be suspected clinically, it is extremely uncommon and one should be reluctant to make this diagnosis in a patient with dextroversion or levoversion. It has been suggested that the electrocardiogram will aid in determining inversion of the atria. However, we as well as others have found the electrocardiogram to be inconsistent in this respect.[6,251] Other electrocardiographic findings depend on the associated anomalies. Cardiac catheterization is often difficult to interpret, but the combination of cardiac catheterization and venous and selective angiocardiography may be of great help in defining the lesions and directing surgical therapy. Multiple splenic masses or splenic agenesis may occur. Absence of the spleen should be suspected if there are Howell-Jolly bodies in the peripheral blood.[252,253]

REFERENCES

1. MacMahon, B., McKeown, T., and Record, R. G.: The Incidence and Life Expectation of Children with Congenital Heart Disease, *Brit. Heart J.,* **15:**121–129, 1953.
2. Richards, M. R., et al.: Congenital Malformations of the Cardiovascular System in Series of 6,053 Infants, *Pediatrics,* **15:**12–32, 1955.
3. Mustacchi, P., Sherins, R. S., and Miller, M. J.: Congenital Malformations of the Heart and the Great Vessels, *J.A.M.A.,* **183:**241–244, 1963.
4. Carlgren, L.: The Incidence of Congenital Heart Disease in Children Born in Gothenburg 1941–1950, *Brit. Heart J.,* **21:**40–50, 1959.
5. Nadas, A. S.: "Pediatric Cardiology," 2d ed., W. B. Saunders Company, Philadelphia, 1963.
6. Keith, J. D., Rowe, R. D., and Vlad, P.: "Heart

Disease in Infancy and Childhood," The Macmillan Company, New York, 1958.

7. Abbott, M. E. S.: "Atlas of Congenital Cardiac Disease," The American Heart Association, New York, 1936.

8. Wood, P. H.: "Diseases of the Heart and Circulation," 2d ed., J. B. Lippincott Company, Philadelphia, 1956.

9. McKeown, T., MacMahon, B., and Parson, C. G.: The Familial Incidence of Congenital Malformations of the Heart, *Brit. Heart J.*, **15**:273–277, 1953.

10. Burnard, E. D.: Changes in Heart Size in the Dyspnoeic Newborn Baby, *Brit. M. J.*, **1**:1495–1500, 1959.

10a. Stahlman, M., et al.: Cardiovascular Assessment in Hyaline Membrane Disease, Program and Abstracts, Am. Pediat. Soc., May 6, 7, 8, 1965, p 58.

11. Martin, J. F., and Friedell, H. L.: The Roentgen Findings in Atelectasis of the Newborn: With Special Reference to Changes in the Cardiac Silhouette, *Am. J. Roentgenol.*, **67**:905–923, 1952.

12. Smith, C. H.: "Blood Diseases of Infancy and Childhood," The C. V. Mosby Company, St. Louis, 1960, pp. 141–142.

13. Morgan, C. L., and Nadas, A. S.: Sweating and Congestive Heart Failure, *New England J. Med.*, **268**:580–585, 1963.

14. Joos, H. A., et al.: Arterial Blood Pressure in Infancy and Childhood Measured by Direct and Indirect Methods, *A.M.A. J. Dis. Child.*, **100**:526–527, 1960.

15. Braudo, M., and Rowe, R. D.: Auscultation of the Heart—Early Neonatal Period, *Am. J. Dis. Child.*, **101**:575–586, 1961.

16. Castle, R. F., and Craige, E.: Auscultation of the Heart in Infants and Children, *Pediatrics*, **26**:511–561, 1960.

17. Craige, E., and Harned, H. S., Jr.: Phonocardiographic and Electrocardiographic Studies in Normal Newborn Infants, *Am. Heart J.*, **65**:180–189, 1963.

18. McNamara, D. G.: Prevention of Infant Deaths from Congenital Heart Disease, *Pediat. Clin. North America*, **10**:127–144, 1963.

19. Keith, J. D.: Congestive Heart Failure, *Pediatrics*, **18**:491–500, 1956.

20. Hauck, A. J., and Nadas, A. S.: Cardiac Failure in Infants and Children, *Pediat. Clin. North America*, **5**:1125–1141, 1958.

21. McCue, C. M., and Young, R. B.: Cardiac Failure in Infancy, *J. Pediat.*, **58**:330–341, 1961.

22. Neill, C. A.: Recognition and Treatment of Congestive Failure in Infancy. I. Diagnosis. II. Treatment *Mod. Concepts Cardiovas. Dis.*, **28**:499–512, 1959.

23. Engle, M. A.: Cardiac Failure in Infancy: Recognition and Management, *Mod. Concepts Cardiovas. Dis.*, **32**:825–830, 1963.

24. Hauck, A. J., and Nadas, A. S.: Heart Failure in Infants and Children: A Survey of Recent Literature, Etiologic Considerations and Recommendations for Therapy, *Postgrad. Med.*, **34**:244–250, 1963.

25. Fruthaler, G. J., and Snyder, C. H.: Poisoning in Children, *Pediat. Clin. North America*, **9**:41–66, 1962.

26. Hastreiter, A. R., et al.: Secundum Atrial Septal Defects with Congestive Heart Failure during Infancy and Early Childhood, *Am. Heart J.*, **64**:467–472, 1962.

26a. Nakamura, F. F., Hauck, A. J. and Nadas, A. S.: Atrial Septal Defect in Infants, *Pediatrics*, **34**:101–106, 1964.

27. Besterman, E.: Atrial Septal Defect with Pulmonary Hypertension, *Brit. Heart J.*, **23**:587–598, 1961.

28. Wood, P.: The Eisenmenger Syndrome or Pulmonary Hypertension with Reversed Central Shunt. I and II, *Brit. M. J.*, **2**:701–709, 755–762, 1958.

29. Leatham, A., and Gray, I. R.: Auscultatory and Phonocardiographic Signs of Atrial Septal Defect. *Brit. Heart J.*, **18**:193–208, 1956.

30. Evans, J. R., Rowe, R. D., and Keith, J. D.: The Clinical Diagnosis of Atrial Septal Defect in Children, *Am. J. Med.*, **30**:345–356, 1961.

31. Lopez, J. F., Linn, H., and Shaffer, A. B.: The Apical First Heart Sound as an Aid in Diagnosis of Atrial Septal Defect, *Circulation*, **26**:1296–1301, 1962.

32. Lee, Y., and Scherlis, L.: Atrial Septal Defect: Electrocardiographic, Vectorcardiographic and Catheterization Data, *Circulation*, **25**:1024–1041, 1962.

33. Sodi-Pallares, D., et al.: The Mean Manifest Electrical Axis of the Ventricular Activation Process ($\hat{A}QRS$) in Congenital Heart Disease: A New Approach in Electrocardiographic Diagnosis, *Am. Heart J.*, **55**:681–700, 1958.

34. Dow, J. D.: The Radiological Diagnosis of the Sinus Venosus Type Atrial Septal Defect, *Guy's Hosp. Rep.*, **108**:305–313, 1959.

35. Brock, R., and Ross, D. N.: The Sinus Venosus Type of Atrial Septal Defect; Surgical Treatment, *Guy's Hosp. Rep.*, **108**:291–304, 1959.

36. Gorlin, R., and Gorlin, S. G.: Hydraulic Formula for Calculation of Area of the Stenotic Mitral Valve, Other Cardiac Valves and Central Circulatory Shunts. I, *Am. Heart J.*, **41**:1–29, 1951.

37. Leatham, A., and Segal, B.: Auscultatory and Phonocardiographic Signs of Ventricular Septal Defects with Left-to-right Shunts, *Circulation*, **25**:318–327, 1962.

38. Roger, H.: Recherches cliniques sur la communication congenitale des deux coeurs, part inocclusion du septum interventriculaire, *Bull. Acad. méd. Paris*, **8**:1074, 1879.

39. Wood, P., Magidson, O., and Wilson, P. A. O.: Ventricular Septal Defect, with Note on Acyanotic

Fallot's Tetralogy, *Brit. Heart J.*, **16**:387–406, 1954.

40. Van der Hauwaert, L., and Nadas, A. S.: Auscultatory Findings in Patients with a Small Ventricular Septal Defect, *Circulation*, **23**:886–891, 1961.

41. Vince, D. J., and Keith, J. D.: The Electrocardiogram in Ventricular Septal Defect, *Circulation*, **23**:225–240, 1961.

42. Fyler, D. C. et al.: Ventricular Septal Defect in Infants and Children: A Correlation of Clinical, Physiologic and Autopsy Data, *Circulation*, **18**:833–851, 1958.

43. Katz, L. N., and Wachtel, H.: The Diphasic QRS Type of Electrocardiogram in Congenital Heart Disease, *Am. Heart J.*, **13**:202–206, 1937.

44. Levy, M., and Lillihei, C. W.: Left Ventricular–Right Atrial Canal, *Am. J. Cardiol.*, **10**:623–633, 1962.

45. Braunwald, E., and Morrow, A. G.: Left Ventriculo–Right Atrial Communication, *Am. J. Med.*, **28**:913–920, 1960.

46. Gerbode, F., et al.: Syndrome of Left Ventricular–Right Atrial Shunt, *Ann. Surg.*, **148**:433–446, 1958.

47. Lynch, D. L., et al.: Congenital Ventriculo-atrial Communication with Anomalous Tricuspid Valve, *Am. J. Cardiol.*, **1**:404–409, 1958.

48. Bloomfield, D. K.: The Natural History of Ventricular Septal Defect in Patients Surviving Infancy, *Circulation*, **29**:914–955, 1964.

49. Nadas, A. S., et al.: Spontaneous Functional Closing of Ventricular Septal Defects, *New England J. Med.*, **264**:309–316, 1961.

50. Evans, J. R., Rowe, R. D., and Keith, J. D.: Spontaneous Closure of Ventricular Septal Defects, *Circulation*, **22**:1044–1054, 1960.

51. Engle, M. A.: Ventricular Septal Defect in Infancy, *Pediatrics*, **14**:16–27, 1954.

52. Sirak, H. D., Hosier, D. M., and Clatworthy, H. W., Jr.: Defects of the Interventricular Septum in Infancy, *New England J. Med.*, **260**:147–151, 1959.

53. Arcilla, R. A., et al.: Further Observations on the Natural History of Isolated Ventricular Septal Defects in Infancy and Childhood: Serial Cardiac Catheterization Studies in 75 Patients, *Circulation*, **28**:560–571, 1963.

54. Gasul, B. M., et al.: Ventricular Septal Defects: Their Natural Transformation into Those with Infundibular Stenosis or into the Cyanotic or Noncyanotic Type of Tetralogy of Fallot, *J.A.M.A.*, **164**:847–853, 1956.

55. Stanton, R. E., and Fyler, D. C.: The Natural History of Pulmonary Hypertension in Children with Ventricular Septal Defects Assessed by Serial Right-heart Catheterization, *Pediatrics*, **27**:621–626, 1961.

56. Weidman, W. H., and DuShane, J. W.: Some Observations Concerning Progressive Pulmonary Vascular Obstructive Disease in Children with Ventricular Septal Defect, *Am. J. Dis. Child.*, **102**:778–779, 1961.

57. Kaplan, S., et al.: Natural History of Ventricular Septal Defect, *Am. J. Dis. Child.*, **105**:581–587, 1963.

58. Rowe, R. D., Vlad, P., and Keith, J. D.: Atypical Tetralogy of Fallot: A Non-cyanotic Form with Increased Lung Vascularity. *Circulation*, **12**:230–238, 1955.

59. Rudolph, A. M., Nadas, A. S., and Goodale, W. T.: Intracardiac Left-to-right Shunt with Pulmonic Stenosis, *Am. Heart J.*, **48**:808–816, 1954.

60. Nadas, A. S., Hauck, A. J., and Gross, R. E.: Ventricular Septal Defect with Aortic Regurgitation, *Circulation*, **26**:766, 1963.

61. Scott, R. C., et al.: The Syndrome of Ventricular Septal Defect with Aortic Insufficiency, *Am. J. Cardiol.*, **2**:530–553, 1958.

62. Keck, E. W. O., et al.: Ventricular Septal Defect with Aortic Insufficiency: A Clinical and Hemodynamic Study of 18 Proved Cases, *Circulation*, **27**:203–218, 1963.

63. Wakai, C. S., and Edwards, J. E.: Developmental and Pathologic Considerations in Persistent Common Atrioventricular Canal, *Proc. Staff Meet. Mayo Clin.*, **31**:487–508, 1956.

64. Blount, S. G., Jr., Balchum, O. J., and Gensini, G.: The Persistent Ostium Primum Atrial Septal Defect, *Circulation*, **13**:499–509, 1956.

65. Paul, M. H.: Endocardial Cushion Defects, *Pediat. Clin. North America*, **5**:1011–1028, 1958.

66. Rowe, R. D., and Uchida, I. A.: Cardiac Malformation in Mongolism: A Prospective Study of 184 Mongoloid Children, *Am. J. Med.*, **31**:726–735, 1961.

67. Scott, L. P., Hauck, A. J., and Nadas, A. S.: Endocardial Cushion Defect with Pulmonic Stenosis, *Circulation*, **25**:653–662, 1962.

68. Tascano-Barbosa, E., Brandenburg, R. O., and Burchell, H. B.: Electrocardiographic Studies of Cases with Intracardiac Malformations of Atrioventricular Canal, *Proc. Staff Meet. Mayo Clin.*, **31**:513–523, 1956.

69. Burchell, H. B., DuShane, J. W., and Brandenburg, R. O.: The Electrocardiogram of Patients with Atrioventricular Cushion Defects, *Am. J. Cardiol.*, **6**:575–588, 1960.

70. Harrison, D. C., and Morrow, A. G.: Electrocardiographic Evidence of Left-axis Deviation in Patients with Defects of the Atrial Septum of the Secundum Type, *New England J. Med.*, **269**:743–745, 1963.

71. Baron, M. G., et al: Endocardial Cushion Defects: Specific Diagnosis by Angiocardiography, *Am. J. Cardiol.*, **13**:162–175, 1964.

72. Neufeld, H. N., et al.: Isolated Ventricular Septal Defect of the Persistent Common Atrioventricular Canal Type, *Circulation* **23**:685–696, 1961.

73. Talner, N. S., Stern, A. M., and Sloan, H. E., Jr.:

Congenital Mitral Insufficiency, *Circulation,* **23:** 339–349, 1961.

74. Brockenbrough, E. C., et al.: Partial Persistent Atrioventricular Canal Simulating Pure Mitral Regurgitation, *Am. Heart J.,* **63:**9–17, 1962.

75. Macleod, C. A.: Endocardial Cushion Defects with Severe Mitral Insufficiency and Small Atrial Septal Defect, *Circulation,* **26:**755, 1962.

76. Scott, L. P., et al.: Endocardial Cushion Defect: Preoperative and Postoperative Survey, *Circulation,* **26:**218–227, 1962.

76a. Levy, M. J., et al.: Atrioventricularis Communis: Clinical Aspects and Surgical Treatment, *Am. J. Cardiol.,* **14:**587–598, 1964.

77. Lev, M.: Architecture of the Conduction System in Congenital Heart Disease. I. Common Atrioventricular Orifice, *A.M.A. Arch. Path.,* **65:**174–191, 1958.

78. Umansky, R., and Hauck, A. J.: Factors in Growth of Children with Patent Ductus Arteriosus, *Pediatrics,* **30:**540–551, 1962.

79. Wood, P., McDonald, L.; and Emanuel, R.: The Clinical Picture Correlated with Physiological Observations in the Diagnosis of Congenital Heart Disease, *Pediat. Clin. North America,* **5:**981–1010, 1958.

80. Watson, D. G., and Keith, J. D.: The Q Wave in Lead V₆ in Heart Disease of Infancy and Childhood, with Special Reference to Diastolic Loading, *Am. Heart J.,* **63:**629–635, 1962.

81. Hultgren, H., et al.: The Syndrome of Patent Ductus Arteriosus with Pulmonary Hypertension, *Circulation,* **8:**15–35, 1953.

82. Sellors, T. H.: Surgery of Persistent Ductus Arteriosus, *Lancet,* **1:**615–617, 1945.

83. Hodgson, C. H., et al.: Hereditary Hemorrhagic Telangiectasia and Pulmonary Arteriovenous Fistula, *New England J. Med.,* **261:**625–636, 1959.

84. Heiner, D. C., Hara, M., and White, H. J.: Cardioaortic Fistula and Aneurysms of Sinus of Valsalva in Infancy: A Report of Aortic–Left Atrial Communication Indistinguishable from a Ruptured Aneurysm of the Aortic Sinus, *Pediatrics,* **27:**415–426, 1961.

85. Magidson, O., and Kay, J. H.: Ruptured Aortic Sinus Aneurysms, *Am. Heart J.,* **65:**597–606, 1963.

86. Taussig, H. B.: "Congenital Malformations of the Heart," vols. 1, 2, 2d ed., Harvard University Press, Cambridge, 1960.

87. Neufeld, H. N., et al.: Aorticopulmonary Septal Defect, *Am. J. Cardiol.,* **9:**12–25, 1962.

88. D'heer, D. A. H., and Van Nieuwenhuizen, C. L. C.: Diagnosis of Congenital Aortic Septal Defects, *Circulation,* **13:**58–62, 1956.

89. Lyon, R. A., and Kaplan, S.: Patent Ductus Arteriosus in Infancy, *Pediatrics,* **13:**357–362, 1954.

90. Ash, R., and Fischer, D.: Manifestations and Results of Treatment of Patent Ductus Arteriosus in Infancy and Childhood: An Analysis of 138 Cases, *Pediatrics,* **16:**695–703, 1955.

91. Ziegler, R. F.: The Importance of Patent Ductus Arteriosus in Infants, *Am. Heart J.,* **43:**553–572, 1952.

92. Dammann, J. F., Jr., and Sell, C. G. R.: Patent Ductus Arteriosus in the Absence of a Continuous Murmur, *Circulation,* **6:**110–124, 1952.

93. Gray, I. R.: Paradoxical Splitting of the Second Heart Sound, *Brit. Heart J.,* **18:**21–28, 1956.

94. Keith, J. D., and Forsyth, C.: Aortography in Infants, *Circulation,* **2:**907–914, 1950.

95. Gregg, N. M.: Congenital Cataract Following German Measles in the Mother, *Tr. Ophth. Soc. Australia,* **3:**35, 1941.

96. Swan, C., et al.: Congenital Defects in Infants Following Infectious Diseases during Pregnancy, with Special Reference to the Relationship between German Measles and Cataract, Deaf-mutism, Heart Disease and Microcephaly, and to the Period of Pregnancy in Which the Occurrence of Rubella Is Followed by Congenital Anomalies, *M. J. Australia,* **2:**201–210, 1943.

97. Rudolph, A. J., et al.: Transplacental Rubella Infection in Newly Born Infants, *J.A.M.A.,* **191:**843–845, 1965.

97a. Rowe, R. D.: Maternal Rubella and Pulmonary Artery Stenosis, *Pediatrics,* **32:**180–185, 1963.

98. Campbell, M.: The Place of Maternal Rubella in the Aetiology of Congenital Heart Disease, *Brit. M. J.,* **1:**691–696, 1961.

99. Gasul, B. M., Fell, E. H., and Casas, R.: The Diagnosis of Aortic Septal Defect by Retrograde Aortography: Report of a Case, *Circulation,* **4:** 251–254, 1951.

100. Sodi-Pallares, D., et al.: Electrocardiography in Infants and Children, *Pediat. Clin. North America,* **5:**871–905, 1958.

101. Anderson, R. C., Obarta, W., and Lillihei, C. W.: Truncus Arteriosus: Clinical Study of Fourteen Cases, *Circulation,* **16:**586–598, 1957.

101a. Morgan, A. D., Brinsfield, D., and Edwards, F. K.: Persistent Truncus Arteriosus: An Unusual Variant with Atresia of the Aortic Arch, *Am. J. Dis. Child.,* **109:**74–79, 1965.

102. Blake, H. A., and Manion, W. C.: Thoracic Arterial Arch Anomalies, *Circulation,* **26:**251–265, 1962.

103. Edwards, J. E.: Anomalies of the Derivation of the Aortic Arch System, *M. Clin. North America,* July, 1948, 925–949.

104. Gross, R. E., and Neuhauser, E. B. D.: Compression of the Trachea or Esophagus by Vascular Anomalies: Surgical Therapy in 40 Cases, *Pediatrics,* **7:**69–88, 1951.

105. Bahnson, H. T., Cooley, R. N., and Sloan, R. D.: Coarctation of the Aorta at Unusual Sites, *Am. Heart J.,* **38:**905–913, 1949.

106. McGregor, M., and Medalie, M.: Coarctation of the Aorta, *Brit. Heart J.,* **14:**531–533, 1952.

107. Haddad, H. M., and Wilkins, L.: Congenital

Anomalies Associated with Gonadal Aplasia: Review of 55 Cases, *Pediatrics*, 23:885–902, 1959.

108. Edwards, J. E.: Congenital Bicuspid Aortic Valve, *Circulation*, 23:485–488, 1961.

109. Reifenstein, G. H., Levine, S. A., and Gross, R. E.: Coarctation of the Aorta: Review of 104 Autopsied Cases of "Adult Type," 2 Years of Age or Older, *Am. Heart J.*, 33:146–168, 1947.

110. Rosenthal, L.. Coarctation of the Aorta and Pregnancy; Report of Five Cases, *Brit. M. J.*, 1:16–18, 1955.

111. Crafoord, C., and Nylin, G.: Congenital Coarctation of the Aorta and Its Surgical Treatment, *J. Thoracic Surg.*, 14:347–361, 1945.

112. Schuster, S. R., and Gross, R. E.: Surgery for Coarctation of Aorta: Review of 500 Cases, *J. Thoracic & Cardiovas. Surg.*, 43:54–70, 1962.

113. Campbell, M., and Bayliss, J. H.: The Course and Prognosis of Coarctation of the Aorta, *Brit. Heart J.*, 18:475–495, 1956.

114. Deboer, A., et al.: Coarctation of Aorta, *Arch. Surg.*, 83:801–812, 1961.

115. Harris, J. S., et al.: The Treatment of Paradoxical Hypertension and Necrotizing Arteriolitis Following Resection of Coarctation of the Aorta, *A.M.A. J. Dis. Child.*, 94:423, 1957.

116. Mustard, W. T., Rowe, R. D., and Keith, J. D.: Coarctation of the Aorta with Special Reference to First Year of Life, *Ann. Surg.*, 141:429–436, 1955.

117. Glass, I. H., Mustard, W. T., and Keith, J. D.: Coarctation of the Aorta in Infants: A Review of Twelve Years' Experience, *Pediatrics*, 26:109–121, 1960.

118. Freundlich, E., Engle, M. A., and Goldberg, H. P.: Coarctation of the Aorta in Infancy: Analysis of 10 Year Experience with Medical Management, *Pediatrics*, 27:427–440, 1961.

119. Braunwald, E., et al.: Congenital Aortic Stenosis. I. Clinical and Hemodynamic Findings in 100 Patients. II. Surgical Treatment and Results of of Operation, *Circulation*, 27:426–462, 1963.

120. Ongley, P. A., et al.: Aortic Stenosis in Infants and Children, *Pediatrics*, 21:207–221, 1958.

121. Lees, M. H., et al.: Congenital Aortic Stenosis: Operative Indications and Surgical Results, *Brit. Heart J.*, 24:31–38, 1962.

122. Goldblatt, A., Aygen, M. M., and Braunwald, E.: Hemodynamic-Phonocardiographic Correlations of the Fourth Heart Sound in Aortic Stenosis, *Circulation*, 26:92–98, 1962.

123. Reynolds, J. L., et al.: Critical Congenital Aortic Stenosis with Minimal Electrocardiographic Changes: A Report on Two Siblings, *New England J. Med.*, 262:276–282, 1960.

124. Hugenholtz, P. G., Lees, M. H., and Nadas, A. S.: The Scalar Electrocardiogram, Vectorcardiogram and Exercise Electrocardiogram in the Assessment of Congenital Aortic Stenosis, *Circulation*, 26:79–91, 1962.

124a. Hugenholtz, P. G., and Gamboa, R.: Effect of Chronically Increased Ventricular Pressure on Electrical Forces of the Heart: A Correlation between Hemodynamic and Vectorcardiographic Data (Frank System) in 90 Patients with Aortic or Pulmonic Stenosis, *Circulation*, 30:511–530, 1964.

125. Nadas, A. S., et al.: Combined Aortic and Pulmonic Stenosis, *Circulation*, 25:346–355, 1962.

126. Brent, L. B., et al.: Familial Muscular Subaortic Stenosis: Unrecognized Form of "Idiopathic Heart Disease" with Clinical and Autopsy Observations, *Circulation*, 21:167–180, 1960.

127. Mengis, H., Jr., Brandenberg, R. O., and Brown, A. L., Jr.: The Clinical, Hemodynamic and Pathologic Diagnosis of Muscular Subvalvular Aortic Stenosis, *Circulation*, 24:1126–1136, 1961.

128. Pare, J. A. P., et al.: Hereditary Cardiovascular Dysplasia, *Am. J. Med.*, 31:37–62, 1961.

129. Manchester, G. H.: Muscular Subaortic Stenosis, *New England J. Med.*, 269:300–306, 1963.

129a. Braunwald, E., et al.: Idiopathic Hypertrophic Subaortic Stenosis. I. A Description of the Disease Based upon an Analysis of 64 Patients, *Circulation*, 30 (supplement no. 4): 3–119, 1964.

130. Brachfeld, N., and Gorlin, R.: Subaortic Stenosis: Revised Concept of the Disease, *Medicine*, 38:415–433, 1959.

131. Braunwald, E., and Ebert, P. A.: Hemodynamic Alterations in Idiopathic Hypertrophic Subaortic Stenosis Induced by Sympathomimetic Drugs, *Am. J. Cardiol.*, 10:489–495, 1962.

132. Braunwald, E., Brockenbrough, E. C., and Frye, R. L.: Studies on Digitalis. V. Comparison of Effects of Ouabain on Left Ventricular Dynamics in Valvular Aortic Stenosis and Hypertrophic Subaortic Stenosis, *Circulation*, 26:166–173, 1962.

133. Braunwald, E., Brockenbrough, E. C., and Morrow, A. G.: Hypertrophic Subaortic Stenosis: A Broadened Concept, *Circulation*, 26:161–165, 1962.

133a. Braudo, M., Wigle, E., and Keith, J. D.: A Distinctive Electrocardiogram in Muscular Subaortic Stenosis Due to Ventricular Septal Hypertrophy, *Am. J. Cardiol.*, 14:599–607, 1964.

134. Williams, J. C. P., Barratt-Boyes, B. G., and Lowe, J. B.: Supravalvular Aortic Stenosis, *Circulation*, 24:1311–1318, 1961.

135. Beuren, A. J., Aptiz, J., and Harmjanz, D.: Supravalvular Aortic Stenosis in Association with Mental Retardation and a Certain Facial Appearance, *Circulation*, 26:1235–1240, 1962.

136. Wooley, C. F., et al.: Supravalvular Aortic Stenosis, *Am. J. Med.*, 31:717–725, 1961.

137. McGoon, D. C., et al.: The Surgical Treatment of Supravalvular Aortic Stenosis, *J. Thoracic Surg.*, 41:125–133, 1961.

138. Franch, R. H., and Oran, E.: Asymmetric Arm and Neck Pulses: A Clue to Supravalvular Aortic Stenosis (Abstract). *Circulation*, 28:722–723, 1963.

139. Wooley, C. F., et al.: Supravalvular Aortic Stenosis: An Emerging Clinical Entity, *Circulation,* **28:** 827–828, 1963.

140. Bourassa, M. G., and Campeau, L.: Combined Supravalvular Aortic and Pulmonic Stenosis, *Circulation,* **28:**572–581, 1963.

140*a.* Gracia, R. E., et al.: Idiopathic Hypercalcemia and Supravalvular Aortic Stenosis: Documentation of a New Syndrome, *New England J. Med.,* **271:** 117–120, 1964.

140*b.* Shumacker, H. B., and Mandelbaum, I.: Surgical Considerations in the Management of Supravalvular Aortic Stenosis, *Circulation,* **31** (supplement no. 1): 36–43, 1964.

141. Hastreiter, A. R., et al.: Congenital Aortic Stenosis Syndrome in Infancy, *Circulation,* **28:**1084–1095, 1963.

142. Edwards, J. E.: Editorial on the Etiology of Calcific Aortic Stenosis, *Circulation,* **26:**817–818, 1962.

143. Noonan, J. A., and Nadas, A. S.: The Hypoplastic Left Heart Syndrome, *Pediat. Clin. North America,* **5:**1029–1056, 1958.

144. Friedman, S., Murphy, L., and Ash, R.: Aortic Atresia with Hypoplasia of Left Heart and Aortic Arch, *J. Pediat.,* **38:**354–368, 1951.

145. Currarino, G., Edwards, F. K., and Kaplan, S.: Hypoplasia of the Left Heart Complex: Report of Two Cases Showing Premature Obliteration of the Foramen Ovale and Differential Cyanosis, *A.M.A.J. Dis. Child.,* **97:**839–844, 1959.

146. Friedman, S., Murphy, L., and Ash, R.: Congenital Mitral Atresia with Hypoplastic Nonfunctioning Left Heart, *A.M.A. J. Dis. Child.,* **90:**176–188, 1955.

147. Kleinerman, J., et al.: Absence of the Transverse Aortic Arch, *A.M.A. Arch. Path.,* **65:**490–498, 1958.

148. Daoud, G., et al.: Congenital Mitral Stenosis, *Circulation,* **27:**185–196, 1963.

149. Ferencz, C., Johnson, A. L., and Wiglesworth, F. W.: Congenital Mitral Stenosis, *Circulation,* **9:** 161–179, 1954.

150. Baker, C. G., et al.: Congenital Mitral Stenosis, *Brit. Heart J.,* **24:**498–504, 1962.

151. Starkey, G. W. B.: Surgical Experience in the Treatment of Congenital Mitral Stenosis and Mitral Insufficiency, *J. Thoracic & Cardiovas. Surg.,* **38:** 336–352, 1959.

152. Slade, P. R., Tubs, O. S., and Wells, B. G.: Cor Triatriatum: A Case Successfully Corrected by Surgery, *Brit. Heart J.,* **24:**233–236, 1962.

153. Anderson, R. C., and Varco, R. L.: Cor Triatriatum: Successful Diagnosis and Surgical Correction in a Three Year Old Girl, *Am. J. Cardiol.,* **7:**436–440, 1961.

154. Andersen, D. H., and Kelly, J.: Endocardial Fibroelastosis. I. Endocardial Fibro-elastosis Associated with Congenital Malformations of the Heart. II. A Clinical and Pathologic Investigation of Those Cases without Associated Cardiac Malformations,

Including Report of Two Familial Instances, *Pediatrics,* **18:**513–555, 1956.

155. Blumberg, R. W., and Lyon, R. A.: Endocardial Sclerosis, *A.M.A.J. Dis. Child.,* **84:**291–308, 1952.

156. Lambert, E. C., and Vlad, P.: Primary Endomyocardial Disease, *Pediat. Clin. North America,* **5:** 1057–1085, 1958.

157. Vlad, P., Rowe, R. D., and Keith, J. D.: Electrocardiogram in Primary Endocardial Fibroelastosis, *Brit. Heart J.,* **17:**189–197, 1955.

158. Lynfield, J., et al.: Right-and-left Heart Catheterization and Angiocardiographic Findings in Idiopathic Cardiac Hypertrophy with Endocardial Fibroelastosis, *Circulation,* **21:**386–400, 1960.

159. Linde, L. M., Adams, F. H., and O'Loughlin, B. J.: Endocardial Fibroelastosis: Angiocardiographic Studies, *Circulation,* **17:**40–45, 1958.

160. Wood, P.: Pulmonary Hypertension, *Mod. Concepts Cardiovas. Dis.,* **28:**513–518, 1959.

161. Dammann, J. F., Jr., and Ferencz, C.: Significance of the Pulmonary Vascular Bed in Congenital Heart Disease: Defects between Ventricles or Great Vessels in Which Both Increased Pressure and Blood Flow May Act upon the Lungs and in Which There Is a Common Ejectible Force, *Am. Heart J.,* **52:**210–231, 1956.

162. Edwards, J. E.: Conner Memorial Lecture: Functional Pathology of the Pulmonary Vascular Tree in Congenital Cardiac Disease, *Circulation,* **15:** 164–196, 1957.

163. Silverman, B. K., et al.: Pulmonary Stenosis with Intact Ventricular Septum: Correlation of Clinical and Physiologic Data with Review of Operative Results, *Am. J. Med.,* **20:**53–64, 1956.

164. Kjellberg, S. R., et al.: "Diagnosis of Congenital Heart Disease," The Year Book Medical Publishers, Inc., Chicago, 1955.

165. Dimond, E. G., and Lin, T. K.: The Clinical Picture of Pulmonary Stenosis (without Ventricular Septal Defect), *Ann. Int. Med.,* **40:**1108–1124, 1954.

166. Marquis, R. M.: Ventricular Septal Defect in Early Childhood, *Brit. M. J.,* **12:**265–276, 1950.

167. Crevasse, L., and Logue, R. B.: Valvular Pulmonic Stenosis: Auscultatory and Phonocardiographic Characteristics, *Am. Heart J.,* **56:**898–907, 1958.

168. Leatham, A., and Vogelpoel, L.: Early Systolic Sound in Dilatation of Pulmonary Artery, *Brit. Heart J.,* **16:**21–33, 1954.

169. Leatham, A.: Auscultation of the Heart, *Lancet,* **2:**703–708, 757–765, 1958.

169*a.* Gamboa, R., Hugenholtz, P. G., and Nadas, A. S.: Accuracy of the Phonocardiogram in Assessing Severity of Aortic and Pulmonic Stenosis, *Circulation,* **30:**35–46, 1964.

170. Cabrera, E., and Monroy, J. R.: Systolic and Diastolic Loading of the Heart. II. Electrocardiographic Data. *Am. Heart J.,* **43:**669–686, 1952.

171. Caylor, G. G., Ongley, P., and Nadas, A. S.: Re-

lation of Systolic Pressure in the Right Ventricle to the Electrocardiogram, *New England J. Med.*, **258**:979–982, 1958.

172. Bassingthwaighte, J. B., et al.: The Electrocardiographic and Hemodynamic Findings in Pulmonic Stenosis with Intact Ventricular Septum, *Circulation*, **28**:893–905, 1963.

173. Namin, E. P., et al.: Vectorcardiographic Criteria (Frank System) for Right Ventricular Overwork in Children (Abstract), *Circulation*, **28**:776–777, 1963.

174. Johnson, R. P., and Johnson, E. E.: Congenital Pulmonic Stenosis with Open Foramen Ovale in Infancy: Report of Five Proved Cases, *Am. Heart J.*, **44**:344–359, 1952.

175. Engle, M. A., and Taussig, H. B.: Valvular Pulmonic Stenosis with Intact Ventricular Septum and Patent Foramen Ovale: Report of Illustrative Cases and Analysis of Clinical Syndrome, *Circulation*, **2**:481–493, 1950.

176. Paul, M. H., and Rudolph, A. M.: Pulmonary Valve Obstruction during Cardiac Catheterization, *Circulation*, **18**:53–59, 1958.

177. Johnson, A. M.: Hypertrophic Infundibular Stenosis Complicating Simple Pulmonary Valve Stenosis. *Brit. Heart J.*, **21**:429–439, 1959.

178. Engle, M. A., et al.: Regression after Open Valvotomy of Infundibular Stenosis Accompanying Severe Pulmonic Stenosis, *Circulation*, **17**:862–873. 1958.

179. Harris, P.: Some Variations in the Shape of Pressure Curve in Human Right Ventricle, *Brit. Heart J.*, **17**:173–182, 1955.

180. Gyllenwärd, A., et al.: Congenital, Multiple Peripheral Stenosis of the Pulmonary Artery, *Pediatrics*, **19**:399–410, 1957.

181. Van Epps, E. F.: Primary Pulmonary Hypertension in Brothers, *Am. J. Roentgenol.*, **78**:471–482, 1957.

182. Loehr, H., Loogen, F., and Vieten, H.: Peripheral Pulmonary Stenosis, *Fortschr. Geb. Roentgenstrahlen*, **94**:285–304, 1961.

183. Agustsson. M. H., et al.: The Diagnosis of Bilateral Stenosis of the Primary Pulmonary Artery Branches Based on Characteristic Pulmonary Trunk Pressure Curves: A Hemodynamic and Angiocardiographic Study, *Circulation*, **26**:421–427, 1962.

184. Davignon, A. L., et al.: Congenital Pulmonary Atresia with Intact Ventricular Septum: Clinicopathologic Correlation of Two Anatomic Types, *Am. Heart J.*, **62**:591–602, 1961.

184a. Lauer, R. M. et al.: Angiographic Demonstration of Intramyocardial Sinusoids in Pulmonaryvalve Atresia with Intact Ventricular Septum and Hypoplastic Right Ventricle, *New England J. Med.*, **271**:68–72, 1964.

185. White, P. D., and Sprague, H. B.: The Tetralogy of Fallot: Report of a Case in a Noted Musician Who Lived to His Sixtieth Year, *J.A.M.A.*, **92**:787–791, 1929.

186. Hoffman, J. I. E., et al.: Pulmonic Stenosis, Ventricular Septal Defect, and Right Ventricular Pressure above Systemic Level, *Circulation*, **22**:405–411, 1960.

187. Noonan, J. A., et al.: Transposition of the Great Arteries: A Correlation of Clinical, Physiologic and Autopsy Data, *New England J. Med.*, **263**:592–596, 637–642, 684–692, 739–744, 1960.

188. Mirowski, M., Mehrizi, A., and Taussig, H. B.: The Electrocardiogram in Patients with Both Great Vessels Arising from the Right Ventricle Combined with Pulmonary Stenosis: An Analysis of 22 Cases with Special Reference to the Differential Diagnosis from the Tetralogy of Fallot, *Circulation*, **28**:1116–1127, 1963.

189. Neufeld, H. N., et al.: Origin of Both Great Vessels from the Right Ventricle. I. Without Pulmonary Stenosis. II. With Pulmonary Stenosis, *Circulation*, **23**:399–412, 603–612, 1961.

190. Schiebler, G. L., et al.: Congenital Corrected Transposition of the Great Vessels: A Study of 33 Cases, *Pediatrics*, **27**: (Suppl.), 849–888, 1961.

191. Tandon, R., Hauck, A. J., and Nadas, A. S.: Persistent Truncus Arteriosus: A Clinical, Hemodynamic, and Autopsy Study of Nineteen Cases, *Circulation*, **28**:1050–1060, 1963.

192. Martelle, R. R., and Linde, L. M.: Cerebrovascular Accidents with Tetralogy of Fallot, *Am. J. Dis. Child.*, **101**:206–209, 1961.

193. Banker, B. Q.: Occlusive Vascular Disease Affecting the Central Nervous System in Infancy and Childhood, *Tr. Am. Neurol. A.*, **84**:38–46, 1959.

194. Paine, R. S.: Emergencies of Cerebral Origin, *Pediat. Clin. North America*, **9**:67–100, 1962.

195. Newton, E. J.: Hematogenous Brain Abscess in Cyanotic Heart Disease, *Quart. J. Med.*, **25**:201–220, 1956.

196. Cohen, M. M.: The Central Nervous System in Congenital Heart Disease, *Neurology*, **10**:452–456, 1960.

197. Matson, D. D., and Salom, M.: Brain Abscess in Congenital Heart Disease, *Pediatrics*, **27**:772–789, 1961.

198. Rich, A. R.: A Hitherto Unrecognized Tendency to the Development of Widespread Pulmonary Vascular Obstruction in Patients with Congenital Pulmonary Stenosis (Tetralogy of Fallot), *Bull. Johns Hopkins Hosp.*, **82**:389–401, 1948.

199. Heath, D., et al.: The Etiology of Pulmonary Thrombosis in Cyanotic Congenital Heart Disease with Pulmonary Stenosis, *Thorax*, **13**:213–217, 1958.

200. Fragoyannis, S., and Kandalenos, A.: Congenital Heart Disease with Pulmonary Ischemia: A Study of the Pulmonary Vascular Lesions before and after Systemic Pulmonary Anastomosis, *Am. Heart J.*, **63**:335–345, 1962.

201. Rudolph, A. M., Nadas, A. S., and Borges, W. A.:

Hematologic Adjustments to Cyanotic Congenital Heart Disease, *Pediatrics,* **11**:454–463, 1953.

202. Hartmann, R. C.: A Hemorrhagic Disorder Occurring in Patients with Cyanotic Congenital Heart Disease, *Bull. Johns Hopkins Hosp.,* **91**:49–67, 1952.

203. Verel, D., et al.: Thrombocytopenia in Congenital Heart Disease, *Brit. Heart J.,* **24**:92–94, 1962.

204. Somerville, J.: Gout in Cyanotic Congenital Heart Disease, *Brit. Heart J.,* **23**:31–34, 1961.

205. Nadas, A. S., et al.: Tetralogy of Fallot with Unilateral Pulmonary Atresia: A Clinically Diagnosable and Surgically Significant Variant, *Circulation,* **8**:328–336, 1953.

206. Miller, R. A., Lev., M., and Paul, M. H.: Congenital Absence of the Pulmonary Valve: The Clinical Syndrome of Tetralogy of Fallot with Pulmonary Regurgitation, *Circulation,* **26**:266–278, 1962.

207. Steinberg, I.: Left-sided Patent Ductus Arteriosus and Right-sided Aortic Arch: Angiocardiographic Findings in Three Cases, *Circulation,* **28**: 1138–1142, 1963.

208. Campbell, M., and Hills, T. H.: Angiocardiography in Cyanotic Congenital Heart Disease, *Brit. Heart J.,* **12**:65–95, 1950.

209. Dekker, A., Mehrizi, A., and Vengsarkar, A. S.: Corrected Transposition of the Great Vessels with Ebstein Malformation of the Left Atrioventricular Valve: An Embryologic Analysis and Two Case Reports, *Circulation,* **31**:119–126, 1965.

210. Mayer, F. E., Nadas, A. S., and Ongley, P. A.: Ebstein's Anomaly: Presentation of 10 Cases, *Circulation,* **16**:1057–1069, 1957.

211. Engle, M. A., et al.: Ebstein's Anomaly of the Tricuspid Valve: Report of 3 Cases and Analysis of Clinical Syndrome, *Circulation,* **1**: 1246–1260, 1950.

212. Arcilla, R. A., and Gasul, B. M.: Congenital Aplasia or Marked Hypoplasia of the Myocardium of the Right Ventricle (Uhl's Anomaly): Clinical, Angiocardiographic, and Hemodynamic Findings, *J. Pediat.,* **58**:381–388, 1961.

212a. Reeve, R., and Macdonald, D.: Partial Absence of the Right Ventricular Musculature: Partial Parchment Heart, *Am. J. Cardiol.,* **14**:415–419, 1964.

213. Blount, S. G., Jr., McCord, M. C., and Gelb, I. J.: Ebstein's Anomaly, *Circulation,* **15**:210–224, 1957.

214. Yim, B. J. B., and Yu, P. N.: Value of an Electrode Catheter in Diagnosis of Ebstein's Disease, *Circulation,* **17**:543–548, 1958.

215. Hernandes, F. A., Rochkind, R., and Cooper, H. R.: The Intracavitary Electrocardiogram in the Diagnosis of Ebstein's Anomaly, *Am. J. Cardiol.,* **1**:181–190, 1958.

216. McCredie, R. M., et al.: Ebstein's Disease: Diagnosis by Electrode Catheter and Treatment by Partial Bypass of the Right Side of the Heart, *New England J. Med.,* **267**:174–179, 1962.

217. Scott, L. P., et al.: A Surgical Approach to Ebsteins' Disease, *Circulation,* **27**:574–577, 1963.

217a. Bahnson, H. T., Bauersfeld, S. R., and Smith, J. W.: Pathological Anatomy and Surgical Correction of Ebstein's Anomaly, *Circulation,* **31** (supplement no. 1): 3–8, 1965.

218. Elliott, L. P., et al.: Complete Transposition of the Great Vessels. II. An Electrocardiographic Analysis, *Circulation,* **27**:1118–1127, 1963.

219. Abrams, H. L., Kaplan, H. S., and Purdy, A.: Diagnosis of Complete Transposition of the Great Vessels, *Radiology,* **57**:500–513, 1951.

220. Taussig, H. B. and Bing, R. J.: Complete Transposition of the Aorta and a Levoposition of the Pulmonary Artery, *Am. Heart J.,* **37**:551–559, 1949.

221. Beuren, A.: A Differential Diagnosis of the Taussig-Bing Heart from Complete Transposition of the Great Vessels with a Posteriorly Overriding Pulmonary Artery, *Circulation,* **21**:1071–1087, 1960.

222. Engle, M. A., et al.: Acyanotic Ventricular Septal Defect with Both Great Vessels from the Right Ventricle, *Am. Heart J.,* **66**:755–766, 1963.

223. Witham, A. C.: Double Outlet Right Ventricle: A Partial Transposition Complex, *Am. Heart J.,* **53**: 928–939, 1957.

224. Neufeld, H. N., et al.: Origin of Both Great Vessels from the Right Ventricle without Pulmonary Stenosis, *Brit. Heart J.,* **24**:393–408, 1962.

225. Levy, M. J., et al.: Accessory Valvular Tissue Causing Subpulmonary Stenosis in Corrected Transposition of Great Vessels, *Circulation,* **27**: 494–502, 1963.

226. De la Cruz, M. V., Polansky, B. J., and Novarro-Lopez, F.: The Diagnosis of Corrected Transposition of the Great Vessels, *Brit. Heart J.,* **24**:483–497, 1962.

227. Anderson, R. C., Lillehei, C. W., Lester, R. G.: Corrected Transposition of the Great Vessels of the Heart, *Pediatrics,* **20**:626–646, 1957.

228. Honey, M.: Anatomical and Physiological Features of Corrected Transposition of the Great Vessels, *Guy's Hosp. Rep.,* **111**:250–275, 1962.

229. Lev, M., Licata, R. H., and May, R. C.: The Conduction System in Mixed Levocardia with Ventricular Inversion (Corrected Transposition), *Circulation,* **28**:232–237, 1963.

229a. Edwards, J. E., et al.: "Congenital Heart Disease: Correlation of Pathologic Anatomy and Angiocardiography," vol. I, W. B. Saunders Company, Philadelphia, 1965, p. 179.

230. Darling, R. C., Rothney, W. B., and Craig, J. M.: Total Pulmonary Venous Drainage into the Right Side of the Heart, *Lab. Invest.,* **6**:44–64, 1957.

231. Guntheroth, W. G., Nadas, A. S., and Gross, R. E.: Transposition of the Pulmonary Veins, *Circulation,* **18**:117–137, 1958.

232. Hastreiter, A. R., et al.: Total Anomalous Pulmonary Venous Connection with Severe Pulmonary

Venous Obstruction, Circulation, **25**:916–928, 1962.

233. Kauffman, S. L., Ores, C. N., and Andersen, D. H.: Two Cases of Total Anomalous Pulmonary Venous Return of the Supracardiac Type with Stenosis Simulating Infradiaphragmatic Drainage, *Circulation*, **25**:376–382, 1962.

234. Sepulvedo, G., Lukas, D. S., and Steinberg, I.: Anomalous Drainage of Pulmonary Veins: Clinical, Physiologic and Angiocardiographic Features, *Am. J. Med.*, **18**:883–899, 1955.

235. Snellen, H. A., and Dekker, A.: Anomalous Pulmonary Venous Drainage in Relation to Left Superior Vena Cava and Coronary Sinus, *Am. Heart J.*, **66**:184–196, 1963.

236. Gott, V. L., et al.: Total Anomalous Pulmonary Return: Analysis of Thirty Cases, *Circulation*, **13**:543–552, 1956.

237. Ryan, N. J., et al.: Total Anomalous Pulmonary Venous Drainage, *Am. J. Dis. Child.*, **105**:42–52, 1963.

238. Rowe, R. D., Glass, I. H., and Keith, J. D.: Total Anomalous Pulmonary Venous Drainage at Cardiac Level: Angiocardiographic Differentiation, *Circulation*, **23**:77–80, 1961.

239. Harris, G. B., Neuhauser, E. B., and Geedion, A.: Total Anomalous Pulmonary Venous Return below the Diaphragm, *Am. J. Roentgenol.*, **84**:436–441, 1960.

240. Bruwer, A.: Roentgenologic Findings in Anomalous Pulmonary Venous Connection, *Proc. Staff Meet. Mayo Clin.*, **28**:480–485, 1953.

241. Ferencz, C.: Congenital Abnormalities of Pulmonary Vessels and Their Relation to Malformations of the Lung, *Pediatrics*, **28**:993–1010, 1961.

242. Swan, H. J. C., Buchell, H. B., and Wood, E. H.: Symposium on Anomalous Pulmonary Venous Connection (Drainage): Differential Diagnosis at Cardiac Catheterization of Anomalous Pulmonary Venous Drainage Related to Atrial Septal Defects or Abnormal Venous Connections, *Proc. Staff Meet. Mayo Clin.*, **28**:452–462, 1953.

243. Davis, W. H., Jordan, F. R., and Smyman, H. W.: Persistent Left Superior Vena Cava Draining into the Left Atrium, as an Isolated Anomaly, *Am. Heart J.*, **57**:616–622, 1959.

244. Gardner, D. L., and Cole, L.: Long Survival with Inferior Vena Cava Draining into Left Atrium, *Brit. Heart J.*, **17**:93–97, 1955.

245. Campbell, M., and Deuchar, D. C.: Left Sided Superior Vena Cava, *Brit. Heart J.*, **16**:423–439, 1954.

246. Anderson, R. C., Adams, P., and Burke, B.: Anomalous Inferior Vena Cava with Azygos Continuation (Infrahepatic Interruption of the Inferior Vena Cava), *J. Pediat.*, **59**:370–383, 1961.

247. Downing, D. F.: Absence of the Inferior Vena Cava, *Pediatrics*, **12**:675–680, 1953.

248. Grant, R. P.: The Syndrome of Dextroversion of the Heart, *Circulation*, **18**:25–36, 1958.

249. Arcilla, R. A., and Gasul, B. M.: Congenital Dextrocardia: Clinical, Angiocardiographic, and Autopsy Studies on 50 Patients, *J. Pediat.*, **58**:39–58, 251–262, 1961.

250. Rosenbaum, H. D., Pellegrino, E. D., and Treciokas, L. J.: Acyanotic Levocardia, *Circulation*, **26**:60–72, 1962.

251. Mirowski, M., Neill, C., and Taussig, H. B.: Left Atrial Ectopic Rhythm in Mirror-image Dextrocardia and in Normally Placed Malformed Hearts: Report of 12 Cases with "Dome and Dart" P Waves, *Circulation*, **27**:864–877, 1963.

252. Bush, J. A., and Ainger, L. E.: Congenital Absence of Spleen with Congenital Heart Disease, *Pediatrics*, **15**:93–99, 1955.

253. Ruttenberg, H. D., et al.: Syndrome of Congenital Cardiac Disease with Asplenia: Distinction from Other Forms of Congenital Cyanotic Cardiac Disease, *Am. J. of Cardiol.*, **13**:387–406, 1964.

21 SURGICAL TREATMENT OF CONGENITAL HEART DISEASE

John W. Kirklin, M.D., Robert B. Wallace, M.D., and James W. DuShane, M.D.

SURGICAL SIGNIFICANCE OF PULMONARY VASCULAR DISEASE

The life history, ability to be operated on, and response to operation of many patients with congenital heart disease is determined by the status of their pulmonary vasculature.

Patients with lesions allowing communication between the systemic and pulmonary circulations or producing pulmonary venous hypertension may develop mild, moderate, or severe pulmonary vascular disease. The pathologic features of pulmonary vascular disease have been studied by Dammann and Ferencz,[1] Heath and Edwards,[2] and others, and a correlation between the pathologic changes and the calculated value for pulmonary vascular resistance has been made by Heath and associates.[3] An estimate of pulmonary artery pressure and pulmonary blood flow can often be made with reasonable accuracy on the basis of physical examination, electrocardiogram, and roentgenogram of the thorax. Thus, some deductions can be made concerning the extent of pulmonary vascular disease.[4] The most precise evaluation is obtained by relating pulmonary vascular resistance to systemic arterial resistance, these values being calculated from data obtained by catheterization of the heart of the un-

Table 21-1. DATA OBTAINED AT CARDIAC CATHETERIZATION IN A PATIENT WITH ATRIAL SEPTAL DEFECT*

	At rest	After exercise
Femoral artery pressure, mm Hg	120/68	138/80
Pulmonary artery pressure, mm Hg	88/34	113/54
Systemic index, L/min/m²	2.7	4.1
Pulmonary index, L/min/m²	3.4	2.6
Systemic resistance, units/m²	32	24
Pulmonary resistance, units/m²	15	28
P/S resistance ratio	0.47	1.17

* Note that pulmonary flow fell and pulmonary resistance rose with exercise. Systemic flow rose but only by right-to-left shunting across the atrial septal defect. It can be inferred that with the atrial septal defect closed this patient would be unable to increase systemic flow. Operation is contraindicated.

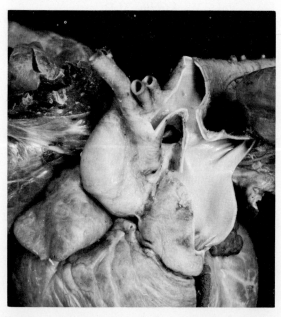

Fig. 21-1. Patent ductus arteriosus in the typical position (extending from the upper part of the descending thoracic aorta to the main pulmonary artery at the point of its bifurcation). (*Reproduced with permission from J. E. Edwards, T. J. Dry, R. L. Parker, H. B. Burchell, E. H. Wood, and A. H. Bulbulian: "An Atlas of Congenital Anomalies of the Heart and Great Vessels," Charles C Thomas, Publisher, Springfield, Ill., 1954, 202 pp.*)

anesthetized patient who is breathing air spontaneously. Additional information can be obtained by studies during exercise (Table 21-1).

Normally, the ratio between pulmonary vascular resistance and systemic arterial resistance (P/S resistance ratio) is about 0.25. When this ratio is between 0.25 and 0.45, the pulmonary vascular disease is considered mild. It is considered moderate when the ratio is between 0.45 and 0.75, and severe when the ratio is greater than 0.75. Generally, severe pulmonary vascular disease does not regress significantly after repair of systemic-pulmonary artery communication, although exceptions occur (notably after repair of patent ductus arteriosus).[5] Actually, following repair of ventricular septal defect in some patients with severe pulmonary vascular disease (i.e., with P/S resistance greater than 0.75), an increase in P/S resistance is seen.

When the P/S resistance ratio approximates 1, operation for repair of systemic-pulmonary artery communications is considered inadvisable because of the severity of the pulmonary vascular disease. Operative risk is high, the severe pulmonary vascular disease rarely if ever regresses under these circumstances, and pulmonary artery pressure remains high postoperatively. The clinical state of the patient and his tolerance for exercise may actually be worsened by repair. With the communication open, systemic blood flow can be augmented during exercise by right-to-left shunting across the defect, albeit at the expense of decreased oxygen saturation of arterial blood.[6] When the defect has been closed in a patient with severe pulmonary vascular disease, pulmonary artery pressure rises still farther on exercise and systemic flow can increase only slightly.[7] Exercise tolerance is thereby severely limited, and fatal ventricular fibrillation sometimes develops suddenly.

PATENT DUCTUS ARTERIOSUS

Surgical Pathology (Fig. 21-1) and Diagnosis. The diagnosis of patent ductus arteriosus in children and young adults can usually be made on clinical grounds, the most specific sign being a continuous murmur best heard anteriorly over the second left interspace. The roentgenogram of the thorax may be normal or may show pulmonary plethora, enlargement of the pulmonary artery, and enlargement of the aortic arch (this last finding being in contrast to the finding in cases of atrial and ventricular septal defects). The electrocardiogram may be normal or may reflect increased left ventricular work. Infants present a special situation, for the murmur of patent ductus arteriosus is usually not continuous in the first year of life.[8] Yet the diagnostician must be alert to the possibility that this correctable lesion may be present in any infant presenting with growth failure or recurrent pulmonary congestion.[9,10] On some occasions older patients may exhibit a murmur which is atypical in location or quality (the latter occurring particularly in the presence of pulmonary hypertension, when only a diastolic murmur may be audible or, rarely, there may be no murmur). Cardiac catheterization and occasionally angiocardiography are then indicated, for a similar clinical picture can be produced by aortopulmonary window, coronary arteriovenous fistula, ruptured aneurysm of the sinus of Valsalva, or ventricular septal defect with aortic insufficiency.

Life History and Indications for Operation. Some patients with a large patent ductus arteriosus die from it in infancy. Others develop pulmonary vascular disease, which in a few instances becomes so severe that the P/S resistance becomes greater than 1, the shunt reverses to become right-to-left, and the condition becomes inoperable. The majority of patients suffer neither of these fates but may fail to grow. It has been shown that individuals 17 years of age with patent ductus arteriosus have a life expectancy only one-half that of the general population of that age.[11]

Because of these facts and the negligible operative mortality rate, the mere presence of a patent ductus arteriosus is generally considered an *indication* for operation.[12] The optimal age is 3 to 6 years. Patients exhibiting cardiac failure or severe growth retardation as infants should undergo operation promptly, and the results even at this young age are excellent.[13] When there has been bacterial infection in the region of the ductus arteriosus, the patient is given appropriate antimicrobial therapy, and operation is performed about 6 weeks later. *Contraindication* to operation is severe pulmonary vascular disease, with a P/S resistance ratio of about 1 or greater.

Surgical Treatment. Operation is performed by us through a posterolateral thoracotomy (Fig. 21-2). The ductus arteriosus is dissected out essentially by the method of Jones.[14] The vagus nerve is reflected medially, thus avoiding the need for dividing its pulmonary branches. The ductus is divided between appropriate clamps (usually Potts's fine-tooth clamps),[15] and aortic and pulmonary ends are oversewn with No. 5-0 silk.[16,17]

Results. Hospital mortality for closure of uncomplicated patent ductus arteriosus by experienced hands is essentially zero. In patients with moderate or severe pulmonary vascular disease, severe hypertension in the pulmonary artery renders dissection and division of the ductus more hazardous than usual. This, plus residual pulmonary hypertension,

renders the risk approximately 5 per cent in such cases.

Late complications from operation are rare. Results are excellent, and in those patients without pulmonary vascular disease a cure is obtained. In children with growth failure from the patent ductus arteriosus, growth accelerates after repair. If operated on prior to 8 years of age[18] patients usually reach normal percentiles for growth. Results are unsatisfactory for patients with a P/S resistance greater than 1, virtually all patients dying within a year or two after operation.[19] When the P/S resistance ratio is 0.45 to 0.9 or thereabouts, surgical closure of the defect is not literally curative because of residual pulmonary vascular disease, but it is beneficial.

AORTOPULMONARY WINDOW

Surgical Pathology (Fig. 21-3). Aortopulmonary window is a communication between the aorta and the pulmonary artery just above the semilunar valves. Such communications are usually large (although occasionally as small as 2 mm), and severe pulmonary artery hypertension and varying degrees of pulmonary vascular disease usually are present.

Diagnosis. The diagnosis should be considered in patients who have a continuous murmur suggestive of patent ductus arteriosus but who have signs of severe hypertension in the pulmonary arteries. In most patients, however, the murmur is systolic only. Cardiac catheterization and angiocardiographic study are indicated in all patients in whom this condition is suspected, in order to define the anatomic features and the operability (i.e., the P/S resistance ratio). Particular care must be taken to differentiate this condition, which is essentially an incomplete form of truncus arteriosus, from true truncus arteriosus.

Life History and Indications for Operation. The lesion is uncommon, and a clear account of the life history of patients with it has not been given. Some patients die in infancy of cardiac failure, and in those surviving this period the development of severe pulmonary vascular disease and its sequelae seems the usual result. It is said that all patients with defects 1 cm or larger are dead before the age of 20 years.[20]

Operation is clearly indicated in all patients in whom the P/S resistance ratio indicates operability (i.e., less than 1).

Surgical Treatment. Operation has been successfully performed in a few patients by a closed technique, but the use of cardiopulmonary bypass is now clearly the method of choice.[21] Median sternotomy is carried out. Cardiopulmonary bypass is established, and if possible, the defect is digitally

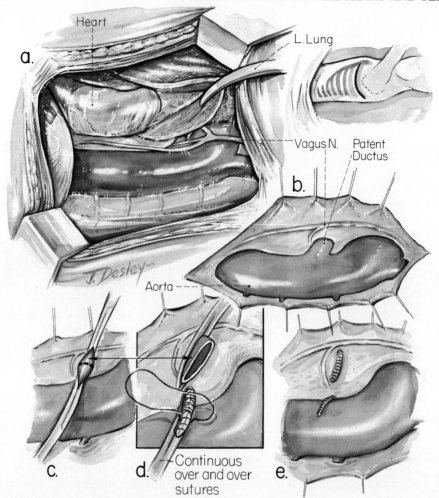

Fig. 21-2. Division of patent ductus arteriosus. *a.* Mediastinal pleura is opened over the upper part of the descending thoracic aorta and pleural flaps are retracted with fine silk sutures. *b.* Ductus arteriosus is nicely exposed as the vagus and recurrent laryngeal nerves are reflected medially. *c* and *d.* Ductus is appropriately clamped (*c*) and divided (*d*). *e.* Aortic and pulmonary ends are oversewn with two rows of continuous No. 5-0 silk sutures.

occluded while the heart is cooled by the perfusate and external cardiac cooling.[22] The aorta is cross-clamped downstream to the window, and the pulmonary artery is opened opposite the aortopulmonary window. From within the pulmonary artery the window is closed by direct suture or by use of a piece of intracardiac knitted polytetrafluoroethylene (Teflon) or pericardium, a method first suggested to us by Bjork[23] (Fig. 21-4). The older technique of dividing the aortopulmonary communication and suturing the resultant defect in aorta and pulmonary artery (which can be inordinately difficult and time-consuming at times) is now used by us only in the rare cases in which the communication has some length, is well downstream to the semilunar valves, and is of moderate size.

Results. The results of operation for aortopulmonary window at present are good, but the small number of patients operated on by any one clinic makes statistical evaluation impossible. Hospital mortality rate at present is about 5 to 10 per cent; this figure is as high as it is because most of these patients have some pulmonary vascular disease. Late results have been good, compromised only if there is significant residual pulmonary vascular disease.

VENTRICULAR SEPTAL DEFECT

Surgical Pathology (Figs. 21-5 to 21-7) and Diagnosis. The diagnosis of ventricular septal defect is usually made on the basis of the characteristic regurgitant type of systolic murmur that is best heard in the third and fourth left interspaces and often extends into the axilla,[24] the electrocardiogram,[25] and the chest roentgenogram. The degree of pulmonary vascular disease can often be evaluated on clinical grounds also[4,26] (Fig. 21-8). When it seems moderate or severe, cardiac catheterization is usually indicated in order that the most precise possible estimate can be made of the P/S resistance ratio and thus of operability (see "Surgical Significance of Pulmonary Vascular Disease," at the start of this chapter).

Life History. The life history of patients with ventricular septal defect has become of great interest since the advent of surgical therapy. It is clear that some infants with large defects, large left-to-right shunts, and mild pulmonary vascular disease die from their lesion in the early months of life;[27] that in some patients pulmonary vascular disease develops and progresses so that by the age of 2 to 5 years their P/S resistance ratio has become 1 or greater, rendering their condition inoperable;[28] and that some continue to live without progression of the pulmonary vascular disease but with growth failure. Some infants with apparently large ventricular septal defects, large left-to-right shunting, and mild pulmonary vascular disease improve after the age of about 9 months, and the defect in some cases appears to become smaller. In a few such patients, the defects undergo spontaneous, complete closure.[29-31] Infundibular pulmonary stenosis develops in certain infants with large ventricular septal defect and large left-to-right shunting as they age, and in some, the stenosis becomes sufficiently severe that the malformation becomes typically a tetralogy of Fallot.[32]

Infants with moderate-sized defects (distinctly smaller than the aortic orifice) rarely have significant symptoms early in life, rarely have progressing pulmonary vascular disease, and rarely die of cardiac failure during infancy or childhood. In childhood they usually present large left-to-right shunting and no hypertension, or mild hypertension, in the pulmonary artery (pressure in the pulmonary artery is 45 per cent, or less, of that in the aorta). Symptoms of easy fatigability sometimes develop in such patients late in childhood or early in adult life, and a few at least follow a course like that of patients with atrial septal defect in that chronic right-sided heart failure develops in adult life.[29] A few patients with moderate-sized defects probably experience spontaneous closure of the defect.

Small ventricular septal defects result in small left-to-right shunts and do not produce pulmonary vascular disease. The only hazard that appears to challenge patients with such defects is bacterial endocarditis. Probably about 20 per cent of defects

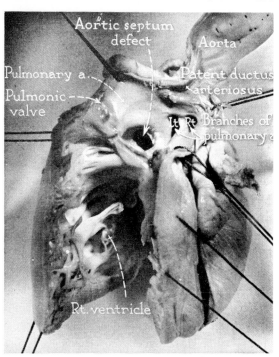

Fig. 21-3. Necropsy specimen of aortopulmonary window ("aortic septum defect"). Defect is just downstream to the pulmonary valve and is large. (*Reproduced with permission from R. A. Sprengel and A. F. Brown: Aortic Septum Defect, Am. Heart J., 48:796–798, 1954.*)

of this size undergo spontaneous closure.[29]

Some young children with moderate-sized or small ventricular septal defects (usually high defects located somewhat more anteriorly than usual) develop incompetence of the aortic valve.[33] The prolapse of the right aortic cusp seems to result in elongation of the cusp and worsening of the incompetence as the years pass[34] (Fig. 21-9).

Indications for Operation. The indications for operation in patients with ventricular septal defects are based on the foregoing and on the results which can be obtained by properly executed surgical procedures. For young children with small ventricular septal defects and small left-to-right shunts (which result in no demonstrable cardiac enlargement, no apical diastolic murmur, no evidence on chest roentgenogram of increased pulmonary blood flow, and no evidence of left ventricular overload on the electrocardiogram), repair is not ordinarily advised by us.

Most infants less than 6 months old who exhibit congestive heart failure from a large ventricular septal defect respond well to medical management; thus, deferral of operation is possible. The few infants who fail to respond are treated at present by the surgical creation of moderate pulmonary

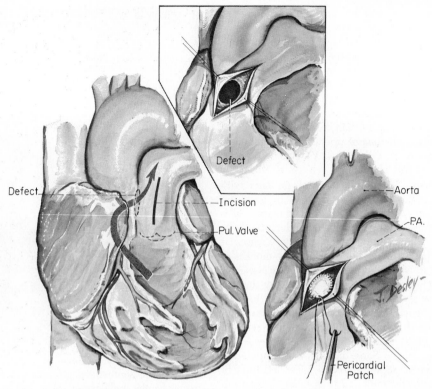

Fig. 21-4. Steps in repair of aortopulmonary window from within the pulmonary artery. After cardiopulmonary bypass has been established and the heart has been thoroughly cooled, a left ventricular vent is inserted and the aorta is cross-clamped. Defect is exposed by incision in the pulmonary artery. It is usually repaired by insertion of a patch of pericardium or Teflon.

stenosis (banding of the pulmonary artery).[35] The band should be removed and the defect repaired when the child has reached the age of 3 to 6 years. When infants more than 6 months of age remain in chronic heart failure from a large ventricular septal defect or exhibit marked growth failure or evidence of progressing pulmonary vascular disease, intracardiac repair is indicated[4] (see "Results," p. 461). Children with large defects that are well tolerated, or with moderate-sized defects, are ordinarily not operated on until the age of about 5½ years, which seems to be an ideal age for withstanding most types of intracardiac surgery. Patients with such lesions who are older than this when first seen are advised to have operations at their early convenience.

Patients with large ventricular septal defect with mild pulmonary vascular disease (some of whom have severe hypertension in the pulmonary artery) are advised to have operation in the knowledge that the end results are excellent and hospital risks are low. Those with moderate pulmonary vascular disease (P/S resistance ratio between 0.45 and 0.75) are advised to have operation, although the

hospital mortality rate is a little higher and the end results usually are marred by persistence of moderate hypertension in the pulmonary artery. Patients with ventricular septal defect and severe pulmonary vascular disease are considered to have clearly inoperable conditions when the P/S resistance ratio is 1 or greater. At present, operation is usually advised when the P/S resistance ratio is 0.75 to 0.9, although the beneficial effects of successful repair in this circumstance have not been firmly established.

Patients with ventricular septal defect and pulmonary stenosis (in whom systolic pressure in the inflow portion of the right ventricle is less than that in the left ventricle, in contrast to that in tetralogy of Fallot) are advised to have operation, since results are excellent. Those with ventricular septal defect and established incompetence at the aortic valve present a difficult decision. Repair of the ventricular septal defect alone is unsatisfactory. Attempts at relieving the incompetence at the aortic valve by a plication procedure or cusp replacement, although initially encouraging, have not proved satisfactory in our hands for most patients.

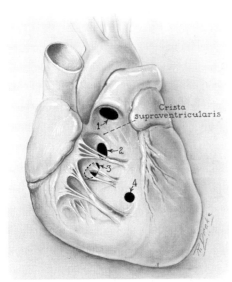

Fig. 21-5. Diagrammatic representation of types of ventricular septal defects. 1. A high defect immediately under the pulmonary valve. 2. The typical high ventricular septal defect. 3. The atrioventricular canal type of ventricular septal defect. 4. A defect in the muscular portion of the septum. (*Reproduced with permission from J. W. Kirklin, H. G. Harshbarger, D. E. Donald, and J. E. Edwards: Surgical Correction of Ventricular Septal Defect: Anatomic and Technical Considerations, J. Thoracic Surg., 33:45–57, 1957.*)

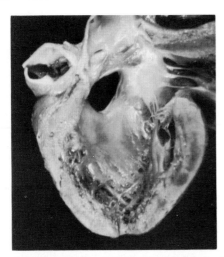

Fig. 21-6. Typical high ventricular septal defect viewed from left ventricular side. Note intimate relation of defect to the aortic valve cusps and anterior leaflet of the mitral valve. (*Reproduced with permission from J. W. Kirklin, H. G. Harshbarger, D. E. Donald, and J. E. Edwards: Surgical Correction of Ventricular Septal Defect: Anatomic and Technical Considerations, J. Thoracic Surg., 33:45–57, 1957.*)

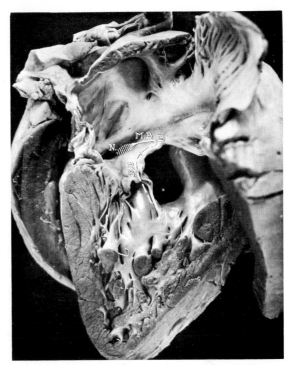

Fig. 21-7. Atrioventricular canal type of ventricular septal defect, located beneath the septal leaflet of the tricuspid valve. *N.*, atrioventricular node; *M.B.* and *B.*, main bundle and branching point. (*Reproduced with permission from H. N. Neufeld, J. L. Titus, J. W. DuShane, H. B. Burchell, and J. E. Edwards: Isolated Ventricular Septal Defect of the Persistent Common Atrioventricular Canal Type, Circulation, 28:685–696, 1961.*)

At present, repair of the defect and insertion of a total aortic valve prosthesis appears to be the only procedure assuring an excellent hemodynamic response. Such patients, therefore, are not subjected to operation unless they have significant and progressing symptoms.

Surgical Treatment. Surgical methods have now been developed to the point that complete repair usually results and heart block is rare.[36,37] The high-lying ventricular septal defect is the most commonly encountered and the most difficult to repair.[38] Direct suture is employed for many moderate-sized defects in this area, while closure of large defects is made with a knitted Teflon prosthesis or occasionally with pericardium. Knowledge of the course of the main bundle of His allows the stitches to be placed without injury to it.[39] The area between each stitch is palpated with a fine probe in order to assure complete closure. If even a tiny aperture is found, an additional stitch is placed. Those high defects that lie anteriorly, and

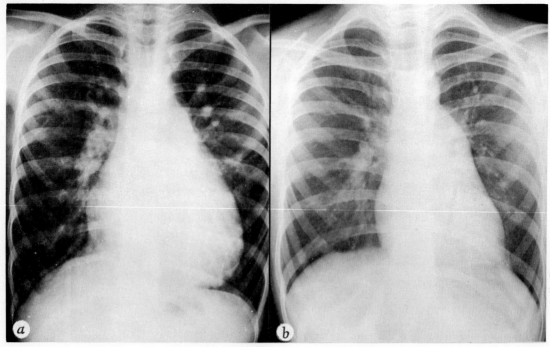

Fig. 21-8. *a.* Large left-to-right shunt and moderate pulmonary hypertension. Note cardiac enlargement and evidence of large pulmonary blood flow. Condition is operable since pulmonary vascular resistance must be significantly less than systemic resistance. (This and subsequent roentgenograms and angiocardiograms are presented with the assistance of Dr. Owings Kincaid, Section of Roentgenology, Mayo Clinic.) *b.* Ventricular septal defect, severe pulmonary hypertension, pulmonary flow similar to systemic flow and severe pulmonary vascular disease; condition is inoperable. Note large pulmonary artery shadow, tapering of branches of the pulmonary arteries, absence of evidence of pulmonary plethora, and normal-sized heart. (*Reproduced with permission from J. W. Kirklin and J. W. DuShane: Indications for Repair of Ventricular Septal Defects, Am. J. Cardiol., 12:75–79, 1963.*)

thus immediately beneath the pulmonary valve ring, are closed by suture or a patch, and the stitches may be placed without fear of injury to the bundle of His, which is well posterior to the defect. The cusps of the aortic valve must be visible during the placement of each stitch along the cephalad border of the defect, lest they be injured. Defects in the muscular portion of the septum can usually be closed by direct suture. Ventricular septal defects of the atrioventricular canal type[40] are triangular and should always be closed with a patch.

A median sternotomy and cardiopulmonary bypass are used.[41,42] Since a precise, atraumatic repair requires excellent exposure, which is best obtained by temporary interruption of coronary flow, the myocardium is thoroughly cooled by the perfusate and external cardiac cooling prior to aortic cross-clamping to minimize the ill effects of the period of ischemia. The defect is routinely approached through a transverse incision in the anterior wall of the right ventricle.

Postoperative care must be precisely managed, with prime attention being given to maintenance of optimal cardiac performance.[43,44]

Results of Operation. A recent review of experience at the Mayo Clinic since 1960 with repair in 689 cases of ventricular septal defect (isolated and as part of the tetralogy of Fallot) indicates the incidence of *permanent heart block* to be 0.9 per cent.[37] This confirms our previous observations[36] that a proper surgical technique can nearly prevent the occurrence of this catastrophic complication. *Recurrent or residual shunts* occur in 5 to 10 per cent of the cases of large ventricular septal defects in spite of meticulous technique, but they are rarely of sufficient magnitude to require reoperation.

Hospital Mortality. This has been zero following repair of small or moderate-sized ventricular septal defects since 1960 in our clinic. All the patients (100 per cent) with large defects survived the period of hospitalization when pulmonary vascular disease was mild; 90 per cent survived when it

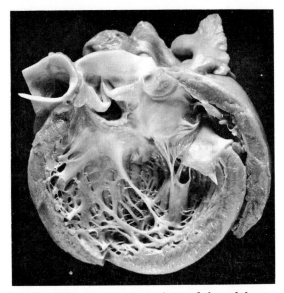

Fig. 21-9. Necropsy specimen (viewed from left ventricular aspect) from a patient with ventricular septal defect and aortic valve incompetence. Note prolapse and deformity of right aortic cusp. (*Reproduced wtih permission from F. H. Ellis, Jr., P. A. Ongley, and J. W. Kirklin: Ventricular Septal Defect with Aortic Valvular Incompetence: Surgical Considerations, Circulation, 27:789–795, 1963.*)

was moderate; and 85 per cent when it was severe; these figures are based on our experience since 1960.[37] Infants less than age 6 months are at present treated by pulmonary artery banding, since open repair was associated with a 63 per cent mortality in this group.[45] Pulmonary artery banding can be accomplished at a risk of about 15 per cent. The mortality for repair of large ventricular septal defects in infants between 7 and 24 months of age has been 7 per cent, a rate sufficiently low that primary repair is considered by us the treatment of choice when operation is required at these ages.

Late Results. These have been excellent in patients with no or mild pulmonary vascular disease. Those with moderate pulmonary vascular disease have usually been improved by operation, although their exercise tolerance is often not normal. This is probably related to the residual hypertension in the pulmonary artery. The results, both early and late, have been uniformly poor in patients with severe pulmonary vascular disease and a P/S resistance ratio of about 1 or greater. Insufficient data are at present available to decide about the value of repair in patients with severe pulmonary vascular disease and a P/S resistance ratio between about 0.75 and 0.9. Regression of the pulmonary vascular disease under these circumstances has not been docu-

mented; in a few cases it appears to have progressed. Yet closure of the defect may prevent progression of the disease in some patients.

COMMON ATRIOVENTRICULAR CANAL

Surgical Pathology (Fig. 21-10) and Diagnosis. Diagnosis of the *partial* form of common atrioventricular canal is based in part on the physical and roentgenologic signs of right ventricular dilatation and increased pulmonary blood flow. In contrast to patients with ostium secundum defects, these individuals usually have in addition apical systolic murmur and an electrocardiogram characterized by a counterclockwise QRS loop in the frontal projection.[46–48]

Patients with the *complete* form of common atrioventricular canal have the signs of severe pulmonary hypertension in early life, and they usually exhibit significant symptoms.

The clinical diagnosis of partial or complete forms of atrioventricular canal is confirmed by demonstration of the typical "goose-neck" outflow tract of the left ventricle in the left ventricular angiocardiogram (Fig. 21-11).[49]

Life History. Patients with a *partial* form of atrioventricular canal on occasion have severe incompetence at the mitral valve. Such patients usually have significant symptoms within the first two decades of life. With only mild or moderate incompetence at the mitral valve, patients are often without symptoms (other than growth failure) until the second or third decade, when fatigue and exercise intolerance appear. In the third and fourth decades, chronic heart failure appears, and on occasion pulmonary vascular disease develops. Some patients with the partial form of atrioventricular canal do develop congestive heart failure in infancy. Patients with the *complete* form of common atrioventricular canal often die in infancy or childhood in congestive heart failure. Severe hypertension in the pulmonary artery is the rule, and pulmonary vascular disease has often progressed to a severe degree in those children surviving to the second decade.

Indications for Operation. In view of the results of operation for this condition and the life history without operation, surgical treatment is believed advisable for all patients with the partial form of common atrioventricular canal and no, mild, or moderate incompetence of the mitral valve. The ideal age for operation is between 5 and 6 years. Individuals with this lesion and severe incompetence at the mitral valve (occurring in only 7 per cent of·cases) have been difficult to treat surgically; therefore, operation is deferred at the present unless significant symptoms appear.[50]

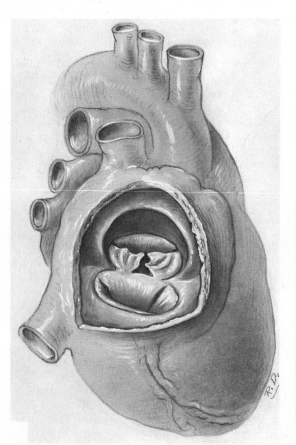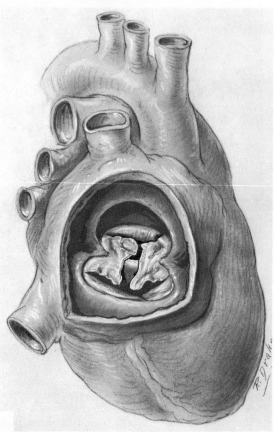

Fig. 21-10. Diagrammatic representation of common atrioventricular canal. *a*. Partial form. There are an inter-atrial communication of the ostium primum type and a cleft in the anterior leaflet of the mitral valve. Note absence of interventricular communication. *b*. Complete form, identified by the interventricular communication and the cleft in the septal leaflet of the tricuspid valve as weyy as in the anterior leaflet of the mitral valve. (*Reproduced with permission from J. C. Cooley, J. W. Kirklin, and H. G. Harshbarger: The Surgical Treatment of Persistent Common Atrioventricular Canal, Surgery, 41:147–152, 1957.*)

All patients with the complete form of this malformation should be operated on unless the P/S resistance ratio puts them into an inoperable category. Operative risks are high (see p. 463), but the prognosis in such cases makes surgical treatment nonetheless advisable. Operation is sometimes necessary in the first few years of life because of serious symptoms.

Surgical Treatment. The operation for repair of the *partial form* is done with cardiopulmonary bypass. A prosthesis is necessary for closure of the interatrial communication in nearly all cases, and we believe that the pericardium is clearly the material of choice for this. If no or mild incompetence is present at the mitral valve, the notch or cleft in the anterior leaflet of the mitral valve or any accessory orifices in the leaflets may be left undisturbed.

If moderate incompetence is present, the cleft is closed with interrupted No. 5-0 silk sutures.[51] If the incompetence is severe and repair in this fashion does not afford significant improvement, replacement of the valve with a prosthesis may be required.

Repair of the *complete form* of common atrioventricular canal is not yet a standardized procedure, since no one technique has yielded a high incidence of satisfactory results. Insufficient leaflet tissue often frustrates attempts to achieve competence of the atrioventricular valves. Because of the anatomy of the subaortic region of the left ventricle, significant stenosis results in this area from repair of the interventricular communication unless particular care is taken to avoid it. Complete heart block is an ever-present hazard, the incidence of which can be minimized, however, by bearing in mind the location of the bundle of His as sutures are being placed. The most satisfactory technique at present employs the creation of a separate anterior mitral leaflet and septal tricuspid leaflet by suture of the clefts and then by appropriate incisions in the common atrioventricular valve, a pericardial patch to close the interventricular and interatrial communications, and reattachment of the newly created anterior leaflet of the mitral valve to the left side of the pericardial septum and of the newly created septal leaflet of the tricuspid valve to the right side.

Results. Hospital mortality rates have been low (3.9 per cent of the 123 patients operated on in our clinic) following repair of the *partial form* of common atrioventricular canal. Actually in our institution there have been no deaths among patients with no or mild incompetence at the mitral valve. Heart block has not occurred in the last 92 consecutive cases. Late results have been excellent, except in that small group of cases with severe incompetence at the mitral valve. In this group, some patients have shown persistent severe incompetence after operation.

Hospital mortality has been high in the *complete form*, being more than 50 per cent in most series. The chief cause of death is low cardiac output,

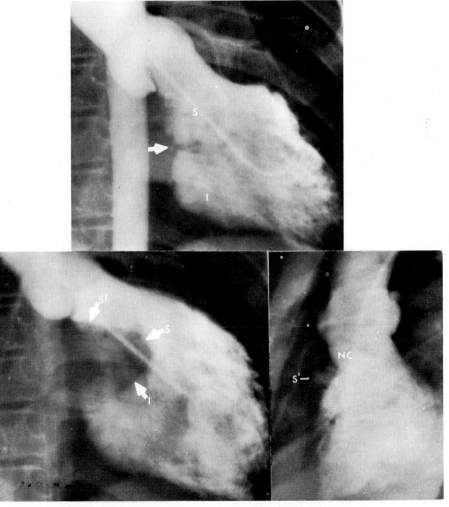

Fig. 21-11. Left ventricular angiocardiogram of a patient with partial form of common atrioventircular canal. The gooseneck-like appearance of outflow tract of left ventricle is caused by the mode of attachment of the anterior leaflet of the mitral valve in this malformation. (*Reproduced with permission from M. G. Baron, B. S. Wolf, Leonard Steinfeld, and L. H. S. Van Mierop: Endocardial Cushion Defects: Specific Diagnosis by Angiocardiography, Am. J. Cardiol.,* **13:**162–175, 1964.)

which is related largely to incompetence of the atrioventricular valves after repair and to the usual presence of significant degrees of pulmonary vascular disease. All survivors have some incompetence of atrioventricular valves, but most of them have obtained a good result.

ATRIAL SEPTAL DEFECT

Surgical Pathology (Fig. 21-12) and Diagnosis. The diagnosis of a large left-to-right shunt at the atrial level can usually be made clinically on the basis of the fixed splitting of the second heart sound at the base, the soft ejection type of murmur in the second and third left interspaces, the right ventricular lift, and the characteristic chest roentgenogram. Defects of the atrioventricular canal type are excluded with a high degree of accuracy by the electrocardiographic findings.[48] We do not use cardiac catheterization routinely prior to operation in

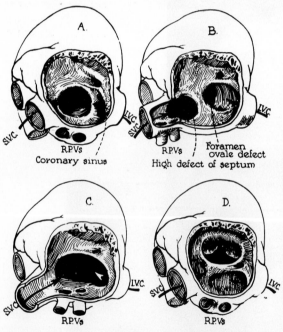

Fig. 21-12. Types of interatrial communications. *A.* Large ostium secundum type of atrial septal defect. *B.* So-called sinus venosus type of defect—one high in the atrial septum associated with anomalous connection of the right superior pulmonary vein to the junctional area of the superior vena cava and right atrium. *C.* Very large ostium secundum type of atrial septal defect with absence of the posterior rim. *D.* Partial form of common atrioventricular canal with cleft mitral valve. (*Reproduced with permission from F. J. Lewis, Paul Winchell, and F. A. Bashour: Open Repair of Atrial Septal Defects: Results in Sixty-three Patients, J.A.M.A.,* **165:**922–927, 1957.)

uncomplicated cases. It is prudent, however, to advise cardiac catheterization prior to operation in cases without classic findings. When there is evidence of hypertension in the pulmonary artery, values for pulmonary and systemic resistance should be obtained by cardiac catheterization so that operability can be assessed.

Life History. In rare instances of atrial septal defect, chronic heart failure and severe retardation of growth develop in infancy. Commonly no symptoms are present in early life, but when the shunt is large, some degree of growth failure is evident. Some patients have no symptoms until the fourth, fifth, or sometimes sixth decade, when fatigue, retention of fluid, and hepatomegaly become apparent and progress slowly until they cause invalidism and death.[52] In such patients, interestingly, significant pulmonary vascular disease has not ordinarily developed. Yet rapidly progressing pulmonary vascular disease does develop in the occasional patient with atrial septal defect; this seems to occur most often in females in the second or third decade of life and after pregnancy.

Indications for Operation. The risks are low and the results excellent after repair of atrial septal defect (see "Results"). This plus knowledge of the life history of the disease indicates that repair should be advised for all patients with uncomplicated atrial septal defect of such a size as to produce clinical evidence of hemodynamic derangement (which occurs when the left-to-right shunt is about 30 per cent or greater). The ideal age for operation is about 5 or 6 years. Operation, however, can yield excellent results in patients as old as 68 years.

Severe pulmonary vascular disease, with a P/S resistance ratio of more than about 0.9, is a contraindication to operation (see above). Special attention must be given in adult patients to the status of the mitral valve. Repair of atrial septal defect in the presence of uncorrected stenosis or incompetence at the mitral valve results in sudden left atrial and pulmonary venous hypertension. An asymptomatic patient thus may be converted into a severely symptomatic one. Patients with atrial septal defect and moderate or severe incompetence at the mitral valve should be advised against operation until signs or symptoms are severe enough to justify replacement of the mitral valve with a prosthesis should such an extreme measure be necessary to correct the lesion.

Surgical Treatment. Various methods have been used to repair these lesions, but our preference in recent years has been the use of cardiopulmonary bypass with normothermic whole-body perfusion. The only absolute protection against air embolism is the prevention of cardiac action while the left side of the heart is open, i.e., while the defect is open. Therefore, ventricular fibrillation is induced electrically prior to opening the heart, the left atrium is not emptied of blood, and the atrial septal defect is closed before the heart is allowed to beat.

Ostium secundum and foramen ovale defects can usually be closed by suture. High atrial septal defects,[53] associated with anomalous pulmonary venous connection of the right superior pulmonary vein to the junctional area between the superior vena cava and the right atrium, can often be repaired by suture in children; in adults a patch of pericardium is usually employed (Fig. 21-13).

Results. The hospital mortality rate is low, and results are excellent after these operations in uncomplicated cases. A number of clinics, including our own, have experienced no deaths in a large series of these operations on children and young adults and have reported a mortality rate of about 5 per cent among patients who are more than 40 years of age. Late results in uncomplicated cases are superb.

Adult patients sometimes have chronic heart failure with moderate incompetence at mitral and tricuspid valves, which is presumed to be secondary to ventricular dilatation. Mild pulmonary vascular disease may be present. Repair of the atrial septal defect and of the incompetent atrioventricular valve, if the incompetence is marked, usually eradicates the signs and symptoms of chronic heart failure, although in some patients ventricular failure

(used here to designate a state in which the ventricular function curve is chronically depressed) continues after operation. Obviously, repair of the defect prior to this stage is desirable.

Patients with pulmonary vascular disease respond to operation in a manner similar to that outlined for other lesions.

TOTAL ANOMALOUS PULMONARY VENOUS CONNECTION

Surgical Pathology (Fig. 21-14) and Diagnosis. The diagnosis can often be suspected from a history of persistent mild cyanosis and physical findings of precordial bulge and left sternal lift from an enlarged right ventricle, fixed splitting of the second sound at the base, and a normal or mildly accentuated pulmonary second sound. The electrocardiographic evidence usually allows the distinction of this lesion from common atrium. The chest roentgenogram is often diagnostic when the connection is to the left brachiocephalic vein via a persistent left vertical vein (Fig. 21-15). Cardiac catheterization is advisable in many cases for confirmation of the diagnosis and estimation of the P/S resistance ratio.

Life History. Death may occur in infancy in patients with total anomalous pulmonary venous connection, particularly when the connection is to the left brachiocephalic vein, to the portal vein, or to the inferior vena cava. Children with these

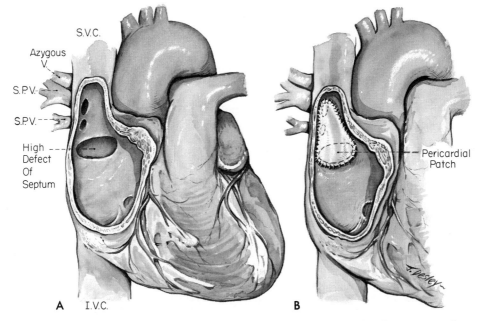

Fig. 21-13. A. High atrial septal defect associated with anomalous connection of right superior pulmonary vein. B. Repair is effected with a pericardial patch, so placed as to divert pulmonary venous blood across the defect into the left atrium and to divert superior vena caval blood to the right atrium.

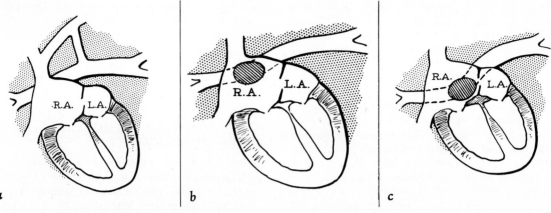

Fig. 21-14. Schematic representation of drainage of common pulmonary venous sinus. *a.* To left innominate vein via a persistent left vertical vein. *b.* Directly to right atrium. *c.* To coronary sinus. (*Reproduced with permission from Kirklin, J. W.: Corrective Surgical Treatment for Cyanotic Congenital Heart Disease, in A. D. Bass and G. K. Moe, "Congenital Heart Disease," American Association for the Advancement of Science, Washington, 1960, pp. 329–344.*)

lesions often exhibit marked growth retardation and limitation of exercise tolerance, but some survive into young adult life. Progressing pulmonary vascular disease may render some patients progressively more cyanotic[54] and ultimately make their condition inoperable.

Indications for Operation. In view of the significant and progressing nature of the disability from this lesion, and the good results from surgical treatment (except in infants), the lesion is considered an indication for operation. The optimal age for operation is 5 to 6 years, but excellent results have been obtained in some patients operated on in adult life.

Infants in trouble from this lesion pose a particularly difficult problem (see "Results"); yet some type of operative intervention is clearly necessary.

Surgical Treatment. Rerouting the pulmonary venous return to the left atrium is rendered feasible in most cases by the presence of a common pulmonary venous sinus posterior to the pericardium.[55] The pulmonary veins usually converge into it, and the common sinus in turn drains to the left brachiocephalic vein, coronary sinus, right atrium, superior vena cava, inferior vena cava, or portal vein. An atrial septal defect exists in all cases.

When the connection is to the coronary sinus, repair is made by a procedure which closes the interatrial communication in such a way that the coronary sinus now drains to the left atrium. Similarly, a direct anomalous connection to the right atrium is treated by closing the interatrial communication in such a way that the orifice of the anomalous connection drains to the left atrium.[56] When the anomalous connection is via a left vertical vein to the left brachiocephalic vein, an anastomosis is made between the common pulmonary venous sinus behind the heart and the left atrium. The persistent vertical vein is ligated, and the interatrial communication is closed. A similar

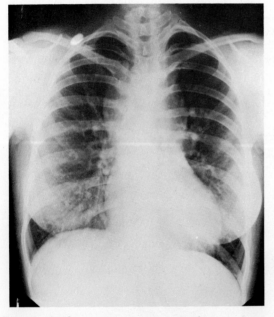

Fig. 21-15. Characteristic roentgenographic appearance produced by total anomalous pulmonary venous connection to the left innominate vein. Note shadows along each side of the superior mediastinum, produced on the left by the large persistent left vertical vein, and on the right by the markedly enlarged superior vena cava. (*Reproduced with permission from O. W. Kincaid: Approach to the Roentgenologic Diagnosis of Congenital Heart Disease, J.A.M.A., **173**:637–647, 1960.*)

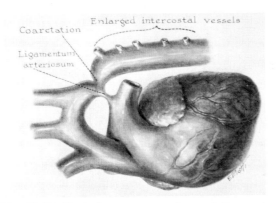

Fig. 21-16. Typical appearance of coarctation aorta at level of ligamentum arteriosum. (*Reproduced with permission from R. E. Gross: "The Surgery of Infancy and Childhood: Its Principles and Techniques," W. B. Saunders Company, Philadelphia, 1953, 1,000 pp.*)

type of repair can be accomplished for patients with drainage to the portal vein.[57]

Results. In patients more than about 1 year of age, results of operation for total anomalous pulmonary venous connection are good. The hospital mortality rate has been low, and the late results are excellent.[58] Unless significant pulmonary vascular disease has been present, these patients can be considered to be cured by operation.

The problem is much more difficult in sick, very young infants. The pulmonary veins usually drain into the left brachiocephalic or a subdiaphragmatic vein. Pulmonary venous hypertension may be severe, and pressure in the pulmonary artery may be higher than in a systemic artery. The mortality rate following surgical correction has been high. In view of this, Mustard and associates[59] have recommended a two-stage operation. The first stage consists of making an anastomosis between the common pulmonary venous sinus and left atrium and closing the atrial septal defect. The second stage consists of ligation of the left vertical vein several years later. Another method of staging employed in a few cases by McGoon consists of enlarging the atrial septal defect, which is usually very small in infants critically ill from this malformation. Definitive repair then can be done as a second stage several years later. Success has been obtained with both one-stage and two-stage operations for total anomalous pulmonary venous connection in some sick small infants. The mortality rate remains relatively high, however, in this particular group regardless of the procedure performed. Additional knowledge of the factors leading to the extreme pulmonary venous hypertension and improvements in the techniques for open-heart surgery in very young infants will be required for more satisfactory management of this particular problem.

COARCTATION OF AORTA

Surgical Pathology (Figs. 21-16 and 21-17) and Diagnosis. Absence or marked dimunition of pulsations in the femoral arteries of young patients is the basic clue to the diagnosis of coarctation of the aorta. Arterial hypertension in the upper part of the body and evidence on physical examination and in the chest roentgenogram of collateral circulation around the coarctate area are confirmatory signs, although the latter usually are not present until the patient is about 8 to 10 years of age.

In patients with the classic findings, confirmation of the diagnosis by aortography is unnecessary. In infants and other patients in whom associated lesions or unusual forms of coarctation are suspected, special study is useful, including visualization of the upper part of the thoracic aorta by angiographic techniques.

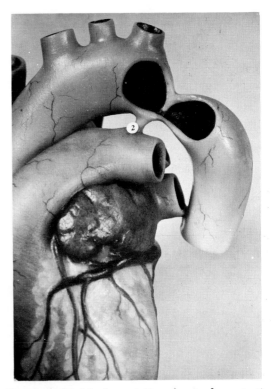

Fig. 21-17. Model of coarctation of aorta demonstrating that the lumen through the coarctate area is always smaller than would be suspected from the external appearance. (*Reproduced with permission from J. E. Edwards, T. J. Dry, R. L. Parker, H. B. Burchell, E. H. Wood, and A. H. Bulbulian: "An Atlas of Congenital Anomalies of the Heart and Great Vessels," Charles C Thomas, Publisher, Springfield, Ill., 1954, 202 pp.*)

Life History. On occasion infants with coarctation of the aorta have congestive heart failure in the early weeks of life. Relief can be given to some by medical management, but others will die if surgical intervention is not instituted.[60] Most patients with only coarctation of the aorta do not have symptoms in early life and enter adolescence well developed and in good health. Death usually occurs in the second and third decades of life from the complications of hypertension (cerebral hemorrhage or cardiac failure) or from rupture of aneurysm in the area of coarctation.[61]

Indications for Operation. The presence of coarctation of the aorta is an indication for surgery. The ideal age for this is between 8 and 12 years. Operation is advised even at 5 or 6 years of age

if hypertension or cardiomegaly is unusually marked. Some relief of hypertension can be accomplished even in the sixth decade of life, and unless degenerative disease is advanced in the region of the coarctation, operation at this age should be advised. Infants with coarctation of the aorta and congestive heart failure in the first few weeks of life should be treated by operation when prompt relief of cardiac failure is not effected by a strict medical regimen. The high incidence of associated cardiac lesions, however, should be recognized, particularly in causes of preductile coarctation.[62]

Surgical Treatment. Resection and end-to-end anastomosis can be accomplished in most patients[63,64] (Figs. 21-18 and 21-19). In 5 to 10 per cent of patients, usually those with aneurysm

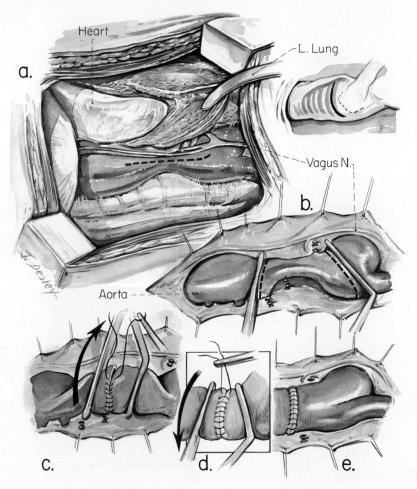

Fig. 21-18. Steps in operative repair of coarctation of aorta. *a.* Mediastinal pleura is opened over the upper part of the descending thoracic aorta. *b.* After appropriate mobilization of coarctate area and division of ligamentum arteriosum, appropriate clamps are placed above and below the stricture. At times the distal clamp must be placed more downstream than in the illustration, and then the intercostal arteries are temporarily controlled with bulldog clamps. *c, d,* and *e.* End-to-end anastomosis is made with interrupted simple sutures of No. 5-0 silk.

secondary to the coarctation, adequate resection of the coarctate area in the presence of the pathologic anatomy precludes direct anastomosis, and a tubular prosthesis (usually of knitted Dacron) is required for restoration of continuity. In a few older patients, in whom the pathologic anatomy appears to make resection unusually hazardous, the procedure of bypassing the obstruction, suggested by Morris, Cooley, De Bakey, and Crawford,[65] is useful.

In children, particularly, the surgeon must assure himself of a well-developed collateral circulation around the coarctation before operation. If it is not clearly present, it should be searched for by aortography. When it is not present (as the result of only moderate aortic obstruction or of a patent ductus arteriosus supplying the distal aorta), paraplegia may result unless the patient is cooled to about 33°C to protect the spinal cord from ischemia during aortic cross-clamping.[66]

Results. Hospital mortality rates are low, and early results are excellent. Schuster and Gross[67] reported a hospital mortality rate of 2.1 per cent in a large series of cases. Hospital mortality rate can be low even for small infants.

Late results also are excellent.[68] Normotension is established in most patients. When the operation is necessary in infancy, relief of congestive heart failure is dramatic. A few patients operated on at this early age require reoperation at about 12 years of age because of recurrence of the coarctation due to inadequate growth of the anastomosis.

CONGENITAL AORTIC STENOSIS

Surgical Pathology (Figs. 21-20 to 21-23) and Diagnosis. The characteristic loud systolic murmur of the stenotic type in the second and third interspaces to the left and right of the sternum, which usually extends to the neck, is the basis for the diagnosis of congenital aortic stenosis. A narrow pulse pressure is often present. There may or may not be clinical, roentgenographic, or electrocardiographic evidence of left ventricular hypertrophy.

The association of a peculiar facies and mental retardation with such findings suggests that the stenosis is supravalvular,[69] although many patients with supravalvular aortic stenosis have normal facies and normal mental development. Patients with supravalvular stenosis sometimes have diminished femoral and left brachial pulsations, compared to right brachial pulsation. The commonest form of congenital aortic stenosis is valvular stenosis. A soft, short diastolic murmur over the base of the heart raises the suspicion of localized subvalvular stenosis. A family history of congenital

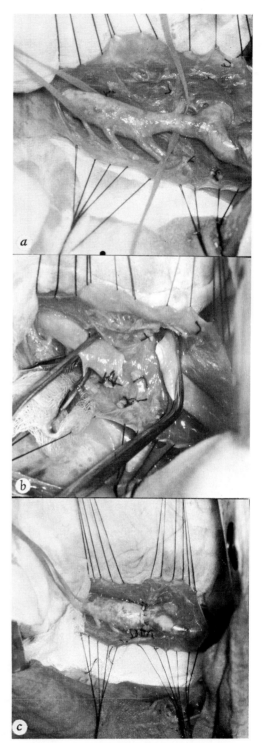

Fig. 21-19. *a.* Exposure of coarctate area, ligamentum arteriosum, and intercostal arteries. *b.* Occluding devices are in place and the coarctate area has been excised. *c.* End-to-end anastomosis has been established.

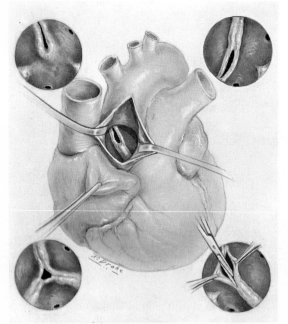

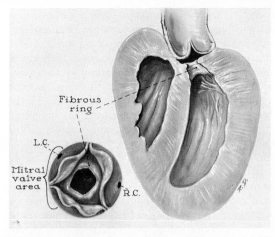

Fig. 21-21. Localized subvalvular aortic stenosis. Obstruction is immediately upstream from the aortic valve. (*Reproduced with permission from J. W. Kirklin and F. H. Ellis, Jr.: Surgical Relief of Diffuse Subvalvular Aortic Stenosis, Circulation, 24:739–742, 1961.*)

Fig. 21-20. Types of valvular deformity in patients with congenital valvular aortic stenosis. (*Reproduced with permission from F. H. Ellis, Jr., and J. W. Kirklin: Congenital Valvular Aortic Stenosis: Anatomic Findings and Surgical Technique, J. Thoracic Surg., 43:199–202, 1962.*)

cardiac defect that might be aortic stenosis, a murmur best heard in the third and fourth left interspaces, evidence of mild mitral valve incompetence, and extreme left ventricular hypertrophy suggest diffuse subvalvular aortic stenosis.[70,71]

The severity of the stenosis can be judged by measurement of the systolic pressure difference

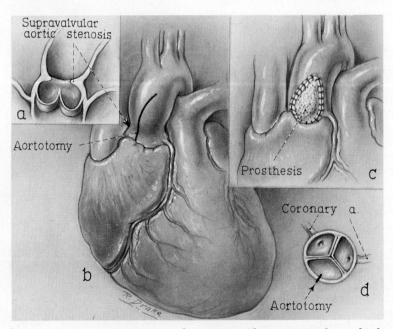

Fig. 21-22. *a* to *d*. Supravalvular aortic stenosis and its repair. Obstruction is almost diaphragmatic in nature (*a*) and is not easily recognized externally (*b*). *c*. The complete repair. (*Reproduced with permission from D. C. McGoon, H. T. Mankin, Peter Vlad, and J. W. Kirklin: The Surgical Treatment of Supravalvular Aortic Stenosis, J. Thoracic Surg., 41:125–133, 1961.*)

between the left ventricle and the ascending aorta.[72] Measurement of cardiac output at this time lends additional confidence in interpretation of these measurements. Angiocardiography can help in distinguishing between the various types of stenoses but is usually considered by us unnecessary.

Life History. A few patients with congenital aortic stenosis have acute left ventricular failure in infancy and die unless surgical treatment is undertaken promptly. In some patients chronic left ventricular failure develops in childhood. Syncope and angina may occur. A few patients die suddenly, presumably from ventricular fibrillation, in the first or second decade of life. Many live into adult life, when increasingly severe obstruction may develop as the malformed valve calcifies in those with valvular stenosis.

Indications for Operation. Operation is clearly indicated for the infant, child, or adult with syncope, angina, or evidence of left ventricular failure from congenital aortic stenosis. Decision is more difficult in patients without symptoms, but it has seemed reasonable to base advice on the adjudged severity of the stenosis and thus the probability of trouble from it. It has been our practice to consider operation rather urgently indicated when the difference in systolic pressures in the left ventricle and the ascending aorta is more than 80 mm Hg. When it is between 50 and 80 mm, operation is felt to be indicated at a time of election. When it is less than 50 mm, operation is considered unnecessary.

Surgical Treatment. Operation is done with a cardiopulmonary bypass. The heart is thoroughly cooled prior to aortic cross-clamping to protect it

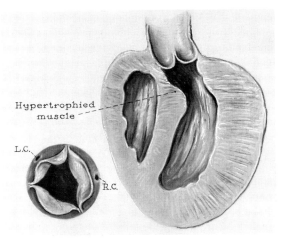

Fig. 21-23. Diffuse subvalvular aortic stenosis. Obstruction is diffuse and is a centimeter upstream from the aortic valve. When viewed surgically through an aortotomy, it usually cannot be seen. (*Reproduced with permission from J. W. Kirklin and F. H. Ellis, Jr.: Surgical Relief of Diffuse Subvalvular Aortic Stenosis, Circulation,* **24**:739–742, 1961.)

against ischemia while there is no coronary flow. The aorta is cross-clamped, and its root is opened to allow assessment and correction of the condition.[73,74] When the stenosis is valvular, the fused commissures are opened. When this is done precisely, incompetence does not result. A rudimentary raphe cannot always be opened without producing incompetence, and judgment must be used in differentiating the raphes to be incised from those to be left alone. Resection for localized subvalvular stenosis can be effected through the aortotomy. The anterior leaflet of the mitral valve must be

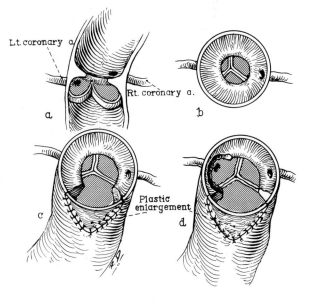

Fig. 21-24. *a* to *d*. Repair of supravalvular aortic stenosis. Since the intimal ridge partially obstructs the left sinus of Valsalva (*b* and *c*), that portion of the ridge overlying this sinus must be removed (*d*). The longitudinal aortotomy, made through the obstructing area, is then closed by insertion of a patch of pericardium or Teflon. This effectively enlarges the orifice and relieves the obstruction.

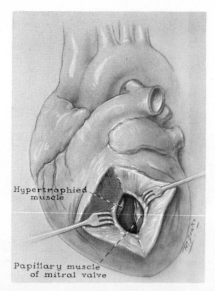

Fig. 21-25. Repair of diffuse subvalvular aortic stenosis. The approach is via left ventriculotomy, through which the hypertrophied muscle along the septum and anteriorly can be resected. (*Reproduced with permission from J. W. Kirklin and F. H. Ellis, Jr.: Surgical Relief of Diffuse Subvalvular Aortic Stenosis, Circulation,* **24:** 739–742, 1961.)

visualized and protected, and the resection must not be carried into the area occupied by the bundle of His. Special measures are necessary for the relief of supravalvular stenosis[75] and diffuse subvalvular stenosis[76] (Figs. 21-24 and 21-25).

Results. In general, hospital mortality rates are low and early results are satisfactory, but long-term results · are uncertain for patients with congenital valvular aortic stenosis.

Several centers have reported hospital mortality rates of less than 10 per cent following operation for congenital valvular and localized subvalvular aortic stenosis.[73,74,77] There have been no deaths at the Mayo Clinic following these procedures since 1960. We have operated on 12 patients with diffuse subvalvular aortic stenosis by the transventricular approach, with one death, and on 13 patients for supravalvular stenosis, with one death.

Following operations for localized subvalvular and supravalvular aortic stenosis, the systolic pressure gradient across the area is usually eliminated. Rarely, operations for localized subvalvular aortic stenosis have resulted in complete heart block. When the commissures are opened accurately and judiciously in the repair of congenital valvular stenosis, significant incompetence does not result. The severity of the stenosis is reduced by the commissurotomy, but some patients have persisting, significant differences in systolic pressure between

the left ventricle and the ascending aorta. This may be in part because of secondary subvalvular narrowing (which in some cases seems to regress following valvulotomy) and in part because of residual obstruction from the deformed cusps of the aortic valve. It seems likely that with the passage of years these deformed cusps may undergo further degenerative changes, including calcification, and significant stenosis may again be present.

STENOSIS OF PULMONARY VALVE WITH INTACT VENTRICULAR SEPTUM

Surgical Pathology (Figs. 21-26 and 21-27) and Diagnosis. Patients with this lesion are acyanotic when the atrial septum is intact but may become cyanotic when there is a patent foramen ovale. A prominent systolic murmur of the stenotic type is heard in the second and third interspaces to the left of the sternum.[78] Prominence of the left precordium, the electrocardiogram, and giant A waves in the venous pulse give evidence of right ventricular hypertrophy.[79] Poststenotic dilatation of the pulmonary artery is usually visible in the chest roentgenogram. The diagnosis can be confirmed by cardiac catheterization, although this is not necessary in many cases.

There is merit, from a surgical standpoint, in obtaining a right ventricular angiocardiogram prior

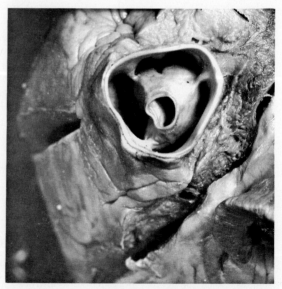

Fig. 21-26. Necropsy specimen illustrating classic features of stenosis of pulmonary valve. The valve is dome-shaped and there is fusion of the three commissures. (*Reproduced with permission from R. L. Parker: Pulmonary Stenosis: Tetralogy of Fallot, M. Clin. North America,* **32:**855–877, 1948.)

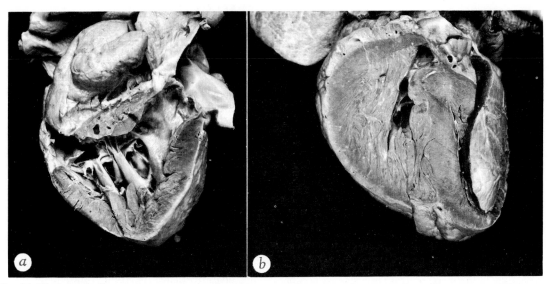

Fig. 21-27. Subvalvular area in patients with stenosis of pulmonary valve. *a.* Wide outflow tract of right ventricle. *b.* Massive subvalvular obstruction. In this case relief of valvular stenosis alone clearly would be inadequate. (*Reproduced with permission from J. W. Kirklin, D. C. Connolly, F. H. Ellis, Jr., H. B. Burchell, J. E. Edwards, and E. H. Wood: Problems in the Diagnosis and Surgical Treatment of Pulmonic Stenosis with Intact Ventricular Septum Circulation,* 8:849–863, 1953.)

to operation.[80] When it gives evidence of a wide subvalvular area and obstruction limited to the pulmonic valve itself, operation can be done through an incision in the pulmonary artery. When the subvalvular area is narrow, the approach should be through the right ventricle (see "Surgical Treatment").

Life History. Death may occur from this lesion in the first few days of life. Many patients tolerate it well until progressing severity, resulting usually from increase in subvalvular as well as valvular narrowing, causes massive right ventricular hypertrophy. Then hepatomegaly, retention of fluid, progressing invalidism, and death ensue—a series of events which often occurs late in the second decade of life. Cyanosis, polycythemia, and resultant progressing disability and death develop in patients with associated atrial septal defect.

The life history of children with mild pulmonary stenosis is not clearly understood at present. In some, progressively more severe obstruction probably does not develop.

Indications for Operation. Patients with cyanosis clearly require operation. Acyanotic patients with right ventricular systolic hypertension of more than about 70 mm Hg are advised to have operation, since it is likely their life expectancy is compromised. The decision for operation can best be made after studying during exercise patients whose systolic pressure in the right ventricle at rest is about 70 mm Hg, for a few such patients show

marked increase in pressure with exercise.[81] These should be operated on.

Surgical Treatment. Although some surgeons continue to employ simpler methods, it has been for some years our practice to use cardiopulmonary bypass in operations for pulmonic stenosis with essentially intact ventricular septum. When an atrial septal defect is present, even though small, it is closed via right atriotomy. The pulmonic valve is approached through a short vertical incision in the pulmonary artery when the stenosis is known from preoperative study to be limited to the valve. The rudimentary commissures are opened accurately with a small knife. The incision should be carried down on the ventricular side of the valve to the ring itself, in order that a complete opening can be made. When preoperative study or inspection at operation indicates that the pulmonary valve ring is small or that there is significant subvalvular narrowing during ventricular systole, a transverse incision is made in the outflow tract of the right ventricle. Pulmonary valvulotomy can be done accurately through this, essentially as described. The hypertrophied musculature of the right ventricle (which produces the subvalvular obstruction) extending up to the valve ring is excised. Often small incisions in the ring itself allow its enlargement by forceful dilation with curved forceps. Early in our experience enlargement of the outflow tract and valve ring by insertion of a plastic or pericardial patch seemed necessary on occasions. In recent years satisfactory results have been obtained without this.

Rarely, there is isolated infundibular pulmonary stenosis. In such cases, the hypertrophied septal and parietal bands of the crista and its body are excised through a transverse incision in the right ventricle. Complete relief of the stenosis usually results. A very small ventricular septal defect often exists in such cases and should be searched for and closed if present.[82]

Results. The hospital mortality rate in children with stenosis of the pulmonary valve and intact ventricular septum is low; 57 such patients have been operated on by us since 1960, without a death. The hospital mortality rate is somewhat higher in older patients because of the marked impairment in right ventricular performance that is usually present and often is associated with incompetence of the tricuspid valve.

Although in some patients there is evidence of regression of infundibular narrowing after valvulotomy alone, others fail to show this, and right ventricular hypertension persists. For this reason the associated subvalvular obstruction should be relieved surgically. Results are generally excellent when valvulotomy alone is done for *isolated* pulmonary stenosis, and valvulotomy *plus infundibular resection*, for valvular and subvalvular narrowing.[83-85] Relief of symptoms is usually complete, even though some incompetence of the pulmonary valve may result from even the most carefully performed pulmonary valvulotomy.[86]

TETRALOGY OF FALLOT

Surgical Pathology. Tetralogy of Fallot is a form of congenital heart disease in which there is a large ventricular septal defect with pulmonary stenosis of such severity that systolic pressure in the two ventricles is the same. The aorta is usually dextroposed and originates in part from the right ventricle. The wall of the right ventricle is hypertrophied (Fig. 21-28).

Diagnosis. Typically, patients with tetralogy of Fallot are cyanotic, although some with the same basic malformation and slightly less severe pulmonary stenosis are acyanotic. The heart is small and not hyperactive, and there is no evidence of pulmonary congestion, hepatomegaly, or retention of fluid. A harsh systolic murmur is usually present to the left of the sternum and is best heard in the second and third interspaces. The electrocardiogram gives evidence of right ventricular hypertrophy. There are usually polycythemia and clubbing of the fingers. Most of these patients squat after any exertion.

When clinical features are typical, patients can undergo operation without special studies. When features are atypical, cardiac catheterization and angiocardiography should be performed prior to operation (Fig. 21-29).

Life History. Occasionally, patients with tetralogy of Fallot have severe anoxic episodes in the early months of life, and death may occur in such an episode. Many patients with tetralogy of Fallot

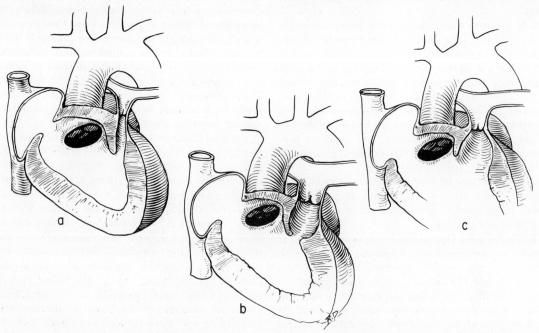

Fig. 21-28. Diagrammatic representation of tetralogy of Fallot and associated conditions. *a.* Valvular and subvalvular pulmonary stenosis. *b.* Isolated infundibular pulmonary stenosis. *c.* Isolated valvular pulmonary stenosis.

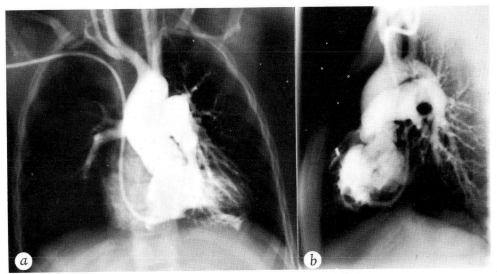

Fig. 21-29. Angiocardiogram made after injection of radiopaque medium into right ventricle. Note the simultaneous opacification of the markedly enlarged aorta (via the ventricular septal defect) and the pulmonary artery. *a.* Anteroposterior view showing narrow infundibulum of right ventricle. *b.* Lateral view again demonstrating narrow infundibulum. The aorta is moderately dextroposed.

exhibit *no* cyanosis in the early months or first few years of life. Actually, some individuals who are cyanosed from the typical malformation of tetralogy of Fallot at age 6 years have in early life evidence of a large ventricular septal defect, left-to-right shunt, and mild pulmonary stenosis (see "Ventricular Septal Defect," earlier in this chapter). Cyanosis and polycythemia usually increase gradually as time passes, primarily because of increasing severity of the pulmonic stenosis.

If the patient survives early infancy, death may occur late in the first decade or early in the second decade of life. Anoxic episodes, pulmonary hemorrhages, and cerebral infarction or abscess are the commonest causes of death. An occasional patient lives into adult life with only moderate cyanosis; very few have survived into the fifth and sixth decades of life.

Indications for Operation. Open intracardiac repair is advisable for all patients with tetralogy of Fallot, in view of the life history of patients with the malformation and the good results that can now be obtained by operation. It is performed as the primary procedure in patients who have reached the age of about 5 to 6 years, including those who are deeply cyanosed. Operation is deferred until about this age when patients seen earlier in childhood are in satisfactory condition. If cyanosis or symptoms are marked before the age of about 5 years, operation is performed promptly and usually consists of an anastomotic procedure. Open operation and closure of the anastomosis is then performed at about 6 years of age.

Surgical Treatment. *Anastomotic Operation.* Infants needing operative intervention before the age of about 1½ years are usually treated by us by the construction of a side-to-side aortopulmonary anastomosis (Potts's operation).[87] Body temperature is reduced to 33°C by surface cooling, and the left side of the thorax is entered through a posterolateral incision. An exclusion clamp of the Derra or Cooley type is placed across the aorta without mobilizing it. No attention need be paid to maintaining blood flow beyond the clamp as the baby is protected against paraplegia by the surface cooling. Side-to-side anastomosis then is made, with an internal diameter of about 4 mm between the aorta and the left pulmonary artery.

When the child is about 18 months or more of age, or whenever the aortic arch is on the right, end-to-side subclavian-pulmonary artery anastomosis (the Blalock operation)[88,89] is performed (Fig. 21-30). The subclavian artery originating from the brachiocephalic artery is chosen for anastomosis to the side of the corresponding pulmonary artery (the right if the aortic arch is on the left, and the left if the arch is on the right).

Open Intracardiac Repair. The repair is done through a median sternotomy with the aid of a pump-oxygenator.[90] The heart is protected against the ill effects of anoxia by thorough cooling, and the aorta is cross-clamped. The right ventricle is opened by a transverse incision. In about 85 per cent of cases the pulmonary stenosis can be effectively treated by excision of the hypertrophied crista supraventricularis with its septal and parietal

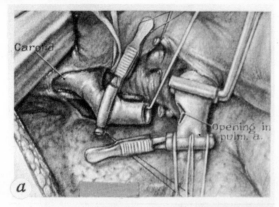

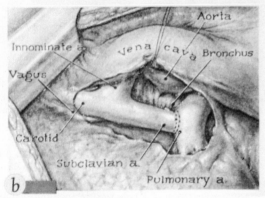

Fig. 21-30. Blalock operation on the right side. *a.* Previously divided right subclavian artery ready for anastomosis. Note the lack of angulation at the point of origin of the right subclavian artery from the innominate artery. (*Reproduced with permission from Alfred Blalock: Surgical Procedures Employed and Anatomical Variations Encountered in the Treatment of Congenital Pulmonic Stenosis, Surg. Gynec. & Obst.*, **87**:385–409, 1948.)

bands and mobilization of the free wall of the right ventricle.[91] Pulmonary valvulotomy is done also when there is obstruction at this level. In about 15 per cent of cases narrowing of the infundibulum and pulmonary valve ring requires enlargement by a patch of pericardium. The ventricular septal defect is nearly always repaired with a Teflon prosthesis. Care and precision must be used to achieve complete repair without the production of heart block.

A previously established aortopulmonary anastomosis must be closed prior to opening the heart or to the heart's becoming ineffective. When the anastomosis is of the Blalock type, it is dissected out before cardiopulmonary bypass is established, and ligation is done immediately after establishing bypass.[92] When the anastomosis is of the Potts type, it is closed from within the pulmonary artery after hypothermia and temporary total circulatory

arrest are induced.[93] Then the intracardiac repair is accomplished as usual.

Results. In general, the results of proper open repair of tetralogy of Fallot are now excellent. In early years, hospital mortality was high, but in the past 2 years (1963 and 1964) the hospital mortality rate among cyanotic patients at the Mayo Clinic has been 9 per cent. Patients with previous anastomotic operations (of either the Blalock or Potts type) have been subjected to operation at the same relatively low risk, unless they are more than about 15 years of age; the risk then is a little greater. This is because extensive collateral circulation has usually developed in those with Blalock's anastomoses, and pulmonary vascular disease may have developed in those with Potts's anastomoses. Permanent heart block occurred with disturbing frequency in the early years of definitive surgery. Since 1960, however, the incidence of this complication in our clinic has been reduced to 0.9 per cent because of the technique employed for repair of the ventricular septal defect. Complete and permanent repair of the ventricular septal defect and adequate relief of the pulmonary stenosis can be accomplished in nearly all cases.

Long-term results are superb after complete repair. Nearly all patients are asymptomatic and participate in strenuous physical activity. A number have become parents of normal children.

TRANSPOSITION OF GREAT ARTERIES

Surgical Pathology (Fig. 21-31). An atrial septal defect, ventricular septal defect, or patent ductus arteriosus is essential for survival in patients with transposition of the great arteries. Thus, in surgical correction, attention must be given to these associated lesions. Coarctation of the aorta may coexist with transposition, as may valvular or subvalvular pulmonic stenosis.

Diagnosis. The diagnosis should be suspected in deeply cyanotic infants and small children whose chest roentgenograms show cardiomegaly and varying degrees of pulmonary plethora (Fig. 21-32. Auscultation reveals no murmur in some patients; in others there is a short harsh precordial murmur over the left precordium from the associated ventricular septal defect or pulmonic stenosis. The characteristic electrocardiogram gives evidence of right ventricular hypertrophy in all cases, reflecting the fact that the right ventricle is the systemic ventricle. Left ventricular hypertrophy is associated in those patients with large ventricular septal defects or significant pulmonary stenosis.

The diagnosis of transposition can be confirmed by retrograde aortography. Mere confirmation of the basic diagnosis is no longer sufficient, however,

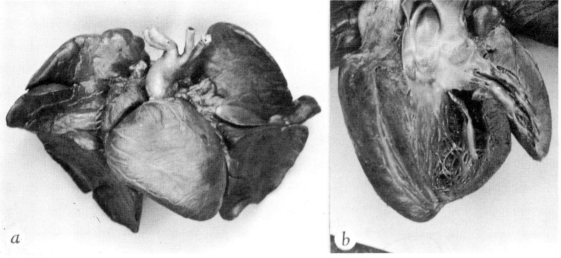

Fig. 21-31. Transposition of great arteries (aorta arising from right ventricle; pulmonary artery arising from left ventricle). *a.* Anterior external view. Aorta arises directly in front of the pulmonary artery which is hidden in this view. *b.* Left ventricle and base of pulmonary artery have been opened. Note relation of pulmonary valve to anterior leaflet of mitral valve. (*Reproduced with permission from J. E. Edwards, T. J. Dry, R. L. Parker, H. B. Burchell, E. H. Wood, and A. H. Bulbulian: "An Atlas of Congenital Anomalies of the Heart and Great Vessels," Charles C Thomas, Publisher, Springfield, Ill., 1954, 202 pp.*)

for every infant with this malformation should be considered for operation. Therefore, cardiac catheterization and angiocardiography are indicated for delineation of the anatomic features, identification of associated defects, and whenever possible, assessment of the extent of pulmonary vascular disease.

Life History. Many infants with transposition of the great arteries die in the first month of life, and 50 per cent are dead by the age of 6 months.[94] A few survive into childhood, and rarely a patient survives into young adult life. Those who do survive have, as a rule, either an atrial septal defect alone or a ventricular septal defect and pulmonic stenosis as the associated defects.

Pulmonary vascular disease exists in a high percentage of patients with transposition of the great arteries.[95] It is often severe by the age of 1 year and may in some instances render the patient's condition inoperable. The somewhat more favorable prognosis for patients who have as their associated lesion atrial septal defect or ventricular septal defect associated with pulmonic stenosis is due in large part to the lesser degree of pulmonary vascular disease ordinarily present.

Indications for Operation. In view of their very poor prognosis, all patients with transposition of the great arteries are candidates for operation. Since many die in the early weeks and months of life, the surgical approach must embrace techniques applicable to the very sick, very small baby.

Patients with transposition of the great arteries,

severe pulmonary vascular disease, and P/S resistance ratios of about 1 have inoperable conditions insofar as the present state of our knowledge goes. A palliative operation, such as creation of an atrial septal defect, can be accomplished but is not recommended by us in view of the poor prognosis for such patients no matter what the treatment.

Patients with associated pulmonary stenosis must be studied by angiocardiography to determine the correctability of the pulmonary stenosis. When the obstruction is in the valve between the left ventricle and the pulmonary artery, complete correction, including valvulotomy, may be accomplished successfully. When the obstruction is well localized beneath the valve, surgical relief should be possible. When the angiocardiogram reveals a long subvalvular narrowing and transposition of the great arteries, however, complete correction has been considered impossible. A subclavian-pulmonary artery anastomosis plus creation of an atrial septal defect may give some palliation.

Surgical Treatment. In infants 1 year of age or older, without a P/S resistance ratio of more than 0.9 or diffuse obstruction beneath the "pulmonary" valve, complete intracardiac repair is indicated. A number of successes have been obtained by surgically rearranging venous return so that systemic and coronary venous blood passes through the mitral valve and left ventricle to the pulmonary artery, and pulmonary venous blood passes through the tricuspid valve and right ventricle to the aorta. The principles of this operation were first described

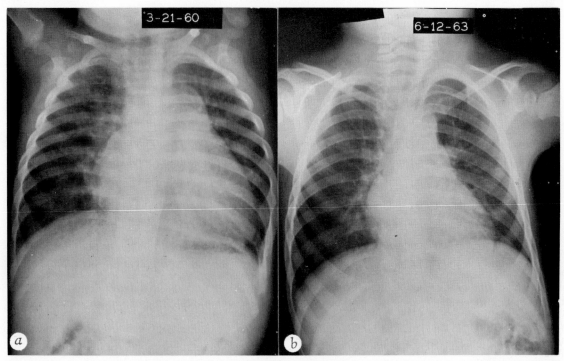

Fig. 21-32. Transposition of great arteries and ventricular septal defect. *a.* Note the cardiac enlargement of pulmonary plethora before repair in a 9-month-old infant. *b.* Same patient, 3 years after complete repair.

by Albert[96] and were first successfully applied clinically by Senning[97] in a 4-year-old child with atrial septal defect as the only associated lesion. Subsequently the operation was successfully performed in small infants with other associated lesions.[98] These defects, such as ventricular septal defect, patent ductus arteriosus, or pulmonary valvular stenosis, are repaired at the same time. The hospital mortality rate from complete repair among infants who are more than 1 year of age has been 56 per cent in our experience (until May 1, 1964). One of the patients operated on early by us is now 5 years of age and remains in excellent health (Fig. 21-32*b*). Mustard[99] has recently reported a modification of the technique of venous rearrangement, with only 2 deaths in the 8 cases in which he has employed it. We have now adopted his procedure and agree that it is safer and simpler than the Senning operation.

The mortality rate from complete intracardiac repair for transposition of the great arteries in infants *less than* 1 year of age has been 78 per cent in our hands. This excessive mortality must be related in large measure to subtle inadequacies in methods for cardiopulmonary bypass in the sick, small infant. At present, therefore, babies less than 1 year of age in urgent need of help because of transposition of the great arteries are treated by us by creation of an atrial septal defect or enlarge-

ment of the one present. This is done by open cardiotomy during moderate hypothermia induced by surface cooling and inflow stasis or by the Blalock-Hanlon operation[100] (Fig. 21-33). Complete repair is then performed when the patient is about the age of 18 to 24 months.

Comment. Surgical experience with complete intracardiac repair for transposition has indicated (1) that complete repair can be performed successfully, (2) that the long-term results can be good, and (3) that hospital mortality rates are decreasing. In view of these considerations and the lethal nature of this malformation, all babies with transposition of the great vessels should be considered for operation.

CORRECTED TRANSPOSITION OF GREAT ARTERIES

Surgical Pathology. The phrase "corrected transposition of the great arteries" describes a group of congenital malformations having in common the following characteristics: (1) The ascending aorta lies anterior and usually to the left of the pulmonary artery (the aorta is levotransposed). (2) The aorta arises nonetheless from the ventricle receiving pulmonary venous blood and lying to the left (i.e., the left ventricle) and the pulmonary artery from the ventricle receiving systemic venous blood and lying anteriorly and to the right (i.e., the right ventricle). Thus the transposition is physiologically "corrected." (3) The interior of the left ventricle morphologically resembles a normal right ventricle, and vice versa. (4) The left atrioventricular valve is tricuspid, and the right atrioventricular valve is bicuspid.

The malformation as described would not impair cardiac performance. Additional lesions are common,[101] however, including ventricular septal defect, ventricular septal defect and pulmonic stenosis, left atrioventricular valve incompetence, and single ventricle. The last is by definition a malformation in which both atrioventricular valves empty into the same ventricle;[102] there also may be a second rudimentary ventricle.

Diagnosis. The diagnosis is often first suspected from examination of the chest roentgenogram (Fig. 21-34). The electrocardiogram may afford further evidence of the lesion, since inversion of the ventricles alters the depolarization pattern in most instances. Deep Q waves in lead III and Q-R complexes in the right and R-S patterns in the left precordial leads probably reflect the abnormal distribution of the bundle of His. The infundibulum is not located in the right ventricle; thus the lack of a terminal R wave in a lead VR, particularly in the presence of right ventricular hypertension, might be expected.

Angiocardiography often is the definitive study

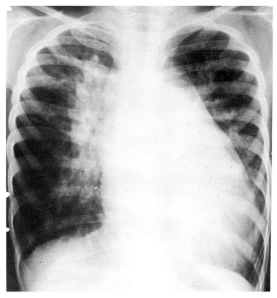

Fig. 21-34. Corrected transposition and ventricular septal defect. An oblique upper left border to the cardiac silhouette should always suggest corrected transposition.

(Fig. 21-35); it and catheterization of the right side of the heart are usually required to elucidate the sometimes complex anatomy.

Life History. The life history of patients with corrected transposition of the great arteries is in large part that of the associated lesions. In these

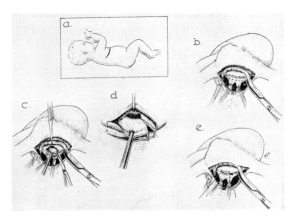

Fig. 21-33. *a* to *e*. Steps in the Blalock-Hanlon operation. By the use of an occluding clamp and an incision into the right atrium (*b* and *c*) anterior to the interatrial groove, and an incision into the left atrium posteriorly (*b* and *c*), a generous portion of the posterior aspect of the atrial septum is excised (*d*). Anterior lip of the right atrial incision is then sutured to posterior lip of left atrial incision (*e*). (*Reproduced with permission from J. L. Ochsner, D. A. Cooley, L. C. Harris, and D. G. McNamara: Treatment of Complete Transposition of the Great Vessels with the Blalock-Hanlon Operation, Circulation, 24:51–57, 1961.*)

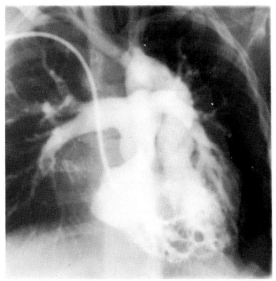

Fig. 21-35. Angiocardiogram made after injection of radiopaque medium into right ventricle, in a patient with corrected transposition of great arteries and ventricular septal defect. The aorta lies to the left of the pulmonary artery (i.e., it is levotransposed).

patients also there is a strong tendency toward a spontaneous gradual increase in the length of the P-R interval and finally to complete atrioventricular dissociation. Fatal Stokes-Adams episodes may then occur.

Indications for Operation. Theoretically, indications for operation for the associated lesions, such as ventricular septal defect or ventricular septal defect and pulmonary stenosis, are the same as those for the same lesions in patients without corrected transposition. Several facts negate such an approach, however:

1. The incidence of complete heart block after an operative procedure is relatively high in these patients, probably because of the same factors that lead to the spontaneous development of AV dissociation in them.

2. Many patients with corrected transposition and ventricular septal defect have associated significant incompetence of the left-sided atrioventricular valve, that cannot usually be corrected by a plastic procedure.

3. Pulmonary stenosis, when it exists in patients

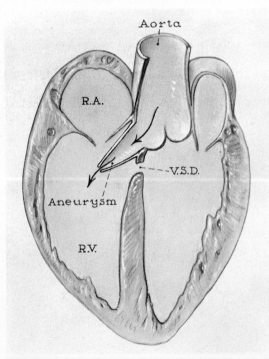

Fig. 21-36. Coronal section of heart showing aneurysm of the right sinus of Valsalva rupturing into the right ventricle. In this case there was an associated small ventricular septal defect. Note typical wind-sock appearance of the aneurysm and perforation at its tip. (*Reproduced with permission from D. C. McGoon, J. E. Edwards, and J. W. Kirklin: Surgical Treatment of Ruptured Aneurysm of Aortic Sinus, Ann. Surg., 147: 387–392, 1958.*)

with corrected transposition, is often subvalvular, is not easily relieved by simple resection, and cannot be corrected by insertion of a patch like that used in some cases of tetralogy of Fallot.

Thus patients are required to have considerably more disability before being submitted to operation than are those with similar defects but without corrected transposition. If operation is undertaken for patients with pulmonary stenosis as a part of their malformation, the angiocardiogram should show the stenosis to be at the valve and the subvalvular area to be wide.

Surgical Treatment. Experience is small and is primarily with the repair of ventricular septal defect in patients with corrected transposition of the great arteries. The defect is usually easily exposed; and the relation of the bundle of His to it is not well understood. In view of these facts and the great tendency of these patients toward complete atrioventricular dissociation with even minor cardiac manipulation, the repair is usually carried out at normothermia and with the heart beating. The defect is approached through an oblique incision in the right ventricle, which parallels the abnormal course of the coronary arteries.

Pulmonary valvulotomy, through an incision in the pulmonary artery, has been done successfully in a few patients, as have other miscellaneous procedures.

Comment. In recent years, good results have been obtained in the few patients with corrected transposition of the great arteries undergoing repair of the associated defects. Caution is indicated in selection of patients for operation and the technique of operation because of the special conditions presented by patients with this group of defects.

ANEURYSMS OF SINUS OF VALSALVA

Surgical Pathology (Fig. 21-36) and Diagnosis. Aneurysms of the sinus of Valsalva are asymptomatic and usually undetected until they rupture. Thereafter, a continuous murmur is present, heard variously over the left precordium but usually heard best in the third and fourth interspaces near the sternum. In some patients the heart is overactive, venous pressure is elevated, and fluid is retained. Rapid runoff of blood from the aorta, including wide pulse pressure and at times a collapsing pulse, is usually evident. The chest roentgenogram may be normal or may give evidence of increased pulmonary blood flow. The right atrium, right ventricle, or left ventricle may appear enlarged, depending on the site of rupture. Electrocardiographic findings mirror the same basic disturbance.

Although the diagnosis can often be strongly

suspected from the history of the sudden appearance of a continuous murmur, special studies are usually necessary before this entity can be distinguished positively from patent ductus arteriosus, aortopulmonary window, coronary arteriovenous fistula, or ventricular septal defect and aortic valve incompetence. Cardiac catheterization discloses arterialization of blood in the right atrium (rupture of aneurysm of noncoronary sinus of Valsalva) or right ventricle (rupture of aneurysm of right sinus of Valsalva). In the latter case there is often a small difference in systolic pressure in the inflow and outflow portions of the right ventricle, produced by the wind sock of the aneurysm. Aortography, with injection of radiopaque medium into the ascending aorta just downstream from the aortic valve, gives the most definitive information.

Life History. The life history of these patients is variable, and the prognosis depends presumably on the size of the rupture in the aneurysm and the resultant magnitude of the aortic runoff. Patients without rupture are asymptomatic. A few patients have no symptoms at the time of rupture and remain asymptomatic for a long period. Other patients, with presumably large ruptures and large shunts, become symptomatic at the time of rupture and pursue a rapidly progressing course until death. Others have symptoms soon after rupture but stabilize promptly, with resultant cardiac performance which remains adequate for a variable period.

Indications for Operation. The presence of a ruptured aneurysm of the sinus of Valsalva with or without symptoms is considered an indication for operation. The risk of operation is low, and the correction is complete.

Surgical Treatment. Surgical repair is based on the concept of pathogenesis proposed by Edwards and Burchell.[103] The aneurysm results from a defect in the attachment of the aortic root to the upper end of the ventricular septum. Thus, after excision of the aneurysm, the resultant defect is closed by reattaching the aortic wall to the upper end of the ventricular septum, either directly or with use of a patch.

When rupture has been into the right atrium, cardiopulmonary bypass is established, the ascending aorta is cross-clamped, and the right atrium is opened. The aneurysm with its perforation is visualized, and the base is clamped with right-angled forceps. The aortic root may now be unclamped without loss of blood through the ruptured aneurysm of the noncoronary sinus of Valsalva, and internal and external cooling of the heart is accomplished. The aorta is again cross-clamped. The aneurysm is excised, with care to viewing and protecting the aortic cusp. Closure is then made in a line transverse to that of the long axis of the aorta,

with one layer of interrupted silk sutures which grasp both the atrial and the aortic walls. Rarely a patch (pericardium) is necessary. When the aneurysm presents into the right ventricle, an essentially similar procedure is followed after exposure of the aneurysm through a transverse incision in the anterior wall of the right ventricle.

Results. Since only a small number of such cases have come to surgery, statistically significant numbers of cases managed by modern methods are not available for analysis. However, the hospital mortality in cases in which the aneurysm ruptures into the right atrium or the right ventricle is in most centers less than 5 per cent, and the results of operation are excellent.[104,105]

ORIGIN OF BOTH VESSELS FROM THE RIGHT VENTRICLE

Surgical Pathology (Fig. 21-37) and Diagnosis. The clinical picture in cases in which both vessels originate from the right ventricle without pulmonic stenosis is similar to that in cases of large ventricular septal defect. There are evidences of mild, moderate, or severe pulmonary vascular disease. The patients are usually acyanotic, because of the high degree of streamlining of flow of blood from the left ventricle across the outflow tract of the

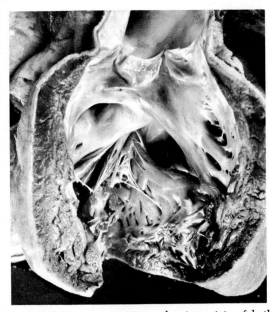

Fig. 21-37. Necropsy specimen showing origin of both vessels from right ventricle and large ventricular septal defect. The right ventricle and pulmonary artery have been opened. The orifice at the right of the specimen leads into the aortic root. Just to the left of this lies the ventricular septal defect. Both great vessels clearly originate *in toto* from right ventricle.

right ventricle to the aorta. On angiocardiography it is not always possible to distinguish between an ordinary ventricular septal defect and origin of both vessels from the right ventricle, but this procedure usually provides the most definitive diagnostic information.[106] Patients with this malformation plus pulmonary stenosis present clinical features usually indistinguishable from those of patients with the severe form of tetralogy of Fallot. Again, angiocardiography may suggest the exact pathologic anatomy.

Some patients will continue to appear in the operating room with the preoperative diagnosis of ventricular septal defect or tetralogy of Fallot. The surgeon, therefore, must always be prepared to identify the anatomy and carry out an appropriate repair.

Life History and Indications for Operation. These are ordinarily the same as for patients with large ventricular septal defects. For patients with origin of both vessels from the right ventricle plus pulmonary stenosis, however, they are the same as for patients with a severe form of the tetralogy of Fallot.

Surgical Treatment. When the pericardium is opened, the finding of the aorta in a slightly more anterior position than usual with the pulmonary artery in essentially normal position should make one suspect the malformation under discussion. The branches of the right coronary artery sometimes pursue an abnormal, rather oblique course across the anterior wall of the right ventricle, and the incision into the right ventricle must parallel them. When the ventricle is opened, the aorta is identified as arising entirely from the right ventricle, and the aortic valve cusps accordingly lie far to the right of the ventricular septal defect.[107,108] Repair is accomplished by creating a tunnel of pericardium which conducts left ventricular blood from the ventricular septal defect to the aorta while isolating it from the right ventricle.[109]

Surgical treatment of patients with pulmonary stenosis is similar to that of patients with tetralogy of Fallot, except that the interventricular communication must be managed as just described. The pulmonary stenosis, which is usually severe, can sometimes be relieved by valvulotomy and resection, but in some cases enlargement with a pericardial patch is necessary. Because of this, the location of the coronary arteries must be carefully assessed prior to cardiotomy. In a few cases, branches from the right coronary artery will traverse the outflow tract of the right ventricle in a manner which precludes the use of a pericardial patch in this area. If the coronary arteries are so arranged, and if external inspection indicates the high probability of the need for a pericardial patch,

open repair is contraindicated and an anastomotic operation is all that can be offered.

Comment. Origin of both vessels from the right ventricle has been treated surgically in too few cases to allow an accurate statistical estimate of the hospital mortality and late results. Suffice it to say that we have operated on 16 patients. In the early years, the mortality rate was high, particularly in patients with associated pulmonary stenosis. Since 1960, however, 4 patients without pulmonary stenosis and 4 with pulmonary stenosis have been operated on without any mortality. Long-term results have been good and are quite comparable to those obtained with isolated ventricular septal defect with comparable degrees of pulmonary vascular disease, and in severe forms of the tetralogy of Fallot.

CONGENITAL MITRAL VALVE DISEASE

Surgical Pathology. Congenital malformations of the mitral valve result in stenosis of the mitral orifice, incompetence of the valve, or a combination of both. The stenosis results from thickening of deformed leaflets and fusion of the commissures. The chordae tendineae are also thickened and shortened. Valvular incompetence results from an absolute or relative lack of valve substance. This may be a result of clefts in the valve leaflets, anomalous attachments of chordae tendineae, or accessory orifices.[110]

In 50 per cent of cases there is evidence of endocardial fibroelastosis.[111] Other lesions commonly associated with congenital mitral valve disease are patent ductus arteriosus, aortic stenosis, coarctation of the aorta, and abnormalities of the cusps of the aortic valve.

Diagnosis. Mitral valve lesions manifest themselves similarly whether the lesion is congenital or the result of acquired disease. The degree of cardiomegaly is often severe, as are the symptoms of pulmonary venous hypertension. The electrocardiogram reflects left atrial enlargement as well as right ventricular hypertrophy. In cases of mitral incompetence there is evidence of left ventricular hypertrophy. Cardiac catheterization and angiocardiography are helpful in determining the presence of associated defects and also in evaluating the character of the left ventricle when surgical correction is indicated.

Life History. Patients with severe malformation of the mitral valve usually become critically ill in infancy and often do not survive the first decade.[112] Patients with mild congenital mitral valve disease, particularly those in whom the main defect is valvular incompetence, may live into adult life.[113]

Indications for Operation. The indications for operation are tempered by knowledge of the frequent association of fibroelastosis and by the fact that congenitally diseased mitral valves are often highly abnormal and not amenable to simple reparative procedures. Thus patients with congenital mitral valve disease are ordinarily not subjected to operation unless the symptoms and signs are advanced and indicate that survival for more than a year or two is unlikely. Under these circumstances, the radical procedure of total replacement of the mitral valve, which might be required, is justified.

Surgical Treatment. Surgical techniques are similar to those for operations for acquired mitral disease. When a cleft or an accessory orifice is found to be the cause of incompetence, it is sutured. Annuloplasty is occasionally useful. Unfortunately, there is often a combination of stenosis and incompetence, and then only replacement of the valve seems effective. Fortunately, even relatively small children requiring the insertion of a mitral valve prosthesis have immense hearts that will usually accommodate an adult-size valve.

Comment. Relatively few patients with congenital mitral valve disease have been treated surgically. In a few instances in which reparative operation has proved feasible, the apparent result is good, although in most cases some residual mitral valve incompetence remains. The long-term results of the use of the Starr valve prosthesis in this situation are not known as yet.

VASCULAR RINGS

Surgical Pathology. Abnormalities in the embryologic development of the aortic arch may result in vascular rings capable of producing obstruction of the esophagus and trachea. Although several varieties are possible,[114] the commonest are double aortic arch and right aortic arch with retroesophageal segment and left-sided ligamentum arteriosum (Figs. 21-38 and 21-39).

Diagnosis. Noisy respiration, recurrent pulmonary infections, and dysphagia in the early months of life are suggestive of a vascular ring.[115] The diagnosis is usually made by fluoroscopic examination of the barium-filled esophagus. Bronchoscopy and esophagoscopy are unnecessary and hazardous.

In recent years it has become apparent that an exact delineation of the vessels comprising the vascular ring can be made by aortography. Since this has allowed more precise planning of operation prior to thoracotomy, it is considered advisable to perform this examination prior to operation.

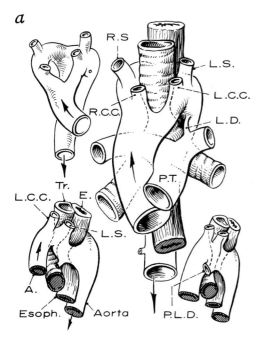

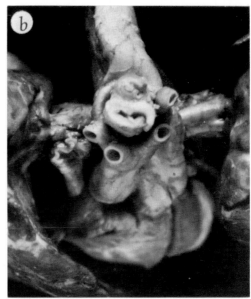

Fig. 21-38. *a.* Double aortic arch producing tight vascular ring around the trachea and esophagus. *L.C.C.* and *R.C.C.*, left and right common carotid arteries; *L.S.* and *R.S.*, subclavian arteries; *P.T.*, pulmonary trunk; *L.D.* and *P.L.D.*, ligamentum arteriosum and posterior ligamentum. *b.* Specimen with this malformation illustrated in *a.* (*Reproduced with permission from J. R. Stewart, O. W. Kincaid, and J. E. Edwards: "An Atlas of Vascular Rings and Related Malformations of the Aortic Arch System," Charles C Thomas, Publisher, Springfield, Ill., 1964, 171 pp.*)

a

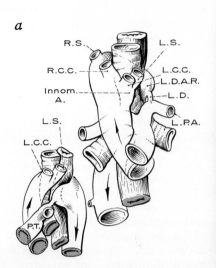

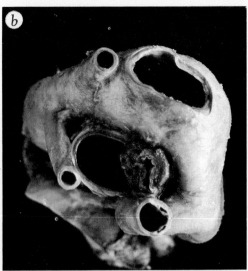

Fig. 21-39. *a*. Right aortic arch, retroesophageal segment, and ligamentum arteriosum *L.D.* extending from left side of upper portion of descending aorta *L.D.A.R.* to left pulmonary artery. This closes the vascular ring around the trachea and esophagus. *b*. Specimen with this malformation. (*Reproduced with permission from J. R. Stewart, O. W. Kincaid, and J. E. Edwards: "An Atlas of Vascular Rings and Related Malformations of the Aortic Arch System," Charles C Thomas, Publisher, Springfield, Ill., 1964, 171 pp.*)

Life History and Indications for Operation. Many patients appear to have congenital vascular rings without significant symptoms. In these the diagnosis is made incidentally, often in adult life, by fluoroscopic examination of the thorax and barium contrast studies of the esophagus.[114] Symptoms, when present, do not seem to disappear spontaneously in infants, and operation is required. It is, of course, unnecessary in the absence of symptoms.

Surgical Treatment. Virtually all types of congenital vascular rings are best approached through a left posterolateral thoracotomy.[116,117] Study of the preoperative aortogram correlated with the findings at operation will indicate the procedure of choice. When a double aortic arch is present, the smaller of the two arches is normally divided. When division of the posterior or right arch is elected, the absence of an atretic zone in the anterior arch should be ascertained. When there are a right aortic arch and a retroesophageal segment, the ring is usually adequately interrupted by ligation and division of the left-sided ligamentum arteriosum. It is important to divide any fibrous bands accompanying the great vessels in order that a thorough break is made in the ring surrounding and compressing the trachea or esophagus.

Results. Hospital mortality rates are low, and results of operation in general are good. During the first few postoperative months, however, noisy respirations may persist, presumably because of

softening of the tracheal cartilages in the region of the ring. These gradually subside, and the child is left with an excellent long-term result.

CONGENITAL CORONARY ARTERIO-VENOUS FISTULA

Surgical Pathology. This term is applied to an anomaly in which a large branch of a coronary artery empties directly into the vena cava, right atrium, right ventricle, or pulmonary artery (Fig. 21-40). This arteriovenous fistula produces a left-to-right shunt. Rarely, the opening may be into the left ventricle.

Diagnosis. The diagnosis is usually first suspected by auscultation of a continuous murmur. The chest roentgenogram may show cardiac enlargement. The electrocardiogram usually is not diagnostic. Cardiac catheterization reveals arterialization in the appropriate chamber if the communication is to the right side of the heart.[118] A definitive diagnosis is made by angiographic study after injection of radiopaque dye into the aortic root.

Life History and Indications for Operation. Many patients with these lesions have no symptoms, since many of the left-to-right shunts are about 30 per cent. Large shunts have been reported,[119] and then there may be symptoms, including growth failure, limitation of exercise tolerance, and dyspnea. Angina may occur as a result of impoverished coronary blood flow to portions of the ventricle from rapid runoff of blood through the fistula.[120] The lesion is considered to be an indication for operation.

Surgical Treatment and Results. The surgical treatment is ligation of the anomalous coronary artery as close as possible to its entrance into the cardiac chamber.[120,121] Normally no arrhythmia or cardiac dysfunction results.[122]

Operations have been performed in too few cases to allow a statistical analysis of the hospital mortality rates and end results. The operation, however, seems simple and safe, and the long-term results appear to be excellent.

ORIGIN OF LEFT CORONARY ARTERY FROM PULMONARY ARTERY

Surgical Pathology (Fig. 21-41) and Diagnosis. The diagnosis is suggested by the clinical course and electrocardiographic pattern. The characteristic clinical picture is that of an infant who was well at birth but began to have signs and symptoms of congestive heart failure when 2 to 3 months of age. Marked cardiac enlargement is present, and the

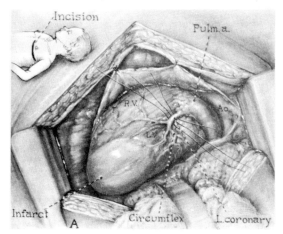

Fig. 21-41. Left coronary artery originating from pulmonary artery as seen at operation. (*Reproduced with permission from D. C. Sabiston, Jr., Catherine A. Neill, and Helen B. Taussig: The Direction of Blood Flow in Anomalous Left Coronary Artery Arising from the Pulmonary Artery, Circulation,* **22:**591–597, 1960.)

electrocardiographic pattern is similar to that seen in adults with anterior myocardial infarction. Aortography with injection into the aortic root shows a large right coronary artery but fails to demonstrate a left coronary artery.[123]

Life History. Patients in whom the left coronary artery arises from the pulmonary artery usually have symptoms within the first few months of life and succumb within the first year. No patient in the series of Sabiston and associates[124] reached 1 year of age without surgical intervention. However, rare cases of this anomaly in adults have been reported.[125]

Surgical Treatment and Results. Studies reported by Sabiston and associates[126] indicate that the anomalous vessel acts as an arteriovenous fistula, with blood flowing from the coronary artery into the pulmonary artery. Surgical therapy, based on these findings, is ligation of the anomalous coronary artery at its origin, pericardiectomy, and de-epicardialization.

Too few patients have been treated surgically to allow assessment of the results of the operative procedures.

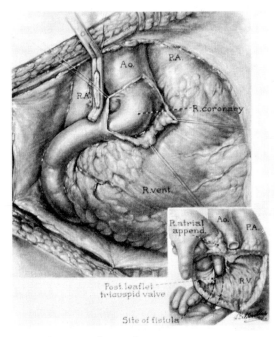

Fig. 21-40. Anomalous right coronary artery emptying into the right ventricle immediately beneath the septal leaflet of the tricuspid valve (coronary arteriovenous fistula). (*Reproduced with permission from D. C. Sabiston, Jr., R. S. Ross, J. M. Criley, R. A. Gaertner, Catherine A. Neill, and Helen B. Taussig: Surgical Management of Congenital Lesions of the Coronary Circulation, Ann. Surg.,* **157:**908–924, 1963.)

TRICUSPID ATRESIA

Surgical Pathology. Constant features of this complex malformation include atresia of the tricuspid orifice, patency of the atrial septum, and a large mitral orifice leading into a large left ventricular cavity and a diminutive right ventricle.[127]

Diagnosis and Life History. Patients with tricuspid atresia are usually cyanotic at birth or become cyanotic within the first months of life. The chest roentgenogram reveals a heart of normal size or slightly enlarged, with a rounded left border. The pulmonary vasculature is usually diminished. The electrocardiogram shows evidence of left axis deviation, left ventricular hypertrophy, and peaked P waves.

The prognosis for children with this deformity is extremely poor; many die in the first few weeks or months of life. Riker and Miller[128] reported that 80 per cent of those not operated on die before 3 years of age, but some do survive into the second decade and even into adult life.

Surgical Treatment and Results. Tricuspid atresia does not lend itself to complete surgical correction at present. Surgical efforts have been directed toward palliation. Systemic-pulmonary anastomosis in the form of a Blalock anastomosis or an aortopulmonary artery anastomosis has been performed in many patients and has given fair results.[128] Recently, anastomosis of the side of the superior vena cava to the distal end of the right main pulmonary artery has gained acceptance as the most satisfactory palliative procedure in this condition.[129] In some cases in which the main pulmonary arteries are small, a systemic-pulmonary anastomosis with conversion later to a caval-pulmonary anastomosis, as advocated by Bopp and coworkers,[130] may be warranted.

The hospital mortality from these palliative procedures is low, and in some cases the palliation achieved has been excellent.

EBSTEIN'S MALFORMATION

Surgical Pathology. Downward displacement of the tricuspid valve with the posterior and septal leaflets of the valve arising from the right ventricular wall and septum results in a part of the right ventricle's being continuous with the right atrium.[131] The tricuspid valve is usually incompetent, and there is frequently a patent foramen ovale.

Diagnosis and Life History. This condition is well tolerated for many years by some patients. Ultimately, however, in most patients either progressing cyanosis from the right-to-left shunt across the foramen ovale or gradually progressing symptoms from systemic venous hypertension develop.[132,133]

Surgical Treatment. A few patients have been treated by closure of the foramen ovale, thus abolishing the right-to-left shunt. Generally, this procedure is unsatisfactory because the problem of systemic venous hypertension remains. Anastomosis of the superior vena cava to the right pulmonary artery has been carried out in some patients, with good palliation reported in a few.[134]

Recently several reports of cases have appeared in which the basic malformation has been attacked. These direct attacks are based on the premise that the right ventricle is capable of propelling blood through the pulmonary artery, and that a good result will be obtained if the receptive volume of the right ventricle can be increased, incompetence of the tricuspid valve corrected, and right ventricular outflow obstruction by abnormal attachment of the valve leaflets relieved. Barnard and Schrire[135] reported two cases in which the abnormally displaced valve was excised and replaced with a prosthetic valve. Hardy and associates[136] plicated the markedly dilated inflow portion of the right ventricle in such a manner as to narrow the tricuspid annulus. This procedure yielded a satisfactory result in the one patient in which it was tried.

Further experience is needed before it can be determined whether these are truly satisfactory approaches to this problem.

REFERENCES

1. Dammann, J. F., Jr., and Ferencz, C.: The Significance of the Pulmonary Vascular Bed in Congenital Heart Disease. III. Defects between the Ventricles or Great Vessels in Which Both Increased Pressure and Blood Flow May Act upon the Lungs and in Which There Is a Common Ejectile Force, *Am. Heart J.,* 52:210–231, 1956.
2. Heath, D., and Edwards, J. E.: The Pathology of Hypertensive Pulmonary Vascular Disease: A Description of Six Grades of Structural Changes in the Pulmonary Arteries, with Special Reference to Congenital Cardiac Septal Defects, *Circulation,* 18:533–547, 1958.
3. Heath, D., Helmholz, H. F., Jr., Burchell, H.B., DuShane, J. W., and Edwards, J. E.: Graded Pulmonary Vascular Changes and Hemodynamic Findings in Cases of Atrial and Ventricular Septal Defect and Patent Ductus Arteriosus, *Circulation,* 18:1155–1166, 1958.
4. Kirklin, J. W., and DuShane, J. W.: Indications for Repair of Ventricular Septal Defects, *Am. J. Cardiol.,* 12:75–79, 1963.
5. Braunwald, N. S., Braunwald, E., and Morrow, A. G.: The Effects of Surgical Abolition of Left-to-right Shunts on the Pulmonary Vascular Dynamics of Patients with Pulmonary Hypertension, *Circulation,* 26:1270–1278, 1962.
6. Swan, H. J. C., Marshall, H. W., and Wood, E. H.: The Effect of Exercise in the Supine Position on Pulmonary Vascular Dynamics in Patients with Left-to-right Shunts, *J. Clin. Invest.,* 37:202–213, 1958.

7. Beck, W., Swan, H. J. C., Burchell, H. B., and Kirklin, J. W.: Pulmonary Vascular Resistance after Repair of Atrial Septal Defects in Patients with Pulmonary Hypertension, *Circulation,* **22:** 938–946, 1960.

8. Dammann, J. F., Jr., and Sell, C. G. R.: Patent Ductus Arteriosus in Absence of a Continuous Murmur, *Circulation,* **6:**110–124, 1952.

9. Ziegler, R. F.: The Importance of Patent Ductus Arteriosus in Infants, *Am. Heart J.,* **43:**553–572, 1952.

10. Rudolph, A. M., Mayer, F. E., Nadas, A. S., and Gross, R. E.: Patent Ductus Arteriosus: A Clinical and Hemodynamic Study of 23 Patients in the First Year of Life, *Pediatrics,* 22:892–904, 1958.

11. Keys, A., and Shapiro, M. J.: Patency of the Ductus Arteriosus in Adults, *Am. Heart J.,* **25:**158–186, 1943.

12. Gross, R. E.: The Patent Ductus Arteriosus: Observations on Diagnosis and Therapy in 525 Surgically Treated Cases, *Am. J. Med.,* **12:**472–482, 1952.

13. Pate, J. W., and Ainger, L. E.: Aggressive Approach to Malignant Patent Ductus Arteriosus, *Surgery,* 53:811–815, 1963.

14. Jones, J. C.: The Surgery of Patent Ductus Arteriosus, *Ann. Surg.,* 130:174–185, 1949.

15. Potts, W. J., Gibson, S., Smith, S., and Riker, W. L.: Diagnosis and Surgical Treatment of Patent Ductus Arteriosus, *A.M.A. Arch. Surg.,* **58:**612–622, 1949.

16. Gross, R. E., and Hubbard, J. P.: Surgical Ligation of Patent Ductus Arteriosus: Report of First Successful Case, *J.A.M.A.,* 112:729–731, 1939.

17. Gross, R. E.: Complete Division for the Patent Ductus Arteriosus, *J. Thoracic Surg.,* 16:314–322, 1947.

18. Umansky, R., and Hauck, A. J.: Factors in the Growth of Children with Patent Ductus Arteriosus, *Pediatrics,* **30:**540–551, 1962.

19. Ellis, F. H., Jr., Kirklin, J. W., Callahan, J. A., and Wood, E. H.: Patent Ductus Arteriosus with Pulmonary Hypertension: Analysis of Cases Treated Surgically, *J. Thoracic Surg.,* 31:268-282, 1956.

20. Morrow, A. G., Greenfield, L. J., and Braunwald, E.: Congenital Aortopulmonary Septal Defect: Clinical and Hemodynamic Findings, Surgical Technic, and Results of Operative Correction, *Circulation,* 25:463–476, 1962.

21. Cooley, D. A., McNamara, D. G., and Latson, J. R.: Aorticopulmonary Septal Defect: Diagnosis and Surgical Treatment, *Surgery,* 42:101–120, 1957.

22. Hufnagel, C. A., Conrad, P. W., Schanno, J., and Pifarré, R.: Profound Cardiac Hypothermia, *Ann. Surg.,* 153:790–796, 1961.

23. Bjork, V.: Personal communication to the authors.

24. Leatham, A., and Segal, B.: Ausculatatory and Phonocardiographic Signs of Ventricular Septal Defect with Left-to-right Shunt, *Circulation,* **25:** 318–327, 1962.

25. Toscano-Barboza, E., and DuShane, J. W.: Ventricular Septal Defect: Correlation of Electrocardiographic and Hemodynamic Findings in 60 Proved Cases, *Am. J. Cardiol.,* 3:721–732, 1959.

26. DuShane, J. W., and Kirklin, J. W.: Selection for Surgery of Patients with Ventricular Septal Defect and Pulmonary Hypertension, *Circulation,* **21:**13–20, 1960.

27. Morgan, B. C., Griffiths, S. P., and Blumenthal, S.: Ventricular Septal Defect. I. Congestive Heart Failure in Infancy, *Pediatrics,* 25:54–62, 1960.

28. Weidman, W. H., DuShane, J. W., and Kincaid, O. W.: Observations Concerning Progressive Pulmonary Vascular Obstruction in Children with Ventricular Septal Defects, *Am. Heart J.,* **65:**148–154, 1963.

29. Bloomfield, D. K.: The Natural History of Ventricular Septal Defect in Patients Surviving Infancy, *Circulation,* 24:914–955, 1964.

30. Nadas, A. S., Scott, L. P., Hauck, A. J., and Rudolph, A. M.: Spontaneous Functional Closing of Ventricular Septal Defects, *New England J. Med.,* 264:309–316, 1961.

31. Evans, J. R., Rowe, R. D., and Keith, J. D.: Spontaneous Closure of Ventricular Septal Defects, *Circulation,* 22:1044–1054, 1960.

32. Gasul, B. M., Dillon, R. F., Vrla, V., and Hait, G.: Ventricular Septal Defects: Their Natural Transformation into Those with Infundibular Stenosis or into the Cyanotic or Noncyanotic Type of Tetralogy of Fallot, *J.A.M.A.,* **164:**847–853, 1957.

33. Keck, E. W. O., Ongley, P. A., Kincaid, O. W., and Swan, H. J. C.: Ventricular Septal Defect with Aortic Insufficiency: A Clinical and Hemodynamic Study of 18 Proved Cases, *Circulation,* **27:**203–219, 1963.

34. Nadas, A. S., Thilenius, O. G., LaFarge, C. G., and Hauck, A. J.: Ventricular Septal Defect with Aortic Regurgitation: Medical and Pathologic Aspects, *Circulation,* 29:862–873, 1964.

35. Muller, W. H., Jr., and Dammann, J. F., Jr.: The Treatment of Certain Congenital Malformations of the Heart by the Creation of Pulmonic Stenosis to Reduce Pulmonary Hypertension and Excessive Pulmonary Blood Flow: A Preliminary Blood Flow, *Surg. Gynec. & Obst.,* 95:213–219, 1952.

36. Lauer, R. M., Ongley, P. A., DuShane, J. W., and Kirklin, J. W.: Heart Block after Repair of Ventricular Septal Defect in Children, *Circulation,* 22:526–534, 1960.

37. McGoon, D. C., Ongley, P. A., and Kirklin, J. W.: Surgically Induced Heart Block, *Ann. New York Acad. Sc.,* 111:830–834, 1964.

38. Kirklin, J. W., Harshbarger, H. G., Donald, D. E., and Edwards, J. E.: Surgical Correction of Ventricular Septal Defect: Anatomic and Technical

Considerations, *J. Thoracic Surg.*, **33**:45-57, 1957.

39. Lev, M.: The Architecture of the Conduction System in Congenital Heart Disease. III. Ventricular Septal Defect, *Arch. Path.*, **70**:529-549, 1960.

40. Neufeld, H. N., Titus, J. L., DuShane, J. W., Burchell, H. B., and Edwards, J. E.: Isolated Ventricular Septal Defect of the Persistent Common Atrioventricular Canal Type, *Circulation*, **23**:685-696, 1961.

41. Kirklin, J. W., and Theye, R. A.: Whole-body Perfusion from a Pump-oxygenator for Open Intracardiac Surgery, in J. H. Gibbon, Jr., "Surgery of the Chest," W. B. Saunders Company, Philadelphia, 1962, pp. 694-707.

42. Theye, R. A., Moffitt, E. A., and Kirklin, J. W.: Anesthetic Management during Open Intracardiac Surgery, *Anesthesiology*, **23**:823-827, 1962.

43. Lyons, W. S., DuShane, J. W., and Kirklin, J. W.: Postoperative Care after Whole-body Perfusion and Open Intracardiac Operations: Use of Mayo-Gibbon Pump-oxygenator and Browns-Emmons Heat Exchanger, *J.A.M.A.*, **173**:625-630, 1960.

44. Kirklin, J. W., and Theye, R. A.: Cardiac Performance after Open Intracardiac Surgery, *Circulation*, **28**:1061-1070, 1963.

45. Kirklin, J. W., and DuShane, J. W.: Repair of Ventricular Septal Defect in Infancy, *Pediatrics*, **27**:961-966, 1961.

46. Toscano-Barbosa, E., Brandenburg, R. O., and Burchell, H. B.: Electrocardiographic Studies of Cases with Intracardiac Malformations of the Atrioventricular Canal, *Proc. Staff Meet. Mayo Clin.*, **31**:513-523, 1956.

47. Burchell, H. B., DuShane, J. W., and Brandenburg, R. O.: The Electrocardiogram of Patients with Atrioventricular Cushion Defects (Defects of the Atrioventricular Canal), *Am. J. Cardiol.*, **6**:575-588, 1960.

48. DuShane, J. W., Weidman, W. H., Brandenburg, R. O., and Kirklin, J. W.: Differentiation of Intra-atrial Communications by Clinical Methods: Ostium Secundum, Ostium Primum, Common Atrium, and Total Anomalous Pulmonary Venous Connection, *Circulation*, **21**:363-371, 1960.

49. Baron, M. G., Wolf, B. S., Steinfeld, Leonard, and Van Mierop, L. H. S.: Endocardial Cushion Defects: Specific Diagnosis by Angiocardiography, *Am. J. Cardiol.*, **13**:162-175, 1964.

50. Blondeau, P., Piwnica, A., Guilmet, P., and Dubost, C.: Problèmes posés par la cure chirurgicale du canal atrioventriculaire partiel, à propos de 46 interventions, *Ann. chir. thorac. cardiovas.*, **2**:295-298, 1963.

51. McGoon, D. C., DuShane, J. W., and Kirklin, J. W.: The Surgical Treatment of Endocardial Cushion Defects, *Surgery*, **46**:185-196, 1959.

52. Mark, Herbert: Natural History of Atrial Septal Defect with Criteria for Selection for Surgery, *Am. J. Cardiol.*, **12**:66-74, 1963.

53. Kirklin, J. W., Ellis, F. H., Jr., and Wood, E. H.: Treatment of Anomalous Pulmonary Venous Connections in Association with Interatrial Communications, *Surgery*, **39**:389-398, 1956.

54. Burchell, H. B.: Total Anomalous Pulmonary Venous Drainage: Clinical and Physiologic Patterns, *Proc. Staff Meet. Mayo Clin.*, **31**:161-167, 1956.

55. Kirklin, J. W.: Corrective Surgical Treatment for Cyanotic Congenital Heart Disease, in A. D. Bass and G. K. Moe (eds.), "Symposium on Congenital Heart Disease," American Association for the Advancement of Science, Washington, D.C., 1960, pp. 329-344.

56. Burroughs, J. T., and Kirklin, J. W.: Complete Surgical Correction of Total Anomalous Pulmonary Venous Connection: Report of Three Cases, *Proc. Staff Meet. Mayo Clin.*, **31**:182-188, 1956.

57. Woodwark, G. M., Vince, D. J., and Ashmore, P. G.: Total Anomalous Pulmonary Venous Return to the Portal Vein: Report of a Case of Successful Surgical Treatment, *J. Thoracic Surg.*, **45**:662-666, 1963.

58. Cooley, D. A., and Balas, P. E.: Total Anomalous Pulmonary Venous Drainage into Inferior Vena Cava: Report of Successful Surgical Correction, *Surgery*, **51**:798-804, 1962.

59. Mustard, W. T., Keith, J. D., and Trusler, G. A.: Two Stage Correction for Total Anomalous Pulmonary Venous Drainage in Childhood, *J. Thoracic Surg.*, **44**:477-485, 1962.

60. Glass, I. H., Mustard, W. T., and Keith, J. D.: Coarctation of the Aorta in Infants: A Review of Twelve Years' Experience, *Pediatrics*, **26**:109-121, 1960.

61. Reifenstein, G. H., Levine, S. A., and Gross, R. E.: Coarctation of the Aorta: A Review of 104 Autopsied Cases of the "Adult Type," 2 Years of Age or Older, *Am. Heart J.*, **33**:146-168, 1947.

62. Malm, J. R., Blumenthal, S., Jameson, A. G., and Humphreys, G. H., II.: Observations on Coarctation of the Aorta in Infants, *Arch. Surg.*, **86**:96-103, 1963.

63. Gross, R. E.: Surgical Correction for Coarctation of the Aorta, *Surgery*, **18**:673-678, 1945.

64. Crafoord, C., and Mylin, G.: Congenital Coarctation of the Aorta and Its Surgical Treatment, *J. Thoracic Surg.*, **14**:347-361, 1945.

65. Morris, G. C., Jr., Cooley, D. A., De Bakey, M. E., and Crawford, E. S.: Coarctation of the Aorta with Particular Emphasis upon Improved Techniques of Surgical Repair, *J. Thoracic Surg.*, **40**:705-721, 1960.

66. Pontius, R. G., Brockman, H. L., Hardy, E. G., Cooley, D. A., and DeBakey, M. E.: The Use of Hypothermia in the Prevention of Paraplegia Following Temporary Aortic Occlusion: Experimental Observations, *Surgery*, **36**:33-38, 1954.

67. Schuster, S. R., and Gross, R. E.: Surgery for Coarctation of the Aorta: A Review of 500 Cases, *J. Thoracic Surg.*, **43**:54-68, 1962.

68. Wright, J. L., Burchell, H. B., Wood, E. H., Hines, E. A., Jr., and Clagett, O. T.: Hemodynamic and Clinical Appraisal of Coarctation Four to Seven Years After Resection and End-to-end Anastomosis of the Aorta, *Circulation,* 24:806–814, 1956.

69. Williams, J. C .P., Barratt-Boyes, B. G., and Lowe, J. B.: Supravalvular Aortic Stenosis, *Circulation,* 24:1311–1318, 1961.

70. Brachfeld, N., and Gorlin, R.: Subaortic Stenosis: A Revised Concept of the Disease, *Medicine,* 38:415–433, 1959.

71. Goodwin, J. F., Hollman, A., Cleland, W. P., and Teare, D.: Obstructive Cardiomyopathy Simulating Aortic Stenosis, *Brit. Heart J.,* **22**:403–414. 1960.

72. Braunwald, E., Goldblatt, A., Aygen, M. M., Rockoff, S. D., and Morrow, A. G.: Congenital Aortic Stenosis. I. Clinical and Hemodynamic Findings in 100 Patients, *Circulation,* **27**:426–462, 1963.

73. Ellis, F. H., Jr., Ongley, P. A., and Kirklin, J. W.: Results of Surgical Treatment for Congenital Aortic Stenosis, *Circulation,* 25:29–38, 1962.

74. Morrow, A. G., Goldblatt, A., and Braunwald, E.: Congenital Aortic Stenosis. II. Surgical Treatment and the Results of Operation, *Circulation,* 27:426–462, 1963.

75. McGoon, D. C., Mankin, H. T., Vlad, P., and Kirklin, J. W.: The Surgical Treatment of Supravalvular Aortic Stenosis, *J. Thoracic Surg.,* 41:125–133, 1961.

76. Kirklin, J. W., and Ellis, F. H., Jr.: Surgical Relief of Diffuse Subvalvular Aortic Stenosis, *Circulation,* 24:739–742, 1961.

77. Lees, M. H., Hauck, A. J., Starkey, G. W. B., Nadas, A. S., and Gross, R. E.: Congenital Aortic Stenosis, Operative Indications and Surgical Results, *Brit. Heart J.,* 24:31–38, 1962.

78. Leatham, A., and Weitzman, D.: Auscultatory and Phonocardiographic Signs of Pulmonary Stenosis, *Brit. Heart J.,* 19:303–317, 1957.

79. Bassingthwaighte, J. B., Parkin, T. W., DuShane, J. W., Wood, E. H., and Burchell, H. B.: The Electrocardiographic and Hemodynamic Findings in Pulmonary Stenosis with Intact Ventricular Septum, *Circulation,* 28:893–905, 1963.

80. Little, J. B., Lavender, J. P., and DeSanctis, R. W.: The Narrow Infundibulum in Pulmonary Valvular Stenosis: Its Preoperative Diagnosis by Angiocardiography, *Circulation,* 28:182–189, 1963.

81. Lewis, J. M., Montero, A. C., Kinard, S. A., Jr., Dennis, E. W., and Alexander, J. K.: Hemodynamic Response to Exercise in Isolated Pulmonic Stenosis, *Circulation,* 29:854–861, 1964.

82. McGoon, D. C., and Kirklin, J. W.: Pulmonic Stenosis with Intact Ventricular Septum: Treatment Utilizing Extracorporeal Circulation, *Circulation,* 17:180–186, 1958.

83. Kirklin, J. W., Connolly, D. C., Ellis, F. H., Jr., Burchell, H. B., Edwards, J. E., and Wood, E. H.: Problems in the Diagnosis and Surgical Treatment of Pulmonic Stenosis with Intact Ventricular Septum, *Circulation,* 8:849–863, 1953.

84. Gilbert, J. W., Morrow, A. G., and Talbert, J. L.: The Surgical Significance of Hypertrophic Infundibular Obstruction Accompanying Valvular Pulmonic Stenosis, *J. Thoracic Surg.,* 46:457–466, 1963.

85. Johnson, A. M.: Hypertrophic Infundibular Stenosis Complicating Simple Pulmonary Valve Stenosis, *Brit. Heart J.,* 21:429–439, 1959.

86. Talbert, J. L., Morrow, A. G., Collins, N. P., and Gilbert, J. W.: The Incidence and Significance of Pulmonic Regurgitation after Pulmonary Valvulotomy, *Am. Heart J.,* 65:590–596, 1963.

87. Potts, W. J., Smith, S., and Gibson, S.: Anastomosis of the Aorta to a Pulmonary Artery: Certain Types in Congenital Heart Disease, *J.A.M.A.,* 132:627–631, 1946.

88. Blalock, A., and Taussig, H. B.: The Surgical Treatment of Malformations of the Heart in Which There Is Pulmonary Stenosis or Pulmonary Atresia, *J.A.M.A.,* 128:189–202, 1945.

89. Blalock, A.: Surgical Procedures Employed and Anatomical Variations Encountered in the Treatment of Congenital Pulmonic Stenosis, *Surg. Gynec. & Obst.,* 87:385–409, 1948.

90. Lillehei, C. W., Cohen, M., Warden, H. E., Read, R. C., Aust, J. B., DeWall, R. A., and Varco, R. L.: Direct Vision Intracardiac Surgical Correction of the Tetralogy of Fallot, Pentalogy of Fallot, and Pulmonary Atresia Defects: Report of First Ten Cases, *Ann. Surg.,* 142:418–442, 1955.

91. Kirklin, J. W., and Payne, W. S.: Tetralogy of Fallot, in C. D. Benson, W. T. Mustard, M. A. Ravitch, W. H. Snyder, Jr., and K. J. Welch, "Pediatric Surgery," The Year Book Medical Publishers, Inc., Chicago, 1962, vol. 1, pp. 462–471.

92. Kirklin, J. W., and Payne, W. S.: Surgical Treatment for Tetralogy of Fallot after Previous Anastomosis of Systemic to Pulmonary Artery, *Surg. Gynec. & Obst.,* 110:707–713, 1960.

93. Kirklin, J. W., and Devloo, R. A.: Hypothermic Perfusion and Circulatory Arrest for Surgical Correction of Tetralogy of Fallot with Previously Constucted Potts' Anastomosis, *Dis. Chest,* 39:87–91, 1961.

94. Toole, A. L., Glenn, W. W. L., Fisher, W. H., Whittemore, R., Ordway, N. K., and Vidone, R. A.: Operative Approach to Transposition of the Great Vessels: I. Classification and Review of 32 Cases with and 40 Cases without Operation, *Surgery,* 48:43–57, 1960.

95. Ferguson, D. J., Adams, P., and Watson, D.: Pulmonary Arteriosclerosis in Transposition of the Great Vessels, *A.M.A. J. Dis. Child.,* 99:653–661, 1960.

96. Albert, H. M.: Surgical Correction of Transposition of the Great Vessels, *S. Forum,* 5:74–77, 1954.

97. Senning, Å.: Surgical Correction of Transposition

of the Great Vessels, *Surgery,* **45**:966–980, 1959.

98. Kirklin, J. W., Devloo, R. A., and Weidman, W. H.: Open Intracardiac Repair for Transposition of the Great Vessels: Eleven Cases, *Surgery,* **50**:58–66, 1961.

99. Mustard, W. T.: Successful Two-stage Correction of Transposition of the Great Vessels, *Surgery,* **55**:469–472, 1964.

100. Blalock, A., and Hanlon, C. R.: Interatrial Septal Defect: Its Experimental Production under Direct Vision without Interruption of the Circulation, *Surg. Gynec. & Obst.,* **87**:183–187, 1948.

101. Schiebler, G. L., Edwards, J. E., Burchell, H. B., DuShane, J. W., Ongley, P. A., and Wood, E. H.: Congenital Corrected Transposition of the Great Vessels: A Study of 33 Cases, *Pediatrics,* **27**:851–888, 1961.

102. Van Praagh, R. V., Ongley, P. A., and Swan, H. J. C.: Anatomic Types of Single or Common Ventricle in Man: Morphologic and Geometric Aspects of 60 Necropsied Cases, *Am. J. Cardiol.,* **13**:367–386, 1964.

103. Edwards, J. E., and Burchell, H. B.: The Pathological Anatomy of Deficiencies between the Aortic Root and the Heart, Including Aortic Sinus Aneurysms, *Thorax,* **12**:125–139, 1957.

104. Gerbode, F., Osborn, J. J., Johnston, J. B., and Kerth, W. J.: Ruptured Aneurysms of the Aortic Sinuses of Valsalva, *Am. J. Surg.,* **102**:268–278, 1961.

105. Dubost, C., Blondeau, P., and Piwnica, A.: Right Aorta–Atrial Fistulas Resulting from a Rupture of the Sinus of Valsalva, *J. Thoracic Surg.,* **43**:421–433, 1962.

106. Engle, M. A., Holswade, G. R., Campbell, W. G., and Goldberg, H. P.: Ventricular Septal Defect with Transposition of Aorta Masquerading as Acyanotic Ventricular Septal Defect (Abstract), *Circulation,* **22**:745, 1960.

107. Neufeld, H. N., DuShane, J. W., Wood, E. H., Kirklin, J. W., and Edwards, J. E.: Origin of Both Great Vessels from the Right Ventricle. I. Without Pulmonary Stenosis, *Circulation,* **23**:399–412, 1961.

108. Neufeld, H. N., DuShane, J. W., and Edwards, J. E.: Origin of Both Great Vessels from the Right Ventricle. II. With Pulmonary Stenosis, *Circulation,* **23**:603–612, 1961.

109. Kirklin, J. W., Harp, R. A., and McGoon, D. C.: Surgical Treatment of Origin of Both Vessels from Right Ventricle, Including Cases with Pulmonary Stenosis, *J. Thoracic Surg.,* **48**:1026–1036, 1964.

110. Berghuis, J., Kirklin, J. W., Edwards, J. E., and Titus, J. L.: The Surgical Anatomy of Isolated Congenital Mitral Insufficiency, *J. Thoracic Surg.,* **47**:791–798, 1964.

111. Barcia, A., Titus, J. L., Swan, H. J. C., Ongley, P. A., and Calene, J. G.: Congenital Mitral Stenosis: A Case Studied by Selective Angiocardiog-raphy and Necropsy, *Proc. Staff Meet. Mayo Clin.,* **37**:632–639, 1962.

112. Mata, L. A., Anselmi, G., Velasco, J. R., Monroy, G., and Vela, J. E.: Estenosis mitral congenita: Estudio de dos nuevos casos y revesion de la literatura. *Arch. Inst. cardiol. México,* **30**:318–341, 1960.

113. Prior, J. T.: Congenital Anomalies of the Mitral Valve: Two Cases Associated with Long Survival, *Am. Heart J.,* **46**:649–656, 1953.

114. Stewart, J. R., Kincaid, O. W., and Edwards, J. E.: "An Atlas of Vascular Rings and Related Malformations of the Aortic Arch System," Charles C Thomas, Publisher, Springfield, Ill., 1964.

115. Blumenthal, S., and Ravitch, M. M.: Seminar on Aortic Vascular Rings and Other Anomalies of the Aortic Arch, *Pediatrics,* **20**:896–906, 1957.

116. Gross, R. E.: Surgical Relief for Tracheal Obstruction from a Vascular Ring, *New England J. Med.,* **233**:586–590, 1945.

117. Gross, R. E.: Arterial Malformations Which Cause Compression of the Trachea or Esophagus, *Circulation,* **11**:124–134, 1955.

118. Gasul, B. M., Arcilla, R. A., Fell, E. H., Lynfield, J., Bicoff, J. P., and Luan, L. L.: Congenital Coronary Arteriovenous Fistula: Clinical, Phonocardiographic, Angiocardiographic and Hemodynamic Studies in Five Patients, *Pediatrics,* **25**:531–560, 1960.

119. Neufeld, H. N., Lester, R. G., Adams, P., Jr., Anderson, R. C., Lillehei, C. W., and Edwards, J. E.: Congenital Communication of a Coronary Artery with a Cardiac Chamber on the Pulmonary Trunk ("Coronary Artery Fistula") *Circulation,* **24**:171–179, 1961.

120. Sabiston, D. C., Jr.: Surgery of the Coronary Circulation, *J. Roy. Coll. Surgeons Edinburgh,* **8**:105–121, 1963.

121. Abbott, O. A., Rivarola, C. H., and Logue, R. B.: Surgical Correction of Coronary Arteriovenous Fistula, *J. Thoracic Surg.,* **42**:660–672, 1961.

122. Barcia, A., Kincaid, O. W., Swan, H. J. C., Weidman, W. H., and Kirklin, J. W.: Coronary-artery-to-right-ventricle Communication: Report of Two Cases Studied by Selective Angiocardiography, *Proc. Staff Meet. Mayo Clin.,* **37**:623–631, 1962.

123. Keith, J. D.: The Anomalous Origin of the Left Coronary Artery from the Pulmonary Artery, *Brit. Heart J.,* **21**:149–161, 1959.

124. Sabiston, D. C., Jr., Pelargonio, S., and Taussig, H. B.: Myocardial Infarction in Infancy: The Surgical Management of a Complication of Congenital Origin of the Left Coronary Artery from the Pulmonary Artery, *J. Thoracic Surg.,* **40**:321–335, 1960.

125. Kaunitz, P. E.: Origin of Left Coronary Artery from Pulmonary Artery: Review of the Literature and Report of Two Cases, *Am. Heart J.,* **33**:182–206, 1947.

126. Sabiston, D. C., Jr., Neill, C. A., and Taussig, H. B.: The Direction of Blood Flow in Anomalous Left Coronary Artery Arising from the Pulmonary Artery, *Circulation*, **22**:591–597, 1960.

127. Edwards, J. E., and Burchell, H. B.: Congenital Tricuspid Atresia: A Classification, *M. Clin. North America*, **33**:1177–1196, 1949.

128. Riker, W. L., and Miller, R.: The Diagnosis and Treatment of Tricuspid Atresia, *Surgery*, **38**:886–902, 1955.

129. Glenn, W. W. L., and Patiño, J. F.: Circulatory By-pass of the Right Heart. I. Preliminary Observations on the Direct Delivery of Vena Caval Blood into the Pulmonary Arterial Circulation: Azygos Vein–Pulmonary Artery Shunt, *Yale J. Biol. & Med.*, **27**:147–151, 1954.

130. Bopp, R. K., Larsen, P. B., Caddell, J. L., Patrick, J. R., Hipona, F. A., and Glenn, W. W. L.: Surgical Considerations for Treatment of Congenital Tricuspid Atresia and Stenosis: With Particular Reference to Vena Cava–Pulmonary Artery Anastomosis, *J. Thoracic Surg.*, **43**:97–111, 1962.

131. Kilby, R. A., DuShane, J. W., Wood, E. H., and Burchell, H. B.: Ebstein's Malformation: A Clinical and Laboratory Study, *Medicine*, **35**:161–185, 1956.

132. Mayer, F. E., Nadas, A. S., and Ongley, P. A.: Ebstein's Anomaly: Presentation of Ten Cases, *Circulation*, **16**:1057–1069, 1957.

133. Blount, S. G., Jr., McCord, M. C., and Gelb, I. J.: Ebstein's Anomaly, *Circulation*, **15**:210–224, 1957.

134. Gasul, B. M., Weinberg, M., Jr., Luan, L. L., Fell, E. H., Bicoff, J., and Steiger, Z.: Superior Vena Cava–Right Main Pulmonary Artery Anastomosis: Surgical Correction for Patients with Ebstein's Anomaly and for Congenital Hypoplastic Right Ventricle, *J.A.M.A.*, **171**:1797–1803, 1959.

135. Barnard, C. N., and Schrire, V.: Surgical Correction of Ebstein's Malformation with Prosthetic Tricuspid Valve, *Surgery*, **54**:302–308, 1963.

136. Hardy, K. L., May, E. A., Webster, C. A., and Kimball, K. C.: Ebstein's Anomaly: A Functional Concept and Successful Definitive Repair, *J. Thoracic Surg.*, **48**:927–940, 1964.

Section B: Acute Rheumatic Fever and Acquired Valvular Heart Disease

22 ETIOLOGY OF RHEUMATIC HEART DISEASE

Thomas F. Sellers, Jr., M.D.

The specific etiology of acute rheumatic fever and the subsequent lesions of rheumatic heart disease are only poorly understood. At least two distinct yet intimately related etiologic factors appear to be involved—an initial group A streptococcal infection and a specifically susceptible host.

STREPTOCOCCAL INFECTION

There appears to be almost universal agreement that acute rheumatic fever requires infection by the β-hemolytic, group A streptococcus for its initiation. At first suspected by random clinical observation, this relationship has been confirmed by recent epidemiologic studies employing large numbers of subjects and advanced serologic techniques.[1,2]

The evidence for the relationship of group A streptococcal infection and acute rheumatic fever may be summarized as follows.

1. About 3 per cent of patients with infection of the throat with group A streptococci will develop rheumatic fever.[1] A large number of acute rheumatic patients give a history of symptomatic sore throat approximately 2 weeks before onset.

2. Epidemics of streptococcal infections (such as scarlet fever) are frequently followed by epidemics of acute rheumatic fever. Curiously—and no doubt significantly—streptococcal infection not involving the upper respiratory tract rarely, if ever, gives rise to acute rheumatic fever. This is not true for other poststreptococcal diseases, such as acute glomerulonephritis, which, for example, often follow skin infection with group A streptococci.

3. Seasonal variations in incidence of streptococcal infection are paralleled by the incidence of

rheumatic fever. Both streptococcal infection and rheumatic fever are diseases of winter and early spring and have their lowest incidence in summer and early fall.[3]

4. Recurrences of rheumatic activity frequently follow infection by group A streptococci in persons with previous attacks of rheumatic fever.

5. Specific prophylaxis of β-streptococcal infection or its early treatment is highly effective in reducing the incidence of recurrences of rheumatic fever. This, of course, is the basis for the extensive program of sulfonamide or penicillin prophylaxis in persons who have rheumatic fever or rheumatic heart disease.

6. Elevated or rising titers of antistreptococcal antibodies are found in virtually every patient with acute rheumatic fever. Although antibody to a specified streptococcal antigen may be present only in about 85 per cent of cases, streptococcal antibodies will be found in nearly 100 per cent when several streptococcal antigens are used.[2] Although untreated streptococcal infection gives rise to antibodies in almost every individual whether rheumatic fever develops or not, the level of antibody which ensues is distinctly higher in rheumatic patients.[4]

How the streptococcus causes rheumatic fever is much more difficult to determine, and no clear answer can be given to such a seemingly simple question as whether streptococci must continue to live in the body for rheumatic fever to develop.[5] Many patients show no clinical evidence of streptococcal infection at the time rheumatic fever develops and have negative throat cultures. Furthermore, the histologic appearance of rheumatic fever lesions is unlike that of acute streptococcal infection, and appropriate antibiotic treatment does not seem to affect the course of acute rheumatic fever once symptoms have begun. On the other hand, before the antibiotic era, some investigators reported recovery of hemolytic streptococci from heart valves of patients dying of rheumatic fever. More recently Catanzaro et al.[6] have shown that delayed penicillin treatment begun as late as 9 days after onset of streptococcal infection is effective in preventing most of the expected rheumatic fever. This has been cited as evidence that streptococcal infection does not produce rheumatic fever until the organisms have been present for a considerable period of time. In another study it was found that 42 days of penicillin treatment for acute rheumatic fever reduced the incidence of rheumatic valvular disease observed 1 year later, even though no beneficial effect was noted during the acute phase.[7] This study has raised speculation that persistent living streptococci are significant in the development of valvulitis but not in the other manifestations of the rheumatic

state. Because streptococci are so often difficult to isolate from the nasopharynx of patients with rheumatic fever and because some investigators before the antibiotic era reported isolations of β-hemolytic streptococci from the valves themselves,[8–10] it has been suggested that rheumatic heart disease represents a form of β-streptococcal bacterial endocarditis. This evidence, however, does not preclude the possibility that living streptococci might influence the heart valves from a more distant point without being actually present in the valve.

Other streptococci than group A have also been implicated in the development of rheumatic fever. Marienfeld et al.[11] have carefully reviewed a rather numerous but largely ignored group of reports which describe the recovery of a "short-chain" or "diplo"-streptococcus from the heart or blood of patients with rheumatic fever. In this report Marienfeld also describes the recovery of a similar organism now classed as enterococcus from two-thirds of patients with acute rheumatic fever and smaller percentages of convalescent and inactive rheumatic patients. There are a number of possible explanations of this finding, but the one favored by the authors is that the enterococcus shares a number of antigens with the group A streptococcus and perpetuates a local tissue sensitivity to streptococcal antigen. Just why the enterococcus is able to invade the blood or the heart in such patients is unexplained.

That more than streptococcal infection must be involved in rheumatic fever is obvious from the fact that only a very small percentage of persons infected with β-streptococci ever develop the disease. Yet once a person develops rheumatic fever, recurrent attacks following subsequent streptococcal infections are much more common. Thus the concept has been widely accepted that altered host susceptibility must also be present for rheumatic fever to develop.

ANTIBODY

There is considerable evidence to suggest that rheumatic fever may be an antibody disease. The incubation period after streptococcal infection is comparable to the time required for development of antibody and is similar to the incubation period of known antibody diseases such as serum sickness. Moreover, the incubation period is shortened after later streptococcal infections, in keeping with the presence of an established antibody mechanism.

It has been suggested that rheumatic subjects are hyperactive antibody formers and respond excessively to the stimulus of streptococcal infection. Studies on this point are contradictory. Studies with many nonstreptococcal antigens, however, have revealed no strikingly increased antibody responses by rheumatic subjects.[12,13]

Acute streptococcal infection or injection of various streptococcal products can be shown to cause a variety of cardiac lesions in experimental animals, but these develop more quickly and do not resemble rheumatic carditis histologically.[14,15] It is possible, however, that such damaged cardiac tissue may become antigenic in itself and cause the host immunologic mechanism to react to it; this is the concept of autoimmunity. The heart has not been shown to be a source of organ-specific antigen as have the thyroid, brain, lens, or testis.[*]

Many studies have been performed in experimental animals by injecting various preparations of cardiac tissue alone or in combination with such items as killed streptococci, tuberculin, or Freund's adjuvant. Although cardiac lesions result in some of these animals, their histologic appearances are not identical to and are often quite dissimilar from those of rheumatic carditis.

Kaplan[16] demonstrated by immunofluorescence that auricular appendages from some patients with rheumatic heart disease showed specific deposition of human gamma-globulin whereas similar nonrheumatic tissue did not. Moreover, the serums from certain rheumatic patients were shown to react with normal and rheumatic heart tissue.

The demonstration that "anti-heart" antibody can be produced experimentally or detected in rheumatic serum does not prove, of course, that rheumatic carditis is caused by such antibodies. They may be the result rather than the cause of damaged cardiac tissue. Indeed, similar antibodies may be produced by nonrheumatic myocardial injury, such as mitral commissurotomy or myocardial infarction.

Kaplan[17] has also demonstrated that antigenic materials from certain strains of streptococci when injected into rabbits give rise to antibodies which in turn react with human cardiac myofibers and smooth-muscle cells. The presence of the antibody was demonstrated by immunofluorescence and complement fixation. It is not clear, however, whether the characteristic rheumatic lesions such as Aschoff's bodies or valvulitis are related to the deposition of this antibody.

HEREDITY

Susceptibility to rheumatic fever also appears to have an inherited basis. Wilson[18] has shown by

[*] Autoantiboides have been implicated in specific diseases involving these organs. Unlike cardiac tissue, there appears to be a separation of these organs from the circulation in the normal state, and it may be a breakdown in this "barrier" which releases the organ-specific antigen.

genetic analysis of families having at least one rheumatic individual that there is a clear increase in rheumatic fever among other members. When families having a rheumatic parent were compared with comparable control families, it was found that the incidence of rheumatic fever among the offspring was consistent with a genetic mechanism of recessive inheritance. Thus all children of two rheumatics, half the children of a rheumatic and a carrier, one-fourth of the children of two carriers, and none of the children of two noncarriers would be susceptible to rheumatic fever. Unfortunately, there is no way to determine which individuals are susceptible and which nonsusceptible except to express a statistical estimate based on the family history of rheumatic fever.

In another genetic approach, studying secretors and nonsecretors of blood group substances into the saliva, it has been found that the incidence of rheumatic fever is higher among nonsecretors than among secretors. These data are compatible with the concept that individuals who are homozygous for secretion of ABO substance are immune and that only those heterozygous or homozygous for the nonsecretor gene are susceptible.[19] More study is needed to determine the significance of this association.

RACIAL AND SOCIOECONOMIC STATUS

The etiology of rheumatic fever has also been tied into certain racial and socioeconomic influences, though these have not always been substantiated by convincing evidence. The incidence of rheumatic fever is clearly highest among the lowest socioeconomic groups and falls progressively as higher income groups are considered. The frequency of rheumatic fever among the Irish immigrants living in cities of the Northeast has been frequently cited as an example of racial predisposition to the disease.[20] Yet the poverty of this group, resulting in poor nutrition and crowded, miserable living conditions, may be more of a determining factor than their racial inheritance. Crowding together of susceptible persons is thought to be at least partly responsible for the winter peaks of streptococcal infection, and this influence would be at its greatest in crowded slums exposed to a northern winter. Negroes are said to be more likely than whites to develop rheumatic heart disease, although the incidence of rheumatic fever is similar in the two groups.[20]

Over the past 40 years at least, the mortality from acute rheumatic fever has been declining.[21] This trend cannot be explained solely by antibiotics, since it preceded even sulfa drugs. It may be explained by a relative increase in socioeconomic status which has been going on over this period or perhaps by a change in the rheumatic fever potential of the prevalent group A streptococcal strains.

Another characteristic of a low socioeconomic environment is the poor nutritional status of its population. Coburn[22] has proposed that a specific dietary deficiency may be involved and suggests that a genetically controlled error in lipid metabolism is responsible for susceptibility to rheumatic fever. His evidence is largely circumstantial and is based in part on the low serum-lipid levels among rheumatic susceptibles.

At present the cause of rheumatic fever cannot be explained without bringing together a combination of circumstances, and even then many unknowns still exist. It appears that the full explanation of rheumatic fever, if ever it can be given, will have to include the role of the group A streptococcus, the genetically susceptible host, the role of antibodies, and the possible influences of race and nutrition.

REFERENCES

1. Rammelkamp, C. H., et al.: Studies on the Epidemiology of Rheumatic Fever in the Armed Services, in L. Thomas (ed.), "Rheumatic Fever: A Symposium," The University of Minnesota Press, Minneapolis, 1952, pp. 72–89.
2. Wannamaker, L. W., and Ayoub, E. M.: Antibody Titers in Acute Rheumatic Fever, *Circulation,* 21: 598–614, 1960.
3. Paul, J. R.: "Epidemiology of Rheumatic Fever and Some of Its Public Health Aspects," 2d ed., Metropolitan Life Insurance Company, New York, 1943, p. 163.
4. Stollerman, G. H.: Factors Determining the Attack Rate of Rheumatic Fever, *J.A.M.A.,* 177:823–828, 1961.
5. McCarty, M.: Nature of Rheumatic Fever, *Circulation,* 14:1138–1143, 1956.
6. Catanzaro, F. J., et al.: Role of the Streptococcus in the Pathogenesis of Rheumatic Fever, *Am. J. Med.,* 17:749–756, 1954.
7. Mortimer, E. A., et al.: Effect of Penicillin on Acute Rheumatic Fever and Valvular Heart Disease, *New England J. Med.,* 260:101–112, 1959.
8. Green, C. A.: Researches into Etiology of Acute Rheumatism. I. Rheumatic Carditis: Post-mortem Investigation of Nine Consecutive Cases, *Ann. Rheumat. Dis.,* 1:86–98, 1939.
9. Collis, W. R. F.: Bacteriology of Rheumatic Fever, *Lancet,* 2:817–820, 1939.
10. Thomson, S., and Innis, J.: Haemolytic Streptococci in Cardiac Lesions of Acute Rheumatism, *Brit. M. J.,* 2:733–736, 1940.
11. Marienfeld, C. J., Scheff, G., Hackett, E., and Jones,

D.: Studies on the Occurrence of Bacteremia in Rheumatic Fever, *J. Chron. Dis.,* 9:334–352, 1959.
12. Stetson, C.: The Relation of Antibody Response to Rheumatic Fever, in Maclyn McCarty (ed.), "Streptococcal Infections," Columbia University Press, New York, 1954, pp. 208–218.
13. Crawford, Y. E., and McNamara, M. J.: The Antibody Response of Rheumatic Fever Subjects to Respiratory Viruses, *Ann. Int. Med.,* 56:389–396, 1962.
14. Glaser, R. J., Thomas, W. A., Morse, S. I., and Darnell, J. E. Jr.: The Incidence and Pathogenesis of Myocarditis in Rabbits after Group A Streptococcal Pharyngeal Infections, *J. Exper. Med.,* 103: 173–187, 1956.
15. Char, D. F. B., and Wagner, B. M.: The Cardiac Effects of Group A Streptococcal Sonicates in Rabbits, *Ann. New York Acad. Sc.,* 86 (article 4): 1009–1024, 1960.
16. Kaplan, M. H.: Concept of Autoantibodies in Rheumatic Fever and in the Postcommissurotomy State, *Ann. New York Acad. Sc.,* 86:974–991, 1960.
17. Kaplan, M. H., and Meyeserian, M.: An Immunologic Cross Reaction between Group A Streptococcal Cells and Human Heart Tissue, *Lancet,* 1:706–710, 1962.
18. Wilson, M. G.: "Advances in Rheumatic Fever, 1940–1961," Hoeber Medical Division, Harper & Row, Publishers, Incorporated, New York, 1962.
19. Glynn, L. E., and Holborow, E. J.: Relation between Blood Groups, Secretor Status and Susceptibility to Rheumatic Fever, *Arthritis & Rheumatism,* 4:203–207, 1961.
20. Paul, J. R.: "Clinical Epidemiology," The University of Chicago Press, Chicago, 1958.
21. Bland, E. F.: Declining Severity of Rheumatic Fever: A Comparative Study of the Past Four Decades, *New England J. Med.,* 262:597–599, 1960.
22. Coburn, A. F.: Susceptibility to Rheumatic Disease, *J. Pediat.,* 58:448–451, 1961.

SUGGESTED READING

Hess, E. V., Fink, C. W., Taranta, A., and Ziff, M.: Heart Muscle Antibodies in Rheumatic Fever and Other Diseases, *J. Clin. Invest.,* 43:886, 1964.
McCarty, M.: Missing Links in the Streptococcal Chain Leading to Rheumatic Fever, *Circulation,* 29:488, 1964.
Murphy, G. E.: Nature of Rheumatic Heart Disease with Special Reference to Myocardial Disease and Heart Failure, *Medicine,* 39:289, 1960.
Rantz, L. A.: Hemolytic Streptococcal Infection and Rheumatic Fever, *Progr. Cardiovascular Diseases,* 4:483, 1962.
Watson, R. F., and Rothbard, S.: Experimental Studies in Rheumatic Fever, *Progr. Cardiovascular Diseases,* 4:464, 1962.

23 PATHOLOGY OF RHEUMATIC HEART DISEASE

Robert S. Eliot, M.D., and
Jesse E. Edwards, M.D.

Rheumatic involvement of the heart may be divided into two stages, the acute and the healed, although characteristically, recurrence of activity occurs in patients with healed lesions of earlier acute attacks. It is, nevertheless, convenient to consider the active and healed stages separately.

ACTIVE RHEUMATIC CARDITIS

Rheumatic fever has the potential for involving each layer of the heart, the endocardium, myocardium, and pericardium. Any one or all three of these layers may be involved in any given individual.

Endocardial involvement in acute rheumatic fever classically involves the valvular endocardium; the mural endocardium generally is spared. The primary process may be swelling of the valve leaflets, and an early secondary change is erosion along the lines of contact of the leaflets. At such sites elements of the blood, platelets and fibrin, are deposited as vegetations. Characteristically, the vegetations are small (usually less than 1 mm), beadlike deposits, uniformly distributed (Fig. 23-1). There is a strong tendency for the vegetations to be restricted to the line of closure, although, in the case of the atrioventricular valves, some vegetations may be deposited on the surfaces of the chordae. The mitral valve is most commonly affected, and in order of decreasing frequency is involvement of the aortic and tricuspid valves. Only rarely is the pulmonary valve involved.

Histologically, the lesion of the valves is nonspecific. Beneath the vegetative material the cells of the leaflet, particularly macrophages and fibroblasts, are mobilized. The latter type of cells tends to be arranged at right angles to the surface of the leaflet, and together they yield a pattern of palisading. In the valvular endocardium Aschoff bodies are uncommon, but they may be observed in the mural endocardium, particularly of the left atrium.

The myocardial lesions of acute rheumatic carditis represent the basis on which histologic confirmation of acute rheumatic carditis depends. The specific lesion is the Aschoff body (Fig. 23-2). This is characterized primarily by swelling, eosinophilia, and fragmentation of interstitial collagen, particularly common in the perivascular supporting connective tissue. Cellular reaction to the altered collagen yields a nodule, the so-called Aschoff body. The body contains a variety of cells, including the multinucleated Aschoff cells, the "owl-eyed" Anitschkow myocardial monocytes, and fibroblasts. As the lesion ages it becomes progressively less cellular and more fibrous. In a given patient with active rheumatic carditis, at any one time, Aschoff bodies of varying age may be observed. It is to be emphasized that the Aschoff body is fundamentally a lesion of interstitial tissue and that there is only little evidence for loss of myocardial fibers, even in cases with extensive involvement of the myocardial layer.

Uncommonly, acute inflammation of intramyocardial branches of the coronary arteries may occur in acute rheumatic carditis. In involved arteries, luminal narrowing may result from cellular infiltration, from thrombosis, or from a combination of the two. Occlusive lesions so derived may be responsible for foci of acute myocardial infarction. These are, fortunately, uncommon and appear to be associated with cases of fulminating acute rheumatic carditis.

The pericardial lesion of acute rheumatic carditis by itself is not specific for rheumatic fever. It takes the form of a serofibrinous effusion. The amount of fluid compared to the amount of fibrin varies. The exterior of the heart has deposited upon it shaggy elements of fibrin, which has led to the unappetizing name of "bread-and-butter" heart.

HEALING OF RHEUMATIC CARDITIS

The lesions of acute rheumatic carditis heal in a way that is peculiar to the healing of acute lesions

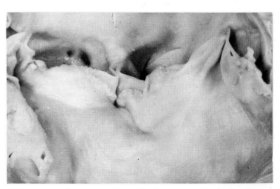

Fig. 23-1. Acute rheumatic endocarditis of the aortic valve. The vegetations form a beadlike row of deposits which tends to conform to the line of closure.

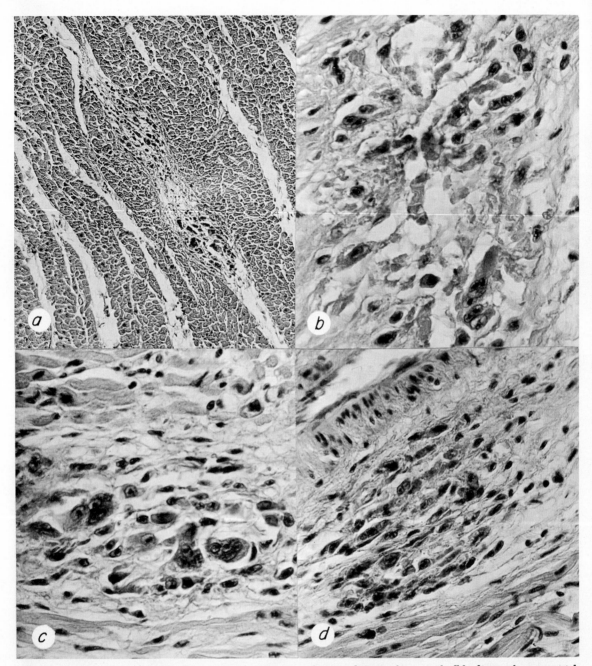

Fig. 23-2. Myocardial Aschoff bodies. *a.* Low-power view showing deposit of two Aschoff bodies in the interstitial tissue between muscle bundles (H & E; ×120). *b.* High-power magnification of an early Aschoff body showing eosinophilic necrosis of collagen and mobilization of tissue cells (H & E; ×460). *c.* A classical Aschoff body with multinucleated giant cells (H & E; ×460). *d.* A late Aschoff body lying in a perivascular position. A tendency for the cells to be predominantly fibroblastic is evidence of the healing stage (H & E; ×400).

in other organs, i.e., by scar formation and/or by resolution.

In the endocardium and myocardium, healing by scar formation predominates. In the pericardium either resolution of the inflammatory process may occur, leaving a normal pericardium, or the fibrin may become organized, resulting in pericardial adhesions. As the two processes may occur simultaneously in some individuals, there are examples of healed rheumatic pericarditis in which part of the

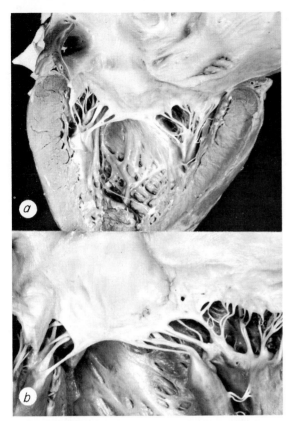

Fig. 23-3. Two examples of minor residual changes of rheumatic endocarditis involving the mitral valve. *a.* Thickening of the valvular tissue, particularly in relation to the line of closure. Mild thickening of some chordae. Vascularization of the leaflet. *b.* Minor degree of thickening of the leaflets and of the chordae. There is minor fusion of the leaflets at the commissures.

pericardium is normal while adhesions occur focally in other portions.

HEALED RHEUMATIC CARDITIS

One attack or a limited number of attacks of acute rheumatic carditis leaves relatively little residual change. In the valves, at the sites where vegetations had been present, there is a beadlike row of tiny fibrous elevations, and removed from this zone the leaflets may exhibit slight degrees of fibrosis. Vascularization of valve leaflets, particularly the anterior leaflet of the mitral valve, is still another minor residual effect. The chordae of the atrioventricular valves may exhibit minor degrees of thickening or may be normal (Fig. 23-3).

The myocardium may appear normal or show small perivascular scars as the only residua of previous Aschoff bodies. The pericardial changes have been mentioned.

It is evident that the description just given does not conform to the cardiac changes of patients with clinical chronic rheumatic heart disease. The minor residua described are usually not associated with significant cardiac dysfunction except that the valves may be more susceptible to bacterial infection than are the valves of persons who have had no attacks of rheumatic carditis.

Clinical chronic rheumatic heart disease, commonly referred to pathologically as healed rheumatic heart disease, represents the compound effects of many recurrent attacks of active rheumatic carditis and of the associated healing. It is commonly recognized that clinically evident recurrent acute rheumatic carditis may follow known streptococcal infections of the respiratory tract. Less commonly appreciated is that many episodes of active rheumatic carditis are without obvious clinical counterparts. The high incidence of histologically proved acute rheumatic carditis in subjects coming to necropsy with "healed" rheumatic heart disease was emphasized by Gross.[1]

The more recent experience on the high incidence (average of about 40 per cent) of Aschoff bodies in amputated left atrial appendages from patients with mitral stenosis but without clinical evidence of active rheumatic carditis is additional evidence of the strong tendency for rheumatic patients to experience recurrent episodes of active carditis (Fig. 23-4).

HEALED RHEUMATIC CARDITIS OF SIGNIFICANT NATURE

Under this heading are considered those valvular lesions of rheumatic origin which cause significant alteration in the cardiac dynamics. The pulmonary

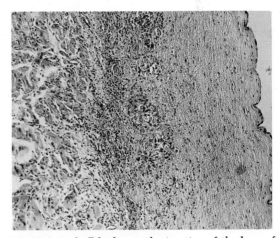

Fig. 23-4. Aschoff bodies at the junction of the base of the thickened endocardium and the myocardium of left atrium. From a patient with chronic, recurrent, acute rheumatic endocarditis.

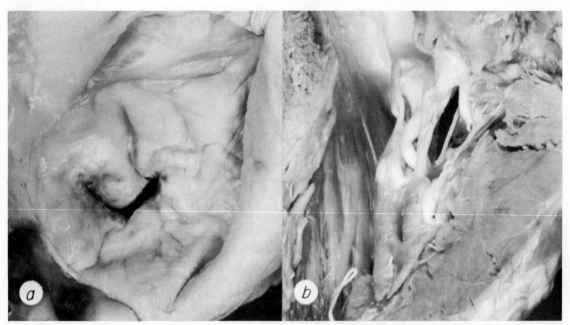

Fig. 23-5. Mitral stenosis. *a.* Unopened mitral valve from above. The inlet to the funnel-like deformity which characterizes mitral stenosis is wider than the outlet which lies in the left ventricle, below. *b.* The mitral valve from the left ventricular aspect. The valve has been converted into a funnel-shaped structure with a narrow orifice (containing probe).

valve, for practical purposes, may be considered immune from significant involvement and will not be considered further. Reference will now be made to each of the other valves according to the functional alteration that rheumatic endocarditis may cause in them.

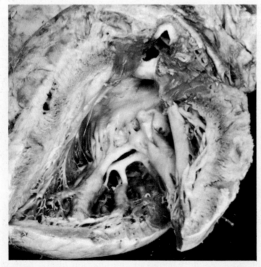

Fig. 23-6. Mitral valve from below in a case of mitral stenosis. The valve is converted into a funnel-shaped structure, the apex of which is in the left ventricle and is narrow.

Mitral Stenosis. The end result of recurrent rheumatic endocarditis is that the valvular leaflets and the chordae tendineae are affected by the addition of fibrous tissue, with concomitant contracture. An additional feature is that at each of the two junctional areas (the commissures) between the two major leaflets there is interadhesion between the two leaflets. This process, along with concomitant shortening of the chordae, causes the two interadherent leaflets to be held downward. The entire process is manifested by the leaflets' forming a funnel-shaped structure (Figs. 23-5 and 23-6). The inlet to the funnel is at the level of the left atrial floor and is wider than the apex, which presents in the left ventricular cavity. The anterior leaflet of the stenotic mitral valve frequently exhibits an interesting deformity. Near its basal aspect the leaflet is convex toward the left atrium. It is possible that during left ventricular diastole, the deformity is buckled in the opposite direction and may account for the "opening snap" of mitral stenosis. Such movement does not affect the caliber of the effective orifice, which lies at a lower level. The deformity may contribute to closure of the valve as it is pressed against the base of the opposite leaflet during ventricular systole.

Certain observations may be made regarding the structure of the stenotic valve as they pertain to present-day surgical procedures for relieving mitral stenosis.

It is to be realized in the first place that the structure of the stenotic mitral valve is such that a "successful" commissurotomy does not cure mitral stenosis. It simply opens the valve enough to make the stenosis less severe.

Two major factors in the alteration of the stenotic mitral valve contribute to "restenosis" following commissurotomy. These are calcification of the leaflets and short chordae. Calcified material, even if broken at the time of commissurotomy, tends to leave the leaflets fixed, allowing them to re-fuse. Short chordae also tend to keep the leaflets relatively immobile, favoring union of one with the other, following commissurotomy.

Mitral Insufficiency. The same fundamental processes which result in mitral stenosis may cause mitral insufficiency. The differences depend, in part, on fortuitous differences in physical orientation of the leaflets. While changes which tend to maintain the valve in a closed position cause mitral stenosis, those which cause the valve to be held open are associated with incompetence of the valve. The following structural patterns are found among cases of mitral insufficiency of rheumatic origin: (1) calcification of commissures, (2) fibrous contracture of valvular tissue, and (3) minor intrinsic valvular shortening with secondary distortion of the valve. That calcification which causes mitral insufficiency extends from one leaflet into the other across one or both of the commissures. The C-shaped plate of calcium is oriented across the commissure in such a way as to keep the two leaflets apart at the involved commissure (Fig. 23-7).

Fibrous contracture as a cause of mitral insufficiency is usually dominant at one commissure, with shortening of valvular tissue so great that the two leaflets cannot make contact. The shape of the deformity has been compared to a teardrop.

Perhaps the most interesting type of mitral insufficiency of rheumatic origin is that in which only minor scarring and shortening of the leaflets are present, while the valve is grossly incompetent. In such cases it is presumed that a series of circumstances is set into play.

The first step is intrinsic shortening of the leaflets, which causes a mild degree of mitral insufficiency. The left atrium responds to this valvular dysfunction by dilating. As the left atrium dilates it tends to pull the posterior leaflet of the mitral valve away from the anterior leaflet. As this process increases, the degree of mitral insufficiency increases and the left atrium dilates further and causes ever-increasing tension on the posterior mitral leaflet. While this process is in operation, the posterior leaflet is restrained at the opposite extremity by the chordae which insert into it. In the final stage the posterior mitral leaflet is immobilized over the base of the left ventricular wall as it is pulled in a posterior

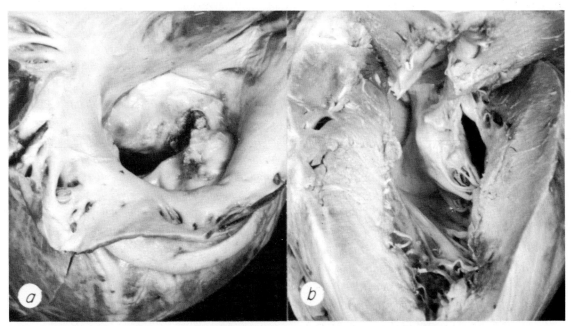

Fig. 23-7. Mitral insufficiency resulting from shortening of leaflets and commissural calcification. *a*. Unopened mitral valve from above. At the posteromedial commissure is a plate of calcium which crosses from the anterior to the posterior leaflets. In the left side of the illustration the valvular tissue is short, making the two leaflets incapable of apposition. *b*. Mitral valve from below. The fixed orifice imparted by short valvular tissue and calcification of a commissure causes the valve orifice to be fixed in an open state, thus causing the valve to be incompetent.

direction by the large left atrium and concomitantly restrained by the chordae inserting into it.

The views expressed about the series of events in the third type of rheumatic mitral insufficiency conform to the concept that "mitral insufficiency begets mitral insufficiency.".[2]

Aortic Insufficiency. Incompetence of the aortic valve of rheumatic origin is perhaps the simplest process to understand. In its pure form, there are scarring and contracture of the cusps, while no adhesions between the cusps at the commissures are present.

The normal aortic valve closes by virtue of the fact that each cusp is sufficiently long for its center to extend to the center of the aortic orifice during ventricular diastole. When the cusps become shortened as a result of fibrous contracture, each is incapable of extending to the center of the aortic orifice and thus each lacks the ability to make full contact with the other two cusps. An illustration of this is the characteristic triangular defect at the center of the aortic orifice when the valve is in a "closed" position (Fig. 23-8).

Aortic Stenosis. The crucial change of rheumatic endocarditis which leads to aortic stenosis is interadhesion between adjacent cusps at the commissures. As there are three aortic valvular commissures, the degree of obstruction caused primarily by the effects of rheumatic endocarditis depends on the number of commissures involved (Fig. 23-9).

When commissural adhesion occurs only at one commissure, the valve is converted into a bicuspid one (acquired bicuspid valve). In a valve so affected, the orifice is somewhat reduced, but usually not to such a degree that an obstructive effect may be demonstrated. Such valves, while not intrinsically stenotic, offer (as do congenital bicuspid valves) the tendency for acquired calcification of the leaflets. This tendency in bicuspid aortic valves (whether congenital or acquired) is the usual basis for the appearance of calcific aortic stenosis.

At the opposite extreme in functional effect from rheumatic fusion of one aortic commissure is the situation in which there is fusion at each of the commissures. In such valves, each cusp is prevented from lateral excursion during ventricular systole and the valve is stenotic. In valves so affected, the presence of any opening in the valve is dependent on shortening of the cusps. When there is fusion at each of the three commissures, therefore, the valve has a restricted orifice that cannot change its caliber. Incompetence of the valve accompanies this type of stenosis.

Fusion at two commissures results in a variable effect, depending on the degree of shortening and the degree of rigidity of the valvular tissue. When the valvular tissue on each side of the one remaining normal commissure is pliable and but little shortened, incompetence of the valve may not be present, and though the orifice is reduced in size, a stenotic effect may not be measurable. Such valves present the same potential problems as the acquired bicuspid valve, i.e., tendencies for calcification with secondary stenosis or for bacterial endocarditis.

Most commonly, when fusion occurs at two commissures, the effects are fundamentally like those of

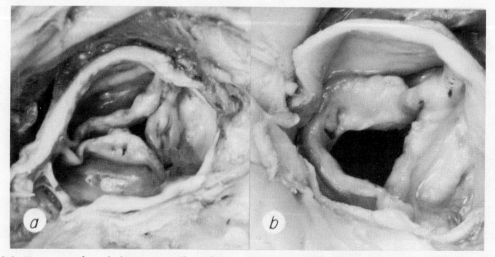

Fig. 23-8. Two examples of rheumatic endocarditis with aortic insufficiency. *a.* The valve leaflets are thickened and shortened to a relatively minor degree. The latter change is responsible for a small triangular-shaped orifice being present in the center of the aortic valve during diastole. *b.* The aortic valve leaflets are significantly reduced in size, causing a wide triangular-shaped orifice to be present and the valve to be competent.

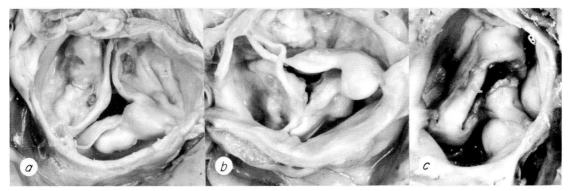

Fig. 23-9. Aortic valve in rheumatic endocarditis. *a.* Fusion between two adjacent leaflets at one commissure, creating an acquired bicuspid valve. Such valves are probably not stenotic but are subject to secondary calcification and also are susceptible to bacterial endocarditis. *b.* In this case there is fusion at two commissures, causing reduction in flexibility of the valve leaflets and an absolute reduction in size of the orifice during ventricular systole. *c.* Fusion at each of the three aortic commissures causing an absolute reduction in size of the orifice. The orifice is now fixed and is both stenotic and incompetent.

fusion at each commissure but the degree of stenosis may be less than when three commissures are fused.

SECONDARY EFFECTS ON THE MITRAL VALVE IN AORTIC VALVULAR DISEASE OF RHEUMATIC ORIGIN

In the patient with rheumatic aortic valvular disease in whom the mitral valve is incompetent, two pathologic processes are possible. The first is that this valve may also be involved by changes of rheumatic origin and exhibit alterations like those already described. The other possibility is that enlargement of the left ventricle, on the basis of the aortic valvular disease, has caused the mitral valve to become secondarily incompetent. Under such circumstances the mitral insufficiency appears to be dependent on displacement of the papillary muscles. In some cases, as the left ventricle elongates, the papillary muscles move downward, away from the mitral orifice. In such cases the chordae tendineae may show compensatory elongation. A stage may be reached beyond which chordal elongation is insufficient and as the papillary muscles continue to be shifted downward with the enlarging ventricle, undue restraint is imposed on the mitral leaflets and incompetence occurs.

The other process which may lead to secondary mitral insufficiency is left ventricular dilatation. This process causes the papillary muscles to shift away from each other. This results in loss of efficiency for restraint of the mitral leaflets by the chordae-papillary muscle systems. During ventricular systole the mitral leaflets may overshoot the level of optimal efficiency for closure of the valve, and mitral insufficiency results.

TRICUSPID INVOLVEMENT

Significant sequelae of rheumatic involvement of the tricuspid valve exhibit rather uniform changes from case to case. The major change is obliteration of each of the commissures. In the valve so affected, the distinction between one leaflet and the adjacent one is lost, and separate flaps, characteristic of the normal, are no longer identifiable. Chordal shortening and contracture of valvular tissue are usually only of minor degree. The important change of commissural fusion results in a relatively fixed orifice which is more narrow than the original tricuspid orifice, and varying degrees of stenosis may be measurable (Fig. 23-10). Incompetence, because

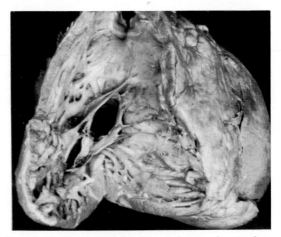

Fig. 23-10. Tricuspid valve from below in chronic rheumatic endocarditis. Although the chordae are relatively uninvolved, there is fusion of the leaflets at the commissures, creating a narrowed and fixed orifice. The valve is both stenotic and incompetent.

of fixation of the orifice, is inevitable. Tricuspid incompetence owing to right ventricular failure may also occur.

REFERENCES

1. Gross, L.: Lesions of the Left Auricle in Rheumatic Fever, *Am. J. Path.*, **11**:711–735, 1935.
2. Edwards, J. E., and Burchell, H. B.: Pathologic Anatomy of Mitral Insufficiency, *Proc. Staff Meet. Mayo Clin.*, **33**:497–509, 1958.

24 ALTERED CARDIOVASCULAR FUNCTION IN RHEUMATIC HEART DISEASE

Robert C. Schlant, M.D.

The changes in cardiovascular function in rheumatic heart disease may be divided into two types: the changes occurring during acute rheumatic fever and the chronic changes persisting and/or developing afterwards. Often there is no sharp demarcation between the two categories, particularly in patients with "smouldering" rheumatic fever.

ACUTE RHEUMATIC FEVER

During acute rheumatic fever, there may be a pancarditis, with evidence of inflammation in virtually all of the heart, including the pericardium. The acute inflammatory process in the atria and ventricles interferes with their normal function. This alteration is reflected in their depressed "function curves." It may result in "failure" of either the right or left ventricle or both, although more frequently the left ventricle fails and produces pulmonary congestion. It is uncertain whether myocardial function is depressed by interference with cellular metabolic processes or by interference with the process of energy utilization and muscular contraction, or both. That myocardial function is depressed is often apparent from the weak force of myocardial contraction of the ventricles, which may be extremely dilated, and from the cardiac output, which may be decreased despite elevation of left ventricular end-diastolic and atrial mean pressures. Patients with less severe depression of myocardial function may have normal cardiac output at rest but frequently have an elevation of left ventricular end-diastolic pressure. These patients are often unable to increase their cardiac output during exercise despite further elevation of left ventricular end-diastolic pressure. Whenever there is an elevation

of left atrial mean pressure, pulmonary venous and pulmonary capillary pressures are similarly elevated. If pulmonary capillary pressure exceeds the oncotic pressure of blood (25 to 30 mm Hg), pulmonary transudation of fluid occurs. In addition to the myocardial element in acute rheumatic fever, there is usually valvular dysfunction, which further burdens the heart. While some of the acute valvular dysfunction is caused by the acute valvulitis, mitral regurgitation may also be caused by the rather acute development of ventricular dilatation. This "functional" mitral regurgitation may be caused by several mechanisms. As a result of acute left ventricular dilatation, the mitral valve ring may be significantly dilated and may not be narrowed as much as normal during ventricular systole. Furthermore, acute left ventricular dilatation may interfere with the normal function of the papillary muscles and chordae tendineae in maintaining normal valve function. Although murmurs associated with stenosis of the mitral or aortic valve may occur during acute rheumatic fever, hemodynamically significant valvular stenosis is rarely, if ever, present during the initial acute attack. At times, the murmur of mitral stenosis is the consequence of several factors: a high flow across the mitral valve during diastole necessitated by the mitral regurgitation, a mitral valve deformed by rheumatic valvulitis, and a large, dilated left ventricle.

The moderate prolongation of AV conduction frequently present in acute rheumatic fever probably does not by itself interfere significantly with cardiac performance. Very high degrees of first-degree block or second-degree block may decrease the efficiency of the atrial booster-pump function. Complete heart block is rare during acute rheumatic fever.

Despite the frequent presence of large amounts of fluid in the pericardium associated with the pericarditis of acute rheumatic fever, it rarely, if ever, produces cardiac tamponade. It is thought that the relatively slow rate of accumulation of the fluid allows the pericardium to stretch without a significant elevation of pericardial pressure. Rheumatic pericarditis probably never produces chronic constrictive pericarditis.

CHRONIC RHEUMATIC HEART DISEASE

Cardiac dysfunction in chronic rheumatic heart disease is principally the consequence of altered function of the cardiac valves. It is likely that in some cases there is also a myocardial or muscular factor[1-4] which results from the acute rheumatic fever process and contributes to the derangement of function of the atria, the ventricles, or both.

The normal valves of a human being offer minimal resistance to forward flow, yet they are able to close abruptly with minimal leakage and minimal displacement. Although there must be some pressure difference across heart valves for blood to flow, the pressure difference across the valves of a normal heart is probably not greater than 1 to 3 mm Hg and is therefore usually too small to be measured accurately. With any form of significant obstruction to flow across a heart valve, there are three basic adjustments which may occur: (1) the pressure proximal to the obstruction may rise in an attempt to maintain the same quantity of flow; (2) the amount of flow may decrease and hence require less pressure difference across the obstruction; (3) the duration of flow past the obstruction may be prolonged, as systolic ejection is prolonged with aortic and pulmonic valve obstruction.

The basic relationship between valve area, blood flow, and pressure difference across stenotic valves and orifices is shown by the Gorlin and Gorlin[5] modification of standard hydraulic orifice formulas:

$$\text{Valve area} = \frac{\text{blood flow}}{K \times 44.5 \times \sqrt{P_1 - P_2}}$$

Valve area is in square centimeters; blood flow is in milliliters per second (for the mitral and tricuspid valves, milliliters per second of diastole; for the aortic and pulmonic valves, milliliters per second of systole); K is an empirical constant to correct for hydraulic losses through the valve orifice, the conversion of millimeters of mercury to centimeters of water, and errors introduced by the usual methods of measuring the periods of systole and of diastole; 44.5 equals $\sqrt{2g}$, where g equals the acceleration factor; and P_1 and P_2 represent the mean pressures in millimeters of mercury during the period of flow in the chambers or vessels on each side of the valve. As usually applied, K is 0.7 for the mitral valve and 1.0 for other stenotic valves and orifices. Estimations of valve area by this formula usually agree well with surgical and autopsy findings when the mitral orifice is less than 2.0 cm² or the aortic valve is less than 1.2 cm² and when there is a significant pressure difference across the valve. The presence of regurgitation makes it impossible to know the *total* amount of blood flowing across the valve during forward flow and therefore impossible to calculate valve area except by assuming various amounts of regurgitation. When accurate methods become available for measuring the amount of regurgitation, this difficulty will be overcome.

Mitral Stenosis. Following the initial acute attack of rheumatic fever, it is probable that the mitral valve becomes progressively narrowed over a period of time, usually 20 to 30 years. As this occurs the normal orifice of the mitral valve, which is normally 4 to 6 cm² in the adult, becomes smaller and smaller.

During most of this time, however, the narrowing of the valve orifice produces no significant hemodynamic alterations. In fact, the effective valve area must be reduced very markedly before it seriously interferes with cardiovascular hemodynamics. The narrowing is probably insignificant down to 2.6 cm². Between 2.1 to 2.5 cm² the narrowing is usually responsible for symptoms only with extreme exertion. Between 1.6 to 2.0 cm² mitral stenosis may produce symptoms with moderate exertion but rarely produces severe interference with light physical activity if it is uncomplicated by other factors such as mitral regurgitation, thyrotoxicosis, tachycardia, pregnancy, etc. The severity of the altered hemodynamics of pure stenosis of the mitral valve increases rapidly as the valve area becomes narrowed to 1.5 cm² or less. By the time the valve area is 1.0 cm², the patient will usually experience symptoms with very mild exertion. A mitral area of about 0.3 to 0.4 cm² is the minimal size compatible with life.

In most patients with significant mitral stenosis (i.e., with a valve orifice of 1.5 cm² or less), the flow across the valve is decreased and the left atrial pressure is increased. Occasionally, when the stenosis is not extreme, one of these factors may change proportionately much more than the other. Figure 24-1 illustrates the normal pressures and flow in the heart and the alterations present in severe mitral stenosis with and without severe pulmonary vascular disease. It is apparent that the rise in the left atrial mean pressure is accompanied by a rise in mean pressure in the pulmonary veins and capillaries and in the systolic pressure in the pulmonary artery. At a valve area of about 1.0 cm² the left atrial mean pressure, and hence pulmonary capillary pressure, is about 25 to 30 mm Hg at rest. This is about the level at which the oncotic pressure of blood is exceeded and pulmonary transudation occurs. If the rate of pulmonary transudation exceeds the rate of pulmonary lymphatic drainage, progressive pulmonary congestion will occur. In patients with milder degrees of stenosis, elevation of left atrial pressure and hence pulmonary edema may occur with exertion, emotion, or shortening of diastole with tachycardia.

The basic hemodynamic finding in mitral stenosis is a pressure difference between the left atrium and left ventricle during diastole. When the stenosis is severe the pressure gradient persists throughout diastole, but in mild stenosis it may be present only during the initial phase of rapid ventricular filling and/or during the increased flow across the valve during atrial contraction. In addition to the measurement of diastolic pressure gradient, however, it is essential to measure the flow across the valve, since alterations in flow markedly influence the pres-

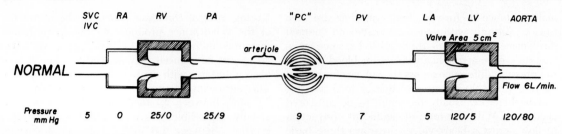

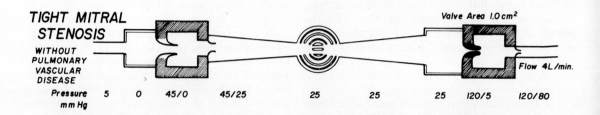

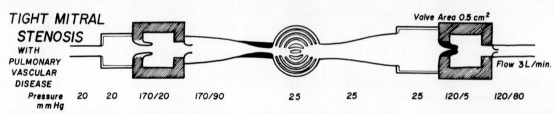

Fig. 24-1. Circulatory schemata of the pressures and flows in a normal individual (top), a patient with tight mitral stenosis without severe pulmonary vascular disease (middle), and in a patient with tight mitral stenosis with severe pulmonary vascular disease (bottom). Note that patients with tight mitral stenosis complicated by severe pulmonary vascular disease have two areas of obstruction to blood flow. See text for details. (*Adapted from the publications of L. Dexter et al.*)

sure difference across a stenotic valve. Some important relationships between mitral valve area, flow, and pressure difference are shown in Fig. 24-2. It is apparent that with a severely stenotic mitral valve, the heart is unable to increase the forward flow significantly by elevation of the gradient across the mitral valve, since the pulmonary edema threshold of left atrial pressure is rapidly exceeded. It is also apparent that remarkable improvement in hemodynamics can be achieved by relatively slight increases in mitral valve orifice.

During exercise, patients with mitral stenosis usually increase their left atrial, pulmonary capillary, pulmonary artery, and right ventricular pressures. If the stenosis is relatively mild, the cardiac output may be normal at rest and may increase with exercise. If the stenosis is severe, however, the resting cardiac output is low and exercise may produce no change or even a decrease in cardiac output, particularly if there is severe pulmonary vascular disease with right ventricular failure and tricuspid regurgitation. Since the stenotic valve area does not alter, the failure of the cardiac out-

put to rise despite the elevation of left atrial pressure is caused by the shortening of the total period of diastole available for flow across the mitral valve. Tachycardia from other causes may also result in a decreased cardiac output and/or elevation of left atrial pressure. Right ventricular failure and tricuspid regurgitation secondary to mitral stenosis with severe pulmonary vascular disease may contribute to the decrease in cardiac output during exercise in these patients.

In patients with severe stenosis, usually with a valve orifice of 1.0 cm[2] or less, pulmonary vascular changes often occur and markedly modify both the hemodynamics and the clinical symptoms. In the normal person large volumes of blood pass through the lung under low pressure and with little pressure difference across the lungs. In severe mitral stenosis, the resistance offered by the pulmonary vasculature may increase as a result of (1) structural changes in the arterioles and arteries, and (2) vasoconstriction of the small arteries. This vasoconstriction has been said to function as a "protective" mechanism, preventing the pulmonary capillaries from being flooded by sudden surges of right ventricular output. The anatomic changes in the pulmonary vessels may markedly decrease the lumen of the vessels and thereby increase the vascular resistance. Further, vessels with medial muscular hypertrophy may respond with proportionately greater further narrowing of the lumen to local hypoxic or other vasoconstrictive stimuli. As a result of the increase in pulmonary vascular resistance, which may be fifteen to twenty times normal and be associated with a pulmonary artery pressure exceeding systemic pressure, the patient may have *two* areas of relatively fixed severe obstruction to flow: the mitral valve and the pulmonary vasculature. Patients who develop high pulmonary vascular resistance often have fewer respiratory complaints than previously, since the right ventricle cannot pump blood into the lungs faster than it can escape through the mitral valve. These patients also frequently have associated right ventricular failure with tricuspid regurgitation. Although severe exertional dyspnea may persist in these patients, attacks of acute pulmonary edema are uncommon and many of the symptoms are related to the extremely low cardiac output and systemic venous congestion. At times patients with severe mitral stenosis and severe pulmonary vascular disease may even have *lower* left atrial pressures than patients with severe mitral stenosis but lower pulmonary vascular resistance.

In normal individuals at rest in the upright position the upper portions of the lungs have significantly less perfusion than the basal portions because of the effect of gravity on the perfusing pressure of the upper and lower areas of the lung.[6-7] This hydrostatic difference and the unequal distribution of blood flow is abolished when the person lies flat. In normal individuals in the vertical position, exercise is associated with a decrease in normal difference between upper and lower lobe blood flow. Patients with moderately severe mitral stenosis and moderate pulmonary hypertension tend to have relatively more perfusion of the upper areas of the lungs as compared to the lower areas.[8-11] If the pulmonary hypertension and pulmonary vascular resistance are extremely high, there may even be more perfusion in the upper zones as compared to the lower zones. Patients in left ventricular failure from other causes may also reverse the normal distribution of pulmonary blood flow. This shift of blood flow to the upper lobes in severe mitral stenosis is in part related to the greater degree of pulmonary arterial vasoconstriction and pulmonary vascular disease, including arterial medial hypertrophy, present in the dependent portions.

The mechanism of the pulmonary vasoconstriction in mitral stenosis is not clear. It is also not known

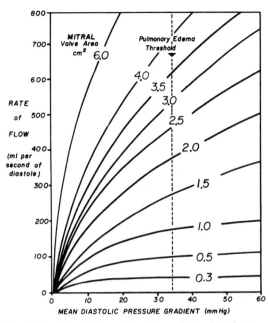

Fig. 24-2. Chart illustrating the relationship between mean diastolic gradient across the mitral valve and rate of flow across the mitral valve per second of diastole, as predicted by the Gorlin and Gorlin formula. Note that when the mitral valve area is 1.0 cm² or less, very little additional flow can be achieved by an increased pressure gradient. Transudation of fluid from the pulmonary capillaries and the development of pulmonary edema begins when pulmonary capillary pressure exceeds the oncotic pressure of plasma, which is about 25 to 35 mm Hg. It is also apparent that *severe* mitral regurgitation is incompatible with very tight mitral stenosis.

why some patients have more marked vasoconstriction and more marked pulmonary vascular disease than other patients with similar hemodynamics. The pulmonary vascular resistance in patients with mitral stenosis is often found to be markedly elevated in patients with a resting mean left atrial pressure of 20 to 25 mm Hg, which usually corresponds to a mitral valve area of about 1.0 cm². When the left atrial pressure is *acutely* elevated, increased pulmonary vascular resistance is usually much less apparent. The vasoconstriction, as well as the vascular disease changes in the pulmonary vasculature, in mitral stenosis is more marked in the dependent portions of the lungs. In these areas the vascular pressures are greater because of the effect of gravity and there is a greater likelihood for transudation of fluid from the pulmonary capillaries into the interstitial spaces. There is also probably more "reactive" hypertrophy of the arterial smooth muscle in these zones. Although it has been suggested that pulmonary vasoconstriction is produced by a reflex initiated by elevation of pressure in the left atrium, pulmonary veins, or pulmonary capillaries, it is perhaps more likely related to regional vasoconstriction produced by alveolar hypoventilation which occurs as the consequence of chronic excessive transudation of fluid from pulmonary capillaries. The pulmonary arteries may also be more responsive and more effective vascular sphincters as a result of the medial hypertrophy secondary to chronic pulmonary arterial hypertension.

In mitral stenosis the characteristic left atrial pressure tracing (Fig. 24-3) has an elevated mean pressure level with a prominent, or even giant, a wave, usually a good x descent, and occasionally a prominent v wave, followed by a slow descent of the y wave with an absent diastasis. At times the c wave is also prominent. If atrial fibrillation is present, the a wave is absent and the x descent is less pronounced whether or not stenosis is present. Unfortunately, the many variables affecting left atrial pressure tracings preclude accurate estimations of the degree of stenosis and/or regurgitation from the pressure tracing alone (see below).

In association with the decreased cardiac output produced by mitral stenosis, certain peripheral adjustments take place. Of particular value are a

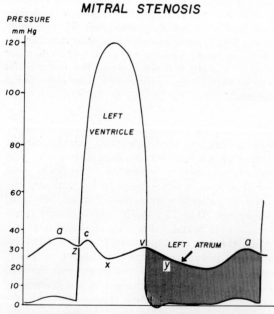

Fig. 24-3. Simultaneous left atrial and left ventricular pressure tracings in mitral stenosis. The diastolic pressure gradient is indicated by the cross-hatched area. The left atrial pressure tracing has good a and c waves and a good x descent. The y descent following the opening of the mitral valve has a slow rate of descent. These findings are in contrast with the typical findings in "pure" mitral regurgitation (see Fig. 24-4).

greater oxygen extraction per unit of blood flow to tissues, resulting in a greater systemic arteriovenous oxygen difference; the utilization of anaerobic metabolism, particularly during exertion; and an increase in total peripheral resistance.

Mitral Regurgitation. Mitral regurgitation when due to rheumatic fever usually coexists with some degree of narrowing of the mitral valve orifice. As a consequence, not only is the left ventricle burdened by the extra volume of blood regurgitated back across the mitral valve, but the left atrium is burdened to get this volume of blood across the mitral valve during diastole in addition to the volume which the ventricle pumps out of the aorta. Both left atrium and left ventricle are therefore doing "high-volume" work. Consequently, both chambers are dilated and usually hypertrophied. The net amount delivered out of the aorta may be normal if the regurgitation is mild or moderate but is usually decreased if the regurgitation is marked. Since there are two orifices—the aortic valve and the regurgitant mitral valve—through which blood may flow as a result of ventricular systole, anything which increases resistance to flow out of the aortic valve (peripheral arterial vasoconstriction, aortic stenosis, etc.) will increase the relative amount of blood flowing backward across the mitral valve. The peripheral vasodilatation and decrease in peripheral resistance usually associated with exercise may be one mechanism by which patients with mild or moderate mitral regurgitation are able to increase their peripheral output with exercise. Because of the large pressure gradient during systole between the left ventricle and left atrium, a very small mitral regurgitant orifice permits a large regurgitant flow. It is likely that the amount of regurgitant flow at times is three to five times the flow out of the aortic valve.

In patients with mitral regurgitation and some degree of mitral stenosis causing a diastolic pressure gradient across the mitral valve, an elevation of left ventricular diastolic pressure caused by left ventricular "failure" will be reflected in an increase in left atrial, pulmonary venous, and pulmonary capillary pressures. As in pure mitral stenosis or other conditions with chronic elevation of pulmonary venous pressure, the pulmonary artery pressure also increases. Although occasional patients with severe mitral regurgitation may have marked increases in pulmonary artery pressure and pulmonary vascular resistance leading to right ventricular failure, this sequence is not so frequently encountered in the severe degree often found in "pure" mitral stenosis.

In mitral regurgitation the left atrial pressure tracing (Fig. 24-4) may reveal no apparent distinct c wave since the x descent is absent and there is an early onset of a giant regurgitant *v* wave. When the mitral valve opens very slightly after the peak of the *v* wave, there is a rapid *y* descent of the pressure tracing. When the regurgitant wave is very marked, the left atrial pressure pulse resembles the ventricular pressure tracing in form. This is referred to as "ventricularization" of the atrium. Occasionally, the giant regurgitant *v* wave may be reflected back to the pulmonary artery pressure tracing, where it produces a notch—the "mitral insufficiency shoulder"—shortly after the peak systolic pressure.[12] In most patients with rheumatic mitral disease with predominant or even clinically "pure" mitral regurgitation, there is a pressure gradient between the left atrium and left ventricle during diastole. Because of the large flow during diastole, the diastolic gradient and the left atrial pressure are often as high as in "pure" mitral stenosis of equal clinical severity. In patients with massive amounts of mitral regurgitation, the stenotic mitral valve area is usually over 1.8 cm². Patients with only mild to moderate mitral regurgitation may have stenotic mitral valve areas as small as 0.9 to 1.6 cm²; however, hemodynamically severe mitral stenosis is incompatible with severe regurgitation. In "pure" mitral regurgitation, the left ventricular end-diastolic pressure may be normal at rest even with marked left ventricular dilatation, although the end-diastolic pressure usually increases abnormally with exercise. Rarely, patients are encountered with significant symptoms from "pure" rheumatic mitral regurgitation in whom left ventricular diastolic and left atrial mean pressures are normal at rest and in whom there is no pressure gradient across the mitral valve in diastole.[13]

Gorlin and Dexter[14] derived a formula for the calculation of the mitral regurgitant area in patients with combined mitral stenosis and regurgitation. The formula utilized the preoperative measurement of cardiac output and pressure gradient across the stenotic mitral valve together with the estimation of the stenotic valve orifice at the time of surgery. Several methods of analysis of left atrial pressure tracings have also been used to estimate the severity of mitral regurgitation.[15–28] Because of the many variables affecting the atrial pressure tracing, these methods are of limited value in an individual patient except in an approximate, qualitative fashion. Estimations of regurgitation from "PC" or wedged pulmonary artery pressure tracings are of even less value in an individual patient. Clinically useful estimations of mitral regurgitation may be obtained from left ventricular angiography[29–39] and from analysis of indicator-dilution curves.[40–77] In some techniques, the indicator (dye, hydrogenated saline, ascorbic acid, saline, etc.) is introduced in the chamber immediately beyond the regurgitant valve

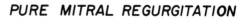

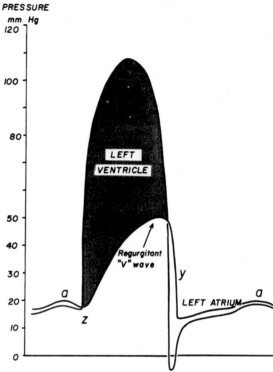

Fig. 24-4. Simultaneous left atrial and left ventricular pressure tracings in severe "pure" mitral regurgitation. The left atrial pressure tracing is characterized by a *regurgitant wave* which begins in early systole and obscures the *c* wave and obliterates the *x* descent. The regurgitant wave is produced by the flow of blood into the left atrium from both the pulmonary veins and the left ventricle, in contrast to the normal *v* wave. In extremely severe mitral regurgitation, the regurgitant wave resembles the ventricular systolic pressure tracing ("ventricularization" of the left atrium). The *y* descent of the left atrial pressure tracing following opening of the mitral valve shows a rapid fall in pressure, since the mitral valve offers relatively little resistance to the flow of blood into the left ventricle. These findings are in contrast with the typical findings in "pure" mitral stenosis (Fig. 24-3). Although little diastolic gradient between left atrium and left ventricle is present in this example, more commonly there is a moderate or high diastolic gradient. This is produced by a very high flow across a mitral valve which is only mildly or moderately stenotic. See text for details.

(left ventricle) and indicator-dilution curves are obtained from the chamber proximal to the regurgitant valve (left atrium) as well as from a peripheral artery. Other techniques employ injection proximal to the regurgitant valve (pulmonary artery or left atrium) and analysis of the indicator-dilution curve obtained from a peripheral artery. Most of the techniques used have been of considerable clinical value in 90 to 95 per cent of cases, but none of the available methods has been proved to provide an accurate measurement of the actual amount of blood regurgitated. Similarly, selective angiography has not yet been proved to provide a consistent quantitative measurement of the amount of regurgitant flow actually present under normal conditions.

Aortic Stenosis. Aortic stenosis produces predominantly a resistance or pressure load on the left ventricle, which responds with marked hypertrophy but relatively little or no dilatation. Normally, there is probably a 1 to 3 mm Hg pressure difference between the left ventricle and the aorta during systole. This pressure difference changes relatively little until the effective aortic valve area is markedly decreased. Although the effective cross-sectional area of the orifice of the aortic valve in the average adult is 2.6 to 3.5 cm^2, the "critical" aortic valve area at which patients develop pulmonary congestion, angina pectoris, or syncope is only 0.5 to 0.7 cm^2. Figure 24-5 illustrates the basic relationships between aortic valve area, blood flow, and mean systolic gradient across the aortic valve. Naturally, aortic stenosis of less severe degree will contribute to ventricular dysfunction and clinical symptoms if there is associated disease, such as aortic regurgitation or coronary artery disease. Many patients with pure stenosis of the aortic valve will maintain a relatively normal cardiac output by means of left ventricular hypertrophy, even though this may be associated with a left ventricular sys-

tolic pressure of about 300 mm Hg, which is about the maximum the left ventricle can generate for any length of time. If the stenosis is severe, however, the cardiac output usually does not rise on exertion even though the left atrial and pulmonary capillary pressures rise. The thick, hypertrophied ventricle in aortic stenosis is less distensible than normal, and the diastolic pressure is frequently elevated even at rest. The final filling and the final increase in end-diastolic fiber length and pressure of the ventricle are normally accomplished by atrial contraction (see Fig. 19-2, Chap. 19, p. 383). In aortic stenosis, this "atrial kick" is more forceful and is reflected in an increased amplitude of the left atrial *a* wave. It is also apparent from a marked increase in left ventricular pressure just prior to ventricular contraction. This momentary increase in stretch and pressure produced by left atrial contraction increases the force of the subsequent ventricular contraction. Since the left atrial pressure is elevated for only a brief period, pulmonary edema may not be produced even though the height of the left atrial *a* wave may be 30 to 35 mm Hg. If, however, the *mean* pressure in the left atrium becomes elevated above 25 to 30 mm Hg, pulmonary edema is imminent.

When left ventricular failure occurs in the late stages of aortic stenosis, the cardiac output may decrease and there may be an increase in left ventricular pressure throughout diastole and in the pressures back through the left atrium to the right ventricle. Only rarely are pulmonary artery and right ventricular pressures more than moderately elevated in pure aortic stenosis.

As a consequence of the obstruction at the aortic valve, the arterial pressure pulse is damped in aortic stenosis. Classically, the pulse wave is of low amplitude, with a slow rate of rise and a prominent anacrotic shoulder on the ascending limb, and has a low, rounded, delayed peak (Fig. 5-26, Chap. 5). The incisura and the dicrotic notch, which are delayed by the prolongation of systole, are less prominent than normal, or absent, particularly with severe stenosis. This pulse wave is sometimes referred to as *parvus et tardus*. There is a tendency for the anacrotic shoulder, or notch, to occur earlier on the upstroke when the stenosis is more severe. Although the rate of increase of arterial pressure, the duration of systolic ejection, and the period from the onset of the pulse wave to the peak pressure are prolonged in aortic stenosis, these measurements do not give an accurate estimation of the effective area of the stenotic aortic valve.

Patients with severe aortic stenosis may demonstrate *pulsus alternans*, with an alternation of the left ventricular systolic pressure and, to a lesser extent, the arterial systolic pressure. In most in-

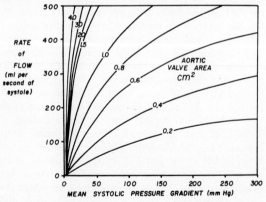

Fig. 24-5. Chart illustrating the relationship between mean systolic pressure gradient across the aortic valve and the rate of flow across the aortic valve per second of systole, as predicted by the Gorlin and Gorlin formula. Although the effective area of the aortic valve in the adult is about 2.6 to 3.5 cm^2, there is relatively little obstruction to blood flow until the area is markedly reduced. At the "critical" valve area, about 0.5 to 0.7 cm^2, relatively little further increase in flow is achieved even with marked increases in mean systolic gradient.

stances the weak beat is initiated from a shorter end-diastolic fiber length than is the strong beat, whether the end-diastolic pressure is lower, the same, or higher. Pulsus alternans in itself is frequently evidence of ventricular myocardial failure.

Ischemic heart pain in aortic stenosis is the consequence of many factors: increased myocardial requirements for oxygen associated with the high left ventricular tension-time index; relatively fewer capillaries per gram of myocardium as a result of hypertrophy; relatively low pressure in the aorta during diastole, when most coronary flow to the left ventricle occurs, and during systole, when the high intramyocardial pressure may impede the lesser amount of coronary flow normally occurring during systole; relative shortening of diastole; and the frequent occurrence of associated coronary atherosclerosis. The mechanism of exertional syncope is usually said to be a decrease in peripheral vascular resistance combined with a fixed cardiac output, producing a fall in arterial pressure. Other possible mechanisms are the occurrence of asystole or transient arrhythmias or a reflex decrease in peripheral resistance and pressure produced by a marked increase in left ventricular systolic pressure.

Combined Mitral and Aortic Stenosis. Hemodynamically significant mitral stenosis and aortic stenosis may exist together in the same patient. In this situation, the cardiac output is limited by the mitral stenosis. As a result the left ventricle is spared or "protected" from much of the markedly excessive work and hypertrophy usually produced by aortic stenosis, since the low flow across the aortic valve requires considerably less left ventricular systolic pressure. This is in contrast to pure aortic stenosis, in which the cardiac output is usually normal or even slightly elevated until the terminal, decompensated phase of the disease is reached. When combined aortic stenosis and mitral stenosis is suspected, it is imperative to obtain measurements of both pressure and flow and to calculate valve areas, since the mean systolic gradient across the aortic valve may be only 20 to 25 mm Hg even though the aortic valve is severely stenotic. In patients with both aortic and mitral stenosis, the hemodynamic changes across the mitral valve, in the left atrium, pulmonary circuit, and right side of the heart are similar to those in pure mitral stenosis. In most instances the left ventricle tolerates the limited increase in pressure work with only moderate elevation of its systolic pressure and without significant elevation of its diastolic pressure. If, however, the mitral stenosis is less severe and more blood enters the left ventricle or if the left ventricle should "fail" from other causes, the diastolic as well as the systolic pressures may become elevated. In the presence of mitral stenosis any elevation of left

ventricular diastolic pressures causes an increase in the left atrial and pulmonary capillary pressures. Similarly, if mitral regurgitation is present in addition to mitral and aortic stenosis, the elevation of left ventricular *systolic* pressure (produced by the aortic stenosis) results in more regurgitation back across the mitral valve during systole. In combined mitral and aortic stenosis the arterial pressure pulse wave may be less strikingly abnormal than in pure aortic stenosis. In most instances, however, it is still characterized by a small pulse wave having a prolonged systolic upstroke wave with an anacrotic shoulder, a delayed systolic peak, and a delayed incisura or dicrotic notch. The central incisura and peripheral dicrotic notch may be indistinct or even absent.

Aortic Regurgitation. Aortic regurgitation, like mitral regurgitation, imposes a large volume load upon the left ventricle. The amount of blood regurgitated may be estimated by several indicator-dilution techniques[78-82] or by angiocardiography,[38,83] but no readily applicable method has been proved to be quantitatively accurate in human beings. A very large amount of aortic regurgitation can occur across regurgitant valve areas of less than 1.0 cm^2, because of the relatively high pressure gradient between the aorta and the left ventricle during diastole. Initially, the ventricle accomplishes this increase in stroke volume with dilatation and an end-diastolic pressure which is within normal limits or only slightly elevated. Unless ventricular failure occurs, the pressure wave of the left ventricle is characterized by a rapid rise of pressure during systole to an early peak which is frequently higher than normal and by a rapid decline in pressure late in systole, the "systolic collapse." Later, as ventricular myocardial "failure" occurs (see Chap. 11, p. 224), the total output of the left ventricle may decrease, despite an elevation of left ventricular diastolic pressure and fiber length. The elevation of left ventricular diastolic pressure is reflected in a similar change in left atrial pressure and thence back to the pulmonary capillaries, perhaps producing pulmonary edema. At times the elevation of ventricular diastolic pressure may *decrease* the diastolic regurgitant pressure difference across the aortic valve and therefore the amount of regurgitation. Even the murmur of aortic regurgitation may disappear.

The arterial pressure pulse in aortic regurgitation is characterized by a wide pulse pressure with a rapid rate of rise of pressure to a high systolic peak and by a low diastolic pressure. At times coarse vibrations, which may be associated with a thrill, are present just prior to the peak. Following the early peak of the pulse wave there is a rapid fall of pressure, much of which actually occurs during systole and continued ejection. In aortic regurgitation the central incisura, or peripheral dicrotic notch, and the dicrotic wave are often lost completely. If they are present, they are usually less prominent and occur at lower levels than normal. The low arterial diastolic pressure in severe aortic regurgitation may surprisingly return towards normal, at times even to normal values, if there is severe left ventricular failure.

In the presence of aortic regurgitation, it is apparent that at the end of ventricular ejection, the relative amounts of blood passing to the periphery and passing back through the regurgitant valve during diastole will depend on (1) the pressures in the aorta and left ventricle, (2) relative resistances of the peripheral arterial system and of the regurgitant aortic valve and left ventricle, and (3) the duration of diastole. Thus, anything which increases peripheral vascular resistance tends to increase the amount of regurgitant flow. In many patients with aortic regurgitation there is apparent peripheral vasodilatation. This aids the rapid runoff of blood to the periphery and lessens the relative amount regurgitated into the left ventricle. The beneficial effect of tachycardia in aortic regurgitation is explained by the associated shortening of the total period of diastole per minute. When the left ventricle is markedly dilated because of aortic regurgitation, functional mitral regurgitation may occur because of dilatation of the mitral valve ring and interference with the function of the chordae tendineae and papillary muscles. The development of mitral regurgitation is an important factor contributing to the rapid downhill course of patients with aortic regurgitation when left ventricular "failure" develops.

Aortic Stenosis and Aortic Regurgitation. Aortic stenosis together with regurgitation is a vicious combination. In addition to the pressure work from the stenosis, the left ventricle has the added load of pumping an even greater volume of blood across the valve. From the basic relationships of hydraulic flow across a stenotic valve, it is apparent that if the flow is to double, the mean pressure difference must increase fourfold. It should also be kept in mind that, as in mitral valvular disease, *severe* stenosis is hemodynamically impossible in the presence of *severe* regurgitation although their contributory effects may be nearly balanced if both are moderate. The carotid or aortic pulse pressure tracing may often suggest which lesion predominates, although catheterization of the left side of the heart with measurement of the systolic gradient across the aortic valve and of the net cardiac output and estimation of aortic regurgitation by aortic angiography and/or special dilution techniques are frequently required. When a *bisferiens* carotid or

arterial pressure tracing is encountered in mixed aortic stenosis and regurgitation, aortic regurgitation is usually the predominant lesion. This characteristic pulse consists of a rapid rise of pressure to an initial peak (the "percussion" wave), followed by a brief fall or dip in the pulse wave, and a slower rise in the pulse wave (the "tidal" wave) to a delayed second peak usually of about the same magnitude as the first peak. The central incisura and the peripheral dicrotic notch and wave tend to be less prominent than usual or may even be absent.

Pulmonary Stenosis and Pulmonary Regurgitation. Pulmonary stenosis and pulmonary regurgitation rarely result from rheumatic fever, although occasionally patients with long-standing pulmonary hypertension secondary to chronic rheumatic disease of the mitral, or rarely of the aortic, valve may develop "functional" pulmonary regurgitation. Pulmonary regurgitation in these circumstances is usually ascribed to pulmonary hypertension and dilatation of the pulmonary valve ring. The volume of pulmonary regurgitation can be estimated semiquantitatively by special indicator-dilution techniques.[84-86] When pulmonary regurgitation is very severe, the pressures in the pulmonary artery and in the right ventricle may be equal or nearly equal at the end of diastole. Isolated pulmonary regurgitation seems to be clinically tolerated remarkably well in young persons or in experimental animals. Pulmonary stenosis, which is usually congenital, is discussed further in Chap. 20, p. 429.

Tricuspid Stenosis. Tricuspid stenosis is usually found in association with severe mitral valvular disease. Occasionally tricuspid stenosis may be the predominant lesion. Only rarely is it the only valvular lesion. The basic finding in tricuspid stenosis is a pressure difference across the tricuspid valve during diastole. The mean right atrial and venous pressures are frequently elevated to 10 to 20 mm Hg. If the atrial septum is intact, the *a* wave of atrial contraction is accentuated, or even "giant." The rate of fall of the *y* descent is slow because of the obstruction to forward flow across the tricuspid valve. Usually the mean diastolic pressure differences across the stenotic tricuspid valve are less (5 to 15 mm Hg) than those measured across the mitral valve in severe mitral stenosis. A very large *a* wave may also be found in right ventricular hypertrophy caused by pulmonary stenosis or pulmonary hypertension from any cause. It is therefore essential for the diagnosis of tricuspid stenosis to demonstrate a diastolic gradient between right atrium and ventricle. Most patients with tricuspid stenosis begin to develop peripheral edema or even ascites when the mean right atrial pressure is above 10 mm Hg. The cardiac output tends to be low at rest, and it does not increase normally with exercise, particularly if the valve orifice is below 1.5 cm².

Tricuspid Regurgitation. Tricuspid regurgitation most frequently occurs because of right ventricular dilatation and failure secondary to right ventricular hypertension resulting from (1) elevation of left atrial pressure from any cause, (2) pulmonary hypertension from cor pulmonale, or (3) pulmonary stenosis. At times, it is the result of bacterial endocarditis or of valvular damage from rheumatic fever, when it is often associated with some degree of tricuspid stenosis. The regurgitation into the right atrium produces a prominent "regurgitant" *v* wave in right atrial and internal jugular pulse recordings. When the regurgitation is marked, it causes a positive wave in the right atrium beginning with ventricular systole, obliterating the distinct *c* wave and the normal *x* descent, and reaching a very high peak. The *y* descent following opening of the tricuspid valve is rapid if there is no associated tricuspid stenosis. The large atrial wave which begins during early ventricular systole is perhaps better referred to as a *regurgitant wave* rather than a *v* wave, since much of its genesis is different from that of the normal *v* wave. Like the murmur of tricuspid regurgitation, the right atrial regurgitant wave may be increased by inspiration. The character of the regurgitant wave is affected by many factors, particularly the volume of regurgitation and venous inflow into the right atrium and the pressure-volume characteristics of the right atrium. At times, massive regurgitation into a flabby, giant right atrium may produce a relatively small regurgitant wave. Although indicator-dilution techniques have been used to estimate the amount of tricuspid regurgitation,[84,85] the available methods do not give a consistently reliable and accurate measurement of the volume of regurgitation.

REFERENCES

1. Harvey, R. M., Ferrer, M. I., Samet, P., Bader, R. A., Bader, M. E., Cournand, A., and Richards, D. W.: Mechanical and Myocardial Factors in Rheumatic Heart Disease with Mitral Stenosis, *Circulation,* 11:531, 1955.

2. Soloff, L. A., Zatuchni, J., and Mark, G. E.: Myocardial and Valvular Factors in Rheumatic Heart Disease with Mitral Stenosis: An Analysis Based upon the Combined Techniques of Cardiac Catheterization and Sequential Venous Angiocardiography, *Am. J. M. Sc.,* 233:518, 1957.

3. Fleming, H. A., and Wood, P.: The Myocardial Factor in Mitral Valve Disease, *Brit. Heart J.,* 21: 117, 1959.

4. Murphy, G. E.: The Characteristic Rheumatic Lesions of Striated and of Non-striated or Smooth Muscle Cells of the Heart, *Medicine,* 42:73, 1963.

5. Gorlin, R., and Gorlin, S. G.: Hydraulic Formula for Calculation of the Area of the Stenotic Mitral Valve, Other Cardiac Valves, and Central Circulatory Shunts, I., *Am. Heart J.,* 41:1, 1951.

6. West, J. B., and Dollery, C. T.: Distribution of Blood Flow and the Pressure-Flow Relations of the Whole Lung, *J. Appl. Physiol.,* 20:175, 1965.

7. West, J. B.: Regional Differences in Gas Exchange in the Lung of Erect Man, *J. Appl. Physiol.,* 17: 893, 1962.

8. Doyle, A. E., Goodwin, J. F., Harrison, C. V., and Steiner, R. E.: Pulmonary Vascular Patterns in Pulmonary Hypertension, *Brit. Heart J.,* 19:353, 1957.

9. Dollery, C. T., and West, J. B.: Regional Uptake of Radioactive Oxygen, Carbon Monoxide and Carbon Dioxide in the Lungs of Patients with Mitral Stenosis, *Circulation Res.,* 8:765, 1960.

10. Dollery, C. T., West, J. B., Goodwin, J. F., Hugh-Jones, P., and Wilckens, D. E. L.: Regional Pulmonary Blood Flow in Mitral and Congenital Heart Disease, in A. V. S. de Reuck and M. O'Connor (eds.), "Problems of Pulmonary Circulation," Little, Brown and Company, Boston, 1961, p. 17.

11. Dollery, C. T., and Hugh-Jones, P.: Distribution of Gas and Blood in the Lungs in Disease, *Brit. M. Bull.,* 19:59, 1963.

12. Levinson, D. C., Wilburne, M., Meehan, J. P., Jr., and Shubin, H.: Evidence for Retrograde Transpulmonary Propagation of the V (or Regurgitant) Wave in Mitral Insufficiency, *Am. J. Cardiol.,* 2: 159, 1958.

13. Braunwald, E., and Awe, W. C.: The Syndrome of Severe Mitral Regurgitation with Normal Left Atrial Pressure, *Circulation,* 27:29, 1963.

14. Gorlin, R., and Dexter, L.: Hydraulic Formula for Calculation of the Cross-sectional Area of the Mitral Valve during Regurgitation, *Am. Heart J.,* 43:188, 1952.

15. Allison, P. R., and Linden, R. J.: The Bronchoscopic Measurement of Left Auricular Pressure, *Circulation,* 7:669, 1953.

16. Owen, S. G., and Wood, P.: New Method of Determining the Degree or Absence of Mitral Obstruction: An Analysis of Diastolic Part of Indirect Left Atrial Pressure Tracings, *Brit. Heart J.,* 17:41, 1955.

17. Kent, E. M., Ford, W. B., Fisher, D. L., and Child, T. B.: The Estimation of the Severity of Mitral Regurgitation, *Ann. Surg.,* 141:47, 1955.

18. Ankeney, J. S., Fishman, A. P., and Fritts, H. W., Jr.: An Analysis of Normal and Abnormal Left Atrial Pressure Pulse in Man, *Circulation Res.,* 4: 95, 1956.

19. Haring, O. M., Liu, C. K., and Trace, H. D.: The Left Atrial Pressure in Experimental Mitral Valve Lesions, *Circulation Res.,* 4:381, 1956.

20. Connolly, D. C., and Wood, E. H.: Hemodynamic Data during Rest and Exercise in Patients with Mitral Valve Disease in Relation to the Differenti-

ation of Stenosis and Insufficiency from the Pulmonary Artery Wedge Pressure Pulse, *J. Lab. & Clin. Med.*, 49:526, 1957.

21. McMichael, J., and Shillingford, J. P.: The Role of Valvular Incompetence in Heart Failure, *Brit. M. J.*, 1:537, 1957.

22. Morrow, A. G., Braunwald, E., Haller, J. A., and Sharp, E. H.: Left Atrial Pressure Pulse in Mitral Valve Disease: A Correlation of Pressures Obtained by Transbronchial Puncture with the Valvular Lesion, *Circulation*, 16:399, 1957.

23. Marshall, H. W., Woodward, E., Jr., and Wood, E. H.: Hemodynamic Methods for Differentiation of Mitral Stenosis and Regurgitation, *Am. J. Cardiol.*, 2:24, 1958.

24. Braunwald, E., Welch, G. H., Jr., and Morrow, A. G.: The Effects of Acutely Increased Systemic Resistance on the Left Atrial Pressure Pulse: A Method for the Clinical Detection of Mitral Insufficiency, *J. Clin. Invest.*, 37:35, 1958.

25. Hancock, E. W.: Assessment of Mitral Valve Disease by Left Heart Catheterization, *Brit. Heart J.*, 21:389, 1959.

26. Neustadt, J. E., and Shaffer, A. B.: Diagnostic Value of the Left Atrial Pressure Pulse in Mitral Valvular Disease, *Am. Heart J.*, 58:675, 1959.

27. Hamer, N. A. J., Roy, S. B., and Dow, J. W.: Determinants of the Left Atrial Pressure Pulse in Mitral Valve Disease, *Circulation*, 19:257, 1959.

28. Fairley, K. F.: The Influence of Atrial Size and Elasticity on the Left Atrial Pressure Tracing, *Brit. Heart J.*, 23:512, 1961.

29. Arvidsson, H., and Karnell, J.: Quantitative Assessment of Mitral and Aortic Insufficiency by Angiocardiography, *Acta Radiol.*, 2:105, 1964.

30. Uricchio, J. F., Lehman, J. S., Lemmon, W. M., Boyer, R. A., and Likoff, W.: Cardiac Ventriculography in the Selection of Patients for Mitral Valve Surgery, *Am. J. Cardiol.*, 3:22, 1959.

31. Sellers, R. D., Levy, M. J., Amplatz, K., and Lillehei, C. W.: Left Retrograde Cardioangiography in Acquired Cardiac Disease. Technic, Indications, and Interpretations in 700 Cases, *Am. J. Cardiol.*, 14:437, 1964.

32. Björk, V. O., Lodin, H., and Malers, E.: The Evaluation of the Degree of Mitral Insufficiency by Selective Left Ventricular Angiocardiography, *Am. Heart J.*, 60:691, 1960.

33. Dodge, H. T., Sandler, H., Ballew, D. W., and Lord, J. D., Jr.: The Use of Biplane Angiocardiography for the Measurement of Left Ventricular Volume in Man, *Am. Heart J.*, 60:762, 1960.

34. Starobin, O. E., Littmann, D., Sanders, C. A., and Turner, J. D.: Retrograde Catheterization of the Left Ventricle and Angiography in the Diagnosis of Mitral Valve Disease, *New England J. Med.*, 265:462, 1961.

35. Kjellberg, S. R., Nordenström, B., Rudhe, U., Björk, V. O., and Malmström, G.: Cardioangiographic Studies of the Mitral and Aortic Valves, *Acta radiol.*, Suppl. 204, pp. 1–85, 1961.

36. Gray, I. R., Joshipura, C. S., and Mackinnon, J.: Retrograde Left Ventricular Cardioangiography in the Diagnosis of Mitral Regurgitation, *Brit. Heart J.*, 25:145, 1963.

37. Sandler, H., Dodge, H. T., Hay, R. E., and Ruckley, C. E.: Quantitation of Valvular Insufficiency in Man by Angiocardiography, *Am. Heart J.*, 65:501, 1963.

38. Aker, U. T., Friedenberg, M. J., and Parker, B. M.: Retrograde Left Ventricular Angiocardiography and Aortography, *Circulation*, 29:34, 1964.

39. Miller, G. A. H., Brown, R., and Swan, H. J. C.: Isolated Congenital Mitral Insufficiency with Particular Reference to Left Heart Volumes, *Circulation*, 29:356, 1964.

40. Korner, P. I., and Shillingford, J. P.: The Quantitative Estimation of Valvular Incompetence by Dye Dilution Curves, *Clin. Sc.*, 14:553, 1955.

41. Korner, P. I., and Shillingford, J. P.: Further Observations on the Estimation of Valvular Incompetence from Indicator-dilution Curves, *Clin. Sc.*, 15:417, 1956.

42. Keys, J. R., Swan, H. J. C., and Wood, E. H.: Dye-dilution Curves from Systemic Arteries and Left Atrium of Patients with Valvular Heart Disease, *Proc. Staff Meet. Mayo Clin.*, 31:138, 1956.

43. Wood, E. H., Woodward, E., Jr., Swan, H. J. C., and Ellis, F. H., Jr.: Detection and Estimation of Mitral Regurgitation by Indicator-dilution Technics, *J. Clin. Invest.*, 35:745, 1956.

44. Woodward, E., Jr., Burchell, H. B., and Wood, E. H.: Dilution Curves Associated with Valvular Regurgitation, *Proc. Staff Meet. Mayo Clin.*, 32:518, 1957.

45. Woodward, E., Jr., Swan, H. J., and Wood, E. H.: Evaluation of a Method for Detection of Mitral Regurgitation from Indicator-dilution Curves Recorded from the Left Atrium, *Proc. Staff Meet. Mayo Clin.*, 32:525, 1957.

46. Wood, E. H., and Woodward, E., Jr.: A Simple Method for Differentiating Mitral Regurgitation from Mitral Stenosis by Means of Indicator-dilution Curves, *Proc. Staff Meet. Mayo Clin.*, 32:536, 1957.

47. Shillingford, J.: Simple Method for Estimating Mitral Regurgitation by Dye Dilution Curves, *Brit. Heart J.*, 20:229, 1958.

48. Lange, R. L., and Hecht, H. H.: Quantitation of Valvular Regurgitation from Multiple Indicator-dilution Curves, *Circulation*, 18:623, 1958.

49. Levison, W. H., and Sherman, H.: The Measurement of Mitral Regurgitation by Indicator-dilution Techniques, *Mass. Inst. Tech. Rep.*, 20-0020 (Dec), 1959, 58 pp.

50. Korner, P. I., Thorburn, G. D., and Edwards, A. W. T.: Limiting Conditions in the Application of the Dye Dilution Method to the Quantitative Estimation of Valvular Incompetence, *Clin. Sc.*, 18:321, 1959.

51. Thorburn, G. D., Korner, P. I., and Stephens, J.: The Effect of Volume Dimensions and Type of Flow on the Dispersion of Dye in Normal Dye Curves, *Clin. Sc.*, 18:345, 1959.

52. Shillingford, J. P., and Zoob, M.: Dye Dilution Curves in the Clinical Assessment of Mitral Valve Disease, *Brit. Heart J.*, 19:589, 1959.

53. Emanuel, R. W., Lacy, W. W., and Newman, E. V.: Relative Effects of Heart Chambers, Lungs and Mitral Insufficiency on the Shape of Indicator Dilution Curves, *Circulation Res.*, 7:141, 1959.

54. Lacy, W. W., Goodson, W. H., Wheeler, W. G., and Newman, E. V.: Theoretical and Practical Requirements for the Valid Measurement by Indicator-dilution of Regurgitant Flow across Incompetent Valves, *Circulation Res.*, 7:454, 1959.

55. McClure, J. A., Lacy, W. W., Latimer, P., and Newman, E. V.: Indicator Dilution in an Atrioventricular System with Competent or Incompetent Valves: A Complete Analysis of the Behavior of Indicator Injected Instantaneously or Continuously into Either Chamber, *Circulation Res.*, 7:794, 1959.

56. Carleton, R. A., Levinson, G. E., and Abelmann, W. H.: Assessment of Mitral Regurgitation by Indicator Dilution: Observations of the Principle of Korner and Shillingford, *Am. Heart J.*, 58:663, 1959.

57. Levinson, G. E., Carleton, R. A., and Abelmann, W. H.: Assessment of Mitral Regurgitation by Indicator Dilution: An Analysis of the Determinants of Abnormal Dilution Curve, *Am. Heart J.*, 58:873, 1959.

58. Hoffman, J. I. E., and Rowe, G. G.: Some Factors Affecting Indicator Dilution Curves in the Presence and Absence of Valvular Incompetence, *J. Clin. Invest.*, 38:138, 1959.

59. Eich, R. H., Staib, I., and Enerson, D.: An Experimental Evaluation of the Indicator Dilution Technique for the Measurement of Mitral Regurgitation, *J. Clin. Invest.*, 38:2035, 1959.

60. Conn, H. L., Jr.: Use of Indicator-dilution Curves in the Evaluation of Acquired Heart Disease, *Progr. Cardiovas. Dis.*, 2:166, 1959.

61. Novack, P., and Schlant, R. C.: Korner-Shillingford Method for Estimating Regurgitant Flow, *Methods M. Res.*, 7:76, 1958.

62. Carleton, R. A., Levinson, G. E., and Abelmann, W. H.: Assessment of Mitral Regurgitation by Indicator Dilution: A modification of the Variance Method of Korner and Shillingford, *Am. Heart J.*, 60:396, 1960.

63. Jose, A. D., McGaff, C. J., and Milnor, W. R.: The Value of Injections of Dye into the Left Heart in the Study of Mitral and Aortic Valvular Disease by Catheterization of the Left Heart, *Am. Heart J.*, 60:408, 1960.

64. Yu, P. N., Finlayson, J. K., Luria, M. N., Stanfield, C. A., Schreiner, B. F., and Lovejoy, F. W., Jr.: Indicator-dilution Curves in Valvular Heart Disease: After Injection of Indicators into the Pulmonary Artery and the Left Ventricle, *Am. Heart J.*, 60:503, 1960.

65. Sinclair, J. D., Newcombe, C. P., Donald, D. E., and Wood, E. H.: Experimental Analysis of an Atrial Sampling Technic for Quantitating Mitral Regurgitation, *Proc. Staff Meet. Mayo Clin.*, 35:700, 1960.

66. Arditi, L. I., Pearce, C. W., Winston, A. L., and Lukas, D. S.: Experimental Assessment of Technique for Measurement of Valvular Regurgitation by Constant Infusion of Indicator, *Circulation Res.*, 9:146, 1961.

67. Lukas, D. S., Arditi, L. I., Winston, A. L., and Pearce, C. W.: Effects of Quantitatively Controlled Left Ventricular-atrial Regurgitation on Indicator-dilution Curves in the Dog, *Circulation Res.*, 9:375, 1961.

68. Polissar, M. J., and Rapaport, E.: Some Theoretical Aspects of Quantification of Mitral Valve Regurgitation by the Indicator-dilution Method: Sufficient and Insufficient Experiments, *Circulation Res.*, 9:639, 1961.

69. Levison, W. H., Jackson, W. D., Sherman, H., and McQuire, L. B.: Measurement of Mitral Regurgitation by Indicator-dilution Techniques, *Circulation Res.*, 9:1109, 1961.

70. Newcombe, C. P., Sinclair, J. D., Donald, D. E., and Wood, E. H.: Detection and Assessment of Mitral Regurgitation by Left Atrial Indicator-dilution Curves, *Circulation Res.*, 9:1196, 1961.

71. Wilson, W. S., Brandt, R. L., Judge, R. D., Morris, J. E., and Clifford, M. E.: An Appraisal of the Double Indicator-dilution Method for the Estimation of Mitral Regurgitation in Human Subjects, *Circulation*, 23:64, 1961.

72. Levinson, G. E., Stein, S. W., Carleton, R. A., and Abelmann, W. H.: Measurement of Mitral Regurgitation in Man from Simultaneous Atrial and Arterial Dilution Curves after Ventricular Injection, *Circulation*, 24:720, 1961.

73. Resnekov, L.: Assessment of Mitral Regurgitation by Dye Dilution Curves, *Brit. Heart J.*, 24:17, 1962.

74. Nixon, P. G. F., and Snow, H. M.: Indicator Dilution Curves in Mitral Valvular Disease, *Brit. Heart J.*, 24:637, 1962.

75. Marshall, R. J.: Factors Modifying the Contours of Indicator-dilution Curves, *Circulation Res.*, 10:123, 1962.

76. Gorelick, M. M., Lenkei, S. C. M., Heimbecker, R. O., and Gunton, R. W.: Estimation of Mitral Regurgitation by Injection of Dye into Left Ventricle with Simultaneous Left Atrial Sampling: A Clinical Study of 60 Confirmed Cases, *Am. J. Cardiol.*, 10:62, 1962.

77. Levinson, G. E., Frank, M. J., Palman, R. S., and Hellems, H. K.: Studies in a Cardiovascular Model

on the Arterial Dilution Curve of Valvular Regurgitation, *Am. Heart J.,* **66:**767, 1963.

78. Warner, H. R., and Toronto, A. F.: Quantitation of Backflow in Patients with Aortic Insufficiency Using an Indicator Technique, *Circulation Res.,* **6:**29, 1958.

79. Braunwald, E., and Morrow, A. G.: A Method for the Detection and Estimation of Aortic Regurgitant Flow in Man, *Circulation,* **17:**505, 1958.

80. Snow, H. M., and Nixon, P. G. F.: Arterial Indicator-dilution Curves in Aortic Incompetence, *Thorax,* **18:**354, 1963.

81. Armelin, E., Michaels, L., Marshall, H. W., Donald, D. E., Cheesman, R. J., and Wood, E. H.: Detection and Measurement of Experimentally Produced Aortic Regurgitation by Means of Indicator-dilution Curves Recorded from the Left Ventricle, *Circulation Res.,* **12:**269, 1963.

82. Armelin, E., Donald, D. E., and Wood, E. H.: Comparison of Dilution Technics Using Aortic Injection with Upstream Sampling for Assessment of Aortic Regurgitation, *Circulation Res.,* **15:**287, 1964.

83. Arcilla, R. A., Agustsson, M. H., Steiger, Z., and Gasul, B. M.: An Angiocardiographic Sign of Aortic Regurgitation: Its Utilization for the Measurement of Regurgitant Flow, *Circulation,* **23:**269, 1961.

84. Bajec, D. F., Birkhead, N. C., Carter, S. A., and Wood, E. H.: Localization and Estimation of Severity of Regurgitant Flow at the Pulmonary and Tricuspid Valves, *Proc. Staff Meet. Mayo Clin.,* **33:**569, 1958.

85. Collins, N. P., Braunwald, E., and Morrow, A. G.: Detection of Pulmonic and Tricuspid Valvular Regurgitation by means of Indicator Solutions, *Circulation,* **20:**561, 1959.

86. Wanzer, S. H., Cudkowicz, L., and Daley, R.: Diagnosis of Pulmonary Regurgitation by a Dye Method, *Brit. Heart J.,* **22:**720, 1960.

SUGGESTED READING °

General

Allan, G. A.: A Schema of the Circulation with Experiments to Determine the Additional Load in the Apparatus Produced by Conditions Representing Valvular Lesions, *Heart,* **12:**181, 1925.

Anderson, M. W., and Marshall, H. W.: Acquired Valvular Heart Disease, in B. L. Gordon (ed.), "Clinical Cardiopulmonary Physiology," 2d ed., Grune & Stratton, Inc., New York, 1960, p. 249.

Bayliss, W. M.: On the Local Reactions of the Arterial Wall to Changes in Internal Pressure, *J. Physiol.,* **28:**220, 1902.

Besterman, E. M.: The Cardiac Output in Acute Rheumatic Carditis, *Brit. Heart J.,* **16:**8, 1954.

Braunwald, E., and Sarnoff, S. J.: The Hemodynamics of Valvular Regurgitation, in A. A. Luisada (ed.),

"An Encyclopedia of the Cardiovascular System," McGraw-Hill Book Company, New York, 1959, vol. 3, pp. 7–63.

Dexter, L., Dow, J. W., Haynes, F. W., Whittenberger, J. L., Ferris, B. G., Goodale, W. T., and Hellems, H. K.: Studies of the Pulmonary Circulation in Man at Rest: Normal Variations and the Interrelations between Increased Pulmonary Blood Flow, Elevated Arterial Pressure, and High Pulmonary "Capillary" Pressures, *J. Clin. Invest.,* **29:**602, 1950.

Dock, D. S., Kraus, W. L., McGuire, L. B., Hyland, J. W., Haynes, F. W., and Dexter, L.: The Pulmonary Blood Volume in Man, *J. Clin. Invest.,* **40:**317, 1961.

Donald, K. W., Bishop, J. M., and Wade, O. L.: A Study of Minute to minute Change of Arteriovenous Oxygen Content Difference, Oxygen Uptake and Cardiac Output and Rate of Achievement of a Steady State During Exercise in Rheumatic Heart Disease, *J. Clin. Invest.,* **33:**1146, 1954.

Folkow, B.: Intravascular Pressure as a Factor Regulating the Tone of Small Vessels, *Acta physiol. scandinav.,* **17:**289, 1949.

Gorlin, R.: Calculation of Orifice Areas within the Cardiovascular System, *Methods M. Res.,* **7:**102, 1958.

Gorlin, R.: Shunt Flows and Valve Areas, in H. A. Zimmerman (ed.), "Intravascular Catheterization," Charles C Thomas, Publisher, Springfield, Ill., 1959, p. 140.

Heath, D., and Whitaker, W.: Hypertensive Pulmonary Vascular Disease, *Circulation,* **14:**323, 1956.

Keys, A., Friedell, H. L., Garland, L. H., and Madrazo, M. F.: The Valvular Efficiency in Mitral and Aortic Insufficiency, *Am. J. Physiol.,* **129:**397, 1940.

Rapaport, E., and Dexter, L.: Pulmonary "Capillary" Pressure, *Methods M. Res.,* **7:**58, 1958.

Rodrigo, F. A.: Estimation of Valve Area and "Valvular Resistance": A Critical Study of the Physical Basis of the Methods Employed, *Am. Heart J.,* **45:**1, 1953.

Shepherd, J. T., and Wood, E. H.: The Role of Vessel Tone in Pulmonary Hypertension, *Circulation,* **19:**641, 1959.

Snellen, H. A.: Estimation of Valve Area and "Valvular Resistance," *Am. Heart J.,* **45:**1, 1963.

Werkö, L.: The Dynamics and Consequences of Stenosis or Insufficiency of the Cardiac Valves, in W. F. Hamilton and P. Dow (eds.), "Handbook of Physiology," sec. 2, "Circulation," vol. 1, American Physiological Society, Washington, D.C., 1962, p. 645.

Wiggers, C. J.: Dynamics of Ventricular Contraction under Abnormal Conditions, *Circulation,* **5:**321, 1952.

Wood, P.: Selection of Patients for Surgery in Acquired Heart Disease, *Brit. M. Bull.,* **11:**203, 1955.

Wood, P.: "Diseases of the Heart and Circulation," 2d ed., J. B. Lippincott Company, Philadelphia, 1956.

° See references following chapter on Congenital Heart Disease, Chapter 19.

Wood, P.: A Physician's Responsibility in Respect of the Surgical Treatment of Acquired Valvular Disease of the Heart, *Progr. Cardiovas. Dis.*, 1:28, 1958–59.

Wright, J. L., and Wood, E. H.: Value of Central and Peripheral Intra-arterial Pressures and Pulse Contours in Cardiovascular Diagnosis, *Minnesota Med.*, 41:215, 1958.

Yu, P. N., Glick, G., Schreiner, B. F., Jr., and Murphy, G. W.: Effects of Acute Hypoxia on the Pulmonary Vascular Bed of Patients with Acquired Heart Disease: With Reference to the Demonstration of Active Vasomotion, *Circulation*, 27:541, 1963.

Mitral Stenosis

Arnott, W. M.: The Lungs in Mitral Stenosis, *Brit. M. J.*, 2:765, 1963.

Ball, J. D., Kopelman, H., and Witham, A. C.: Circulatory Changes in Mitral Stenosis at Rest and on Exercise, *Brit. Heart J.*, 14:363, 1952.

Basu, A. K., and Sen Gupta, D.: Haemodynamics in Mitral Stenosis before, during, and after Valvotomy, *Brit. Heart J.*, 24:445, 1962.

Bayliss, R. I. S., Etheridge, N. J., and Hyman, A. L.: Pulmonary Hypertension in Mitral Stenosis, *Lancet*, 2:899, 1950.

Bishop, J. M., and Wade, O. L.: Relationships between Cardiac Output and Rhythm, Pulmonary Vascular Pressures and Disability in Mitral Stenosis, *Clin. Sc.*, 24:391, 1963.

Björk, V. O., and Mamström, G.: The Diastolic Pressure Gradient between the Left Atrium and Left Ventricle in Cases of Mitral Stenosis, *Am. Heart J.*, 58:486, 1959.

Braunwald, E., Moscovitz, H. L., Amram, S. S., Lasser, R. P., Sapin, S. O., Himmelstein, A., Ravitch, M. M., and Gordon, A. J.: The Hemodynamics of the Left Side of the Heart as Studied by Simultaneous Left Atrial, Left Ventricular, and Aortic Pressures; Particular Reference to Mitral Stenosis, *Circulation*, 12:69, 1955.

Brock, R. C.: The Surgical and Pathological Anatomy of the Mitral Valve, *Brit. Heart J.*, 14:489, 1952.

Carman, G. H., and Lange, R. L.: Variant Hemodynamic Patterns in Mitral Stenosis, *Circulation*, 24:712, 1961.

Clowes, G. H. A., Jr., Hackel, D. B., Mueller, R. P., and Gillespie, D. G.: Relationship of Pulmonary Functional and Pathological Changes in Mitral Stenosis, *A.M.A. Arch. Surg.*, 67:244, 1953.

Connolly, D. C., Thompkins, R. G., Lev., R., Kirklin, J. W., and Wood, E. H.: Pulmonary-artery Wedge Pressures in Mitral Valve Disease: Relationship to Left Atrial Pressures, *Proc. Staff Meet. Mayo Clin.*, 28:72, 1953.

Dexter, L.: Physiologic Changes in Mitral Stenosis, *New England J. Med.*, 254:829, 1956.

Dexter, L.: Pathologic Physiology of Mitral Stenosis and Its Surgical Implications, *Bull. New York Acad. Med.*, 28:90 1952.

Dexter, L., Gorlin, R., Lewis, B. M., Haynes, F. W., and Harken, D. E.: Physiological Evaluation of Patients with Mitral Stenosis before and after Mitral Valvuloplasty, *Tr. Am. Clin. & Climatol. A.*, 62:170, 1950.

Dexter, L., McDonald, L., Rabinowitz, M., Saxton, G. A., Jr., and Haynes, F. W.: Medical Aspects of Patients Undergoing Surgery for Mitral Stenosis, *Circulation*, 9:758, 1954.

Donald, K. W.: Pulmonary Vascular Resistance in Mitral Valve Disease, in W. R. Adams and I. Veith, (eds.), "Pulmonary Circulation," Grune & Stratton, Inc., New York, 1959, p. 285.

Eliasch, H.: The Pulmonary Circulation at Rest and on Effort in Mitral Stenosis, *Scandinav. J. Clin. & Lab. Invest.*, 4, Suppl. 4, 1952.

Eliasch, H., Wade, G., and Werkö, L.: The Effects of Work on the Pulmonary Circulation in Mitral Stenosis, *Circulation*, 5:271, 1952.

Ellis, L. B., Bloomfield, R. A., Graham, G. K., Greenberg, D. J., Hultgren, H. N., Krans, H., Maresh, G., Mebane, J. G., Pfeiffer, P. H., Seilverstone, L. A., and Taylor, L. A.: Studies in Mitral Stenosis, I., *A.M.A. Arch. Int. Med.*, 88:515, 1951.

Goodwin, J.: Mitral Valve and Left Atrial Disease, in R. Daley, J. F. Goodwin and R. E. Steiner (eds.), "Clinical Disorders of the Pulmonary Circulation," Little, Brown and Company, Boston, 1960, p. 197.

Gorlin, R., Lewis, B. M., Haynes, F. W., Spiegl, R. J., and Dexter, L.: Factors Regulating Pulmonary "Capillary" Pressure in Mitral Stenosis, IV, *Am. Heart J.*, 41:834, 1951.

Gorlin, R., Haynes, F. W., Goodale, W. T., Sawyer, C. G., Dow, J. W., and Dexter, L.: Studies of the Circulatory Dynamics in Mitral Stenosis, II, *Am. Heart J.*, 41:30, 1951.

Gorlin, R., Sawyer, C. G., Haynes, F. W., Goodale, W. T., and Dexter, L.: Effects of Exercise on Circulatory Dynamics in Mitral Stenosis. III, *Am. Heart J.*, 41:192, 1951.

Harrison, C. V.: Pathology of Pulmonary Vessels in Pulmonary Hypertension, *Brit. J. Radiol.*, 31:217, 1958.

Harrison, D. C., and Dexter, L.: Evaluation of Patients Who Develop Recurrent Cardiac Symptoms after Mitral Valvuloplasty, *Am. Heart J.*, 65:583, 1963.

Hugenholtz, P. G., Ryan, T. J., Stein, S. W., and Abelman, W. H.: The Spectrum of Pure Mitral Stenosis: Hemodynamic Studies in Relation to Clinical Disability, *Am. J. Cardiol.*, 10:773, 1962.

Larrabee, W. F., Parker, R. L., and Edwards, J. E.: Pathology of Intrapulmonary Arteries and Arterioles in Mitral Stenosis, *Proc. Staff Meet. Mayo Clin.*, 24:316, 1949.

Lewis, B. M., Gorlin, R., Houssay, H. E. J., Haynes, F. W., and Dexter, L.: Clinical and Physiological Correlation in Patients with Mitral Stenosis, *Am. Heart J.*, 43:2, 1952.

Lukas, D. S., and Dotter, C. T.: Modifications of the

Pulmonary Circulation in Mitral Stenosis, *Am. J. Med.*, 12:639, 1952.

Lutembacher, R.: De la stenose mitrale avec communication interauriculaire, *Arch. mal. coeur,* 9: 237, 1916.

Milne, E. N. C.: Physiological Interpretation of the Plain Radiograph in Mitral Stenosis Including a Review of Criteria for the Radiological Estimation of Pulmonary Arterial and Venous Pressures, *Brit. J. Cardiol.*, 36:902, 1963.

Moore, C. B., Kraus, W. L., Dock, D. S., Woodward, E., Jr., and Dexter, L.: The Relationship between Pulmonary Arterial Pressure and Roentgenographic Appearance in Mitral Stenosis, *Am. Heart J.,* 58: 576, 1959.

Parker, F., Jr., and Weiss, S.: The Nature and Significance of the Structural Changes in the Lungs in Mitral Stenosis, *Am. J. Path.,* 12:573, 1936.

Rapaport, E., Kuida, H., Haynes, F. W., and Dexter, L.: The Pulmonary Blood Volume in Mitral Stenosis, *J. Clin. Invest.,* 35:1393, 1956.

Rowe, G. G., Maxwell, G. M., Castillo, C. A., Huston, J. H., and Crumpton, C. W.: Hemodynamics of Mitral Stenosis with Special Reference to Coronary Blood Flow and Myocardial Oxygen Consumption, *Circulation,* 22:559, 1960.

Semler, H. J., Shepherd, J. T., and Wood, E. H.: The Role of Vessel Tone in Maintaining Pulmonary Vascular Resistance in Patients with Mitral Stenosis, *Circulation,* 19:386, 1959.

Werkö, L.: The Use of Digitalis in Mitral Stenosis without Right Heart Failure, *Progr. Cardiovasc. Dis.,* 7:284, 1964.

Wood, P.: An Appreciation of Mitral Stenosis, *Brit. M. J.*, 1:1051, 1954.

Yu, P. N. G., Simpson, J. H., Lovejoy, F. W., Jr., Joos, H. A., and Nye, R. E., Jr.: Studies of Pulmonary Hypertension. IV. Pulmonary Circulatory Dynamics in Patients with Mitral Stenosis at Rest, *Am. Heart J.,* 47:330, 1954.

Yu, P. N., Nye, R. E., Jr., Lovejoy, F. W., Jr., Macias, J. DeJ., Schreiner, B. F., and Lux, J. J.: Studies of Pulmonary Hypertension. VIII. Effects of Acetyl Strophanthidin on Pulmonary Circulation in Patients with Cardiac Failure and Mitral Stenosis, *Am. Heart J.,* 54:235, 1957.

Mitral Stenosis and Regurgitation

Dogliotti, G. C., Angelino, P. F., Brusca, A., Garbagni, R., Gavosta, F., Magri, G., and Minetto, E.: Pulmonary Function in Mitral Valve Disease: Hemodynamic and Ventilatory Studies, *Am. J. Cardiol.,* 3:28, 1959.

Draper, A., Heimbecker, R., Daley, R., Carroll, D., Mudd, G., Wells, R., Falholt, W., Andrus, E. C., and Bing, R. J.: Physiologic Studies in Mitral Valvular Disease, *Circulation,* 3:531, 1951.

Eliasch, H., Lagerlöf, H., and Werkö, L.: Pulmonary and Renal Circulatory Adjustments to the Upright

Position in Patients with Mitral Valvular Disease, *Am. Heart J.,* 62:519, 1961.

Ferrer, M. I., Harvey, R. M., Cathcart, R. T., Cournand, A., and Richards, D. W., Jr.: Hemodynamic Studies in Rheumatic Heart Disease, *Circulation,* 6:688, 1952.

Harvey, R. M., and Ferrer, I.: A Consideration of Hemodynamic Criteria for Operability in Mitral Stenosis and in Mitral Insufficiency, *Circulation,* 20: 442, 1959.

Haynes, F., Novack, P., Schlant, R., Phinny, A., and Dexter, L.: Hemodynamics of Mitral Stenosis and Regurgitation, *Fed. Proc.,* 16:56, 1957.

Luisada, A. A., and Liu, C. K.: Left Atrial Electrokymograms and Pressure Pulses in Mitral Valve Disease, *Am. J. Cardiol.,* 1:68, 1958.

McDonald, L., Dealy, J. B., Jr., Rabinowitz, M., and Dexter, L.: Clinical, Physiological and Pathological Findings in Mitral Stenosis and Regurgitation, *Medicine,* 36:237, 1957.

MacCallum, W. G., and McClure, R. D.: On the Mechanical Effects of Experimental Mitral Stenosis and Insufficiency, *Bull. Johns Hopkins Hosp.,* 17: 260, 1906.

Sosman, M. C.: Symposium on the Diagnosis and Treatment of Mitral-valve Disease, *New England J. Med.,* 254:825-837, 1956.

Mitral Stenosis and Aortic Stenosis

Honey, M.: Clinical and Hemodynamic Observations on Combined Mitral and Aortic Stenosis, *Brit. Heart J.,* 23:545, 1961.

Katznelson, G., Jreissaty, R. M., Levinson, G. E., Stein, S. W., and Abelmann, W. H.: Combined Aortic and Mitral Stenosis: A Clinical and Physiological Study, *Am. J. Med.,* 29:242, 1960.

Morrow, A. G., Awe, W. C., and Braunwald, E.: Combined Mitral and Aortic Stenosis, *Brit. Heart J.,* 24:606, 1962.

Reid, J. M., Stevenson, J. G., Barclay, R. S., and Welsh, T. M.: Combined Aortic and Mitral Stenosis, *Brit. Heart J.,* 24:509, 1962.

Uricchio, J. F., Goldberg, H., Sinah, K. P., and Likoff, W.: Combined Mitral Aortic Stenosis: Clinical and Physiologic Features and Results of Surgery, *Am. J. Cardiol.,* 4:479, 1959.

Zitnik, R. S., Piemme, T. E., Messer, R. J., Reed, D. P., Haynes, F. W. and Dexter, L.: The Masking of Aortic Stenosis by Mitral Stenosis, *Am. Heart J.,* 69:22, 1965.

Mitral Regurgitation

Becker, D. L., Burchell, H. B., and Edwards, J. E.: Pathology of the Pulmonary Vascular Tree. II. The Occurrence in Mitral Insufficiency of Occlusive Pulmonary Vascular Lesions, *Circulation,* 3:230, 1951.

Braunwald, E., Welch, G. H., Jr., and Sarnoff, S. J.: Hemodynamic Effects of Quantitatively Varied Experimental Mitral Regurgitation, *Circulation,* **5:** 539, 1957.

Brigden, W., and Leatham, A.: Mitral Incompetence, *Brit. Heart J.,* **15:**55, 1953.

Daley, R., McMillan, I. K. R., and Gorlin, R.: Mitral Incompetence in Experimental Auricular Fibrillation, *Lancet,* **2:**18, 1955.

Dexter, L.: Valvular Regurgitation, *Proc. Inst. Med. Chicago,* **21:**219, 1957.

Dexter, L., Novack, P., Schlant, R. C., Phinney, A. O., Jr., and Haynes, F. W.: Mitral Insufficiency, *Tr. A. Am. Physicians,* **70:**262, 1957.

Edwards, J. E., and Burchell, H. B.: Pathologic Anatomy of Mitral Insufficiency, *Proc. Staff Meet. Mayo Clin.,* **33:**497, 1958.

Friedman, B., Daily, W. M., and Wilson, R. H.: Studies on Mitral Valve Function: Effect of Acute Hypervolemia, Premature Beats and Other Arrhythmias, *Circulation Res.,* **4:**33, 1956.

Gorlin, R., Lewis, B. M., Haynes, F. W., and Dexter, L.: Studies of the Circulatory Dynamics at Rest in Mitral Valvular Regurgitation with and without Stenosis, *Am. Heart J.,* **43:**357, 1952.

Marshall, H. W., and Wood, E. H.: Hemodynamic Considerations in Mitral Regurgitation, *Proc. Staff Meet. Mayo Clin.,* **33:**517, 1958.

Nixon, P. G. F., and Wooler, G. H., Rapid Left Ventricular Filling and Stasis in Mitral Regurgitation, *Brit. Heart J.,* **23:**161, 1961.

Nixon, P. G. F., and Wagner, G. R.: The Duration of Left Ventricular Systole in Mitral Incompetence, *Brit. Heart J.,* **24:**464, 1962.

Rodbard, S., and Williams, F.: The Dynamics of Mitral Insufficiency, *Am. Heart J.,* **48:**521, 1954.

Ross, J., Jr., Braunwald, E., and Morrow, A. G.: Clinical and Hemodynamic Observations in Pure Mitral Insufficiency, *Am. J. Cardiol.,* **2:**11, 1958.

Shapiro, H. A., and Weiss, D. R.: Mitral Insufficiency Due to Ruptured Chordae Tendinae Simulating Aortic Stenosis, *New England J. Med.,* **261:**272, 1959.

Wiggers, C. J., and Feil, H.: The Cardio-dynamics of Mitral Insufficiency, *Heart,* **9:**149, 1921–1922.

Aortic Valve Disease

Bramwell, C.: Arterial Pulse in Health and Disease, *Lancet,* **2:**239, 301, 336, 1937.

Feil, H. S., and Gilder, M. D. D.: Pulse in Aortic Disease as Felt and Graphically Inscribed, *Heart,* **8:**4, 1921.

Goldberg, H., Bakst, A. A., and Bailey, C. P.: The Dynamics of Aortic Valvular Disease, *Am. Heart J.,* **47:**527, 1954.

Gorlin, R., Matthews, M. B., McMillan, I. K. R., Daley, R., and Medd, W. E.: Physiological and Clinical Observations in Aortic Valvular disease, *Bull. New England M. Center,* **16:**13, 1954.

Gorlin, R., McMillan, I. K. R., Medd, W. E., Matthews, M. B., and Daley, R.: Dynamics of the Circulation

in Aortic Valvular Disease, *Am. J. Med.,* **18:**855, 1955.

Moscovitz, H. L., and Wilder, R. J.: The Pressure Events of the Cardiac Cycle in the Dog: Aortic Valve Lesions, *Am. Heart J.,* **54:**572, 1957.

Sancetta, S. M., and Kleinerman, J.: Effect of Mild, Steady State Exercise on Total Pulmonary Resistance of Normal Subjects and Those with Isolated Aortic Valvular Lesions, *Am. Heart J.,* **53:** 404, 1957.

Björk, V. O., Cullhed, I., and Lodin, H.: Aortic Stenosis: Correlations between Pressure Gradient and Left Ventricular Angiocardiography, *Circulation,* **23:**509, 1961.

Braunwald, E., and Morrow, A. G.: Obstruction to Left Ventricular Outflow: Current Criteria for the Selection of Patients for Operation, *Am. J. Cardiol.,* **12:** 53, 1963.

Buteler, B. S.: The Relation of Systolic Upstroke Time and Pulse in Aortic Stenosis, *Brit. Heart J.,* **24:**657, 1962.

Castenfors, H., Porje, I., and Rudewald, B:. The Hydrodynamics of Aortic Valve Stenosis: Experiments with a Special Model, *Cardiologia,* **25:**37, 1954.

Cooper, T., Braunwald, E., and Morrow, A. G.: Pulsus Alternans in Aortic Stenosis: Hemodynamic Observations in 50 Patients Studied by Left Heart Catheterization, *Circulation,* **18:**64, 1958.

Dexter, L., Harken, D. E., Cobb, L. A., Jr., Novack, P., Schlant, R. C., Phinney, A. O., Jr., and Haynes, F. W.: Aortic Stenosis, *A.M.A. Arch. Int. Med.,* **101:**254, 1958.

Dow, P.: Development of Anacrotic and Tardus Pulse of Aortic Stenosis, *Am. J. Physiol.,* **131:**432, 1940.

Epstein, E. J., and Coulshed, N.: Assessment of Aortic Stenosis from the External Carotid Pulse Wave, *Brit. Heart J.,* **26:**84, 1964.

Feil, H. S., and Katz, L. N.: The Transformation of the Central into the Peripheral Pulse in Patients with Aortic Stenosis, *Am. Heart J.,* **2:**12, 1926.

Hammarsten, J. F.: Syncope in Aortic Stenosis, *A.M.A. Arch. Int. Med.,* **87:**274, 1951.

Hancock, E. W., and Fleming, P. R.: Aortic Stenosis, *Quart. J. Med.,* **29:**209, 1960.

Hancock, E. W., and Abelman, W. H.: A Clinical Study of the Brachial Arterial Pulse Form, with Special Reference to the Diagnosis of Aortic Valvular Disease, *Circulation,* **16:**572, 1957.

Katz, L. N., Ralli, E. P., and Cheer, S.: The Cardiodynamic Changes in the Aorta and Left Ventricle Due to Stenosis of Aorta, *J. Clin. Invest.,* **5:**205, 1928.

Katz, L. N., and Siegel, M. L.: The Cardiodynamic Effects of Acute Experimental Stenosis, *Am. Heart J.,* **6:**672, 1931.

Kraus, W. L., Schlant, R. C., Moore, C. B., Dock, D. S., Woodward, E., Jr., Haynes, F. W., and Dexter, L.: The Hemodynamic Results of Surgery for Aortic Stenosis, *Am. Heart J.,* **58:**174, 1959.

Morrow, A. G., Sharp, E. H., and Braunwald, E.: Congenital Aortic Stenosis, *Circulation,* 18:1091, 1958.

Raber, G., and Goldberg, H.: Left Ventricular, Central Aortic, and Peripheral Pressure Pulses in Aortic Stenosis, *Am. J. Cardiol.,* 1:572, 1958.

Robinson, B.: The Carotid Pulse. I. Diagnosis of Aortic Stenosis by External Recordings, *Brit. Heart J.,* 25: 51, 1963.

Soulié, P., Degeorges, M., Joly, F., Caramanian, M., and Carlotti, J.: Une cause d'erreur dans le diagnostic hémodynamique des rétrécissements aortiques, *Arch. mal. coeur,* 52:1002, 1959.

Tjong, O. S., and Verheugt, A. P. M.: Peripheral and Central Arterial Pressure Pulse in the Estimation of the Severity of Aortic Stenosis, *Am. Heart J.,* 62:180, 1961.

Wood, P.: Aortic Stenosis, *Am. J. Cardiol.,* 1:553, 1958.

Aortic Regurgitation

Austen, W. G., Bender, H. W., Wilcox, B. R., and Morrow, A. G.: Experimental Aortic Regurgitation: The Magnitude and Acute Hemodynamic Effects of Regurgitant Flows Associated with Valvular Defects of Various sizes, *J. Surg. Res.,* 3:466, 1963.

Frahm, C. J., Braunwald, E., and Morrow, A. G.: Congenital Aortic Regurgitation: Clinical and Hemodynamic Findings in Four Patients, *Am. J. Med.,* 31: 63, 1961.

Goldstein, S., and Killip, T., III: Comparison of Direct and Indirect Arterial Pressures in Aortic Regurgitation, *New England J. Med.,* 267:1121, 1962.

Gorlin, R., and Goodale, W. T.: Changing Blood Pressure in Aortic Insufficiency: Its Clinical Significance, *New England J. Med.,* 255:77, 1956.

Meadows, W. R., Van Praagh, S., Indreika, M., and Sharp, J. T.: Premature Mitral Valve Closure. A Hemodynamic Explanation for Absence of the First Sound in Aortic Insufficiency, *Circulation,* 28:251, 1963.

Rees, J. R., Epstein, E. J., Criley, J. M., and Ross, R. S.: Haemodynamic Effects of Severe Aortic Regurgitation, *Brit. Heart J.,* 26:412, 1964.

Regan, T. J., DeFazio, V., Binak, K., and Hellems, H. K.: Norepinephrine Induced Pulmonary Congestion in Patients with Aortic Valve Regurgitation, *J. Clin. Invest.,* 38:1564, 1959.

Schenk, W. G., Jr., Portin, B. A., Leslie, M. B., and Anderson, M. N.: Hemodynamics of Experimental Acute Aortic Insufficiency, *Ann. Surg.,* 150:104, 1959.

Segal, B. L., Likoff, W., and Kaspar, A. J.: "Silent" Rheumatic Aortic Regurgitation, *Am. J. Cardiol.,* 14:628, 1964.

Warner, H. R., and Toronto, A. F.: Effect of Heart Rate on Aortic Insufficiency as Measured by a Dye-dilution Technique, *Circulation Res.,* 9:413, 1961.

Welch, G. H., Jr., Braunwald, E., and Sarnoff, S. J.: Hemodynamic Effects of Quantitatively Varied Experimental Aortic Regurgitation, *Circulation Res.,* 5:546, 1957.

West, J. W., Wendel, H., and Foltz, E. L.: Effects of Aortic Insufficiency on Circulatory Dynamics of the Dog: With Special Reference to Coronary Blood Flow and Cardiac Oxygen Consumption, *Circulation Res.,* 7:685, 1959.

Wiggers, C. J.: The Magnitude of Regurgitation with Aortic Leaks of Different Sizes, *J.A.M.A.,* 97:1359, 1931.

Pulmonic Valve Disease

Camp, F. A., McDonald, K. E., and Schenk, W. G., Jr.: Hemodynamics of Experimental Pulmonic Insufficiency, *J. Thoracic & Cardiovas. Surg.,* 47:372, 1964.

Ellison, R. G., Brown, W. J., Jr., Hague, E. E., Jr., and Hamilton, W. F.: Physiologic Observations in Experimental Pulmonary Insufficiency, *J. Thoracic Surg.,* 30:633, 1955.

Fish, R. G., Takaro, T., and Crymes, T.: Prognostic Considerations in Primary Isolated Insufficiency of the Pulmonic Valve, *New England J. Med.,* 261: 739, 1959.

Kahout, F. W., and Katz, L. N.: Pulmonic Valvular Regurgitation, *Am. Heart J.,* 49:637, 1955.

Kay, J. H., and Thomas, V.: Experimental Production of Pulmonary Insufficiency, *A.M.A. Arch. Surg.,* 69:646, 1954.

Lendrum, B. L., and Shaffer, A. B.: Isolated Congenital Pulmonic Valvular Regurgitation, *Am. Heart J.,* 57:298, 1959.

Price, B. O.: Isolated Incompetence of the Pulmonic Valve, *Circulation,* 23:596, 1961.

Silber, E. N., Prec, O., Grossman, N., and Katz, L. N.: Dynamics of Isolated Pulmonary Stenosis, *Am. J. Med.,* 10:21, 1951.

Tricuspid Valve Disease

Ferrer, M. I., Harvey, R. M., Kuschner, M., Richards, D. W., Jr., and Cournand, A.: Hemodynamic Studies in Tricuspid Stenosis of Rheumatic Origin, *Circulation Res.,* 1:49, 1953.

Kilip, T., and Lukas, D. S.: Tricuspid Stenosis, *Circulation,* 16:3, 1957.

Kitchen, A., and Turner, R.: Diagnosis and Treatment of Tricuspid Stenosis, *Brit. Heart J.,* 26:354, 1964.

McCord, M. C., and Blount, S. G., Jr.: The Hemodynamic Pattern in Tricuspid Valve Disease, *Am. Heart J.,* 44:671, 1952.

McCord, M. C., Swan, H., and Blount, S. G., Jr.: Tricuspid Stenosis: Clinical and Physiologic Evaluation, *Am. Heart J.,* 48:405 1954.

Rubeiz, G. A., Nassar, M. E., and Dagher, I. K.: Study of the Right Atrial Pressure Pulse in Functional Tricuspid Regurgitation and Normal Sinus Rhythm, *Circulation,* 30:190, 1964.

Smith, J. A., and Levine, S. A.: The Clinical Features of Tricuspid Stenosis, *Am. Heart J.,* 23:739, 1942.

Yu, P. N., Harken, D. E., Lovejoy, F. W., Jr., Nye, R. E., Jr., and Mahoney, E. B.: Clinical and Hemodynamic Studies of Tricuspid Stenosis, *Circulation,* 13:680, 1956.

25 CLINICAL RECOGNITION AND MEDICAL MANAGEMENT OF RHEUMATIC FEVER AND VALVULAR HEART DISEASE

B. Woodfin Cobbs, Jr., M.D.

RHEUMATIC FEVER

The Disease Pattern and Incidence

The true disease pattern of rheumatic fever is hard to ascertain because of the large percentage of persons with undiagnosed cases who, nonetheless, later develop evidence of obvious rheumatic heart disease. If the minor valve lesions and chordal thickening seen at postmortem examinations can be attributed to rheumatic fever, the disease must be very common indeed and largely subclinical. In general it appears that severe, clinically recognizable, acute rheumatic fever with carditis often leads to marked valvular deformities characterized by mitral and aortic regurgitation or by the early development of mitral stenosis. Milder and often clinically inapparent carditis seems more likely to produce slighter degrees of valvular involvement, such as simple fusion of the leaflets, which may lead to delayed mitral stenosis or minor degrees of insufficiency. Recognizable rheumatic fever occurs in discrete episodes which usually last less than 6 or 8 weeks.[1] Under conditions of modern institutional care and antibiotic therapy, all but 4 per cent of cases have subsided in 7 months; truly chronic rheumatic fever lasting a year or more is a rare but definite syndrome.[1-3] Each acute episode of rheumatic fever follows infection with M-typable β-hemolytic streptococci.[2,4,5] Yet clinical rheumatic fever afflicts only a small percentage of those who experience this ubiquitous disease (0.3 per cent in ordinary pediatric experience[6] but up to 2 per cent during epidemics of unusually severe streptococcosis in closed military populations[7]).

The characteristics of rheumatic fever and the percentage of clinical recognition vary greatly with geography and other environmental factors.[8-11] Certain areas of the world, notably Greece, Israel, and central Mexico, at present have the highest incidence and the most severe disease. The experience in Army camps in this country during World War II suggests that such endemic pockets are due to epidemic streptococcosis.[7,12] The present account of rheumatic fever describes a different and milder disease, its streptococcal factor at least partly controlled. Over the past 30 years in the United States and northern Europe, clinically obvious rheumatic fever has become less common and a great deal less severe.[13,14] The death rate in the first 5 years of the disease has fallen to well under 4 per cent.[15] This favorable trend began before the antibiotic era and has been attributed to less virulent streptococcal infection (fewer M-typable strains) and to less re-kindling of infections as crowded living conditions have been improved.[2,6] In specific instances, however, adequate antibiotic therapy has been of proved value in drastically reducing the incidence of rheumatic fever, both by shortening the course of streptococcosis and by decreasing the size of the reservoir of infection.[2,4] Treatment must be prompt and thorough.[4,5] Shotgun antibiotic therapy for undiagnosed respiratory infection as usually given in doses inadequate for treatment of streptococcosis is rightly condemned. About 45 per cent of the first attacks of rheumatic fever in a recent study developed despite such treatment.[16]

Now that it is possible at least partly to control the streptococcal factor, we are in a better position to appreciate the true importance of other variables. It has long been known that a tendency to rheumatic fever is often familial, but studies with twins indicate that the gene must have low penetrance.[17] More important is an individual host factor which cannot yet be evaluated in genetic terms. Once a patient has had rheumatic fever, streptococcosis is much more likely to produce a subsequent attack; the likelihood is further increased if he has had previous carditis, and it approaches 50 per cent in the patient whose heart disease is already severe.[18] Clinically, succeeding attacks tend to be replicas of the first one; and if the patient is spared early heart disease, he seems to be unlikely to acquire it with later episodes.[19] This has led to the proposal that some rheumatic fever is essentially "noncardiac." Long follow-up studies on some patients with "noncardiac" rheumatic fever, however, have shown an appreciable incidence of definite rheumatic heart disease, apparent only after 20 years.[20,21] This discrepancy may be due to the fact that clinical signs of carditis may have subsided before the patient is brought under observation, whereas the residual valvular damage may gradually and silently progress. More important is the fact that rheumatic fever may also be "non-rheumatic," manifested only by carditis, and the insidious development of valvular stenosis.

Acute rheumatic fever seldom occurs outside the age limits of 2 to 25 years; but age alone is never sufficient to exclude the diagnosis. The incidence of first attacks is highest in children between the ages of 7 and 14. Recurrences are most common in the first 3 years after the initial attack, and the incidence falls quite rapidly after 5 years and as the child advances into adolescence.[7,22] First attacks of rheumatic fever, however, are common in teenagers.[18,19,22,23] These older patients are somewhat less likely to develop carditis; but if they do, mitral involvement is somewhat less common and aortic valve disease far more frequent than in patients whose disease begins early in life.[19,24]

Signs and Symptoms

Streptococcal Infection. In only about two-thirds of the patients with first attacks of rheumatic fever has there been a history of a respiratory infection; this is often merely a "cold" rather than a sore throat and has occurred a few days to 6 weeks before, rather than at the classical 2 weeks' interval.[5,19] The history is an unreliable way of diagnosing streptococcosis and becomes even more useless as the age of the patient increases. The first symptoms of rheumatic fever may overlap with those of streptococcal infection, causing diagnostic confusion. Streptococcosis itself may produce arthralgias, fever, rash, and laboratory signs of systemic infection, including increased sedimentation rate and elevation of the C-reactive protein. A 5-year follow-up of patients with prolonged P-R intervals during streptococcal infection and a moderately protracted course (with vague pains in the extremities, borderline fever, postexercise tachycardia, and increased sedimentation rate) did not reveal any delayed appearance of heart murmurs.[2] Whether or not these patients will be as free from rheumatic heart disease 20 or 30 years later is a question to be answered by long-term follow-up only.

Systemic Signs. A fever of 100.4°F or higher, of the relapsing type, is encountered in the great majority of patients with carditis or arthritis.[11,25,26] However, it is rare to find the extremely high, spiking fever seen commonly in juvenile rheumatoid arthritis, and chills are most unusual. Fever is nonspecific but important as a diagnostic flare. Importantly, the patient with rheumatic fever does not necessarily feel very sick. Carditis would often be overlooked if prolonged and unexplained fever did not bring the child to a physician and lead to the discovery of significant murmurs.[19] When fever or malaise seem disproportionate to other signs in a patient who already has valvulitis from a previous attack, blood cultures should be drawn because of the possibility of bacterial endocarditis, even in a young child.[28]

Arthritis. Arthritis is the most common presenting complaint, appearing in one-half to three-fourths of the cases; without suppressive treatment it usually runs its course in 3 weeks or less,* though it may rebound briefly after the withdrawal of suppressive therapy.[19] Characteristically, two or more joints are involved simultaneously or in succession, but the arthritis is not uncommonly monoarticular.[19] The joints most commonly affected are the knees and ankles; the wrists, shoulders, hands, and feet are also frequently involved; spinal arthritis is uncommon.[19,29] The joints are usually extremely tender and hurt on the slightest movement so that the child is often unable to walk. Objectively, in the typical case there are swelling, often redness, and evidence of effusion.

The arthritis of rheumatic fever is sometimes confused with harmless "growing pains," which, however, are worse at night, likely to involve predominantly muscles and tendons, and may be relieved by massage—in marked contrast to exquisitely tender rheumatic joints.[25] The briefness of the rheumatic arthritis and the lack of residual deformity usually serve to distinguish it from rheumatoid disease, but these characteristics allow confusion with disseminated lupus erythematosus. Sickle-cell anemia more commonly produces bone than joint pain: it is associated with a low or normal sedimentation rate, characteristic hematologic findings, and a distinctive pattern on hemoglobin electrophoresis. Septic arthritis may be hard to distinguish in its early stages, and its diagnosis often requires a needle aspiration of the involved joint. Serum sickness is likely to be especially confusing because it may follow penicillin therapy given for a streptococcal infection; urticaria and marked eosinophilia are features distinguishing it from most cases of rheumatic fever.

The joint involvement does not have to be florid or disabling in order to be significant.[19] Arthralgia and myalgia are common in patients with previous rheumatic fever; their significance is yet undetermined. It is the writer's opinion that persistent pains which are definitely in the joints (not merely in muscles), which are brought on by physical exertion, weight bearing, or fatigue, and which cause

---

* Jaccoud's arthritis is an exception. Rarely after severe and recurrent rheumatic arthritis progressive periarticular fibrosis develops. The changes are most pronounced in the hands, especially the metacarpophalangeal joints. At first there is only ulnar deviation; later there is subluxation, but usually little pain or loss of mobility. This disease is unlikely to be a variant of rheumatoid arthritis, because in spite of the prolonged course, the rheumatoid factor is absent from the serum.[30]

the child to limp or favor an extremity may be valid grounds for considering the diagnosis of mild rheumatic arthritis. If carefully sought, slight but cyclic and objective changes may often be found in such joints. Naturally, trauma is the commonest cause of a limp, but the child often mistakenly adduces an injury to explain unaccountable symptoms. Any hint that the process is polyarticular or inappropriate to the alleged injury should arouse suspicion. The unusually rapid response of rheumatic arthritis to salicylates is not sufficiently specific to provide a very useful key to diagnosis. The proposition "suspected rheumatic arthritis" is not an invitation to treatment but rather a impetus to look carefully for other signs of rheumatic fever.

Heart Disease. Inflammation of the pericardium, the myocardium, and the valves may occur, but the latter are by far the most susceptible to damage. The involved valves are mitral, aortic, or both. Acute tricuspid valvulitis does not occur without severe involvement of the other two and cannot be recognized clinically. The natural trauma to which the mitral valve is subjected (the force of the systolic blood pressure) exceeds that applied to the aortic valve (the diastolic blood pressure) and is much higher than the forces acting on the tricuspid valve. These facts may explain selective localization of valvular damage from a process that undoubtedly involves the entire heart.[29] At present, clinical carditis is apparent in about one-half the cases of recognized acute rheumatic fever and is usually obvious within the first week or two.[19] Carditis, however, may occur in the absence of rheumatic symptoms sufficient to cause the patient to consult a physician, and possibly inadequate for firm diagnosis even under medical supervision.

Pericarditis. Pericarditis in rheumatic fever may be entirely missed. Clinically it is diagnosed in about 10 per cent of present-day cases, always in the severe ones and generally with other definite evidence of pancarditis.[11,19,26,29] The most valuable sign is a friction rub which usually has components synchronous with atrial systole, ventricular systole, and often the early stage of rapid diastolic filling. The rub is out of phase with the heart sounds and thus produces a syncopated effect; when just developing or subsiding it may have only a systolic component and be mistaken for a murmur. The rub may be evanescent but often lasts a week or two in the untreated case. Anterior chest pain attributable to pericarditis may occur in adolescents and adults with active cardiac involvement but is rare in children.[19,29] *Pericardial effusion* is now rare but remains an important cause for the sudden development of apparent cardiomegaly. True cardiac dilatation usually requires at least 3 or 4 months to develop and usually implies some permanent valve deformity; on the other hand, a large pericardial effusion can accumulate within a week and subside in less than a month.[29] Special fluoroscopic technique makes possible the detection of pericardial effusion by visualization of the pulsating, radiolucent epicardial fatpads 1 or 2 cm *inside* the apparent border of the cardiac silhouette; but the method is less reliable in children.[31] Cardiac tamponade practically never occurs in rheumatic carditis. Nowadays, effusion seldom becomes manifest,[19] probably partly because of the readiness with which it responds to corticosteroid therapy for rheumatic fever. Rheumatic pericarditis is generally accompanied by fever and leukocytosis and occasionally by S-T and T-wave changes in the electrocardiogram.

Myocarditis and Valvulitis. Accurate diagnosis requires some care. Many signs are not specific. Persistent tachycardia often occurs but usually is not disproportionate to fever, anxiety, or obvious congestive heart failure. Even tachycardia persisting during sleep is not an infallible sign of cardiac involvement. In severe disease, precordial activity is usually far more tumultuous than in other types of myocarditis. Damping of the apex impulse and muffling of the heart sounds are uncommon and usually due to pericardial effusion. These observations are probably the clinical corollary of the facts that (1) valvular regurgitation is usually present in severe cases and (2) the patient's resting cardiac output is more frequently high than low, although he is incapable of raising his blood flow with exercise.[32] Sometimes the first heart sound is indeed disproportionately faint; often, however, this merely reflects a prolonged P-R interval, which occurs in about 20 per cent of cases.[11,25]

The most distinctive aspect of rheumatic carditis is its ability to produce *new mitral and aortic murmurs* (a trait which it shares, however, with endocardial fibroelastosis). Persistent cardiomegaly or failure *without murmurs* is either mainly pericardial or not rheumatic at all.[25] The most common murmur in cases of rheumatic fever is apical, systolic, and due mainly to *mitral regurgitation*.[29,33] It occupies all or most of systole and is high-pitched (blowing or harsh), although it may have medium-frequency musical overtones during the most acute phase of the illness.[34] The murmur often radiates to the left beyond the apex impulse. It is never evanescent and varies little with respiration or from beat to beat; once established, however, it may gradually fade over a period of weeks or months.[24,34]

Much confusion about rheumatic carditis has resulted from the misinterpretation of common, innocent systolic murmurs, which are accentuated by increased cardiac output and which, since their intensity parallels the course of any febrile illness, are likely to be seized upon as evidence of carditis.[19,24,35,36] Such innocent murmurs are often quite variable and are rarely, if ever, consistently pansystolic. They are often medium-pitched and "vibratory" in quality, slightly twanging.[37,42] Usually they are loudest medial to the cardiac apex. Other innocent murmurs seem perhaps to be apical transmissions of normal pulmonary, aortic, and carotid murmurs.[38] Brief systolic murmurs, even when loud and easy to hear, are usually irrelevant to the question of rheumatic carditis.[35] On the other hand, a soft but definitely high-pitched and pansystolic murmur almost always means disease.[39] Phonocardiography may be helpful. A sometimes useful test may be done with 0.2 mg intravenous Neo-Synephrine, which can temporarily convert a borderline murmur into one that is clearly pansystolic. Some systolic murmurs remain indeterminate, and serial evaluation is required to assess them.

In diastole a *loud third heart sound* is common in normal children, especially in the presence of febrile illness. However, when one observes the rheumatic patient over a period of days, what seems at first to be an unusually loud third heart sound may gradually broaden into a short, *middiastolic rumble.*[34] The boundary between a sound and a brief rumble may be hard to define. Aftervibrations following a normal third heart sound are not so common in children with nonspecific fevers. Of course, even a pronounced middiastolic rumble does not mean that organic mitral stenosis is present. Yet definite presystolic accentuation indicates that the patient has some mitral narrowing.[19,24] The mitral diastolic murmur of acute rheumatic fever is rarely very prominent without an associated systolic murmur.[19,24] Perhaps an inconspicuous mitral diastolic murmur early in the patient's course is due mainly to swelling and stiffening of the mitral leaflets, but is later augmented by the diastolic reentry of regurgitated blood as mitral insufficiency develops. In general, it is a mistake to make a firm diagnosis of mitral stenosis solely on the basis of a brief isolated middiastolic rumble, which can usually be expected to clear, leaving no apparent residual of carditis.[24]

Both systolic and diastolic mitral murmurs are often an *early* sign of carditis when the heart itself is not obviously enlarged;[34] they are most often seen to appear in the first week or two of the illness.[19,25,34] Murmurs of active carditis not uncommonly improve or completely clear after recovery from an acute episode.[19,20,24] Mitral murmurs which are undoubtedly organic disappear in one-half the cases without cardiomegaly, but they usually persist if the heart is definitely enlarged.[19,24] If one is less rigorous about the definition of organic systolic murmurs, he will find a spuriously high disappearance rate. An associated mitral diastolic murmur or especially an aortic diastolic murmur means that evidence of carditis is unlikely to disappear.[23] The silencing of significant murmurs may mean that the patient has escaped functionally significant disease but does not guarantee that he may not later insidiously develop severe valvular deformity.[20,40,41] Whether these late effects are due to healing of the rheumatic lesion or to covert rheumatic activity is not known. Evidence from a recent 10-year follow-up study of patients on streptococcal prophylaxis suggests that mitral stenosis does not develop insidiously in cases of rheumatic fever without evidence of carditis early in their course.[24] Such experience probably is not applicable in isolated chorea, perhaps because clinical evidence of carditis may have subsided before this delayed neurological manifestation brings the child to the doctor. It should be remembered that a child with no murmur when first seen two or three months after his rheumatic fever has not necessarily been spared delayed mitral stenosis or the risk of carditis with a subsequent attack.

Aortic diastolic murmurs are distinctly less common and are most likely to develop in males and in patients who are older than average at the time of their first attack of rheumatic carditis.[19,24] The aortic diastolic murmur of acute carditis occasionally does not begin in the expected way coincident with the second heart sound, but may be delayed by a brief interval.[42] Such murmurs disappear in about one-fourth of present-day cases,[19,24] a considerably higher percentage than formerly. Some of these changing murmurs may be spurious; for undoubtedly with careless auscultation one may mistake the early diastolic part of a pericardial rub for the murmur of aortic regurgitation. On the other hand, because of spontaneous variation in audibility of such soft, brief murmurs (whether due to human error or to real changes in the noise level), one should always listen carefully and repeatedly before deciding that the murmur has indeed cleared. Aortic systolic murmurs are not a recognized feature of acute rheumatic fever; carotid bruits sometimes mistaken for such murmurs are common in normal children because of the hyperkinetic circulation.[38] Yet even a slight aortic diastolic murmur, especially if persistent, raises the specter of progressively severe aortic valve disease—stenosis, insufficiency, or a compound aortic valve lesion—later in life.[20,24] Fortunately, there is reason to believe that this unhappy sequence can be avoided, to some extent, by assiduous antistreptococcal prophylaxis.

Congestive heart failure itself is often an important sign of rheumatic carditis but does not invariably mean activity.[27] The signs and symptoms of failure in the 8- to 14-year age group, when rheumatic fever is most common, are more like those of adulthood than those of infancy but are sufficiently distinctive to require comment.[43-45] Not uncommonly failure is asymptomatic and is suspected clinically because of inappropriate tachycardia, increasing heart size, hepatomegaly, or edema.

Left ventricular failure is always part of the picture but is often missed. The majority of patients have dyspnea or a curious, persistent, dry cough either when first seen or as they are observed.[43] Inappropriate tachypnea, which may be mistaken for nervous hyperventilation, is especially important but quite easy to overlook. As in adulthood the traditional physical findings of left ventricular failure are often absent, but expertly interpreted serial roentgenograms usually leave little doubt about the diagnosis.[46] Relative freedom from paroxysmal symptoms of left ventricular failure is a noteworthy feature of this age group.

By contrast, one or more signs of *right ventricular failure* are usually easily observed:[43,44] (1) An abnormal level to the pulsating venous column in the neck (hard to detect in young, short-necked children); (2) unaccountable weight gain which often precedes obvious edema; (3) an enlarged or tender liver; and (4) nausea and vomiting. Nausea and liver tenderness are especially common signs of rapidly evolving heart failure in this age group. The latter may be elicited by palpation or by slapping over the right side of the lower part of the chest or over the upper part of the abdomen (using the left side as a control).[43] Facial edema, albuminuria, oliguria, and nocturia may result in a mistaken diagnosis of renal disease, especially in the younger child.

Now that recurrent rheumatic fever can be prevented, the effects of acute carditis can be more readily distinguished from those of late and permanent valvular deformity. Death from acute carditis is now extremely rare in centers devoted to the care of rheumatic fever in this country. Yet even when subsequent attacks are prevented, cardiac damage from the first one may be enough to cause eventual death.[19,24] Juvenile mitral stenosis or mitral regurgitation may be severe enough to produce symptoms in its own right, without any contribution from myocarditis.[47,48] These are distinct entities, more common in areas where rheumatic fever is unusually severe, but also clearly recognized in this country. Severe and permanent mitral regurgitation may be established within a few weeks; mitral stenosis usually takes longer to mature.[22,24] The symptoms are much the same as in adults, often with prominent paroxysmal dyspnea and orthopnea.

Skin Lesions. A number of toxic erythemas are associated with acute streptococcal infections; erythema nodosum and erythema multiforme may be later consequences of streptococcal sensitization.

Yet none of these has any intimate relation to rheumatic fever. *Erythema marginatum* is an exception.[49] This migratory, annular, flat, and non-pruritic eruption is usually evanescent but may be striking and recurrent. Typically, lesions affect the warm areas of the body, the intertriginous folds, and (after bedrest) the back. Often the patient is best examined after a hot bath. The lesions are not merely red splotches. Their margins are irregular but sharply demarcated, even though the pattern may change completely within a quarter of an hour. Erthema marginatum occurs in about 5 per cent of present-day cases, most often in association with carditis; sometimes it may appear or recur as other manifestations are subsiding.[19] Petechiae and splinter hemorrhages rarely occur during acute rheumatic fever and may cause confusion with bacterial endocarditis.

Rheumatic nodules average about 3 mm in diameter but vary from imperceptibility to the size of a peanut.[29,50] They are painless, usually attached to tendon sheaths (so that the skin rides over them freely), and are best seen on the knuckles, elbows, wrists, knees, or the back of the head.[29] They last a few days or a few weeks. Though these nodules are usually not so obvious or permanent as those of rheumatoid arthritis, the distinction is not always obvious. Rheumatic nodules almost always mean carditis; but in exceptional cases they have been an isolated manifestation with no sequelae.[51] As the severity of rheumatic fever has waned in the past two decades, the incidence of nodules has dropped from a former 20 per cent to 1 to 4 per cent.[19] Rheumatic nodules also must be distinguished from the nodular panniculitis which occasionally occurs after withdrawal of prolonged corticosteroid therapy.[52]

Sydenham's Chorea. Chorea may be a late manifestation, often occurring 2 and sometimes 6 months after the streptococcal infection. Thus it begins during or after convalescence from other manifestations of rheumatic fever. Therefore, *isolated* chorea is often associated with no clear-cut evidence of recent streptococcosis, no elevation of the sedimentation rate, and no systemic signs.[53] In first attacks of rheumatic fever, chorea affects 10 to 15 per cent of girls and 3 per cent of boys.[19] The onset often takes a week or two, and the symptoms and signs may be unilateral. In its early stages the condition is often misdiagnosed as nervousness or habit tic;[26] however the movements are never so stereotyped or repetitive as in the latter condition. Because of awkwardness or grimacing the child is usually punished before she is treated. There are multiple purposeless movements, which deform all muscular activity and often make it impossible to hold still. Small ordered movements are catapulted into gross disordered flings and swoops. Often the patient tries to disguise her predicament by continuing to move voluntarily in the direction in which she has been projected; since she cannot hold still, she may deliberately engage in pseudo-purposeful repetitive activity. The movements themselves are predominantly writhing (relatively slow) but are punctuated by sudden jerks. Mild chorea is best brought out by asking the patient to perform a task which requires maintenance of a sustained posture and a fine balance between opposing muscle groups. For instance, the rigidly extended arms soon begin to move uncontrollably; and as the child is vigorously urged to hold still, the movements may worsen. Often maintaining a steady grip on the examiner's hand becomes impossible. In severe cases talking and walking are badly affected. In milder ones the diagnosis may be overlooked unless the signs are carefully sought. The average case lasts 1 to 3 months, subsiding gradually. There is no satisfactory therapy. Sedatives such as phenobarbital help somewhat; $\frac{1}{2}$ to 1 gr of the latter drug four times daily may be required to control the symptoms. Diphenhydramine (Benadryl) has also been used. Phenothiazines probably should not be given because they may sometimes produce confusing and often painful extrapyramidal manifestations. Sydenham's chorea never leaves permanent neurologic residuals, but 20 per cent of patients *without apparent carditis* have developed rheumatic heart disease (usually mitral stenosis) after 20 years.[21] Chorea developing during convalescence from other manifestations should be recognized as a later evidence of the present attack and not be mistaken for recrudesence of rheumatic fever. Chorea apparently indistinguishable from that of rheumatic fever may occasionally appear in pregnant women and tends to recur during subsequent confinements.

Other Manifestations. 1. *Abdominal pain* is an important symptom of acute rheumatic fever although it occurs in only about 10 per cent of patients.[19] The mechanism is not necessarily hepatic congestion; for in many cases there is no congestive heart failure, and the pain involves the lower quadrants so that appendicitis may be mistakenly suspected.[54] Abdominal pain may precede other complaints and is associated with obvious carditis in about three-quarters of the cases.[19]

2. *Epistaxis*, if unaccountable, and especially if recurrent, may be a sign of rheumatic fever, most commonly occurring in patients with carditis.[19] Formerly more common, it is now seen in fewer than 10 per cent of patients. When one is attempting to obtain a retrospective history of rheumatic fever, nosebleeds may provide a useful, easily remembered beacon, which may lead to the recall of other symptoms. Undue emphasis should not be placed on such a history. Nose picking remains the commonest cause of epistaxis.

3. *Chest pain* of several types occurs in rheumatic fever. The most common is anterior chest or shoulder ache, often pleuritic but not always clearly attributable to pericarditis, pulmonary infarction, or pneumonia.[19]

4. Some manifestations seen in earlier times are now extremely rare. Rheumatic pneumonia, distinct from the effects of pulmonary infection or left ventricular failure, is now almost never recognized. Some previously supposed manifestations of rheumatic fever, such as thyroiditis and the "typhoidal forms," were probably due to errors in diagnosis. Lymphadenopathy and splenomegaly, however, may occasionally be so striking as to suggest lymphoma.

Laboratory Findings

An increased sedimentation rate and increased C-reactive protein levels may be expected in most cases of active rheumatic fever except those with isolated chorea.[55,56] C-reactive protein may appear before the sedimentation rate goes up but may subside earlier during the convalescent phase.[57]

Congestive heart failure does not usually produce a falsely low sedimentation rate except occasionally when it is quite severe.[27] Both tests are valuable in screening patients for rheumatic activity.[28] They are, however, quite nonspecific. Any respiratory infection, including streptococcosis, will produce an elevation in the level of C-reactive protein.[56] Some patients continue to have increased sedimentation rates for many years without any other signs of rheumatic activity. These limitations notwithstanding, the test remains a very valuable screening device. *A mild illness associated with minor or transient elevation of the level of C-reactive protein and the sedimentation rate usually should not be diagnosed as rheumatic fever.* Moderate polymorphonuclear leukocytosis is usual but not invariable in rheumatic fever; the white count is an insensitive index of rheumatic activity.

Since in many cases the streptococcal infection may have subsided before the rheumatic fever has been diagnosed, *throat cultures* are not necessarily helpful and may be misleading because some patients are in a benign carrier state.[57] Properly performed *serologic examinations* fill a great need. Ninety-five per cent of patients with rheumatic fever seen in the first 2 months (except those with isolated chorea) show an elevated titer of an antibody to one or more streptococcal antigens: antistreptolysin-O, antistreptokinase, antihyaluronidase, anti-DPNase, and the anti-DNAases.[28,59-62] The height of the titer probably has something to do with both the antigenicity of the organism and the duration of the infection. Infection with mildly elevated antistreptococcal titers is unlikely to produce recurrence of rheumatic fever, unless the patient has had carditis with his previous attack.[28] On the other hand, high antistreptococcal titers are associated with a recurrence rate of one-third in patients with previous mild rheumatic fever and of two-thirds in patients with previous carditis.[19,28] It is important not to confuse data from a battery of antistreptococcal tests with results of studies for a single antibody performed in an ordinary laboratory. After streptococcal infection about one patient in four never develops a diagnostic antistreptolysin-O titer and acquires antibodies only to other products of the organism.[59,62] Unfortunately in many hospital laboratories the antistreptolysin-O test is the only one done, and even this may not be accurately performed. In any case a normal antistreptolysin-O titer is never grounds for excluding active rheumatic fever, especially a recurrent attack. A single test is often useless. Usually diagnosis of recent streptococcal infection requires the demonstration of a changing titer.[63]

The electrocardiogram rarely provides any new information but may help round out the diagnosis of carditis. Atrioventricular dissociation and other nodal rhythms are not uncommon but are usually episodic. Prolongation of the P-R interval is quite common (it is found in about 20 per cent of cases) and likely to be transient. The likelihood of finding a long P-R interval depends on the frequency of electrocardiographic recording. It is helpful to record the electrocardiogram when the first heart sound becomes faint, since this is when the P-R interval is more likely to be prolonged. Higher degrees of AV block are uncommon, and complete block is most rare. There is controversy about how heavily prolongation of the P-R interval should be weighted in the diagnosis of rheumatic fever.[11,28] Certainly the finding is nonspecific and may be congenital or a temporary consequence of both streptococcal and other childhood diseases. It seems to have no prognostic significance.[15,28] The prolongation may persist after acute carditis has subsided, and this does not necessarily indicate continued rheumatic activity. Atrial fibrillation is unusual and is generally seen only in patients who have previously acquired mitral disease. Electrocardiographic changes of pericarditis seldom occur without other unmistakable clinical findings and may be absent even when a rub is obvious.

Problems of Diagnosis

Fully developed rheumatic fever with all the manifestations listed above is exceedingly rare. The disease is protean and sometimes largely concealed.

Important carditis often occurs in patients with little or no arthritis. Unfortunately there is no specific laboratory test. The demonstration of antistreptococcal antibodies bound to cardiac muscle[64] has suggested an avenue for the development of a diagnostic test, but none has yet been devised.

One of the pioneer attempts at "computer medicine" was made by the late T. Duckett Jones, whose criteria for the diagnosis of rheumatic fever were later revised by a committee of the American Heart Association.[65] The Jones criteria are an effort to weight the various manifestations as to their importance in aiding recognition of the disease— so as to minimize confusion with other conditions and to prevent overdiagnosis. Thus an orderly approach was obtained to what remains sometimes an insoluble problem. There are five major criteria: (1) arthritis, (2) carditis, (3) chorea, (4) erythema marginatum, and (5) rheumatic nodules. Six minor criteria were proposed: (1) fever, (2) arthralgia (pain in the joints without objective findings), (3) increased sedimentation rate and presence of C-reactive protein or leukocytosis, (4) evidence of preceding β-hemolytic streptococcal infection, (5) a previous history of rheumatic fever or the presence of inactive rheumatic heart disease, (6) a prolonged P-R interval in the electrocardiogram. According to the committee: *The presence of two major criteria or one major and two minor criteria indicates a high probability of the diagnosis of acute rheumatic fever.* This formula has imperfections and needs revision. For instance, isolated Sydenham's chorea with typical findings and clinical course is by itself sufficient evidence for a firm diagnosis of rheumatic fever.[19] The formula does not exploit the importance of negative findings: for instance, fever though listed as a minor manifestation, is found in 90 per cent of clinically recognized rheumatic episodes;[19] therefore, its absence makes a rather strong point against the diagnosis although its presence is a nonspecific sign. The sedimentation rate is a similar case in point.[28] If a complete battery of tests for antistreptococcal antibodies is normal early in the patient's course and on follow-up, rheumatic fever is an unlikely explanation for his symptoms.[59,66] The triad of polyarthritis, fever, and elevated sedimentation rate is the weakest of all combinations of major and minor criteria: rheumatoid arthritis, gonococcal arthritis, lupus erythematosus, subacute bacterial endocarditis, viral pericarditis, leukemia, serum sickness (including manifestations of penicillin sensitivity), and many other conditions may produce this set of findings.[64] One minor manifestation, prolongation of the P-R interval, is considered too nonspecific by some workers to be useful.[19,24] Certainly it should never be the sole basis for a diagnosis of carditis. Subcutaneous nodules and erythema marginatum are quite specific, but unfortunately are rarely present except in cases which are easily diagnosed on other grounds.[19] Finally, and most important, the Jones formula and similar methods are valid only if clinical evaluation of the various signs is reliable. The formula is not a substitute for clinical acumen or repeated examinations. For instance, the difference between arthritis (a "major" criteria) and arthralgia (a "minor" one) may be merely that of a circumspectly recorded history versus careful and serial observations of the actual joint manifestations. Similar pitfalls in the diagnosis of carditis have been mentioned previously (see Fig. 25-1). The Jones criteria obviously cannot help in the recognition of patients who insidiously develop mitral stenosis over a period of years without other manifestations of activity.

Recurrent rheumatic fever often presents a difficult diagnostic problem. There is never recurrence without a new streptococcal infection, which, however, may be missed if the patient is not carefully followed.[22,28,59] The history is not very helpful: Many sore throats are not streptococcal, and many streptococcal throats are not sore.[28] Frequently the clinical features of a recurrence are not so obviously expressed as in the first attack. The severity of arthritis and carditis may be inversely related;[28] the latter may not produce any symptoms and may be overlooked, unless the patient is under careful observation.[19,24] Furthermore, it is often hard to detect or interpret changes in cardiac findings; sometimes a "new" murmur is really an old one newly heard.[67] Increasing heart size and even heart failure do not always correlate with other signs of rheumatic activity. The patient with previous carditis may gradually become decompensated without any acute or obvious reason. The sedimentation rate and C-reactive protein have been advocated as reliable screening tests to distinguish

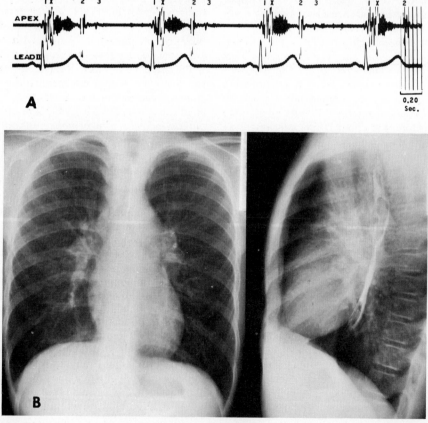

Fig. 25-1. An innocent murmur mistaken for evidence of rheumatic valvulitis. An 8-year-old girl received 1 week of oral penicillin for a sore throat proved by culture to be streptococcal. Two weeks later she developed painful ankles and sore lumps on the shin. A loud, musical murmur was heard (*A*) depicted by phonocardiogram. Since the chest film (*B*, frontal and lateral views) was abnormal, a diagnosis of rheumatic carditis was made. Actually she had a typical innocent vibratory murmur, which was quite variable from day to day. The radiologic changes were due to hilar adenopathy, most likely related to her erythema nodosum, which in turn might have been caused by penicillin therapy.

true from false recurrence;[28] but they are often not abnormal in patients who develop unaccountable congestive failure.[27] Whether most such cases are due to otherwise inapparent carditis or to other factors is a matter of spirited controversy.[11,25,27] This point can never be satisfactorily settled until a specific test for rheumatic activity has been devised.

Rheumatic fever in adults may be severe but often lacks some of the distinctive features seen in childhood.[68,69] This is no justification for making the diagnosis promiscuously; for the condition is rare in adults and the chance of a simulating illness, such as disseminated lupus erythematosus or rheumatoid arthritis, is also greatly increased.[70]

In general, rheumatic fever is probably overdiagnosed at present.[71] Overdiagnosis is an increasing temptation to the conscientious physician who recognizes the importance and efficacy of antistreptococcal prophylaxis and is aware of the fact that much rheumatic fever is missed. The real question is whether patients with borderline manifestations of rheumatic fever (not quite satisfying the Jones criteria) are more likely to develop rheumatic heart disease than the general population and, therefore, deserve antibiotic prophylaxis. A 5-year follow-up of such patients has not shown any such tendency.[2] However, until more definitive data are available, each physician is likely to reach his own conclusion on the subject, often on somewhat emotional grounds.

Treatment

Antibiotic Therapy

The first duty of the physician is to see that the present streptococcal infection is eradicated and that continuous chemo-prophylaxis is maintained.[2,72]

For the eradication of streptococcal infections, any one of four treatment schedules may be used: (1) penicillin (G or V) orally in divided doses of at least 800,000 units per day for 10 days; (2) 600,000 units of procaine penicillin intramuscularly daily for 10 days; (3) a single injection of 1.2 million units of benzathine penicillin (600,000 units in small children); (4) for patients sensitive to penicillin, 10 days of erythromycin.[2] Somewhat smaller doses of penicillin were recommended by a committee of the American Heart Association in 1960.[73]

Treatment with benzathine penicillin has the advantages of simplicity and of requiring less cooperation from the patient. Unfortunately, it often causes considerable local pain. The incidence of anaphylaxis is low and probably not appreciably higher than with the other injectable penicillins; but this problem is greater in older patients.[74,75]

Massive and prolonged penicillin therapy at the onset of rheumatic fever has been recommended,[76] but proof of its efficacy is lacking.[77]

Prevention of first attacks of rheumatic fever obviously would be highly desirable. Within a week or two of the onset of the disease about 50 per cent of children have acquired valvulitis.[16,19] Prospective studies suggest that prompt and adequate treatment of all cases of streptococcosis in pediatric practice can prevent rheumatic fever.[6] Even in the severe military epidemics during World War II, diagnosis and treatment of infection within the first week greatly reduced the incidence of rheumatic fever.[78] Routine administration of benzathine penicillin to all incoming recruits eliminated one previously severe pocket of disease.[79] The problem is far more complicated in civilian populations, where streptococcosis is more sporadic. Here the only hope of success rests on prompt recognition and treatment of infection. Unfortunately many patients never feel sick enough to consult a physician, and furthermore, clinical diagnosis is woefully inadequate. Adequate penicillin treatment of all patients with clinical findings of exudative pharyngitis and polymorphonuclear leukocytosis would probably reach many of the younger patients with streptococcosis who happened to consult their physicians. It would also miss many others and reach a number with irrelevant illnesses. Shot-gun therapy with benzathine penicillin has not come into vogue among pediatricians because it is painful and very occasionally produces anaphylaxis. Throat cultures by mail may soon become more widely available in larger cities,[80] but the delay perhaps inherent in this method will have to be eliminated. Sometimes the clinical manifestations of rheumatic fever begin within a few days of the apparent onset of the streptococcal infection. Mass survey programs for the detection of inapparent streptococcal infection are cumbersome and not worthwhile in areas with a low natural incidence of infection.[81]

For long-term chemoprophylaxis, sulfadiazine in the dose of 0.5 Gm twice daily has been proved to be just as effective as penicillin G in the dosage of 200,000 units twice daily.[82] Sulfadiazine is also cheaper and definitely safer if precautions are taken to avoid severe dehydration during intercurrent illnesses. Neither currently used method for oral prophylaxis is really satisfactory. Part of the difficulty is that pill taking is monotonous, without clear-cut immediate benefit, and often considered a badge of disability; hence, a program of oral prophylaxis is seldom consistently followed.[58] Even in carefully supervised patients, the annual streptococcal recurrence rate is about 20 per cent, most of the infections being asymptomatic and detected only by culture or serologic tests.[82] It might be anticipated that larger and intermittently bactericidal doses of oral penicillin will be more satisfactory. Without question the most effective way of avoiding streptococcal infection is by administering monthly injections of benzathine penicillin (Bicillin 1.2 million units), which produces bactericidal levels for the first week.[83] No method prevents all streptococcal infections, and any suspicious illness is reason enough for obtaining a throat culture and making serologic studies.

The proper time to stop chemoprophylaxis is not known.[84] Most authorities believe that it should be continued indefinitely[73] or at least until the patient is well into his twenties. One group of older adolescent patients free of symptoms of active rheumatic fever for at least 5 years were taken off continuous prophylaxis and treated only when they had symptomatic streptococcal infections.[2,22] Three-quarters of the infections proved by specific immune responses, however, were asymptomatic. The overall annual recurrence rate of rheumatic fever on this program was only 1.3 per cent.[22] In determining the proper duration of prophylactic treatment, climate, age, occupation, household situation, cardiac status, and length of time since the previous attack are all significant variables which make arbitrary recommendations relatively meaningless for the individual case.[2] Even isolated chorea, however, is sufficient grounds for long-term chemoprophylaxis.

Regulation of Physical Activity

In the absence of carditis, strict bed rest is unnecessary after the first few weeks of the disease provided the acute manifestations are suppressed or have abated.[85] Spontaneous reactivation of acute rheumatic fever after a period of 2 months probably does not occur unless new streptococcal infection has intervened.[1,2,19] Thus the patient without clinical carditis on adequate antistreptococcal therapy may resume full activity 2 months after the attack has ended.[2] If carditis was present but murmurs have disappeared, full activity may be resumed after 6 months of observation has confirmed the continued absence of significant heart disease.[2] Premature resumption of exercise may cause a relapse of heart failure.[43] There is now partial experimental backing for the strong traditional clinical feeling that exercise is undesirable during the course of active myocarditis.[86] However, bed rest has been overused in the past. The author has encountered patients confined for a year after rheumatic fever, which had produced no evidence of carditis whatsoever; often slavish attention to a persistently elevated sedimentation rate has caused this error. Usually, prolonged bed rest

means the loss of a year's schooling and all too often sets in motion a pattern which eventually results in the patient's dropping out of school altogether. Such an outcome is particularly unfortunate in the child with rheumatic heart disease, who should learn to live by his brain rather than his brawn. In a borderline case, it is probably better to get the patient back to school a little prematurely rather than run the risk of creating impossible dilemmas for him later in life. An important advantage of many specialized institutions for the treatment of rheumatic fever is the availability of good schooling for bed-fast patients.

Suppressive Therapy

To avoid endless confusion, it is best not to give corticosteroid or salicylate until the diagnosis has been firmly established.[2] Sometimes it is necessary simply to wait a few days until the clinical picture is more completely developed. Suppressive therapy (combined with antibiotics) will often produce a favorable response, regardless of the diagnosis, and make it impossible to determine whether the patient really had rheumatic fever. Neither corticosteroid nor aspirin alters the duration of the rheumatic attack or has any effect on the course of Sydenham's chorea. Both, however, are valuable in controlling the toxic manifestations of the disease and in contributing to the comfort of the patient. In the management of acute carditis with severe congestive heart failure, however, corticosteroid may be life-saving and should always be used along with diuretics and digitalis. Clinical evidence leaves no doubt of its efficacy in tilting the balance in favor of some critically ill patients.[2,88] The increased sedimentation rate and C-reactive protein are restored to normal by corticosteroid, but not by salicylates.

Whether or not corticosteroid suppression reduces the ultimate cardiac scarring is a question which is far more difficult to answer.[89,90] Two short-term studies have been organized to try to settle this matter.[15,87] In neither did corticosteroid suppression reduce the incidence of murmurs in a follow-up examination. In spite of this negative evidence, some competent investigators believe that corticosteroids do have an important effect in preventing residual valvular deformity.[88] More evidence is needed to prove their contention.

In general, the best current practice seems to be to use salicylates when no evidence of carditis is present, but to add corticosteroids if signs and symptoms are not adequately suppressed. Currently most patients with even mild carditis receive corticosteroids, but the basis for such treatment is not so surely grounded as in the severe cases. Huge doses of salicylates, such as were employed in earlier times, are no longer justifiable and may cause dangerous salicylate intoxication with hyperventilation, metabolic acidosis, and ultimately coma. In some cases, congestive heart failure seems to be brought on by such treatment.[91] The oral dose of salicylates may be 60 mg per lb body weight daily for the first days but should be rapidly reduced to about 30 mg per lb for the next 5 weeks. No arbitrary dose of corticosteroids can be recommended. Most patients will respond to an initial dose of 30 to 40 mg prednisone rather rapidly reduced to 20 to 30 mg and continued for 4 to 6 weeks in the presence of carditis. If symptoms are not well controlled with six aspirin tablets (1.8 Gm) daily in the average 6-year-old, corticosteroids probably should be used instead. The duration of corticosteroid therapy is also an individual matter. In 80 per cent of the patients the attack lasts only 6 to 8 weeks[1] and steroids may be tapered after that time; unfortunately, it is impossible to tell except by trial and error which patients belong to the less fortunate 20 per cent.

Rebound of rheumatic activity after withdrawal of steroid therapy is common and usually occurs within 2 weeks (occasionally as late as 4 weeks) after suppressive therapy has been stopped. If no relapse is evident within 1 or 2 months, the attack may be considered to have ended.[2,19,92] Rebounds usually can be controlled by the administration of salicylates for joint symptoms and diuretics for congestive failure. Rebounds may be mistakenly diagnosed as recurrences unless the patients have been carefully followed with serial cultures and (accurately performed) antistreptolysin titers, which will detect most cases of streptococcal infection. Relapses most commonly occur in patients who have had carditis and in whom remission was induced by steroid therapy. Salicylates used during the withdrawal period help to prevent rebound. If nothing becomes abnormal except the sedimentation rate, the rebound is not significant.

Management of Heart Failure. Corticosteroids are part of the treatment whenever there is good evidence for rheumatic activity.[2,88] The supposed intolerance of patients with active carditis to digitalis is largely a myth based on the fact that ordinary doses will sometimes not slow the tachycardia and higher doses merely produce intoxication. Digitalis is useful if not "pushed." Diuretics, however, are the cornerstone of therapy, and deserve the primary emphasis.[43] Nausea, vomiting, and even ectopic beats are common results of juvenile heart failure itself; thus, the diagnosis of digitalis intoxication is not always easy. Rigid salt restriction is hard to enforce and seldom necessary with the potent oral diuretics presently available.

MITRAL VALVE DISEASE

Rheumatic mitral valve disease is not so simple as it was once thought to be. Although physiologically either stenosis or insufficiency is usually predominant, there are many important anatomic variations.[93–97] It is important and usually possible from clinical evidence to specify the dominant physiologic defect. Recent work points the way toward a better correlation between clinical signs and certain features of valvular anatomy.

Mitral Stenosis

Disease Mechanisms

The basic problem in tight mitral stenosis is getting blood out of the blocked left atrium and into the left ventricle during diastole. The price of moving blood rapidly is inevitably an increase in the left atrial pressure, which must be shared by the pulmonary venous reservoir.[98,99] However, at low rates of flow the most tightly stenotic valve may raise the pressure surprisingly little. For mysterious reasons, some patients set themselves rather modest flow requirements and, except during unusual exertion, may dodge many of the problems of mitral stenosis.[98,100]

Two events contribute to the left atrial pressure and hence to the important task of squeezing blood through the stenotic valve into the left ventricle:

1. Atrial systole is the more directly applied effort but unfortunately is quite brief. It may not shrink the atrium greatly[101] but nonetheless delivers a larger than normal and very significant fraction of the ventricle's ration of blood.[102] Atrial contraction obviously must be an important compensatory mechanism during exercise, when tachycardia reduces the ventricular diastolic filling time but provides a greater number of atrial systoles per minute.

2. More important is the *vis a tergo*, the leftover force of right ventricular contraction damped more or less by its transmission through the pulmonary vascular bed. Unfortunately, this is rather like trying to inflate a truck tire through a Penrose drain tube. Before it can help the problem of left atrial emptying, the force of right ventricular contraction must balloon the delicate pulmonary capillary bed and dilate the pulmonary veins. The vulnerability of the pulmonary conduit tends to limit the pressure that can be generated in the left atrium and, therefore, to put a ceiling on blood flow in mitral stenosis.

Severe mitral block almost always dilates the left atrium, this being usually apparent by x-ray.[103,104] In a few patients susceptible to sudden rises of the pulmonary venous pressure, gross hemoptysis (pulmonary apoplexy) may come from varices of the endobronchial veins, which act as collaterals draining from the distended pulmonary venous reservoir.[105,106] Such varices are not always grossly visible on bronchoscopy,[107] but the bright-red, nonfrothy appearance of the hemoptysis is most compatible with a source in rather direct contact with a sizable reservoir of oxygenated blood.

Dyspnea is the most important symptom in mitral stenosis.[99,108–110] Very likely, it somehow originates in the delicate pulmonary capillary bed, where the onslaught of the right ventricle and the mitral block may keep the hydraulic pressure close to or above the oncotic pressure of the blood.[98,99] The distribution of this pressure, however, is most important.[111] The critical pulmonary capillary pressure leading to transudation is only 25 to 30 mm Hg. This amounts to a column of water (or blood) only 11 to 14 in. high, whereas the height of the average chest is about 20 in. Thus it is obvious that the shape of the human thorax and the position of the body are crucial factors in the allotment of this pressure. In the sitting position a "critical" left atrial pressure of 30 mm Hg reaches the upper lobes and capillaries at an effective level of less than 5 mm Hg (which is harmless) but floods the lower lobes with its full destructive force. [111,112] Inevitably the changes are much more marked in the lower lobes, in spite of an often intense compensatory constriction of all the arteries and veins attached to them.[112,113] In severe mitral stenosis often one of the earliest radiographic signs is dilatation of the low-pressure, upper lobe veins, which are obviously carrying more than their share of blood.[114] In the lower lobes there is chronic interstitial edema;[115–117] plasma water leaks out of the capillaries, perhaps nearly continuously in severe cases and during exertion in the milder ones. Crammed with dilated vessels and transudated fluid, the alveolar walls probably become more rigid and the bronchioles may swell and narrow.[110] Such high pressures always increase the flow of pulmonary lymph.[118] The prime causes of the transverse costophrenic lines of Kerley seen on the chest x-ray are interlobular edema and huge interlobular lymphatics busily draining off the constant seepage.[115,116] Variations in the function of the pulmonary lymphatics may well be decisive in the symptoms of mitral stenosis.

The human chest is generally half again as tall as it is thick; therefore, recumbency instantly converts larger areas of the lung into high pressure zones, often immediately accentuating the symptoms of mitral stenosis. Recumbency also leads to rapid redistribution of blood from the periphery to the pulmonary bed, producing a prompt rise in the left atrial pressure.[119] Prolonged recumbency also allows the mobilization of peripheral edema, further aggravating the problem.[120]

Despite the considerable number of studies on the dyspnea of mitral stenosis, it is not yet possible to define its pathogenesis in a completely satisfactory manner for all patients.[109,110] Dyspnea is clearly related to increased left atrial pressure and improves when this pressure is brought down.[110,121] In symptomatic patients, although at rest hyperventilation is often not noticeable, exercise usually produces an inappropriate and prolonged increase in respiration; and the most consistent effect of successful valvulotomy is improvement in this response.[110,122] Close analysis, however, becomes more difficult. The disabled patient's vital capacity is reduced and his residual volume is increased, but not critically.[110] Abnormally low pulmonary compliance (distensibility) and diffusing capacity, especially during exercise, are part of the picture;[110,123] but often neither improves a great deal in spite of a good result from valvulotomy.[124,125] A disturbed ratio between ventilation and perfusion (uneven distribution of inspired air) may be due to the selective damage mitral stenosis inflicts on the lung bases.[126]

Respiratory complaints, even though we may not fully understand their pathogenesis, are the main concern of both the symptomatic patient and his physician. Chronic interstitial edema of his lower lobes keeps the patient miserable with coughing and dyspnea—brought on sometimes by exertion and sometimes by recumbency. Occasionally, with sudden increases in the pulmonary venous congestion, interstitial fluid bursts into the alveoli and the patient has frank acute pulmonary edema, during which he may die.

Atrial fibrillation is a common but often late complication of mitral stenosis; it always imposes additional problems.[127] Aside from the loss of atrial contraction, it usually causes inappropriate tachycardia, with a shortened diastolic filling interval, and hence aggravates the task of atrial emptying. In mitral stenosis, time is of the essence. A leisurely diastole allows good atrial drainage; an abbreviated one may cause pulmonary edema.[29] With digitalis one may slow the ventricular rate in atrial fibrillation and undo much of the damage. Even so, the cardiac output is usually significantly cut, especially during exercise.[128] In its early stages, atrial fibrillation is often paroxysmal and may be the explanation for sudden reversible cardiac decompensation.[29,99] Eventually, it usually becomes fixed. Chronic atrial fibrillation in itself tends to enlarge the left atrium disproportionately and greatly increases the risk of atrial thrombosis and consequent systemic embolization.[129,130] Such emboli may occur, however, when atrial fibrillation has never been documented and may be the first and only symptom of the disease.[99]

Secondary obstruction in the pulmonary vascular

bed is one of the most common but unpredictable complications of mitral stenosis.[99,108,131,132] It may occur at any stage of the disease and is of crucial importance in the course of the patient. Its earliest cause is probably active vasoconstriction, rather than the structural changes in the small pulmonary vessels described by Parker and Weiss.[133] A high pulmonary resistance may often be momentarily reversed by the intrapulmonary infusion of acetyl-choline.[134] Dexter and his colleagues introduced the concept that adjustments in the pulmonary arterial resistance protect the patient with mitral stenosis from drowning during moments when an overzealous right ventricle might otherwise pump blood into the lung considerably faster than it could be removed.[98] Yet, if pulmonary vascular constriction is initiated by some benevolent reflex, its long-range effect is nonetheless always destructive. It does not even prevent the patient from having symptoms of pulmonary congestion.[108,121,135] A sustained increase in pulmonary vascular resistance simply forces the right ventricle to do more work in order to produce the same amount of left atrial emptying and leads to a more rapid downhill course. A rare patient, however, presents with evidence chiefly of pulmonary vascular obstruction and right ventricular failure, never having had orthopnea or paroxysmal dyspnea at any stage of his career.[99,136]

Chronic right ventricular failure manifested by distended, pulsating neck veins and hepatomegaly is usually a late and needless complication preventable by early treatment.[99] Most but not all of the patients have atrial fibrillation. There are three possible causes: (1) the commonest is some degree of pulmonary vascular obstruction and atrial fibrillation; (2) sometimes repeated pulmonary embolization plays an important role; (3) associated organic tricuspid disease must also be considered. At times all three factors are important, and the proper role of each may be difficult to assess.

In isolated mitral stenosis rheumatic fever is especially likely to have been mild and has been overlooked completely in nearly half the cases.[99] If rheumatic fever has been apparent, there is always a latent period, averaging about 12 years but sometimes as brief as 3 or as long as 25 years.[20,99] Rheumatic valvular deformity, especially stenosis, is probably not static and is likely to be capable of progressing in adult life long after rheumatic fever has apparently subsided. Whether this is because of covert rheumatism is unknown.[137] It seems likely that once a valve is misshapen (whether congenitally or by the rheumatic process) hemodynamic factors can advance the lesion to its ultimate deformity.[138,139] In tight mitral stenosis, the period from the onset of symptoms to the complete incapacity has been said to average 7 years;[29] but such figures are probably weighted toward the gloomy side because many of them are obtained from patients who have already gotten into serious difficulties. Among patients with pure isolated mitral stenosis there is a 2:1 preponderance of women.

Symptoms

In general, the liability to the symptoms in mitral stenosis correlates rather well with the severity of the lesion. Except when there are added burdens (such as thyrotoxicosis, pregnancy, other valvular disease, or the idiopathic hyperkinetic state[140]), patients with mitral valve areas over 1.5 cm^2 usually have no disability.[98] However, there is often no distinction in symptoms between patients who have valve areas of this size and those who have extreme stenosis.[131] The author believes that different individual susceptibilities to tachycardia explain much of this otherwise unaccountable variation. Unusual bradycardia is often associated with a very favorable course. Though symptoms may be amazingly slight even in the severe cases, such patients are in constant jeopardy of sudden deterioration.[141] Usually pulmonary infection[142] or the onset of atrial fibrillation[99] seems to be the triggering event. Influenza can lead to death within 24 hr in a patient with little previous difficulty.[143] Pulmonary embolization[144] and, rarely, coronary embolization[145] are other causes of sudden worsening. The patient, especially if a woman, may reach a rather advanced state of incapacity without being clearly aware of it because of the gradual compromises she has made with her disability.[146]

Respiratory Symptoms. The commonest early symptom is dyspnea on exertion, often vaguely described as fatigue, "asthma," or "chronic bronchitis."[99,108] Orthopnea and paroxysmal nocturnal dyspnea or cough, however, sometimes occur even before the patient is aware of much exertional difficulty. Recumbency and exercise aggravate the symptoms even when the patient describes them in an atypical way. Beware of a nocturnal "cigarette cough"! Frank pulmonary alveolar edema with diffuse rales, pink, foamy sputum, and a butterfly pattern of hilar clouding by x-ray is rather unusual, but it is especially likely to occur in younger patients with sinus rhythm.[98,99] Gross, bright-red hemoptysis may appear without warning after a nonchalant cough in a patient with few previous difficulties.[99] This terrifying symptom is likely to be recurrent but usually causes little immediate danger. Less dramatic bleeding may streak the sputum after fits of cough when the pulmonary venous congestion is severe. Hemoptysis may also result from pulmonary embolization but is not so sudden and massive as in pulmonary apoplexy.[99]

Chronic Right Ventricular Failure. Chronic right

ventricular failure causes edema and occasionally a painful, nauseating drag in the right upper quadrant from an engorged liver. Elevation of the serum-bilirubin level and sometimes frank jaundice may result from severe, prolonged hepatic congestion alone.[147,148] Pulmonary infarction will, of course, increase this tendency but will not produce jaundice by itself. With prolonged failure, most of the clinical and laboratory manifestations of hepatic cirrhosis may appear, including prolongation of the prothrombin time; less frequently, disordered serum proteins; and rarely, elevation of the serum alkaline phosphatase.[147,148] The serum-transaminase level is a sensitive but nonspecific index of hepatic congestion.[149]

Atrial Fibrillation. The longer the duration of the illness, the older the patient, and the larger the left atrium, the more likely fibrillation is to be present.[99,150] Palpitation is not universal. Some patients can give the date and the hour when their arrhythmia began. Others can slip in and out of pulmonary edema, triggered each time by the onset of atrial fibrillation, and remain completely unconscious of the heart. The proneness to fibrillation in the postoperative period after mitral valvulotomy has recently been clarified by the observation that the blood supply to the sinus node is very superficial and may therefore be jeopardized by pericarditis.[151]

Systemic Embolization. Systemic embolization is not uncommon in tight mitral stenosis, and the risk is greatly increased by atrial fibrillation. Provided there is fibrillation, emboli may occur even with mild stenosis.[152] Once the process begins it is likely to be recurrent.[153] The diagnosis is often difficult. Cerebrovascular accidents are the most commonly detected. This is probably because the brain reveals its damage more transparently than most other organs. Minor neurologic episodes properly interpreted are a great aid to early diagnosis, which is important because long-term anticoagulant therapy is rather effective prophylaxis.[153] The prognosis for return of function is rather good.[154] Convulsive seizures are distinctly more common among patients with mitral stenosis than in the general population, and are probably due to embolization, which, more than other types of cerebrovascular accidents, is likely to set up an epileptogenic focus.[155] Repeated seizures may occur after a single embolus, and postictal paralyses may give the false impression of repeated vascular accidents. On the other hand, an embolus may land in a silent area and not be detected clinically except as a convulsive seizure or a typical psychomotor attack (often misinterpreted as temporary psychosis). Coronary embolization is not uncommon in pathologic studies and may occasionally cause obvious acute myocardial infarction.[145] Renal or splenic in-

farcts may produce episodes of obscure abdominal or back pain; in the great majority of such cases the diagnosis is missed.[153] Superior mesenteric embolization produces midabdominal pain, often crampy, but associated with well-preserved peristalsis and often with no outstanding tenderness so that the diagnosis is often not made until gangrene has set in. Endarterectomy may save the patient's life if undertaken soon enough.[156] The physician's awareness of the possibility of this complication and his willingness to advise early laparotomy are the only means of lowering the high mortality. Saddle embolus is usually misinterpreted by the patient as a "stroke" because of numbness and inability to move his legs. The aortic obstruction may also be chronic, clinically closely mimicking the Leriche syndrome.[157]

Atypical chest pain is rather common in mitral disease and is indistinguishable from that occurring in anxiety neurosis.[99]

Classical angina pectoris appears in 10 per cent or more of patients with tight mitral stenosis, which appears to be somehow responsible for it.[99,108,158] The angina is usually relieved by successful mitral valvulotomy. Such angina has been attributed to (1) dilation of the pulmonary artery;[159] (2) pulmonary vascular obstruction with right ventricular ischemia (such as has been postulated in congenital heart disease[160]); (3) left ventricular ischemia because of a poor cardiac output;[161,162] (4) coronary embolization, which careful pathologic studies have shown is far more common and significant than is clinically recognized.[145] The first two explanations seem unlikely in mitral stenosis because neither factor can be closely correlated with the occurrence of angina. The third is in considerable vogue and is supported by the fact that electrocardiographic changes may appear in the left precordial leads after exercise. Unfortunately, some published examples of this phenomenon seem to have been obtained in patients probably receiving digitalis, which is known to produce false-positive reactions in exercise electrocardiography; in others junctional S-T changes[163,164] were mistakenly interpreted as indicating ischemia.[162] Most important, a disproportion between left ventricular work and coronary blood flow has not been demonstrated in mitral stenosis, and angina may occur in patients whose resting and exercise outputs are not greatly reduced.[165] The fourth explanation is perhaps the most appealing—although it would not necessarily explain improvement after valvulotomy, and to the author's knowledge, persistent embolic occlusion of a major coronary artery, capable of producing repeated anginal attacks, has not been proved by serial coronary angiograms.

As a practical point: confusion with coronary

artery disease can often be avoided if one remembers that in mitral stenosis angina is rarely an isolated symptom, but usually occurs simultaneously and parallel with dyspnea. When the valvular lesion is apparently mild or dyspnea is slight, angina should probably be attributed to coronary artery disease or to concurrent aortic valve disease. The problem in the elderly patient may be difficult. It is possible to have both tight mitral stenosis and significant atherosclerotic coronary disease. The accurate diagnosis of coronary embolization awaits studies carefully correlating symptoms with coronary angiograms.

Physical Findings

There is usually nothing about the *general aspect* of the patient to suggest the diagnosis as he comes to his physician complaining of his "chronic bronchitis" or "asthma." [79,108] The classic mitral facies is pallid, with red, slightly dusky cheeks and lips in startling contrast; but this appearance is actually rather unusual and is encountered chiefly in patients with very low cardiac outputs and severe pulmonary vascular obstruction in whom cyanosis of the fingers and toes is also common.[99,136] At rest the patient who has severe symptoms can often be seen to be hyperventilating slightly, but the rapidity and difficulty of respiration are likely to be much less than that of a patient with a comparable amount of chronic lung disease and, except during alveolar pulmonary edema, there is much less likely to be an obstructive element in the breathing. Even marked interstitial pulmonary edema does not guarantee any apparent respiratory difficulty at rest,[46] However, the patient who has had recent symptoms of pulmonary vascular congestion often finds it inconvenient to lie flat for very long on the examining table.

Examination of the chest is generally not very helpful because the signs are non-specific.° Wheezing and ausculatory rhonchi frequently accompany chronic interstitial edema—and may cause the physician to concur with the patient's mistaken diagnosis of lung disease. Basal rales are often present. Yet the chest may appear practically clear even in a severe case.

The venous pressure may be assessed reliably by physical examination. It is completely normal in uncomplicated cases but may become temporarily elevated during episodes of tachycardia and intense pulmonary venous congestion. Unless there is also rheumatic tricuspid valve disease, chronic elevation of the venous pressure generally means an element

° A considerably enlarged left atrium may compress a segment of lung, producing dullness and egophony under the left scapula (Ewart's sign) but the same findings may be produced by pericardial effusion.

of pulmonary vascular obstruction, since prolonged right ventricular failure does not usually occur otherwise.[99] The venous pressure is elevated when with the patient propped· at 30° the top of the oscillating column of venous blood in the neck is 5 cm or more above the level of the sternal angle.[29,99]

The Cardiac Impulse. Analysis of the left ventricular impulse provides an important and sensitive way of assessing the disordered physiology in mitral valvular disease.[166-169] Disregarding the information it provides usually results in misdiagnosis.[99,170,171] In pure mitral stenosis the left ventricular impulse at the apex is often completely normal. Sometimes it is brief and tapping or simply unaccountably hard to feel in a patient who lacks obesity or a thick chest wall. The impulse should not occupy an area larger than that of a 50 cent piece and should never fill more than two-thirds of systole.[172] The first sound may be delayed until quite appreciably after the onset of the systolic wave.°

Because of the hindrance to filling, the early diastolic expansion of the left ventricle is greatly slowed; but this fact can be recorded only indirectly and with special apparatus such as the apex cardiogram or the kinetocardiogram.[166-168] Clinically one can usually appreciate only the quietness of the total impulse, the briefness of the systolic thrust, and the absence of any obvious early diastolic movement. If the patient is obese or emphysematous he should be turned into the lateral decubitus position so that the left ventricular impulse can be brought into contact with the chest wall and its duration studied.[166] If the systolic portion of the impulse has a wide excursion and is prolonged, one should strongly suspect an important complicating factor such as mitral regurgitation or aortic valve disease even if the other clinical evidence is not very impressive. Rarely a clinically overactive left ventricle does occur in pure mitral stenosis, but it is usually associated with equally mysterious left ventricular hypertrophy when such exceptional patients come to operation.[99] Occasionally a grossly dilated right ventricle may simulate left ventricular hypertrophy, but in these cases the electrocardiographic changes are usually so obvious that no confusion need arise.[99]

° Normally the mitral component of the first sound occurs 0.02 sec after the onset of the apex impulse. In tight mitral stenosis it may be delayed by 0.07 sec.[173] With practice these relations are easy to detect clinically. It is rare for the presystolic portion of the impulse to be very large in mitral stenosis unless there is also some mitral insufficiency. Large presystolic impulses associated often with a presystolic (fourth) sound, however, are common in patients with severe disease of either ventricle.[174,175] Probably in every case they are associated with giant atrial contraction.

A parasternal lift is good clinical evidence of right ventricular hypertrophy but does not prove that the rheumatic lesion is stenosis, as the lift is also not uncommon in predominant mitral regurgitation.[99,108,176] Regardless of the mitral lesion the presence of a well-marked right ventricular lift means considerable pulmonary vascular obstruction, rheumatic tricuspid insufficiency, or both. Properly used, the clinical assessment of ventricular activity should be more reliable than the electrocardiogram; newer recording techniques have confirmed the potentialities of the method.[177]

Auscultation. The three hallmarks of mitral stenosis heard on *auscultation* are a loud snapping first sound (S-1),[99,178] an opening snap (OS),[179,180] and a diastolic rumble,[181] which in patients with sinus rhythm has presystolic (atriosystolic) accentuation.[99] Unfortunately, in special instances any one or all of these signs may be missing. Absence of an expected sound, however, often has important implications. Attention to auscultatory detail can pay rich dividends.

Accentuation of the first sound (S-1) is often the first clue to the diagnosis of mitral stenosis and should always make one listen carefully for the more subtle signs. Though it may be absent in the most trivial cases, it is otherwise of little use in assessing the severity of the lesion.[99] Tachycardia, a short P-R interval, systemic hypertension, and thyrotoxicosis may also sharpen S-1.[178]

The opening snap (OS) is usually a brief and often high-pitched, popping sound. Occasionally, however, it is not at all easy to hear and seems like an echo of the second heart sound on another plane from the rest of the auscultatory phenomena. Sometimes it may be missed because it is buried in the end of a split second heart sound or not distinguished from an unusually loud diastolic rumble closely following it.[173] For accurate recognition and timing of the snap one should listen at a point where the rumble is less obvious. Listening at the lower or even upper sternal area is preferable and allows proper identification of the components of the second heart sound. Opening snaps usually occur from 0.03 to 0.12 sec after the onset of the second sound (S-2)—earlier with tachycardia and later with slower rates. At rates of 70 to 90, a S-2-OS interval of 0.07 to 0.08 sec is the most common[182,183] and may be approximated by saying the word "da-tah" as fast as possible.*

* The "d" and "t" sounds are produced in rapid sequence by moving the ti of the tongue quickly back from behind the gum to the fore part of the palate. "Da-da" said as fast as possible with two quick motions of the lower jaw (the tip of the tongue being held rigid) is about 0.10 sec. "Bruh" is about 0.03 sec. It is important to recognize brief time intervals accurately.

Because of their proximity to the second heart sound and easy audibility over the upper portion of the heart, loud opening snaps are often confused with a delayed pulmonary closure sound, i.e., the second heart sound is thought to be widely and persistently split.[178,184] On the other hand, a widely split second sound may be mistaken for an S-2 and OS complex. These mistakes need not be made if one remembers that:

1. Wide splitting of the S-2 (unless there is right ventricular failure) may open still further with deep inspiration and close somewhat with expiration, but is very little affected by heart rate.[185] By contrast the opening snap interval tends to vary as a function of the length of the previous diastole and is not usually affected by respiration.[178,182,186] Thus during atrial fibrillation one may readily study the effects both of respiration and of variations in the length of the cardiac cycle. Here phonocardiography is valuable both to conform clinical impressions and to provide a permanent record.

2. Except in children, wide, persistent splitting of S-2 can never be physiologic and always demands an explanation such as right bundle branch block, atrial septal defect, moderate pulmonic stenosis, or severe mitral regurgitation.[185]

3. Inspiration will often split the second heart sound enough to uncover the fact that there are really three events instead of the two previously suspected.[178]

4. Unlike the pulmonary closure sound, the opening snap is usually, but not always, louder midway between the apex and the lower margin of the sternum.[178,180]

5. Standing will almost always widen the 2-OS interval (unless it speeds the heart rate considerably);[187,188] it will usually allow the physiologically split S-2 to close completely in expiration; it may not affect the interval when S-2 is pathologically split.[189] Sometimes, especially during tachycardia, a snap may be so close that it can be missed, and standing may provide a valuable way of separating and unmasking it.[187]

Opening snaps may sometimes be confused with third heart sounds (S-3).[99] The distinction is important because a well-defined S-3 is most unusual in mitral stenosis and implies some additional process.[173] The snap may be most reliably differentiated by its relationship to the left ventricular impulse.[166,181] The snap occurs when the left ventricle is smallest, therefore, coinciding with the nadir of a record of the left ventricular impulse. By contrast a third sound occurs a moment later as the ventricle swells during the rapid inflow of blood. With practice these distinctions can be appreciated

The above method is analogous to solfeggio used by musicians to recognize pitch.

clinically—by *simultaneous* auscultation and palpation—but they sometimes need verification by a simultaneous record of heart sounds and apex impulse. The interval from the onset of S-2 to S-3 is seldom under 0.12 sec. There may be some overlap between the timing of late snaps and premature third sounds; but the timing of the snap in mitral stenosis is usually much affected by changes in heart rate while the S-2 to S-3 interval usually is not much altered. The location and quality of the sound are also important. With the patient in the left lateral decubitus position, the S-3 is usually low-pitched and always clearly maximal directly over the apical impulse. The OS is not only sharper and more clicking but often maximal somewhat medially.

Physiologic Correlates of the Accentuated First Sound and Opening Snap. The normal mitral valve is subjected to sudden and violent reversals of pressure. Often the rheumatic process merely glues the edges of the cusps together, converting the valve into a limp diaphragm, its outer rim relatively immobile.[93,94] The bellies of the cusps, however, may pop "like wet sails" in the upward (closing snap or loud first heart sound) and downward (opening snap) excursions.[42] During systole the billowing redundant valve cusps are in contact like a pair of parachutes over a broad area above the stenotic mitral orifice, producing an important suprastenotic seal against mitral regurgitation.[190] Palpation of the valve at operation and recent angiographic studies suggest that the snap is produced by sudden tensing of the valve at the bottom of its diastolic descent.[191,192] Probably neither snap nor first sound is produced by opening or closure of the valve;[42] they follow the pressure "crossover" by a small but appreciable interval[193] and therefore are likely to be made by subsequent tensing of the mobile cusps. The opening snap occurs during or just after the brief but violent moment of active ventricular expansion in early diastole,[194] which also may contribute to the rapid descent of the valve. Exactly why the first sound is accentuated is not known. The author agrees with those[99,178] who believe that the usual mechanism largely depends on an abnormal position of the fused valve cusps, which normally have risen somewhat by the end of diastole but are kept in a downwardly tented position by the presence of mitral stenosis.

The effects of cardiac cycle length and body position on the timing of the opening snap may be correlated with changes in the left atrial pressure, which is higher after a short diastole than after a long one—and drops when the patient goes from the recumbent to the standing position.[119,195] Though accentuation of the first sound and the opening snap are probably produced by reciprocal forces acting on the aortic cusp of the mitral valve, the sounds are not of strictly parallel intensity. The first sound almost always is more intense because the systolic force is more violent than the diastolic. When the presystolic murmur is obliterated by atrial fibrillation, the first sound may be audibly split, the first (tricuspid) component becoming quite sharp during tachycardia.[173] In appraising the typical case of mitral stenosis one should expect both the loud first sound and the opening snap and should be concerned about the absence of either. Both are usually present in the presence of the simple anatomic arrangement just described.[196]

The Diastolic Murmur. The middiastolic rumble is the feature of mitral stenosis which is easiest to miss.[184] Often the sharp first sound or the opening snap makes the listener hone his ears for a previously missed murmur. Although occasionally the noise may be of almost blowing quality, as a rule it deserves to be called a rumble. At least its beginning (usually 0.02 to 0.04 sec after the opening snap) is usually quite low pitched and may be easily ignored if one is focusing only on sharper sounds. This portion of the murmur has been evocatively described as the "thunder of a distant oxcart rumbling over a loose wooden bridge." Atrial systole produces sharpening and intensification: presystolic accentuation which may be audible even when the rest of the murmur is not.[181] If one pronounces "uh-ah-ah-rup" (using broad *a*'s and trilling the *r*) he approximates (1) the early diastolic rumble ("uh-uh-ah"); (2) the presystolic accentuation (the trilled *r*); (3) the sharp first heart sound (*p*). Perhaps the most important reason that rumbles are missed is that they may be sharply localized to the cardiac apex and quite inaudible even an inch away. Thus the murmur will not be imparted to a sloppily placed stethoscope heavily mashed against the chest wall. Furthermore, the amount of sound is often genuinely variable and may be rather slight most of the time, though often considerably augmented for a few moments after the patient has exercised, the heart rate has speeded, and the velocity of mitral flow has temporarily increased. The lateral decubitus position throws the cardiac apex against the chest wall and improves transmission of the murmur. The act of turning sometimes provides enough exercise to bring out the rumble momentarily, but if one fails to believe his ears at first, the sound will often dissolve into limbo.[184] More vigorous exercise will bring out the murmur for longer periods. Yet, when there are already sounds in diastole, exercise may be misleading. For example, exercise in a person with a loud third heart sound will increase its intensity and abbreviate diastole (by increasing the heart rate). A shortened diastole more filled with sound may give the erroneous impression of a diastolic rumble, when actually only a loud third heart sound is present. When the P-R interval is very short, the presystolic murmur of severe stenosis may be quite abbreviated and indistinguishable from a fourth heart sound or from the brief crescendo effect commonly associated with the first heart sound in persons without mitral lesions.[178,197] The distinction between a fourth sound and a presystolic rumble is not always easy. Indeed, a moderate Valsalva maneuver can easily reduce the murmur to the proportions of a single sound.[181] A deep breath has been claimed to clear away the buildup to a crescendo first heart sound but not to affect the mitral presystolic murmur.[197] The author has not found this as useful as (1) prior inspection of the electrocardiogram to see if the P-R interval is short enough to abbreviate presystolic accentuation; (2) simultaneous palpation of the apex impulse (in the lateral decubitus position), which may reveal that a supposed first heart sound is really an ejection click occurring 0.05 to 0.06 sec after a normal or soft sound of mitral closure.° Atrial fibrillation obliterates atrial contraction and inevitably causes loss of presystolic accentuation of the murmur. Since, however, the diastolic rumble of tight mitral stenosis is often itself quite long, the noise may continue up to the first heart sound, especially when the heart rate is fast. The machine gun rattle produced by tetany of the chestwall muscles has also been mistaken for a diastolic rumble. Such auscultatory static can be eliminated by warming the room or by asking the patient voluntarily to tense and then to relax his pectoral muscles.

In general, the diastolic murmur is produced by high-velocity flow past a shelf of mitral tissue which does not retract properly in diastole. The loudness of the murmur does not correlate well with the severity of stenosis.[99] Yet variations in an individual patient's rumble are a useful means of gauging changes in the velocity of his mitral flow. Exercise and tachycardia, by reducing the duration of diastole and sometimes by increasing cardiac output, augment the flow velocity and hence the murmur. If flow is sufficiently reduced for any reason, the rumble may be extremely hard to hear. Amyl nitrite may sometimes accentuate the murmur more strikingly than does exercise.[198]

° The normal apex impulse begins to ascend practically coincident with the first sound. Before using the apex impulse to time the onset of ventricular systole, however, one must make sure that there is no presystolic impulse. A preliminary check for this is made by simultaneous palpation of cardiac apex and carotid artery. An unusual "delay" in the onset of the carotid upstroke often means a presystolic impulse, which in itself is good evidence against tight mitral stenosis.

X-ray Findings

The left atrium takes the burden of mitral stenosis and is dilated in all but the mildest cases.[104,199] Therefore radiologic assessment is a useful screening test. The earliest sign is usually provided in the lateral view: the middle one-third of the barium-filled esophagus, instead of continuing straight down, bulges posteriorly behind a line connecting its upper and lower thirds.[103,104,199,200] Backward displacement of the lower two-thirds of the esophagus is nonspecific and may be due to any combination of ventricular or atrial enlargement, or to adherence of the esophagus to an ectatic aorta.[200,201] In the frontal view of the chest, enlargement of the left atrium often produces prominence of the auricular appendage, which reaches around from behind like a chubby hand clasping the waist of the heart between the pulmonary artery segment and the ventricle. Thus the normally concave upper left border of the heart becomes a straight line or even acquires moderate convexity.[104] The barium-filled esophagus is often displaced to the right by a considerably enlarged left atrium,[200] occasionally when the posterior displacement is not obvious.

The left atrium is really a midline structure, so that on enlarging it commonly spreads to both the right and the left, remaining in some patients still a rather flat ovoid. Hence: (1) esophageal displacement in the lateral view (checked against angiographic techniques) often fails to give a true impression of the large left atrium;[201] (2) the rounded right edge of the enlarged left atrium can often be seen shining through the thin structures of the right side of the heart in the well penetrated frontal view.[104] Sometimes the entire circular atrial silhouette can be made out with the aid of an overpenetrated grid film or tomography. Once the left atrium is definitely dilated, its size has no useful relationship to the severity of the stenosis and is importantly affected by other factors, including the duration of the process, atrial fibrillation, and associated mitral regurgitation, which tend to enlarge it disproportionately.[99,101,202,203] Unfortunately, the greatest limitation of radiographic diagnosis is that the amount of esophageal displacement may be borderline and the important distinction between a normal and a slightly enlarged left atrium may be impossible to make.[204] Recumbency and incomplete inspiration tend to exaggerate the esophageal curve.[104] Thus a diagnosis of mitral valve disease should never be made solely from a borderline esophagram.

Enlargement of the right side of the heart is a more indirect consequence of mitral stenosis, usually occurring only when the pulmonary vascular resistance is considerably increased. In severe cases on the lateral film the dilated anterior structures may fill the normal clear space between the heart silhouette and the sternum.[103,104]

It is well to remember that the overall heart size assessed on the usual posteroanterior film is commonly normal even in tight mitral stenosis. When gross cardiomegaly occurs, it is usually from aneurysm of the left atrium or from pulmonary vascular obstruction with dilatation of the right side of the heart.

Calcification of the mitral valve is rare in patients under 30 years of age.[205] Often it is slight and detectable only by its characteristic movement seen during image-intensifier fluoroscopy. Heavy calcification is more obvious and is clinically important. The mitral and aortic valves are quite close together and may be confused.[103] Figure 7-21, p. 159, shows their relative positions.

The pattern of the pulmonary vasculature is of great importance and may give valuable information about the degree of physiologic disorder.[112,113] Dilated superior veins project upward in each lung like the antlers of a stag, in vivid contrast to the constricted lower lobe veins, whose caliber is reduced about 20 per cent.[114] This radiologic pattern indicates one of the most sensitive early stages of pulmonary venous hypertension; changes often begin when the left atrial pressure is not much over 15 mm Hg and are usually obvious in patients with pressures in excess of 25 mm Hg. However, with the development of pulmonary vascular obstruction, venous engorgement may become appreciably less. At the lung bases the transverse costophrenic lines clearly testify to chronic basal interstitial edema[115,116] and usually a mean left atrial pressure of 20 mm Hg or more.[112,113,117] These lines, however, are not always obvious even in tight mitral stenosis, and they may be simulated by interlobular thickening of pulmonary fibrosis, cancer, or acute vitral pneumonitis.[46] To the uninitiated, the "B lines" are rather easier to see than the venous pattern; but for firm diagnosis they must be quite definite continuous lines and some at least must extend all the way to the periphery of the lung. Borderline changes may be confused with normal variants.[206]

Pulmonary artery dilatation is diagnosed when the right descending branch is over 17 mm wide in an average adult[207] (though this measurement is perhaps best related to the transverse diameter of the chest.[208] Dilatation is always found in patients with severe pulmonary hypertension but does not guarantee its presence; dilated central arteries with rapidly tapering peripheral branches always mean severe pulmonary vascular obstruction.[113] A profusion of small vessels at the periphery of the lung and an overall fuzziness of outline both of the hilar and peripheral structures (as if the patient had moved or breathed during the exposure

of the film) provide a very useful index of interstitial edema.[115*] When interstitial edema is not obvious on a single film, a follow-up after the patient has had a diuretic often provides a convincing diagnosis in retrospect.

Such a venous pattern, septal lines, and perihilar haze are, of course, not peculiar to mitral stenosis and may occur whenever there is pulmonary venous hypertension.[115] With the prolonged venous congestion of mitral disease a fine miliary pattern of pulmonary hemosiderosis may develop, especially in the midzone of the lung. Rarely, and almost exclusively in males, small pulmonary nodules of bone may simulate the findings in chronic histoplasmosis.[209]

Angiographically the only entirely specific sign of mitral stenosis is persistent doming of the mitral valve into the left ventricle during diastole, at which time the negative shadow of the valve normally has disappeared.[210,211] Another very useful and more obvious sign is holdup of contrast material in an enlarged and densely opacified left atrium, which contrasts vividly with a poorly opacified and normal-sized left ventricle.[211,212]

The Electrocardiogram of Mitral Stenosis

As noted, the left atrium is selectively affected by mitral stenosis. Therefore, the most characteristic electrocardiogram, while usually displaying a QRS axis further to the right than +60°, often shows nothing but P-wave changes.[99,108,213] These are most striking because they are *unassociated* with evidence of left ventricular disease (hypertrophy or myocardial infarction), which is the usual cause of left atrial embarrassment. Unfortunately, the definition of "P mitrale" is not so clear is it should be. There are many different grades of abnormality, some quite ambiguous, others more clearly diagnostic; even the heart rate has an effect.[213,214] At present the interpretation of such electrocardiographic subtleties often has a strong subjective flavor. Since the P wave probably deserves to be scrutinized in more detail than is possible with the average electrocardiograph machine, newer amplification techniques may help.[215] At present the true incidence of P-wave abnormalities in tight mitral stenosis is hard to come by. Values of 90 per cent,[213] 80 per cent[216] and 20 per cent[217] have been reported.

The best available profile of left atrial hypertrophy seems to include both the following features:

1. The P wave is notched and commonly at least 0.12 sec in duration (as usually measured without amplification techniques); the widening is

---

* The fact that he has *not* breathed is established by the fact that the diaphragms and other structures are in sharp focus.

mainly due to a secondary hump caused by continuing atrial depolarization after the right atrial portion is completed.[218–220] Widening, however, may not be apparent.[216] Unfortunately, much of the P wave may be isoelectric in many leads; hence even previously quoted "normal values" may be too low.[221]

2. The axis of the P wave (sometimes only its second half) is shifted to the back, to the left, or in both directions.[219,220] In the standard electrocardiogram, backward deflection means that in V_1 and V_2 the P wave is either negative or biphasic with an impressively negative second half.[220,223] Leftward (upward) deflection means that in V_5 and V_6 the P wave is often more easily seen than normal and may be clearly notched, while in the limb leads the second peak is often broad and tall and more pronounced in lead I than in lead III.[219,220] Leftward deflection and backward deflection of the second peak are not always both apparent in the same patient. For accurate diagnosis, both widening of the P wave and the abnormal axis of its second half should be required. Attempts to simplify the criteria by focusing on a single aspect of the abnormal P wave are probably not satisfactory.[224] It is most important to remember that a completely normal P wave does not exclude the diagnosis of tight mitral stenosis.[216] Furthermore, any cause of an increased left ventricular end-diastolic pressure—hypertension even when relatively asymptomatic, aortic valve disease, and left ventricular failure—may cause "mitral" P waves.[214] Fortunately in these cases there are almost always other clinical or electrocardiographic signs of left ventricular involvement. Some perfectly normal persons, however, have moderately broad and notched P waves, which are perhaps associated at times with a tendency to paroxysmal tachycardia.[214,225]

In the presence of atrial fibrillation the size of the fibrillatory wave in V_1 has been claimed to be distinctively larger in rheumatic heart disease.[226] Unfortunately there is important overlap. Rather large fibrillatory waves have been encountered by the writer in hypertensive patients and by other investigators in idiopathic paroxysmal atrial fibrillation.[226] Yet a flat base line usually means coronary disease, while unusually coarse waves are pretty good evidence for valvular disease or thyrotoxicosis. About 10 per cent of patients with tight mitral stenosis have low-voltage fibrillatory waves, and this group apparently includes many of those who cannot be kept in sinus rhythm even after successful mitral valvulotomy.[227]

The Ventricular Complex. After the left atrium, the right ventricle receives the burden of mitral stenosis, but it will be recalled that the right ventricle does not hypertrophy greatly unless its job is further augmented by pulmonary vascular obstruction. Therefore, even in severe mitral stenosis, there are no QRS abnormalities in many cases.[99,108] In fact, a totally normal electrocardiogram is quite compatible with tight mitral stenosis even when it is complicated by moderate pulmonary vascular obstruction.[99,213,228] The most sensitive index of right ventricular hypertrophy is the mean axis in the frontal plane.[108,228] An axis further to the right than $+100°$ is rather unusual in the normal population but is common in mitral stenosis and often the sole electrocardiographic clue to the presence of right ventricular hypertrophy.[213] Almost all patients with mitral stenosis and definite right axis deviation do indeed have significant pulmonary arterial hypertension. Standard electrocardiographic criteria for right ventricular hypertrophy (in the presence of normal QRS duration) include both an axis of 100° or more and an R/S ratio in V_1 greater than unity. In fact either of these criteria alone probably would suffice.[229] In mitral stenosis, such classic right ventricular hypertrophy almost always indicates a mean pulmonary artery pressure over 35 mm Hg and a range up to 80 mm or above.[228] Stated vectorially, the deviation of the QRS axis in the right ventricular hypertrophy of mitral stenosis is likely to be more rightward than anteriorly—except in extreme cases, when it is both. After mitral valvulotomy the more severe grades of right ventricular hypertrophy regress slowly, sometimes not at all.[230]

In summary the electrocardiogram is usually an inadequate way of assessing the severity of mitral stenosis. Though relatively insensitive, it often helps in gauging the degree of pulmonary vascular obstruction and right ventricular hypertrophy.[108,213,228] As a screening test the electrocardiogram may be useful; normal or right axis deviation of the QRS complex associated with P mitrale or coarse atrial fibrillation may lead the clinician back to the bedside to check more carefully for previously missed physical findings. Conversely, the most important role of the electrocardiogram is in the detection of left ventricular disease, which almost always means the presence of some other lesion (such as mitral insufficiency or aortic valve disease). Though the accuracy of the electrocardiographic diagnosis or left ventricular hypertrophy is far from satisfactory,[231] a florid pattern with both voltage and ST-T changes is extremely unusual in uncomplicated mitral stenosis.[99] Unfortunately even high-grade mitral regurgitation often does not produce electrocardiographic signs of left ventricular hypertrophy.[232] Serial electrocardiograms after mitral valvulotomy have aided in the detection of restenosis.[233]

Estimation of the Severity of Mitral Stenosis

As noted, symptoms are not always a reliable guide to the severity of a mitral lesion.[99,141] Formerly, cardiac catheterization was often needed to assess the severity of mitral stenosis. At present an accurate judgment can usually be made from a careful clinical examination.[171,234]

Auscultatory Details. *Timing of the Heart Sounds.* A delay of the mitral component of the first heart sound (Q-1 time) and a brief space between the second sound and the opening snap (2-OS interval) are common in tight mitral stenosis and classically have been attributed to the high left atrial pressure, which delays upward movement of the mitral valve in systole and hastens its descent in early diastole.[182]* Various attempts have been made to correlate phonocardiographic findings with the severity of mitral stenosis.[182,183,237-241]

In order to compensate for the effect of different valve mobilities, Wells devised an index obtained by subtracting the 2-OS interval from the Q-1 time (compensating for the effect of heart rate by "correcting" these figures according to a previously constructed nomogram).[183] If the result (expressed without decimals) was −1 to +5 he felt that tight mitral stenosis could be predicted. At present the writer seldom uses the Q-1 time or the Wells index. These measurements require that the onset of the mitral component of the first sound be clearly identified. Defining this point is not always possible, though two ingenious and often workable methods have been suggested.[173,242] Furthermore, other clinically unmeasurable factors play a role in the Q-1 time; perhaps most importantly the rate of ascent of the early part of the ventricular pressure curve.[241] It is possible that the P-R interval and the vigor of atrial systole may also have an effect. Delay of the first sound is also not confined to mitral stenosis and has been encountered in systemic hypertension, ventricular septal defect, and other conditions.[243-245] The 2-OS interval, on the other hand, may be more accurately measured, and in the only satisfactorily planned study it correlated quite well with the simultaneously meas-

* The Q-1 time is usually measured from the onset of the Q wave of the electrocardiogram to the first high frequencies of the mitral component of the first heart sound (if this can be accurately identified).[182,183,235] The range is 0.04 to 0.08 sec, depending somewhat on the size of the individual [236] but not correlating clearly with any easily assessed clinical factor. The 2-OS interval is measured from the onset of the second heart sound to the beginning of the opening snap. The curious differences in the Q-1 times reported by different workers are due to different methods of measurement. [173,183,235,239,241] Probably none of these methods gives consistent results.

ured pulmonary wedge pressure.[237] At best, however, the 2-OS interval is no more than a rough index of the relation between the aortic closing and the mitral opening pressures. If it is to be used intelligently, five important facts must be kept in mind:

1. The level of the aortic closing pressure must be considered; this is not a fixed landmark. Systemic diastolic hypertension causes aortic closure to occur higher along the curve of left ventricular relaxation and therefore produces apparent delay of the opening snap.[237,241] An unusually low diastolic blood pressure, on the other hand, makes the snap disproportionately premature.[237]

2. The timing of the snap has no logical relation to the average left atrial pressure and can be related only to the atrioventricular gradient at the onset of diastole.[216] Though commonly the left atrial pressure at this moment is a fair index of the average level, sometimes it may be a good deal higher. A disproportionately large atrial V wave seems especially likely to occur when the atrial wall is relatively noncompliant and the mitral curtain is unusually ample so that it rises piston-like into the atrium during systole, encroaching somewhat on the volume of the chamber (Fig. 25-2). A small amount of mitral regurgitation may also augment the atrial V wave. Physical characteristics of the valve have been thought to affect the timing of the snap through yet other mechanisms.[182]

3. Variations in the shape of the ventricular pressure curve probably may occasionally produce atypical timing of the snap.*

4. Even if the timing of the heart sounds were a direct and sensitive pressure gauge, it could no more provide a completely reliable index of the severity of mitral stenosis than do pressure measurements obtained at cardiac catheterization when considered without regard to the mitral flow.[98]

5. The 2-OS interval, like the mitral pressure gradient, may be considerably affected by the heart rate.[182] As the left atrial pressure falls during bradycardia,[195] the interval may widen greatly.[183] On the other hand, as the left atrial pressure rises during tachycardia,[195] the opening snap may occasionally almost fuse with the second heart sound. However, the pattern of response is rather variable. Attempting to "correct" the 2-OS interval for faster or slower rates seems as illogical in phonocardiography as it would be in cardiac catheteriza-

* One patient with tight mitral stenosis and chronic complete heart block had an A-2 to OS interval of 0.12 sec even when paced at a rate of 90 from a right ventricular catheter which produced a left bundle branch configuration and paradoxic splitting of the second heart sound.

tion. With exercise or vagal stimuli (such as a deep breath or carotid sinus massage) one can often vary the heart rate as desired.

In tight mitral stenosis with a normal systemic blood pressure and a pulse between 70 and 90, the 2-OS interval is usually about 0.08 sec, commonly varying from 0.06 to 0.09 sec.[173,182] During extreme bradycardia the interval may widen to 0.12 in spite of tight mitral stenosis.[183] Standing reduces venous return, lowers the left atrial pressure, and hence widens the 2-OS interval, provided there is not considerable acceleration of the rate. Widening of the 2-OS interval following successful mitral valvulotomy occurs in most patients,[183,230] but the improvement is commonly much better appreciated by comparison of findings obtained in the standing position. Pre- and postoperative phonocardiograms done at similar heart rates are needed to detect the change. The snap disappears in fewer than one-third of cases.[99]

When the 2-OS interval is borderline at rest (0.09 sec or more), the study should be repeated

after exercise.[247] Tight mitral stenosis may permit a nearly normal left atrial pressure during rest and a slow heart rate. Exercise and its associated tachycardia, however, will promptly raise the pressure. In our experience, if there is important mitral stenosis, the 2-OS interval can easily be narrowed with exercise to 0.08 sec or less. On the other hand, if a patient is studied only during extreme tachycardia (e.g., uncontrolled atrial fibrillation), the severity of the valve lesion is likely to be overestimated. An identical problem, however, is encountered with cardiac catheterization or any method of defining the functional significance of mitral stenosis. Uncontrollable tachycardia may render even moderate mitral stenosis physiologically intolerable—just as bradycardia may obviate many of the difficulties of the severest lesions. When the mitral valve area is calculated by the Gorlin formula, the effect of heart rate is taken into consideration (see Chap. 24).

Varying opinions exist about the accuracy of the 2-OS interval in the assessment of the severity of

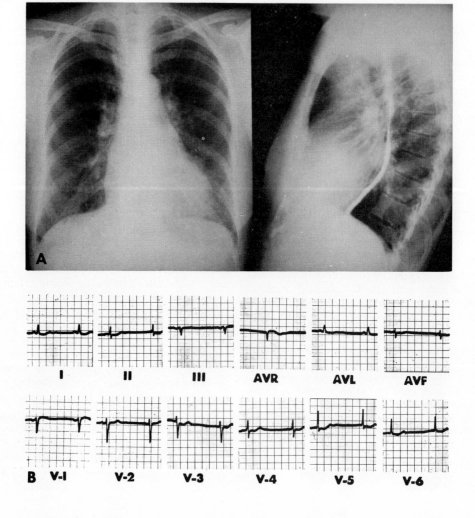

mitral stenosis.[237,183,239] Certainly it should never be the sole basis, especially if there are other valve lesions. Yet if proper allowance is made for the effect of the aortic diastolic pressure and if the patient is studied in different stages of activity and at different heart rates, one may obtain an approximate idea of how the early diastolic mitral pressure gradient varies in response to a number of physiologic stimuli. To help in the evaluation of mitral valvulotomy, preoperative and postoperative phonocardiograms should be obtained in all cases. Serial records may help to diagnose re-stenosis. The intensity of the pulmonic component of the second sound (if this separates enough during inspiration to be identified) bears a rough relation to the pulmonary artery pressure.[99] The pulmonic (latter) half of the split second sound if normal should be softer than the aortic (first) component at the lower left sternal border. If the accent is on the "second syllable" of the second sound, one should suspect pulmonary hypertension or unusual dilatation of the right side of the heart and pulmonary artery.

Evidence for Right Ventricular Hypertrophy. Whether palpable or electrocardiographic, evidence of right ventricular hypertrophy is a sign of advanced mitral stenosis and is helpful, though not encountered in all such patients.[99,108]

The X-ray. Various attempts have been made to correlate radiographic findings with the degree of mitral stenosis assessed by cardiac catheterization or at operation.[112,113,115,248] Details of such correlations have already been given. Definite atrial enlargement is almost always present with hemodynamically significant mitral disease; but otherwise, atrial size does not correlate with the severity of the lesion. Radiographic signs of pulmonary interstitial edema are more directly relevant to the patient's immediate symptoms than is any other single clinical test. A patient with marked and clinically obvious dyspnea at rest practically always has such x-ray signs. However, when current symptoms are not severe, absence of interstitial edema does not exclude tight mitral stenosis. A diuretic will often wash away the perihilar haze and some of the Kerley's lines; yet later a paroxysm of atrial fibrillation may bring them back. The vascular pattern tends to be more fixed. For example, films taken in recumbency do not show any change in the venous ratio between upper and lower lobes.[249] After strenuous exercise sufficient to raise the pulmonary pressure, there is usually no immediate change in

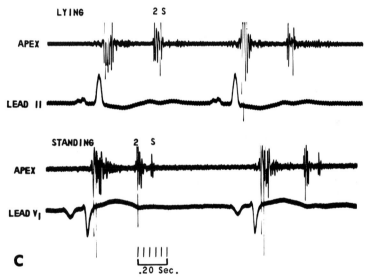

Fig. 25-2. Mitral stenosis with unusual timing of the opening snap. A 30-year-old female with moderately severe disability had typical left atrial enlargement and costophrenic lines (Kerley) at the lung bases on her chest x-ray (A, opposite page, frontal and lateral views). The electrocardiogram (B, opposite page) showed small but broad, leftwardly directed P waves but was otherwise nondescript. On the initial examination she was thought to have a loud first heart sound and a split second sound, but no opening snap. This anomalous situation was clarified when a phonocardiogram (C), made with the patient in recumbent and standing positions, showed that the second half of the "split" second sound was really a premature opening snap. The blood pressure was 100/60, and the left atrial pressure rose to 35 with each ventricular systole. The closeness of aortic closing and mitral opening pressures probably explains the unusually short snap interval. At operation the mitral valve was tightly stenosed but extremely mobile, rising far into the atrium with each systole. There was a small but strong regurgitant jet. A satisfactory valvulotomy was obtained.

the caliber of any of the pulmonary vessels seen on the ordinary roentgenogram. Patients who know they have mitral stenosis may develop cardiac neuroses. Here the x-ray has special relevance in the interpretation and validation of symptoms. A person who reports only of effort dyspnea may legitimately have no radiographic findings except enlargement of the left atrium and an abnormal pulmonary vascular pattern. Yet if he complains of orthopnea or dyspnea at rest—and is observed to be hyperventilating during the examination—the radiologic corrolary should be nothing less than interstitial pulmonary edema.

If the entire x-ray picture is correlated intelligently with the history and is double-checked against the auscultatory evidence, the clinical assessment of the severity of mitral stenosis is rarely mistaken. In the difficult case when physiologic studies are needed because of contradictory findings, pressure measurements and angiocardiography complement each other and should be done together.[250]

Atypical Mitral Stenosis

Mild Mitral Stenosis. This produces no physiologic disadvantage. The diagnosis is often missed, since it usually must be made solely on the basis of auscultatory findings which are not necessarily easy to detect. The patient has no genuine cardiac symptoms and no electrocardiographic abnormality; the x-ray shows nothing except perhaps borderline left atrial enlargement as revealed by the barium swallow in the lateral view. The first clue is often an unaccountable sharpness of the first heart sound.[99] The early diastolic murmur at rest is frequently absent. The presystolic murmur is often the only one heard and may be quite brief; however, with exercise it often becomes longer and is therefore more easily distinguished from the crescendo effect so often associated with a normal first heart sound.[173,180] There is often no opening snap. If the snap is present, it is quite delayed and often low-pitched, disappearing altogether on standing. The 2-OS interval fails to shorten significantly after exercise. Many patients have a soft pansystolic murmur of mild associated mitral regurgitation.

Tight Mitral Stenosis with an Apical Systolic Murmur. A brief apical systolic murmur is common and of no consequence in tight mitral stenosis.[252,253] Also, not uncommonly, stiffness of the mitral aperture, local chordal traction, or partial immobilization of a cusp may allow *jet regurgitation* in tight mitral stenosis with otherwise mobile leaflets.[254] The latter murmur is pansystolic, maximal at the apex, and sometimes grade II or III. Yet the sharp S-1, opening snap, quiet apical impulse, and long diastolic murmur testify to typical tight mitral ste-

nosis. The surgeon will probably find a reasonably favorable situation for blind valvulotomy or for open reconstruction without the need for valve replacement. Any hint of left ventricular hypertrophy is reason to abandon this diagnosis.

A *tricuspid systolic murmur* may also be well heard at the midclavicular line in those cases with marked right ventricular dilatation.[255] The distinction, especially from mitral insufficiency, can usually be made. The mitral systolic murmur is almost always louder beyond and to the left of the apex impulse than at the lower left sternal border. The tricuspid murmur, if well heard at the apex, is just as obvious in the lower sternal area. There may not be an obviously abnormal cervical venous pulse. Not all tricuspid systolic murmurs are augmented by inspiration, but Carvallo's sign, if definite, is pathognomonic. Sometimes both mitral and tricuspid systolic murmurs may be present. Here pharmacologic auscultation is most useful.[256] Amyl nitrite reduces and sometimes almost obliterates the murmur of mitral insufficiency but tends to increase that of tricuspid incompetence. Phenylephrine (Neosynephrine)* given intravenously in amounts sufficient to raise the systemic blood pressure 40 mm Hg augments mitral insufficiency and accentuates the murmur; it has no effect on tricuspid insufficiency.

Mild Mitral Stenosis with Serious Symptoms. Mitral stenosis of less than critical severity may of course occur and be diagnosed in a patient whose main difficulty is coronary disease or hypertension. There is, also, a small group of severely symptomatic patients, mainly women, who have most of the hallmarks of mild stenosis unaccountably associated with chronic atrial fibrillation[257] (Fig. 25-3). Moderate cardiomegaly and occasionally considerable enlargement of the left atrium may occur. These patients have repeated episodes of failure and peripheral embolization for many years but do fairly well in between times and respond to medical treatment. They are not benefited by operations on the mitral valve. A myocardial factor seems likely in this group; however, there is really remarkably little clinical or pathologic evidence bearing on the nature of the left ventricular disease. Angiographically, impaired left ventricular emptying has been demonstrated in patients whose symptoms were disproportionate to their valvular disease.[258] Usually atrial fibrillation seems an integral part of the disability. At cardiac catheterization the most impressive finding is a low cardiac output. Under such conditions of low flow, however, the mitral gradient is minimized and catheterization of

* A sympathomimetic amine which increases peripheral resistance but which has little or no effect upon myocardial contractility.

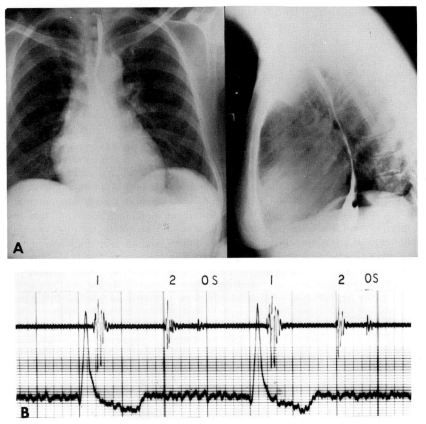

Fig. 25-3. Mitral stenosis with a predominant myocardial factor. A 55-year-old woman with chronic atrial fibrillation had had episodes of mild congestive failure for 15 years. In spite of several peripheral emboli, however, she did well on digitalis and regular oral diuretic therapy and remained active. The electrocardiogram showed only nonspecific ST-T abnormalities. The chest film (*A*, frontal and lateral views) showed moderate cardiomegaly. There was a short middiastolic murmur at the apex. In phonocardiogram (*B*), study of the opening snap at the lower sternal border showed that the 2-OS interval exceeded 0.12 sec at a heart rate of 70 beats per minute. The calculated mitral orifice was 2.8 cm².

the right side of the heart is not enough to exclude tight mitral stenosis. Catheterization and angiography of the *left* side of the heart should be done in all such cases before the diagnosis of tight mitral stenosis is discarded.[250,259]

Severe Mitral Stenosis with a Rigid Valve. In a large percentage of cases of mitral stenosis, stricture of the subvalvular apparatus and shrinkage of the leaflets destroy the mitral "parachutes" and convert the valve into a fibrous funnel aimed at the left ventricle—an arrangement not very amenable to the older surgical techniques.[260] In extreme cases the valve is altogether rigid, and the sharp first sound and opening snap are usually reduced or obliterated.[150,261] The opening snap is often the first to go;[262] the loud first sound may persist, especially if the patient also has systemic hypertension (Fig. 25-4). The rumble is unaffected by the process. If, however, the diastolic murmur is absent or soft for any other reason, the mitral stenosis may

be totally silent. Because of rigidity of the leaflets and loss of the suprastenotic seal, a mitral pansystolic murmur is not uncommon even in critical stenosis.[263] Fluoroscopically there is often, but not always, heavy calcification of the valve.[263] Unfortunately, radiographic techniques cannot yet outline the distribution of the calcium and the extent to which it immobilizes the cusps.

Heavy calcification by x-ray may be due to localized excrescences which do not critically interfere with valve function; on the other hand, a valve may be practically of the consistency of cartilage and show little or nothing by image-intensifier fluoroscopy. The writer believes that the significance of calcification is best evaluated together with the auscultatory evidence. Certainly if the snap is absent and there is also heavy calcification, one may confidently predict that the valve is virtually destroyed. Blind commissurotomy will not help and may lead to embolization of the cerebral and coronary vessels with calcium particles.[171] Even without obvious calcium, definite absence of the opening snap (confirmed by careful phonocardiographic study) should lead one to recommend only an open heart procedure. There is probably a rigid mitral apparatus which will function no better—and probably will be worse—after a blind valvulotomy.[261] Heavy calcification is distinctly more common in males, being found in about one-third of men referred for mitral valvulotomy.[264] Unfortunately, typical snaps may also be produced by valves too severely diseased to be greatly benefited by closed operation.[171] Failure of the first sound and opening snap to become louder and sharper during the tachycardia 30 sec after the administration of amyl nitrite has been proposed as evidence for impaired valvular mobility in these cases.[198]

Mitral Stenosis with Extreme Pulmonary Vascular Obstruction. This is a rare but very important syndrome because it can be confused with primary pulmonary hypertension and the patient may be condemned to the therapeutic neglect implicit in the latter diagnosis.[136,265] The pulmonary pressure is in the systemic range, and the cardiac output is usually quite low. Electrocardiographic evidence of right ventricular hypertrophy is obvious, and by x-ray the pulmonary arteries are grossly dilated, with amputation of the most peripheral branches characteristic of severe pulmonary vascular obstruction. The patients are always very severely dyspneic and often have a deep cyanotic flush. A right ventricular heave, a ringing, widely transmitted pulmonic component of the second sound (unfortunately S-2 often fails to split enough for proper analysis), and sometimes a Graham Steell murmur all testify to serious pulmonary hypertension. Right ventricular failure is common. A curious feature of these extreme cases is that sinus rhythm is almost universal.[79,136] The mitral diastolic murmur is often absent and if present is likely to be atypically confined to middiastole. Some workers have claimed that a sharp first sound and opening

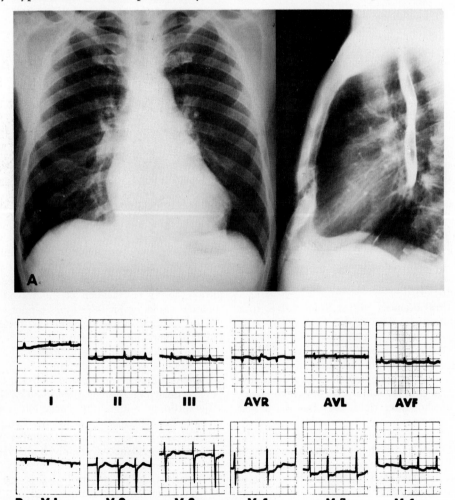

snap may be absent even in cases with mobile mitral leaflets.[136,266] The most important clues to proper diagnosis are (1) Kerley's lines or dilated pulmonary veins and left atrial enlargement by x-ray (such findings may not be striking); (2) the residue of auscultatory evidence. In some cases no clue is present. To further complicate the matter, some cases of primary pulmonary hypertension have combined third and fourth sounds which may be mistaken for a mitral murmur.[267] Because of these facts no case of severe unexplained pulmonary hypertension has been completely studied until mitral stenosis has been excluded by cardiac catheterization. Many of these patients can be totally rehabilitated by mitral valvulotomy.[136,268] In others pulmonary vascular obstruction persists.[136]

Silent Mitral Stenosis. In most cases the problem is not silence but deafness.[42] Perhaps more properly, it is the failure to listen directly over the apex impulse, immediately after exercise, with the patient in the left lateral decubitus position.[184] Emphysema and obesity may greatly attenuate the findings of mitral stenosis.[42] In the obese woman with heavy breasts the apex impulse may be temporarily lost during the act of turning into the lateral position, and the diastolic murmur may have disappeared by the time the proper auscultatory

site has been relocated. Here it is better to prop the recumbent patient on her side with pillows and after clearly locating the apex impulse ask her to exercise by pretending to bicycle. Often an opening snap or an unaccountably sharp first sound is the vital clue in otherwise silent mitral stenosis. Complete and genuine silence may occur when the first sound and opening snap are reduced owing to severe valvular immobility and when mitral flow and hence the rumble are curtailed by atrial fibrillation and right ventricular failure. Severe pulmonary vascular obstruction and sometimes massive atrial thrombosis can also probably produce genuine silence.[136,269,270] Tachycardia may make diastole very hard to analyze in many cases. Therefore no search for mitral stenosis is complete until follow-up examination is done after failure has been cleared as much as possible and the heart rate has been slowed to under 100 beats per minute. The ease and safety with which the d-c countershock apparatus accomplishes the conversion of atrial fibrillation make this a valid diagnostic maneuver;[271] restoration of sinus rhythm will often bring out a previously inapparent rumble and will restore presystolic accentuation. Amyl nitrite inhalation is usually a most effective means of bringing out the diastolic rumble.[198]

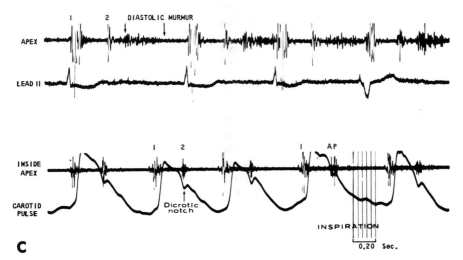

C

Fig. 25-4. Mitral stenosis with a rigid valve. An elderly male with rather severe long-standing diastolic hypertension was discovered to have mitral stenosis after he developed congestive failure and paroxysmal atrial fibrillation. The x-ray (A, opposite page, frontal and lateral views) showed left atrial enlargement and moderate cardiomegaly. Even with careful image-intensifier fluoroscopy there was no trace of mitral valvular calcification. The electrocardiogram (B, opposite page) showed atrial fibrillation and ST-T changes characteristic of digitalis effect. On auscultation, depicted by phonocardiogram (C), there was a sharp first heart sound, a loud diastolic rumble, but definitely no opening snap. At operation the surgeon encountered extreme mitral stenosis and an atrium full of mushy clot. A good split was obtained, but unfortunately the valve was so rigid that its function was not greatly improved. Death occurred from cerebral embolization. At postmortem the valve was studied with the tenometer. In no area did a pressure less than 100 mm Hg produce any deflection of the rigid cartilage-like structure. Therefore, the absence of an opening snap was not surprising. Perhaps the persistence of the sharp first heart sound was related to the systemic hypertension.

Mitral Stenosis with Aortic Valve Disease. A good many patients with tight mitral stenosis have mild aortic regurgitation, which in the past has often been mistaken for a Graham Steell murmur.[272] Provided there is no left ventricular hypertrophy or marked cardiomegaly or unusually wide pulse pressure and the aortic diastolic murmur is brief, one can usually safely assume that the leak is small. In fact, pure tight mitral stenosis is uncommonly associated with severe aortic regurgitation.[132,273] The differentiation of pulmonary and aortic regurgitation, however, is of some importance. The diagnosis of a Graham Steell murmur in mitral stenosis should never be seriously considered unless there is gross dilatation of the pulmonary artery together with the other clinical and radiographic signs of severe pulmonary hypertension. Amyl nitrite is often useful. This drug produces striking peripheral vasodilatation but raises the cardiac output. Hence it softens the murmur of aortic insufficiency but may increase an authentic Graham Steell murmur.[274]

Any plans for mitral valvulotomy should always include the knowledge that a coincident aortic lesion is always partly disguised by mitral stenosis and almost always becomes more manifest after operation.[132,273,275] Patients with moderately severe combined mitral and aortic lesions, though somewhat disabled by symptoms of mitral stenosis, may still survive in reasonable comfort for many years on medical therapy. In these cases mitral stenosis seems to have a genuinely protective effect on the left ventricle. When aortic stenosis has been underestimated, correction of the mitral stenosis has led to progressive left ventricular dilatation and failure within a few months or a year.[275] On the other hand, even moderate pure aortic insufficiency does not prevent good results from valvulotomy. Operation should not be deferred in a patient with symptomatic tight mitral stenosis merely because of the presence of an aortic diastolic murmur.[273] Unfortunately, at times the diagnostic problem may be far from simple. By interfering with normal early diastolic ventricular filling but reducing cardiac output, mitral stenosis tends to bring out the murmur of aortic insufficiency and to conceal that of aortic stenosis. Hence, patients with high-grade aortic stenosis have been mistakenly thought to

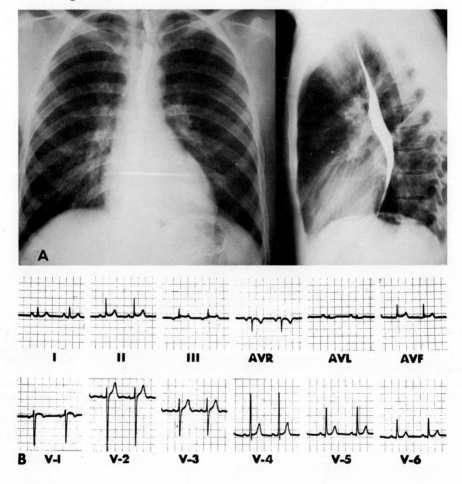

have nothing but minor aortic insufficiency.[150] When the aortic lesion is hard to evaluate, retrograde aortography should always be done in hopes of outlining the function of the aortic valve more clearly. In a borderline case, however, such studies cannot always predict the capabilities of the left ventricle once removal of the mitral block has further increased its diastolic filling. Furthermore, even moderate surgically induced mitral incompetence may be disastrous in the face of left ventricular systolic hypertension.[132] In cases with a significant element of aortic stenosis, it is better to treat medically until the patient's condition justifies the risk of definitive operations on both valves.

The interaction between mitral stenosis and aortic regurgitation may also lead to a mistaken estimate of the mitral lesion by standard auscultatory techniques. A diastolic pressure of 50 to 60 mm Hg is common both in moderate and severe aortic regurgitation; in the former case the lower diastolic pressure brings the second sound and the opening snap closer together and, hence, may give a false impression of tight mitral stenosis (Fig. 25-5). In severe aortic insufficiency, however, the large leak tends to dampen the early diastolic downward motion of the mitral valve and therefore may delay and sometimes obliterate the opening snap.[99,276] An early diastolic sound 0.11 or 0.12 sec from the onset of the aortic component of the second sound in an otherwise typical case of tight mitral stenosis* often means that any concomitant aortic regurgitation is too severe to be ignored during an operation on the mitral valve. The first sound is usually quiet in severe aortic regurgitation, but an early systolic click sometimes heard at the apex can lead to gross overestimation of the Q-1 time.[277]

The syndrome of combined mitral and aortic stenosis is treated in a later section.

Mitral Stenosis with Pulmonary Embolization. This is not an uncommon syndrome producing sudden, unaccountable, and usually reversible decompensation.[278] In mitral stenosis pulmonary embolization is especially likely to produce hemoptysis,

---

* Studied at a heart rate between 75 and 90 beats per minute.

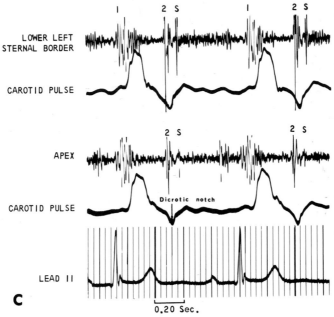

Fig. 25-5. The effect of moderate aortic insufficiency on the auscultatory findings in mitral stenosis. The patient, a youth of 20, had mild cardiac disability compounded by emotional factors. The chest film (A, opposite page, frontal and lateral views) showed slight left ventricular and left atrial enlargement and was compatible with aortic and mitral lesions. The electrocardiogram (B, opposite page) showed increased QRS voltage. On auscultation, depicted in phonocardiogram (C), a prominent murmur of aortic insufficiency was heard along the left sternal border, and the blood pressure was 100/50. An opening snap was noted also 0.09 sec after the onset of the second heart sound. The snap was hard to hear because it was buried in the loud aortic diastolic blow, but was easily recorded on the phonocardiogram. Such a 2-OS interval would ordinarily be compatible with tight mitral stenosis. However, the patient had only moderate aortic insufficiency and only mild mitral stenosis with a normal left atrial pressure when studied with catheterization and cineangiography. The rather short 2-OS interval was probably due to the low aortic diastolic pressure, which made the aortic closure sound fall closer to the mitral opening snap.

which, however, is far from a specific symptom.[99] The character and amount of hemoptysis as well as the setting in which it occurs must be considered. Pleurisy or pulmonary infiltrates are likely to be called pneumonia. Yet, unless there is clear-cut relation to an infection of the respiratory tract and obvious purulent sputum early in the clinical course, the proper diagnosis is often pulmonary embolization. Occasionally suppuration may occur in older pulmonary infarcts. The diagnosis of repeated pulmonary embolization should be suspected in any patient with an intractable course, especially if there are uncontrollable atrial fibrillation and pleural effusion.[279] Chronic consolidation and pleural effusion lasting a month or two may follow a single pulmonary infarction.[171,273] Ordinarily pulmonary embolism produces infarction in only approximately 10 per cent of cases. The percentage is probably higher in mitral stenosis. Some infarcts are probably at least partly due to local thrombosis rather than to embolism.[280] The syndrome is an indication for valvulotomy,[273] but other measures may also be needed.

Mitral Stenosis with Atrial Septal Defect. This rare combination was formerly much overdiagnosed because of the presence of a diastolic rumble in many cases of atrial septal defect.[281] Depending on the dominant lesion, true Lutembacher's syndrome may appear as either mitral or atrial septal defect, usually, however, with some atypical features.[282,283] Striking cardiomegaly and pulmonary hypertension result if both lesions are severe. When mitral stenosis is tight and the atrial defect is tiny, a curious continuous musical murmur at the left lower sternal border may be encountered. This has appeared following transseptal catheterization of patients with critical disease.[284] Larger atrial defects often produce incomplete right bundle branch block, which may occur in combined mitral and tricuspid disease, but should always cause uneasiness about the diagnosis of uncomplicated mitral stenosis.

Mitral Stenosis with a Dominant Myocardial Factor. In the author's opinion, this condition is rare. Frequently the diagnosis conceals diagnostic error—and is offered as an excuse for failure of the patient to improve after mitral valvulotomy. More common causes for such bad results are given on p. 567.

There remains, however, an undoubted residue of "myocardial mitrals." These are usually drawn from the group of patients with considerable cardiomegaly, chronic atrial fibrillation, and long-standing right ventricular failure, many of whom do poorly after mitral valvulotomy.[286] Unfortunately, none of the physiologic studies advocated to detect the myocardial factor has stood the test of time.[287-289] Some of them may give frankly misleading re-

sults.[290] Impairment of left ventricular emptying, as determined angiographically, is a logical and more specific criterion.[258] Its relation to operative results has not yet been established.

The nature of the myocardial factor remains mysterious. Probably it is most usually rheumatic myocarditis. Clinically there is nothing to indicate coronary embolization, which pathologic studies suggest.[145] Many cases are undoubtedly due to important but unrelated heart disease: coronary atherosclerosis or systemic hypertension.

Ball-valve and Massive Atrial Thrombus. One of these complications occurs in perhaps 3 per cent of patients, the incidence increasing with prolonged atrial fibrillation and advancing age.[291] A thrombus lying relatively free in the left atrial cavity may intermittently or partly occlude the stenotic mitral valve, with disastrous effects. Unfortunately the symptoms may not be distinctive and the diagnosis may not be considered until sudden death has occurred.[292] Usually such patients have signs of severe pulmonary congestion, and often left atrial thrombi may be suspected because of recent or past peripheral embolization.[269,270] Sometimes sitting up and leaning forward helps the dyspnea.[292] A fulminating course is suggestive, particularly if there are intervals of sudden unaccountable improvement.[291] Syncope may occur in uncomplicated mitral stenosis; yet in a case with rapidly progressing pulmonary congestion, it should always suggest a ball-valve thrombus. There is often persistent tachycardia, so that changing murmurs are hard to evaluate.[270,291] Occasionally, distinctive episodes of cyanosis, coldness, and numbness of the hands or feet have been described. Many of these clinical features are indistinguishable from those produced by myxoma of the left atrium. Massive left atrial thrombosis with no ball-valve effect is more common but even less distinctive clinically.[291] An acceleration in the downhill course and the presence of atrial fibrillation, especially if there is also peripheral embolization, are enough indication for angiocardiography (from the right side of the heart) in any case of mitral stenosis.[293] It has been claimed that the opening snap may be muffled by massive left atrial thrombosis, but in many of the examples reported the absent snap seems to have been associated also with rigid, immobile mitral valves.[270] From the writer's experience, however, it appears that the snap may persist in spite of massive thrombosis, provided the valve is mobile. Radiographically a line of calcification along the left atrial wall on the ordinary chest x-ray is associated with a high incidence of atrial clots. Massive atrial thrombosis may extend into or occlude a pulmonary vein, producing persistent unilateral pleural effusion.[113,269]

The Differential Diagnosis of Mitral Stenosis[42,295]

Congenital mitral stenosis produces signs and symptoms similar to those of the rheumatic variety except that it usually affects children under age 4.[294] It is associated with a high incidence of both fibroelastosis and ventricular septal defect or ductus arteriosus with reversed shunt. Excellent simulation of mitral stenosis is produced by left atrial myxoma or sarcoma. Though in some myxomas the course is chronic, the most important clue is a rapidly progressive decline in a patient with documented previous absence of heart disease. (Old x-rays should always be obtained if possible.) An unaccountably late opening snap and an unusually small left atrium in a patient with serious symptoms has led to consideration of the proper diagnosis.[296] Repeated peripheral embolization in the absence of atrial fibrillation is another clue. Occasionally marked changes in both auscultatory findings and symptoms may occur from day to day or with changes in body position; if the symptoms and signs vary in parallel fashion, useful diagnostic information is obtained. Malignant tumors which fill the left atrium can produce typical auscultatory mitral stenosis with a close opening snap.[296]

Good simulation of mitral stenosis is produced by the following:

1. Some cases of predominant mitral regurgitation. A pansystolic apical murmur is usually present, though sometimes quite unimpressive[297] compared with the loud diastolic rumble which is a common feature even of "pure" high-grade mitral insufficiency. One reason for the apparent lack of the systolic murmur and an abnormal apex impulse may be that the examiner never listens over the true left ventricular apex, which is displaced much further to the left than he realizes. In patients with a pansystolic murmur and an obvious opening snap the predominance of mitral regurgitation may be recognized from the character of the systolic apex thrust and from the patterns of the diastolic murmur and the diastolic filling wave. In the occasional case without an impressive apical systolic murmur, the definite absence of an opening snap and a brief, loud diastolic rumble should arouse suspicion that something is amiss. Failure of an accentuated first sound to remain sharp after a long pause in atrial fibrillation is unusual in mitral stenosis and may mean important regurgitation[169] or a rigid valve. A common source of error is physical examination conducted during tachycardia or bigeminal rhythm, which may make the proper analysis of diastole impossible. No examination is complete until the patient has been studied under more favorable conditions. The really difficult case is found in a patient has marked obesity or a barrel chest, which both obscure left ventricular hypertrophy and dampen the murmurs. Such cases should be recognized as sources of diagnostic difficulty and studied carefully with left ventricular angiography before surgical therapy is undertaken.

2. Atrial septal defect. Usually the simulation is more auscultatory than radiographic. The widely split second heart sound may be mistaken for the 2-OS complex but may be differentiated by the method previously described. The tricuspid opening snap sometimes found in a large atrial septal defect provides a complex of three sounds at the junction of systole and diastole.[298] At the apex the first heart sound is often sharp, and there is a diastolic rumble. The murmur, however, is often initiated by a loud third heart sound and at slower heart rates rarely has presystolic accentuation. The pulmonary systolic flow murmur in the second left interspace is not necessarily loud but often (particularly in the older patient) has a curious scratchy quality, which is quite distinctive and with the other findings should immediately lead one to suspect atrial septal defect.

3. A variety of other conditions associated with increased mitral or tricuspid flow. These have been called "high-flow rumbles" but in fact often do not begin until after the rate of ventricular filling has somewhat slowed as the result of the (partly papillochordal) check to unusually rapid diastolic expansion of the ventricle.[299,300] This check is commonly associated with an audible tug on the mitral valve signaled by the third heart sound. Under such circumstances it seems most logical to suppose that the succeeding diastolic rumble is largely due to tensing and partial coaptation of the mitral or tricuspid leaflets produced by their attachment to the suddenly elongated ventricle.[301] Thus, the murmur often follows in the train of the most abrupt ventricular diastolic expansion in a still rapidly swelling ventricle; it is usually brief and does not often crescendo with atrial contraction except when tachycardia (115 beats per minute or over) or a prolonged P-R interval produces a summation effect. By contrast the murmur of mitral stenosis begins sooner, usually within 0.02 sec of the opening snap (if present) or the "O point" of the apex cardiogram (if no opening snap is heard); it never starts with a loud, low-pitched thud which imparts a wiggle of rapid diastolic movement to the stethoscope. Instead the stenotic rumble follows an even course, is associated with no obvious diastolic thrust, and except at very slow heart rates almost always crescendos in presystole (provided the heart rhythm is sinus and the P-R interval is not extremely short). "High-flow" murmurs are encountered in all large left-to-right shunts, in severe anemia, and occasionally when there are other causes of an un-

usually high cardiac output. In these cases genuine opening snaps are extremely rare.

4. Some conditions associated with unusual ventricular hypertrophy. Of these, the most important is probably primary pulmonary hypertension, which is best distinguished by the absence of left atrial enlargement radiographically. On auscultation a loud, ringing, early systolic click may be mistaken for the first sound of mitral stenosis but is maximal at the base of the heart.[42] Furthermore there is no trace of an opening snap. Diastolic murmurs may occur and apparent presystolic accentuation is not uncommon. Phonocardiographically such murmurs frequently turn out to be the combination of a broad third and fourth heart sound in a patient with a rapid ventricular rate. The diastolic rumbles heard in some patients with congenital aortic ste-

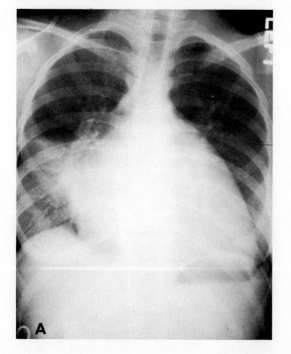

nosis and coarctation of the aorta[29] are probably similar.

5. The Austin Flint murmur of aortic insufficiency, discussed elsewhere (p. 111).

6. Ventricular dilatation (under certain circumstances). The Carey Coombs murmur of acute rheumatic fever is an early and middiastolic rumble, usually quite low pitched, sometimes rather long but often amounting to little more than "reduplication" of the third heart sound. Diastolic murmurs may also appear in diffuse myocardial disease and after myocardial infarction. In all the above cases there is either an associated systolic murmur or clear-cut clinical evidence of left ventricular failure.

7. Tricuspid stenosis. This condition rarely occurs in the absence of mitral disease, and hence the diagnosis may be difficult to make. The murmur is best differentiated by the fact that it is maximal over the lower sternum and is frequently augmented by inspiration. Sometimes it is so high pitched that it is more likely to be confused with aortic insufficiency than with mitral stenosis. Other signs of tricuspid disease should also be present.

Radiographically mitral stenosis may be simulated to some extent by congenital enlargement of the left atrial appendage.[304] This rare condition is sometimes associated with a localized defect of the parietal pericardium and has occasionally led to repeated peripheral embolization. It does not cause the characteristic backward displacement of the middle one-third of the esophagus.

Mitral Insufficiency

Disease Mechanisms

Mechanism and Pattern of the Disease. Mitral incompetence causes the shunting back and forth of blood between the left atrium and the left ventricle, both of which share the liabilities of this futile exchange. Mild regurgitation may occur from trivial rheumatic valvulitis. A sizable leak in rheumatic disease usually means one or more of the follow-

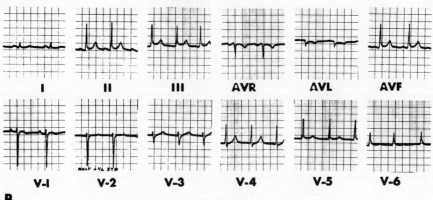

PRECORDIAL LEADS RECORDED AT ½ STANDARDIZATION

ing:[96,97,262,253,305,306] (1) severe destruction of the posterior leaflet; (2) stiffening and loss of substance in the anterior leaflet; (3) fibrous ankylosis of subvalvular structures; (4) loss of support of the valve because of ruptured chordae tendineae or disease of papillary muscle; (5) excessive downward traction owing to shortened chordae; (6) holes in the valve from bacterial endocarditis (nowadays the infection sometimes having been cured without benefit of diagnosis).[307] Often in severe valvulitis the lateral portions of the commissures fuse and there is some stenosis as well.[169,170,305,308] Regurgitation occurs in the "stenotic" cases because of a rigid mitral aperture and the loss of slack and mobility of leaflets so that all or part of the suprastenotic seal is destroyed.[190,305] Because of the complexities of mitral function the systolic regurgitant orifice is not always the same as the diastolic opening through which blood reenters the ventricle.[253] Furthermore, the amount of mitral regurgitation may fluctuate somewhat, being dependent in part on certain properties of ventricular function[309] as well as the systemic resistance.[311]

The hallmark of mitral regurgitation is a systolic murmur usually maximal over the area of the left ventricular apex and transmitted to the axilla.[39,310,311] With intracardiac phonocardiography, it is maximal inside the left atrium.[312] The murmur is usually pansystolic because a left ventricular pressure high enough to cause the first heart sound is usually enough to begin rapid flow into the low-resistance area provided by the left atrium, and to maintain retrograde flow throughout systole, sometimes even for an instant after the aortic valve is closed.[308,313,314] The first portion of the murmur may not be conspicuous, but the latter part almost always blurs into the second heart sound.[311] An audible murmur is probably produced mainly because of some systolic impedance to backward flow. This "retrograde stenosis" may be anything from an almost intact set of normal mitral cusps to a narrow shelf of unrecognizably shriveled valve tissue, either of which can cause vibrations in the wake of the jet being forced back into the left atrium.[315]

The high velocity imparted by left ventricular contraction to the systolic jet makes the murmur "harsh" or "blowing," its essential feature being a considerable content of high-frequency sound.[316] The intensity is usually greater even lateral to the apex than over the sternum, but localization and radiation in certain special situations may be atypical.[317–319] As might be expected, though loud murmurs often mean big leaks, there is no consistent correlation between the severity of the regurgitation and the amount of systolic murmur.[170,297,315,330] Only the pansystolic shape is of crucial importance.

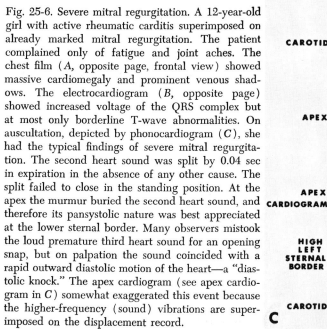
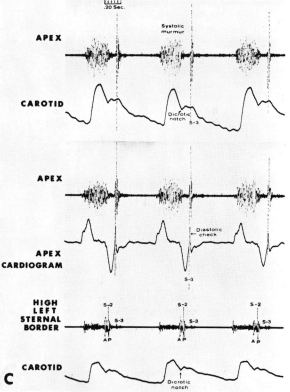

Fig. 25-6. Severe mitral regurgitation. A 12-year-old girl with active rheumatic carditis superimposed on already marked mitral regurgitation. The patient complained only of fatigue and joint aches. The chest film (A, opposite page, frontal view) showed massive cardiomegaly and prominent venous shadows. The electrocardiogram (B, opposite page) showed increased voltage of the QRS complex but at most only borderline T-wave abnormalities. On auscultation, depicted by phonocardiogram (C), she had the typical findings of severe mitral regurgitation. The second heart sound was split by 0.04 sec in expiration in the absence of any other cause. The split failed to close in the standing position. At the apex the murmur buried the second heart sound, and therefore its pansystolic nature was best appreciated at the lower sternal border. Many observers mistook the loud premature third heart sound for an opening snap, but on palpation the sound coincided with a rapid outward diastolic motion of the heart—a "diastolic knock." The apex cardiogram (see apex cardiogram in C) somewhat exaggerated this event because the higher-frequency (sound) vibrations are superimposed on the displacement record.

Failure of the murmur to reach the second heart sound makes severe rheumatic mitral regurgitation unlikely.

Flow through an incompetent mitral valve is bidirectional; and when the leak is large, noise is often made by blood going both ways. The diastolic inflow operates under the lower head of pressure but is augmented by the boomerang of regurgitated blood. The diastolic murmur, therefore, is usually a loud but low-pitched rumble,[313] rarely extending past the first 0.25 sec of diastole, and often initiated by a third heart sound.[169,299,300,313]

A loud, often premature and high-pitched third heart sound is a common and distinctive feature of severe mitral regurgitation.[299,311] The mechanism probably is as follows.[299] The violent, high-pressure gush of blood entering the ventricle rapidly expands the chamber to the point at which the internal reins provided by the chordae and papillary muscles suddenly give an abrupt jerk. This tug rapidly tenses the mitral leaflets, producing the loud diastolic sound and, at the same time, a sharp momentary check to the wantonly rapid diastolic filling wave (as recorded externally) (see Fig. 25-6). In extreme cases a palpable shock is produced by this violent encounter between the expanding ventricular wall and its internal rigging—the event being called an "early diastolic knock."[331]

The rumble is probably a complex event requiring high flow and caused by whatever diastolic valve shelf rheumatic deformity provides, usually only after the valve remnant has been tensed (after the first surge of diastolic inflow) by papillochordal attachments to the elongating ventricular apex;*[300] Though diastolic rumbles are most likely in cases with some commissural fusion, they are heard in a sizable percentage of the group with no significant stenosis, and are increased by physiologic maneuvers which accentuate the mitral leak.[311]

On clinical grounds it is often possible not only to grade the severity of a mitral leak and the amount of commissural fusion, but also to gain useful information about valvular anatomy. Correlations of the latter sort at present are not precise enough to serve as anything but screening techniques; yet such information is helpful in figuring out the complex case and anticipating how difficult surgical correction may be.

The sex incidence of pure or predominant mitral regurgitation is preponderantly female,[311,314,321] though perhaps not so strikingly as in mitral stenosis.[99,310] On the other hand the incidence of severe compound mitral lesions, which generally re-

---

* From a consideration of the anatomic features it can be seen that sudden ventricular diastolic dilatation pulls the mitral valve into a rigid, partly closed position.[301]

flect the severest grade of rheumatic deformity, is probably higher in males.[264] Mitral insufficiency greatly increases susceptibility to bacterial endocarditis,[20,29,310] though the extraordinary incidence in some series[311] is probably due to factors in the selection of patients. Patients with severe rheumatic mitral insufficiency—in contrast to pure stenosis—usually have had clinically obvious rheumatic fever.[176,314]

Mild Mitral Regurgitation

The great majority of cases of rheumatic mitral regurgitation are mild, the result of slight valvular damage, usually with some rolling under or shortening of a cusp or chorda.[20,322] The pathologic changes probably persist for life, even though the murmur may disappear in a child or a young adult. The murmur is usually pansystolic and, in contrast to that of mitral stenosis, often dates back to the time of rheumatic fever (if this has been diagnosed). Such mitral regurgitation causes no physiologic difficulty and no symptoms.[323] Medically the patient's career is likely to be long and uneventful, except for the furor created by routine health examinations and the disappointment caused by his exclusion from jobs of which he is physically perfectly capable. The only danger is bacterial endocarditis, the incidence of which, however, is impossible to obtain from present data.

In mild mitral regurgitation, except for the systolic murmur, the heart sounds are perfectly normal.[317,322,323] An ordinary third heart sound is as common in the youthful patient as in the general population but is rare over the age of 25. There is never a diastolic rumble; a rumble in a patient with a small heart usually means significant mitral stenosis in spite of the systolic murmur. Splitting of the second heart sound is normal. Some patients have evidence of slight left atrial or, rarely, overall cardiac enlargement by x-ray.[323] There is never definite evidence of left ventricular hypertrophy by electrocardiogram.

When a suspected murmur is soft or atypical, "pharmacologic auscultation" may help in its analysis.[256] The murmur of mild as well as of severe mitral regurgitation is affected by changes in the systemic resistance. Phenylephrine (Neo-synephrine) causes a rise in the systemic resistance, which increases the retrograde pressure against an incompetent mitral valve, augmenting the leak and hence the murmur and sometimes converting it from an atypical form to a typical pansystolic configuration. Amyl nitrite lowers the peripheral resistance and has an opposite effect.* In contrast, amyl

---

* Unfortunately, the effect is not invariable. Therefore, if one is using the amyl nitrite test, it is important to have an assistant follow the blood pressure and

nitrite, by lowering the systemic resistance, may sometimes augment the murmur of aortic stenosis. Patients with mild rheumatic mitral deformity who acquire systemic hypertension may develop an apical pansystolic murmur that disappears when the blood pressure is brought down.

Mild mitral regurgitation with a purely late systolic murmur seems usually to be due to disease of the supporting structures of the valve.[317,325,326] Such a murmur is sometimes initiated by a click which may be due to sudden traction on a single short chorda.[325] Angiography often shows an abrupt protrusion of the mural cusp of the mitral valve into the left atrium during systole.[317] Some, but probably not all, of these cases are rheumatic. In two of our own cases studied with phonocardiography, a murmur occupying only the latter two-thirds of systole became pansystolic in the standing position. Amyl nitrite usually accentuates the first part of the murmur.[311] Some late systolic murmurs are alleged to be contact sounds, attributable to previous pericarditis and associated with lingering S-T and T-wave abnormalities on the electrocardiogram.[318] The author does not share this view. Mitral regurgitation occurs in many advanced cases of subvalvular muscular aortic stenosis which distorts the mitral ring during left ventricular systole. The mitral murmur is often atypical and in some cases may be purely late systolic.[317] A congenital aneurysm of the mitral valve is another cause for such a murmur. Patients with a late systolic murmur due to mild mitral regurgitation probably have an increased risk of developing bacterial endocarditis.[310]

Severe Mitral Regurgitation (Fig. 25-6)

When there is little block to the interchange of blood between the left atrium and ventricle, the stroke volume of the ventricle greatly increases and the atrium and ventricle must dilate by at least the amount of the leak. Yet the pressure-volume relationships of the left side of the heart are far more complex than has been suggested by the preceding statement.[327] In acute mitral insufficiency and sinus rhythm, the atrium may be comparatively small while its pressure is very high. An unyielding atrial wall may even tend to limit the amount of regurgitation.[176] A high peripheral resistance will exaggerate the leak. Atrial fibrillation develops sooner or later in most of the advanced cases and is often followed by a rapid increase in atrial size. In chronic mitral insufficiency gradual dilatation of both atrium and ventricle has been thought to create a vicious cycle by putting more traction on

pulse. Considerable tachycardia and hypotension should develop within 30 to 60 sec of the inhalation if the test is valid.[324]

shortened chordae and mitral cusps, thereby exaggerating the degree of regurgitation.[305] This phenomenon may perhaps explain progressively increasing mitral regurgitation after damage to the valve during closed operation for mitral stenosis. In some chronic cases, massive mitral regurgitation which drains off half the ventricular stroke volume and raises the atrial pressure briefly in each systole to 30 to 40 mm Hg may produce no pulmonary congestion and few, if any, symptoms. It is not known whether the lungs are perhaps partly protected by a compliant left atrium,[328] with perhaps a throttle-valve mechanism at the sites of entry of the pulmonary veins,[329] or whether the intermittency of the pressure surge renders it relatively innocuous.[330] The ventricle may pump with a virtually normal end-diastolic pressure in spite of impaired systolic emptying and great dilatation.[327] In some severely disabled patients with long-standing complaints, a large, compliant, fibrillating atrium so well cushions the systolic surge that free regurgitation may occur without any increase in left atrial or pulmonary artery pressure.[203] Thus, the central circulation in advanced mitral insufficiency may operate either as a low- or high-pressure system. Finally, progressive pulmonary vascular obstruction may complicate and even dominate the disease picture.[176,203] The variability in the physiologic patterns of severe mitral insufficiency may explain some of the variability in the clinical findings; this area needs more exploration.

Symptoms of severe mitral regurgitation at first are easy fatigability, dyspnea on exertion, and sometimes palpitation.[29,170,176,314] In many patients, weakness is the only complaint. Disability is often surprisingly mild in proportion to the striking findings on physical examination and x-ray. Yet pulmonary congestive symptoms, once they appear, are likely to be steadily progressive, so that the patient rapidly becomes dependent on careful medical treatment. Perhaps the crucial factor in this rapid deterioration is failure of the left ventricle, which is no longer able to operate at a low diastolic pressure.[314] With the onset of progressive symptoms, the patient usually acquires severe exertional and sometimes paroxysmal nocturnal dyspnea. He experiences atrial fibrillation, chest pain, and right ventricular failure just as frequently as a person with mitral stenosis.[29,170,176] Hemoptysis, systemic emboli, and acute pulmonary edema are somewhat less common. Yet for the purpose of diagnosis, there is no really reliable distinction between the symptoms of mitral stenosis and those of pure mitral regurgitation.[170,176]

Clinical examination should usually allow one to make a clear-cut diagnosis and to grade the severity of the regurgitation with reasonable accuracy.

1. As a screening test, the most reliable and nearly invariable clue to severe mitral regurgitation is a pansystolic *murmur* of any grade from II to VI. Such a murmur must be distinguished from that of tricuspid insufficiency, the most important point being that it is never maximal at the lower sternal border or augmented by inspiration.[255]

2. The second clue is an easily felt *left ventricular impulse* which is prolonged (lasts over two-thirds of systole), abnormally wide (over the size of a 50-cent piece), and often displaced downward and to the left.[99,172] The fraction of systole occupied by the left ventricular impulse is best calculated by listening at the lower sternal border, to outline the boundaries of systole, while simultaneously palpating the apex impulse. An associated sternal lift is not uncommon.[176] In an exceptional case there is no left ventricular systolic thrust and one encounters only right ventricular heave, coupled with right ventricular hypertrophy on the electrocardiogram.[176]

3. The third set of clues comes from the *analysis of diastole*, if possible by simultaneous auscultation and palpation. This correlation can be done fairly well by paying attention to the wiggles of the stethoscope over the apex impulse as one listens with the patient in the left lateral decubitus position. Inspection will show that part of the heaving left ventricular impulse is due to a rapid diastolic filling wave and that the diastolic sounds occur during the time when the heart is rapidly swelling with blood. In doubtful cases the crucial correlation of the diastolic sounds and movements can be recorded with special apparatus.[166,167]

As previously noted, it can be seen that the third heart sound of mitral regurgitation is often a built-in fixture of the disease and may not imply the same degree of ventricular malfunction as the ventricular gallop in other conditions. Except in a young person, however (where it may be normal), a third sound maximal over the left ventricular apex always implies a large leak, and if loud and sharp usually means left ventricular decompensation.[317] A third sound may occasionally be missing in high-grade mitral regurgitation,[310,311] perhaps as a result both of peculiarities of the valve and of left ventricular function. Production of sound is probably only a byproduct. The crucial event is likely to be exceptionally gross and rapid early diastolic filling.[300] This filling pattern is incompatible with isolated tight mitral stenosis, which impedes ventricular diastolic inflow and produces a slow ascent of the diastolic wave.[167]*

* None of the current methods for recording apex impulses is universally accepted. The "apex cardiogram," which is the only one easily and commercially available, may be considerably affected by improper placement of the microphone and by idiosyncrasies of

The third heart sound often ushers in a loud diastolic rumble which begins explosively and then fizzles out within 0.25 sec.[311,318,334] Its presence does not prove any physiologic stenosis; indeed unusually loud rumbles may occur when there is very little commissural fusion. The hallmarks of such murmurs are (1) their very loud beginning and relatively rapid dissolution; their lack of presystolic accentuation at heart rates between 70 and 90 beats per minute; (2) their occurrence in a rapidly swelling ventricle. Among the minority of patients with sinus rhythm, a loud fourth heart sound occasionally is heard; it often originates on the left side of the heart and angiographically correlates best with a small, rigorously contracting atrium.[317] Clinically the writer has not confused such a fourth sound with a presystolic murmur because most such sounds are first recognized phonocardiographically.

Common Mistakes. Since the third heart sound in mitral regurgitation may be quite sharp and occur as early as 0.11 or 0.12 sec after the onset of the second heart sound, it can be mistaken for the latter at the apex; in this case the systolic murmur will be erroneously diagnosed as being of the ejection type. The second sound is often inaudible, being buried by the murmur at the apex. The proper relation of the second sound to the end of the murmur is best established at the left lower sternal border, the impression being double-checked by "inching" toward the apex. A more forgivable error is to mistake a sharp premature third sound for an opening snap. The snap occurs, however, at the moment when the imprint of the left ventricle against the chest wall is smallest—at the nadir of the apex impulse and at the very beginning of the

the crystal pickup.[332,333] It records only the difference between the amount of movement in the center and the rim of the recording microphone cup. Under the best of circumstances the size of the waves is affected somewhat by their velocity as well as by the actual displacement. With the usual equipment it is also not possible to adjust the microphone area for differences in the size of the apex impulse. Present apparatus could certainly be easily improved. Devices such as the kinetocardiogram which record absolute movement may be inherently superior.[168] However, no record of the external movements of the chest can be expected to have an altogether linear relationship to the diastolic movements of the heart itself. Even cardiac pulses directly recorded are a function not only of ventricular filling but also of movements of the apex. Detailed mathematic analysis of this type of crude record is probably not justified. Yet, if their limitations are kept in mind, the apex cardiogram and kinetocardiogram remain of great clinical usefulness as the only simple indirect ways of assessing diastolic events on the left side of the heart.[166]

diastolic expansion of the ventricle.[166] The third heart sound, on the other hand, occurs during unusually rapid diastolic expansion and as a momentary check to it (Fig. 25-6). The impact of the "knock" is quite unlike the quiet click imparted to the chest by the loudest opening snap. Furthermore, the left ventricular third sound is loudest over the left ventricular apex, while the opening snap is often maximal closer to the sternum.

4. Otherwise unaccountably *wide expiratory splitting of the second heart sound* is a frequent badge of really severe mitral regurgitation.[310,311,317] This sign is apparently due to shortening of left ventricular systole.[310,311] Left ventricular systole, however, is not always shortened and may actually be prolonged.[335] Distinctions between the two types of ventricular response should be clinically important but have not yet been made. During inspiration the second sound in some cases may open as widely as 0.06 to 0.08 sec. Therefore, when respiratory mobility is ignored, such a widely split second sound can easily be mistaken for the sequence of a fused second sound and an opening snap.[311] Right ventricular failure may destroy the respiratory mobility of the split second sound, freezing the two components into widely separated positions.[336] This creates more genuine diagnostic difficulty. Even so, full use of the techniques already given usually makes possible a reliable distinction between snap and widely split second sound.

5. The first sound in severe mitral regurgitation has been variously described.[42,99,310,331] It is usually perfectly normal or even accentuated[311,317] unless the anterior mitral cusp is rigid or destroyed.[331] Apparent softness of the first sound is sometimes an auscultatory illusion due to its merging with the loud systolic murmur. In severe mitral regurgitation there may be diastasis—rapid disappearance of the mitral pressure gradient and a secondary rise in atrial pressure due to near-maximal ventricular filling—and hence, virtual cessation of mitral flow before the completion of diastole.[338] Lack of an end-diastolic pressure gradient should prevent the abnormal delay of the first sound which is often associated with mitral stenosis and is probably partly caused from persistence of a mitral gradient throughout diastole.[311] Unfortunately, however, delay of the mitral component of the first sound (authentically identified) may occur in compound mitral lesions with severe regurgitation.[169] Accurate clinical recognition of diastasis would be useful.

The Electrocardiogram. The electrocardiogram of severe mitral regurgitation is usually not of pivotal diagnostic importance unless it happens to show unequivocal evidence of left ventricular hypertrophy in a patient who is not receiving digitalis. Cases meeting both these requirements are the exception rather than the rule. There are many conflicting opinions on this subject, owing largely to the unsatisfactory nature of the electrocardiographic diagnosis of left ventricular hypertrophy,[231] which makes it always subject to a partly unconscious reinterpretation after other more useful findings are gathered. Definite left ventricular hypertrophy with both voltage and S-T criteria occurs in less than one-half the patients and is commonly associated with a rightward or normal axis in the frontal plane.[232,339] Anterior displacement of the left ventricle by a grossly enlarged left atrium has been thought to contribute to the increased voltage of the QRS complex.[339] Cases of severe mitral regurgitation confirmed at operation may show anything from clear-cut right ventricular hypertrophy to definite left ventricular "strain."[232,314] In a good many, however, the electrocardiogram is nondescript. With sinus rhythm, the "left atrial" P wave is likely to be present. Atrial fibrillation occurs in the majority of long-standing cases.

X-ray. The x-ray often adds no crucial information from that already gleaned from clinical examination.[340] The left atrium is usually definitely bigger than normal, and the degree of enlargement is usually greater than in mitral stenosis,[99,320,321,340] though sometimes in severe acute mitral regurgitation the degree of enlargement may be unimpressive,[203,341] and the differentiation of left atrial enlargement may be difficult when there is considerable cardiomegaly. The left ventricle is necessarily dilated by severe mitral regurgitation, but enlargement is not always obvious on the x-ray. Often nothing about the heart size or contour serves reliably to distinguish mitral regurgitation from mitral stenosis.[340] A prudent radiologist will palpate the apical impulse and glance at the electrocardiogram before making his pronouncement. Aneurysmal enlargement of the left atrium is more likely in mitral regurgitation[342] but may occur in pure stenosis.[328] Rarely the chamber may extend to the right wall of the chest and occasionally the condition may be mistakenly diagnosed and treated as pericardial or pleural effusion. In such cases attempted pericardiocentesis has given spectacular if unexpected results.*

* There are no distinctive symptoms of an aneurysmal left atrium except sometimes for a curious right posterior chest pain, worsened by fatigue and often affected by changes in body position. A rocking-chair motion of the right and left sides of the chest may occur. Gross enlargement does not aggravate the course of severe mitral disease.[328,342] Indeed many such patients do surprisingly well, and the incidence of severe pulmonary vascular obstruction may be lower than average.[328]

In spite of considerable cardiomegaly, the pulmonary vascularity of severe mitral regurgitation may be surprisingly normal. There is yet no systemic study correlating venous patterns with hemodynamics; this might provide more understanding of the special effect of mitral regurgitation on the lungs. Septal lines probably do not develop until there is left ventricular failure. As in mitral stenosis, these lines testify to chronic basal interstitial edema and severe disease, but they are more likely to clear up completely with treatment. The classic x-ray findings of pulmonary vascular obstruction may be encountered in an occasional patient. Easily visible calcification of the mitral leaflets is rather unusual in the patient with high-grade mitral regurgitation associated with little commissural fusion. Left ventricular angiography is the definitive means of quantitating mitral regurgitation.

Estimation of the Severity of Mitral Regurgitation

Signs of a severe lesion are (1) left ventricular hypertrophy by palpation; an overactive apex impulse displaced downward and to the left; (2) a loud and frequently premature third heart sound, often initiating a brief diastolic rumble; (3) definite cardiomegaly and left atrial enlargement by x-ray in all but the most acute cases; (4) often, but not always, wide splitting of the second heart sound; (5) authentic symptoms (though there may be no apparent disability in some cases).

Signs of a mild lesion are (1) absence of left ventricular overactivity and of electrocardiogram abnormalities; (2) no diastolic sounds except those normal for the patient's age; (3) normal size of the heart and left atrium by x-ray; (4) normal splitting of the second sound for the patient's age; (5) no genuine symptoms.

Atypical Mitral Regurgitation

The Syndrome of the Mobile Anterior Cusp. Normally the larger anterior (aortic) leaflet closes all of the mitral orifice except for a posterolateral crescent, which is covered by the smaller mural cusp.[93,96] Serious regurgitation may occur from deficiencies mainly in the smaller cusp, whether they are due to actual shrinkage or to its being tacked down to the side of the ventricle by shortened chordae.[96,305,337,343] In such cases there may be some degree of commissural fusion, producing a diastolic opening of 1.2 to 3.0 cm^2. A distinguishing feature of the syndrome is that the aortic cusp retains some degree of mobility and pliancy. Therefore, it omits opening and closing snaps during its downward and upward movements.[337] Clinically such patients all have serious mitral disease, often with high left atrial pressures, and almost all are women. This is the only condition which allows

high-grade mitral regurgitation in the presence of a loud opening snap, and it may account for as many as 10 per cent of patients with serious mitral disease.[337] Surgically the presence of an opening snap means that mitral insufficiency may often be benefited by annuloplasty or other procedures short of total valvular replacement, which, however, is being increasingly used even in this group with "favorable" valves.

This syndrome may be simulated by those cases of serious mitral insufficiency with a widely split second sound. The matter is further complicated when a loud, premature third sound is present. The most meticulous auscultation and phonocardiography are essential to dissect away the four closely related sounds and to reach the proper diagnosis* (Fig. 25-7). Recognizing the "mobile anterior cusp syndrome" does not tell one whether stenosis or regurgitation is dominant. This question must be settled by other methods (see "Compound Mitral Lesions," p. 563). Failure of the 2-OS interval to vary with rate has been proposed as a sign of dominant regurgitation.[344] This effect is probably due to the fact that in mitral regurgitation the left ventricular thrust (rather than mitral block) is the main factor elevating the early diastolic pressure in the left atrium. We, like others, have not found this sign dependable.[169,321] Perhaps this inconsistency is due to the fact that patients with similar valvular anatomy may have greatly different contours of the atrial pulse.[345] Variation of the 2-OS interval with heart rate is not the same in every patient with tight mitral stenosis; and normal variation of the interval may be encountered in patients with rather severe compound mitral lesions.

Mitral Regurgitation Due to an Improperly Supported Valve Segment. A common hallmark of this condition is mitral regurgitation with an atypical systolic murmur. There are at least two causes: (1) ruptured or locally shortened chordae tendineae;[305,346] (2) disease affecting the papillary muscle.[347]

Ruptured chordae tendineae may convert a mild

---

* In general, the principles are as follows: (1) the split of the second sound, though wide, is still affected by respiration; (2) the timing of the opening snap is affected by heart rate and body position; (3) the timing of the left ventricular third sound is affected neither by respiration nor by the heart rate, and the sound is always maximal over the left ventricular apex, coinciding with a check on the upstroke of the diastolic filling wave; (4) occasionally the widely split second sound and the snap of severe mitral regurgitation may overlap. Auscultation in the standing position is most helpful in dissecting the sounds apart by widening the snap interval and increasing expiratory closure of the split second sound.

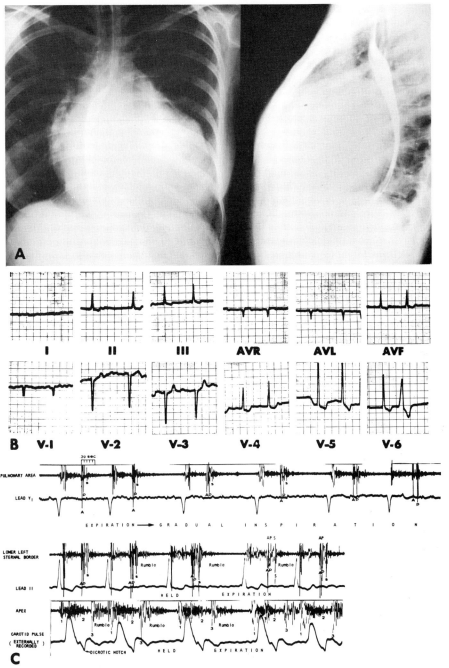

Fig. 25-7. Mitral insufficiency with a mobile anterior cusp. A 32-year-old woman completely disabled with severe mitral regurgitation had responded extremely well to a mitral annuloplasty until the sutures pulled out 18 months after operation. When she was admitted to the hospital for the insertion of a Starr-Edwards prosthesis, the x-ray (A, frontal and lateral views) showed gross cardiomegaly and left atrial enlargement. The electrocardiogram (B) showed atrial fibrillation, digitalis effect, and left ventricular hypertrophy with an axis of +90°. On auscultation, depicted in phonocardiogram (C), the second heart sound was thought by some observers to be persistently split. Actually the latter half of the supposed split was an opening snap with a 2-OS interval of 0.08 sec. The second heart sound, though closed on inspiration, split abnormally with inspiration, the pulmonic component merging into the opening snap. As was anticipated because of the loud opening snap, the surgeon found that the mitral regurgitation was due to destruction of the posterior cusp. The anterior leaflet was well preserved and mobile, though its chordae were shortened. These findings explained the patient's original favorable response to mitral annuloplasty.

rheumatic lesion into a severe one, but they are not always related to rheumatic valvulitis.[346] The cause is most commonly bacterial endocarditis but may be a curious idiopathic attenuation which stretches the chrodae like taffy candy until they break. The heart disease may begin suddenly and lead to a rapid downhill course. On the other hand, insidious progression of symptoms and of murmur may be due to successive chordal ruptures (Fig. 25-8). The degree of mitral regurgitation is often massive. Characteristic of such regurgitation is that the size of the regurgitant orifice varies. For instance, the leaflet may be competent in early systole and then suddenly prolapse into the atrium.[317] The configuration of the murmur may closely mirror the dynamics of left ventricular contraction[348] and the capacity of the atrial reservoir, sometimes reaching a midsystolic peak and decreasing again in late systole. The murmur is not really typically diamond-shaped, however, but genuinely pansystolic,[349] the high-frequency noise continuing into and enveloping the sound of aortic closure. Therefore, even though such a murmur may be quite loud in the high sternal area, it should not be mistaken for the ejection murmur of aortic stenosis, which loses its high frequencies about 0.04 sec before the second heart sound.[39] A loud and sharp apical third heart sound, however, is common and may compound the confusion if carelessly mistaken for the second heart sound when the latter is buried in the murmur. Simultaneous phonocardiograms at the base and apex of the heart timed with the carotid pulse will often be needed to characterize the situation properly.

The murmur of a poorly supported cusp often has atypical radiation, possibly because the regurgitant jet is sharply focused in an unusual direction.[319]

It has been thought that the flail portion of the leaflet forms a hood, directing blood in the opposite direction. Thus eventration of the posterior cusp hoses the jet forward against the left atrium adjacent to the roots of the great vessels. Prolapse of the anterior leaflet hoses the jet backwards. Pathologically the sites of endocardial plaques produced by such jets correlate to some extent with unusual radiation of the murmur.[346]

However, atypical radiation is not confined to cases with chordal disease; it may even occur when angiography shows no jet effect (perhaps because of the massiveness of the leak.[211,317] The author has observed predominant radiation of the murmurs to the back in a case of the "intact anterior leaflet syndrome" where the posterior cusp was nailed to the ventricular wall by chordopapillary shortening. Atypical radiation has also been associated with a giant left atrium.[318]

Except in the setting of bacterial endocarditis, the diagnosis of ruptured chordae tendineae is often extremely difficult. A reliable history of sudden onset or dramatic change in the murmur, symptoms, and heart size is the cardinal point in the diagnosis. Physical examination may be inconclusive. With careful auscultation the most common mistake is to conclude that the patient has both aortic stenosis and mitral regurgitation.[317,319] A fine point of considerable importance on the phonocardiogram is that the late systolic vibrations which envelop the second heart sound may be louder at the upper left sternal border than at the apex. This finding is unusual in ordinary mitral regurgitation. Indeed an apparently pansystolic murmur maximal at the base of the heart is an oddity compatible also with some cases of patent ductus arteriosus or coarctation of the pulmonary artery.[350] Another

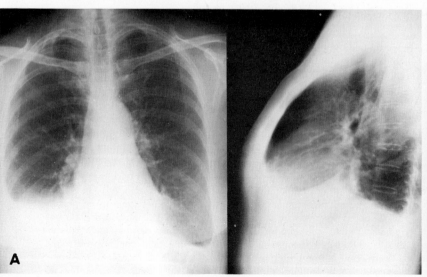
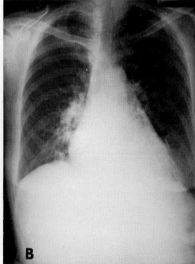

A   B

source of difficulty is muscular subaortic stenosis, which often produces superimposed ejection and late systolic murmurs.[317] Mitral regurgitation with a purely late systolic murmur also appears to be a special example of the syndrome, in which support of the mitral cusps suddenly becomes abnormal during the course of systole, probably usually because of diseased chordae.

Ordinary chest x-rays and electrocardiograms have no special contribution to make to the diagnosis. Systolic expansion of the left atrium is an old and somewhat discredited radiologic sign of mitral regurgitation. However, patients who have massive acute mitral insufficiency without any impedance to the ventricular reentry of the regurgitated blood often have striking systolic expansion and diastolic collapse of an only mildly enlarged atrium[343]—a useful sign if the murmur is atypical and the very presence of mitral regurgitation is being questioned. By angiography one may often see the site of the prolapsed cusps and often observe a curious midsystolic hesitation in aortic flow corresponding to the maximal regurgitation into the left atrium.[351]

Malfunction of the papillary muscle apparatus in

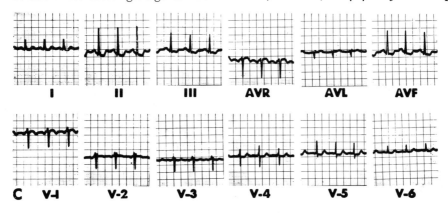

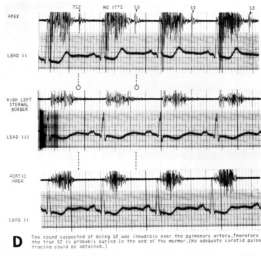

Fig. 25-8. Mitral insufficiency due to ruptured chordae tendineae. A 50-year-old woman had an abrupt onset of unexplained congestive heart failure shown in the frontal and lateral views of the chest (*A,* opposite page). Six months later (*B,* opposite page, frontal view) the heart was much larger and the symptoms had become intractable in spite of careful medical therapy. The electrocardiogram (*C*) showed digitalis effect. At the onset of the illness the soft pansystolic murmur was noted which became much louder as the illness progressed (phonocardiogram, *D*). Some observers thought that the murmur was of the ejection type, but careful auscultation showed that it completely buried the second heart sound. Confusion occurred because (1) a loud, premature third sound, heard only at the apex, was mistaken for the second heart sound, and (2) the murmur frequently had a diamond shape. With correlated angiography the midsystolic peak of the murmur corresponded with a midsystolic hesitation in the advancement of contrast material in the aorta, suggesting that regurgitation was greatest in midsystole. At operation, four chordae were ruptured and several others severely attenuated.

coronary artery disease may also cause mitral regurgitation.[347] For example, if the papillary muscle inserts into an area of ventricular aneurysm, it tugs the edge of the mitral valve down into the ventricle, causing leakage. If, on the other hand, a papillary muscle fails to contract properly, there will be partial prolapse of one or more of the leaflets into the atrium. These murmurs sometimes have bizarre timing and may not be obviously pansystolic. Although the amount of mitral regurgitation has not yet been measured in such cases, it probably can be large and may sometimes persist for months or years.

Actual rupture of a papillary muscle may occur in acute myocardial infarction and may produce mitral regurgitation because of inadequate support of the cusps.[352] The rupture usually occurs about a week after the onset of the pain, and the posterior papillary muscle is the one most likely involved. Patients usually survive only a few hours or days, succumbing in acute intractable pulmonary edema. Survival for as long as a year has been reported in one or two cases. The murmur is usually not extremely loud and is very rarely associated with a thrill. The diagnosis is made by the sudden onset of the murmur coincident with severe pulmonary edema and shock usually on the fourth to tenth day following a myocardial infarction. The condition is much rarer than papillary muscle dysfunction, which may also have a delayed onset.

Calcification of the Mitral Annulus. This lesion, probably often a nonrheumatic process, is common in the elderly and usually is silent or causes only an asymptomatic apical systolic murmur. It can occasionally produce heart block by extending into the neighboring septum. A small group of elderly women with massive annular calcification suffer serious physiologic handicaps.[353] A broad shelf projects from under the mitral cusps, elevating the base of the leaflets. During ventricular contraction this shelf curtails the effective width of the valve curtain; in diastole it adds an element of stenosis as well. The rigid annular skeleton also prevents contraction of the mitral ring, which very likely is a factor in normal valve closure. In the functionally severe cases there are also shrinkage and stiffening of the cusps and shortening of chordae.[354]

The symptoms, even in severe disease, are quite variable. Some patients are not disabled, others ultimately develop symptoms of progressive pulmonary congestion and finally right ventricular failure, the course of symptoms extending from 4 to 8 years.[353] The heart sounds are often unremarkable. The systolic murmur may be grade II to IV. In the severe cases it is *pansystolic* (or it can be rendered so with Neo-synephrine) and not uncommonly associated with a brief diastolic rumble. The character of

the systolic murmur is frequently not only harsh but somewhat musical. Its cooing quality may cause it to be mistaken for aortic stenosis. In fact, sclerosis of the aortic leaflets is probably common in these cases and though physiologically harmless may contribute a great deal to the general noise level [355] (Fig. 25-9).

The x-ray is the cornerstone of the diagnosis. The knob of the aorta is often ectatic and calcified. The frequently associated aortic valve sclerosis does not produce detectable calcification by x-ray. The hallmark of the condition is a thick line of calcification lying just to the left of the midline in the frontal projection and in the posterior third of the heart on the lateral projection. This density has a J, U, or oval shape (Fig. 25-9). Unfortunately, even in severe cases, calcification is often not obvious on an ordinary chest x-ray. An overpenetrated film made with a short exposure time and the use of a grid technique is better. Fluoroscopy with the image intensifier is perhaps the definitive method.

In summary, the typical patient is an elderly female who has no distinctive physical findings except for an apical murmur, which may be pansystolic. The condition, though often asymptomatic, may produce unexplained congestive heart failure, which is mistakenly diagnosed as being due to rheumatic or coronary artery disease. The main clue to the diagnosis is obtained only after careful radiographic examination.

Silent Mitral Insufficiency. This is a rare but well-established syndrome which has never been completely explained.[297,320] It seems most likely to occur (1) when mitral insufficiency is due to ventricular dilatation, coronary disease, or cardiomyopathy; (2) when rheumatic mitral insufficiency is massive. The characteristic of some of these latter cases seems to be complete absence of commissural fusion, uniform shrinkage of the mitral leaflets, and a remarkable shortening of the chordae—so that with each systole the cusps are probably flattened against the ventricular wall[320,343] and perhaps only annular contraction serves to reduce the size of the mitral orifice. Ordinarily the regurgitating blood develops vibrations because of the interposition of some residual shelf or valve tissue. Otherwise it might be expected to be as silent as normal systolic flow through the aortic valve. Silent mitral regurgitation has also been associated with severe right ventricular failure and with pulmonary emphysema.[42] As a rule, however, the murmur of mitral regurgitation is little reduced by curtailment of forward cardiac output.[169]

In general, mitral regurgitation is much less often silent than it is ignored. The patient may never have been examined over the true cardiac apex when this is greatly displaced to the left. The mur-

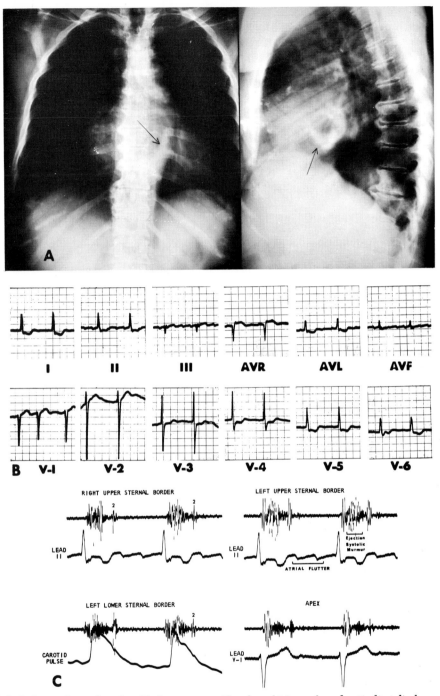

Fig. 25-9. Calcified mitral annulus. An elderly woman with a long history of moderate diastolic hypertension and rather marked typical angina pectoris had two previously documented myocardial infarctions. At the time of examination she had mild congestive heart failure. On x-ray (A, frontal and lateral views) there was striking C-shaped calcification on the mitral annulus. The electrocardiogram (B) showed left ventricular hypertrophy, with atrial flutter, and digitalis effect. The murmur, depicted on phonocardiogram (C), was of the ejection type and very probably due to sclerosis of the aortic valve leaflets. Thus the outstanding x-ray findings and the auscultatory signs were not directly related to each other or to the patient's symptoms. In some cases mitral annular calcification produces no auscultatory findings. Often it is associated with an asymptomatic and atypical murmur. Occasionally it seems to cause severe mitral regurgitation.

mur may have been soft; but its location, its high pitch, and pansystolic duration should have reminded one that some mitral regurgitation was present and that, as usual, factors other than the intensity of the systolic murmur were needed to estimate the size of the leak. Sometimes, however, a systolic thrill over the left atrium may be felt at operation or the murmur recorded with an intracardiac phonocardiogram (taken in the left atrium[312]) when absolutely nothing has been heard or recorded clinically. The first hint may be provided by the x-ray, which shows unaccountable

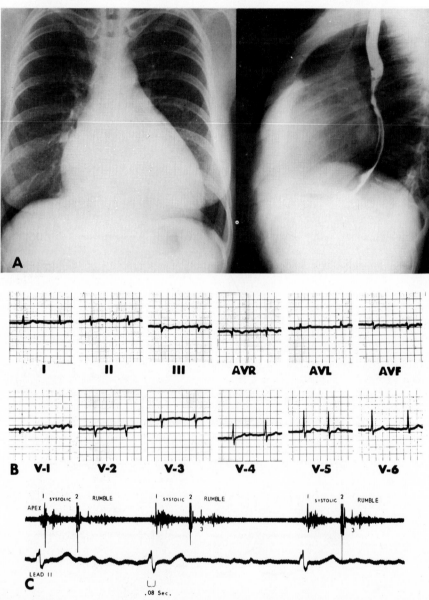

Fig. 25-10. Mitral insufficiency with a predominantly diastolic murmur. A 35-year-old woman had had a murmur since rheumatic fever at age 10. In spite of chronic atrial fibrillation and great cardiomegaly she was able to do light housework, and on digitalis and oral diuretics she had no serious complaints. The x-ray (A, frontal and lateral views), showed great enlargement of the heart but no evidence of interstitial pulmonary edema. The electrocardiogram (B) showed atrial fibrillation. In spite of free mitral regurgitation she had little systolic murmur. The pattern of her diastolic murmur shown in phonocardiogram (C), provided the best insight into the abnormal physiology. The rumble began explosively with the third heart sound, 0.13 sec after the onset of the second heart sound. By palpation the left ventricular systolic impulse was also found to be abnormally prolonged.

enlargement of the left atrium. This finding, however, unless quite disproportionate, is not especially suggestive of mitral disease and is common to many afflictions of the aortic valve and the left ventricle.[202] The electrocardiogram is often nondescript except for abnormal P waves.

Very occasionally the diastolic murmur of mitral regurgitation may persist even when the systolic is absent or inconspicuous (Fig. 25-10). In these cases there is a very real danger of making an erroneous diagnosis of pure or predominant mitral stenosis. The vital clue is often provided by the palpation of a left ventricular type of apex impulse and careful analysis of the diastolic murmur, which must be studied at a heart rate between 70 and 90 beats per minute. In some cases phenylephrine (Neo-synephrine) will help to bring out the systolic murmur and reveal the masquerade.

Differential Diagnosis

Rheumatic mitral regurgitation may be simulated by several conditions already described: (1) active or healed bacterial endocarditis; (2) spontaneous rupture of chordae tendineae; (3) calcified mitral annulus; (4) mitral regurgitation associated with muscular subaortic stenosis; (5) papillary muscle malfunction or rupture.

Severe left ventricular dilatation is a surprisingly unusual cause of mitral insufficiency; but this may be because cases are missed since the murmur is not striking. Mitral insufficiency has been documented in gross ventricular dilatation associated with aortic regurgitation,[356] and in the diffuse myocardial fibrosis caused by anomalous origin of the left coronary artery.[357]

Congenital mitral regurgitation is often not difficult to distinguish because of the earlier onset of both the murmur and the clinical manifestations and because most patients, having associated atrioventricular canal malformations, display very characteristic electrocardiographic and clinical findings. However, in an exceptional group with small interatrial communications, the helpful electrocardiographic signs are missing.[358] In these cases cardiac catheterization is necessary to make the diagnosis.

Mitral regurgitation occurs also occasionally in both Marfan's and Ehlers-Danlos syndrome.[359,360] Rarely it has been seen in the cardiac involvement of rheumatoid arthritis. As previously noted, other murmurs may be mistaken for that of mitral insufficiency. The murmurs of ventricular septal defect and coarctation of the pulmonary artery differ in their more basal location.[350] The murmur of the latter condition may straddle the second sound. At present angiocardiography is the only reliable method of diagnosis for the latter condition.

Compound Mitral Lesions

A stenotic mitral valve with well-preserved leaflets billows together during systole, functioning like a pair of parachutes sewn together with an opening in the middle of the fused area.[94,190] Combined mitral stenosis and insufficiency may result from (1) partial commissural fusion associated with predominant disease of the posterior leaflet (described under "The Syndrome of the Mobile Anterior Cusp," earlier in this chapter); or (2) more frequently, shrinkage and immobilization of both "parachutes," producing a diaphragm or funnel which has a rigid aperture, lacks a suprastenotic seal, and therefore leaks.[190,305] A rigid valve with almost identical systolic and diastolic apertures explains most cases of "mixed" stenosis and regurgitation. Physiologically these lesions are particularly unfortunate. A left atrium gorged simultaneously with blood from the pulmonary veins and from the left ventricle may not properly decompress itself even through an orifice of 1.5 to 2.0 cm^2.[170,314,334] Thus mitral regurgitation converts moderate stenosis into a critical degree of block, the effect being magnified whenever there is tachycardia. Symptoms and physical signs may considerably mimic those of tight stenosis and have lured cardiologists into advising operation on the basis of this mistaken diagnosis. However, even when stenosis predominates, opening the commissures in the traditional way by an ordinary blind valvulotomy is likely to produce severe mitral regurgitation. To differentiate this condition from pure mitral stenosis several hints are usually available. Their significance is additive.

1. An authentic mitral (not tricuspid[251]) pansystolic murmur is usually present but may occasionally be absent, especially in the case with mitral insufficiency induced by previous valvulotomy.

2. An unaccountably soft first sound and absent opening snap associated with any degree of pansystolic apical murmur and a diastolic rumble are good evidence for an immobile valve with identical systolic and diastolic orifices.

3. Fluoroscopic evidence of heavy mitral calcification, if present, in addition to auscultatory evidence makes the diagnosis of a destroyed and ankylosed valve virtually certain. Unfortunately, the converse of this statement is not true. Absent calcium does not guarantee that the leaflets have not been immobilized by subvalvular disease or by shrinkage and calcification too fine to be visible by x-ray.

4. Another set of clues has to do with the amount of regurgitation.[299,300,334] These become especially important in the patient with a well-preserved first heart sound and opening snap: (a) An easily felt

left ventricular impulse which seems inappropriately active for mitral stenosis is sometimes an important clue to significant regurgitation. This sign, however, may be absent, and a frank right ventricular heave may be palpated even when regurgitation is severe. (*b*) The character and the length of the diastolic murmur are also useful. Simultaneous palpation and auscultation often help one to form the clearest mental image of the disturbance. Prolongation of the left ventricular systolic impulse often goes hand in hand with telescoping of the diastolic noises into a third heart sound and a brief explosive rumble. As previously emphasized, the patient must be studied when the heart rate is between 70 and 90 beats per minute. In spite of tight mitral stenosis, extreme bradycardia or severe right ventricular failure appreciably shortens the diastolic murmur.[331] Tachycardia is the plague of diagnosis, hiding the important diastolic relationships and spuriously sharpening the first sound. The pansystolic murmur, however, is not affected by heart rate.

5. Selective cineangiography, particularly when combined with measurements of flow and pressure, is the definitive way of assessing complex mitral disorders.

Injections into the left ventricular cavity provide the best available estimate of the amount of regurgitation; occasionally even the size and direction of the systolic jet may be seen.[211] Injections into the left atrium or pulmonary artery also give a great deal of information.[210–212] In severe mitral insufficiency dilatation of the left ventricle and behavior of the atrium and ventricle as a "common opacification chamber" are apparent. With dominant mitral stenosis there is hold-up of contrast material in the left atrium and comparatively poor opacification of a normal-sized left ventricular cavity. In these cases the downwardly bulging plane of the mitral valve can be seen in diastole, well delineated because of the difference in opacification of atrium and ventricle. In normal and severely insufficient mitral valves, the plane of the mitral valve disappears in diastole. Angiographic studies should not be undertaken casually; the information they provide may be often obtained from clinical examination, and, at present, they also entail a small but appreciable risk.

In patients with recurrent difficulty after previous blind mitral valvulotomy, the evaluation of mitral physiologic status from clinical evidence is often inaccurate.[361] Specifically, (1) there may be palpatory evidence of left ventricular overactivity in cases with severe mitral stenosis; (2) the pansystolic murmur of surgically induced mitral regurgitation is more likely to be inconspicuous or absent; (3) x-ray and electrocardiographic signs of

right ventricular hypertrophy are meaningless since they frequently persist or worsen regardless of whether the postoperative physiologic abnormality is pure mitral stenosis or a compound mitral lesion. It has been suggested that most, if not all, such patients require detailed catheterization and angiographic studies for proper evaluation. However, it is often possible clinically to make a diagnosis of a destroyed mitral valve, which is the main information needed by the surgeon.

From the standpoint of surgical treatment a decision about whether mitral stenosis or regurgitation is the dominant lesion is no more important than an estimation of the degree of valvular disease. Immobilization of the valve bellies (which may be predicted clinically with fair accuracy and sometimes further documented with meticulous cineangiography) means severe anatomic destruction and a small chance of successful surgical reconstruction without total valvular replacement.

Medical Therapy of Mitral Valve Disease

Although the definitive therapy of severe mitral valve disease is surgical, many of its aspects require careful medical management. In the past the generally unsatisfactory nature of surgical treatment for mitral regurgitation and for mitral stenosis with clinical signs of an immobile valve or heavy calcification by fluoroscopy made prolonged periods of medical therapy advisable in these patients. However, the group consigned to medical therapy progressively shrinks as safer methods are devised for surgical replacement of hopelessly diseased valves.

Episodes of acute pulmonary edema in mitral stenosis are a real emergency requiring all the physician's skill in the use of opiates, positive-pressure oxygen, phlebotomy (or its equivalents), and intravenous diuretics. The exciting causes of each episode should also be sought and treated.

Pulmonary apoplexy is rarely fatal or exsanguinating and usually requires only bed rest and opiates.[99]

Paroxysmal atrial fibrillation in mitral stenosis requires prompt and carefully monitored digitalization to prevent the especially grave acute consequences of an uncontrolled ventricular rate. Direct current defibrillation[271] offers a new and very effective way of coping with this problem, obviating the use of potentially toxic doses of quinidine. Once sinus rhythm is restored, however, maintenance quinidine sulfate—often in considerable doses—is usually needed to prevent recurrence. Very considerable improvements in exercise tolerance can often be gained by restoration of sinus rhythm even when fibrillation is long-standing.[362] There is a small but definite risk of embolization at or soon after conversion in such patients.[363] Preoperative conversion may be used to gain a temporary respite and improvement in cardiac function. Yet once a certain stage is reached in the course of severe mitral valvular disease, sinus rhythm cannot be maintained even with heavy doses of quinidine.

For control of chronic atrial fibrillation larger doses of digitalis are needed than will suffice for ordinary congestive heart failure. Therefore, it is important to clock the patient's pulse after exercise in order to assess the adequacy of digitalization— while at the same time checking carefully for evidence of digitalis intoxication: nausea, anorexia, blurring of vision (occasionally yellowing), and frequent coupled ventricular ectopic beats. Though there is evidence that "atrial failure" can occur, the effect of digitalis on the symptoms of cases of mitral stenosis with sinus rhythm is negligible,[364] whereas diuretics produce prompt and striking benefit. Digitalis, however, is an important part of the treatment of the patient with severe mitral regurgitation, even when symptoms are mild. Cardiac glycosides should be temporarily omitted before d-c electrical conversion, which may otherwise trigger digitalis intoxication. Because of the ever-present possibility of bacterial endocarditis, any febrile patient with valvular disease deserves at least one blood culture before antibiotics are begun, even if he has an obvious cause for fever.

Whenever there is unaccountable deterioration, pulmonary infection should be suspected because it is common and not always clinically obvious. All sputum should be saved and carefully examined. If the secretions appear purulent, penicillin should probably be used even if there is no distinctive bacteriologic flora.

In the therapy of chronic heart failure it is important to remember: (1) the problems of electrolyte imbalance in the prolonged use of a diuretic agent; (2) the (not always obvious) role of pulmonary emboli. The author believes that most patients taking as much as 1 Gm chlorothiazide (or an equivalent drug) per day should also receive 3 Gm potassium chloride, which is often most conveniently and palatably administered as a concentrated solution, 1 Gm at a time, dissolved in 3 to 4 oz tomato or grapefruit juice or sweet fruit syrup. In advanced cases not suitable for surgical treatment an aldosterone inhibitor can significantly prolong life; but it is wasteful to use such a drug except in conjunction with full doses of a chlorothiazide diuretic.[365] Because of the threshold effect of the aldosterone antagonists, no less than 75 to 100 mg aldactone-A should be used per day. Potassium supplements should not as a rule be given to a patient receiving spironolactone; in very sick patients or those with renal disease, spontaneous and occasionally dangerous rises in the serum-potassium level should be anticipated, and if for any reason the patient does poorly, the serum electrolytes should immediately be checked. Maintaining a mild metabolic acidosis by the administration of ammonium chloride or 1-arginine hydrochloride may be helpful in patients with advanced cases who do poorly on spironolactone alone.[366] The latter drug is the more palatable but is quite expensive. Forcing ammonium chloride (in doses of 6 to 10 G serum daily) should never be done except for short periods and with close supervision of the electrolytes. Otherwise, dangerous and even fatal metabolic acidosis may result.

For the patient with peripheral or pulmonary embolization, anticoagulant therapy with coumarin derivatives offers an appreciable degree of protection, which is further increased by valvulotomy in mitral stenosis.[153,367] Unfortunately, long-term anticoagulant therapy presents many problems.[368] Furthermore, embolization commonly occurs in patients with hepatic congestion, as a result of which the prothrombin time is already prolonged and, ironically, sometimes in the "therapeutic" range.[369] Confronted with such a case one may consider the use of heparin and subsequent valvulotomy for the case with peripheral embolization, or ligation of the inferior vena cava for pulmonary embolization. Such clinical situations are desperate enough to justify bold and decisive treatment. The Starr-Edwards valvular prosthesis to date, however, has created its own problems with postoperative peripheral embolization—a point to be remembered when the only satisfactory operation will entail total valvular replacement.[370] The chief barrier to effective treatment remains timid and tardy diagnosis. Before the disabling hemiparesis there are often minor neurologic episodes.[153] Unaccountable digitalis intoxication, unresponsive congestive failure, and an uncontrollable ventricular rate may be the chief manifestation of repeated pulmonary embolization.[279] Anticonvulsant drugs may be needed for the epilepsy of mitral stenosis secondary to previous cerebral emboli.[155]

The Selection of Patients for Surgical Treatment

In general, patients who are symptomatic and have isolated tight mitral stenosis, a good opening snap, and a loud first heart sound with little or no mitral calcification by image-amplifier fluoroscopy are good candidates for closed mitral valvulotomy. However, the results of blind valvulotomy are never entirely predictable; hence when the pump oxygenator becomes less cumbersome, it will undoubtedly be kept on standby for use as needed even in these "favorable" cases. Because of the present risk of mitral valve replacement and the definite incidence of late peripheral embolization in cases with the Starr-Edwards prosthesis, the patient with an absent opening snap, heavy valvular calcification, or predominant mitral regurgitation probably should be treated medically as long as he is asymptomatic or his course is stable. Operations on patients with "unfavorable" mitral valves and multivalvular disease are certainly safer and more satisfactory when open-heart techniques are used. Ultimately probably two-thirds of the cases of mitral stenosis and all those of mitral regurgitation will be so managed. However, at present, the added dangers of the open-heart technique more than cancel out its advantages in the "favorable" cases of mitral stenosis. Definite and sustained systemic hypertension (especially in an older person) or considerable cardiomegaly generally means that the risk of operation will be high and the chance of a good result low.[286] Either factor should make one hesitate to recommend a blind operation on the mitral valve. One should also not advise operation on a patient thought also to have significant aortic valve disease unless there are facilities for replacing both valves if necessary.

The symptoms which may be benefited by operations on the mitral valve are (1) dyspnea, including exertional, nocturnal, and paroxysmal symptoms; (2) peripheral embolization, the risk of which can be materially reduced but not always eliminated;* (3) uncontrollable atrial fibrillation, which may often be successfully converted after satisfactory correction of the valvular lesion; (4) congestive hemoptysis; (5) chronic right ventricular failure provided there is no organic tricuspid disease or (very rarely) irreversible pulmonary vascular obstruction; (6) fatigability, provided it is genuinely cardiac. This last symptom is the hardest to evaluate. Anxiety neurosis (neurasthenia) also produces fatigability, heart consciousness, and a tendency to nervous hyperventilation; the patient's obvious excitability and sighing respirations help to make the diagnosis. Mental depression produces lassitude, which, however, is frequently associated with a sleep disorder and is usually worse on arising in the morning; basically it causes loss of drive and initiative rather than genuine fatigue; most important, it is accompanied by an unaccountable sense of sadness, boredom, or desperation, which has many guises but can be readily detected by an experienced observer. The most difficult cases are those who have two genuine sources of difficulty. For example, (1) patients whose psychiatric disease submerges or distorts definite cardiac symptoms; (2) patients with a severe

ventilatory disorder (e.g., pulmonary emphysema) in addition to mitral lung disease; (3) patients with both mitral and coronary artery disease. In the selection of patients with complex causes of disability the entire picture must be carefully considered. In complex cases it is important to spend some time with the patient, to exercise him as vigorously as possible, and to observe carefully his responses both physiologic and emotional. Often it is important to have him come back again later. For whereas the first history may be atypical and contradictory, the second is often readily deciphered. In general, a severe psychiatric disorder is no contraindication to mitral valve surgery provided the indications for operation are clear otherwise. Persons accustomed to using their heart disease as an emotional crutch, however, cannot be expected to be altogether enthusiastic and grateful after successful surgery.

The risk of closed mitral valvulotomy in some hands is only 2 per cent. Unfortunately, the risk of restenosis in 10 years is 20 per cent.[264,273] Thus surgery may be advised without fear whenever it is needed; but it is wrong to recommend prophylactic operation to a patient with borderline mitral stenosis and no genuine cardiac symptoms. Unfortunately, symptoms are not always a reliable guide in severe mitral stenosis.[131,141] Apparent disability may have been mild in the patient who suddenly develops fulminating pulmonary edema during a respiratory infection, an episode of atrial fibrillation, or a pregnancy—or who suffers a devastating cerebral embolus.[141] If there is definite clinical evidence for severe "favorable" mitral stenosis and the patient has enough genuine cardiac symptoms to bring him to a physician, early surgical treatment should be advised. If there is clinical evidence for pulmonary hypertension, one should suspect important symptoms even if the patient is not clearly aware of his disability. A patient should not be denied the benefits of surgery because of his stoicism; nor should an excitable or demanding person be allowed to stampede his physician into an unwise or premature decision. At present the approach to lesions requiring open-heart operation is more conservative.

Medical Problems Associated with Surgical Treatment

In the preparation of patients for operation, there is some evidence that a prolonged period of digitalization is beneficial.[371] Cardiac compensation should be restored, but overdiuresis should be avoided. A patient depleted of potassium and plasma volume is a poor surgical risk. Closed valvulotomy should be delayed for 2 months after the last clinically obvious peripheral embolus, because

---

* After operation a few patients without a history of previous difficulty develop peripheral embolization.[286]

of the excellent chance of surgically dislodging further clots when there have been more recent emboli.[372] Anti-coagulants may be used profitably during this waiting period. Though some investigators believe that coumarin derivatives are best continued even through the operative period,[373] this practice has not become widely accepted. Open-heart techniques make it possible to operate with relative safety on the patient with probable atrial thrombosis. The presence of atrial clots, however, should be confirmed by angiography, if this is to be the main indication for the use of the pump oxygenator. Conversion of atrial fibrillation is usually pointless in the preoperative period.

Following operation, atrial fibrillation may be expected to develop in 20 to 30 per cent of patients, including some who have been known not to have it previously.[286,374] Prophylactic quinidine can probably reduce this incidence. Reversion is spontaneous in some patients. When evidence of pericarditis has subsided, conversion using d-c countershock can be effected in most cases. (It is usually advisable to wait 1 or 2 months.) Congestive heart failure appearing or intensifying after operation is an unfavorable sign, for which a cause should be sought (see below). Moderate venous distension, however, probably may result from pericardial effusion, and mild congestive phenomena for the first postoperative week are not uncommon. Tricuspid incompetence may be unmasked by successful mitral valvulotomy, but such patients have been found to do well even after several years' follow-up.[375] Unexplained fever or tachycardia in the early postoperative period is frequently due to pulmonary complications and responds well to bronchoscopy. A persistently rapid pulse and restlessness, however, may also be the first warning of wound infection. Routine administration of penicillinase resistant penicillin will prevent most of the local infections as well as postoperative bacterial endocarditis, which is usually staphylococcal.

The *postcardiotomy syndrome* at present is underdiagnosed and undertreated. The incidence is probably about 30 per cent.[376] From 2 weeks to many months after operation, symptoms (not always signs) of pericarditis occur, and there may be repeated episodes which may dwarf the patient's original postoperative discomfort. Fever is often but not always present. The condition must be distinguished from pulmonary embolization, for anticoagulant therapy mistakenly given can aggravate hemopericardium.[377] As already noted, atrial fibrillation often is triggered by the recurrent pericarditis, and sinus rhythm can seldom be maintained until the inflammation has subsided or been suppressed. Sometimes pulmonary congestive phenomena or pleural effusion may occur, just as in more severe cases of postmyocardial infarction syndrome.[378] Corticosteroid will rapidly erase most of the evidence of the syndrome, but large and sometimes prolonged dosage is required. The medication should not be witheld in the severely symptomatic patient. Salicylates occasionally help the milder case.

Evaluation of the Surgical Result

This can usually be made clinically but in special instances requires cardiac catheterization and angiography. Often with older techniques of valvulotomy the chief objective evidence of improvement is a change in the patient's course and symptoms. The murmur is often not greatly altered. Sometimes the only auscultatory change is delay of the opening snap.[183,195] Even this difference may not be obvious unless one studies the patient under several different conditions, including standing and exercise. Electrocardiographic evidence of right ventricular hypertrophy when present preoperatively has often been surprisingly permanent, and roentgenographic findings have often not cleared up completely.[361] Preliminary experience with prosthetic valves suggests that many lingering abnormalities were due to incomplete correction of the underlying disease.[366] If mitral insufficiency is corrected, there should be no pansystolic mitral murmur. Unfortunately, important leaks around the Starr-Edwards prosthesis may sometimes be practically silent.[379] Angiographic studies are often required to evaluate the patient who is doing poorly in such a circumstance.

Patients with recurrent complaints after mitral valvulotomy greatly tax the diagnostic ingenuity of the physician.[361] Causes of difficulty may be (1) uncorrected or aggravated disease of the mitral valve; (2) important, uncorrected disease of the aortic valve which may create progressive difficulty (and since there are shortened chordae in most cases of mitral stenosis, any cause of left ventricular dilatation may create a vicious circle, leading to progressive traction on the mitral leaflets and increasing mitral insufficiency); (3) postopericardiotomy syndrome, which fortunately has only a temporary effect; (4) pulmonary embolization or pulmonary venous thrombosis; (5) continuing tricuspid incompetence from right ventricular dilatation in advanced cases, especially when there is delayed or only partial regression of pulmonary vascular obstruction (annuloplasty of the tricuspid valve may help some of these patients over the hump); (6) recurrent stenosis; (7) a myocardial factor—which should never be diagnosed except by the most rigid process of exclusion; (8) rarely, acute rheumatic fever; (9) psychiatric illness.

Mitral restenosis and surgically induced mitral insufficiency are the most important causes of lasting difficulty. The problem of evaluating the status of patients with recurrent complaints is sometimes so complex that the physician should not tackle it without the aid of cardiac catheterization and angiography of the left side of the heart. Incomplete or technically inadequate studies, however, are worse than none at all.

AORTIC VALVE DISEASE

Disease Mechanisms

Aortic valve disease, if severe, greatly taxes the left ventricle, which, however, may sustain the circulation for some time without the development of any progressive symptoms. In rheumatic heart disease, aortic valvular involvement is commonly associated with some mitral lesion.[20] Any compilation of cases of isolated pure aortic stenosis inevitably includes a large number of congenitally deformed valves. Also, there are many non-rheumatic causes of pure aortic insufficiency. Rheumatic fever, however, is the distinctive cause of a compound aortic valve lesion, in which there is severe commissural fusion but a rigid orifice that allows a large leak in diastole.[20]

The "critical" systolic orifice in simple aortic stenosis is 0.8 to 1.0 cm^2 (in an average-sized adult). In this range there is a pressure gradient at ordinary rates of flow.[380] Because of the high pressure in the normal aorta, a diastolic orifice of only 0.3 to 0.5 cm^2 may permit regurgitation into a compliant ventricle of 2 to 5 liters per min, more than doubling the necessary volume of blood to be handled.[381] A severe compound lesion—which easily results from a fused valve with a rigid orifice—imposes the painful price of stenosis upon the necessity of moving a large volume of blood.

The peripheral resistance probably has an important effect on the course of aortic valve disease. A high resistance may augment the pressure work in aortic stenosis or increase the leak in aortic regurgitation. There is suggestive evidence that peripheral vasodilatation during exercise may be an important compensatory device[382] and, conversely, that increases in peripheral resistance can be very damaging.[383] With a cooperative peripheral vasculature the patient with aortic stenosis can probably raise his cardiac output without much increase in the work of his left ventricle. This physiologic bargain—the smallness of the extra load imposed by exercise—is in distinct contrast to the immediate aggravation of the physiologic difficulty in mitral stenosis. Severe dyspnea in aortic valve disease, however, means left ventricular failure and implies more advanced disease than do comparable symptoms in mitral stenosis.

The correlation between symptoms and valvular anatomy is not perfect. The duration of the lesion is surely important. An increased peripheral resistance may explain many of the unaccountable cases who deteriorate in spite of a less than critical valve lesion. The clinical recognition of this syndrome is probably not as simple as it may seem. For example, the usual method of estimating the peripheral resistance (measuring the blood pressure) is rendered unreliable by significant aortic regurgitation. In aortic stenosis, hypertrophy of the left ventricular outflow tract can occasionally add an additional functional obstruction, which may be severe in some cases.

The line separating ventricular competence from failure is often not clearly drawn in severe aortic valve disease. In aortic stenosis, pulsus alternans of the left ventricle (never clearly transmitted to the peripheral pulse) is rather common in patients with severe symptoms, but no clinical signs of decompensation.[385] Even in patients without symptoms, the diastolic pressure in the small, thick-walled ventricle may be high, and especially during exertion, it may be further augmented by giant atrial contraction.[385,386] It is quite possible that such pressure changes can produce mild temporary embarrassment to the lungs, especially during exercise tachycardia, long before left ventricular failure becomes clinically recognizable.

In severe aortic insufficiency there is striking reversal of flow in the aorta during diastole; normal ventricular filling competes with the backward gush.[381] In extreme cases with little "retrograde stenosis," premature closure of the mitral valve serves to protect the lungs from the rapidly rising ventricular diastolic pressure.[387]

In general, clinical detection of aortic disease is by the characteristic murmurs and physical signs. Yet accurate estimation of the severity of the lesion must include a careful history. Because of the inadequacies of clinical diagnosis, catheterization of the aorta and left ventricle and angiocardiography may be needed in special cases, but the present risk of the procedure does not justify its use in lieu of careful clinical evaluation—or until surgical treatment is being considered.

In the following discussion, aortic valve lesions are treated for the most part without proper regard for the mitral disease which commonly coexists with them and complicates their physiology. This deficit is regrettable but simply due to a lack of knowledge. Multivalvular disease is less understood both because its physiology is more complex and because such cases were systematically excluded from most earlier studies which were naturally more concerned with the simpler lesions amenable to closed operative techniques.

Aortic Stenosis

Symptoms

A history of rheumatic fever is obtained in only about one-third of the cases.[388,389] If proper allowance could always be made for the congenitally stenotic valves, a previous diagnosis of rheumatic fever would probably be about as common as in mitral stenosis. In aortic stenosis without mitral disease there is a 3:1 or 4:1 predominance of males, a reversal of the sex ratio in rheumatic lesions of the other valves.[388,389] There is surprisingly little information about the evolution of severe rheumatic aortic stenosis. In the patient under 40 years of age it is likely to be associated with a history of rheumatic fever and evidence of mitral disease as well.[389] Isolated aortic stenosis in this age group has a reasonably good chance of being congenital. Isolated severe aortic stenosis, however, is often first detected in old age, the rheumatic fever, if any, having occurred 40 years or so before. Although there are few long-term follow-ups, stenosis probably can and does progress considerably during adult life—whether by covert rheumatism or by hemodynamic factors.[138,139,390] A grade I (but indisputably aortic) systolic murmur followed for 10 to 30 years may metamorphose into high-grade aortic obstruction.[388,390] There is evidence that the aggravating factor may not be entirely rheumatic but may be superimposed atherosclerosis.[391] In mild mitral insufficiency there is much less evidence that the lesion may progress;[323] in rheumatic aortic insufficiency, although worsening occurs, it is not common except from rheumatic activity or bacterial endocarditis. Yet stenotic lesions of both aortic and mitral valves seem to have the faculty for insidious progression.

Even in tight aortic stenosis there is probably a long stable period nearly or completely without symptoms, which begins at an average age of 45 to 50 years.[388,389,392] The earliest complaints are usually of increased fatigability and dyspnea on unusual exertion.[392,393] There are often vaguely described dizzy spells, but if careful inquiry proves that they are brought on by exertion, this complaint becomes considerably more specific.

The appearance of any one of a characteristic triad of symptoms means a turning point in the course of the illness:[380,388,393-395] (1) effort syncope, (2) angina pectoris, (3) left ventricular failure. Sudden death, which accounts for 20 per cent of the fatalities, may occur even in previously asymptomatic patients, especially the younger ones, and there is no reliable way to predict it. There is reason to believe, however, that most such patients have had hemodynamic evidence of left ventricular failure even though many of them have been asymptomatic.[393] Once any of the classic symptoms appear, an abrupt decline in the patient's status may occur at any time and the chances of sudden death are increased.[389,394] Sudden death almost always occurs during the waking hours but otherwise cannot be significantly correlated with exertion.

Angina, breathlessness, and syncope are common presenting complaints in younger patients. Left or even right ventricular failure is often the first sign of trouble in the aged.[389] Failure is the most serious of the classic triad of symptoms and always injects an element of urgency lacking in the corresponding stage of mitral disease. The average length of life after the onset of heart failure in pure aortic stenosis has been found to be 2 to 3 years,[389,394] but the interval varies from 1 week to a decade, making any "average" rather meaningless. With the recent improvement in the treatment for congestive failure, longer reprieves can probably be granted. Effort syncope and angina are usually rather earlier symptoms, with "average" life expectancies of 3 to 4 years.[389,394] Grave portent is attached not only to a specific symptom but to any evidence of an acceleration of the disease process: increasing frequency of attacks or the addition of any new member of the triad.

Effort Syncope. There are three different kinds of syncope in aortic stenosis. (1) Near-syncope, "graying out," on exertion is the commonest. It often occurs in the early stages of the disease and has been attributed to sudden vasodilatation.[381] The author believes, however, that its mechanism may be the same as in the third type described below. (2) About 10 per cent of elderly patients with aortic stenosis have involvement of the AV node,[396,397] very likely by extension of calcium into the septum. Even without severe stenosis they may develop stable or episodic complete heart block, which has no consistent relation to exertion and has been relieved by removing an offending spicule during aortic valvulotomy. (3) Complete loss of consciousness brought on by effort (the classic syncope of aortic stenosis) occurs in about one-third of patients with aortic stenosis with serious symptoms and is commonly associated with angina pectoris.[388,389,397,398] Sometimes occasional attacks may occur for many years before other symptoms appear. By contrast, syncopal spells beginning after the onset of left-sided heart failure are often brought on by little, if any, effort and are of the gravest significance. Sometimes a patient has definite premonitory symptoms and be able to avoid an attack by rest.[397,398] Occasionally, however, even if he lies down, he steadily worsens, loses consciousness completely, and may develop generalized convulsions. At times the first signs of syncope appear a few minutes after the patient stops exercise. Some episodes are undoubtedly due to a rhythm disorder. Yet continuous electrocardiograms have shown that the patient has often fainted before the rhythm disorder begins. During the unconsciousness the pulse, the murmur, and the heart sounds may disappear for as much as several minutes, though the electrocardiogram and sometimes a feeble apex impulse certify that a potentially useful cardiac rhythm and indeed some ventricular activity continue.[398,399] Vasodilatation seems insufficient to explain such an attack. Temporarily, ventricular power to eject blood seems to be lost. Sudden reversible subaortic obstruction is a possible explanation. During recovery a momentary overshoot of the systolic blood pressure to levels of 200 has been recorded,[397] which is perhaps analogous to the blood pressure overshoot seen after the pharmacologic relief of hypertrophic subvalvular stenosis with methoxamine (Vasoxyl).[400] It is important to distinguish the classic effort syncope of aortic stenosis from Stokes-Adams attacks. The latter are sometimes brought on after effort, but the relation is never so consistent or striking as in aortic stenosis.[389,393]

Angina Pectoris. Atypical chest pain is common in aortic stenosis, but on closer questioning it often turns out to be associated with angina pectoris. Classical angina occurs in up to two-thirds of patients with severe aortic stenosis and in all age groups.[388,389,393] It is a sign of well-matured disease and does not occur in mild or early cases. It may be classical in its character, radiation, and being provoked by effort or recumbency. It may follow severe exertion immediately or by an appreciable interval. The absence of angina does not indicate mild stenosis; some patients with end-stage congestive heart failure have never had any chest or arm discomfort. Angina is very frequently associated with effort syncope—sometimes as a premonitory symptom. In some cases prolonged episodes occur without relation to effort. When failure appears, angina may occasionally improve; it usually becomes even more intractable. Nitroglycerin may provide relief, but there is a less satisfactory response than in coronary artery disease and also a definitely increased risk of nitrite syncope.[388] The explanation for angina pectoris is commonly thought to be that the hard-working ventricle has outgrown its blood supply.[388,389] Embolization of particles from the aortic valve[401] undoubtedly explains some cardiac pain in aortic stenosis. Regardless of the mechanism of angina, there is no doubt that it sometimes signals myocardial necrosis. Multiple discrete areas of myocardial fibrosis and occasionally even sizable areas

of infarction may occur without any coronary disease whatsoever.[402] Advanced changes of this sort may explain the course of occasional patients who fail to respond to definitive operations on the aortic valve.

In the elderly, trivial aortic stenosis or aortic valve sclerosis may produce an aortic ejection murmur[355] and coronary disease may be responsible for angina or Stokes-Adams attacks. Therefore angina in the setting of aortic stenosis always deserves careful scrutiny. For intelligent treatment two questions should be asked: (1) Is the aortic stenosis severe enough to be responsible for angina? (2) Does the patient have coronary artery disease (with or without severe aortic stenosis)? In general, the angina of aortic stenosis is known by the company it keeps: (*a*) Frequent association with effort or post-effort syncope (which must be distinguished from the Stokes-Adams attacks of coronary artery disease); (*b*) unmistakable evidence compatible with severe stenosis on clinical examination (not always easy to detect even when present). Catheterization and angiography of the left side of the heart are justified in cases where aortic stenosis is of dubious severity.[403] If angina is disproportionate or if the patient is elderly, coronary arteriography should probably be done before aortic valve surgery. Severe aortic stenosis confers no immunity to atherosclerotic coronary disease. Indeed the advancement of both lesions may be by the same process.[391]

Congestive Heart Failure. This is a most sinister occurrence in pure aortic stenosis, and reliance on the traditional signs will often result in underdiagnosis, especially in the younger patient.[385,393] Dyspnea on exertion does not necessarily mean failure, but a valid history of progressive dyspnea may prove to be due to pulmonary interstitial edema when an x-ray is taken. Paroxysmal nocturnal dyspnea is very serious unless the patient's predominant lesion is mitral stenosis. Commonly patients do not survive to reach the end stage of gross right ventricular decompensation, which in itself usually means death within a year. Manifest failure as an isolated symptom is more likely to occur in older patients. Once failure has occurred, even when compensation is apparently restored, the threat of sudden death remains greatly increased.[394] Patients with advanced failure not uncommonly have abrupt crises of restlessness, flushing, cyanosis, heavy sweating, and shock.[404] These spells are not explainable by arrhythmia or pulmonary embolization. Death often comes in such a crisis.

Other Symptoms. Palpitation with exercise is not uncommon. However, atrial fibrillation in aortic stenosis usually means either associated mitral disease or a very advanced stage of the illness, usually with death not very far away.[393] Embolization occurs chiefly from associated mitral stenosis, which should be suspected in any patient with occlusion of a large or medium-sized peripheral vessel. Calcareous emboli from the aortic valve itself are usually asymptomatic but can produce a distinctive kind of sudden occlusion in smaller vessels.[401] As noted, these undoubtedly include some of the episodes of myocardial infarction[402] as well as sudden spells of quadrantic blindness, analogous to that caused by Hollenhorst plaques. Bacterial endocarditis may occur[406] but is probably less common in pure aortic stenosis than in cases with some element of insufficiency.[393] Dissection of the aorta is a rare complication, perhaps in a congenitally disposed individual, and is not dependent on severe stenosis.[407] The medionecrosis in such rare cases is confined to the area of the ascending aorta. Rupture of an aortic sinus also associated with medionecrosis has also occurred several months after the insertion of a Starr-Edwards aortic valve prosthesis.

Physical Examination

Murmur. The distinctive finding of aortic stenosis is a diamond-shaped ejection murmur, its high frequencies ending about 0.02 to 0.06 sec before the second heart sound.[39,388] Usually the murmur is loudest in the aortic area and occasionally is so poorly transmitted that failure to listen to the right of the upper sternum (a common error) may cause a missed diagnosis. Not uncommonly one can palpate a thrill, which may be transmitted to the carotid arteries in the neck. On the other hand the murmur may seem maximal at the apex.[388] In either case it retains its characteristic diamond shape. The intensity of the murmur usually varies from grade II to V but bears no useful relation to the severity of the lesion. It may be rather loud in trivial aortic stenosis and quite hard to hear in a severe lesion, provided the chest is thick or the aortic flow is greatly reduced by advanced congestive heart failure or concomitant mitral stenosis. In emphysematous patients sometimes when the murmur is hard to hear over the chest it still may be audible at the base of the neck. A grade I or II murmur of minor aortic insufficiency is common[388] and may persist even when the major systolic murmur has been all but obliterated by severe failure.[150]

When the murmur of aortic stenosis is loud or maximal at the apex, it may be mistaken for mitral regurgitation. On the other hand murmurs of mitral insufficiency due to improper support of the valve (ruptured chordae tendineae or papillary muscle dysfunction after myocardial infarction) may be diamond-shaped and maximal at the upper left sternal border. The diagnosis of an "ejection" or "pansystolic" murmur should usually imply that

the observer has positively identified the first and second heart sounds and is sure of the relation of the murmur to each. Unfortunately, this is not always easy to do. At the left ventricular apex in mitral insufficiency both heart sounds may be buried in the murmur; whereas in calcific aortic stenosis the second sound may be inaudible and the first sound difficult to hear. A better place to study the relationship of murmur and heart sounds is at the lower sternal border, where the sound is more likely to be heard and the murmur is not deafeningly loud. The murmur of moderate or severe aortic stenosis is characteristic in that it is nearly, but not quite, pansystolic; the difference between a blurred and a clean onset of the second heart sound is usually perfectly obvious if one listens carefully. Sometimes in severe calcific stenosis the aortic component of the second sound is missing altogether. Here it is useful to time the murmur against the carotid pulse; the aortic murmur lasts only to the peak, whereas the pansystolic murmur continues after the pulse has begun to fall. When clinical distinction is not certain or the presence of both murmurs is suspected, phonocardiography timed against the electrocardiogram and carotid pulse will settle the diagnosis. The administration of amyl nitrite will help by decreasing the murmur of mitral insufficiency[256] and, less consistently augmenting the murmur of aortic stenosis. A long pause in atrial fibrillation or after an ectopic beat considerably increases ventricular diastolic filling, sometimes increasing the murmur of aortic valvular stenosis, reducing that of hypertrophic subvalvular stenosis, and not affecting that of mitral regurgitation.[169] Effects of changes in the duration of diastole, however, are not always clean-cut.

Ejection Click. An aortic ejection click occurs 0.03 to 0.06 sec after the onset of the sharp portion of the first heart sound and, being maximal at the apex, may stimulate a loud or split first heart sound.[411] Such clicks are probably usually caused from resonance of aortic valve tissue and coincide with the ultimate upward tensing of a mobile diaphragm.[408]* Hence clicks are common in congenital aortic stenosis, rather unusual in rheumatic stenosis, and are progressively rare after the third decade because of the increasing incidence of heavy valvular calcification.

The Second Heart Sound. This sound in the average adult case is soft and pure (incapable of inspiratory splitting). Moderate normal splitting on inspiration, however, is not incompatible with a

---

* Newer evidence is against the older view that aortic ejection clicks are due to sudden hosing of the jet of blood against the aortic wall.

severe lesion. Paradoxic splitting, the result of pro-longation of left ventricular systole, occasionally can be detected.[185,400] It is probably commoner than is appreciated. In severe aortic stenosis the pulmonic component of the second sound may be buried in the end of the murmur. Thus paradoxic splitting may explain some cases of an unaccountably pure second sound. In 20 per cent of patients the aortic component is absent,[388] and in many of these the entire second sound is thought clinically to be missing. Good audibility of the second sound at left ventricular apex and left lower sternal border usually means that the aortic component is present. In the young patient with congenital aortic stenosis and a mobile valve diaphragm, the aortic component is usually of normal intensity and always well separated from the end of the murmur. Softness or inaudibility of the second sound in the aortic area—the traditional absent "A_2"—is often partly an auscultatory illusion owing to the observer's slight physiologic deafness immediately following a loud murmur.

Fourth Heart Sound. A fourth heart sound and a presystolic heave are common but not invariable findings in severe stenosis.[400,409] Unless the patient is young, a third sound appears only with the onset of left ventricular failure.

The character of the *carotid pulse* is frequently distinctive.[388,393,410] Classically it is small, slow rising, and often prolonged; in some extreme cases it is almost as immobile as a tendon, vibrating with the transmitted aortic thrill. Uses and limitations of the pulse as an index of aortic stenosis will be discussed later.

Apex Impulse. The apex impulse is not usually significantly displaced unless there is failure.[388,393] It is not hyperkinetic, as in mitral or aortic regurgitation, though the outward thrust usually occupies more than two-thirds of systole.[172,174] It is a quiet but authoritative heave, sometimes beginning in presystole.[411] There is no rapid early diastolic movement. In a few cases no obvious abnormality of any sort can be made out—but concomitant mitral stenosis should be suspected in such instances.

Because of the relative quietness of the apex impulse, its character and duration are best appreciated when it is in closest contact with the chest wall, with the patient in the left lateral decubitus position. Simultaneous auscultation (to outline the boundaries of systole) is helpful in defining the normality of the duration of the apex thrust.

Blood Pressure. The blood pressure is very helpful in the diagnosis of aortic stenosis if used intelligently and if properly related to the other findings.[388] Classical cases with a narrowed pulse pressure of 30 mm Hg or less are common and

almost always can be counted as indicating severe disease. More frequently the blood pressure is perfectly normal. Certain outside limits are clinically useful: A sustained systolic blood pressure over 175 mm Hg is most unusual and especially if associated with a pulse pressure over 60 mm Hg is very strong evidence against tight aortic stenosis. The pulse pressure may be wide, however, when the systolic level is normal. These observations do not mean that marked hypertension is incompatible with symptomatic aortic stenosis. Rather, the added load of systemic hypertension can probably convert moderate aortic valve disease into an intolerable lesion.

X-ray Findings

A calcified aortic valve lies in the midline in the frontal view and in the middle third of the heart in the lateral projection.[103,104] In most cases of severe isolated rheumatic aortic stenosis over age 35, calcification can be seen by x-ray or with image-intensified fluoroscopy. Indeed one should be reluctant to diagnose isolated valvular stenosis in this age group without such a finding.[384,412] As in mitral disease, there is a sex difference, calcification being somewhat less common in females.

Except in advanced cases the heart size is usually normal or nearly so, the apex perhaps hugging the diaphragm a little more than normally.[388,400] This benign appearance is deceptive, for angiocardiography shows that the left ventricular wall is exceedingly thick, encroaching greatly on a small cavity. The left atrium may be definitely enlarged (as demonstrated by barium swallow in the lateral position) even when failure has not been clinically diagnosed.[393,400] X-ray evidence of interstitial pulmonary edema often precedes the traditional signs of left ventricular failure. Gross cardiomegaly means congestive failure in the past or present and carries a very bad prognosis.[412]

Poststenotic dilatation may produce a selective rightward bulge of the ascending aorta which often is in considerable contrast to a normal-sized aortic knob.[400,413] More sensitive and frequently encountered signs (which we believe to be present in most cases) may be detected with the aid of image-intensifier fluoroscopy.[414,415]

1. Often a small area in the root of the aorta (just above its junction with the right atrial shadow) will be seen to bulge actively for a moment in early systole. This is undoubtedly because of hosing of the jet from the stenotic valve against the right or posterior aortic wall, and is the physiologic counterpart of the jet lesions described pathologically.[356] Detecting this curious aortic pulse takes practice. Usually unless the pa-

tient is in the far right anterior oblique position, it will be missed.

2. Diffuse increase of pulsation of the ascending aorta with much less pulsation of the descending portion—differential pulsation—is seen in most patients with a jet pulse. Pathologically the jet lesion is occasionally noted in the far posterior aspect of the aortic wall,[356] and this may explain the absence of a directly visible jet effect in some cases. Differential pulsation is a less specific sign of aortic stenosis, being practically indistinguishable from that seen in coarctation of the aorta.

When present, these fluoroscopic signs strongly imply that the anatomy of stenosis is present. They do not occur in the elderly patient with noisy flow from a sclerotic valve. Thus far, however, they have not separated moderate from severe stenosis, and they do not always accurately characterize compound aortic valve lesions.

Electrocardiogram

In severe aortic stenosis there is usually some evidence of left ventricular hypertrophy.[388,393,385] Especially in the younger patient, however, this may be merely increased voltage of the QRS complex, which is always an ambiguous finding.[411] Lack of S-T and T-wave abnormalities, however, is encountered with increasing frequency as one diagnoses the condition in younger patients and at earlier stages of symptoms. In the young or middle-aged patient the axis is more commonly not leftward in the frontal plane and often is about $+60°$.[339] Left axis deviation becomes increasingly common with advancing age or with increasing amounts of aortic regurgitation. In the great majority of symptomatic adult patients there is depression of the S-T segment, with total or partial T-wave inversion in V_5 and V_6. Such signs commonly precede the development of symptoms,[380, 388,412] but occasionally the electrocardiogram remains normal in a dangerously ill patient. The left atrial type of P wave is common in severe cases.[416] Electrocardiographic evidence of previous myocardial infarction is occasionally seen. It is not known how often this occurs in the absence of associated coronary atherosclerosis. Severe left ventricular hypertrophy may simulate an old antero-septal myocardial infarction; but a predominant S wave persisting in V_6 in patients with Q-S complexes in V_1 and V_2 is usually associated with vectorcardiographic and pathologic evidence of infarction.[417] Left bundle branch block is compatible with uncomplicated aortic stenosis, usually in the elderly or in the more extreme degrees of left ventricular hypertrophy.[418] Yet its presence should make one consider associated coronary artery disease. Atrial fibrillation is rare in simple

aortic stenosis and should suggest associated mitral stenosis.[383]

In the younger patient with severe aortic stenosis and a normal scalar electrocardiogram, it has been claimed that vectorcardiography (using the cube system) can detect left ventricular hypertrophy in many cases.[419] The most characteristic finding is marked posterior displacement of the terminal portion of the QRS loop.

Unfortunately in the elderly patient left ventricular hypertrophy is hard to diagnose for other reasons. Voltage of the QRS complex may normally decline with age. S-T and T-wave abnormalities become much less specific for left ventricular hypertrophy and may be due to coronary artery disease. Even clear-cut left ventricular hypertrophy does not always prove to be related to the patient's murmur.

Estimation of the Severity of Aortic Stenosis

The signs and symptoms of tight aortic stenosis (Fig. 25-11) are frequently not altogether typical and can be simulated by other conditions.[412] There are patients chiefly over the age of 50 years in whom there is only trivial aortic stenosis despite a very suggestive clinical picture. There may be severe symptoms, usually due to coronary artery disease, although in some instances mitral valve disease has been the chief disorder.[412] In these older patients dilatation of the aorta and T-wave abnormalities in the electrocardiogram are much less specific evidence of aortic stenosis than in young patients. In fact it has been suggested that the severity of aortic stenosis cannot be reliably predicted by clinical examination.[395] This is probably overstating the case. Once symptoms have appeared their characteristic behavior and interplay may sometimes allow the diagnosis of tight aortic stenosis to be made almost from a skillfully taken history. Yet it is desirable that the condition be recognized before the patient is in an advanced stage of symptoms. Furthermore clinical examination does provide objective evidence of the severity of the aortic lesion. The following nine signs are most useful. No single clue is infallible or applicable in every case, but careful consideration of all the evidence usually allows accurate diagnosis and intelligent selection of patients for cardiac catheterization and operation.

Left Ventricular Hypertrophy. Otherwise unaccountable left ventricular hypertrophy, manifested by prolongation of the left ventricular impulse, is the basic quantitating sign. It should be detected by physical examination in almost every patient in whom the chest contour makes accurate palpation possible—and may precede definite electrocardiographic signs.[411] Undeniable electrocardiographic evidence is also present in the great majority of symptomatic adults. Limitations of the electrocardiogram in the diagnosis of left ventricular hypertrophy should be recalled, and great reliance should not be placed on an incomplete picture: isolated S-T and T-wave abnormalities in the older patient, or borderline QRS voltage in the younger or slender person who has no other signs. A "left atrial" P wave is a nonspecific sign usually present, however, in severe disease.[416]

Presystolic Heave. Sometimes resulting from giant atrial contraction against the rigid diastolic ventricle, presystolic heave strongly implies that the aortic valve lesion is severe.[400] The obvious problem with such a heave is distinguishing it from the systolic thrust itself. This can be done fairly reliably by simultaneous palpation of the carotid pulse and the left ventricular apex. Normally the onset of the carotid pulse occurs about 0.04 sec after the onset of the apex thrust.* If the P-R interval

* This interval is about that between the "c" and the "l" when one pronounces the word "clock."

is not unusually short, the presystolic heave can often be distinguished by the fact that it considerably precedes the onset of the carotid upstroke, which therefore seems delayed. The presence of a presystolic impulse may also be verified by the apex cardiogram or kinetocardiogram.[168,400]

Fourth Heart Sound (S_4). A fourth heart sound practically always accompanies the presystolic heave but is considerably more common; it also usually means considerable left ventricular hypertrophy and perhaps physiologic embarrassment.[420] Therefore, when other findings are suggestive, the fourth heart sound validates severe stenosis and is but rarely absent in critical cases.[409] Occasional exceptions are probably due to the fact that the fourth sound reflects not only the rigidity of the ventricle, but also the vigor of atrial systole, which may be reduced in very advanced disease. Unfortunately under the best of circumstances the clinical diagnosis of the S_4 is often unreliable. The sound is usually brief and low pitched. Especially when the P-R interval is short, the S_4 may be

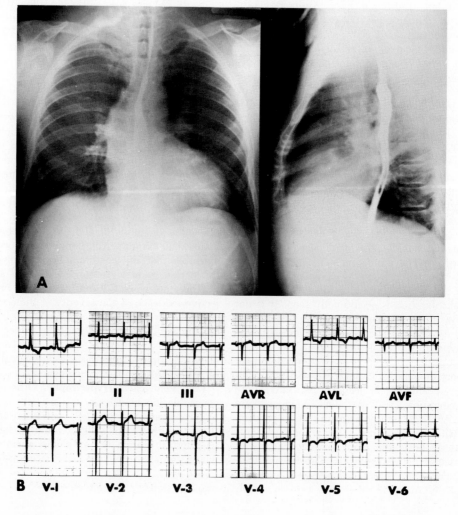

almost impossible to distinguish from the beginning of a normal crescendo first heart sound. It is also likely to be overlooked when one is deafened by the loud systolic murmur, although in extreme cases it is obvious and may resemble a short presystolic murmur. Improvement in the accuracy of clinical diagnosis may be gained by the following two-step method: (1) At first one simultaneously palpates the apex impulse and the carotid pulse. If, after due consideration of the P-R interval, one concludes that there is a presystolic apical impulse, it is not necessary to go any further. Often in aortic stenosis, the onset of the carotid pulse may be very quiet, but with care this point may be recognized. (2) If no presystolic pulse is present, the onset of the apex impulse may be used to demarcate the onset of systole and the presystolic nature of the fourth sound may be recognized. The fourth sound may also be recognized by its cadence: The sequence of a fourth heart sound leading into a first heart sound almost never causes two sharp, brief noises. The first heart sound closely followed by an early systolic aortic ejection click, however, may produce just such a sequence and be mistaken by the uninitiated for a fourth heart sound. Because of the difficulties of clinical diagnosis and the importance of the fourth sound in aortic stenosis, a phonocardiogram should be made when possible. In general the sooner the S_4 occurs after the onset of the P wave, the graver its physiologic significance.[421]

Carotid Pulse. The character of the carotid pulse

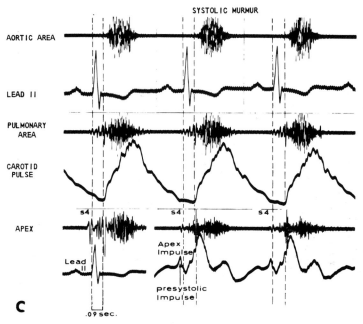

Fig. 25-11. Advanced calcific aortic stenosis. A 35-year-old man, whose lesion was very likely congenital rather than rheumatic, had an 8-month history of very severe symptoms of congestive heart failure, angina, and effort syncope. Clinical findings allowed an accurate prediction of the disease process. The x-ray (*A,* opposite page, frontal and lateral views) showed unusual left ventricular enlargement for isolated aortic stenosis and strongly implied an advanced stage of symptoms. By fluoroscopy there was heavy calcification in the aortic valve, also seen on the lateral film in the middle of the heart. The electrocardiogram (*B,* opposite page) showed severe left ventricular hypertrophy, the electrical axis being somewhat more horizontal than usual for pure aortic stenosis, also implying that important left ventricular dilatation (the end stage of the disease) had begun to occur. A thrill was felt over the aortic area corresponding with the maximum intensity of a diamond-shaped murmur. In the illustration (*C*), however, different sensitivities were used in recording the heart sounds, so that the size of the murmur would be about the same in all three areas of auscultation and its identical shape, regardless of transmission, could be appreciated. The slowly ascending carotid pulse continued to rise through the entire duration of the murmur. Even at high sensitivity no evidence of a second heart sound was found at the lower sternal border. Therefore, the aortic component was probably absent. A loud fourth heart sound (certifying left ventricular hypertrophy) is recorded at the apex, synchronous with a presystolic thrust, which was suspected clinically because the onset of the apex impulse quite appreciably preceded that of the carotid upstroke. Thus the character of the carotid pulse and the apex thrust implied critical aortic stenosis. The x-ray calcification and genuinely absent aortic component of the second sound certified severe stenosis with a rigid valve. At operation the valve was found to be calcified, 6 mm thick, with an orifice 0.3 cm².

is an important but not infallible guide to the severity of aortic stenosis. It is worthwhile to consider the limitations of this sign: The pressure pulse midway up the ascending aorta is strikingly uniform in every adult case of aortic valvular stenosis of at least moderate severity.[385] Instead of the usual rise and fall during the ejection period (which is a faithful replica of left ventricular pulse), there is a gradual and steady ascent to a peak pressure at the very end of systole. There is also often a hesitation on the upstroke, because of the Venturi (suction) effect of the aortic jet during the period of its maximal velocity.[385,422] A central aortic pressure pulse whose ascent fills all of systole is virtually pathognomonic of moderate or severe fixed, discreet obstruction to left ventricular outflow (whether valvular, subvalvular, or supravalvular). Unfortunately peripheral transmission always tends to hide the character of this pulse, making its ascent sharper and its excursion wider.[385,410] Examination of the brachial artery is almost worthless, since its pulse is often nondescript and there is much overlap with the normal.[380,384] The carotid pulse is much less deformed,[384] but often it has a flat top and seems more "slowly moving" than "slowly ascending." Indirect carotid tracings in the majority of cases will have a grossly prolonged upstroke time, and the diagnosis can be made with reasonable accuracy from this feature alone.[410,423]

Usually the carotid pulse continues to rise or plateaus for almost the entire interval between the first and second sound. The systolic excursion is not often large, and the duration of the pulse is usually prolonged in proportion to its height.

An abnormal pulse is strong evidence for moderate or severe aortic stenosis. Yet an apparently normal pulse does not always exclude the diagnosis: (1) The rigid aorta of an elderly person accepts even small net volume changes with wide variations in pressure; instead of providing an expandable systolic reservoir, it immediately transmits blood to its branches, tending to widen their movement and pulsation. Therefore, an occasional elderly person with tight aortic stenosis may have an actively rising and falling carotid pulse.[380,393] (2) Congenital valvular aortic stenosis in children is often not reliably evaluated by carotid palpation.[424] Tachycardia and a very rapid rate of initial ventricular contraction are probably important factors. (3) With reduction of stroke output by severe left ventricular failure, tachycardia, or associated mitral stenosis, the pulse duration may be abbreviated and the slow ascent is often not obvious. Yet the immobility of the pulse in such cases is usually striking.

Good records of the pulse movements may be hard to obtain and are seldom more reliable than the trained finger.[410] Even the best externally recorded carotid pulse may not be linear, is very difficult to calibrate, and sometimes is affected by changes of velocity as well as of displacement.[384,410] Diastolic events are never faithfully recorded.[410] Furthermore, displacement of a pulse, no matter how detected, does not always clearly reflect the pressure events occurring within the vessel. In systemic hypertension, for instance, the intraarterial pressure may rapidly rise toward the limits of carotid distensibility, producing a flattening of the top of the pulse and spurious delay in the upstroke of the displacement record.[410] If one remembers the limitations of the method, externally recorded carotid pulses, however, are useful as a permanent and objective record.

It is recommended that each examiner accumulate his own series of controls by palpating many normal and abnormal carotids at different heart rates. He may use his own carotid pulse as a control provided his heart rate is not too dissimilar from the patient's. Simultaneous auscultation of the heart and palpation of the pulse are helpful.

In summary, the pulse is not infallible in the recognition of severe aortic stenosis. Yet a normal contour in a suspected adult case should suggest either a mild valvular lesion or subvalvular functional hypertrophic stenosis.

The Murmur. The diamond shape of an ejection murmur is a mirror of changing left ventricular ejection velocities.[348] Often in trivial aortic valve lesions, only the peak flow in the first half of systole may produce high-frequency sound. Usually a brief early systolic murmur can be dismissed as unimportant[355] unless the patient is in severe congestive heart failure. Unfortunately, the pitch of a murmur is also dependent on factors other than ejection velocity,[315] and many trivial lesions can produce harsh noise. Simultaneous auscultation of the heart and palpation of the carotid pulse are most helpful in visualizing the abnormal physiology. Persistence of both the ejection murmur and the pulse ascent into later systole implies a strong left ventricular effort dampened by fixed outflow obstruction. Musical ("cooing") overtones to the murmur are irrelevant to the severity of the valve lesion.

The Blood Pressure. This is chiefly of use as a factor of exclusion. Sustained hypertension (as already noted) is strong evidence against tight stenosis.

Valvular Calcification. If aortic stenosis is severe, valvular calcification easily visible by image-intensifier fluoroscopy should be expected in almost all males over the age of 30 and in most older females.[412] It is most likely to be missing in younger females, in patients with combined mitral stenosis, and also in patients with trivial aortic valve lesions. Conversely, heavy aortic valvular calcification usually means important stenosis. Jet effects by fluoroscopy are very useful signs of the stenotic condition, but their significance in quantitating the lesion has not been established.

Paradoxic Splitting of the Second Sound. Genuinely documented and occurring without left bundle branch block, this always means severe stenosis. Unfortunately it is rarely detectable in adults.

Estimation of the Mobility of the Aortic Valve Diaphragm. This estimation can be made clinically. In the writer's experience a very soft or absent aortic component of the second sound is the most sensitive sign of immobility. The finding should always be verified phonocardiographically with simultaneous recording of the second sound at the aortic, pulmonary, and apex areas during deep respiration. An absent ejection click seems always to mean a rigid valve, but presence of some sound does not guarantee a flexible aortic diaphragm. Sometimes the systolic click may persist when the aortic component of the second sound is obliterated. This observation is probably explained by the fact that the systolic forces directed against the valve are more violent than the diastolic.

Heavy calcification seen by x-ray, especially if associated with auscultatory evidence, usually means a badly destroyed valve, which the majority of surgeons now prefer to replace with a prosthesis.

Atypical Aortic Stenosis

Combined Aortic Stenosis and Mitral Stenosis

This syndrome is not uncommon, perhaps amounting to 5 per cent of severe rheumatic cases.[425,426] It is presented under the category of aortic stenosis because the patient's auscultatory signs commonly suggest this diagnosis, and the mitral stenosis is sometimes missed.[425-427] The mitral lesion, however, is often the more important cause of symptoms.[425,428] It often limits the cardiac output and may soften the aortic murmur.[428,429] In other cases, however, the mitral murmur may be the more prominent so that the severity of aortic stenosis may be underestimated.[429,430] Distinctively the patient's aortic stenosis, though perhaps severe, is in an early phase at the time symptoms appear.[428] Some patients also have the pansystolic murmur of mitral regurgitation, which may be loud. However, high-grade mitral regurgitation combined with severe aortic stenosis is unusual and probably, in fact, very badly tolerated.[428,429] By increasing the

left ventricular systolic pressure (though often only moderately), aortic valve obstruction probably increases the likelihood of an audible mitral leak, even in the presence of tight mitral stenosis.*

The history in such a case has the definite stamp of mitral stenosis.[425,429] There is a 3:1 preponderance of females. A past history of rheumatic fever is unusually common, occurring in two-thirds or more of the cases. The average patient gets into difficulty in her late thirties or early forties, as does the person with solitary mitral stenosis—sooner than the average patient with isolated aortic stenosis. Symptoms are likely to be chronic and remitting. Dyspnea, fatigue, palpitation, and nocturnal dyspnea are common. Atrial fibrillation and its complications were found in two-thirds of the patients in one series[425] but rarely in another.[428] Peripheral emboli occur in about one-third of the patients; angina and effort syncope are less common.

On auscultation the murmur of aortic stenosis and perhaps of mild aortic regurgitation may dominate the picture. In one series better than one-half the patients lacked an opening snap or an accentuated first sound, and in a considerable number the diastolic rumble was missing[425] (Fig. 25-12). The reason for the relative silence of this mitral stenosis is not altogether clear. In the writer's experience and that of others, the lack of an opening snap even in combined cases has usually been attributed to a calcified and immobilized mitral valve.

Palpation of the chest usually suggests that the diagnosis of isolated aortic stenosis is mistaken.[425] Left ventricular hypertrophy is often not evident, and a right ventricular lift is noted in some of the cases. The blood pressure and pulse pressures are normal. The characteristically abnormal pulse contour of aortic stenosis is often somewhat disguised by abbreviation of the left ventricular stroke output. In our experience, however, the "slow-moving" quality of the carotid pulse has remained even when the pulse duration was shortened.

The electrocardiogram is usually nondescript except for atrial fibrillation or "left atrial" P waves; it usually does not show left ventricular hypertrophy.[426,428] By x-ray there is usually evidence of pulmonary venous hypertension and left atrial enlargement. Calcification of the aortic valve has been found in less than half the patients, a much lower incidence than in isolated aortic stenosis.[426,429] This

---

* With careless auscultation the apical transmission of the aortic systolic murmur may be mistaken for a pansystolic murmur, especially when the second sound is not audible at the apex. A technique for avoiding this mistake has been described (see "Murmur," under "Aortic Stenosis," earlier in this chapter).

probably chiefly reflects the lower age of the patients and the preponderance of females.

Isolated aortic stenosis sometimes causes signs which may be confused with mitral stenosis. A loud fourth sound may be mistaken for a presystolic murmur, and a systolic ejection click maximal at the apex may simulate a loud first sound. Careful auscultation or phonocardiography will make the distinction.

To conclude, if a patient with apparent aortic stenosis has severe respiratory symptoms, atrial fibrillation, and evidence of pulmonary venous hypertension on x-ray, he is usually very far along in the course of his disease and always has marked left ventricular hypertrophy. The lack of left ventricular hypertrophy in such a pattern of clinical findings should always make one suspect hidden mitral stenosis. Absence of aortic valve calcification also suggests the syndrome. Clinical suspicions are not enough in such cases, and careful catheterization of the left side of the heart with calculation of both mitral and aortic valve areas should be done in all patients with combined stenosis whose symp-

toms are severe enough to justify consideration of surgery. If both lesions are severe, surgical correction should not be done unless both can be safely and completely corrected. Only open-heart procedures are acceptable, since even trivial postoperative mitral insufficiency is greatly aggravated by incompletely relieved aortic stenosis.

Aortic Valve Sclerosis

Any thin abrupt shelf, even a narrow one, provided it is perpendicular to the direction of blood flow, is an efficient producer of murmurs, which are a more sensitive gauge of minor obstruction than the pressure gradient obtained at cardiac catheterization.[315] Ejection murmurs in the aortic area of grade I to III intensity are common in the elderly and seem usually to be due to mere atherosclerotic stiffening of the aortic leaflets so that they do not fold back as much as normally.[355] In the past such basal murmurs have been commonly attributed to aortic dilatation, which, however, seems to be an inefficient producer of sound. The audible high-frequency portion of this murmur is always briefer

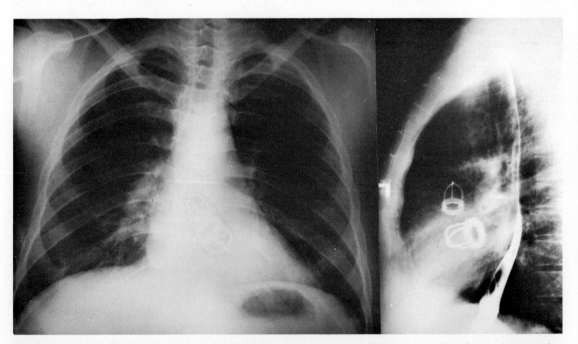

Fig. 25-12. Combined aortic stenosis and mitral stenosis after insertion of double Starr-Edwards prostheses. Before operation the patient, a 32-year-old male, had experienced angina pectoris, dyspnea on effort, and severe nocturnal paroxysmal dyspnea. Yet left ventricular hypertrophy by palpation and electrocardiogram was only borderline. Physical examination revealed nothing except the murmur of aortic stenosis, and there was no evidence of mitral stenosis, which was strongly suspected, however, because of genuine paroxysmal dyspnea in the absence of signs of marked left ventricular hypertrophy. Fluoroscopically the radiologist could not be sure that all the heavy calcification seen was in the aortic valve. The reason for the difficulty can be appreciated from the postoperative film, frontal and lateral views, which shows how closely the mitral and aortic rings lie together, especially in the frontal plane. The silence of the mitral stenosis in this case correlated with an altogether rigid mitral valve in the presence of tight aortic stenosis.

than that of aortic stenosis, corresponding only to the period of peak ejection velocity, usually occupying less than three-fifths of systole and rarely, if ever, approaching within 0.06 sec of the second sound.[355] This timing should be confirmed phonocardiographically. Pathologically there is often calcification of such valves, which, however, usually cannot be seen even with image-intensifier fluoroscopy. The x-ray provides an important differential point, because severe valvular aortic stenosis in the older age group almost invariably produces visible calcification. On the other hand, visible calcification of the proximal coronary arteries is not uncommon in association with valve sclerosis. The lesion does not produce left ventricular hypertrophy, which, if present, is caused by associated hypertension or coronary artery disease.

Carotid or subclavian bruits may also simulate aortic stenosis but may be distinguished by their localization and by the fact that gentle pressure with the stethoscope over the involved vessel sharply increases the murmur.

Mild Aortic Stenosis

The pressure-flow relationship over the aortic valve is such that anatomically significant fusion may occur without any significant pressure gradient, and hence probably without any important physiologic effect.[431] This may occur in any age group, and in children, if isolated, is much more likely to be from a congenitally deformed (perhaps bicuspid) valve than from rheumatic heart disease. Many cases are missed earlier in their course because it is not appreciated that the murmur is maximal in the aortic area and is of the ejection type. Once the lesion is of moderate severity the murmur usually acquires the "not-quite-pansystolic" duration characteristic also of tight aortic stenosis. In the absence of other complicating lesions left ventricular hypertrophy is absent, however. In a person under age 60 no systolic ejection murmur maximal in the aortic area, regardless of length or intensity, is ever "innocent."[388,390] Some persons many years after correction of coarctation of the aorta, have developed severe stenosis of the commonly associated bicuspid aortic valve, which had been clinically inapparent in the earlier phase.

Mild Aortic Stenosis with Serious Symptoms

As noted, disability in mild aortic stenosis may be due to associated coronary disease, to mitral stenosis, or to chronic anxiety. There is also a group of patients (of whom the writer has seen three) with definite but only moderate aortic valve lesions proved at postmortem study or operation. Nonetheless, they have extreme left ventricular hypertrophy and congestive heart failure without obvious cause and finally die of their cardiac disease. Perhaps many of these patients have aortic stenosis complicated by obstructive hypertrophy of the left ventricular outflow tract. Others may have had myocarditis which might have remained silent except for the extra load imposed by the valve defect. A few patients with mild aortic stenosis are definitely hypertensive, and the two sources of strain on the left ventricle are certainly additive.

Supravalvular Stenosis and Discreet Subvalvular Stenosis

These are congenital lesions which may closely mimic valvular stenosis and are discussed on pp. 422 and 423. They both may be associated with mild aortic regurgitation. Discrete (membranous) subvalvular stenosis is often indistinguishable from congenital valvular stenosis.[411]

Functional Hypertrophic Subaortic Stenosis

This is probably a common condition affecting all age groups and producing any of the symptoms of valvular stenosis (Fig. 25-13). Probably under the proper circumstances hypertrophic stenosis can complicate any lesion, producing severe thickening of the wall and encroachment of the cavity of the left ventricle.[432,433] It is probably present in about 10 per cent of patients with severe aortic valvular stenosis; however, usually it is not apparent until the time of operation and sometimes not until the postoperative course has shown that the patient has not been benefited and has acquired new and distinctive physical signs.[384,434] Such subvalvular stenosis may regress spontaneously,[434] but it probably increases the immediate postoperative death rate.

Most cases of hypertrophic stenosis have no obvious cause, and some may have a congenital *anlage*.[432,433,435] There is always generalized cardiac hypertrophy, especially of the septum, which bulges into the area of the left ventricular outflow tract. Commonly associated with this is apparent drawing of the anterior mitral leaflet across the posterior aspect of the aortic outflow.[436] This latter process is thought by some investigators to be due to a congenitally anomalous valve insertion but seems more likely to be due to acquired distortion of the septum.[435,436] In either case the anterior mitral leaflet probably contributes to aortic outflow obstruction, and at least in the latter part of systole, mitral insufficiency often occurs.[317,437]

In some cases there is a family history of a murmur or of sudden death in early life.[433,435] Sometimes there is a personal background of moderate hypertension.[317] The electrocardiogram often shows extreme left ventricular hypertrophy and occasionally seems diagnostic of previous myocardial infarction even when none is present pathologically.[438] Prominent A waves in the neck may be the result of associated right ventricular involvement.[435] The pressure gradient over the left ventricular outflow tract and often the murmur vary strikingly from day to day, being aggravated by anything that makes the muscle-bound heart pump in a more contracted state. Examples of such factors include[432,439,440] inotrophic catecholamines (including those endogenously produced by normal exercise and standing), the Valsalva maneuver, digitalis, and nitrites.

There are several distinguishing features of the condition.

1. The diamond-shaped ejection murmur is maximal at the lower sternal border or apex, rather than in the aortic area.[432,433]

2. Often there is a superimposed murmur of mitral regurgitation so that high frequencies continue into the second sound, especially in the pulmonary area. These auscultatory findings somewhat resemble those of ventricular septal defect and may be almost identical with the murmur produced by many cases of ruptured chordae tendineae. An important characteristic of the auscultatory findings is the disagreement they cause among examining physicians.[319] With careful and repeated auscultation the murmur sometimes appears pansystolic and sometimes not, while its intensity may change for no apparent reason. This behavior, of course, is due to spontaneous variation in the functional abnormality. Hypertrophic subaortic stenosis should always be considered whenever the clinician is tempted to diagnose combined aortic stenosis and mitral insufficiency.

When the murmur blurs into the second heart sound, i.e., appears pansystolic, pharmacologic auscultation may help: Methoxamine or phenylephrine tend to increase ordinary mitral regurgitation by dilating the heart, but this same effect may greatly reduce the aortic outflow gradient in subvalvular obstruction[439] and erase the murmurs. The amyl nitrite test produces a converse effect and is especially useful in patients with softer murmurs. From 30 to 60 sec after the inhalation of this drug, the murmur of the usual case of mitral regurgitation is much reduced;[256] by contrast, in subaortic

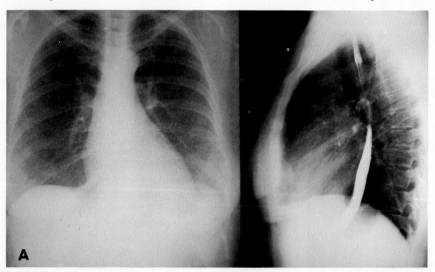

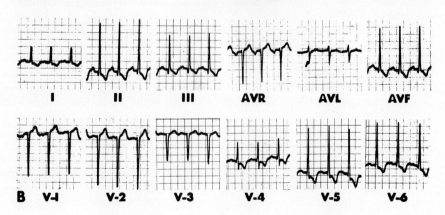

stenosis the murmur, especially its late systolic portion, is greatly augmented. The two tests may be combined.

3. A clear-cut aortic ejection click is never present, but this merely certifies the lack of a mobile or resonant aortic diaphragm. An ejection click is often absent in adults with aortic valvular stenosis.

4. A diastolic murmur of 'aortic insufficiency is never present.

5. The most important feature distinguishing hypertrophic from valvular aortic stenosis is a fast-rising pulse, sometimes with a midsystolic collapse and a definitely smaller second hump[441] (Fig. 25-14). This contour is due to the fact that the obstruction is not critical in early systole but suddenly becomes so about one-half way through the course of left ventricular contraction. At the same moment the mitral leak, when present, seems also to begin or to worsen, producing a late systolic murmur. A late systolic bulge of the apex impulse sometimes coincides with the second hump of the carotid pulse.[434]

6. On x-ray the ascending aorta is seldom dilated. The conspicuous absence of valvular calcification on image-intensifier fluoroscopy should lead

to serious questioning of the diagnosis of severe valvular aortic stenosis in a patient over 40.[384] The heart size is normal in about half the patients and only moderately enlarged in many of the others.[433,435]

7. A patient with aortic stenosis should either have an early systolic ejection click (certifying the presence of a mobile valve diaphragm)[408] or show valvular calcification by fluoroscopy (to explain why the click is absent). If both click and calcium are missing in undoubtedly severe stenosis, a muscular lesion is probable.

Finally, there is a group of patients with idiopathic myocardial hypertrophy who remain asymptomatic and may have ejection murmurs of slight or moderate intensity along with striking and unexplained left ventricular hypertrophy.[442] At cardiac catheterization there is no pressure gradient over the left ventricular outflow tract. These patients seem to have myocardiopathy with only potential or intermittent obstruction. In such instances the amyl nitrite test should be done. In the writer's experience an insignificant murmur may rise to grade IV intensity, becoming a loud systolic diamond, often with a superimposed late systolic mur-

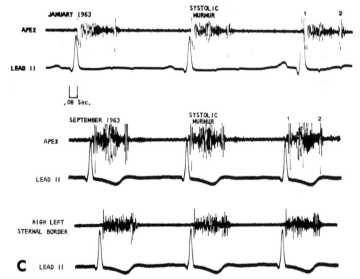

Fig. 25-13. Functional hypertrophic subaortic stenosis. The patient, a 34-year-old female, had a history of curious episodes of prolonged chest pain and effort dyspnea which had been attributed to severe coronary artery disease. The chest film (A, opposite page, frontal and lateral views) showed moderate cardiomegaly, but the electrocardiographic evidence of left ventricular hypertrophy was striking and disproportionate (B, opposite page). The patient had experienced mild labile hypertension, probably due to intermittent relaxation of her subaortic stenosis. The murmur, shown in the phonocardiogram (C), at first was soft (grade II) and was ignored. During the 6-month period after the institution of therapy with large doses of long-acting nitrites and digitalis she deteriorated rapidly and developed severe syncopal episodes. The murmur was then found to be of grade IV intensity, diamond-shaped, and maximal at the apex; however, without question it was frequently pansystolic at the high left sternal border. These findings caused much disagreement among different examiners. A clinical diagnosis of ruptured chordae tendineae was finally made, but cardiac catheterization proved the diagnosis (which in retrospect should have been obvious.)

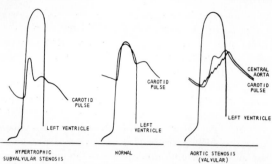

HYPERTROPHIC SUBVALVULAR STENOSIS   NORMAL   AORTIC STENOSIS (VALVULAR)

Fig. 25-14. The differentiation of valvular and hypertrophic subvalvular stenosis by carotid palpation (functional hypertrophic subaortic stenosis). In valvular stenosis (right side of diagram) the gradual ascent of the aortic pulse is to a large degree reflected in the carotid record, which shows an anacrotic notch probably related to the Venturi effect during maximum systolic flow velocity. The pulse contour continues to rise until the occurrence of the second heart sound and does not have the normal rounded top which should clearly reflect the left ventricular pulse. By contrast in subvalvular stenosis (functional hypertrophic subaortic stenosis), depicted in the diagram on the left, the initial rise is often abnormally rapid and the pulse falls away in late systole as subsequent contraction of the left ventricular outflow tract increases the obstruction. The unusually rapid upstroke alone should be enough evidence to indicate that the patient does not have uncomplicated severe valvular aortic stenosis.

mur of mitral regurgitation continuing into the second heart sound. It seems likely that physiologic stress or catechol discharge can have acute and very damaging effects in such cases.

Aortic Insufficiency

Symptoms

Mild rheumatic aortic insufficiency is common both as an isolated lesion (often without a history of rheumatic fever) and in association with overt valve defects.[20,443] In general, a mild lesion does not modify the patient's course except by increasing the risk of bacterial endocarditis.[20,444] No data are available on the natural history of moderate aortic regurgitation. We believe from personal experience, however, that some such patients may develop symptoms of congestive heart failure after many years. The sex incidence, even of minor isolated aortic regurgitation, is predominantly male.

Free aortic insufficiency in rheumatic heart disease is most commonly established early in life.[444-446] The murmur is often first noted during or just after an attack of rheumatic fever, and the average patient has had several attacks.[447] In one series 80 per cent of the patients had had previous

obvious rheumatic fever.[445] There is a 2:1 or 3:1 male sex ratio.[445] The average patient has been observed to have rheumatic fever in his teens (often with recurrent attacks) and to have developed progressively severe aortic insufficiency over a 7- to 10-year period, so that he has advanced valve disease by the time of his early twenties. He still often has no symptoms, however, for perhaps as long as 10 years. In one carefully followed group, about 25 per cent of patients with free aortic regurgitation survived for 20 years almost or completely asymptomatic.[444] The majority, however, succumb to recurrent rheumatic fever, subacute bacterial endocarditis, or heart failure; some die unexpectedly. Nearly 40 per cent of the patients are dead at 10 years and over half of them in 20 years.[444] The more proximate relation of the lesion to rheumatic fever and the rapid evolution to a severe but often stable stage is in distinct contrast to the picture in predominant aortic stenosis.

It is important that the symptoms of severe aortic insufficiency be recognized in their early stages.[445,448] The first symptom may be palpitation due to marked overactivity of the heart and pulse, which can at times cause visible throbbing in the neck or rhythmic splashing noises of the stomach—sources of considerable embarrassment to some patients. Dyspnea on exertion is the commonest early symptom and ultimately will develop in practically every severe case. Once dyspnea begins to occur with ordinary activity, a progressive downhill course can be expected. The onset of left ventricular failure is often ill defined. Excessive sweating and heat intolerance are common early complaints and generally worsen as failure becomes more definitely established.

Angina pectoris may sometimes be an isolated symptom occurring only with heavy exertion for a decade or more.[444,445] Angina coinciding with the onset of heart failure is much more serious, especially when prolonged, atypical, or worse at night. Coronary flow is actually increased in severe aortic insufficiency, but the myocardial oxygen extraction is high, probably indicating relative ischemia.[449] There is a strong tendency for symptoms to cluster, and appearance of one increases the likelihood of another. In the late stages of the illness a distinctive syndrome may appear, characterized by nightmares and a striking vasomotor discharge with tachycardia, marked sweating, flushing, and paroxysmal hypertension; these symptoms generally are closely followed by severe chest pain which requires narcotics for relief.[444] Death may be expected usually within a few months. Sudden death, often at night, may occur, usually in the patient who has developed obvious congestive failure or has severe angina pectoris.

Bacterial endocarditis contributed to the valve damage in one-fourth of the patients in one series of severe aortic regurgitation.[445] Cardiac symptoms may be the main complaint of a patient with endocarditis. Therefore, when any patient with aortic insufficiency first comes to the physician with congestive heart failure or progressive symptoms, it is the duty of his physician to consider the possibility of bacterial endocarditis carefully and to follow up his suspiscions with blood cultures.

Carotid sheath pain is an unusual but rather distinctive symptom of severe aortic regurgitation.[448] It is usually bilateral and often begins acutely with the severe throbbing along the sternomastoid muscles in the neck; the discomfort commonly lasts several days. There is marked tenderness over the involved vessels. Corticosteroids in high dosage usually provide quick relief. The condition seems most likely to be due to acute arteritis. After one attack recurrent episodes are not uncommon.

Abdominal pain is a problem for some patients, particularly in the later stages of the disease.[448] It cannot be explained by the hepatic congestion of heart failure. The location is usually epigastric, and the quality is poorly described. The discomfort has simulated peptic ulcer, gallbladder disease, pancreatitis, and even renal colic. Radiographically and even pathologically no basis has been found for it. The author believes that such pain is often referred cardiac pain. However, spontaneous infarction of the bowel has occurred in association with severe aortic regurgitation.

Physical Examination

The Peripheral Circulation. Although auscultation leads to the diagnosis of aortic insufficiency, the best idea of its physiologic importance can be gained from examination of the peripheral circulation.[451] Trivial aortic insufficiency does not affect the blood pressure. Moderate aortic insufficiency always widens the pulse pressure but not necessarily in direct proportion to the severity of the lesion.[451,452] In severe aortic regurgitation, there is usually a rapidly rising and collapsing pulse.[445,451] The excursion of the wave is often large so that the carotid pulses may be readily visible and obviously bounding. The diastolic collapse is caused not only by the aortic valve leak but often by marked compensatory peripheral vasodilatation. The rapid systolic ascent is produced by the left ventricle, primed with a large end-diastolic volume and discharging into a relatively lax and easily distensible aorta. Various aspects of the pulse have attracted attention. The sharp tap provided by the rapid upstroke has been compared fancifully with that produced by a "water hammer," a Victorian child's toy consisting of a vacuum tube partly filled with water.[42] Pistol shot sounds may be encountered over any of the larger arteries.[453] They are possibly analogous to Korotkoff sounds produced by the blood pressure cuff, occur at the onset of the pulse wave, and probably are correlated as much with the degree of peripheral vasodilatation (and hence also with the shape of the carotid upstroke[453]) as with the amount of aortic regurgitation.[42,453,454] Pistol shot sounds may also be heard in thyrotoxicosis, anemia, pregnancy, and some severe anxiety states. Duroziez's murmur is a biphasic bruit detected with mild pressure of the stethoscope bell over any large artery.[42] Duroziez and others more recently have proposed that all such double murmurs are caused by systolic advancement and diastolic retreat of the arterial blood.[455] The diastolic component heard in severe anemia thyrotoxicosis, however, may perhaps be caused by unusually rapid forward diastolic flow, due to peripheral vasodilatation and the elastic recoil of an overdistended aorta.[42,456] The effect of vasodilatation and diastolic flow reversal may also be seen in abnormal capillary pulsation: alternate paling and flushing of the skin, best appreciated by applying gentle pressure with a glass slide or compressing the nail bed slightly by pushing downward on the free edge of the nail.[445] A host of other redundant signs has been described, all of which merely demonstrate that the circulation is hyperdynamic and usually vasodilated; none is specific for aortic regurgitation.

The blood pressure in free aortic regurgitation often offers a reasonably clear picture of the physiologic derangement. The pulse pressure is wide; there may be systolic hypertension; the diastolic pressure is under 80 and often close to 40.[445,457] One might suppose that the amount of widening of the pulse pressure and lowering of the diastolic pressure would be proportional to the severity of the leak—the diastolic pressure in particular reflecting how closely the aorta and left ventricular pressure equilibrate. This is probably roughly true in the young, perfectly compensated patient with pure aortic regurgitation. It is not true in other cases. The systolic pressure is greatly affected by the rigidity of the aorta and, hence, tends to be higher in the older patient. The diastolic pressure is a function not only of the equilibration of aortic and left ventricular pressures, but also of the peripheral resistance. Therefore, in order to assess the significance of a given level one would have to know both the left ventricular late diastolic pressure and the peripheral resistance. Peripheral vasodilatation is certainly present in many cases of aortic insufficiency and is apparently unrelated to the severity of the lesion. Unfortunately, at present there is no good clinical way to guess the height of the diastolic pressure in the ventricle, which may rise as high as 60 mm Hg in occasional cases.[457] Suffice to say that a blood pressure of 130/65 is compatible with either moderate or extreme regurgitation. Also during severe congestive heart failure the pulse pressure may narrow and the diastolic level may rise. If compensation is restored, the blood pressure often returns to its old levels.[452] During such severe decompensation the patient's cool pale extremities suggest vasoconstriction. This syndrome is always most ominous.

Although the true diastolic blood pressure in free aortic insufficiency is almost never less than 35, the pistol shot sounds over the brachial artery may give a false impression that the level is zero. A change in quality of the sound ("the muffle" point) usually indicates the true value.[458] An observant patient can also recognize the level of his own diastolic pressure as the cuff is progressively deflated by noting the point at which the pulsations in his arm cease and a mild steady ache begins. Aortic insufficiency associated with diastolic hypertension is common, almost never severe, and produces only a very brief murmur which is easily missed.[459] If hypertension is severe and long-standing, the aortic leak is sometimes due to an aortic cusp with fenestrated edges, which began to leak after hypertension had distended the aorta.[460] The leak (and the murmur) often may be eliminated by reducing the blood pressure.

The Heart. Rhythm. The cardiac rhythm is usually regular, and atrial fibrillation should lead one to look for hidden mitral stenosis.

Palpation. The heart in severe aortic regurgitation is hyperdynamic, with a prolonged systolic apex thrust and often a rapid diastolic filling wave. The excursions are wide, and the apex impulse is at least moderately displaced downward and to the left—even in the asymptomatic patient.[29,445] This is in distinct contrast to pure aortic stenosis, in which displacement of the apex usually means an advanced stage of symptoms. In aortic insufficiency of intermediate severity—and in patients with thick chests or advanced failure—the palpatory evidence may not be clean-cut.

Murmurs. A *high-pitched decrescendo diastolic murmur*, beginning with a normal or sometimes accentuated second heart sound, characterizes aortic insufficiency. Short murmurs may simply give the impression that the second sound is blurred. Sometimes, especially in mild aortic insufficiency, there is a brief gap between sound and murmur. At times the murmur may have a musical overtone in addition to its predominant harsh high-frequency content.[42] A strongly musical or low-pitched murmur, however, should suggest syphilitic eversion of an aortic cusp or possibly regurgitation through a smooth hole caused by bacterial endocarditis or

a fenestrated valve.[42] The usual murmur is maximal at the left lower or midsternal border; at the apex it may be loud but is always lower pitched. If the murmur is best heard to the right of the lower sternum, one should suspect unusual dilatation of the ascending aorta, bringing it into close contact with the chest wall in this area.[461] Such dilatation is more likely due to Marfan's syndrome, dissection of the aorta, or syphilis than to rheumatic heart disease. The ability to hear the murmur of aortic regurgitation varies from person to person and from time to time; it is much affected by mild, high-frequency deafness, which is common with advancing age. Grade I intensity to one examiner may be grade III to another. If one is a little deaf, it is often best to listen over the sternum as well as alongside it, since bone is an excellent conductor of high-frequency sound.[462] Listening with the patient leaning forward or on all fours may bring out a previously inaudible murmur; but some murmurs are louder with the patient recumbent.[355] The patient must stop breathing; otherwise a soft murmur will be buried in the breath sounds, which is noise of very similar quality. An amplifying stethoscope is sometimes useful.

A *systolic ejection murmur* of grade II to V intensity (sometimes with a thrill) is the rule in severe aortic regurgitation—but it may fade with the onset of failure.[445,452] Systole may be silent if the aortic leak is small or if the leaflets are particularly flexible. With the augmented systolic flow produced by free aortic regurgitation, however, the most trivial rolling of an aortic cusp may generate considerable sound. Thus the presence of systolic murmur does not necessarily mean that stenosis is present.

Sounds. The first heart sound is normal in mild or moderate cases of aortic regurgitation. It is strikingly reduced in intensity or absent in the extreme cases if the heart rate is normal but may sharpen during tachycardia.[387] A fourth heart sound is rare, perhaps because of the lack of left ventricular rigidity in moderate aortic insufficiency and the nullification of atrial systole by premature mitral closure in the severe cases. A third heart sound is the rule in free aortic regurgitation, even in the absence of symptomatic heart failure, and may initiate a diastolic (Austin Flint) rumble. The Flint rumble is occasionally augmented by atrial contraction in late diastole so that it crescendos into the first heart sound.

An *early systolic click* is common in moderate or severe aortic regurgitation; it simulates the second half of a widely split first heart sound. The phonocardiogram shows, however, that it is too late (usually 0.10 sec after the QRS) to be due to either mitral or tricuspid closure. The author believes that it is a "pistol shot" sound of the central arteries.

Moderate or severe aortic regurgitation commonly creates the *illusion of concomitant mitral stenosis*, especially during tachycardia[276,463] (Fig. 25-15). Superficially the ejection click and an unusually sharp third heart sound may be mistaken for the loud first sound and opening snap of mitral stenosis. Careful auscultation and phonocardiography will readily make these distinctions. The diastolic rumble is a more difficult problem. Combined mitral and aortic lesions are common, and the signs of mitral stenosis may be much altered by concomitant aortic insufficiency (see Mitral Stenosis earlier in this chapter). It has been stated that the only definitive diagnosis of a Flint murmur is at the autopsy table or in the cardiac catheterization laboratory. Statistically the Flint murmur may be diagnosed when other clinical features are absolutely typical of moderate or severe aortic regurgitation, and there are no other auscultatory signs of mitral stenosis or mitral calcification by x-ray. There remains a significant gray zone. A valuable and crucial test is provided by the inhalation of amyl nitrite.[464] This substance produces an increase of the heart rate and cardiac output but marked peripheral vasodilatation. It greatly reduces both the murmur of aortic insufficiency and the Flint rumble but strikingly augments the murmur of mitral stenosis. Amyl nitrite also often allows the distinction of aortic insufficiency and pulmonary insufficiency.

Clinical-physiologic Correlation. At present the full spectrum of possible diastolic events produced by aortic insufficiency has not been clearly related with clinical findings. However, physiologic and cineangiographic studies suggest that:

1. In *mild aortic regurgitation* the leak is largest in early diastole and quickly tapers. This is perhaps the result of a higher initial aortic tension in early diastole and a slightly larger initial opening caused by maximal traction on the valve ring from systolic distension of the aorta. The briefer murmurs may sound like a blur on the end of the second heart sound. Leaks of a little greater severity are likely to cause murmurs of more definite duration. On listening with an amplifying stethoscope, one may be surprised to find that the length of the murmur is somewhat greater than previously appreciated, and cineangiography often shows a small continuing leak when no sound is audible. Unfortunately, quantitative observations are hard to make because soft, high-frequency sounds are much better heard than recorded with present equipment.

2. In *moderate and severe aortic regurgitation*, the flow, though maximal in early diastole, continues at considerable velocity throughout the filling period of the ventricle. In spite of an aperture of

perhaps 0.3 cm², the valve remains an important obstruction to backflow and never allows any close approximation of aortic and left ventricular diastolic pressures. Here the murmur, in spite of a decrescendo shape, often quite audibly fills diastole at a heart rate of 70 beats per minute because of persistence of a diastolic gradient over the aortic valve. The duration of diastole (and hence the heart rate) is an important determinant of how much blood leaks.[465] Exercise tachycardia, therefore, is comparatively well tolerated. In spite of the competition between left atrial and aortic influx, left ventricular pressure never rises high enough to close the mitral valve,[457] and therefore atrial contraction can interact with the aortic regurgitation. Occasionally atrial systole may appear to interrupt the aortic diastolic murmur.[42] This is especially likely to happen if there is giant atrial contraction excited by concomitant aortic stenosis. At other times the atrial contraction (especially if the P-R interval is prolonged) may actually augment the intensity of the aortic diastolic murmur, as well as the apical diastolic rumble.[42,463] Differentiation of the two murmurs at the apex is not easy, for transmission of the aortic murmur lowers its pitch.[42,315] A typical Flint rumble with presystolic accentuation probably occurs most commonly in this type of case. Pathologically jet lesions on the anterior mitral cusp indicate that aortic leak may sometimes be directed against it.[356] In these cases it has been thought that a pandiastolic rumble may be produced because the anterior leaflet is held in the middle of two opposing streams from atrium and aorta (like the reed of an oboe) throughout diastole.[463]

Regardless of the mechanism of the Flint rumble, when the P-R interval is normal, any atrial effect on the murmurs gives useful information, implying that the ventricular end-diastolic pressure is not too high to nullify the effect of atrial systole. The first sound is normal in moderately severe aortic regurgitation unless the P-R interval is prolonged.

3. In *extreme aortic regurgitation* and in cases where the ventricle is noncompliant the pressure in the chamber may rapidly rise toward aortic levels. If it exceeds left atrial pressure before the onset of left ventricular contraction, it produces premature upward tensing of the mitral curtain and, perhaps for this reason, great attenuation of the first heart sound.[387] If the ventricular pressure rises even faster, it may actually equilibrate with the aortic pressure at a normal heart rate.[457] Such cases are rare but explain some instances in which the diastolic murmur of severe aortic regurgitation is rather brief, lasting only for the first half of diastole at a heart rate of 70 beats per minute. Such patients have usually had clinical signs of failure, but

restoration of clinical compensation does not restore the ventricular diastolic pressure to normal.[457]

X-ray Findings. In severe aortic insufficiency the apex of the heart is usually elongated, producing a boot-shaped configuration in the frontal projection.[104,414] The posterior extent of the dilated left ventricle may also be considerable, so that cardiac size may be greatly underestimated unless a lateral film is also taken. Often the apex projects even behind the barium-filled esophagus. Left atrial enlargement is not uncommon but may be hard to distinguish in the presence of marked left ventricular dilatation.

Even with the use of image-intensifier fluoroscopy, valvular calcification is considerably less commonly detected than in cases with a significant element of stenosis. It is seen in only about one-fifth of the patients with severe aortic regurgitation.[414] Increased left ventricular pulsation produces a "rocking heart," with large systolic and diastolic excursions. There should also be a diffuse increase in the entire aortic pulsation, involving both the ascending and descending portions. If dif-ferential pulsations and disproportionate dilatation of the ascending aorta are definitely present, the diagnosis of free aortic rheumatic regurgitation is usually mistaken. In such a case there is (1) an important element of stenosis, or (2) aortic wall disease, usually caused by Marfan's syndrome or syphilis.

X-ray findings are not always striking or directly proportional to the severity of the lesion; duration of the condition probably has an important effect.

The Electrocardiogram. The electrocardiogram in moderate aortic insufficiency is often not distinctive, but in free aortic regurgitation usually shows some abnormality.[466] It has been claimed that the earliest changes consist of increased voltage of both QRS and T waves in the lateral precordial leads.[467] In actual fact, this is uncommon, and electrocardiographic changes once they appear are usually the traditional ones of left ventricular hypertrophy.[339,466] Left axis deviation in aortic insufficiency appears earlier in the course of the disease than in aortic stenosis but is not necessarily present. Left ventricular parietal block (with a wide angle

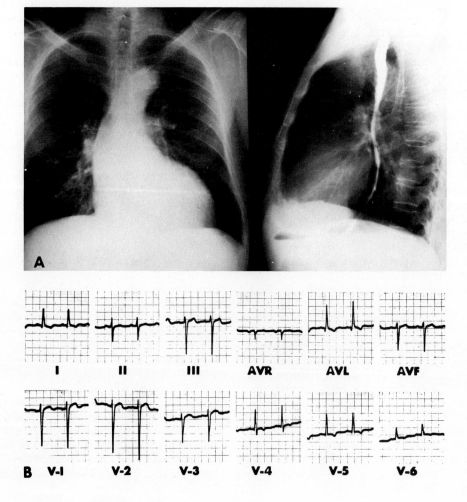

between the initial and terminal 0.04 sec of the QRS) is found in about one-third of the patients.[466] A widened QRS complex is occasionally seen, but the classic left bundle branch block is not usual. Severe ST-T abnormalities are present in the great majority of severe or symptomatic cases. P-wave abnormalities of the left atrial type are rather common[466] and may precede obvious left ventricular failure. This fact is not surprising in view of the enormous atrial pressure sometimes generated in contracting against the high left ventricular end-diastolic pressures produced by the abnormal communication with the aortic reservoir. The P-R interval is commonly prolonged in severe aortic regurgitation. Atrial fibrillation is very rare and should suggest either terminal disease or associated mitral stenosis. If there are definite symptoms, the electrocardiogram practically always shows some evidence for left ventricular hypertrophy, though not necessarily enough to make a firm diagnosis. Vectorcardiographic techniques may improve its specificity.[417]

Estimation of the Severity of Aortic Insufficiency. Inconsequential aortic insufficiency is easy to recognize from the soft, very brief diastolic blow and the normal pulse pressure.

Severe aortic insufficiency is also frequently obvious from (1) the loud diastolic murmur lasting at least one-half of diastole, (2) the bounding pulse and wide pulse pressure, (3) the presence of an S_3

(ventricular gallop), (4) dampening of the first sound in the occasional cases with exceptionally high left ventricular end-diastolic pressure (a prolonged PR interval is a common and much more innocuous cause for this finding), (5) an abnormal difference between the blood pressures in the arm and leg (Hill's sign). Normally the pressures in arm and leg are identical; the higher pressures commonly recorded in the leg are spurious and due to use of a small arm cuff which inadequately compresses the vessels.[468] If one uses a smaller cuff, it should be applied to the ankle. According to a recent angiographic correlation study, Hill's sign is the most reliable clinical index of the severity of aortic regurgitation. If the systolic pressure in the leg is less than 20 mm above that in the arms, the aortic insufficiency is mild; if the differential is 20 to 40 mm, the insufficiency is moderate; if it is over 60 mm, there is gross regurgitation.[469] The author believes that Hill's sign (and perhaps other tests) underestimate the size of the aortic regurgitant orifice when there is significant concomitant mitral insufficiency.

In the older patient with a murmur of aortic insufficiency and a wide pulse pressure, careful fluoroscopy of the aorta will help to decide if there is truly a hyperdynamic circulation. The sclerotic aorta of the aged produces a wide pulse pressure but does not pulsate actively on fluoroscopy.

It should be recalled again that a clinically meas-

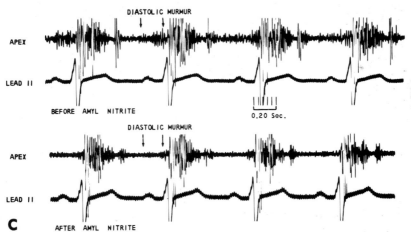

Fig. 25-15. Severe aortic insufficiency with mild cardiac symptoms and an Austin Flint murmur. The patient, a man of 55, had a history of two episodes of bacterial endocarditis in 10 years, but his only cardiac medication was digitalis. His x-ray (A, opposite page, frontal and lateral views) showed diffuse dilatation of the ascending aorta, a classic boot-shaped silhouette, and left atrial impression on the esophagus. A fluoroscopy, pulsation of the entire thoracic aorta was greatly increased. The electrocardiogram (B, opposite page) showed left ventricular hypertrophy. The blood pressure was 160/60. Superimposed on a loud transmitted murmur of aortic insufficiency at the apex was a lower-frequency diastolic rumble with presystolic accentuation (see phonocardiogram C). For 1 minute after peripheral vasodilatation with amyl nitrite the diastolic blow virtually disappeared and the rumble was also considerably decreased, strongly implying that the latter was related to the aortic insufficiency rather than to associated mitral stenosis. Tachycardia was induced by exercise for the control tracing.

ured diastole blood pressure of 60 or 70 mm Hg is as compatible with extreme regurgitation as with mild. It is not always possible to guess clinically whether a given diastolic pressure is mainly a question of peripheral vasodilatation or of an exceptionally high late diastolic pressure in the left ventricle. Congestive failure tends to elevate the diastolic blood pressure and thus hide the significance of the aortic leak.[452,457]

For surgical purposes one would like to know the size of the abnormal diastolic orifice in the aortic valve. Elaborate and ingenious methods have been devised for measuring regurgitant flow, but these may not allow an accurate prediction of the size and fixity of the opening. Backflow is also affected considerably by the peripheral resistance, perhaps by the diastolic compliance (distensibility) of the left ventricle, and very likely by co-existing lesions such as mitral regurgitation, which provides competition for diastolic filling during the early phase of rapid inflow. Cineangiography is the best available method for demonstrating the anatomic cause of aortic insufficiency and estimating the extent of valve damage. Yet it is least reliable where it is most needed—in the evaluation of combined aortic and mitral disease. At present the surgeon must approach many such cases with an open mind; the decision whether to replace one or both valves often cannot be made except at the operating table.

Less Common Causes of Aortic Regurgitation

1. Bacterial endocarditis is the first diagnosis to consider in any patient with the abrupt onset of aortic regurgitation or the sudden aggravation of an existing lesion. The clinical spectrum of the disease is wide. If blood cultures have been drawn and the physician is not quite sure whether endocarditis is present, he should regard his uncertainty as grounds for beginning treatment.

2. Rheumatoid aortic regurgitation may be distinguished by its classic relationships to the course of spondylitis.[471] It may occasionally occur in purely peripheral rheumatoid arthritis.

3. Syphilitic aortic insufficiency is often associated with disproportionate dilatation of the ascending aorta (and sometimes tell-tale calcification confined to this area).[472] A predominantly right-sided murmur of aortic insufficiency correlates well with such roentgenologic evidence. Eversion of a cusp, producing a musical or a groaning diastolic murmur, is a rather distinctive but unusual result of syphilis.[42] The ordinary serologic tests are often negative, but in many cases the treponema immobilization test or the fluorescent treponema antibody test is still positive.[473]

4. Marfan's syndrome may cause aortic regurgitation by producing dilatation of the aortic sinuses

and the base of the aorta.[474] This may occur early in the disease and without any obvious roentgenographic signs. Selective transmission of the murmur to the right lower sternal area and localized fluoroscopic pulsation to the base of the aorta may sometimes cause one to suspect the diagnosis even in its early stage. As the disease progresses, dilatation may extend up the entire acending aorta, producing disproportionate enlargement and pulsation of this segment. These findings in a patient with free aortic insufficiency should always suggest either syphilis or Marfan's syndrome. In the latter condition, murmurs may be confusing because of the frequent association of mitral regurgitation due to abnormal redundancy of the mitral leaflets.

5. An aortic dissection may produce aortic insufficiency both in Marfan's syndrome and in other cases of cystic necrosis. Such patients only occasionally survive to the chronic stage, but in such instances the pain may have been atypical or absent. Fluoroscopically the intramural hematoma often produces a sharply demarcated zone of abscence or markedly decreased pulsation in an enlarged aorta.

6. Congenital aortic insufficiency may sometimes be distinguished by a long history of a murmur. Its origin is not clearly established, but it may be due to unusual behavior of a bicuspid valve, which, however, as an isolated lesion rarely leaks.[476] On the other hand, aortic regurgitation due to an associated bicuspid valve is common in the presence of aortic coarctation because of the high pressure and distention of the ascending aorta. Though usually mild, such regurgitation can be severe enough to produce active femoral pulses and help conceal the presence of the coarctation. Aortic regurgitation associated with a ventricular septal defect is likely to be confused with conditions causing a continuous murmur.

7. An unruptured congenital aneurysm of the sinus of Valsalva, if large enough to put traction on the aortic ring, may cause the valve to leak.[477,478] Rupture of the sinus into the left ventricle has an identical effect. The diagnosis requires aortography but is suggested by the sudden onset of aortic regurgitation in a patient with a longstanding systolic murmur or with a history of no previous murmurs.

8. Mild aortic insufficiency is not uncommon among older hypertensive patients (5 per cent).[459] Usually the lesion is a minimal shortening of the edge of a cusp, likely rheumatic, and surprisingly trivial—until one recalls how much the leak of aortic insufficiency may be augmented by raising the peripheral resistance.

9. Fenestration of the aortic valve is another cause of the very brief, soft aortic diastolic murmur

heard in long-standing hypertensives.[459] Even normotensive individuals may develop large fenestrations and significant leaks, usually in association with dilatation of the aorta from cystic medionecrosis.[479] A hypertensive patient who suddenly acquires free aortic regurgitation and drops his diastolic pressure to 50 or 60 mm Hg has probably ruptured a fenestrated cusp.[460]

10. Traumatic rupture has rarely occurred after blows to the chest or heavy lifting,[445] perhaps sometimes in a congenitally predisposed individual.

11. Aortic insufficiency is also reported occasionally in other conditions. These include disseminated lupus erythematosus, relapsing polychondritis, pseudo-xanthoma elasticum, Reiter's syndrome, and a curious chronic nonsyphilitic aortitis.[480–483] Aortic insufficiency may also be disproportionately common among patients with idiopathic retinal detachment.

Compound Aortic Valve Lesions

Even with major insufficiency, the rheumatic process has a strong tendency to produce commissural fusion;[97] therefore, there are many gradations from tight stenosis to major incompetence and there is a large area of overlap in all the signs and physiologic manifestations. This presents a fascinating prospect to the clinician interested in clinical-physiologic correlations. Yet all these lesions represent badly shrunken and immobilized aortic valves. To quote an extreme example: with a rigid orifice of 0.5 cm² in both systole and diastole, either stenosis or insufficiency would be critical in the absence of the other lesion. Even if one type of valvular dysfunction predominates, the presence of the other greatly multiplies its effect. Now that the surgical approach has taken the course of complete replacement rather than valvuloplasty, defining the predominant disorder of a badly destroyed aortic valve has become relatively unimportant. What should be established is whether the valvular deformity is severe and is the cause of the patient's symptoms. Sometimes the latter point may be difficult to settle. Prolonged clinical observation, cardiac catheterization, angiocardiography, and even coronary arteriography may be needed.

Although loudness of both systolic and diastolic aortic murmurs does not necessarily mean a destroyed valve with a fixed orifice, certain other features help confirm the diagnosis. Heavy calcification added to these auscultatory findings is very good evidence. Gross regurgitation through a moderately stenotic fixed orifice is probably the clinical situation most likely to produce a "carotid shudder" —a heavily vibrating but active carotid pulse.[484]

The pulse contour in compound lesions may have a surging collapsing quality owing to a large but rather slow upstroke and rapid diastolic descent. In cases where insufficiency is predominant, a pulsus bisferiens is often apparent on palpation of the carotid.[422] This pulse rises very rapidly, falls away briefly in midsystole, and then reaches a second peak before collapsing in diastole. It may be easier to appreciate the quick-rising, broad-topped, and rapidly falling character of such a pulse than the sharp notch in its center. The notch is important, however, because it implies a Venturi effect from an unusually forceful systolic flow which has been converted into a jet by perhaps a modicum of stenosis and is powerfully augmented by the blood that has regurgitated into the ventricle during diastole;[422] in fact, the effect requires very little commissural fusion. The pulsus bisferiens is not confined to aortic regurgitation.[319] A somewhat similar pulse (with, however, a smaller second peak) may occur in functional hypertrophic subaortic stenosis. A briefer and much smaller pulse, also with a midsystolic collapse, can be felt in severe mitral regurgitation, and this fact can be convincingly documented by angiocardiography.

The routine x-ray and electrocardiogram are not of much help in evaluating compound aortic lesions, except to help establish that the disease is severe.

The development of a large systolic gradient obviously implies that the valve lesion is severe—regardless of its exact nature. Cineangiocardiography provides the best available assessment of the disturbed physiology.

Once congestive failure has developed, patients with compound aortic valve lesions may present a very confusing clinical picture. The systolic murmur softens, and the significance of the diastolic murmur may be underestimated because of the narrowing of the pulse pressure produced by failure. It is a good rule to pay special attention to any aortic murmur detected during cardiac decompensation and to remember that an iceberg of disease may be concealed under it.

Medical Treatment

Aortic Stenosis

The only satisfactory treatment of severe aortic stenosis is surgical, but at present the risk of operation is too high and the long-range effects are too uncertain for it to be recommended for asymptomatic patients. The most important aspect of medical care is intelligent observation of the patient's course early in the disease to make sure that he is genuinely asymptomatic and to detect the point when acceleration of the disease process begins. At each follow-up visit the electrocardiogram is checked and the patient is asked to recount all unusual exertion and his response to it. The physician must constantly reweigh the risk of continued inaction versus the danger of the presently available surgical operations. The patient who first comes to the physician with heart failure must be digitalized, given diuretics, and returned if necessary to electrolyte balance before he is presented to the surgeon. Surgical treatment should be considered for all patients with any sign of left ventricular failure and for all those with more than mild angina or occasional effort syncope. Former reservations about the use of artificial valves are falling away because of the success with the Starr-Edwards prosthesis.

Prolonged medical treatment of advanced aortic stenosis is generally unsatisfactory, amounting to a holding operation for patients who for one reason or another cannot have surgical therapy. Severe aortic stenosis in the elderly associated also with severe occlusive coronary artery disease (proved if possible by coronary angiography) seems to be the prime example of such a case. Yet with the combination of chlorothiazide and spironolactone, even severe congestive heart failure can often be controlled surprisingly well, and the present prospect for aortic stenosis is probably less gloomy than any available data imply. Angina may often be helped with nitrites, but one should be on the lookout for nitrite syncope. Although hypertension may compound the physiologic disorder in moderate aortic stenosis, most of our present therapies for hypertension tend to reduce stroke output rather than the peripheral resistance itself, and the writer's own experience indicates that they are not helpful.

When a diagnosis of asymptomatic aortic stenosis is made in a young person clinical clues will often tell whether it is very mild or moderate to severe. It is not proper or honest to reassure a patient with mild aortic stenosis that he has a "functional murmur," since there is a definite possibility that his lesion may ·progress. Rather, the patient should be told in explicit terms that he has a minor aortic valve condition, which though likely never to be of importance, may perhaps someday cause fatigue or dyspnea (these being the commonest early complaints) and will require both strict annual follow-up and prompt reporting of symptoms. The patient with senile aortic valve sclerosis should be reassured about his murmur; but a general search should be made for reduced pulses or for arterial bruits; alertness should be maintained for symptoms of atherosclerosis.

In cases with combined mitral and aortic stenosis, surgical therapy should not be recommended until both lesions can be safely corrected using open-heart techniques. Clinical assessment of valve mobility is relevant. If one or both valves appear mobile and well preserved (as is not uncommonly the case), operation may be more readily undertaken, since direct-vision valvuloplasty (rather than insertion of a prosthesis) may suffice.

The patient with asymptomatic but probably severe aortic stenosis presents a special problem. The possibility of sudden death is a constant worry. Yet the physician should not confide his disquietude to the patient until the time comes when he feels that operative treatment is indicated. Then he may use all the facts at his disposal to help persuade the patient of the proper course. It is a little comfort to remember that (after childhood) there is usually some warning period before sudden death in aortic stenosis. Unfortunately, this is not always true. No drugs are required for the patient without symptoms. Though digitalis improves some parameters of left ventricular function in persons without failure,[485] it serves clinically only to confuse interpretation of the electrocardiogram. Curtailing exercise, except for the most strenuous, is probably a useless precaution and serves only to compound the patient's anxieties. It is the physician's duty to see that no such patient is lost to follow-up. The problem will become much simpler when we can advise prophylactic replacement of the aortic valve without the fear of a 20 per cent incidence of significant late complications.

Aortic Insufficiency

In mild or moderate aortic insufficiency, the only important treatment is prophylaxis of bacterial endocarditis and education of the patient to recognize the early symptoms of this disease so as to make his own diagnosis, if possible. He should be impressed with the importance of (1) 4 days of penicillin therapy after any oral procedure; (2) penicillin and streptomycin therapy after any urologic procedure; (3) avoiding antibiotics until obtaining blood cultures when he suspects that he has developed bacterial endocarditis. Early self-diagnosis by an intelligent patient is the best way to reduce the death toll. In severe aortic insufficiency medical therapy is probably of little benefit before symptoms develop, although prophylactic digitalization has been recommended. Once the stage of advancing symptoms has begun, surgical replacement of the aortic valve should be advised. In patients who do not have operation, careful therapy of congestive heart failure often gets very good symptomatic results for some years. Concomitant coronary artery disease seems to be a rather uncertain problem in patients with severe aortic insufficiency. Yet if surgery is being considered and angina seems disproportionate to the other findings, coronary angiograms should probably be done.

TRICUSPID DISEASE

Pathologically tricuspid valvular disease is present in 20 to 30 per cent of patients with severe rheumatic heart lesions.[486] Clinically important organic tricuspid disease, however, is far less common, probably amounting to no more than 5 or 10 per cent of such patients. The clinical diagnosis of tricuspid lesions is complicated by the facts that (1) they are seldom isolated and usually occur in combination with severe mitral or aortic disease; (2) they are very much affected by the functional stage of the right side of the heart. Postmortem inspection will show that the competence of the tricuspid valve is dependent on effective contraction of the right ventricle and tricuspid ring and that dilatation of the ventricle much more readily produces functional incompetence than on the left side of the heart.[487] Dilatation of the right ventricle is extremely common as a consequence of pulmonary hypertension from mitral or aortic valve disease. Therefore, any lesion of the tricuspid valve (except tight stenosis) is likely to be compounded by functional tricuspid insufficiency, which may vary from time to time.[285]

Tricuspid Insufficiency

Isolated tricuspid insufficiency is well tolerated, but pulmonary vascular obstruction increases the right ventricular systolic pressure and greatly aggravates the effect of the tricuspid leak. Advanced deformity of the tricuspid valve is not nearly so common as that of the mitral or aortic valve, and there is usually some commissural fusion as part of the abnormality.[486] In general, if the functional component is dominant, the lesion improves with treatment for cardiac failure or mitral or aortic valve surgery. Organic tricuspid insufficiency, however, tends to be more obvious after the improvement of the left-sided lesion, and in some cases the diagnosis can be delayed until after successful mitral or aortic valvulotomy has increased the cardiac output.[375]

The patient's symptoms are usually those of his left-sided lesion, although in some cases the development of tricuspid insufficiency and severe right-sided congestion seems to relieve some of the paroxysmal pulmonary symptoms and orthopnea. Jaundice, pain in the right upper quadrant from an engorged liver, and cyanosis are classical signs of tricuspid insufficiency compounded with right ventricular hypertension. If the patient is a female and has severe disease of the mitral and aortic valves with a history of prolonged, recurring venous stasis, there is also very likely to be an element of organic tricuspid disease.[486] Symptoms usually

begin relatively early, often in the late twenties.

Clinical Examination. Significant tricuspid insufficiency always elevates the venous pressure, producing a systolic jugular pulse which extends above the level of the cricoid cartilage of the neck with the patient propped 45° above the horizontal.[488] One may use the pulsating venous column as a manometer to calculate the pressure in the right atrium, which lies 4 cm beneath and along an imaginary plumb line dropped from the sternomanubrial angle. If the venous pressure is very high, the patient's head should be gradually elevated until the top of the oscillating venous column can be seen. The predominant venous pulse wave is systolic and therefore might be mistaken for the carotid pulse. The venous wave, however, rises and falls much more slowly than does the carotid, a fact which can be easily appreciated by simultaneous palpation of the left carotid and observation of the right jugular pulse. It is best not to base deductions about the venous pressure on the appearance of the left jugular pulse, because dilatation of the aorta may distend the vessel.[490] Auscultation of the heart is less useful in the diagnosis of tricuspid insufficiency. Both organic and predominantly functional tricuspid leaks may produce a systolic murmur maximal at the lower sternal border and augmented by inspiration.[302,486] A mild leak, however, may produce a loud murmur, while severe tricuspid insufficiency may be silent.[488] If a murmur is present, it is often but not always augmented by inspiration which selectively increases the filling of the right ventricle. At present there is no satisfactory hemodynamic method to separate functional and organic tricuspid insufficiency. Clinical and radiographic signs of pulmonary hypertension very strongly suggest an important functional component. The electrocardiogram usually shows the effects of a dominant left-sided lesion. Atrial fibrillation is usually present in severe cases. The x-ray is likely to show marked generalized cardiomegaly. Right atrial enlargement may produce considerable prominence of the cardiac silhouette to the right of the midline. It should be remembered that a giant left atrium may project similarly to the right, though at a lower level, touching the diaphragm.[342]

Tricuspid Stenosis

Moderate degrees of tricuspid stenosis in association with other valve lesions are probably of clinical importance in 3 to 5 per cent of rheumatic patients.[302,303,486,489] Critical tricuspid stenosis is unusual, and isolated tricuspid stenosis is extremely rare and often possibly congenital or related to metastatic carcinoid. Rheumatic tricuspid stenosis occurs more often in females than in males. The average patient is about 30 years old and has a definite history of rheumatic fever with involvement of both mitral and aortic valves. In about one-third of patients with readily diagnosable cases the tricuspid lesion is even more important than the mitral.[302] The history should suggest tricuspid stenosis when a patient with mitral stenosis or aortic valve disease, though perhaps dyspneic and orthopneic, seems unusually free of paroxysmal pulmonary symptoms. This freedom is perhaps due to the attenuating effect of tricuspid obstruction on abrupt increases of blood flow into the lesser circulation. In advanced cases the patient's recurrent hepatomegaly, ascites, and edema seem out of proportion to the rest of his illness.

Clinical Examination. The diagnosis of tricuspid stenosis can usually be strongly suspected from physical examination, although its degree may not always be accurately predicted. The jugular venous pulse provides the most important clinical evidence, especially in the presence of sinus rhythm, which may persist in one-third to one-half of cases. The examination should be conducted with the patient propped up halfway in bed, the examiner palpating the left carotid and observing the right internal jugular pulse. The distinctive finding is a large A wave which sometimes is brief and sharp enough to be mistaken for an arterial pulse. With simultaneous carotid palpation, it is very easy to recognize the presystolic nature of the A wave. In the presence of atrial fibrillation the A wave is wiped out; the contour of the pulse is much less specific, and trivial associated insufficiency may produce large systolic waves, falsely suggesting major incompetence.[489] Severe tricuspid stenosis may be excluded, however, if one observes a surging and collapsing venous pulse of the type commonly seen in severe right-sided failure or tricuspid insufficiency.[302] A rapid early diastolic fall cannot occur in the presence of severe tricuspid stenosis; in fact, slowness of the Y descent (from the apex of the systolic wave at the second heart sound) can often be appreciated on clinical examination, provided one carefully times the venous pulse by simultaneous palpation of the carotid.

In examination of the heart the character of the apex and parasternal impulse is usually too much modified by other valve disease to be of much help to the diagnosis.

Auscultation of the heart, however, frequently allows a firm diagnosis to be made. The characteristic murmur of tricuspid stenosis is maximal at the lower left sternal border and is sometimes considerably higher pitched than that of mitral stenosis.[303] In the presence of sinus rhythm, it is almost always concentrated in the period of atrial

systole and its augmentation by inspiration is obvious. It is important that the patient be asked to breathe deeply and freely. The characteristic augmentation of the murmur (Carvalho's sign) is usually most marked during active inspiration and diminishes as the breath is held, particularly if the patient performs a slight involuntary Valsalva maneuver.[302] Since the P-R interval is commonly prolonged in tricuspid stenosis, the presystolic murmur is often remarkably discrete and separate from the first sound.[302] In the presence of atrial fibrillation the murmur follows closely after the second heart sound, and since it is sometimes scratchy or high pitched, it may be mistaken for an aortic-diastolic murmur or a Graham Steele murmur.[303] Careful auscultation or phonocardiography will show that its onset is separated from the second heart sound by at least 0.05 sec, a pattern which is rare in significant aortic insufficiency. The murmur is not always augmented by inspiration and is dependent on many factors, including the thickness of the patient's chest and the character of his respiration. When Carvalho's sign is noted, however, it is almost pathognomonic of a right-sided murmur. The opening snap of tricuspid disease can only rarely be distinguished from that of concomitant mitral stenosis.[302] If the mitral valve is heavily calcified and the first heart sound is diminished at the apex, an opening snap sound may be reasonably attributed to the tricuspid lesion. If inspiration definitely augments the snap, the diagnosis is on firmer ground.

The electrocardiogram in severe tricuspid stenosis usually shows (1) large, narrowly peaked P waves, downwardly directed (best seen in lead AVF and III but positive in V—the "right atrial configuration," a valuable sign erased of course by atrial fibrillation); (2) no right ventricular hypertrophy unless produced by concomitant tight mitral stenosis. Correlation of the electrocardiogram and the venous pulse is useful.[302] "Right atrial" P waves and giant jugular A waves may also be due to severe right ventricular hypertrophy with a marked right ventricular heave and clinical and radiographic signs of severe pulmonary hypertension. Isolated signs of overactive right atrial contraction are probably due to tricuspid obstruction. Since associated severe mitral stenosis and pulmonary hypertension are common, however, frank right ventricular hypertrophy not uncommonly does occur in spite of severe tricuspid stenosis.[489]

The x-ray is often not diagnostic because of left-sided valvular disease. If the tricuspid stenosis is a dominant lesion, however, a striking finding is prominence of the right border of the heart which is out of proportion to the size of the pulmonary arteries or other evidence of pulmonary hypertension.

Problems in the Diagnosis of Tricuspid Disease

1. Sometimes tricuspid disease may be overestimated (see Fig. 25-16). If a low cardiac output and severe valvular calcification have obliterated many of the signs of mitral and aortic stenosis, the tricuspid murmurs and sounds may be given a false prominence. Assessment of the entire picture, with emphasis on the radiographic demonstration of pulmonary venous congestion and aortic and mitral valve calcium, should help to keep the proper perspective.

2. The interaction of functional and organic factors in tricuspid disease may produce a confusing picture. The best way to solve this problem is by serial observations of the patient during the course of treatment. If the venous pressure comes down to normal after diuresis and bed rest, it is unlikely that the tricuspid lesion is critical. In cases where the murmurs persist or become louder after the venous pressure has been lowered considerably, one should suspect that there is definite tricuspid valve disease, compounded by the effects of right ventricular failure.

3. Tricuspid stenosis may be simulated by other conditions. (a) Right atrial myxoma should be excluded by angiocardiography in every patient with an apparently isolated tricuspid lesion. (b) Constrictive pericarditis has been mistakenly diagnosed in some cases. However, it produces no murmurs and an altogether different venous pulse. Constriction oscillations at the top of the venous column are small in proportion to the height of the pressure, and the diastolic descent of the venous pulse (which may be timed because it begins roughly with the second heart sound) is a mere flicker. In tricuspid stenosis the diastolic descent is slow and prolonged, and A waves (during sinus rhythm) stand out in bold relief from the rest of the pulse.

4. Tricuspid stenosis may also be produced by carcinoid, endocardial fibroelastosis, and possibly by systemic lupus erythematosus.

In suspected but doubtful cases cardiac catheterization supplemented with angiocardiography should be performed, especially in the presence of atrial fibrillation; the tricuspid gradient may be small even with severe stenosis. Holdup of contrast material in the right atrium, a relatively small right ventricle, and the absence of tricuspid regurgitation are all valuable clues that may be provided by angiocardiography. The diastolic gradient, like the murmur, is much augmented by inspiration.[489]

Unless tricuspid stenosis is of proved critical severity, one should hesitate to advise surgical treatment. Since there is very likely to be an associated element of tricuspid insufficiency, most tricuspid valves are not really suitable for ordinary closed valvulotomy. A tricuspid valve stenotic enough to cause symptoms is best handled quite conservatively by the surgeon or replaced outright; valvuloplasties have given disappointing results. On the other hand, surgical palliation of severe tricuspid insufficiency by annuloplasty often improves the chances of a severely and chronically ill patient with multivalvular disease.[285]

RHEUMATOID HEART DISEASE

Rheumatoid Spondylitis

Severe ankylosing spondylitis, especially if also associated with peripheral joint involvement,* may produce three kinds of heart lesions (almost always in males):[471,491–493]

1. Pericarditis always parallels severe arthritic symptoms and clinically is often overshadowed by them[494]—but in children may sometimes lead to cardiac tamponade.

2. Occasionally nodules in the heart are grossly and pathologically very similar to those encountered peripherally under the skin in ordinary rheumatoid arthritis.[493] These are rarely of any clinical significance, although one case of mitral regurgitation seems to have resulted from a strategically placed nodule.

3. An important and distinctive aortitis and aortic valvulitis is a third possibility (mitral valvular thickening occurs but usually is not clinically significant). Among patients with only peripheral rheumatoid arthritis, the incidence of aortic insufficiency is only 0.2 per cent. Yet if there is severe rheumatoid spondylitis, it seems likely that 10 per cent of patients may acquire an aortic valve lesion if followed over a 30-year period [492] and an even higher percentage will be found at postmortem.[493] Aortic insufficiency usually develops during a time when the arthritis is active and requiring therapy, usually only after severe disease has been present for 10 years or more. The average duration of the spondylitis was about 20 years in one series, but the interval has been as short as 4 years and as long as 30 years. The duration may be hard to establish because even severe spondylitis sometimes may be asymptomatic for long periods. Intractable spondylitis, especially if associated with swelling in peripheral joints or with signs of involvement of nonarticular tissues (iritis, rheumatoid nodules, pericarditis), seems to be associated with a more rapid evolution.[471,492] Sometimes carditis may be sus-

---

* Acute peripheral arthritis is common, especially in the early stages of spondylitis; chronic deformity of peripheral joints is rare.

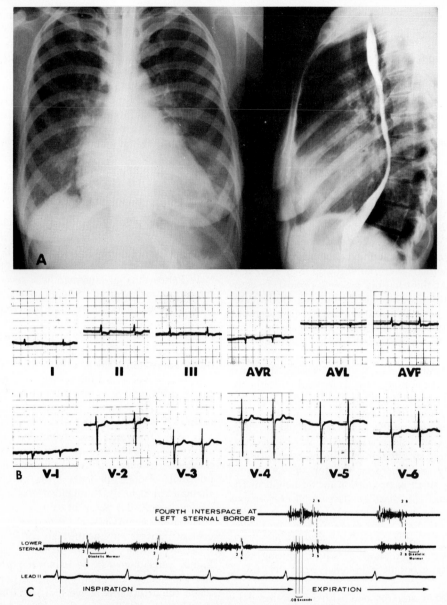

Fig: 25-16. Trivalvular disease with misleading auscultatory signs. The subject was a class IV cardiac patient who had had previous mitral valvulotomy; at the second operation, tightly stenotic and altogether rigid mitral and aortic valves were found. The x-ray (*A,* frontal and lateral views) showed left atrial and general cardiac enlargement. The electrocardiogram (*B*) showed atrial fibrillation, slight digitalis effect, and perhaps combined ventricular hypertrophy. The murmur of aortic stenosis was only grade II. The first heart sound was soft and no mitral rumble could be heard even though the patient was slender and easy to examine. Along the lower sternal border, however (phonocardiogram *C*), there were typical auscultatory findings of tricuspid stenosis; a rather high-pitched early diastolic murmur greatly augmented by inspiration. The murmur began after an opening snap, S. Since the snap was similarly augmented by inspiration and the mitral valve was utterly destroyed, the sound in this case probably came from the tricuspid valve. In spite of these auscultatory findings the tricuspid valve was only moderately stenotic and not appreciably insufficient at operation. The mildness of the tricuspid lesion was clinically suspected because with diuresis and improvement in the patient's condition the venous pressure (estimated from observation of the neck veins) had fallen almost to normal while the auscultatory findings had persisted.

pected before the appearance of the murmur because of chest pain, cardiac enlargement, and unaccountable tachycardia.[492] Associated mitral valve involvement is not uncommon but is usually not clinically significant.[493] Amyloidosis with involvement of the heart is a rare complication.

Clinical Signs. *Aortitis.* The effect of spondylitis on the aorta seems to be chiefly of pathologic interest.[491,493] There are grossly visible plaques and wrinkled scars; microscopic evidence of destruction of muscle and elastic tissue with replacement by collagen and, distinctively, marked fibromuscular obliteration of the vasa vasorum. The pathologic similarity of the aortic lesion to syphilis has been repeatedly commented on. Clinically, however, rheumatoid arthritis does not produce radiologic evidence of disproportionate enlargement of the ascending aorta with calcification, abnormal "aneurysmal" pulsation, or other signs of syphilitic aortitis.

Aortic Valvulitis. The aortic valve cusps are shortened, with the greatest disease at the bases rather than at the edges, which are never extensively fused.[493] The coronary ostia may be distorted, but this is probably not of great importance in most cases. The patient's symptoms seem to coincide with the development of free aortic insufficiency, and the manifestations of this condition are entirely similar to those produced by rheumatic heart disease. The murmur of aortic insufficiency is maximal at the lower left sternal border. The electrocardiogram has been abnormal in all the severe cases, showing definite left ventricular hypertrophy and often also a prolonged P-R interval.[471,492] An increased sedimentation rate and anemia are often found and probably indicate continuation of the activity of the basic process.

Medical therapy of such free aortic regurgitation is only a holding operation. Fortunately in some cases the disease ceases to progress and the patient is left with quite significant but stable disease.[492] At this writing it is not known how suitable the condition will be for the insertion of prosthetic aortic valves. Involvement of the aortic wall, however, has not prevented the successful use of the Hufnagel prosthesis in times past. The patient with prolonged or unusually severe activity of rheumatoid spondylitis (manifested not only by pain but also by increased sedimentation rate and often by anemia and the nonarthritic clinical signs) should be carefully watched for the development of the soft, aortic diastolic murmur. In the writer's opinion the appearance of a murmur in these circumstances is an indication for a prolonged course of the most potent suppressive therapy for rheumatoid spondylitis available at the time. In spite of this opinion it is not known whether corticosteroids can delay the evolution of the aortic lesion.

Chest pain in rheumatic spondylitis may be a complex problem.[495] Pericarditis occurs fairly often in the severer cases; neither the pericordial rub nor the typical clinical pain pattern is invariably present (there may be no pain). Patients with spondylitis may also have severe burning or aching chest-wall discomfort, which is often in the left precordial area or occasionally over the sternomanubrial point, but not usually substernal. It has been confused with angina pectoris but is less connected with effort than aggravated by trivial movements of the shoulder girdle or hypertension of the thoracic spine. There are more valid grounds for confusion with pericarditis. Genuine angina may occur in the patient with free aortic insufficiency.

Peripheral Rheumatoid Arthritis

Rheumatoid arthritis involving only peripheral joints is also associated with a variety of cardiac lesions. Rheumatoid granulomas, obliterative pericarditis, coronary arteritis, as well as mitral and aortic valve deformities may occur.[496] Congestive failure and even death may result from such lesions. A spectrum of diseases between classic rheumatic fever and rheumatoid arthritis has been proposed.[497] In spite of these interesting and important conditions the commonest cause of cardiac disability in the patient with rheumatoid arthritis remains atherosclerotic coronary artery disease.[498]

REFERENCES

1. Feinstein, A. R., and Spagnuolo, M.: The Duration of Activity in Acute Rheumatic Fever, *J.A.M.A.,* **175:**1117, 1961.
2. Stollerman, G. H.: Current Evaluation of the Diagnosis, Treatment and Prevention of Rheumatic Fever, *Bull. Rheumat. Dis.,* **13:**293, 1962.
3. Taranta, A., Spagnuolo, M., and Feinstein, A. R.: "Chronic" Rheumatic Fever, *Ann. Int. Med.,* **56:** 367, 1962.
4. Rammelkamp, C. H., Jr.: Rheumatic Heart Disease, a Challenge. *Circulation,* **17:**842, 1958.
5. Zagala, J. G., and Feinstein, A. R.: The Preceding Illness of Acute Rheumatic Fever, *J.A.M.A.,* **179:** 863, 1962.
6. Siegal, A. C., Johnson, E. E., and Stollerman, G. H.: Controlled Studies of Streptococcal Pharyngitis in a Pediatric Population. 1. Factors Related to the Attack Rate of Rheumatic Fever. 2. Behavior of the Type-specific Immune Response, *New England J. Med.,* **265:**559, 566, 1961.
7. Mortimer, E. A., and Rammelkamp, C. H., Jr.:

Prophylaxis of Rheumatic Fever, *Circulation,* **14:** 1144, 1956.

8. Stollerman, G. H., and Sackett, S. J.: Factors That Predispose to Rheumatic Fever, *M. Clin. North America,* **44:**17, 1960.

9. Diehl, A. M., Lode, R. I., and Hamilton, T. R.: Epidemiology of Rheumatic Fever, *Am. J. Cardiol.,* **1:**423, 1958.

10. Epidemiology and Control of Rheumatic Fever, *Lancet,* **2:**989, 1956.

11. Nadas, A.: Acute Rheumatic Fever and Rheumatic Heart Disease, in "Pediatric Cardiology," W. B. Saunders Company, Philadelphia, 1963, pp. 171–213.

12. Denny, F. W., Wannamaker, L. W., Brink, W. R., Rammelkamp, C. H., Jr., and Custer, E. A.: Prevention of Rheumatic Fever: Treatment of Preceding Streptococcic Infection, *J.A.M.A.,* **143:**151, 1950.

13. Bland, E. F.: Declining Severity of Rheumatic Fever: A Comparative Study of the Past Four Decades, *New England J. Med.,* **262:**597, 1960.

14. Wilson, M. G., Lim, W. N., and Birch, A. McA.: The Decline of Rheumatic Fever. Recurrent Rate of Rheumatic Fever among 782 Children for Twenty-one Consecutive Calendar Years, 1936–1956, *J. Chron. Dis.,* **7:**183, 1958.

15. The Evolution of Rheumatic Heart Disease in Children: Five Year Report of a Cooperative Clinical Trial of ACTH, Cortisone, and Aspirin, *Circulation,* **22:**503, 1960.

16. Grossman, B. J., and Stamler, J.: Potential Preventability of First Attacks of Acute Rheumatic Fever in Children, *J.A.M.A.,* **183:**985, 1963.

17. Taranta, A., Torosdag, S., Metrakas, J. D., Jegier, W., and Urchida, I.: Rheumatic Fever in Monozygotic and Dizygotic Twins, *Circulation,* **20:**778, 1959.

18. Taranta, A., Kleinberg, E., Feinstein, A. R., Wood, H. F., Tursky, E., and Simpson, R.: Rheumatic Fever in Children and Adolescents. V. Relation of the Rheumatic Fever Recurrence Rate per Streptococcal Infection to Pre-existing Clinical Features of the Patients, *Ann. Int. Med.,* **60:**58, (Feb. suppl. #5), 1964.

19. Feinstein, A. R., and Spagnuolo, M.: The Clinical Patterns of Acute Rheumatic Fever: A Reappraisal, *Medicine,* **41:**279, 1962.

20. Bland, E. F., and Jones, T. D.: Rheumatic Fever and Rheumatic Heart Disease: A Twenty Year Report on 1,000 Patients Followed Since Childhood, *Circulation,* **4:**836, 1951.

21. Bland, E. F.: Chorea as a Manifestation of Rheumatic Fever: A Long-term Perspective, *Tr. Am. Clin. & Climatol. A.,* **73:**209, 1961.

22. Johnson, E. E., Stollerman, G. H., Grossman, B. J., and McCulloch, H.: Streptococcal Infections in Adolescents and Adults after Prolonged Freedom from Rheumatic Fever. 1. Results of the First 3 Years of Disease Study, *New England J. Med.,* **263:**105, 1960.

23. Bywaters, E. G. L., and Thomas, G. T.: Prevention of Rheumatic Fever Recurrences, *Brit. M. J.,* **2:**350, 1958.

24. Feinstein, A. R., Wood, H. F., Spagnuolo, M., Taranta, A., Jonas, S., Kleinberg, E., and Tursky, E.: Rheumatic Fever in Children and Adolescents. VII. Cardiac Changes and Sequelae, *Ann. Int. Med.,* **60:**87, (suppl. #5), 1964.

25. Massell, B. F., Fyler, D. C., and Roy, S. B.: The Clinical Picture of Rheumatic Fever: Diagnosis, Immediate Prognosis, Course and Therapeutic Implications, *Am. J. Cardiol.,* **1:**436, 1958.

26. Keith, J. D., Rowe, R. D., and Vlad, P.: "Heart Disease in Infancy and Childhood," The Macmillan Company, New York, 1958, p. 611.

27. Spagnuolo, M., and Feinstein, A. R.: Congestive Heart Failure and Rheumatic Activity in Young Patients with Rheumatic Heart Disease, *Pediatrics,* **33:**653, 1964.

28. Feinstein, A. R., Spagnuolo, M., Wood, H. F., Taranta, A., Tursky, E., and Kleinberg, E.: Rheumatic Fever in Children and Adolescents. VI. Clinical Features of Streptoccocal Infections and Rheumatic Recurrences, *Ann. Int. Med.,* **60:**68, (suppl. #5), 1964.

29. Wood, R. H.: "Diseases of the Heart and Circulation," 2d ed., J. B. Lippincott Company, Philadelphia, 1956.

30. Zvaifler, N. J.: Chronic Postrheumatic-fever (Jaccoud's) Arthritis, *New England J. Med.,* **267:**10, 1962.

31. Jorgens, J., Kundel, R., and Lieber, A.: The Cinefluorographic Approach to the Diagnosis of Pericardial Effusion, *Am. J. Roentgenol.,* **87:**911, 1962.

32. Besterman, E. M. M.: The Cardiac Output in Acute Rheumatic Carditis, *Brit. Heart J.,* **16:**8, 1954.

33. Lessof, M., and Brigden, W.: Systolic Murmurs in Healthy Children and in Children with Rheumatic Fever, *Lancet,* **2:**673, 1957.

34. Besterman, E. M. M.: Phonocardiography in Acute Rheumatic Carditis, *Brit. Heart J.,* **17:**360, 1955.

35. Fogel, D. H.: The Innocent Systolic Murmur in Children: A Clinical Study of Its Incidence and Characteristics, *Am. Heart J.,* **59:**844, 1960.

36. Marienfeld, C. J., Telles, N., Silvera, J., and Nordsieck, M.: A 20-year Follow-up Study of Innocent "Murmurs," *Pediatrics,* **30:**42, 1962.

37. Castle, R. F., and Craige, E.: Auscultation of the Heart in Infants and Children, *Pediatrics,* **26:**511, 1960.

38. Stapleton, J. S., and El-Hajj, M. M.: Heart Murmurs Simulated by Arterial Bruits in the Neck, *Am. Heart J.,* **61:**178, 1961.

39. Leatham, A.: Systolic Murmurs, *Circulation,* **17:** 601, 1958.

40. Bland, E. F., and Jones, T. D.: The Delayed

Appearance of Heart Disease after Rheumatic Fever, *J.A.M.A.*, **113**:1380, 1939.

41. Harris, T. N., Friedman, S., and Tang, J.: Appearance of New Cardiac Murmurs in Patients Having Rheumatic Heart Disease with no Concommitant Evidence of Rheumatic Activity, *Am. J. Med.*, **23**:748, 1957.

42. McKusick, V. A.: "Cardiovascular Sound in Health and Disease," The Williams & Wilkins Company, Baltimore, 1958.

43. Feinstein, A. R., and Arevale, A. C.: Manifestations and Treatment of Congestive Heart Failure in Young Patients with Rheumatic Heart Disease, *Pediatrics*, **33**:661, 1964.

44. Kreidberg, M. B., Chernoff, H. L., and Lopez, W. L.: Treatment of Cardiac Failure in Infancy and Childhood, *New England J. Med.*, **268**:23, 1963.

45. Petry, E. L., Tauer, R. M., and Diehl, A. M.: Heart Failure in Childhood, *Pediat. Clin. North America*, **9**:113, 1962.

46. Logue, R. B., Rogers, J. V., Jr., and Gay, B. B.: Subtle Roentgenographic Signs of Left Ventricular Failure, *Am. Heart J.*, **65**:464, 1963.

47. Castle, R. F., and Baylin, G. J.: Severe Acquired Mitral Stenosis in Childhood and Adolescence, *J. Pediat.*, **58**:404, 1961.

48. Reale, A., Colella, C., and Bruno, A. M.: Mitral Stenosis in Childhood: Clinical and Therapeutic Aspects, *Am. Heart J.*, **66**:15, 1963.

49. Burke, J. B.: Erythema Marginatum, *Arch. Dis. Childhood*, **30**:359, 1955.

50. Baldwin, J. S., Kerr, J. M., Kuttner, A. G., and Doyle, E. F.: Observations on Rheumatic Nodules over a 30 Year Period, *J. Pediat.*, **56**:465, 1960.

51. Taranta, A.: Occurrence of Rheumatic-like Subcutaneous Nodules without Evidence of Joint or Heart Disease, *New England J. Med.*, **266**:13, 1962.

52. Taranta, A., Mark, H., Haas, R. C., and Cooper, N. S.: Nodular Panniculitis after Massive Prednisone Therapy, *Am. J. Med.*, **25**:52, 1958.

53. Taranta, A.: Relation of Isolated Recurrences of Syndenham's Chorea to Preceding Streptococcal Infections, *New England J. Med.*, **260**:104, 1959.

54. Friedberg, C. K.: "Diseases of the Heart," 2d ed., W. B. Saunders Company, Philadelphia, 1956.

55. Eastham, R. D., Szekely, P., and Davison, K.: C-reactive Protein in Rheumatic Heart Disease, *Ann. Rheumat. Dis.*, **17**:314, 1958.

56. Eastham, R. D., Szekely, P., and Davison, K.: Comparison of the Erythrocyte Sedimentation Rate, C-reactive Protein, Serum Diphenylamine and Tetramonium Tests in Rheumatic Fever and Rheumatic Heart Disease, *Ann. Rheumat. Dis.*, **17**:319, 1958.

57. Wood, H. F., and McCarty, M.: Laboratory Aids in the Diagnosis of Rheumatic Fever and in Evaluation of Disease Activity, *Am. J. Med.*, **17**:768, 1954.

58. Wood, H. F., Feinstein, A. R., Taranta, A., Epstein, J. A., and Simpson, R.: Rheumatic Fever in Children and Adolescents. III. Comparative Effectiveness of Three Prophylaxis Regimens in Preventing Streptococcal Infections and Rheumatic Recurrences, *Ann. Int. Med.*, **60**:31, (suppl. #5), 1964.

59. Stollerman, G. H., Lewis, A. J., Schultz, I., and Taranta, A.: Relationship of Immune Response to Group A Streptococci to the Course of Acute Chronic and Recurrent Rheumatic Fever, *Am. J. Med.*, **20**:163, 1956.

60. Taranta, A., and Stollerman, G. H.: The Relationship of Sydenham's Chorea to Infection with Group A Streptococci, *Am. J. Med.*, **20**:170, 1956.

61. Wannamaker, L. W., and Ayoub, E. M.: Antibody Titers in Acute Rheumatic Fever, *Circulation*, **21**:598, 1960.

62. Ayoub, E. M., and Wannamaker, L. W.: Evaluation of the Streptococcal Desoxyribonuclease B and Diphosphopyridine Nucleotidase Antibody Tests in Acute Rheumatic Fever and Acute Glomerulonephritis, *Pediatrics*, **29**:527, 1962.

63. Taranta, A., Wood, H. F., Feinstein, A. R., Simpson, R., and Kleinberg, E.: Rheumatic Fever in Children and Adolescents. IV. Relation of the Rheumatic Fever Recurrence Rate Per Streptococcal Infection to the Titers of Streptococcal Antibodies, *Ann. Int. Med.*, **60**:47, (suppl. #5), 1964.

64. Kaplan, M. H.: Immunologic Relationship of Group A Streptococcal Strains and Human Heart Tissue: Possible Significance for the Pathogenesis of Rheumatic Fever, *Am. Heart J.*, **65**:426, 1963.

65. American Heart Association: Report of Committee on Standards and Criteria for Programs of Care of Council on Rheumatic Fever. Jones Criteria (Modified) for Guidance in Diagnosis of Rheumatic Fever. *Mod. Concepts Cardiovas. Dis.*, **24**:291, 1955.

66. Feinstein, A. R.: Current Status of Prophylaxis Against Rheumatic Fever, *Progr. Cardiovas. Dis.*, **3**:204, 1960–61.

67. Feinstein, A. R., and DiMassa, R.: The Unheard Diastolic Murmur in Acute Rheumatic Fever, *New England J. Med.*, **260**:1331, 1959.

68. Malpas, J. S., and Landon, J.: Rheumatic Fever in the Young Adult, *Ann. Rheumat. Dis.*, **19**:262, 1960.

69. Pader, E., and Elser, S. K.: Studies of Acute Rheumatic Fever in Adults. I. Clinical and Laboratory Manifestations in 30 Patients, *Am. J. Med.*, **26**:424, 1959.

70. Friedberg, C. K.: Rheumatic Fever in the Adult: Criteria and Implications, *Circulation*, **19**:161, 1959.

71. Grossman, D. J., and Athreya, A.: Sources of Errors in the Diagnosis of Acute Rheumatic Fever in Children, *J.A.M.A.*, **182**:830, 1962.

72. Keith, J. D.: Modern Trends in Rheumatic Fever, *Canad. M. A. J.*, **83**:789, 1960.

73. American Heart Association: Committee on Prevention of Rheumatic Fever and Bacterial Endocarditis. Prevention of Rheumatic Fever and Bacterial Endocarditis through Control of Streptococcal Infections, *Circulation*, **21**:151, 1960.

74. Hsu, I., and Evans, J. M.: Untoward Reactions to Benzathine: Penicillin G in a Study of Rheumatic Fever Prophylaxis in Adults, *New England J. Med.*, **259**:581, 1958.

75. Bernstein, S. H., and Hauser, H. B.: Sensitivity Reactions to Intramuscular Injections of Benzathine Penicillin, *New England J. Med.*, **260**:747, 1959.

76. Mortimer, E. A., Vaisman, S. B., Vignau, A. I., Guasch, J. L., Schuster, A. C., Rakita, L., Krause, R. M., Roberts, R., and Rammelkamp, C. H., Jr.: The Effect of Penicillin on Acute Rheumatic Fever and Valvular Heart Disease, *New England J. Med.*, **260**:101, 1959.

77. Carter, M. E., Bywater, E. G. L., and Thomas, G. T. G.: Rheumatic Fever Treated with Penicillin and Bacteriacidal Dosage for Six Weeks: Report of a Small Controlled Trial, *Brit. M. J.*, **2**:965, 1962.

78. Catanzaro, F. J., Stetson, C. A., Morris, A. J., Chamovitz, R., Rammelkamp, C. H., Jr., Stolzer, B. L., and Perry W. D.: The Role of the Streptococcus in the Pathogenesis of Rheumatic Fever, *Am. J. Med.*, **17**:749, 1959.

79. Frank, P. F., Schultz, E. I., Eeklund, A. M., and Miller, quoted by Stollerman, G. H.: Current Evaluation of the Diagnosis, Treatment and Prevention of Rheumatic Fever, *Bull. Rheumat. Heart Dis.*, **13**:293, 1962.

80. Lattimer, A. D., Siegel, A. C., and De Celles, J.: Evaluation of the Recovery of Beta Hemolytic Streptococci from Two Mail-in Methods, *Am. J. Pub. Health*, **53**:1594, 1963.

81. Saslaw, M. S., Jablon, J. M., and Jenks, J. A.: Problems Associated with the Use of Antibiotics for the Prevention of Primary Episodes of Rheumatic Fever, *Am. J. Cardiol.*, **5**:777, 1960.

82. Feinstein, A. R., Wood, H. F., Spagnuolo, M., Taranta, A., Tursky, E., and Kleinberg, E.: Oral Prophylaxis of Recurrent Rheumatic Fever: Sulfadiazine vs. a Double Daily Dose of Penicillin, *J.A.M.A.*, **188**:489, 1964.

83. Stollerman, G. H.: The Use of Antibiotics for the Prevention of Rheumatic Fever, *Am. J. Med.*, **17**:757, 1954.

84. Miller, J. M., Freemont-Smith, P., and Breihahn, R. L.: Incidence and Nature of Streptococcal Infection in Adult Rheumatic Heart Disease as a Basis for Penicillin Prophylaxis, *Circulation*, **22**:789, 1960.

85. Feinstein, A. R., Taube, H., Cavalier, R., Schultz, S. C., and Koyle, L.: Physical Activities and Rheumatic Heart Disease in Asymptomatic Patients, *J.A.M.A.*, **180**:1028, 1962.

86. Tilles, J. O., Elson, P., Shaka, J. A., and Ferner, A. M.: Effects of Exercise on Coxsackie Myocarditis in Mice, *Fed. Proc.*, **12**:246, 1964.

87. Combined Rheumatic Fever Study Group: A Comparison of the Effect of Prednisone and Acetylsalicylic Acid on the Incidence of Residual Rheumatic Heart Disease, *New England J. Med.*, **262**:895, 1960.

88. Czoniczer, G., Amezena, F., Pelorgonio, A., and Massell, B. F.: Therapy of Severe Rheumatic Carditis: Comparison of Adrenocortical Steroids and Aspirin, *Circulation*, **29**:813, 1964.

89. Feinstein, A. R.: Standards, Stethoscopes, Steroids and Statistics: The Problem of Evaluating Treatment in Acute Rheumatic Fever, *Pediatrics*, **27**:819, 1961.

90. Stollerman, G. H.: Prognosis and Treatment of Acute Rheumatic Fever: The Possible Effect of Treatment on Subsequent Cardiac Disease, *Progr. Cardiovas. Dis.*, **3**:611, 1960–61.

91. Bywaters, E. G. L., and Thomas, G. T.: Bedrest, Salicylates, and Steroid in Rheumatic Fever, *Brit. M. J.*, **1**:1628, 1961.

92. Feinstein, A. R., and Spagnuolo, M.: Rebound Phenomenon in Acute Rheumatic Fever, *Circulation*, **22**:747, 1960.

93. Brock, R. C.: The Surgical and Pathological Anatomy of the Mitral Valve, *Brit. Heart J.*, **14**:489, 1952.

94. Harken, D. E., Dexter, L., Ellis, L. B., Farrand, R. E., and Dickson, J. F.: The Surgery of Mitral Stenosis. III. Finger Fracture Valvuloplasty, *Ann. Surg.*, **134**:722, 1951.

95. Rusted, I. E., Sheifley, C. H., and Edwards, J. E.: Studies of the Mitral Valve. II. Certain Anatomic Features of the Mitral Valve and Associated Structures in Mitral Stenosis, *Circulation*, **14**:398, 1956.

96. Davila, J. C., and Trevelyan, E. P.: The Mitral Valve: Anatomy and Pathology for the Surgeon, *Arch. Surg.*, **84**:174, 1962.

97. Amador, E., Thrower, W. B., and Dammin, G. J.: Dynamics of Normal and Diseased Cardiac Valves, *Am. Heart J.*, **66**:777, 1963.

98. Lewis, B. M., Gorlin, R., Houssay, H. E. J., and Dexter, L.: Clinical and Physiological Correlations in Patients with Mitral Stenosis, *Am. Heart J.*, **43**:2, 1952.

99. Wood, P.: An Appreciation of Mitral Stenosis. I. Clinical Features. II. Investigations and Results, *Brit. M. J.*, **1**:1051, 1113, 1954.

100. Carman, G. H., and Lange, R. L.: Variant Hemodynamic Patterns in Mitral Stenosis, *Circulation*, **24**:712, 1961.

101. Lukas, D. S., Mahrer, P. R., and Steinberg, I.: Angiocardiographic and Physiologic Correlations in Mitral Stenosis, *Circulation*, **17**:567, 1958.

102. Pugh, D., Dodge, H., and Figley, M.: Obser-

vations on Left Atrial Function in Mitral Stenosis, *Clin. Res.,* 12:105, 1964.

103. Sosman, M. C.: Roentgenological Aspects of Acquired Valvular Heart Disease, *Am. J. Roentgenol.,* 42:47, 1939.

104. Amplatz, K.: The Roentgenographic Diagnosis of Mitral and Aortic Valvular Disease, *Am. Heart J.,* 64:556, 1962.

105. Gilroy, J. C., Marchand, P., and Wilson, V. J.: The Role of Bronchial Veins in Mitral Stenosis, *Lancet,* 2:957, 1952.

106. Lunger, M., Abelson, D. S., Elkind, A. H., and Kantrowitz, A.: Massive Hemoptysis in Mitral Stenosis: Control by Emergency Commissurotomy, *New England J. Med.,* 261:393, 1959.

107. Thompson, A. C., and Stewart, W. C.: Hemoptysis in Mitral Stenosis, *J.A.M.A.,* 147:21, 1951.

108. Goodwin, J. F., Hunter, J. D., Cleland, W. P., Davis, L. G., and Steiner, R. E.: Mitral Valve Disease and Mitral Valvotomy, *Brit. M. J.,* 2:573, 1955.

109. Donald, K. W.: Disturbances in Pulmonary Function in Mitral Stenosis and Left Heart Failure, *Progr. Cardiovas. Dis.,* 1:298, 1958–59.

110. Arnott, W. M.: The Lungs in Mitral Stenosis, *Brit. M. J.,* 2:765, 1963.

111. Dock, W.: The Clinical Significance of Some Peculiarities of the Circulation in the Kidneys, Liver, Lungs and Heart, *New England J. Med.,* 236:773, 1947.

112. Simon, M.: The Pulmonary Veins in Mitral Stenosis, *J. Fac. Radiologists,* 9:25, 1958.

113. Steiner, R. E.: Radiology of Pulmonary Circulation: Chamberlain Lecture, *Am. J. Roentgenol.,* 91:259, 1964.

114. Dollery, C. T., and West, J. B.: Regional Uptake of Radioactive Oxygen, Carbon Monoxide and Carbon Dioxide in Lungs of Patients with Mitral Stenosis, *Circulation Res.,* 8:765, 1960.

115. Short, D. S.: Radiology of the Lung in Severe Mitral Stenosis: Radiology of the Lung in Left Heart Failure, *Brit. Heart J.,* 17:33, 1955; 18:233, 1956.

116. Trapnell, D. H.: The Peripheral Lymphatics of the Lung, *Brit. J. Radiol.,* 36:660, 1963.

117. Grainger, R. G.: Interstitial Pulmonary Edema and Its Radiological Diagnosis: A Sign of Pulmonary Venous and Capillary Hypertension, *Brit. J. Radiol.,* 31:201, 1958.

118. Uhley, H. N., Leeds, S. E., Sampson, J. J., and Friedman, M.: Role of Pulmonary Lymphatics in Chronic Pulmonary Edema, *Circulation Res.,* 11:966, 1962.

119. Cardus, D., Mackinnon, J., and Wade, G.: Effect of Tilting on Intracardiac Pressures, *Brit. Heart J.,* 20:233, 1958.

120. Finlayson, J. K., Luria, N. N., Stanfield, C. A., and Yu, P. N.: Hemodynamic Studies in Acute Pulmonary Edema, *Ann. Int. Med.,* 54:244, 1961.

121. Bishop, J. M., and Wade, O. L.: Relationships between Cardiac Output and Rhythm, Pulmonary Venous Pressure and Disability in Mitral Stenosis, *Clin. Sc.,* 24:391, 1963.

122. Stock, J. P. P., and Kennedy, M. C. S.: Ventilatory Cost of Exercise before and after Mitral Valvotomy, *Thorax,* 14:238, 1959.

123. Reid, J. M., and Stevenson, J. G.: Pulmonary Diffusing Capacity in Mitral Valve Disease, *Brit. Heart J.,* 25:741, 1963.

124. Saxton, G. A., Jr., Rabinowitz, M., Dexter, L., and Haynes, F.: The Relationship of Pulmonary Compliance to Pulmonary Vascular Pressures in Patients with Heart Disease, *J. Clin. Invest.,* 35:611, 1956.

125. MacIntosh, D. J., Sinnott, J. C., Milne, I. G., and Reid, E. G. S.: Some Aspects of Disordered Pulmonary Function in Mitral Stenosis, *Ann. Int. Med.,* 49:1294, 1958.

126. Raine, J., and Bishop, J. M.: The Distribution of Alveolar Ventilation in Mitral Stenosis, at Rest and after Exercise, *Clin. Sc.,* 24:63, 1963.

127. Rowe, J. C., Bland, E. F., Sprague, H. B., and White, P. D.: Course of Mitral Stenosis without Surgery: Ten and Twenty-year Perspectives, *Ann. Int. Med.,* 52:741, 1960.

128. Selzer, A.: Effects of Atrial Fibrillation upon the Circulation in Patients with Mitral Stenosis, *Am. Heart J.,* 59:518, 1960.

129. Daley, R., Mattingly, T. W., Holt, C. L., Bland, E. F., and White, P. D.: Systemic Arterial Embolism in Rheumatic Heart Disease, *Am. Heart J.,* 42:566, 1951.

130. Wood, P.: Systemic Embolism, *Brit. M. J.,* 1:1056, 1954.

131. Hugenholtz, P. G., Ryan, T. H., Stein, S. W., and Abelman, W. H.: The Spectrum of Pure Mitral Stenosis: Hemodynamic Studies in Relation to Clinical Disability, *Am. J. Cardiol.,* 10:773, 1962.

132. Soloff, L. A.: The Failing Rheumatic Heart Mechanisms and Present Day Therapy, *Am. J. Med.,* 240:1, 1960.

133. Parker, F., Jr., and Weiss, S.: The Nature and Significance of the Structural Changes in the Lungs in Mitral Stenosis, *Am. J. Pathol.,* 12:573, 1936.

134. Wood, P.: Pulmonary Hypertension with Special Reference to the Vasoconstrictive Factor, *Brit. Heart J.,* 20:557, 1958.

135. Holling, H. E., and Venner, A.: Disability and Circulatory Changes in Mitral Stenosis, *Brit. Heart J.,* 18:103, 1956.

136. Mackinnon, J., Wade, E. G., and Vickers, C. F. H.: Mitral Stenosis with Very High Pulmonary Vascular Resistance and Atypical Features, *Brit. Heart J.,* 13:449, 1956.

137. Hargreaves, I.: Rheumatic Mitral Valve Disease in the Elderly: Incidence Found at Necropsy, *Brit. M. J.,* 2:342, 1961.

138. Rodbard, S.: Physical Factors in the Progression of Stenotic Vascular Lesions, *Circulation,* **17**:410, 1958.

139. Smith, D. E., and Matthews, M. B.: Aortic Valvular Stenosis with Coarctation of the Aorta: With Special Reference to the Development of Aortic Stenosis upon Congenital Bicuspid Valves, *Brit. Heart J.,* **17**:198, 1955.

140. Gorlin, R.: The Hyperkinetic Heart Syndrome, *J.A.M.A.,* **182**:823, 1962.

141. Short, D., and Brunnel, P. L.: The Case for Ignoring Symptoms in Assessing the Severity of Mitral Stenosis, *Brit. Heart J.,* **25**:695, 1963.

142. Robin, E. D., and Thomas, E. R.: Some Relations between Pulmonary Edema and Pulmonary Inflammation (Pneumonia), *A.M.A. Arch. Int. Med.,* **93**:713, 1954.

143. Newcombe, C. P., Nixon, P. G. F., and Thompson, H.: Influenzal Pneumonia in Mitral Stenosis, *Acta med. Scandinav.,* **162**:441, 1958.

144. Dexter, L., Dock, D. S., McGuire, L. B., Hyland, J. W., and Haynes, F. W.: Pulmonary Embolism, *M. Clin. North America,* **44**:1251, 1960.

145. Oakley, C., Yusuf, R., and Hollman, A.: Coronary Embolism and Angina in Mitral Stenosis, *Brit. Heart J.,* **23**:357, 1961.

146. Hurst, J. W.: Mitral Stenosis: A Clinical-Pathophysiological Correlation, in B. L. Segal (ed.), "The Theory and Practice of Auscultation," F. A. Davis Company, Philadelphia, 1964, p. 367.

147. Sherlock, S.: Liver in Heart Failure: Relation of Anatomical, Functional and Circulatory Changes, *Brit. Heart J.,* **13**:273, 1951.

148. Felder, L., Mund, A., and Parker, J. G.: Liver Function Tests in Chronic Congestive Heart Failure, *Circulation,* **2**:286, 1950.

149. Killip, T., III, and Payne, M. A.: High Serum Transaminase Activity in Heart Disease: Circulatory Failure and Hepatic Necrosis, *Circulation,* **21**:646, 1960.

150. Mounsey, P.: Determination of Success after Mitral Valvotomy: Role of Circulatory Obstruction of Myocardium and of Other Factors, *Brit. M. J.,* **2**:311, 1957.

151. James, T. N.: Pericarditis and the Sinus Node, *Arch. Int. Med.,* **110**:305, 1962.

152. Fleming, H. A., and Wood, P.: Myocardial Factor in Mitral Valve Disease, *Brit. Heart J.,* **21**:117, 1959.

153. Askey, J. M., and Bernstein, S.: The Management of Rheumatic Heart Disease in Relation to Systemic Arterial Embolism, *Progr. Cardiovas. Dis.,* **3**:220, 1960.

154. Keen, G., and Leveaux, V. M.: Prognosis of Cerebral Emboli in Rheumatic Heart Disease, *Brit. M. J.,* **2**:91, 1958.

155. Finnegan, T. R. L., and Baker, C. G.: Epilepsy in Mitral Stenosis, *Brit. Heart J.,* **19**:159, 1957.

156. Shaw, R. S., and Rutledge, R. H.: Superior Mesenteric Artery Embolectomy in the Treatment of Massive Mesenteric Infarction, *New England J. Med.,* **257**:595, 1957.

157. Starer, F., and Sutton, D.: Aortic Occlusion (Leriche's Syndrome) in Mitral Stenosis: Report of 76 Cases, *Brit. M. J.,* **2**:644, 1960.

158. Logan, A., and Turner, R.: Mitral Stenosis, Diagnosis and Treatment, *Lancet,* **1**:1007, 1953.

159. Viar, W. N., and Harrison, T. R.: Chest Pain in Association with Pulmonary Hypertension: Its Similarity to the Pain of Coronary Disease, *Circulation,* **5**:3, 1952.

160. Ross, R. S.: Right Ventricular Hypertension as a Cause of Precordial Pain, *Am. Heart J.,* **61**:134, 1961.

161. Stuckey, D.: Cardiac Pain in Association with Mitral Stenosis and Congenital Heart Disease, *Brit. Heart J.,* **17**:397, 1955.

162. Ramsey, L. H., and Beeble, J.: Electrocardiographic Response to Exercise in Patients with Mitral Stenosis, *Circulation,* **19**:424, 1959.

163. Caskey, T. D., and Estes, E. H., Jr.: Deviation of the S-T Segment, *Am. J. Med.,* **36**:424, 1964.

164. Simonson, E., "Differential between Normal and Abnormal in Electrocardiography," The C. V. Mosby Company, St. Louis, 1961.

165. Rome, G. G., Maxwell, G. M., Costello, C. A., Huston, J. H., and Crumpton, C. W.: Hemodynamics of Mitral Stenosis with Special Reference to Coronary Blood Flow and Myocardial Oxygen Consumption, *Circulation,* **22**:559, 1960.

166. Coulshed, N., and Epstein, E. J.: The Apex Cardiogram: Its Normal Features Explained by Those Found in Heart Disease, *Brit. Heart J.,* **25**:697, 1963.

167. Benchimol, A., Dimond, E. G., Waxman, D., and Shen, G.: Diastolic Movements of the Precordium in Mitral Stenosis and Regurgitation, *Am. Heart J.,* **60**:417, 1960.

168. Eddleman, E. E., Hefner, L., Reeves, T. J., and Hanson, T. R.: Movements and Forces of the Human Heart: The Genesis of the Apical Impulses, *A.M.A. Arch. Int. Med.,* **99**:401, 1957.

169. Hultgren, H., and Leo, T.: Phonocardiographic Features of Combined Mitral Stenosis and Insufficiency, *Medicine,* **38**:103, 1959.

170. McDonald, L., Dealy, J. B., Jr., Rabinowitz, M., and Dexter, L.: Clinical, Physiological and Pathological Findings in Mitral Stenosis and Regurgitation, *Medicine,* **36**:237, 1957.

171. Turner, R. W. D., and Fraser, H. R. L.: Mitral Valvotomy: A Progress Report, *Lancet,* **2**:526, 1956.

172. Deliyannis, A. A., Gillam, P. M. S., Mounsey, P. D., and Steiner, R. E.: The Cardiac Impulse and the Motion of the Heart, *Brit. Heart J.,* **26**:396, 1964.

173. Leo, T., and Hultgren, H.: Phonocardiographic Characteristics of Tight Mitral Stenosis, *Medicine,* **38**:85, 1959.

174. Beilen, L., and Mounsey, P.: The Left Ventricu-

lar Impulse in Hypertensive Heart Disease, *Brit. Heart J.*, **24**:409, 1962.

175. Weitzman, D.: The Mechanism and Significance of the Auricular Sound, *Brit. Heart J.*, **17**:70, 1955.

176. Bentivoglio, L., Uricchio, J., and Goldberg, H.: Clinical and Hemodynamic Features of Advanced Rheumatic Mitral Regurgitation: Review of Sixty-five Patients, *Am. J. Med.*, **30**:372, 1961.

177. Eddleman, E. E., and Thomas, H. D.: The Recognition and Differentiation of Right Ventricular Pressure and Flow Loads: A Correlative Study of Kinetocardiograms, Electrocardiograms, Fluoroscopy, and Cardiac Catheterization Data in Patients with Mitral Stenosis, Septal Defect, Pulmonic Stenosis and Isolated Pulmonary Hypertension, *Am. J. Cardiol.*, **4**:652, 1959.

178. Leatham, A.: Auscultation of the Heart, *Lancet*, **2**:703, 757, 1958.

179. Margolis, A., and Wolferth, C. C.: Opening Snap (*claquement d'ouverture de la mitrale*) in Mitral Stenosis: Its Characteristic Mechanism of Production and Diagnostic Importance, *Am. Heart J.*, **7**:433, 1932.

180. Mounsey, P.: The Opening Snap of Mitral Stenosis, *Brit. Heart J.*, **15**:135, 1953.

181. Ongley, P. A., Sprague, H. B., and Rappaport, M. B.: Diastolic Murmur of Mitral Stenosis, *New England J. Med.*, **253**:1049, 1955.

182. Wells, B.: The Assessment of Mitral Stenosis by Phonocardiography, *Brit. Heart J.*, **16**:261, 1954.

183. Craige, E.: Phonocardiographic Studies in Mitral Stenosis, *New England J. Med.*, **257**:650, 1957.

184. Harvey, W. P.: Clinical Aspects of Mitral Stenosis, *Mil. Med.*, **120**:282, 1957.

185. Leatham, A.: Splitting of the First and Second Heart Sounds, *Lancet*, **2**:607, 1954.

186. Messer, A. L., Counihan, T. B., Rappaport, M. B., and Sprague, H. B.: The Effect of Cycle Length on the Time of Occurrence of the First Heart Sound and the Opening Snap in Mitral Stenosis, *Circulation*, **4**:576, 1951.

187. Surawicz, B.: Effect of Respiration and Upright Position on the Interval Between the Two Components of the Second Heart Sound and That between the Second Sound and Mitral Opening Snap, *Circulation*, **16**:422, 1957.

188. Rodin, P., and Tabatznik, P.: The Effect of Posture on Added Heart Sounds, *Brit. Heart J.*, **25**:69, 1963.

189. Breen, W. J., and Rekate, A. C.: Effect of Posture on Splitting of the Second Heart Sound, *J.A.M.A.*, **173**:1326, 1960.

190. Van Der Spuy, J. C.: The Functional and Clinical Anatomy of the Mitral Valve, *Brit. Heart J.*, **20**: 471, 1958.

191. Cobbs, B. W., Jr., and Abbott, O. A.: Personal observation.

192. Criley, J. M., Neda, K., de Souza, A. D., and Ross, R. S.: Functional Anatomy of the Stenotic Mitral Valve, *Clin. Res.*, **10**:170, 1962.

193. Di Bartolo, G., Nunez-Dey, D., and Bendezu-Prieto, J.: Left Heart Studies in Mitral Stenosis with Special Reference to Intracardiac Phonocardiograph, *Am. J. Cardiol.*, **10**:93, 1962.

194. Dodge, H. T., Hay, R. E., and Sandler, H.: Pressure Volume Characteristics of the Diastolic Left Ventricle in Man with Heart Disease, *Am. Heart J.*, **64**:503, 1962.

195. Silverman, L. M., Samet, P., Bernstein, W. H., and Litwak, R. S.: Effect of Variations in Cardiac Output and Diastolic Filling Period on the Mitral Diastolic Gradient, *Circulation*, **22**:811, 1960.

196. Sellors, T. H., Bedford, D. E., and Somerville, W.: Valvotomy in the Treatment of Mitral Stenosis, *Brit. M. J.*, **2**:1059, 1953.

197. Phillips, J. H., and Burch, G. E.: Selected Clues in Cardiac Auscultation, *Am. Heart J.*, **63**:1, 1962.

198. Bousvaros, G. A.: Response of Phonocardiographic and Hemodynamic Features of Mitral Stenosis to Inhalation of Amyl Nitrite, *Am. Heart J.*, **63**:101, 1962.

199. Kirsh, I. E., and Kinney, J. F.: The Roentgenologic Diagnosis of Mitral Stenosis, *A.M.A. Arch. Surg.*, **79**:785, 1959.

200. Evans, W.: The Course of the Esophagus in Health and in Disease of the Heart and Great Vessels, M. Res. Council Report no. 208, H.M. Stationery Office, London, 1936.

201. Soloff, L. A., and Zatuchni, J.: the Relationship of Displacement of the Esophagus to Left Atrial Volume and Heart Size in Persons with Mitral Stenosis, *Am. J. Med.*, **21**:551, 1956.

202. Sauter, H. J., Dodge, H. T., Johnston, R. R., and Graham, T. T.: Relationship of Left Atrial Pressure and Volume in Patients with Heart Disease, *Am. Heart J.*, **67**:635, 1964.

203. Braunwald, E., and Awe, W. C.: Syndrome of Severe Mitral Regurgitation with Normal Left Atrial Pressure, *Circulation*, **27**:29, 1963.

204. Frieden, J., Feinstein, A. R., Shapiro, H., and Di Massa, R.: Evaluation of Heart Size in Children and Adolescents Who Have Had Rheumatic Fever, *Circulation*, **20**:697, 1959.

205. Links, E., and Sysimetsa, E.: Clinical and Radiological Aspects of Calcification of the Mitral Valve, *Brit. Heart J.*, **20**:329, 1958.

206. Felson, B.: "Fundamentals of Chest Roentgenology," W. B. Saunders Company, Philadelphia, 1960.

207. Chang, J.: The Normal Roentgenographic Measurement of the Right Descending Pulmonary Artery: 1085 Cases, *Am. J. Roentgenol.*, **87**:929, 1962.

208. Moore, C. B., Kraus, W. L., Dock, D. S., Woodward, E., Jr., and Dexter, L.: The Relationship between Pulmonary Artery Pressure and Roentgenographic Appearance in Mitral Stenosis, *Am. Heart J.*, **58**:576, 1959.

209. Galloway, R. W., Epstein, E. G., and Coulshed,

N.: Pulmonary Ossific Nodules in Mitral Valve Disease, *Brit. Heart J.*, 23:297, 1961.

210. Arvidson, H.: Angiocardiographic Observations in Mitral Disease: With Special Reference to Volume Variation in the Left Atrium, *Acta radiol.*, Suppl. 158, 1958.

211. Ross, R. S., and Criley, J. M.: Contrast Radiography in Mitral Regurgitation, *Progr. Cardiovas. Dis.*, 5:195, 1962–63.

212. Aetis-Dato, A., Angeline, P. F., and Brisca, A.: An Angiopulmographic Study of the Lesser Circulation in Mitral Stenosis, *Am. Heart J.*, 52:1, 1956.

213. Fraser, H. R. L., and Turner, R.: Electrocardiography in Mitral Valvular Disease, *Brit. Heart J.*, 17:459, 1955.

214. Abildskov, J. A.: The Atrial Complex of the Electrocardiogram, *Am. Heart J.*, 57:930, 1959.

215. Ziegler, R. F.: Importance of Amplification Techniques in Routine Clinical Electrocardiography, *Circulation*, 24:1076, 1961.

216. Mounsey, P.: The Atrial Electrocardiogram as a Guide to Prognosis after Mitral Valvotomy, *Brit. Heart J.*, 22:617, 1960.

217. Hayward, J., and Selvester, R. H.: Vectorcardiographic and Electrocardiographic Analysis of Atrial Enlargement, *Circulation*, 28:734, 1963.

218. Reynolds, G.: The Atrial Electrocardiogram in Mitral Stenosis, *Brit. Heart J.*, 15:250, 1953.

219. Katz, L. N.: "Electrocardiography," Lea & Febiger, Philadelphia, 1946.

220. Martens de Oliveira, J., and Zimmerman, H. A.: Auricular Overloadings: Electrocardiographic Analysis of 193 Cases, *Am. J. Cardiol.*, 3:453, 1959.

221. Caceres, C. A., and Xelser, G. A., Jr.: Duration of the Normal P Wave, *Am. J. Cardiol.*, 3:449, 1959.

222. Sano, T., Hellerstein, H. K., and Vaughn, E.: P Vector in Health and Disease as Studied by the Technique of Electrical Dissection of the Vectorcardiogram (Differential Vectorcardiography), *Am. Heart J.*, 53:854, 1957.

223. Morris, J. J., Jr., Estes, E. H., Jr., Whalen, R. E., Thompson, H. K., Jr., and McIntosh, H. D.: P-wave Analysis in Valvular Heart Disease, *Circulation*, 29:242, 1964.

224. Kahn, M., Scheuer, J., Wachtel, F., Grishman, A. J., and Donosco, E.: An Evaluation of the Ratio of P-wave Duration to PR Segment in the Diagnosis of Atrial Enlargement, *Am. Heart J.*, 60:23, 1960.

225. Davies, L. G., and Ross, I. P.: Abnormal P Waves and Paroxysmal Tachycardia, *Brit. Heart J.*, 25:570, 1963.

226. Culler, M. R., Boone, J. A., and Gazes, P. C.: Fibrillatory Wave Size as a Clue to Etiological Diagnosis, *Am. Heart J.*, 66:435, 1963.

227. Aber, C. T.: Quinidine Therapy after Mitral Valvotomy, *Thorax*, 17:274, 1962.

228. Semler, H. J., and Pruett, R. D.: An Electro-

cardiographic Estimation of Pulmonary Vascular Obstruction in 80 Patients with Mitral Stenosis, *Am. Heart J.*, 59:541, 1960.

229. Milner, W. R.: Electrocardiogram and Vectorcardiogram in Right Ventricular Hypertrophy and Right Bundle Branch Block, *Circulation*, 16:348, 1957.

230. Rodrigues Torres, R. V. R., Mackinnon, J., Wade, E. G., and Vickers, F. H.: Persistence of Right Ventricular Hypertrophy Following Mitral Valvotomy, *Brit. Heart J.*, 23:81, 1959.

231. Selzer, A., et al.: Reliability of Electrocardiographic Diagnosis of Left Ventricular Hypertrophy, *Circulation*, 17:255, 1958.

232. Bentivoglio, L. G., Uricchio, J. F., Waldow, A., Litsoff, W., and Goldberg, H.: An Electrocardiographic Analysis of 65 Cases of Mitral Regurgitation, *Circulation*, 18:572, 1958.

233. Demerdash, H., and Goodwin, J. T.: The Cardiogram of Mitral Re-stenosis, *Brit. Heart J.*, 25:474, 1963.

234. Goodwin, J.: Mitral Valve and Left Atrial Disease, in "Clinical Disorders of the Pulmonary Circulation," Little, Brown and Company, Boston, 1960.

235. Kelly, J. J., Jr.: Diagnostic Value of Phonocardiography in Mitral Stenosis: Mode of Production of the First Heart Sound, *Am. J. Med.*, 54:684, 1957.

236. Stroberm, M., Martinez, F., and Kelly, J. J., Jr.: Factors Influencing the Time of Onset of the First Heart Sound in Normal Subjects, *Am. Heart J.*, 54:684, 1957.

237. Bayer, O., Loogen, F., and Wolter, H. H.: The Mitral Opening Snap in the Quantitative Diagnosis of Mitral Stenosis, *Am. Heart J.*, 51:234, 1956.

238. Julian, D., and Davies, L. G.: Heart Sounds and Intracardiac Pressures in Mitral Stenosis, *Brit. Heart J.*, 19:486, 1957.

239. Proctor, M. H., Walker, R. P., Hancock, E. W., and Abelmann, W. H.: The Phonocardiogram in Mitral Valvular Disease: A Correlation of the Q-1 and 2-OS Intervals with Findings at Catheterization of the Left Side of the Heart and at Mitral Valvuloplasty, *Am. J. Med.*, 24:861, 1958.

240. Donnelly, G. L., Mako, G. E., and Orgain, E. S.: The Phonocardiogram as a Method for Evaluating Mitral Stenosis: Correlation with Operative Findings, *J. Thoracic Surg.*, 37:200, 1959.

241. Rich, C. B.: The Relation of Heart Sounds to Left Atrial Pressure, *Canad. M. A. J.*, 81:800, 1959.

242. Heintzen, P.: The Genesis of the Normally Split First Heart Sound, *Am. Heart J.*, 62:332, 1961.

243. Weissler, A. M., Leonard, J. J., and Harvey, J. V.: Observations on the Delayed First Sound in Mitral Stenosis and Hypertension, *Circulation*, 18:165, 1958.

244. Karnegis, J. N., and Wang, Y.: The Q-1 Interval

of the Phonocardiogram in Patients with Ventricular Septal Defect, Patent Ductus Arteriosus and Blalock Anastomosis, *Am. J. Cardiol.*, 11:452, 1963.

245. Gibney, J., Sutton, G., and McEwen, E.: Time Intervals of the Cardiac Cycle in Several Forms of Organic Heart Disease Other than Mitral Stenosis, *Am. J. M. Sc.*, 241:503, 1961.

246. Wells, B. G.: Prediction of Mitral Pressure Gradient from Heart Sounds, *Brit. M. J.*, 1:551, 1957.

247. Castle, R. F.: The Opening Snap in Mitral and Tricuspid Disease, in B. L. Segal (ed.), "The Theory and Practice of Auscultation," F. A. Davis Company, Philadelphia, 1963.

248. Milne, E. N. C.: Physiological Interpretation of the Plain Radiograph in Mitral Stenosis, Including a Review of Criteria for Radiological Estimation of Pulmonary Arterial and Venous Pressure, *Brit. J. Radiol.*, 36:902, 1963.

249. Dulfano, M. J., and Adler, H.: Tomographic Evaluation of Hemodynamic Changes in Mitral Stenosis with a Statistical Note on Normal Tomographic Findings, *Circulation*, 23:177, 1961.

250. Sommer, L. S., and Gosselin, A. J.: Apparent Discrepancies between Hemodynamic and Angiocardiographic Findings in Mitral Stenosis, *Circulation*, 28:809, 1963.

251. Walsh, B. J., Bland, E. F., and Jones, I. D.: Pure Mitral Stenosis in Young People, *A.M.A. Arch. Int. Med.*, 61:161, 1938.

252. Mounsey, P., and Brigden, W.: The Apical Systolic Murmur in Mitral Stenosis, *Brit. Heart J.*, 16:255, 1954.

253. Janton, O. H., Heidorn, G., Soloff, L. A., O'Neill, T. J. E., and Glover, R. P.: The Clinical Determination of Mitral Insufficiency when Associated with Mitral Stenosis, *Circulation*, 10:207, 1954.

254. Peel, A. A. F.: Mitral Stenosis with Jet Regurgitation, *Scot. M. J.*, 3:422, 1958.

255. Schilder, D. P., and Harvey, W. P.: Confusion of Tricuspid Incompetence with Mitral Insufficiency: A Pitfall in the election of Patients for Mitral Surgery, *Am. Heart J.*, 54:352, 1957.

256. Beck, W., Schrire, V., Vogelpoel, L., Nellen, M., and Swanepoel, A.: Hemodynamic Effects of Amyl Nitrite and Phenophyphrine on the Normal Human Circulation and Their Relation to Changes in Cardiac Murmurs, *Am. J. Cardiol.*, 8:341, 1961.

257. Fleming, H. A., and Wood, P.: The Myocardial Factor in Mitral Valve Disease, *Brit. Heart J.*, 21: 117, 1959.

258. Criley, J. M., and Ross, R. S.: Mitral Valve Function in Man, *Circulation*, 24:911, 1961.

259. Samet, P., Litwak, R. S., Bernstein, W. H., Fierer, E. M., and Silverman, L. M.: Clinical and Physiologic Relationships in Mitral Valve Disease, *Circulation*, 19:517, 1959.

260. Bailey, C. P., Hirosi, T., and Morse, D. P.: Mitral Stenosis: New Concept of Correction by Rehinging of the Septal Leaflet: Neo-strophingic Mobilization, *Am. J. Cardiol.*, 11:81, 1963.

261. Taber, R. E., and Lam, C. R.: Indications for Open Operations for Mitral Stenosis, *Am. J. Cardiol.*, 12:30, 1963.

262. Belcher, J. R.: The Influence of Mitral Regurgitation on the Results of Mitral Valvotomy, *Lancet*, 2:7, 1956.

263. Wynn, A.: Gross Calcification of the Mitral Valve, *Brit. Heart J.*, 15:214, 1953.

264. Ellis, L. B., and Harken, D. E.: Closed Valvuloplasty for Mitral Stenosis: A Twelve-year Follow-up Study of 1571 Patients, *New England J. Med.*, 270:643, 1964.

265. Brachfeld, J., Reals, A., and Goldberg, H.: Pitfalls in the Diagnosis of Pulmonary Hypertension, *Am. Heart J.*, 55:905, 1958.

266. Dack, S., Bleifer, S., Grishman, A., and Donoso, E.: Mitral Stenosis: Auscultatory and Phonocardiographic Findings, *Am. J. Cardiol.*, 5:815, 1960.

267. Goodwin, J. F., Harrison, C. V., and Wilcken, D. E. L.: Obliterative Pulmonary Hypertension and Thrombo-embolism, *Brit. M. J.*, 1:701, 777, 1963.

268. Emanuel, R.: Valvotomy in Mitral Stenosis with Extreme Pulmonary Vascular Resistance, *Brit. Heart J.*, 25:119, 1963.

269. Dorney, E. R., and Cabaud, P. G.: Massive Left Atrial Thrombosis and Recurring Pleural Effusion, *Am. Heart J.*, 48:459, 1954.

270. Surawicz, B., and Nierenberg, M. A.: Association of Silent Mitral Stenosis with Massive Thrombi in the Left Atrium, *New England J. Med.*, 263:423, 1960.

271. Lown, B., Perlroth, M. G., Kaidbey, A., Tadaaki, A., and Harken, D. E.: "Cardioversion" of Atrial Fibrillation: A Report on the Treatment of 65 Episodes in 50 Patients, *New England J. Med.*, 269:325, 1963.

272. Runco, V., Molnar, W., Meckstroth, C. V., and Ryan, J. M.: The Graham Steele Murmur versus Aortic Regurgitation in Rheumatic Heart Disease: Results of Aortic Valvulography, *Am. J. Med.*, 31: 71, 1961.

273. Lowther, C. P., and Turner, R. W. D.: Deterioration after Mitral Valvotomy, *Brit. M. J.*, 1:1027, 1102, 1962.

274. Suh, S. K.: Differentiation of the Murmur of Aortic Regurgitation and Pulmonary Regurgitation with Amyl Nitrite, *Circulation*, 22:820, 1960.

275. Uricchio, J., and Likoff, W.: Effect of Mitral Commissurotomy on Coexisting Aortic Valve Lesion, *New England J. Med.*, 256:199, 1957.

276. Segal, J. P., Harvey, W. P., and Corrado, M. A.: The Austin Flint Murmur: Its Differentiation from the Murmur of Rheumatic Mitral Stenosis, *Circulation*, 18:1025, 1958.

277. Segal, B. L.: Diagnosis of Aortic Regurgitation, in "The Theory and Practice of Auscultation," F. A. Davis Company, Philadelphia, 1964.

278. Hampton, H. O., and Castleman, B.: Correlation of Postmortem Chest Teleroentgenograms with Autopsy Findings with Special Reference to Pulmonary Embolism and Infarction, *Am. J. Roentgenol.*, 43:305, 1940.

279. Tench, W. R.: Triad of Tachycardia, Digitalis Toxicity and Mercurial-fast Edema in Congestive Heart Failure Complicated by Pulmonary Embolism, *Am. J. Med.*, 19:869, 1955.

280. Harrison, C. V.: Pathology in "Clinical Disorders of the Pulmonary Circulation," Little, Brown and Company, Boston, 1960, p. 136.

281. Nadas, O. S., and Alimurung, M. M.: Apical Diastolic Murmurs in Congenital Heart Disease: The Rarity of Lutembacher's Syndrome, *Am. Heart J.*, 43:691, 1952.

282. Espino-Vela, J.: Rheumatic Heart Disease Associated with Atrial Septal Defect: Clinical and Pathologic Study of 12 Cases of Lutembacher's Syndrome, *Am. Heart J.*, 57:185, 1959.

283. Marshall, R. J., and Warden, H. E.: Mitral Valve Disease Complicated by Left-to-right Shunt at Atrial Level, *Circulation*, 29:432, 1964.

284. Ross, J., Braunwald, E., Mason, D. T., Friedman, M., Graunwald, N. S., and Morrow, A. G.: Interatrial Communication and Left Atrial Hypertension: A Cause of Continuous Murmur, *Circulation*, 28:853, 1963.

285. Kay, J. H., and Tsuji, H. K.: Surgical Treatment of Tricuspid Insufficiency Secondary to Mitral Valve Disease, Thirteenth Annual Meeting, American College of Chest Physicians, June 18–22, 1964.

286. Keith, T. A., Fowler, N. O., Helmsworth, J. A., and Gralnick, H.: The Course of Surgically Modified Mitral Stenosis, *Am. J. Med.*, 34:308, 1963.

287. Harvey, R. M., and Ferrer, M. I.: A Consideration of Hemodynamic Criteria for Operability in Mitral Stenosis and in Mitral Insufficiency. *Circulation*, 20:442, 1959.

288. Soloff, L. A., Zatuchni, J., and Mark, G. E.: Myocardial and Valvular Factors in Rheumatic Heart Disease with Mitral Stenosis: An Analysis Based upon the Combined Techniques of Cardiac Catheterization and Sequential Venous Angiocardiography, *Am. J. M. Sc.*, 233:518, 1957.

289. Cox, A. R., Cobb, L. A., and Bruce, R. A.: Differential Hemodynamic Effects of Isoproterenol on Mitral Stenosis and Left Ventricular Disease, *Am. Heart J.*, 65:802, 1963.

290. Selzer, A.: Hemodynamic Sequelae of Sustained Elevation of Left Atrial Pressure, *Circulation*, 20:243, 1959.

291. Bubray, E. R., and Pomerantz, H. Z.: Mass Thrombus of the Left Auricle, *Canad. M. A. J.*, 84:258, 1961.

292. Case Records of the Massachusetts General Hospital, *New England J. Med.*, 264:820, 1961.

293. Soloff, L. A., and Zatuchni, J.: Angiocardiographic

294. Daoud, G., Kaplan, S., Perrin, E. U., Dorst, J. P., and Edwards, F. K.: Congenital Mitral Stenosis, *Circulation*, 27:185, 1963.

295. Hurst, J. W., and Cobbs, B. W., Jr.: Diastolic Rumbles, in B. L. Segal (ed.), "The Theory and Practice of Auscultation," F. A. Davis Company, Philadelphia, 1963, p. 395.

296. Abbott, O. A., Warshawski, F. E., and Cobbs, B. W., Jr.: Primary Tumors and Pseudotumors of the Heart, *Ann. Surg.*, 155:855, 1962.

297. Schrire, V., Vogelpoel, L., Nellen, M., Swanepoel, A., and Beck, W.: Silent Mitral Incompetence, *Am. Heart J.*, 61:723, 1961.

298. Aravanis, C.: Opening Snap in Relative Tricuspid Stenosis: Report of 2 Cases of Atrial Septal Defect, *Am. J. Cardiol.*, 12:408, 1963.

299. Nixon, P. G. F.: The Third Heart Sound in Mitral Regurgitation, *Brit. Heart J.*, 23:677, 1961.

300. Nixon, P. G. F., and Wooler, G. H.: Left Ventricular Filling Pressure Gradient in Mitral Insufficiency: Phases of Diastole in Various Syndromes of Mitral Valvular Disease, *Brit. Heart J.*, 25:382, 393, 1963.

301. Rushmer, R. F.: "Cardiac Diagnosis: A Physiologic Approach," W. B. Saunders Company, Philadelphia, 1955, p. 338.

302. Perloff, J. K., and Harvey, W. P.: Clinical Recognition of Tricuspid Stenosis, *Circulation*, 22:346, 1960.

303. Bousvaros, G. A., and Stubington, D.: Some Auscultatory and Phonocardiographic Features of Tricuspid Stenosis, *Circulation*, 29:26, 1964.

304. Williams, W. G.: Dilatation of the Left Atrial Appendage, *Brit. Heart J.*, 25:637, 1963.

305. Levy, M. J., and Edwards, J. E.: Anatomy of Mitral Insufficiency, *Progr. Cardiovas. Dis.*, 5:119, 1962–1963.

306. Ray, E. B., Mendelsohn, D., Jr., and Zimmerman, H. A.: The Role of Surgery in the Treatment of Mitral Regurgitation, *Progr. Cardiovas. Dis.*, 4:259, 1961–1962.

307. Hepper, N. G. G., Burchell, H. B., and Edwards, J. E.: Mitral Insufficiency in Healed Unrecognized Bacterial Endocarditis, *Proc. Staff Meet. Mayo Clin.*, 31:659, 1956.

308. Perloff, J. K.: Combined Mitral Stenosis and Regurgitation: An Auscultatory Evaluation of Their Relative Significance, in B. L. Segal (ed.), "The Theory and Practice of Auscultation, F. A. Davis Company, Philadelphia, 1963.

309. Braunwald, E., Welch, G., and Sarnoff, S.: Hemodynamic Effects of Quantitatively Varied Experimental Mitral Regurgitation, *Circulation Res.*, 5:539, 1957.

310. Brigden, W., and Leatham, A.: Mitral Incompetence, *Brit. Heart J.*, 15:55, 1953.

311. Perloff, J. K., and Harvey, W. P.: Auscultatory

and Phonocardiographic Manifestations of Pure Mitral Regurgitation, *Progr. Cardiovas. Dis.*, **5**: 172, 1962–1963.

312. Segal, B. L., Novack, P., and Kasparian, H.: Intracardiac Phonocardiography, *Am. J. Cardiol.*, **13**: 188, 1964.

313. Hubbard, T. F., Dunn, F. L., and Neis, D. D.: A phonocardiographic Study of the Apical Diastolic Murmurs in Pure Mitral Insufficiency, *Am. Heart J.*, **57**:223, 1959.

314. Ross, J., Jr., Braunwald, E., and Morrow, A. G.: Clinical and Hemodynamic Observations on Pure Mitral Insufficiency, *Am. J. Cardiol.*, **2**:11, 1958.

315. Bruns, D. L.: A General Theory of the Causes of Murmurs in the Cardiovascular System, *Am. J. Med.*, **27**:360, 1959.

316. Leatham, A.: The Value of Auscultation in Cardiology, *A.M.A. Arch. Int. Med.*, **105**:349, 1960.

317. Humphries, J. O'N.: Diagnosis of Pure Mitral Regurgitation, in B. L. Segal (ed.), "The Theory and Practice of Auscultation," F. A. Davis Company, Philadelphia, 1963.

318. Humphries, J. O'N., and McKusick, V. A.: The Differentiation of Organic and "Innocent" Systolic Murmurs, *Progr. Cardiovas. Dis.*, **5**:152, 1962–63.

319. Burchell, H. B.: Possibly Unrecognized Forms of Heart Disease, *Circulation*, **28**:1153, 1964.

320. Logan, A., and Turner, R.: The Diagnosis of Mitral Incompetence Accompanying Mitral Stenosis: Review of 11 Cases Treated Surgically, *Lancet*, **2**:593, 1952.

321. Abelmann, W. H., Ellis, L. B., and Harken, D. E.: The Diagnosis of Mitral Regurgitation: An Evaluation of Clinical Criteria, Fluoroscopy, Phonocardiography, Auricular Esophagogram and Electrokymogram, *Am. J. Med.*, **15**:5, 1953.

322. Wilson, M. G.: The Life History of Systolic Murmurs in Rheumatic Heart Disease, *Progr. Cardiovas. Dis.*, **5**:145, 1962.

323. Jhaveri, S., Czoniezer, G., Reider, R. B., and Massell, B. F.: Relatively Benign "Pure" Mitral Regurgitation of Rheumatic Origin: A Study of Seventy-four Adult Patients, *Circulation*, **22**:39, 1960.

324. Endrys, J., Belobradek, M. P., and Steinhart, L.: Diagnosis of Dominant Mitral Stenosis or Regurgitation Using Amyl Nitrite, *Brit. Heart J.*, **26**: 250, 1964.

325. Barlow, J. B., Pocock, W. A., Marchand, P., and Denny, M.: The Significance of Late Systolic Murmurs, *Am. Heart J.*, **66**:443, 1963.

326. Segal, B. L., and Likoff, W.: Late Systolic Murmurs of Mitral Regurgitation, *Am. Heart J.*, **67**: 757, 1964.

327. Jones, J. W., Rackley, C. E., Bruce, R. A., Dodge, H. T., Cobb, L. A., and Sandler, H.: Left Ventricular Volumes in Valvular Heart Disease, *Circulation*, **29**:887, 1964.

328. Best, R. V., and Heath, D.: The Right Ventricle

and Small Pulmonary Arteries in Aneurysmal Dilatation of the Left Atrium, *Brit. Heart J.*, **26**:312, 1964.

329. Burch, G. E., and Romney, R. B.: Functional Anatomy and "Throttle Valve" Action of the Pulmonary Veins, *Am. Heart J.*, **47**:58, 1954.

330. Donald, K. W.: Pulmonary Vascular Resistance in Mitral Valvular Disease, in "Pulmonary Circulation," International Symposium Sponsored by the Chicago Heart Association, Grune & Stratton, Inc., New York, 1959, p. 285.

331. Harvey, W. P., Corrado, M., and Perloff, J. K.: Some Newer or Poorly Recognized Auscultatory Findings of the Heart: Symposium on Cardiovascular Sound, *Circulation*, **16**:414, 1957.

332. Rappaport, M. B., and Sprague, H. B.: The Graphic Registration of the Normal Heart Sounds, *Am. Heart J.*, **23**:591, 1942.

333. Johnston, F. D., and Overy, D. C.: Vibrations of Low Frequency over the Precordium, *Circulation*, **3**:579, 1951.

334. Nixon, P. G. F., and Wooler, G. H.: Clinical Assessment of Mitral Orifices in Patients with Regurgitation, *Brit. M. J.*, **2**:1122, 1960.

335. Nixon, P. G. F., and Wagner, G. R.: The Duration of Left Ventricular Systole in Mitral Incompetence, *Brit. Heart J.*, **24**:464, 1962.

336. Perloff, J. K., and Harvey, W. P.: Mechanisms of Fixed Splitting of the Second Heart Sound, *Circulation*, **18**:998, 1958.

337. Nixon, P. G. F., Wooler, G. H., and Radigan, L. R.: Mitral Incompetence Caused by Lesions of the Mural Cusp, *Circulation*, **19**:839, 1959.

338. Morrow, A. G., Braunwald, E., Haller, J. A., and Sharp, E. H.: Left Atrial Pressure Pulse in Mitral Valve Disease, *Circulation*, **16**:399, 1957.

339. Grant, R. P.: "Clinical Electrocardiography: The Spatial Vector Approach," McGraw-Hill Book Company, New York, 1957.

340. Priest, E. A., Finlayson, J. K., and Short, D. S.: The X-ray Manifestations of the Heart and Lungs of Mitral Regurgitation, *Progr. Cardiovas. Dis.*, **5**: 219, 1962–63.

341. Khalat, J. D., Chapman, C. B., and Ernst, R.: The Cinefluorographic Approach to the Diagnosis of Mitral Regurgitation, *Progr. Cardiovas. Dis.*, **5**: 631, 1962–63.

342. DeSanctis, R. W., Dean, D. C., and Bland, E. F.: Extreme Left Atrial Enlargement: Some Characteristic Features, *Circulation*, **29**:14, 1964.

343. Douglas, D. M.: Mitral Regurgitation with Mobile Valve Cusps, *Brit. M. J.*, **1**:191, 1953.

344. Schillig, R.: The Significance of Rate and Output Related Variations in the A2–OS Interval, *Am. Heart J.*, **66**:645, 1963.

345. Hamer, M. B., Sujoy, B. R., and Dow, J. W.: Determinants of Left Atrial Pressure Pulse in Mitral Valve Disease, *Circulation*, **19**:257, 1959.

346. Osmundson, P. J., Callahan, J. A., and Edwards,

J. E.: Ruptured Mitral Chordae Tendineae, *Circulation*, 23:42, 1961.

347. Phillips, J. H., Burch, G. E., and De Pasquale, N. P.: The Syndrome of Papillary Muscle Dysfunction: Its Clinical Recognition, *Ann. Int. Med.*, 59:508, 1963.

348. Spencer, M. P., and Greiss, F. C.: Dynamics of Ventricular Ejection, *Circulation Res.*, 10:274, 1962.

349. Sleeper, J. C., Orgain, E. S., and McIntosh, H. D.: Mitral Insufficiency Simulating Aortic Stenosis, *Circulation*, 26:429, 1962.

350. Franch, R. H., and Gay, B. B., Jr.: Congenital Stenosis of the Pulmonary Artery Branches: A Classification, with Postmortem Findings in Two Cases, *Am. J. Med.*, 35:512, 1963.

351. Cobbs, B. W., Jr., Gay, B. B., and Sorsdahl, O.: Personal observation.

352. Breneman, G. M., and Drake, E. H.: Ruptured Papillary Muscle Following Myocardial Infarction with Long Survival: Report of Two Cases, *Circulation*, 25:862, 1962.

353. Korn, D., De Sanctis, R. W., and Sell, S.: Massive Calcification of the Mitral Annulus: A Clinicopathological Study of Fourteen Cases, *New England J. Med.*, 267:900, 1962.

354. DeSanctis, R. W., Tomchik, F. S., and Scully, R. E.: Case Records of the Massachusetts General Hospital, *New England J. Med.*, 269:969, 1963.

355. Bruns, D. L., and Van Der Hauwaert, L. G.: The Aortic Systolic Murmur Developing with Increasing Age, *Brit. Heart J.*, 20:370, 1958.

356. Edwards, J. E., and Burchell, H. B.: Endocardial and Intimal Lesions (Jet Impact) as Possible Sites of Origin of Murmurs, *Circulation*, 28:946, 1958.

357. Burchell, H. B., and Brown, A. L.: Anomalous Origin of Coronary Artery from Pulmonary Artery Masquerading as Mitral Insufficiency, *Am. Heart J.*, 63:388, 1962.

358. Brockenbrough, E. C., Braunwald, E., Roberts, W. C., and Morrow, A. G.: Partial Persistent Atrioventricular Canal Simulating Pure Mitral Regurgitation, *Am. Heart J.*, 63:9, 1962.

359. Bowers, D.: An Electrocardiographic Pattern Associated with Mitral Valve Deformity in Marfan's Syndrome, *Circulation*, 23:30, 1961.

360. Madison, W. M., Bradley, E. J., and Costello, A. J.: Ehlers-Danlos Syndrome with Cardiac Involvement, *Am. J. Cardiol.*, 11:689, 1963.

361. Harrison, D. C., and Dexter, L.: The Evaluation of Patients Who Develop Recurrent Cardiac Symptoms after Mitral Valvuloplasty, *Am. Heart J.*, 65:583, 1963.

362. Varnauskas, E., Cramer, G., Malmcrona, R., Dahl, L. E., Nystrom, W. B., and Werko, L.: Restoration of Normal Sinus Rhythm in Patients with Mitral Valve Disease and Atrial Fibrillation, *Nord. med.*, 62:1109, 1959.

363. Goldman, M. J.: Management of Chronic Atrial

Fibrillation: Indications for and Method of Conversion to Sinus Rhythm, *Progr. Cardiovas. Dis.*, 2:465, 1960.

364. Greene, M. A., Gordon, A., and Boltax, A. J.: Effects of Intravenous Lanatoside-C upon Cardiodynamics in Patients with Mitral Stenosis and Regular Sinus Rhythm, *Am. Heart J.*, 61:622, 1961.

365. Seller, R. H., Swartz, C. D., Raminez-Muxo, O., Brest, A. H., and Mayer, J. H.: Aldosterone Antagonists in Diuretic Therapy: Their Effect in the Refractory Phase, *Arch. Int. Med.*, 113:350, 1964.

366. Ogden, D. A., Scherr, L., Spritz, N., Rubin, A. L., and Luckey, E. H.: The Management of Resistant Fluid-retention States with Intravenous L-arginime Monohydrochloride in Combination with Mercurial Diuretics, *Am. Heart J.*, 61:16, 1961.

367. Ellis, L. B., and Adler, L. N.: Criteria for Surgery in Mitral Valvular Disease, *Am. J. Cardiol.*, 12:17, 1963.

368. Pollard, J. W., Hamilton, M. J., Christensen, N. A., and Achor, R. W.: Problems Associated with Long-term Anticoagulant Therapy: Observations in 139 Cases, *Circulation*, 25:311, 1962.

369. Sherlock, S., Barber, K. M., Bell, G. L., and Watt, P. J.: Anticoagulants and the Liver, in G. W. Pickering (ed.), "Symposium on Anticoagulant Therapy," Harvey and Blythe, London, 1961.

370. McKenzie, M. B., and Ellis, F. H., Jr.: Current Concepts in Surgical Correction of Acquired Mitral Insufficiency, *Circulation*, 28:603, 1963.

371. Burack, B.: The Optimal Time for Cardiac Surgery, *Am. J. Cardiol.*, 12:4, 1963.

372. Ellis, L. B., and Harken, D. E.: Arterial Embolization in Relation to Mitral Valvuloplasty, *Am. Heart J.*, 62:611, 1961.

373. Dahlgren, S., and Bjork, V. O.: Thromboembolic Complications in Connection with Mitral Commissurotomy after Discontinuation of Anticoagulant Therapy, *J. Thoracic & Cardiovas. Surg.*, 43:780, 1962.

374. Bloom, V. R.: The Prognosis of Atrial Fibrillation Following Mitral Valvotomy, *Brit. Heart J.*, 25:595, 1963.

375. Mounsey, P.: Determination of Success after Mitral Valvotomy: The Role of Circulatory Obstruction, the Myocardium and Other Factors, *Brit. M. J.*, 2:311, 1957.

376. Engle, M. A., and Ito, T.: The Post-pericardiotomy Syndrome, *Am. J. Cardiol.*, 7:73, 1961.

377. Smith, W. G.: Postcardiotomy Syndrome: Anticoagulants and Hemopericardium, *Lancet*, 1:750, 1961.

378. Weiser, N. J., Kantor, M., Russell, H. K., and Murphy, L.: The Post-myocardial Infarction Syndrome: The Non-specificity of the Pulmonary Manifestations, *Circulation*, 25:643, 1962.

379. Morrow, A. G., Harrison, D. C., Ross, J., Jr., Braunwald, N. S., and Clark, W. D.: The Surgical

Management of Mitral Valve Disease: A Symposium on Diagnostic Methods, Operative Techniques, and Results, *Ann. Int. Med.*, **60**:1073, 1964.

380. Dexter, L., Harken, D. E., Cobb, L. A., Jr., Novack, P., Schlant, R. C., Phinney, A. O., Jr., and Haynes, T. W.: Aortic Stenosis, *A.M.A. Arch. Int. Med.*, **181**:754, 1958.

381. Gorlin, R., McMillan, I. K. R., Medd, W. E., Matthews, M. B., and Daley, R.: Dynamics of the Circulation in Aortic Valvular Disease, *Am. J. Med.*, **18**:858, 1955.

382. Samet, P., Bernstein, W. H., and Litwak, R. S.: The Effect of Exercise upon the Mean Systolic Left Ventricular-brachial Artery Gradient in Aortic Stenosis, *Dis. Chest*, **40**:665, 1961.

383. Regan, T. J., De Fazio, V., Binals, K., and Hellenic, H. K.: Neosynephrine Induced Pulmonary Congestion in Patients with Aortic Valve Regurgitation, *J. Clin. Invest.*, **38**:1564, 1959.

384. Hancock, E. W.: Differentiation of Valvar, Subvalvar and Supravalvar Aortic Stenosis, *Circulation*, **20**:709, 1959.

385. Hancock, E. W., and Fleming, P. R.: Aortic Stenosis, *Quart. J. Med.*, **29**:209, 1960.

386. Braunwald, E., and Ross, J., Jr.: The Ventricular End Diastolic Pressure: Appraisal of Its Value in the Recognition of Ventricular Failure in Man, *Am. J. Med.*, **34**:147, 1963.

387. Meadows, W. R., Van Pragh, S., Indreika, M., and Sharp, J. T.: Premature Mitral Valve Closure, an Explanation for Absence of the First Sound in Aortic Regurgitation, *Circulation*, **28**:251, 1963.

388. Wood, P.: Aortic Stenosis, *Am. J. Cardiol.*, **1**:553, 1958.

389. Mitchell, A. M., Sackett, C. H., Hunzicker, W. J., and Levine, S. A.: The Clinical Features of Aortic Stenosis, *Am. Heart J.*, **48**:684, 1954.

390. Daoud, G., Reppert, E. H., Jr., and Butterworth, J. S.: Basal Systolic Murmurs and the Carotid Pulse in the Diagnosis of Calcareous Aortic Stenosis, *Ann. Int. Med.*, **50**:323, 1959.

391. Edwards, J. E.: The Etiology of Calcific Aortic Stenosis, *Circulation*, **26**:817, 1962.

392. Anderson, M. W.: The Clinical Course of Patients with Calcific Aortic Stenosis, *Proc. Staff Meet. Mayo Clin.*, **36**:439, 1961.

393. Baker, C., and Somerville, J.: Clinical Features and Surgical Treatment of Fifty Patients with Severe Aortic Stenosis, *Guy's Hosp. Rep.*, **108**:101, 1959.

394. Takeda, J., Warren, R., and Holzman, D.: Prognosis of Aortic Stenosis, *Arch. Surg.*, **87**:931, 1963.

395. Abelman, W. H., and Ellis, L. B.: Severe Aortic Stenosis in Adults: Evaluation by Clinical and Physiologic Criteria and Results of Surgical Treatment, *A.M.A. Arch. Int. Med.*, **51**:449, 1959.

396. Zoob, M., and Smith, K. S.: The Etiology of Complete Heart Block, *Brit. M. J.*, **2**:1149, 1963.

397. Warshawsky, H., and Abramson, W.: Complete Heart Block in Calcareous Aortic Stenosis, *Ann. Int. Med.*, **27**:1040, 1947.

398. Hammarsten, J. G.: Syncope and Aortic Stenosis, *A.M.A. Arch. Int. Med.*, **87**:274, 1951.

399. Leak, D.: Case Report: Effort Syncope in Aortic Stenosis, *Brit. Heart J.*, **21**:289, 1959.

400. Braunwald, E., Roberts, W. C., Goldblatt, A., Aygen, M. M., Rockoff, D., and Gilbert, J. W.: Aortic Stenosis: Physiological, Pathological, and Clinical Concepts (Clinical Staff Conference at the National Institutes of Health), *Ann. Int. Med.*, **58**:494, 1963.

401. Holley, K. E., Bahn, R. C., McGoon, D. C., and Markin, H. T.: Spontaneous Calcific Embolization Associated with Calcific Aortic Stenosis, *Circulation*, **27**:197, 1963.

402. Wigle, E. D.: Myocardial Fibrosis and Calcareous Emboli in Valvular Heart Disease, *Brit. Heart J.*, **19**:539, 1957.

403. Hamer, N. A. J., and Dow, J. W.: The Indications for Measurement of Left Heart Pressures in Mitral and Aortic Valvular Disease, *Am. Heart J.*, **62**:344, 1961.

404. Kumpe, C. W., and Bean, W. B.: Aortic Stenosis: A Study of the Clinical and Pathologic Aspects of 107 Cases, *Medicine*, **27**:139, 1948.

405. Hollenhorst, R. W.: Significance of Bright Plaques in the Retinal Arterioles, *J.A.M.A.*, **178**:23, 1961.

406. Lillington, G. A., Connolly, D. C., and Kavanaugh, G. J.: Coronary Embolism Secondary to Subacute Bacterial Endocarditis in a Case of Calcific Aortic Stenosis, in Symposium on Unusual Manifestations of Aortic Stenosis, *Proc. Staff Meet. Mayo Clin.*, **33**:216, 1958.

407. Heath, D., Edwards, J. E., and Smith, L. A.: The Rheologic Significance of Medial Necrosis and Dissecting Aneurysm of the Ascending Aorta in Association with Calcific Aortic Stenosis, *Proc. Staff Meet. Mayo Clin.*, **33**:228, 1958.

408. Ross, R. S., Criley, J. M., and Epstein, E. J.: Cinecardiographic Studies of Sound Production by Diseased and Prosthetic Aortic Valves, in B. L. Segal (ed.), "The Theory and Practice of Auscultation," F. A. Davis Company, Philadelphia, 1963. p. 500.

409. Goldblatt, A., Aygen, M. M., and Braunwald, E.: Hemodynamic Phonocardiographic Correlations of the Fourth Heart Sound in Aortic Stenosis, *Circulation*, **25**:92, 1962.

410. Robinson, B.: The Carotid Pulse. I. Diagnosis of Aortic Stenosis by External Recordings: II. Relation of External Recordings to Carotid, Aortic, and Brachial Pulses, *Brit. Heart J.*, **25**:51, 61, 1963.

411. Braunwald, E., Goldblatt, A., Aygen, M. M., Rockoff, S. D., and Morrow, A. G.: Congenital Aortic Stenosis. I. Clinical and Hemodynamic Findings in 100 Patients, *Circulation*, **27**:426, 1963.

412. Ellis, L. B. J., and Hancock, E. W.: Evaluation of Surgical Treatment of Acquired and Congenital

Aortic Stenosis, *Progr. Cardiovas. Dis.*, 3:247, 1960.

413. Straube, K. R., McMillan, J. C., Menashe, V. D., and Dotter, E. P.: Post-stenotic Aortic Dilatation as a Roentgenographic Sign in Congenital Valvular Aortic Stenosis. *Am. J. Roentgenol.*, 90:571, 1963.

414. Klatte, E. C., Tampas, J. P., Campbell, J. A., and Lurie, P. R.: The Roentgenographic Manifestations of Aortic Stenosis and Aortic Valvular Insufficiency, *Am. J. Roentgenol.*, 88:57, 1962.

415. Gay, B. B.: Personal communication.

416. Sutnick, A. I., and Soloff, L. A.: P-wave Abnormalities as an Electrocardiographic Index of Hemodynamically Significant Aortic Stenosis, *Circulation*, 28:814, 1963.

417. Wolff, L., Wolff, R., Samartzis, M. D., Mazzoleni, A., Soffe, A. M., Reiner, L., and Matsuoka, S.: Vectorcardiographic Diagnosis: A Correlation with Autopsy Findings in 167 Cases, *Circulation*, 23:861, 1961.

418. Abdin, Z. H.: The Electrocardiogram in Aortic Stenosis, *Brit. Heart J.*, 20:31, 1958.

419. Hugenholtz, P. G., Lees, M. M., and Nadas, A. S.: The Scalar Electrocardiogram, Vectorcardiogram, and Exercise Electrocardiogram in the Assessment of Congenital Aortic Stenosis, *Circulation*, 26:79, 1962.

420. Kontos, H. A., Shapiro, W., and Kemp, V. E.: Observations on the Atrial Sound in Hypertension, *Circulation*, 28:877, 1963.

421. Kincaid-Smith, P., and Barlow, J.: The Atrial Sound in Hypertension and Ischaemic Heart Disease: With Reference to Its Timing and Mode of Production, *Brit. Heart J.*, 21:479, 1959.

422. Fleming, P. R.: The Mechanism of the Pulsus Bisferiens, *Brit. Heart J.*, 19:519, 1957.

423. Benchimol, A., Dimond, E. G., and Shen, Y.: Ejection Time in Aortic Stenosis and Mitral Stenosis: Comparison between the Direct and Indirect Arterial Tracings, with Special Reference to Pre- and Postoperative findings, *Am. J. Cardiol.*, 5:728, 1960.

424. Lees, M., Hauck, A. J., Rudolph, A. M., Nadas, A. S., and Gross, R. E.: Pre- and Postoperative Assessment of Aortic Stenosis, *Circulation*, 22:776, 1960.

425. Katznelson, G., Jreissaty, R. M., Levinson, G. E., Stein, S. W., and Abelmann, W. H.: Combined Aortic and Mitral Stenosis, *Am. J. Med.*, 29:242, 1960.

426. Uricchio, J. F., Sinba, K. P., Bentivoglio, L., and Goldberg, H.: Combined Mitral and Aortic Stenosis, *Ann. Int. Med.*, 51:668, 1959.

427. Uricchio, J. F., Goldberg, H., Sinah, K. P., and Likoff, W.: Combined Mitral and Aortic Stenosis: Clinical and Physiologic Features and Results of Surgery, *Am. J. Cardiol.*, 4:479, 1959.

428. Morrow, A. G., Awe, W. C., and Braunwald, E.: Combined Mitral and Aortic Stenosis, *Brit. Heart J.*, 24:606, 1962.

429. Honey, M.: Clinical and Hemodynamic Observations on Combined Mitral and Aortic Stenosis, *Brit. Heart J.*, 23:545, 1961.

430. Reid, J. M., Stevenson, J. G., Barclay, T. S., and Welsh, T. M.: Combined Aortic and Mitral Stenosis, *Brit. Heart J.*, 24:509, 1962.

431. Hancock, E. W., Madison, W. M., Jr., Proctor, M. H., Abelmann, W. H., and Starkey, G. W. B.: Aortic Stenosis of No Physiologic Significance, *New England J. Med.*, 258:305, 1958.

432. Braunwald, E., Morrow, A. G., Cornell, W. P., Aygen, M. M., and Hilbish, T. F.: Idiopathic Hypertrophic Subaortic Stenosis: Clinical, Hemodynamic, and Angiographic Manifestations, *Am. J. Med.*, 29:924, 1960.

433. Manchester, G. H.: Muscular Subaortic Stenosis, *New England J. Med.*, 269:300, 1963.

434. Benchimol, A., Legler, J. F., and Dimond, E. G.: The Carotid Tracing and Apexcardiogram in Subvalvular Stenosis and Idiopathic Myocardial Hypertrophy, *Am. J. Cardiol.*, 11:427, 1963.

435. Cohen, J., Effat, H., Goodwin, J. F., Oakley, C. M., and Steiner, R. E.: Hypertrophic Obstructive Cardiomyopathy, *Brit. Heart J.*, 26:16, 1964.

436. Bjork, V. O., Hultquist, G., and Lodin, H.: Subaortic Stenosis Produced by an Abnormally Placed Anterior Mitral Leaflet, *J. Thoracic & Cardiovas. Surg.*, 41:659, 1961.

437. Humphries, J. O.'N., and McKusick, V. A.: Murmur of Late Systole, *Circulation*, 26:735, 1962.

438. Prescott, R., Quinn, J. S., and Littman, D.: Electrocardiographic Changes in Hypertrophic Aortic Stenosis Which Simulate Myocardial Infarction, *Am. Heart J.*, 66:42, 1963.

439. Braunwald, E., and Ebert, P. A.: Hemodynamic Alterations in Idiopathic Hypertrophic Subaortic Stenosis Induced by Sympathomimetic Drugs, *Am. J. Cardiol.*, 10:489, 1962.

440. Braunwald, E., Oldham, H. N., Ross, J., Kinhart, J. W., Mason, D. T., and Fort, L., III: The Circulatory Response of Patients with Idiopathic Hypertrophic Subaortic Stenosis to Nitroglycerin and to the Valsalva Maneuver, *Circulation*, 29:422, 1964.

441. Wigle, E. D.: The Arterial Pressure Pulse in Muscular Subaortic Stenosis, *Brit. Heart J.*, 25:92, 1963.

442. Braunwald, E., and Aygen, M. M.: Idiopathic Myocardial Hypertrophy without Congestive Heart Failure or Obstruction to Blood Flow, *Am. J. Med.*, 35:7, 1963.

443. Magida, M. G., and Roseman, D. M.: Long-term Course of Patients with a Basal Diastolic Murmur and Predominant Mitral Stenosis, *New England J. Med.*, 265:118, 1961.

444. Bland, E. F., and Wheeler, E. O.: Severe Aortic Regurgitation in Young People: A Long-term Perspective with Reference to Prognosis and Prosthesis, *New England J. Med.*, 256:667, 1957.

445. Segal, J., Harvey, W. P., and Hufnagel, C.: A

Clinical Study of One Hundred Cases of Severe Aortic Insufficiency, *Am. J. Med.*, 21:200, 1956.

446. Kay, E. B., Suzuki, E., and Zimmerman, H. E.: Criteria for Surgery in Aortic Valvular Disease, *Am. J. Cardiol.*, 12:40, 1963.

447. Wilson, M. G., and Lim, W. N.: The Natural History of Rheumatic Heart Disease in the Third, Fourth, and Fifth Decades of Life, *Circulation*, 16:700, 1957.

448. Harvey, W. P., Segal, J. P., and Hufnagel, C. A.: Unusual Clinical Features Associated with Severe Aortic Insufficiency, *Ann. Int. Med.*, 47:27, 1957.

449. West, J. W., Wendel, H., and Foltz, E. L.: Effects of Aortic Insufficiency on Circulatory Dynamics of the Dog, *Circulation Res.*, 7:685, 1959.

450. Hoffman, F. G., Zimmerman, S. L., and Cardwell, E. S., Jr.: Massive Intestinal Infarction without Vascular Occlusion Associated with Aortic Insufficiency, *New England J. Med.*, 263:436, 1960.

451. Gorlin, R., and Case, R. B.: Clinical Diagnosis of Aortic Valve Disease, *New England J. Med.*, 255:368, 1956.

452. Gorlin, R., and Goodale, W. T.: Changing Blood Pressure in Aortic Insufficiency, *New England J. Med.*, 255:77, 1956.

453. Lange, R. L., and Hecht, H. H.: Genesis of Pistol-shot and Korotkoff Sounds, *Circulation*, 18:975, 1958.

454. Rodbard, S.: Mechanisms, Significance and Alterations of Korotkoff Sounds, in B. L. Segal (ed.), "The Theory and Practice of Auscultation," F. A. Davis Company, Philadelphia, 1964.

455. Rowe, G. G., and Afonso, S.: Investigation of Durozier's Murmur, *J. Clin. Invest.*, 41:1395, 1962.

456. Blumgarth, H. L., and Ernstene, A. C.: Two Mechanisms in the Production of Durozier's Sign: Their Diagnostic Significance and Clinical Test for Differentiating between Them, *J.A.M.A.*, 100:173, 1933.

457. Rees, J. R., Epstein, E. J., Criley, J. M., and Ross, R. S.: Haemodynamic Effects of Severe Aortic Regurgitation, *Brit. Heart J.*, 26:412, 1964.

458. Goldstein, S., and Killip, T., III: Comparison of Direct and Indirect Arterial Pressures in Aortic Regurgitation, *New England J. Med.*, 267:1121, 1962.

459. Puchner, T. C., Huston, J. H., and Hellmuth, G. A.: Aortic Valve Insufficiency in Arterial Hypertension, *Am. J. Cardiol.*, 5:758, 1960.

460. Friedman, B., and Hathaway, B. M.: Fenestration of the Semilunar Cusps, and "Functional" Aortic and Pulmonic Valve Insufficiency, *Am. J. Med.*, 24:549, 1958.

461. Harvey, W. P., and Perloff, J. K.: Some Recent Advances in Clinical Auscultation of the Heart, *Progr. Cardiovas. Dis.*, 2:97, 1959.

462. Faber, J. J.: Sound Damping as Found on the Chest Surface, *Circulation Res.*, 13:352, 1963.

463. Currens, J. H., Thompson, W. B., Rappaport, M. B., and Sprague, H. B.: Clinical and Phono-

cardiographic Observations on the Flint Murmur, *New England J. Med.*, 248:583, 1953.

464. Kiger, R. C.: Differentiation of Austin Flint and Mitral Stenosis Murmurs by Amyl Nitrite, *Clin. Res.*, 11:24, 1963.

465. Aldridge, H. E.: The Estimation of Aortic Insufficiency, *Canad. M. A. J.*, 87:941, 1962.

466. Singer, D. H., and Perloff, J. K.: Electrocardiogram of Free Aortic Insufficiency, *Circulation*, 26:786, 1962.

467. Sodi-Pallares, D.: "New Bases of Electrocardiography," R. M. Colder (ed.), The C. V. Mosby Company, St. Louis, 1956.

468. Pascarelli, E. F., and Bertrand, C. A.: Comparison of Blood Pressures in the Arms and Legs, *New England J. Med.*, 270:693, 1964.

469. Frank, M. J., Casanegra, T., and Levinson, G. E.: Evaluation of Aortic Insufficiency, *Circulation*, 28:723, 1963.

470. Sandler, H., Dodge, H. T., Hay, R. E., and Rackley, C. E.: Quantitation of Valvular Insufficiency in Man by Angiocardiography, *Am. Heart J.*, 65:501, 1963.

471. Schulder, D. G., Harvey, W. P., and Hufnagel, C. A.: Rheumatic Spondylitis and Aortic Insufficiency, *New England J. Med.*, 255:11, 1956.

472. Heggtveit, H. A.: Syphilitic aortitis: A Clinicopathologic Autopsy Study of 100 Cases, *Circulation*, 29:346, 1964.

473. Friedman, B., and Olansky, S.: Diagnosis of Syphilitic Cardiovascular Disease with Special Reference to Treponemal Immobilization Tests, *Am. Heart J.*, 50:323, 1955.

474. McKusick, V. A.: The Cardiovascular Aspects of Marfan's Syndrome: A Heritable Disorder of Connective Tissue, *Circulation*, 11:321, 1955.

475. Headley, R. N., Carpenter, H. M., and Sawyer, C. G.: Unusual Features of Marfan's Syndrome Including Two Postmortem Studies, *Am. J. Cardiol.*, 11:259, 1963.

476. Segal, J. P.: Diagnosis of Aortic Regurgitation, in B. L. Segal (ed.), "The Theory and Practice of Auscultation," F. A. Davis Company, Philadelphia, 1963, p. 477.

477. Steinberg, I., and Finby, N.: Clinical Manifestations of the Unperforated Aortic Sinus Aneurysm, *Circulation*, 14:115, 1956.

478. London, S. B., and London, R. E.: Production of Aortic Regurgitation by Unperforated Aneurysm of the Sinus of Valsalva, *Circulation*, 24:1403, 1961.

479. Levy, M. J., Siegal, D. L., Wang, Y., and Edwards, J. E.: Rupture of Aortic Valve Secondary to Aneurysm of Ascending Aorta, *Circulation*, 27:422, 1963.

480. Csonkna, G. W., Litchfield, J. W., Otis, J. W., and Willcox, R. R.: Cardiac Lesions in Reiter's Disease, *Brit. M. J.*, 1:243, 1961.

481. Coffman, J. D., and Sommers, S. C.: Familial Pseudoxanthoma Elasticum and Valvular Heart Disease, *Circulation*, 19:242, 1959.

482. McGuire, J., Scott, R. C., and Goll, I. A.: Chronic Aortitis of Undetermined Cause with Severe and Fatal Aortic Insufficiency, *Am. Clin. & Climatol. A. J.,* **69**:61, 1957.

483. Logue, R. B.: Personal communication.

484. Evans, W., and Lewis, D.: The Carotid Shudder, *Brit. Heart J.,* **7**:171, 1945.

485. Adler, L. W., Yankopoulous, N. A., Federici, E. E., and Abelmann, W. H.: Hemodynamic Effects of Ouabain upon the Hypertrophied Left Ventricle in Aortic Stenosis, *J. Clin. Invest.,* **42**:912, 1963.

486. Aceves, S., and Carral, R.: The Diagnosis of Tricuspid Valve Disease, *Am. Heart J.,* **34**:114, 1947.

487. Goodale, F., and Shaw, R. S.: Functional Examination of the Heart at Autopsy, *New England J. Med.,* **253**:719, 1955.

488. Muller, O., and Shillingford, J.: Tricuspid Incompetence, *Brit. Heart J.,* **16**:194, 1954.

489. Kitchin, A., and Turner, R.: Diagnosis and Treatment of Tricuspid Stenosis, *Brit. Heart J.,* **26**:354, 1964.

490. Sleight, P.: Unilateral Elevation of the Internal Jugular Pulse, *Brit. Heart J.,* **24**:726, 1962.

491. Clark, W. S., Kulka, J. P., and Bauer, W.: Rheumatic Aortitis with Aortic Regurgitation: An Unusual Manifestation of Rheumatoid Arthritis (Including Spondylitis), *Am. J. Med.,* **22**:580, 1957.

492. Graham, D. C., and Smythe, H. A.: The Carditis and Aortitis of Ankylosing Spondylitis, *Bull. Rheumat. Dis.,* **9**:171, 1958.

493. Davidson, P., Baggenstoss, A. H., Slocumb, C. H., and Daugherty, G. W.: Cardiac and Aortic Lesions in Rheumatoid Spondylitis, *Proc. Staff Meet. Mayo Clin.,* **38**:427, 1963.

494. Wilkinson, M.: Rheumatoid Pericarditis: Report of Four Cases, *Brit. M. J.,* **2**:1723, 1962.

495. Good, A. E.: The Chest Pain of Ankylosing Spondylitis, *Ann. Int. Med.,* **58**:926, 1963.

496. Lebowitz, W. B.: Heart in Rheumatoid Arthritis (Rheumatoid Disease): Clinical and Pathological Study of Sixty-two Cases, *Ann. Int. Med.,* **58**:102, 1963.

497. Weintraub, A. M., and Zvaifler, N. J.: The Occurrence of Valvular and Myocardial Disease in Patients with Chronic Joint Deformity, *Am. J. Med.,* **35**:145, 1963.

498. Sokoloff, L.: Cardiac Involvement in Rheumatoid Arthritis and Allied Disorders: Current Concepts, *Mod. Concepts Cardiovas. Dis.,* **32**:847, 1964.

26 SURGICAL TREATMENT OF ACQUIRED VALVULAR HEART DISEASE

John W. Kirklin, M.D.,
Robert B. Wallace, M.D., and
Howard B. Burchell, M.D.

MITRAL STENOSIS

Pathology and Etiology

Rheumatic fever is considered the usual cause of mitral stenosis. A documented episode of it is apparent historically in 60 to 65 per cent of cases.[1,2] The initial rheumatic involvement ordinarily occurs along the free edges of the valve leaflets, where thickening and loss of pliability develop. Progressive scarring and deformity of the valve follow. Fusion at the anterolateral and posteromedial commissures causes narrowing of the valve orifice. Valve function frequently is further impaired by fusion and contraction of the chordae tendineae. Calcium deposits, either localized or generalized, are found in the valve leaflets in approximately 40 per cent of operative cases[3] (Fig. 26-1).

Life History

Patients with mitral stenosis usually suffer gradual progression of disability, although temporary plateaus of remarkable exercise tolerance occur. Concomitant with advancing valvular obstruction, the end-diastolic pressure difference between left atrium and left ventricle increases and results in elevated left atrial and pulmonary venous pressure. Episodes of pulmonary edema occur, frequently initiated by the onset of atrial fibrillation. Later, pulmonary vascular disease develops in many patients, and resultant pulmonary artery hypertension increases the work load of the right ventricle. Right ventricular function may decrease, tricuspid valve

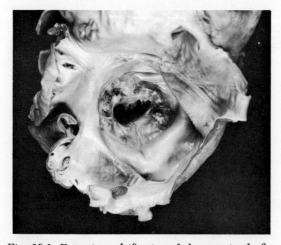

Fig. 26-1. Extensive calcification of the anterior leaflet and both commissural areas. (Necropsy specimen of a calcified, stenotic, incompetent mitral valve.) Leaflets are immobile, and surgical correction obviously requires replacement of such a valve.

incompetence develop, and fluid retention and hepatomegaly result.

Olesen[2] reported that 20 per cent of patients with mitral stenosis died within 1 year from the time that they were first seen. Sixty per cent were dead within 10 years. In the survivors there was progressive cardiac disability.

Surgical Treatment by Closed Technique

Operation

A closed operation is the authors' preference at present in the initial surgical treatment of the stenotic, pliable mitral valve. The approach used is similar to that described by Souttar[4] in 1925 and later advocated by Bailey[5] and Harken and associates.[6] About 1960 the technique was modified to include the use of a dilator introduced transventricularly as described by Logan and Turner.[7]

An anterolateral thoracotomy is utilized. The pericardium is incised longitudinally, anterior to the phrenic nerve. The left atrial appendage is incised without clamping it (to avoid dislodgement of an atrial thrombus), and a small amount of blood is allowed to gush out in order that any loose thrombus may be extruded. The surgeon's right index finger is introduced into the atrium through the appendage with bleeding controlled by a previously positioned Rumel tourniquet. If adequate mobilization of the valve leaflets can be achieved with minimal digital manipulation, which is possible in about 10 per cent of cases, this is all that is done. In the remaining cases the dilator, introduced transventricularly, is used [8,9] (Fig. 26-2A and B).

Postoperative Care

The postoperative care in general is the same as that for any patient who has undergone thoracotomy. If the patient has been receiving digitalis preoperatively, this is continued. If a thrombus was present in the left atrium, anticoagulant therapy (warfarin) is started 24 hr after operation and continued for 10 days.

Prophylactic quinidine therapy is employed for patients in sinus rhythm before operation. It has been shown that this practice reduces the incidence of postoperative atrial fibrillation by 50 per cent.[10]

Hospital Mortality and Morbidity

At the Mayo Clinic, since 1960, the mortality rate for primary closed mitral commissurotomy has been 1.8 per cent. This is similar to rates reported from other centers during the same period.[11] It is lower than the mortality rate of 10 to 12 per cent reported in earlier periods.[8] In previous series the deaths occurred primarily among patients with markedly thickened, nonpliable, calcified valves[12]

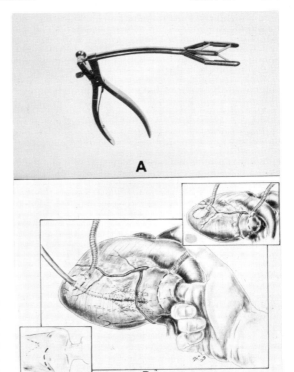

Fig. 26-2. A. Tubbs's mitral valve dilator. In practice either this dilator or the one described by Gerbode[8] is used. B. Transventricular mitral valvotomy. It is important to advance the dilator into the mitral valve under digital control by the right index finger. (*Reproduced from D. A. Cooley and J. M. Stoneburner: Transventricular Mitral Valvotomy, Surgery, 46:414–420, 1959, with permission of authors and publisher.*)

and among patients with multivalvular disease. Both groups are now treated by open operation. Patients treated by closed operation, therefore, are better selected. This is probably the most important factor in the reduced mortality from closed operation.

The most frequently encountered postoperative complication is the postcommissurotomy syndrome, characterized by numerous symptoms and signs including chest pain and fever. This occurred in 30 per cent of patients in the series of Ellis, Harken, and Black.[13] The condition is usually self-limiting and is not thought in and of itself to lead to a poor result. Atrial fibrillation develops after operation in 24 to 44 per cent of patients who are in sinus rhythm preoperatively,[10] unless quinidine is employed prophylactically. The previously reported incidence of arterial embolization of 2.1 per cent in class III patients and 8.0 per cent in class IV patients[13] (New York Heart Association classification) has been reduced considerably with the present criteria for selection of patients and technique of operation.

The development of a degree of mitral regurgitation during transventricular mitral commissurotomy was reported by Björk and Malers[14] in 14 per cent of cases (12 out of 83 patients operated on). In two cases the complication was thought to contribute to an operative mortality.

Results

Initial good results can be expected in 80 to 85 per cent of the patients who survive closed mitral commissurotomy.[13,15] Hemodynamic correlation with symptomatic improvement can be demonstrated by postoperative catheterization studies. Morrow and Braunwald [16] reported that the mean postoperative diastolic-pressure gradient across the mitral valve is 6 mm Hg, a 62 per cent reduction from the mean preoperative gradient of 16 mm Hg.

Follow-up studies over a 5- to 10-year period after operation reveal deterioration in some patients who initially had a good result. This deterioration is reported to be at the rate of about 5 per cent per year.[17] It is usually associated with restenosis or the development of incompetence at the mitral valve. This observation supports the concept that the scarring and deformity from rheumatic valvulitis are a continuing, progressive process. Embolization occurs in the late follow-up period at a rate of 0.5 to 0.7 per cent per patient year. This complication accounts for 10 per cent of the deaths in the follow-up period.[13]

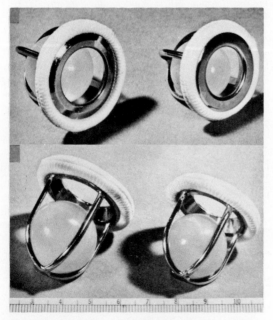

Fig. 26-3. Starr-Edwards ball-valve prosthesis for replacement of mitral or tricuspid valve.

Present Indications for Closed Mitral Commissurotomy

The present low mortality and morbidity and the early and late results following closed mitral commissurotomy form the basis for determining the indications for operation. On the basis of these, mitral commissurotomy is considered advisable for patients whose daily activities are impaired by the symptoms of mitral stenosis. Symptoms should not be allowed to progress to an advanced degree before surgical treatment is advised. It may be recommended for some patients with minimal or no symptoms in whom there is evidence of pulmonary vascular disease and an obstructive mitral valve.

Closed mitral commissurotomy is not indicated when physical findings or x-ray studies indicate gross multivalvular disease, mitral regurgitation, or nonpliable or heavily calcified mitral leaflets. If symptoms warrant, such patients should be considered for open operation. Usually, open operation is preferred also for patients who have previously undergone closed commissurotomy.

Surgical Treatment by Open Operation

Some surgeons have advocated that an open technique be used in all operations for mitral stenosis.[18,19] At present the authors reserve open operation for the patients just described as being unsuited to commissurotomy by a closed technique. In these circumstances, adequate repair often necessitates excision of the valve and replacement with a prosthesis.

Operative Technique and Postoperative Care

At present the authors employ a median sternotomy routinely for open operations on the mitral valve, because it provides adequate exposure of the valve and good conditions for establishing cardiopulmonary bypass and for preventing air embolization. Defects of other valves can be studied and corrected also. After extracorporeal circulation is instituted, ventricular fibrillation is established by cardiac cooling, and the mitral valve is approached through an incision in the right wall of the left atrium anterior to the entrance of the right pulmonary veins. Commissurotomy is performed with a knife if the findings indicate that good function can be so achieved. Usually such is not the case, and the valve is excised. The authors' present preference for mitral valve replacement is the Starr-Edwards ball-valve prosthesis (Fig. 26-3),[20] which is sutured in place with multiple interrupted sutures of Tevdak.

Postoperatively, blood replacement is determined by arterial pressure and left atrial pressure.[21] If cardiac output is low in spite of adequate ventricular filling pressure, attention is directed toward maintaining optimal blood levels of oxygen by tracheostomy and utilization of intermittent positive-pressure breathing.[22] Digitalis is useful primarily in the presence of atrial fibrillation with rapid ventricular rate. Oliguria persistent through the first postoperative day is treated with mannitol in those patients who show a favorable response to a test dose. (Renal shutdown has been rare in the authors' experience following any type of open intracardiac surgery.) Methicillin (Staphcillin) is given preoperatively and for 5 days postoperatively. Anticoagulant therapy (warfarin) is begun on the fourth postoperative day and continued indefinitely in patients with prosthetic valves.

Results

The mortality rate reported from centers that employ open operation for correction in all cases of mitral stenosis is 6.5 to 10 per cent.[18,19] Kay[23] reported improvement in 93 per cent of patients surviving operation. Sixty per cent are said to have normal hemodynamics postoperatively.[23] The follow-up on these patients has not been sufficiently long to compare results with those of patients treated by closed technique.

The operative mortality for mitral valve replacement in a series of 72 patients operated on at the Mayo Clinic from January, 1962, to February 1, 1964, is 19 per cent. In the patients surviving operation, the initial results have been excellent. Insufficient time has passed for evaluation of the long-term results of this procedure.

MITRAL VALVE INCOMPETENCE

Etiology and Pathology

Competence of the mitral valve depends on the integrity of the valve leaflets, chordae tendineae, and papillary muscles and the size of the valve ring. Inflammatory changes associated with rheumatic valvulitis may produce retraction of valve leaflets, particularly the posterior one, and fusion and contraction of the chordae tendineae, thus preventing apposition of the leaflets during systole. Dilatation of the valve ring may produce incompetence, there being a relative decrease in the amount of valve tissue. Calcification of the valve is present in 8 to 10 per cent of cases in which the primary hemodynamic deficit is incompetence.[24] In such cases, the valve is usually somewhat stenotic as well.

Subacute bacterial endocarditis with chordal rupture and destruction of leaflet tissue may result in incompetence of the mitral valve. Myocardial infarction or ischemia involving the posterior wall and the anterolateral or posterior papillary muscles can lead to sudden development of incompetence of the mitral valve due to rupture of the papillary muscle or the chordae tendineae.[25] Incompetence also can follow surgical correction of mitral stenosis.

Life History

Pure rheumatic mitral valvular incompetence, mild to moderate in degree, may be well tolerated for a long time. Onset and progression of symptoms are often gradual. The acute onset of gross mitral regurgitation, which occurs on rupture of chordae tendineae or a papillary muscle, quickly produces severe symptoms, including severe dyspnea and weakness, and is tolerated poorly. In the presence of incompetence of the mitral valve, congestive heart failure may be precipitated by the onset of atrial fibrillation, pulmonary embolism, or bronchopulmonary infection.

Surgical Treatment

Operation and Postoperative Care

At present an open operative technique is used exclusively. A limiting factor in all these operations except total valvular replacement is the difficulty of ascertaining the precise anatomic cause of the incompetence when the mitral valve is exposed and of assessing the *completeness* of repair while the left atrium is still open.

Annuloplasty[26] has been the most successful procedure short of total mitral valve replacement and has the obvious advantages of a procedure utilizing the patient's own tissues. Results are best when there is annular dilatation and the valve leaflets are pliable and without chordal elongation or rupture. A commonly used surgical approach for annuloplasty is a right anterolateral thoracotomy, with entrance into the left atrium from its right side. The mitral valve then can be studied to good advantage, because it is not distorted by efforts to expose it. However, the authors prefer median sternotomy for *all* open operations on the mitral valve because of the advantages indicated earlier. When annuloplasty is performed, the technique of Merendino et al. is employed [26] (Fig. 26-4).

Numerous other techniques have been described for plastic reconstruction of the incompetent mitral valve. In the authors' experience they are often unsatisfactory. An exception is the repair of a solitary perforation of the anterior leaflet resulting from bacterial endocarditis (Fig. 26-5). This procedure has given good results for a long period to the few patients on whom the authors have performed it. Plication of the leaflet when incompetence is due to isolated chordal rupture can also give good results in properly selected cases.[27]

In practice, the authors now employ total replacement of the mitral valve for most patients with incompetent mitral valves. The incision and approach have been described. The valve is totally excised. The Starr-Edwards ball-valve prosthesis[20] is sutured in place with Tevdak sutures in such a way that the sewing ring lies on the atrial side of the annulus. When the ring is jammed into position on the ventricular side of the annulus, left ventricular performance is sometimes severely impaired for the first few postoperative days, probably because the sewing ring in this position interferes with ventricular systole. Particular attention must be paid to the prevention of entrapment and later embolization of air in the large left atrium and ventricle of these patients. Excision of the valve and insertion of the prosthesis, therefore, are done during hypothermically induced ventricular fibrillation. The aorta may be cross clamped for short

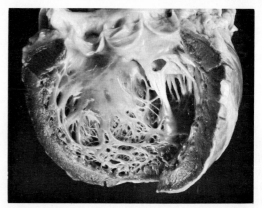

Fig. 26-5. Solitary perforation of the anterior leaflet of the mitral valve. This could be repaired with a patch of pericardium.

periods to facilitate exposure. After the left atrium is closed, all air is aspirated from the left side of the heart via the suction line that has previously been inserted into the left ventricle through a stab wound in its tip. Only then are the ventricles defibrillated.

Postoperative care is accomplished in a fashion similar to that described under Mitral Stenosis.

Hospital Mortality and Morbidity

Mortality rates for annuloplasty have now become low (7 per cent in the authors' hands since January, 1962),[28] primarily because of the limitation of its use to patients in whom it is clearly indicated. Mortality after total replacement of the mitral valve has been 21 per cent in the authors' hands. Similar results are reported by others.[29]

Although mortality and morbidity have occurred in the past from air embolization, with present techniques this has not occurred and should not occur. Embolization of thrombotic material has been rare in the authors' experience. Infection has not become manifest in the early postoperative period in their cases but is an ever-present threat in all situations where a prosthesis is utilized. The chief cause of mortality has been low cardiac output, which in most cases has been associated with a high left atrial pressure and a low right atrial pressure. It is believed that the sewing ring and cage of the Starr-Edwards prosthesis interfere with left ventricular systole and contribute to mortality. If the patient survives the first few postoperative days, adaptation of the ventricle seems to occur, and the hemodynamic state becomes good.

Results

Good long-term results from annuloplasty in properly selected cases have been documented by

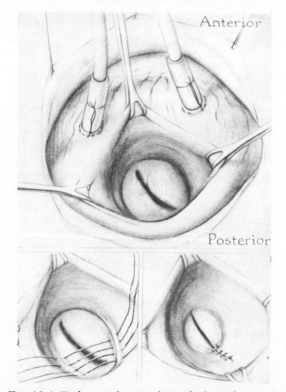

Fig. 26-4. Technique for mitral annuloplasty described by Merendino and associates in 1959.[26] Heavy silk sutures are utilized for the narrowing of the annulus in the region of the medial commissure. (*Reproduced from K. A. Merendino, G. I. Thomas, J. E. Jesseph, P. W. Herron, L. C. Winterscheid, and R. R. Vetto: The Open Correction of Rheumatic Mitral Regurgitation and/or Stenosis with Special Reference to Regurgitation Treated by Posteromedial Annuloplasty Utilizing a Pump-oxygenator, Ann. Surg., 150:5–22, 1959, with permission of authors and publisher.*)

Anderson and associates[30] and by Bigelow and associates.[31]

The follow-up period after mitral valve replacement with the Starr-Edwards prosthesis is limited to about 2½ years at present. During this time 10 per cent of the authors' patients who have left the hospital have died, in nearly all instances from infection or embolization (all were on anticoagulant treatment). The result in surviving patients has been superb, with nearly all becoming virtually asymptomatic in spite of their advanced degree of disability before operation. If the passage of more years does not witness further complications such as infection, thrombosis, embolization, or dehiscence, total valve replacement promises to be an excellent therapeutic procedure.

Present Indications for Operation

Significant and progressing symptoms must be present in a patient who is to be subjected to surgical treatment for incompetence of the mitral valve, for long-term results of total valvular replacement are not yet known. Whenever possible, symptoms should not be allowed to progress to the stage of chronic intractable heart failure before operation is advised. The presence of defects at other valves and of chronic intractable heart failure increase the risk of operation but are *not* a contraindication for it. Operation is urgently indicated for patients in whom significant incompetence of the mitral valve has developed suddenly.

AORTIC STENOSIS

Pathology

The appearance of the valve in adult patients with aortic stenosis may not permit distinction between congenital and acquired disease. However, a history of rheumatic fever in 51 per cent of cases[32] and involvement of the mitral valve in approximately 50 per cent of cases[33] suggest that rheumatic fever is frequently causative in aortic stenosis. There are many examples of isolated calcific aortic stenosis that suggest a degenerative process superimposed on a congenitally bicuspid valve.

Calcification is present in a high percentage of cases. In female patients calcification occurs somewhat less frequently, and the basic architecture of the cusps is often preserved (Fig. 26-6). When the aortic valve is heavily calcified, the commissure between the left and right coronary cusps is usually unrecognizable, and there is only a slit-like orifice (Fig. 26-7). In the most advanced examples of the disease the calcification involves and distorts all cusps (Fig. 26-8) and may extend down into the anterior leaflet of the mitral valve or into the ven-

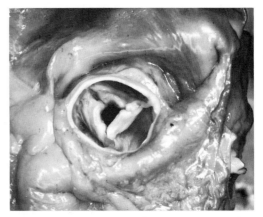

Fig. 26-6. Stenotic aortic valve with thickened but noncalcified cusps. The commissures, now fused, are easily identified.

tricular septum. Complete heart block may result from the latter. Because of the rigidity of the cusps, varying degrees of incompetence of the valve may be present.

Arteriosclerosis of the coronary arteries is present in a significant number of patients with aortic stenosis and may complicate the therapeutic problem. Calcific emboli dislodged spontaneously from the aortic valve may produce coronary artery obstruction. Such emboli may go also to brain and kidney.[34]

Life History

Aortic stenosis may be well tolerated for long periods without symptoms. Sudden death, without significant preexisting symptoms, occurs in about

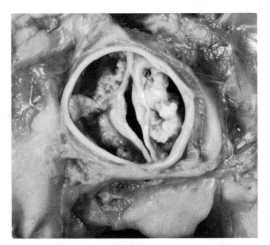

Fig. 26-7. Stenotic, calcified aortic valve. The right and left coronary cusps (to the viewer's left) appear as an essentially single cusp because of the complete fusion of their commissure.

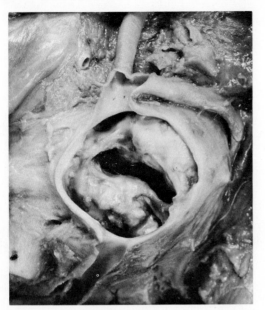

Fig. 26-8. Heavily calcified aortic valve in which normal architecture of the valve cusps has been completely destroyed.

20 per cent of untreated patients, presumably from cardiac arrhythmia resulting from myocardial ischemia. Angina develops in some patients as the first symptom and, although of serious import, may be present years before additional symptoms develop.[35] Syncopal attacks are more ominous. Symptoms of pulmonary venous hypertension (dyspnea, orthopnea, and paroxysmal nocturnal dyspnea) indicate reduction of left ventricular function and are often the prelude to death. Signs and symptoms of right ventricular dysfunction indicate that the end stage of the disease has been reached.

Surgical Treatment

The pathologic alterations in the valve are such that a satisfactory result can be obtained in only a few patients from incision of fused commissures and debridement of cusps. The operation of choice is usually excision and replacement of the valve. The authors' experience with replacement of individual cusps by Teflon cusps has been unsatisfactory,[36] and at present a Starr-Edwards ball-valve prosthesis is used to replace the entire valve. A median sternotomy is used. Normothermic cardiopulmonary bypass is established (Fig. 26-9), a sucker is inserted into the left ventricle through a stab wound in its apex, and a longitudinal incision is made in the ascending aorta above the aortic valve. The valve is excised, during which great pains are taken to prevent the dislodgement of

any calcific particles and their loss into the left ventricle,[37] whence they would subsequently embolize. Direct perfusion of the left and right coronary arteries is then begun at about 150 ml per min each (Figs. 26-10 and 26-11). A Starr-Edwards ball-valve prosthesis (Fig. 26-12) is sutured into place with multiple interrupted sutures of Tevdak. Normothermic perfusion of the coronary arteries is continued until about 10 min before closure of the aortotomy; then the coronary perfusate is cooled to 15°C. The myocardium is thus cooled, and the coronary cannulas are removed before starting closure of the aortotomy. The incision in the aortic root is closed, and the aortic clamp is released. Air must be completely evacuated from the left side of the heart via the *sucker* in the left ventricle. Because of the previous myocardial cooling, there is ventricular fibrillation, which is terminated by electric shock. The remainder of the procedure is completed as usual.

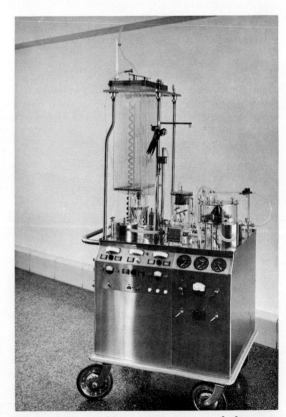

Fig. 26-9. Mayo-Gibbon stationary vertical sheet oxygenator employed in the authors' institution. Several types of pump oxygenators have been proved to be satisfactory for the long perfusions necessary in replacement of a valve, including this particular pump oxygenator. Use of this equipment results in minimal blood trauma, adequate arterial gas levels, and adequate blood flow.

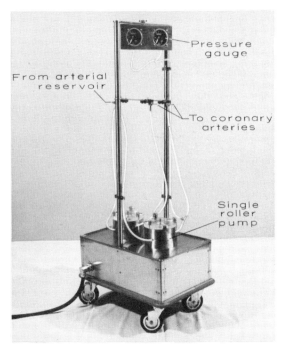

Fig. 26-10. Equipment for direct perfusion of coronary arteries (see also Fig. 26-11). Separate pumps are employed for perfusion of each coronary artery, with pressure gauges for monitoring the pressure within the line leading to the coronary perfusion cannulas.

Postoperative Care

This is managed in a fashion similar to that for replacement of the mitral valve. Arrhythmias, including atrial fibrillation, are common after replacement of the aortic valve; thus quinidine is employed prophylactically if sinus rhythm is present immediately after operation. Anticoagulant therapy, begun on the fourth postoperative day, is usually discontinued after 3 months.

Results

The mortality rate for aortic valve replacement with the Starr-Edwards ball-valve prosthesis in 133 patients operated on at the Mayo Clinic between January, 1963, and April 15, 1964, has been 4 per cent. Patients with chronic heart failure have not had a higher mortality rate than others.[39] The deaths have been from myocardial infarction, infection, and low cardiac output. There have been seven known late deaths among the 127 patients who left the hospital alive. In surviving patients the symptomatic improvement has been striking, and in many there is objective evidence of reduction in size of the left ventricle. The longest period of follow-up of a patient with a ball-valve prosthesis in the aortic area is 2½ years.[40]

Indications for Operation

Asymptomatic patients with aortic stenosis should not be subjected to operation at present. Patients with symptoms from pulmonary venous hypertension should be advised to have operation promptly, as should those with hepatomegaly and fluid retention. Patients with a history of repeated syncope are advised to have operation. Patients whose only symptom is significant angina are usually advised to have operation, although it does not seem so urgently necessary in these. When symptoms are not clearly on the basis of aortic stenosis, assessment of the difference in systolic pressure between left ventricle and ascending aorta and measurement of cardiac output are helpful. When angina is a prominent symptom, consideration must be given to the possible coexistence of coronary artery disease. If there is significant obstruction at the aortic

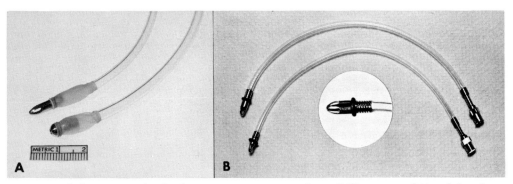

Fig. 26-11. A. Cuffed King cannulas for direct coronary artery perfusion.[38] These are so designed that the pressure within the cannula itself inflates the silastic cuff. (*Reproduced from B. J. King: An Improved Coronary Artery Perfusion Cannula, J. Thoracic Surg.*, **45**:667–669, 1963, *with permission of author and publisher.*) B. Cannulas of Albertal type with O-rings. Occasionally in small coronary artery ostia these are more easily utilized than the King cannulas.

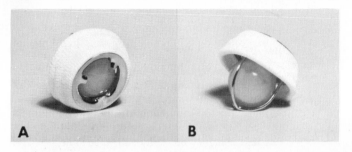

Fig. 26-12. Recent model of Starr-Edwards ball-valve prosthesis for replacement of the aortic valve.

valve, operation is usually advised even though coronary artery disease of mild or moderate degree is known to be present.

AORTIC VALVE INCOMPETENCE

Pathology

Acquired incompetence of the aortic valve may result from deformity or loss of substance of the aortic cusps or from dilatation of the aortic annulus. Rheumatic valvulitis, syphilitic aortitis, bacterial endocarditis, and aneurysms involving the ascending aorta may produce such deformities. The incidence of proximal aortic dilatation due to lesions of medionecrosis cystica type appears to be increasing, perhaps owing to greater awareness. Cases of traumatic rupture of aortic cusps either from strenuous effort or chest wall trauma have been recorded.[41]

Commonly, at operation for severe, noncalcific incompetence of the aortic valve, the cusps appear at first glance to be normal. Close inspection reveals that they are slightly thickened, the free edges are

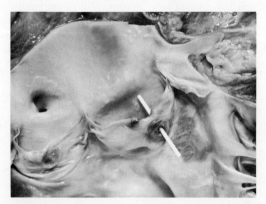

Fig. 26-13. Ruptured aneurysm of an aortic cusp secondary to subacute bacterial endocarditis. Notice the rather discrete perforation in the noncoronary cusp with minimal distortion in the remainder of the cusps. (*Reproduced from J. E. Edwards: "An Atlas of Acquired Diseases of the Heart and Great Vessels: Diseases of the Valves and Pericardium," W. B. Saunders Company, Philadelphia, 1961, vol. 1, p. 331, with permission of author and publisher.*)

rolled, and the distance from the free margin to the aortic wall is shortened. Varying degrees of incompetence are found in patients with calcified, stenotic valves whose cusps are sometimes shortened and immobile. Syphilitic aortitis with aortic insufficiency is now uncommon. In this condition, the ascending aorta becomes flaccid and dilated because of destruction of muscle and elastic fibers in the media. Dilatation of the valve ring, shortening of valve cusps, and widening of the commissures between the cusps produce valvular incompetence. Coronary artery flow may be impaired by involvement of the coronary ostiums. Discrete perforation from bacterial endocarditis may render severely incompetent an otherwise only mildly deformed cusp (Fig. 26-13). Aneurysms of the ascending aorta, with or without Marfan's syndrome, may produce aortic incompetence by dilatation of the valve ring.[42] Dissecting aneurysms of the ascending aorta may result in the sudden onset of incompetence of the aortic valve. The dissection proceeds down toward the sinuses of Valsalva, loosens the attachment of the cusps, and thus renders them deformed and incompetent.[43]

Life History

An asymptomatic period for as long as 10 years usually occurs in patients whose aortic valve incompetence has appeared gradually. Most patients die within 5 years after onset of symptoms. Although sudden death, attributed to myocardial ischemia and arrhythmia, occurs in 5 per cent of cases, the general course of rheumatic aortic insufficiency is relatively slow and predictable.[44] In cases of acute onset of aortic regurgitation, as may occur in a dissecting aneurysm or rupture of a cusp, the course is rapid, and the response to medical management is poor.[45]

Surgical Treatment and Results

In most cases a deformed and incompetent aortic valve is best treated by excision and replacement. The Starr-Edwards ball-valve prosthesis appears to be the best type of replacement at present. The technique was described earlier.

The incompetence resulting from aneurysmal

enlargement of the annulus has been successfully treated in some cases by transforming the valve into a bicuspid one.[46] The result is somewhat uncertain in the individual case, however, and the authors now usually employ the ball-valve prosthesis in such cases. In cases of dissecting aneurysm, complete competence can sometimes be restored by obliteration of the false channel, which relieves the deformity of the cusps resulting from their loss of proper suspension[47,48] (Fig. 26-14).

Results of the use of the ball-valve prosthesis in replacement of the aortic valve at the Mayo Clinic have been described.

Indications for Surgical Treatment

Patients with chronic aortic valve incompetence are advised at present to undergo operation only when symptoms are present. Cardiomegaly without symptoms is not considered an indication for surgical treatment. When incompetence of the aortic valve develops suddenly, operation should be performed promptly.

TRICUSPID STENOSIS AND INCOMPETENCE

Intrinsic disease of the tricuspid valve, in association with involvement of the aortic or mitral valve, occurs in 10 to 15 per cent of patients with chronic rheumatic heart disease.[49] The valve leaflets are thickened; the commissures are fused and usually ill-defined. The chordae may be fused and shortened. The tricuspid valve is usually rendered both stenotic and incompetent thereby.

Patients with disease of the mitral valve commonly exhibit signs and symptoms of tricuspid valve incompetence. In many such cases the leaflets of the tricuspid valve appear normal, and the incompetence is believed to be caused by malfunction of the valve due to severe right ventricular hypertension or dilatation of the right ventricle.[50] When regurgitation at the tricuspid valve is mild or moderate, correction of the defect at the *mitral* valve usually produces a good result and regression of the malfunction at the tricuspid valve. When regurgitation is severe, the patient is usually far along in the course of his disease, and true reduction in myocardial function is often present. The authors' experience indicates that the operative procedure in such a patient must include correction of the incompetence at the tricuspid valve. Annuloplasty has given good results in a few patients, but replacement of the valve with a Starr-Edwards ball-valve prosthesis is the procedure used at present.

A few surgeons[51,52] have reported good results from closed commissurotomy for rheumatic ste-

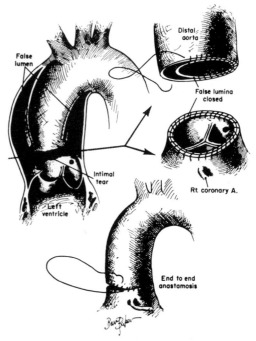

Fig. 26-14. Incompetence of aortic valve due to dissecting aneurysm. Note the loss of attachment of the valve cusps. The aorta is transected just downstream of the aortic valve, and the false lumen is closed both proximally and distally. The aortic cusps are thereby resuspended and again are competent. End-to-end anastomosis then reestablishes continuity. (*Reproduced from C. A. Hufnagel and P. W. Conrad: Dissecting Aneurysms of the Ascending Aorta: Direct Approach to Repair, Surgery,* **51**:84–88, 1962, *with permission of authors and publisher.*)

nosis of the tricuspid valve. In the authors' experience such a procedure always increases the incompetence of the valve and, therefore, is generally unsatisfactory. When patients with significant disease at the mitral or aortic valve have intrinsic disease at the tricuspid valve (which usually produces both stenosis and incompetence), the authors use an open technique and include replacement of the tricuspid valve with a prosthesis.

COMBINED MITRAL AND AORTIC VALVE DISEASE

A number of patients with severe and progressing symptoms exhibit evidence of disease at both mitral and aortic valves. The authors' experience indicates that replacement of both valves with Starr-Edwards prostheses can be accomplished at an acceptable hospital mortality rate. Of 26 patients so treated at the Mayo Clinic, 5 have died in the hospital, a mortality rate of 19 per cent. There has been marked subjective and objective improvement in surviving patients, but for most the follow-up period is less than 18 months.

When hemodynamic derangement is significant at both valves, the decision to repair both is easily made, and the principles of surgical treatment are the same as when one valve alone requires attention. Median sternotomy is performed. After cardiopulmonary bypass is established and the ascending aorta is cross clamped, the root of the aorta is opened, the aortic valve excised, and direct coronary artery perfusion begun. The left atrium is opened from the right side, and the mitral valve repair is accomplished as described earlier (usually by its excision and replacement). After the left atrium is closed, the aortic valve prosthesis is sewed into place, and the procedure is completed as described earlier.

When the aortic valve is severely diseased and only about grade II incompetence (on the basis of I to VI) is evident at the mitral valve, without stenosis, attention to the mitral valve seems unnecessary. This is true even if left atrial pressure is very high, since such pressure can result solely from severe pressure or volume overload of the left ventricle. After repair of the aortic valve disease, such mild incompetence of the mitral valve usually regresses. When there is incompetence at the aortic valve of about grade II, in the presence of severe disease at the mitral valve, the aortic valve incompetence often appears to be of greater magnitude after repair of the mitral valve only and may contribute to poor cardiac performance postoperatively. In these situations, therefore, repair of both mitral and aortic valves seems indicated.

REFERENCES

1. Wood, Paul: An Appreciation of Mitral Stenosis. Part I. Clinical Features. *Brit. M. J.*, 1:1051–1063, 1954.

2. Olesen, K. H.: "Mitral Stenosis: A Follow-up of 351 Patients," Ejnar Munksgaard, Copenhagen, 1955.

3. Baden, Helge: "Surgical Treatment of Mitral Stenosis," Store Nordiske Videnskabsboghandel, Copenhagen, 1958.

4. Souttar, H. S.: The Surgical Treatment of Mitral Stenosis, *Brit. M. J.*, 2:603–606, 1925.

5. Bailey, C. P.: The Surgical Treatment of Mitral Stenosis (Mitral Commissurotomy), *Dis. Chest*, 15:377–393, 1949.

6. Harken, D. E., Ellis, L. B., Ware, P. F., and Norman, L. R.: The Surgical Treatment of Mitral Stenosis. I. Valvuloplasty, *New England J. Med.*, 239:801–809, 1948.

7. Logan, A., and Turner, R.: Surgical Treatment of Mitral Stenosis, with Particular Reference to the Transventricular Approach with a Mechanical Dilator, *Lancet*, 2:874–880, 1959.

8. Gerbode, F.: Transventricular Mitral Valvotomy, *Circulation*, 21:563–567, 1960.

9. Cooley, D. A., and Stoneburner, J. M.: Transventricular Mitral Valvotomy, *Surgery*, 46:414–420, 1959.

10. Black, H., Lown, B., and Bartholomay, A. F.: The Value of Quinidine in the Prevention of Atrial Fibrillation after Mitral Valvuloplasty, *Circulation*, 23:519–524, 1961.

11. Johnson, J., Kirby, C. K., Blakemore, W. S., Zinsser, H. F., Joyner, C. R., and Helwig, J.: Present Indication for the Use of Cardiopulmonary Bypass in Surgical Treatment of Mitral Stenosis, *Ann. Surg.*, 157:902–907, 1963.

12. Stewart, H. J., and Glenn, F.: "Mitral Valvulotomy," Charles C Thomas, Publisher, Springfield, Ill., 1959.

13. Ellis, L. B., Harken, D. E., and Black, H.: A Clinical Study of 1,000 Consecutive Cases of Mitral Stenosis Two to Nine Years after Mitral Valvuloplasty, *Circulation*, 19:803–820, 1959.

14. Björk, V. O., and Malers, E.: Traumatic Mitral Insufficiency Following Transventricular Dilatation for Mitral Stenosis, *J. Thoracic Surg.*, 46:84–93, 1963.

15. Ellis, F. H., Jr., Connolly, D. C., Kirklin, J. W., and Parker, R. L.: Results of Mitral Commissurotomy: Follow-up of Three and One-half to Seven Years, *A.M.A. Arch. Int. Med.*, 102:928–935, 1958.

16. Morrow, A. G., and Braunwald, N. S.: Transventricular Mitral Commissurotomy: Surgical Technique and a Hemodynamic Evaluation of the Method. *J. Thoracic Surg.*, 41:225–235, 1961.

17. Baker, C., and Hancock, W. E.: Deterioration after Mitral Valvotomy, *Brit. Heart J.*, 22:281–294, 1960.

18. Nichols, H. T., Blanco, G., Morse, D. P., Adam, A., and Baltazar, N.: Open Mitral Commissurotomy: Experience with 200 Consecutive Cases, *J.A.M.A.*, 182:268–270, 1962.

19. Kay, E. B., and Zimmerman, H. A.: Surgical Treatment of Mitral Stenosis: Open Versus Closed Techniques, *Am. J. Cardiol.*, 10:1–4, 1962.

20. Starr, A., and Edwards, M. L.: Mitral Replacement: Clinical Experience with a Ball-valve Prosthesis, *Ann. Surg.*, 154:726–740, 1961.

21. Kirklin, J. W., and Theye, R. A.: Cardiac Performance after Open Intracardiac Surgery, *Circulation*, 28:1061–1070, 1963.

22. Dammann, J. F., Jr., Thung, N., Christlieb, I. I., Littlefield, J. B., and Muller, W. H., Jr.: The Management of the Severely Ill Patient after Open-heart Surgery, *J. Thoracic Surg.*, 45:80–89, 1963.

23. Kay, E. B.: Discussion, *J. Thoracic Surg.*, 43:32, 1962.

24. Ross, J., Jr., Braunwald, E., and Morrow, A. G.: Clinical and Hemodynamic Observations in Pure Mitral Insufficiency, *Am. J. Cardiol.*, 2:11–23, 1958.

25. Edwards, J. E., and Burchell, H. B.: Pathologic Anatomy of Mitral Insufficiency, *Proc. Staff Meet. Mayo Clin.*, 33:497–509, 1958.

26. Merendino, K. A., Thomas, G. I., Jesseph, J. E., Herron, P. W., Winterscheid, L. C., and Vetto, R. R.: The Open Correction of Rheumatic Mitral Regurgitation and/or Stenosis, with Special Reference to Regurgitation Treated by Posteromedial Annuloplasty Utilizing a Pump-oxygenator, *Ann. Surg.*, 150:5–22, 1959.

27. McGoon, D. C.: Repair of Mitral Insufficiency Due to Ruptured Chordae Tendineae, *J. Thoracic Surg.*, 39:357–362, 1960.

28. Ellis, F. H., Jr., McGoon, D. C., Brandenburg, R. O., and Kirklin, J. W.: Clinical Experience with Total Mitral Valve Replacement with Prosthetic Valves, *J. Thoracic Surg.*, 46:482–492, 1963.

29. Effler, D. B., and Groves, L. K.: Mitral Valve Replacement: Clinical Experience with the Ball-valve Prosthesis, *Dis. Chest*, 43:529–538, 1963.

30. Anderson, A. M., Cobb, L. A., Bruce, R. A., and Merendino, K. A.: Evaluation of Mitral Annuloplasty for Mitral Regurgitation: Clinical and Hemodynamic Status Four to Forty-one Months after Surgery, *Circulation*, 26:26–38, 1962.

31. Bigelow, W. G., Kuypers, P. J., Heimbecker, R. O., and Gunton, R. W.: Clinical Assessment of the Efficiency and Durability of Direct Vision Annuloplasty, *Ann. Surg.*, 154:320–328, 1961.

32. Anderson, M. W.: The Clinical Course of Patients with Calcific Aortic Stenosis, *Proc. Staff Meet. Mayo Clin.*, 36:439–444, 1961.

33. Mitchell, A. M., Sackett, C. H., Hunzicker, W. J., and Levine, S. A.: The Clinical Features of Aortic Stenosis, *Am. Heart J.*, 48:684–720, 1954.

34. Holley, K. E., Bahn, R. C., McGoon, D. C., and Mankin, H. T.: Spontaneous Calcific Embolization Associated with Calcific Aortic Stenosis, *Circulation*, 27:197–202, 1963.

35. Ellis, L. B., and Hancock, E. W.: Evaluation of Surgical Treatment of Acquired and Congenital Aortic Stenosis, *Progr. Cardiovas. Dis.*, 3:247–262, 1960.

36. Larson, R. E., and Kirklin, J. W.: Early and Late Results of Partial and Total Replacement of the Aortic Valve with Individual Teflon Cusps, *J. Thoracic Surg.*, 47:720, 1964.

37. Morrow, A. G., and Austen, W. G.: A Technique for Preventing Calcific Emboli Following Aortic Valvuloplasty, *Surg. Gynec. & Obst.*, 114:635, 1962.

38. King, B. J.: An Improved Coronary Artery Perfusion Cannula, *J. Thoracic Surg.*, 45:667–669, 1963.

39. McGoon, D. C., Mankin, H. T., and Kirklin, J. W.: Results of Open-heart Operation for Acquired Aortic Valve Disease, *J. Thoracic Surg.*, 45:47–61, 1963.

40. Starr, A.: Discussion, *J. Thoracic Surg.*, 45:63–64, 1963.

41. Howard, C. P.: Aortic Insufficiency Due to Rupture by Strain of a Normal Aortic Valve, *Canad. M. A. J.*, 19:12–24, 1928.

42. Bahnson, H. T., and Spencer, F. C.: Excision of Aneurysm of the Ascending Aorta with Prosthetic Replacement During Cardiopulmonary Bypass, *Ann. Surg.*, 151:879–888, 1960.

43. Spencer, F. C., and Blake, H.: A Report of the Successful Surgical Treatment of Aortic Regurgitation from a Dissecting Aortic Aneurysm in a Patient with the Marfan Syndrome, *J. Thoracic Surg.*, 44:238–245, 1962.

44. Segal, J., Harvey, W. P., and Hufnagel, C.: A Clinical Study of One Hundred Cases of Severe Aortic Insufficiency, *Am. J. Med.*, 21:200–210, 1956.

45. Spurny, O. M., and Hara, M.: Rupture of the Aortic Valve Due to Strain, *Am. J. Cardiol.*, 8:125–129, 1961.

46. Garamella, J. J., Schmidt, W. R., Jensen, N. K., and Lynch, M. F.: Clinical Experiences with the Bicuspid Operation for Aortic Regurgitation, *Ann. Surg.*, 157:310–313, 1963.

47. Hufnagel, C. A., and Conrad, P. W.: Dissecting Aneurysms of the Ascending Aorta: Direct Approach to Repair, *Surgery*, 51:84–88, 1962.

48. Morris, G. C., Jr., Henly, W. S., and DeBakey, M. E.: Correction of Acute Dissecting Aneurysm of Aorta with Valvular Insufficiency, *J.A.M.A.*, 184:63–64, 1963.

49. Cooke, W. T., and White, P. D.: Tricuspid Stenosis: With Particular Reference to Diagnosis and Prognosis, *Brit. Heart J.*, 3:147–165, 1941.

50. Salazar, E., and Levine, H. D.: Rheumatic Tricuspid Regurgitation: The Clinical Spectrum, *Am. J. Med.*, 33:111–129, 1962.

51. Yu, P. N., Harken, D. E., Lovejoy, F. W., Jr., Nye, R. E., Jr., and Mahoney, E. B.: Clinical and Hemodynamic Studies of Tricuspid Stenosis, *Circulation*, 13:680–691, 1956.

52. Sapirstein, W., and Baker, C. B.: Isolated Tricuspid-valve Stenosis: Report of a Surgically Treated Case, *New England J. Med.*, 269:236–240, 1963.

Section C: Coronary Artery Disease

27 ETIOLOGY OF CORONARY ATHEROSCLEROSIS *

Robert E. Olson, Ph.D., M.D.

Definition of Atheroma

Coronary atherosclerosis is a disease of the coronary arteries in which fatty granulomatous lesions develop in the arterial wall and undergo a series of changes which may lead to hardening and/or

* The material contained in this chapter is somewhat similar to a chapter written by Dr. Olson and contained in Cecil & Loeb, "A Textbook of Medicine," 11th ed. The material has been modified and updated. We wish to thank W. B. Saunders Company, publishers, and Paul B. Beeson, M.D., and Walsh McDermott, M.D., editors, for their permission to use the material here.

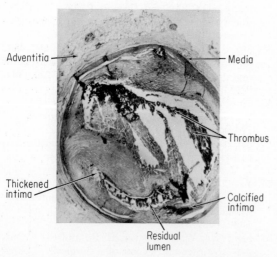

Fig. 27-1. Advanced atherosclerosis with thrombus. This photomicrograph of a coronary artery shows extensive atherosclerosis including marked intimal thickening, reduction in lumen, thinning and dilatation of the media, and calcification with fibrosis. The thrombus shown has apparently arisen by dissection of blood into the necrotic center of the atheroma. Subintimal hemorrhage could also have contributed to the massive thrombus beneath the surface of the intima. (*Courtesy of Dr. R. H. Fennell, Jr., Professor of Pathology, University of Pittsburgh School of Medicine.*)

occlusion of the vessel. The lesions, known as *atheromas* (Greek for *gruel*), are characterized by focal intimal thickening, variable amounts of intimal and subintimal lipid deposition, deformation and fragmentation of the internal elastic membrane, and, in advanced cases, fibrosis and calcification, as shown in Fig. 27-1. Coronary arteries are particularly susceptible to atheromatosis because of the turbulence of flow at branch points and rhythmic torsion of the vessels which occurs with every heart beat.

Coronary atherosclerosis is usually most advanced in the proximal parts of the main vessels extending for some 5 cm into the anterior descending and circumflex branches of the left trunk and 6 to 8 cm into the right coronary artery. Plaques tend to be localized at points of branching, giving it the characteristic x-ray appearance of "nipping."

Atheromas have two major constituents from a pathologic point of view, i.e., fat and fibrous tissue. Sometimes the one element may predominate, sometimes the other does, but both are always represented. This spectrum of relative predominance has given rise to the terms *fatty plaques* and *pearly plaques*, which are used to describe given atheromas. The fat is principally in macrophages, although free lipid appears in old or necrotic lesions. The fibrous tissue develops from marked intimal proliferation and thickening. Ulceration of a plaque, subintimal hemorrhage into a plaque, or progressive thrombin deposition upon the surface of a plaque in a greatly narrowed vessel may lead to thrombosis and total occlusion of the vessel. As a result the well-known constellation of ischemic signs and symptoms occurs.

Incidence and Prevalence of Coronary Artery Disease

Coronary artery disease and its complications are presently the leading causes of death in North America and Western Europe. The crude rate, for all ages and both sexes, from arteriosclerotic heart disease alone is approximately 3 per thousand a year in the United States and Britain, 2 per thousand a year in Denmark, the Netherlands, and Germany, and less than 0.5 per thousand in Japan, China, Chile, Ceylon, Central America, and the Indonesian Islands. In men forty to fifty-nine years of age, the rates in these same countries vary from

8 to less than 1 per thousand.[1] Most authorities agree that there has been a genuine increase in the incidence of clinical coronary heart disease over the past 50 years in the high-incidence countries, although the evidence for an increase in atheromatosis itself is somewhat controversial. There seems little doubt that improvements in diagnostic skill and increased rates of thrombosis, as well as increased rates of atherogenesis, have contributed to the current high rates of coronary heart disease. In 1956 in Great Britain, 45,000 deaths of males were reported as due to arteriosclerotic heart disease, whereas in 1921, only 800 were reported. The low rates observed in the Orient cannot be attributed to race alone, since Japanese living in United States show rates of coronary disease approaching those of the Caucasians in this country. The incidence of the disease rises with age, being practically absent before the age of puberty and moderate to high (70 to 80 per cent) in subjects reaching the age of seventy. Forty per cent of well-nourished young men twenty to thirty years of age may show some involvement of the coronary arteries as revealed by studies of American soldiers killed in Korea. Women during the childbearing period are less susceptible than men. Most atheromas are clinically silent, so that the extent of atherosclerosis in ostensibly healthy subjects or even in those with some clinical evidence of its complications is extraordinarily difficult to evaluate. Studies of the incidence and prevalence of coronary artery disease in men from different socioeconomic strata in this country have not revealed marked differences which could be attributed to such factors.

Host-Agent Interaction

Numerous hypotheses regarding the causes of atherosclerosis have been proposed. It seems clear that coronary atherosclerosis is a disease of multiple causes in which various factors may have different relative values in different individuals and populations. In contradistinction to many microbial and chemical diseases, the agent for the disease appears to arise within the host as a result of host-environment interaction. Since atheromas develop in a two-phase system involving the lining of the artery and the plasma, a search of factors in both plasma and artery which satisfy the definition of agent, i.e., a cause which is essential but not necessarily sufficient to induce disease, seems indicated. Theories of the causes of atherosclerosis may be clearly divided among those that postulate that the primary change is in the artery and those that insist that the primary change is in the plasma. Of possible factors in the plasma, the lipids have claimed attention of investigators more prominently than any other component, (1) because the earliest lesion the pathologist sees is an accumulation of lipids in intimal and subintimal cells, (2) because of greater prevalence of atheroma in patients with disturbed lipid metabolism, (3) because patients suffering from atherosclerosis taken as a group have higher plasma-lipid levels than those not suffering from the disease, and (4) because the only means by which a lesion simulating human atheroma may be produced in experimental animals thus far is by producing an elevation of plasma lipids. Another group of humoral factors are the heparinoid polysaccharides which act to clear lipids and prevent coagulation.

Local factors impinging upon, or intrinsic to, the artery are (1) hemodynamic factors relating to blood flow, turbulence, and pressure; (2) metabolic factors intrinsic in the arterial tissue which control its respiration, lipogenesis, and lipoprotein transformations; (3) structural factors relating to differentiation of intima, internal elastic membrane, and other components of the arterial wall such as mucopolysaccharides and mucoproteins; and (4) traumatic factors secondary to injury, ulceration, and repair. The data from experimental studies of atherogenesis suggest that these local factors are important but not essential factors in the genesis of atheroma. Furthermore, in the light of modern knowledge, it seems unlikely that lipids per se are the agents of the disease, since unbound lipids do not exist in plasma.

The study of the physiology of lipid transport in the past few years has convincingly shown that the physiologic form of all plasma lipids is that of a lipoprotein complex. It is therefore important to review the theories of lipid causation of coronary atheroma in the light of this more recent physiologic evidence and to consider the facts that link one or another lipoprotein form to the disease. Four groups of lipoproteins in plasma have been identified: (1) the chylomicrons, (2) the low-density β-lipoproteins, (3) the high-density α-lipoproteins, and (4) the albumin–nonesterified fatty acid (albumin-NEFA) complexes. Cholesterol, cholesterol ester, phospholipid, and triglyceride are distributed through the first three classes of lipoproteins in various proportions as shown in Table 27-1.[2,3]

Cholesterol is distributed throughout all the lipoprotein fractions of the plasma except the albumin-NEFA complex and stands in various relationships to cholesterol ester in these same lipoproteins. Cholesterol has no physiologically unique role to play in the plasma other than that of the lipoproteins with which it is associated. The preoccupation with cholesterol as a "cause" of coronary atheromatosis has possibly been attributed to the fact that it is relatively easy to measure

Table 27-1. MAIN VEHICLES FOR FAT TRANSPORT IN MAN

| | | | | | Lipoprotein composition | | | | | | |
| | | | | | Pro-tein, per cent | Lipid, per cent | Lipid composition as per cent total lipid | | | | |
Form	Average concentrations, mg/100 ml*	Density	S_f†	$-S$†			TG‡	PL§	Choles-terol ester	Choles-terol	NEFA
Chylomicrons	0–50	<0.96	10^4–10^5		1	99	88	8	3	1	
Low-density β-lipoproteins:											
LDF 1	150	0.96–1.006	20–400	>70	7	93	56	20	15	8	1
LDF 2	50	1.006–1.019	12–20	40–70	11	89	29	26	34	9	1
LDF 3	350	1.019–1.063	0–12	20–40	21	79	13	28	48	10	1
High-density α-lipoproteins:											
HDL 2	50	1.063–1.125		4–20	33	67	16	43	31	10	
HDL 3	300	1.125–1.210		0–4	57	43	13	46	29	6	6
Albumin-NEFA	4,000	....		.....	99	1	0	0	0	0	100

* Concentrations are average postabsorptive values for a healthy and well-nourished forty-year-old male.
† S_f = Svedberg flotation units ($-S \times 10^{-13}$ sec) at density 1.063 and $t = 26°$; $-S$ = Svedberg flotation units at density 1.21 and $t = 26°$.
‡ TG = triglyceride.
§ PL = phospholipid.

and does to a certain extent reflect the concentration of the β-lipoproteins in plasma. The triglycerides[4] equally well reflect the concentration of β-lipoproteins. In fact, neither lipid is important by itself but only to the extent that it reflects the concentration of the β-lipoprotein family. It can be stated at this point that the studies of the physiologically significant lipoprotein families in relation to atherosclerosis have clearly shown that neither α-lipoproteins, chylomicrons, nor albumin-NEFA

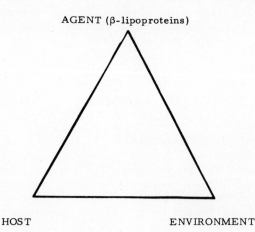

Fig. 27-2. Epidemiologic triangle illustrating the interaction of certain host and environmental factors and their relationship to β-lipoproteins.

complexes bear any correlation at all with the incidence or prevalence, experimental or clinical, of atherosclerosis. The β-lipoproteins may be regarded as the "agent" of the disease on the basis of mounting evidence including that satisfying Koch's postulates.[5] The incidence of atherosclerosis is a function of the average β-lipoprotein concentration operating over the lifetime in a wide range of different species. The rates are lowest for rats, dogs, and cats; intermediate for birds, rabbits, and monkeys; and highest in man. In the low-incidence group, the β-lipoprotein concentration is of the order of 50 mg/100 ml, whereas in man it averages about 500 mg/100 ml.

If one accepts this evidence in favor of the view that the β-lipoproteins may be considered the agent for atherosclerosis, all other factors known to be involved in the etiology may be viewed to determine whether they influence the concentration of the agent in the plasma or whether they influence the reactivity of the arterial wall to the agent. Host and environmental factors may then be grouped according to the epidemiologic triangle shown in Fig. 27–2. Since the β-lipoproteins are known to be synthesized and catabolized in the liver, this organ can be viewed as the source of the agent. Changes in its capacity to synthesize or degrade the β-lipoproteins may have marked effects upon the plasma concentration.

Environmental Factors

Diet

Many studies[6–11] of diet in relationship to degenerative heart disease have shown that populations with high rates of coronary artery disease generally have high average plasma–β-lipoprotein (and cholesterol) concentrations and eat diets rich in animal protein, fat, and calories. Some statisticians[12, 13] have suggested that a stronger association exists between dietary animal-protein intake and mortality from coronary heart disease than exists between dietary fat intake and that of mortality. The association between animal-protein intake and mortality from coronary disease may in part reflect the association of relatively saturated fat with most animal protein as well as a "protective" effect of animal-protein deficiency at the low end of the scale. The plotting of hard fat/liquid fat ratios as an index of relative saturation of the dietary fat improved the correlation with coronary mortality at the high end of the scale.[14]

Strong evidence that the key to this association is an effect of diet upon serum–β-lipoproteins in man has been provided by intensive studies of human subjects, in which diet and other variables were strictly controlled for long periods.[15] It has been shown that reducing the total fat from 40 to 10 per cent of calories without change in fatty acid at a constant caloric intake or composition or increasing the concentration of polyunsaturated fatty acids from 4 to 20 per cent of calories at a constant total fat and calorie intake will appreciably lower the β-lipoprotein cholesterol in man. These effects appear to be maintained as long as the diets are kept constant. Low-protein diets have also been shown to decrease serum–β-lipoproteins in human beings.[16]

It is, of course, clear that great individual variation occurs within populations. Some subjects living in Western countries with a high standard of nutrition may have low serum–β-lipoprotein concentrations due to inherent metabolic pathways that govern synthesis and catabolism of β-lipoproteins. Conversely, in certain hyperlipidemias, dietary intake may have little, if any, effect.

Obesity arises from ingestion of more calories than required for normal energy exchange. Insurance actuaries and pathologists have observed for many years that coronary artery disease and other forms of atherosclerosis are more prevalent in the obese than in the nonobese. In the recent prospective study of heart disease in Framingham, Massachusetts[17], it was found that obesity, hypercholesterolemia, and hypertension were factors associated with proneness to coronary disease. The unsettled problem is whether increased body fat per se is related to atherosclerosis or whether obese persons, as a group, have other traits favoring atherogenesis. Both hypertension and hypercholesterolemia are somewhat more prevalent in obese than in nonobese persons. Weight reduction of 10 to 20 per cent in middle-aged men and women has been found to have some effect upon hypertension but relatively little permanent effect upon serum cholesterol and β-lipoproteins.[18]

The effect of exercise, occupation, and culture on atherogenesis is still under study.

Host Factors

Racial, Ethnic, and Hereditary Factors

These intrinsic host factors are extraordinarily complicated and difficult to differentiate from environmental and cultural factors in population studies. Some variables may be polygenic, giving continuous distributions, and others may be due to single genes which show discontinuous distributions according to Mendelian laws. It is probable that both types of genetic influence operate in determining susceptibility to coronary artery disease. Genetic factors may influence the concentration of β-lipoproteins in the plasma by controlling the activity of enzymes concerned with β-lipoprotein metabolism. Similarly, they may operate to increase or decrease susceptibility of the artery to permeation by these lipoproteins and subsequent chronic inflammatory change through effects on the structure and metabolism of the artery.

Specific hereditary disorders which increase the incidence of coronary atheromatosis are the hyperlipidemias. Familial hypercholesterolemia is characterized by elevated serum-cholesterol levels and β-lipoproteins, clear fasting serum, tendon nodules (xanthoma tendinosum), xanthelasma, and (less frequently) skin xanthoma of the tuberous type. The β-lipoprotein spectrums in these patients are increased mainly in the S_f* 0 to 12 range with significant but somewhat lesser increases in the S_f 12 to 400 range. The increase in serum β-lipoproteins in this disorder appears to be due to hepatic overproduction of cholesterol and possibly other constituents of the β-lipoproteins. A favorable response of hypercholesterolemia to increased dietary polyunsaturated fat is noted in many of these patients.

The second hyperlipidemia is familial hyperlipemia. It appears to be due to a single gene with incomplete dominance. The homozygotes have milky plasma, delayed clearance of ingested fat, hepatosplenomegaly, abdominal crises, childhood atherosclerosis, and xanthomatosis, and they usually die in childhood. The heterozygotes survive childhood to develop early atherosclerosis and coronary artery disease as adults. The lipid disorder in this disease is characterized by a great elevation of plasma-triglyceride levels and lesser increases in cholesterol and phospholipid levels. The β-lipoprotein spectrum is distinctive in that the S_f 0 to

* S_f = Svedberg flotation units ($-S \times 10^{-13}$ sec) at density 1.063 and $t = 26°$.

12 fraction is reduced as much as 50 per cent with several-fold increases in the lower-density S_f 12 to 400 group. Chylomicrons are poorly cleared after a fatty meal, and a biochemical lesion featuring a lack of lipoprotein lipase has been suggested. Low-fat diets may improve the hyperlipemia in some cases. In others, in whom carbohydrate feeding exaggerates the hyperlipemia, diets high in polyunsaturated fat may lower plasma lipids.

Age

In general, atherosclerosis is more prevalent in aged subjects than in young ones. Children eight or nine years of age with serum lipidoses, however, may suffer from severe atherosclerosis. Conversely, very old people may die with relatively little evidence of the disease. At least two factors appear to contribute to the effect of age: one is the effect of aging itself, and the other is the effect of time. Experimental studies have shown that the uptake of sudanophilic material by arteries is a function of the concentration of β-lipoproteins and time of exposure to that concentration. In human material it has been found that fatty streaks develop in the aortas of infants regardless of environment at about the same rate up to the time of puberty. Beyond puberty, the well-nourished North American male develops atheromas at twice the rate of the Central American, but both increase fairly linearly with time. The average concentration of β-lipoproteins in the plasma of North American males also increases from puberty to about sixty years. In the individual, the influences of aging upon the metabolism and flexibility of the artery is a factor that will affect the rate of atheroma formation.

Sex

Women of childbearing age suffer fewer complications of atherosclerosis than men of the same age. After the menopause, however, the incidences in men and women rapidly approach one another, and, in fact, in the latter decades of life the rates for women exceed those for men. This appears to be related to estrogen secretion. One effect of estrogen is to decrease the ratio of β- to α-lipoproteins at a given serum-cholesterol value, and the other is to increase the resistance of the coronary arteries to atheroma formation.

Hemodynamic Factors

Local hemodynamic factors play a significant role in the development of individual lesions. Increased lateral pressure on the arterial wall generated in hypertensive states increases the frequency and severity of atherosclerosis. In the Framingham study, arterial pressures in excess of 160/95 were associated with a threefold increase

in the incidence of coronary artery disease in middle-aged subjects.

Arterial sites exposed to turbulence of flow also appear to be more susceptible to atheroma. This is evident at branch points and bifurcations of major vessels. The coronary arteries may be particularly susceptible because they undergo torsion with every heart beat.

Endocrine Factors

Certain of the hormones affect the rate of development of atherosclerosis in man. The most important of these appear to be insulin, thyroxin, epinephrine, estrogen, and androgen. They may act to modify lipid metabolism or to affect the artery itself.

Atherosclerosis appears more frequently and more extensively in diabetes mellitus. Diabetic patients in ketosis usually demonstrate some lipemia, featuring a preferential increase in triglycerides and the lower-density S_f 20 to 400 β-lipoproteins. This defect may be visible even in well-controlled diabetic patients, and cyclic changes in the concentration of lower-density β-lipoproteins in relation to insulin dosage are noticed in many. In addition, the increased tendency to degeneration of connective tissue in diabetic patients may increase the proneness to atheroma formation. Hypercholesterolemia occurs in myxedema, although in this disorder both α- and β-lipoproteins increase. Patients with long-standing myxedema may have extensive coronary atheromatosis.

Epinephrine and norepinephrine stimulate the release of nonesterified fatty acids from adipose tissue. If this effect is brisk or prolonged enough, it may increase the output of β-lipoproteins by the liver and increase their concentration in the plasma. It has been observed that certain hypercholesterolemic and coronary-prone men in stressful occupations excrete more catecholamines than control subjects during the waking hours. It is possible that the medullary hormones may be playing a role in aggravating the vascular disorders of these men.

Pathogenesis

Atheromatosis of the coronary artery with its sequelae is of multiple causation. It is suggested that the β-lipoproteins of the plasma may be regarded as the agent of the disease. Nonetheless, the events characterizing the interaction of the agent with the arterial wall to produce the discrete lesion under many different modifying circumstances constitutes the sinuous chain of pathogenesis. Virchow first visualized atheroma formation as beginning with intimal proliferation in selected areas determined by local factors followed by imbibition of plasma and subintimal deposition of lipid. This "filtration hypothesis" was strengthened by Anitschkow's discovery[19] that feeding cholesterol to rabbits (which massively increases the β-lipoproteins) produced atheromatosis. The belief that the lipid which accumulates in the atheroma is derived largely (but probably not exclusively) from the agent, i.e., the β-lipoproteins, is based upon (1) demonstrated filtration of macromolecules through endothelium, (2) isolation of low-density lipoproteins from atheromatous but not from normal aorta, (3) chemical similarity of the lipids in the plaques and those of the β-lipoproteins, and (4) transfer of isotopic cholesterol from plasma to the lesion in man.

The earliest atheromatous patch consists of a slightly raised yellow streak of lipid consisting mainly of cholesterol ester, phospholipid, neutral fat, carotene, and protein, roughly in the proportions that occur in the β-lipoproteins. This lipid is in the subintima, partly in the ground substance and partly in macrophages which appear as foam cells. At this stage, the lesion appears to be reversible. If the connective tissue and intima in the fat-laden areas undergo proliferation, plaque formation begins. The intimal proliferation may be so great as to produce a raised, hyaline, pearly plaque, or lipid deposition may predominate to result in a soft, yellow plaque. Hydrolysis of cholesterol esters to yield free cholesterol occurs in more advanced lesions, necrosis occurs, vasa vasorum may invade the area from the media, and a chronic inflammatory lesion is produced. Fibrin may be deposited on these plaques minutely or massively with resulting occlusion. It has been suggested by Duguid that minute thrombi play a significant role in the generation of the primary atheroma. Recent electron microscopic studies, however, have shown in both animals and man[21,22] that fibrin is conspicuous by its absence in the earliest lesions detectable either in human beings or in animals fed diets which elevate β-lipoprotein concentrations. Lesions of basement membrane and internal elastic lamina were easily identified by this technique as well as the active transformation of various reticuloendothelial cells, including some smooth muscle cells, into lipid-engulfing foam cells in the subendothelial space. It would appear therefore that although thrombogenic factors and thrombosis itself play an important role in the causation of the ischemic complications of atherosclerosis, current evidence suggests that fibrin deposition is not critical in the initiation of the earliest intimal lesion.

Coronary atherosclerosis is thus viewed as a metabolic disease featuring interaction of one family of macromolecules (the β-lipoproteins) with another (those of the intimal cell). Metabolic and dietary factors influence both the concentration of

β-lipoproteins and the resistance of the intima and its adjoining subintimal compartment to change. Much of what the pathologist views in a diseased artery and much of what the patient with coronary artery suffers in the course of his disease are the result of secondary biologic responses set into play by the primary interaction of macromolecules at the plasma-intimal interface.

REFERENCES

1. Keys, A.: Diet and the Epidemiology of Coronary Heart Disease, *J.A.M.A.*, **164:**1912, 1957.
2. Oncley, J. L.: Plasma Lipoproteins, in I. H. Page (ed.), "Chemistry of Lipides as Related to Atherosclerosis," Charles C Thomas, Publisher, Springfield, Ill., 1958, pp. 114–133.
3. Olson, R. E., and Vester, J. W.: Nutrition-Endocrine Interrelationships in the Control of Fat Transport in Man., *Physiol. Rev.*, **40:**677, 1960.
4. Albrink, M. J., Lavietes, P. H., and Man, E. B.: Relationship between Serum Lipids and the Vascular Complications of Diabetes from 1931 to 1961, *Tr. A. Am. Physicians*, **75:**235, 1962.
5. Olson, R. E.: Prevention and Control of Chronic Disease. I. Cardiovascular Disease: With Particular Attention to Atherosclerosis, *Am. J. Pub. Health*, **49:**1120, 1959.
6. Keys, A., Kimura, N., Kusukawa, A., Bronte-Stewart, B., Larsen, N., and Keys, M. H.: Lessons from Serum Cholesterol Studies in Japan, Hawaii, and Los Angeles, *Ann. Int. Med.*, **48:**83, 1958.
7. Gupta, K. K., Iyer, P. V., and Nath, H. P.: Studies of Serum Cholesterol and Lipid Phosphorus in Coronary Heart Disease, *Metabolism*, **7:**349, 1958.
8. Groen, J. J.: The Effect of Diet on the Serum Lipids of Trappist and Benedictine Monks, in "Essential Fatty Acids," Academic Press, Inc., New York, 1958, p. 147.
9. Keys, A., and Grande, F.: Role of Dietary Fat in Human Nutrition. III. Diet and the Epidemiology of Coronary Heart Disease., *Am. J. Pub. Health*, **47:**1520, 1957.
10. Bronte-Stewart, B., Keys, A., and Brock, J. F.: Serum-cholesterol, Diet, and Coronary Heart Disease: An Inter-racial Survey in the Cape Peninsula, *Lancet*, **2:**1103, 1955.
11. Roine, P., Pekkarinen, M., Karvonen, M. J., and Kihlberg, J.: Diet and Cardiovascular Disease in Finland, *Lancet*, **2:**173, 1958.
12. Yerushalmy, J., and Hilleboe, H. E.: Fat in the Diet and Mortality from Heart Disease: A Methodologic Note, *New York J. Med.*, **57:**2343, 1957.
13. Yudkin, J.: Diet and Coronary Thrombosis Hypothesis and Fact. *Lancet*, **2:**155, 1957.
14. Bronte-Stewart, B.: The Effect of Dietary Fats on the Blood Lipids and Their Relation to Ischaemic Heart Disease, *Brit. M. Bull.*, **14:**243, 1958.

15. Ahrens, E. H., Jr.: Nutritional Factors and Serum Lipid Levels, *Am. J. Med.,* **23:**928, 1957.

16. Olson, R. E., Vester, J. W., Gursey, D., Davis, N., and Longman, D.: The Effect of Low-protein Diets upon Serum Cholesterol in Man, *Am. J. Clin. Nutrition,* **6:**310, 1958.

17. Dawber, T. R., Moore, F. E., and Mann, G. V.: Measuring the Risk of Coronary Heart Disease in Adult Population Groups (The Framingham Study), *Am. J. Pub. Health,* **47:**4, 1957.

18. Olson, R. E.: Obesity as a Nutritional Disorder, *Fed. Proc.,* **18:**58, 1959.

19. Anitschkow, N.: In "Arteriosclerosis: A Survey of the Problem," The Macmillan Company, New York, 1954.

20. Duguid, J. B.: Thrombosis as a Factor in the Pathogenesis of Coronary Atherosclerosis, *J. Path. & Bact.,* **58:**207, 1946.

21. Buck, R. C.: The Fine Structure of the Aortic Endothelial Lesions in Experimental Cholesterol Atherosclerosis of Rabbits, *Am. J. Path.,* **34:**897–910, 1958.

22. Buck, R. C.: Electron Microscopic Observation on Capillaries of Atherosclerotic Aorta, *A.M.A. Arch. Path.,* **67:**656–659, 1959.

28 ANATOMY OF THE CORONARY ARTERIES AND VEINS *

Thomas N. James, M.D.

Although the anatomy of the coronary arteries aroused the curiosity of Vieussens 350 years ago, it was only after a relation between disease of the coronary arteries and chest pain was established in this century that knowing about these vessels assumed pragmatic significance. In more recent years the rapid advances in cardiac surgery and in coronary angiography have stimulated further interest in the coronary arteries. In this chapter the typical course as well as the important variations of each major artery will be presented, followed by anatomy of the coronary veins and of arterial anastomoses. The concluding section will deal with the blood supply of special regions of the heart.

* The work on which this chapter is based has been supported in part by grants from the United States Public Health Service and the Michigan Heart Association.

All the figures in the chapter except the drawings in Figs. 28-7*A*, 28-8*A*, and 28-14*A* are reproduced (some slightly modified) from T. N. James, "Anatomy of the Coronary Arteries," 1961, with permission of the publisher, Paul B. Hoeber, Inc., New York.

The Left Coronary Artery

In nearly all human hearts the left coronary artery arises from a single ostium located in the middle of the upper half of the left coronary sinus of the aorta, which protrudes between the main pulmonary artery and the body of the left atrium (Fig. 28-1). There are virtually never any branches of the main left coronary artery proximal to its division into anterior descending and circumflex arteries. This stout vessel, which varies from a few millimeters to a few centimeters in length, lies free in epicardial fat. During systolic filling of the coronary arteries, it buckles easily, because it is not held down to myocardium by branches like those of the anterior descending artery.

Although the division of the main left coronary artery is usually referred to as a bifurcation, it is much more common for there to be three or more equally large divisions at this point (Fig. 28-2). The large branch which courses down the anterior interventricular sulcus becomes the left anterior

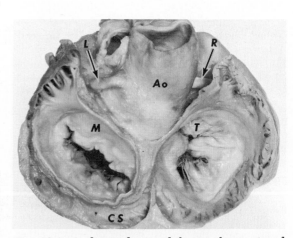

Fig. 28-1. A dissected normal human heart viewed from above demonstrating the origins of the left coronary artery (arrow with *L*) and right coronary artery (arrow with *R*) from the sinuses of Valsalva in the root of the aorta (*Ao*). The noncoronary sinus of the aorta bulges posteriorly into the anterior margin of the interatrial septum, dividing the left atrium and mitral valve (*M*) from the right atrium and tricuspid valve (*T*). The left coronary sinus bulges slightly between the root of the aorta and the main pulmonary artery, which is cut flush with the right ventricle just anterior to the aorta. The right coronary sinus is not seen in this view, but with the two other sinuses occupying two-thirds of the circumference of the aortic root its position is easy to infer. The upper half of the coronary sinus (*CS*) has been removed to demonstrate its course behind the left atrium; its entrance into the right atrium is marked by the inefficient semilunar Thebesian valve which protrudes in an anterior direction.

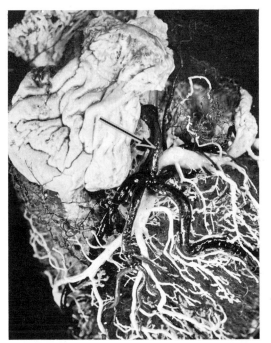

Fig. 28-2. A Vinylite cast of the left coronary artery (arrow) appears dark. The frequently complex division conventionally designated a "bifurcation" is seen. Here the left coronary artery divides into four almost equal trunks, the left anterior descending artery, two diagonal branches, and the left circumflex artery, indicated in order from the left. The left circumflex artery immediately twists beneath the great cardiac vein, which is cast white along with all other veins and the right cardiac chambers; the left atrium and ventricle are uncast.

descending artery, while the one which courses into the left atrioventricular sulcus becomes the left circumflex artery. The intervening branches of the main left coronary artery distribute diagonally over the free wall of the left ventricle and are usually proportionately spaced between the anterior descending and circumflex arteries; these are commonly referred to as *diagonal* or *straight* left ventricular branches, are often one to three in number, and course between the anterior interventricular sulcus and the obtuse margin toward the apex of the heart.

The Left Anterior Descending Artery

Viewed frontally, the left anterior descending artery appears to be a direct continuation of the main left coronary artery, the two together forming a reverse-S curve,[1] the initial turn being around the base of the pulmonary artery into the anterior interventricular sulcus and the second turn being around the apex cordis into the posterior interven-

tricular sulcus (Fig. 28-3). The anterior descending artery gives off major branches in two directions: those which course over the free wall of the left ventricle and those which penetrate and curve posteriorly into the interventricular septum. Lesser branches are distributed to the adjacent wall of the right ventricle, although in rare instances a single major vessel arises from the anterior descending artery to cross diagonally over the anterior wall of the right ventricle. At the level of the pulmonary valves there is a constant small artery which curves about the pulmonary conus to meet a similar branch from the right side. Together these two form an important anatomic landmark first described by Vieussens.[2]

Branches of the left anterior descending artery arise at an acute angle from the parent trunk, whether distributing to the free wall of the left ventricle or to the interventricular septum. The septal branches of the anterior descending artery (numbering three to five in different hearts) fix it to the epicardium and limit its range of excursion

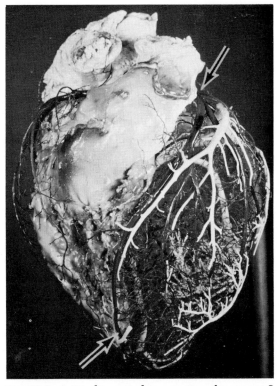

Fig. 28-3. A Vinylite cast demonstrating the reverse-S curve of the left anterior descending coronary artery, indicated by the two arrows; the upper arrow indicates the origin of the artery, and the lower indicates its course near the apex cordis. Again the right cardiac chambers and veins are cast white, while the left chambers are uncast.

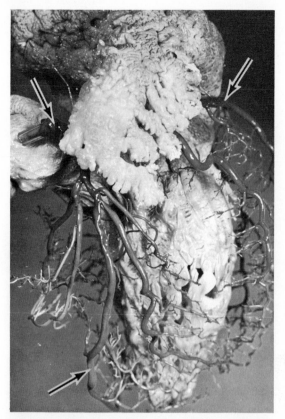

The Left Circumflex Artery

In contrast to the left anterior descending branch, which characteristically arises as a direct continuation of the main left coronary artery, the left circumflex branch typically arises at an angle of 90° or more and occasionally courses in an almost opposite direction from the main left coronary artery. The proximal portion of the left circumflex artery, as well as most of the area of the "bifurcation" of the main left coronary artery, is normally covered by the overlying left atrial appendage (Fig. 28-4). Because of the proximity of the atrial appendage and because the left circumflex artery sometimes courses directly in myocardium of the base of the appendage, this artery is not infrequently injured during surgical procedures which ligate or amputate the left atrial appendage.

From its origin near the aorta and pulmonary

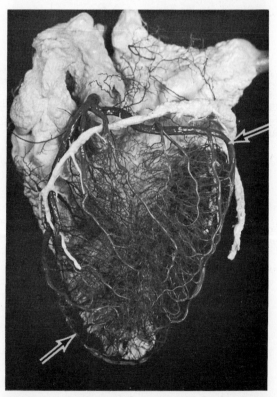

Fig. 28-4. A Vinylite cast demonstrating the close relationship between the left atrial appendage, seen protruding down the center of the upper half of the picture, and the division of the main left coronary artery (left upper arrow) into left circumflex (right upper arrow) and left anterior descending (lower arrow) rami. Branches into the interventricular septum may be seen curving from the anterior descending artery to the viewer's left and then posteriorly. The arrow on the left circumflex artery indicates the termination of its course in the atrioventricular sulcus, just as it begins to turn down the margo obtusus. Note that most of the proximal course of the circumflex artery is covered by the atrial appendage. In this heart the left cardiac chambers are cast white, and the right chambers and veins are uncast.

during systolic filling. The branches to the free wall of the left ventricle (also usually three to five in number) course parallel to diagonal branches of the main left coronary artery. It is not generally appreciated that the anterior descending artery rarely terminates on the anterior surface of the apex but nearly always curves around to the posterior interventricular sulcus and ascends for 2 to 5 cm, distributing branches to the posterior surfaces of the apex of the left and right ventricles.[1] It is met at its termination by the distal branches of the posterior descending artery.

Fig. 28-5. A Vinylite cast demonstrating the distribution of left ventricular branches from the left circumflex (right upper arrow) and left anterior descending (left lower arrow) arteries. The right cardiac chambers are cast white, but the left chambers and many of the veins are uncast. The root of the aorta, from which the main left coronary artery emerges, is also cast white and is joined with an artificial plastic bridge to the root of the pulmonary artery in the left upper corner of the photograph.

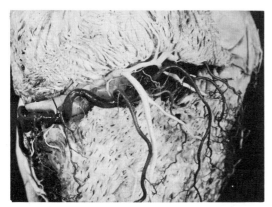

Fig. 28-6. A Vinylite cast demonstrating the course of the right coronary artery (dark plastic) in the right atrioventricular sulcus, with the right atrium above and the right ventricle below. The pulmonary valves may be seen in the right upper corner of the picture. Anterior cardiac veins and a subintimal collecting vein are cast white and course near the artery. Note that the right coronary artery lies deep in fat of the atrioventricular sulcus, with the ventricular branches looping out to the epicardial surface.

artery, the left circumflex artery ascends into the left atrioventricular sulcus and courses to the obtuse margin of the left ventricle. Just proximal to the obtuse margin it emerges from beneath the lateral margin of the atrial appendage and is then covered only by epicardial fat. At the obtuse margin it usually turns down the left ventricle toward the apex of the heart. It always provides stout branches to the posterior (diaphragmatic) surface of the left ventricle from its course along the obtuse margin, including one or more fairly large branches which continue in the atrioventricular sulcus toward the posterior interventricular sulcus, where they are met by terminal branches of the right coronary artery. In about 10 per cent of human hearts the left circumflex artery itself continues in the posterior half of the left atrioventricular sulcus and crosses the crux of the heart, from which it turns down into the posterior interventricular sulcus to form the posterior descending artery; in such hearts branches of the left coronary artery supply the entire left ventricle and interventricular septum.

Branches of the left circumflex artery supply most of the left atrium and the lateral and part of the posterior walls of the left ventricle (Fig. 28-5). The two significant atrial branches are the one supplying the sinus node in about 45 per cent of human hearts (discussed later in this chapter) and the left atrial circumflex artery.[1] This latter vessel courses parallel to the main left circumflex artery but above it, lying in the lower portion of the left atrium; it is often 1 or 2 mm in diameter, and in

some hearts is larger than the ventricular counterpart. Occasionally the left atrial circumflex artery, which usually terminates on the posterior wall of the left atrium, crosses back over the atrioventricular sulcus to supply the upper portion of the posterior left ventricle. The ventricular branches of the left circumflex artery arise at acute angles from the parent vessel in the same way as the branches of the anterior descending artery. These ventricular branches course toward the obtuse margin from the atrioventricular sulcus and are roughly parallel to the diagonal branches of the main left coronary artery and similar branches arising from the left anterior descending artery.

The Right Coronary Artery

Whereas the left coronary artery nearly always arises from a single ostium, in approximately half of human hearts there are two ostiums in the right coronary sinus, which normally bulges from the aorta in a direction between the base of the pulmonary artery and the body of the right atrium. The smaller of these two ostiums is rarely more than 1 or 2 mm from the larger and is usually 1 mm or less in diameter. It gives rise to the conus artery,[3] which forms the right half of Vieussens's ring at the level of the pulmonary valves. When the conus artery does not arise from the aorta directly, it is the first branch of the main right coronary artery. The potential importance of the conus artery as an alternate route of collateral arterial circulation is apparent.

The right coronary artery courses from the aorta into the right atrioventricular sulcus, lying more deeply in the fat of the sulcus than the left circumflex artery (Fig. 28-6). In 90 per cent of human hearts it continues past the acute margin of the right ventricle in the posterior right atrioventricular sulcus to cross the crux of the heart and divide terminally in two directions; two or more branches descend in or near the posterior interventricular sulcus toward the apex of the heart, while another stout branch continues in the left atrioventricular sulcus about half way to the obtuse margin, with its descending branches supplying nearly half of the diaphragmatic surface of the left ventricle (the other half usually supplied by terminal branches of the left circumflex artery). Nearly all right ventricular branches of the right coronary artery arise perpendicular to the parent vessel, and those from the right atrioventricular sulcus to the anterior wall of the right ventricle have a looping exit as they emerge from their deep position in fat. The anterior right ventricular branches are three or four in number, the one coursing along the acute margin being the dominant of these; all these branches are roughly parallel to the acute margin of the heart,

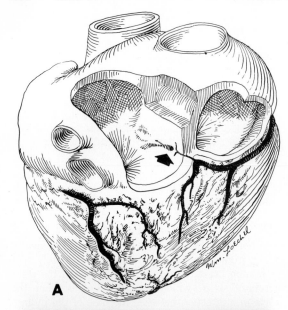

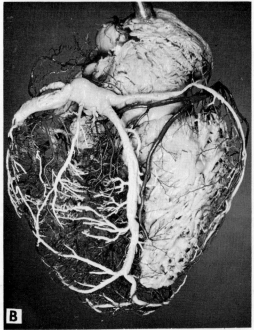

Fig. 28-7. A drawing (*A*) and Vinylite cast (*B*) demonstrating the arterial supply to the posterior (diaphragmatic) surface of the human heart as it occurs in about 90 per cent of instances. The left circumflex artery terminates at or near the margo obtusus, while branches of the right coronary artery cross the crux and supply the A-V node (arrow). The crux is the arbitrary point at which the A-V sulci cross the posterior margin of the interatrial and interventricular sulci. Note the penetrating U turn of the artery crossing the crux of the heart, which here is the right coronary artery. The value of this U turn as an angiographic landmark is discussed in the text.

coursing toward the apex and anterior interventricular sulcus. In about 55 per cent of human hearts the right coronary artery provides the sinus node's arterial supply (see below), but other atrial branches are smaller and less constant.

It is the reciprocal lengths of the right coronary and left circumflex in the posterior atrioventricular sulci—one being longer as the other is shorter—which led Bianchi[4] and Spalteholz[5] to classify coronary distribution in this region as right or left predominant. Thus if the right coronary (Fig. 28-7) crossed the crux of the heart (as it does in 90 per cent of human beings), it predominated, while the left circumflex did so in only 10 per cent (Fig. 28-8). They did not intend this classification to refer to arterial supply of the entire heart, which is the unfortunate way the classification is now commonly used. It is frequently stated in describing angiograms, for example, that the heart may be classified as a "right coronary–predominant heart," implying that the right coronary artery supplies most of the heart. Actually this is so rarely the case, considering the mass of ventricular and atrial myocardium normally supplied by the left coronary artery, that the misused terminology becomes grossly misleading. It would seem simpler and more accurate to say that the right or left coronary artery crosses the crux, as the case may be, or that the right coronary is as usual (90 per cent) the longer, and to abandon the misleading terms "preponderant" or "predominant."

The Coronary Veins

There are three systems of veins in the human heart. The smallest of these is comprised of the *Thebesian veins,* which neither are large nor account for much of the volume of venous drainage. They occur primarily in the right atrium and right ventricle but are occasionally demonstrable in the left side of the heart. In both sides of the heart they are more numerous near the septums than in the free walls. The intermediate system of veins is larger and more important, providing most of the venous drainage of the right ventricle. These are the *anterior cardiac veins* (Fig. 28-9), which, over the anterior wall of the right ventricle, form two or three large trunks draining in the direction of the anterior right atrioventricular sulcus, which they cross either deep or superficial to the main right coronary artery to empty directly into the right atrium. In some hearts there is a collecting subintimal vein in the base of the right atrium, into which the anterior cardiac veins drain.

Venous drainage of the left ventricle is under normal circumstances primarily through the *coronary sinus and its tributaries,* which together form the third and largest system of coronary veins (Fig.

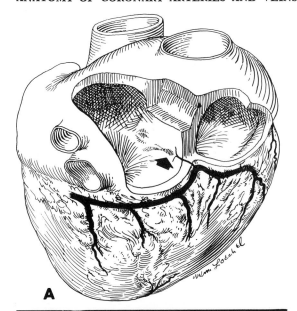

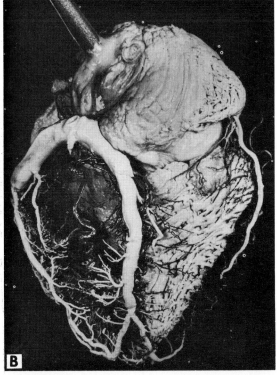

Fig. 28-8. A drawing (A) and Vinylite cast (B) of the arterial supply to the posterior surface as seen in about 10 per cent of human hearts. The left circumflex artery crossing the crux makes a deep U turn and supplies the A-V node (arrow).

28-10). Although there are equally large tributaries further along its course, it is convenient to think of this system as originating with the anterior interventricular vein, which courses parallel to the left

anterior descending artery in most of the anterior interventricular groove (blood flow in the two vessels being in opposite directions, however). Near the origin of the anterior descending artery, the anterior interventricular vein diverges toward the atrioventricular sulcus. At this point it becomes known as the great cardiac vein, receiving smaller tributary veins from the left ventricle. About midway in the course of this vein within the left atrioventricular sulcus it receives the curving entrance of a small but very important left atrial vein known as the *oblique vein of Marshall*.[6] Opposite the entrance of this vein there is commonly a loose fold of endothelium forming an incompetent valve. Together this valve and the point of entrance of the oblique vein of Marshall mark the anatomic division between the great cardiac vein and the coronary sinus (Fig. 28-11), which then extends to the point of entrance into the right atrium. Embryologically the oblique vein of Marshall represents the residual of the left superior cardinal vein and left superior vena cava, and the coronary sinus itself is the remains of the terminal portion of the left superior vena cava.

Near the junction of the great cardiac vein and coronary sinus, one or more large tributary veins enter from the lateral and posterior surfaces of the left ventricle. A large vein along the obtuse margin is the left marginal vein, while a similar vein between this margin and the posterior interventricular sulcus is the left posterior ventricular vein. Frequently one or the other of these veins is absent or replaced by a number of smaller tributaries. The last major tributary of the coronary sinus is the

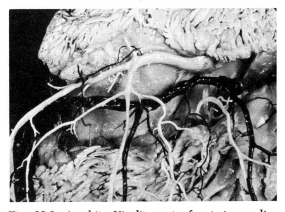

Fig. 28-9. A white Vinylite cast of anterior cardiac veins. The corresponding course of the right coronary artery (dark plastic) closely follows the veins. Some veins pass beneath the artery and others over it to merge in a subintimal collecting vein, which then drains anteriorly to enter the right atrium directly beneath the atrial appendage, seen in the right upper corner of the photograph.

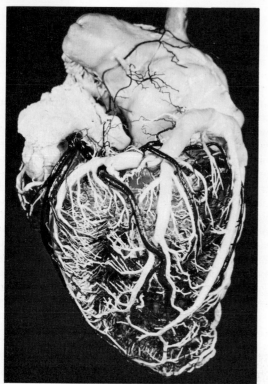

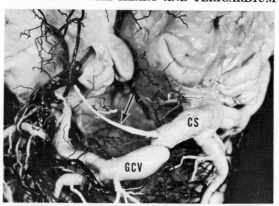

Fig. 28-11. A Vinylite cast of the great cardiac vein (*GCV*) and coronary sinus (*CS*). The indentation at the juncture of these two structures is caused by the valve of Vieussens, and directly adjacent to this is the entrance of the oblique vein of Marshall (arrow), which descends along the posterior wall of the uncast left atrium. The embryologic and anatomic importance of this area is discussed in the text.

Fig. 28-10. A Vinylite cast of the veins of the left ventricle, which unite to form the great cardiac vein and coronary sinus. All the veins and the right cardiac chambers are cast white, with the left chambers uncast. The anterior interventricular vein courses parallel to the anterior descending artery along the left margin of the photograph. Near the middle of the cast the left marginal vein is seen ascending along the margo obtusus. At the right margin of the photograph the posterior vein of the left ventricle ascends to the coronary sinus. Only the apical portion of the posterior interventricular vein is well seen. Although much of the course of the venous branches is in relation to arteries, at some points there is considerable divergence, as in the region of the margo obtusus.

are similar anastomoses between each of the various large veins over the free walls of the right and left ventricles. Although venous flow from right ventricular myocardium is generally through the anterior cardiac veins and that of the left ventricular myocardium generally through the coronary sinus, there is no anatomic reason why, with the least resistance occurring in either of these two venous systems, the flow could not go in the opposite direction via the large anastomoses. For example, if flow in the coronary sinus were impeded, as with an intracardiac catheter, a variable but pos-

posterior interventricular vein, which joins it just proximal to the right atrial ostium of the coronary sinus and sometimes drains separately into the right atrium directly adjacent to the ostium of the coronary sinus. The entrance of the coronary sinus into the right atrium is guarded by an incompetent semilunar fold of endothelium known as the Thebesian valve. A number of venous lacunas or Thebesian veins drain the region of the interatrial septum directly into the right atrium, their ostiums being near the coronary sinus ostium.

Anastomoses between the anterior cardiac veins and the tributaries of the coronary sinus are numerous and large, frequently measuring 1 or 2 mm in diameter in normal hearts (Fig. 28-12). There

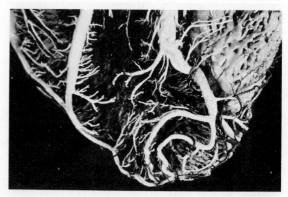

Fig. 28-12. Venous anastomoses of the human heart are numerous and large, often 1 or 2 mm in internal diameter, as in this photograph. The view is toward the posterior surface of the apex cordis, with white plastic filling the veins and right ventricle; the left ventricle is uncast. These normal venous anastomoses join the apical ends of the posterior interventricular and posterior left ventricular veins.

sibly large volume of the left ventricular venous flow could shift into the anterior cardiac veins. It is of further anatomic significance in physiologic studies that the tip of a catheter cannot be placed sufficiently deep into the coronary sinus in vivo to avoid right atrial mixing without being well past the entrance of the posterior interventricular vein as well as one or more of the major veins draining the posterior left ventricle.

Arterial Anastomoses

Much has been made of the size of anastomoses between the coronary arteries of the normal human heart, and too little attention has been paid to the fact that almost no one questions the existence of such anastomoses. The weight of present evidence indicates that arterial anastomoses in the normal human heart are commonly over one hundred microns in diameter and that some are several hundred microns. This has been demonstrated by injection of radiographic dyes,[7–11] by perfusion of small calibrated spheres,[12] and by the classic injection and corrosion technique.[1,13] In view of this demonstration by a variety of investigators employing a number of different techniques, it seems likely that the often quoted criterion of 40 μ as the upper limit of size of normal coronary arterial anastomoses[14] is too conservative.

Arterial anastomoses occur throughout the human heart, but they are particularly numerous within the interventricular and interatrial septums, at the apex of the heart, at the crux of the heart, over the anterior surface of the right ventricle, and between the sinus node artery and other atrial arteries. The anastomoses in right ventricular epicardium become particularly important and large following an occlusion of either the left anterior descending or right coronary artery (Fig. 28-13). Although there are anastomoses in the region of the endocardium of both ventricles, these are not as numerous or large as those in the epicardium. Epicardial anastomoses on the left ventricle connect all three major coronary trunks. These epicardial anastomoses over the surfaces of both ventricles appear from an anatomic standpoint to be among the most important routes for collateral circulation, and it is therefore incongruous that a number of surgical procedures devised for "revascularizing" the heart make a particular point of producing extensive epicardial fibrosis by abrasion, talc powder, or phenol, which must of necessity obliterate a large number of the major normal routes of anastomosis.

Demonstration of the presence of anastomoses does not of course establish their functional importance. However, the excellent functional recovery of most patients who suffer coronary occlusion indicates that the collateral arterial circulation is in

most patients capable of functioning efficiently. Since all human hearts possess an abundant number of coronary arterial anastomoses (of various sizes), the critical question is why some patients who develop coronary occlusion fail to utilize the anastomoses efficiently for collateral circulation. A number of quickly apparent factors contribute to such failure, including the speed of development of the occlusion, its location more distally or more proximally in the artery, and the presence or absence of occlusions in neighboring arteries; but there are probably still other factors which are presently less clearly defined. Among these may be the maintenance of adequate arterial pressure to ensure a sufficient gradient across the anastomosis to permit flow from an unoccluded artery into the distal segment of the occluded artery.[15]

There is one anatomic characteristic of coronary arterial anastomoses which may be a crude indication of whether the anastomosis functioned during life to carry collateral circulation, and this is the shape of the anastomotic artery. Coronary anastomoses in normal human hearts are generally straight or gently curving, regardless of their diameter, while those in hearts with coronary occlusion (Fig. 28-13B) are extensively twisted and commonly corkscrew in shape.[1,13] It seems likely that the normal anastomoses (not regularly participating in coronary flow) are not under much stress, while those connecting a low-pressure occluded artery with a high-pressure unoccluded artery do participate in flow, the stress of higher pressure and pulsation causing them to become elongated, enlarged, and tortuous. If this consideration is correct, then the gross shape of coronary anastomoses may be a reasonable indication of whether they were functioning for collateral flow in vivo.

Blood Supply of Special Areas of the Heart

Most special areas of the heart either have a dual arterial supply or have a single primary supply with important secondary sources. Presenting the anatomy of the course of each branch of the coronary arteries in sequence still leaves the reader with a task of synthesizing in his mind how these branches distribute in a single area. To simplify such a synthesis, this section will deal with special areas of the heart and describe their usual blood supply. As a corollary, the effect of coronary occlusion at various locations will be discussed in relation to the effect on each special area.

The Interventricular Septum

Contrary to frequent descriptions of the blood supply of the interventricular septum as almost equally supplied by the anterior and posterior descending arteries, in man this supply is provided

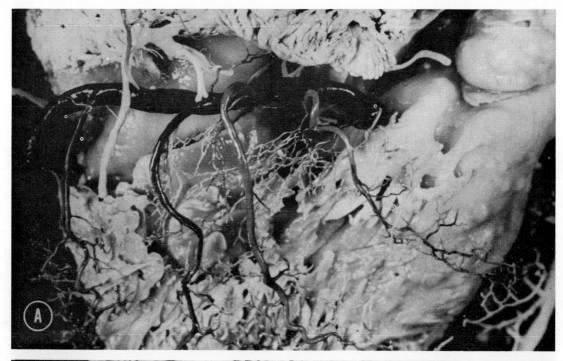
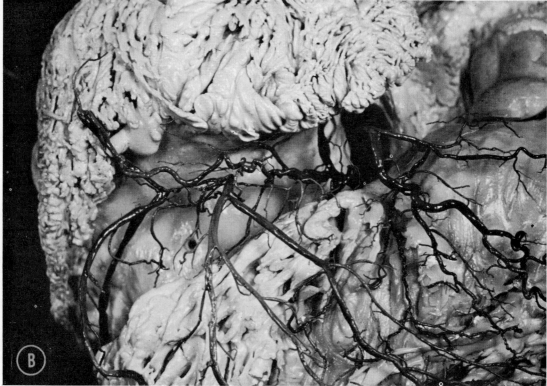

Fig. 28-13. Two Vinylite casts presenting a comparison of the same region of the right coronary artery in normal (A) and atherosclerotic (B) hearts. Note the smooth configuration of the dark plastic in the normal right coronary artery and gradual termination of its branches in relatively straight or gently curving descent over the surface of the right ventricle. By contrast, the branches of the occluded right coronary artery are thicker distally and become extremely twisted into corkscrew shapes. A complete occlusion of the main trunk of the right coronary artery is bridged by intracoronary anastomoses, while the branches over the right ventricle course toward the anterior interventricular sulcus, where they anastomosed with the left anterior descending artery (not shown).

predominantly by branches from the anterior descending artery (Fig. 28-14). These large septal arteries in most of their course lie very close to the right ventricular endocardium, with their terminal ramifications penetrating the septum itself. Only a small portion of the posterior margin of the muscular septum is supplied by the posterior descending artery. However, in the event of occlusion of the anterior descending artery, the posterior artery becomes the principal route of collateral circulation. It follows logically, therefore, that most instances of perforation of the interventricular septum due to myocardial infarction occur in patients in whom both these arteries are occluded, although one .occlusion may be an old one and may or may not have been associated with a previous clinically recognizable episode. When the posterior descending artery is a terminal branch of the left circumflex artery, as it is in 10 per cent of human hearts, the entire septum is supplied by branches of the left coronary tree.

The Crista Supraventricularis

The crista supraventricularis abuts into the interventricular septum directly under the proximal portion of the right coronary artery and is nourished by penetrating branches from it. These are usually small branches and naturally not visible on the surface of the heart nor in ordinary dissection, as at a necropsy table. Occasionally there is a large branch of the right coronary artery which descends directly into the crista supraventricularis and courses through it into the interventricular septum, where it may terminate by supplying a small local area of septal myocardium. In three hearts studied by the author, this branch was sufficiently large to continue through the interventricular septum anteriorly

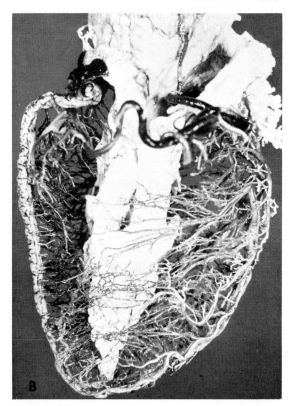

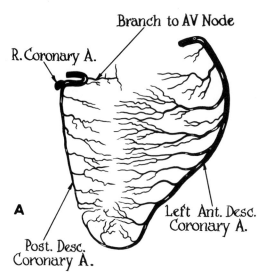

Fig. 28-14. A drawing (*A*) and Vinylite cast (*B*) demonstrating the normal blood supply of the human interventricular septum. The lighter branches of the left anterior descending artery in the cast correspond to those labeled such in the drawing, as do the dark but much shorter branches of the posterior descending branch of the right coronary artery. The U turn of the right coronary artery is obscured in the cast by the posterior interventricular vein, identified by its wrinkled surface. Right ventricular branches of the right coronary artery have been cut away in the cast to reveal the septal arteries, which are seen to be predominantly branches of the left anterior descending ramus. White plastic fills the left atrium and left ventricle; the right chambers are uncast. (*The drawing in A is from T. N. James and G. E. Burch: Blood Supply of the Human Interventricular Septum, Circulation, 17:391, 1958, and is reproduced by permission of Grune & Stratton, Inc., New York.*)

and emerge to the surface in the anterior interventricular sulcus, where it descended and distributed branches to neighboring right and left ventricular myocardium. In one of these three hearts there was no conventional left anterior descending artery, so the branch through the crista supraventricularis supplied a major portion of the left ventricle as well as the interventricular septum. In addition to being an interesting anomalous distribution, this provides a point of functional significance in that the patient died with progressively increasing myocardial insufficiency and ischemia. Anomalous coronary branches distributing to the left ventricle from the right coronary artery commonly follow one of three routes: in epicardium curving behind the aorta, in epicardium coursing across the pulmonary conus, or deep in myocardium via the crista supraventricularis. Since the course of most large coronary arteries is normally epicardial, this intramyocardial course by the third route may be a singularly inefficient one because of the compression of a large coronary trunk during ventricular systole, preventing its normal filling at a time when most coronary trunks are filled. Thus although some anomalous courses for major coronary arteries may be of primarily academic interest, a course deep through the crista supraventricularis may be a slowly lethal anomaly.

Papillary Muscles of the Left Ventricle

The anterior papillary muscle is virtually always supplied by branches of the left coronary artery, while the posterior papillary muscle is usually supplied by branches of both the right and left coronary artery. One of the diagonal branches of the main left coronary artery commonly descends over the anterior papillary muscle, but there are always major additional branches to this area from both the anterior descending artery and the marginal termination of the left circumflex artery. When the right coronary supplies half or more of the diaphragmatic surface of the left ventricle, as it usually does, its terminal branches end directly over the posterior papillary muscle; but again there are additional branches coursing to that area from the marginal termination of the left circumflex artery and occasionally from the posterior apical termination of the left anterior descending artery. Because both papillary muscles receive regularly multiple sources of blood supply, occlusion of a single major coronary artery rarely deprives them of all their circulation. Complications of myocardial infarction such as ruptured papillary muscle are usually due to occlusion of more than one major artery.

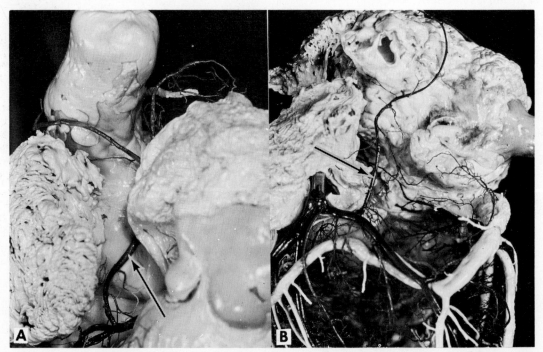

Fig. 28-15. Two inylite casts showing the usual course of the sinus node artery when it originates from the right (A) and from the left (B). In A the sinus node artery (arrow) arises from the proximal portion of the right coronary artery, as it does in 55 per cent of human hearts, and courses between the right atrial appendage and root of the aorta along the medial surface of the body of the right atrium to the base of the superior vena cava, which protrudes upward in the left upper corner of the picture. As the right sinus node artery curves about the vena cava, it enters the sulcus terminalis and penetrates the sinus node. An additional large branch is seen coursing into the dorsal wall of the uncast left atrium. In B the sinus node artery (arrow) arises from the proximal left circumflex artery and crosses beneath the uncast left atrial appendage to the base of the superior vena cava, which protrudes toward the viewer. Here it circles counterclockwise to enter the sulcus terminalis and penetrate the sinus node.

The Sinus Node

In man the artery supplying the sinus node originates from the proximal few centimeters of the right coronary artery in about 55 per cent of instances and from the proximal few millimeters of the left circumflex artery in about 45 per cent (Fig. 28-15). Collateral circulation to the sinus node is provided by neighboring atrial arteries, but the primary supply is virtually always a single unilaterally derived artery.[1] Despite its proximity to the main left coronary artery and anterior descending ramus, the left sinus node artery virtually never arises from any but the left circumflex ramus. From either right or left origin the sinus node artery courses in the adjacent atrial epicardium to the base of the superior vena cava, which it encircles as it penetrates the center of the sinus node (see Chap. 29). In addition to being the primary supply of the sinus node, this artery is also the largest atrial artery and distributes to a major portion of the atrial myocardium and interatrial septum. It regularly provides almost the entire supply to the thickest portion of atrial myocardium, the crista terminalis. All but the smallest atrial infarctions are associated with occlusion of flow into the sinus node artery. Such occlusions also cause infarction of the sinus node and lead to atrial arrhythmias.[16] An occlusion of this type is rarely in the sinus node artery itself, however, but usually in the main coronary artery proximal to the origin of the sinus node branch. Most posterior myocardial infarctions being due to right coronary occlusion, the concurrent onset of an atrial arrhythmia indicates that the occlusion must be in the proximal few centimeters of the right coronary artery in order to block flow into the sinus node branch. Similarly, lateral myocardial infarctions due to left circumflex artery occlusion and associated with the onset of atrial arrhythmias carry a grave prognosis,[17] for the occlusion must be in the first few millimeters of the left circumflex artery and any proximal propagation of the occlusion would block the main left coronary artery.

The Atrioventricular (A-V) Node

The artery supplying the A-V node regularly arises from the apex of the penetrating U turn made by the artery (either right or left coronary) crossing the crux of the heart (Fig. 28-16). This deep turn is a useful angiographic landmark,[18] being easily visualized on good-quality coronary angiograms, and marks the posterior junction of the interatrial and interventricular septums. The U turn additionally lies just below the ostium of the coronary sinus, and its apex is only a few millimeters from the A-V node. A line drawn from the apex of this turn to the noncoronary sinus of the

aorta separates the right from the left atrioventricular orifices and the interatrial septum above from the interventricular septum below. The U turn and A-V node artery are provided by the right coronary artery in 90 per cent of human beings and by the left circumflex artery in 10 per cent. The coronary anatomy of the dog, of which space does not permit discussion, is quite different in this region.[1] Some collateral circulation to the A-V node is provided by Kugel's artery (arteria anastomotica auricularis

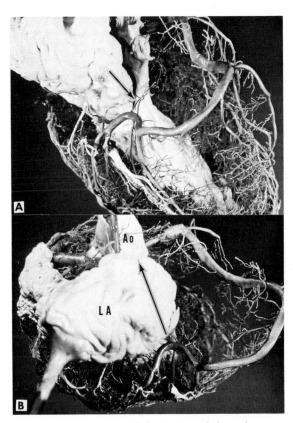

Fig. 28-16. Two views of the U turn of the right coronary artery at the crux of the heart. In *A* the view is from above and behind the uncast right atrium, showing the sweep of the right coronary artery as well as the A-V node artery itself (arrow), originating from the apex of the U turn. In *B* the same cast is viewed from directly above, with the uncast right atrium to the right and the left atrial cast (*LA*) to the left. *Ao* is the root of the aorta. The long arrow lies directly over the normal position of the interatrial septum. The left atrial cast bulges over this line because the right atrium is uncast. The usefulness of a line drawn from the apex of the U turn to the noncoronary sinus of the aorta is apparent for the interpreter of coronary angiograms. Such a line divides the right atrioventricular valve from the left and the interatrial septum above from the interventricular septum below, thus forming almost a central axis for the heart.

magna),[19] which arises from the proximal right or left coronary artery and courses posteriorly through the base of the interatrial septum. Coronary occlusions which produce posterior myocardial infarction necessarily deprive the A-V node of its primary blood supply. Fainting and syncope during angina or during an acute infarct are characteristic clinical features of acute posterior infarcts,[20-21] because of transient ischemia of the A-V node.

The A-V Bundle and Bundle Branches

Terminal branches of the A-V node artery (in 90 per cent of human beings a branch of the right coronary artery) supply the A-V bundle and the proximal few millimeters of the right and left bundle branches, as well as neighboring septal myocardium. These arterial branches coursing inward from the posterior surface of the heart are met by the terminal branches of Kugel's artery, which enters from the anterior portion of the heart. Distal to the inferior margin of the membranous portion of the interventricular septum, the bundle branches on both sides are supplied by the septal arteries arising from the left anterior descending artery. Since the right bundle branch is a single small bundle of fibers while the left branches occur in a large sheet of fibers, vascular and other lesions producing focal damage can more readily lead to right bundle branch block than to left bundle block. Conversely, the presence of left bundle branch block indicates damage to a larger associated area of myocardium.

The Little Coronary Arteries

Although not generally supplying a single special area (the sinus node and A-V node are exceptions), the little coronary arteries have been so frequently neglected in studies of the heart that they deserve special mention. It is customary at necropsies to dissect only the larger trunks of the coronary tree and neglect small branches. Recent histopathologic studies have indicated that these little arteries (0.1 to 1.0 mm diameter) may be the site of important changes.[22-25] When it is the sinus node or A-V node arterial supply which is involved, the consequences in disturbed cardiac rhythm or conduction are predictable. Perhaps equally important, however, is that these little arteries seem to be involved rather diffusely in a number of the so-called myocardiopathies[22-24] and may be the basis of previously poorly understood instances of cardiac enlargement and failure, especially if such cases are additionally associated with frequently documented examples of arrhythmia or heart block. Knowledge of how frequently pathologic conditions in such small arteries are responsible for these myocardiopathies will await the results of additional, more careful examinations than are currently routine.

REFERENCES

1. James, T. N.: "Anatomy of the Coronary Arteries," Hoeber Medical Division, Harper & Row, Publishers, Incorporated, New York, 1961.
2. Vieussens, R.: "Nouvelles découvertes sur le coeur," Paris, 1706.
3. Schlesinger, M. J., Zoll, P. M., and Wessler, S.: The Conus Artery: A Third Coronary Artery, *Am. Heart J.*, 38:823, 1949.
4. Bianchi, A.: Morfologia delle arteriae coronariae cordis, *Arch. ital. anat. e embriol.*, 3:87, 1904.
5. Spalteholz, W.: "Die Arterien der Herzwand," S. Hirzel Verlag, Leipzig, 1924.
6. Marshall, J.: "On the Development of the Great Anterior Veins in Man and Mammalia, Including an Account of Certain Remnants of Foetal Structure Found in the Adult: A Comparative View of These Great Veins in the Different Mammalia, and an Analysis of Their Occasional Peculiarities in the Human Subject, *Phil. Tr. Roy. Soc. London, 140:* 133, 1850.
7. Vastesaeger, M. M., Van Der Straeten, P. P., Friart, J., Candaele, G., Ghys, A., and Bernard, R. M.: Les anastomoses intercoronariennes telles qu'elles apparaissent á la coronarographie post mortem, *Acta cardiol.*, 12:365, 1957.
8. Laubry, C. H., Soulie, P., and Thys, H.: Les anastomoses septales., *Arch. mal. coeur*, 141:1, 1948.
9. Laurie, W., and Woods, J. D.: Anastomosis of the Coronary Circulation, *Lancet*, 2:812, 1958.
10. Pepler, W. J., and Meyer, B. J.: Interarterial Coronary Anastomosis and Coronary Arterial Pattern, *Circulation*, 22:14, 1960.
11. Bellman, S., and Frank, H. A.: Intercoronary Collaterals in Normal Hearts, *J. Thoracic Surg.*, 36:584, 1958.
12. Prinzmetal, M., Simkin, B., Bergman, H. C., and Kruger, H. E.: Studies on the Coronary Circulation. II. The Collateral Circulation of the Normal Human Heart by Coronary Perfusion with Radioactive Erythrocytes and Glass Spheres, *Am. Heart J., 33:* 420, 1947.
13. Baroldi, G., Mantero, O., and Scomozoni, G.: The Collaterals of the Coronary Arteries in Normal and Pathologic Hearts, *Circulation Res.*, 4:223, 1956.
14. Blumgart, H. L., Schlesinger, M. J., and Davis, D.: Studies on the Relation of the Clinical Manifestations of Angina Pectoris, Coronary Thrombosis, and Myocardial Infarction to the Pathologic Findings, *Am. Heart J.*, 19:1, 1940.
15. Kattus, A. A., and Gregg, D. E.: Some Determinants of Coronary Collateral Blood Flow in the Open-chest Dog, *Circulation Res.*, 7:628, 1959.
16. James, T. N.: Myocardial Infarction and Atrial Arrhythmias, *Circulation*, 24:761, 1961.
17. Wood, F. C., Wolferth, C. C., and Ballet, S.: In-

farction of the Lateral Wall of the Left Ventricle: Electrocardiographic Characteristics, *Am. Heart J.,* **16:**387, 1938.

18. James, T. N.: A Useful Landmark for Interpreting Angiocardiograms, *Radiology,* **75:**804, 1963.

19. Kugel, M. A.: Anatomical Studies on the Coronary Arteries and Their Branches. I. Arteria Anastomotica Auricularis Magna, *Am. Heart J.,* **3:**260, 1927.

20. James, T. N.: Posterior Myocardial Infarction, *J. Michigan M. Soc.,* **60:**1409, 1961.

21. James, T. N.: Arrhythmias and Conduction Disturbances in Acute Myocardial Infarction, *Am. Heart J.,* **64:**416, 1962.

22. James, T. N.: Observations on the Cardiovascular Involvement, Including the Cardiac Conduction System, in Progressive Muscular Dystrophy, *Am. Heart J.,* **63:**48, 1962.

23. James, T. N., and Fisch, C.: Observations on the Cardiovascular Involvement in Friedreich's Ataxia, *Am. Heart J.,* **66:**164, 1963.

24. James, T. N.: Degenerative Arteriopathy with Pulmonary Hypertension: A Revised Concept of Socalled Primary Pulmonary Hypertension, *Henry Ford Hosp. M. Bull.,* **9:**271, 1961.

25. James, T. N.: An Etiologic Concept Concerning the Obscure Myocardiopathies, *Progr. Cardiovascular Diseases,* **7:**43, 1964.

29 ANATOMY OF THE CONDUCTION SYSTEM OF THE HEART *

Thomas N. James, M.D.

Man has been fascinated by the spontaneous beating of the heart throughout recorded history, and many ancient rites of worship included excision of the living heart. Despite this long history of curiosity, factual knowledge about the structures actually responsible for the heart beat is relatively recent. The classic studies of His the younger,[1] Tawara,[2] and Keith and Flack[3] were performed only near the start of this century. It is remarkable in studying their papers to see how clearly the sinus node, the atrioventricular (A-V) node, and the A-V bundle and its branches were described. It makes all the more puzzling the current aura of mystery which seems to pervade most discussions of the conduction system of the heart.

In this chapter on the anatomy of the cardiac conduction system there will be four divisions: the

* The work on which this chapter is based has been supported in part by grants from the United States Public Health Service and the Michigan Heart Association.

sinus node, the A-V node, the A-V bundle with its branches and peripheral arborization, and the internodal and interatrial pathways. In each division the description of normal anatomy will be combined with a brief consideration of the pertinent pathologic anatomy.

The Sinus Node

Since the pacemaker of the heart is near the junction of superior vena cava and sinus intercavarum with both atrium and auricle, neither *sinoatrial* nor *sinoauricular* is a completely accurate term. It seems more suitable, as initially proposed by Walmsley,[4] to refer to this structure by the less restrictive term of *sinus node,* a name which has the additional attractive advantage of brevity.

It has been suggested by Patten[5] that embryologically the sinus node and A-V node are analogous structures, arising at the junctions of right and left superior cardinal veins, respectively, with the sinus venosus. Then as the sinus venosus ultimately becomes the medial half of the right atrium and part of the interatrial septum, the A-V node migrates to the internal position it occupies in the heart of the human adult. The sinus node, on the other hand, even in the adult heart remains more nearly in its primitive position. Whether Patten's explanation is correct or not, it is a sufficiently useful concept to retain unless clearly disproved. In lower animals the entire region of the sinus venosus has been demonstrated to have special electrophysiologic properties,[6] and one may think of the two nodes as representing the opposite poles of this special region of the heart.

Grossly the sinus node lies near the junction of the superior vena cava and right atrium (Fig. 29-1), its anterior margin being a few millimeters posterior to the crest formed by the junction of the anterior margin of the atrial appendage with superior vena cava.[7-8] From this point the sinus node extends posteriorly for 10 to 20 mm, lying just beneath the sulcus terminalis, so that its posterior margin is at the junction of atrium with sinus intercavarum instead of superior vena cava. The shape of the node is roughly a flattened ellipse, and it does not have a head or tail, as so commonly alleged. Being located a millimeter or less beneath the epicardium (Fig. 29-2), it is heir to all the diseases which afflict that surface, most notably pericarditis.[9] The opposite surface of the node is slightly farther from the endocardium, but the inferior margin of the node joins the free wall of the right atrium directly over the recess between the crista terminalis and lateral wall of atrium, an area known as the *antrum atrii dextri.*[10] On cross section the sinus node has an approximate triangular shape with the apex pointing toward the superior vena

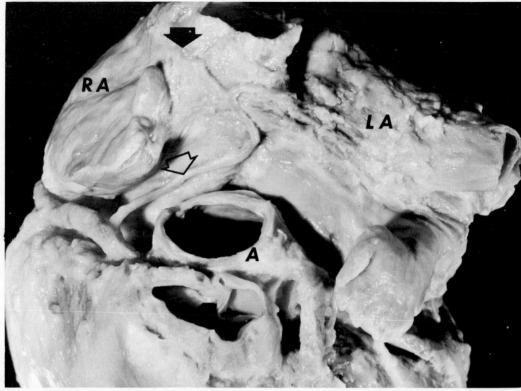

Fig. 29-1. Dissection of a normal human heart demonstrating the course of a right sinus node artery (open arrow) and the location of the sinus node (black arrow) between the superior vena cava and right atrium (*RA*). Although the caliber of the sinus node artery remains the same, the artery disappears when it enters the sinus node, because it becomes invested by a dense collagen matrix which is the framework of the node. *LA*, left atrium; *A*, aorta. (*Adapted from an illustration in T. N. James, "Anatomy of the Coronary Arteries," 1961, and reproduced with permission of the publisher, Paul B. Hoeber, Inc., New York.*)

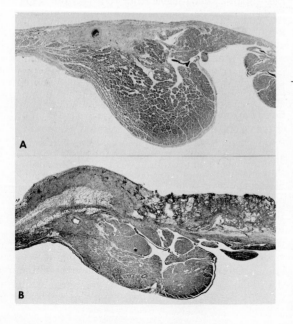

cava and sinus intercavarum, while the base is astride the antrum atrii dextri, with angular extensions into both the free wall of the right atrium and the crista terminalis. Disease of the sinus node is commonly associated with extensive thrombus formation in the antrum atrii dextri.

Fig. 29-2. *A.* Low-power (× 7) photomicrograph showing the normal sinus node, which is the pale-staining area about a centrally located artery. Note its proximity to the epicardium above. The free wall of the right atrium extends to the right, and the sinus intercavarum extends to the left from the node. The large mass of atrial myocardium extending to the right and below the node is a cross section of the crista terminalis. The interspaces between the crista terminalis and free wall of right atrium are the antrum atrii dextri. *B.* Relationship of pericarditis to the sinus node (× 7). Because of its proximity to the epicardium, the node is virtually always involved during pericarditis. Orientation of structures in *B* is the same as in *A*. *A* is stained with the Goldner modification of the Masson trichrome stain, and *B* with Verhoeff–Van Gieson stain.

Internally the most intriguing feature of the sinus node is its constant relationship to a disproportionately large centrally located artery (Fig. 29-3). While some small lateral branches of this artery function to nourish the node, the large artery itself passes directly through the center of the node as if en route elsewhere. This close anatomic relationship prompted Söderström to describe the sinus node as resembling an enormous adventitia of its artery.[10] Since the sinus node artery is regularly one of the first branches of the coronary arteries, which are in turn the first branches of the aorta, the sinus node is in an admirable position to monitor central aortic pressure and pulsation. The possibility of a functional relationship between pulsation and caliber of the intranodal artery and pacemaking by the sinus node has led to a number of physiologic and pharmacologic studies.[11–15] Observations to the present time indicate that those drugs and procedures which accelerate the sinus node may decrease the caliber of the artery, while those which slow the node may be associated with increased caliber of the artery. Though further studies are necessary

concerning this functional hypothesis, anatomically the structure of the node is entirely compatible with this reasoning.

The framework of the sinus node is dense collagen which is closely attached to the entire circumference of the central artery. Within this collagen lattice there are interlacing bundles of fibers which also attach to this framework. These fibers are of smaller diameter and stain paler than ordinary myocardium with almost all dyes (Fig. 29-4). Nearest the central artery, the bundles of sinus node fibers tend to encircle the vessel, while farther out into the substance of the node the bundles interweave more at random. At the margins of the node in nearly all directions the sinus node fibers converge into exiting Purkinje tracts. Some sinus node fibers unite to form large Purkinje fibers, but occasionally a single small fiber may be seen progressively to enlarge as it leaves the node.

There are numerous nerve endings but no ganglions within the sinus node. At the anterior and posterior margins of the sinus node there are many ganglions, however. Within the midportion of the sinus node there are a variable number of

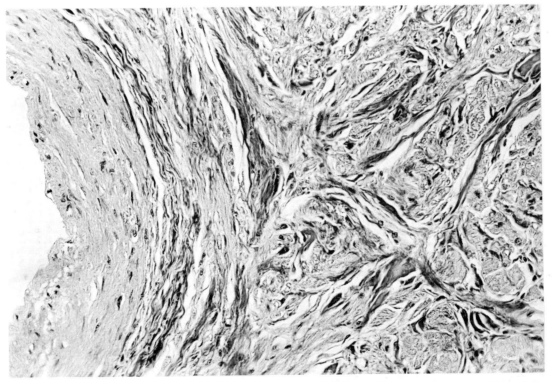

Fig. 29-3. Photomicrograph demonstraing the internal structure of the normal human sinus node and the relationship between the centrally located disproportionately large artery and the node. The darker-staining tissue is collagen, and the lighter-staining tissue consists of sinus node fibers, except for smooth muscle in the wall of the artery (left margin of the picture). The sinus node fibers occur in interlacing bundles, except for those nearest the artery, which encircle it. (Goldner trichrome stain, × 325.)

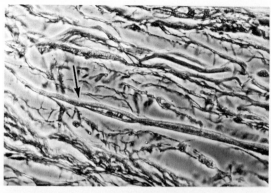

Fig. 29-4. Photomicrograph showing details of individual sinus node fibers. The fiber indicated by the arrow demonstrates the perinuclear bulge and clear zone, which resemble those of the larger conventional Purkinje fibers elsewhere in the heart. (Goldner trichrome stain, × 160 with phase illumination.)

stellate or syncytial cells which have a large round nucleus (Fig. 29-5). Sinus node fibers commonly distribute from these syncytial cells, which are often near nerve endings. It has been suggested that these primitive-appearing cells may be the site of actual pacemaking within the sinus node.[8] Their close resemblance to the "leading cells" shown by Harary to be dominant pacemakers in myocardial fiber tissue cultures[16] is intriguing.

Pathology of the sinus node is closely related to two of its anatomic features, the proximity to the epicardium and the centrally located artery. Peri-

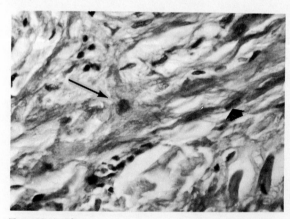

Fig. 29-5. Photomicrograph of a syncytial cell (long arrow) found in the central portion of the normal human sinus node. Compare the round, relatively large nucleus with that of a conventional sinus node fiber (short arrow). Another sinus node fiber is faintly shown connected to the right upper margin of the syncytial cell and coursing toward the right upper corner of the picture, almost parallel to the indicated (short arrow) sinus node fiber. (Goldner trichrome stain, × 160.)

carditis almost invariably involves at least the epicardial surface of the node and often even deeper portions.[9] Vascular lesions are generally of two types: those caused by occlusion of the main coronary artery proximal to the sinus node branch and those involving small arteries directly. The former vascular lesions are usually associated with acute ventricular myocardial infarction and commonly atrial arrhythmias; in these there is characteristically hemorrhage at the junction of the sinus node and right atrium.[17] The lesions of the small arteries include all the diseases affecting such arteries, e.g., lupus erythematosus and polyarteritis nodosa. Additionally, there are a number of heritable disorders commonly associated with myocardiopathy and arrhythmias or conduction disturbances which have surprisingly exhibited widespread lesions of the small arteries of the heart, including those of the sinus node and A-V node.[18-20]

The A-V Node

Located at a critical vantage point guarding the only normal conduction path between the atria and ventricles, the A-V node is in a peculiarly strategic position. One A-V nodal function is "triage" of atrial signals for transmission to the ventricles. Another function, according to current electrophysiologic concepts, is a delay of approximately 0.04 sec in A-V transmission which occurs at or near the atrionodal junction.[21] There are two advantages to this normal delay: one is postponement of ventricular excitation until the atria have had time to eject their contents into the ventricles, and the second is a coincident limitation in the maximum number of signals which can be accommodated for transmission by the A-V node. An appreciation of the anatomic location and internal structure of the A-V node is essential to an accurate concept of its electrophysiologic function.

The human A-V node is situated just beneath the right atrial endocardium directly above the insertion of the septal leaflet of the tricuspid valve and just anterior to the ostium of the coronary sinus.[22] The surface it presents toward the right atrium is convex, and the opposite surface (concave) rests on the collagenous base of the mitral annulus (Fig. 29-6). At its posterior and superior margins the A-V node receives fibers from the interatrial septum and eustachian ridge, which are the terminal portion of the internodal tracts (discussed later). In addition to these fibers which enter the margins of the A-V node, there are a number of similar fibers which course past the margins to enter the node at various points along its convex surface, including some which enter near the region at which the node begins to form A-V bundle (Fig. 29-7). If the anatomic location of the point of nor-

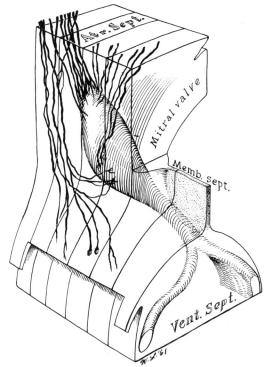

Fig. 29-6. Schematic drawing of the human A-V node, showing its relationship to the two atrioventricular valves and the interatrial and interventricular septums, including the membranous portion of the interventricular septum. As the node courses medially and inferiorly along the lower margin of the membranous interventricular septum, it gives rise early to a single right bundle branch but continues providing multiple left bundle branches, which form virtually a sheet of fibers down the left septal endocardium. Only a few fibers from the internodal tracts are shown, to avoid obscuring details of the A-V node, but these may be seen entering the superior and posterior margins of the node as well as the lower portion of the convex right atrial surface of the node. A few internodal fibers terminate in the base of the tricuspid valve, and rarely (almost exclusively in infants) a few may penetrate directly to the interventricular septum. The potential electrophysiologic significance of these multiple entrances into the A-V node is discussed in the text.

mal electrophysiologic delay in A-V transmission is at the proximal (marginal) atrionodal junction, then these fibers entering the lateral surface of the node may function to bypass the point of normal delay.[22] The anatomy of this region therefore provides anatomic support for the concept of dual A-V transmission proposed on the basis of physiologic studies by Moe et al.[23] Although electrocardiographic phenomena such as the Wolff-Parkinson-White complexes are commonly attributed to aberrant conduction through lateral A-V connec-

tions, there are good reasons to doubt this explanation:

1. Cases with accelerated conduction have been found which had no lateral atrioventricular bundles, and conversely cases with such bundles demonstrable do not always exhibit accelerated conduction.

2. Even the demonstrations of lateral A-V bundles have shown only ordinary myocardium, which may or may not be capable of rapid conduction.

3. If dual A-V conduction does occur in the

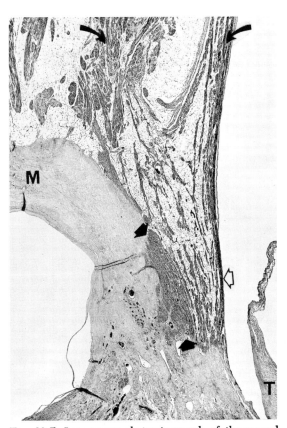

Fig. 29-7. Low-power photomicrograph of the normal human A-V node near its midportion. Decussation of internodal fibers as they approach the node from above is shown, the fibers in the central interatrial septum (curved arrow on the left) entering predominantly the superior margin of the node while those in the bypass region (curved arrow on the right and open arrow adjacent to the node) circumvent the margins to enter the convex surface of the node. The body of the A-V node lies between the two short black arrows, lying on the annulus of the mitral valve (*M*). *T* = a deflected leaflet of the tricuspid valve. (Goldner trichrome stain, × 15.) (*From T. N. James: The Connecting Pathways between the Right and Left Atrium in the Human Heart, Am. Heart J., 66:498, 1963, and reproduced with permission of The C. V. Mosby Company, St. Louis.*)

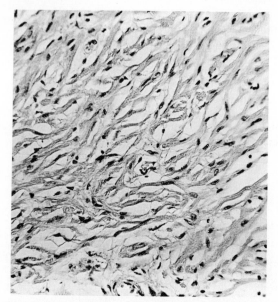

Fig. 29-8. Photomicrograph showing details of the internal structure of a human A-V node. The fibers are slightly shorter than those of the sinus node, and there is much less supporting collagen. A central artery sometimes is seen in the A-V node but is not a constant feature, whereas it is in the sinus node. Fibers of the A-V node interweave and interconnect abundantly. (Goldner trichrome stain, × 325.)

region of the A-V node, there are more tenable explanations for intermittent occurrence of accelerated conduction, e.g., the influence of the rich innervation of the node but not of lateral A-V bundles. On the basis of present anatomic and electrophysiologic evidence, it seems unlikely that lateral atrioventricular bundles are of any functional significance and that phenomena such as the Wolff-Parkinson-White complexes are best explained by altered conduction in or very near the A-V node.

Internally the A-V node exhibits both similarities to and differences from the sinus node. Like those of the sinus node, fibers of the A-V node interweave to form a meshwork, but there is much less collagen between fibers (Fig. 29-8). Although there is some variation in the size and length of A-V node fibers from one heart to another, in general they are slightly thicker and shorter than those of the sinus node but not as thick as those of ordinary myocardium. Throughout the upper and middle portions of the A-V node the fibers frequently connect with each other and interweave at random, but in the anterior and inferior portion of the node they begin to orient into a longitudinal axis as they form the A-V bundle. There is no anatomic feature of the A-V node to suggest a morphologic basis

for the commonly used electrocardiographic terms of *upper, lower,* and *middle A-V nodal rhythm,* and the history of the origin of these terms casts even greater doubt on their validity.[24] Similarly, the electrocardiographic term *coronary sinus rhythm* may serve some useful didactic purpose, but anatomically it seems unlikely that a signal originating in the coronary sinus (if indeed it does) could inscribe a significantly different peripherally recorded electrocardiographic complex from a signal originating in A-V node, since the coronary sinus and the A-V node are only a few millimeters apart.

Behind the A-V node, in the small area between it and the coronary sinus, there are a number of autonomic ganglions. These are presumably vagal ganglions, and it has been suggested they may have a receptor function[25] as well as being the probable route by which afferent vagal stimuli arrive at the A-V node. The commonest pathologic condition of the A-V node is ischemic infarction or fibrosis due to occlusion of the main coronary artery supplying the A-V node branch (Fig. 29-9). In 90 per cent of human beings the A-V node is supplied by the right coronary artery, the occlusion of which is associated with posterior myocardial infarction as well as A-V nodal ischemia or infarction.

In addition to syncope or more prolonged loss of consciousness during angina pectoris preceding a posterior infarction, or during the actual infarction, other clinical features of this type of infarction include an uncommonly high incidence of nausea and vomiting, unusual diaphoresis, sialorrhea, tenesmus, and intense sinus bradycardia. All these symptoms can be caused by excess vagal discharge, and in the patient with acute posterior myocardial

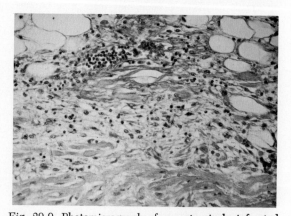

Fig. 29-9. Photomicrograph of an extensively infarcted A-V node from a patient with acute posterior myocardial infarction and heart block. Hemorrhage and necrosis are evidence of very recent damage, while the fat spaces and young connective tissue suggest older injury. (Goldner trichrome stain, × 192.)

infarction most of them can be promptly abolished with atropine. There has been some question as to the origin of this vagotonia, but the demonstration by Juhasz-Nagy and Szentivanyi of vagal receptor sites in or near the wall of the coronary sinus[26] suggests that the ganglions observed near the posterior margin of the human A-V node may be this site.[25] If this is so, the vagal reflex phenomenon of acute posterior myocardial infarction may be a human counterpart of the von Bezold-Jarisch reflex, which has heretofore been recognized and extensively studied only in experimental animals.[27,28]

The A-V Bundle and Its Proximal and Distal Branches

Formed by convergence of fibers at the anterior and inferior margin of the A-V node, the parallel fibers of the A-V bundle veer from the right atrial endocardial location of the A-V node into the middle of the central fibrous body. At the same time the A-V bundle descends along the posterior margin of the membranous interventricular septum to the crest of the muscular septum. The A-V bundle is initially triangular in cross section, and the two lower corners of the triangle give rise to the right and left bundle branches (Fig. 29-10). The right bundle branch is a single slender group of fibers which leave the common bundle shortly after it reaches the muscular crest of the interventricular septum. The left bundle branch is a virtual sheet of fibers cascading down from the left margin of the common bundle through most of its course. The difference in size of the two bundle branches is a striking anatomic feature which probably accounts for the clinical observation that right bundle branch block is more often an innocuous finding in the electrocardiogram, since it can be produced by such a small focal lesion, whereas blocking the left bundle branches requires a much more extensive lesion.

From their origin near the membranous septum the two bundle branches both course generally in an anterior and apical direction along the endocardium, rapidly fanning out in all directions to cover the ventricular endocardium. The left bundle branches form two relatively direct pathways to the anterior and posterior papillary muscles in addition to spreading more diffusely. Presumably this permits delivery of a slightly earlier signal to these two structures, since their effective contraction should slightly precede contraction of the ventricular free walls in order to prevent mitral regurgitation. Peripheral divisions of the right bundle branch are fairly evenly distributed, but because the right bundle branch originates at a level considerably below the crista supraventricularis, this

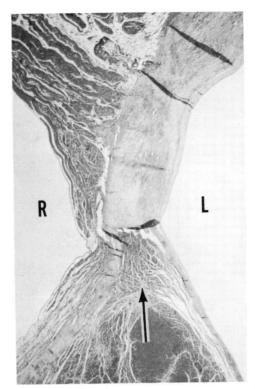

Fig. 29-10. Photomicrograph of a human A-V bundle (arrow). Note the triangular shape of this cross section, with right and left bundle branches originating from its two lower corners. *R*, right side of the heart; *L*, left. The mitral annulus and valve course from the center of the picture to the right upper corner. The tricuspid valve base is in the left lower corner, the interatrial septum above, and interventricular septum below. (Goldner trichrome stain, × 12.)

structure is some distance removed and therefore activated relatively late.

The noncoronary sinus of the aorta protrudes into the interatrial septum just above the membranous interventricular septum, so that its posterior margin is in close proximity to the common A-V bundle (Fig. 29-11). It is hardly surprising, therefore, that lesions causing aortic valvulitis so commonly are associated with disruption of A-V conduction, because of associated inflammation or other pathology of the A-V bundle. During aortic bacterial endocarditis the A-V bundle may even be destroyed, as it may also be in extensive calcification of the aortic valve. Occasionally inflammation of the mitral annulus may extend to involve either the A-V bundle or A-V node (which are directly adjacent to the annulus), and calcification or abscesses of the mitral ring are particularly prone to do so. Whether inflammation of the mitral annulus may contribute to heart block sometimes

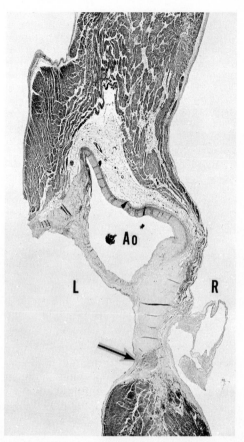

Fig. 29-11. Photomicrograph demonstrating the proximity of the noncoronary sinus of the aorta (*Ao*) to the A-V bundle (arrow). The septal leaflet of the tricuspid valve is attached to the left upper margin of the noncoronary sinus. The interatrial septum extends upward and the interventricular septum down. *L*, left side of the heart; *R*, right. (Goldner trichrome stain, × 4.)

branches are composed exclusively of Purkinje fibers in the human heart and that there are many fibers which are directly continuous with such fibers but which are morphologically indistinguishable (at least by present methods) from ordinary myocardium. This occurs not only at the points of transition from bundle branch area to definite ordinary myocardium but also within the main course of the bundle branch area itself. More peripherally there are commonly areas of right and left ventricular subendocardium where many Purkinje fibers occur in a layer or small groups, but there are also areas of subendocardium where such fibers cannot be identified. Much confusion has resulted from the implication by some that rapid conduction is an exclusive property of Purkinje fibers. The presence of fibers of ordinary appearance within the bundle branches themselves strongly suggests that some such fibers also conduct rapidly. As recently discussed by Truex,[29] it is probable that rapidly conducting fibers in the human heart often exhibit classic Purkinje characteristics similar to those in ungulates but that some fibers which we now consider morphologically as ordinary myocardium must also possess the ability to conduct rapidly.

Internodal and Interatrial Connecting Pathways

Largely because of the erroneous assumption that rapid conduction is exclusively a property of fibers with Purkinje characteristics, it is frequently stated that there is no pathway of specialized tissue between the sinus node and A-V node. Since electrophysiologic studies have established beyond doubt that the impulse from the sinus node arrives at the A-V node more rapidly than it could in ordinary myocardium,[21] the question is really not whether

seen in acute rheumatic fever may also be considered, although pathologic studies of this stage of the disease are understandably uncommon.

Fibers in the A-V bundle are similar in size to those in the A-V node, but their arrangement is parallel and therefore entirely different from the thickly interwoven fibers of the node. Shortly after bifurcation of the bundle into its right and left branches, the fibers not only become enlarged but are then of even greater diameter than ordinary myocardial fibers. Most of the fibers in the bundle branches have thicker myofibrils, with rectangular or oblong nuclei, and a perinuclear clear zone and bulge, thus resembling the classic Purkinje fibers (Fig. 29-12), which are much better seen and were originally described in ungulates, not in man. It is important to realize that not even the bundle

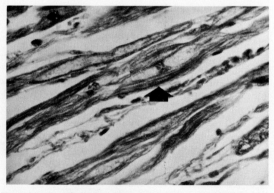

Fig. 29-12. Photomicrograph showing several human Purkinje fibers. In addition to the coarse myofibrils, note the rectangular nucleus with a perinuclear bulge and clear zone (arrow). (Goldner trichrome stain, × 480.)

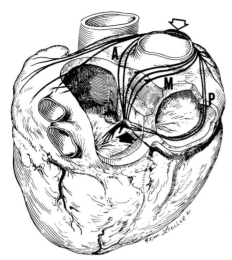

Fig. 29-13. Location and course of the three internodal tracts of the human heart. The heart is viewed from above and behind the left atrium. The open arrow indicates the sinus node, at the junction of superior vena cava and right atrium, while the black arrow indicates the A-V node, lying near the junction of inter-atrial and interventricular septums and between the ostium of the coronary sinus behind and membranous interventricular septum ahead. *A*, the anterior internodal tracts and the predominant interatrial tracts, the division occurring as they course in Bachmann's bundle; these interatrial fibers were first described by Bachmann. *M*, the middle internodal tracts, first described by Wenckebach. *P*, the posterior internodal tracts, first described by Thorel See text for further discussion.

such pathways exist but where they are. On gross dissection there are three potential pathways between the sinus node and A-V node (Fig. 29-13), the continuity of fibers being demonstrable with serial sectioning. These pathways are similar in man[30] and the dog,[31] and correspond in part to areas previously described by Wenckebach,[32,33] Thorel,[34,35] and Bachmann.[36] The pathway originally described by Bachmann, on the basis of both physiologic and anatomic studies, was concerned primarily with interatrial conduction, and he made no mention of its function in internodal conduction.

The *anterior internodal tract* extends from the anterior margin of the sinus node to curve about the superior vena cava and enter the anterior interatrial myocardial band (Bachmann's bundle). Fibers in this bundle divide near the anterior margin of the interatrial septum (Figs. 29-13, 29-14), some continuing into the left atrium and others descending obliquely and posteriorly within the interatrial septum behind the noncoronary sinus of the aorta to enter the upper margin of the A-V node. This is a well-developed pathway in almost all human hearts and can easily be demonstrated throughout

its course by careful dissection. It is composed of both ordinary and Purkinje fibers, with a large number of the latter but frequent continuity of both types. The initial portion of this pathway and

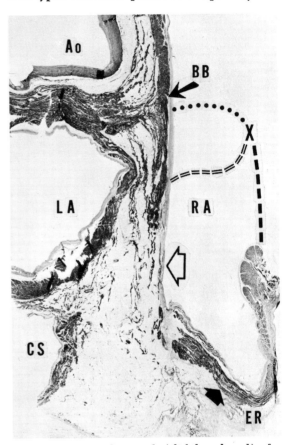

Fig. 29-14. Gross photograph (slightly enlarged) of a horizontal section through the atria and interatrial septum of a human heart, demonstrating the general location of the three internodal tracts. *X* indicates the location of the sinus node, which is above the plane of this section; the open arrow indicates the approximate location of the A-V node, which is below the plane of this section. The short black arrow indicates fibers in the posterior internodal tract as they approach the A-V node from the eustachian ridge (*ER*). Bachmann's bundle is indicated by the narrow black arrow and the letters *BB*. Note its division into fibers which continue into the left atrium and others which descend obliquely in the interatrial septum to the A-V node. The dots indicate the course of fibers in the anterior internodal tract, the thin double dashes those in the middle internodal tract, and bold single dashes those in the posterior internodal tract. *Ao*, aorta; *CS*, coronary sinus; *RA*, right atrium; *LA*, left atrium. (*From T. N. James: The Connecting Pathways between the Right and Left Atrium in the Human Heart, Am. Heart J.*, 66:498, 1963, *and reproduced with permission of the C. V. Mosby Company, St. Louis.*)

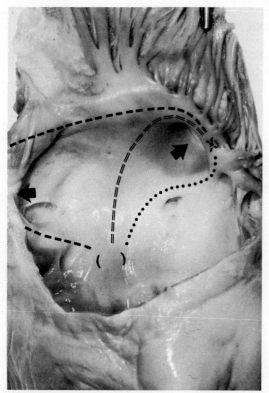

Fig. 29-15. Interior of the right atrium, showing the relation of the three internodal tracts to internal structures. Dots and dashes indicate the same courses of fibers as in Fig. 29-14. The arrow on the right is in the ostium of the superior vena cava, while that on left indicates the inferior vena cava, which has been cut open as the free wall of the right atrium was reflected upward from the atrioventricular sulcus. The parentheses indicate the approximate location of the A-V node just anterior to the ostium of the coronary sinus. The broken X indicates the location of the sinus node, which is epicardial. The anterior internodal tracts curve anteriorly about the superior vena cava through Bachmann's bundle into the interatrial septum, where they descend to the A-V node. The middle internodal tracts curve behind the superior vena cava across the sinus intercavarum to the top of the interatrial septum and then descend to the A-V node. The posterior internodal tracts follow the crista terminalis to the posterior margin of the interatrial septum and A-V node, crossing the top of the ostium of the coronary sinus. (*From T. N. James: The Connecting Pathways between the Right and Left Atrium in the Human Heart, Am. Heart J.,* 66:498, 1963, *and reproduced with permission of The C. V. Mosby Company, St. Louis.*)

its continuity into the left atrium are the tract described by Bachmann, who did not indicate awareness of the division descending to the A-V node.

The *middle internodal tract* was first described by Wenckebach, who suggested it was the route of conduction not only from node to node but also between the two atria. These fibers leave the superior and posterior margins of the sinus node to curve behind the superior vena cava and cross the sinus intercavarum to the crest of the interatrial septum. There they divide into a few sparse fibers continuing into the left atrium and a much larger number which descend within the interatrial septum to enter the top of the A-V node (Figs. 29-13, 29-15). The connections with the left atrium by this route are inconstant and seldom very extensive, suggesting that Wenckebach's concept of interatrial conduction by this route is important only in exceptional hearts.

The *posterior internodal tract* was first described by Thorel and was more recently emphasized by Söderström[10] as a major pathway for internodal conduction. These fibers leave the posterior margin of the sinus node and continue along the crista terminalis to the eustachian ridge, in which they sweep into the interatrial septum directly above the posterior margin of the A-V node (Figs. 29-13–29-15). There they curve down to enter the node. Like the anterior internodal tract, this pathway is fairly constant and easily demonstrable by gross dissection, especially in hearts with a prominent eustachian ridge. When the eustachian ridge is diminutive, appearing as a thin fold, it is composed almost exclusively of fibers with Purkinje characteristics. The route of conduction in this posterior internodal tract in man is similar to that in the dog, but in the rabbit there is an important difference. Instead of entering the interatrial septum above the coronary sinus and thence connecting with the A-V node, the fibers in the rabbit descend farther in the crista terminalis to the level of the tricuspid ring and then course medially to enter the interatrial septum *beneath* the ostium of the coronary sinus. It is important to note this difference because of its potential significance in experimental electrophysiologic studies, which commonly employ the rabbit. An additional important anatomic difference exhibited by the rabbit heart is its constant left superior vena cava, a feature first reported by Marshall.[37] In view of Patten's theory about the embryologic origin of the sinus node and A-V node, the lack of attrition of the left superior vena cava in the rabbit may suggest a more primitive state of associated structures, including the A-V node. Finally, the large size of the ostium of the coronary sinus in the rabbit (because it drains the left superior vena cava as well as the cardiac veins) leads to a more anterior intracardiac displacement of the A-V node in the rabbit than in man or the dog.

As fibers of all three internodal tracts approach the A-V node, some merge with each other while others enter the node directly. Some fibers of all three tracts additionally bypass the marginal atrionodal junctions and enter the A-V node at various points along its convex surface. The general outline of the area encompassed by the internodal tracts indicates most of the residuum of the primitive sinus venosus, another reason to anticipate that fibers within this area may have specialized conduction properties, whether these are morphologically identifiable by current methods or not. Furthermore, when one considers the merging of the three tracts in the vicinity of the A-V node as well as their common origin in the sinus node, a reasonable route is presented for the circus movement so often employed in electrocardiographic theory but rarely defined anatomically.

Interatrial conduction may occur along any one of the three internodal tracts but under normal circumstances in most hearts is probably preferentially through Bachmann's bundle (Figs. 29-14, 29-16), beginning along the anterior internodal tract. Fibers in the middle internodal tract are so sparse and inconstant as to make them unlikely to be of much importance in interatrial conduction. Fibers from the posterior internodal tract have such a long interatrial route, spreading from the A-V node up the left atrial side of the interatrial septum, that they probably participate little if at all in normal interatrial conduction. During ectopic rhythm originating in the A-V node, however, the posterior internodal tract may become the major pathway of spread to both atria. Conduction to the right atrium from the sinus node is virtually direct,

radiating mainly from the inferior margin of the node into the trabeculae of the free wall of the right atrium and extending into the crista terminalis, from which more distal radiation may occur. Just as in the ventricles, there are many fibers in both atria which exhibit Purkinje characteristics, particularly in the regions of the internodal and interatrial pathways.

Although it may reasonably be presumed that normal spread of excitation is radial from the sinus node into the right atrium and through Bachmann's bundle to the left atrium, what the normal pathway is for internodal conduction is not so apparent. For example, one internodal tract may function selectively under normal conditions, the others providing alternate routes in the case of disease. On the other hand, two or more tracts may function normally with some means of cancellation of late-arriving impulses at the A-V node or of synchronization of conduction between the various pathways just prior to arrival of an impulse at the A-V node. Future studies on the electrophysiology of these regions will doubtless explain how what we see functions.

REFERENCES

1. His, W., Jr.: Die Thatigkeit des embryonalen Herzens und deren Bedeutung für die Lehre von der Herzbewegung beim Erwachsenen, *Arb. med. Klin.,* 14, 1893.
2. Tawara, S.: "Das Reizleitungssystem des Saugetierherzens," Jena, Fischer, 1906.
3. Keith, A., and Flack, M.: The Form and Nature of the Muscular Connections between the Primary Di-

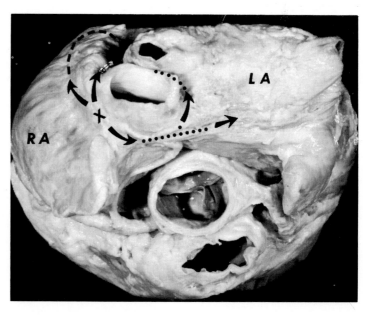

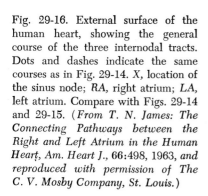

Fig. 29-16. External surface of the human heart, showing the general course of the three internodal tracts. Dots and dashes indicate the same courses as in Fig. 29-14. *X*, location of the sinus node; *RA*, right atrium; *LA*, left atrium. Compare with Figs. 29-14 and 29-15. (*From T. N. James: The Connecting Pathways between the Right and Left Atrium in the Human Heart, Am. Heart J.,* 66:498, 1963, *and reproduced with permission of The C. V. Mosby Company, St. Louis.*)

visions of the Vertebrate Heart, *J. Anat. & Physiol.*, **41**:172, 1907.

4. Walmsley, T.: Comparative Anatomy of the Heart, in Quain's "Elements of Anatomy," Part III, Longmans, Green & Co., London, 1929, vol. 4, p. 3.

5. Patten, B. M.: "Human Embryology," 2d ed., McGraw-Hill Book Company, New York, 1953.

6. Weidmann, S.: Resting and Action Potentials of Cardiac Muscle, *Ann. New York Acad. Sc.*, **65**:663, 1957.

7. Hudson, R. E. B.: The Human Pacemaker and Its Pathology, *Brit. Heart J.*, **2**:153, 1960.

8. James, T. N.: Anatomy of the Human Sinus Node, *Anat. Rec.*, **141**:109, 1961.

9. James, T. N.: Pericarditis and the Sinus Node, *Arch. Int. Med.*, **110**:305, 1962.

10. Söderström, N.: Myocardial Infarction and Mural Thrombosis in the Atria of the Heart, *Acta med. scandinav.*, **132** (Suppl. 217):114, 1948.

11. James, T. N., and Nadeau, R. A.: Sinus Bradycardia during Injections Directly into the Sinus Node Artery, *Am. J. Physiol.*, **204**:9, 1963.

12. James, T. N., and Nadeau, R. A.: Effects of Sympathomimetic Amines Studied by Direct Perfusion of the Sinus Node, *Am. J. Physiol.*, **204**:591, 1963.

13. James, T. N., and Nadeau, R. A.: Selective Cholinergic Stimulation and Blockade of the Sinus Node by Direct Perfusion through Its Artery, *J. Lab. & Clin. Med.*, **62**:40, 1963.

14. James, T. N., and Nadeau, R. A.: Relation of Retrograde Pressure in the Sinus Node Artery to Sinus Tachycardia from Stellate Stimulation, *J. Lab. & Clin. Med.*, **62**:777, 1963.

15. James, T. N., and Nadeau, R. A.: The Effects of Vagal Stimulation, Eserine and Atropine on Retrograde Pressure in the Sinus Node Artery, *Henry Ford Hosp. M. Bull.*, **12**:23, 1964.

16. Harary, I.: Heart Cells in Vitro, *Scient. Am.*, **206**: 141, 1962.

17. James, T. N.: Myocardial Infarction and Atrial Arrhythmias, *Circulation*, **24**:761, 1961.

18. James, T. N.: Observations on the Cardiovascular Involvement, Including the Cardiac Conduction System, in Progressive Muscular Dystrophy, *Am. Heart J.*, **63**:48, 1962.

19. James, T. N.: Degenerative Arteriopathy with Pulmonary Hypertension: A Revised Concept of So-called Primary Pulmonary Hypertension, *Henry Ford Hosp. M. Bull.*, **9**:271, 1961.

20. James, T. N., and Fisch, C.: Observations on the Cardiovascular Involvement in Friedreich's Ataxia, *Am. Heart J.*, **66**:164, 1963.

21. Hoffman, B. F., and Cranefield, P. F.: "Electrophysiology of the Heart," McGraw-Hill Book Company, New York, 1960.

22. James, T. N.: Morphology of the Human Atrioventricular Node, with Remarks Pertinent to Its Electrophysiology, *Am. Heart J.*, **62**:656, 1961.

23. Moe, G. K., Preston, J. B., and Burlington, H.: Physiologic Evidence for a Dual A-V Transmission System, *Circulation Res.*, **4**:357, 1956.

24. Brumlik, J. V.: The Sinoatrial Node, the Atrioventricular Node and Atrial Dysrhythmias, in Charles E. Kossman (ed.), "Advances in Electrocardiography," Grune & Stratton, Inc., New York, 1958, p. 252.

25. James, T. N.: Arrhythmias and Conduction Disturbances in Acute Myocardial Infarction, *Am. Heart J.*, **64**:416, 1962.

26. Juhasz-Nagy, A., and Szentivanyi, M.: Localisation of the Receptors of the Coronary Chemoreflex in the Dog, *Arch. internat. pharmacodyn.*, **131**:39, 1961.

27. Dawes, G. S.: Studies on Veratrum Alkaloids. VII. Receptor Areas in the Coronary Arteries and Elsewhere as Revealed by the Use of Veratridine, *J. Pharmacol. & Exper. Therap.*, **89**:325, 1947.

28. Dawes, G. S.: Cardiovascular Reflexes and Myocardial Infarction, in T. N. James and J. W. Keyes (eds.), "The Etiology of Myocardial Infarction," Little, Brown and Company, Boston, 1961.

29. Truex, R. C.: Comparative Anatomy and Functional Considerations of the Cardiac Conduction System, in A. P. De Carvalho (ed.), "Specialized Tissues of the Heart," Elsevier Publishing Company, New York, 1962, pp. 22–43.

30. James, T. N.: The Connecting Pathways between the Sinus Node and the A-V Node and between the Right and the Left Atrium in the Human Heart, *Am. Heart J.*, **66**:498, 1963.

31. James, T. N.: Anatomy of the Sinus Node of the Dog, *Anat. Rec.*, **143**:251, 1962.

32. Wenckebach, K. F.: Beitrage zur Kenntnis der menschlichen Herztätigkeit, *Arch. Anat. Physiol.*, **1–2**:1, 1907.

33. Wenckebach, K. F.: Beitrage zur Kenntnis der menschlichen Herztätigkeit, *Arch. Anat. Physiol.*, **3**:53, 1908.

34. Thorel, C.: Vorläufige Mitteilung über eine besondere Muskel verbindung zwischen der Cava superior und dem Hisschen Bündel, *München. med. Wchnschr.*, **56**:2159, 1909.

35. Thorel, C.: Über den Aufbau des Sinusknotens und seine Verbindung mit der Cava superior und den Wenckebachschen Bündeln, *München. med. Wchnschr.*, **57**:183, 1910.

36. Bachmann, G.: The Inter-auricular Time Interval, *Am. J. Physiol.*, **41**:309, 1916.

37. Marshall, J.: On the Development of the Great Anterior Veins in Man and Mammalia; Including an Account of Certain Remnants of Foetal Structure Found in the Adult: A Comparative View of These Great Veins in the Different Mammalia, and an Analysis of Their Occasional Peculiarities in the Human Subject, *Phil. Tr. Roy. Soc. London*, **140**: 133, 1850.

30 PHYSIOLOGY OF THE CORONARY CIRCULATION

Richard Gorlin, M.D.

Knowledge of the physiology of the coronary circulation is essential in understanding some aspect of almost every disease of the heart. This chapter will attempt to cover fundamentals of coronary physiology. Situations peculiar to the various cardiac ailments which affect or are influenced by the coronary circulation will be described when pertinent.

Normal Values

Coronary flow is subject to change from moment to moment to an extraordinary degree, as is cardiac output. The reasons for this will be discussed below. Some estimate may be made, however, of average values. Coronary blood flow has been determined in man almost solely by diffusible indicators, and only for the left ventricle (because coronary sinus blood is the only venous effluent readily accessible for analysis). Most workers report a flow of between 0.7 and 0.9 ml per Gm left ventricular muscle per min.[1,2] The weight of the left ventricle in grams is approximate to the body weight of the human subject in pounds.[1] Thus, normal resting left ventricular coronary flow in a subject of 150 lb lies between 105 and 135 ml per min. Under experimental conditions, values up to two and one-half times the resting coronary flow have been recorded in man[3] and up to five times the resting flow in the dog.[4]

The arteriovenous oxygen difference averages 0.12 ml per ml coronary flow,[1] giving an average cardiac oxygen consumption per gram of 0.8 and 1.0 ml per min. The normal heart is completely aerobic and does not exhibit anaerobic energy metabolism at rest or with various stresses.[5]

Vascular resistance, usually calculated as mean pressure gradient divided by mean flow, is not readily estimated for the coronary system, because in the left ventricle the small vessels are closed in systole yet in the right ventricle they are open (cf. below). The author has employed an empirical calculation which considers only the resistance in small vessels of the left ventricle.[1] This is expressed as:

$$CVR = \frac{P \times T \times 1332}{CF}$$

where CVR = coronary diastolic vascular resistance

P = arterial diastolic mean–coronary venous pressure
T = coronary diastolic filling time
CF = coronary flow

Thus, the pressure and cycle time directly affecting left ventricular coronary flow can be entered into the assessment of small-vessel resistance.

In order to find any pattern in the response of the coronary circulation, one must distinguish between *hydraulic* factors mechanically responsible for any given flow and *metabolic* or other factors initiating a need for a certain quantity of flow.

Hydraulic Factors

Coronary blood flow (Fig. 30-1) is phasic in nature, first because it is dependent on phasic aortic pressure and secondly because the myocardium offers a variable degree of resistance to flow during systole. For those branches of the coronary arteries which supply the right ventricle, this latter factor is usually insignificant because of the low intramyocardial pressure in relation to the aortic pressure. For those branches which plunge through the left ventricular myocardium the situation is quite different, however. The heart is a thick-walled shell, and intramyocardial tension must always be greater than intracavity pressure[6] with a steady increase from the epicardium to the endocardium. Thus, left ventricular coronary flow is virtually all diastolic in phase.[7] This places a certain premium on the time available for left ventricular coronary flow. This time can be encroached upon by either prolongation of systole or increase in cardiac rate. The effect of perfusion pressure alone

MECHANISMS CHANGING CORONARY FLOW

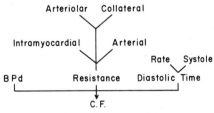

Fig. 30-1. The mechanical factors which can mechanically affect the volume of coronary flow (CF). Diastolic blood pressure (BPd) is critical to left ventricular flow and mean blood pressure to right ventricular flow. The duration of diastole, so important to left ventricular flow, is shortened by increase in heart rate or duration of systole (as in aortic stenosis). Resistance to flow can occur in the large arteries, in the myocardium during its contraction, and in the collateral and other small vessels of the coronary tree. Change in arteriolar resistance is probably the most important regulator of coronary flow.

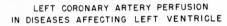
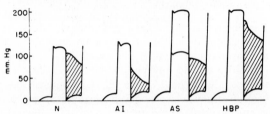

LEFT CORONARY ARTERY PERFUSION
IN DISEASES AFFECTING LEFT VENTRICLE

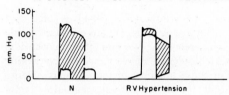

RIGHT CORONARY ARTERY PERFUSION
IN DISEASES AFFECTING RIGHT VENTRICLE

Fig. 30-2. In the upper figure are seen the pressure-time relationships in normal individuals (N) and in those with aortic insufficiency (AI), aortic stenosis (AS), or hypertension (HBP). In the lower figure are seen the pressure-time relationships in the normal subject (N) and the subject with right ventricular (RV) hypertension. The hatched area represents effective perfusion pressure–time.

is also influenced by right atrial or coronary venous exit pressure. From these simple facts, one can readily appreciate the effect which different diseases and conditions have on mechanical coronary perfusion (Fig. 30-2). Hypertension is self-compensating, whereas aortic stenosis is not. Aortic insufficiency, through low aortic diastolic pressure, and tachycardia, through lessened diastolic coronary filling time, place mechanical disadvantages upon the coronary perfusion system at a time when the work load may be greatly augmented by these very conditions. Similarly, right ventricular hypertension, if severe, can interfere with the normal pancyclic right coronary flow and predispose to right-sided coronary insufficiency.[1] Impedance to coronary venous exit by significant right atrial pressure elevation,[8] as with right ventricular failure or tricuspid stenosis, rarely seems to be clinically important.

In addition to being dependent on aortic pressure, coronary flow is regulated by changes in small-vessel resistance, primarily at the arteriolar level. These arterioles are greatly responsive to many stimuli (cf. below) and exhibit both constriction and dilatation. It has been estimated that these vessels can dilate to a degree sufficient to increase coronary flow five times without changes

in any other mechanical supply factor.[4] Large-artery resistance can also occur, as in coronary atherosclerosis, although it is generally necessary to decrease vessel lumen by greater than two-thirds to cause a significant pressure loss under resting conditions. With conditions requiring augmented flow, as with physical exercise, the moderately compromised large-vessel cross-sectional area, adequate for transmission of a resting flow requirement, may seriously impede adequate delivery of coronary flow.

No discussion of coronary vessel resistance would be complete without mention of collateral vascular pathways. These structures are anatomically present from early life but become large and significant only if the need for coronary flow exists in some region of the heart. They serve as alternative and sometimes as solitary routes of blood flow around stenotic or occluded arteries.

Metabolic Factors (Fig. 30-3)

Oxygen Requirement

The heart extracts approximately 70 per cent of the oxygen in every milliliter of blood, leaving

FACTORS REGULATING CORONARY FLOW

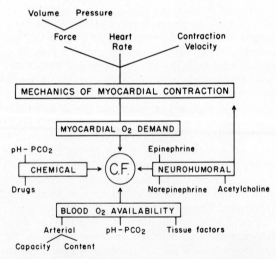

Fig. 30-3. Factors affecting coronary flow (CF) through neurometabolic pathways. The factors are arranged in four groups: chemical, blood oxygen availability, neurohumoral, and myocardial oxygen demand. These are further broken down into subcategories. Note in particular the factors which affect myocardial mechanics. Note also that neurohumoral agents (the catecholamines in particular) exert effects on the coronary circulation both directly in the arteriole and indirectly through induced changes in·mechanical modalities of contraction.

venous blood about 30 per cent saturated at a pO_2 of 18 to 20 mm Hg.[9] This is the lowest value for venous oxygen in the body and is matched only by exercising skeletal muscle (Fig. 30-4). The heart functions almost solely on aerobic metabolic pathways (contrary to skeletal muscle), and the deprivation of oxygen for more than 2 min results in total cessation of mechanical activity. As a result, the most urgent stimulus to increased coronary flow (regionally or throughout the heart) is myocardial hypoxia.[8] Hypoxia invariably produces prompt vasodilatation. This is evident from the fact that coronary venous oxygen saturation remains remarkably constant in a given patient over a wide range of spontaneous or induced hemodynamic variables.[10] The "hypoxic feedback" may be initiated in the following situations:

I. Regional—decreased oxygen tension distal to an obstruction or stenosis can cause local vasodilatation and restoration of flow.[8]
II. General—reduced oxygen tension can result from:
   A. Reduced arteriovenous extraction as with arterial hypoxia or anemia. Change in pH and pCO_2 can have minor but definite effects on oxygen extraction through change in the oxygen dissociation curve.
   B. Increase in mechanical activity of the heart. Energy consumption of any pump is usually related directly to the work done, with a fixed efficiency. This does not appear to be true for the heart, primarily for two reasons: (1) heart size, and therefore the pump itself, is constantly changing, and (2) external work (i.e., that volume of blood moved out of the heart at any pressure) is not necessarily the same as internal work (i.e., that performed by the contractile element itself).[11] Muscle shortening is not directly equatable with contractile-element shortening, because there is an elastic component acting in series with the contractile element.[12] Despite these theoretical problems, certain empirical variables of cardiac action seem to relate well to changes in cardiac oxygen requirement, and hence to affect coronary flow. These are:
   1. Time integral of ventricular systolic pressure. Acute changes in blood pressure can affect oxygen consumption and, hence, coronary flow. This is also seen with aortic stenosis and systemic hypertension. However, in the latter condition, some self-compensation occurs solely through increased diastolic coronary perfusion pressure (Fig. 30-2).

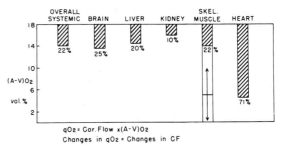

OXYGEN EXTRACTION BY THE HEART AND OTHER ORGANS

Fig. 30-4. Arteriovenous oxygen difference and per cent extraction (of original arterial oxygen concentration) for each of the various organs at rest. Note the high myocardial and exercising skeletal muscular extractions (clear bar). The two-headed arrow on the skeletal muscle bar represents the somewhat greater variability seen in venous oxygen content here as compared to heart.

2. Heart rate.[15] Tachycardia, by increasing time spent in contraction, increases oxygen consumption and the need for coronary flow. The product of items 1 and 2, variously called *tension-time index*[13] and *pressure time per minute*,[14] correlate well with oxygen consumption in most situations.
3. Cardiac size.[16] Increased cardiac size results in increased ventricular wall tension per unit systolic pressure developed. With increased cardiac volume, oxygen consumption increases, and usually out of proportion to the increase in mechanical work induced by increased fiber length.
4. Cardiac fiber–shortening velocity.[17] There appears to be an energy cost associated with this factor, although at present it is the least understood. Increased contraction velocity occurs particularly with sympathetic or catecholamine stimulation and is the mechanism for increasing or maintaining stroke volume at unchanged end-diastolic cardiac size. This kinetic change has an energy cost of its own (to be differentiated from the increased stroke volume which occurs with increased cardiac end-diastolic volume. This has been shown to be a relatively "cheap" action and has given rise to a distinction between costly "high-pressure" and efficient "high-flow" work. This probably occurs because when heart size is increased by increased stretch, more blood will be ejected per unit fiber shorten-

ing.[*][18] Thus, stroke volume can increase with relatively minor changes in mean systolic cardiac volume and tension and no change in kinetics of fiber shortening —therefore, little increase in oxygen consumption or coronary flow).

In this regard, it is perhaps relevant to point out that catecholamines affect oxygen consumption only in relation to an induced change in mechanical activity.[17] With norepinephrine, for example, if blood pressure rises, then oxygen consumption follows this change; if fiber shortening increases also, then energy cost will be proportionately greater, and so on.

C. Chemical uncoupling of oxidative phosphorylation, as with dinitrophenol or cytochrome enzymatic block as with cyanide, can greatly increase coronary flow. Neither the naturally occuring catechols[19] nor thyroid hormone[20] act upon the heart through these mechanisms.

Local or Circulating Metabolites

Coronary flow is increased and oxygen extraction decreased in beri beri[21] and to some extent in thyrotoxicosis.[22] Rather than a metabolic block to oxygen uptake,[23] this may be the participation of the coronary system in a generalized circulatory vasodilatation, possibly induced by some metabolic substance.

Neurohumoral Factors

The coronary system can be made to dilate or constrict irrespective of metabolic influences. This can be accomplished through autonomic nervous system stimulation and through circulating catecholamines. A likely example of neural regulation is seen in chronic low output failure where coronary flow at rest is lower and oxygen extraction is higher than in the normal output subject.[10] Norepinephrine is a primary coronary vasconstrictor[24,25] and almost invariably causes an increase in oxygen extraction and a drop in coronary venous oxygen saturation.[25] The increased mechanical activity of the heart induced by norepinephrine acts as a secondary and competing dilator stimulus through the *hypoxic* mechanism.[24] Norepinephrine activates *alpha*, or vasoconstrictor, receptors. On the other hand, isoproterenol, which affects only *beta*, or dilator, receptors, causes a rise in coronary venous oxygen saturation.[3] Epinephrine has a milder pri-

mary dilator action. Pitressin is another naturally occurring hormone which has a profound constrictor influence on the coronary circulation.[26]

One can see, then, that analysis of any given coronary blood-flow response becomes extremely complex. A catecholamine, for example, can change from one to four mechanical variables of cardiac action and therefore oxygen requirements. Satisfaction of these increased coronary flow requirements will be mechanically aided if catechol action induces diastolic hypertension but will be hindered if a primary vasoconstrictor action is exerted upon the coronary arterioles themselves. By contrast, during physical exercise, apparently only the hypoxic feedback from the working myocardium is initiated. Coronary venous oxygen saturation and oxygen extraction remain constant, and coronary flow rises *pari passu* with cardiac oxygen requirements.[10,27] The flow increment occurs primarily through dilatation of arterioles, because the diastolic perfusion pressure–time factor usually remains constant.[27]

Coupling of Supply-Demand Mechanisms

In certain situations, increased demand is met directly by the involved variable. Specifically, in hypertension, the increase in coronary flow and oxygen consumption needed to keep up the increased systolic pressure load is brought about directly by the simultaneous increase in diastolic perfusion pressure.

In most circumstances, however, there is believed to be a direct chemical mediator which acts either through the neural receptors, as with norepinephrine, epinephrine, and acetylcholine, or directly on the arteriolar wall, as has been suggested for bradykinin,[28] lactic acid,[29] or the adenine nucleotides.[30] With the exception of Berne's work,[24] relatively little information has been forthcoming to indicate the link between demand and supply on the heart. Berne has suggested that with hypoxia there is an immediate local breakdown of adenine nucleotides. Some of these are known potent vasodilators. A new steady state with increased flow and no hypoxia is established and maintained by local biochemical feedback. It may even be that the myocardium is peculiarly responsive because pO_2 is about 18 to 20 mm Hg, or only 10 mm Hg above the level[31] at which anaerobic metabolism sets in (presumably because of shift in cell redox potential).

Coronary Insufficiency

Coronary insufficiency results whenever the demand for energy exceeds the supply. As described earlier, this can be generalized or localized within the heart. Whether generalized, as in the patient

---

[*] $dv = 4\pi r^2 \ dr$ where $v =$ stroke volume and $r =$ ventricular radius. Thus, small changes in radius have exponential effects on stroke volume.

with aortic valvular disease, or localized, as in coronary atherosclerosis, coronary insufficiency manifests itself physiologically in the following ways: (1) reduction in coronary venous oxygen saturation and increase in oxygen extraction over previous values;[10] (2) appearance of myocardial anaerobic metabolism[32] (Fig. 30-5). There are other abnormalities peculiar to the patient with coronary heart disease, due to the patchy distribution of ischemia and scarring. Often the mixed coronary venous oxygen saturation is *higher* than normal at rest, possibly from shunts through scar tissue or inappropriate vasodilatation.[10] Also, coronary blood-flow determinations may vary, depending on the region of the heart studied. This, in all probability, does not represent varying rates of perfusion* as much as staggered or sequential onset of perfusion of different parts of the myocardium because of the devious collateral pathways. A particular characteristic of the coronary heart disease condition is that stress evokes a greater than normal increase in coronary flow, presumably as a result of inefficient contractile mechanisms in the ischemically damaged myocardium.[33] This, of course, uses up the available coronary reserve for lesser degrees of stress than in the normal, thus potentiating coronary insufficiency.

In summary, the human coronary circulation is unique in that (1) flow through a part of the system occurs only during one phase of the cardiac cycle; (2) oxygen extraction is high and flow relatively low; (3) flow is exquisitely sensitive to change in oxidative energy need and therefore to any change in cardiac mechanical activity; and (4) flow requirements and supply mechanisms can be simultaneously affected, and often in opposite directions by a single variable.

REFERENCES

1. Gorlin, R.: Measurement of Coronary Blood Flow in Health and Disease, in A. Morgan Jones (ed.), "Modern Trends in Cardiology," Butterworth & Co. (Publishers), Ltd., London, 1960, p. 191.
2. Rowe, G. G.: Nitrous Oxide Method for Determining Coronary Blood Flow in Man, *Am. Heart J.*, 58:268, 1959.
3. Krasnow, N., Rolett, E. L., Yurchak, P. M., Hood, W. B., Jr., and Gorlin, R.: Isoproterenol and Cardiovascular Performance, *Am. J. Med.* 37:514, 1964.
4. Case, R. B., Berglund, E., and Sarnoff, S. J.: Ventricular Function. VII. Changes in Coronary Resistance and Ventricular Function Resulting from

* A persistent difference in perfusion should lead ultimately to local necrosis. This probably occurs sporadically and not as a day-to-day process.

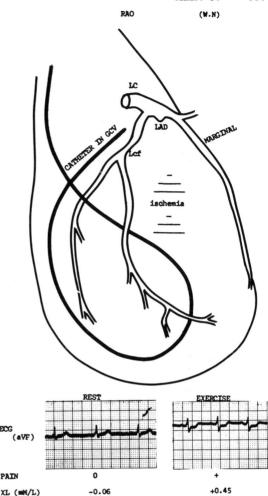

Fig. 30-5. Integrated study of myocardial ischemia: the heart of a patient in the right anterior oblique projection. The catheter and coronary artery were drawn directly from the selective left coronary arteriogram. The catheter is in the great cardiac vein (GCV). LC, left coronary artery; LCF, left circumflex; LAD, stump of left anterior descending branch. The catheter is draining venous blood from the anterior surface of the heart labeled "ischemia." Note the occurrence of pain, ST-segment depression, and excess lactate (XL) formation at this time. It should be noted that the blood samples on which excess lactate was obtained were drawn in close proximity to the region of local ischemia.

Acutely Induced Anemia and the Effect Thereon of Coronary Stenosis, *Am. J. Med.*, 18:397, 1955.
5. Krasnow, N., Neill, W. A., Messer, J. V., and Gorlin, R.: Myocardial Lactate and Pyruvate Metabolism, *J. Clin. Invest.*, 41:2075, 1962.
6. Pflugge, W.: "Stresses in Shells," Springer-Verlag, Berlin, 1960, pp. 18–27.
7. Laszt, L., and Muller, A.: Pressure and Velocity Conditions in the Coronary Circulation of the Dog, *Helvet. physiol. acta*, 15:38, 1957.

8. Gregg, D. E.: "Coronary Circulation in Health and Disease," Lea & Febiger, Philadelphia, 1950.

9. Brachfeld, N., Bozer, J., and Gorlin, R.: Action of Nitroglycerin on the Coronary Circulation in Normal and in Mild Cardiac Subjects, *Circulation*, **19:** 697, 1959.

10. Messer, J. V., Wagman, R. J., Levine, H. J., Neill, W. A., Krasnow, N., and Gorlin, R.: Patterns of Myocardial Oxygen Extraction during Rest and Exercise, *J. Clin. Invest.*, 41:725, 1962.

11. Britman, N. A., and Levine, H. J.: Contractile Element Work: A Major Determinant of Myocardial Oxygen Consumption, *J. Clin. Invest.*, 43:1397, 1964.

12. Hill, A. V.: The Abrupt Transition from Rest to Activity in Muscle. *Proc. Roy. Soc., London, ser. B*, **136:**399, 1949.

13. Sarnoff, S. J., Braunwald, E., Welch, G. H., Jr., Case, R. B., Stainsby, W. N., and Macruz, R.: Hemodynamic Determinants of Oxygen Consumption of the Heart with Special Reference to the Tension Time Index, *Am. J. Physiol.*, **192:**148, 1958.

14. Neill, W. A., Levine, H. J., Wagman, R. J., and Gorlin, R.: Left Ventricular Oxygen Utilization in Intact Dogs: Effect of Systemic Hemodynamic Factors, *Circulation Res.*, 12:163, 1963.

15. Gorlin, R.: Studies on the Regulation of the Coronary Circulation in Man. I. Atropine Induced Changes in Cardiac Rate, *Am. J. Med.*, 25:37, 1958.

16. Rolett, E. L., Yurchak, P. M., Cohen, L. S., Elliott, W. C., and Gorlin, R.: Relation between Ventricular Force and Oxygen Consumption, *Fed. Proc.*, 22:345, 1963.

17. Gorlin, R., Yurchak, P. M., Rolett, E. L., Elliott, W. C., and Cohen, L. S.: Inferential Evidence for the Fenn Effect in the Human Heart, *J. Clin. Invest.*, 42:939, 1963.

18. Gorlin, R., Rolett, E. L., Yurchak, P. M., and Elliott, W. C.: Left Ventricular Volume in Man Measured by Thermodilution, *J. Clin. Invest.*, 43: 1244, 1964.

19. Lianides, S. P., and Beyer, R. E.: Oxidative Phosphorylation in Liver Mitochondria Prepared from Adrenal-demedullated and Epinephrine-treated Rats, *Biochim. et biophys. acta*, 44:356, 1960.

20. Lee, C. W.: Effect of Hyperthyroidism on Oxidative Phosphorylation in the Rat Heart, Master's Thesis, University of Pittsburgh Graduate School of Public Health, 1958.

21. Hackel, D. B., and Kleinerman, J.: Effects of Thiamin Deficiency on Myocardial Metabolism in Intact Dogs, *Am. Heart J.*, 46:1, 1953.

22. Leight, L., Defazio, V., Talmers, F. N., Regan, T. J., and Hellems, H. K.: Coronary Blood Flow, Myocardial Oxygen Consumption and Myocardial Metabolism in Normal and Hyperthyroid Human Subjects, *Circulation*, 14:90, 1956.

23. Olson, R. E.: Myocardial Metabolism in Congestive Heart Failure, *J. Chron. Dis.*, 9:442, 1959.

24. Berne, R. M.: Effect of Epinephrine and Norepinephrine on the Coronary Circulation, *Circulation Res.*, 6:644, 1958.

25. Yurchak, P. M., Rolett, E. L., Cohen, L. S., and Gorlin, R.: Effects of Norepinephrine on the Coronary Circulation in Man, *Circulation*, 30:180, 1964.

26. Green, H. D.: Effects of Pitressin, the Nitrites, Epinephrine and the Xanthines on Coronary Flow in Mammalian Hearts, in "Blood, Heart and Circulation," Publication 13, American Association for the Advancement of Science, 1940, pp. 105–113.

27. Gorlin, R., Krasnow, N., Levine, H. J., and Messer, J. V.: Effect of Exercise on Cardiac Performance in Human Subjects with Minimal Heart Disease, *Am. J. Cardiol.*, 13:293, 1964.

28. Hilton, S. M., and Lewis, G. P.: Relationship between Glandular Activity, Bradykinin Formation and Functional Vasodilatation in the Submandibular Salivary Gland, *J. Physiol.*, 134:471, 1956.

29. Lundholm, L.: Mechanism of the Vasodilator Effect of Adrenaline. I. Effect on Skeletal Muscle Vessels, *Acta physiol. scandinav.*, 39, Suppl. 133, 1956.

30. Berne, R. M.: Nucleotide Degradation in the Hypoxic Heart and Its Possible Relation to Regulation of Coronary Blood Flow, *Fed. Proc.*, 20:101, 1961.

31. Shea, T. M., Watson, R. M., Piotrowski, S. F., Dermksian, G., and Case, R. B.: Anaerobic Myocardial Metabolism, *Am. J. Physiol.*, 203:463, 1962.

32. Krasnow, N., and Gorlin, R.: Myocardial Lactate Metabolism in Coronary Insufficiency, *Ann. Int. Med.*, 59:781, 1963.

33. Messer, J. V., Levine, H. J., Wagman, R. J., and Gorlin, R.: Effect of Exercise on Cardiac Performance in Human Subjects with Coronary Artery Disease, *Circulation*, 28:404, 1963.

31 PATHOLOGY OF CORONARY ATHEROSCLEROSIS AND ITS COMPLICATIONS

Richard P. Lynch, M.D., and Jesse E. Edwards, M.D.

Intrinsic disease of the coronary arteries is overwhelmingly atherosclerotic in nature. Uncommon forms of significant coronary disease include ostial stenosis from primary disease of the aorta, coronary embolism, coronary arterial involvement by inflammatory disease, of which periarteritis is the most common, and congenital states in which part of the coronary arterial system makes gross communication with the pulmonary trunk, a cardiac chamber or a thoracic vein.

In this chapter we are concerned primarily with coronary atherosclerosis.

Nature and Distribution of Coronary Atherosclerosis

Controversy still exists as to the nature of the earliest change in atherosclerosis. A commonly held theory, which is based upon histologic observations, is that first lipid-filled macrophages are localized in the arterial intima. The distribution is of interest in that often it does not follow a circumferential pattern. Rather, the lesion of atherosclerosis is focal. In cross section it is often apparent that one arc of the vessel is involved while the remainder is immune to the lesion (Fig. 31-1A). This phenomenon lends support to the opinion that whatever the various factors are that stimulate atherogenesis, one of these is local and may represent stress. The tendency for concentration of greatest atherogenic effect at bifurcations of arteries is also in support of local mechanical factors as playing roles either in stimulating or retarding atherogenesis.

Following the accumulation of lipid-laden macrophages the intima is further thickened (at the expense of the lumen) by a fibrous reaction to the fatty material. The new fibrous tissue tends to encapsulate the foci of lipid-filled cells. Following the earliest stage, cells containing lipid disintegrate, and the lipid material is extruded into the extracellular areas of the intima. Crystallization and calcification of this material follow, as does progressive increase in the amount of encapsulating fibrous tissue. In the fibrous wall of the atheroma capillaries are formed. Medial atrophy and the presence of stainable neutral fat in the muscle cells beneath the atheroma are commonly observed.

Histologically, evidence for an episodic tendency toward atherogenesis may be observed. This evidence takes the following form: In arteries with "old" atheromas (that is, extracellular lipids associated with crystallization and/or calcification) one may observe one or several more superficial accumulations of lipid-filled macrophages. These accumulations suggest an atheroma of more recent onset than the deeper "burned-out" lesion.

Intraarterial Complications of Atherosclerosis

The major intraarterial complications of atherosclerosis are (1) luminal narrowing by the fundamental process, (2) intramural hemorrhage, and (3) thrombosis. Embolism of atheromatous tissue and aneurysm formation are considered less common, although the incidence of embolism of material from an atheroma in one segment to a second segment of the same coronary artery is unknown.

Intramural (intimal) hemorrhage is a common

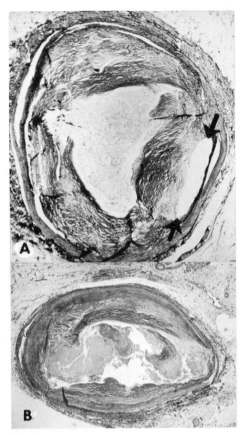

Fig. 31-1. A. Cross sections of an atherosclerotic coronary artery. The intima is greatly thickened by fibrous and atheromatous material, some of which is calcified. The remaining lumen is narrow and appears between the arrows. It is significant that that arc of the intima related to one portion of the narrowed lumen is devoid of atherosclerosis. The focal nature of atherosclerotic lesions, even in single cross sections, is common and is represented by this illustration. B. Photomicrograph of an atherosclerotic coronary artery. At the right and left extremes of the illustration are foci of hemorrhage within the atherosclerotic intima. There has been rupture of the overlying connective tissue with extrusion of atheromatous material into the lumen of the vessel. Such material may embolize. Also, the process of the intimal hemorrhage with rupture of the overlying tissue may serve as a nucleus for thrombosis.

phenomenon in well-established atheromas, as these lesions are supplied with capillaries. Opinions are not uniform as to the functional significance of such hemorrhages. That these, per se, are common causes of acute coronary arterial occlusion seems doubtful. The basis for this opinion is the fact that even in instances of extensive intimal hemorrhage, the arterial lumen maintains a circular shape in cross section. One would expect flattening of the lumen were the hemorrhage directly responsible for narrowing of the lumen.

That intimal hemorrhages with associated rupture of the overlying intima may be the cause of acute coronary arterial thrombosis must be accepted. That this process is not uncommonly observed in chance single sections of thrombosed coronary arteries suggests that it may indeed be a fairly common phenomenon in cases of acute coronary thrombosis. Hemorrhages with rupture of the lining may cause extrusion of atheromatous material into the lumen and set the stage for embolism of atheromatous material (Fig. 31-1*B*).

Yet another possible effect of intramural hemorrhage is that the hemorrhage is an irritant and sets into operation a reflex, the end result of which is spasm of collateral arteries.

Coronary thrombosis when present is usually observed in segments of arteries with established atherosclerotic lesions, supplying evidence for the opinion that atherosclerosis is the main underlying factor favoring thrombosis. It has already been mentioned that intramural hemorrhage with rupture of the intima may precipitate thrombosis. Thrombosis may occur over an atheroma in the absence of rupture of the atheroma. The classic thrombus within a coronary artery involves but a short length of the involved segment, usually less than 1 cm of the length of the vessel.

The usual appearance of the thrombus is uniform, suggesting that the process which occludes the lumen occurs within a very short period of time. In some instances, however, one may observe only a mural thrombus, or if the lumen is occluded, the thrombotic material may suggest several ages, as though the initial stage was mural thrombosis followed by one or several additional episodes until the process of luminal occlusion was complete.

The reaction to a thrombus in a coronary artery is like that which occurs in thrombi in any vessel or cardiac chamber. Encapsulation and organization occur, but it is to be recognized that the process of organization of thrombi in atherosclerotic vessels proceeds at a considerably slower pace than in thrombi which occur, for one reason or another, in fundamentally normal arteries. So delayed may organization be in atherosclerotic coronary arteries that when there is an associated myocardial infarct, the latter may be completely healed while organization of the underlying arterial thrombus is far from complete. Such observations have suggested the theory that in some cases of myocardial infarction and coronary thrombosis the former precedes the latter.

The process by which a thrombus becomes replaced by fibrous and vascular tissue has been called *organization, recanalization,* or *organization and recanalization.* The term *recanalization* with regard to coronary arterial thrombi needs special consideration. While the term may suggest that the original lumen is restored, this is far from reality. In arteries harboring "recanalized" thrombi the vessels in the original lumen are usually narrow. Even if these communicate with the parent lumen, both proximal and distal to the thrombus, the channels are so narrow that they do not appear capable of carrying any significant volume of blood. Therefore, a segment of an artery at the level of a "recanalized" thrombus is, as a practical matter, an occluded segment (Fig. 31-2*A*).

Occasionally an atheroma within a coronary artery may become dislodged, flow as an embolus peripherally, and become impacted at a distal point within the artery of origin. Here it may serve to cause myocardial ischemia, as the newly occluded segment may lie at a level distal to the level of entrance of collateral vessels that had bypassed the initially narrowed segment. Such emboli may also serve as nuclei upon which thrombosis occurs.

Atherosclerosis of coronary arteries commonly is

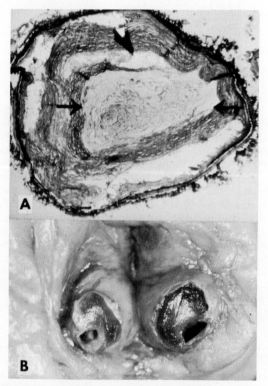

Fig. 31-2. *A.* Coronary atherosclerosis and organized thrombosis. Between the arrows the lumen, narrowed by fundamental atherosclerosis, is filled with loose vascular tissue representing organized (so-called recanalized) thrombosis. *B.* Gross sections of an atherosclerotic coronary artery with aneurysm formation.

associated with atrophy of the media underlying the intimal lesion. In spite of the common occurrence of medial atrophy and possibly because of splinting by the atheroma, aneurysms only rarely occur in atherosclerotic coronary arteries (Fig. 31-2*B*). Such aneurysms are usually saccular, and laminated thrombi are present within them. Usually, however, an effective lumen for the flow of blood remains. The main complication of coronary aneurysms of atherosclerotic origin is that portions of the contained thrombus may become dislodged and embolize.

Myocardial Complications of Coronary Atherosclerosis

The major significance of coronary atherosclerosis is that the lesion, either alone or in association with acute coronary occlusion, is a cause of myocardial ischemia. Myocardial ischemia, in turn, is responsible for a variety of clinical states including angina pectoris, sudden death, status anginosus, and acute myocardial infarction. In the material that follows the authors will consider these within the framework of the pathologic processes that underlie these clinical states.

Angina Pectoris

It is firmly established that in angina pectoris organic coronary arterial disease is almost universally present. In the overwhelming number of instances coronary atherosclerosis is widely distributed. Organized thrombi may also be present as causes of coronary arterial narrowing.

The myocardium may be normal, it may show evidence of a healed classic myocardial infarct, and/or there may be small scars which, from case to case, vary in number from a few to innumerable ones. These small scars have by some been considered the lesions of *chronic infarction*. This term implies that chronic coronary arterial disease is responsible for "slow death" of muscle fibers with ultimate fibrous replacement. Such an explanation is not inviting to the authors. One would prefer to deny the concept of "slow death." Rather, the authors would consider that in the patient with clinical angina pectoris there occurs from time to time typical acute myocardial infarction which involves small areas of the myocardium. Such changes are not associated with typical signs of classic clinical acute myocardial infarction, but the lesions go through the usual pathologic stages, ending as scars.

Sudden Death

It is recognized that among patients who die while convalescing from acute myocardial infarction, sudden death is not uncommon. A more common circumstance among subjects with coronary atherosclerosis is sudden and unexpected death in the absence of acute myocardial infarction. This phenomenon has had relatively little emphasis in the literature dealing with the pathology of coronary arterial disease, as the latter is mostly derived from hospital experience. A broader view of the serious complications of coronary arterial disease should include data relating to deaths from coronary disease which occur outside the hospital. When this is done, as in the survey of one community by Spiekerman and associates,[1] sudden death in the absence of acute myocardial infarction is the largest single type of death from coronary disease and in fact is the largest single type of death from all causes.

Pathologic examination of subjects who die suddenly outside the hospital reveals several significant features: Acute coronary occlusion is uncommon, as is acute myocardial infarction. Signs of earlier myocardial infarction, either that typical of an antecedent classic clinical attack or that characterized by small variously distributed scars, are common, but some cases show no signs of organic myocardial disease.

Such observations suggest that the greatest single cause of death in coronary arterial disease is not a problem in thrombosis but rather is a problem in myocardial rhythm. Ventricular fibrillation is usually assumed to be the mechanism through which sudden death occurs under these circumstances.

In the minority of cases of sudden death without an antecedent suspicion of an acute coronary arterial problem acute myocardial infarction is found. These are examples of silent myocardial infarction.

Coronary Insufficiency without Myocardial Infarction

Patients with chronic coronary disease may experience certain episodes which are indistinguishable from acute myocardial infarction. Electrocardiographically, signs of acute myocardial ischemia may be observed, but with this method of study necrosis of muscle cannot be established. Other laboratory studies do not indicate conclusive signs of acute myocardial infarction. Among such cases there are some in which circumstances permit a pathologic examination at such a time as to allow correlation with the clinical episodes. In some of these, the pathologic evidence is that focal subendocardial myocardial infarction had occurred when the patient presented with the clinical episode. In others, on the contrary, there are no signs of acute myocardial infarction having occurred at the time when the patient complained. In such cases a state of *coronary insufficiency without myocardial infarction* may be said to have been present. In those cases where the episode of thoracic pain had been present over a protracted period the term *status anginosis* may be applied.

There are cases with the clinical picture mentioned in which acute myocardial infarction is observed pathologically but in which the age of infarction clearly represents a shorter period between the time of its occurrence and death than between the onset of the clinical episode and death. Such are to be interpreted as examples of coronary insufficiency without infarction in which myocardial infarction represented a delayed complication of myocardial ischemia.

The pathologic evidence is that in most cases of those clinical states variously designated as coronary insufficiency without myocardial infarction, or

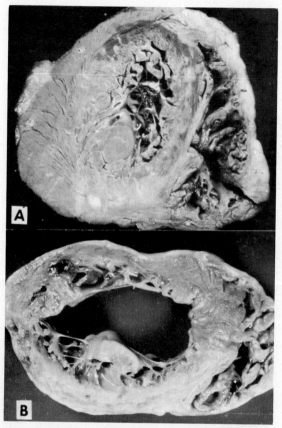

Fig. 31-3. *A.* Acute anteroseptal myocardial infarction in an early stage. The darker zone of the myocardium was purple in the fresh state and represents myocardial infarction of less than 1 day's duration. *B.* Acute posterior myocardial infarction in the posterior wall of the left ventricle (lower part of illustration) and of the ventricular septum. The pallor of the muscle represents extensive acute myocardial infarction of several days' duration. In the fresh state this area was yellow. In the opposite wall there is focal thinning representing healed anterior subendocardial myocardial infarction.

status anginosis, there is no acute coronary arterial occlusion.

Acute Myocardial Infarction

Pathologic Processes. Necrosis of cardiac muscle as a complication of ischemia is infarction. The ischemia may be precipitated by acute coronary occlusion (usually thrombotic in nature). Indeed, many hold to the concept that acute coronary occlusion is a prerequisite for acute myocardial infarction. That this is an untenable view is supported by the fact that in many cases (perhaps the majority) of acute myocardial infarction there is no acute arterial occlusion. In these, only old narrowing or occlusion, either by atherosclerosis or by atherosclerosis and organized thrombosis, is found in the coronary arteries. In some of these cases a basis for ischemia may be identified in a hypotensive episode or in demands upon the heart by unusual levels of work or emotional stress. In many instances no basis for ischemia can be identified, however.

Whether or not acute myocardial infarction is attended by acute coronary occlusion is related to the type of myocardial infarct present.[2] In cases wherein infarction involves the entire (or almost the entire) thickness of the muscle in the involved segment, so-called *transmural* infarction, there is a great tendency for acute coronary arterial occlusion to be present. When infarction is confined to a restricted segment of the myocardium (usually muscle in the endocardial half of the left ventricular wall), acute coronary occlusion is usually not present. In such infarcts, often termed *subendocardial infarcts,* there is a tendency for infarcted and noninfarcted muscle bundles to alternate.

The pathologic stages in acute myocardial infarction as described by Mallory and associates[3] will now be traced.

In the earliest stage of acute myocardial infarction, both the gross and histologic appearances may reveal no change that may be considered abnormal, even though the electrocardiographic picture is specific and results of serum transaminase studies are incontrovertible.

At about 12 hr the involved myocardium grossly may possess a bluish hue (Fig. 31-3A), while histologically the myocardial fibers may be somewhat more eosinophilic than are fibers in the uninvolved parts of the myocardium.

By 18 hr, there may be some clumping of the cytoplasm of myocardial fibers. The capillaries tend to be dilated, and early interstitial exudation of leukocytes, predominantly neutrophils, takes place. Grossly, the myocardium has lost its bluish hue, and there is either no remarkable appearance or a shade of yellow.

After 24 hr have elapsed, the stage of leukocytic infiltration is well-established. The infiltration is derived mainly from the tissues around the infarcted zone and is, therefore, concentrated at the periphery of the infarct. Within the depths of the infarct lesser concentrations of leukocytic infiltration may occur around blood vessels. The corresponding picture grossly is that of an obvious yellow discoloration of the infarct. The demarcation between infarcted and noninfarcted muscle is fairly sharp (Fig. 31-3*B*).

The appearances in the second and third days are elaborations of the leukocytic infiltrate of the first day. The nuclei of the myocardial fibers tend to become indistinct. While the cross striations become altered, they do not disappear, contrary to common teaching. The cross striations become more coarse but continue to be demonstrable as long as infarcted fibers are demonstrable.

The stage of removal of muscle fibers follows the stage of leukocytic infiltration. First, identifiable by the end of the third day, removal of fibers continues for days or weeks until usually all necrotic fibers are removed. The stage of removal dominates the picture during the second week. As the leukocytic infiltration begins at the periphery of the infarct, so does the removal of necrotic fibers. Here, there is fragmentation of muscle fibers and interstitial infiltration of macrophages and lymphocytes, while the stroma, composed of the capillaries and supporting connective tissue, remains. Deeper within the infarct the neutrophils, which had infiltrated earlier, show various stages of disintegration.

As the removal starts at the periphery of the infarct, the gross characteristics of removal of muscle are noted in the same area. Here, between the yellow infarcted muscle on one side and the normal muscle more peripherally, there lies a band of reddish purple. On cut section of the myocardium this band is depressed.

The stage of removal of muscle fibers affords one an opportunity to appreciate the variation in effect of ischemia upon the myocardium. At the junction of the periphery of the zone of infarction with the intact muscle, even in large, seemingly well-demarcated infarcts, there is an irregular border between the necrotic and viable muscle. In this zone, even though elsewhere there may be conglomerate masses of infarcted muscle, characteristically there is alternation between small masses of viable muscle and areas of infarction (Fig. 31-4). This picture suggests that in the junctional zone ("the twilight zone") between obviously viable and obviously necrotic muscle myocardial ischemia has a variable effect upon the myocardium.

Some affected muscles become necrotic while others survive. Survival of fibers in this area is,

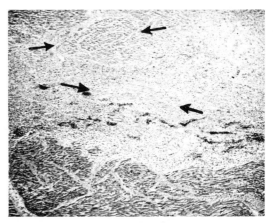

Fig. 31-4. Photomicrograph of healing acute myocardial infarction. In the lower portion of the illustration is intact muscle. In the upper portion is a zone of removal of muscle fibers peripheral to a large area of myocardial infarction. Between the facing arrows are collections of viable muscle fibers demonstrating that at the periphery of a mass of infarcted myocardium, zones of intact muscle fibers alternate with infarcted ones.

however, not necessarily to be taken as an ideal situation, when one recalls that though these fibers survive, they are ischemic. During the early stages of infarction their ischemia may be reflected in certain of the electrocardiographic abnormalities of repolarization. Throughout the course of the clinical state of infarction and recovery, these fibers may be responsible for clinical episodes of myocardial ischemia and even for the initiation of ventricular fibrillation.

With the beginning of the third week, following infarction, the stage of scar formation becomes apparent (Fig. 31-5*A*). At the periphery of the infarct where removal is proceeding and which is represented by a depressed red band during the second week, a change in color becomes apparent. This is characterized by the appearance of a ground-glass gray hue to the depressed zone. Histologically, it is characterized by activity of fibroblasts and by the appearance of widening bundles of collagen. Some of the latter substance is undoubtedly of new origin, while some may simply represent consolidation of preexisting supporting collagenous fibers.

Removal of muscle is responsible, in part, for obvious thinning of the cardiac wall at the site of the infarct. It is to be emphasized, however, that thinning of the wall may occur early in myocardial infarction, before significant removal of muscle has taken place. The basis for this is that in large infarcts with paradoxical motion of the infarcted area the necrotic muscle is stretched, cannot recoil, and gradually becomes thin.

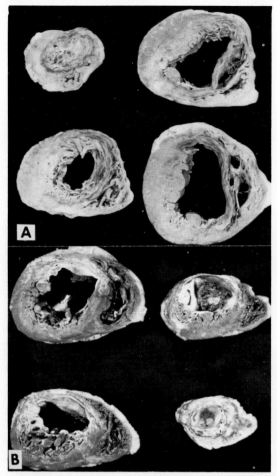

Fig. 31-5. *A.* Healing anterior and septal myocardial infarction. In the anterior and septal walls of the left ventricle, thinning represents myocardial infarction of extensive nature from which a considerable past of the necrotic muscle has been removed. In the two right-hand sections the pale area in the ventricular septum was yellow in the fresh state and represents necrotic, as yet unremoved, muscle. The age of this infarct is about 3 weeks. *B.* Healed anterior and septal myocardial infarction. The main involvement is in the anteroseptal region, which is scarred and markedly thinned. The regional endocardium is thickened. Mural thrombosis is present over the infarct (particularly apparent in the right upper unit of this illustration).

In most instances of myocardial infarction, regardless of the size of the lesion, the major portion of the necrotic muscle has been removed by the end of the fourth week. At the site of the previously necrotic muscle the process of scar formation proceeds so that in the case of large infarcts only a thin portion of the cardiac wall is represented, and this is formed principally by preexisting stroma and new connective tissue. Along with the healing

that occurs within the infarct itself the overlying endocardium shows gradual increase in thickness, ultimately leading to obvious gray opaque thickening of the endocardium over the infarcted area (Fig. 31-5*B*).

Causes of Death. Among patients who fail to survive from acute myocardial infarction, a number of pathologic states are evident.[4] Some may be related to certain mechanisms, while in other instances the exact mechanism of death is a matter of conjecture. It is to be emphasized that in many instances of acute myocardial infarction the death of the patient results not from a direct complication of the presence of necrotic muscle but rather from a complication which occurs within that muscle that survives. One of the common causes of death is considered to be acute coronary failure or acute coronary insufficiency wherein the mechanism of death is either ventricular fibrillation or cardiac arrest. In all probability, of the latter two conduction disturbances ventricular fibrillation is the more common.

Pathologically, these cases are represented by myocardial infarction which conforms in appearance with the clinical age of the infarct, and no more recent infarction is identifiable; nor is there coronary thrombosis of any more recent age than the myocardial infarct. In many instances, as indicated earlier, a coronary occlusion is not even identifiable as related to the infarct that is present. In such cases there is usually a clinical history of recurrent episodes of thoracic pain during the period of convalescence and often unexpected sudden death. The lungs show a variable appearance. In some instances there is no evidence of pulmonary edema, while in others there is pulmonary edema, a process that may develop rapidly during the terminal stages in patients who evidently die with serious conduction disturbances.

Congestive cardiac failure with acute pulmonary edema is yet another cause of death in acute myocardial infarction. In some, the congestive cardiac failure is of the classic right-sided variety with accumulation of fluid in the serous cavities, edema, and hepatomegaly. This follows unrecognized left ventricular failure. In such cases, coexistent hypertension is not infrequent, and often the myocardial infarct is large and/or associated with signs of preceding episodes of myocardial infarction.

Another major cause of death among patients dying with acute myocardial infarction is rupture of the heart. This type of death occurs decidedly more commonly among women than men. The prevalent type of rupture is that which occurs through the so-called free wall of the left ventricle leading to a fatal hemopericardium (Figs. 31-6 and 31-7). Less common types are rupture of the ven-

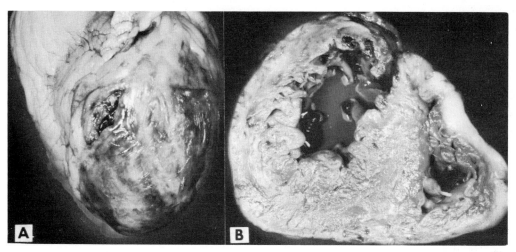

Fig. 31-6. Acute anterior myocardial infarction with rupture of the heart. *A*. Exterior of the heart viewed from in front. A laceration is present in the epicardium. *B*. Cross section of the ventricular portion of the heart. The rupture represents a laceration in the anterior wall at the periphery of the infarct (near the ventricular septum).

tricular septum (Figs. 31-8 and 31-9) and rupture of a papillary muscle (Fig. 31-10), particularly the posteromedial muscle. The latter complication leads to acute and often massive mitral insufficiency. It is significant that when rupture of the myocardium occurs as a complication of myocardial infarction, the site of rupture has a peculiar localization. This occurs in the periphery of the infarct near the healthy muscle. The basis for the rupture is probably that, during contraction, there is paradoxical motion of the infarcted area compared to the noninfarcted heart muscle. This motion causes a shearing action. With a tear of the endocardium and the endocardial aspect of the myocardium, there then follows a dissection of blood through the

myocardium and ultimately through the epicardium into the pericardial sac. The channel which the rupture takes may be an undulating one. In instances of rupture of the heart, histologic examination usually shows a heavy infiltration with leukocytes, and it is possible that uncommonly active proteolytic action upon the cardiac muscle

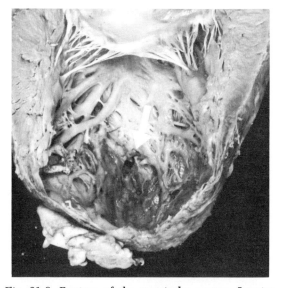

Fig. 31-8. Rupture of the ventricular septum. Interior of the left ventricle. Below the arrow is the rupture site. This lies at the junction of uninfarcted muscle and the zone of extensive infarction, which occupies the apical one-third of the left ventricle. Tissue attached to the apical portion of the left ventricle represents pericardium adherent by process of organizing pericarditis.

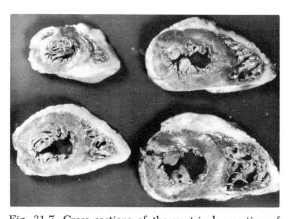

Fig. 31-7. Cross sections of the ventricular portion of the heart in an example of acute lateral myocardial infarction (left side of each section) with rupture of the heart. The rupture site is seen in the right lower segment of the illustration. It is between the two papillary muscles and at the periphery of the infarct.

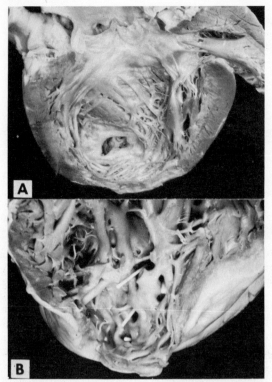

Fig. 31-9. Healed myocardial infarction with old rupture of the ventricular septum in a patient who had suffered an acute attack considered to have been that of acute myocardial infarction about 3 months before death from congestive cardiac failure. A. Left ventricular aspect. Near the apical region of the left ventricle is a large opening representing an old rupture of the ventricular septum. B. Right ventricle. In the apical region three probes lead from the single rupture seen in A. Muscle bundles of the right ventricle obscure the single rupture.

tends to underlie the factor of rupture. Rupture of the heart does not occur in so-called subendocardial myocardial infarcts but is restricted to those cases in which the infarct is of the transmural variety.

Contrary to earlier teaching, the peak of occurrence of rupture of the heart is not during the second week following the onset of myocardial infarction but is at an earlier period. In the majority of instances, rupture of the heart occurs at the third or fourth day after the onset of myocardial infarction.

Additional sequelae of acute myocardial infarction are the so-called thromboembolic complications. Two major sources for thrombosis occur in patients with acute myocardial infarction. The first is the left ventricular cavity; the second, the systemic veins. When left ventricular mural thrombosis occurs as a complication of myocardial infarc-

tion, the thrombus tends to involve the apical portion of the left ventricle, even though the infarct may be at a different location. In general, the larger the infarct, the more likely is left ventricular thrombosis to occur, and, indeed, in examples of transmural myocardial infarction, left ventricular mural thrombosis is more commonly present than not. Left ventricular mural thrombosis is a potential source for systemic arterial embolism to such important sites as the brain (Fig. 31-11), the coronary arterial system itself, and the mesenteric system, among others (Fig. 31-12). It is significant that sudden death without any specific anatomic lesions is a much more common type of death than is that resulting from embolism.

In some instances of embolism the latter process may be the first objective abnormal clinical sign in a patient with a silent myocardial infarct (Fig. 31-11).

Systemic venous thrombosis is important as a potential site for pulmonary embolism.

Pericarditis is a complication of acute myocardial infarction which is restricted to those cases in which the infarct is of the transmural variety. Usually the pericarditis is of passing interest and of no major functional significance. In a few cases, however, the pericarditis assumes importance. This occurs when during the stage of organization of the fibrinous pericarditis, hemorrhagic effusion occurs into the pericardium, with resulting cardiac tamponade. It is recognized that in patients receiving anticoagulant therapy there may be a greater risk for hemorrhage from coexistent pericarditis than among patients in whom no anticoagulants are administered. In the latter group, however, there is

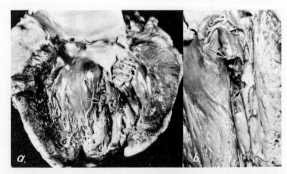

Fig. 31-10. Partial rupture of the posterior papillary muscle complicating acute posterior myocardial infarction. A. The posterior papillary muscle is lacerated (point of arrow). B. Between the arrows is a defect in the posterior papillary muscle, but continuity of this structure is still maintained. Beyond the point of the lower arrow, necrotic muscle, which was yellow in the fresh state, is identified. (*From Levy and Edwards, Prog. in Cardiovas. Dis.,* **5**:119, 1962, *with permission.*)

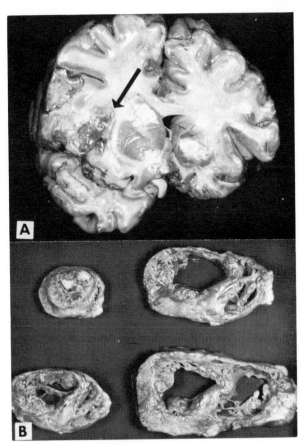

Fig. 31-11. Acute myocardial infarction with cerebral embolism and cerebral infarction. *A.* Brain. Recent cerebral infarction represented the primarily apparent medical problem of the patient who had suffered from a so-called acute silent myocardial infarction. *B.* Mural thrombus in the apical region of the left ventricle, the site of a healing acute myocardial infarct. The spleen also exhibited infarcts.

no absolute immunity from the hemorrhage of organizing pericarditis.

Healed Myocardial Infarction: Fate of the Patient

The patient who recovers from acute myocardial infarction has open to him a wide variety of circumstances. Some continue without complications. The majority are subject to recurrent problems, either from the fact that considerable muscle has been lost or from peculiar localization of the infarction in the papillary muscles (Fig. 31-13) so as to cause mitral insufficiency. Others suffer from the effects of existing coronary arterial disease and experience either recurrent myocardial infarction or acute ischemic attacks which become complicated either by ventricular fibrillation or cardiac standstill.

The combined reviews of Achor and associates[5] and of Juergens and associates[6] involved 329 patients with healed myocardial infarction observed at necropsy. Approximately one-third of these patients had succumbed to noncardiac causes, while two-thirds had died of cardiac disease, including embolism (Fig. 31-14) but usually a form of coro-

nary disease. Sudden death without recurrent acute myocardial infarction was the most common mode of death (38 per cent) among the latter group. The remaining deaths were distributed among congestive cardiac failure (27.5 per cent) or problems related to recurrent acute myocardial infarction (34.5 per cent).

Among patients harboring extensive healed myocardial infarcts *ventricular aneurysm* may be observed. The aneurysm is characterized by extreme thinning of the cardiac wall with a convex deformity of the external surface corresponding to the zone of infarction (Fig. 31-15). Intraaneurysmal thrombosis is common, and the tendency toward systemic embolism is greater than average for all patients with healed myocardial infarction.[7]

Calcification may be observed in the wall of some aneurysms. This may be located either in nonremoved necrotic muscle or in unorganized thrombotic material near the wall of the aneurysm.

While some patients with ventricular aneurysm exhibit no significant disturbance of myocardial efficiency, others may manifest congestive cardiac failure. This complication may simply be an expres-

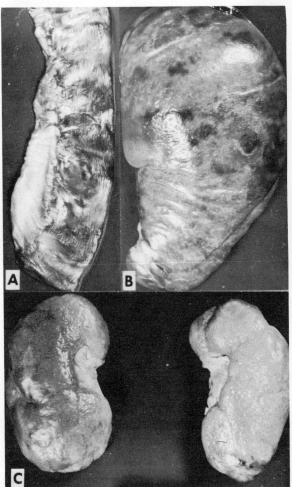

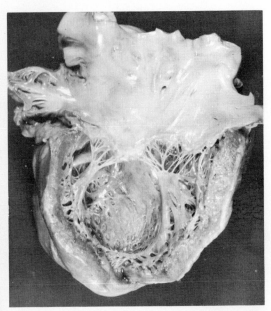

Fig. 31-13. Healed myocardial infarction with involvement of papillary muscles and mitral insufficiency. The left atrium is dilated. The two papillary muscles of the left ventricle are atrophic as a result of myocardial infarction, now healed. It is considered that mitral insufficiency had resulted from deficient action of the papillary muscles.

Fig. 31-12. Sites of systemic embolism with infarction representing complications of acute myocardial infarction. *A*. Small intestine. Discoloration of serosa is representative of changes in entire wall. *B*. Spleen. Multiple areas of discoloration represent acute infarction. *C*. Depressed areas on the surfaces of the kidneys are sites of infarction.

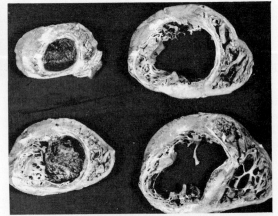

Fig. 31-14. Healed myocardial infarction and mural thrombosis. Cross sections of the ventricular portion of the heart. In these sections the anterior wall is toward the upper aspect of the illustration, the posterior wall toward the lower. There is healed infarction both of the septal and the lateral regions. A large mural thrombus is present at the apical region and represents a potential site for embolism. At the sites of healed infarction there is obvious thinning of the ventricular wall.

sion of extensive loss of muscle, or it may have alternative explanations. Among these is the problem of paradoxical motion of the aneurysm during systole with loss of efficiency of the cardiac beat for the forward propulsion of blood. Another alternative is that the aneurysm may be so located as to cause mitral insufficiency.

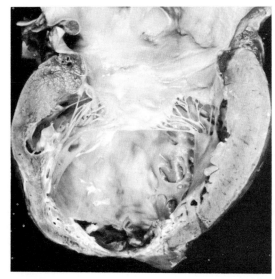

Fig. 31-15. Extensive healed anteroseptal myocardial infarction with early aneurysm formation. A mural thrombus is present in the apical region of the left ventricle. Thrombi in this location represent sites for systemic embolism.

REFERENCES

1. Spiekerman, R. E., Brandenburg, J. T., Achor, R. W. P., and Edwards, J. E.: The Spectrum of Coronary Heart Disease, *Circulation,* **25**:57, 1962.
2. Miller, R. D., Burchell, H. B., and Edwards, J. E.: Myocardial Infarction with and without Acute Coronary Occlusion, *A.M.A. Arch. Int. Med.,* **88**:597, 1951.
3. Mallory, G. K., White, P. D., and Salcedo-Salgar, J.: The Speed of Healing of Myocardial Infarction, *Am. Heart J.,* **18**:647, 1939.
4. McQuay, N. W., Edwards, J. E., and Burchell, H. B.: Types of Death in Acute Myocardial Infarction, *A.M.A. Arch. Int. Med.,* **96**:1, 1955.
5. Achor, R. W. P., Futch, W. D., Burchell, H. B., and Edwards, J. E.: The Fate of Patients Surviving Acute Myocardial Infarction, *A.M.A. Arch. Int. Med.,* **98**: 162, 1956.
6. Juergens, J. L., Edwards, J. E., Achor, R. W., and Burchell, H. B.: Prognosis of Patients Surviving First Clinically Diagnosed Myocardial Infarction, *A.M.A. Arch. Int. Med.,* **105**:444, 1960.
7. Phares, W. S., Edwards, J. E., and Burchell, H. B.: Cardiac Aneurysms: Clinicopathologic Studies, *Proc. Staff Meet. Mayo Clin.,* **28**:264, 1953.

32 CLINICAL RECOGNITION OF CORONARY ATHEROSCLEROSIS AND ITS COMPLICATIONS

R. Bruce Logue, M.D., and
J. Willis Hurst, M.D.

Atherosclerosis of the coronary arteries is the most common cause of heart disease in the adult in the United States.[1] Below the age of sixty it is more common in the male.[2] The knowledge that in the female it is statistically more common after the menopause does not exclude the diagnosis in the younger female.[3] The peak incidence is at about fifty to sixty years of age in the male and sixty to seventy in the female. It is common in the male between the ages of forty and fifty. It occurs not infrequently between the ages of thirty and forty and was a common cause of death in young American soldiers in World War II.[4,5] When coronary heart disease appears in the family, it is more significant if both parents have it, the occurrence in father and sibling(s) or mother and sibling(s) being of less predictive value.[6]

The majority of male patients with coronary atherosclerosis are normotensive. The presence of hypertension is an accelerating factor, and the incidence is higher in the hypertensive population.[7] The incidence of hypertension in females with coronary atherosclerosis is greater than in male patients. Diabetes and, to a lesser extent, myxedema also predispose to atherosclerosis.[7] Familial hypercholesterolemia is associated with a high incidence of the disease, but this occurs in only a small percentage of patients.[7] Clinical evidence of coronary disease is commonly manifest in the patient with what is currently considered a normal level of serum cholesterol. The knowledge that the serum cholesterol level is higher than normal in a population group with clinical evidence of coronary atherosclerosis is of no help in the immediate diagnosis of the disease in an individual patient. Recent evidence that the incidence of coronary disease is higher in the heavy smoker does not give license to diagnose the disease in the smoker nor to eliminate its presence in the nonsmoker (see Chap. 65). It occurs in the lean as well as in the obese. Although many have emphasized the "masculine male" as being coronary-prone,[3] the disease may occur with any type of body build.

Although the factors mentioned above are extremely important epidemiologically and may be important in long-term management, they are of limited value in the immediate clinical diagnosis of coronary disease.

CLINICAL SPECTRUM

When the pathologist examines the coronary arteries with great care, he is likely to find evidence of atherosclerosis in the majority of adult males in the United States.[1] The pathologist cannot look at the coronary arteries and determine which patients had symptoms during life. The disease process may be so slight that the impairment of blood flow in the coronary arteries is negligible. On the other hand, the disease process may be quite extensive, but its development so gradual that adequate collateral circulation develops in parallel with the obstructive process and symptoms do not occur.[8–10] The clinician does not make a diagnosis of coronary atherosclerosis merely because the pathologist is likely to find evidence of the disease. The clinician makes the diagnosis of coronary atherosclerosis when the disease process has reached the state at which there is clinical evidence of cardiac disease.[11,12] This evidence may be found in the patient's history, the physical examination, the electrocardiogram, the laboratory, or the routine x-ray of the heart. The technique of cine coronary arteriography may identify the presence of disease in the coronary arteries (Chap. 33). The mere presence of the disease, which is present in many adults, does not necessarily prove that the patient's symptoms are secondary to coronary atherosclerosis. Coronary arteriography cannot be done routinely, and great skill, such as that attained by Sones, is required to perform a satisfactory examination. Accordingly, even though cine coronary arteriography represents a giant step forward, it does not eliminate the physician's need to understand the clinical expressions of coronary atherosclerosis.

The initial manifestation of coronary artery disease may be *sudden death* due to cardiac standstill or ventricular fibrillation (see Chap. 16). These arrhythmias may be transient and represented by an episode of *syncope* (see Chap. 17). *Angina pectoris* and *myocardial infarction* are the most common expressions of coronary atherosclerosis; they are the most specific and more readily recognized. Ischemia of specialized tissue such as the sinoatrial node, the atrioventricular node, and the bundle of His and bundle branches may produce *arrhythmias* and *atrioventricular* and *intraventricular conduction disturbances* without angina pectoris or myocardial infarction. These are less reliable evidence of coronary atherosclerosis. Complete heart block, ventricular tachycardia, and left bundle branch block—while not pathognomonic—are statistically more often associated with coronary atherosclerosis than other types of heart disease. Coronary atherosclerosis is the most common cause of right bundle branch block; however, the frequency of noncoronary causes limits its diagnostic significance. Atrial fibrillation, atrial flutter, and paroxysmal atrial tachycardia may also be related to coronary disease; but the diverse causes of these arrhythmias limit their usefulness in diagnosis. *Acute pulmonary edema* may be the presenting manifestation of myocardial infarction due to coronary disease, with or without a prior history of angina pectoris, and may occur in the absence of chest pain. *Chronic congestive heart failure* in the absence of angina pectoris, myocardial infarction, or some other sign of coronary atherosclerosis is rare. In some patients with chronic heart failure, which is said to be due to coronary disease without angina or infarction, the experienced clinician can often elicit a history of angina pectoris, identify satisfactory electrocardiographic evidence compatible with old myocardial infarction, or find another cause for failure such as aortic stenosis or cor pulmonale. On the other hand, certain diseases, such as amyloidosis, may be associated with angina pectoris and electrocardiographic changes ordinarily considered diagnostic of myocardial infarction. *Ventricular aneurysm*—with or without *myocardial wall calcification*—is a specific but relatively uncommon manifestation of coronary atherosclerosis which may be found on physical examination or demonstrated by fluoroscopic or x-ray examination in patients without a history of angina pectoris or infarction, although there is usually other evidence of the disease (see p. 158). *Calcification of the coronary arteries* detected by fluoroscopy or x-ray examination may indicate the presence of disease but gives no evidence of whether the disease is symptomatic (see p. 155).

DIAGNOSIS

Coronary atherosclerosis is a ubiquitous disease, insidious in onset, without signs or symptoms for many years until the disease process attains a degree of obstruction that interferes with the arterial blood supply to the atrial and ventricular myocardium. If the obstructive process is gradual over a period of years, intercoronary collateral circulation may develop, and clinical evidence of disease may be long deferred or never occur. In this instance, although there is marked obstructive disease, the myocardial cells receive adequate oxygen, regardless of demands. On the other hand, even when the disease is not advanced, inadequate oxygen may be delivered to the myocardial cells under the following circumstances:

1. When the atherosclerotic process in the coronary arteries progresses more rapidly than the collateral circulation,[8] adequate oxygen may not reach the myocardial cells, and ischemia may occur under the increased demands of effort, emotion, meals, etc., or may occur spontaneously.

2. Coronary thrombosis or subintimal hemorrhage in a coronary artery may suddenly alter blood flow to a local area of myocardium, and the collaterals may be inadequate to compensate for the abrupt change.[8]

3. Arteriographic studies have shown that an apparently normal coronary artery may undergo spasm when stimulated by an arterial catheter.[13] The blood flow distal to the area of spasm is still evident and adequate. No recognizable ischemia develops, and pain does not occur. Such studies have also shown that spasm may occur at the site of atherosclerotic narrowing, and in this instance the flow distal to the narrowing may become significantly reduced or stop, and ischemic signs may develop. Arterial spasm may or may not play a significant role in the production of symptoms and disease under more natural circumstances. The fact, however, that it can occur, even during artificial circumstances, demands additional investigation.

4. Hypotension, however induced, may reduce mean arterial pressure and coronary arterial blood flow.[14–16]

5. There are additional factors which determine when symptoms occur. Myocardial cellular hypertrophy increases the demand for oxygen but is not associated with an increase in size and number of coronary arteries and capillaries. Valve disease, such as aortic stenosis, aortic insufficiency, and mitral stenosis, may interfere with effective coronary perfusion through impairment of cardiac output with poor filling of the coronary arteries in addition to the results of hypertrophy. These are generally aggravating factors superimposed upon underlying atherosclerosis.[16]

Tachycardia, either sinus or ectopic, may precipitate symptoms in patients with coronary atherosclerosis (see pp. 287–288).

The oxygen-carrying capacity of the blood is an important determinant of effective delivery of oxygen to the cell, and anemia may induce myocardial ischemia in patients with coronary atherosclerosis.

The metabolic demands of cells, including those of the myocardium, for oxygen may be increased by thyrotoxicosis or fever. Atherosclerosis of the coronary arteries may prevent sufficient blood flow to meet the increased needs of the myocardial cells under these circumstances, and the clinical signs of disease may appear.[17] Coronary atherosclerosis can be diagnosed by cine coronary arteriography. This technique is discussed in Chap. 33. The clinical application of selected coronary arteriography is discussed in Chap. 34.

SPECIFIC CLINICAL SYNDROMES

Angina Pectoris

The diagnosis of angina pectoris is made from characteristic history.[18–36] In eliciting a history of angina pectoris, one should not merely inquire about pain, since pain may be denied. The discomfort may be described as a sense of constriction, tightness, aching, squeezing, pressing, heaviness, expanding sensation, choking in the throat, indigestion, or burning. The location of the discomfort in the overwhelming majority of patients is the substernal region. The discomfort may be confined to the chest, or there may be associated aching in one or both arms, more often the left. The discomfort is often mild, rather than severe. Occasionally it is confined to the elbow, forearm, jaw, throat, neck, back, or epigastrium without anterior chest location, or it may radiate to these areas. The pain tends to be diffuse and is seldom accompanied by localized tender areas in the chest wall. It is helpful to have the patient localize the site of distress by pointing to the area with his finger.

During an attack, the patient may remain motionless; at times he may experience a feeling of impending doom. The clenched fist over the sternum may graphically depict the constricting nature of the discomfort (Fig. 32-1). The sign has been attributed to Dr. Samuel Levine. Of more importance than the location is the duration of the pain and the circumstances under which it occurs. Angina pectoris lasts only a few minutes, usually 3 to 5 minutes if the precipitating factor is relieved. Frequently, attacks are induced by effort and tend to occur during, rather than after, the exertion. Exertion following meals is particularly prone to produce pain, and the sedentary individual may experience discomfort only after meals. Exposure to cold, cold wind, or cold bed sheets and drinking iced drinks may excite discomfort.

Of great importance is the intimate relation of

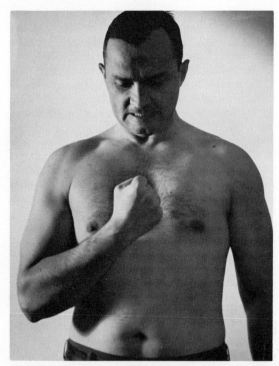

Fig. 32-1. The "clenched-fist sign" (attributed to Dr. Samuel Levine) of myocardial ischemia. The manner in which the patient "tells" his story of discomfort, the way he looks when he tells it, and the motions of his hands at the time are as important as the story itself in the diagnosis of angina pectoris or myocardial infarction.

emotional tension and pain. Disturbing thoughts, smoking, stressful life situations, worry, anger, hurry, and excitement are common causes of pain. A not infrequent story is that discomfort first occurred while hurrying to catch a bus or while carrying a bag to and from a train or plane. Parking a car in close places, driving in heavy traffic, shaving, bathing, painful stimuli, sexual intercourse, micturition,[37] or straining at stool may produce pain.

Relief of angina pectoris may come with rest. Sublingual nitroglycerin may produce prompt and dramatic relief of discomfort, usually within 2 to 3 min. Patients with chest pain from other causes may report relief with nitroglycerin, but careful questioning may reveal that relief was partial and only occurred over a longer period—perhaps 30 min. Carotid sinus massage, applied during an attack, as emphasized by Levine, may give prompt relief if heart rate is slowed. In order to evaluate the response properly, one should ask the patient if the pain is made worse by the maneuver rather than asking whether the pain was lessened.[38]

The classic manifestations of angina pectoris are well known and occur in approximately 80 per cent of patients, but the wide range of symptoms is less well appreciated. There is an appalling rigidity of thought when symptoms and findings are less typical. Much diagnostic blindness is due to lack of suspicion of discomfort which occurs in less common locations of the body but which is otherwise typical in relation to precipitating factors, duration, and relief. Many diagnostic errors are due to an unholy reliance on the electrocardiogram.

It may be difficult for the patient to express verbally the sensation due to myocardial ischemia. He may be unable to put into words a description which the physician can recognize. One patient described a "good feeling" in the chest like the one you had when you ran as a boy, while another described a "feeling like a red-hot poker."

It is a notorious fact that the patient with coronary disease rarely relates his symptoms to the heart but is more likely to attribute them to the digestive tract. Thus a complaint of "indigestion," "gas on the stomach," "heartburn," "belching," or "fullness in the stomach" is readily dismissed by the patient and physician unless it is noted that the symptom occurs in the upper abdomen, radiates to the substernal region or is confined to this area, is related to effort and emotional tension, as well as meals, or is relieved by rest or nitroglycerin. The fact that belching may relieve angina pectoris heightens the diagnostic difficulty. The sensation of abdominal fullness may lead to the diagnosis of the syndrome of aerophagia and excessive belching when the patient seeks relief. Furthermore, such symptoms may appear on recumbency, be relieved by the upright position, and therefore falsely attributed to the common, nonsymptomatic hiatal hernia detected by x-ray examination. The unwary physician may pounce on this objective finding, only to be dismayed when sudden death or infarction ensues. People of sedentary habits may note distress only after meals, and the inability to relate the discomfort to the usual forms of physical effort may obscure the diagnosis. The frequent association of gallbladder disease and peptic ulcer with coronary artery disease may produce overlapping symptoms.

There is a small group of patients who develop symptoms upon first exerting themselves but whose symptoms disappear if activity is continued—so-called "second-wind" angina. Some patients experience pain at rest but not during effort.

Many teeth are sacrificed on the altar of ignorance when coronary pain is referred to the mandible or maxilla. Pain or burning sensation in the tongue or hard palate, induced by effort or emotional tension and relieved by rest or nitroglycerin, has also been noted. Pain in the front or back of the neck may trip the unwary. Aching in the left interscapular region may occur. The distress may rarely be noted in the right side of the chest or axillary region. Aching confined to the shoulder, wrist, elbow, or forearm becomes significant when reproduced by effort which does not involve the shoulder or arm. Curiously, mild work utilizing the arms above shoulder level may precipitate angina in patients in whom walking sometimes may be done in comfort. Stooping over is another unusual precipitating factor. Drying oneself with a towel may precipitate angina pectoris. This may surprise the patient and physician when the patient is able to engage in more strenuous effort without symptoms. In a rare patient, talking may induce pain, whereas physical effort may not. The symptoms of breathlessness during effort may replace the complaint of pain in some patients in whom there is no overt evidence of heart failure. On the other hand, nocturnal angina is occasionally associated with mild interstitial pulmonary edema. Nightmares may precipitate angina, as may micturition. Syncope or sudden death may occur during angina pectoris. In the natural history of coronary disease, the location of angina may occasionally change; the reason for this, although unknown, is presumably involvement of a new area of myocardium.

The results of the *physical examination* of the cardiovascular system are usually normal in most patients with angina pectoris due to coronary atherosclerosis. Evidence of hypertension, valve disease, cardiac enlargement, peripheral vascular disease, and retinal arterial abnormalities may be present, but none of these findings are specific for coronary atherosclerosis. In some patients exertion produces significant hypertension which may contribute to the subsequent development of angina pectoris. Inspection of the patient *during* an attack may show either no alteration in appearance or the presence of pallor and cold, clammy sweating. The apical impulse may become abnormal during angina pectoris.[39-41] (See p. 100).

Categories

The categories of angina pectoris are (1) stable angina pectoris, (2) initial onset of angina pectoris, (3) progressive angina pectoris, (4) angina decubitus.

Stable angina is characterized by recurring pattern of discomfort brought about by predictable precipitating factors over a period of months. This suggests that the collateral circulation, though inadequate, is able to compensate for the obliterative process, as long as the demands for coronary flow are not increased.

The initial onset of angina pectoris usually means an abrupt change in the coronary circulation with inadequate collaterals. Even though discomfort is brief, one occasionally finds evidence of myocardial necrosis. As a rule, the patient has experienced several episodes before he consults the physician.

Progressive angina pectoris is characterized by an increase in frequency and severity of attacks which occur with less provocation, and at times, under new circumstances. This suggests either that the obstructive process is outstripping the collateral circulation or that extracardiac factors increasing the demands on the coronary circulation are present.

Angina decubitus occurs only in a small percentage of patients and always signifies life-threatening advanced disease, which often presages myocardial infarction or cardiac arrest. The exact mechanism of this type of angina, which may recur throughout the day and night for weeks or months, is unknown.

Differential Diagnosis

Anxiety states are the most common cause of confusion with angina pectoris[42] (see Chap. 63). Complaints are often multiple with predominance of symptoms such as weakness, giddiness, and breathlessness. The chest discomfort is of several types: (1) sharp, intermittent lancinating, or stabbing precordial or apical pain often associated with local areas of hyperesthesia of the chest wall; (2) precordial aching pain which lasts hours or days and is unrelated to effort; (3) substernal tightness of variable duration, unrelated to exercise and associated with hyperventilation. There may be a choking sensation in the throat due to globus hystericus which may be difficult to distinguish from myocardial ischemia. Palpitation and extrasystoles may occur. Claustrophobia and the occurrence of symptoms in crowded places, such as in church, may be related. A clue on inspection, while recording the history, may be the presence of sighing respiration.

Usually the patient with anxiety neurosis is certain that he has heart disease. Indeed, these may be the disabling symptoms in the patient with known coronary disease—as, for example, following acute myocardial infarction. Furthermore, while the functional complaints may have brought the patient to the physician on occasion, one may uncover true angina pectoris. The exact reproduction of the patient's symptoms with forced hyperventilation may identify the nature of the complaints. Hyperventilation for 2 min is usually sufficient; indeed, many patients with chronic hyperventilation become troubled after a few deep breaths.[43] One cannot invariably reproduce symptoms by hyperventilation, perhaps because of the sense of security in the physician's presence, in contrast to the fear and terror engendered when the patient awakens at night with an attack. The common occurrence in these patients of junctional type of ST depression in the electrocardiogram taken at rest or during exercise only accentuates the problem of recognition. *If one cannot diagnose angina pectoris with reasonable certainty, it is better to miss the diagnosis.* It is perhaps in this group of patients that coronary arteriography, by demonstrating a normal coronary tree, will make its greatest contribution.

Pain in the chest and arm can be produced by many *musculoskeletal disorders.*[44] These conditions, grouped under the general term of thoracic outlet syndrome, produce discomfort by involvement of nerves, muscle, and bone in a local area. Examples are the scalenus anticus, cervical rib, and hyperabduction syndromes. In many patients the primary disorder arises from disk degeneration or arthritis of the cervical spine. Reproduction of discomfort by movement of the arm and head through a full range of motion may aid diagnosis. While x-rays of the cervical spine may reveal abnormalities, these may or may not be the cause of symptoms, and the crucial evidence is the reproduction of the complaints by appropriate maneuvers or the relief of symptoms by a therapeutic trial of cervical traction. The occurrence of symptoms during effort, such as carrying a suitcase or a golf bag, may be a source of confusion unless it is realized that the identical symptoms can be produced at rest by manipulation of the extremity and neck.

In rare instances *arthritis of the thoracic spine* may give rise to chest wall discomfort that is neuromuscular in origin.[45] It may be reproduced by movements of the trunk at rest, tends to occur at night, and may respond to salicylates.

Local pain and swelling of *costochondral* or *chondrosternal* joints (Tietze's syndrome) or of the *xiphosternal* joint may occur for unknown reasons.[46–49] Pain and tightness may be reproduced by palpation of local areas; the patient is generally unaware of the superficial and local nature of the involvement and may wrongly attribute these to the heart. Local procaine infiltration and salicylates may control symptoms. The *shoulder-hand syndrome* is discussed in the section dealing with complications of myocardial infarction.[50] Superficial thrombophlebitis of the veins of the precordial area may occur rarely and produce a confusing clinical picture (Mondor's syndrome).[51–53] The tender cordlike vein is often palpable and is the clue to the diagnosis.

Patients with anxiety may complain of pain in the chest in the absence of demonstrable disease of the spine or thoracic outlet.[54,55] There may be tenderness of the muscles of the chest wall, with production of pain or tightness on palpation of these areas, and the discomfort may be reproduced by movements of the thoracic cage, such as bending, stooping, twisting, turning, or swinging the arms while walking. In contrast to angina pectoris, the pain may last for seconds or for hours, and prompt relief is not afforded by nitroglycerin. Local infiltration of the involved areas with procaine or hydrocortisone at times may relieve musculoskeletal pain.

Reflux esophagitis closely mimics the discomfort of myocardial ischemia.[56–59] The discomfort is generally confined to the lower substernal area. It may be gripping, squeezing, or burning in character and at times is associated with regurgitation. It tends to wax and wane. Like angina pectoris, the discomfort may be precipitated by recumbency or meals. More often it follows the ingestion of highly seasoned foods and alcohol—particularly after excessive intake—and is prone to occur in association with constipation. It is probable that the presence of pylorospasm is an important determinant of symptoms. Sitting upright may give variable relief; nitroglycerin gives no predictable relief; milk and antacids may be helpful. It should be emphasized that there may or may not be a demonstrable hiatal hernia but that the symptoms usually are not due to the hernia itself. Although the mechanism of esophageal pain has been studied using distension with balloons and recordings of motility, the exact mechanism has not been clearly delineated, and a reliable diagnostic test is still to be developed.

The vast majority of small *hiatal hernias*[60] produce no symptoms; even when symptomatic they rarely, if ever, produce pain on effort. Occasionally they may produce substernal or precordial discomfort when the patient is bending or lying on the left side. It is probable that most symptoms attributed to hiatal hernia are actually due to reflux esophagitis.

Distension of the splenic flexure[61] may give rise to pain in the left hypochondrium and precordial region with referred pain to the left arm. The lack of relationship to effort, relief by bowel movements or passage of flatus, and reproduction of the pain by distension of the colon through a colon tube may clarify the nature of the symptoms. The splenic flexure syndrome is more common in the patient with irritable colon and spastic constipation. Typical peptic ulcer rarely mimics angina pectoris; however, coronary disease may at times simulate peptic ulcer.

In the authors' opinion, "pulmonary hypertensive pain" is not due to distension of the pulmonary artery, nor is it critically related to the height of the pulmonary arterial pressure.[62–64] Although it is frequently associated with diseases that produce pulmonary hypertension, the authors believe it is due to myocardial ischemia. This pain may occur with lesions such as mitral stenosis, atrial septal defect, Eisenmenger's syndrome due to left-to-right shunt, primary pulmonary hypertension, pulmonary embolism, and cor pulmonale due to chronic lung disease. It may occur in the presence of a lowered pulmonary arterial pressure, i.e., severe valvular pulmonic stenosis with right ventricular hypertension. The pain is believed to be caused by inadequate coronary profusion due to a limitation in cardiac output, reduced mean aortic pressure, reduced coronary flow, increased right ventricular oxygen needs, and, in the patient with right ventricular hypertrophy and heart failure, perhaps impaired myocardial venous return to the coronary sinus. It is not clear whether the ischemia is confined to the right or left ventricle. Usually the response to nitroglycerin is not as sharp as it is in ordinary angina pectoris. Since the discomfort may be self-limited and may disappear within a few minutes without therapy, the response to this drug may be difficult to evaluate. When pain can be reproduced by a given amount of exercise and can be prevented by prophylactic administration of nitroglycerin, associated coronary atherosclerosis is the most likely cause. The traditional response of "pulmonary (right ventricular) hypertensive pain" to intravenous aminophylline may be due to its positive inotropic effect of improving cardiac output. In contrast to angina pectoris this form of chest pain is almost invariably associated with dyspnea, which may be the dominant symptom. Many patients may have a "positive" electrocardiographic exercise-test result.

Patients with heart failure may have pain in the right upper quadrant during exercise. This discomfort is due to *paroxysmal hepatic engorgement* and is rarely confused with angina pectoris.[65]

Informed individuals who have various reasons for self-pity, including those seeking sympathy or financial gain from pensions or insurance, or individuals who are morphine addicts can fool the experienced physician. This is especially true of patients with a previous well-documented myocardial infarction, since in such a patient even coronary arteriography cannot clarify the issue. Often the physician has a feeling that the patient's discomfort is not due to ischemia, but he may be unable to translate this impression into effective management in these emotionally ill patients.

Electrocardiogram[66-70]

Seventy per cent of patients with angina pectoris and no prior myocardial infarction have normal electrocardiograms at rest.[71] The remaining 30 per cent of patients may show nonspecific ST-T changes, A-V block, bundle branch block, left ventricular hypertrophy, changes of previously unsuspected old healed infarction, or, perhaps, an arrhythmia such as atrial fibrillation. If a tracing is recorded during pain, there may be ST-segment depression, which is usually most marked in unipolar leads from the left precordium. Unfortunately, such changes do not always occur, and a normal tracing under such circumstances does not rule out angina pectoris (Fig. 32-2). In one study ST-segment depression occurred in only 50 per cent of 30 patients' electrocardiograms taken during pain.[71] Exercise

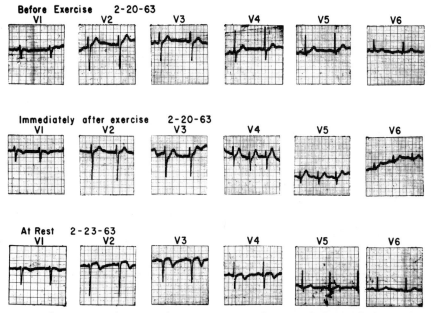

Fig. 32-2. Patient, age forty-two, with angina pectoris. Note normal tracings before and after exercise on February 20, 1963. The patient experienced a prolonged period of chest discomfort the following day. Electrocardiogram on February 23, 1963, shows acute anteroseptal myocardial infarction.

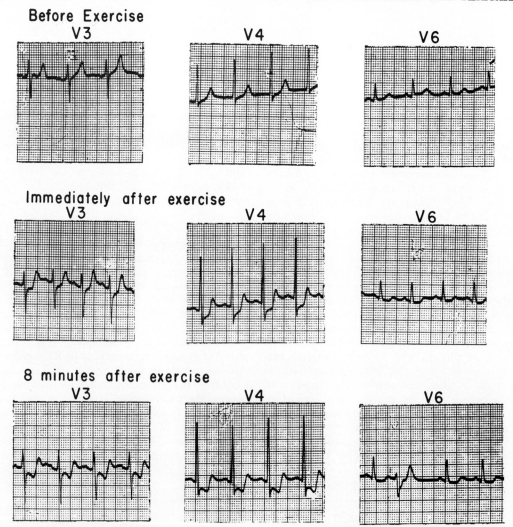

Fig. 32-3. Positive exercise-test result in a patient with classic angina pectoris. Note the downward-sloping ST segment ending in upright pointed T wave, most noticeable in lead V₄. The ST segment is depressed 3.5 mm below J point and is of the flat ischemic type immediately after exercise and of the downward-sloping type 8 min after exercise.

tests may not produce pain in 60 per cent of patients with classic histories of angina pectoris.[72] There may be false-negative and false-positive exercise tests. Friedberg,[73] using a double-blind technique in 100 patients with angina and nonanginal pain, found an incidence of 39 per cent false-positive and 43 per cent false-negative tests using Master's old criterion of 1-mm ST-segment depression. When the newer criterion of 2-mm ST depression was used, there were 32 per cent false-positive tests among the nonanginal patients and 27 per cent false-negative tests among the anginal patients. Using Q-X/Q-T ratio greater than 50 per cent, 8 per cent of the nonanginal group gave a false-positive test, whereas 58 per cent of patients with angina showed a false-negative test.[73] (Q-X represents origin of Q wave and X the point of return of the depressed ST to the isoelectric line.) Furthermore, the ischemic type of ST depression may be seen in patients without symptomatic coronary disease. Master has emphasized that false-positive tests may occur among neurotic patients, women at the menopause, and patients with tachycardia, particularly those of asthenic build with vasomotor instability.[74] Positive tests have been noted as frequently in patients with rheumatic heart disease as among patients with coronary disease.[75] The patient receiving digitalis often has a false-positive exercise test, and under these circumstances the test has no value. Numerous errors have been made because of this fact. Criteria for a positive test vary widely among many authors, and the results are variable.

Our present criteria for a positive exercise test are (1) flat "ischemic" type of ST depression of 2 mm or more with ST extending horizontally at least 0.12 sec (Fig. 32-3) or (2) downward-sloping ST segment with upright T wave (Fig. 32-3). Occasionally the ST segment becomes elevated rather than depressed after exercise, suggesting an acute infarction. This variation of response was described by Prinzmetal[75a] (Fig. 32-4). Some authors have considered a J type of depression of 2 mm or more as a positive test, but there may be overlap with response of normal individuals (Fig. 32-5). Inversion of T waves in the left precordial leads occurs in one third of the tests during exercise in patients with angina pectoris, and deep inversion of T waves are occasionally noted, but these changes are not reliable signs of myocardial ischemia. Premature beats occurring after effort should not be considered as a positive exercise test, since these are commonly seen in apparently normal individuals.[76] The development of A-V block or of bundle branch block during exercise may be seen in diffuse myocardial disease or other types of noncoronary disease.

One of the major problems in the evaluation of the electrocardiogram during exercise is the observer's bias. There may be difficulty in differentiating the J type of ST-segment depression from ischemic depression. One electrocardiographic lead may show one type of depression and another lead another type. A drifting base line may be a source of confusion. Tachycardia incident to exercise commonly produces an atrial T wave with striking shifts of the J segment (Fig. 32-5). Although changes may occur several minutes after exercise rather than immediately, recent studies have emphasized the changes during exercise. Using radioelectrocardiography in 70 patients, Bellet et al. found positive tests in 37 patients (53 per cent) during a single Master test but positive tests in only 24 patients (34 per cent) after exercise.[77] He estimated that one-third of the positive tests recorded during exercise would have been missed by conventional techniques. At the moment, there is inadequate data to determine whether tracings taken during exercise will be superior to those recorded after exercise. In fact, electrocardiographic changes made during exercise may not reflect the same disturbance that occurs after exercise.

Angina pectoris is a clinical diagnosis, and electrocardiographic exercise tests are mere adjunct to the recognition of disease where symptoms are less than classic. All too often when the clinical picture is typical, the exercise response may be equivocal, and the observer must make a judgment in the light of the total findings. The wide range of findings in the exercise tests limits sharply its use in diagnosis of the individual patient suspected of hav-

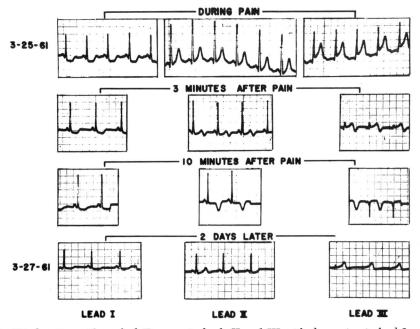

Fig. 32-4. Note ST elevation with peaked T waves in leads II and III with depression in lead I recorded during anterior chest pain. Three minutes after pain, the T waves have become inverted in leads II and III. Ten minutes after pain, there is a QRS deflection in lead III with deeply inverted T waves in II and III suggesting acute diaphragmatic infarction. A follow-up tracing taken 2 days later shows very slight ST-segment displacement. The changes typify those emphasized by Prinzmetal.

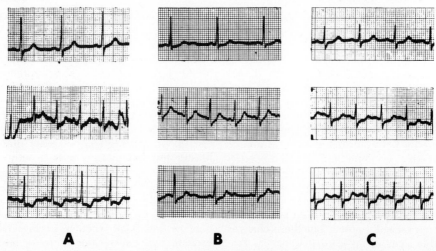

A   **B**   **C**

Fig. 32-5. All leads are V₄. The top row was taken at rest, the middle row immediately after exercise, and the lower row 5 min after exercise. *A.* Patient with classic angina pectoris. Note the junctional displacement immediately after exercise, whereas there is the downward-sloping segment characteristic of a positive response at 5 min. Note the difficulty of interpretation due to a wandering stylus immediately after exercise, i.e., ST elevation when the stylus is moving upward and ST depression when the stylus is moving downward. *B.* Patient with anxiety and functional chest pain and no evidence of coronary disease. Note the displacement of the base line at the junction of the QRS with the ST segment (J point). The ST segment immediately slopes upward to the T wave. This may be due to repolarization of the atrium, the Ta-segment displacement being noted between the end of the P wave, extending through the QRS, and the beginning of the ST segment. This is a negative exercise-test result. *C.* Patient with typical angina pectoris and a positive exercise-test result demonstrating the flat ischemic type of ST depression, which extends horizontally for 0.12 sec before joining the T wave.

ing coronary artery disease. When the history is not reliable—as in the military service, with airline pilots, or for insurance or pension purposes—it has found some use as a screening procedure. It has been used in determining functional recovery after myocardial infarction and in predicting mortality with or without symptoms of coronary disease. Long-term follow-up of a group of 1,236 insurance applicants showed a mortality rate four times greater in subjects with a positive test as compared with those with negative tests.[78] The group included those with a history of chest pain (57 per cent). Healed infarction or an abnormal electrocardiogram was evident in 30 per cent; ischemic depression was noted in 16 per cent; junctional depression, in 27.3 per cent; and T-wave changes or arrhythmias, in 2.5 per cent. The exercise test was negative in 54.5 per cent. There was no difference in mortality in those with negative tests and those with junctional displacement.

Typical pain may be reproduced by exercise tests without the development of electrocardiographic changes and may constitute a positive response. At times walking the patient briskly up an incline and producing characteristic pain relieved by nitroglycerin may afford confirmation of angina pectoris.

At the time of this writing, many clinical in-

vestigators have voiced their dissatisfaction with the interpretation of the exercise electrocardiogram and are reevaluating its relationship to ischemic heart disease in an effort to clarify many of the confusing aspects of the problem. Reeves[78a] of Birmingham, Alabama, and Bruce[78b] of Seattle, Washington, and others are utilizing graded exercise or maximal exercise as a technique of stressing the cardiovascular system rather than the technique described by Master. The value of this approach is now under active study.

Coronary Insufficiency ("Coronary Failure" or "Intermediate Coronary Syndrome")[16,79–89]

The various terms applied to prolonged discomfort without conventional evidence of myocardial infarction have led to confusion. In this syndrome pain is more prolonged than in angina pectoris and frequently lasts as long as an hour. Nitroglycerin may give transient relief or no relief; the pain may persist and require opiates. The longer duration of pain suggests the occurrence of acute changes in the coronary circulation, such as subintimal hemorrhage or thrombosis, increased myocardial demands for oxygen, or impaired myocardial perfusion due to extracardiac factors.

The majority of episodes are not produced by unusual effort but develop at rest without the precipitating factor discussed below. An acute change in the coronary arteries, producing significant occlusion, is likely to be the cause of the "discomfort" under these circumstances.[16] Prolonged emotional upheaval may be an inciting factor on occasion; angiographic studies indicate that spasm proximal to a partially occluded vessel is possible, and one might speculate that this may be one type of precipitating factor, perhaps associated with endogenous release of catecholamines due to anxiety. The sudden increase in demands for oxygen or a change in myocardial perfusion may lead to ischemia of a local area, inadequately supplied through obstructed vessels. Examples of precipitating factors are hemorrhage, shock, anesthesia, drugs increasing the work of the heart such as Apresoline hydrochloride (hydralazine hydrochloride), fever, ectopic tachycardia, thyrotoxicosis, severe anemia, hypoglycemia, and pulmonary embolism.

Although the electrocardiogram on occasion may show the ST depression of subendocardial ischemia or alterations of the T waves, these may occur only during pain, or there may be no alterations. The QRS alterations of infarction are lacking in the electrocardiogram. Since the electrocardiogram is commonly normal—and even when abnormal, does not fit the physician's rigid requirement for diagnostic change—a diagnosis of infarction is often not made. The authors feel that most instances are indeed associated with infarction at the time of this syndrome or else have preceded definite infarction (preinfarction syndrome).[16,90] This is especially true when the precipitating and aggravating factors mentioned above are not present. It should be noted that small areas of necrosis may occur without deforming the electrocardiogram. This is especially likely to occur in the papillary muscles, the subendocardium, certain areas of the septum, atria, right ventricle, and base of the heart and, occasionally, the apex of the heart. Furthermore, the necrosis may be confined to small intramural areas without producing alterations. Occasionally, the sole evidence of infarction may be the development of persistently abnormal T waves, the appearance of which may be delayed for 7 to 10 days. One might ask how many dead myocardial cells must be present before the changes of infarction occur on the electrocardiogram. A smaller number of cells situated toward the epicardial surface might produce alterations, whereas a larger number toward the endocardial region might produce no changes. To produce alterations of the leukocyte count, sedimentation rate, serum enzymes, and fever, a sufficient number of myocardial cells must be destroyed. Since the areas of necrosis in coronary insufficiency are generally small, these ancillary aids to diagnosis are generally not helpful.

There may be subtle differences in the natural history of the patient in whom prolonged ischemic pain develops spontaneously, as contrasted to the person in whom the syndrome is precipitated by one of the extracardiac factors mentioned above. Often, when such factors are relieved, there may be no recurrence of pain, even though infarction in a small area may have occurred. In others the same course may develop as in those with the spontaneous variety, in whom there may be episodes of prolonged pain or troublesome angina decubitus. Under these circumstances the outcome is uncertain, and the course may vary as follows: (1) gradual improvement of angina over a long period, presumably due to development of collaterals; (2) sudden death due to ventricular standstill or fibrillation, which occurs in a small per cent; (3) conventional myocardial infarction occurring days to weeks later (paradoxically, improvement in symptoms may occur following this event); (4) no recurrences of pain and no angina on effort following the episode (there may be complete freedom of symptoms for months to years).

Prinzmetal has emphasized the syndrome of recurrent prolonged pain, which is usually unrelated to effort or emotion, requires opiates for relief, and is accompanied by elevation of the ST segments during the attack with return of the ST segments to normal after relief of pain.[75a] The location of the ST segment identifies the area of future myocardial infarction. When infarction occurs, the attacks may cease. A high incidence of arrhythmias, usually ventricular in origin, may be noted.

Myocardial Infarction[21,91–96]

Pain is the presenting symptom in the majority of patients with myocardial infarction. It may occur anywhere in the anterior chest, back, epigastrium, jaw, neck, shoulder, elbow, forearm, or wrist. The usual location is substernal. The patient may describe it as heaviness, burning, indigestion, choking, constriction, tightness, pressure, aching, or expanding sensation. Expressions such as "like a red-hot poker," "like hot smoke," "like someone sitting on my chest," "like a belt tightening around my chest," "an elephant stepped on me," or "feeling as if my forearms would break" may be used, or weakness or numbness of arm may be described. There may be minimal or no discomfort in the anterior chest, and the symptoms may be confined to one of the other areas listed above. In exceptional instances the distress may last no longer than 5 min; however, in the majority of patients, the duration of pain is 1 hr or more until it is relieved spontaneously or, more often, by the administration of opiates. Al-

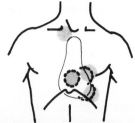

A. ABNORMAL PULSATIONS

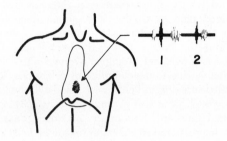

B. FRICTION RUB

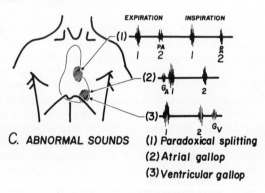

C. ABNORMAL SOUNDS   (1) *Paradoxical splitting*
(2) *Atrial gallop*
(3) *Ventricular gallop*

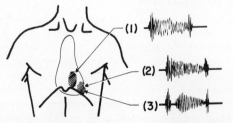

D. ABNORMAL MURMURS   1) *Septal rupture*
2) *Papillary muscle rupture*
3) *Papillary muscle dysfunction*

Fig. 32-6. The physical findings associated with myocardial infarction. (The vast majority of myocardial infarcts are not associated with definite and specific physical abnormalities of the heart when first seen by the physician.) *A.* Abnormal pulsations. Abnormal precordial pulsations due to "physiologic aneurysms" secondary to myocardial ischemia may be located anteriorly, at the apex, and in ectopic positions (below the

though the distress may progress in intensity during the early stages, it is constantly present and not intermittent. Rarely one may elicit slight aggravation by deep breathing, perhaps due to associated pericarditis in patients in whom infarction has preceded the onset of pain. The pain may begin during the day while the patient is sitting at a desk or while he is walking, or may awaken the patient from a sound sleep. Most patients are content to sit or lie quietly, but a few may be restive and walk the floor clutching the chest (Fig. 32-1). The patient may or may not give a history of prior angina pectoris. Some may have experienced previous symptoms of coronary origin which were ignored.

When observed during pain, the patient may have pallor, cold, clammy sweating, or an ashen appearance; but the majority of patients when seen by the physician appear relatively normal. An observer, often the wife, may describe alteration in appearance at onset. The blood pressure is usually normal, but transient hypotension or hypertension may occur. The pulse rate may be normal, but there may be sinus bradycardia—especially with occlusion of the right coronary artery—or slight sinus tachycardia. Various cardiac arrhythmias may be detected (see Chap. 16). The physical examination of the heart at this time is frequently normal. A "physiologic aneurysm" at the apex or over the precordium, a ventricular diastolic gallop rhythm, or an atrial gallop may be detected.[97] Paradoxical splitting of the second heart sound may occur (Fig. 32-6). Many patients do not have fever following infarction. When present, it occurs after several days and is seldom more than 101°F. Rarely, fever of 103°F may be present for periods of up to a week. Chills do not occur.

Atypical Presentations

In about 15 per cent of patients myocardial infarction develops without symptoms.[98–105] Many

area of pulmonary artery pulsation, away from the apex and lateral to the sternum). The circle drawn at the right sternoclavicular joint indicates the area of pulsation occasionally found in patients with dissecting aneurysm of the aorta. This sign, when present, suggests the diagnosis of dissection of the aorta rather than myocardial infarction. *B.* Friction rub. A pericardial friction rub may be heard over the precordium. The "classic" rub has three components as shown. A rub may have only one or two components. *C.* Heart sounds. An atrial gallop, ventricular gallop, and paradoxical splitting of the second sound may occur after myocardial infarction. *D.* Abnormal murmurs. New murmurs may appear after myocardial infarction. They may be due to septal rupture, papillary muscle rupture, or papillary muscle dysfunction.

patients experience no pain with myocardial infarction; in some, pain is obscured by anesthesia,[106] cerebral vascular accident, diabetic acidosis, insulin shock, etc. Some patients may present with signs of peripheral vascular collapse, nausea, and vomiting. Others present with acute pulmonary edema or arrhythmias such as ventricular tachycardia, whereas syncope due to hypotension, transient cardiac arrest, ventricular fibrillation, or onset of complete heart block may be the presenting symptom in a few. Rarely, the sudden onset of profound weakness may herald infarction. Cerebral infarction incident to reduced cardiac output may obscure the recognition of the underlying myocardial infarction. An extremely rare mode of presentation is unexplained fever. Peripheral arterial embolism may lead to the recognition of unsuspected "silent" infarction.[107] Finally, myocardial infarction may be recognized for the first time on a "routine" electrocardiogram.

Differential Diagnosis

An *acute anxiety state* may produce prolonged discomfort and, when coupled with peripheral vasoconstriction and mild stasis-type cyanosis, may be mistaken for myocardial infarction (see Chap. 63). Overt fear may necessitate prompt therapy. Opiates and oxygen may be administered, and this may further cloud the clinical picture and subsequent observations. The emotional reaction of the physician when this occurs in a close friend compounds differential diagnosis and has led to the term *friendship syndrome*.

Acute pericarditis may produce precordial and substernal pain which is characteristically aggravated by deep inspiration (see Chap. 49), change of position, and, occasionally, swallowing. Stimulation of sensory fibers involving the pericardium and diaphragmatic pleura produce radiation of pain to the precordium, the trapezius muscle area, the back of the neck, or the upper part of the abdomen. Confusion occurs when discomfort is confined to the neck, shoulder, or abdomen unless the clear relation to breathing and turning is noted. The pain of pericarditis may diminish if the breath is held. It tends to be sharp or cutting and may recur with intermittent bursts, which are usually precipitated by change of body position. At times, the patient may be more comfortable in the upright position leaning forward. The patient with myocardial infarction may infrequently present with a pericardial friction rub when first seen by the physician; in this instance painless infarction may have preceded the onset of pericardial pain by several days. Classically, the early appearance of fever and pericardial friction rub suggests pericarditis rather than myocardial infarction, in which these are usually delayed for several days. In pericarditis the electrocardiographic abnormalities are confined to the ST segment, and T waves and QRS changes do not occur except for occasional lowering of amplitude due to effusion. In general, the ST-segment vector due to epicardial injury is located between 30 and 90° in the frontal plane and is often directed slightly posteriorly in the sagittal plane, so that ST-segment changes are best recorded in the lateral precordial leads. Reciprocal changes are generally absent. The ST-T abnormalities of apical infarction may simulate pericarditis when significant Q waves are absent. T-wave inversion of considerable magnitude may occur with infarction but is less likely with pericarditis. There may be no alterations of the electrocardiogram, even in the presence of a pericardial friction rub. A pericardial friction rub is not invariably present in acute pericarditis. A small pleural effusion which obscures the left costophrenic angle may occur. Modest elevation of serum transaminase may at times occur, especially when pericardial effusion results in venous hypertension and hepatic congestion, and values up to 90 units have been reported. The clinical differentiation from infarction depends on the total synthesis of the history, physical findings, and serial electrocardiographic changes.

Dissecting aneurysm of the aorta, although far less common than myocardial infarction, is not rare (see Chap. 56). A prior history of angina or infarction favors new infarction but does not exclude dissecting aneurysm. The pain of dissecting aneurysm often has its peak intensity at the onset in contrast to a more gradual buildup in patients with infarction. Although back pain occurs with infarction, wide radiation to the back, flank, abdomen, or legs suggests dissecting aneurysm. If the patient appears to be in shock but there is hypertension, dissection is likely. The diagnosis of dissecting aneurysm is suggested in a patient with chest pain who has any of the following signs and symptoms: syncope, weakness or transient paralysis of legs, hemiplegia, aortic insufficiency, sternoclavicular joint pulsation (Fig. 32-6), wide differences in pulses or in blood pressure between arms or carotid arteries, left pleural effusion, and significant widening of the aortic shadow by x-ray. Pericarditis occurs with both myocardial infarction and dissecting aneurysm and is of little differential value. Since hypertension is commonly associated with dissecting aneurysm, the electrocardiogram commonly reveals the pattern of left ventricular hypertrophy. The demonstration of serial electrocardiographic changes may be diagnostic of myocardial infarction; however, very rarely these may occur with dissection of the coronary ostia. The serum transaminase is not helpful, since modest elevations occur in both conditions. Aortographic studies may be necessary to confirm the presence of dissecting aneurysm.

The syndrome of massive *pulmonary embolism* without infarction of the lung may closely simulate myocardial infarction, since impaired coronary perfusion is present in both conditions. The diagnosis of pulmonary embolism is favored by the presence of intense cyanosis and profound dyspnea and tachypnea from the onset of chest pain (see Chap. 47). Syncope may be the presenting or sole complaint of embolism. Referred pain in the arms or jaw favors myocardial infarction. The clinical setting of the patient may furnish a clue to diagnosis; for example, pulmonary embolism is more likely in the postoperative or postpartum period, following trauma, fractures, or amputations, and in the presence of thrombophlebitis. The development of acute relative tricuspid regurgitation, which may be reflected as a deep systolic jugular venous pulse in addition to prominent A waves, may be noted following a pulmonary embolus. The diagnosis of pulmonary embolus is favored by the following physical signs: fixed splitting of the second heart sound, a systolic murmur at the second and third left intercostal space, a contact sound in systole and diastole at this area (perhaps due to dilatation of the outflow tract of the right ventricle) simulating a pericardial friction rub, and, rarely, the presence of a systolic bruit over an obstructed large pulmonary artery which may be heard in the back or over the lateral thorax. A systolic impulse over the pulmonary artery area or a systolic lifting of the sternal or parasternal area may occur. Sinus tachycardia, atrial tachycardia, or atrial fibrillation may be recorded. The electrocardiogram may exhibit evidence of myocardial ischemia and intraventricular conduction abnormalities; furthermore, on occasion myocardial infarction may be precipitated by pulmonary embolism. Sinus tachycardia with ST-segment depression of variable degree is common; in fact, the pulse rate is seldom below 100 following an acute pulmonary embolus. There may be a conduction defect characterized by a shift of the terminal portion of the QRS force to the right, which produces an S wave in lead I, V_6, and a terminal R wave in AVR and V_1. Along with these there may be a Q wave in leads II, III, and AVF, which suggests inferior infarction. Anterior myocardial ischemia with inverted T waves and transient loss of R waves in the right precordial leads may simulate anterior myocardial infarction. The ST-segment depression may be of the flat ischemic type and may be identical to the changes of subendocardial infarction; indeed, the latter may be precipitated by a pulmonary embolus.

The determination of serum transaminase levels will not routinely separate pulmonary embolism and infarction from myocardial infarction (see section on laboratory findings). The x-ray with massive pulmonary embolism is commonly normal, although an increase of radiolucency of an area of lung associated with a dilated pulmonary artery having an abrupt decrease in size may be suggestive of the proper diagnosis. It should be reemphasized that only approximately 10 per cent of pulmonary emboli produce infarction; however, the detection of an area of infarction by x-ray may clinch the diagnosis. Conventional pulmonary infarcts with pleuritic pain and rub offer little diagnostic problem, but many do not have these features and are difficult to identify. Intercostal muscle spasm over the area of infarction with tenderness on palpation may occur. Selective pulmonary angiography or pulmonary scanning using radioactive substances may confirm the diagnosis (see Chap. 47).

Acute gallbladder colic may produce epigastric and lower substernal pain; the discomfort may be steady and constant and simulate myocardial infarction. Reference of pain to the back and right scapular area may be a clue as cholecystitis develops. Pain and hyperesthesia over the gallbladder area may help to differentiate the pain from that of myocardial infarction. A history of previous attacks with chilliness and fever may be helpful. Although pain in the right shoulder area may be noted, pain in the arm or jaw does not occur. Gallbladder disease is not uncommonly associated with coronary disease; however, the demonstration of gallstones does not indicate whether or not they are symptomatic. Gallbladder colic can precipitate angina pectoris in a patient with coronary disease, and this heightens the diagnostic difficulties. When pain is suspected of arising in the gallbladder, roentgenographic demonstration of the absence of disease of this structure is helpful; however, stones may occasionally be missed on cholecystography. When stones are found and when, after a period of observation, the symptoms cannot be clearly attributed to coronary disease which may be known to be present, one faces the dilemma of surgical removal of the gallbladder. Levine[108] has reported that cholecystectomy in such patients decreases the frequency and severity of attacks of angina pectoris; it is probable that the mechanism is nonspecific painful stimuli that induce angina.

Mediastinal emphysema (Hamman's disease) due to rupture of alveoli with dissection of air along periarterial tissue may present with chest pain, mediastinal crepitation, which is often noticed by the patient, air in the mediastinum and left pleural space, and occasionally subcutaneous emphysema of the neck and upper thorax.[109] The mediastinal crunch heard on auscultation is characteristic even to the uninitiated. The lateral roentgenogram of the chest and neck is of great help in confirming the diagnosis.

Spontaneous pneumothorax with pleuritic pain over the lateral thorax associated with dyspnea may be suspected from physical findings and confirmed by x-ray examination.[110]

Cervical disk degeneration or arthritis and other thoracic outlet syndromes may simulate the discomfort of myocardial ischemia, as previously pointed out.

Perforation of a peptic ulcer may occur without previous symptoms; the pain is usually confined to the epigastrium or upper abdominal region and is associated with tenderness and muscle spasm.[111] Demonstration of air under the diaphragm by x-ray in the upright position is usually, but not always, present. Bleeding from peptic ulcer may produce hypotension, syncope, or shock.[112] Tachycardia is usually present, but some patients at the onset have a slow pulse which simulates occlusion of the right coronary artery. Depression of the ST segments secondary to shock may cause confusion. The reduction of hematocrit, demonstration of blood in the stools, and gastrointestinal x-rays identify the cause of the symptoms. Where there is a typical history of peptic ulcer, there may be no difficulty in diagnosis, although the presence of both diseases may cause confusion; rarely peptic ulcer with atypical symptoms may be mistaken for coronary disease. It is more likely that coronary disease with the syndrome of bloating, belching, and aerophagia after meals may raise the possibility of peptic ulcer.

Rupture of the esophagus closely mimics myocardial infarction. Vomiting from diverse causes prior to onset is a strong diagnostic clue. Recognition is afforded by the presence of air in the mediastinum extending upward to the neck.[113,114] Barium swallowing using a water-soluble contrast material may show the area of disruption. The Mallory-Weiss syndrome of gastroesophageal tear is less often a source of confusion.

Necrotizing pancreatitis presents as an acute condition within the abdomen with pain and shock.[115] Pain may radiate into the substernal region and lower part of the chest on occasion and may be mistaken for myocardial infarction. Pronounced changes in the ST-T segments of the electrocardiograms associated with shock may be a source of confusion. ST-segment and T-wave changes suggestive of pericarditis are rare. QRS changes have been reported but probably represent associated myocardial infarction. Recurrent attacks of pancreatitis in the alcoholic, with or without pancreatic calcification, may pose a problem of differentiation. Elevations in the serum- and urinary amylase levels give confirmatory evidence of pancreatitis. Elevations in the serum-transaminase levels may cause confusion with myocardial infarction. Hyperglycemia may develop acutely during an episode of pancreatitis, but this abnormality may also occur in some patients with myocardial infarction.

Laboratory Findings

Sedimentation Rate. The sedimentation rate[116,117] of red blood cells has been used as a laboratory sign of myocardial infarction. The authors do not believe that this test has diagnostic or prognostic value and therefore do not use it.

Leukocytosis. Although the white blood cell count frequently increases after myocardial infarction, it has little diagnostic value. The white cell count may become elevated by the second and third day and usually reaches a maximum in a few more days, after which the count rapidly declines to normal. The peak white blood cell count is usually between 12,000 and 15,000 cells per cubic centimeter. On rare occasions the count may be as high as 20,000. The differential white blood cell count shows an increase of polymorphonuclear leukocytes with an increase in young forms. Many have reported that leukocytosis occurs in virtually all cases of myocardial infarction.[116] The authors believe that small infarcts occur without stimulating a significant increase in white blood cells. Certainly a normal white blood cell count should not be used as evidence against the diagnosis of myocardial infarction.

Glycosuria and Hyperglycemia. When a myocardial infarct occurs in a patient with controlled diabetes mellitus, the blood sugar may become elevated, and glycosuria may occur. Diabetic acidosis may be precipitated in such patients. Glycosuria and hyperglycemia may also occur in patients who are not diabetic. This has been attributed to adrenal stimulation secondary to stress and shock. Some patients who have glycosuria and hyperglycemia probably have latent diabetes; even though these findings may disappear shortly after the infarction, some of these patients will have abnormal glucose tolerance curves when checked some months later, and in a few obvious diabetes mellitus will develop.[118]

Miscellaneous Findings. The C-reactive protein may become positive as a result of large myocardial infarction. *Azotemia* may develop, secondary to shock or heart failure. Red blood cells may occur in the *urine* as a result of renal infarction secondary to an embolus originating from a left ventricular mural thrombus. *Oliguria* and *anuria* may occur in patients with severe shock.

Serum Enzymes. Certain enzymes are produced by certain tissues. When the tissues are damaged, the enzymes may be liberated into the blood stream. The development of simple techniques useful in measuring these enzymes have encouraged the study of these substances in patients with myocardial infarction. Unfortunately, these new diagnostic techniques are not as valuable as they were first thought to be, and many problems may be created by their misuse. Despite the difficulties currently dulling the glitter of these tests, a new field has been opened, and the future may well be brighter.

The test for serum glutamic oxalacetic transaminase (SGOT) was developed in 1954.[119] The test has been used widely since then, and the SGOT level has been correlated with many disease states.[120-128] After a patient sustains an acute myocardial infarction, the SGOT level becomes elevated above the normal value of 8 to 40 units in 6 to 8 hr and usually reaches peak levels in 24 to 48 hr and returns to normal in 4 to 8 days. An exceedingly high SGOT level indicates a poor prognosis. The test is often misused, for unfortunately the test is considered by some to be a test for coronary disease and many patients with definite angina pectoris are reassured when the SGOT is normal. The SGOT level may be normal in a patient with changing angina, and this has led to confusion and poor advice. Even small infarcts may not be associated with a significant rise in the SGOT level. The statement that 98 per cent of patients with acute transmural infarcts have elevated SGOT levels may be correct, but many infarcts are not transmural. Furthermore, many disorders other than myocardial infarction may be associated with elevated SGOT levels:

1. Acute hepatocellular damage after alcohol ingestion in patients with chronic liver disease.

2. Congestive heart failure. Some reports indicate that the SGOT level is normal in mild failure. The clinician is usually unable to draw a line between mild and moderate failure and is therefore not comfortable with this test whenever there is any heart failure.

3. Arrhythmias when the ventricular rate is above 160 beats per minute.

4. Pericarditis. Reports indicate elevated SGOT levels are not found in patients with mild pericarditis but are found in patients with pericarditis associated with sanguinous effusion and epicarditis. Where "mild" stops and "moderately severe" begins is arbitrary, and the test may be confusing in this setting, especially when there is increased venous pressure and hepatomegaly.

5. Dissecting aneurysm.

6. Pulmonary infarction. The SGOT level becomes elevated several days after pulmonary infarction. This delay has been said to help separate pulmonary infarct from myocardial infarct. The au-

thors question this because so many pulmonary infarcts go unrecognized and it is not always easy to date the onset of this disorder.

7. Unaccustomed vigorous exercise, trauma, cerebral infarction, acute cholecystitis, pancreatitis, renal infarction, splenic infarction, neuromuscular disease such as dermatomyositis and muscular dystrophy, hemolytic crisis, and certain drugs such as narcotics and anticoagulants.

Since SGOT can be released from many tissues other than the heart and since small infarcts do not produce diagnostic levels of the enzyme, the test has limited value. Interest in SGOT, however, stimulated the work on lactic dehydrogenase (and its five isoenzymes), which may prove to be of more diagnostic value.[129] Patients with acute myocardial infarction have an increase in fraction 4 and, especially, in fraction 5 (Fig. 32-7). This is demonstrable within 12 hr after the clinical history of myocardial infarction and may be present in the serum for as long as 10 days. The only other patients who have had an increase in fractions 4 and 5 are those with megaloblastic anemias.[130]

Electrocardiogram. The electrocardiographic abnormalities related to myocardial infarction will be only briefly mentioned here, and the reader should consult Chap. 6 of this book and textbooks of electrocardiography for more detailed discussion.

The majority of myocardial infarcts involve the left ventricle and septum. After myocardial infarction the initial portion of the QRS complex, or vector loop, becomes abnormal. The forces generated during the initial 0.02 to 0.04 sec tend to be directed away from the area of dead myocardial tissue. The ST segment becomes displaced from the base line. When represented as a mean vector it tends to be directed toward the area of epicardial injury which surrounds the dead zone or to be directed away from an area of subendocardial injury.[131] The T waves become abnormal and when represented as a mean vector tend to be directed away from the area of epicardial ischemia which surrounds the area of injury.

In order to understand how myocardial infarction alters the electrocardiogram and vectorcardiogram it is necessary to have the following information:

1. The normal anatomic position of the left ventricle and septum in the chest

2. How the forces generated by the heart are projected onto, and recorded from, the body surface

3. The normal sequence of ventricular activation and how it is changed by myocardial infarction

4. The normal sequence of repolarization and how it is changed by myocardial infarction

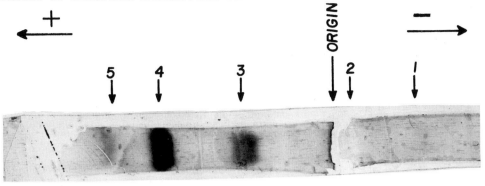

NORMAL

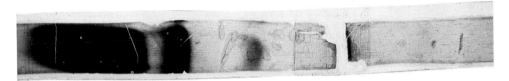

MYOCARDIAL INFARCT

Fig. 32-7. Starch-gel electrophoresis of isozymes of lactic dehydrogenase. (The starch gel has been dried and then mounted between two pieces of Scotch tape and is then run through a densitometer. The finished preparation can then be placed on the patient's chart.) The upper strip is from a normal individual and exhibits the three bands (3, 4, and 5) usually found in a normal patient. The lower strip shows a marked increase in bands 4 and 5 found in acute myocardial infarction. (*This figure was supplied by Dr. Edwin Galler of Atlanta, Georgia. His work in this field was done during his tenure at the Atlanta Veterans Hospital.*)

5. How to recognize the new ST forces produced by injury.

When these are understood as a unified concept, it is possible to assume that an infarct is located in any portion of the left ventricle and septum and to predict, within reasonable limits, what the electrocardiogram and vectorcardiogram will show or vice versa (see Fig. 32-8).

The following discussion highlights the limitations of electrocardiography as it relates to myocardial infarction and emphasizes certain aspects of the technique that have been neglected (Figs. 32-9–32-14).

The technique of electrocardiography does not identify coronary atherosclerosis per se. Unfortunately the electrocardiogram can be normal at one moment, and the patient can have a myocardial infarct in the next. The electrocardiogram becomes abnormal only after the disease process in the coronary artery has reached a certain stage at which time significant myocardial ischemia, injury, and necrosis develop.

Myocardial infarction may be present, and the expected QRS, ST, and T abnormalities may not be present in the electrocardiogram. A certain number of myocardial cells must die before the electrocardiogram becomes altered. The exact number is unknown, but it is likely that 1 cm^2 myocardium may be necrotic without deforming the QRS complex. Of even greater importance is the location of the infarction, since there are "silent" areas in the myocardium. For example, QRS changes may not develop when there is an infarction of the endocardial area, the central portion of the ventricular wall, the back of the left ventricle, the cardiac apex (Fig. 32-13), the papillary muscles, the septum, the right ventricle, or the atrium (Fig. 32-14). On rare occasion a patient may die of shock or myocardial rupture secondary to myocardial infarction, and the tracing still may not show diagnostic changes. After a secondary myocardial infarct, the electrocardiogram may no longer show the classic changes of the first infarct. In fact, at times, the electrocardiogram may even "improve" after the second infarct. Subsequent infarcts—the third and fourth—rarely deform the QRS complex. Standard electrocardiographic teaching which has emphasized that QRS, ST, and T changes must be present in order to diagnose a myocardial infarction has led to such rigidity that

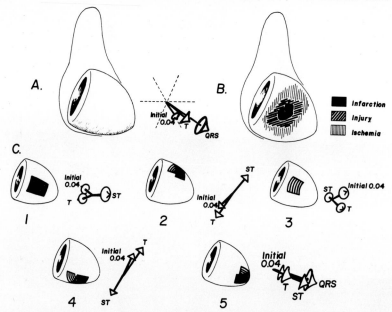

Fig. 32-8. Most myocardial infarcts are located in the left ventricle and septum. (Right ventricular and atrial infarcts also occur.) Seen here are the location of the left ventricle in the chest, the usual locations of infarcts that occur in this structure, and how the altered electrical forces are reflected on the electrocardiogram. A. The anatomic position of the left ventricle and septum viewed from the front. The normal mean QRS vector is located to the left and is directed inferiorly and slightly posteriorly. The normal mean T vector lies very near the mean QRS vector but is slightly anterior to it. The forces generated during the first portion (initial 0.04 sec) of the QRS, when represented as a mean vector, also lie very near the mean QRS vector but is slightly anterior to it. The forces generated during the first portion (initial 0.04 sec) of the QRS, when represented as a mean vector, also lie very near the mean QRS vector. B. Diagram of a myocardial infarction, zone of injury, and zone of ischemia. The mean dead-zone vector (initial QRS forces) points away from the infarct, the mean injury vector (ST-segment forces) points toward the area of epicardial injury, and the mean ischemia vector (T-wave forces) points away from the area of epicardial ischemia. C. (1) Anteroseptal infarction. The electrocardiogram would show abnormal Q waves in leads I, AVL, V₁, V₂, V₃, V₄, abnormal ST-segment elevation in leads I, AVL, and the anterior precordial leads, and abnormal T-wave inversion in leads I, AVL, and the anterior precordial leads. (2) Lateral infarction. The electrocardiogram would show abnormal Q waves, abnormal ST-segment elevation and abnormal T-wave inversion in leads I, AVL, V₄, V₅, V₆. (3) True posterior infarction. The electrocardiogram would show an abnormally tall R wave in lead V₁, and perhaps an abnormal Q wave in lead AVF, abnormal ST-segment depression in leads V₁, V₂, and V₃, and tall T waves in leads V₁, V₂, and V₃. (4) Inferior infarction. The electrocardiogram would show abnormal Q waves in leads II, III, and AVF, abnormal ST elevation in leads II, III, and AVF; and abnormally inverted T waves in leads II, III, and AVF. (5) Apical infarction. The dead-zone vector ("abnormal Q waves") may or may not appear. The mean ST and mean T vector may increase in size and point toward the apex. (The illustrations in this figure are shown to illustrate a concept. They are not designed to illustrate all the variables that must be considered in the theory and practice of electrocardiography.)

it has not been adequately appreciated that an infarct can occur without such changes. Specifically, a myocardial infarction can occur and the electrocardiogram show only T-wave changes. Obviously T-wave abnormalities are not specific for infarction, and these changes must be correlated with the clinical features in an individual case. The T-wave abnormality associated with infarction may be delayed and may not develop until 3 to 10 days after the onset of the chest pain. Accordingly, multiple tracing may be needed, and a single electro-

cardiogram is virtually worthless in ruling out an acute infarct.

The electrocardiographic abnormalities due to myocardial infarction may disappear. The ST-segment abnormality frequently returns to normal after myocardial infarction, and the T wave occasionally returns to normal. As a rule, the QRS abnormality (initial 0.04 abnormality—"Q wave") persists, but it too may shrink in size until the tracing returns to normal. In such cases subtle changes may be detected only when the tracing is compared with the preinfarction normal tracing. In patients who may have had a previous infarction, it is especially prudent to examine the tracing taken at the time of the previous episode before doubting, on the basis of current normal tracing, that such occurred.

Certain QRS conduction defects such as left bundle branch may obscure the QRS changes of myocardial infarction. The ST- and T-wave ab-

normalities of infarction may be identified when there is left bundle branch block, although these are usually more difficult to recognize in the presence of the block. Right bundle branch block ordinarily does not obscure the findings of infarction.

Many other diseases can produce electrocardiographic abnormalities which mimic those of myocardial infarction (Figs. 32-15–32-17). The patient

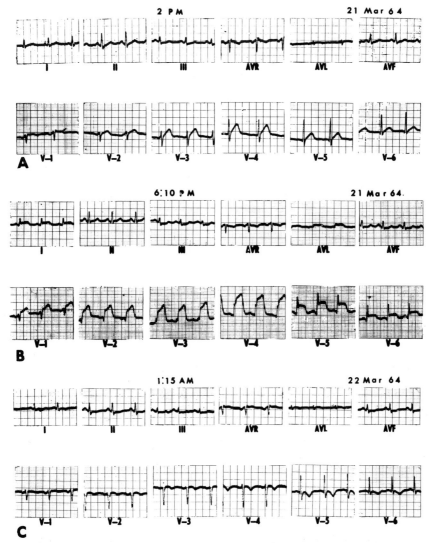

Fig. 32-9. A. One hour prior to this electrocardiogram the patient developed severe substernal "indigestion." Electrocardiogram shows slight ST- and T-wave abnormalities especially in V₂, V₃, V₄, V₅, and V₆. There appears to be slight ST-segment elevation blending into a prominent T wave in the above leads. This type of abnormality is not infrequent in the early course of myocardial infarction, but it is often overlooked. B. Four hours and ten minutes later the electrocardiogram shows extensive anterior epicardial injury with only slight QRS changes. C. Electrocardiogram five hours and five minutes after B shows T-wave abnormality consistent with anterolateral ischemia and disappearance of the giant-sized ST-segment elevation. The QRS abnormality is now clearly seen, indicating anterior dead zone.

The electrocardiogram has remained unchanged for the past 6 months. This series of tracings illustrates the difficulty in judging the age of an infarction by noting the configuration of QRS, ST, and T waves. (This one "evolved" in 12 hr and has remained the same since.)

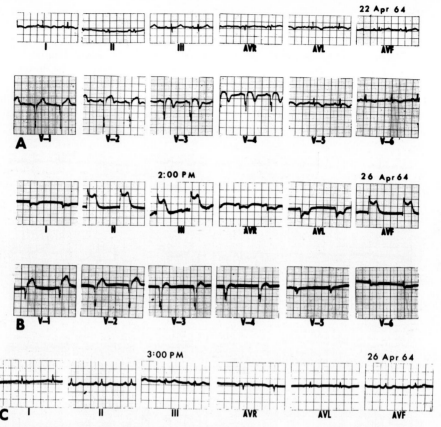

Fig. 32-10. A sixty-eight-year-old man with a history of two previous myocardial infarctions noted increasing angina pectoris for 4 days prior to admission. On the day of admission he had severe prolonged substernal pain. *A.* QRS-, ST- and T-wave abnormalities indicative of massive anterior myocardial infarction. *B.* Four days after the initial tracing the patient had a paroxysm of coughing followed by hypotension. Electrocardiogram shows nodal rhythm, change in QRS, and marked ST elevation compatible with epicardial injury of the inferior wall of the left ventricle. *C.* One hour later, when the blood pressure returned to normal following 5 mg metaraminol (Aramine) injected parenterally, the ST segments returned to base line.

This series of tracings illustrates the relationship of severe paroxysms of coughing and hypotension with abnormalities of the electrocardiogram in certain patients with severely compromised coronary circulation. It is imperative to restore blood pressure promptly in this type of patient.

with advanced emphysema often exhibits a QRS abnormality that suggests myocardial infarction. Patients with left ventricular hypertrophy may have a posteriorly directed QRS loop which produces absence of the R wave in leads V_1 V_2, V_3, and occasionally in lead V_4. (The absence of R waves in these leads may be produced by infarction, but this finding is not as specific for infarction as when the R wave is absent in V_1, V_2 and there is a QR pattern in V_3. In this situation the QRS loop is not smooth, and the initial QRS forces are posterior to the subsequent QRS forces. A "dead-zone" effect in the electrocardiogram may occur as a result of amyloid in the myocardium, scleroderma,

Fig. 32-11 (opposite page). A fifty-seven-year-old male was admitted to the hospital with prolonged substernal chest pain. No previous history of heart disease was obtained. *A.* Electrocardiogram on admission. The initial 0.002 sec of the mean QRS is directed to the left and indicates a small dead zone. The ST-segment displacement represented as a mean vector is directed inferiorly, to the right, and posteriorly indicating inferoposterior injury. The T waves are prominent. This is often the case in the hyperacute stage of myocardial infarction. *B.* Vectorcardiogram on admission. The frontal (F), horizontal (H), and left sagittal (S) views of the vectorcardiogram show a large abnormal ST-T loop consistent with inferoposteriorepicardial injury. *C.* Prior to this tracing, the patient was pain-free, normotensive, and without detectable abnormality on physical examination. One hour after admission, while turning in bed, the onset of ventricular fibrillation was observed on the oscilloscope.

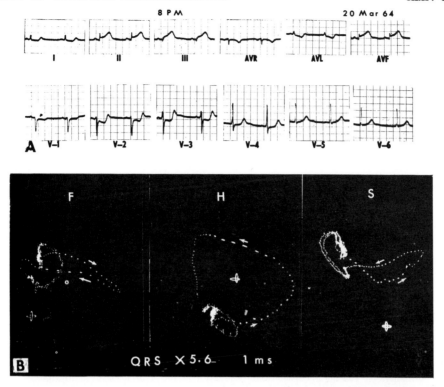

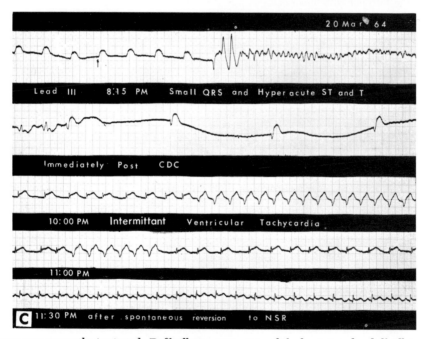

External massage was promptly instituted. Defibrillation was accomplished using a d-c defibrillator. (Ventricular fibrillation recurred nine times with successful defibrillation in the first 24 hr.) The patient has now returned to hard manual labor as a welder and is symptom-free. Some of the arrhythmias seen in the first 24 hr in this patient are depicted here.

This case illustrates that a patient with myocardial infarction may appear stable and comfortable and suddenly develop treacherous arrhythmia. The case also illustrates the modern technique of management of myocardial infarction.

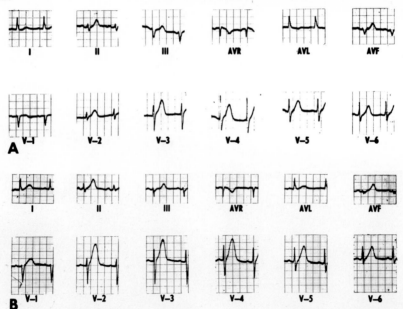

Fig. 32-12. An eighty-four-year-old woman was admitted to the orthopedic service with a fractured hip. Five days after surgical treatment she had sudden collapse and hypertension and was transferred to the medical service with a diagnosis of massive pulmonary embolism. *A.* Electrocardiogram recorded several hours after symptoms began. The tracing shows prominent T waves. The QRS axis is rotated to the left because of terminal QRS-force abnormality. *B.* Tracing recorded four days after *A* and 1 hr prior to death. The T waves are more prominent, and the terminal QRS abnormality is less obvious.

Autopsy revealed a large apical myocardial infarction, but no evidence of pulmonary emboli. This tracing is shown to illustrate that large infarctions may be present in certain areas of the heart (the apex, in this case) without classic QRS-, ST-, or T-wave changes.

diffuse myocardial disease, metastatic neoplasm, or sarcoid of the heart, and with certain conduction defects which may be associated with Wolff-Parkinson-White syndrome, acute pulmonary embolism, myotonia atrophica or Friedreich's ataxia.

ST-segment and T-wave abnormalities may be caused by many conditions. Pericarditis and digitalis are perhaps the best examples of this group of conditions.

The electrical activity of the heart does not

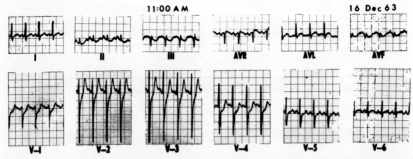

Fig. 32-13. A fifty-four-year-old man. Seven days prior to admission the patient had severe substernal chest pain lasting 15 min and relieved by rest. Two days prior to admission the patient had mild substernal discomfort radiating to the back and lasting 1 to 2 hr. Thirty minutes prior to the above tracing the patient experienced sudden onset of severe chest pain, became dyspneic, and collapsed while climbing stairs.

The electrocardiogram shows sinus tachycardia. The initial portion of the QRS is suggestive of an inferior dead zone. ST-segment displacement is consistent with subendocardial injury, and there are tall, peaked T-waves in V_2, V_3, and V_4.

Autopsy revealed hemopericardium and rupture of the posterior wall of the left ventricle from massive inferoposterior myocardial infarction.

This case illustrates that cardiac rupture can occur without classic ST- and T-wave abnormalities.

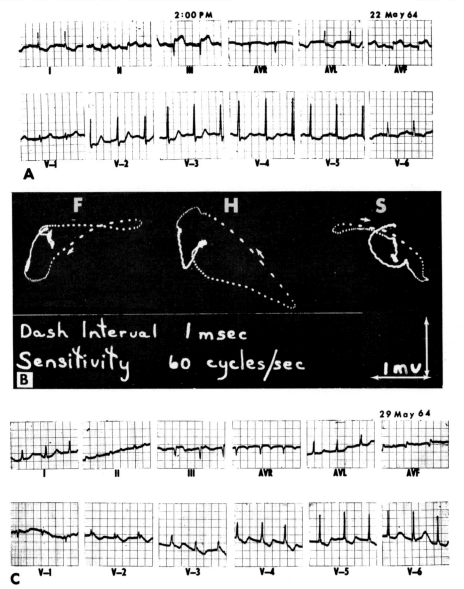

Fig. 32-14. A sixty-four-year-old man with 2 hr duration of severe substernal chest pain and moderate hypotension. *A.* Electrocardiogram reveals first-degree heart block and QRS-, ST-, and T-wave changes consistent with inferolateral myocardial infarction. *B.* Vectorcardiogram (dash interval = 1 msec). The frontal (F), horizontal (H), and left sagittal (S) views of the vectorcardiogram show inferoposterior infarction. *C.* One day prior to this tracing the patient developed complete heart block, and a catheter pacemaker was inserted. The complete heart block disappeared, and the catheter pacemaker was discontinued. This tracing shows nodal rhythm, inferoinfarction, and a change in the T wave.

The patient died from ventricular fibrillation the day following the last tracing. Autopsy revealed a 7- to 8-day-old inferior posterior infarction of the left ventricle and a fresh hemorrhagic infarction of the entire right ventricle and right atrium.

This tracing is shown to illustrate that massive destruction of the right ventricle can occur without diagnostic electrocardiographic abnormalities.

necessarily parallel cardiac function. It is true that when there is no electrical activity of the heart, there is no function. It does not follow that electrical activity indicates normal function. This needs emphasis today, since the cardiac activity (electrical) of many patients with myocardial infarction is monitored for long periods of time. Electrical monitoring does not replace the blood pressure cuff.

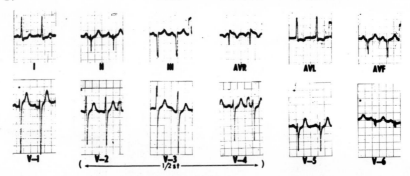

Fig. 32-15. Electrocardiogram of a twenty-four-year-old woman with functional hypertrophic subaortic and subpulmonic stenosis. Note the QRS complex abnormality suggesting lateral myocardial infarction. This type of abnormality is commonly observed in patients with functional hypertrophic subaortic stenosis.

The value of electrocardiography in the diagnosis of myocardial infarction has been firmly established. We must not forget, however, that electrocardiography does not solve all problems and that some problems are created by its use.

Complications[132-134]

The average patient with myocardial infarction pursues an untroubled course after the pain is controlled. However, there are many complications which add to the morbidity and mortality of this common problem. One must anticipate these problems, since proper management may be crucial to recovery and rehabilitation.

Arrhythmias.[135] Ventricular premature beats are common and constitute the most frequent disturbance of rhythm; they may be the forerunner of ventricular tachycardia. These may be related to myocardial ischemia, hypotension, myocardial insufficiency, impaired pulmonary ventilation, or even drug therapy. On occasion, ventricular tachycardia may be the presenting manifestation of acute myocardial infarction. This catastrophic event is associated with a high incidence of shock, congestive heart failure, and ventricular fibrillation. Sudden death due to ventricular fibrillation or standstill accounts for many deaths due to coronary disease with or without acute myocardial infarction. Many patients die before diagnostic histologic changes in the myocardium have a chance to develop. Yater et al. noted that in 75 per cent of 250 deaths occurring in patients under the age of forty the patient died early of "coronary insufficiency" and did not show infarction at autopsy.[4] The Seattle study showed that two-thirds of 122 males died within 1 hr and only 33 per cent lived long enough to be seen by a physician.[136] Hartenauer et al. noted abrupt death in 58 out of 1,104 hospitalized cases (5.3 per cent).[137] Spain et al., in a study of 1,329 consecutive autopsies, noted coronary disease as a cause of sudden death (less than 1 hr) in 422 of 463 adult males and 32 of 66 white females.[138] Coronary disease was thought to be the cause of death in 90 per cent of witnessed sudden deaths in men surviving less than 1 hr. McQuay, Edwards, and Burchell noted 23 per cent of 133 hospital deaths due to myocardial infarction as due to "coronary failure."[134] Hellerstein and Turell and

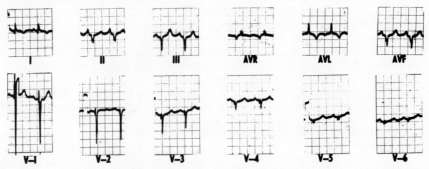

Fig. 32-16. A thirteen-year-old boy with dextroversion and transposition of the great vessels. The QRS abnormality suggests anterior dead zone, and the T-wave inversion in lead I might be interpreted as ischemia. This tracing is shown to emphasize that "dead-zone effects" can be produced by heart disease other than myocardial infarction.

others have observed the types of arrhythmias occurring at the time of death in patients with myocardial infarction.[139]

Atrial tachycardia, atrial flutter, or atrial fibrillation may follow impairment of the blood supply to the atria. This may occur after occlusion of either the left coronary or the circumflex coronary proximal to its first branch, which often (45 per cent) supplies an artery to the sinus node. It also occurs after occlusion of the right coronary artery proximal to the sinus node artery, which originates from the right coronary in 55 per cent of patients[140–142] (see p. 639). It is probable that the presence of these arrhythmias is associated with a high incidence of atrial infarction, particularly of the region of the sinus node, although they may occur as a result of vagal stimulation without infarction of the atria. The arrhythmia may either result from shock or be followed by shock.

Prolonged P-R interval, Wenckebach phenomenon, 2:1 A-V block, and complete heart block may follow occlusion of the right coronary artery proximal to the artery to the A-V node[142–144] (see p. 639). Stokes-Adams attacks may occur. The A-V conduction disturbances are generally transient and last from hours to days. Sinus bradycardia is more common with occlusion of the right coronary artery and posterior infarction.

Nonparoxysmal nodal tachycardia and A-V dissociation may also follow occlusion of the proximal right coronary artery. Digitalis administration may accentuate many of these disturbances of rhythm and conduction. Anxiety, retching, and straining at the stool may also precipitate arrhythmia. Occasionally drugs which impair pulmonary ventilation are precipitating factors.

The exact incidence of arrhythmia after myocardial infarction is unknown, but the introduction of intensive-care units with constant cardiac monitoring will undoubtedly furnish more reliable data. In a study employing continuous monitoring, Spann et al. recorded an incidence of 73 per cent in 30 patients.[145] Only 12 of 40 arrhythmias (30 per cent) were detected by the usual clinical methods; thus 70 per cent of the documented arrhythmias would have gone unnoticed without electrical monitoring. Forty-seven per cent either had ventricular tachycardia or a slow ectopic ventricular rhythm. The majority of disturbances of rhythm occurred within the first 24 hr.

Shock. Shock at onset of infarction is frequent but is transient in most instances.[146] In about 10 to 15 per cent of patients clinical shock develops which persists at least $\frac{1}{2}$ to 1 hr. The patient appears pale and sweaty with cool, clammy skin, and there is tachycardia with a weak, thready pulse and lowered blood pressure. There may be restlessness, confusion, or obtundation. The mortality remains high in this group, being approximately 80 per cent without pressor therapy and 60 per cent with treatment. Arrhythmias and congestive heart failure are frequently found in association with shock. There may be several mechanisms in the production of shock, including decreased cardiac output, peripheral vascular collapse, or even outflow tract obstruction in the presence of marked hypovolemia, particularly if catecholamine therapy has been used.[147–150] Hypovolemia may at times be a precipitating or aggravating factor when the patient has veen under prolonged therapy with chlorothiazide derivatives.

Left Ventricular Failure. This is common during the course of myocardial infarction, and of all patients who die, 30 per cent die from this complication.[134] It may occur in the patient whose heart size is within normal limits by physical examination and x-ray, particularly after an initial myocardial infarction. It may be present with a

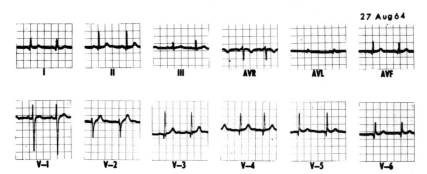

Fig. 32-17. A fourteen-year-old asymptomatic boy with slight valvular aortic stenosis who participates without difficulty in active sports, including basketball. The initial portion of the QRS complex is prominent and produces deep Q waves, especially in V_3, V_4, V_5, and V_6. This case is presented to show that Q waves do not always equate with dead zone. Electrocardiogram must always be interpreted in light of all other clinical information.

pulse rate that is not unduly accelerated and can occur in the absence of symptoms and in the absence of a ventricular diastolic gallop rhythm, pulsus alternans, pulmonary rales, or abnormal distension of the neck veins. In this phase interstitial pulmonary edema may be demonstrated by the portable chest x-ray.[151] Pulmonary rales occurring during the first week after infarction are commonly overlooked or are attributed to hypostasis, chronic bronchitis, etc. For every case of alveolar pulmonary edema there are probably 20 cases of unrecognized interstitial pulmonary edema.

In this setting the development of either atrial or ventricular gallop rhythm suggests myocardial insufficiency. Slightly abnormal neck vein pulsations detected with the patient at an angle of 30 to 45° are often overlooked (see p. 90). If the early manifestations of left ventricular failure are unrecognized and untreated, disastrous alveolar pulmonary edema may follow in a few hours or days. There is a high incidence of interstitial pulmonary edema during shock or uncontrolled arrhythmia lasting an hour or longer and even with persistent sinus tachycardia with a rate of 120 or greater.

Pulmonary Embolism. This may precipitate angina, myocardial infarction, arrhythmia, or congestive heart failure. It is one of the major complications of myocardial infarction. Since infarction of the lung occurs in less than 10 per cent of pulmonary emboli, the clinical and x-ray recognition of embolus is difficult. This difficulty in diagnosis is responsible for the wide difference between the clinical and autopsy incidence (see Chap. 47). Pulmonary emboli should be suspected in patients with recurrent bouts of congestive failure, particularly if cyanosis is present and in patients in whom heart failure does not respond to treatment; it should be suspected when there is pleural effusion confined to the left chest.

Systemic Arterial Embolism. Systemic arterial embolism from mural thrombi in the left ventricle or left atrium may produce cerebral vascular accident, vascular occlusion of the bifurcation of the aorta or of a peripheral artery, mesenteric, splenic, or renal. Systemic arterial embolism may be the major manifestation of silent infarction.[107, 152, 153]

Rupture of the Heart. This causes about 10 per cent of the deaths of patients who die in the hospital after an acute myocardial infarction.[154-161] The peak incidence is within the first week: rupture is rare after 2 weeks. Rupture is almost always due to transmural infarction, particularly of the free wall of the left ventricle. Rupture is more common in the anterolateral region near the apex than with inferior or posterior myocardial infarction. Clinically, this catastrophe may be recognized by sudden worsening of the patient's condition with dyspnea, shock, and strutted neck veins accompanied by pulsus paradoxicus. Death shortly ensues from tamponade. The appearance of a systolic murmur and thrill has occasionally been noted, but these do not generally occur. Death may be sudden and unexpected. Although pericarditis at the site of necrosis has been observed prior to rupture, this finding is of no significant value in predicting rupture. Rupture has been reported to be more common when there has been inadequate rest.

Rupture of the Septum. This occurs in about one-fourth of all cases of myocardial rupture (1 to 20 per cent).[162-166] Although septal rupture is less frequent than external rupture, it is more readily recognized by the abrupt appearance of a pansystolic murmur and thrill characteristic of a ventricular septal defect. Heart failure develops or increases abruptly. About 50 per cent of patients die within 1 week, and only 13 per cent survive 2 months, with rare survival up to 5 years.[167]

Rupture of a Papillary Muscle. This is heralded by the sudden appearance of an apical pansystolic murmur which begins with the first sound and is characteristic of mitral insufficiency.[168-171] It may be rough or musical and may or may not be accompanied by a diastolic rumble. A systolic thrill may be present. There is generally severe congestive failure, and death ensues within a few hours.

Papillary Muscle Dysfunction. Burch has emphasized that papillary muscle dysfunction due to infarction of the anterolateral papillary muscle or its anchoring adjacent myocardium may also produce a systolic murmur at the apex.[172] In this instance, however, the murmur generally has an onset delayed after the first sound, and the murmur may be crescendo-decrescendo in type. This ejection type of murmur serves to differentiate it from the murmur due to rupture of a papillary muscle. It may be transmitted to the second right interspace, where this diamond-shaped murmur may be wrongly attributed to aortic stenosis. In the past, many such murmurs probably due to this syndrome were thought to be due to dilatation of the mitral valve ring. These murmurs may vary in intensity during the course of myocardial infarction, and occasionally they disappear. In other patients the murmur may appear initially during infarction and persist thereafter. Burch has also emphasized that infarction of the anterolateral wall with involvement of the papillary muscle may be accompanied by depression of the ST segment and prominent U waves in the electrocardiogram. However, the syndrome may occur in the presence of conventional transmural infarction patterns.

Ventricular Aneurysm. Ventricular aneurysm of the anatomic type occurs in 20 per cent of cases at autopsy.[173] It more often includes the anterior than the posterior surface. Rupture occasionally occurs during the stage of acute myocardial necrosis, but once healing and scar-tissue formation have occurred, delayed rupture does not occur unless reinfarction develops. Mural thrombi and embolism from the aneurysm produce death in about one-third of patients, whereas, about one-half of patients subsequently die of congestive heart failure with this as a contributory factor in about one-fifth of patients.[173] Contrary findings were reported in a recent study of 65 patients, in whom there was no difference in survival between the groups with and without aneurysm and in whom peripheral embolism was not found as a cause of death. Only one patient showed persistent ST elevation in the electrocardiogram, and only four were diagnosed during life.[174] In only 13.8 per cent of patients could death be attributed to the aneurysm.

Ventricular aneurysm is more common in the presence of diastolic hypertension and perhaps inadequate rest. It is often associated with a visible or palpable systolic sustained thrust at the apex or adjacent area (see p. 100). It may be detected on routine x-ray, but more often fluoroscopy is required to demonstrate the paradoxical movement. Calcification may be detected in the wall of the aneurysm (see p. 157). The patient's electrocardiogram often has ST-segment elevation, inverted T waves, and Q-wave changes which persist in an unvarying pattern for months or years.

The trained observer may detect an ischemic, kinetic, or physiologic aneurysm by inspection and palpation in up to 10 per cent of cases of acute infarction. Such changes may be detected in the majority by the use of the kinetocardiogram (see p. 100). This type of aneurysm may occur transiently during angina pectoris but is more common after infarction. It usually disappears in 2 or 3 weeks. This type of aneurysm can rarely be demonstrated at autopsy, since it depends upon the presence of systolic ventricular pressure. Rarely the abnormal impulse may occur in diastole at the time of rapid ventricular filling.

Pericarditis. This may appear in about 10 per cent of patients after acute myocardial infarction.[132] It usually appears transiently several days after the infarction and often disappears in a few hours to a few days. It may be localized with anterior infarction, but it may be diffuse with either anterior or posterior infarction. Occasionally, a pericardial rub may persist for several weeks. In the circumscribed type the electrocardiographic changes of infarction are not altered; however, when pericarditis is extensive, there may be classic changes of pericarditis superimposed on those due

to infarction. Rarely the accumulation of significant pericardial effusion may produce lowering of amplitude of all complexes. Hemorrhagic pericardial effusion may complicate pericarditis with or without anticoagulant therapy, and, rarely, it produces tamponade. Gross hemopericardium follows rupture of the external myocardium, and peaked T waves have been reported as a sign of this complication.[175]

Post-myocardial Infarction Syndrome. The postmyocardial infarction syndrome,[176-180] as emphasized by Dressler, occurs in a small percentage of patients. The cause is unknown, but it has been attributed to a hypersensitivity reaction in which the antigen is necrotic cardiac muscle. It usually occurs a few weeks or months after myocardial infarction. The syndrome is recognized by the pericardial type of pain, pericardial friction rub, fever, occasionally pneumonitis, left pleural effusion, and leukocytosis, and rarely pericardial effusion with tamponade. It may last days to weeks. It must be differentiated from recurrent myocardial infarction and pulmonary infarction.

Shoulder-Hand Syndrome of Periarthritis. The shoulder-hand syndrone of periarthritis occasionally occurs, but it is distinctly less common than the 15 per cent incidence reported in the past when therapy with rigid rest was in vogue.[181,182] Symptoms include tenderness, stiffness, and discomfort on abduction of the shoulder, usually on the left but occasionally bilaterally. The skin over the hands and fingers may be tense, shiny, and swollen. There may be swelling of the hands and fingers with discoloration. Palmar nodules and Dupuytren's contractures are not infrequent. This neurotrophic disorder may persist for many months and may be mistaken by patients for recurrent angina or infarction.

Chest Wall Syndrome. The chest wall syndrome with localized pain and tenderness is probably of similar origin to the shoulder-hand syndrome, and it may be difficult to differentiate from similar symptoms due to anxiety neurosis.[183]

Hiccups, Retching, Nausea, and Vomiting. These are occasionally troublesome complications. Hiccups are more common with diaphragmatic infarction and may prevent rest. Although nausea and vomiting may be due to myocardial infarction, these symptoms are more frequently due to the administration of opiates or related drugs. Retching is an ominous sign and is associated with a high incidence of arrhythmia. Severe gastric distension, which may induce hypotention, is more common with intranasal oxygen administration. Reflex ileus with abdominal distension and troublesome constipation and fecal impaction may be produced by opiates or potassium depletion following diuresis.

Hemorrhagic disease of the bowel follows prolonged shock.[184] Gastrointestinal hemorrhage due to peptic ulcer may be precipitated by the stress reaction and may be complicated by administration of anticoagulants.[185]

Bladder distension is particularly common in the male with prostatic hypertrophy; it is usually induced by bedrest, opiates, sedatives, or atropine derivatives. The need for an indwelling catheter may predispose to urinary tract infection and rarely to catastrophic Gram-negative septicemia.

Cerebral Infarction. Cerebral infarction due to an abrupt decrease in cardiac output and cerebral blood flow may occur at onset of infarction, particularly if there is atherosclerotic obstruction of the carotid or basilar-vertebral arteries.[107,152] Cerebral infarction due to embolism from mural thrombi in the left ventricle or atrium occurs later during the course of infarction, usually after an interval of several weeks but occasionally after a period of months. Embolism can develop with a normal sinus mechanism, but occasionally atrial fibrillation may be an additional predisposing factor.

Complications. The authors have seen one patient with bacterial endocarditis superimposed on a septal rupture due to infarction, one patient with an infected mural thrombus, and one patient with a myocardial abscess occurring as a result of myocardial infarction in a patient with septicemia.

Sudden numbness, pain, or coldness in an extremity suggests embolic occlusion from a mural thrombus in the left heart. The bifurcation of the aorta is a particularly common site of lodgment, and the iliac and femoral pulses may be diminished or absent bilaterally. Mesenteric, renal, or splenic infarction are less common complications. Renal infarction may produce pain in the renal area, hematuria, and rarely, acute hypertension.

The emotional response of the patient to myocardial infarction is quite variable. To a degree it is conditioned by the approach of the physician. Anxiety of varying degree is common, and a few patients develop depression.

Amnesia, confusion, and personality changes due to a combination of hypotension, impaired cerebral blood flow, and drug administration are rare complications during the early days following infarction.

REFERENCES

1. Enos, W. F., Holmes, R. H., and Beyer, J.: Coronary Disease among United States Soldiers Killed in Action in Korea, *J.A.M.A.,* **152**:1090, 1953.
2. Dock, W.: Why Are Men's Coronary Arteries so Sclerotic? *J.A.M.A.,* **170**:90, 1959.
3. Gertler, M. M., Driskell, M. M., Bland, E. F.,

Garn, S. M., Lerman, J., Levine, S. A., Sprague, H. B., and White, P. D.: Clinical Aspects of Coronary Heart Disease, *J.A.M.A.,* **146**:1291, 1951.
4. Yater, W. M., Traum, A. H., Brown, W. G., Fitzgerald, R. P., Geisler, M. A., and Wilcox, B. B.: Coronary Artery Disease in Men 18 to 39 Years of Age: Report of 866 Cases, 450 with Necropsy Examination, *Am. Heart J.,* **36**:334, **481**, 683, 1948.
5. Poe, W. D.: Fatal Coronary Artery Disease in Young Men, *Am. Heart J.,* **33**:76, 1947.
6. Gertler, M. M., Woodbury, M. A., Gottsch, L. G., White, P. D., and Rusk, H. A.: The Candidate for Coronary Heart Disease: Discriminating Power of Biochemical Hereditary and Anthropometric Measurements, *J.A.M.A.,* **170**:87, 1959.
7. Seminar on Atherosclerosis, *Am. J. Med.,* **23**:120, 269, 463, 653, 769, 928, 1957.
8. Blumgart, H. S., Schlesinger, M. J., and Davis, D.: Studies on the Relation of the Clinical Manifestations of Angina Pectoris, Coronary Thrombosis, and Myocardial Infarction to the Pathological findings, *Am. Heart J.,* **19**:1, 1940.
9. Blumgart, H. L., Schlesinger, M. J., and Zoll, P. M.: Angina Pectoris, Coronary Failure and Acute Myocardial Failure, *J.A.M.A.,* **116**:91, 1941.
10. Zoll, P. M., Wessler, S., and Blumgart, H. L.: Angina Pectoris: A Clinical and Pathologic Correlation, *Am. J. Med.,* **11**:331, 1951.
11. Plotz, M.: "Coronary Heart Disease: Angina Pectoris; Myocardial Infarction," Hoeber Medical Division, Harper & Row, Publishers, Inc., New York, 1957.
12. The Criteria Committee of the New York Association: *Diseases of the Heart and Blood Vessels. Nomenclature and Criteria for Diagnosis,* 6th ed., Little, Brown and Company, Boston, 1964.
13. Sones, F. M.: Personal communication.
14. Master, A. M., et al.: Acute Coronary Insufficiency Due to Acute Hemorrhage: An Analysis of One Hundred and Three Cases, *Circulation,* **1**:1302, 1950.
15. Costantin, L.: Extracardiac Factors Contributing to Hypotension during Coronary Occlusion, *Am. J. Cardiol.,* **11**:205, 1963.
16. Proger, S., and Selverstone, L. A.: The Diagnosis of Coronary Heart Disease, in M. A. Jones (ed.), "Modern Trends in Cardiology," Hoeber Medical Division, Harper & Row, Publishers, Incorporated, New York, 1961.
17. Somerville, W., and Levine, S. A.: Angina Pectoris and Thyrotoxicosis, *Brit. Heart J.,* **12**:245, 1950.
18. Heberden, W.: Some Account of a Disorder of the Heart, *Med. Tr. Roy. Coll. Physicians,* **2**:59, 1768.
19. Williams, F. A., and Keys, T. E.: "Cardiac Classics," The C. V. Mosby Company, St. Louis, 1941, p. 267.
20. Osler, W.: The Lumleian Lectures on Angina Pectoris, *Lancet,* **1**:839, 1910.

21. Herrick, J. B.: Clinical Features of Sudden Obstruction of the Coronary Arteries, *J.A.M.A.,* **59:** 201, 1912.

22. MacKenzie, J.: "Angina Pectoris," Oxford University Press, New York, 1924.

23. Keefer, C. S., and Resnik, W. H.: Angina Pectoris: A Syndrome Caused by Anoxia of the Myocardium, *A.M.A. Arch. Int. Med.,* **41:**769, 1928.

24. Bourne, G., and Scott, R. B.: Angina of Effort: A Clinical Study, *Brit. M. J.* 1:55, 1938.

25. Spillane, J. D., and White, P. D.: Atypical Pain in Angina Pectoris and Myocardial Infarction, *Brit. Heart J.,* 2:123, 1940.

26. Harrison, T. R.: The Clinical Aspects of Pain in the Chest. I. Angina Pectoris, *Am. J. M. Sc.,* **207:** 561, 1944.

27. Hecht, H. H.: Concepts of Myocardial Ischemia, *A.M.A. Arch. Int. Med.,* **84:**711, 1949.

28. Rinzler, S. H.: "Cardiac Pain," Charles C Thomas, Publisher, Springfield, Ill., 1951, p. 139.

29. Riseman, J. E. F.: Differential Diagnosis of Angina Pectoris, *Circulation,* 14:422, 1956.

30. Ernstene, A. C.: Differential Diagnosis of the Pain of Coronary Heart Disease, *Ann. Int. Med.,* **46:**247, 1957.

31. Prinzmetal, M., Kennamer, R., Merliss, R., Wada, T., and Bor, N.: Angina Pectoris. I. A Variant Form of Angina Pectoris: Preliminary Report, *Am. J. Med.,* 27:375, 1959.

32. Harrison, T. R.: Some Clinical and Physiologic Aspects of Angina Pectoris, *Bull. Johns Hopkins Hosp.,* **104:**275, 1959.

33. Andrus, E. C.: Diagnosis of Angina Pectoris, *Circulation,* 22:979, 1960.

34. Prinzmetal, M., Ekmekci, A., Kennamer, R., Kwoczynski, J. K., Shubin, H., and Toyoshima, H.: Variant Form of Angina Pectoris: Previously Undelineated Syndrome, *J.A.M.A.,* **174:**1094, 1960.

35. Burwell, C. S.: A Commentary on Professor John Warren's Paper, "Remarks on Angina Pectoris," *New England J. Med.,* **266:**7, 1962.

36. Katz, L. N., Silber, E. N., Kossman, C. E., Burch, G. E., and Blumgart, H. L.: Pitfalls in Diagnosing Coronary Artery Disease, *Circulation,* **28:**274, 1963.

37. Morris, J. J., and McIntosh, H. D.: Angina of Micturition, *Circulation,* **27:**85, 1963.

38. Levine, S. A.: Carotid Sinus Massage: A New Diagnostic Test for Angina Pectoris, *J.A.M.A.,* **182:**1331, 1962.

39. Dock, W.: "Heart Sounds, Cardiac Pulsations, and Coronary Disease," University of Kansas Press, Lawrence, Kan., 1956.

40. Skinner, N. S., Jr., Leibeskind, R. S., Phillips, H. L., and Harrison, T. R.: Angina Pectoris: Effect of Exertion and Nitrites on Precordial Movements, *Am. Heart J.,* **61:**250, 1961.

41. Dimond, E. G.: Precordial Vibrations: Clinical Clues from Palpitation, *Circulation,* **30:**284, 1964.

42. Wood, P.: Da Costa's Syndrome (or Effort Syndrome), *Brit. M. J.,* 1:767, 1941.

43. Okel, B. B., and Hurst, J. W.: Prolonged Hyperventilation in Man, *Arch. Int. Med.,* **108:**757–762, 1961.

44. Davis, D.: Radicular Syndromes, with Emphasis on Chest Pain Simulating Coronary Heart Disease, Year Book Publishers, Chicago, 1957.

45. Good, A. E.: The Chest Pain of Ankylosing Spondylitis: Its Place in the Differential Diagnosis of Heart Pain, *Ann. Int. Med.,* **58:**926, 1963.

46. Kayser, H. L.: Tietze's Syndrome: A Review of the Literature, *Am. J. Med.,* 21:982, 1956.

47. Wehrmacher, W. H.: Significance of Tietze's Syndrome in Differential Diagnosis of Chest Pain, *J.A.M.A.,* **157:**505, 1955.

48. Ausubel, H., Cohen, B. D., and LaDue, J. S.: Tietze's Disease of Eight Years' Duration, *New England J. Med.,* **261:**190, 1959.

49. Barnes, N., and Graham, J.: Parasternal Chondrodynis (Tietze's Syndrome), *Ann. Int. Med.,* **50:** 57, 1959.

50. Russek, H. I.: Shoulder-Hand Syndrome Following Myocardial Infarction, *M. Clin. North America,* **42:**1555, 1958.

51. Mondor, H.: Tronculite sous-cutanée subaiguë de la paroi thoracique antéro-latérale, *Mém. Acad. chir. Paris,* **65:**1271, 1939.

52. Mondor, M. H.: Phlébite en cordon de la paroi thoracique, *Mém. Acad. chir. Paris,* **70:**96, 1944.

53. Castleton, K. B., Cloud, R. S., and Ward, J. R.: Anterior Chest Wall: Superficial Thrombophlebitis, *Arch. Surg.,* **88:**1010, 1964.

54. Miller, A. J., and Texidor, T. A.: The "precordial catch": A Syndrome of Anterior Chest Pain, *Ann. Int. Med.,* **51:**461, 1959.

55. Wehrmacher, W. H.: The Painful Anterior Chest Wall Syndromes, *M. Clin. North America,* **42:**111, 1958.

56. Harrison, T. R.: The Clinical Aspects of Pain in the Chest. II. Pain Arising from the Esophagus, *Am. J. M. Sc.,* **209:**765, 1945.

57. Harrison, T. R.: The Clinical Aspects of Pain in the Chest. III. Pain Arising from the Stomach, *Am. J. M. Sc.,* **209:**771, 1945.

58. Kramer, P., and Hollander, W.: Comparison of Experimental Esophageal Pain with Clinical Pain of Angina Pectoris and Esophageal Disease, *Gastroenterology,* **29:**719, 1955.

59. Bernstein, L. M., Fruin, R. C., and Pacini, R.: Differentiation of Esophageal Pain from Angina Pectoris: Role of the Esophageal Acid Perfusion Test, *Medicine,* **41:**143, 1962.

60. Alder, R. H.: Hiatal Hernia and Esophagitis, *Surg. Gynec. & Obst.,* **116:**1, 1963.

61. Reeves, T. J., and Harrison, T. R.: Diagnostic and Therapeutic Value of the Reproduction of Chest Pain, *A.M.A. Arch. Int. Med.,* **91:**8, 1953.

62. Viar, W. V., and Harrison, T. R.: Chest Pain in Association with Pulmonary Hypertension: Its

Similarity to the Pain of Coronary Disease, *Circulation*, **5**:1, 1952.

63. Ross, R. S.: Right Ventricular Hypertension as a Cause of Precordial Pain, *Am. Heart J.*, **61**:134, 1961.

64. Braun, K.: Pulmonary Artery Dilatation as a Cause of Chest Pain, *Am. Heart J.*, **62**:715, 1961.

65. Boyer, N. H., and White, P. D.: Right Upper Quadrant Pain on Effort: Early Symptom of Failure of Right Ventricle, *N. England J. Med.*, **226**: 217–220, 1942.

66. Feil, H., and Siegel, M. L.: Electrocardiographic Changes during Attacks of Angina Pectoris, *Am. J. M. Sc.*, **175**:256, 1928.

67. Lepeschkin, E.: Exercise Tests in the Diagnosis of Coronary Heart Disease, *Circulation*, **22**:986, 1960.

68. Scherf, D., and Schaffer, A. I.: The Electrocardiographic Exercise Test, *Am. Heart J.*, **43**:927, 1952.

69. Mattingly, T. W., Robb, G. P., and Marks, H. H.: Stress Tests in the Detection of Coronary Disease, *Postgrad. Med.*, **24**:4, 1958.

70. Simonson, E.: Use of the Electrocardiogram in Exercise Tests, *Am. Heart J.*, **66**:552, 1963.

71. Wood, P. W., McGregor, M., Mogidson, O., and Whittaker, W.: The Effort Test in Angina Pectoris, *Brit. Heart J.*, **12**:363, 1950.

72. Dimond, E. G.: "The Exercise Electrocardiogram in Office Practice," Charles C Thomas, Publisher, Springfield, Ill., 1961.

73. Friedberg, C. K., Jaffe, H. L., Pordy, L., and Chesky, K.: The Two-step Exercise Electrocardiogram: A Double-blind Evaluation of Its Use in the Diagnosis of Angina Pectoris, *Circulation*, **26**: 1254, 1962.

74. Master, A. M.: Chest Pain and the Master "Two-step" Exercise Test: Indications and Criteria, in W. Likoff and J. H. Moyer (eds.),"The Seventh Hahnemann Symposium," Grune & Stratton, Inc., New York, 1963, pp. 209–214.

75. Hellerstein, H. K., Prozan, G. B., Liebow, I. M., Doan, A. E., and Henderson, J. A.: Two-step Exercise Test of Cardiac Function in Chronic Rheumatic Heart Disease and in Arteriosclerotic Heart Disease with Old Myocardial Infarction, *Am. J. Cardiol.*, **7**:234, 1961.

75a. Ekmekci, A., Toyoshima, H., Kwoczynski, J. K., Nagaya, T., and Prinzmetal, M.: Angina Pectoris. IV. Clinical and Experimental Difference between Ischemia with ST Elevation and Ischemia with ST Depression, *Am. J. Cardiol.*, **7**:412, 1961.

76. Lamb, L. E., and Hiss, R. G.: Influence of Exercise on Premature Contractions, *Am. J. Cardiol.*, **10**:209, 1962.

77. Bellet, S., Eliakim, M., Deliyiannis, S., and LaVan, D.: Radioelectrocardiography during Exercise in Patients with Angina Pectoris, *Circulation*, **25**:5, 1962.

78. Robb, G. P., and Marks, H. H.: The Post-exercise Electrocardiogram in the Detection of Coronary Disease: A Long Term Evaluation, *Tr. A. Life Insurance M. Directors America*, **45**:81, 1962.

78a. Sheffield, L. T., and Reeves, T. J.: Graded Exercise in the Diagnosis of Angina Pectoris. *Modern Concepts of Cardiovascular Disease*, **34**:1, 1965.

78b. Bruce, R. A., Jones, J. W., and Strait, G. B.: Anaerobic Metabolic Responses to Acute Maximal Exercise in Male Athletes, *Am. Heart J.*, **67**:643, 1964.

79. Feil, H.: Preliminary Pain in Coronary Thrombosis, *Am. J. M. Sc.*, **193**:42, 1937.

80. Blumgart, H. L., Schlesinger, M. J., and Zoll, P. M.: Angina Pectoris, Coronary Failure and Acute Myocardial Infarction: The Role of Coronary Occlusion and Collateral Circulation, *J.A.M.A.*, **116**:91–97, 1941.

81. Freedberg, A. S., Blumgart, H. L., Zoll, P. M., and Schlesinger, M. J.: Coronary Failure: The Clinical Syndrome of Cardiac Pain Intermediate between Angina Pectoris and Acute Myocardial Infarction, *J.A.M.A.*, **138**:107, 1948.

82. Mounsey, P.: Prodromal Symptoms in Myocardial Infarction, *Brit. Heart J.*, **13**:215, 1951.

83. Scherf, D., and Golbey, M.: Critique: An Evaluation of the Term "Coronary Insufficiency," *Am. Heart J.*, **47**:928, 1954.

84. Graybiel, A.: The Intermediate Coronary Syndrome, *U.S. Armed Forces M. J.*, **6**:1, 1955.

85. Master, A. M., et al.: Acute Coronary Insufficiency: Its Differential Diagnosis and Treatment, *Ann. Int. Med.*, **45**:561, 1956.

86. Feil, H.: The Problems of Acute Coronary Attacks without Classic Electrocardiographic Signs of Acute Myocardial Infarction, *Progr. Cardiovas. Dis.*, **1**:165, 1958.

87. Vakil, R. J.: Intermediate Coronary Syndrome, *Circulation*, **24**:557, 1961.

88. Resnik, W. H.: The Significance of Prolonged Anginal Pain (Preinfarction Angina), *Am. Heart J.*, **63**:290, 1962.

89. Resnik, W. H.: Preinfarction Angina. II. An Interpretation, *Mod. Concepts Cardiovas. Dis.*, **31**: 757, 1962.

90. Snow, P. J. D., Morgan Jones, A., and Daber, K. S.: A Clinico-pathological Study of Coronary Disease, *Brit. Heart J.*, **18**:435, 1956.

91. Hurst, J. W., and Schlant, R. C.: Acute Phases: Infarction in *The Heart and Circulation*, 2nd National Conference on Cardiovascular Disease, vol. 1, part 1, p. 816. American Heart Association and U.S. Public Health Service, Washington, D.C., 1964.

92. Herrick, J. B.: Thrombosis of Coronary Arteries, *J.A.M.A.*, **72**:387, 1919.

93. Levine, S. A.: Coronary Thrombosis: Its Various Clinical Features, *Medicine*, **8**:245, 1929.

94. Wood, P.: Acute and Subacute Coronary Insufficiency, *Brit. M. J.*, **1**:1779, 1961.

95. Master, A. M.: Acute Coronary Diseases, *Am. J. Med.*, **2**:501, 1947.

96. Selzer, A.: Clinical Observations in Cases of Massive Myocardial Infarction, *A.M.A. Arch. Int. Med.*, 82:196, 1948.

97. Butterworth, J. S., and Reppert, E. H., Jr.: Auscultatory Findings in Myocardial Infarction, *Circulation*, 22:448, 1960.

98. Lindberg, H. A., Berkson, D. M., Stamler, J., and Poindexter, A.: Totally Asymptomatic Myocardial Infarction: An Estimate of Its Incidence in the Living Population, *Arch. Int. Med.*, 106:628, 1960.

99. Rosemen, M. D.: Painless Myocardial Infarction. A Review of the Literature and Analysis of 220 Cases, *Ann. Int. Med.*, 41:118, 1954.

100. Evans, W., and Sutton, G. C.: Painless Cardiac Infarction, *Brit. Heart J.*, 18:259, 1956.

101. Marchand, W. E.: Occurrence of Painless Myocardial Infarction in Psychotic Patients, *New England J. Med.*, 254:307, 1956.

102. Stokes, J., III, and Dawber, T. R.: The "Silent Coronary": The Frequency and Clinical Characteristics of Unrecognized Myocardial Infarction in the Framingham Study, *Ann. Int. Med.*, 50:1359, 1959.

103. Wróblewski, F., and LaDue, J. S.: Myocardial Infarction as a Postoperative Complication of Major Surgery, *J.A.M.A.*, 150:1212, 1952.

104. Landman, M. E., Anhalt, H. S., and Angrist, A.: Asymptomatic Myocardial Infarction, *A.M.A. Arch. Int. Med.*, 83:665, 1949.

105. Evans, W., and Sutton, G. C.: Painless Cardiac Infarction, *Brit. Heart J.*, 18:259, 1956.

106. Driscoll, A. C., Hobika, J. H., Etsten, B. E., and Proger, S.: Clinically Unrecognized Myocardial Infarction Following Surgery, *New England J. Med.*, 264:633, 1961.

107. Harrison, C. E., Jr., Spittel, J. A., Jr., and Mankin, H. T.: Sudden Arterial Occlusion: A Clue to Silent Myocardial Infarction, *Proc. Staff Meet. Mayo Clin.*, 37:293, 1962.

108. Levine, S. A.: "Clinical Heart Disease," 5th ed., W. B. Saunders Company, Philadelphia, 1958.

109. Hamman, L.: "Spontaneous Mediastinal Emphysema, *Bull. Johns Hopkins Hosp.*, 64:1, 1939.

110. Ruttenberg, T. A., and Golden, R.: Spontaneous Pneumothorax: Study of 105 Cases, *Radiology*, 53:157, 1949.

111. Bloomfield, A. L.: Mechanism of Pain with Peptic Ulcer, *Am. J. Med.*, 17:165, 1954.

112. Jones, F. A.: Hematemesis and Melena: With Special Reference to Causation and to Factors Influencing the Mortality from Bleeding Peptic Ulcers, *Gastroenterology*, 30:166, 1956.

113. Gay, B. B., and Priviteri, C. A.: Spontaneous Rupture of the Esophagus with Report of Five Cases, *Radiology*, 57:48, 1951.

114. Clain, A., and Heffernan, S. J.: Spontaneous Rupture of the Esophagus: Diagnosis and Successful Management, *Lancet*, 2:1284, 1956.

115. Riceman, A.: Acute Pancreatitis, *Am. J. Med.*, 21:246, 1956.

116. Shillito, F. H., Chamberlain, F. L., and Levy, R. L.: Cardiac Infarction: The Incidence and Correlation of Various Signs, with Remarks on Prognosis, *J.A.M.A.*, 118:779, 1942.

117. Plotz, M.: Sedimentation Rate in Myocardial Infarction, *Am. J. M. Sc.*, 224:23, 1952.

118. Goldberger, E., Alesio, J., and Woll, F.: Significance of Hyperglycemia in Myocardial Infarction, *New York J. Med.*, 45:391, 1945.

119. LaDue, J. S., Wroblewski, F., and Karmen, A.: Serum Glutamic Oxaloacetic Transaminase Activity in Human Acute Transmural Myocardial Infarction, *Science*, 120:497, 1954.

120. Friedberg, C. K.: Cardiac Pain, the Electrocardiogram, Serum Transaminase and the Diagnosis of Myocardial Infarction, Subendocardial Necrosis or Myocardial Ischemia, *Progr. Cardiovas. Dis.*, 1:109, 1958.

121. Sampson, J. J.: Serum Transaminase and Other Enzymes in Acute Myocardial Infarction, *Progr. Cardiovas. Dis.*, 1:187, 1958.

122. Agress, C. M.: Evaluation of the Transaminase Test, *Am. J. Cardiol.*, 3:74, 1959.

123. Symposium on Diagnostic Enzymology, *Am. J. Med.*, 27:849, 1959.

124. Wróblewski, F.: The Clinical Significance of Transaminase Activities of Serum, *Am. J. Med.*, 27:911, 1959.

125. Killip, T., III, and Payne, M. A.: High Serum Transaminase Activity in Heart Disease, *Circulation*, 21:646, 1960.

126. Agress, C. M., and Kim, J. H. C.: Evaluation of Enzyme Tests in the Diagnosis of Heart Disease, *Am. J. Cardiol.*, 6:641, 1960.

127. Hamolsky, M. W., and Kaplan, N. O.: Measurements of Enzymes in the Diagnosis of Acute Myocardial Infarction, *Circulation*, 23:102, 1961.

128. Meyers, F., and Evans, J. M.: The Serum Transaminase (S-Got) and Electrocardiogram in Autopsy-confirmed Acute Myocardial Infarction, *Am. Heart J.*, 67:15, 1964.

129. Wróblewski, F., Ross, C., and Gregory, K.: Isoenzymes and Myocardial Infarction, *New England J. Med.*, 263:531, 1960.

130. Galler, E.: Personal communication.

131. Levine, H. D., and Ford, R. V.: Subendocardial Infarction: Report of Six Cases and Critical Survey of the Literature, *Circulation*, 1:246, 1950.

132. Pearson, H. E.: The Early Complications of Cardiac Infarction, *Brit. M. J.*, 2:4, 1953.

133. Ernstene, A. C.: Complications and Sequelae of Acute Myocardial Infarction, *J.A.M.A.*, 150:1069, 1952.

134. McQuay, N. W., Edwards, J. E., and Burchell, H. B.: Types of Death in Acute Myocardial Infarction, *A.M.A. Arch. Int. Med.*, 96:1, 1955.

135. Johnson, C. C., and Miner, P. F.: The Occurrence of Arrhythmias in Acute Myocardial Infarction, *Dis. Chest*, 33:414, 1958.

136. Bainton, C. R., and Peterson, D. R.: Death from

Coronary Heart Disease in Persons 50 Years of Age and Younger: A Community-wide study, *New England J. Med.*, **268**:569, 1963.

137. Hartenauer, G., Dewees, R. L., and Krieger, E. M.: Acute Myocardial Infarction, *Delaware M. J.*, **35**:167, 1963.

138. Spain, D. M., Brodess, V. A., and Mohr, C.: Coronary Atherosclerosis as a Cause of Unexpected and Unexplained Death, *J.A.M.A.*, **174**:384–388, 1960.

139. Hellerstein, H. K., and Turell, D. J.: Mode of Death in Coronary Artery Disease: Electrocardiographic and Clinical-pathologic Correlation, *Circulation*, **18**:735, 1958.

140. James, T. N., and Hershey, E. A.: Experimental Studies on the Pathogenesis of Atrial Arrhythmias in Myocardial Infarction, *Am. Heart J.*, **63**:196, 1962.

141. James, T. N.: Myocardial Infarction and Atrial Arrhythmias, *Circulation*, **24**:761, 1961.

142. James, T. N.: Arrhythmias and Conduction Disturbances in Acute Myocardial Infarction, *Am. Heart J.*, **64**:416, 1962.

143. Cohen, D. B., Doctor, L., and Pick, A.: The Significance of Atrioventricular Block Complicating Acute Myocardial Infarction, *Am. Heart J.*, **55**:215, 1958.

144. Courter, S. R., Moffat, J., and Fowler, N. O.: Advanced Atrioventricular Block in Acute Myocardial Infarction, *Circulation*, **27**:1034, 1963.

145. Spann, J. F., Jr., Moellering, R. C., Jr., Haber, E., and Wheeler, E. O.: Arrhythmias in Acute Myocardial Infarction: A Study Utilizing Electrocardiographic Monitor for Automatic Detection and Recording of Arrhythmias, *New England J. Med.*, **271**:427, 1964.

146. Sampson, J. J.: Shock of Cardiac Origin, *Mod. Concepts Cardiovas. Dis.*, **26**:379, 1957.

147. Agress, C. M., and Binder, M. J.: Cardiogenic Shock, *Am. Heart J.*, **54**:458, 1957.

148. Guzman, S. V., Swenson, E., and Mitchell, R.: Mechanism of Cardiogenic Shock, *Circulation Res.*, **10**:746, 1962.

149. Heyer, H. E.: A Clinical Study of Shock Occurring during Acute Myocardial Infarction: An Analysis of 58 Cases, *Am. Heart J.*, **62**:436, 1961.

150. Friedberg, C. K.: Cardiogenic Shock in Acute Myocardial Infarction (Editorial), *Circulation*, **23**:325, 1961.

151. Logue, R. B., Rogers, J. V., Jr., and Gay, B. B., Jr.: Subtle Roentgenographic Signs of Left Heart Failure, *Am. Heart J.*, **65**:464, 1963.

152. Glathe, J. P., and Achor, R. W. P.: Frequency of Cardiac Disease in Patients with Strokes, *Proc. Staff Meet. Mayo Clin.*, **33**:417, 1958.

153. Hellerstein, H. K., and Martin, J. W.: Incidence of Thromboembolic Lesions Accompanying Myocardial Infarction, *Am. Heart J.*, **33**:443, 1947.

154. Jetter, W. W., and White, P. D.: Rupture of the Heart in Patients in Mental Institutions, *Ann. Int. Med.*, **21**:783, 1944.

155. Wessler, S., Zoll, P. M., and Schlesinger, M. J.: The Pathogenesis of Spontaneous Cardiac Rupture, *Circulation*, **6**:334, 1952.

156. Oblath, R. W., Levinson, D. C., and Griffith, G. C.: Factors Influencing Rupture of the Heart after Myocardial Infarction, *J.A.M.A.*, **149**:1276, 1954.

157. Maher, J. F., Mallory, G. K., and Laurenzi, C. A.: Rupture of the Heart after Myocardial Infarction, *New England J. Med.*, **225**:1, 1956.

158. Kohn, R. M.: Mechanical Factors in Cardiac Rupture, *Am. J. Cardiol.*, **4**:440, 1959.

159. Sigler, L. H.: Rupture of the Heart in Myocardial Infarction, *Am. J. Cardiol.*, **5**:14, 1960.

160. Zeman, F. D., and Rodstein, M.: Cardiac Rupture Complicating Myocardial Infarction in the Aged, *A.M.A. Arch. Int. Med.*, **105**:431, 1960.

161. Griffith, G. C., Hegde, B., and Oblath, R. W.: Factors in Myocardial Rupture: An Analysis of Two Hundred and Four Cases at Los Angeles County Hospital between 1924 and 1951, *Am. J. Cardiol.*, **8**:792, 1961.

162. Bond, V. F., et al.: Perforation of the Interventricular Septum Following Myocardial Infarction, *Ann. Int. Med.*, **38**:706, 1953.

163. Shickman, M. D., Fields, J., and Pearce, M. L.: Repair of Ruptured Interventricular Septum Complicating Acute Myocardial Infarction, *A.M.A. Arch. Int. Med.*, **103**:140, 1959.

164. Bohan, J. L., and Stansbury, F.: Myocardial Infarction Followed by Septal Perforation, *J.A.M.A.*, **173**:1004, 1960.

165. Landale, D. G., and Schlappi, J. C.: Thirteen-year Survival with Acquired Interventricular Septal Defect after Myocardial Infarction, *Am. Heart J.*, **64**:33, 1962.

166. Lee, W. Y., Cardon, L., and Slodki, S. J.: Perforation of Intraventricular Septum, *Arch. Int. Med.*, **109**:731, 1962.

167. Sanders, R. J., Kern, W. H., and Blount, S. G., Jr.: Perforation of the Interventricular Septum Complicating Myocardial Infarction, *Am. Heart J.*, **51**:736, 1956.

168. Craddock, W. L., and Mahe, G. A.: Rupture of Papillary Muscle of Heart Following Myocardial Infarction: Differential Criteria from Perforation of Interventricular Septum, *J.A.M.A.*, **151**:884, 1953.

169. Sanders, R. J., Neuberger, K. T., and Ravin, A.: Rupture of Papillary Muscles: Occurrence of Rupture of the Posterior Muscle in Posterior Myocardial Infarction, *Dis. Chest*, **31**:316, 1957.

170. Beaghler, R. L., and Laurain, A. R.: Rupture of Cardiac Papillary Muscle, *Arch. Path.*, **76**:609, 1963.

171. Breneman, G. M., and Drake, E. H.: Ruptured Papillary Muscle Following Myocardial Infarction with Long Survival: Report of Two Cases, *Circulation*, **25**:862, 1962.

172. Burch, G. E., DePasquale, N. P., and Phillips,

J. H.: Clinical Manifestations of Papillary Muscle Dysfunction, *Arch. Int. Med.,* **112:**112, 1963.

173. Schlichter, J., Hellerstein, H. K., and Katz, L. N.: Aneurysm of the Heart: A Correlated Study of 102 Proved Cases, *Medicine,* **33:**43, 1954.

174. Abrams, D. L., Edelist, A., Luria, M. H., and Miller, A. J.: Ventricular Aneurysm: A Reappraisal Based on a Study of Sixty-five Consecutive Autopsied Cases, *Circulation,* **27:**164, 1963.

175. London, R. E., and London, S. B.: The Electrocardiographic Sign of Acute Hemopericardium, *Circulation,* **25:**780, 1962.

176. Dressler, W., and Leavitt, S. S.: Pericarditis after Acute Myocardial Infarction, *J.A.M.A.,* **173:**1225, 1960.

177. Dressler, W.: A Post-myocardial Infarction Syndrome, *J.A.M.A.,* **160:**1379, 1956.

178. Dressler, W.: The Post-myocardial Infarction Syndrome: A Report on Forty-four Cases, *A.M.A. Arch. Int. Med.,* **103:**28, 1959.

179. Weiser, N. J., Kantor, M., and Russell, H. K.: Postmyocardial Infarction Syndrome, *Circulation,* **20:** 371, 1959.

180. Weiser, N. J., Kantor, M., Russell, H. K., and Murphy, L.: The Post-myocardial Infarction Syndrome: The Nonspecificity of the Pulmonary Manifestations, *Circulation,* **25:**643, 1962.

181. Russek, H. I.: Shoulder-hand Syndrome Following Myocardial Infarction, *M. Clin. North America,* **42:**1555, 1958.

182. Johnson, A. C.: Disabling Changes in the Hands Resembling Aclerodactylia Following Myocardial Infarction, *Ann. Int. Med.,* **19:**433, 1943.

183. Edwards, W. L.: Musculoskeletal Chest Pain Following Myocardial Infarction, *Am. Heart J.,* **49:** 713, 1955.

184. Bachrach, W. H., and Thorner, M. C.: Hemorrhagic Enteropathy Complicating Myocardial Infarction, *Am. J. Cardiol.,* **11:**89, 1963.

185. Shipp, J. C., Sidel, V. W., Donaldson, R. M., Jr., and Gray, S. J.: Serious Complications of Peptic Ulcer after Acute Myocardial Infarction, *New England J. Med.,* **261:**222, 1959.

33 CINE CORONARY ARTERIOGRAPHY *

F. Mason Sones, Jr., M.D.

During the past 6 years, the technique of cine coronary arteriography has been developed in an effort to provide a more objective and precise

* Revision of F. M. Sones, Jr., and E. K. Shirey: Cine Coronary Arteriography, *Mod. Concepts Cardiovas. Dis.,* vol. 31, no. 7, July, 1962. Printed with permission of American Heart Association, Inc.

standard of diagnosis for human coronary artery disease. Heretofore, the diagnosis of coronary atherosclerosis has been primarily dependent on the physician's interpretation of the efforts of distressed patients to describe chest pain and upon recognition of transient or chronic electrocardiographic changes which usually indicate the presence of myocardial ischemia or necrosis. Although conscientious, knowledgeable history taking and electrocardiographic study require no apologies for their contributions to understanding, their limitations have been responsible, even in the hands of experts, for the production of iatrogenic disability on the one hand and unjustified reassurance on the other in a significant number of patients. A safe and dependable method for demonstrating the physical characteristics of the human coronary artery tree, which could be applied in any phase of the natural history of coronary artery disease, was needed to supplement available diagnostic methods.

Direct coronary artery catheterization has been used for deliberate selective opacification of individual coronary arteries in more than 4,200 patients.

Preliminary studies performed in the author's laboratory from 1956 through the first 6 months of 1958 on dogs and human beings without clinical evidence of coronary artery disease demonstrated that dependable opacification of the normal coronary artery tree could not be achieved by conventional aortographic techniques. Doses of contrast mediums, ranging from 40 to 60 ml, were injected into the aortic root under pressures of 10 kg per cm² with a Gidlund pressure syringe and provided adequate visualization of major branches of the right and left coronary arteries in fewer than 70 per cent of the patients studied.[1]

The use of acetylcholine to produce asystole and facilitate improved coronary perfusion with smaller doses of contrast medium was explored by Lehman and associates.[2] In the author's laboratory this seemed undesirable because of the variable response of different patients to similar doses of the drug and because the consequences of its use in patients with unknown degrees of myocardial ischemia were feared.

Dotter and associates[3] proposed the introduction of a balloon catheter into the ascending aorta to produce temporary aortic occlusion while injecting a small dose of contrast substance above the aortic valve. While this undoubtedly resulted in effective concentrations of dye reaching the coronary circulation, the combined hazards of sudden obstruction to left ventricular outflow and accidental displacement of the balloon made routine application seem undesirable.

In October of 1958, the first deliberate efforts

to perform "selective" coronary arteriography were made in the author's laboratory. Serial doses of 20 to 30 ml contrast medium were injected under a pressure of 4 kg per cm² into a catheter after its tip was carefully placed in first one and then the other anterior sinus of Valsalva. This ensured the introduction of a large volume of dye into the immediate vicinity of each coronary orifice during the interval of three to six heart cycles. In a series of 137 patients studied by this method, visualization of each coronary artery was considered to be adequate in more than 90 per cent. Ventricular arrhythmias, which had been feared as a consequence of transient asymmetrical myocardial hypoxia with this method of delivery, failed to materialize in this group of patients. During this experience, clear-cut demonstration of intercoronary collateral channels was first observed in the living human being. It was also noted that coronary artery orifices could occasionally be catheterized without causing injury to the patient.

In April, 1959, a special catheter was fabricated at the author's request by the United States Catheter and Instrument Company for this specific purpose. The shaft of this thin-walled radiopaque woven catheter is 2.7 mm in external diameter (8 French) to provide enough rigidity for dependable manipulation in the systolic jet immediately above the aortic valve. The tip is open, and four side openings are arranged in opposed pairs within 7 mm of its distal end. The shaft is sharply tapered to an external diameter of 1.6 mm (5 French) at a point 5 cm from its tip. This provides an extremely flexible "fingertip," which may be curved upward into the coronary orifices by pressure of the more rigid shaft against the aortic valve cusps. It has been possible to enter both coronary arteries in 99 per cent of the 4,200 patients studied. In no instance has failure to enter at least one vessel occurred. Since each artery is routinely photographed in multiple projections, a total of more than 35,000 individual arteriograms was recorded in this group of patients.

Technique

General anesthesia is never used. One hour before the procedure the patient is given a single injection of 1.2 million units of Bicillin C-R 300 (benzathine penicillin G and procaine penicillin G). If the patient gives a history of sensitivity to penicillin, 500 mg erythromycin is administered 2 hr before the procedure, and the drug is maintained in doses of 250 mg four times daily for 2 days.

All patients are given 180 mg sodium phenobarbital by hypodermic 1 hr before the procedure.

The right brachial artery is exposed by a small cutdown immediately above the skin crease in the right antecubital fossa following infiltration of the area with 2 per cent procaine hydrocloride. Two soft umbilical tapes are looped beneath the artery. Thirty milligrams of heparin in 6 ml normal saline solution is slowly instilled into the artery below the tapes to prevent thrombosis in distal radicals of the artery. Under direct vision, the vessel is catheterized through the smallest possible arteriotomy between the umbilical tapes. Slight traction on the distal tape below the arteriotomy prevents backbleeding. If bleeding occurs around the catheter from above the arteriotomy, a sterile rubber band is passed around the artery and the indwelling catheter immediately above the arteriotomy and secured under slight tension with a small forceps. This does not interfere with catheter manipulation.

The catheter tip is passed through the brachial, subclavian, and brachiocephalic arteries to the ascending aorta at the level of the aortic valve. The patient is asked to roll toward the operator onto his right side. This places him in a comfortable position in the left anterior oblique position. In this projection, the left coronary sinus of Valsalva lies in the aortic root, above the aortic annulus in a position closest to the shadow of the spine. The right coronary sinus of Valsalva lies opposite the aortic root in a position which appears closest to the anterior chest wall. The posterior noncoronary sinus of Valsalva occupies an intermediate position above the aortic annulus between the right and left coronary sinuses, and its lower border extends slightly farther caudad than that of either the right or left coronary sinus.

The catheter tip is directed into either the right or left coronary sinus of Valsalva. Small injections of 3 to 5 ml contrast medium, performed manually with a 10-ml syringe and observed through the optical system of an adequate 5-in. image amplifier, will demonstrate the orifice of the right or left coronary artery arising from the cephalic aspect of its respective sinus. Once the orifice is so demonstrated, it may, with a little practice, be readily catheterized with a flexible catheter tip like the one described above.

The electrocardiogram is monitored throughout the procedure with an oscilloscope. Pressure from the catheter tip must be monitored constantly, except during momentary periods when contrast medium is being injected through the catheter, in order to recognize instantly mechanical damping of arterial pressure which occurs if the catheter tip obstructs the coronary artery. This provides ample time to correct inadvertent obstruction of the artery, since such mechanical obstruction must persist for a minimum of 10 sec and usually as long as 30 sec before acute obstruction may cause the development of a metabolic defect in the myocardium perfused by the artery.

A P-23-Db Statham transducer, attached to the side arm of a three-way stopcock locked to the hub of the catheter, is used for this purpose. The side arms of two additional three-way stopcocks, soldered to the first in series, provide connections to reservoirs containing 5 per cent glucose in water and contrast medium. Either of these solutions may be used to fill the syringe, attached to the distal stopcock, for intermittent flushing of the catheter or contrast visualization without interfering with constant pressure measurements transmitted through the proximal side arm to the pressure transducer. It is essential to keep all connections of the system completely airtight, since a small air bubble injected directly into a coronary artery may cause serious arrhythmias or myocardial injury.

When the catheter tip has been satisfactorily positioned in the orifice of the coronary artery, the patient is asked to take a deep breath and stop breathing in full inspiration. The Valsalva maneuver is avoided. From 2 to 6 ml contrast medium is injected manually into the artery over a period of 3 to 5 sec. Its passage through the vessel is observed directly through the optical system of the image amplifier and is simultaneously recorded with a 35-mm motion-picture camera at a rate of 60 photographs per second.

When contrast medium enters the coronary veins and begins to empty into the right atrium by way of the coronary sinus, the patient is asked to exhale. Bradycardia frequently occurs during the capillary and venous phases of the passage of contrast medium through the coronary circulation. When this occurs, the patient is immediately asked to cough two or three times. This causes a marked elevation of aortic pressure when the ventricles are relaxed in diastole, facilitating prompt washout of the small remaining quantity of contrast medium. There is invariably a prompt return to normal sinus rhythm at approximately the rate previously maintained.

The procedure causes no pain. The patient is subjectively unaware that an injection of contrast medium has been made if all of it enters the coronary artery. If a small amount flows backward from the orifice of the coronary artery into the aortic root, he may experience a barely perceptible sense of burning in the episternal notch which persists for 1 or 2 sec.

The conduct of individual examinations must be flexible to permit adequate solution of the infinite variety of problems encountered in patients who may exhibit any phase of the natural history of coronary artery disease. Severe obstructions or total occlusions in major radicals of the coronary artery tree are usually clearly recognized immediately during momentary periods of observation while the vessels are being photographed. It is much more difficult to be certain that no obstructive lesions are present. For this reason, each vessel must be photographed in multiple projections in an attempt to view all segments of major radicals of both coronary arteries in a plane perpendicular to that of the x-ray beam. This may usually be accomplished by photographing the left coronary artery in three left anterior oblique projections ranging from 30 to 60° and two right anterior oblique projections ranging from 10 to 30°. The right coronary artery may usually be adequately demonstrated by two left anterior oblique projections at 40 to 60° and a right anterior oblique projection at 20 to 30°. The exact planes selected will depend upon the configuration of the individual heart under study and upon the presence or absence of ventricular dilatation. It should be emphasized that the exact projections selected in each individual patient are determined by the operator on the basis of the intracardiac anatomy of the individual patient rather than upon fixed projections related to external body planes.

Functional segmental constriction may be encountered particularly in the upper and middle thirds of the right coronary artery. This may be mistaken for fixed organic obstruction. For this reason, it is essential to photograph the right coronary artery 5 to 10 min after sublingual administration of a potent coronary dilator such as fresh nitroglycerin or isosorbide dinitrate (Isordil), if an obstruction is recognized in this area. This technique is also helpful in causing minor variations in lumen diameter in any branch of the coronary circulation to become more apparent, because uninvolved segments of such vessels appear to dilate more than adjacent sclerotic segments.

In many instances, the use of a potent coronary dilator will increase the diameter of extremely small intercoronary collateral arteries in patients with obstructive lesions, providing a better understanding of their origin, distribution, and functional importance in individual patients. Such intercoronary collateral vessels are never visualized by these techniques when the coronary circulation is normal.

When both coronary arteries have been adequately demonstrated, the left ventricle may be selectively opacified with 30 to 40 ml contrast medium to demonstrate or rule out complications of coronary atherosclerosis, such as myocardial aneurysm, diffuse myocardial fibrosis, septal perforation, or mitral regurgitation due to rupture of papillary muscle or chordae tendineae. This is particularly important if implantation of the internal mammary artery into the anterolateral wall of the left ventricle (Vineberg technique) is contemplated in patients with obstructive lesions in major radicals of the left anterior descending coronary artery. Such implants will not function in an area of myocardium which has been replaced by scar tissue.

The catheter is withdrawn. The brachial artery is allowed to bleed briskly from above and below the arteriotomy for a few moments. If adequate backflow distal to the arteriotomy does not occur, gentle probing of its lumen immediately distal to the arteriotomy usually reveals a soft clot which is readily extracted. The arteriotomy is closed with one or two small mattress sutures of 5-0 white braided Dacron (Decnatel-1338). The skin is closed with two silk vertical mattress sutures.

The patient is asked to exercise his arm by full flexion and extension of the elbow, wrist, and hand, fifteen to twenty times per hour beginning 1 hour after the procedure. In all but exceptional circumstances, patients are discharged from the hospital on the morning following the procedure. Skin sutures are removed 4 or 5 days later.

Materials and Equipment

The contrast mediums most frequently employed have been 90 per cent Hypaque and 85 per cent Cardiografin. More than seven thousand arteriograms have been performed by direct injection of each of these compounds into human coronary arteries. Although they are difficult to handle because of high viscosity, adequate opacification of individual vessels is constantly achieved with doses of 2 to 5 ml, and they cause less frequent side effects than other available mediums.

For routine clinical study, all coronary arteriograms performed in the author's laboratory are photographically recorded on 35-mm Eastman Double X negative film with Arriflex cameras at a rate of 60 frames per second. The cameras are equipped with color-corrected f 2.0 lenses with a focal length of 75 mm to photograph the output of 5-in. Philips image amplifiers capable of amplifying light from 1,200 to 3,000 times. After a prolonged experience with 11-, 9-, and 8-in. image amplifiers equipped with 16- and 35-mm cameras, the author is convinced that the 5-in. amplifier and 35-mm camera described above are the best combination of equipment commercially available for this purpose. The 5-in. field is large enough to cover adequately the distribution of individual coronary arteries by moving the amplifier no more than 2 in. during each exposure. Its small area ensures a homogeneous background density within the heart silhouette, which simplifies the problem of obtaining dependable light measurement for precise photographic exposure. It ensures the smallest possible x-ray dose to the patient and provides better photographic reproduction of small structures than any other combination of equipment available for high-speed x-ray motion-picture recording. Paradoxically, the 5-in. amplifier is considerably less expensive than its larger counterparts.

Exposed film is processed immediately in a Fisher Processall model S-XR-6, using Ethol-90 developer and Kodak Rapid x-ray fixer at a speed of 4 ft per min. Processed 35-mm negative film is routinely available for viewing within 1 hr of exposure. A Tage-Arno 35-mm viewer is used for this purpose and has been satisfactory for all routine diagnostic study. It provides a projected image which can be comfortably observed by one to four persons at any desired speed, from still projection of individual frames to a rate of 50 frames per second. It does not scratch or tear film.

Although still photographs cannot provide the information imparted to the observer by careful motion study, individual frames which most clearly demonstrate the anatomic characteristics of each arteriogram are selected. These are reproduced as enlarged positive prints on 2- by 3-in. photographic paper. These prints are mounted and incorporated in duplicate reports for the hospital chart, the referring physician, and the laboratory file.

Standard of Performance

Using the techniques, equipment, and materials described, the following standard of performance may be anticipated, during motion study of projected images:

1. All branches of the coronary artery tree should be visualized down to distal radicals with a lumen diameter of 100 to 200 μ.

2. Total occlusion and partial segmental narrowing which obstructs the lumen diameter by more than 20 per cent should be clearly defined in all vessels with an internal diameter larger than 1 mm.

3. The origin and distribution of functioning intercoronary collateral arterial channels larger than 100 μ should be defined. Collateral channels arising above obstructed arterial segments which perfuse distal branches of the same vessel should be recognized.

4. Segmental narrowing due to functional coronary artery constriction should be distinguishable from fixed organic obstructions by repeated visualization before and after the use of amyl nitrite or nitroglycerin.

5. Functional segmental arterial obstructions due to extrinsic pressure by perivascular myocardial bands, which constrict during ventricular systole, should be distinguishable from fixed organic intraluminal obstructions.

6. Calcification in the coronary artery tree should be defined.

7. When the internal mammary arteries are se-

lectively opacified, the presence of extracoronary myocardial perfusion from distal radicals of these vessels should be demonstrable.

8. Coronary arteriovenous fistulas and fistulous tracts into cardiac chambers are demonstrable when they exist.

9. When left ventriculography is performed, the presence and physical characteristics of myocardial aneurysms, septal perforations, and mitral regurgitation, due to myocardial infarction, are recognized.

Figures 31-1 through 31-4 illustrate the normal coronary arterial tree, the effect of nitroglycerin on the coronary arteries, obstructive disease of the coronary arteries, and one example of surgical correction.

Indications for Coronary Arteriography

Clinical application of cine coronary arteriography is indicated when a problem is encountered which may be resolved by objective demonstration of the coronary artery tree, provided competent personnel and adequate facilities are available and the potential risks are acceptable to the patient and his physician. The largest group of patients which may be studied with benefit are those in whom the diagnosis of coronary artery disease is suspected but ill-defined or questioned because of atypical clinical features.

The pitfalls encountered in the assessment of such problems are so numerous that diagnostic errors are usually accepted with stoic resignation when they are uncovered by the passage of time. Instances of sudden death or acute myocardial infarction due to unrecognized coronary artery disease occur with distressing frequency within a month following the reassurance of a "complete checkup and normal electrocardiogram." On the other hand, patients with chest pain accompanied by minor electrocardiographic changes may pursue a restricted existance for years in anticipation of "a heart attack," following the sincere, but mistaken, diagnosis of angina pectoris or coronary insufficiency.

Normal coronary arteriograms have been demonstrated in a number of such patients following years of well-intentioned treatment with vasodilators, sedatives, or anticoagulant drugs. In some, the combination of pain, unresolved hopelessness, and personality maladjustment, compounded by poor medical management, has led to narcotic addiction. In others, pericardial poudrage, internal mammary artery ligation, or the production of myxedema with radioactive iodine has been needlessly performed.

Cine coronary arteriography has been routinely performed on patients with aortic valve disease who gave a history of syncopal attacks or retrosternal distress. This has made it possible to rule out coronary disease as a possible cause of symptoms in some patients. In others, only mild valve obstruction associated with severe and unrecognized coronary artery disease was demonstrated. In these patients, an unnecessary and potentially lethal surgical attack on the aortic valve was avoided. Accidental division of anomalous major coronary artery branches has been observed in patients with congenital heart disease during right ventriculotomy. For this reason, cine coronary arteriograms are made routinely to define the origin and distribution of major branches of the coronary artery tree during the course of heart catheterization and cine cardioangiography in these patients.

As surgical techniques directed toward improving myocardial perfusion evolve to a stage of clinical application, cine coronary arteriography has provided an anatomic basis for the selection of patients to whom specific surgical procedures may be helpful. It has also been of value in demonstrating the success or failure of such procedures in postoperative patients. Recently, it has been possible to demonstrate that left internal mammary arteries implanted into the left ventricular wall by the method of Vineberg[4] were effectively perfusing the left ventricle 6 months to 7 years after operation. In a series of more than thirty patients, it has been impossible to demonstrate myocardial perfusion from branches of the internal mammary arteries following pericardial poudrage and partial coronary sinus legation. Similar negative results have been encountered in patients after internal mammary artery ligation.

Serial studies performed on patients in all phases of the natural history of coronary atherosclerosis will ultimately provide a better understanding of its complications and the evolution of compensatory mechanisms which permit survival.

Complications

Ventricular fibrillation occurred in 84 of 4,200 patients. Prior to June, 1960, two of three patients treated by emergency thoracotomy and open-chest cardiac massage expired. The third survived after a stormy postoperative course. Since June, 1960, 81 patients have been treated with external cardiac massage by the method of Kouwenhoven and associates.[5] One spontaneously reverted to normal sinus rhythm after 20 sec of massage. The remaining 80 required one to three shocks with an external defibrillator to restore normal rhythm. In all these, subsequent coronary arteriograms were performed as soon as functional stability was reestablished. Left ventriculograms were also made of 28 of these patients who had valvular heart disease

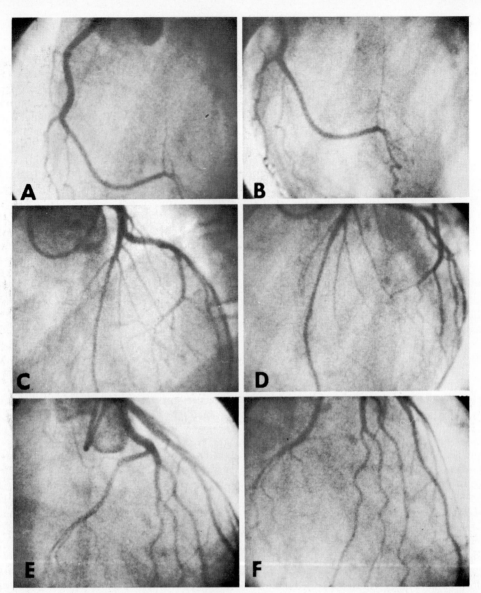

Fig. 33-1. Normal coronary artery tree in a healthy young adult. A. Early phase of right coronary artery filling in the left oblique projection. The main trunk passes around the right atrioventricular (A-V) sulcus. It gives off numerous small branches to the right atrium and ventricle. B. Distal radicals of the right coronary artery reveal a normal appearance. The large trunk passing diagonally to the central portion of the frame lies in the right A-V sulcus. It curves sharply downward as the posterior descending coronary artery. A small radical passes upward from the point of sharp curvature. This is the branch to the A-V node. (See Chap. 10.) Small marginal branches which are distributed over the epicardial surface of the right ventricle are seen passing down the left side of the frame. C. Early phase of left coronary artery filling with the patient in the left anterior oblique projection. The large branch passing straight down the center of the frame is the main anterior descending coronary artery. The branch passing obliquely toward the right lower corner of the frame is the left circumflex coronary artery. D. A late phase of left coronary artery filling in the left oblique projection shows distal radicals of the anterior descending and circumflex coronary arteries. Diagonal branches of the anterior descending trunk pass downward to the right of the main anterior descending coronary artery. Small perforating branches pass into the septum slightly to the left of the main anterior descending trunk. E. The left coronary artery as seen with the patient rotated 15° into the right anterior oblique projection. The proximal anterior descending trunk lies above and slightly to the right of the short main circumflex coronary artery. The latter divides into an A-V branch passing toward the left lower corner of the frame in the left A-V sulcus and three posterolateral branches which pass downward over the posterolateral wall of the left ventricle. F. Distal radicals of the left coronary artery are seen in the right oblique projection. The large anterior descending trunk is seen at the right side of the frame. The posterolateral branches of the circumflex trunk pass down the central area, and the A-V branch of the left circumflex coronary artery is seen at the left side of the frame.

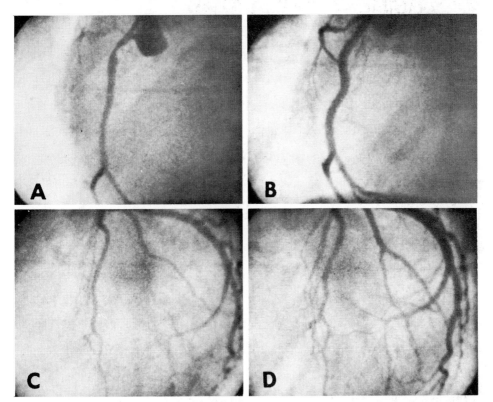

Fig. 33-2. *A.* The early phase of right coronary artery filling before administration of nitroglycerin. Note segmental narrowing in the upper segment of the right main coronary artery immediately beyond its orifice at the right anterior sinus of Valsalva. *B.* Two minutes after sublingual administration of 1/150 gr nitroglycerin the segmental narrowing has disappeared, and all distal radicals of the right coronary artery are significantly dilated. The narrowing in the proximal segment of the vessel was due to functional constriction rather than organic disease. *C.* The normal left coronary artery as seen in the left anterior oblique projection before administration of nitroglycerin. *D.* Three minutes after administration of nitroglycerin very significant dilatation of all major radicals of the left coronary artery has occurred, and distal radicals not noted before use of the drug are readily visualized.

subsequent to defibrillation. The arrhythmia did not recur. Except for first-degree burns on the chest wall from the defibrillator electrodes, there were no complications; all 80 patients have survived. Effective treatment, promptly applied under adequate control, has reduced this formidable complication to the status of a reversible incident without residual injury.

Death due to ventricular asystole followed sudden functional constriction of the left coronary artery in a third patient, whose right coronary artery was totally obstructed.

The fourth death occurred 30 min after completion of the procedure. The patient was a fifty-seven-year-old physician in medically intractable congestive failure. The preceding study demonstrated total occlusion near the origins of his right main and left circumflex coronary arteries and more than 90 per cent obstruction in the proximal left anterior descending coronary artery. The

dilated left ventricle had been largely replaced by scar tissue. His resting left ventricular diastolic pressure was 46 mm Hg. After the catheter had been withdrawn and the brachial arteriotomy closed, ventricular asystole suddenly developed. All attempts at resuscitation failed.

The mortality rate attributed to cine coronary arteriography in 4,200 patients has been 0.09 per cent. Three of four deaths occurred among the patients of whom the first 1,000 coronary arteriograms were made. One occurred among the ensuing 1,800, and none has occurred which could be attributed to the procedure during or after the last 2,400 studies performed.

Acute posterior myocardial infarction occurred in one patient with severe generalized coronary atherosclerosis, as a result of dissection of the right coronary artery. This developed 10 min after the catheter was removed from its orifice and was verified by subsequent opacification of the vessel.

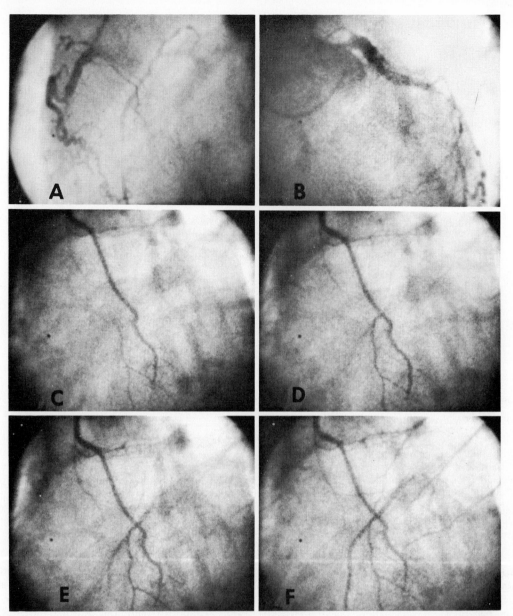

Fig. 33-3. *A*. Heavy opacification of the right coronary artery of a fifty-six-year-old man who previously had suffered acute anteroseptal and posterior myocardial infarctions and had recovered. The right coronary artery is completely obstructed. Immediately above the point of obstruction a large, tortuous vessel arises which passes across the right ventricle to the lower central portion of the frame, where it faintly opacifies the anterior descending branch of the left coronary artery. During motion study this is easily seen to fill from the lower central portion of the frame back upward to its right upper corner. This is an example of intercoronary arterial collateral circulation from the right coronary artery to the left anterior descending coronary artery. *B*. Heavy opacification of the left main coronary artery. The main anterior descending trunk fails to fill from its orifice at the top of the frame. The distal radicals of the circumflex trunk are very severely narrowed. *C*. Early filling of the internal mammary artery 11 months after the internal mammary artery and vein were implanted as a pedicle graft into the anterolateral wall of the left ventricle by the Sewell modification of Vineberg's procedure in the patient whose vessels are demonstrated in *A* and *B*. The internal mammary artery is seen passing obliquely across the center of the frame. It is beginning to fill a small tertiary branch of the occluded left anterior descending coronary artery extending obliquely toward the left from the distal extremity of the implant. *D*. A moment later there is heavy filling of a diagonal branch of the anterior descending coronary artery back to its point of origin from the main anterior descending trunk. *E* and *F*. Later phases of opacification of the entire anterior descending system from the internal mammary artery implant. This is an example of successful extracoronary perfusion of the myocardium by implantation of the internal mammary artery into an ischemic left ventricle.

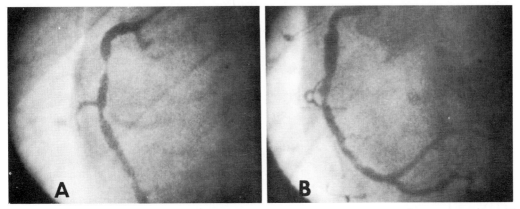

Fig. 33-4. *A.* Severe organic segmental obstruction in the proximal segment of a right coronary artery. *B.* The same vessel 3 months after successful endarterectomy and closure of the vessel with a pericardial patch graft. This led to complete remission of anginal symptoms. The patient remained asymptomatic 1 year following the operation by Drs. Donald B. Effler and Laurence Groves.

The patient recovered. There have been no other instances of myocardial injury due to coronary arteriography.

In one patient with severe generalized atherosclerosis, an elongated aorta, and unusually tortuous brachiocephalic and subclavian arteries, a plaque distal to the origin of the right vertebral artery was partially dislodged by the catheter tip. This completely occluded the subclavian trunk, causing severe pain, numbness, and pallor of the right arm. Obliteration of arterial pulsations in the distal subclavian and axillary arteries was demonstrated with the catheter tip. Small injections of contrast medium localized and confirmed the nature of the obstruction. Prompt subclavian endarterectomy by a well-qualified member of the surgical staff relieved the obstruction. The patient recovered completely with excellent peripheral pulses.

Segmental occlusion at the site of brachial arteriotomy has occurred in 6 to 7 per cent of the patients. It must be emphasized that if occlusion occurs at the antecubital fossa in the absence of proximal occlusions, collateral circulation around the elbow will always be adequate to prevent major disability or tissue loss. This is not true if the axillary artery is selected as the site for arteriotomy. Following occlusion of the brachial artery at the antecubital fossa, a few patients have complained of claudication and sensitivity to cold. More than 90 per cent have become completely asymptomatic 3 months after the procedure if they were encouraged to exercise the arm and hand and avoid exposure to cold. Mild urticaria has been encountered occasionally following repeated small injections of contrast medium. This is promptly controlled by 25 to 30 mg diphenhydramine hydro-

chloride (Benadryl hydrochloride) administered slowly through the catheter into the aortic root. Anaphylaxis has never occurred.

With increasing experience, the potential risks of coronary arteriography have been reduced by improved technical performance. The hazards have seemed acceptable in view of the objectives attained. The use of cine coronary arteriography in the immediate future will be limited by the availability of adequately trained and equipped personnel to perform the procedure safely and interpret it reliably. These limitations will be gradually overcome by the human and technical resources available. It must be emphasized, however, that inept performance, inadequate instrumentation, and overimaginative or undiscerning interpretation provide the means of opening a Pandora's box of misinformation which may plague the physician, harm his patients, and retard evolution of a better understanding of human coronary artery disease. These hazards can be minimized only by the exercise of our best judgment, care, and technical skill in the application and further refinement of the techniques described. If this is done, we and our patients will profit by the availability of an objective diagnostic standard for defining the presence of coronary atherosclerosis.

REFERENCES

1. Sones, F. M.: Cinecardioangiocgraphy, in B. L. Gordon (ed.), "Clinical Cardiopulmonary Physiology," 2d ed., Grune & Stratton, Inc., New York, 1960, pp. 130–144.
2. Lehman, J. S., Boyer, R. A., and Winter, F. S.: Coronary Arteriography, *Am. J. Roentgenol.,* **81**:749, 1959.

3. Dotter, C. T., and Frische, L. H.: An Approach to Coronary Arteriography, in H. L. Abrams (ed.), "Angiography," Little, Brown and Company, Boston, 1961, vol. 1., pp. 259–273.

4. Vineberg, A.: Surgery of Coronary Artery Disease, *Progr. Cardiovas. Dis.*, 4:391, 1962.

5. Kouwenhoven, W. B., Jude, J. R., and Knickerbocker, G. G.: Closed-chest Cardiac Massage, *J.A.M.A.*, **173**: 1064, 1960.

34 CLINICAL APPLICATION OF SELECTIVE CINE CORONARY ARTERIOGRAPHY

William L. Proudfit, M.D.

It is commonly accepted that the symptoms of coronary disease, in the absence of complicating conditions, are associated with anatomic changes in the coronary arteries. Pathologic studies have confirmed this relationship. If coronary arteriography is a valid technique, there must be a close correlation between the classic syndromes of coronary arterial disease and the presence of significant angiographic abnormalities. One thousand selective coronary cine arteriographic studies performed by Sones, Shirey, and associates were reviewed to test this conclusion (see Chap. 33). Excluded from the series were patients who had rheumatic valvular heart disease. Almost all patients had been told by one or more physicians that coronary disease was present or suspected. The clinical diagnoses were made independently of the arteriographic diagnoses. The accuracy of clinical diagnoses is dependent to some extent on the ability and experience of the evaluator.

Typical angina pectoris was considered to be pain, pressure, or tightness which was induced by physical exertion and was relieved by rest within 5 or 10 min; in most patients there were other precipitating or potentiating factors. The location of the pain was considered to be not critical, provided it was in the upper half of the body. Patients who also had rest pain were considered separately. In about 94 per cent of patients who had typical exertional distress, there were moderate or severe arteriographic abnormalities in major vessels. Ninety-eight per cent of patients who had QRS abnormalities diagnostic of myocardial infarc-

tion had significant disease; in all the patients the disease was severe. In about 16 per cent major disease was confined to one vessel in patients who had evidence of myocardial infarction. Angina at rest as well as on exertion was associated with abnormalities in about 87 per cent of patients. It has been found to be difficult to exclude anginal pain in some patients who have psychosomatic problems; almost always the pain is severe in these cases and occurs at rest as well as with activity. Rest pain alone and prolonged ("coronary insufficiency") pains were associated with significant arterial obstruction in about 80 per cent of instances, but in atypical chest pain thought to be of coronary origin the percentage declined to 65.

On the other hand, in only about 15 per cent of patients thought to have noncoronary pain was significant disease demonstrated. Some coronary disease is to be expected in even asymptomatic patients in the age group studied. It is significant that more than one-fourth of the entire series of patients had no demonstrable disease, and more than one-third had no disease thought to be dynamically significant. Subsequent to study, reassurance of these patients was usually of remarkable therapeutic value.

Patients who had congestive heart failure generally had extensive coronary disease in multiple major vessels, ventricular aneurysm, mitral insufficiency, or a concomitant cardiac or circulatory disease.

Electrocardiographic abnormalities were encountered in about 55 per cent of patients who had no, or only slight, arteriographic abnormalities and no coronary symptoms. Frequently the association of chest pain with electrocardiographic changes was the basis for previous diagnosis of coronary disease. The resting electrocardiogram was abnormal in 58 per cent of patients who had typical angina pectoris and arteriographic abnormalities. The exercise tolerance test, evaluated by the criteria of Mattingly, appeared to be a specific, but insensitive, index of disease, even when involvement of several major vessels was encountered. The criteria of Master were more sensitive but less specific.

It is concluded that the accuracy of clinical diagnosis in patients who had typical angina pectoris of mild or moderate severity and in patients who have myocardial infarction manifested by definite QRS abnormalities is excellent, but errors are common in diagnosing other conditions in which coronary arterial disease is clinically suspected.

35 MANAGEMENT OF CORONARY ATHEROSCLE-ROSIS AND ITS COMPLICATIONS

R. Bruce Logue, M.D., and
J. Willis Hurst, M.D.

The management of coronary atherosclerosis has undergone considerable change during the last two decades. Not only has the treatment of specific clinical syndromes such as angina pectoris and myocardial infarction changed, but anticoagulants, special diets, and drugs designed to lower the serum cholesterol have made their appearance. The effect of tobacco on coronary atherosclerosis has been partially clarified during the last few years, and the effect of exercise and stress is still under study. The treatment of the complications of myocardial infarction has improved enormously during the last decade. The rehabilitation of patients after myocardial infarction has been revolutionized during the last few years, and the prognosis is far better today than it has been in the past. Unfortunately, the absolute prevention of coronary atherosclerosis is not yet possible, but certain factors thought to be etiologic in nature may be altered under certain circumstances. Hopefully, all the etiologic factors may be identified and modified in the future.

Anticoagulants

It was natural that anticoagulants would be used in the prevention of the complications of coronary atherosclerosis, since thrombosis is a common cause of myocardial infarction and since other thromboembolic disorders are not infrequent. Anticoagulants were first used for this disease approximately twenty years ago.[1-4] It is noteworthy that even after this period of time and after an enormous amount of study the controversy regarding the value of anticoagulant therapy still rages. Usually a new therapeutic measure which is of definite value can be evaluated in a short period of time. For example, the value of treating pneumococcal pneumonia with penicillin or congestive heart failure with digitalis and diuretics is not debated today, because the answer is clear. It is more difficult to evaluate therapy in diseases which are recurrent or chronic, but even in such disorders one may sometimes obtain definite answers. For example, the prophylactic value of penicillin and sulfonamides in the prevention of rheumatic fever is not questioned. The fact that there is still no universal acceptance of the place of anticoagulants in the therapy of coronary atherosclerosis suggests one or more of the following possibilities:

1. That therapy with anticoagulants is not clearly superior to treatment without anticoagulants.

2. That other improvements in therapy have influenced the more recent statistics of treated and untreated groups. For example, a decrease in thromboembolism has probably occurred as a result of more prompt treatment of heart failure and earlier ambulation and the avoidance of prolonged periods of strict bed rest. The evaluation of therapy in patients with angina pectoris is clouded, because an optimistic physician enhances the placebo effect of any therapy.

3. That the risk of hemorrhagic complications, although small, may influence the widespread use of the drug. The present authors suspect that fatal complications from hemorrhage may not be accurately reported from the population at large.

The use of anticoagulants in the treatment of acute myocardial infarction was first reported by Wright in 1945,[2] and a group study authorized by the American Heart Association under his leadership gave a progress report in 1948.[5] The latter study showed a mortality of 23.4 per cent in 442 control cases and of 16 per cent in 589 treated cases. Forty-two per cent of control patients and twenty-three per cent of treated patients developed clinically recognized thromboembolic complications. When cases were separated into "good risk" cases approximating the criteria of Russek, there was a death rate below 2 per cent in both treated and control groups; however, thromboembolism occurred in 29 per cent in the control group and only 9 per cent in the treated group.[6] Wright's recent conclusions regarding the value of anticoagulants is as follows:[7]

In summary, the total world evidence suggests that in the absence of compelling contraindications and with the availability of satisfactory laboratory and clinical facilities, patients suffering with acute myocardial infarction should receive adequate anticoagulant therapy during the first month, and that the risk of reinfarction and death is reduced if this is continued for 1 to 2 years after the first month. More long-term studies should be conducted to evaluate this treatment in succeeding years. This form of therapy presents certain difficulties that must be weighed against the possible gains in deciding whether or not to continue it.

Hilden and associates, who have recently challenged Wright's views, reported no significant difference in mortality between their treated and control groups.[8,9] There was, however, a difference in thromboembolism, detected clinically or at autopsy, with a 15 per cent incidence in the treated group and a 25 per cent incidence in the control group. Patients who died showed pulmonary embolism or infarction in 5 per cent of the treated and 28 per cent of the control patients, and mural thrombosis was found in 24 per cent of the treated and 58 per cent of the control patients. Death from thromboembolism occurred in 1.4 per cent of the treated and in 4 per cent of the control patients. The total mortality rate was 33 per cent in the treated group and 40 per cent in the control group. Hilden believes that by proper mobilization of patients the incidence of thromboembolism can be reduced almost as much as with the use of anticoagulants, which have the associated risk of bleeding.[9] He calls attention to the published decrease in clinically recognized thromboembolism in both treated and untreated patients reported by various authors since 1948. After evaluating the studies of Wright and of Hilden, which represent diverse viewpoints, and the studies of others, the present authors advise the use of anticoagulants in the treatment of acute myocardial infarction when the diagnosis is definite, when there are no contraindications, and when adequate laboratory facilities are available. At the same time they recognize that the benefit derived from the type of therapy is probably less today than it was 20 years ago.

Anticoagulants are customarily given during the period of hospitalization which averages 3 to 4 weeks. While many recommend a gradual reduction of dosage to minimize the so-called rebound phenomenon, the authors have customarily stopped therapy abruptly.[10–12] There is no evidence that heparin is superior to bishydroxycoumarin (Dicumarol) derivatives in the treatment of acute myocardial infarction, and the incidence of hemorrhage may be higher. Indeed, some studies have no difference in mortality from the control group.[13]

The authors have not divided their patients into good and poor risk groups. They formerly used bishydroxycoumarin but have used warfarin sodium (Coumadin) in recent years. Even though the current incidence of thromboembolism in untreated groups is now lower than formerly, the authors use anticoagulants to lessen the risk of this complication. Although the data is extremely controversial, they also use anticoagulants for patients with preinfarction angina during hospitalization.[14,15] Resnick reports that in approximately 50 per cent of patients with preinfarction angina infarction

developed without anticoagulants, whereas it developed in only 5 per cent of patients on anticoagulants.[10]

Long-term anticoagulant therapy has been claimed to reduce the incidence of reinfarction.[17–20] Bjerkelund in a study of 237 patients noted protection for 1 year, with a mortality of 30 per cent in the control group and of 20 per cent in the treated group. In his group of 118 treated cases there were four fatal cases of cerebral hemorrhage.[21] The study of the British Medical Research Council found protection for 2 years with a reduction of reinfarction from 26 per cent in the controls to 13 per cent in the treated group.[22] Seaman et al. in a 7-year study noted no difference in morbidity or mortality among three groups of patients:[23] one group of 66 patients treated with anticoagulants, one group of 67 treated with a placebo, and a group of 63 patients who served as controls. Harvald et al. found no difference in reinfarction in treated and control groups with a total of 315 patients studied over a period of several years.[24] Borchgrevink, in one significant long-term study on the effect of anticoagulants on patients with angina pectoris of less than 2 years' duration without prior infarcts, found there was a reduction of infarction in those treated with therapeutic doses compared to the group treated with low dosage.[25] After evaluating all data Hilden concludes: "As matters stand today, I cannot advise long-term anticoagulant therapy as a routine after myocardial infarctions."[9]

Lest we forget the controversial claims regarding the use of anticoagulants in coronary disease we should recall the following:

Some authors claim benefit only in preinfarction angina, some for acute myocardial infarction and long-term therapy under the age of sixty, and some at younger ages as well as over the age of sixty. In long-term therapy, some note protection of patients from reinfarction for only 1 year, whereas, others claim benefit for 2 years. Some noted beneficial effects in acute myocardial infarction with prothrombin levels of 25 to 50 per cent of normal, whereas others recommend levels of 10 to 25 per cent.[26]

It is curious that most authors favor heparin for venous thrombosis and pulmonary embolism, yet one group study of myocardial infarction found Coumadin superior to heparin, which gave no better results than in controls; furthermore, there was a higher incidence in bleeding in patients receiving heparin.[13] Therefore, a judgment must be made with these factors in the background. The present authors choose to use anticoagulants (Coumadin) in preinfarction angina and acute myocardial infarction but do not routinely use long-term anticoagulant therapy. Long-term anti-coagulant therapy is used only if there has been recurrent thromboembolism and if there are no contraindications.

To date fibrinolysis therapy has been totally in-effective in the treatment of myocardial infarction. Furthermore, the occurrence of toxic reactions such as chills, fever, and homologous serum hepa-titis increase the morbidity with preparations cur-rently available.[27-32]

The anticoagulation controversy should not divert the physician's attention from other facets of therapy that are more important, including the proper management of arrhythmias, heart block, and cardiac arrest, the early recognition and treat-ment of heart failure and shock, and the proper use, rather than abuse, of rest.

Diet

There has been uniform agreement that obesity adversely affects the symptoms of angina pectoris and is detrimental to patients who have experi-enced myocardial infarction. In both instances obesity increases the work load of the heart, and weight reduction is clearly indicated.[33] The bene-fit derived from weight reduction in such cases may be explained as removing the extra baggage (fat) which imposes a greater burden on the heart. The relationship of obesity to the causes of coronary atherosclerosis is not quite so clear. Obese sub-jects are more susceptible to the development of myocardial infarction and angina pectoris.[34-36] The exact reasons why this is so have not yet been determined. Dawber and Kannel[36] have sum-marized the problem as follows:

Data from life insurance companies have for many years indicated increased death rates from cardiovas-cular disease associated with obesity. Data from epide-miological studies tend to corroborate this finding. In the most obese, there is a slightly higher rate in both morbidity and mortality of coronary heart disease. There is a slight positive correlation between body weight, blood pressure, and serum cholesterol level. When these factors are taken into consideration, the independent contribution of excess weight to the risk of development of coronary heart disease becomes small indeed. However, because of the association between the easily identified characteristic of weight and the important factors of blood pressure and serum choles-terol level, reduction in weight is advisable because of a possible favorable effect on the other factors.

The relationship of the diet to the development of coronary atherosclerosis has been studied exten-sively during the last 20 years.[37-48] Most investi-gators claim that the high fat content of the diet is detrimental, while some believe that the high

carbohydrate content of the diet is the culprit.[49,50] Although much work has been done in the field, the absolute scientific proof that coronary disease may be prevented or altered by modifying the diet is still lacking. Indirect evidence, however, sug-gests potential beneficial effect of diet. The caloric intake should be restricted according to need. This should be accomplished by the restriction of total fat to about 30 per cent of the caloric require-ment, with the polyunsaturated fatty acids pre-dominating. Stamler has written the following:[34]

In the language of nutrition, they* involve diets moderate in total calories, total fats, polyunsaturated fatty acids and carbohydrates; low in saturated fatty acids and cholesterol; and high in all essential nutrients (proteins, amino acids, vitamins, minerals). In terms of foodstuffs this means:

Emphasizing the low-fat dairy products (skim milk, buttermilk, cottage cheese), and de-emphasiz-ing the high-fat (sweet cream, sour cream, ice cream, whipped cream, cheeses, butter).
Emphasizing the lean cuts of meat and poultry, and de-emphasizing the fat cuts, with trimming off fat before cooking, cooking so as to get rid of fat (broiling, rotisseriering, roasting with discarding of drippings, letting stews and soups stand in the refrigerator overnight and skimming off congealed fat); use of vegetable oils in braising meats, etc.; moderation of meat portion size (four to six ounces, not twelve to sixteen!).
Emphasizing fish, and sea food; de-emphasizing eggs.
Emphasizing vegetable oils, and de-emphasizing solid table spreads (butter, margarines) and solid shortenings (lard, suet, hydrogenated vegetable fats, drippings).
Emphasizing fruit desserts (citrus and non-citrus), and de-emphasizing commercial cakes, pastries, shortcakes, cookies and pies.
Emphasizing green and yellow vegetables and legumes (peas, beans).
Emphasizing moderation in the use of starches (potatoes, rice, spaghetti, breads, cereals), carbo-hydrate-rich spreads (jellies, jams, honey, marma-lade), alcoholic beverages.

The Prudent Diet (a recipe book) published by the Department of Health of the New York City Bureau of Nutrition[51] is a worthwhile booklet for patient use.[52,53]

If the evidence were clear that an *extremely* low-fat diet would routinely prevent coronary atherosclerosis, then the present authors would ob-viously recommend its use. Until the evidence is clearer, it would seem wise to recommend a diet

---

* Referring to dietary approaches to the prevention of coronary atherosclerosis.

such as that recommended in *The Prudent Diet,* since it is far more acceptable to the patient. Accordingly, this diet is recommended for patients with angina pectoris and myocardial infarction. Asymptomatic patients who are coronary-prone, especially those with a strong family history of coronary disease, may also be motivated to try such a diet. The emotional reaction of an occasional patient to a stringent change in diet may temper its use. While most observers claim that serum cholesterol can be lowered by this diet, excessive emphasis on the exact level of cholesterol from time to time is not justified and, indeed, may create additional emotional problems. The diet is not indicated in elderly patients with coronary atherosclerosis. Such patients eat poorly, their dietary habits are not easy to break, and the benefit of the diet in such a setting is very questionable.

A study on the prevention of coronary atherosclerosis by the long-term use of diet is now under way in the United States ("The National Diet-Heart Study" [54]). The results of the study are needed in order to consider the advisability of strongly urging the wide-scale use of a diet designed to prevent this common disease. In the meantime it may be wise for persons who eat excessive fat to alter their diet along the lines suggested above. It must be realized by all concerned that absolute proof of benefit is not yet available. It must also be understood that multiple etiologic factors act in concert in the production of this disease (see Chap. 27).

Exercise

Exercise is beneficial in aiding weight reduction and creating physical fitness. Obviously, the amount and type of exercise recommended for patients with clinical evidence of coronary atherosclerosis must be individualized and guided by the patient's physician. The authors wish to emphasize the value of this neglected aspect of rehabilitation.[55,56] It is literally true that many patients may be allowed to be more active after coronary disease is recognized than they were prior to symptoms. This is true because many people live inactive sedentary lives prior to the development of symptoms. The treatment of angina pectoris occurring for the first time, angina pectoris that is getting worse, and acute myocardial infarction includes rest. Following the initial phase of treatment for these disorders, it is usually possible to begin a program of rehabilitation that includes the intelligent use of exercise. [55,56] Epstein has pointed out that exercise affects a number of physiologic processes, apart from its possible stimulating effect on coronary anastomoses.[57] For example,

thrombolytic activity of the blood is enhanced by physical activity.[58]

The psychologic benefit of having the patient walk up a flight or so of stairs following recovery from myocardial infarction is immeasurable. The knowledge by the patient that most heart attacks occur at rest or during normal activity is strong positive reassurance.

Is the lack of exercise an etiologic factor in the development of coronary atherosclerosis? This question has not been answered at this point. Certainly the disease develops in active individuals and may not in inactive people. On the other hand the findings of some investigators who have studied large groups of subjects suggest that physical activity might protect against the development of clinically recognizable coronary disease.[59-61] Until this is settled, it seems prudent, for many reasons, for healthy individuals to remain active throughout their lives.

Drugs Used in Lowering Serum Cholesterol

Many drugs have been employed to lower the serum cholesterol in an effort to prevent the progression of coronary atherosclerosis. Desiccated thyroid extract was used in the past.[62] The use of Triparanol (MER 29) was abandoned because of toxicity. Estrogens are not popular because of troublesome side effects and the question of possible deleterious effects when instituted within 2 months of myocardial infarction.[62,63] Nicotinic acid preparations may produce reversible liver damage and hyperglycemia. The dextro isomer of thyroxin has calorigenic effects that may aggravate the symptoms of angina pectoris.[62] β sitosterol is bulky and unpalatable. Most workers rely solely on diet and do not use medication to lower serum cholesterol. Some confine the use of such drugs to patients with familial hypercholesterolemia.

Tobacco

See Chap. 65.

Alcohol

Alcohol adds to the caloric intake and therefore plays its role in the development of obesity. The serum cholesterol rises in some patients following the ingestion of alcohol. The role this plays, if any, in atherogenesis is not clear. Alcohol, used in moderation, may be helpful to selected patients with angina pectoris. The mechanism of action is not known with certainty. It probably acts as a sedative rather than as a coronary dilator, since it does not prevent the ST-segment abnormality from occurring after exercise.[64,65]

Management of Angina Pectoris

General Advice[65,66]

An attempt should be made to have patients with angina pectoris live with a *minimum of restrictions*. Patients soon identify factors which precipitate their angina, such as toweling after a bath; first exercising in the morning; parking in close spaces; walking up an incline to work; exposure to cold wind; meals, or exercise following meals; anger; anxiety; excitement, whether pleasurable or not; watching television; pain of extracardiac origin; smoking; first lying down at night; and either winning or losing at cards. Once these are pinpointed, the patient should be instructed either to avoid these events or to use nitroglycerin *before* possibly experiencing them. Sedatives and tranquilizers may be useful but should not be used routinely. Phenobarbital is usually adequate, but other drugs may be used, depending upon the individual's response.

Exercise

The scientific value of exercise in the therapy of *stable angina pectoris* is undetermined (see earlier section of this chapter). Although patients and family are often fearful of any exercise, moderate exercise *short of producing discomfort* is not harmful and often produces a sense of well-being. It also aids in weight control and in the establishment of good muscular reflexes, even though there is no definite proof that exercise improves collateral circulation in the myocardium. Patients are instructed to avoid vigorous sustained activity and sudden bursts of exercise such as changing a tire, mowing the lawn with a hand mower, lifting heavy objects such as a motor for a boat, playing tennis, running to catch a bus or train, hurrying to catch a plane, or going on tiring shopping trips. Walking is excellent exercise, because it is easily controlled by the patient. It is recommended that patients walk on level ground at a leisurely pace when weather is not unduly hot or cold. This activity should be performed regularly and should be increased gradually over a period of weeks or months. Many can graduate from walking to playing golf and swimming in warm water. If at any time discomfort occurs, the program of activity should be decreased. By such a regimen, many sedentary businessmen actually become more physically active than they were before angina pectoris developed.

Diet

Patients with angina pectoris should eat a low-fat diet. No more than 30 per cent of the total calorie intake should be made up of fat. The fat eaten should be predominantly of the unsaturated variety. Aside from the possible relation of the composition of the diet to the causes of atherosclerosis, it is clear that the frequency and severity of attacks of angina frequently lessen with weight reduction, which decreases the work load of the heart. An increased sense of well-being may also accompany such weight reduction. In some patients a small meal may be well tolerated, whereas a large meal may be followed by angina; this has been attributed to the increased work of the heart in shunting extra blood to the gastrointestinal tract. It is also possible that postprandial hyperlipemia may interfere with the delivery of oxygen to myocardial cells.

(See also the earlier section on Diet in this chapter.)

Smoking

Angina pectoris is occasionally precipitated by smoking, perhaps due to nicotine-induced catecholamine release. All patients with angina are advised to stop smoking, whether or not a relationship to angina has been identified. The patient with angina is not doing his part to obtain maximum comfort until he has undergone a trial period without smoking. The frustrations of withdrawal and the ensuing rapid weight gain must be balanced against the advantages gained. In the authors' experience, the advice to cut down on smoking is futile; those who successfully stop usually do so abruptly. Beware of creating guilt feelings over this issue. Once the patient understands the need for cessation of smoking, the physician and family should forgo further harrassment.

(See also Chap. 65.)

Drugs

The most important drug in the management of angina pectoris is *nitroglycerin*.[65,66] The patient and the family must be instructed in its use; often members of the family become anxious when it is used by the patient, and the patient may either forgo its use or resort to using it surreptitiously. The family should know that the mere use of nitroglycerin does not indicate another "heart attack." It should be clearly stated that the drug is not habit-forming and that it does not become ineffective with repeated use. The sublingual dose of nitroglycerin should be small, either 0.16 mg (1/400 gr) or 0.32 mg (1/200 gr) in order to minimize side effects such as headache. If too large a dose is used initially, the patient may subsequently refuse to take the drug. Instructions should include its use for such symptoms as heaviness, substernal pressure, and indigestion, as well as for pain. Many patients are denied benefit because they were instructed to use nitroglycerin for "pain," when all the while they are troubled by the more usual symptoms of pressure or constriction. Nitroglycerin should be used prophylactically when angina can be predicted by experience to occur during or after precipitating events such as emotional tension, sexual intercourse, meals, assuming the recumbent position, walking up an incline, or undergoing unusual stress or effort. It may be repeated after 5 min. In the occasional patient who may deny relief of symptoms by nitroglycerin one should be certain that a nitrite effect with fullness and throbbing of the head has occurred, since the particular preparation may have lost its potency. It is a good general rule to replenish the supply every 6 months. The relief of symptoms by nitroglycerin should be prompt and complete by the end of 5 min; when patients relate that relief occurred after 15 to 30 min, it is clear either that the discomfort was not of coronary origin or that simple angina pectoris was not present. Not every patient with angina obtains prompt and complete relief, but it is effective in perhaps 90 per cent of patients. The drug may give transient or equivocal effects in cardiospasm, pylorospasm, and cholecystitis. Rarely nitrite syncope may occur following excessive amounts if the patient is in the upright position. The postural hypotension is more likely to occur in such situations as when the patient is standing in line, when he is overheated, with hyperventilation, and when other drugs such as chlorothiazide or phenothiazide derivatives have been administered. On rare occasions angina pectoris is precipitated by nitroglycerin; some of these patients may be found to have functional hypertrophic subaortic muscular stenosis.

Methemoglobinuria from excessive use of nitroglycerin is virtually nonexistent.

Long-acting drugs, claimed to be useful in the prevention of angina pectoris, are numerous.[67–72] They do not substitute for sublingual nitroglycerin. Along with various placebos, these may be beneficial in some patients. Double-blind studies of their value have usually given inconclusive results. Physicians have learned to be wary of unwarranted claims for various preparations. Sustained-action Isordil (Isordil Tembids) is the authors' current choice. It should be started in doses of 20 mg every 12 hr and increased as tolerated. Many patients develop severe headache with 40 mg as an initial dose. The authors have not seen impressive and reproducible benefit with the following: pentaerythritol tetranitrate (Peritrate tetranitrate), trolnitrate phosphate (Metamine), dipyridamole (Persantin). In contrast to these medications, nitroglycerin ointment is useful when applied at bedtime where nocturnal pain occurs or when there are frequent episodes during the day.[73]

Long-term anticoagulants are not routinely recommended for stable angina pectoris (see the earlier section of this chapter).

Angina pectoris may be aggravated by anemia. Therefore, the cause of anemia must be determined and approximate therapy instituted. Thyrotoxicosis aggravates angina pectoris and must be considered in all patients when routine management is not adequate. Patients with angina pectoris and heart failure may be improved following digitalization and diuretic therapy. Patients with nocturnal angina should routinely be given a trial on digitalis. Mild failure must not be overlooked in this clinical situation. Patients with angina pectoris and atrial fibrillation may have less angina after the arrhythmia has been reverted to normal [74] (see Chap. 16).

The production of hypothyroidism in the euthyroid patient by administering radioactive iodine is useful for the group of patients who are *disabled by frequent attacks of angina pectoris* which are not controlled by customary therapy.[75–81] It should be reserved for those whose angina has been stable for a period of 3 months. Benefit from this form of treatment usually takes 2 to 3 months to be apparent. The hypothyroidism is usually permanent, and one usually needs small increments of thyroid to maintain the patient at the optimum level at which angina is improved but the side effects of hypometabolism are at a minimum.

Patients in whom angina pectoris appears for the first time without other clinical abnormality require a period of modified rest for 2 to 3 weeks at home while allowing collateral circulation to develop. Patients are allowed up and about the house. The initial appearance of angina pectoris is often the forerunner of obvious infarction; indeed, electrocardiographic evidence of infarction may occur with discomfort lasting no longer than 5 min. Anticoagulants should be used if the practical problems associated with their use can be solved.

When stable angina undergoes a sudden change with an increase in the frequency and severity of attacks or when attacks occur with less provocation, a period of modified rest and anticoagulants are also indicated.

Angina decubitus may require a prolonged period of rest. Long-acting nitrites, sedation, and a trial of digitalization may be helpful. Frequent small meals should be tried if discomfort follows eating. Narcotic addiction is a constant threat when repeated opiate administration is necessary. Hospitalization is essential, and many authorities advocate anticoagulants for these patients. The usual duration of angina decubitus is 1 to 3 months unless the patient sustains a myocardial infarction, which is often followed by improvement of pain. Some patients have only a gradual lessening of symptoms over an agonizing period of time; others die suddenly from ventricular fibrillation or cardiac arrest. Ordinarily patients in this category are not candidates for I_{131} administration or surgical procedures designed to improve blood flow to the myocardium.

Surgical Procedures

Revascularization procedures including instillation of talc or asbestos into the pericardial sac, application of phenol to the epicardium, and partial ligation of the coronary sinus have been largely abandoned.[82-84] Internal mammary artery ligation was of no value.[85] Neurosurgical treatment of angina pectoris is no longer employed.[86,87] Clinical improvement has followed the Vineberg procedure, in which an internal mammary artery is implanted into a tunnel in the myocardium, and the Sewell modification, in which a pedicle containing artery, vein, muscle, and connective tissue is implanted in the myocardium.[88-91] The latter two procedures are applicable only where selective coronary arteriography shows the blood supply to the anterior or lateral wall to be significantly decreased. These procedures are the only ones in which Sones has been able to demonstrate patent vessels and increased blood flow to the involved area.[92] Patients with disabling angina pectoris without a recent history of myocardial infarction are now being operated on with this technique. This approach is still in the developmental phase but at this writing offers more hope than was offered by the surgical procedures that preceded it.

If coronary arteriography reveals localized obstruction of a coronary artery at or near its origin, coronary endarterectomy may be feasible.[93,94] Unfortunately, only a very small percentage of patients are suitable for the procedure. This surgical approach is definitely experimental at the present time.

Management of Myocardial Infarction[95-98]

The management of myocardial infarction includes the relief of pain, oxygen, anticoagulants, the proper use of rest, the frequent search for, and treatment of, complications, and the emotional and physical rehabilitation of the patient. The majority of patients should be admitted to the hospital, and many aspects of therapy are carried out simultaneously.

Relief of Pain

Prompt relief of pain is essential. This can be obtained only by the administration of opiates.[99] One should not make futile attempts to relieve prolonged discomfort by the use of nitroglycerin. Morphine sulfate, 10 to 15 mg ($\frac{1}{6}$ to $\frac{1}{4}$ gr), may be given intramuscularly and repeated in 4 hr if there is no respiratory depression. Although the majority of patients obtain relief with this dosage, some require additional small increments which may be given intravenously. The latter route of administration affords quicker relief with smaller dosage. If respiratory depression occurs, it can be promptly recognized and managed, whereas the delayed onset of hypoventilation following intramuscular injection may not be recognized. The drug may be diluted in 10 to 20 ml saline solution and given 2 ml at a time; one should pause several minutes between increments to be certain that respiratory depression does not occur. It is advisable to have morphine antagonists such as N-allylnormorphine hydrochloride (Nalline hydrochloride) available. Decreased alveolar ventilation follows the administration of every opiate and may occur at any dosage level regardless of the route of administration. It should be emphasized that the amplitude of respiratory excursions may be diminished when the respiratory rate is normal. The pain of infarction must be relieved, but beware of doing so at the risk of hypoxia. The hypoxia which occurs predisposes to ventricular fibrillation and standstill. Since morphine sulfate is vagotonic, atropine sulfate, 0.5 to 1.0 mg, is advised when there is bradycardia, nausea and vomiting, A-V block, nodal rhythm, or A-V dissociation. These complications are especially likely to occur if the infarction is posterior or inferior in location (see Chap. 29). Meperidine hydrochloride (Demerol hydrochloride) has an anticholinergic effect, and on occasion it may increase the ventricular rate in patients with atrial flutter or fibrillation. All opiates and derivatives may produce hypotension and even shock. Caution is always needed in the patient with respiratory disease or myxedema. Meperidine hydrochloride (75 to 100 mg) is widely used because it is convenient to administer and is thought to produce less nausea and respiratory depression as compared to morphine. Since these possible advantages are not so apparent to the authors, they prefer morphine sulfate because of its superior ability to relieve pain; furthermore, meperidine is more irritating to the tissues.

Addiction to opiates must be avoided, but at times it is wise to give average amounts of opiates every 4 to 6 hr for 2 or 3 days when it becomes obvious that recurrent pain is a problem. When pain is recurrent, it may be difficult to relieve even when a private-duty nurse is at the bedside prepared to give an opiate intramuscularly.

Patients may have chest pain due to pericarditis and anxiety (see Treatment of Complications, below) following myocardial infarction. Opiates are not needed for many of the nonischemic causes of chest pain. Furthermore, after analyzing the patient's discomfort it is proper to explain to him that he is not having a "new heart attack."

Oxygen

Most patients with acute myocardial infarction do not require oxygen. It is given for respiratory depression, shock, cyanosis, mild dyspnea, cough, and wheezing, and when the respiratory rate is increased. It is of dubious value in relieving pain. Oxygen is preferably given by nasal route with care to avoid gastric dilatation. If it is still needed after 28 to 48 hr, one may shift to an oxygen tent to avoid prolonged irritation and drying of the upper respiratory tract. When this is done, special care must be instituted in order to guarantee proper observation on the part of the physician and nurse, since the oxygen tent serves as a barrier to frequent examination. It is rare for oxygen therapy to be required for more than a few days. Patients who have myocardial infarction and also have advanced emphysema may develop profound respiratory depression following the administration of barbiturates, opiates, or oxygen, and such patients challenge the ingenuity of the physician. The role of hyperbaric oxygen in the treatment of myocardial infarction remains to be determined.[100]

Rest

The patient should be allowed to assume the position in which he is most comfortable, including the upright position. Motion in bed is not restricted. When pain has been relieved, the effects of opiates have subsided, and there is no hypotension in the upright position, patients may be allowed the use of a bedside commode, and the male patient may be allowed to void while standing by the bed. Periodic dorsiflexion of the feet and movements of the knees and hips are encouraged to minimize a phlebothrombosis. Immobility of the shoulders should be avoided and full range of movement of the shoulder joints encouraged to lessen peritendinitis and the shoulder-hand syndrome. The patient may usually be helped to a large, comfortable chair by the side of the bed for ½ hr or longer three to four times daily beginning on the second or third day.[101–103] The recurrence of pain, hypotension, or arrhythmias may delay the institution of rest in the chair. By the end of the first week, the patient with uncomplicated infarction may be

sitting in the chair many hours per day. This modified rest is progressively increased by trial and error during his hospital stay, which averages 3 or 4 weeks. The patient may walk to the toilet in his room during the latter part of his hospitalization. Most patients are allowed to go home in a car. At home he is allowed progressive increase in activity for the next several weeks.[104] At the end of this time he may take short rides and walk outside in mild weather. He may be allowed to walk up a flight of steps. He is usually able to return to work by the end of 2 or 3 months. It is preferable to begin working a few hours daily and increasing the time weekly as tolerated. If there is no angina or congestive heart failure, he should be encouraged to take mild forms of exercise such as walking. Many are able to return to playing golf and swimming. Many asymptomatic patients are able to do more after myocardial infarction than they did prior to infarction. This is true because many patients were inactive prior to their attack. Discussion of sexual intercourse should be initiated by the physician; it may be resumed by 6 to 8 weeks if there has been no angina; prophylactic nitroglycerin is recommended.

Diet

A liquid or soft diet should be given during the first 24 to 48 hr after a myocardial infarction. This period of time may be extended when complications are present. As a rule the patient can and should feed himself. After a few days a general diet can be allowed. Sodium restriction is not needed as a routine measure. The total caloric intake should be restricted so that normal weight can be achieved, keeping in mind that the patient is likely to be inactive for 2 to 3 months. No more than 30 per cent of the total calories of the diet should consist of fat. The majority of the fat should be made up of the unsaturated variety.

(See the earlier section on Diet in this chapter.)

Anticoagulants

Anticoagulants should be given to all patients in whom the diagnosis of myocardial infarction is definite and when no contraindication to such therapy exists. The authors use 3-(1-phenylpropyl)-4-oxycoumarin warfarin (Coumadin) at the present time. It is effective in 24 to 48 hr, and its duration of action is about a week. The initial dose is said to be 1 mg per kg body weight. In the authors' experience the initial dose is about 40 mg for most patients. No drug is given the subsequent day, and 2.5 to 12.5 mg is given daily thereafter, depending upon the prothrombin time, which should be maintained at 10 to 20 per cent of normal. Anticoagulants should be continued for

3 to 4 weeks (the period of hospitalization). Long-term anticoagulant therapy is not routinely recommended at this time.

(See also the earlier section on Anticoagulants in this chapter.)

Other Aspects of Management

Intensive-care cardiac units are useful in the care of patients with myocardial infarction. The units can be designed so that several patients can be seen from a central nursing desk. The *electrical activity of the heart* of several patients can be *monitored* at one time from the central observation area. When the alarm system indicates than an arrhythmia, such as cardiac standstill or ventricular fibrillation, has occurred, resuscitative measures can be initiated promptly. The personnel in such units are taught to be alert for certain dangers common to patients in this group. Routine care in such a unit should not be neglected. For example, the electrical activity of the heart may be satisfactory, but the blood pressure may be dangerously low. The environment of the intensive-care unit can reek with anxiety, the personnel may appear frantic, and the noise level may be high. The majority of hospitals do not have intensive-care units. Therefore the hospital room should be equipped with oxygen, portable monitoring equipment should be available, and floor personnel should be familiar with resuscitative techniques. In the future it is likely that all patients with myocardial infarction will have the electrical activity of the heart, blood pressure, and respiration continuously monitored with simplified electronic equipment. When this day comes, we must not forget that no amount of equipment can substitute for the good judgment of the physician.

A *permanent electrocardiogram* should be made as soon as possible after the onset of myocardial infarction. If the initial tracing is abnormal and supports the diagnosis, it is not necessary to make another tracing until about the third day. A final tracing should be made a day or so prior to discharge from the hospital. When the initial tracing is not diagnostic, serial tracings for 7 to 10 days may be needed before changes occur. When a cardiac arrhythmia is suspected during physical examination, a long "rhythm strip" should be obtained. Cardiac arrhythmias are quite common during the first 24 to 48 hr after myocardial infarction.[105] It is for this reason that continuous monitoring of the electrical activity of the heart is desirable. When an arrhythmia is detected on the monitor, it is then necessary to make a permanent electrocardiogram, so that the rhythm disturbance can be studied more easily.

Smoking is often prohibited during the early stage of acute myocardial infarction because of sedation and oxygen administration. The patient should be advised not to restart smoking during the period of convalescence.

The period of rest following a myocardial infarction should be pleasant for the patient, and *anxiety, fear,* and *anger should be prevented or alleviated when possible.* Proper management of the individual patient in this regard varies greatly from patient to patient. Business worries should not be brought to the patient. On the other hand, certain compulsive patients may not be able to rest until urgent business decisions have been made. The number of visitors, the viewing of television, and reading are determined on an individual basis. The morning visit of the technician assigned to draw blood for prothrombin determination may be disturbing to a patient. On rare occasions it may be necessary for the physician to do the venipuncture or omit the procedure. *Mild sedation* with phenobarbital may be used for several days but should not be continued indefinitely if all goes well.

Rehabilitation

Years ago a patient with a heart attack remained in bed for weeks or months, resigned from his job, and lived the remainder of his restricted life with fear and unhappiness. Dr. Paul White deserves the credit for reversing this approach and teaching physicians and patients that total rehabilitation is usually possible and desirable. The rehabilitation of the patients with myocardial infarction must be in the physician's mind when he first sees the patient. As a general rule it is wise to tell the patient the nature of his illness when the diagnosis is established. At the same time it is essential to indicate to the patient and his family that he is *expected* to return to his job after a period of convalescence. The intelligent patient will ask many questions during the early period of convalescence. These questions should be answered with an optimistic outlook, since the vast majority of patients have few complications and are able to return to work. The usual plan of rehabilitation may be altered later if complications such as congestive heart failure or disabling angina pectoris occur and persist.

Treatment of Complications[106]

It is important to anticipate the development of certain complications that may follow myocardial infarction in order be prepared to institute treatment promptly.

Shock is responsible for many deaths[107–118] (see Chap. 17). It is often transient and self-limited at the onset of infarction; when it persists for an hour or more, the mortality approaches 80 per cent. Perfusion of vital organs such as the heart, brain, and kidney is impaired, and arrhythmias, congestive heart failure, cerebral vascular accident, confusion, psychosis, and oliguria may ensue. Gangrene of the bowel has been noted in extreme instances. Shock is treated with oxygen, digitalis, and pressor amines. The patient should be placed in the recumbent position. When alveolar pulmonary edema is also present, it may be necessary to elevate the head of the bed in order to relieve dyspnea. Oxygen is given by nasal catheter with due care to avoid air swallowing and gastric distension. One is often faced with the problem of relieving persistent pain in the patient with shock, when additional drugs may enhance peripheral vascular collapse. The management of such problems must be individualized weighing the fact that the price of pain relief of many may be additional hypotension and respiratory depression, which increase the risk of cardiac arrest. Pain relief in this setting is best accomplished by the cautious administration of small doses of morphine sulfate intravenously. The case against the intramuscular administration of morphine sulfate is the delayed absorption incident to shock and the fact that one may be tempted to repeat the dose before optimum effect has been reached from the first one. With a rise in blood pressure there may be rapid absorption of an excessive dose of the drug with attendant respiratory depression. The mere presence of hypotension unaccompanied by clinical evidence of shock does not require pressor drug therapy. An exception is the occurrence of an arrhythmia, such as atrial fibrillation or ventricular tachycardia, which may be reverted by raising the blood pressure and increasing effective coronary perfusion. With mild shock, meteraminol (Aramine) is preferred as initial therapy, and often the blood pressure may stabilize after a single dose of 2.5 to 5.0 mg intramuscularly. It may be repeated at intervals as needed. If shock is not controlled by this drug, *l*-norepinephrine (Levophed) should be given by intravenous drip. Four to eight micrograms should be diluted in 1,000 ml 5 per cent glucose in distilled water and given in the arm vein at a rate of 1 ml per min or less to avoid circulatory overloading. The technique of administering this drug requires the skill of a physician. This drug produces cutaneous arteriolar constriction, which leads to cold, clammy, cyanotic skin; rarely the arterial constriction may produce gangrene of digits as well as necrosis of tissue at the site of administration. Phentolamine methanesulfonate (Regitine) may be injected into the perivenous tissue when extravasation occurs to decrease the possibility of tissue slough. Inadvertent abrupt increase in the administration of the drug may produce hypertension, pulmonary edema, treacherous arrhythmias, and further infarction of

the myocardium.[119] There is risk of subendocardial hemorrhage when a large concentration of norepinephrine is used. Gauer et al. have shown that these lesions develop because the ventricular pressure may exceed aortic pressure and that shearing forces produced by cardiac contraction are applied to the endocardium when there is no residual volume in the heart.[120] Although these drugs have an inotropic effect on the myocardium with increased contractility and stroke output, these beneficial effects may be outweighed by the marked increase in peripheral resistance and consequent increase in cardiac work. Furthermore, tachyphylaxis rapidly occurs, so that it is difficult to withdraw the drug without subsequent hypotension. These side effects are generally outweighed by the beneficial effects, and some reduction in mortality can be obtained. Rapid digitalization by vein is indicated for virtually all cases of shock secondary to myocardial infarction (see Chap. 15). It is beneficial where there is sinus tachycardia but may be dramatically beneficial when atrial fibrillation or flutter is present. Ventricular tachycardia in the undigitalized patient is no contraindication to its use. There is a high incidence of interstitial pulmonary edema in persistent shock, and alveolar pulmonary edema is not uncommon. Whereas shock may precipitate cardiac arrhythmias, the latter may precipitate shock. While the elevation of blood pressure produced by pressor amines may eliminate certain arrhythmias, it is often necessary to use more specific antiarrhythmic drugs and measures. Accordingly, therapy with lidocaine, procaine amide, and quinidine may be needed (see Chap. 16). These drugs are frequently used for ventricular tachycardia, but they may produce hypotension. If there is not a prompt response to their use, the d-c converter may be used at the bedside with morphine analgesia (see Chap. 16). It should be recalled in the management of shock that most monitoring devices measure electrical activity and give no information regarding blood pressure. Therapy such as intraarterial or intravenous transfusion is generally contraindicated; however, infusion of plasma may restore the blood pressure to normal in the patient with hypovolemia due to prior therapy with chlorothiazide drugs and in the patient who has received catecholamines over a period of time. Corticosteroids are not of predictable value. The use of adrenergic blocking drugs or epidural analgesia in an effort to increase tissue perfusion is under investigation.

Congestive heart failure occurs during the acute stage of myocardial infarction more often than is generally appreciated. Basal rales, often thought to be due to "hypostasis," in reality indicate failure of the left side of the heart in the absence of chronic lung disease. This can be verified by the x-ray demonstration of interstitial pulmonary edema. The latter may be present in the absence of rales, ventricular diastolic gallop rhythm, neck vein distension, and symptoms such as dyspnea. Sinus tachycardia of 120 or greater in the absence of shock is often associated with interstitial pulmonary edema. Digitalis is indicated when any one or a combination of these findings is present (see Chap. 15). The authors have observed no harmful effects from the cautious use of digitalis in this setting. Appropriate diuretic therapy is given in conjunction with digitalization (see Chap. 15). Alveolar pulmonary edema is treated by propping the patient upright, administering morphine sulfate intravenously (while observing the blood pressure and respiratory amplitude), oxygen, rotating tourniquets, and digitalis. Phlebotomy may be helpful when there is not a prompt response. The success of therapy may depend upon controlling a cardiac arrhythmia. Atrial fibrillation or flutter is usually controlled by digitalis. Ventricular tachycardia should be reversed to normal using procaine amide (Pronestyl hydrochloride), lidocaine hydrochloride, quinidine sulfate, or the d-c converter.

While the use of constant monitoring devices has shown a greater incidence of *arrhythmias* than previously suspected,[105] the routine administration of quinidine sulfate prophylactically has not altered the mortality rate. When frequent atrial or ventricular premature beats occur each minute, 0.2 gm quinidine sulfate may be given orally every 4 hr (see Chap. 16). Atrial tachycardia is treated by pressor amines, digitalis, or quinidine sulfate. Carotid sinus massage, ordinarily useful in this arrhythmia, carries a small risk with myocardial infarction. Atrial fibrillation and flutter are treated by digitalization and usually revert to normal within a few hours or a few days (see Chap. 16). Ventricular tachycardia responds to lidocaine hydrochloride (Xylocaine hydrochloride), quinidine sulfate, or procaine amide intravenously (see Chap. 16). In urgent situations the d-c converter should be employed.

Atrioventricular block, usually associated with occlusion of the right coronary artery, is generally transient, and no therapy is indicated for simple P-R prolongation. When 2:1 A-V block is present, it is necessary to monitor the rhythm continuously. The external cardiac pacemaker should be set to stimulate the heart should arrest occur. If the external pacemaker is used a single time, it seems advisable to insert a catheter pacemaker in the outflow tract of the right ventricle in order to take over pacing of the heart. The catheter pacemaker is not employed in every case because of the problems associated with inserting the catheter in the jugular vein, the need to transport the patient for fluoroscopy, and the rare stimulation of ectopic ventricular arrhythmia by the catheter tip. Its use is justified after a need has been demonstrated, since the external pacemaker is not as satisfactory and its use is associated with pain and anxiety.

Complete heart block is an indication for a catheter pacemaker whether a Stokes-Adams attack has occurred or not. The rate is usually set at about 60 per min. It not only prevents standstill but may prevent or effectively control heart failure. The internal catheter pacemaker is usually required no more than a few days, but occasionally complete heart block persists and periods of ventricular standstill or fibrillation may be present in spite of the use of isopropyl norepinephrine and other drugs. Permanent implantation of a pacemaker may be required, and this may be done several weeks after infarction.

Complete heart block and Stokes-Adams attacks commonly occur in the absence of acute myocardial infarction (see Chap. 16).

Sudden death due to ventricular standstill or fibrillation may occur unpredictably.[121] Immediate external cardiac massage and pulmonary ventilation is required for this catastrophic event. Electrical defibrillation is usually required when ventricular fibrillation is present. Many lives have been saved by using these techniques.

Thromboembolism may involve the venous or arterial system.[122]

Pulmonary emboli may originate in the right side of the heart as mural thrombi or in the peripheral venous system. They may produce sudden death, precipitate myocardial ischemia, cardiac arrhythmias, and congestive heart failure. Treatment consists of anticoagulation with heparin followed later by Coumadin. If the patient has already been given anticoagulant therapy with coumarin derivatives, it may be wise to change to heparin therapy for 7 to 10 days. The risk associated with ligation of the inferior vena cava in the wake of an acute myocardial infarction usually prohibits the use of this procedure.

Peripheral arterial embolism, arising from mural thrombi in the left side of the heart, may occlude the bifurcation of the aorta, iliac, femoral, popliteal, or occasionally the brachial arteries.[123] (See Chap. 59 for discussion of the surgical treatment of peripheral emboli.) Cerebral, mesenteric, splenic, and renal artery occlusion may also occur. Except in cerebral infarction, with its attendant risk of hemorrhage, heparin is used in acute occlusion in the hope of preventing propagation of the clot. Anticoagulant therapy should be continued for several months in an effort to decrease the chance of recurrence.

The transient type of *pericarditis* usually makes

its appearance from the second to fifth day after myocardial infarction, disappears in a few days, and usually requires no therapy unless pain is prominent, in which event salicylates or corticosteroids are used. Anticoagulants can be continued with reasonable safety when this type of pericarditis is present. On the other hand, diffuse pericarditis with persistent friction rub contraindicates anticoagulants because of the risk of pericardial hemorrhage. Cardiac tamponade has occurred under these circumstances.[124] Post-myocardial-infarction pericarditis, as described by Dressler, may be delayed in appearance several weeks to several months.[125] It is often associated with pneumonitis, pleuritis, leukocytosis, pericardial effusion, and rarely cardiac tamponade. Anticoagulants are contraindicated in the syndrome. Salicylates and corticosteroids may give dramatic relief. A tendency to recurrence is notable. Occasionally pericardial aspiration is necessary.

The *shoulder-hand syndrome* is thought to be a neurotrophic disorder.[126] It makes its appearance one to several months after infarction and is associated with pain on abduction of the arm at the shoulder. There may be pain, stiffness, swelling, and discoloration of the skin of the hand. Palmar nodules and Dupuytren's contractures are not uncommon. The incidence of this disorder has decreased since earlier mobilization of the patient and active motion of the shoulders have supplanted immobility. The condition usually affects the left shoulder and hand but may be bilateral. It is treated by physiotherapy, heat, and a program of gentle exercise of the shoulder. The course may be a protracted one lasting many months. Some patients develop the rotator-cuff syndrome because of calcific tendinitis. In selected cases, the intraarticular injection of hydrocortisone may give relief. Dupuytren's contractures and palmar nodules may on occasion require surgical excision.

Prostatic obstruction with retention of urine in the bladder may occur in the elderly male who is placed at bed rest and is given opiates. If the patient cannot void standing by the bed, catheterization of the bladder may be needed. If the symptoms recur, an indwelling catheter may be needed for a short period of time. If an indwelling catheter is required, a constant slow drip of 0.25 per cent acetic acid or dilute neomycin and polymyxin solution through a three-way (continuous-flow) catheter in the bladder has been shown to be capable of preventing bacteremia (40 mg neomycin and 20 mg polymyxin are mixed in 1,000 ml isotonic saline solution and dripped into the bladder at a rate of 40 ml per hr, or 1 liter per day[127]). Refractory congestive heart failure may be due to inapparent bladder obstruction. Rarely, an indwelling catheter

may be necessary for 3 months until prostatic resection can be done safely.

Fecal impaction is catastrophic and may induce recurrent myocardial ischemic pain, abdominal distension, and abdominal pain. It should be avoided by the use of appropriate laxatives such as Dulcolax, colace, or milk of magnesia, or by the use of rectal suppositories. It is more common in women.

Pulmonary infection in the patient with congested lungs may be wrongly attributed to heart failure. While bronchopneumonia is an uncommon complication of myocardial infarction, it should be promptly recognized and treated with appropriate antibiotics. Pulmonary infarction is commonly misdiagnosed as pneumonia.

Both *gout* and *diabetes* may be precipitated by myocardial infarction and are occasionally brought to light by the administration of chlorothiazide drugs. Patients with a history of frequent attacks of gout should receive colchicine or Benemid as a prophylactic measure.

Surgical treatment for *rupture of the interventricular septum* should be considered for those patients who survive several weeks. Successful cures have been reported.[128] External rupture of the heart commonly produces sudden death and is not amenable to surgical treatment. Selected cases of *ventricular aneurysm* associated with refractory heart failure may be resected surgically with restoration of cardiac compensation.[129-133]

Virtually all patients with myocardial infarction have some degree of *anxiety*, either suppressed or overt. Although certain aspects of this problem have been discussed earlier in this chapter, a few points are repeated here for emphasis: A confident optimistic attitude by the physician may greatly allay apprehension. The various types of chest pain which the patient may experience must be deciphered and explained, so that those of noncardiac origin are not misinterpreted by the patient as new "heart attacks." Early mobilization in a chair, as described earlier, affords reassurance. The knowledge imparted at onset to the patient that he will be expected to return to his usual occupation has psychologic virtue. Mild sedatives are useful during the illness. Mild depression is not infrequent. The majority of such cases can be, and should be, satisfactorily handled by the internist. Drugs such as imipramine hydrochloride (Tofranil), 25 mg four times daily, may be helpful. *Psychotic depression* is a rare complication, and psychiatric help may be required.

Prognosis of Patients with Angina Pectoris and Myocardial Infarction

The prognosis of patients with angina pectoris and myocardial infarction cannot be stated with certainty. Numerous studies of large groups of patients have been reported with conflicting results. The trend during the last two decades has been toward less mortality and greater longevity. This more favorable outlook is undoubtedly due to the fact that milder cases are recognized more readily today and that treatment has improved considerably (especially that of myocardial infarction).

The prognosis of patients with angina pectoris depends upon associated complications of coronary disease such as myocardial infarction and congestive heart failure. Other factors adversely influencing long-range prognosis include hypertension, cardiac enlargement, atrial fibrillation, diabetes mellitus, and valvular heart disease.[134] Many patients with angina pectoris live 20 years after the onset of symptoms, and some live as long as 30 years.[136] Richards, Bland, and White noted an average survival of between 9 and 10 years in a large group of patients.[135,136] Another study of 6,882 cases followed for 5 to 23 years indicated a mortality of 15 per cent in the first year and a 9 per cent death rate per year thereafter.[137] *The true prognosis is undoubtedly better than most published figures, since many patients have unrecognized angina pectoris and do not seek medical advice.* Angina pectoris may lessen or disappear as the result of the development of collateral circulation or as the result of myocardial infarction.

The data on mortality from myocardial infarction are customarily weighted by inclusion of only those who live to be hospitalized; furthermore, it is usual to include only patients with myocardial infarction documented by electrocardiogram, which would exclude many patients. Data from large public institutions are weighted to exclude patients with mild symptoms who do not seek advice or who are not admitted.

Bainton and Peterson found that 63 per cent of men who died from coronary disease did so within *1 hr* and 85 per cent within *24 hr*.[138] Only 23 per cent of patients who died lived long enough to be seen by a physician. Spain, in reviewing the cause of sudden death, found that a witnessed fatal episode lasting less than an hour was due to coronary disease in over 90 per cent of the cases.[139] These studies indicate that sudden death is usually due to coronary disease. They also indicate that sudden death is not a rare manifestation of the disease. A recent study by Hagstrom et al. indicates that in patients who have experienced myocardial infarction, even though they survive and are in good health, the risk of dying suddenly is seven times greater than that of the general population.[140]

Mortality rates for initial attacks of myocardial infarction vary widely from 12 per cent to 40 per cent, 25 per cent being a common figure. *Death is usually due to congestive heart failure, cardiac arrhythmia, shock, cardiac rupture, or pulmonary embolus.* Dividing patients into "good-risk" and "poor-risk" groups has merit in prognosis, if one allows for the fact that perhaps up to one-fourth of patients classified as good risk on admission need reclassification into the poor-risk group during the course of the illness. Russek and Zohman in a retrospective study of myocardial infarction noted a mortality of 3.1 per cent of 489 hospitalized good-risk patients.[141] Almost one-half of those dying did so in the first *48 hr*. The poor-risk group (558 patients) included patients with previous myocardial infarctions, intractable pain, extreme degree of persistent shock, significant enlargement of the heart, gallop rhythm, congestive heart failure, diabetic acidosis, marked obesity, prior pulmonary embolism, varicose veins in lower extremities, thrombophlebitis (old or recent), or other states predisposing to thrombosis. The mortality of the poor-risk group was 60 per cent.[141]

The published mortality rates for women following myocardial infarction are higher than for men, but most attribute this to the fact that infarction occurs on the average 10 years later in women than men. Mortality is greater in the older age group than in the younger age group; it is higher when there is overt diabetes. Patients with prior infarctions have a more serious outlook, reflecting perhaps a greater loss of myocardial function due to the loss of contractile units from prior scarring plus the additional acute loss of myocardium. Persistent pain unrelieved by opiates is a poor prognostic sign and is associated with a higher mortality rate and a higher incidence of cardiac arrest. The mortality will obviously be higher in patients with occlusion of the vessel which provides the major blood supply to the heart, whether it be the right coronary artery, which is more often dominant, or the left coronary artery, which less often supplies the major part of the coronary circulation. Furthermore, when the right coronary is occluded proximal to its first branch, there is a high incidence of infarction of both the sinoatrial (S-A) node and the atrioventricular (A-V) node with resultant atrial arrhythmias and A-V conduction disturbances. Similarly, atrial arrhythmias may occur if the left coronary is occluded proximal to the circumflex or to the first branch of the circumflex, which supplies the S-A node in 40 per cent of patients (see Chap. 29). Nonparoxysmal nodal tachycardia or complete heart block may follow occlusion of the right coronary artery, which supplies the A-V node in about 90 per cent of patients. In patients with acute myocardial infarction the mortality rates associated with these disorders approach the mortality rate associated with ventricular tachycardia. James has emphasized the differences in complications and mortality produced by infarction of various parts of the myocardium.[142] Patients with anterior myocardial infarction may lose a large mass of myocardium and develop congestive heart failure, but they are less likely to develop arrhythmias or heart block. With infarction of the lateral wall, there may be a smaller loss of muscle but a greater susceptibility to arrhythmias and heart block, which are associated with a poorer prognosis. Since posterior or inferior infarction is more often associated with arrhythmias and heart block, the acute course is more likely to be fatal or "suddenly stormy"; on the other hand, because of the smaller mass of muscle involved, the long-term prognosis is better once the acute phase is survived.

The true incidence of arrhythmia complicating myocardial infarction is not known, but Hurwitz and Eliot have established the following guidelines:[143] Death occurred in 27 per cent of their patients who had an arrhythmia and in only 12 per cent of those without an arrhythmia. Mortality associated with the more serious arrhythmias was 47 per cent. The mortality of patients with ventricular tachycardia, which may presage ventricular fibrillation, approaches 60 per cent.[143] Transient A-V block is not uncommon with occlusion of the right coronary artery proximal to the artery to the A-V node. Complete heart block with or without Adams-Stokes seizures has been accompanied by a higher mortality; however, electronic monitoring and pacing may reduce the hazards of this complication.

Shock lasting 1 hr or longer is associated with a mortality of approximately 80 per cent, which may be reduced to 50 per cent with pressor therapy.

Congestive heart failure may be responsible for 30 per cent of deaths following acute myocardial infarction. Mild left ventricular failure with interstitial pulmonary edema demonstrated by x-ray is very common, but is not associated with the high mortality of advanced heart failure or alveolar pulmonary edema. On the other hand pulmonary edema at onset of infarction is associated with a mortality approaching 80 per cent.

Thromboembolism involving major pulmonary artery trunks or the bifurcation of the aorta carries a high mortality.

Myocardial rupture occurring within 3 weeks is responsible for 10 to 15 per cent of all deaths in patients hospitalized for acute myocardial infarction. The most common cause of death in patients who survive 2 months or more is *recurrent myocardial infarction.*

One can be lulled into a false sense of security by so-called "mild" coronary attacks with no complications and with limited ECG abnormalities; however, more serious attacks may occur within a few years. Of 100 such patients followed for 5 years, 48 per cent suffered another myocardial infarction with 18 per cent mortality; 54 continued to have angina, and 70 per cent developed reinfarction—50 per cent within 1 year.[144] *The best index of recovery from myocardial infarction is the ability of the patient to resume normal activities without angina or congestive heart failure.*

Feil has recently written on the prognosis of coronary heart disease.[145] A portion of his discussion is reproduced below with the permission of Dr. Feil and the publishers.

The prognosis of coronary heart disease has changed considerably since the days of Heberden. We now recognize the many patients who survive the attack of infarction for many years. From a study of the literature and from his own experience the author believes that the following factors influence prognosis.

Factors influencing prognosis

Previous attacks.—Patients who are experiencing their second or third attack have a more serious outlook.

Pain.—If the pain lasts longer than 24 hours after the infarction, the prognosis is correspondingly poorer.

Shock.—Perhaps the most serious of omens is shock. In spite of oxygen and the pressor drugs the outlook is poor although some patients are tided over. Hypotension may be relative; for example, if the patient was previously normotensive then a systolic pressure of 80 to 90 mm. Hg. is not shock.

Heart failure.—This signifies extensive myocardial injury and few patients survive. But the prognosis is not uniformly bad for an occasional patient lives many years in comfort.

Fever and leukocytosis.—If the temperature is high and persistent and if the leukocytosis is over 15,000 cells per cu. mm. the chances of recovery are less. If the transaminase level is high the prognosis is more grave.

Diabetes mellitus.—This does not add to the gravity of the immediate situation, but the long-range prognosis is less favourable due to the progression of atherosclerosis and the probability of death from other arterial disease.

Arrhythmias.—The most serious complication is that of ventricular tachycardia, if not readily controlled by quinidine or Pronestyl. Atrial fibrillation and flutter are serious only if not readily controlled by digitalis.

Embolism.—This occurs less frequently today with anticoagulant therapy and early ambulation.

Electrocardiogram.—Favourable aspects of the electrocardiogram are rapid return to normal, non-transmural infarcts, absence of frequent premature beats, absence of heart block, normal voltage, and normal rates.

Obesity.—This adds to the gravity of the situation from a long-term point of view.

Severe hypertension.—This decreases life expectancy.

Pulmonary disease.—Severe emphysema and asthma add to the gravity of prognosis.

There is one imponderable factor in determining prognosis, namely the architecture of the coronary arteries. If the coronaries are both well-developed and have an equal share of the available blood supply, the patient will stand a better chance of recovery following infarction. Cardiac enlargement of considerable degree and cardiac aneurysms are unfavourable features.

The findings presaging a favourable long-term prognosis are as follows: The patient should be of average weight, middle age, have normal pulmonary function, have only a moderate reduction in blood pressure, have little fever and that of short duration, have his pain relieved promptly, be free from arrhythmias and congestive failure, and readily respond to the optimism of the attending physician. He should not have had previous infarctions.

The prognosis in myocardial infarction cannot be accurately made; some patients apparently making an uneventful recovery die suddenly; others pass through a stormy convalescence but do well. It is best not to be too precise in judgment. If the patient survives the first year he has a 75 per cent chance of living 5 years; if he lives 5 years and is seemingly well, he has a slightly less than even chance of living 15 years; and then, if well, he has a 41 per cent chance of surviving 20 years.

Sigler studied 255 patients who lived or are still living 10 years or longer following acute myocardial infarction. A good percentage of the patients in the series have surpassed the average life expectancy.[146]

Prevention

The prevention of disease is the ultimate goal of medicine. Coronary atherosclerosis is no exception. Unfortunately we do not have proof that steps taken during early life may prevent the development of the disease. Sufficient information relative to this problem should accrue in the next several years. In the meantime certain high-risk coronary-prone individuals (subject to clinically recognizable coronary disease with greater frequency than others) have been identified and are now being studied.[34] Factors common to this group include being male, hypertension, obesity, high serum cholesterol, cigarette smoking, lack of exercise, history of atherosclerosis occurring prematurely (before age sixty) in members of the family, and diseases such as diabetes and hypothyroidism. Certain of these factors can be altered and some cannot. Our present state of knowledge does not allow us to state that if the factors are controlled, angina pectoris or myocardial infarction will be prevented, thereby returning the patient to the low-risk group. It does seem wise, however, to recognize that the facts point very strongly in certain directions. They indicate the *"possibility* of *prevention"* [34]

The book *Heart Attack! Are You a Candidate?* by Arthur Blumenfeld [147] was written for the layman and should be quite helpful to the coronary-prone individual.

REFERENCES

1. Solandt, D. Y., and Best, C. H.: Heparin and Coronary Thrombosis in Experimental Animals, *Lancet*, **2**:130, 1938.
2. Wright, I. S.: Experiences with Dicumarol in the Treatment of Coronary Thrombosis, *Proc. Am. Fed. Clin. Res.*, **2**:101, 1945.
3. Nichol, E. S., and Page, S. W., Jr.: Dicumarol Therapy in Acute Coronary Thrombosis: Results in Fifty Attacks, *J. Florida M.A.*, **32**:365, 1946.
4. Peters, H. R., Guyther, J. R., and Brambel, C. E.: Dicumarol in Acute Coronary Thrombosis, *J.A.M.A.*, **130**:398, 1946.
5. Wright, I. S., Marple, C. D., and Beck, D. F.: Anticoagulant Therapy of Coronary Thrombosis with Myocardial Infarction, *J.A.M.A.*, **138**:1074–1079, 1948.
6. Russek, H. I., and Zehman, B. L.: Limited Use of Anticoagulants in Acute Myocardial Infarction: Analysis of 1000 "Good Risk" Patients, *J.A.M.A.*, **163**:922, 1957.
7. Wright, I. S.: The Case for Anticoagulant Therapy, *Circulation*, **30**:447, 1964.
8. Hilden, T., Iverson, K., Raaschou, F., and Schwartz, M. M.: Anticoagulants in Acute Myocardial Infarction, *Lancet*, **2**:327, 1961.
9. Hilden, T.: The Case against Anticoagulant Therapy, *Circulation*, **30**:458, 1964.
10. Sise, H. S., Moschos, C. B., Gauthier, Jacques, and Becker, R.: The Risk of Interrupting Long-term Anticoagulant Treatment: A Rebound Hypercoagulable State Following Hemorrhage, *Circulation*, **24**:1137–1142, 1961.
11. Sevitt, S., and Innes, D.: Evidence against "Rebound" Thrombosis after Stopping Oral Anticoagulant Drugs, *Lancet*, **2**:974–975, 1963.
12. Seaman, A. J., Griswold, H. E., Reaume, R. B., and Ritzman, L. W.: Anticoagulants in Coronary Artery Disease, *J.A.M.A.*, **189**:183, 1964.
13. Achor, R. W., et al.: Cooperative Study: Sodium Heparin vs. Sodium Warfarin in Acute Myocardial Infarction, *J.A.M.A.*, **189**:555–562, 1964.
14. Nichol, E. S., Phillips, W. C., and Casten, G. G.: Virtue of Prompt Anticoagulant Therapy in Impending Infarction: Experiences with 318 Patients during a 10-year Period, *Ann. Int. Med.*, **50**:1158, 1959.
15. Wood, P.: Acute and Subacute Coronary Insufficiency, *Brit. M. J.*, **1**:1779, 1961.
16. Resnik, W. H.: Preinfarction Angina. Part II. An Interpretation, *Mod. Concepts Cardiovas. Dis.*, **31**:757–761, 1962.
17. Waaler, B.: The Effect of Permanent Anticoagulant Therapy on Symptoms and Mortality in

Angina Pectoris, *Acta med. scandinav.*, **157**:289, 1957.

18. Manchester, B.: The Value of Continuous (1 to 10 Years) Long-term Anticoagulation Therapy, *Ann. Int. Med.*, **47**:1202, 1957.

19. Suzman, M. M., Ruskın, H. D., and Goldberg, B.: Evaluation of Effect of Continuous Long-term Anticoagulant Therapy on Prognosis of Myocardial Infarction, *Circulation*, **12**:338–352, 1955.

20. Thomes, A. B., Scallen, R. W., and Savage, I. R.: Value of Long-term Anticoagulant Therapy in Coronary Disease, *J.A.M.A.*, **176**:181, 1961.

21. Bjerkelund, C. J.: The Effect of Long Term Treatment with Dicumarol in Myocardial Infarction, *Acta med. scandinav.*, **158** (supp. 330): 1, 1957.

22. Report of the Working Party on Anticoagulant Therapy in Coronary Thrombosis to the Medical Research Council: An Assessment of Long-term Anticoagulant Administration after Cardiac Infarction, *Brit. M. J.*, **1**:803, 1959.

23. Seaman, A. J., Griswold, H. E., Reaume, R. B., and Ritzman, L. W.: Prophylactic Anticoagulant Therapy for Coronary Artery Disease, *J.A.M.A.*, **189**:183–187, 1964.

24. Harvald, B., Hilden, T., and Lund, E.: Long-term Anticoagulant Therapy after Myocardial Infarction, *Lancet*, **2**:327, 1961.

25. Borchgrevink, C. F.: Long-term Anticoagulant Therapy in Angina Pectoris, *Lancet*, **1**:449, 1962.

26. Meltzer, L. E., Palmon, F., Ferrigan, M., Pekover, J., Sauer, H., and Kitchell, J. R.: Prothrombin Levels and Fatality Rates in Acute Myocardial Infarction, *J.A.M.A.*, **187**:986–993, 1964.

27. Symposium on Fibrinolysis, *Am. J. Cardiol.*, **6**: 367–563, 1960.

28. Sherry, S., and Fletcher, A. P.: Thrombolytic Therapy (Editorial), *Am. Heart J.*, **61**:575–578, 1961.

29. Richter, I. H., Cliffton, E. E., Epstein, S., Musacchio, F., Nassar, A., Favazza, A. G., and Katabi, G.: Thrombolysin Therapy in Myocardial Infarction, *Am. J. Cardiol.*, **9**:82, 1962.

30. Dewar, H. A., Stephenson, P., Horler, A. R., Cassells-Smith, A. J., and Ellis, P. A.: Fibrinolytic Therapy of Coronary Thrombosis, *Brit. M. J.*, **1**:915, 1963.

31. Katz, A. M., McDonald, L., Davies, B., and Edgill, M.: Fibrinolysis and Blood Coagulation in Ischaemic Heart Disease, *Lancet*, **1**:801, 1963.

32. Mazel, M. S., Bolton, H. E., Stern, J. R., Riera, R., and Cabral, H.: Coronary Arterial and Other Intravascular Thromboses Treated with Fibrinolysin: Experimented and Clinical Results, *Angiology*, **14**: 88, 1963.

33. Alexander, J. K.: Obesity and Cardiac Performance, *Circulation*, **30**:41, 1964.

34. Stamler, J.: Are Heart Attacks Preventable? *Illinois M. J.*, **123**:145 (Feb.) 1963.

35. Master, A. M., Jaffe, H. L., and Chesky, K.: Relationship of Obesity to Coronary Disease and Hypertension, *J.A.M.A.*, **153**:1499–1501, 1953.

36. Dawber, T. R., and Kannel, W. B.: Susceptibility to Coronary Heart Disease, *Mod. Concepts Cardiovas. Dis.*, **30**:671–676, 1961.

37. Byers. S. O., Friedman, M., and Rosenman, R. H.: Review: On the Regulation of Blood Cholesterol, *Metabolism*, **1**:479–503, 1952.

38. Page, I. H., Stare, F. J., Corcoran, A. C., Pollack. H., and Wilkinson, C. F., Jr.: Atherosclerosis and the Fat Content of the Diet, *Circulation*, **16**:163–178, 1957.

39. Brown. H. B., and Page, I. H.: Lowering Blood Lipid Levels by Changing Food Patterns, *J.A.M.A.*, **168**:1989–1995, 1958.

40. Ahrens, E. J., Jr., Hirsch, J., Insull, W., Tsaltas, T. T., Blomstrand, R., and Peterson, M. L.: The Influence of Dietary Fats on Serum-lipid Levels in Man, *Lancet*, **1**:943, 1957.

41. Bronte-Stewart, B.: The Effect of Dietary Fats on the Blood Lipids and Their Relation to Ischaemic Heart Disease, *Brit. M. Bull.*, **14**:243, 1958.

42. Boyer, P. A., Jr., Lowe, J. T., Gardier, R. W., and Ralston, J. D.: Effect of a Practical Dietary Regimen on Serum Cholesterol Level, *J.A.M.A.*, **170**:257–261, 1959.

43. Jolliffe, N.: Fats, Cholesterol, and Coronary Heart Disease, *Circulation*, **20**:109–127, 1959.

44. Stamler, J.: Current Status of the Dietary Prevention and Treatment of Atherosclerotic Coronary Heart Disease, *Progr. Cardiovas. Dis.*, **3**:56–95, 1960.

45. Report by the Central Committee for Medical and Community Program of the American Heart Association, Dr. A. Carlton Ernstene, Chairman: Ad Hoc Committee on Dietary Fat and Atherosclerosis, Irvine H. Page, M.D., Chairman: Dietary Fat and Its Relation to Heart Attacks and Strokes, *J.A.M.A.*, **175**:389–391, 1961.

46. Report by the Central Committee for Medical and Community Program of the American Heart Association: Dietary Fat and Its Relation to Heart Attacks and Strokes, *Circulation*, **23**:1–5, 1961.

47. Poole, J. C. F.: Effect of Diet and Lipemia on Coagulation and Thrombosis, *Fed. Proc.*, Part 2, Suppl. 11, **21**:20, 1962.

48. Master, A. M., and Jaffe, H. L.: Fads, Public Opinion, and Heart Diseases, *J.A.M.A.*, **183**:102–107, 1963.

49. Yudkin, J.: Diet and Coronary Thrombosis, *Lancet*, **2**:155, 1957.

50. Yudkin, J.: Dietary Carbohydrate and Ischemic Heart Disease, *Am. Heart J.*, **66**:835, 1963.

51. "How to Follow the Prudent Diet," Department of Health, Bureau of Nutrition, City of New York, 1961.

52. Jolliffe, N., Rinzler, S. H., and Archer, M.: The Anti-Coronary Club: Including a Discussion of the Effect of a Prudent Diet on the Serum Cholesterol

Level of Middle-aged Men, *Am. J. Clin. Nutrition,* **7**:451–462, 1959.

53. Dock, W.: Want to Live Dangerously: Try the Prudent Diet! *Arch. Int. Med.,* **113**:613, 1964.

54. Baker, B. M., Frantz, I. D., Keys, A., Kinsell, L. W., Page, I. H., Stamler, J., and Stare, J. J.: The National Diet-Heart Study, *J.A.M.A.,* **185**: 105–106, 1963.

55. Symposium on Rehabilitation in Cardiovascular Disease, *Am. J. Cardiol.,* **7**:315–385, 1961.

56. Newman, L. B.: Total Rehabilitation in Heart Disease, *J.A.M.A.,* **176**:114, 1961.

57. Epstein, F. H.: Epidemiology of Coronary Heart Disease, in A. Morgan Jones (ed.), "Modern Trends of Cardiology" Hoeber Medical Division, Harper & Row, Publishers, Incorporated, New York, 1961.

58. Billimoria, J. D., Drysdale, J., James, D. C. O., and Maclagan, N. F.: Determination of Fibrinolytic Activity of Whole Blood with Special Reference to the Effects of Exercise and Fat Feeding, *Lancet,* **2**:471, 1959.

59. Morris, J. N.: Health and Social Class, *Lancet,* **1**: 1, 69, 1951.

60. Morris, J. N., Heady, J. A., Raffle, P. A. B., Roberts, C. G., and Parks, J. W.: Coronary Heart Disease and Physical Activity of Work, *Lancet,* **2**:1053, 1111, 1953.

61. Morris, J. N., and Crawford, M. D.: Coronary Heart Disease and Physical Activity of Work: Evidence of a National Necropsy Survey, *Brit. M. J.,* **2**:1485, 1958.

62. Stamler, J., Best, M. M., and Turner, J. D.: The Status of Hormonal Therapy for the Primary and Secondary Prevention of Atherosclerotic Coronary Heart Disease, *Progr. Cardiovas. Dis.,* **6**:220–235, 1963.

63. Stamler, J., Pick, R., Katz, L. N., Pick, A., Kaplan, B. M., Berkson, D. M., and Century, D.: Effectiveness of Estrogens for Therapy of Myocardial Infarction in Middle-age Men, *J.A.M.A.,* **183**:632, 1963.

64. Russek, H. I., Naegele, C. F., and Regan, F. D.: Alcohol in the Treatment of Angina Pectoris, *J.A.M.A.,* **143**:355, 1950.

65. Blumgart, H. L.: Current Status of Angina Pectoris, in "The Heart and Circulation, Preprint Report Second National Conference on Cardiovascular Disease," Washington, D.C., 1964, vol. 1, part I, pp. 806–812.

66. Proudfit, W. L.: Treatment of Angina Pectoris and Coronary Insufficiency, *M. Clin. North America,* **45**:1409–1414, 1961.

67. Russek, H. I. et al.: Long-acting Coronary Vasodilator Drugs Metamine, Paveril, Nitroglyn, and Peritrate, *Circulation,* **12**:169, 1955.

68. Towers, M. K., and Wood, P.: Use of Iproniazid in Ischaemic Angina Pectoris, *Brit. M. J.,* **2**:1067, 1958.

69. Russek, H. I., and Funk, E. H.: Comparative Responses to Various Nitrates in the Treatment of Angina Pectoris, *Postgrad. Med.,* **31**:150–155, 1962.

70. Editorial: Drugs in Angina, *Brit. M. J.,* **1**:257–259, 1960.

71. Griffith, C. C.: Amine Oxidase-inhibitors, *Progr. Cardiovas. Dis.,* **3**:119–133, 1960.

72. Cole, S. L., Kaye, H., and Griffith, G. C.: Assay of Anticoagulant Agents. I. A Curve Analysis with Multiple Control Periods, *Circulation,* **15**:405–413, 1957.

73. Davis, J. A., and Wiesel, B. H.: Treatment of Angina Pectoris with a Nitroglycerin Ointment, *Am. J. M. Sc.,* **230**:259, 1955.

74. Corday, E., Gold, H., de Vera, L. B., Williams, J. H., and Fields, J.: Effect of the Cardiac Arrhythmias on the Coronary Circulation, *Ann. Int. Med.,* **50**:535, 1959.

75. Blumgart, H. L., Levine, S. A., and Berlin, D. D.: Congestive Heart Failure and Angina Pectoris: The Therapeutic Effect of Thyroidectomy on Patients without Clinical or Pathological Evidence of Thyroid Toxicity, *A.M.A. Arch. Int. Med.,* **51**:866, 1933.

76. Blumgart, H. L., Freedberg, A. S., and Kurland, G. S.: Treatment of Incapacitated Euthyroid Cardiac Patients with Radioactive Iodine, *J.A.M.A.,* **157**:1, 1955.

77. Paul, O.: Intractable Angina, *Progr. Cardiovas. Dis.,* **6**:212, 1963.

78. Hellerstein, H. K., and Ford, A. B.: Comprehensive Care of the Coronary Patient, *Circulation,* **22**: 1166–1178, 1960.

79. Logue, B.: Treatment of Intractable Angina Pectoris, *Circulation,* **22**:1151–1155, 1960.

80. White, P. D.: The Choice of Therapy in the Management of Refractory Angina Pectoris, *Progr. Cardiovas. Dis.,* **3**:97–107, 1960.

81. Jaffe, H. L., and Corday, E.: The Radioactive Iodine Treatment of Angina Pectoris, *Progr. Cardiovas. Dis.,* **3**:108–118, 1960.

82. Beck, C. S., and Leighninger, D. S.: Scientific Basis for the Surgical Treatment of Coronary Artery Disease, *J.A.M.A.,* **159**:1264–1271, 1955.

83. Bailey, C. P., Truex, R. C., Angulo, A. W., Geckeler, G. D., Likoff, W., Antonius, N., and Neptune, W. B.: The Anatomic (Histologic) Basis and Efficient Clinical Surgical Technique for the Restoration of the Coronary Circulation, *J. Thoracic Surg.,* **25**:143–172, 1953.

84. Bailey, C. P., and Likoff, W.: The Surgical Treatment of Coronary Insufficiency, *Dis. Chest,* **27**: 447, 1955.

85. Dimond, E. G., Kittle, C. F., and Crockett, J. E.: Comparison of Internal Mammary Artery Ligation and Sham Operation for Angina Pectoris, *Am. J. Cardiol.,* **5**:483–486, 1960.

86. White, J. C., and Bland, E. F.: The Surgical Re-

lief of Severe Angina Pectoris, *Medicine*, **27**:1, 1948.

87. Lindgren, I.: Angina Pectoris: A Clinical Study with Special Reference to Neuro-surgical Treatment, *Acta med. scandinav.*, **138**, Suppl. 243, 1950.

88. Vineberg, A.: Experimental Background of Myocardial Revascularization by Internal Mammary Artery Implantation and Supplementary Technics, with Its Clinical Application in 125 Patients: A Review and Critical Appraisal, *Ann. Surg.*, **159**: 185, 1964.

89. Vineberg, A., and Walker, J.: Progress in Cardiovascular Surgery: The Surgical Treatment of Coronary Artery Heart Disease by Internal Mammary Artery Implantation, *Dis. Chest*, **45**:190, 1964.

90. Sewell, W.: Personal communication.

91. Effler, D. B., Groves, L. K., Sones, F. M., Jr., and Shirey, E. K.: Increased Myocardial Perfusion by Internal Mammary Artery Implant: Vineberg's Operation, *Ann. Surg.*, **158**:526, 1963.

92. Sones, F. M.: Personal communication.

93. Hallen, A., Bjork, L., and Bjork, V. O.: Coronary Thromboendarterectomy, *J. Thoracic & Cardiovas. Surg.*, **45**:216, 1963.

94. Effler, D. B.: Surgical Treatment of Coronary Artery Disease, *Heart Bull.*, **13**:89, 1964.

95. Mallory, G. K., White, P. D., and Salcedo-Salgar, J.: The Speed of Healing of Myocardial Infarction: A Study of the Pathologic Anatomy in 72 Cases, *Am. Heart J.*, **18**:647, 1939.

96. Friedberg, C. K.: Atherosclerosis and Myocardial Infarction, *Progr. Cardiovas. Dis.*, **3**:1–95, 1960.

97. Levy, R. L.: A Critique of Certain Measures Presently Employed in Managing Patients with Cardiac Infarction, *Am. Heart J.*, **64**:1, 1962.

98. Lindsay, M. I., Jr., and Spierkerman, R. E.: Reevaluation of Therapy of Acute Myocardial Infarction, *Am. Heart J.*, **67**:559, 1964.

99. Modell, W.: Narcotic Analgesics in Heart Disease, *Am. Heart J.*, **65**:709, 1963.

100. Moon, A. J., Williams, K. G., and Hopkinson, W. I.: A Patient with Coronary Thrombosis Treated with Hyperbaric Oxygen, *Lancet*, **1**:18, 1964.

101. Levine, S. A., and Lown, B.: The "Chair" Treatment of Acute Coronary Thrombosis, *Tr. A. Am. Physicians*, **64**:316–327, 1951.

102. Levine, S. A., and Lown, B.: "Armchair" Treatment of Acute Coronary Thrombosis, *J.A.M.A.*, **148**:1365, 1952.

103. Mitchell, A. M., Fealy, J. B., and Levine, S. A.: Further Observations on the Armchair Treatment of Acute Myocardial Infarction, *J.A.M.A.*, **155**:810, 1954.

104. Cain, H. D., Frasher, W. G., Jr., and Stivelman, R.: Graded Activity Program for Safe Return to Self-care after Myocardial Infarction, *J.A.M.A.*, **177**:111–115, 1961.

105. Spann, J. F., Jr., Moellering, R. C., Jr., Haber, E.,

and Wheeler, E. O.: Arrhythmias in Acute Myocardial Infarction: A Study Utilizing an Electrocardiographic Monitor for Automatic Detection and Recording of Arrhythmias, *New England J. Med.*, **271**:427, 1964.

106. Person, H. E.: The Early Complications of Cardiac Infarction, *Brit. M. J.*, **2**:4–9, 1953.

107. Miller, A. J., Shifrin, A., Kaplan, B. M., Gold, H., Billings, A., and Katz, L. N.: Arterenol in Treatment of Shock, *J.A.M.A.*, **152**:1198, 1953.

108. Gootmick, A., and Knox, F. H., Jr.: Management of Shock in Acute Myocardial Infarction, *Circulation*, **7**:511, 1953.

109. Blumgart, H. L.: Treatment of Acute Myocardial Infarction with Particular Reference to Shock, *J.A.M.A.*, **154**:107, 1954.

110. Binder, M. J., Ryan, J. A., Jr., Marcus, S., Mugler, F., Jr., Strange, D., and Agress, C. M.: Evaluation of Therapy in Shock Following Acute Myocardial Infarction, *Am. J. Med.*, **18**:622, 1955.

111. Gorlin, R., and Robin, E. D.: Cardiac Glycosides in the Treatment of Cardiogenic Shock, *Brit. M. J.*, **1**:937, 1955.

112. Selzer, A., and Rytand, D.: Use of Drugs in Shock Accompanying Myocardial Infarction, *J.A.M.A.*, **168**:762, 1958.

113. Moloch, M., and Rosenberg, B. A.: Acute Myocardial Infarction in a City Hospital. III. Experience with Shock, *Am. J. Cardiol.*, **5**:487–492, 1960.

114. Sampson, J. J.: The Treatment of Shock in Myocardial Infarction, *Dis. Chest*, **33**:667, 1958.

115. Agress, C. M.: Management of Coronary Shock, *Am. J. Cardiol.*, **1**:231, 1958.

116. Bernstein, A., Simon, F., Rothfeld, E. J., Robins, B., Cohen, F. B., and Kaufman, F. G.: Treatment of Shock in Myocardial Infarction, *Am. J. Cardiol.*, **9**:74, 1962.

117. Besterman, E. M. M.: Treatment of Cardiac Shock with Metaraminol, *Brit. M. J.*, **1**:1081–1083, 1959.

118. Bernstein, A., Rothfeld, E. L., Robins, B., Cohen, F., and Simon, F.: The Treatment of Shock Accompanying Myocardial Infarction, *Angiology*, **14**:559, 1963.

119. Szakács, J. E., and Mehlman, B.: Pathologic Changes Induced by *l*-Norepinephrine, *Am. J. Cardiol.*, **5**:619, 1960.

120. Gauer, O. H., and Henry, J. P.: Subendocardial Hemorrhage in Hypotension Treated with Norepinephrine, *Am. Heart J.*, **67**:713, 1964.

121. Surawicz, B., and Pellegrino, E. D.: "Sudden Cardiac Death," Grune & Stratton, Inc., New York, 1964.

122. Miller, R. D., Jordan, R. A., Parker, R. L., and Edwards, J. E.: Thrombo-embolism in Acute and in Healed Myocardial Infarction. II. Systemic and Pulmonary Arterial Occlusion, *Circulation*, **6**:7–15, 1952.

123. Lary, S. G., and de Takats, G.: Peripheral Arterial Embolism after Myocardial Infarction: Occur-

rence in Unsuspected Cases and Ambulatory Patients, *J.A.M.A.*, **155**:10, 1954.

124. Rose, O. A., Ott, R. H., and Maier, H. C.: Hemopericardium with Tamponade during Anticoagulant Therapy of Myocardial Infarct, *J.A.M.A.*, **152**: 1221–1223, 1953.

125. Dressler, W.: The Post-myocardial Infarction Syndrome, *A.M.A. Arch. Int, Med.*, **103**:28–42, 1959.

126. Russek, H. I.: Shoulder-Hand Syndrome Following Myocardial Infarction, *M. Clin. North America*, **42**:1555–1566, 1958.

127. Martin, C. M., and Bookrajian, E. N.: Bacturia Prevention after Indwelling Urinary Catheterization, *Arch. Int. Med.*, **110**:703–711, 1962.

128. Boicourt, O. W., Ritzman, L. W., Chase, J. D., Starr, A., and McCord, C. W.: Rupture of the Infarcted Interventricular Septum: Surgical Repair with Survival, *Circulation*, **26**:1321, 1962.

129. Chapman, D. W., Amad, K., and Cooley, D. A.: Ventricular Aneurysm: Fourteen Cases Subjected to Cardiac Bypass Repair Using the Pump Oxygenator, *Am. J. Cardiol.*, **8**:633–648, 1961.

130. Lillehei, C. W., Levy, M. J., De Wall, R. A., and Warden, H. E.: Resection of Chronic Postinfarction Myocardial Aneurysms, *Geriatrics*, **17**:786, 1962.

131. Cathcart, R. T., Fraimow, W., and Templeton, J. Y., III: Postinfarction Ventricular Aneurysm: Four Years Follow-up of Surgically Treated Cases, *Dis. Chest*, **44**:449, 1963.

132. Effler, D. B., Westcott, R. N., Groves, L. K., and Scully, N. M.: Surgical Treatment of Ventricular Aneurysm, *Arch. Surg.*, **87**:249, 1963.

133. Lam, C. R., Gale, H., and Drake, E.: Surgical Treatment of Left Ventricular Aneurysms, *J.A.M.A.*, **187**:1, 1964.

134. Paul, O.: The Prognosis of Angina Pectoris, in W: Likoff and J. Mayer (eds.), "Seventh Hahnemann Symposium: Coronary Disease," Grune & Stratton, Inc., New York, 1963, pp. 469–472.

135. White, P. D., Bland, E. F., and Muskall, E. W.: The Prognosis of Angina Pectoris: A Long-term Follow-up of 497 Cases Including a Note of 75 Additional Cases of Angina Pectoris Decubitus, *J.A.M.A.*, **123**:801–804, 1943.

136. Richards, D. W., Bland, E. F., and White, P. D.: A Completed Twenty-five-year Follow-up Study of 200 Patients with Myocardial Infarction, *J. Chron. Dis.*, **4**:415–422, 1956.

137. Block, W. J., Crumpaker, E. L., Dry, T. J., and Gage, R. P.: Prognosis of Angina Pectoris, *J.A.M.A.*, **150**:259–264, 1952.

138. Bainton, C. R., and Peterson, D. R.: Deaths from Coronary Heart Disease in Persons Fifty Years of Age and Younger, *New England J. Med.*, **268**: 569–574, 1963.

139. Spain, D. M., Brade, V. A., and Mohr, C.: Coronary Atherosclerosis as a Cause of Unexpected and Unexplained Death, *J.A.M.A.*, **174**:122, 1960.

140. Hagstrom, R. M., Billings, F. T., Chapnick, E. M.,

and Ball, O. T.: Sudden Death in Survivors of Myocardial Infarction, *Circulation*, **30**:91, 1964.

141. Russek, H. I., and Zohman, B. L.: Prognosis in the "Uncomplicated" First Attack of Acute Myocardial Infarction, *Am. J. M. Sc.*, **224**:479–496, 1952.

142. James, T. N.: Arrhythmias and Conduction Disturbances in Acute Myocardial Infarction, *Am. Heart J.*, **64**:416–426, 1962.

143. Hurwitz, M., and Eliot, R. S.: Arrhythmias in Acute Myocardial Infarctions, *Dis. Chest*, **45**:616–626, 1964.

144. Likoff, W., Bender, S., and Dreifus, L.: The Fate of a Patient with So-called Mild Coronary, *J.A.M.A.*, **177**:579–581, 1961.

145. Feil, H.: The Prognosis of Coronary Heart Disease, in A. Morgan Jones (ed.), "Modern Trends in Cardiology," Hoeber Medical Division, Harper & Row, Publishers, Incorporated, New York, 1961.

146. Sigler, L. H.: Long Survival Following Myocardial Infarction, *Am. J. Cardiol.*, **9**:547–557, 1962.

147. Blumenfeld, A.: "Heart Attack! Are You a Candidate?" Paul S. Eriksson, Inc., New York, 1964.

SELECTED READING

Aarseth, S., and Lange, H. F.: The Influence of Anticoagulant Therapy on the Occurrence of Cardiac Rupture and Hemopericardium Following Heart Infarction. I. A Study of 89 Cases of Hemopericardium (81 of Them Cardiac Ruptures). II. A Controlled Study of a Selected Treated Group Based on 1044 Autopsies, *Am. Heart J.*, **56**:250–256, 257–263, 1958.

Abrams, D. L., Edelist, A., Luria, M. H., and Miller, A. J.: Ventricular Aneurysm: Reappraisal Based on Study of 65 Consecutive Autopsied Cases, *Circulation*, **27**:164–169, 1963.

Achor, R. W. P., Berge, K. G., Barker, N. W., and McKenzie, B. F.: Treatment of Hypercholesteremia with Nicotinic Acid, *Circulation*, **16**:499, 1957.

Adams, C. W. M.: Multiple Factors in the Pathogenesis of Atherosclerosis, *Guy's Hosp. Rep.*, **112**:222–253, 1963.

Adlersberg, G. D.: Hormonal Influences on the Serum Lipids, *Am. J. Med.*, **23**:769, 1957.

Ahrens, E. H., Jr., Hirsch, J., Oette, K., Farquhar, J. W., and Stein, Y.: Carbohydrate-induced and Fat-induced Lipemia, *Tr. A. Am. Physicians*, **74**:134–146, 1961.

Ahrens, E. H., Jr., Hirsch, J., Peterson, M. L., Stoffel, W., and Farquhar, J. W.: Symposium on Significance of Lowered Cholesterol Levels, *J.A.M.A.*, **107**:2198–2203, 1959.

Alaupovic, P., Howard, R. P., and Furman, R. H.: Effect of Estrogens and Androgens on the Alpha- and Beta-lipoprotein Composition in Human Subjects, *Circulation*, **28**:647, 1963.

Anitschkow, N. N., Wolkoff, K. G., Kikaion, E. E., and Pzharisski, K. M.: Compensatory Adjustments in the Structure of Coronary Arteries of the Heart with Stenotic Atherosclerosis, *Circulation*, **29**:447, 1964.

Antar, M. A., Ohlson, M. A., and Hodges, R. E.: Changes in Retail Market Food Supplies in the United States in the Last Seventy Years in Relation to the Incidence of Coronary Heart Disease, with Special Reference to Dietary Carbohydrates and Essential Fatty Acids, *Am. J. Clin. Nutrition*, **14**:169–178, 1964.

Bachrach, W. H., and Thorner, M. C.: Hemorrhagic Enteropathy Complicating Myocardial Infarction, *Am. J. Cardiol.*, **11**:89–92, 1963.

Bajusz, E.: Early Metabolic Aberrations through Which Epinephrine May Elicit Myocardial Necrosis, paper delivered at International Conference on Preventive Cardiology, University of Vermont, Burlington, Vt., Aug. 1964.

Berge, K. G., Achor, R. W. P., Christensen, N. A., Mason, H. L., and Barker, N. W.: Hypercholesteremia and Nicotinic Acid: A Long-term Study, *Am. J. Med.*, **31**:24–36, 1961.

Beveridge, J. M. R., and Connell, W. E.: The Effect of Commercial Margarines on Plasma Cholesterol Levels in Man, *Am. J. Clin. Nutrition*, **10**:391–397, 1962.

Blumgart, H. L., and Zoll, P. M.: Pathologic Physiology of Angina Pectoris and Acute Myocardial Infarction, *Circulation*, **22**:301, 1960.

Boas, E. P.: The Natural History of Coronary Artery Disease of Long Duration, *Am. Heart J.*, **41**:323, 1951.

Bradley, R. F., and Bryfogle, J. W.: Survival of Diabetic Patients after Myocardial Infarction, *Am. J. M. Sc.*, **20**:207, 1956.

Branwood, A. W.: "Modern Concepts of the Pathogenesis of Coronary Atherosclerosis," Livingstone, Edinburgh, 1963, pp. 1–14.

Brontë-Stewart, B., Antonis, A., Eales, L., and Brock, J. F.: Effects of Feeding Different Fats on Serum-cholesterol Level, *Lancet*, **1**:521, 1956.

Brown, K. W. G., MacMillan, R. L., Forbath, N., Mel'grano, F., and Scott, J. W.: Coronary Unit: An Intensive-care Center for Acute Myocardial Infarction, *Lancet*, **2**:349–352, 1963.

Brunner, D., Manelis, G., and Loebl, K.: Influence of Normal Labor and Occupation on the 5-year Mortality of Middle-aged Patients with Initial Myocardial Infarction, *Circulation*, **26**:693, 1962.

Charm, S., McComis, W., Tejada, C., and Kurland, G.: Effect of a Fatty Meal on Whole Blood and Plasma Viscosity, *J. Appl. Physiol.*, **18**:1217–1220, 1963.

Clarkson, F. B., and Lofland, H. B.: Effect of Age on Response to Atherogenic Diets, *Fed. Proc.*, **22**:386, 1963.

Cliffton, E. E.: Fibrinolytic Agents, *M. Clin. North America*, **45**:917–933, 1961.

Cohen, D. B., Doctor, L., and Pick, A.: The Significance of Atrioventricular Block Complicating Acute Myocardial Infarction, *Am. Heart J.*, **55**:215–219, 1958.

Cole, D. R., Singian, E. B., and Katz, L. N.: The Long-term Prognosis Following Myocardial Infarction, and Some Factors Which Affect It, *Circulation*, **9**:321, 1954.

Cole, S. L., Kaye, H., and Griffith, G. C.: Assay of Antianginal Agents: A Long-acting Nitrate, Psychic Energizers, and a Tranquilizer, *Am. J. Cardiol.*, **11**:639–645, 1963.

Cossio, P.: The Treatment of Angina Pectoris and Other Muscular Pain Due to Ischemia with Iproniazid and Isoniazid, *Am. Heart J.*, **56**:113, 1958.

Council on Foods and Nutrition, A.M.A.: The Regulation of Dietary Fat, *J.A.M.A.*, **181**:411–429, 1962.

Dayton, S., Pearce, M. L., Hashimoto, S., Fakler, L. J., Hiscock, E., and Dixon, W. J.: A Controlled Clinical Trial of a Diet High in Unsaturated Fat, *New England J. Med.*, **266**:1017–1023, 1962.

Dimond, E. G.: Assessment of Functional Recovery of Men Surviving First Myocardial Infarction, *Am. Heart J.*, **65**:832–838, 1963.

Dimond, E. G., and Benchimol, A.: Summary of Current Therapy. The Exercise Apexcardiogram in Angina Pectoris: Its Possible Usefulness in Diagnosis and Therapy, *Dis. Chest*, **43**:92–93, 1963.

Dock, W.: Treatment of Angina Pectoris and Myocardial Infarction, *M. Clin. North America*, **46**:1599–1612, 1962.

Eckstein, R. W.: Effect of Exercise and Coronary Arterial Narrowing on Coronary Collateral Circulation, *Circulation Res.*, **5**:230, 1957.

Edwards, W. L.: Musculoskeletal Chest Pain Following Myocardial Infarction, *Am. Heart J.*, **49**:713–718, 1955.

Epstein, F. H.: Hereditary Aspects of Coronary Heart Disease, *Am. Heart J.*, **67**:445, 1964.

Farquhar, J. W., and Sokolow, M.: Response of Serum Lipids and Lipoproteins of Man to Beta Sitosterol and Safflower Oil: A Long-term Study, *Circulation*, **17**:890–899, 1958.

Fredrickson, D. S.: Essential Familial Hyperlipidemia, in J. B. Stanbury, J. B. Wyngaarden, D. S. Fredrickson (eds.), "Metabolic Basis of Inherited Disease," McGraw-Hill Book Company, New York, 1960, pp. 489–552.

Furman, R. H., and Robinson, C. W., Jr.: Hypocholesterolemic Agents, *M. Clin. North America*, **45**:935–959, 1961.

Gertler, M. M., Driskell, M. M., Bland, E. F., Garn, S. M., Lerman, J., Levine, S. A., and Sprague, H. B.: Clinical Aspects of Coronary Heart Disease, *J.A.M.A.*, **146**:1291, 1951.

Glagov, S., Rowley, D. A., and Kohut, R. I.: Atherosclerosis of Human Aorta and Its Coronary and Renal Arteries: A Consideration of Some Hemodynamic Factors Which May Be Related to the Marked Difference in the Atherosclerotic Involvement of the Coronary and Renal Arteries, *Arch. Path.*, **72**:558–571, 1961.

Gorlin, R.: Modern Treatment of Coronary Occlusion and Insufficiency, *M. Clin. North America,* **46:** 1243–1260, 1962.

Green, J. G., Brown, H. B., Meredith, A. P., and Page, I. H.: Use of Fat-modified Foods for Serum Cholesterol Reduction, *J.A.M.A.,* **183:**5–12, 1963.

Gregg, D. E.: Physiology of the Coronary Circulation, *Circulation,* **27:**1128, 1963.

Griffith, G. C., Hegde, B., and Oblath, R. W.: Factors in Myocardial Rupture: An Analysis of Two Hundred and Four Cases at Los Angeles County Hospital between 1924 and 1951, *Am. J. Cardiol.,* **8:**792–798, 1961.

Gubner, R. S., and Ungerleider, H. E.: Long-term Prognosis and Insurability in Coronary Heart Disease, *Am. Heart J.,* **58:**436, 1959.

Gwinup, G., Byron, R. C., Rousch, W. H., Kruger, F. A., and Hamwi, G. J.: Effect of Nibbling versus Gorging on Serum Lipids in Man, *Am. J. Clin. Nutrition,* **13:**209–213, 1963.

Hellerstein, H. K.: A Primary and Secondary Coronary Prevention Program, Progress Report, International Conference on Preventive Cardiology, University of Vermont, Burlington, Vt., Aug. 1964.

Hollister, L. E., and Arons, W. L.: Effect of Dextroisomers of Thyroid Hormones on Serum Cholesterol Levels in Euthyroid Hypercholesterolemic Patients, *Ann. Int. Med.,* **56:**570–576, 1962.

Honey, G. E., and Truelove, S. C.: Prognostic Factors in Myocardial Infarction, *Lancet,* **1:**1155–1161, 1209–1212, 1957.

Howard, R. P., and Furman, R. H.: Estrogens, Androgens and Serum Lipids, the Enigmatic Triad of Atherogenesis, *Ann. Int. Med.,* **56:**668, 1962.

Hughes, W. L., Kalbfleisch, J. M., Brandt, E. N., and Costiloe, J. P.: Myocardial Infarction Prognosis by Discriminant Analysis, *Arch. Int. Med.,* **111:** 338–345, 1963.

Imperial, E. S., Carballo, R., and Zimmerman, H. A.: Disturbances of Rate, Rhythm and Conduction in Acute Myocardial Infarction: A Statistical Study of 153 Cases, *Am. J. Cardiol.,* **5:**24–29, 1960.

Iversen, K., and Hilden, T.: The Use of Anticoagulants in Coronary Heart Disease, *M. Clin. North America,* **46:**1613–1637, 1962.

Jolliffe, N., Baumgartner, L., Rinzler, S. H., Archer, M., Stephenson, J. H., and Christakis, G. J.: The Anti-Coronary Club, the First Four Years, *New York J. Med.,* **63:**69–79, 1963.

Kaplan, B. M., and Grunes, J.: Emotional Aspects of Estrogen Therapy in Men with Coronary Atherosclerosis, *J.A.M.A.,* **183:**734–736, 1963.

Katz, L. N.: Atherosclerosis: Present Status of the Management of the Disease, *California Med.,* **96:**373–380, 1962.

Kinsell, L. W.: Some Thoughts Regarding the P:S Ratio Concept, *Am. J. Clin. Nutrition,* **12:**228–229, 1963.

Kinsell, L. W.: Unsaturated Dietary Fats, *Am. J. Clin. Nutrition,* **14:**125–127, 1964.

Klein, A. J., and Palmer, L. A.: Plasma Cortisol in Myocardial Infarction: A Correlation with Shock and Survival, *Am. J. Cardiol.,* **11:**332–337, 1963.

Kraus, H., and Raab, W.: "Hypokinetic Disease," Charles C Thomas, Publisher, Springfield, Ill., 1961, pp. 65, 66, 84, 85, 104.

Leak, D., and Julian, D. G.: Iproniazid, Nialamide, and Meprobamate in Angina Pectoris, *Brit. M. J.,* **1:** 1593–1594, 1962.

Lewis, L., Turnbull, R. B., and Page, I. H.: Short Circuiting of the Small Intestine: Effect on Concentration of Serum Cholesterol and Lipoproteins, *J.A.M.A.,* **182:**77–79, 1962.

Luyken, R., Pikaar, N. A., Polman, H., and Schippers, F. A.: The Influence of Legumes on the Serum Cholesterol Level, *Voeding,* **5:**447–453, 1962.

Maher, J. F., Mallory, G. K., and Laurenzi, C. A.: Rupture of the Heart after Myocardial Infarction, *New England J. Med.,* **255:**1–10, 1956.

Master, A. M., Jaffe, H. L., Field, L. E., and Donoso, E.: Acute Coronary Insufficiency: Its Differential Diagnosis and Treatment, *Ann. Int. Med.,* **45:**561–581, 1956.

Master, A. M., Jaffe, H. L., Teich, E. M., and Brinberg, L.: Survival and Rehabilitation after Coronary Occlusion, *J.A.M.A.,* **156:**1552, 1954.

Mathur, K. S., Kashyap, S. K., and Kumar, V.: Correlation of the Extent and Severity of Atherosclerosis in the Coronary and Cerebral Arteries, *Circulation,* **27:**929–934, 1963.

McKusick, V. A., and Murphy, E. A.: Genetic Factors in the Etiology of Myocardial Infarction, in T. N. James and J. W. Keyes (eds.), "The Etiology of Myocardial Infarction," Little, Brown and Company, Boston, 1963, pp. 13–20.

Messer, J., Levine, H. J., Wagman, R. J., and Gorlin, R.: Effect of Exercise on Cardiac Performance in Human Subjects with Coronary Artery Disease, *Circulation,* **28:**404–414, 1963.

Meissner, G. F., and Moehring, C. M.: Synthetic Estrogens in Treatment of Atherosclerosis, *Arch. Int. Med.,* **110:**467–471, 1962.

Millot, J., and Daux, J. L.: Influence de la ménopause précoce, naturelle ou chirurgicale sur le délenchement des coronautes, *Arch. mal. coeur,* **52:**297, 1959.

Morgan, A. D.: The Thrombogenic Hypothesis in Coronary Atherosclerosis, *Cardiologia,* **40:**77, 1962.

National Dairy Council: "Attitudes of Medical Doctors toward Dairy Products and Heart Disease," Chicago, 1963.

Nicholson, J. H., and Leavitt, T., Jr.: Coumadin® (Warfarin) Sodium: New Anticoagulant, *New England J. Med.,* **255:**491–501, 1956.

Oaks, W., Lisan, P., and Moyer, J. M.: Inhibition of Cholesterol Synthesis with the Use of MER-29, *A.M.A. Arch. Int. Med.* **104:**527, 1959.

Oliver, M. F.: Coronary Disease, Hypercholesterolaemia and Its Treatment, *Scot. M. J.,* **3:**225, 1958.

Oliver, M. F., and Boyd, G. S.: Endocrine Aspects of Coronary Sclerosis, *Lancet,* **2:**1273, 1956.

Oliver, M. F., and Boyd, G. S.: Influence of Sex Hormones on Circulating Lipids and Lipoproteins in Coronary Sclerosis, *Circulation*, 13:82, 1956.

Oliver, M. F., and Boyd, G. S.: Reduction of Serum-cholesterol by Dextro-thyroxine in Men with Coronary Heart-disease, *Lancet*, 1:783–785, 1961.

Oliver, M. F., and Boyd, G. S.: The Influence of Reduction of Serum Lipids on Prognosis of Coronary Heart Disease: A Five-year Study Using Estrogen, *Lancet*, 2:499, 1962.

Page, I. H., Allen, E. V., Chamberlain, F. L., Keys, A., Stamler, J., and Stare, F. J.: Dietary Fat and Its Relation to Heart Attacks and Strokes, *Circulation*, 23:1–5, 1961.

Parsons, W. B., Achor, R. W. P., Berge, K. S., McKenzie, B. F., and Barker, N. W.: Changes in Concentration of Blood Lipids Following Prolonged Administration of Large Doses of Nicotinic Acid to Persons with Hypercholesterolaemia, *Proc. Staff Meet. Mayo Clin.*, 31:377, 1956.

Peel, A. A. F., Semple, T., Wang, I., Lancaster, W. M., and Dall, J. L. G.: A Coronary Prognostic Index for Grading the Severity of Infarction, *Brit. Heart J.*, 24:745–760, 1962.

Peyman, M. A.: The Significance of Haemorrhage during Treatment of Patients with the Coumarin Anticoagulants, *Acta med. scandinav.*, 162 Suppl. **339:** 62, 1958.

Pitt, B., Zoll, P. M., Blumgart, H. L., and Freiman, D. G.: Location of Coronary Arterial Occlusions and Their Relation to the Arterial Pattern, *Circulation*, 28:35, 1963.

"Planning Fat-controlled Meals," American Heart Association, New York, 1962, p. 25.

Pomeranze, J., Goalwin, A., and Slobody, L. B.: The Effect of a Corn Oil–Evaporated Milk Mixture on Serum Cholesterol Levels in Infancy, *A.M.A. J. Dis. Child.*, 95:622–625, 1958.

Raab, W.: Prevention of Degenerative Heart Disease by Neurovegetative Reconditioning, *Pub. Health Rep.*, 78:317, 1963.

Raab, W.: The Nonvascular Metabolic Myocardial Vulnerability Factor in "Coronary Heart Disease," *Am. Heart J.*, 66:685, 1963.

Raab, W., Paula e Silva, P. de, Marchet, H., Kimura, E., and Starcheska, Y. K.: Cardiac Adrenergic Preponderance Due to Lack of Physical Exercise and Its Pathogenic Implications, *Am. J. Cardiol.*, 5:300, 1960.

Raab, W., Van Lith, P., Lepeschkin, E., and Herrlich, H. E.: Catecholamine-induced Myocardial Hypoxia in the Presence of Impaired Coronary Dilatability, Independent of External Cardiac Work, *Am. J. Cardiol.*, 9:455, 1962.

Riccitelli, M.: Nutritional Uses of Dietary Fats and Oils in the Aged and Infirm, *J. Am. Geriat. Soc.*, 10:593–603, 1962.

Riseman, J. E. F.: Treatment of Angina Pectoris: Summary of 10 Years Objective Study, *New England J. Med.*, 229:670, 1943.

Ritterband, A. B., Jaffe, I. A., Denson, P. M., Magagna, J. F., and Reed, E.: Gonadal Function and the Development of Coronary Heart Disease, *Circulation*, 27:237, 1963.

Robb, G. P., and Marks, H. H.: What Happens to Men Disabled by Heart Disease, *Statist. Bull. Metrop. Life Insur. Co.*, 34:10, 1953.

Robinson, R. W., Higano, N., and Cohen, W. D.: Increased Incidence of Coronary Heart Disease in Women Castrated Prior to the Menopause, *Arch. Int. Med.*, 104:907, 1959.

Robinson, R. W., Higano, N., and Cohen, W. D.: Long-term Effects of High-dosage Estrogen Therapy in Men with Coronary Heart Disease, *J. Chron. Dis.*, 16:155, 1963.

Robinson, R. W., and LeBeau, R. J.: Dextro-thyroxine as a Cholesterol Lowering Agent in Patients with Angina Pectoris, *Circulation*, 28:531, 1963.

Rushmer, R. F., Smith, O. A., and Lasher, E. P.: Natural Mechanisms of Cardiac Control during Exertion, *Physiol. Rev.*, 40:27, 1960.

Salisbury, P. F., Cross, C. E., and Riebens, P. S.: Acute Ischemia of Inner Layers of Ventricular Wall, *Am. Heart J.*, 66:650, 1963.

Sambhi, M. P. and Zimmerman, H. A.: Progress in the Long-term Management of Coronary Artery Disease. *A.M.A. Arch. Int. Med.*, 101:974–996, 1958.

Schiller, K. F. R.: Rupture of the Interventricular Septum Associated with Acute Myocardial Infarction, *Lancet*, 2:1322–1327, 1960.

Segal, B. L.: The Distribution and Relation of Atherosclerosis to Coronary Heart Disease, in W. Likoff and J. H. Moyer (eds.), "Coronary Heart Disease," Grune & Stratton, Inc., New York, 1963, pp. 140–145.

Sigler, L. H.: Prognosis of Angina Pectoris and Myocardial Infarction, *Am. J. Cardiol.*, 6:252–258, 1960.

Sodi-Pallares, D., Bisteni, A., Medrano, G. A., Testelli, M. R., and De Micheli, A.: Summary of Current Therapy: The Polarizing Treatment of Acute Myocardial Infarction, *Dis. Chest*, 43:424–432, 1963.

Spain, D. M., Nathan, D. J., and Gellis, M.: Weight, Body Type and the Prevalence of Coronary Atherosclerotic Heart Disease in Males, *Am. J. M. Sc.*, 245:63–69, 1963.

Sprague, H. B.: What I Tell My Patients about Smoking, *Mod. Concepts Cardiovas. Dis.*, 33:881, 1964.

Stamler, J.: The Relationship of Sex and Gonadal Hormones to Atherosclerosis, in M. Sandler and G. H. Bourne (eds.), "Atherosclerosis and Its Origin," Academic Press, Inc., New York, 1963, pp. 231–262.

Stamler, J.: Interrelationships between the Two Diseases, Hypertension and Atherosclerosis, *Am. J. Cardiol.*, 9:743–747, 1962.

Stamler, J., Berkson, D. M., Young, Q. D., Linberg, H. A., Hall, Y., Mojonnier, L., and Andelman, S. L.: Diet and Serum Lipids in Atherosclerotic Coronary Heart Disease, *M. Clin. North America*, 47: 3–31, 1963.

Stephenson, H. E., Jr.: "Cardiac Arrest and Resuscitation," The C. V. Mosby Company, St. Louis, 1958, pp. 52–53.

Stock, T. B., Wendt, V. E., Hayden, R. O., Bruce, T. A., and Bing, R. J.: New Concepts of Angina Pectoris, *M. Clin. North America*, 46:1497–1517, 1962.

Sweeney, M. J., Etteldorf, J. N., Dobbins, W. T., Somervill, B., Fischer, R., and Ferrell, C.: Dietary Fat and Concentrations of Lipid in the Serum during the First Six to Eight Weeks of Life, *Pediatrics*, 27: 765–771, 1961.

Vansant, J. H., and Muller, W. H., Jr.: Surgical Procedures to Revascularize the Heart: A Review of the Literature, *Am. J. Surg.*, 100:572–583, 1960.

Vastesaeger, M. M., and Delcourt, R.: The Natural History of Atherosclerosis, *Circulation*, 26:841, 1962.

Wakerlin, G.: Cigarette Smoking and the Role of the Physician (Editorial), *Circulation*, 29:651, 1964.

Walton, R. S.: Successful Cardiac Massage of Cardiac Arrest Following Coronary Thrombosis, *Brit. M. J.*, 1:155, 1960.

Woodruff, C. W., Bailey, M. C., Davis, J. T., Rogers, N., and Coniglio, J. G.: Serum Lipids in Breast-fed Infants and in Infants Fed Evaporated Milk, *Am. J. Clin. Nutrition*, 14:83–90, 1964.

Young, W.: Hemodynamic Aspects of Atherogenesis, *Nature*, 187:425–426, 1960.

36 RARER CAUSES OF CORONARY ARTERY DISEASE

Nanette Kass Wenger, M.D.

Atherosclerosis predominates as the pathologic lesion in coronary heart disease. Less commonly, other etiologic processes involve the coronary arteries, with and without symptoms.

ANATOMIC CAUSES

Anomalous Origin

Anomalies in the embryologic division of the common arterial trunk result in variation in origin, number, distribution, and size of the coronary arteries. Coronary artery anomalies frequently occur in association with transposition of the great vessels and tetralogy of Fallot.[1,2]

In the major symptomatic anomaly, the Bland-White-Garland syndrome,[3] the left coronary artery originates from the pulmonary artery. The clinical picture[4–6] is that of an apparently normal infant at birth, who in the first six months of life has episodic cyanosis, tachycardia, tachypnea, and perspiration, usually associated with feeding. The infant appears well between attacks but usually dies suddenly before the age of two years. On physical examination there is marked cardiac enlargement and a prominent left ventricular impulse, without murmurs and often with evidence of congestive heart failure. The electrocardiogram is indicative of anterolateral myocardial ischemia or true infarction (Fig. 36-1). On x-ray examination (Fig. 36-2) there is an aneurysmal left ventricular bulge, due to myocardial thinning. At autopsy (Fig. 36-3),[5,6] the myocardial degenerative changes mimic adult atherosclerotic coronary artery disease but are greater in magnitude and more widespread, often with secondary calcification.

Retrograde blood flow[7] in the anomalous left coronary artery, as demonstrated by aortography, may produce myocardial ischemia and anoxia. Sabiston et al.[8] consider the lesion a coronary arteriovenous fistula, with blood flow from aorta →

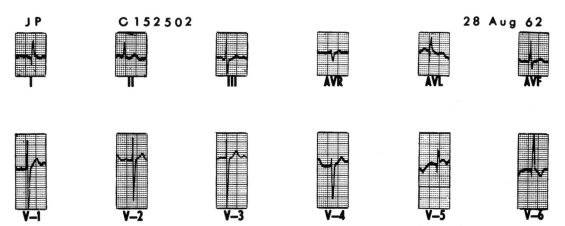

Fig. 36-1. Anomalous origin of the left coronary artery from the pulmonary artery in a three-month-old infant. The electrocardiographic pattern is that of anterolateral myocardial infarction. (*Courtesy of Department of Pediatrics, Emory University School of Medicine, and Grady Memorial Hospital.*)

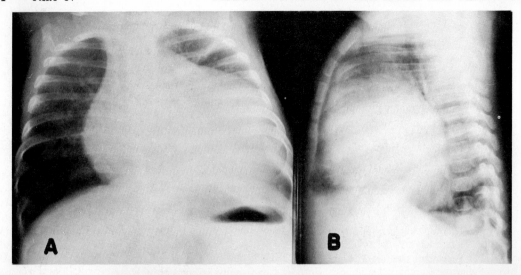

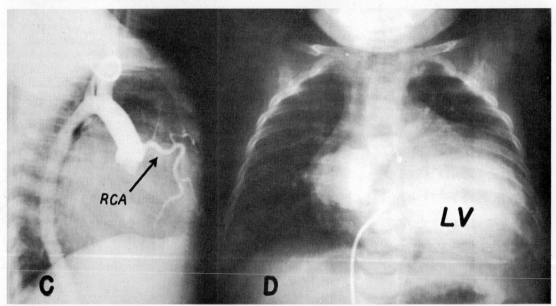

Fig. 36-2. Anomalous origin of the left coronary artery from the pulmonary artery. *A., B.* Roentgenograms of the chest, showing massive cardiomegaly and congestive heart failure. *C.* Retrograde aortogram revealing the presence of a large right coronary artery (RCA) filling from the base of the aorta. There is no visualization of a left coronary artery. *D.* Right ventricular angiocardiogram, showing opacification of the left atrium and left ventricle after contrast-material recirculation. Note the enlarged left ventricular cavity and thin left ventricular wall. (*Courtesy of Department of Radiology, Emory University School of Medicine, and Grady Memorial Hospital.*)

right coronary artery → collaterals → anomalous left coronary artery → pulmonary artery. Edwards[9] proposed that the development of collateral vessels was dependent on the pressure difference between the aorta and pulmonary artery, with collaterals developing after birth, following the fall in pulmonary arterial pressure. Thus the anomalous coronary artery is initially supplied by the pulmonary trunk but, after the development of collateral vessels, actually supplies blood to the pulmonary trunk. The

transitional period is probably the period of maximal myocardial ischemia. Surgical ligation of the left coronary artery at its origin from the pulmonary artery increases left ventricular perfusion if adequate collateral vessels exist; definitive surgical intervention is indicated before irreversible myocardial damage occurs.

Surgical ligation is catastrophic in the infant without adequate collateral vessels. Nadas et al.[10] suggested that banding of the pulmonary artery

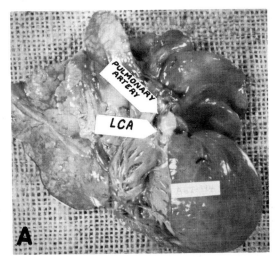
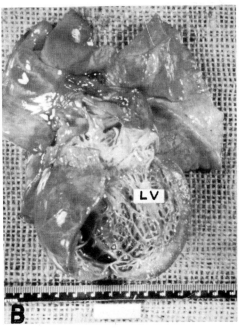

Fig. 36-3. Anomalous origin of the left coronary artery from the pulmonary artery. A. Ostium of the left coronary artery arising from the first portion of the pulmonary artery. B. Marked U-shaped dilatation of the left ventricle. (*Courtesy of Department of Pathology, Emory University School of Medicine, and Grady Memorial Hospital.*)

might increase the perfusion pressure of the poorly oxygenated blood in the anomalous coronary artery; alternatively a Blalock-Taussig operation might provide for increased oxygen content in pulmonary artery blood, which would perfuse at a low pressure.

In the rare patient who reaches adulthood, a continuous murmur is heard along the left sternal border; Massih[11] et al. believe the murmur is due to blood flow in the dilated, tortuous collateral vessels between the right and left coronary arteries.

Anomalous origin of both coronary arteries from the pulmonary artery is invariably fatal.[11a]

Aneurysm

Coronary artery aneurysms occur predominantly in the male and may be single or multiple, fusiform or saccular.[12] They produce no symptoms and are usually unsuspected unless complicated by thrombosis or rupture.[13,14] Crocker et al.[15] suspected the diagnosis in an asymptomatic infant because of the fluoroscopic finding of an asynchronously pulsating mass in the atrioventricular groove. Coronary artery aneurysms occur frequently in polyarteritis nodosa but may also be congenital, traumatic, myocotic-embolic, syphilitic (Fig. 36-4), athero-

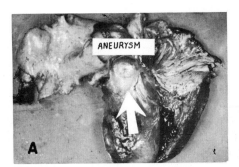
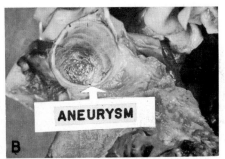

Fig. 36-4. Syphilitic aneurysm of the coronary artery. A. Marked saccular aneurysmal dilatation of the coronary artery due to syphilitic arteritis. B. Cross section of the coronary artery aneurysm. (*Courtesy of Department of Pathology, Emory University School of Medicine, and Emory University Hospital.*)

sclerotic, or rheumatic in origin. Daoud et al.[16] reported frequent association of abdominal aortic aneurysms with atherosclerotic coronary artery aneurysms.

Congenital Arteriovenous Fistula

A coronary arteriovenous fistula[17] is formed by the direct communication of a coronary artery which originates normally from the aorta (right coronary more commonly than left)[18] with the pulmonary artery or with a cardiac chamber; the flow of blood is via a single large vessel or a sinusoidal plexus. In reviewing 73 cases in the literature, Upshaw[19] reported that 89 per cent of coronary arteriovenous fistulas empty into the right side of the heart. There is a disparity between the benign clinical history and the marked physical findings;[20] the patient is characteristically asymptomatic, with a loud, continuous, superficial cardiac murmur in an unusual location found on physical examination.

Gasul et al.[21] noted that when the coronary artery communicates with the pulmonary artery or the right atrium, the systolic component of the continuous murmur is the louder, as blood flow occurs primarily during systole. Blood flow in the coronary artery emptying into the right ventricle is predominantly diastolic, producing diastolic accentuation of the continuous murmur; when the left ventricle is the recipient chamber, blood flow is almost exclusively diastolic, and only a diastolic murmur may be audible.

Electrocardiographic and radiologic examination offers little diagnostic aid in congenital arteriovenous fistulas. A left-to-right shunt is detected at cardiac catheterization, and retrograde aortography delineates the dilated, tortuous coronary artery (Fig. 36-5).

Over the years, the fistula increases in size with resultant high-output left ventricular failure.[22] Carmichael and Davidson[23] advocate surgical ligation to prevent the complications of congestive heart failure, bacterial endocarditis, myocardial ischemia, pulmonary hypertension, aneurysm formation, thrombosis, and coronary sinus rupture.[23a]

Embolism

Coronary emboli most frequently occlude the left coronary artery, particulary its left anterior descending branch, producing the clinical syndrome of acute myocardial infarction: pain, shock, arrhythmia, and pulmonary edema. Embolic occlusion of smaller coronary arteries may not always produce this classic picture. Virchow,[24] in his initial description of coronary embolization in 1856, cited a case of a young woman with bacterial endocarditis who died suddenly from myocardial infarction. Coronary embolization should be suspected among the causes of sudden death in young adults.

Wenger[25] emphasized that bacterial emboli, usu-

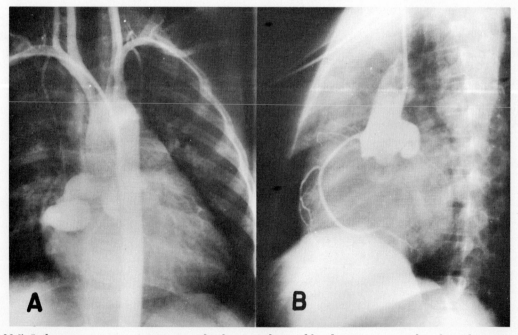

Fig. 36-5. Left coronary artery arteriovenous fistula. *A.* A large, dilated, tortuous vascular channel is opacified during a retrograde aortogram. *B.* Dilatation of the left coronary artery at its origin from the aorta. (*Courtesy of Department of Radiology, Emory University School of Medicine, and Emory University Hospital.*)

ally secondary to bacterial endocarditis, predominate in coronary embolization (Fig. 36-6); vessel wall inflammation secondary to these emboli may result in mycotic coronary artery aneurysms.[26] Less frequently encountered are bland emboli from atherosclerotic plaques, syphilitic plaques, mural thrombi, and fat, air,[27] parasitic, and tumor emboli. Glotzer et al.[28] commented on the increasing frequency of embolization of calcific material to the coronary arteries, associated with cardiac surgical procedures.

Thrombosis

Parasitic

Malarial parasites[29] and parasitized red blood cells usually plug the smaller coronary vessels but occasionally occlude branches of the main coronary arteries. In a case of schistosomiasis, Gazayerli[30] reported an adult *Schistosoma haematobium* in the left circumflex coronary artery, without resultant myocardial infarction.

Hematologic

In thrombotic thrombocytopenic purpura,[31] thrombi commonly involve the myocardial arterioles; however, platelet and fibrin thrombi may occlude larger coronary vessels with resultant myocardial necrosis. Similarly, the agglutination of abnormal red blood cells in sickle-cell anemia has been noted by Oliveira and Gómez-Patiño[32] to produce coronary arterial thrombotic occlusion. Fomina[33] reported a case of leukemic coronary artery thrombosis with resultant fatal myocardial infarction; a similar case was described by Zaitsev and Pokrovskaia.[34]

Patients with polycythemia vera have a high incidence of coronary occlusion,[35] presumably due to increased blood viscosity and a tendency to thrombus formation.[36] Wirth[37] noted that, on occasion, an acute myocardial infarction may be the initial manifestation of polycythemia vera.

Dissecting Aneurysm

In a study of 505 cases of dissecting aneurysm of the aorta, Hirst et al.[38] described 39 cases of associated dissecting aneurysm of the coronary artery. Obliteration of the coronary artery lumen by hemorrhage into the vessel wall may result in myocardial infarction.[39,40] Wainwright[41] attributed the rarity of this lesion to the early fatal extension of a dissecting aortic aneurysm into the pericardial sac, before the dissection could extend to the coronary arteries.

Dissecting aneurysm restricted to the coronary arteries,[42,43] with pathologic evidence of medial

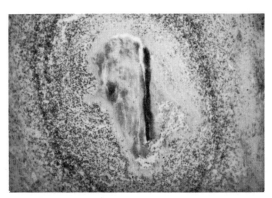

Fig. 36-6. Mycotic aneurysm of the coronary artery due to an infective embolus. The patient had bacterial endocarditis of the mitral valve. (*Courtesy of Department of Pathology, Emory University School of Medicine, and Grady Memorial Hospital.*)

cystic degeneration, has been reported both with and without clinical evidence of Marfan's syndrome.

INFECTIOUS DISEASE

Tuberculosis

Serial electrocardiographic changes in a young patient with active advanced tuberculosis are suggestive of coronary artery or myocardial tuberculosis.

In miliary tuberculosis, tubercles occur in the intima of the coronary arteries, without tuberculous involvement of the media and adventitia. In myocardial tuberculosis, diffuse tuberculous infiltration and noncellular intimal proliferative lesions cause coronary artery occlusion, primarily involving the smaller coronary arteries.[44]

Syphilis

Burch and Winsor[45] described coronary ostial stenosis in about 20 per cent of patients with syphilitic aortitis; the proximal 3 to 4 mm of the coronary arteries are narrowed, with complete sparing of the distal vessels.[46] An obliterative arteritis involves all three layers of the coronary artery; Kobernick[47] attributed the infrequency of myocardial infarction to the gradual progression of the occlusive process, allowing formation of a collateral circulation.

Syphilitic coronary artery involvement is often associated with aortic valve insufficiency and presents the clinical syndrome of angina, cardiac enlargement, and progressive congestive heart failure.

Successful surgical correction of syphilitic coronary ostial obstruction has been reported.[47a]

Less commonly, a syphilitic gumma may occlude a coronary artery, with resultant myocardial necrosis.[47]

Salmonellosis

Purulent thromboarteritis of the coronary vessels due to *Salmonella choleraesuis* has been observed in disseminated salmonellosis. In the cases reported by Barnett and Zimmerman[48] and Hennigar et al.[49] the coronary artery thrombosis caused fatal myocardial infarction.

Typhus

Allen and Spitz[50] described arteritis and thrombosis of the coronary vessels in patients with epidemic typhus (*Rickettsia prowazeki*). These processes usually involve the smaller coronary vessels and are rarely of clinical significance. Arteritis is not a feature of scrub typhus (*R. orientalis*) or of Rocky Mountain spotted fever, in which the lesion is that of myocarditis.

Bacterial Endocarditis

Coronary arterial lesions in bacterial endocarditis are usually secondary to embolization (Fig. 36-6). Saphir et al.,[51] however, described obliterative vascular changes, occasionally with resultant myocardial infarction, in the coronary vessels traversing an inflammatory myocardial focus.

METABOLIC CAUSES

Amyloidosis

Lindsay[52] reported frequent amyloid infiltration of the intima and media of the coronary arteries in primary cardiac amyloidosis (Fig. 36-7). The amyloid deposits may encroach upon the vessel lumen, producing coronary insufficiency and, at times, coronary occlusion.[53-56] Langsch[57] described two patients who presented with chest pain and severe congestive heart failure and who died suddenly; at autopsy the significant cardiac abnor-

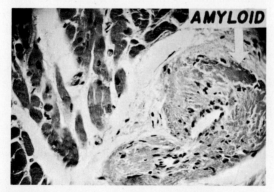

Fig. 36-7. Amyloid deposition in a coronary arteriole (× 250). (*Courtesy of Department of Pathology, Emory University School of Medicine, and Grady Memorial Hospital.*)

mality was severe generalized narrowing and obstruction of the entire coronary arterial tree due to amyloid deposition. In occasional reports, amyloid deposition has been limited to the smaller coronary vessels.[58]

Gout

Traut et al.[59] have observed urate crystals in the intima of the coronary arteries and in organized thrombi in patients with gout, often associated with atherosclerotic changes. The coronary artery walls are hard and gritty,[60] and urate deposition is also seen in the heart valves and myocardium.

Gargoylism (Hurler's Syndrome)

The parenchymal deposition of macromolecular glycoprotein characteristic of gargoylism also involves the coronary arteries.[61] Swollen, vacuolated fibroblasts and dense, wavy, collagenous fibers are seen in the thickened intimal layer; the vessel lumen is narrowed with resultant myocardial ischemia.[62]

COLLAGEN DISEASE

Polyarteritis Nodosa

Lesions of the coronary vessels contribute greatly to the clinical manifestations of polyarteritis nodosa[63] and are often directly responsible for death. An inflammatory, necrotizing, obliterative arteritis[64] involved the large and small coronary vessels in 60 to 70 per cent of cases in the series of Holsinger et al.[65] Aneurysmal dilatation and nodule formation in the coronary arteries produce the characteristic "peas in the pod" [66,67] appearance. Intimal thrombosis or thrombosis of an aneurysm may cause coronary artery occlusion and myocardial necrosis.

The clinical picture in both adults and children is that of coronary insufficiency with or without congestive heart failure. Massive fatal myocardial infarction is rare, as the slow rate of coronary occlusion allows formation of an adequate collateral circulation.[67] However, rupture of an aneurysm, as described by Sinclair and Nitsch[68] may cause sudden death.

The electrocardiographic ischemic changes of polyarteritis nodosa may be due to the coronary artery disease or to the associated myocarditis, pericarditis, or hypertension.

Disseminated Lupus Erythematosus

The vasculitis of disseminated lupus erythematosus usually involves the smaller coronary vessels.[69] Fibrinoid degeneration and fibrosis of the coronary arteries may cause focal myocardial necrosis,[70,71] but these processes are of little clinical importance. Bridgen et al.[72] stated that the cardiac symptoms of lupus erythematosus were attributable to the pericarditis, myocarditis, and hypertension.

Rheumatic Fever

The smaller coronary arteries are conspicuously altered in both active and inactive rheumatic fever;[73-76] however, the inflammatory lesions and fibrinoid degeneration are rarely of clinical significance. Froment et al.[77] described myocardial infarction secondary to obliterative coronary arteritis in a young patient with rheumatic fever.

MISCELLANEOUS CAUSES

Thromboangiitis Obliterans

Patients with Buerger's disease usually have coronary atherosclerosis, but, on occasion, the coronary arteries are sclerosed and thickened by hyalinized, calcified plaques which constrict the lumina. Saphir[78] believed this might be the pathologic basis for sudden cardiac death in young males with thromboangiitis obliterans.

Pulseless (Takayasu's) Disease

Coronary ostial intimal thickening with complete sparing of the distal coronary arteries has been described in Takayasu's disease.[79] The fibrous intimal and subendothelial proliferation is an extension of the aortitis; there is associated round-cell infiltration and adventitial fibrosis.[80] Coronary ostial disease with resultant myocardial infarction was the cause of death in a woman with "pulseless disease" reported by Barker and Edwards.[81]

Medical Calcification of Infancy

Idiopathic medial necrosis and subsequent calcification of the coronary arteries was first described by Bryant and White[82] in 1901; it is one manifestation of a generalized vascular disease of infancy, also involving the pulmonary and renal arteries and large arteries of the extremities and associated with other congenital anomalies.

The symptoms, mimicking those seen with aberrant origin of the left coronary artery from the pulmonary artery, begin in the first weeks of life, sudden death being common before age two. Clinically, there is episodic respiratory distress: dyspnea, cyanosis, tachypnea, with associated feeding difficulty and vomiting.[83] Congestive heart failure is notably absent. The electrocardiogram is compatible with myocardial ischemia or infarction.

Grossly, the coronary arteries are white, opaque, and cordlike, with narrowed lumina. Degeneration and calcification of the media and elastica and fibroblastic intimal proliferation are seen on microscopic examination.[84] The suggested etiologic factors include anoxia, inflammation, abnormalities of calcium metabolism, congenital defect in elastic tissue formation with secondary calcification, and allergic reaction.[85-88] Chipman[89] has observed that medial necrosis occurs in families and suggests that it may be genetically determined. Thomas[90] questioned whether the coronary artery disease was secondary to the frequently associated endocardial fibroelastosis.

Necrotizing Arteritis of Infancy

Monroe-Faure[91] believed that, in the first year of life, necrotizing arteritis has a predilection for the coronary arteries, which are often the only vessels involved. There is destruction of the media and elastica, intimal proliferation, aneurysm formation, and thrombosis, with resultant myocardial necrosis. It has been suggested that this is a hypersensitivity phenomenon.[92]

REFERENCES

1. Reemtsma, K., Longenecker, C. G., and Creech, O., Jr.: Surgical Anatomy of the Coronary Artery Distribution in Congenital Heart Disease, *Circulation*, 24:782, 1961.
2. Rowlatt, U. F.: Coronary Artery Distribution in Complete Transposition, *J.A.M.A.*, **179**:269, 1962.
3. Bland, E. F., White, P. D., and Garland, J.: Congenital Anomalies of the Coronary Arteries: Report of an Unusual Case Associated with Cardiac Hypertrophy, *Am. Heart J.*, **8**:787, 1933.
4. Keith, J. D.: The Anomalous Origin of the Left Coronary Artery from the Pulmonary Artery, *Brit. Heart J.*, **21**:149, 1959.
5. Kaunitz, P. E.: Origin of Left Coronary Artery from Pulmonary Artery, *Am. Heart J.*, **33**:182, 1947.
6. Bassis, M. L., and Sheinkopf, J. A.: Anomalous Origin of the Left Coronary Artery from the Pulmonary Artery, *Ann. Int. Med.*, **42**:983, 1955.
7. Liebman, J., Hellerstein, H. K., Ankeney, J. L., and Tucker, A.: The Problem of the Anomalous Left Coronary Artery Arising from the Pulmonary Artery in Older Children, *New England J. Med.*, **269**:486, 1963.
8. Sabiston, D. C., Neill, C. A., and Taussig, H. B.: The Direction of Blood Flow in Anomalous Left Coronary Artery Arising from the Pulmonary Artery, *Circulation*, **22**:591, 1960.
9. Edwards, J. E.: The Direction of Blood Flow in Coronary Arteries Arising from the Pulmonary Trunk, *Circulation*, **29**:163–166, 1964.
10. Nadas, A. S., Gamboa, R., and Hugenholtz, P. G.: Anomalous Left Coronary Artery Originating from the Pulmonary Artery: Report of Two Surgically Treated Cases with a Proposal of Hemodynamic and Therapeutic Classification, *Circulation*, **29**:167–175, 1964.
11. Massih, N. A., Lawler, J., and Vermillion, M.: Myocardial Ischemia after Ligation of an Anomalous

Left Coronary Artery Arising from the Pulmonary Artery, *New England J. Med.*, **269**:483, 1963.

11a. Colmers, R. A., and Siderides, C. I.: Anomalous Origin of Both Coronary Arteries from Pulmonary Trunk, *Am. J. Cardiol.*, **12**:263, 1963.

12. Scott, D. H.: Aneurysm of the Coronary Arteries, *Am. Heart J.*, **36**:403, 1948.

13. Packard, M., and Wechsler, H. F.: Aneurysm of the Coronary Arteries, *A.M.A. Arch. Int. Med.*, **43**:1, 1929.

14. Weller, S. D. V., and Newstead, S. M.: Aneurysm of Coronary Arteries in an Infant, *Postgrad. M. J.*, **38**:639–640, 1962.

15. Crocker, D. W., Sobin, S., and Thomas, W. C.: Aneurysms of the Coronary Arteries: Report of Three Cases in Infants and Review of the Literature, *Am. J. Path.*, **33**:819, 1957.

16. Daoud, A. S., Pankin, D., Tulgan, H., and Florentin, R. A.: Aneurysms of the Coronary Artery, *Am. J. Cardiol.*, **11**:228, 1963.

17. Edwards, J. E.: Anomalous Coronary Arteries, with Special Reference to Arteriovenous-like Communications, *Circulation*, **17**:1001, 1958.

18. Cooley, D. A., and Ellis, P. R., Jr.: Surgical Considerations of Coronary Arterial Fistula, *Am. J. Cardiol.*, **10**:467–474, 1962.

19. Upshaw, C. B., Jr.: Congenital Coronary Arteriovenous Fistula: Report of a Case with an Analysis of Seventy-three Reported Cases, *Am. Heart J.*, **63**:399, 1962.

20. Engle, M. A., Goldsmith, E. I., Holswade, G. R., Goldberg, H. P., and Glenn, F.: Congenital Coronary Arteriovenous Fistula: Diagnostic Evaluation and Surgical Correction, *New England J. Med.*, **264**:856, 1961.

21. Gasul, B. M., Arcilla, R. A., Fell, E. H., Lynfield, J., Bicoff, J. P., and Luan, L. L.: Congenital Coronary Arteriovenous Fistula: Clinical, Phonocardiographic, Angiocardiographic, and Hemodynamic Studies in Five Patients, *Pediatrics*, **25**:531, 1960.

22. Steinberg, I., Baldwin, J. S., and Dotter, C. T.: Coronary Arteriovenous Fistula, *Circulation*, **17**:372, 1958.

23. Carmichael, D. B., and Davidson, D. G.: Congenital Coronary Arteriovenous Fistula, *Am. J. Cardiol.*, **8**:846, 1961.

23a. Habermann, J. H., Howard, M. L., and Johnson, E. I.: Rupture of the Coronary Sinus with Hemopericardium. A Rare Complication of Coronary Arteriovenous Fistula, *Circulation*, **28**:1143, 1963.

24. Virchow, R.: Ueber capilläre Embolie, *Arch. path. Anat.*, **9**:307, 1856.

25. Wenger, N. K., and Bauer, S.: Coronary Embolism: Review of the Literature and Presentation of Fifteen Cases, *Am. J. Med.*, **25**:549, 1958.

26. Velázquez, T.: Aneurisma micótico de la artèria coronaria: Presentación de un caso y revisión de la literatura, *Arch. Inst. cardiol. México*, **22**:49, 1952.

27. Durant, T. M., Oppenheimer, M. J., Webster, M. R.,

and Long, J.: Arterial Air Embolism, *Am. Heart J.*, **38**:481, 1949.

28. Glotzer, D. J., Shaw, R. S., and Scannell, J. G.: Calcific Coronary Emboli Following Open Valvuloplasty for Aortic Stenosis, *J. Thoracic & Cardiovasc. Surg.*, **43**:434, 1962.

29. Merkel, W. C.: *Plasmodium falciparum* Malaria: The Coronary and Myocardial Lesions Observed at Autopsy in Two Cases of Acute Fulminating *P. falciparum* Infection, *A.M.A. Arch. Path.*, **41**:290, 1946.

30. Gazayerli, M.: Schistosomiasis, *J. Egyptian M. A.*, **22**:34, 1939.

31. Singer, K., Bornstein, F. P., and Wile, S. A.: Thrombotic Thrombocytopenic Purpura: Hemorrhagic Diathesis with Generalized Platelet Thromboses, *Blood*, **2**:542, 1947.

32. Oliveira, E., and Gómez-Patiño, N.: Falcemic Cardiopathy: Report of a Case, *Am. J. Cardiol.*, **11**:686, 1963.

33. Fomina, L. G.: [A Case of Myocardial Infarct in Acute Leukemia], *Sovetskaia med.*, **24**:141, 1960.

34. Zaitsev, V. F., and Pokrovskaia, N. N.: Ostryi gemotsitoblastoz s mnozhestvennymi trombozami, *Klinicheskaia Med.*, **37**:117–121, 1959.

35. Tinney, W. S., Hall, B. E., and Griffin, H. Z.: Cardiac Disease and Hypertension in Polycythemia Vera, *Proc. Staff Meet. Mayo Clin.*, **18**:94, 1943.

36. Miller, H. R.: The Occurrence of Coronary Artery Thrombosis in Polycythemia Vera, *Am. J. M. Sc.*, **198**:323, 1939.

37. Wirth, L.: Myocardial Infarction as the Initial Manifestation of Polycythemia Vera, *Mil. Med.*, **125**:544, 1960.

38. Hirst, A. E., Jr., Johns, V. J., Jr., and Kime, S. W., Jr.: Dissecting Aneurysm of the Aorta: A Review of 505 Cases, *Medicine*, **37**:217, 1958.

39. Whittaker, S. R. F., and Sheehan, J. D.: Dissecting Aortic Aneurysm in Marfan's Syndrome, *Lancet*, **2**:791, 1954.

40. Schatz, I. J., Yaworsky, R. G., and Fine, G.: Myocardial Infarction and Unusual Myocardial Degeneration in Marfan's Syndrome: With Dissection of the Right Coronary Artery and Aorta, *Am. J. Cardiol.*, **12**:553, 1963.

41. Wainwright, C. W.: Dissecting Aneurysm Producing Coronary Occlusion by Dissection of the Coronary Artery, *Bull. Johns Hopkins Hosp.*, **75**:81, 1944.

42. Boschetti, A. E., and Levine, A.: Cystic Medionecrosis with Dissecting Aneurysms of Coronary Arteries, *A.M.A. Arch. Int. Med.*, **102**:562, 1958.

43. McKeown, F.: Dissecting Aneurysm of the Coronary Artery in Arachnodactyly, *Brit. Heart J.*, **22**:434, 1960.

44. Gouley, B. A., Bellet, S., and McMillan, T. M.: Tuberculosis of the Myocardium: Report of Six Cases, with Observations on Involvement of Coronary Arteries, *A.M.A. Arch. Int. Med.*, **51**:244, 1933.

45. Burch, G. E., and Winsor, T.: Syphilitic Coronary Stenosis with Myocardial Infarction, *Am. Heart J.,* **24:**740, 1942.

46. Moritz, A. R.: Syphilitic Coronary Arteritis, *A.M.A. Arch. Path.,* **11:**44, 1931.

47. Kobernick, S. D.: Gumma of the Coronary Artery, Myocardial Infarction and Gumma of the Heart, *A.M.A. Arch. Path.,* **44:**490, 1947.

47a. Sabiston, D. C., Jr.: Direct Surgical Management of Congenital and Acquired Lesions of the Coronary Circulation, *Prog. Cardiovasc. Dis.,* **6:** 299, 1963.

48. Barnett, R. N., and Zimmerman, S. L.: Coronary Arteritis with Fatal Thrombosis Due to *Salmonella Choleraesuis* Variety Kunzendorf, *Am. Heart J.,* **34:** 441, 1947.

49. Hennigar, G. R., Thabet, R., Bundy, W. E., and Sutton, L. E., Jr.: Salmonellosis Complicated by Pancarditis, *J. Pediat.,* **43:**524, 1953.

50. Allen, A. C., and Spitz, S.: A Comparative Study of the Pathology of Scrub Typhus (Tsutsugamushi Disease) and Other Rickettsial Diseases, *Am. J. Path.,* **21:**603, 1945.

51. Saphir, O., Katz, L. N., and Gore, I.: Myocardium in Subacute Bacterial Endocarditis, *Circulation,* **1:** 1155, 1950.

52. Lindsay, S.: The Heart in Primary Systemic Amyloidosis, *Am. Heart J.,* **32:**419, 1946.

53. Hartney, J. B., Biederman, A. A., Blumberg, J. M., and Leedham, C. L.: Primary Systemic Amyloid Disease: Report of a Case Emphasizing Cardiac Involvement, *A.M.A. Arch. Path.,* **47:**598, 1949.

54. Jones, R. S., and Frazier, D. B.: Primary Cardiovascular Amyloidosis: Its Clinical Manifestations, Pathology and Histogenesis, *A.M.A. Arch. Path.,* **50:**366, 1950.

55. Symmers, W. St. C. Amyloidosis: 5 Cases of Primary Generalized Amyloidosis and Some Other Unusual Cases, *J. Clin. Path.,* **9:**212, 1956.

56. Eliot, R. S., McGee, H. J., and Blount, S. G., Jr.: Cardiac Amyloidosis, *Circulation,* **23:**613, 1961.

57. Langsch, H. G.: [Primary Atypical Amyloidosis as an Exceptional Disease of the Coronary Arteries]. *Beitr. path. Anat.,* **125:**123, 1961.

58. Josselson, A. J., Pruitt, R. D., and Edwards, J. E.: Amyloid Localized to the Heart: Analysis of Twenty-nine cases, *A.M.A. Arch. Path.,* **54:**359, 1952.

59. Traut, E. F., Knight, A. A., Szanto, P. B., and Passerelli, E. W.: Specific Vascular Changes in Gout, *J.A.M.A.,* **156:**591, 1954.

60. Pund, E. E., Jr., Hawley, R. L., McGee, H. J., and Blount, S. G., Jr.: Gouty Heart, *New England J. Med.,* **263:**835, 1960.

61. Lindsay, S.: Cardiovascular System in Gargoylism, *Brit. Heart J.,* **12:**17, 1950.

62. Strauss, L.: The Pathology of Gargoylism: Report of a Case and Review of the Literature, *Am. J. Path.,* **24:**855, 1948.

63. Taubenhaus, M., Eisenstein, B., and Pick, A.: Cardiovascular Manifestations of Collagen Diseases, *Circulation,* **12:**903, 1955.

64. Griffith, G. C., and Vural, I. L.: Polyarteritis Nodosa: A Correlation of Clinical and Postmortem Findings in Seventeen Cases, *Circulation,* **3:**481, 1951.

65. Holsinger, D. R., Osmundson, P. J., and Edwards, J. E.: The Heart in Periarteritis Nodosa, *Circulation,* **25:**610, 1962.

66. Rothstein, J. L., and Welt, S.: Periarteritis Nodosa in Infancy and in Childhood: Report of Two Cases with Necropsy Observations: Abstracts of Cases in the Literature, *Am. J. Dis. Child.,* **45:**1277, 1933.

67. Logue, R. B., and Mullins, F.: Polyarteritis Nodosa: Report of 11 Cases with Review of Recent Literature, *Ann. Int. Med.,* **24:**11, 1946.

68. Sinclair, W., Jr., and Nitsch, E.: Polyarteritis Nodosa of the Coronary Arteries: Report of a Case in an Infant with Rupture of an Aneurysm and Intrapericardial Hemorrhage, *Am. Heart J.,* **38:**898, 1949.

69. Harvey, A. M., Shulman, L. E., Tumulty, P. A., Conley, C. L., and Schoenrich, E. H.: Systemic Lupus Erythematosus: Review of Literature and Clinical Analysis of 138 Cases, *Medicine,* **33:**291, 1954.

70. Klemperer, P., Pollack, A. D., and Baehr, G.: Pathology of Disseminated Lupus Erythematosus, *A.M.A. Arch. Path.,* **32:**569, 1941.

71. Shearn, M. A.: The Heart in Systemic Lupus Erythematosus, *Am. Heart J.,* **58:**452, 1959.

72. Brigden, W., Bywaters, E. G. L., Lessof, M. H., and Ross, I. P.: The Heart in Systemic Lupus Erythematosus, *Brit. Heart J.,* **22:**1, 1960.

73. Fraser, A. D.: Coronary Endarteritis in Acute Rheumatism, *Arch. Dis. Childhood,* **9:**267, 1934.

74. Karsner, H. T., and Bayless, F.: Coronary Arteries in Rheumatic Fever, *Am. Heart J.,* **9:**557, 1934.

75. Gross, L., Kugel, M. A., and Epstein, E. Z.: Lesions of the Coronary Arteries and Their Branches in Rheumatic Fever, *Am. J. Path.,* **11:**253, 1935.

76. Rae, M. V.: Coronary Aneurysms with Thrombosis in Rheumatic Carditis, *A.M.A. Arch. Path.,* **24:**369, 1937.

77. Froment, R., Monnet, P., Gallois, P., and Perrin, A.: Les maladies coronariennes tronculaires infantiles et juvéniles: Principaux types anatomo-cliniques, *Arch. mal. coeur,* **50:**55, 1957.

78. Saphir, O.: Thromboangiitis Obliterans of the Coronary Arteries and Its Relation to Arteriosclerosis, *Am. Heart J.,* **12:**521, 1936.

79. Frövig, A. G., and Löken, A. C.: Syndrome of Obliterans of Arterial Branches of Aortic Arch, Due to Arteritis: Post-mortem Angiographic and Pathological Study, *Acta psychiat. et neurol. scandinav.,* **26:**313, 1951.

80. Ask-Upmark, E., and Fajers, C. M.: Further Observations on Takayusu's Syndrome, *Acta med. scandinav.* **155:**275, 1956.

81. Barker, N. W., and Edwards, J. E.: Primary Arteritis of the Aortic Arch, *Circulation,* 11:486, 1955.

82. Bryant, J. H., and White, W. H.: A Case of Calcification of the Arteries and Obliterative Endarteritis, Associated with Hydronephrosis, in a Child Aged Six Months, *Guy's Hosp. Rep.,* **40** (s. 3):17, 1901.

83. Moran, J. J., and Becker, S. M.: Idiopathic Arterial Calcification of Infancy: Report of 2 Cases Occurring in Siblings and Review of the Literature, *Am. J. Clin. Path.,* 31:517, 1959.

84. Kissane, R. W., and Fidler, R. S.: Congenital Medial Sclerosis of the Coronary Artery, *Am. Heart J.,* 7:133, 1931–32.

85. van Creveld, S.: Coronary Calcification and Thrombosis in Infant, *Ann. paediat.,* **157**:84, 1941.

86. Stryker, W. A.: Coronary Occlusive Disease in Infants and Children, *Am. J. Dis. Child.,* 71:280, 1946.

87. Stryker, W. A.: Arterial Calcification with Special Reference to the Coronary Arteries, *Am. J. Path.,* 22:1007, 1946.

88. Traisman, H. S., Limperis, N. M., and Traisman, A. S.: Myocardial Infarction Due to Calcification of the Arteries in an Infant, *Am. J. Dis. Child.,* **91**:34, 1956.

89. Chipman, C. D.: Calcific Sclerosis of Coronary Arteries in an Infant, *Canad. M. A. J.,* 83:955, 1960.

90. Thomas, W. A., Lee, K. T., McGavran, M. H:, and Rabin, E. R.: Endocardial Fibroelastosis in Infants Associated with Thrombosis and Calcification of Arteries and Myocardial Infarcts, *New England J. Med.,* **255**:464, 1956.

91. Munro-Faure, H.: Necrotizing Arteritis of the Coronary Vessels in Infancy: Case Report and Review of the Literature, *Pediatrics,* **23**:914, 1959.

92. Newton, W. A., and Misugi, K.: Partial Obliteration of Coronary Arteries in a Newborn Infant, *Yokohama M. Bull.,* **11**:59, 1960.

Section D: Systemic Hypertension

37 THE ETIOLOGY AND PATHOGENESIS OF SYSTEMIC HYPERTENSION

Elbert P. Tuttle, Jr., M.D.

The problems posed by the study of hypertension extend across the entire range of circulatory investigation. The mechanisms of regulation of the blood pressure are the subject of so vast a literature that only a selective and interpretive summary can serve the purpose of the present discussion. No effort has been made to be exhaustive in the review of reports. The author has attempted to provide a schematic formulation to include the observations of a considerable number of active investigators. It will serve its purpose if an adequate mnemonic for the supporting observations is provided or if it is challenging enough to provoke disproof.

Systemic hypertension arises from many different initial disturbances of the circulation which increase cardiac output or peripheral resistance or both, or one relative to the other, so that for the biologic situation under consideration the blood pressure is higher than would be expected in a normal population. This elevation of blood pressure may entail compensatory readjustments or reinforcement and enhancement by other elements of the circulation. If the elevation be frequent, prolonged, and great enough, it will induce hypertrophy of heart and blood vessels, so that greater pressure can be generated with no increase in the stimulus. Progressive hypertrophy leads to progressive elevation of the blood pressure until vascular damage occurs and the course of the disease is secondarily accelerated. The morbidity of hypertension derives from the work load imposed upon the heart and the injury to blood vessels at their points of least resistance.

Five recent international symposiums[1–4] provide extensive compendiums of current thought regarding the causes and pathogenesis of hypertension. To make available continuing group discussion of new developments the reports[5] of the Council for High Blood Pressure Research of the American Heart Association have brought selected topics to print each year. Additional symposiums and reviews on special topics pertaining to hypertension have recently been published dealing with angiotensin,[6,7] the juxtaglomerular apparatus,[8] the central nervous system control of circulation,[9] hemodynamics,[10] and the kidney.[11] A readable, balanced, and informative brief summary of recent concepts of hypertension is Page's presentation of his "mosaic theory" of hypertension.[12]

Hypertension is recognized as a state of abnormally elevated blood pressure, frequently associated with anatomic and physiologic abnormalities of many organs, particularly of the blood vessels, heart, kidneys, nervous system, and adrenal glands. Since pressure varies directly with flow, any change in blood flow or cardiac output will be associated with a change in blood pressure unless some other compensatory change occurs. The stability of the blood pressure within a range of 50 per cent above or below its usual resting value in healthy man in spite of changes in cardiac output to one-third to five times its usual rate is indication that blood pressure regulation is normally present.

Hypertension in its manifold forms can be understood only if all types are examined to ascertain where and how the normal regulatory mechanisms are circumvented. Special efforts must be made to distinguish the differences in physiology among the hypertensions of known cause so as to throw light on those of unknown cause.

Blood Pressure Control as a Regulated System

The concept of a regulated system in its simpler forms has been outlined by Peterson[13] in a discussion of the feedback regulation of the mechanical properties of blood vessels. In a regulated system of this type a negative feedback consists in the use of a portion of the energy associated with a physical force as a signal to a control mechanism to minimize the "error signal," or the deviation of the force from some basal value. An example is the use of a portion of the energy associated with a rise in blood pressure to stimulate neural receptors which induce reflexes to return the pressure toward normal. Negative feedback tends to stabilize a system provided it is appropriately sensitive. Positive feedback, on the contrary, utilizes a portion of the energy associated with a force to increase any deviation from some initial value. This occurs, for instance, if a rise in blood pressure causes hypertrophy of blood vessels, which causes a further rise in blood pressure.

The complexity of blood pressure regulation can only be hinted at, as the regulatory mechanisms are multiple, are hierarchically arranged, regulate each other, are distributed in space at different points in the circulation, and change in time. Figure 37-1 is a schematic representation of some of the circuits and components which regulate blood pressure.

The basic effector organs determining the blood pressure are the heart, both ventricles and atria,

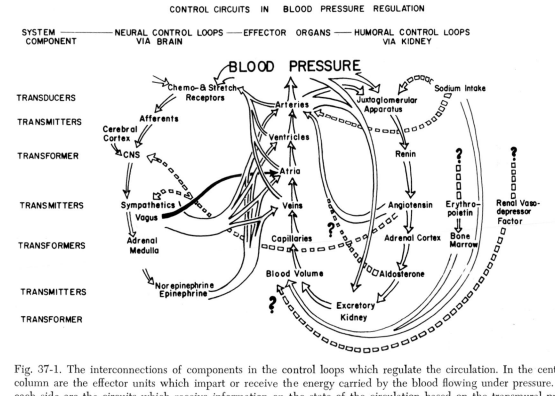

CONTROL CIRCUITS IN BLOOD PRESSURE REGULATION

Fig. 37-1. The interconnections of components in the control loops which regulate the circulation. In the central column are the effector units which impart or receive the energy carried by the blood flowing under pressure. At each side are the circuits which receive information on the state of the circulation based on the transmural pressure differential and the elastic and viscous properties of the vessel walls. This information is transformed and transmitted back to the effector units to regulate the blood pressure.

the blood vessels, including arteries, capillaries, and veins, and the blood. Their functional characteristics arise from their mechanical properties of elasticity, viscosity, and their dimensions: area of lumen, thickness of wall, and length of the blood vessels and heart chambers, and volume of the blood. There are also basic time-related biologic characteristics of the heart, including rate, rhythm, contractility, and synchronization, which are regulated. Each of these components may be varied to produce a resultant blood pressure.

Complex feedback loops regulate each organ, and whether any functional characteristic of any one of the organs acts to stabilize or disturb the system depends on the properties of the whole regulatory system as well as on the characteristics of the effector organ. The logic of the circuit, the sensitivity of the transducers, the transmission and transformation of information, as well as the power of the effector organs all determine how precise regulation will be and how the system will react to a disturbing force.

As illustrated in Fig. 37-1, two major control loops regulate cardiovascular function in man. The neural loop comprises signals traversing the central nervous system. The humoral loop operates through the kidney, which acts as both an endocrine and excretory organ. Each loop contains a number of parallel pathways activating effector organs in series. The two loops are semi-independent, but the control of renal artery tone by sympathetic nerves and the effects of angiotensin on elements of the neural loop allow them on occasion to operate synergistically.

In the diagram no effort has been made to indicate the direction of influence of each component of the loops. It is apparent that disturbance at some points will produce a widespread integrated response; at others, an isolated change. In either case these may be compensated for by more or less extensive negative feedback or exacerbated by positive feedback. The major process of cardiac and vasomuscular *hypertrophy* is a positive feedback of major importance which could not be included in the diagram. It potentiates cardiovascular response to stimulus by strengthening the effector organ.

Insufficient information is available to state with certainty the role of each component in each clinical and experimental form of hypertension. A definite state of operation must be assignable to each component, however, and only when these are known will hypertension be comprehensible.

This complexity accounts for the fact that the natural histories of hypertensive diseases are extremely varied. Some patients survive for years with little progression. Others deteriorate rapidly. It places the debate over the existence of the entity of *essential* hypertension in context. As investigative tools are sharpened and interpretation becomes more sophisticated, new critical malfunctions of the regulatory and effector machinery of the circulation will be found. These become *nonessential* hypertension. This has been the case with pheochromocytoma, aldosterone-secreting tumors, large renal artery stenosis, and coarctation of the aorta. As more "causes" are elucidated, the residual pool of hypertensive patients will increasingly be found to have multiple minor malfunctions which in summation produce a high resistance-flow product. These patients should have a distribution and hereditary pattern of blood pressures similar to other multifactored biologic variables, such as height, and will fall at the upper end of a unimodel distribution curve.

A number of corollaries derive from the recognition of blood pressure as a complexly regulated variable. First is the understanding that abnormal function of a portion of the circulatory system need not manifest itself in an abnormal blood pressure. For example, the onset of atrial fibrillation need not necessarily change either cardiac output or blood pressure. Second is that elevation of the blood pressure always means that some regulatory or effector mechanisms have been driven to function outside their physiologic range. The cardiac output, the peripheral resistance, or the blood volume or its viscosity must be abnormal. A third corollary is that simultaneous abnormalities may compensate for or reinforce each other. It is quite as possible for the slow progression of high blood pressure to be the result of gradual loss of negative feedback as for it to result from progression of the initial abnormality. Fourth, if in a regulated system of this type any of the feedback mechanisms become positive, i.e., tend to increase rather than minimize a change of pressure, then an unstable system results with progressive and accelerating disturbance of blood pressure. This occurs both in malignant hypertension and "irreversible" shock.

With these preliminary remarks about the point of view from which the data regarding hypertension have been examined, it will now be appropriate to turn to a consideration of some of the specific mechanisms involved in hypertension. The major areas to be considered are (1) nervous, (2) renal, (3) endocrine and metabolic, and (4) cardiovascular.

Neural Factors

Neural causes of hypertension may be conceived of at every point in the reflex arcs which regulate the blood vessels. Decreased sensitivity of stretch receptors,[14] interruption of the parasympathetic outflow,[15] or stimulation of sympathetic outflow[16] can all theoretically and experimentally lead to an integrated response increasing cardiac output and vasomotor tone. Direct intracranial stimuli in focal areas,[16] from generalized increase of intracranial pressure,[17] or from intrathecal injection of vasodilators[18] have also been found to produce a rise in blood pressure. There is no evidence that pathologic lesions activating any of these mechanisms cause essential hypertension or any large number of cases of hypertension, though an occasional hypoventilation syndrome, subarachnoid hemorrhage, or cerebral vascular thrombosis can produce hypertension.

A large body of data, especially from the Russian literature, indicates that psychologic and emotional stimuli of various sorts impinging on central nervous system components of the cardiovascular reflex arcs can produce hypertension.[19] This is considered to be the cause of essential hypertension by the Russians. Following Pavlov, Magakian et al., made nonhuman primates hypertensive by inducing experimental neuroses.[20,21] The pattern of hypertension thus induced has not been fully described.

Brod et al. have studied much more carefully a group of hypertensive human beings and a group of normal individuals under experimental emotional stress.[22] He found in both a pattern of hypertension with either increased total peripheral resistance or increased cardiac output or both. Both groups showed increased vascular resistance in kidney and skin but vasodilatation and increased flow in muscular vascular beds. The similarity of this pattern of flow to that seen in muscular exercise or the emotional preparation for it has led Brod to consider essential hypertension a psychogenically induced response to stress. Neurologically this can be imagined as introduced by cortical or reflex inhibition of the depressor relay stations in the brain or by direct stimulation of the sympathetic centers, including the vasodilator centers described by Uvnäs.[23]

The confidence which can be placed in Brod's highly derived estimates of distribution of blood flow is somewhat limited. Cumulative errors in measurement of cardiac output, para-aminohippuric acid (PAH) clearance, skin blood flow, and estimates of skin/muscle volume ratios are large. For this reason, though the hypothesis has much to make it plausible, it must be considered so far unproved.

Of great interest in support of the presence of a neurogenic component in renal hypertension are the effectiveness of sympathetic blocking agents in renal hypertension, the drop to control-animal pressures after pithing in renal-hypertensive rats and dogs,[24] and the well-documented resetting of the carotid sinus to regulate pressure at the new high level in chronic hypertension of both renal and unknown origin.[25] Destruction or severe depression of the nervous system will usually reduce elevated blood pressure of whatever origin, and this is accomplished without the peripheral ischemia which would be anticipated if the total effect were from depression of cardiac output. This does not necessarily imply that the neural outflow of the pressor type to the circulation is greater than normal in hypertension. It may well mean only that the circulatory effector organs are responding more vigorously to a normal level of stimulation. Under these conditions, reduction of nervous outflow below normal would still have the effect of depressing blood pressure.

It is highly probable that normal or abnormal psychologic stress can produce abnormal elevations of blood pressure in a number of individuals. The initial pathway is through autonomic outflow tracts, but with time, and especially if the malignant phase of hypertension should develop, heart, peripheral vessel structure and the kidneys become involved. The removal of stress at this point may not immediately correct the hypertension.

Renal Factors

The second major integrative system regulating the blood pressure arises in the kidney. Goldblatt et al.[26] in 1934 demonstrated that constriction of the renal arteries would consistently produce hypertension. Later work by Kohlstaedt, Helmer, and Page[27] and Braun-Menendez and his colleagues[28] demonstrated that there was a protein called *renin* released from the kidney and a protein substrate which together produced a nonprotein pressor substance in plasma which caused the hypertension.[29] The name *angiotensin* was agreed upon for the peptide, and it was subsequently characterized and synthesized. The exact mechanism and conditions of renin release and the loci of action of angiotensin are still under investigation. Some of the conditions of release are noted in the discussion of the juxtaglomerular apparatus. The renin-angiotensin system is thought to act by three routes: by direct vasoconstriction,[7] by sodium retention and expansion of plasma volume via stimulation of aldosterone secretion,[30] and by increasing the effect of sympathetic stimulation[31] or by direct stimulation of the sympathetic nervous system.[32]

These mechanisms are thought to be activated acutely in the hypertension of acute glomerulonephritis, though proof of specific elevation of renin-angiotensin in the blood is not at hand. The clinical picture is one of increased blood volume[33] with high cardiac output[34] at high pressure. The uncompensated stress on the circulation accounts for decompensation of cerebral, retinal, and cardiac function with encephalopathy, retinopathy, and congestive heart failure. The decompensation is made more likely because no gradual hypertrophy of the myocardium or blood vessels has prepared the heart or vessels to handle the acute work load. The tachycardia and elevated cardiac output frequently seen and the exquisite sensitivity to reserpine support the notion that the sympathetic system is also stimulated by this renal disease.

A similar set of circumstances is seen in acute bilateral renal vascular hypertension and in the malignant phase of chronic hypertension.[35] It has recently been shown that the first effect of elimination of renal artery stenosis is a fall in cardiac output.[36] In malignant chronic hypertension myocardial hypertrophy may offer some protection from congestive heart failure, so that decompensation of cerebral and renal function are more common.

In chronic experimental renal hypertension the secretion and role of renin have recently been documented by sensitive assays of renal vein pressor substance.[37] Antirenin has been shown to correct chronic renal hypertension in dogs years after its induction.[38] For reasons not entirely clear the hypertension of midstage chronic pyelonephritis and glomerulonephritis does not have the totally devastating quality of that in acute glomerulonephritis and malignant hypertension. The loss of oncotically active material preventing expansion of plasma volume in the nephrotic phase of glomerulonephritis and the salt-wasting character of the pyelonephritic kidney may offer partial explanation.

The demonstration by Edelman and Hartroft with fluorescent antibodies[39] and by Bing and Kazimierczak with microseparation techniques[40] that renin is found in or near the juxtaglomerular apparatus and that hypergranulation of these cells generally correlates with chronic conditions releasing angiotensin[41] provides a histologic technique for estimating renin secretion. It has been shown that conditions causing high kidney perfusion pressure[42] or increased body sodium stores[43] suppress juxtaglomerular apparatus hypergranularity. Conversely, low kidney perfusion pressures,[42] contracted blood volume,[44] and decreased body sodium stores[45] stimulate renin secretion. It is unfortunate that not all types of renal disease have been studied so far, and the relationship of renin to acute glomerulonephritis and chronic nephritis has not been clearly worked out.

Of great interest is the demonstration of a possible link between renin and the autonomic nervous system. McCubbin and Page have shown[31] that although infusion of angiotensin does not increase the pressor response to infusion of norepinephrine, it does increase the response to maneuvers that stimulate the release of endogenous norepinephrine.

The responses to injected tyramine and a sympathetic ganglion-stimulating agent (DMPP, dimethyl-phenyl-piperazium iodide) are enhanced. This may account for evidence of increased sympathetic activity in renal hypertension and prevent a fully effective negative-feedback response on the part of the nervous system to renal hypertension.

In addition to the well-documented and characterized mechanism of the renal pressor system, a renal depressor system has also been postulated. Renoprival hypertension was demonstrated in the nephrectomized dog by Grollman and his colleagues.[46] He found it to be aggravated by salt and protein in the diet of the totally nephrectomized dog sustained by chronic dialysis. Ureterocaval anastomosis, producing an "endocrine kidney," showed that protection against hypertension was not related to external excretion of urine. Muirhead, Stirman, and Jones showed that the major antihypertensive action was derived from the medulla rather than the cortex of the dog kidney.[47]

Booth et al.[48] and Hickler and his colleagues[49] have partially isolated low-molecular-weight extracts from rat kidneys which have powerful vasodepressor actions. The fall in pressure in the experimental renal hypertensive rats of Wilson when their clipped kidneys were repaired occurred only when a functioning, though not necessarily an excreting, kidney was preserved.[50] This suggests that renal inactivation of some extrarenal hypertensive factor or the release of a substance acting to reduce vasomotor tone may well play a role in keeping blood pressure down. If this be so, then hypertension in renal disease may result from loss of secretion of this factor instead of, or in addition to, stimulation of renin release.

It has been observed by Kolff[51] and Merrill[52] in bilaterally nephrectomized man that persistence of hypertension is not inevitable without kidneys but pressure can be kept down only on a rigorously restricted sodium intake. Transplantation of a normal kidney into these patients makes them normotensive on normal sodium intake.

It thus appears that both a renin and a renoprival hypertension might exist, but at present the renin mechanism seems better understood and wider in its effects.

An important unanswered question in understanding the mechanisms of renal hypertension is the nature of intrarenal blood flow. Marked differences in distribution of blood flow in the kidney in the experimental animal[53] and in the diseased kidney of man[54] explain the difficulties hitherto encountered in interpreting the function of the kidney, both as an excretory and a secretory organ, on the basis of total renal blood flow.

Endocrine and Metabolic Factors

The relationship of endocrine and metabolic factors to hypertension is complex. Humoral agents from the kidney fall in this category but have already been considered. Specific agents from the adrenal glands have especially been incriminated.

Adrenal Hormones

The adrenal medullary hormones, norepinephrine and epinephrine, are causes of hypertension in pheochromocytoma. Interesting aspects of this type of hypertension are the apparent compensations made by the body which give certain unique characteristics to the physiology of pheochromocytoma. In contrast to patients with essential hypertension, patients with pheochromocytoma often have a fall in blood pressure in changing from a lying to a standing position.[55] This indicates suppression of the carotid and similar regulatory reflexes. A second phenomenon which may be considered compensatory is the reduction of blood volume and extracellular fluid volume usually seen.[56] The urgent necessity of expanding blood volume to prevent shock after removal of a pheochromocytoma has been clearly demonstrated.[56] Experimental data from the author's laboratory indicate that prolonged infusion of norepinephrine induces, after transient sodium retention, a negative sodium balance and positive potassium balance compatible with suppression of aldosterone secretion.[57] These evidences of compensation suggest that negative-feedback loops are at work protecting the body from the malfunction of a single mechanism with distributed effect.

Oversecretion of aldosterone is a second adrenal cause of hypertension. Hypertension is a frequent concomitant of primary hyperaldosteronism.[58] The mechanism of the effect of this hormone on the blood pressure is not clearly understood. It most resembles the effect of massive sodium loading, producing an increase in extracellular volume, blood volume, and intracellular and vascular sodium content. It may have a positive inotropic action on the heart. The hemodynamics of this syndrome have not been extensively studied, so that data relating the hypertension to the basic circulatory variables and the various control mechanisms are not available. The effects may be attributable entirely to the disturbance of sodium and potassium content and distribution. Large loads of sodium in some experimental animals, especially the rat,[59] and occasionally described in man[60] produce a syndrome generally similar in its cardiovascular aspects. Evidence for attempted physiologic compensation for high levels of mineralocorticoids is the depletion of renin granules in the kidneys of animals given deoxycorticosterone[41] pointing to suppression of renal pressor mechanisms. Conn has recently suggested that oversecretion of aldosterone may lead to hypertension in the absence of the classical findings of primary aldosteronism. In this group renin secretion is low. He attributes this type of hypertension to the adrenal cortical adenomas previously thought to be non-functioning which have been found in up to 20 per cent of hypertensive patients at autopsy.[58a] A pressor response to ganglionic blockade in patients with primary aldosteronism is evidence that neural mechanisms are likewise acting in a protective manner.

Critical to the understanding of the mechanism of hypertension is information on the level of aldosterone secretion in the various types of the disease. It has already been suggested that in pheochromocytoma its secretion may be suppressed, providing negative feedback. There is little doubt that in malignant hypertension it is elevated, providing a positive feedback.[61] This may constitute the critical difference between benign and malignant hypertension. There has been long debate as to whether aldosterone secretion is elevated or not in benign essential hypertension.[61] The difficulty is in part due to the many factors of diet that affect aldosterone secretion and in part to the difficulty of the measurement. The problem is made worse by the lack of definite criteria for differentiation between renal and essential hypertension and for diagnosis of the malignant phase of the disease. All the cardiovascular features of malignant hypertension, i.e., retinopathy, encephalopathy, heart failure, rise in pressure, can be induced in the patient with benign hypertension by loading him with sodium.[62] Only the azotemia and the high aldosterone secretion will be missing to complete the picture. On the other hand, rigorous sodium depletion in the patient with malignant hypertension will relieve him of the malignant circulatory manifestations, while only renal insufficiency and high aldosterone output remain.

Two sets of aldosterone measurements suggest that aldosterone secretion *at comparable sodium intakes* are normal or lower in the patient with benign essential hypertension than in normal man. Cope et al.[63] and Laragh et al.[61] have presented data compatible with, but not statistically proving, this hypothesis. Ancillary data on the accelerated excretion of sodium loads in benign essential hypertension[64] suggest that depressed tubular sodium reabsorption may be present.

It is the author's hypothesis that in benign essential hypertension aldosterone secretion is reduced and that this produces a protective effect by minimizing sodium retention. With the onset of the malignant phase of the disease, probably the consequence of renal vascular damage, activation of the renin-angiotensin-aldosterone mechanism sets in motion a powerful positive feedback which makes the hypertension worse and damages renal vessels more. This creates a malignant accelerated disease. If this hypothesis is correct, it is an argument against a renin-angiotensin origin of benign essential hypertension.

Other endocrine and metabolic factors may on occasion produce hypertension. Hyperadrenocorticism[65] and adrenal regeneration in the experimental rat[66] can lead to hypertension by poorly understood pathways.

Sodium

The role of the external balance of sodium in hypertension has received much consideration. Meneely and Dahl [59] and Dahl and Love[67] have emphasized the hypertensogenic potentialities of sodium in rats and man. Dahl [68] has recently selected and bred two strains of rats, one of which develops hypertension on high sodium intake and one of which does not. Widespread clinical and experimental experience from the work of Kempner[69] and Grollman and Harrison[70] document that in the hypertensive patient sodium intake is a major determinant of blood pressure. In a person predisposed to hypertension, a high sodium intake will induce clinical manifestations earlier and in more severe degree. The rarity of hypertension in patients with Addison's disease is also thought to be in part due to the reduced body stores of sodium.

A number of epidemiologic studies of populations have endeavored to detect a correlation between

blood pressure and sodium intake.[71] In general, a positive correlation has been found, but the difficulties in estimating sodium intake for large groups is formidable, and many discrepancies in the correlation have been disclosed. These may well be due to other environmental circumstances or to group differences in the excretion of sodium loads.

Little evidence is available on differences in man's ability to handle a sodium load. There is little question that if disease states are included, the sodium titration curve, i.e., the total body sodium content required to excrete a given daily load of sodium, varies widely in individuals. Preliminary studies in the author's laboratory indicate that the weight which must be reached at steady state to excrete increasing sodium intake follows a sigmoid shape (Fig. 37-2). Variations in the slope and intercept of this curve in a large number of individuals have not been evaluated, and genetic and racial differences of this sort have not been explored in man. Variations in the excretion of sodium, as well as variations in intake, may well be a significant determinant of hypertension in individuals and in groups.

The mechanism of the effect of sodium on blood pressure is obscure. In hypertension restriction of sodium intake and diuretics which induce negative sodium balance cause contraction of plasma volume transiently, but even after restoration of plasma volume[72] the pressure remains down. Recently note has been taken of the fact that in hypertension, blood vessels have increased sodium and water content.[8,3] An increase in vascular stiffness is also found.[73] There is no evidence for differentiating between the change in mechanical properties of vessels due to change in sodium and water content, and the entrapment of sodium secondary to the dimensional change with vasospasm. The hypothesis that body sodium content influences the reactivity of cardiovascular muscle to neural or humoral stimuli on the basis of a dimensional or a biochemical change has been frequently advanced. This has been difficult to support with quantitative data which cannot be otherwise explained, but an effect of sodium on blood pressure greater than can be exclusively attributed to changes in blood volume seems to be present.

The author's interpretation of the role of sodium in hypertension is that in any condition where circulatory regulation is impaired, whether from hypertension or from autonomic insufficiency, as studied by Wagner,[74] blood pressure is inordinately sensitive to changes in blood volume, varies directly with body sodium content, and varies more widely than in one with normal feedback. Overload of sodium, by raising the blood pressure, may cause hypertension only in people with very heavy intake,

SODIUM TITRATION CURVE

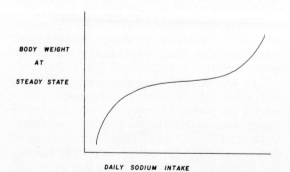

Fig. 37-2. A curve representing the concept of a sodium-titration curve in the intact organism, derived from preliminary studies in man. The slope and level of this curve vary markedly among individuals and between health and disease. The characteristics of the curve depend upon the integrated function of heart, vessels, kidneys, endocrine glands, and metabolic factors such as carbohydrate intake. It has not been studied in the various types of hypertension.

with impaired sodium-handling mechanisms, or with impaired circulatory regulation. In hypertension blood vessels contain excess sodium and water, but it is not clear whether this is cause or effect of the increased stiffness of the vessel walls.

Catabolism of Pressor Substances

Derangement of the metabolism of catecholamines has been considered possibly to account for essential hypertension.[75] Evidence suggesting the delayed breakdown of norepinephrine has not been widely accepted.[76] From the control mechanism standpoint, one would postulate that failure to destroy norepinephrine, for instance, would suppress its secretion.

Angiotensin is rapidly destroyed in normal plasma. Evidence for delay in its destruction or sensitivity to lower levels in some people has been presented by Wood.[77] Individuals showing this trait in a nonhypertensive state have relatives with significantly more hypertension than controls. These and related data will be discussed in Chap. 39.

Other studies on the inactivation of angiotensin by human hypertensive plasma in bioassay in the rat show marked differences in the rate of inactivation in various types of hypertension.[78] Marked differences in the blood pressure response to injected angiotensin have also been found in various types of hypertension.[79] Studies of this type are still in too early a phase to fit any clear-cut pattern, but certainly from data currently available it is clear that there are marked differences in the physiology of angiotensin between the various forms of hypertension, especially between benign and malignant forms.

Cardiovascular Factors

Characteristics of the cardiovascular system itself, rather than disturbance originating in external control organs, may cause hypertension. The cardiovascular system is the source of information which is the basis of blood pressure regulation. Strain or stretch of the blood vessel wall is detected by neural stretch receptors. This is the major type of information on which regulation of the blood pressure is based.

The stretch or strain of the arterial wall has been studied in detail by Peterson.[80] It is the result of the transmural pressure differential, roughly equaling the blood pressure at that point, and of the dimensions and viscoelastic properties of the vessel wall. Thus if a vessel becomes hypertrophied and resistant to stretch or if it actively participates in contraction as blood pressure rises, there may be little added stretch to signal that rise in blood pressure has taken place. It has been shown that application of norepinephrine to the wall of the carotid sinus will cause it to constrict in a manner which will cause reflex changes in blood pressure.[81] It has been stated by Peterson that in normal anesthetized dogs the carotid sinus is the most distensible portion of the arterial tree.[81] Whether this is true in hypertensive man and what his carotid sinus vasomotor innervation is has not been clearly ascertained. If in vasoconstriction in man receptor sites constrict as effectors in a manner to prevent stretch under the higher pressure, as has been shown in the dog,[80] then the negative-feedback loop will not be adequately activated. It has indeed been shown that by some mechanism the carotid sinus mechanism does become adapted in hypertensive man so that it begins to regulate blood pressure about a new higher level.[14]

The cardiovascular system is also the *effector* which generates the blood pressure. Anatomic and metabolic properties of the heart and blood vessels determine the work which will be done upon the blood. The force and rate of myocardial contraction and the mechanical properties of the vessel walls are final determinants of the blood pressure. If the effector organs hypertrophy, they may execute more work with the same neural or hormonal stimulus. Like the muscles of the athlete in training, the myocardium and peripheral vascular muscles undergoing progressive hypertrophy are capable of doing more work, raising the blood pressure even higher, though the stimulus remains the same.

A combination of increased resistance of receptor sites to stretch and increased strength of effector organ contraction in response to a given stimulus would provide the positive feedback to make hypertension a progressive disease. This combination is provided by the muscular hypertrophy of heart and blood vessels. This does not account for the original elevation of blood pressure but may well explain the observation that in the population as a whole, it is those whose blood pressure is originally high in whom progressively rising pressure develops with age.[82]

Many observations support the concept that in spite of the hypertrophy of blood vessels in hypertension, the lumen is not irrevocably diminished but that continued neurologic stimulation is required to sustain the increased peripheral resistance. The rapid relief of correctible forms of hypertension frequently seen, even after long duration, when the cause, such as a pheochromocytoma or renal artery stenosis, is relieved, the response of the experimental animal to pithing, and the marked drop in pressure to hypotensive levels occasionally seen with parenteral sympathetic blocking agents all support the concept that in benign essential hypertension the vascular caliber is not irreversibly reduced. It can be postulated that in benign hypertension the increased peripheral resistance is attributable to hypertrophied vessels responding to stimulation and not to simple encroachment on the lumen by the thickened wall.

In summary, the blood pressure is a regulated complex variable with at least two identifiable control systems which are partially interlocked. Depending upon the point of pathologic disturbance, certain negative-feedback loops can counteract a force tending to elevate the blood pressure. In most situations when elevation of blood pressure reaches a certain point, slow-moving positive feedback makes it progressive. Ultimately, more powerful positive feedback may make it accelerated or malignant.

The stimulus to hypertension may come from outside the control loops as from the cerebral cortex, chemoreceptors, or excessive sodium intake, or from within the control loops by change in activity of one or more components damaged by disease. The causes of hypertension are multiple; they include psychogenic, neurogenic, nephrogenic, hormonal, metabolic, and cardiovascular causes. The initial pathologic change of function need be only minimal and may be unmeasurable, but over a long period of time hypertrophy of heart and vessels allows greater responses to the same stimulus, so that the disease progresses. At a point damage to renal vessels triggers off the release of renal substances which rapidly lead to accelerated rise of pressure and decompensation of brain, heart, and kidneys.

Keeping the blood pressure down, by controlling sodium balance, the autonomic nervous system, renin secretion, and/or hormonal output, should stop the progression of the disease by interrupting positive feedback. The apparent cure of a few patients after long-term careful control of their blood pressure may be an illustration of reversal of changes which lead to progression of hypertension.[12]

REFERENCES

1. "Hypertension: The First Hahneman Symposium on Hypertensive Disease," J. H. Moyer (ed.), W. B. Saunders Company, Philadelphia, 1959.
1a. "Hypertension—Recent Advances: The Second Hahneman Symposium on Hypertensive Disease," A. N. Brest and J. H. Moyer (eds.), Lea & Febiger, Philadelphia, 1961.
2. "Essential Hypertension," Ciba Foundation International Symposium, 1960, K. D. Bock and P. T. Cottier (eds.), Springer-Verlag, Berlin, 1960.
3. "The Pathogenesis of Essential Hypertension," Proceedings of the Prague Symposium, 1960, J. H.

Cort, V. Fencl, Z. Hejl, and J. Jirka (eds.), The Macmillan Company, New York, 1962.
4. "International Symposúm on Angiotensin, Sodium, and Hypertension," *Canad. M. A. J.*, **90**:153, 344, 1964.
5. "Hypertension," *Proc. Council for High Blood Pressure Res.*, vols. 1–13, American Heart Association, New York, 1953–1965.
6. "Symposium on Angiotensin," J. E. Wood and R. P. Ahlquist (eds.), *Circulation*, **25**:167 (part 2), 1962.
7. Page, I. H., and Bumpus, F. M.: Angiotensin, *Physiol. Rev.*, **41**:331, 1961.
8. Tobian, L.: Interrelationship of Electrolytes, Juxtaglomerular Cells and Hypertension, *Physiol. Rev.*, **40**:280, 1960.
9. "Symposium on Central Nervous System Control of Circulation," L. W. Eichna and D. E. McQuarrie (eds.), *Physiol. Rev.*, **40** (Suppl. 4, part 2), 1960.
10. Freis, E. D.: Hemodynamics of Hypertension, *Physiol. Rev.*, **40**:27, 1960.
11. Peart, W. S.: Hypertension and the Kidney. I. Clinical, Pathological, and Functional Disorders, Especially in Man, *Brit. M. J.*, **2**:1353, 1959; II. Experimental Basis of Renal Hypertension, *Brit. M. J.*, **2**:1421, 1959.
12. Page, I. H.: The Mosaic Theory of Hypertension (in ref. 2, p. 1).
13. Peterson, L. H.: Systems Behavior, Feedback Loops, and High Blood Pressure Research, *Circulation Res.*, **12**:585 (part 2), 1963.
14. Kezdi, P.: Sinoaortic Regulatory System, *A.M.A. Arch. Int. Med.*, **91**:26, 1953.
15. Gorten, R., Gunnells, J. C., Weissler, A. M., and Stead, E. A., Jr.: Effects of Atropine and Isoproterenol on Cardiac Output, Central Venous Pressure, and Mean Transit Time of Indicators Placed at Three Different Sites in the Venous System, *Circulation Res.*, **9**:979, 1961.
16. Manning, J. W., Jr., and Peiss, C. N.: Cardiovascular Responses to Electrical Stimulation in the Diencephelon, *Am. J. Physiol.*, **198**:366, 1960.
17. Cushing, H.: Some Experimental and Clinical Observations Concerning States of Increased Intracranial Tension, *Am. J. M. Sc.*, **124**:375, 1902.
18. Kaneko, Y., McCubbin, J. W., and Page, I. H.: Mechanism by Which Serotonin, Norepinephrine, Reserpine Cause Central Vasomotor Inhibition, *Circulation Res.*, **8**:1228, 1960.
19. Simonson, E., and Brozek, J.: Russian Research on Arterial Hypertension, *Ann Int. Med.*, **50**:129, 1959.
20. Magakian, G. O., Miminoshvili, D. I., and Kokaia, G. Ia: Experimental Study of the Pathogenesis of Hypertension and Coronary Insufficiency, *Klinicheskaia Med.*, **37**(7):30, 1956 (ref. in 19 above).
21. Miminoshvili, D. I., Magakian, G. O., and Kokaia, G. Ia: Experimental Production of Arterial Hypertension and Coronary Insufficiency in Monkeys, *Teor. prakt. voprosy med. i biol. eksper. na obezianakh*, **85**, 1956 (ref. in 19 above).
22. Brod, J., Fencl, V., Hejl, Z., and Jirka, J.: Circula-

tory Changes Underlying Blood Pressure Elevation During Acute Emotional Stress (Mental Arithmetic) in Normotensive and Hypertensive Subjects, *Clin. Sc.*, 18:269, 1959.

23. Uvnäs, B., Sympathetic Vasodilator Outflow, *Physiol. Rev.*, 34:608, 1954.

24. Taquini, A. C., Jr.: Neurogenic Control of Peripheral Resistance in Renal Hypertension, *Circulation Res.*, 12:562 (part 2), 1963.

25. McCubbin, J. W., Green, J. H., and Page, I. H.: Baroreceptor Function in Chronic Renal Hypertension, *Circulation Res.*, 4:205, 1956.

26. Goldblatt, H., Lynch, J., Hanzal, R. F., and Summerville, W. W.: Studies on Experimental Hypertension. I. Production of Persistent Elevation of Systolic Blood Pressure by Means of Renal Ischemia, *J. Exper. Med.*, 59:347, 1934.

27. Kohlstaedt, K. G., Helmer, O. M., and Page, I. H.: Activation of Renin by Blood Colloids, *Proc. Soc. Exper. Biol. & Med.*, 39:214, 1938.

28. Braun-Menendez, E., Fasciolo, J. C., Leloir, L. F., and Munoz, J. M.: The Substance Causing Renal Hypertension, *J. Physiol.*, 98:283, 1940.

29. Braun-Menendez, E.: Pharmacology of Renin and Hypertensin, *Pharmacol. Rev.*, 8:25, 1956.

30. Biron, P., Koiw, E., Nowaczynski, W., Brouillet, J., and Genest, J.: Effects of Intravenous Infusions of Valine-5-Angiotensin II and Other Pressor Agents on Urinary Electrolytes and Corticosteroids, Including Aldosterone, *J. Clin. Invest.*, 40:338, 1961.

31. McCubbin, J. W., and Page, I. H.: Renal Pressor System and Neurogenic Control of Arterial Pressure, *Circulation Res.*, 12:553 (part 2), 1963.

32. Bickerton, R. K., and Buckley, J. P.: Evidence for a Central Mechanism in Angiotensin Induced Hypertension, *Proc. Soc. Exper. Biol. & Med.*, 106:834, 1961.

33. Eisenberg, S.: Blood Volume in Patients with Acute Glomerulonephritis, *Am. J. Med.*, 27:241, 1959.

34. DeFazio, V., Christensen, R. C., Regan, T. J., Baer, L. J., Morita, Y., and Hellems, H. K.: Circulatory Changes in Acute Glomerulonephritis, *Circulation*, 20:190, 1959.

35. Tuttle, E. P., Jr.: Unpublished observations.

36. Ledingham, J. M., and Cohen, R. D.: Circulatory Changes during Reversal of Experimental Hypertension, *Clin. Sc.*, 22:69, 1962.

37. Helmer, O. M.: Presence of Renin in Plasma of Patients with Arterial Hypertension, *Circulation*, 25:169, 1962.

38. Wakerlin, G. E.: Antibodies to Renin as Proof of the Pathogenesis of Sustained Renal Hypertension, *Circulation*, 17:653, 1958.

39. Edelman, R., and Hartroft, P. M.: Localization of Renin in Juxtaglomerular Cells of Rabbit and Dog through the Use of the Fluorescent-Antibody Technique, *Circulation Res.*, 9:1069, 1961.

40. Bing, J., Kazimierczak, J.: Renin Content of Different Parts of the Juxtaglomerular Apparatus, *Acta path. et microbiol. scandinav.*, 54:80, 1962.

41. Hartroft, P. M.: Juxtaglomerular Cells, *Circulation Res.*, 12:525 (part 2), 1963.

42. Hartroft, P. M.: Studies on Renal Juxtaglomerular Cells. III. The Effects of Experimental Renal Disease and Hypertension in the Rat, *J. Exper. Med.*, 105:501, 1957.

43. Hartroft, P. M., and Hartroft, W. S.: Studies on Juxtaglomerular Cells. I. Variations Produced by Sodium Chloride and Desoxycorticosterone Acetate, *J. Exper. Med.*, 97:415, 1953.

44. Hirashima, K., and Takaku, F.: Experimental Studies on Erythropoietin. II. The Relationship between Juxtaglomerular Cells and Erythropoietin, *Blood*, 20:1, 1962.

45. Hartroft, P. M., Newmark, L. N., and Pitcock, J. A.: Relationship of Renal Juxtaglomerular Cells to Sodium Intake, Adrenal Cortex, and Hypertension (in ref. 1, p. 24).

46. Grollman, A., Muirhead, E. E., and Vanatta, J.: Role of the Kidney in Pathogenesis of Hypertension as Determined by a Study of the Effects of Bilateral Nephrectomy and Other Experimental Procedures on the Blood Pressure of the Dog, *Am. J. Physiol.*, 157:21, 1959.

47. Muirhead, E. E., Stirman, J. A., and Jones, F.: Renal Autoexplantation and Protection against Renoprival Hypertensive Cardiovascular Disease and Hemolysis, *J. Clin. Invest.*, 39:266, 1960.

48. Booth, E., Hinman, J. W., Daniels, E. G., Kosinski, M., and Muirhead, E. E.: Antihypertensive Renal Factor, *J. Clin. Invest.*, 42:918, 1963 (Abstract).

49. Hickler, R. B., Saravis, C. A., Mowbray, J. F., Lauler, D. P., Vagnucci, A. I., and Thorn, G. W.: Reno Medullary Vasodepressor Factor, *J. Clin. Invest.*, 42:942, 1963 (Abstract).

50. Wilson, C.: The Kidney and Essential Hypertension (in ref. 3, p. 405).

51. Kolff, W. J., Nakamoto, S., Peutasse, E. F., Straffon, R. A., and Figueroa, J. E.: The Effect of Bilateral Nephrectomy and Transplantation on Hypertension in Man, *Circulation*, 30 (supp. 2): 23, 1964.

52. Merrill, J. P., and Schupak, E.: Mechanisms of Hypertension in Renoprival Man, *Canad. M. A. J.*, 90: 328, 1964.

53. Thorburn, G. D., Kopald, H. H., Herd, J. A., Hollenberg, M., O'Morchoe, C. C. C., and Barger, A. C.: Intrarenal Distribution of Nutrient Blood Flow Determined with Krypton-85 in the Unanesthetized Dog, *Circulation Res.*, 13:290, 1963.

54. Tuttle, E. P., and Sadler, J. H.: Measurement of Renal Tissue Fluid Turnover Rates by Thermal Washout Technique. *Proc. Council for High Blood Pressure Res.*, American Heart Association, 13, 1965. (In press.)

55. Smithwick, R. H., Greer, W. E. R., Robertson C. W., and Wilkins, R. W.: Pheochromocytoma: A Discussion of Symptoms, Signs and Procedures of Diagnostic Value, *New England J. Med.*, 242:252, 1950.

56. Brunjes, S., Johns, V. J., and Crane, M. G.: Pheo-

chromocytoma: Post Operative Shock and Blood Volume, *New England J. Med.*, **262**:393, 1960.

57. Tuttle, E. P., Jr.: Saluresis and Potassium Retention Induced by Pressor Amines, *Clin. Res.*, **8**:89, 1960 (Abstract).

58. Conn, J. W.: Aldosteronism and Hypertension: Primary Aldosteronism versus Hypertensive Disease with Secondary Aldosteronism, *Arch. Int. Med.*, **107**:813, 1961.

58a. Conn, J. W.: Plasma Renin Activity in Primary Aldosteronism, *J.A.M.A.*, **190**:222, 1964.

59. Meneely, G. R., and Dahl, L. K.: Electrolytes in Hypertension: The Effect of Sodium Chloride, *M. Clin. North America*, **45**:271, 1961.

60. McDonough, J., and Wilhelmj, C. M.: The Effect of Excess Salt Intake on Human Blood Pressure, *Am. J. Digest. Dis.*, **21**:180, 1954.

61. Laragh, J. H., Ulick, S., Januszewicz, V., Deming, Q. B., Kelly, W. G., and Lieberman, S.: Aldosterone Secretion and Primary and Malignant Hypertension, *J. Clin. Invest.*, **39**:1091, 1960.

62. Tuttle, E. P., Jr.: Unpublished observations.

63. Cope, C. L., Harwood, M., and Pearson, J.: Aldosterone Secretion in Hypertensive Diseases, *Brit. M. J.*, **1**:659, 1962.

64. Birchall, R., Tuthill, S. W., Jacobs, W. S., Trautman, W. J., Jr., and Findley, T.: Renal Excretion of Water, Sodium and Chloride: Comparison of Responses of Hypertensive Patients with Those of Normal Subjects, etc., *Circulation*, **7**:258, 1953.

65. Knowlton, A. I., Loeb, E. N., Stoerk, H. C., White, J. P., and Heffernan, J. F.: Induction of Arterial Hypertension in Normal and Adrenalectomized Rats Given Cortisone Acetate, *J. Exper. Med.*, **96**:187, 1952.

66. Skelton, F. R.: Development of Hypertension and Cardiovascular-Renal Lesions during Adrenal Regeneration in the Rat, *Proc. Soc. Exper. Biol. & Med.*, **90**:342, 1955.

67. Dahl, L. K., and Love, R. A.: Etiological Role of Sodium Chloride Intake in Essential Hypertension in Humans, *J.A.M.A.*, **164**:397, 1957.

68. Dahl, L. K., Heine, M., and Tossi, Nari, L.: The Effects of Chronic Excess Salt Ingestion: Vascular Reactivity in Rats, *Circulation*, **30** (supp. 2): 11, 1964.

69. Kempner, W.: Treatment of Hypertensive Vascular Disease with Rice Diet, *Am. J. Med.*, **4**:545, 1948.

70. Grollman, A., and Harrison, T. R.: Effect of Sodium Restriction on Blood Pressure and Survival of Hypertensive Rats, *Proc. Soc. Exper. Biol. & Med.*, **60**:52, 1945.

71. Dahl, L. K.: Possible Role of Salt Intake in the Development of Essential Hypertension (in ref. 2, p. 53).

72. Wilson, I. M., and Freis, E. D.: The Relationship between Plasma and Extracellular Fluid Volume Depletion and the Anti-hypertensive Effect of Chlorothiazide, *Circulation*, **20**:1028, 1959.

73. Feigl, E. O., Peterson, L. H., and Jones, A. W.: Mechanical and Chemical Properties of Arteries in Experimental Hypertension, *J. Clin. Invest.*, **42**: 1640, 1963.

74. Wagner, H. N.: The Influence of Autonomic Vasoregulatory Reflexes on the Rate of Sodium and Water Excretion in Man, *J. Clin. Invest.*, **36**:1319, 1957.

75. Mendlowitz, M., Gitlow, S., and Naftchi, N.: Cause of Essential Hypertension, *Perspectives Biol. & Med.*, **2**:354, 1959.

76. Sjoerdsma, A.: Relationships between Alterations in Amine Metabolism and Blood Pressure, *Circulation Res.*, **9**:734, 1961.

77. Wood, J. E.: Genetic Control of Neutralization of Angiotensin and Its Relationship to Essential Hypertension, *Circulation*, **25**:225, 1962.

78. Hickler, R. B., Lauler, D. P., and Thorn, G. W.: Plasma Angiotensinase Activity in Patients with Hypertension and Edema, *J. Clin. Invest.*, **42**:635, 1963.

79. Kaplan, N. M., and Silah, J.: Effects of Angiotensin II on the Blood Pressure in Humans with Hypertensive Disease, *J. Clin. Invest.*, **43**:659, 1964.

80. Peterson, L. H.: Properties and Behavior of Living Vascular Wall, *Physiol. Rev.*, **42** (Suppl. 5), 309, 1962.

81. Peterson, L. H., Feigl, E., and Gouras, P.: Properties of the Carotid Sinus Mechanism, *Fed. Proc.*, **19**:40, 1960 (Abstract).

82. Stamler, J., Lindberg, H. A., Berkson, D. M., Shaffer, A. Miller, W., and Poindexter, A.: Epidemiologic Analysis of Hypertension and Hypertensive Disease in the Labor Force of a Chicago Utility Company, *Proc. Council for High Blood Pressure Res.*, American Heart Association, **7**:23, 1958.

38 HEREDITARY AND HUMORAL FACTORS IN ESSENTIAL HYPERTENSION

J. Edwin Wood, M.D.

Essential hypertension is the single largest diagnostic category in explanation of the presence of elevated arterial pressure. This form of hypertension is misnamed. The term was conceived on the basis that patients exhibiting abnormally high diastolic blood pressure for which no explanation could be found had the disorder as an "essential" part of their makeup. More recent studies suggest that the term *genetic* or *familial hypertension* would be better, if terminology were to conform with that generally used in medical science.[1,2]

It has become increasingly apparent that essential hypertension is a familial and very likely a genetic disorder. This is a clinical characteristic of essential hypertension. There are other rare forms of genetically transmitted hypertension, but these are easily distinguished from essential hypertension. Examples are hereditary nephritis associated with hypertension,[3] neurofibramotosis, and hereditary pheochromocytoma[4] and diabetes with its hereditary nature and its complications of renal disease and hypertension.

It is well established that the primary mechanical difficulty in essential hypertension is that of an excessive resistance to the flow of blood from the arterial system to the capillaries and thence to the veins.[5] Numerous factors, discussed both here and elsewhere, determine the caliber of the small arteries and arterioles. However, the neurohumoral systems that are of primary importance in this control are the sympathoadrenal system and the renin-angiotensin system.[6]

The therapy for essential hypertension that has met with the greatest success is an attack upon the sympathetic nervous system by either surgical or pharmacologic means. However, a large body of evidence indicates that excessive activity of the sympathetic nervous system is not responsible for the decrease in caliber of the arterioles. In fact several studies show that the sympathetic nervous system is diminished in activity in patients with hypertension. This finding suggests that the sympathetic nervous system has reduced its activity in the face of another vasopressor stimulus, possibly angiotensin.

Genetic Factors

Physicians who observed families with a high incidence of strokes associated with elevated blood pressure have long been aware of the familial nature of essential hypertension. Aymen first demonstrated this in a systematic manner.[7] Regarding environmental influences, patients with this disease may have a specific personality pattern described as one of "restrained hostility."[8] This observation raises the question of whether hypertension is transmitted from parent to offspring by virtue of exposure of the child to this personality. Proof is certainly lacking for this point of view. The consistency with which the condition is transmitted makes this explanation seem unlikely. The effect of personality is probably an important but not a primary factor.

Recent studies of population groups have utilized methods designed to study possible hereditary patterns of transmission of blood pressure control. There is controversy as to detail, but the concept that essential hypertension is genetically transmitted seems almost inescapable.

The pattern of genetic transmission has been

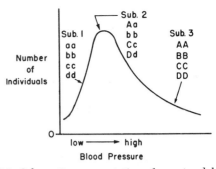

Fig. 38-1. Schematic representation of a unimodal frequency distribution curve, with three examples of individual subjects and their theoretical genetic makeup on the basis of the multifactorial concept.

consistently attributed to that of a dominant gene or genes. Examples of a "skipped generation" in essential hypertension are virtually never seen. This is evidence favoring the dominant- rather than recessive-gene theory.

In carefully delineated population studies of individuals in England, Oldham, Pickering, and their group have observed that the frequency distribution curve for blood pressure was uninterrupted though skewed somewhat toward higher pressures (Fig. 38-1).[9] This led them to the conclusion that excessive blood pressure was transmitted on a genetic basis but that patients considered to have essential hypertension had not been distinguished from others by a single gene. Rather, they had in their genetic makeup a relatively high percentage of dominant genes that somehow resulted in elevated blood pressure. Thus, these individuals were in the upper portion of the normal distribution curve for blood pressure. As an example let us say that four genes, A, B, C, and D, have equal importance in determining the presence of abnormally elevated blood pressure. The blood pressure of the subject in whom all these genes were recessive (subject 1, Fig. 38-1) would appear in the left-hand portion of the frequency distribution curve. An individual who received three dominant genes and five recessive genes (subject 2, Fig. 38-1) would be in the large group near the median of the frequency distribution curve. Finally, if a subject happened to receive eight dominant genes, he would be well to the right in the distribution curve (subject 3, Fig. 38-1). He would be distinctive clinically by virtue of the early ill effects of the high blood pressure upon his arterial system, heart, and kidneys, but he would not be distinctive genetically. He would be an extreme example of a chance distribution of multiple genes. This is the essence of the multifactoral theory.

Platt and coworkers have suggested that if precautions be taken to eliminate patients with the

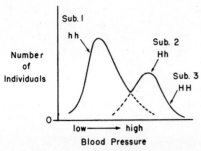

Fig. 38-2. Schematic representation of a bimodal frequency distribution curve, with three examples of individual subjects and their theoretical genetic makeup on the basis of the single-dominant-gene concept.

excessive systolic blood pressure that occurs in older individuals and if subjects who are too young to have developed essential hypertension are eliminated from study, a very different pattern of distribution occurs.[10] Their data were distributed in two groups that overlapped (Fig. 38-2). A single dominant gene was considered as explanatory of these data. It was suggested that all the subjects in the first peak were homozygous recessive for the gene controlling the presence of excessive blood pressure (subject 1, Fig. 38-2). All subjects in the second peak to the right would have at least one dominant gene that has resulted in excessively high diastolic blood pressure (subject 2, Fig. 38-2). A few of the subjects would be homozygous for this gene (subject 3, Fig. 38-2). This pattern of transmission would result in a given subject's having the abnormal gene that potentially could cause clinical hypertension (though not necessarily because of the variable effect of penetrance), or a subject would not have such a gene.

Experience with genetic disorders in human beings would suggest that the homozygote for the dominant gene may be more severely affected than the heterozygote. In clinical terms patients with malignant hypertension might be the homozygotes (subject 3, Fig. 38-2).[2] Studies of one island population support this concept. It was observed that three groups of individuals were present; that is, the frequency distribution curve for blood pressure was trimodal in character.[11] This observation also supports the single-gene theory rather than the multifactorial concept. The observations that some populations experience an extremely high incidence of hypertension while other genetically distinct groups show no hypertension support the genetic theory but shed no light upon the pattern of transmission.[12,13]

Humoral Factors

Clearly the mechanism for elevation of blood pressure in the presence of renal artery obstruction

is that of the abnormal secretion of renin induced by the hemodynamic effect of the obstruction. The classic observations of Goldblatt et al.[14] coupled with the more recent observations of Hartroft and Hartroft[15] and of Tobian et al.[16] establish this pattern. Attempts to link this system with essential hypertension have met with more difficulty. The direct observation of excessive levels of angiotensin (Fig. 38-3) in the renal vein blood of the patients with essential hypertension[17] favors this link. Whether this is primary or secondary in the pathogenic pattern of essential hypertension is the question. Further, hypertension caused by renal vascular disease is associated with much higher levels of angiotensin in renal vein blood than hypertension of similar degree of the essential type.[18] This finding is so consistent that the point is used to differentiate the two disorders.

A second question then arises concerning the participation of the renin-angiotensin system in the causation of essential hypertension. If this system accounts for essential hypertension but is not initially associated with excessive elaboration of renin, then the explanation could lie in retarded degradation of angiotensin.[19] A group of students were investigated with regard to their ability to neutralize the vasopressor quality of synthetic angiotensin and the results evaluated in terms of their parents' blood pressures. Those students who were able to diminish the vasopressor quality of angiotensin most efficiently were also those with normotensive parents. Those less able to do this generally had at least one parent with elevated blood pressure. This study involved the use of whole blood, and a possible explanation lay in the presence of increased enzymatic destruction of angiotensin by the blood. Hickler et al. demonstrated that this is definitely not the case and that in fact patients with essential hypertension have a higher concentration of angiotensinase in whole blood than do normotensive individuals.[20]

These studies suggest that the renin-angiotensin system is somehow involved in the causation of

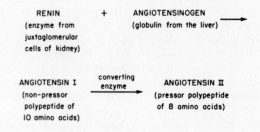

RENIN-ANGIOTENSIN SYSTEM

Fig. 38-3. Major reactions known to take place in the natural production of angiotensin II.

what we call essential hypertension. This aberration of the renin-angiotensin system may be transmitted genetically. It has become clear that if the renin-angiotensin system is involved in the causation of essential hypertension, the mechanism of this involvement is different from that of the hypertension observed in renal vascular disease.

Sympathetic Nervous System

Studies utilizing surgical sympathectomy as the fundamental method of treatment of patients with essential hypertension and more recent studies of patients treated with pharmacologic agents such as guanethidine indicate that reduction of sympathetic nerve activity will reduce arterial blood pressure. The implication of such studies is that the sympathetic nervous system causes essential hypertension. Presently available information indicates the opposite conclusion, however. These results do *not* suggest that presently utilized methods of reduction of sympathetic nerve activity are inappropriate therapy for hypertension.

Studies of vasomotor responses to the upright posture show that hypertensive individuals respond less rapidly to this stimulus than do normotensive subjects.[21] The explanation for this finding might be that the sympathetic nerves of the hypertensive persons were already responding maximally and could not respond more. However, the responses of the catecholamines in the blood were shown by Hickler, Hamlin, and Wells to be normal or low in hypertensive individuals.[22] The 24-hr excretion of catecholamines is less in the patient with essential hypertension than in the normotensive individual.[23] Thus, sympathetic nerve responsiveness as indicated by norepinephrine excretion is in abeyance in the presence of essential hypertension. The more subtle possibility of impaired release of norepinephrine at the nerve endings, with higher concentrations of the material causing excessive end organ response, seems unlikely. The tone of the smooth muscle of the veins is normal in essential hypertension, so that sympathetic nerve activity is not increased here. The responses of veins to infused norepinephrine is normal in the hypertensive subject.[21] This would lead to the unlikely postulate that abnormal release of norepinephrine occurs only on the arterial side of the circulation in essential hypertension.

REFERENCES

1. Wood, J. E., and Battey, L. L.: The Natural History of Diastolic Hypertension and the Effects of Blood Pressure Regulation, *Am. J. Cardiol.,* 9:675, 1962.
2. McKusick, V. A.: Genetics and Nature of Essential Hypertension, *Circulation,* 27:857, 1960.
3. Williamson, D. A. J.: Alport's Syndrome of Hereditary Nephritis with Deafness, *Lancet,* 2:1321, 1961.
4. Smits, M., and Huizinga, J.: Familial Occurrence of Pheochromocytoma, *Acta genet. et statist. med.,* 11:137, 1961.
5. Freis, E. D.: Hemodynamics of Hypertension, *Physiol. Rev.,* 40:27, 1960.
6. Tobian, L.: Relationship of Juxtglomerular Apparatus to Renin and Angiotensin, *Circulation,* 25:189, 1962.
7. Ayman, D.: Heredity in Arteriolar (Essential) Hypertension, *A.M.A. Arch. Int. Med.,* 53:792, 1934.
8. Wolf, S.: Psychosomatic Aspects of Hypertension, *M. Clin. North America,* 45:339, 1961.
9. Oldham, P. D., Pickering, G., Roberts, J. A. F., and Sowry, G. S. C.: Nature of Essential Hypertension, *Lancet,* 1:1085, 1960.
10. Platt, R.: Heredity in Hypertension, *Quart. J. Med.,* 16:111, 1947.
11. Platt, R.: Essential Hypertension: Incidence, Course and Heredity, *Ann. Int. Med.,* 55:1, 1961.
12. Moser, M., Harris, M., Pugatch, D., Ferber, A., and Gordon, B.: Epidemiology of Hypertension. II. Studies of Blood Pressure in Liberia, *Am. J. Cardiol.,* 10:424, 1962.
13. Maddocks, I.: Possible Absence of Essential Hypertension in Two Complete Pacific Island Populations, *Lancet,* 2:396, 1961.
14. Goldblatt, H., Lynch, J., Hanzel, R. F., and Summerville, W. W.: Studies on Experimental Hypertension: I. Production of Persistent Elevation of Systolic Blood Pressure by Means of Renal Ischemia, *J. Exper. Med.,* 59:347, 1934.
15. Hartroft, R. M., and Hartroft, W. S.: Studies on Renal Juxtaglomerular Cells. I. Variations Produced by Sodium Chloride and Deoxycorticosterone Acetate, *J. Exper. Med.,* 97:415, 1953.
16. Tobian, L., Tombonlian, A., and Janecek, J.: The Effect of High Perfusion Pressures on the Granulation of Juxtaglomerular Cells in an Isolated Kidney, *J. Clin. Invest.,* 38:605, 1959.
17. Helmer, O. M., and Judson, W. E.: Presence of Vasoconstrictor and Vasopressor Activity in Renal Vein Plasma of Patients with Arterial Hypertension, *Proc. Council for High Blood Pressure Res.,* American Heart Association, 8, 1960.
18. Morris, R., Langford, H. G., Day, L. H., and Howard, J. E.: In preparation.
19. Wood, J. E.: Genetic Control of Neutralization of Angiotensin and Its Relationship to Essential Hypertension, *Circulation,* 25:225, 1962.
20. Hickler, R. B., Lauler, D. P., and Thorn, G. W.: Plasma Angiotensinase Activity in Patients with Hypertension and Edema, *J. Clin. Invest.,* 42:635, 1963.
21. Wood, J. E.: Peripheral Venous and Arteriolar Responses to Infusions of Angiotensin in Normal and Hypertensive Subjects, *Circulation Res.,* 9:768, 1961.
22. Hickler, R. B., Hamlin, J. T., III, and Wells, R. E.,

Jr.: Plasma Norepinephrine Responses to Tilting in Essential Hypertension, *Circulation,* **20:**422, 1959.

23. Birke, G., Dunér, H., von Euler, U. S., and Plantin, L. O.: Studies on the Adrenocortical, Adreno-medullary and Adrenergic Nerve Activity in Essential Hypertension, *Ztschr. Vitamin- Hormon- u. Fermentforsch.,* 9:41, 1957.

39 PATHOLOGIC SEQUELAE OF SYSTEMIC HYPERTENSION

Robert S. Eliot, M.D., and
Jesse E. Edwards, M.D.

In systemic hypertension, regardless of the cause, initial sites of complication are the myocardium and the systemic arterioles and small arteries. As a result of changes in the arterial vessels, ultimate complications may occur in various organs, particularly the kidneys and the brain. The lungs become affected as a result of changes in the heart, brain, or kidneys. In the following discussion, the complications will be considered according to the anatomic sites at which they occur.

Systemic Arterioles

As systemic hypertension is primarily a vasospastic disease, the arterioles, initially, are histo-

logically normal. The earliest structural change is medial hypertrophy. Later changes include focal hyalinization of the medial layer and intimal fibrous thickening (Fig. 39-1*a*). The latter causes luminal narrowing. In general, there is a relationship between the type of intimal disease and the severity of hypertension. In milder forms of hypertension, the intimal disease is characterized by deposit of relatively acellular connective tissue. In the severe forms of hypertension, especially the rapidly progressive types (malignant hypertension), the intimal thickening is characterized by concentric cellular proliferation (so-called "onion peel" thickening) (Fig. 39-1*b*). Focal necrosis of all layers of the arterial wall occurs in cases of severe hypertension.

Arteriolar changes may occur in all parts of the systemic circulation, including such organs as the myocardium, retina, kidney, pancreas, and brain. The secondary effects of luminal narrowing (and possibly associated vasospasm) may take the form of microinfarcts.

Heart

The primary effect of hypertension upon the heart is concentric hypertrophy of the left ventricle. Also, as hypertension is a factor favoring atherogenesis, coronary atherosclerosis with its own peculiar complications may be observed in the hypertensive subject (Fig. 39-2). The chief complication of hypertension is cardiac failure. This

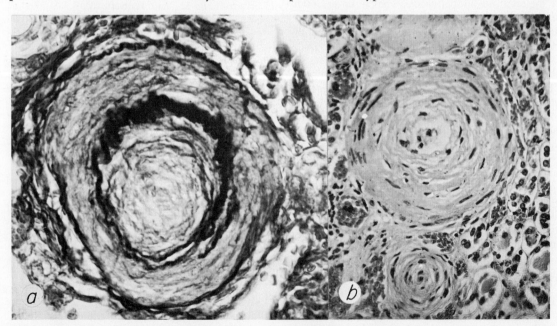

Fig. 39-1. Photomicrographs of a small renal arterial vessel in primary (essential) systemic hypertension. *a.* Medial hypertrophy. Extreme degree of nonspecific intimal thickening causing obliteration of lumen. Elastic tissue stain ($\times$ 450). *b.* A small artery and an arteriole each show concentric intimal fibrous thickening (H & E; $\times$ 250).

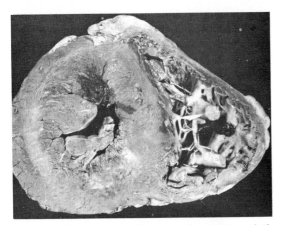

Fig. 39-2. Cross section of ventricular portion of the heart in a hypertensive patient. Left ventricular hypertrophy. Focal myocardial infarcts are also present as signs of the frequent association between hypertension and coronary atherosclerosis.

is attended by left ventricular dilatation. The concomitant elevation of left ventricular diastolic pressure is associated with elevation of pressure in the left atrium (which becomes hypertrophied and dilated) and with pulmonary hypertension. The latter effect of the failing left ventricle is manifested by right ventricular hypertrophy and by structural changes in the pulmonary vascular bed which qualitatively are like those observed in mitral stenosis.

An additional effect of left ventricular failure is the tendency for the development of mural thrombi, particularly in the left atrial appendage and at the apex of the left ventricle. A potential consequence of such thrombi is systemic embolism.

In hypertension, the peripheral manifestations of cardiac failure are like those of right ventricular failure, from any cause. These include hepatic congestion, edema, accumulation of fluid in the serous cavities, ileofemoral venous thrombosis, and pulmonary embolism.

Fibrinous pericarditis occurs uncommonly in those cases of essential hypertension that become complicated by uremia.

Aorta

In hypertensive subjects, cystic medial necrosis of the aorta occurs to a greater degree than in normotensive subjects of comparable age (Fig. 39-3). A consequence of the combined effects of cystic medial necrosis and of hypertension is dissecting aneurysm of the aorta. This lesion may take one of two forms: One is the classic type in which extensive intramural dissection of blood occurs within the aortic wall (Fig. 39-4). The second form, which has received less attention than

the first, is the so-called "incomplete dissecting aneurysm." This lesion is characterized by a tear of the aortic wall like that of the primary tear of classic dissecting aneurysm. The difference between the two conditions is that, in the incomplete variety, no intramural dissection of blood takes place. At the site of the tear, where the aortic wall is consequently weak, a saccular aneurysm may occur. A particular site of predilection for this lesion is the junction of the aortic arch and the descending aorta (Fig. 39-5).

As hypertension stimulates the development of atherosclerosis in the coronary and cerebral arteries, so may it affect the aorta. Aortic atherosclerosis may lead to aneurysm formation, particularly of the abdominal portion. Examples of occlusive thrombosis may occur. Ulceration of aortic atheromas (Fig. 39-6) may lead to widespread embolism of atheromatous material. The latter phenomenon tends to involve small arteries, and because of the disseminated distribution a clinical picture simulating periarteritis nodosa may be obtained.

It is to be emphasized that the atherosclerotic complications in the aorta are not to be confused with the unrelated problem of dissecting aneurysm.

Kidney

The renal complications of hypertension are primarily related to the presence of the small arterial and arteriolar lesions described. These lead to the changes known collectively as nephrosclerosis (Fig. 39-7). As a consequence of chronic focal arterial insufficiency, focal segments of the cortex show structural changes. These are characterized by glomerular hyalinization, by atrophy of associated tubules, and by an increase in surrounding stroma. At the sites of such changes there are depressions of the cortical surface. As the loss of

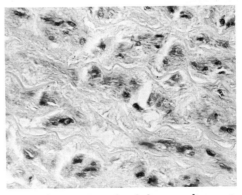

Fig. 39-3. Photomicrograph of the ascending aorta in an example of hypertension with dissecting aneurysm of the aorta. Cystic medial necrosis. (H & E; × 430.)

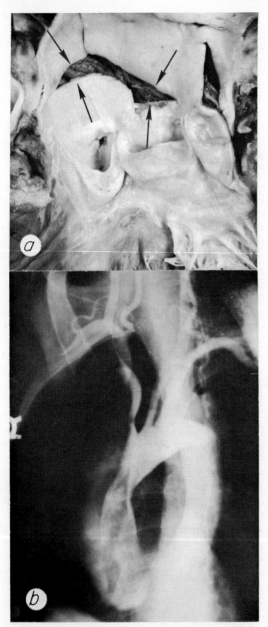

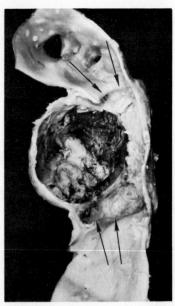

Fig. 39-5. At the junction of the aortic arch and descending aorta is a saccular aneurysm. This is the type of aneurysm that may follow incomplete dissecting aneurysm of the aorta. Sudden interruption in the continuity of the aortic wall is apparent at the arrows.

dilatation of those cortical tubules in zones between atrophic foci occurs. Collections of such tubules bulge above the surface of the kidney and, together with the depressions of atrophy, are responsible for a uniformly granular character of the outer surface of the organ.

Infarction of the kidney may occur as a chance

Fig. 39-4. Classic dissecting aneurysm of the aorta complicating hypertension. *a.* In the ascending aorta is a horizontal tear (between arrows) representing the primary laceration of dissecting aneurysm of the aorta. A typical intramural hematoma extended from this site. *b.* Aortogram in the case shown in *a.* There is distortion of the ascending and descending aorta along with evidence of a false channel in the wall of the vessel. Narrowing of the brachiocephalic artery is also demonstrated.

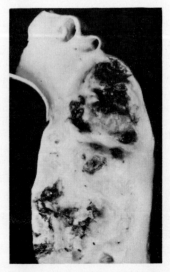

Fig. 39-6. Extensive ulcerative atherosclerosis which occurs in hypertensive patients is demonstrated in this thoracic aorta.

renal substance is of relatively slight order, the kidney of the hypertensive subject is only little reduced in size. If chronic renal failure is present,

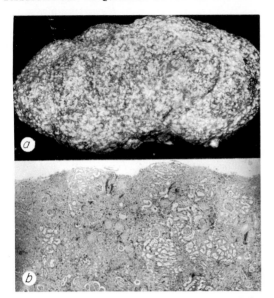

Fig. 39-7. Nephrosclerosis. *a.* Gross specimen of kidney. External view shows fine granularity. Characteristically, the kidney is not greatly reduced in size. *b.* Lower-power photomicrograph showing areas of atrophy of the cortex alternating with zones of relatively intact cortex with dilated tubules.

farction (Fig. 39-8*b*). In other instances, hemorrhage into the substance of the brain appears to be a primary complication. Small but significant hemorrhages involve the substance of the brain stem or cerebellum. Most commonly the primary cerebral hemorrhages are located within the cerebrum, cause extensive destruction of the hemisphere of origin, and frequently rupture into the ventricular septum.

Hypertension is commonly associated with those cases of subarachnoid hemorrhage which result from rupture of a so-called congenital aneurysm of the circle of Willis. In these, the hypertension may have played a role, not only in rupture of the aneurysm, but also in its very development. Classically, rupture of an aneurysm of the circle of Willis is responsible for subarachnoid hemorrhage. If recovery results from such an episode, a subsequent rupture tends to cause hemorrhage into the cerebral substance (Fig. 39-9).

Lung

Pulmonary manifestations are common as late complications in systemic hypertension. Either acute pulmonary edema may occur as a manifestation of left ventricular failure, or it may be a complication either of embolism from intracardiac thrombi or as a manifestation of arterial occlusion from a complicating dissecting aneurysm.

Brain

The cerebral complications of hypertension are numerous and assume a wide variety of appearances.

The simplest changes are of microscopic size and are characterized by perivascular atrophy and/or microinfarction. Gross infarction of the brain occurs commonly in hypertensive subjects (Fig. 39-8*a*). In some instances of cerebral infarction there is clear evidence for the embolism from intracardiac thrombosis or, less commonly, from occlusion of a carotid artery by a dissecting aneurysm. In some cases, in which embolism may be excluded, occlusion of a regional artery by a thrombus developing in an atherosclerotic segment of an artery may be demonstrated. Most often, however, in cerebral infarction no occluded artery is identifiable. It remains to be determined whether, in such circumstances, an organic occlusion or a vasospastic episode is responsible for the ischemia that leads to infarction.

Cerebral hemorrhage may complicate hypertension. This process may assume one of several forms. In some instances (perhaps most commonly) the hemorrhage is secondary within areas of in-

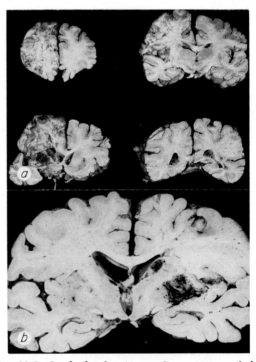

Fig. 39-8. Cerebral infarction. *a.* Cross sections of the brain showing extensive recent infarction of the left hemisphere. *b.* Cross section of a brain showing two areas of discoloration representing infarction with secondary hemorrhage.

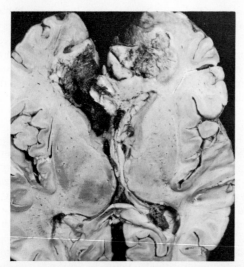

Fig. 39-9. Frontal section of the brain in a patient with a recurrent rupture of an aneurysm of the anterior communicating cerebral artery. As a complication of the second episode of rupture, hemorrhage has extended into each frontal lobe.

phenomenon which stems from the increased intracranial pressure of a cerebral complication.

Pulmonary vascular disease of the type seen in chronic pulmonary venous obstruction may be observed in cases of long-standing left ventricular failure. The various manifestations of pulmonary embolism may be observed as complications of congestive cardiac failure.

If uremia develops, the lungs show signs of this process. These include deposit of hyaline membranes along the surfaces of the alveoli and respiratory bronchioles. Congestion, edema, and bronchopneumonia are common pulmonary findings in uremia.

REFERENCES

1. Castleman, B., and Smithwick, R. H.: The Relation of Vascular Disease to the Hypertensive State. II. The Adequacy of the Renal Biopsy as Determined from a Study of 500 Patients, *New England J. Med.,* **239:**729–732, 1948.
2. Goldblatt, H.: The Renal Origin of Hypertension, *Physiol. Rev.,* **27:**120–165, 1947.
3. Myers, G. B.: Chronic Left Ventricular Dilatation and Hypertrophy, in S. E. Gould, "Pathology of the Heart," 2d ed., Charles C Thomas, Publisher, Springfield, Ill., 1960, p. 999–1001.
4. Koletsky, S.: Role of Salt and Renal Mass in Experimental Hypertension, *A.M.A. Arch. Path.,* **68:** 11–22, 1959.
5. Lynch, R. P., and Edwards, J. E.: Pathologic Aspects of Systemic Hypertension, *Minnesota Med.,* **47:**24–33, 1964.
6. Manlove, F. R.: Retinal and Choroidal Arterioles in Malignant Hypertension: A Clinical and Pathological Study, *A.M.A. Arch. Int. Med.,* **78:**419–440, 1946.
7. Rosenberg, E. F.: The Brain in Malignant Hypertension: A Clinico-pathologic study, *A.M.A. Arch. Int. Med.,* **65:**545–586, 1940.
8. Shennan, T.: Dissecting Aneurysms (Forms No. 193, Spec. Rep. M. Res. Counc., London) H. M. Stat. Off., London, 1934.
9. Smith, D. E., Odel, H. M., and Kernohan, J. W.: Causes of Death in Hypertension, *Am. J. Med.,* **9:** 516–527, 1950.
10. Wagener, H. P., and Keith, N. M.: Diffuse Arteriolar Disease with Hypertension and the Associated Retinal Lesion, *Medicine,* **18:**317–430, 1939.

40 DIAGNOSIS OF HYPERTENSION AND CLUES TO THE CAUSES OF SYSTEMIC HYPERTENSION

Albert N. Brest, M.D., and
John H. Moyer, M.D.

Every patient with hypertension—systolic or diastolic—should have a diagnostic survey to determine the cause of the blood pressure elevation. The ready assumption that diastolic hypertension is essential in origin or that systolic hypertension is due to aortic atherosclerosis is not justified until all other causes have been excluded. Otherwise, potentially correctable lesions will go undetected, and the patient may suffer undue morbidity and mortality.

BLOOD PRESSURE MEASUREMENT

The diagnosis of hypertension per se is made on the basis of the blood pressure reading. Blood pressures lower than 140/90 mm Hg are generally considered normal when found in patients below the age of forty years. Slightly higher systolic and diastolic blood pressures are accepted in older individuals. However, there is less agreement as to the acceptable normal values for elderly subjects. An extensive study of 5,757 apparently healthy individuals between 65 and 106 years of age revealed that after age 65 blood pressure does not show a consistent rise with advancing years as it does below that age.[1] From the findings in this study, it was concluded that blood pressures higher than 160/100 mm Hg should be considered abnormal in elderly male patients whereas levels higher than

170/90 mm Hg are abnormal when found in elderly female subjects. Regardless of age or sex, there is almost universal agreement that diastolic values above 100 mm Hg must be considered abnormal.

In addition to the usual extremity differences, the examiner must also be cognizant of the expected differences between supine and erect blood pressures.[2] Normally, the systolic blood pressure falls and the diastolic pressure tends to rise as the erect position is assumed. However, regardless of position—supine or erect—the blood pressure in the lower extremities is normally higher than that in the upper extremities. The finding of lower blood pressure in the lower extremities, as compared with the upper, suggests aortic coarctation.

Having established that blood pressure elevation exists, it should next be determined whether the hypertension is labile or fixed. This determination is important both from the diagnostic and prognostic standpoints. Labile blood pressure readings may in some cases reflect a prehypertensive state, whereas in others it may represent episodic hypertension such as that associated with pheochromocytoma. Further diagnosis depends upon the clinical history, physical findings, and laboratory studies.

SYSTOLIC HYPERTENSION

Systolic hypertension is a clinical entity which is distinct from that of diastolic blood pressure elevation. It should not be taken for granted that systolic hypertension in an older individual is due necessarily to aortic atherosclerosis, even though this cause is the most frequent. Instead, all other diagnostic considerations should be ruled out by appropriate means.

Various high-output syndromes may be associated with systolic hypertension (see Table 40-1).

Table 40-1. ETIOLOGY OF SYSTOLIC HYPERTENSION

1. High output situations
   a. Anemia
   b. Thyrotoxicosis
   c. Beriberi
   d. Arteriovenous fistula
   e. Idiopathic
2. Increased cardiac stroke volume
   a. Third degree AV heart block
   b. Aortic insufficiency
3. Mechanical
   a. Coarctation of aorta
4. Diminished arterial elasticity
   a. Atherosclerosis

These include anemia, thyrotoxicosis, nutritional deficiency, and arteriovenous fistula. Masked thyro-

toxicosis, in particular, may be overlooked in the older patient, whereas the diagnosis of hyperkinetic heart syndrome should be remembered in the young subject with systolic blood pressure elevation.[3] Clinical situations characterized by increased cardiac stroke volume and accompanying systolic hypertension include complete heart block and aortic regurgitation. Also to be considered in the differential diagnosis, regardless of the age of the patient, is coarctation of the aorta, a mechanical cause for systolic blood pressure elevation.

The diagnosis of systolic hypertension due to aortic atherosclerosis should be made only after all other potential causes for systolic blood pressure elevation have been excluded.

DIASTOLIC HYPERTENSION

As with systolic hypertension, there are numerous known causes for diastolic blood pressure elevation. Responsible lesions can be identified in approximately 10 per cent of the hypertensive population. The most common causes include renal parenchymal and renovascular diseases. Less frequent is hypertension which is adrenal in origin, and the neurogenic types of diastolic hypertension are least common. Differentiation of these disorders is dependent upon the history and physical findings plus appropriate laboratory studies.

CLUES TO THE CAUSES OF SYSTEMIC HYPERTENSION

History and Physical Findings

The age and type of hypertensive onset may provide important clues to the diagnosis of secondary hypertension. Essential hypertension usually becomes manifest after age thirty-five, although it is by no means uncommon for the disease to be initiated earlier. On the other hand, the finding of diastolic blood pressure elevation in younger individuals should heighten the clinical suspicion of secondary hypertension, especially if the hypertension is of moderate or greater severity. Sudden onset of diastolic hypertension in young individuals suggests acute renal parenchymal involvement, e.g., acute glomerulonephritis. In contrast, sudden onset in·middle-aged or older subjects is suggestive of renovascular hypertension. Sudden acceleration of preexistent blood pressure elevation or rapid onset of hypertension with signs and symptoms suggesting renal infarction also infer possible renal arterial occlusive disease.

Although essential hypertension is commonly associated with a positive family history in one or both parents, the absence of a familial background does not negate the diagnosis. Contrariwise, the finding of a positive family history does not exclude secondary blood pressure elevation. Polycystic kidney disease is one of several disorders in which there may be coexisting hypertension and positive family history. Even the familial occurrence of pheochromocytoma has been reported.[4]

The finding of *labile* blood pressure elevation in patients with a strong familial incidence of essential hypertension suggests a so-called prehypertensive state. On the other hand, the occurrence of intermittent hypertension associated with signs and symptoms of catecholamine excess suggests pheochromocytoma. It is noteworthy that symptomatic paroxysms of headache, excessive perspiration, palpitation, nervousness, and/or tremor usually accompany blood pressure elevation in patients with pheochromocytoma, regardless of whether the blood pressure elevation is paroxysmal or sustained.[5]

Hypokalemia-induced muscle weakness may be associated with a host of conditions characterized by coexisting hypertension and hypokalemia.[6] Muscle weakness is particularly prominent in primary aldosteronism. In the latter disorder, the muscle weakness is accompanied typically with nocturnal polyuria and polydipsia, both of which reflect hypokalemia-induced nephrogenic diabetes insipidus.

Pertinent physical findings which have *prognostic* significance include hypertensive alterations in the retina and the finding of cardiomegaly. The fundi usually mirror the degree of accompanying angiospasm and/or arteriolar sclerosis, whereas the finding of left ventricular enlargement suggests that the hypertension has been either severe and/or long-standing. On the other hand, certain physical findings have *diagnostic* value. The existence of a bruit heard in the flanks or anteriorly over the renal vasculature suggests the presence of renal arterial occlusive disease. Postural hypotension may be found as an additional physical finding in patients with renovascular hypertension and in some cases of adrenal hypertension, as well.[7] Palpation of bilateral flank masses in patients with diastolic hypertension suggests polycystic kidney disease, and the absence of femoral pulses infers aortic occlusive disease and possible aortic coarctation. Finally, certain disorders responsible for secondary hypertension (e.g., Cushing's syndrome) may be accompanied by physical findings which are sufficiently characteristic per se to diagnose or at least to suggest strongly the underlying disturbance.

Laboratory Studies

The laboratory investigation of diastolic hypertension can be divided into three categories: routine diagnostic, prognostic, and special diagnostic studies (see Table 40-2). The authors believe that

Table 40-2. DIAGNOSTIC WORKUP FOR PATIENTS WITH DIASTOLIC HYPERTENSION

1. Routine diagnostic studies
   a. Urinalysis
   b. Intravenous pyelogram
   c. Serum potassium
2. Prognostic tests
   a. Electrocardiogram
   b. Chest x-ray
   c. BUN, creatinine
   d. PSP excretion
   e. Urinary concentration
3. Special diagnostic studies
   a. PAH and inulin clearance
   b. Percutaneous renal biopsy
   c. Renal scan
   d. Radiorenogram
   e. Aortography
   f. Differential renal function studies
   g. Histamine or phentolamine test
   h. Catecholamine excretion
   i. Glucocorticoid excretion
   j. Aldosterone (or urinary Na/K excretion)
   k. Retroperitoneal radiography
   l. Skull x-rays, EEG, other cerebral studies

the routine diagnostic tests should be performed in all hypertensive patients. Prognostic studies are employed primarily to provide a measure of the severity and significance of the hypertensive state rather than a diagnostic appraisal. Special diagnostic tests are performed when the history and physical findings and/or routine diagnostic studies suggest the need for further diagnostic evaluation.

Routine Diagnostic Tests

Included in this category are the urinalysis, intravenous pyelogram, and determination of serum potassium level. Each may provide an important diagnostic clue to the underlying hypertensive disorder.

Specific urinary findings may identify or at least suggest the fundamental disorder. For example, red blood cell and white blood cell casts are generally considered pathognomonic of glomerulonephritis and pyelonephritis, respectively. Similarly, an alkaline urine infers the presence of alkalosis, a characteristic finding in primary aldosteronism. On the other hand, proteinuria may occur with either renal hypertension or essential hypertension with accompanying renal functional impairment.

The intravenous pyelogram not infrequently provides an important clue to clinically unsuspected renal disorders.[8] From the hypertensive standpoint, not only is the pelvocalyceal structure important, but also of significance are the comparative lengths of the kidneys as well as the appearance time of dye excretion in the renal pelves.

Difference in the renal lengths of 1.5 cm or more suggests unilateral renal dysfunction. Delayed excretion of dye in one kidney, as compared with its contralateral renal counterpart, also suggests unilateral renal functional impairment. In studying the appearance time and differential excretion of opaque medium by the kidneys during intravenous pyelography, it is important that serial studies be made at 1-min intervals for the first 5 min following rapid injection of contrast medium rather than at the usual 5-min intervals.[9] By this method, minor initial delayed appearance of contrast medium may be detected in an ischemic kidney, whereas this same disparity in renal function may go undetected in the standard 5-, 10-, and 20-min films.

The finding of hypokalemia suggests possible adrenal hypertension, e.g., primary or congenital aldosteronism or Cushing's syndrome. On the other hand, as already mentioned, low serum-potassium levels may be seen with other disorders, as well (see Table 40-3). It is noteworthy, in this regard,

Table 40-3. SYNDROMES CHARACTERIZED BY LOW SERUM POTASSIUM AND HYPERTENSION

1. Primary aldosteronism
2. Congenital aldosteronism
3. Cushing's syndrome
4. Accelerated hypertension with secondary aldosteronism
   a. Renovascular hypertension
   b. Malignant hypertension
5. Potassium-wasting renal parenchymal disease
6. Diuretic-induced hypokalemia in hypertensive patients
7. Pseudo-primary aldosteronism
   a. Chronic licorice ingestion

that a single normal value for serum potassium does not necessarily exclude any of these hypertensive situations.[6]

Prognostic Tests

The electrocardiogram, chest x-ray, and routine renal function studies do not, in general, provide any specific diagnostic clues to the type of diastolic hypertension. On the other hand, they may provide important prognostic indications. Thus the electrocardiogram can indicate whether left ventricular hypertrophy and ischemia are present. Likewise the chest x-ray can confirm the presence of cardiomegaly; however, with the exception of aortic coarctation, in which characteristic aortic and/or rib changes may be found, chest x-ray examination is not helpful in establishing a causal diagnosis. Similarly, routine renal function studies—including blood urea nitrogen (BUN), creatinine, phenolsulfonphthalein (PSP) excretion, and Fishberg's concentration test—can provide information concerning accompanying renal functional impairment, but they are not diagnostic per se.

Special Diagnostic Tests

Additional tests of renal, adrenal, or neurogenic status are indicated when the history and physical findings or the routine diagnostic studies suggest the need for further diagnostic work-up. Also severe unexplained hypertension in the young or malignant hypertension in any age group should be considered further indications for special diagnostic survey studies.

Precise renal function studies (PAH and inulin clearance), percutaneous renal biopsy, and the renal scan may, in some cases, provide definitive clues to hypertensive disorders which are renal parenchymal in origin. For example, the finding of a low filtration fraction* strongly suggests the presence of glomerulonephritis (see Table 40-4). Precise renal hemodynamic measurements may, in fact, be abnormal when routine renal function studies are considered borderline or normal. The renal scintiscanner[10] utilizes mercurial diuretics tagged with Hg^{203}. With the renal scan, the viable renal parenchyma is outlined, and nonviable tissue composed of tumor, cyst, infarction, or atrophy stand out by contrast. Overall, this test appears to have limited application in the diagnosis of hypertension. However,

---

* Filtration fraction =

$$\frac{\text{glomerular filtration rate}}{\text{renal plasma flow}} = \frac{\text{inulin clearance}}{\text{PAH clearance}}$$

Table 40-4. RENAL STUDIES IN A PATIENT WITH DIASTOLIC HYPERTENSION

Pt: C. C.	Age: 19
BUN 21 mg/100 ml	Inulin clearance 67 ml/min (100–125)*
Serum creatinine 1.2 mg/100 ml	PAH clearance 583 ml/min (550–600)*
Urine protein (supine) 0.01 mg/ml	Filtration fraction 0.12 (0.18–0.20)*
Urine protein (walking) 0.75 mg/ml	

* Ranges in parentheses are normal values.

NOTE: Routine renal function studies were not definitive, but the disproportionate reduction in glomerular filtration rate (inulin clearance) and the consequent decrease in filtration fraction strongly suggested glomerular damage in this patient. Percutaneous renal biopsy confirmed the diagnosis of chronic proliferative glomerulonephritis.

in an occasional instance, a specific diagnostic problem, e.g., polycystic kidney disease or renal infarction, may be clarified with the use of this test. Definitive histologic diagnosis of renal parenchymal disease can be established by percutaneous renal biopsy; e.g., the diagnosis of acute proliferative glomerulonephritis or lupus erythematosus may be so established when other diagnostic studies are indefinite.

Renal artery stenosis. is being recognized as an increasingly frequent cause for blood pressure elevation. In addition to the intravenous pyelogram, studies which may be helpful in the diagnosis of renovascular hypertension include radioactive renography, renal arteriography, and differential renal function studies.

The radioactive renogram, utilizing I^{131}-labeled Hippuran, is not a specific diagnostic study, but it does provide a qualitative indication of individual renal functional capacity. Perhaps the chief value of the renogram is the availability of a simultaneous cross-comparison of renal vascular flow. The advantages of this study are as follows: (1) the test is easy to perform, (2) reactions to the test are rare, (3) the study may be completed in 30 min, (4) the test may be repeated several times in a given day, and (5) the cost is reasonable. Many investigators believe that the renogram is superior to the excretory pyelogram for screening hypertensive patients. Morris and DeBakey report that 90 per cent of their patients with proved renovascular hypertension had abnormal renograms,[11] and Hunt found the renogram to be distinctly abnormal in 36 of 37 patients with renovascular hypertension[12] Stewart and Haynie found the renogram to be highly reliable in diagnosing unilateral main artery occlusion but less accurate in the diagnosis of bilateral renal artery occlusion.[13] Whereas positive renograms and excretory pyelograms do not always coincide in the same patient, a combination of the two may identify a renal artery lesion in a larger number of cases than either study used alone.[14]

The definitive diagnosis of unilateral or bilateral renal vascular disease ultimately depends upon renal arteriography. Either translumbar or percutaneous transfemoral and transbrachial arteriography is satisfactory. Although numerous complications of aortography have been described, increasing experiences have indicated that this diagnostic procedure may be consistently performed without fatality or serious complication.[14] It must be recognized that renal arteriography serves only to delineate an anatomic lesion in the renal arteries. Whether or not an occlusive lesion is responsible for the hypertension depends on a correlation of the arteriographic findings with the clinical situation and the data obtained from other diagnostic procedures. In fact, Eyler et al. found that a large number of patients with stenotic lesions of the renal arteries were normotensive.[15] Where it is uncertain whether a lesion is responsible for the patient's hypertension, differential renal function studies should be performed.

The application of differential renal function tests in the diagnosis of renal ischemia is based upon the experimental work of White.[16] He found that constriction of a renal artery in the dog led to marked reduction in the volume and sodium concentration of urine obtained from the involved kidney as compared with urine collected simultaneously from the contralateral kidney. Based on these findings, Howard et al. proposed that a 50 per cent or greater decrease in volume excreted and a 15 per cent or greater decrease in sodium concentration indicated renal artery obstruction and reversible renovascular hypertension.[17] These criteria have proved reliable but too restrictive. Subsequently, Howard and coworkers modified their indications of a "positive" test by the addition of creatinine clearance to the study.[18] An increase in the urine creatinine concentration is felt to be confirmatory evidence of greater water reabsorption as a cause of the decreased volume from the suspected kidney. Modifications of the differential renal function study have been described by Stamey,[19] Birchall et al.,[20] and Rapaport.[21] The practical differences in the results obtained with these methods have been small.

The clinical suspicion of pheochromocytoma should be tested by specific pharmacologic and chemical studies (see Chap. 43).

Adrenal lesions other than pheochromocytoma which may be responsible for diastolic hypertension include Cushing's syndrome and hyperaldosteronism. Cushing's syndrome can be diagnosed by demonstrating an excessive secretion of glucocorticoid hormone. Elevated plasma and/or urine levels of 17-hydroxycorticoid at a time when the patient is not under acute exogenous stress strongly favors the diagnosis. The diagnosis of hyperaldosteronism is made by demonstrating excess secretion of aldosterone. This can be done most accurately by calculation of aldosterone secretion following administration of radioactive aldosterone. Excessive secretion of aldosterone may also be reflected by its physiologic effects. This is best demonstrated by placing the subject on a liberal salt intake and finding high levels of urinary potassium in the presence of abnormally low serum-potassium concentrations. Urinary aldosterone may also be measured but is less definitive, since it accounts for only a small percentage of that secreted.

Retroperitoneal radiography is extremely valuable in the identification of adrenal masses or retroperitoneal tumors which may be responsible for diastolic hypertension. The techniques for performing retroperitoneal pneumography are relatively simple, but interpretation of the results may be quite difficult. Graham's extensive review of the published case reports of pheochromocytoma indicates that the presacral air study gave positive information in only about 50 per cent of unselected cases.[22] It is noteworthy, however, that failure to demonstrate a tumor by retroperitoneal pneumography does not rule out the possibility of demonstration by aortography.[23] The converse of this is also true; i.e., failure to show a tumor by vascular opacification does not mean that such a lesion may not be outlined with gas. Pneumographic and angiographic studies of the abdomen are, in fact, complementary procedures and should be so employed.

Finally, neurogenic lesions including brain tumor, cerebrovascular accident, and diencephalic syndrome may, at times, be responsible for diastolic hypertension. Their presence is generally suspected from the history and/or physical findings. Skull x-rays, electroencephalogram, brain scan, pneumoencephalogram, and/or cerebral angiography may be employed to confirm or deny the presence of these lesions.

In summary, diagnostic surveys should be performed in all patients with blood pressure elevation. Both systolic and diastolic hypertension should be studied until their origins are firmly established. Only in this way will all potentially correctable hypertensive lesions be detected, and only in this manner can an intelligent therapeutic approach be followed.

REFERENCES

1. Master, A. M., and Lasser, R. P.: Blood Pressure Elevation in the Elderly Patient, in "Hypertension: Recent Advances: Second Hahnemann Symposium on Hypertensive Disease," Lea & Febiger, Philadelphia, 1961, p. 24.

2. Burch, G. E., and DePasquale, N. P.: "Primer of Clinical Measurement of Blood Pressure," The C. V. Mosby Company, St. Louis, 1962.

3. Gorlin, R.: The Hyperkinetic Heart Syndrome, J.A.M.A., **182**:823, 1962.

4. Carman, C. T., and Brashear, R. E.: Pheochromocytoma as an Inherited Abnormality, *New England J. Med.*, **263**:419, 1960.

5. Gifford, R. W., Kvale, W. F., Maher, F. T., Roth, G. M., and Priestley, J. T.: Clinical Experiences with Pheochromocytoma: A Review of 71 Cases, in "Hypertension: Recent Advances: Second Hahnemann Symposium on Hypertensive Disease," Lea & Febiger, Philadelphia, 1961, p. 586.

6. Conn, J. W.: Aldosteronism in Man, *J.A.M.A.*, **183**: 169, 1963.

7. Kinsey, D., Whitelaw, G. P., and Smithwick, R. H.: A Screening Test for Adrenal or Unilateral Renal Forms of Hypertension Based upon Postural Change in Blood Pressure, *Angiology*, **11**:336, 1960.

8. Brest, A. N., Hieder, C., and Moyer, J. H.: Diagnosis of Renal Hypertension: Medical Aspects, *J.A.M.A.*, **178**:718, 1961.

9. Maxwell, M. H., and Prozan, G. B.: Renovascular Hypertension, *Prog. Cardiovas. Dis.*, **5**:81, 1962.

10. Sklaroff, D. M.: Photoscanning of Kidney in Hypertension, *Geriatrics*, **17**:423, 1962.

11. Morris, G. C., and DeBakey, M. E.: Diagnosis of Renal Vascular Disease, *Am. J. Cardiol.*, **9**:756, 1962.

12. Hunt, J. C.: Clinical Aspects: Symposium on Hypertension Associated with Renal Disease, *Proc. Staff Meet. Mayo Clin.*, **36**:707, 1961.

13. Stewart, B. H., and Haynie, T. P.: Critical Appraisal of the Renogram in Renal Vascular Disease, *J.A.M.A.*, **180**:454, 1962.

14. Dennis, J. M., Wolfel, D. A., and Young, J. D.: Diagnosis of Renovascular Hypertension: Role of the Radiologist, *Radiol. Clin. North America.*, **1**:61, 1963.

15. Eyler, W. R., Clark, M. D., Garman, J. E., Rian, R. L., and Meininger, D. E.: Angiography of the Renal Areas Including a Comparative Study of Renal Arterial Stenosis in Patients with and without Hypertension, *Radiology*, **78**:879, 1962.

16. White, H. L.: Excretion of Sodium in Relation to Glomerular Filtration, *Tr. Second Conf. on Renal Function*, Josiah Macy, Jr., Foundation, New York, 1950, p. 127.

17. Connor, T. B., Berthrong, M., Thomas, W. C., and Howard, J. E.: Hypertension Due to Unilateral Renal Disease: With a Report on a Functional Test Helpful in Diagnosis, *Bull. Johns Hopkins Hosp.*, **100**:241, 1957.

18. Howard, J. E., and Connor, T. B.: Hypertension Produced by Unilateral Renal Disease, *Arch. Int. Med.*, **100**:62, 1962.

19. Stamey, T. A.: The Diagnosis of Curable Unilateral Renal Hypertension by Ureteral Catheterization, Postgrad. Med., 29:496, 1961.

20. Birchall, R., Batson, H. M., Jr., and Brannan, W.: Contribution of Differential Renal Studies to the Diagnosis of Renal Arterial Hypertension with Emphasis on the Value of $\dfrac{\text{U sodium}}{\text{U creatinine}}$, *Am. J. Med.*, **32**:164, 1962.

21. Rapaport, A.: Modification of the "Howard Test" for the Detection of Renal Artery Obstruction, *New England J. Med.*, **263**:1159, 1960.

22. Graham, J. B.: Pheochromocytoma and Hypertension: An Analysis of 207 Cases, *Internat. Abstr. Surg.*, **92**:105, 1951.

23. Pendergrass, H. P.: Retroperitoneal Radiography: Roentgen Techniques to Demonstrate Pheochromocytomas and Other Retroperitoneal Masses, *Radiol. Clin. North America,* 1:195, 1963.

41 PARENCHYMAL RENAL DISEASES AND THE CIRCULATION

Elbert P. Tuttle, Jr., M.D.

The function of the kidney as an endocrine and an excretory organ in the regulation of blood pressure is indicated in Fig. 37-1. The specific effects of the individual diseases of the kidney on the circulation are conditioned by the precise nature of the disturbances of its function.

Pyelonephritis

Although there is considerable agreement that hypertension and pyelonephritis have a high coincidence in man,[1] it is not clear whether pyelonephritis causes hypertension or hypertension predisposes to pyelonephritis. The situation is clouded by the fact that diagnostic criteria for pyelonephritis are poorly defined. Sterile vascular[2] and obstructive lesions[3] can produce in the kidney anatomic evidence of scarring, tubular dilatation, and inflammation, which are taken by many to be diagnostic of pyelonephritis. Until the definite diagnosis of pyelonephritis is restricted to cases in which bacteria can be proved to be present in the kidney or to

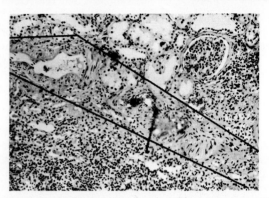

Fig. 41-2. Pyelonephritic scar, near the edge of which can be seen a tortuous arteriole twisting in and out of the plane of section.

have been present in the past, the specificity of the diagnosis will be low, and misinterpretation of clinicopathologic correlations will occur.

Several important phenomena occur in pyelonephritis which may exert strong influence on the circulation: (1) focal scarring of the kidney leads to perivascular fibrosis and distortion of blood vessels; (2) the mass of renal tissue is reduced in chronic pyelonephritis; (3) the kidney of pyelonephritis becomes incapable of maximum sodium conservation or excretion.

The vascular lesion in pyelonephritis is illustrated in studies from the author's laboratory. Figure 41-1 illustrates the proliferation of bacteria, highlighted by staining with specific fluorescent antibodies, in the immediate perivascular area of the kidney. Figure 41-2 shows the edge of a focal pyelonephritic scar in the upper pole of a nephrectomy specimen. The tortuosity of blood vessels in this scarred area is illustrated by the repeated appearance of the medium-sized artery in the plane of the section. Figure 41-3*B* shows a selective renal arteriogram of the same kidney. The tortuous, angulated vessels may be compared with a normal vascular pattern shown in Fig. 41-3*A*.

The possibility that renal ischemia due to renal vascular damage in pyelonephritis may produce hypertension is supported by the reports of relief of hypertension following nephrectomy where unilateral disease was present.[4] The extension of this concept to account for the relationship of pyelonephritis to hypertension has been made most effectively by Kincaid-Smith.[5]

The demonstration of a potent blood pressure-depressing substance from the kidney by several groups[6,7] raises the possibility that loss of renal mass, sufficient, for instance, to produce the anemia of erythropoietin deficiency, would suffice to reduce the blood pressure–lowering action of the kidney significantly. Experimental support for the hypothe-

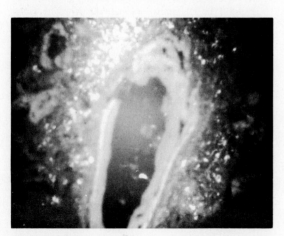

Fig. 41-1. Light spots in the vicinity of the blood vessel are *Escherichia coli* stained by specific antibody labeled with fluorescein.

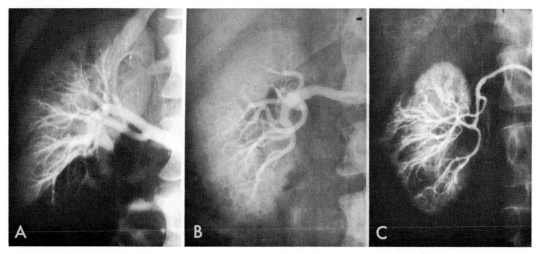

Fig. 41-3. *A.* Normal renal arteriogram. *B.* Arteriogram (from the patient in Fig. 4-2) in acute and chronic pyelonephritis. Note the tortuosity of vessels compared to normal. *C.* Late chronic pyelonephritis. Note the shrunken kidney, atrophy of tissue, and dense crowding of atrophic vessels. (*Photographs courtesy of Dr. Richard S. Foster.*)

sis of renoprival hypertension in animals has been referred to in Chap. 37. Hypertension may thus ensue from lack of an antagonist. The blood pressure–lowering effect of renal transplantation in nephrectomized patients maintained by chronic dialysis supports the hypothesis that this mechanism is physiologically significant in man.[8] Prevention of experimental renoprival hypertension in the dog by implantation of nonexcretory renal tissue in the peritoneum has been demonstrated,[9] but this has not been demonstrated in hypertension with pyelonephritis in man. The vascular pattern in chronic pyelonephritis, with great loss of tissue relative to blood vessel volume, is shown in Fig. 41-3*C*, a selective renal arteriogram in a patient with long-standing disease, hypertension, and azotemia.

One reason for the variability of hypertension in pyelonephritis is the varying state of sodium balance in the disease. In some instances pyelonephritis is a salt-wasting disease and creates a degree of sodium depletion which can mask a marked tendency to hypertension. In many patients with severe chronic pyelonephritis this is achieved deliberately or inadvertently with rigorous restriction of dietary sodium. Conversely many patients with severe pyelonephritis cannot readily excrete large loads of salt. They can be made hypertensive on high sodium intakes. A single patient may be manipulated from one extreme to the other. This unsual sensitivity of the blood pressure to sodium intake in pyelonephritis undoubtedly obscures the relationship of pyelonephritis and hypertension. It is the author's impression that the underlying tendency toward hypertension is present in severe chronic pyelonephritis, in part from vascular dis-

ease, in part from loss of protective renal excretory and secretory mass.

A corollary of these considerations is the action of the pyelonephritic kidney in congestive heart failure. Impairment of maximum sodium conservation in the pyelonephritic kidney constitutes a built-in diuretic which can deplete the patient of salt as required, with careful control of sodium intake. The same may be said of the inability to conserve water in the isosthenuric stage. The impaired ability to manufacture ammonia makes acidifying agents more potent diuretics in many pyelonephritics, but the risk of inducing severe metabolic acidosis is correspondingly increased.

In cardiac patients it is mandatory to endeavor to differentiate between the azotemia resulting from the impaired renal perfusion in severe heart failure or vascular disease and the azotemia from destruction of functioning nephrons by intrinsic renal disease. Toxic effects or overdosage of pharmacologic agents are much more likely in the presence of intrinsic renal disease. Renal concentrating ability, kidney size, excretion of radiographic contrast materials, the power to acidify the urine, sodium excretion on minimum intake, abnormalities of the urine sediment are the clinical tools which aid in this differentiation.

Glomerulonephritis

Acute glomerulonephritis imposes special burdens on the heart and blood vessels. In combination, the water and sodium retention, the attendant increase of circulating blood volume,[10] the dilutional anemia, the increased peripheral resistance, and frequently a high cardiac output[11] increase both pressure work and flow work of the heart to produce a total load which leads to congestive heart failure. With a state of ventricular overload in the absence of hypertrophy and under the biochemical handicap of anemic blood the heart is unable to maintain its compensation.

As has been pointed out in Chap. 37, present evidence suggests that humoral and neurogenic stimuli are active in an integrated response to the renal lesion in acute glomerulonephritis with no evidence of any negative feedback to protect the circulation. A superficially similar situation exists with bilateral renal artery stenosis and with malignant hypertension. Fortunately, in acute glomerulonephritis, except when renal shutdown supervenes, the physiologic derangements are quite sensitive to therapy. Antihypertensive drugs and sodium depletion are dramatically effective.

The circulatory effects of chronic glomerulonephritis depend upon the stage of the disease. In the early or "latent" stages of the chronic disease the circulation is usually normal. In the nephrotic phase of chronic glomerulonephritis, the blood pressure is still often normal, and the edema and abnormalities of electrolyte metabolism result from the abnormal handling of protein, not from heart failure. Late in the course of the disease, though the abnormal permeability of glomerular capillaries to protein often persists, severe reduction of glomerular filtration minimizes albumin loss, and the nephrotic syndrome disappears. Either because of vascular disease or loss of renal mass, or in part because of reconstitution of the intravascular oncotic material, at this stage of the disease hypertension appears or becomes more severe. In the late stages of glomerulonephritis severe hypertension is a major problem. The relative contributions of renal ischemia and of loss of renal vasodepressor function are obscure. Bilateral nephrectomy, followed by chronic dialysis, has resulted in reduction in hypertension in some patients with chronic glomerulonephritis, but they have remained hypertensive until successful transplantation is accomplished.[8]

In chronic renal insufficiency it is possible to utilize cardiovascular reserve to improve renal function by loading patients with sodium, increasing renal perfusion flows and pressures. Limits are imposed by the ability of the heart and blood vessels to tolerate the added work load.

Conversely, renal reserve is frequently encroached upon to relieve the symptoms of congestive heart failure. In severe heart failure diuresis sufficient to relieve pulmonary edema may reduce cardiac output to a point where glomerular filtration rate falls. In these circumstances azotemia may result from, or increase with, the diuretic treatment

of heart failure, but if renal reserve is adequate, it will not be of severe degree. In heart failure with severe renal disease, as in malignant hypertension or that seen in terminal glomerulonephritis, sodium depletion and antihypertensive therapy may induce renal insufficiency incompatible with survival.

A number of less frequent types of renal disease affect the circulation in a manner similar to the renal diseases already mentioned. Disseminated lupus erythematosus, diabetic nephropathy, and pseudoxanthoma elasticum behave in a physiologic manner similar to acute, subacute, or chronic glomerulonephritis. Polycystic renal disease, renal tubular acidosis, and renal injury from analgesic abuse behave like chronic pyelonephritis.

Disease may affect both the excretory and the endocrine functions of the kidney. The intimate effect of both types of function in the circulation make necessary specific measurements of physiologic function to evaluate precisely the effect of kidney disease on the general circulation. Of particular importance in the coming years will be assays of renal vein concentrations of pressor and depressor substances in the various diseases of the kidney.

REFERENCES

1. Brod, J.: Chronic Pyelonephritis, in D. A. K. Black, "Renal Disease," F. A. Davis Company, Philadelphia, 1962, p. 293.
2. Allen, A. C.: "The Kidney," 2nd ed., Grune & Stratton, Inc., New York, 1962, pp. 627–628.
3. Freedman, L. R., Warner, A. S., Beck, D., and Paplanus, S.: Experimental Pyelonephritis. IX. The Bacteriological Course and Morphological Consequences of Staphylococcal Pyelonephritis in the Rat, with Consideration of the Specificity of the Pathological Changes Observed, *Yale J. Biol. & Med,*. **34**:40, 1961.
4. Butler, A. M.: Chronic Pyelonephritis and Arterial Hypertension, *J. Clin. Invest.*, **16**:889, 1937.
5. Kincaid-Smith, P.: Vascular Obstruction in Chronic Pyelonephritic Kidneys and Its Relation to Hypertension, *Lancet*, **2**:1263, 1955.
6. Booth, E., Hinman, J. W., Daniels, E. G., Kosinski, M., and Muirhead, E. E.: Antihypertensive Renal Factor, *J. Clin. Invest.*, **42**:918, 1963 (Abstract).
7. Hickler, R. B., Saravis, C. A. Mowbray, J. F., Lauler, D. P., Vagnucci, A. I., and Thorn, G. W.: Renomedullary Vasodepressor Factor, *J. Clin. Invest.*, **42**:942, 1963 (Abstract).
8. Kolff, W. J., Nakamoto, S., Poutasse, E. F., Straffon, R. A., Figueroa, J. E.: The Effect of Bilateral Nephrectomy and Transplantation on Hypertension in Man, *Circulation*, **30**:23 (suppl. 2) 1964.
9. Muirhead, E. E., Stirman, J. A., and Jones, F.: Renal Autoexplantation and Protection against Re-

noprival Hypertensive Cardiovascular Disease and Hemolysis, *J. Clin. Invest.*, **29**:266, 1960.

10. Eisenberg, S.: Blood Volume in Patients with Acute Glomerulonephritis, *Am. J. Med.*, **27**:241, 1959.

11. De Fazio, V., Christensen, R. C., Regan, T. J., Baer, L. J., Morita, Y., and Hellems, H. K.: Circulatory Changes in Acute Glomerulonephritis, *Circulation*, **20**:190, 1959.

42 UNILATERAL RENAL DISEASE

William C. Waters III, M.D.

Suspicions of a relationship between the kidneys and the systemic arterial blood pressure had been raised by clinical observers as early as the era of Bright, but it has been only in recent years that clinical understanding has progressed to the practical level. Although attempts to document this connection had been made at the turn of the century, it was not until 1934 that the experiments of Goldblatt et al.[1] provided the impetus for what has in recent years become one of the most popular subjects for clinical investigation. Not only has the demonstration of a mechanism for production of hypertension by interference with the arterial supply to one or both kidneys provided a stimulating new concept in pathophysiologic terms; for the clinically oriented investigator it has added a new and reversible cause for a disease process which had traditionally evaded therapeutic efforts. Subsequent research, plagued though it has been by the erratic consequences of varying methodology, has been active and, in sum, highly productive.

Mechanism of Renal Hypertension

Goldblatt's silver clamp, applied to one of the renal arteries of a dog, resulted in blood pressure elevation which appeared within a few days, reached its peak in a week, but usually did not persist indefinitely unless the opposite kidney was removed or its arterial supply compromised; in the rat, the unilateral constriction was sufficient for permanent hypertension.[2] In most species,[3] including man, relief of the one-sided obstruction is often followed by a dramatic disappearance of the hypertension. Although the normal contralateral kidney is subject to the same changes of arteriolar nephrosclerosis seen in spontaneously occurring hypertension, the ischemic kidney appears to be protected[4] from the effects of the elevated blood pressure, much in the same way that the vasculature throughout the body does not suffer hypertensive damage

when hydralazine hydrochloride is used to control mean pressure during such experiments.[5]

The precise sequence whereby interference with renal arterial supply leads to systemic hypertension has not been adequately defined. Reduction in *blood flow* alone seems an insufficient explanation, since the initial fall in perfusion of the affected kidney is soon followed by a return to normal of renal blood flow after hypertension becomes established.[6,7] Likewise, *anoxia* in the renal circulation does not lead to hypertension.[8,9] It has been proposed that a fall in the *blood pressure* distal to the point of obstruction may constitute the stimulus, since wide gradients have been observed in patients at the time of surgical treatment,[10] but a number of experimental studies suggest that hypertension may be produced and sustained even while the tension in the distal renal artery is at control levels.[11,12] More attention has been focused in recent years upon the drop in *pulse pressure* produced by narrowing of the arterial lumen, and the elaboration of pressor substances by the kidney under such conditions.[13,14] The methodology of assay of these substances has, however, been questioned,[14] and others[15] have found that pulse-pressure variation is not critical in the production of hypertension in dogs with renal arterial constriction. Such contradictory results suggest that inadequacies of technique have been the limiting factor in a clear delineation of the pathogenesis of renovascular hypertension; certainly hemodynamic changes, however difficult to measure, must eventually be found to constitute the prime stimulus.

In any event, after interference with the renal vascular supply, physiologic changes take place in the kidney which lead to systemic arterial hypertension, and much evidence indicates that this mechanism is a humoral one. Denervation or removal of the kidney to a remote site in the circulation does not interfere with production of renovascular hypertension;[16,17] on the other hand, interruption of renal venous drainage prevents it.[18] Similarly, as early as 1898, it was demonstrated that when renal cortical extracts with the physical characteristics of protein were injected, they were capable of inducing systemic hypertension.[19] Later work has indicated that extracts of the venous blood from kidneys with arterial constriction have a greater hypertensive effect than blood draining normal kidneys.[20,21] It has been further demonstrated that certain renal extracts (renin) exhibit the biochemical properties of a catalyst,[20,21] with the capacity to accelerate the conversion of a plasma factor to the potent physiologic pressor amine angiotensin. Refinements of investigative approach have now rather clearly elucidated the production of this pressor agent:[22]

Plasma alpha$_2$-globulin $\xrightarrow{\text{renin}}$ angiotensin I (a decapeptide, inactive) $\xrightarrow[\text{enzyme}]{\text{converting}}$ angiotensin II (an octapeptide, highly active vasopressor)

The structure of angiotensin II is now known, and it has been synthesized.[23]

Demonstration of this mechanism has thus posed an attractive hypothesis to explain human renal hypertension and its relief by removal of the offending kidney or repair of the defective arterial supply. The role of this sequence in clinical hypertension is supported by the finding of pressor activity in blood from the systemic circulation or renal vein of animals[22,24] with experimental renal vascular lesions and in renal venous blood from the affected kidney (but not the normal kidney) of patients with renovascular hypertension.[25-27] Further, administration of hog renin in serial doses to dogs with renovascular hypertension results in a rising titer of antirenin and a progressive decline of the blood pressure toward normal.[28]

However attractive this explanation may be, considerable evidence is mounting to suggest that the renin-angiotensin mechanism is not alone responsible for chronic renal hypertension. Dogs with renovascular hypertension often do not maintain their hypertensive levels;[1] experimental animals with chronic renal arterial constriction[29,30] and patients with chronic renovascular hypertension[30,31] exhibit no increase in the renin-angiotensin activity as measured by current techniques. Doubt is cast upon the evidence accumulated through the use of hog renin by the argument that the substance is impure and rabbits do not exhibit the antihypertensive response to serial renin injections.[32] Furthermore, tachyphylaxis to renin occurs in many species;[29,32,33] rabbits with renovascular hypertension do respond initially to renin, and after developing tachyphylaxis, they return to the previous *elevated* pressure rather than to normotensive levels.[32] When renin tachyphylaxis has occurred, angiotensin II is no longer effective.[34] While it appears certain, then, that the renin-angiotensin system participates in the production of experimental and human renovascular hypertension, there is reason to doubt that this mechanism is solely responsible for the sustained blood pressure elevation that ensues. Indeed, the variable clinical results obtained after nephrectomy or vascular repair are consistent with this observation.

An important additional humoral mechanism in the sustained hypertension of renal vascular disease has been brought to light in recent years by the elucidation of what may be referred to as the *renin-angiotensin-aldosterone axis*. A role of renal humoral influences in the regulation of aldosterone production had been suspected since the observation was made that renin administered to rats resulted in hypertrophy of the zona glomerulosa of the adrenal cortex.[35] Subsequently, it has been shown that the customary stimuli for aldosterone secretion (such as inferior vena cava ligation or phlebotomy) are ineffective in the nephrectomized animal.[36,37] Most convincing of all is the observation that administration of renin, renal extract, or angiotensin II causes an increased aldosterone excretion in animals which have previously been hypophysectomized and nephrectomized;[36,37] human subjects respond to angiotensin injection with a striking increase in aldosterone production.[38,39] On the other hand, patients with renal hypertension may[40] or may not[41-43] show increased aldosterone secretion rate; experimental animals tend to exhibit accelerated aldosterone production only when their hypertensive disease is in a malignant phase.[36]

Recent work has brought to light interesting evidence implicating angiotensin in the pathogenesis of essential hypertension. Wolf et al. showed an increased half-life of angiotensin II and increased exchangeable angiotensin in essential hypertension.[44] Wood found a decreased angiotensin in activation rate in patients and relatives of patients with essential hypertension.[45]

Of great academic as well as clinical interest has been the finding by many observers of the antihypertensive action of the kidney.[46,47] Renoprival hypertension develops when bilateral nephrectomy is performed in experimental animals and is corrected by retransplantation; transplantation of a normal kidney to an animal with renovascular hypertension results in improvement of the blood pressure level. The apparently highly important effect of the normal kidney in regulating blood pressure has been most dramatically demonstrated by the variably antihypertensive effect of renal venous blood draining a kidney which is perfused with blood passing through a cannula at different pressures.[48] In this series of experiments, the blood pressure–lowering effect of the kidney was more or less quantitatively related to the height of the perfusing arterial pressure.

Human Hypertension and Unilateral Renal Disease

If constriction of the renal artery or of the kidney itself produces hypertension in experimental animals, it is to be expected that a variety of spontaneously occurring diseases of the kidney will cause blood pressure elevation in man. When the disease is unilateral, the possibility of surgical cure is present, and an impressive number of clinical examples have accumulated. Table 42-1 presents

Table 42-1. CAUSES OF REVERSIBLE HYPERTENSION DUE
TO UNILATERAL RENAL DISEASE

I. Intrinsic unilateral renal disease
   A. Congenital hypoplastic kidney[49]
   B. Pyelonephritis
      1. Pyogenic[50-52]
      2. Tuberculous[53]
   C. Irradiation[54]
   D. Trauma[49]
   E. Renal neoplasm[55]
   F. Unilateral renal vein thrombosis[56]
   G. Obstructive uropathy[57]

II. Renal artery lesions
   A. Intrinsic
      1. Atherosclerotic plaque[58,70]
      2. Thrombosis or embolism[58]
      3. Fibromuscular hyperplasia[58]
      4. Renal artery aneurysm[59]
      5. Other: thromboangiitis obliterans,[60] periarteritis,[61] syphilitic arteritis[62]
   B. Extrinsic compression
      1. Tumor involving renal pedicle[63]
      2. Retroperitoneal fibrosis[64]

those lesions in which favorable results have at times been obtained.

Incidence and Clinical Features

As with any entity under active investigation, the real incidence of curable hypertension due to unilateral renal disease is unknown. Present evidence would suggest that less than 1 per cent of all individuals in the hypertensive population, after thorough diagnostic study, have sufficient findings to warrant nephrectomy or vascular repair. Of this group, only 25 per cent have an unequivocal cure (blood pressure lower than 140/90 for longer than 1 year), and an additional 25 to 35 per cent show definite improvement.[57,65-70]

Clinical suspicion of unilateral renal origin for hypertension may be aroused by a history or findings of the underlying process, such as pyelonephritis or ureteral obstruction (see Table 42-1), but very often such patients are asymptomatic. In the group with renal vascular hypertension, cases reported to date are beginning to suggest a pattern.[57,65-73] Most have been male (possibly 3:1), and a surprising proportion of these patients have reported a recent episode of trauma to the renal area or a spontaneously occurring bout of flank pain. Albuminuria is usual, though not invariable, and bruits, usually confined to systole, may be noted over the anterior abdomen on the affected side. It is the opinion of some observers, including the author, that renovascular hypertension, like that with pheochromocytoma, often exhibits orthostatic variation. The finding of a fall in diastolic blood

pressure of 20 mm or more may thus provide a clinical clue to the presence of "humoral hypertension." Unlike essential hypertension, in which the blood pressure elevation is *usually* benign, and unlike primary aldosteronism, in which it is *almost invariably* benign,[74] renal hypertension may produce malignant grades of hypertensive vascular disease. Indeed, those patients who have exhibited a good response to surgical treatment have in general presented with quite high blood pressure of recent onset, frequently with retinopathy.[75] Whether the selection of such patients has been partially artificial and stimulated by the urgency of their condition or whether malignant progression is in fact characteristic of renovascular hypertension remains to be determined by further experience. Certainly benign hypertension has also responded to surgical intervention, even after intervals of many years since appearance of the elevated blood pressure.[69,76]

Diagnosis

Clinical Criteria

Because of the relative rarity of unilateral renal disease as a cause of hypertension and because of the expense and morbidity associated with definitive investigation, attempts have been made to establish criteria for the selection of hypertensive patients for further study.[67,69,77,78] Most authorities agree that one or more of the following findings warrants a search for curable causation: absence of family history of hypertension; onset before age thirty or after fifty; abrupt appearance of hypertension or acceleration of previously benign hypertension; failure of adequate response to medical therapy of significant hypertension; abdominal bruit; unexplained flank pain; trauma to a kidney; and radiographic evidence of asymmetry of renal outlines, particularly if progressive decrease in renal size has been demonstrated on serial x-ray films.

Ancillary Studies

The advisability of prior selection is made more evident when one considers the fact that no one diagnostic procedure is final in predicting surgical cure; this fact is indicated further by the multiplicity of methods which have been employed. Among the means which have gained clinical acceptance are the plain abdominal film, intravenous urography, radioactive scanning procedures, aortography, and direct differential studies of ureteral urine.

These techniques are discussed below. Recently, an additional technique has been described, the angiotensin infusion test,[79] in which patients with renovascular hypertension exhibit relative insensi-

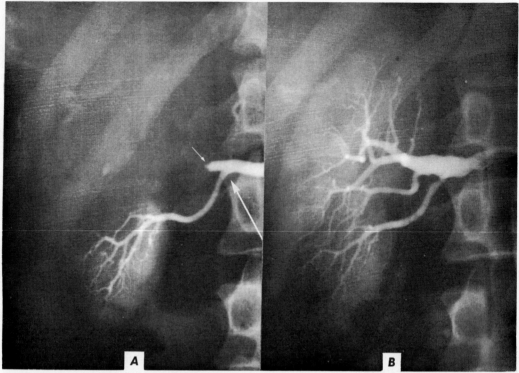

Fig. 42-1. *A.* Selective renal angiography in a man with hypertension demonstrates occlusion of the right main renal artery trunk beyond the point of its first branch. Only the lower renal pole is vascularized. *B.* After surgical repair good opacification of the renal vasculature is obtained. (*R. S. Foster, W. H. Shuford, C. Reiser, E. P. Tuttle, Jr., and M. J. Deitch: Selective Renal Angiography in Clinical Urology, J. Urol.,* **90:**631, 1963, *courtesy J. Urol.*)

tivity to angiotensin as compared with patients with hypertension of other causes. Although initial studies are promising, further study will be necessary to establish validity of this procedure.

In addition, Grollman and associates[80] have described a technique in which renal venous blood is assayed in the rat for pressor activity. Correlations between pressor activity and cure of hypertension have been striking, and further study of the practical value of this method are indicated.

Intravenous Urography. This conventional procedure may reveal, in the hypertensive patient, such obvious lesions as a hypoplastic kidney on one side, a renal tumor, unilateral hydronephrosis, or evidence of preponderantly unilateral pyelonephritis. In renal vascular disease, one or more of the following more subtle findings may be apparent: unilateral reduction in renal mass (greater than 2 cm); delayed appearance of dye on the affected side; greater relative concentration of dye in the collecting system of the diseased side when contrast material does appear; and at times a nephrographic effect on the affected but not the normal side.[80]

False-negative results have been widely reported,[71,73,78,81] and the intravenous pyelogram cannot be taken as final evidence against unilateral renovascular disease; obviously, it will be useless in instances of bilateral renal artery stenosis. On the other hand, and more rarely, apparent false-positive results may occur. Delineation of the anatomy of the urinary tract is nevertheless important in assisting in interpretation of subsequent studies.

Radioactive "Renogram." [82] After injection of radio diodrast or hippuran, a time-curve of appearance and disappearance of radioactivity over each kidney is inscribed and compared. Characteristically, the kidney affected by renovascular hypertension exhibits a delayed appearance and delayed disappearance of dye. Further studies have suggested that osmotic diuresis with mannitol will "wash out" or minimize the difference in these cases when the discrepancy is due to renal vascular disease but will not appreciably shrink the difference when asymmetrical pyelonephritis or a hypoplastic kidney is the basis for the difference in the curves. Preliminary reports indicate a high degree of accuracy as a scanning technique, but in this procedure as in others, segmental arterial occlusion or bilateral renal artery stenosis will predictably be missed. Further study is necessary to establish the place of this procedure.

Radioactive "scanogram." [83] An assessment of renal tubular mass can be accomplished by recording the accumulation of injected radiomercury bilaterally. While results to date suggest this to be a useful and accurate means for estimation of comparative renal size, it does not measure those physiologic disturbances most characteristic of renovascular disease (see next paragraph) and will not distinguish renal vascular disease from other unilateral disease.

Differential Excretion Studies. Much evidence has accumulated to indicate that the kidney affected by renovascular disease exhibits abnormalities of excretory function which may be out of proportion to the reduction in filtration rate or even in renal blood flow. These alterations consist of a fall in the water-excretion rate and an even greater reduction in sodium excretion. Such observations have been taken as evidence that tubular reabsorptive capacity for both water and sodium is augmented,[84] but technical difficulties in measurement of glomerular filtration rate obviate such conclu-

sions. At any rate, the conclusions of Howard and coworkers from bilateral ureteral catheterization data suggest an almost invariable finding of decreased water excretion (50 per cent or greater) and decreased sodium concentration (15 per cent or greater) on the side of the lesion in patients who are later shown to have curable renovascular hypertension.[69] The most serious objections to this procedure have revolved around the false-negative tests in segmental arterial occlusion or bilateral main artery disease[77,85,86] together with the technical problems posed by ureterorenal reflexes[84,85] and bladder leakage.[84] Furthermore, failure to achieve at least 2 ml per min flow from both sides will invalidate a given test.[84] Efforts to improve these failings have centered upon careful positioning of catheters, and infusions of urea, saline solution, and vasopressin. These measures, suggested by Stamey and his coworkers,[84] have been employed with measurements not only of differential urine volumes between the two sides but of differential creatinine concentrations, the latter being higher on the affected side.

Aortography. Visualization of the aorta and renal arteries by means of translumbar puncture or retrograde catheterization of the aorta has made an enormous contribution to the study and disposition

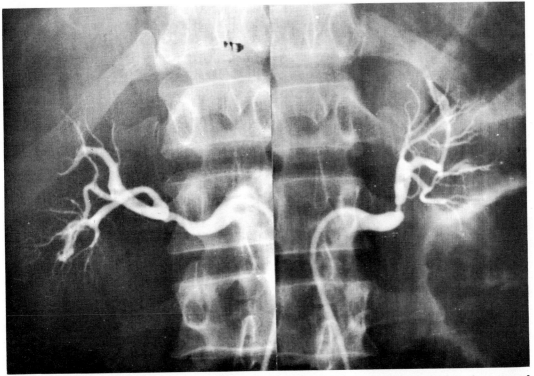

Fig. 42-2 Bilateral renal artery stenosis due to atherosclerotic narrowing is shown by means of selective renal arterial catheterization. Renal mass is reduced bilaterally. *R. S. Foster, W. H. Shuford, C. Reiser, E. P. Tuttle, Jr., and M. J. Deitch: Selective Renal Angiography in Clinical Urology, J. Urol., 90:631, 1963, courtesy J. Urol.*)

of patients with suspected renal vascular disease.[86-90] The chief virtues of this method are direct demonstration of the vascular obstruction, provision of a preoperative "map" of the surgical territory, and the ability to demonstrate segmental arterial or bilateral main arterial disease. However, although reports of false-positive findings are only occasional, it is to be expected that functionally unimportant vascular lesions will be demonstrated,[64,91] especially since such lesions may be present even in the nonhypertensive population.[92] Furthermore, falsely negative results have been obtained in patients who subsequently made a favorable response to surgery. Nonetheless, growing experience with the technique, refinements such as selective renal angiography,[93] and the low mortality-morbidity rates in experienced hands[88-90,94] appear to establish the technique as the most valuable and crucial study now available for patients with suspected reversible hypertension.

Selective renal angiography in particular appears to offer great promise in delineation of segmental renal arterial disease; it also offers an opportunity to evaluate the distal renal arterial tree preoperatively.

Surgical Approach

Some hold to the premise that even in documented unilateral renovascular hypertension a trial of drug therapy is warranted before subjecting patients to surgical intervention, and indeed it appears that previous protestations of the drug-unresponsiveness of renal hypertension may not hold true.[77] In the main, however, authorities are agreed that the risk of surgical intervention is fully warranted by the prospects of cure when the patient has adequate renal function,* the hypertension is producing "target-organ" changes, cerebral and coronary disease are not far advanced, and the surgeon's experience is adequate.[77] Surgical (operative and postoperative) mortality has ranged from 3 to 10 per cent in various centers,[10,76,80] but over half these deaths have derived from nonsurgical causes (e.g., coronary and cerebral vascular disease), so that patients whose only serious affliction is hypertension may be expected to have a far more favorable outlook. Surgical attack has included simple nephrectomy, subtotal nephrectomy, endarterectomy with or without patch graft, splenorenal anastomosis, and bypass grafts. Choice of procedure will be dictated by the lesion present and the patient's condition; it must be recalled that nephrectomy is the simplest operation, though potentiality for preservation of renal tissue often dictates the advisability of the more complicated procedure.

In summary, unilateral renal disease, and particularly that due to renal vascular abnormalities, is a rarely occurring but frequently reversible cause for systemic hypertension which deserves clinical consideration in every hypertensive patient. When the patient has no family history, is outside the age group for essential hypertension, reports a recent onset or acceleration, or presents suggestive physical or radiographic evidence of unilateral renal disease, he should be considered for definitive study, the most prominent aspect of which is likely to be aortography. With adequate confirmation of evidence for a unilateral renal origin for the hypertension, with indications that the hypertension is significant, with assurances of adequate renal function, and with expectations for reasonable surgical risk, the patient should be offered the opportunity to receive the benefit which experienced surgical hands can provide.

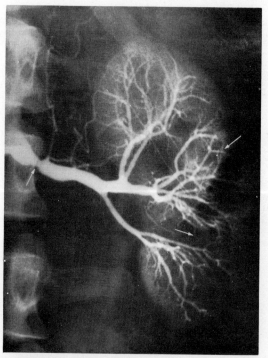

Fig. 42-3. The typical atherosclerotic obstruction of the dye column is indicated by the arrow on the left, followed by an area of poststenotic dilatation. The arrows on the far right indicate abrupt "cut-off" of distal vessels as seen in severe nephrosclerosis. (*R. S. Foster, W. H. Shuford, C. Reiser, E. P. Tuttle, Jr., and M. J. Deitch: Selective Renal Angiography in Clinical Urology, J. Urol.*, **90**:631, 1963, courtesy J. Urol.)

* It should be noted that an occasional patient with bilateral renal vascular disease may exhibit improvement of total renal function after restoration of blood flow[10] and malignant nephrosclerosis, when acute, may be partially reversible by control of blood pressure.

REFERENCES

1. Goldblatt, H., Lynch, J., Hanzal, R. B., and Summerville, W. W.: Studies in Experimental Hypertension. I. The Production of Persistent Elevation of Systolic Blood Pressure by Means of Renal Ischemia, *J. Exper. Med.*, 59:347, 1934.
2. Wilson, C., and Byrom, F. B.: The Vicious Circle in Chronic Bright's Disease: Experimental Evidence from the Hypertensive Rat, *Quart. J. Med.*, 10:65, 1941.
3. Rodbard, S., and Katz, L. N.: The Role of Renal Metabolism in Hypertension and Anemia, *J. Exper. Med.*, 73:357, 1941.
4. Isaacson, C., and Wayburne, S.: Malignant Hypertension in a Child Due to Unilateral Renal Disease, *Arch. Dis. Childhood*, 32:106, 1957.
5. Masson, G. M. C., McCormack, L. J., Dustan, H. P., and Corcoran, A. C.: Hypertensive Vascular Disease as a Consequence of Increased Arterial Pressure, *Am. J. Path.*, 34:817, 1958.
6. Goldblatt, H.: "The Renal Origin of Hypertension," Charles C Thomas, Publisher, Springfield, Ill., 1948.
7. Corcoran, A. C., and Page, I. H.: Renal Blood Flow in Experimental Renal Hypertension, *Am. J. Physiol.*, 135:361, 1941–2.
8. Diory, A.: The Mechanism of the Hypertensive Action of the Kidney, *Arch. internat. physiol.*, 59:211, 1951.
9. Huidobro, F., and Braun-Menendez, E.: The Secretion of Renin by the Intact Kidney, *Am. J. Physiol.*, 137:47, 1942.
10. Spencer, F. C., Stamey, T. A., Bahnson, H. T., and Cohen, A.: Diagnosis and Treatment of Hypertension Due to Occlusive Disease of the Renal Artery, *Am. Surgeon*, 154:674, 1961.
11. Levy, S. E., Light, R. A., and Blalock, A.: The Blood Flow and Oxygen Consumption of the Kidney in Experimental Renal Hypertension, *Am. J. Physiol.*, 122:38, 1938.
12. Mason, M. F., Robinson, C. S., and Blalock, A.: Studies on the Renal Arterial Blood Pressure and the Metabolism of Kidney Tissue in Experimental Hypertension, *J. Exper. Med.*, 72:289, 1940.
13. Hawthorne, E. W., Perry, S. L. C., and Pogue, W. G.: Development of Experimental Renal Hypertension in the Dog Following Reduction of Renal Artery Pulse Pressure without Reducing Mean Pressure, *Am. J. Physiol.*, 174:393, 1953.
14. Kohlstaedt, K. G., and Page, I. H.: The Liberation of Renin by Perfusion of Kidneys Following Reduction of Pulse Pressure, *J. Exper. Med.*, 72:201, 1940.
15. Kolff, W. J.: Discussion, in S. W. Hoobler (guest ed.), Proceedings of the Conference on Basic Mechanisms of Arterial Hypertension, *Circulation*, 17:677, 1958.
16. Blalock, A., and Levy, S. E.: Studies in the Etiology of Renal Hypertension, *Ann. Surg.*, 106:826, 1937.
17. Collins, D. A., Hypertension from Constriction of the Arteries of Denervated Kidneys, *Am. J. Physiol.*, 116:616, 1936.
18. Goldblatt, H.: Studies in Experimental Hypertension. V. The Pathogenesis of Experimental Hypertension Due to Renal Ischemia, *Ann. Int. Med.*, 11:69, 1937–1938.
19. Tigerstedt, R., and Bergman, P. G.: Niere und Kreislauf, *Skandinav. arch. physiol.*, 8:223, 1898.
20. Braun-Menendez, E., Fasciolo, J. C., Leloir, L. F., and Munoz, J. M.: The Substance Causing Renal Hypertension, *J. Physiol.*, 98:283, 1940.
21. Braun-Menendez, E., and Page, I. H.: Suggested Revisions of Nomenclature: Angiotensin, *Science*, 127:242, 1958.
22. Skeggs, L. T., Jr., Kahn, J. R., and Shumway, N. P.: The Isolation and Assay of Hypertensin from Blood, *J. Exper. Med.*, 95:241, 1952.
23. Page, I. H., and Bumpus, F. M.: Angiotensin, *Physiol. Rev.*, 41:331, 1961.
24. Blaguier, P., Bohr, D. F., and Hoobler, S. W.: Evidence against an Increase in Circulating Pressor Material in Renal Hypertensive Rats, *Am. J. Physiol.*, 198:1148, 1960.
25. Judson, W. E., and Helmer, O. M.: Demonstrations of a Pressor Substance in Renal Vein Blood in Patients with Arterial Hypertension, *Circulation*, 20:717, 1959.
26. Judson, W. E.: Pressor Activity of Dialyzed Plasma of Patients with Primary and Secondary (Renal) Hypertension, *Am. J. Physiol.*, 9:710, 1962.
27. Morris, R. E., Jr., Ransom, P. A., and Howard, J. E.: Studies in the Relationship of Angiotensin to Hypertension of Renal Origin, *J. Clin. Invest.*, 41:1386, 1962 (Abstract).
28. Wakerlin, G. E., Bird, R. B., Brennan, B. B., Frank, M. H., Kremen, S., Kuperman, I., and Skorn, J. H.: Treatment and Prophylaxis of Experimental Renal Hypertension with "Renin," *J. Lab. & Clin. Med.*, 41:708, 1953.
29. Peart, W. S.: Hypertension and the Kidney. I. Clinical, Pathological, and Functional Disorders, Especially in Man. II. Experimental Basis of Renal Hypertension, *Brit. M. J.*, 2:1353, 1422, 1959.
30. Taquini, A. C., Blaguier, P., and Taquini, A. C., Jr.: Studies on the Renal Humoral Mechanism of Chronic Experimental Hypertension, in S. W. Hoobler (guest ed.), Proceedings of the Conference on Basic Mechanisms of Arterial Hypertension, *Circulation*, 17:672, 1958.
31. Langford, H. G., and Day, L. H.: Angiotensin and Renal Hypertension, *Clin. Res.*, 9:203, 1961.
32. Taggart, J., and Drury, D. R.: The Action of Renin on Rabbits with Renal Hypertension, *J. Exper. Med.*, 71:857, 1940.
33. Blackett, R. B., Depoorter, A., Pickering, G. W., Sellers, A. L., and Wilson, G. M.: Hypertension Produced in the Rabbit by Long-continued Infusion of Renin, *Clin. Sc.*, 9:223, 1950.
34. Langford, H. G.: Hemodynamic Consequences of

Renin Tachyphylaxis and Norepinephrine Failure of Response, *Am. J. Physiol.*, **198**:561, 1960.

35. Deane, H. W., and Masson, G. M. C.: Adrenal Cortical Changes in Rats with Various Types of Experimental Hypertension, *J. Clin. Endocrinol.*, **11**:193, 1951.

36. Carpenter, C. C. J., Davis, J. O., and Ayers, C. R.: Relation of Renin, Angiotensin II, and Experimental Renal Hypertension to Aldosterone Secretion, *J. Clin. Invest.*, **40**:2026, 1961.

37. Davis, J. O., Carpenter, C. C. J., Ayers, C. R., Holman, J. E., and Bahn, R. C.: Evidence for Secretion of an Aldosterone-stimulating Hormone by the Kidney, *J. Clin. Invest.*, **40**:684, 1961.

38. Biron, P., Koiw, E., Nowaczynski, W., Brouillet, J., and Genest, J.: The Effects of Intravenous Infusions of Saline Without Angiotensin II and Other Pressor Agents on Urinary Electrolytes and Corticosteroids Including Aldosterone, *J. Clin. Invest.*, **40**:338, 1961.

39. Genest, J., Biron, P., Koiw, E., Nowaczynski, W., Chretien, M., and Boucher, R.: Adrenocortical Hormones in Human Hypertension and Their Relation to Angiotensin, *Circulation Res.*, **9**:775, 1961.

40. Laidlaw, J. C., Yendt, E. R., and Gornall, A. G.: Hypertension Caused by Renal Artery Occlusion Stimulating Primary Aldosteronism, *Metabolism*, **9**:612, 1960.

41. Laragh, J. H., Ulick, S., Januszewicz, V., Denning, Q. B., Kelly, W. G., and Liegerman, S.: Electrolyte Metabolism and Aldosterone Secretion in Benign and Malignant Hypertension, *Ann. Int. Med.*, **53**:259, 1960.

42. Laragh, J. H., Ulick, S., Januszewicz, V., Denning, Q. B., Kelly, W. G., and Lieberman, S.: Aldosterone Secretion and Primary and Malignant Hypertension, *J. Clin. Invest.*, **39**:1091, 1960.

43. Samblii, M. P., Levitan, B. A., Beck, J. C., and Venning, E. H.: The Rate of Aldosterone Secretion in Hypertensive Patients with Demonstrable Renal Artery Stenosis, *Metabolism*, **12**:498, 1963.

44. Wolf, R. L., Pick, J., Gitlow, S. E., and Naftchi, N. W.: The Metabolism of Angiotensin II—I$_{131}$, *J. Clin. Invest.*, **40**:1090, 1961.

45. Wood, J. E.: Genetic Control of the Ability of Human Blood to Neutralize Angiotensin and Its Relationship to Essential Hypertension, *J. Clin. Invest.*, **40**:1090, 1961.

46. Muirhead, E. E., Hinman, J. W., Daniels, E. G., Kosinski, M., and Brooks, B.: Refined Antihypertensive Medullorenal Extract and the Protective Action of the Kidney against Hypertension, *J. Clin. Invest.*, **40**:1065, 1961.

47. Floyer, M. A.: Role of the Kidney in Experimental Hypertension, *Brit. M. Bull.*, **13**:29, 1957.

48. Tobian, L., Winn, B., and Janecek, J.: The Influence of Arterial Pressure on the Antihypertensive Action of a Normal Kidney, a Biological Servomechanism, *J. Clin. Invest.*, **40**:1085, 1961.

49. Dunn, J., and Brown, H.: Unilateral Renal Disease and Hypertension, *J.A.M.A.*, **166**:18, 1958.

50. Barker, N. W., and Walters, W.: Hypertension and Chronic Atrophic Pyelonephritis, *J.A.M.A.*, **115**:912, 1940.

51. Butler, A. M.: Chronic Pyelonephritis and Arterial Hypertension, *J. Clin. Invest.*, **16**:889, 1937.

52. Sabin, H. S.: Hypertension in Unilateral Renal Disease, *J. Urol.*, **59**:8, 1948.

53. Richards, G. G.: Unilateral Renal Tuberculosis Associated with Hypertension, *Ann. Int. Med.*, **15**:324, 1941.

54. Dean, A. L., and Abels, J. C.: Study by the Newer Renal Function Tests of an Unusual Case of Hypertension Following Irradiation of One Kidney and the Relief of the Patient by Nephrectomy, *J. Urol.*, **52**:497, 1944.

55. Pincoffs, M. C., and Bradley, J. E.: The Association of Adenosarcoma of the Kidney (Wilms' Tumor) with Arterial Hypertension, *Tr. A. Am. Physicians*, **52**:320, 1937.

56. Gregg, J. A., Shirger, A., and Harrison, E. G., Jr.: Thrombosis of the Renal Veins Associated with Hypertension: Report of a Case, *Proc. Staff Meet. Mayo Clin.*, **36**:550, 1961.

57. Revel, S. T. R., Jr., Borges, F. J., Entwisle, G., and Young, J. D., Jr.: An Appraisal of Certain Tests for the Detection of Hypertension of Unilateral Renal Origin, *Ann. Int. Med.*, **53**:970, 1960.

58. McCormack, L. J., Hazard, J. B., and Poutasse, E. F.: Obstructive Lesions of the Renal Artery Associated with Remediable Hypertension, *Am. J. Path.*, **34**:582, 1958.

59. Howard, T. L., Forbes, R. P., and Lipscomb, W. R.: Aneurysm of the Left Renal Artery in a Child Five Years Old with Persistent Hypertension, *J. Urol.*, **44**:808, 1940.

60. Malisoff, S., and Macht, M. B.: Thromboangiitic Occlusion of the Renal Artery with Resultant Hypertension, *J. Urol.*, **65**:371, 1951.

61. Leiter, L.: Unusual Hypertensive Renal Disease. 1. Occlusion of Renal Arteries (Goldblatt Hypertension). 2. Anomalies of Urinary Tract, *J.A.M.A.*, **111**:507, 1938.

62. Price, R. K., and Skelton, R.: Hypertension Due to Syphilitic Occlusion of the Main Renal Arteries, *Brit. Heart J.*, **10**:29, 1948.

63. Howard, J. E., Berthrong, M., Gould, D. M., and Yendt, E. R.: Hypertension Resulting from Unilateral Renal Vascular Disease and Its Relief by Nephrectomy, *Bull. Johns Hopkins Hosp.*, **94**:51, 1954.

64. Perdue, G., and Waters, W. C.: Unpublished data.

65. Smith, H. W.: Unilateral Nephrectomy in Hypertensive Disease, *J. Urol.*, **76**:685, 1956.

66. Thompson, J. E., and Smithwick, R. H.: Human Hypertension Due to Unilateral Renal Disease, *Angiology*, **3**:493, 1952.

67. Yendt, E. R., Kerr, W. K., Wilson, D. R., and Zaworski, Z. F.: The Diagnosis and Treatment of Renal Hypertension, *Am. J. Med.*, **28**:169, 1960.

68. Spencer, F. C., Stamey, T. A., Bahnson, H. T., and Cohen, A.: Diagnosis and Treatment of Hypertension Due to Occlusive Disease of the Renal Artery, *Ann. Surg.*, **154**:674, 1961.

69. Connor, T. B., Thomas, W. C., Jr., Haddock, L., and Howard, J. E.: Unilateral Renal Disease as a Cause of Hypertension: Its Detection by Ureteral Catheterization Studies, *Ann. Int. Med.*, **52**:544, 1960.

70. Brown, J. J., Owen, K., Peart, W. S., Robertson, J. I. S., and Sutton, D.: The Diagnosis and Treatment of Renal Artery Stenosis, *Brit. M. J.*, **2**:327, 1960.

71. Margolin, E. G., Merrill, J. P., and Harrison, J. H.: Diagnosis of Hypertension Due to Occlusion of the Renal Artery, *New England J. Med.*, **256**:581, 1957.

72. Langley, G. J., and Platt, R.: Hypertension and Unilateral Kidney Disease, *Quart. J. Med.*, **16**:143, 1947.

73. Gellman, D. D., Reversible Hypertension and Unilateral Renal Artery Disease, *Quart. J. Med.*, **27**:103, 1958.

74. Conn, J. W.: Aldosteronism and Hypertension, *Arch. Int. Med.*, **107**:813, 1961.

75. Perera, G. A.: Clinical Characteristics of Hypertension Associated with Unilateral Renal Disease, *Circulation*, **6**:549, 1952.

76. Morris, G. C., Cooley, D. A., Crawford, E. S., Berry, W. B., and DeBakey, M. E.: Renal Revascularization for Hypertension: Clinical and Physiological Studies in 32 Cases, *Surgery*, **48**:95, 1960.

77. Page, I. H., Dustan, H. P., and Poutasse, E. F.: Mechanisms, Diagnosis and Treatment of Hypertension of Renal Vascular Origin, *Ann. Int. Med.*, **51**:196, 1959.

78. Poutasse, E. F., and Dustan, H. P.: Arteriosclerosis and Renal Hypertension: Indications for Aortography in Hypertensive Patients and Results of Surgical Treatment of Obstructive Lesions of the Renal Artery, *J.A.M.A.*, **165**:1521, 1957.

79. Kaplan, N. M., and Silah, J. G.: Angiotensin Infusion: A New Test for Renovascular Hypertension, *Clin. Res.*, **12**:2, 1964 (Abstract).

80. McPhaul, J. J., Jr., McIntosh, D. A., Williams, L. F., Gritti, E. J., Malette, W. G., and Grollman, A.: Pressor Activity of Renal Venous Blood in Hypertension, *Ann. Int. Med.*, **61**:847, 1964.

81. Smithwick, R. H., Porell, W. J., and Whitelaw, G. P.: Diagnosis of Hypertension of Adrenal and Renal Origin, *J.A.M.A.*, **174**:127, 1960.

82. Block, J. B., Hine, G. J., and Burrows, B. A.: I-131 Diodrast Studies in Unilateral Renal Disease, *Circulation*, **22**:913, 1960.

83. Sklaroff, D. M., Berk, N., and Kravitz, C.: The Renal Scintogram in Urologic Workup, *J.A.M.A.*, **178**:418, 1961.

84. Stamey, T. A., Nudelman, I. J., Good, P. H., Schwentker, F. N., and Hendricks, F.: Functional Characteristics of Renovascular Hypertension, *Medicine*, **40**:347, 1961.

85. Hix, E. L.: Uretero-renal Reflex Facilitating Renal Vasoconstrictor Response to Emotional Stress, *Am. J. Physiol.*, **192**:191, 1958.

86. Dustan, H. P., Poutasse, E. F., Corcoran, A. C., and Page, I. H.: Separated Renal Functions in Patients with Renal Arterial Disease, Pyelonephritis, and Essential Hypertension, *Circulation*, **23**:34, 1961.

87. Poutasse, E. F.: Humphries, A. W., McCormack, L. J., and Corcoran, A. C.: Bilateral Stenosis of Renal Arteries and Hypertension, *J.A.M.A.*, **161**:419, 1956.

88. Beall, A. C., Morris, G. C., Crawford, E. S., Cooley, D. A., and DeBakey, M. E.: Translumbar Aortography: Re-evaluation, *Surgery*, **49**:772, 1961.

89. Kincaid, O. W., and Davis, G. O.: Abdominal Aortography, *New England J. Med.*, **259**:1017, 1067, 1958.

90. Page, I. H.: The Mosaic Theory of Hypertension, in K. D. Bock and P. T. Cottier (eds.), "Essential Hypertension: An International Symposium," Springer-Verlag, Berlin, OHG, 1960.

91. Rapoport, A.: Modification of the "Howard Test" for the Detection of Renal Artery Obstruction, *New England J. Med.*, **263**:1159, 1960.

92. Lisa, J. R., Eckstein, D., and Solomon, C.: Relationship between Arteriosclerosis of the Renal Artery and Hypertension: Analysis of 100 Necropsies, *Am. J. M. Sc.*, **205**:701, 1943.

93. Foster, R. S.: Selective Catheterization of the Renal Vessels, *Bull. Emory Univ. Clin.*, **3**:29, 1963.

94. McAfee, J. G.: A Survey of Complications of Abdominal Aortography, *Radiology*, **68**:825, 1957.

43   PHEOCHROMOCYTOMA

Leon I. Goldberg, Ph.D., M.D.

The association of hypertension with tumors of the adrenal gland was first adequately described by Labbé, Tinel, and Doumer[1] in 1922. In 1926 C. H. Mayo[2] successfully removed adrenal tumors associated with hypertension. Pincoffs in 1929[3] made the first correct preoperative diagnosis of pheochromocytoma with successful removal of the tumor. In the same year Rabin[4] demonstrated large quantities of a pressor agent, presumed to be epinephrine, in a pheochromocytoma. Since that time rapid progress has been made in the chemistry, pathology, and diagnosis of this important tumor.

Pheochromocytoma is considered to be a relatively rare cause of hypertension, but its true frequency is unknown. Pheochromocytomas have been found in all age groups, and there does not seem to be a sex difference in their total incidence. A number of familial cases of pheochromocytoma have been reported.[5,6] A higher incidence of the tumor occurs in patients with neurofibromatosis.[5]

Anatomy and Pathology[5,7,8]

Pheochromocytomas arise from chromaffin elements either in the adrenal gland or in the extramedullary chromaffin tissue. The embryonic origin of chromaffin tissue is the sympathogonia, primitive stem cells which arise in the neural crest of the embryo. The sympathogonia develop into both sympathoblasts, from which sympathetic ganglions are derived, and pheochromoblasts, which eventually develop into the adrenal medulla. The separation of these tissues is never complete, and sympathetic ganglion cells are found in the adrenal medulla, and pheochromoblasts are often found in association with sympathetic nervous tissue. Pheochromocytomas may be found in the celiac, renal, adrenal, aortic, and hypogastric plexuses, and elsewhere in the retroperitoneal and paraaortic regions, including the organs of Zuckerkandl. In addition, tumors have been found in the thorax, urinary bladder, testes, ovaries, and elsewhere. Approximately 90 per cent of pheochromocytomas occur in the adrenal gland, and about 10 per cent of these are bilateral. The majority of tumors occur in the right adrenal. Approximately 2 per cent of extramedullary tumors are multiple.

Malignancy is difficult to determine histologically, and it is therefore not possible to assure a patient that removal of the tumor will be curative, particularly since recurrences or metastases may not develop for years. The incidence of malignancy has been variously estimated as being between 8 and 16 per cent of the total number of pheochromocytomas.

Pheochromocytomas may or may not be encapsulated and vary greatly in size. They may weigh less than 3 Gm or more than 3,000 Gm. In recent years "nonchromaffin" tumors, such as ganglioneuromas and neuroblastomas, have been found to secrete catecholamines and in some cases to elevate blood pressure.[9-11] Accordingly, a more appropriate classification of pheochromocytomas and similar

tumors would be on the basis of chemical content rather than on staining characteristics.

Chemical Content[5,7,12-14]

The steps in the biosynthesis of the catecholamines are shown in Fig. 43-1.[15,16] The precursors of catecholamines are found in pheochromocytomas and may be excreted along with catecholamine metabolites in the urine. The metabolic pathways of the catecholamines are shown in Fig. 43-2.[17]

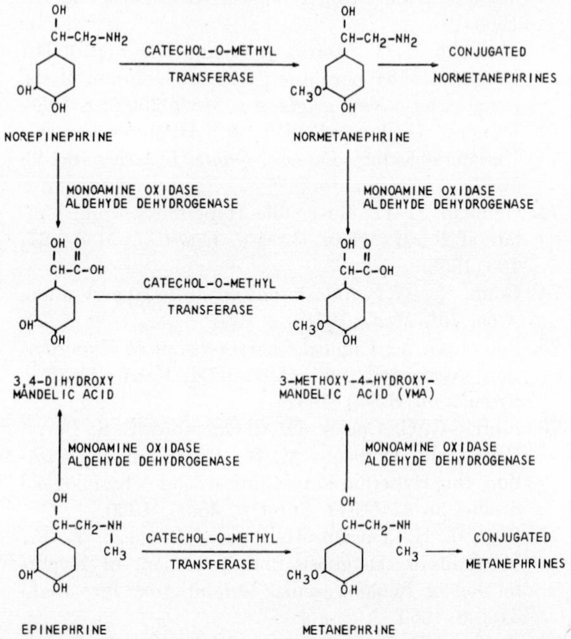

Fig. 43-2. Metabolism of norepinephrine and epinephrine. (*J. Axelrod: The Fate of Adrenaline and Noradrenaline, in J. R. Vane* (ed.), *"Adrenergic Mechanisms," Churchill Ltd., London, 1960, p. 280.*)

These reactions occur in the pheochromocytoma and also in the liver and kidney before the metabolites are excreted into the urine. Because of differing rates of catecholamine production and metabolism by different tumors, the excretion of

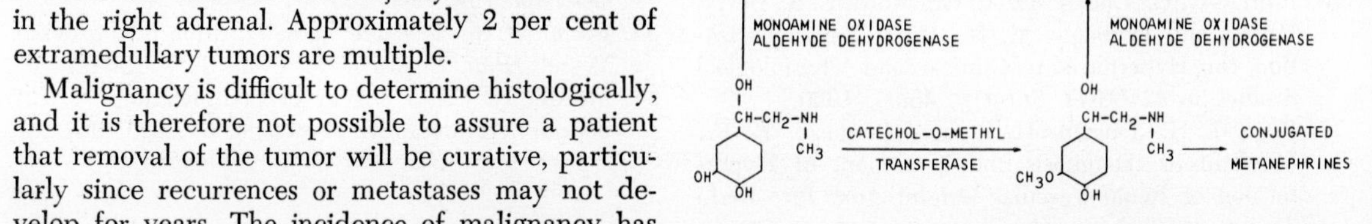

Fig. 43-1. The principal steps in the synthesis of norepinephrine and epinephrine. (*H. Blaschko: The Development of Current Concepts of Catecholamine Formation, Pharmacol. Rev.,* **11**:307, 1959; *H. J. Schümann: Formation of Adrenergic Transmitters, in J. R. Vane, ed., "Adrenergic Mechanisms," Churchill Ltd., London, 1960, p. 6.*)

precursors, catecholamines, and metabolites may vary considerably in patients with pheochromocytoma.[13,18] Norepinephrine is usually the only catecholamine found in extraadrenal tumors, whereas varying amounts of norepinephrine and epinephrine are found in adrenal tumors. Pheochromocytomas containing predominantly epinephrine are extremely rare.[19]

The cardiovascular and metabolic changes produced by pheochromocytoma are considered to be primarily due to the release of norepinephrine and epinephrine. The precursor, dopamine, also has pharmacologic actions,[20] but because of low potency it is difficult to assess its effects in the syndrome. The cardiovascular actions of norepinephrine and epinephrine are described in Chap. 22. The catecholamines produce hyperglycemia by activation of the enzyme phosphorylase, which results in degradation of glycogen to glucose. Epinephrine is more potent in this respect than norepinephrine, but there is little diagnostic significance in this difference, because the massive amount of norepinephrine produced is adequate in many cases of pheochromocytoma to produce hyperglycemia. Norepinephrine and epinephrine have similar actions to increase plasma levels of unesterified fatty acids.[21]

Clinical Aspects[5,8,22]

Pheochromocytomas may be divided into two main types, depending upon whether the hypertension is paroxysmal or persistent. In addition, cases of pheochromocytoma have been discovered without elevation of blood pressure. Patients with paroxysmal hypertension may experience attacks at intervals varying from more than one every hour to one in several months. The duration of the attacks also varies from a few seconds to several days. The attack may be precipitated by such events as change of position, urination, emotional disturbance, intercourse, or heavy eating. More common symptoms described as occuring during the attacks are headache, palpitation, perspiration, pallor, nervousness, tremor, chest and abdominal pain, nausea and vomiting, and visual difficulties. Blood pressure recorded during the attack in these patients almost invariably reaches levels greater than 200 mm systolic and 100 mm diastolic. After an attack the patient may be extremely fatigued and prostrate.

Patients with persistent hypertension usually have fewer symptoms than those with paroxysmal hypertension. In patients without characteristic symptoms it is particularly difficult to differentiate pheochromocytoma from essential or malignant hypertension.

The presence of a pheochromocytoma in a patient is an extremely treacherous and life-threatening situation. Although a few cases of pheochromocytoma have been symptomatic for longer than 30 years,[23,24] there is no way of telling when the release of catecholamines will produce a fatal attack. Patients with pheochromocytoma may die from cerebral vascular accidents, myocardial infarction, cardiac arrhythmias, acute pulmonary edema, intestinal lesions,[25] or shock. It is imperative, therefore, once a pheochromocytoma is diagnosed, that precautions be taken to prevent occurrence of a fatal attack. It is advisable to have the patient watched at all times, with frequent recordings of blood pressure. Intravenous phentolamine (Regitine) should be administered immediately in the event of an attack. Oral administration of phentolamine or other adrenergic blocking agents has been recommended as soon as the condition is diagnosed. The dose of phentolamine needed for this purpose varies from 5 to 100 mg at 2- to 4-hr intervals.[26,27]

Physical Examination and Nondiagnostic Laboratory Tests

The physical examination may be entirely negative. Patients with pheochromocytoma are usually thin, but cases have been described in obese patients. The skin is frequently moist and may be flushed, particularly during an attack. All degrees of hypertensive retinal changes have been observed, including hemorrhages, exudates, and papilledema. The hands may be red or cyanotic. In approximately 10 to 15 per cent of cases the tumor is large enough to be palpated, and the attack may be precipitated by deep palpation. The cardiac examination may be negative or reveal the presence of arrhythmias[28] or cardiomegaly. Orthostatic hypotension is seen in some but not all patients.[29]

Fasting blood sugar is elevated in about half of the patients, usually only slightly above normal values. Glycosuria, if present, is usually intermittent. The basal metabolic rate is also elevated in about half of the patients, but there are no characteristic changes in cholesterol or protein-bound iodine.

Differential Diagnosis

Because of the variety of symptoms and metabolic changes produced by pheochromocytoma, a long list of diseases must be considered. Among the more commonly confused diagnoses are essential and malignant hypertension, thyrotoxicosis, diabetes with hypertension, congestive heart failure, neuroses with anxiety attacks, and acute abdominal emergencies. The condition must be considered in all hypertensive or hypotensive reactions during anesthesia or pregnancy, unexpected hypertensive or hypotensive reactions to antihypertensive agents, and hypotension after administration of phenothiazine tranquilizers.[30]

Diagnostic Tests

Pharmacologic Tests[5,8,31]

Two pharmacologic tests are commonly used in the diagnosis of pheochromocytoma—the phentolamine test for patients with blood pressure elevations above 170/110 and the provocative histamine test for patients with lower blood pressures level. The phentolamine test[32] is based on the principle that this alpha-adrenergic blocking agent will lower the elevated blood pressure by blocking the alpha (vasoconstrictor) effects of the catecholamines. Since the proper execution of this test is imperative for correct interpretation, a detailed summary follows:

An intravenous infusion of 5 per cent glucose in water is started, and the patient is allowed to rest in bed, preferably in a quiet, darkened room, until blood pressure is stabilized at the basal level. Blood pressure recordings should then be obtained at least every 10 min for 30 min. After this period, 5 mg phentolamine is injected rapidly into the rubber tubing of the intravenous set and flushed into the vein. Blood pressure should be recorded immediately after the injection, and at 30-sec intervals for the first 3 min and 60-sec intervals for the following 7 min. An immediate drop in blood pressure of more than 35 mm Hg systolic and 25 mm Hg, diastolic is considered a positive response. Usually a maximal depressor effect is evident within 2 min after the injection, and pressure usually returns to the base line within 15 to 30 min, but a more rapid return is also possible. False-positive tests occur in uremia and in patients taking sedatives, narcotics, anesthetics, antihypertensive agents, sympathomimetic amine nose drops, and a number of other drugs. It is advisable to discontinue sedatives and narcotics at least 48 hr before the test and catecholamine-depleting agents such as reserpine at least 2 weeks prior to the test. False-positive tests may also occur because of release of catecholamines in an anxious patient.

Tachycardia commonly occurs during the phentolamine tests in patients without pheochromocytoma, and the agent must therefore be administered cautiously to patients with known myocardial insufficiency. Severe hypotensive reactions and death have been reported during phentolamine tests, and norepinephrine, metaraminol, or similar sympathomimetic amines should be immediately available.[33]

The histamine test was introduced by Roth and Kvale in 1945.[34] The basis of this test is the provocation of catecholamine release from the tumor by histamine. This release has been related both to direct stimulation of the tumor and to reflex stimulation in response to an initial drop in blood pressure.[35] In this test a cold pressor test is first performed, and after the blood pressure has returned to basal levels, a rapid intravenous injection of 0.025 or 0.05 mg histamine base in 0.25 or 0.5 ml isotonic saline solution is administered. The test is considered positive if the systolic pressure rises 20 mm Hg or more above the highest reading obtained with the cold pressor test. The rise in blood pressure usually becomes evident within 2 min following the injection of histamine and is accompanied by the characteristic symptoms of an attack. The hypertensive response may be immediately terminated by administration of phentolamine, and when the blood pressure is lowered, additional diagnostic significance is provided.

Chemical Methods

A number of chemical methods are available for estimating urinary catecholamines and their metabolites.[5,7,8,36] The normal urinary excretion of free norepinephrine and epinephrine is usually less than 100 μg per 24 hr.[12] Of this amount approximately 75 to 80 per cent is norepinephrine, and the remainder is epinephrine. Most pheochromocytomas excrete more than 300 μg catecholamines per 24 hr. Several have been reported with catecholamine-excretion rates greater than ten times this amount. In general the measurement of total catecholamines is adequate for diagnostic purposes, and the ratio of norepinephrine to epinephrine is valuable only as an aid to localization of the tumor. More recently, measurement of the catecholamine metabolites, metanephrine, normetanephrine, and 3-methoxy-4-hydroxymandelic acid (VMA) have been introduced as diagnostic methods.[18,36–39] These metabolites are excreted in far greater quantity than the catecholamines and can be measured by simple colorimetric techniques rather than by spectrophotofluorimetry. Therefore, relatively simple screening procedures for hospitals without elaborate chemical laboratories have been made available. The upper limits of normal metanephrine plus normetanephrine secretion is considered to be approximately 2.5 mg per 24 hr. The normal values for VMA excretion are usually less than 6 mg per 24 hr, and values above 10 mg per 24 hr are highly suggestive of pheochromocytoma.

There is considerable debate as to whether it is better to measure the excretion of catecholamines or one of the metabolites. This question is largely unanswered, but fortunately each of the tests is adequate for diagnosis of most tumors. It is interesting to note that in a few cases the presence of pheochromocytoma has been diagnosed by measurement of one substance and not by the others.[18] This variance does not necessarily reflect the adequacy of a test but may be the result of variations in metabolism of catecholamines by the tumor.[13] It is important in carrying out all the chemical tests that directions for collections be carried out exactly. Among the substances which either interfere with or alter the urinary content of the catecholamines are bananas and other fruits containing catecholamines,[40] catecholamine-depleting agents such as reserpine and guanethidine, broad-spectrum antibiotics, methyldopa,[41] and the phenothiazines. The VMA test may be altered by monoamine oxidase inhibitors and disulfiram (Antabuse) and by ingestion of coffee, fruit, and items containing vanillin. False-positive reactions may be obtained in conditions other than pheochromocytoma which increase secretion of catecholamines and their metabolites. A partial listing is hypoglycemia, thyrotoxicosis, angina pectoris, myocardial infarction, renal disease, jaundice, lymphoma, and brain tumors. Fortunately many of these conditions do not enter into the differential diagnosis or can be ruled out by clinical means or other laboratory tests.

Plasma Catecholamines[5,7,36]

The measurement of plasma catecholamines is a less satisfactory method for the detection of pheochromocytoma than the measurement of urinary excretion of the amines. However, in cases with low base-line secretions the increase in plasma (and urine) levels of catecholamines after histamine injection may be diagnostic.[18,31] In addition, the measurement of plasma catecholamines may be extremely helpful in localizing a tumor by differential venous catheterization.[5,42]

Roentgen Techniques[43]

Radiologic studies have frequently yielded information leading to the diagnosis and localization of pheochromocytomas. Tumors have been observed in chest x-rays and plain abdominal films. Intravenous urography has resulted in the localization of a number of tumors because of evidence of distortion of the ureters of calyxes and displacement of the kidney. The question as to whether to proceed to more elaborate studies such as retroperitoneal pneumography or aortography is debatable because of the hazards involved.

Fig. 43-3A shows a large calcified tumor which on intravenous urography was found to be distorting the right ureter. Figure 43-3B shows the same tumor with retroperitoneal carbon dioxide insufflation. The patient was a twenty-seven-year-old woman with typical attacks of paroxysmal hypertension. The mass was found on surgical intervention to be a 7- by 5- by 5-cm tumor of the organ of Zuckerkandl, with invasion of the aorta. In removing the tumor, it was necessary to remove a section of the aorta. The patient is normotensive and well 5 years after surgical treatment.[44]

Summary of Diagnostic Techniques

It is now possible to detect pheochromocytoma by a number of adequate methods. Ideally every hypertensive patient and every patient with unexplained "attacks" suggestive of pheochromocytoma should undergo at least one of the screening procedures. The chemical procedures are superior to the pharmacologic methods because of greater safety, but directions concerning collection must be followed precisely. It should be remembered that pheochromocytomas can be missed even by the best screening methods because of low rates of catecholamine secretion and because of errors in collection or technique. Therefore the most important factor in the diagnosis of this disease is the clinical judgment and persistence of the physician. Indeed, many pheochromocytomas have been successfully removed only after repeated diagnostic tests and in some cases after repeated surgical explorations.[45]

Surgical Procedures

Several excellent papers are available which discuss in detail the surgical aspects of pheochromocytoma.[5,8,46]

Surgeons should be prepared to explore both adrenals and the entire abdominal cavity to search for multiple and extraadrenal tumors. Hume[5] recommends a transverse upper abdominal incision, which provides exposure of both adrenal areas, both sympathetic chains, and the abdominal aorta. In addition, the surgeon should be capable of carrying out extensive vascular surgical procedures, since large vessels are sometimes involved.

Preoperative, operative, and postoperative periods are particularly hazardous in these patients, and special precautions are required. It is advisable that the internist or cardiologist be present during the entire procedure. Blood pressure should be recorded frequently, preferably continuously by an intraarterial technique. The electrocardiogram should be monitored because of the dangers of arrhythmias and sudden cardiac arrest. Most anesthesiologists prefer barbiturate anesthesia. Because of the theoretical dangers of arrhythmias produced by cyclopropane or halothane (Fluothane) in the presence of catecholamines, these anesthetics are not recommended. Phentolamine should be administered intravenously whenever the blood pressure rises, including during the period of induction

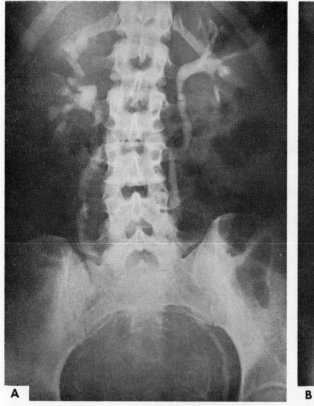
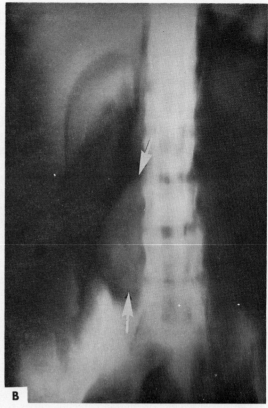

Fig. 43-3. *A.* Intravenous pyelogram demonstrating dislocation of the right ureter by a paraaortic mass. *B.* The same lesion after retroperitoneal carbon dioxide insufflation. Note the calcification of the lesion. (*From Postgraduate Medicine,* 34:25, 1963, *by permission of the publishers; J. R. Amerson and L. I. Goldberg: Pheochromocytoma: Diagnosis and Treatment, Postgrad. Med.,* 34:25, 1963.)

with the anesthetic. Oral administration of phentolamine for several days prior to surgical intervention has also been recommended.[27] Such treatment minimizes the dangers of catecholamine discharge. Since the blood volume is often decreased in patients with pheochromocytoma, plasma volume expanders are useful in prevention and management of postoperative hypotension. Norepinephrine may be required in large quantities after removal of the tumor. Blood loss should be adequately replaced. Finally, in the event of bilateral adrenal surgery, administration of hydrocortisone may be needed.

REFERENCES

1. Labbé, M., Tinel, J., and Doumer, A.: Crises solaires et hypertension paroxystique en rapport avec une tumeur surrenale, *Bull. Soc. méd hôp. Paris,* 46:982, 1922.
2. Mayo, C.: Paroxysmal Hypertension Associated with Tumor of Retroperitoneal Nerve, *J.A.M.A.,* 89:1047, 1927.
3. Pincoffs, U. C.: A Case of Paroxysmal Hypertension Associated with Suprarenal Tumor, *Tr. A. Am. Physicians,* 44:295, 1929.
4. Rabin, C. B.: Chromaffin Cell Tumor of the Suprarenal Medulla (Pheochromocytoma), *Arch. Path.,* 7:228, 1929.
5. Hume, D. M.: Pheochromocytoma in the Adult and in the Child, *Am. J. Surg.,* 99:458, 1960.
6. Tisherman, S. E., Gregg, F. J., and Danowski, T. S.: Familial Pheochromocytoma, *J.A.M.A.,* 182:152, 1962.
7. Straus, R., and Wurm, M.: Catecholamines and the Diagnosis of Pheochromocytoma, *Am. J. Clin. Path.,* 34:403, 1960.
8. Priestley, J. T., Kvale, W. F., and Gifford, R. W., Jr.: Pheochromocytoma: Clinical Aspects and Surgical Treatment, *Arch. Surg.,* 86:778, 1963.
9. Mason, G. A., Hart-Mercer, J., Millar, E. J., Strang, L. B., and Wynne, N. A.: Adrenaline-secreting Neuroblastoma in Infant, *Lancet,* 2:322, 1957.
10. Vorhess, M. L., and Gardner, L. I.: Urinary Excretion of Norepinephrine, Epinephrine and 3-methoxy-4-hydroxymandelic Acid by Children with Neuroblastoma, *J. Clin. Endocrinol.,* 21:321, 1961.

11. von Studnitz, W., Käser, H., and Sjoersma, A.: Spectrum of Catechol Amine Biochemistry in Patients with Neuroblastoma, *New England J. Med.,* 269:232, 1963.

12. Sjoerdsma, A.: Catecholamine Metabolism in Patients with Pheochromocytoma, *Pharmacol. Rev.,* 11:374, 1959.

13. Crout, R. J., and Sjoerdsma, A.: Turnover and Metabolism of Catecholamines in Patients with Pheochromocytoma, *J. Clin. Invest.,* 43:94, 1964.

14. von Euler, U. S.: "Noradrenalin: Chemistry, Physiology, Pharmacology and Clinical Aspects," Charles C Thomas, Publisher, Springfield, Ill., 1956.

15. Blaschko, H.: The Development of Current Concepts of Catecholamine Formation, *Pharmacol. Rev.,* 11:307, 1959.

16. Schümann, H. J.: Formation of Adrenergic Transmitters, in J. R. Vane (ed.), "Adrenergic Mechanisms," Churchill Ltd., London, 1960, p. 6.

17. Axelrod, J.: The Fate of Adrenaline and Noradrenaline, in J. R. Vane (ed.), "Adrenergic Mechanisms," Churchill Ltd., London, 1960, p. 28.

18. Crout, J. R., Pisano, J. J., and Sjoerdsma, A.: Urinary Excretion of Catecholamines and Their Metabolites in Pheochromocytoma, *Am. Heart J.,* 61:375, 1961.

19. Hamrin, B.: Sustained Hypotension and Shock Due to an Adrenaline-secreting Phaeochromocytoma, *Lancet,* 2:123, 1962.

20. Horwitz, D., Fox, S. M., III, and Goldberg, L. I.: Effects of Dopamine in Man, *Circulation Res.,* 10:237, 1962.

21. Mueller, P. S., and Horwitz, D.: Plasma Free Fatty Acid and Blood Glucose Responses to Analogues of Norepinephrine in Man, *J. Lipid Res.,* 3:251, 1962.

22. De Courcy, J. L., and De Courcy, C. B.: "Pheochromocytoma and the General Practitioner," Barclay Newman, Cincinnati, 1952.

23. Bell, M. A., Blakemore, W. S., and Rose, E.: Some Vagaries of Pheochromocytoma: Four Illustrative Cases, *Ann. Int. Med.,* 57:406, 1962.

24. Borch-Johnsen, E.: An Operated Case of Paraganglioma Associated with the Suprarenal Sympathetic Syndrome, *Acta chir. scandinav.,* 80:171, 1937.

25. Brown, R. B., and Borowsky, M.: Further Observation on Intestinal Lesion Associated with Pheochromocytoma, *Ann. Surg.,* 151:683, 1960.

26. Israelski, M., Kendall, A. C., and Shaw, R. E.: A Case of Pheochromocytoma in Childhood, *Arch Dis. Childhood,* 29:18, 1954.

27. Johns, V. J., and Brunjes, S.: Pheochromocytoma, *Am. J. Cardiol.,* 9:120, 1962.

28. Durant, J., and Soloff, L. A.: Arrhythmic Crisis of Phaeochromocytoma, *Lancet,* 2:124, 1962.

29. Smithwick, R. H., Greer, W. E. R., Robertson, C. W., and Wilkins, R. W.: Pheochromocytoma: A Discussion of Symptoms, Signs and Procedures of Diagnostic Value, *New England J. Med.,* 242:252, 1950.

30. Lund-Johansen, P.: Shock after Administration of Phenothiazines in Patients with Pheochromocytoma, *Acta med. scandinav.,* 172:525, 1962.

31. Roth, G. M., Flock, E. V., Kvale, W. F., Waugh, J. M., and Ogg, J.: Pharmacologic and Chemical Tests as an Aid in the Diagnosis of Pheochromocytoma, *Circulation,* 21:769, 1960.

32. Grimson, K. S., Longino, F. H., Kernodle, C. E., and O'Rear, H. B.: Treatment of Patient with Pheochromocytoma: Use of Adrenocytic Drug before and during Operation, *J.A.M.A.,* 140:1273, 1949.

33. Roland, C. R.: Pheochromocytoma in Pregnancy: Report of a Fatal Reaction to Phentolamine (Regitine) Methanesulfonate, *J.A.M.A.,* 171:1806, 1959.

34. Roth, G. M., and Kvale, W. F.: A Tentative Test for Pheochromocytoma, *Am. J. M. Sc.,* 210:653, 1945.

35. Entwistle, G., Stone, C. A., and Loew, E. R.: Pharmacologic Basis of Various Tests Used in the Diagnosis of Pheochromocytoma, *Am. J. Med.,* 11:461, 1951.

36. Krayer, O. (ed.): Symposium on Catecholamines. Sec. I. Measurement of Epinephrine, Norepinephrine, and Related Compounds, *Pharmacol. Rev.,* 11:241, 1959.

37. Sunderman, F. W., Jr., Cleveland, P. D., Law, N. C., and Sunderman, F. W.: A Method for the Determination of 3-methoxy-4-hydroxymandelic Acid ("Vanilmandelic Acid") for the Diagnosis of Pheochromocytoma, *Am. J. Clin. Path.,* 34:293, 1960.

38. Pisano, J. J., Crout, R. J., and Abraham, D.: Determination of 3-methoxy-4-hydroxymandelic Acid in Urine, *Clin. chim. acta,* 7:285, 1962.

39. Gitlow, S. E., Mendlowitz, M., Kruk, E., and Khassis, S.: Diagnosis of Pheochromocytoma by Assay of Catecholamine Metabolites, *Circulation Res.,* 9:746, 1961.

40. Crout, J. R., and Sjoerdsma, A.: The Clinical and Laboratory Significance of Serotonin and Catechol Amines in Bananas, *New England J. Med.,* 261:23, 1959.

41. Gifford, R. W., and Tweed, D. C.: Spurious Elevation of Urinary Catecholamines during Therapy with Alpha-methyl-dopa, *J.A.M.A.,* 182:493, 1962.

42. von Euler, U. S., and Strom, G.: Present Status of Diagnosis and Treatment of Pheochromocytoma, *Circulation,* 15:5, 1957.

43. Pendergrass, H. P., Tristan, T. A., Blakemore, W. S., Sellers, A. M., Jannetta, P. J., and Murphy, J. J.: Roentgen Technics in the Diagnosis and Localization of Pheochromocytoma, *Radiology,* 78:725, 1962.

44. Amerson, J. R., and Goldberg, L. I.: Pheochromocytoma: Diagnosis and Treatment, *Postgrad. Med.,* 34:25, 1963.

45. Effersoe, P., Gertz, T. C., and Lund, A.: Pheochromocytoma: A Case Report of Successful Thoraco-abdominal Operation after Nine Negative Surgical Explorations, *Acta chir. scandinav.,* 103:43, 1952.

46. Cahill, G. F., and Papper, E. M.: Techniques Involved in the Surgical Removal of Pheochromocytoma. *J. Urol.*, **76**:467, 1956.

44 PRIMARY ALDOSTERONISM

William C. Waters III, M.D.

Interest in the relatively small group of patients with curable hypertension received an enormous impetus with the discovery in 1955 of the syndrome of primary aldosteronism. Applying basic physiologic information already obtained by earlier investigators[1-3] to a patient with hypertension, hypokalemia and alkalosis, Conn and his associates demonstrated increased urinary excretion of the potent mineralocorticoid aldosterone and subsequently established the cause to be an adrenal cortical adenoma.[4] Although expectations of a high incidence of this syndrome have not been completely fulfilled, an enthusiastic search has nonetheless been successful in identifying a substantial number of cases, and more are sure to be added as interest in the entity grows.

From a historical point of view, identification of the new syndrome has had the effect of stimulating new interest in the concept of reversible hypertension, in bringing into focus the dynamic influence of aldosterone in a variety of clinical states, and, perhaps most of all, in affirming once again the great importance of an understanding of basic physiologic mechanisms to the progress of clinical research.

Physiology and Pathophysiology

Aldosterone, the 17-aldehyde of corticosterone, is the most physiologically potent mineralocorticoid known. An effect of minute amounts can be demonstrated in the intestine,[5] in sweat glands,[6] in salivary secretions,[7] and possibly even upon transmembrane sodium-potassium transport of muscle cells.[8] By far its most striking effect, however, is in facilitating sodium reabsorption and potassium excretion by the distal renal tubular epithelial cell;[9-11] indeed the entire spectrum of abnormalities found in primary aldosteronism can be traced to its action at this locus.

In the renal tubule, the electrochemical gradient established by the active transport of sodium from tubular urine to peritubular blood must be matched by an equivalent migration of anion (from urine to blood) or by an equivalent exchange of cation (from blood to urine).[12] Thus under the accelerating effect of increased aldosterone activity, chloride may accompany the reabsorbed sodium (with resultant salt and water retention), or potassium and hydrogen may be exchanged for sodium (with resultant potassium depletion and alkalosis). Once potassium depletion has occurred, hydrogen ion loss is further encouraged. The clinical and biochemical disturbances of the full syndrome—hypertension, hypokalemia, and alkalosis—ensue.

A substantial body of data indicate that aldosterone in the human being is normally secreted by the zona glomerulosa of the adrenal cortex[13,14] at a rate of 180 to 330 μg per day[15] and is excreted in the urine both as free aldosterone and as the metabolically inactive degradation product tetrahydroaldosterone.[16] Unlike the secretion of other adrenal hormones, including cortisol, aldosterone is elaborated relatively independently of the influence of adrenocorticotropic hormone.[17,18] On the other hand, its release is exquisitely sensitive to a variety of other stimuli, particularly those involving changes in circulatory dynamics. Inferior vena caval constriction, acute hemorrhage, and salt depletion are known to be regularly associated with increased secretion rates of aldosterone;[19,20] similarly, saline loading or albumin infusion causes a reduction in aldosterone activity.[20] Although earlier work suggested neural[20] or diencephalic[21] control of aldosterone secretion under such circumstances, Carpenter, Davis, and associates[22-24] have now clearly demonstrated the role of angiotensin in stimulating aldosterone release; thus, the renin-angiotensin-aldosterone axis must be recognized as an important homeostatic system in the regulation of extracellular and intravascular volumes.

Considerable information concerning the pathogenesis of primary aldosteronism is contributed by a study of normal subjects given pharmacologic doses of the hormone. Nelson and others[25] found that normal adults receiving large doses of aldosterone daily developed positive salt and water balance, hypokalemia, alkalosis, and hypertension. It is significant that after a 3-kg weight gain a new steady state was attained, and thereafter the patients "escaped" from the effects of the drug. At this level, like patients with the clinical syndrome, these subjects exhibited no edema. Suggested explanations for this "escape phenomenon" have included absence of an adrenal salt-losing factor[26] and hypervolemia with increased renal plasma flow and overload of the distal tubular sodium-reabsorptive mechanism. At any rate, it appears clear that both experimentally and clinically the syndrome of uncomplicated aldosterone excess only very rarely includes edema formation, and the presence of edema in a given case would suggest either complicating heart failure or that the aldosteronism is due to the cause of the edema formation ("secondary aldosteronism"—see Differential Diagnosis).

Incidence

Recently, Conn has proposed that perhaps many cases of "innocent" adrenal cortical tumors found at autopsy may in fact represent incomplete and masked forms of the syndrome; this possibility must await further study.[27]

As of March, 1963, Conn[28] tabulated 145 reported cases of primary aldosteronism and indicated knowledge of some 50 more. Considering the size of the hypertensive population and the apparently intensive search undertaken in many centers, it must still be regarded as an uncommon—if not rare—disease entity. Females have predominated over males in the ratio of 2.7:1, and by far the greatest age incidence falls in the thirty- to forty-year age group (approximately 70 per cent of total cases[28]). Primary aldosteronism is therefore predominately a disease of young and middle-aged females.

Symptomatology

The presenting symptoms of patients with primary aldosteronism can be traced to the underlying disturbance of fluid volume, potassium metabolism, and acid-base equilibrium. By far the most common complaints are *muscle weakness* and *polyuria*, both being present in approximately three-fourths of patients. The muscle weakness may be chronic or episodic and may be responsive in at least some cases to the administration of adequate quantities of potassium salts even prior to surgical intervention. In some cases[28] the weakness has appeared only after administration of thiazide-type diuretics. The polyuria is related to a concentration defect produced in the kidney by potassium depletion. This "potassium-depletion nephropathy" is characterized pathologically by vacuolar degeneration of renal tubular epithelial cells and clinically by a vasopressin-resistant isosthenuria.[29] The nephropathy is not specific for primary aldosteronism but may occur in any disease state attended by significant total body potassium depletion.[29] Other symptoms have included *headache, paresthesias, intermittent paralysis, tetanic manifestations,* including dysesthesias, and a sensation of *fatigue.* In a small percentage of cases (6 per cent in Conn's survey[28]) no symptoms at all have been present, and the diagnosis has been made after the discovery of abnormal serum-electrolyte concentrations in patients being evaluated for hypertension.

Physical Findings

Hypertension has been an invariable finding in all cases reported to date. The elevation of blood pressure has been mild to moderate (160/100 to 200/120) with rare exceptions, and it has been repeatedly emphasized that malignant progression is not a characteristic of primary aldosteronism, although at least one well-documented case has now been reported.[30] *Retinopathy,* usually confined to vascular attenuation and arteriovenous crossing changes has been seen in approximately one-half of cases. While papilledema, as noted below, is almost universally absent, hemorrhages and exudates are occasionally noted. *Cardiomegaly* has been reported in some 40 per cent of cases, although findings of congestive heart failure such as neck vein distension, pulmonary congestion, hepatomegaly, and peripheral edema have been exceptional.[27] Signs of *neuromuscular irritability,* including positive Chvostek and Trousseau signs, or frank tetany, have been demonstrable in approximately 10 to 15 per cent of cases but only very exceptionally in males. Overt *paralysis* has been reported in a few instances and has been confined to females.

Laboratory Findings

Hypokalemia has been present at some time in all patients thus far demonstrated to have a functioning aldosteroma.* The average serum-potassium level is below 3.0 mEq per liter and is usually persistently in this range. However, some patients reach these low levels only episodically. Occasional individuals may show normal serum-potassium concentrations, with paroxysmal drops to hypokalemic levels. A few cases[28] have had their metabolic disturbance unmasked only after therapy with thiazide diuretics, and it has been suggested[28] that suspicion of an aldosteronoma should be aroused by the development of symptoms of muscular weakness occurring within a few days of institution of diuretic therapy. However, mild degrees of hypokalemia are common with thiazide administration in any group, and such slight reductions should of course not be considered diagnostic. *Metabolic alkalosis,* as manifested by an elevated bicarbonate concentration of plasma and normal or elevated blood pH, is present in the majority of cases but is not invariable. Most such patients exhibit a CO_2 content of blood plasma in the range of 32 to 38 mEq per liter. *Hypernatremia* is frequent, though not constant, but hyponatremia is virtually never present[31] and, as noted below, militates against the diagnosis of primary aldosteronism. Serum-*chloride* concentration is depressed reciprocally with the bicarbonate elevation. In a few cases *low serum-magnesium* levels were demonstrated.

Patients with primary aldosteronism can be shown at some time to have increased urinary ex-

* At the time of this writing, one exception to this rule has been documented in a patient with hypertension, hyperaldosteronism, and a functioning aldosteronoma without hypokalemia.[27]

cretion of aldosterone and/or tetrahydroaldoster-one.[31] Double-dilution isotope studies reveal increased endogenous secretion rates of aldosterone; Porter-Silber chromogens (17-hydroxysteroids and 17-ketosteroids), on the other hand, are within normal limits. Potassium-depletion nephropathy is frequently present and is manifested by decreased concentrating ability—resistant to vasopressin—a tendency to alkaluria, and high urinary potassium excretion (usually over 40 mEq per day while the patient is hypokalemic). Other studies have demonstrated low sweat and salivary sodium concentrations, while total body exchangeable sodium is high and body exchangeable potassium is low as determined by radioisotopic measurement methods. An increased plasma volume, with slight decrease of the hematocrit value, is usual. The electrocardiogram may show changes of decreased T vector and prominent U waves consistent with hypokalemia, but diagnostic changes may be absent.

Diagnosis

The diagnosis of primary aldosteronism, in the typical case, will thus not be difficult in the young to middle-aged female with mild to moderate hypertension, hypokalemic alkalosis, increased urinary potassium concentration, alkaline urine, increased aldosterone secretion or excretion, and normal urinary 17-hydroxysteroids and 17-ketosteroids. Further attempts to demonstrate the lesion preoperatively, as by retroperitoneal air or carbon dioxide insufflation, have proved discouraging, since the great majority of tumors weigh less than 6 Gm and generally are less than 3 cm in diameter. The final proof of diagnosis is thus exploration. In the slightly atypical case, however, careful evaluation to exclude other possibilities is essential. Other entities which may produce confusion are discussed in the section on differential diagnosis.

Differential Diagnosis

By far the most common cause of hypokalemic alkalosis in any given hypertensive patient is prior therapy with *thiazide-type diuretics*. Thus, in the evaluation of any hypertensive patient for possible reversible causes, detailed history regarding the many forms of thiazides must be pursued. Even after discontinuation of therapy for a week or more, persistent potassium depletion may perpetuate the hypokalemic alkalosis. Even further confusion may result from an increased urinary aldosterone–secretion rate caused by the extracellular fluid volume depletion which thiazides may produce.[32] It is thus suggested that such patients be given a period of 3 to 4 weeks off thiazide diuretics and that during the first week off therapy adequate provision of potassium chloride, 15 mEq three

times daily, be given. On the other hand, sodium depletion, resulting from either diuretic therapy or dietary salt restriction, may mask the electrolyte abnormalities of primary aldosteronism, and an adequate, or—as some have recommended [28]—increased sodium allowance should be given.

Considerable conceptual as well as diagnostic difficulties may be encountered in the not infrequent patient with *malignant hypertension* and "secondary aldosteronism." A sizable proportion of patients with fulminating hypertensive disease may exhibit hypokalemia, alkalosis, and aldosterone-secretion rates even higher than that seen in primary aldosteronism.[15] Such patients, when explored, have been found to have not adenomas but either bilateral adrenal hyperplasia or normal adrenal glands and have shown either an unfavorable or a poor response to subtotal adrenalectomy; thus the preoperative recognition of this group is of obvious clinical importance. It has been suggested that the presence of malignant hypertension is itself adequate evidence for the absence of an aldosteronoma,[28] but the recent well-documented report of accelerated hypertension cured by removal of a tumor[30] indicates that caution should be used in too rigidly applying this dictum. Other features may serve to distinguish the two groups: the malignant hypertensive generally has a less pronounced hypokalemia (3.2 to 3.8 mEq per liter); alkalosis is less regularly present and less severe; and the patient with accelerated hypertension often has hyponatremia, a rare finding indeed in the patient with adenoma. Similarly, reports of clinical symptoms of muscle weakness and polyuria in the secondary group are scanty. It should be noted that malignant hypertension is not at all uncommon in the juvenile form of primary aldosteronism. This syndrome includes hypokalemia, alkalosis, and greatly increased aldosterone production, is more common in young males, may occur with hyponatremia, is associated with normal or hyperplastic adrenals, and is usually cured by total adrenalectomy.[31]

Patients with hypertension and *incidental potassium depletion* (e.g., individuals with chronic diarrhea) can generally be screened out by an adequate history and by the demonstration of low levels of urinary potassium. Certain patients with unilateral *renal arterial disease* have presented with hypokalemic alkalosis and elevated aldosterone-excretion rates, abnormalities which have responded to unilateral nephrectomy.[33] Although studies suggest that this combination is rare,[34] preoperative exclusion of renovascular hypertension seems desirable before adrenal exploration is carried out. *Potassium-wasting renal disease* in patients with hypertension rarely may serve as a source of confusion, but since most such cases represent aberrant forms of the Fanconi syndrome or instances of primary renal tubular acidosis, evidence for other tubular defects (hyperchloremic acidosis, hypophosphatemia, hypouricemia, renal glycosuria, etc.) will be demonstrable. Patients with *other forms of hyperadrenalism* (Cushing's disease, neoplasms with ACTH production) will exhibit increased urinary 17-hydroxysteroid- and 17-ketosteroid-excretion rates.

A small group of interesting patients with *benign hypertension,* the full biochemical spectrum of primary aldosteronism, but normal adrenal glands has been reported.[35] The hypertension has usually not responded to surgical intervention, but Conn has nonetheless recommended that subtotal adrenalectomy be performed at the time of diagnostic surgical procedure, since a small percentage may be cured but more importantly because the biochemical picture suggests in this group that the renin-angiotensin-aldosterone axis has been activated and malignant progression may be in the offing.[28] Further experience will be necessary to define the status of this group. Chronic ingestion of large amounts of *licorice* has been incriminated in the production of a syndrome of hypokalemic alkalosis and hypertension (but with low aldosterone secretion); it appears that glycyrrhizinic acid is the active ingredient responsible for the metabolic abnormalities.[36]

In the assessment of a patient for adrenal exploration for aldosteronoma, then, the following findings should probably be demonstrated: hypertension, hypokalemic alkalosis, renal potassium wasting, increased secretion and/or excretion of aldosterone, normal 17-hydroxysteroids and 17-ketosteroids; and normal or elevated serum-sodium concentration. Papilledema should be absent, and reasonable suspicion of surgically reversible renal vascular disease should be investigated. Ideally, the suspect should be removed from exposure to thiazide diuretics for several weeks and receive normal or high potassium and sodium intake prior to study. Application of such rigid criteria will, however, fail to identify the juvenile with aldosteronism and may result in inadequate therapy for the rare aldosteronoma which is producing malignant hypertension.

Therapy

Emphasis has been placed on precise diagnosis of the aldosterone-producing tumor, because surgical results have been so encouraging. Agreement among series has been general in that approximately 70 per cent of patients are cured of their hypertension, 25 per cent exhibit improvement, and only a few succumb or are not benefited by extirpation of the adenoma. In the vast majority of instances the tumor has been single, and in nearly all cases the pathology is confined to a single adrenal gland. Since the adenoma appears twice as frequently on the left, it should be explored first; if an adenoma is encountered, unilateral adrenalectomy should be performed and exploration of the contralateral adrenal deferred. Reexploration should be considered only if the metabolic abnormalities and hypertension persist; in this regard it should be noted that hypokalemic alkalosis generally disappears within 1 to 2 weeks, while the hypertension may require months to subside.

Medical considerations in the preoperative preparation of the patient are worthy of note. Attempts to replenish potassium in the patient should be made, employing oral potassium supplements until the serum-potassium level is within a normal range. Furthermore, since the status of the remaining adrenal gland is unknown, stress doses of glucocorticoids should be employed when removal of the adrenal is accomplished. Similarly, since atrophy of mineralocorticoid-producing adrenal tissue occurs with aldosteronoma, postoperative hypoaldosteronism is to be anticipated, and adequate sodium provision together with potassium restriction should be aimed at. Long-acting vasodepressor agents such as reserpine and guanethidine should of course be avoided for a minimum of 3 weeks prior to operation.

REFERENCES

1. Grundy, H. M., Simpson, S. A., and Tart, J. F.: Isolation of Highly Active Mineralocorticoid from Beef Extract, *Nature,* 169:795, 1952.
2. Mattox, V. R., et. al.: Properties of Sodium-retaining Principle from Beef Adrenal Extract, *J. Am. Chem. Soc.,* 75:4869, 1953.
3. Wettstein, A., et. al.: Synthesis of Aldosterone, *Proc. Int. Cong. Pure & Appl. Chem.,* July 22, 1955.
4. Conn, J. W.: Primary Aldosteronism, *J. Lab. & Clin. Med.,* 45:661, 1955.
5. Berger, E. Y., and Steele, J. M.: Suppression of Sodium Excretion by the Colon in Congestive Heart Failure and Cirrhosis of the Liver Demonstrated by the Use of Cation Exchange Resins, *J. Clin. Invest.,* 31:451, 1952.
6. Conn, J. W., and Louis, L. H.: Production of Endogenous "Salt-active" Corticoids as Reflected in Concentrations of Sodium and Chloride of Thermal Sweat, *J. Clin. Endocrinol.,* 10:12, 1950.
7. Simpson, S. A., and Tait, J. F.: Some Recent Advances in Methods of Isolation and the Physiology and Chemistry of Electrocortin, *Recent Progr. Hormone Res.,* 11:183, 1955.
8. Swingle, W. W., DeVanzo, J. P., Crossfield, H. C., Glowister, D., Osborne, M., and Wagle, G.: Effect of Various Adrenal Steroids on Internal Fluid and

Electrolyte Shifts of Fasted Adrenalectomized Dogs, *Proc. Soc. Exper. Biol. & Med.*, 99:75, 1958.

9. Spiers, R. S., Simpson, S. A., and Tait, J. F.: Certain Biological Activities of Crystalline Electrocortin, *Endocrinology*, 55:233, 1954.

10. Gaunt, R., Renzi, A. A., and Chart, J. J.: Aldosterone: A Review, *J. Clin. Endocrinol.*, 15:621, 1955.

11. Bartter, F. C.: The Role of Aldosterone in Normal Homeostasis and in Certain Disease States, *Metabolism*, 4:369, 1956.

12. Berliner, R. W., Kennedy, T. J., Jr., and Orloff, J.: Relationship between Acidification of Urine and Potassium Metabolism: Effect of Carbonic Anhydrase Inhibition on Potassium Excretion, *Am. J. Med.*, 11:274, 1951.

13. Ayres, P. J., Barlow, J., Garrod, O., Kellie, A. E., Tait, S. A. S., Tait, J. F., and Walker, G.: The Metabolism of 16-H³ Aldosterone in Man, in A. F. Muller and C. M. O'Connor (eds.), "International Symposium on Aldosterone," Little, Brown and Company, Boston, 1958, pp. 73–96.

14. Giroud, C. J. P., Stachenko, J., and Venning, E. H.: Secretion of Aldosterone by the Zona Glomerulosa of Rat Adrenal Glands, *Proc. Soc. Exper. Biol. & Med.*, 92:154, 1956.

15. Laragh, J. H., Ulick, S., Januszewicz, V., Deming, O. B., Kelly, W. C., and Lieberman, S.: Aldosterone Secretion and Primary and Malignant Hypertension, *J. Clin. Invest.*, 39:1091, 1960.

16. Ulick, S., Laragh, J. H., and Lieberman, S.: The Isolation of a Urinary Metabolite of Aldosterone and Its Use to Measure the Rate of Secretion of Aldosterone by the Adrenal Cortex of Man, *Tr. A. Am. Physicians*, 71:225, 1958.

17. Lane, N., and de Bodo, R. C.: Generalized Adrenocortical Atrophy in Hypophysectomized Dogs and Correlated Functional Studies, *Am. J. Physiol.*, 168:1, 1952.

18. Rauschkolb, E. W., Farrell, G. L., and Koletsky, S.: Aldosterone Secretion after Hypophysectomy, *Am. J. Physiol.*, 195:55, 1956.

19. Luetscher, J. A., Jr., and Axelrod, B. J.: Increased Aldosterone Output during Sodium Deprivation in Normal Men, *Proc. Soc. Exper. Biol. & Med.*, 87:656, 1954.

20. Bartter, F. C., Mills, I. H., Biglieri, E. G., and Delea, C.: Studies on the Control and Physiological Action of Aldosterone, *Recent Progr. in Hormone Res.*, 15:311, 1959.

21. Farrell, G. H.: The Physiological Factors Which Influence the Secretion of Aldosterone, *Recent Progr. Hormone Res.*, 15:275–297, 1959.

22. Carpenter, C. C. J., Davis, J. O., Ayers, C. R., Holman, J. E., and Bahn, R. C.: Evidence for Secretion of an Aldosterone-secreting Hormone by the Kidney, *J. Clin. Invest.*, 40:684, 1961.

23. Carpenter, C. C. J., Davis, J. O., and Ayers, C. R.: Renal Origin of an Aldosterone-stimulating Hormone in Dogs with Thoracic Caval Constriction and in Sodium-depleted Dogs, *J. Clin. Invest.*, 40:1466, 1961.

24. Carpenter, C. C. J., Davis, J. O., and Ayers, C. R.: Relation of Renin, Angiotensin II, and Experimental Renal Hypertension to Aldosterone Secretion, *J. Clin. Invest.*, 40:2026, 1961.

25. August, J. T., Nelson, D. H., and Thorn, G. W.: Response of Normal Subjects to Large Amounts of Aldosterone, *J. Clin. Invest.*, 37:1549, 1958.

26. August, J. T., and Nelson, D. H.: Adjustments to Aldosterone or Desoxycorticosterone Acetate-induced Sodium Retention in Patients with Addison's Disease, *J. Clin. Invest.*, 38:1964, 1959.

27. Conn, J. W.: Unpublished data.

28. Conn, J. W.: Aldosteronism in Man, part II, *J.A.M.A.*, 183:169, 1963.

29. Relman, A. S., and Schwartz, W. B.: The Kidney in Potassium Depletion, *Am. J. Med.*, 24:764, 1958.

30. Kaplan, N. M.: Primary Aldosteronism with Malignant Hypertension, *New England J. Med.*, 269:1282, 1963.

31. Conn, J. W.: Aldosteronism and Hypertension: Primary Aldosteronism versus Hypertensive Disease with Secondary Aldosteronism, *Arch. Int. Med.*, 107:813, 1961.

32. Venning, E. H., et. al.: Effect of Chlorothiazide upon Aldosterone Excretion and Sodium and Potassium Balance in Essential Hypertension, *J. Lab. & Clin. Med.*, 60:79, 1962.

33. Laidlaw, J. C., Yendt, E. R., and Gornall, A. G.: Hypertension Caused by Renal Artery Occlusion Simulating Primary Aldosteronism, *Metabolism*, 9:612, 1960.

34. Samblii, M. P., Levitan, B. A., Beck, J. C., and Venning, E. H.: The Rate of Aldosterone Secretion in Hypertensive Patients with Demonstrable Renal Artery Stenosis, *Metabolism*, 12:498, 1963.

35. Hill, S. R., Jr., et al.: Studies in Man on Hyper- and Hypoaldosteronism, *A.M.A. Arch. Int. Med.*, 104:982, 1959.

36. Lois, L. H., and Conn, J. W.: Preparation of Glycyrrhizinic Acid, Electrolyte-active Principle of Licorice: Its Effect upon Metabolism and upon Pituitary-adrenal Function in Man, *J. Lab. & Clin. Med.*, 47:20, 1956.

45 TREATMENT OF HYPERTENSION

Edward S. Orgain, M.D.

PRIMARY ARTERIAL (ESSENTIAL) HYPERTENSION

Primary arterial (essential) hypertension is a vascular disorder of complex causation.[1-3] Neurogenic, endocrine, renal, vascular, hormonal, and probably other as yet unidentified mechanisms contribute components which vary in magnitude in different individuals. Since the precise cause of primary hypertensive vascular disease is unknown and the underlying factors numerous, present-day treatment is empiric and nonspecific. Specific and curative therapy will come only when the cause of hypertensive disease is discovered or the importance of each contributing factor is defined.

There is no full agreement among physicians as to what constitutes normal as contrasted to elevated blood pressure, but most will agree that hypertension is present when blood pressure rises above 150 mm Hg systolic and 100 diastolic. The importance of maintaining a normal blood pressure centers upon the following considerations:

1. Insurance statistics[4-6] have amply demonstrated that mortality figures rise and life span is shortened with minimal increments in either systolic or diastolic pressure, and particularly when both are elevated.

2. Mortality in hypertension results primarily from both mechanical factors and vascular complications affecting the brain, heart, and kidney.[7]

3. Arteriosclerosis, although a separate entity, is closely associated with, and accelerated by, the appearance of hypertension;[8,9] the risk for the development of coronary heart disease is increased appreciably in hypertensive individuals.[10]

4. Morbidity and mortality in severe hypertensive states have been reduced by both medical [11-16] and surgical [17] measures.

5. Prolonged medical control of recumbent diastolic blood pressure levels in severe hypertensive patients to levels below 95 mm Hg for periods of 2 to 9 years may reverse the hypertensive process, reset the controlling mechanisms, and allow discontinuance of most or all medication without return of hypertension.[18]

The idealistic aim in therapy, therefore, is to control blood pressure, both systolic and diastolic, at strictly normal levels 24 hr each day in both recumbent and standing positions, and to prevent the onset and progression of vascular damage.

There is little general agreement as to when treatment for hypertension should be instituted.[19-22] Hypertension may be benign, particularly in women, and run a course of 20 years, during three-fourths of which they are asymptomatic.[23] In some patients life expectancy is unaltered and without hypertensive complications.[24] However, follow-up studies of hypertensive patients over a period of 5 or more years indicate a significant mortality of 11 to 22 per cent even in grade I severity groups, with rising mortality rates paralleling each increment in grade severity of hypertensive disease as determined by levels of diastolic pressure and

by changes in brain, fundi, heart, and kidney.[25-28] Although mortality has been reduced by therapy in severe hypertensive states, insufficient time has elapsed to judge the effectiveness of newer drugs in the milder forms of hypertension, either upon the prevention of vascular disease or upon ultimate mortality. Optimism has been expressed that survival time has been extended even for the less severe forms of hypertension.[13,29]

Because of these considerations, some clinicians will not treat mere "figures" during the long asymptomatic phase of benign hypertension, since they regard the value of such therapy as unproved, annoying because of side effects, injurious because of toxic reactions, and expensive because repetitive observations are needed. Opinion regarding the importance of controlling the diastolic blood pressure is changing.[18] Therefore it would appear wise to watch closely those patients whose resting blood pressures repeatedly exceed 140/90 mm Hg and to begin active treatment when the resting diastolic pressure is consistently above 110 mm Hg. The presence of several cardinal prognostic features such as conspicuous family history of hypertension, the youth of the patient, the patient's being male, rapid progression of diastolic pressure, and tissue alterations in the brain, fundi, heart, and kidney, predicates the need of more aggressive treatment at an earlier period in the course of hypertensive disease.

Treatment

The necessity for treating the patient as a whole individual and not merely his blood pressure deserves full emphasis. It is the primary duty of the physician to provide for the patient a regimen of treatment especially tailored to his needs and to his abilities to follow it. Although many patients suffering from hypertension have personality problems (e.g., repressed hostility, aggression and self-assertion, obsessive-compulsive trends, feelings of inadequacy and tension),[30] which make them unusually susceptible to emotional stresses in their environment and in turn create marked fluctuations in blood pressure, detailed psychiatric therapy is only rarely indicated or needed. The average physician can accomplish adequate psychotherapy employing common sense methods devoted to understanding the patient and his problems, allaying his fears, tensions, and anxieties, and repleting his mental and physical reserves. A long-term program must be arranged in which rest, recreation, vacation periods, and work loads are all properly balanced. However, the hypertensive process with its concomitant vascular and tissue changes often demands vigorous attack with every means at one's disposal including rest, diet, drugs, and occasionally sympathectomy.

Dietary Therapy

Table 45-1 presents a variety of dietary programs which have been prescribed for hyperten-

Table 45-1. DIETARY THERAPY

1. Low-caloric diet
2. Low-fat (40–50 Gm) diet
3. Low-protein (20–40 Gm) diet
4. Low-sodium (200–500 mg) diet
5. Low-fat, low-protein, low-sodium diet
6. Low-sodium, low-protein, low-fat, high-carbohydrate, restricted-fluid regimen (Kempner rice-fruit diet)

sive patients according to specific indications. Insurance statistics emphasize the heavy prognostic label carried by obesity,[31] so that weight reduction by simple caloric restriction is universally desirable in the obese patient. Low-fat diets restricted to levels of 40 to 50 Gm per day are prescribed for those who have high blood-cholesterol levels or obvious atherosclerotic disease. When renal disease accompanied by albuminuria, impaired function, and azotemia complicates hypertension, protein should be restricted to 20 to 40 Gm per day. There is little question that the sodium ion plays an important role in hypertension[32] and that sodium restriction to levels of 200 to 500 mg per day may aid in reducing blood pressure.[33–35] The exact mechanisms involved in lowering of blood pressure by sodium restriction are not yet defined. Reduction in extravascular fluid and circulating plasma volumes as well as alterations of blood vessel reactivity have been proposed. Low-sodium diets favor the development of both orthostatic hypotension and postural syncope; particular caution is suggested when ganglionic blocking agents are exhibited concurrently. The introduction of diuretic agents has decreased the necessity for rigid sodium restriction below 1 Gm per day except in severe hypertensive states. Cation-exchange resins possess limited capacity to bind sodium[36] and have been discarded for this purpose. Combinations of low-fat, low-protein and low-sodium diets are reserved for more severe forms of hypertension associated with tissue damage, particularly renal disease, azotemia, retinopathy, and heart failure. The rigid or modified rice-fruit dietary regimen of Kempner,[34] although most difficult for patients to endure for extended periods, finds special usefulness in the initial several weeks of therapy for those who present extensive retinopathy (hemorrhages, exudates, papilledema) and variable degrees of renal failure. Because patients who have renal insufficiency may be salt losers, careful observations

of the blood-electrolyte pattern must be maintained.[37] As the patient's condition improves and hypertension is controlled, rapid adjustment to a more normal and tolerable diet is made.

Drug Therapy

The ideal drug for widespread application to large groups of hypertensive patients must be effective in controlling the systolic and diastolic blood pressure, with the patient standing and recumbent, when administered orally, yet be free of serious toxic or undesirable effects. No drug is available at present which fulfills these requirements. Most of the compounds on the extensive list of those utilized in the past have been discarded for lack of effective hypotensive action. The sedative and tranquilizing drugs, with the recent addition of mebutamate, remain useful for the tense, anxious patient with fluctuating blood pressure levels. The long-acting nitrates, mannitol hexanitrate, erythrol tetranitrate, etc., and the veratrum viride alkaloids are little used because side effects commonly precede and preclude effective lowering of blood pressure.[38] Potassium thiocyanate may control intractable headache in some hypertensive subjects when other drugs are ineffective or undesirable because of varied reactions. During the past two decades the continuous production of new and effective compounds having different pharmacologic actions has revolutionized the treatment of hypertension. These compounds, introduced for clinical trial in this approximate order, comprise the alpha-adrenergic blocking agents, ganglionic blocking agents, hydralazine, *Rauwolfia* and its derivitives, certain diuretics, and adrenergic neuronal blocking agents such as guanethidine, methyl dopa, and monoamine oxidase inhibitors.

Alpha-adrenergic Blocking Agents. Such agents

Table 45-2. ALPHA-ADRENERGIC BLOCKING AGENTS:

1. Tolazoline hydrochloride (Priscoline)
2. Phenoxybenzamine hydrochloride (Dibenzyline)
3. Piperoxan hydrochloride (Benzodioxane)
4. Phentolamine hydrochloride (Regitine)

act at the peripheral receptor areas to block the action of circulating adrenergic hormones, epinephrine and norepinephrine, and sympathetic nervous system stimulation (see Chap. 68). These drugs (Table 45-2) are impractical for the treatment of hypertension, because they tend to induce headache, nausea, vomiting, and tachycardia before satisfactory blood pressure reduction is achieved.

Ganglionic Blocking Agents. These drugs (Table 45-3) produce blockade of both sympathetic and parasympathetic ganglions.[39,40] Pharmacodynamically

Table 45-3. GANGLIONIC BLOCKING AGENTS:

I. Quaternary ammonium compounds
  A. Hexamethonium chloride (Methium)
    1. Oral, 125 mg–1 Gm 4–6 times daily
    2. Parenteral, 2–50 mg IM or IV every 4–6 hr
  B. Pentolinium tartrate (Ansolysen)
    1. Oral, 10–200 mg 4–6 times daily
    2. Parenteral, 1–30 mg IM or IV every 4–6 hr
  C. Chlorisondamine chloride (Ecolid)
    1. Oral, 25–100 mg 1–2 times daily
  D. Trimethidinium methosulfate (Ostensin)
    1. Oral, 10–90 mg 2–3 times daily

II. Tertiary amines
  A. Pempidine bitartrate (Perolysen)
    1. Oral, 2.5–15 mg 3–5 times daily
    2. Parenteral, 1–5 mg IV every 2–6 hr

III. Secondary amines
  A. Mecamylamine hydrochloride (Inversine)
    1. Oral, 2.5–20 mg 3–4 times daily

they lower peripheral vascular resistance, cardiac output, venous pressure, and renal blood flow as blood pressure falls. Although ganglion blockade is always incomplete, these compounds remain the most potent and the most difficult of all the antihypertensive agents to use in clinical practice. Wide fluctuations between recumbent hypertension and postural hypotension are common and frequently prevent drug dosage sufficient to lower supine blood pressure satisfactorily. Unpleasant reactions to these compounds consist principally of weakness, cycloplegia, severe constipation progressing to ileus, bladder atony, impotence, and orthostatic hypotension leading to syncope. Postural fall in blood pressure is enhanced greatly by sodium restriction and by diuretic agents. Fever, hot weather, alcohol, or even a large meal also facilitate orthostatic effects. Weakness and syncope may occur without warning. Constipation is not easily controlled by cathartics, Prostigmine methylsulfate, or pilocarpine, and impotence in young males is not satisfactorily relieved by omission of single or multiple doses of drug before contemplated intercourse.

Excessive hypotension presents the hazards of irreversible uremia in renal disease, and arterial thromboses in the cerebral and coronary circulations, especially in older subjects. These drugs should not be abruptly withdrawn from the therapy of severe diastolic hypertension, since a potentially fatal hypertensive rebound may ensue. Induction of peripheral circulatory stasis and decrease in venous pressure by blocking agents immediately suggest their emergency use parenterally to control acute pulmonary edema (Fig. 45-1).

Each of the ganglionic blocking agents possesses full potency of action when given in sufficient dosage. Hexamethonium is variable in its absorp-

tion from the intestine and difficult to regulate.[41] Chlorisondamine[42] possesses a long duration of action (12 to 24 hr), and when side effects occur, they tend to persist for hours, requiring prolonged bed rest. Mecamylamine[43,44] is uniformly absorbed and the best absorbed of the blocking agents, a characteristic which often adds to its undesirable effects. Tremors, disorders of speech, and mental aberrations have been noted on large doses of mecamylamine.[40,45] Pentolinium[46-48] is very probably the simplest of these compounds to use in oral doses of 10 to 200 mg four to six times daily. Similar enthusiasm is expressed for pempidine,[49] because of its rapid absorption and excretion. Trimethidinium[50] is also potent but presents no distinct advantages.

Ganglionic blocking agents are not satisfactory drugs for hypertension when prescribed alone. Under continued administration tolerance commonly develops perhaps more to the quaternary ammonium group than to the secondary and tertiary amines. Currently, they possess particular utility in severe hypertensive states for combination with other drugs. The physician should obtain thorough familiarity with at least one compound which he may administer with full confidence, both orally and parenterally.

Hydralazine Hydrochloride (Apresoline Hydrochloride). Hydralazine[51-53] possesses complex actions including peripheral vasodilatation, central depression of vasoconstrictor reflexes, adrenergic inhibition, and neutralization of pressor substances. Its hemodynamic effects result in decreased peripheral vascular resistance but elevated heart rate, stroke volume, and cardiac output and increase in renal, coronary, and hepatic circulations.

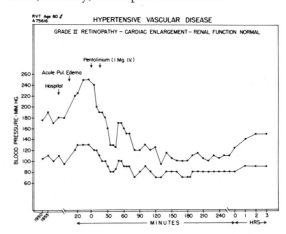

Fig. 45-1. The striking effect on recumbent blood pressure of pentolinium given intravenously for acute pulmonary edema. The drug was considered to be lifesaving in this hypertensive patient, who previously had suffered a myocardial infarction.

This drug should be titrated gradually, beginning with an oral dose of 10 mg four times daily and increasing by 10 to 25 mg per dose, rarely exceeding a total of 200 mg per day except for short periods. It also may be administered parenterally, intramuscularly, or intravenously every 4 hr, in doses of 5.0 to 20 mg with increments depending upon blood pressure response. Small doses often produce mild headache, nasal congestion, tachycardia, nausea, vomiting, numbness, and tingling, which tend to diminish as the drug is continued.

Initially, when larger doses, 300 to 400 mg or more, of the drug were administered daily for prolonged periods, a variety of toxic reactions[54,55] were observed, including fever, pancytopenia, acute psychoses, gastrointestinal bleeding, and a collagenlike illness. In its milder form the condition resembles acute rheumatoid arthritis which subsides spontaneously upon withdrawal of the drug. In more severe form the illness may simulate acute systemic lupus erythematosus (LE) in whole or in part by the presentation of fever, arthralgia, pleurisy, pericarditis with or without effusion, and LE cells in peripheral blood.[55] This reaction may require steroid therapy for its resolution, or it may result in long-term disability[56] and even death.[57] In a sensitive patient even small doses, 10 mg four times daily, of hydralazine will induce recurrence of arthritis or reappearance of LE cells. Serious toxicity has resulted predominantly when drug dosage has exceeded 200 mg per day over a period of several months.

Because hydralazine produces cardiac stimulation, its administration should proceed with appropriate caution in patients who exhibit evidence of coronary arteriosclerosis or congestive heart failure, either overt or impending. When used alone its antihypertensive qualities are weak and limited. Its principal value lies in its ability to potentiate the effects of other drugs, particularly reserpine and the anticholinergic compounds.

Rauwolfia Serpentina Compounds. The whole root of *Rauwolfia serpentina*, used in India for many years, was introduced for the treatment of hypertension in 1952.[58] The compounds it contains deplete the brain, the hypothalamus, and the postganglionic sympathetic fibers of serotonin and catecholamine stores[59,60] and thus reduce effective sympathetic nervous system activity. There is little difference in the antihypertensive effects of the powdered whole root or its derivatives[61] when equivalent doses are given, e.g., whole root 100 to 200 mg, alseroxylon fraction 2.0 to 4.0 mg, and alkaloid 0.25 to 0.5 mg (Table 45-4). Deseripidine perhaps produces fewer side effects than reserpine. Reserpine is more effective than syrosingopine but

Table 45-4. RAUWOLFIA SERPENTINA COMPOUNDS

1. Powdered whole root: Raudixin, 50–100 mg, once or twice daily
2. Alseroxylon fraction: Rauwiloid, 2.0–4.0 mg, once or twice daily
3. Alkaloids: 0.25–0.75 mg, once or twice daily
   a. Reserpine (Serpasil, etc.)
   b. Rescinnamine (Moderil)
   c. Deserpidine (Harmonyl)
4. Synthetic analog: syrosingopine (Singoserp) 0.25–1.0 mg, 3–4 times daily

creates more undesirable central nervous system symptoms.[62] Although tranquilizing and mildly sedative in action, these compounds produce all too frequently unpleasant symptoms of fatigue, loss of energy, nasal congestion, drowsiness, dreams, nightmares, and weight gain. Bradycardia is a useful parasympathomimetic expression of the drug, whereas stimulation of peptic ulcer, colitis, and diarrhea is not. It is important to watch for early signs of parkinsonism or symptoms of mild anxiety, jitteriness, and depression. Continued *Rauwolfia* administration after symptoms develop may result in severe depression necessitating shock therapy for relief.[63] When reserpine is given alone in oral form, 0.25 to 0.75 mg twice daily, its action is usually mild, requiring several weeks to develop fully. Increments in the dosage of reserpine above 1.5 mg per day generally increase symptoms without contributing additional hypotensive effects. Occasional striking effects result from extremely small oral doses, 0.125 to 0.25 mg per day. Parenterally the intramuscular injection of 1.0 to 3.0 mg usually creates a good hypotensive response in 1 to 3 hr, an effect which may last 6 to 24 hr in individual patients. This parenteral effect of reserpine is particularly useful in acute hypertensive states and in those patients unable to ingest oral medication. The *Rauwolfia* compounds should not be administered to patients who already exhibit fatigue states, anxiety, agitation, depression, or an active peptic ulcer. Reactivation of peptic ulcer may be avoided by the use of antispasmodics and liberal ingestion of antacids.

Reserpine seems most suitable for the mildly hypertensive patient suffering from tension, tachycardia, and angina pectoris. It is quite effective when used in combination with other drugs (Fig. 45-2). Unpleasant symptoms may be ameliorated, and reduced dosage of other concurrent hypotensive agents may be permitted. Patients on *Rauwolfia* therapy seem to tolerate anesthesia and operation satisfactorily and at least as well as hypertensive patients not treated with *Rauwolfia*. When blood pressure falls during surgery in a patient receiving *Rauwolfia*, it is likely to be due to the usual causes such as blood loss, speed of anesthetic induction, surgical manipulation, position change, and excessive amounts of anesthetic agents.[64]

Diuretic Compounds (see Chap. 68). The introduction of the benzothiadiazine (thiazide) diuretic compounds in 1957 created a welcome addition to the therapeutic armamentarium of hypertension.[65] The diuretic compounds now available comprise four separate chemical groups, benzothiadiazine (thiazide), phthalimidine (chlorthalidone), quinazoline (quinethazone), and aldosterone antagonist (spironolactone) (Table 45-5). Although the mech-

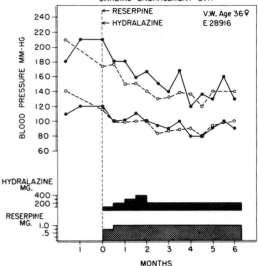

Fig. 45-2. The often satisfactory decline in blood pressure which results from the simple combination of reserpine and hydralazine.

Table 45-5. DIURETIC COMPOUNDS

Generic name	Trademarked name	Dose, mg*
Benzothiadiazine (thiazides):		
Benzthiazide	Exna	50
Benzydroflumethiazide	Naturetin	5.0
Chlorothiazide	Diuril	500
Cyclothiazide	Anhydron	2.5
Hydrochlorothiazide	Esidrix	50
Hydrochlorothiazide	Hydrodiuril	50
Hydrochlorothiazide	Oretic	50
Hydroflumethiazide	Saluron	50
Methyclothiazide	Enduron	2.5
Polythiazide	Renese	2.0
Trichlormethiazide	Metahydrin	2.0
Trichlormethiazide	Naqua	2.0
Phthalimidine:		
Chlorthalidone	Hygroton	100
Quinazoline:		
Quinethazone	Hydromox	50
Aldosterone inhibitor:		
Spironolactone	Aldactone A	25

* For full therapeutic effect these diuretic compounds may be given as follows: (1) thiazides, one or two tablets twice daily; (2) chlorthalidone, 50–100 mg twice daily; (3) quinethazone, 50 mg, one or two tablets daily, and (4) spironolactone, 25 mg 2 to 4 times daily. The diuretic drugs have a maximum dosage range, usually about two to four tablets of a standard dose per day, beyond which further diuretic effects are not obtained. Large doses administered for prolonged periods create electrolyte deficiencies.

anism of hypotensive action is not clearly defined, the thiazide compounds possess powerful diuretic and saluretic activity,[66] apparently decreasing tubular reabsorption of water, sodium, chloride, and potassium, and to a lesser extent bicarbonate. Initial hypotensive effects correlate with diminished blood volume; late effects,[67] evident without disturbance in fluid volumes or blood-electrolyte patterns, are suggestively ascribed to decreased blood vessel reactivity and altered sodium-ion gradients.[51] The thiazide drugs vary in dosage and duration of action, but there is no outstanding superiority of one drug over another either in terms of potency[68] or more favorable sodium/potassium excretion ratios when conventional doses of each drug are prescribed. The electrolyte pattern of the blood must be watched carefully for azotemia, hyponatremia, hypochloremia, hypokalemia, hyperuricemia, and hyperglycemia, particularly when large doses of drug are given for prolonged periods. Salt depletion does not usually occur unless dietary sodium is concomitantly restricted or significant decrease in renal function is present.

The diuretic agents are simple to use and generally well tolerated but may cause dizziness, nausea, weakness, paresthesias, fatigue, gastric irritation, and muscular cramps. Elevation of blood uric acid and glucose may precipitate clinical gout, renal colic, and overt diabetes mellitus.[69] Hyperuricemia can be reversed by uricosuric agents such as probenecid. Hypersensitivity reactions, skin rashes, purpura, thrombocytopenia, leukopenia, agranulocytosis, jaundice, and pancreatitis have rarely occurred.[69]

Chlorthalidone[70] is a potent diuretic drug having the prolonged duration of action of 48 hr as compared to 12 to 24 hr for various thiazide compounds. After doses of 100 to 200 mg per day mild hypokalemia is more often observed than with the thiazides. When sensitivity reactions (e.g., purpura) to a thiazide occur, chlorthalidone, a compound of different chemical structure, may be substituted to avoid interruption of the antihypertensive program.

Diazoxide, which is structurally similar to chlorothiazide, paradoxically causes sodium and water retention yet reduces blood pressure. Orally the drug has produced diabetes mellitus along with other undesirable reactions and has been discarded for clinical use. Administration of the drug, 300 mg rapidly intravenously, produces an immediate hypotensive response in 1 to 2 min which lasts for 4 to 5 hr. Since repetitive injections may be given without undesirable effects, the drug might be useful in acute hypertensive states.[71]

The diuretic drugs are generally useful and effective even when employed alone. Their most valuable characteristic, the potentiation of the action of other drugs, usually permits dose reduction or even discontinuance of one drug when several hypotensive compounds are administered simultaneously. Postural collapse is common when a diuretic is added to a ganglionic blocking agent, or guanethidine, or is administered to a sympathectomized patient. Care must be taken to avoid digitalis intoxication secondary to excessive potassium loss in any patient and electrolyte depletion, which is observed more often in renal disease. Renal insufficiency is generally a contraindication to diuretic therapy.

The aldosterone antagonists (spironolactone), like the thiazides, possess both diuretic and antihypertensive actions dependent upon blocking the renal-sodium-retaining action of aldosterone. When spironolactone is administered in doses of 25 mg two to four times daily, occasional drowsiness is noted, but there are few other side effects, and only rarely is hyperkalemia encountered. Unlike the thiazides, with which it forms a useful hypotensive combination, it does not cause hypokalemia, digitalis intoxication, gout, or diabetes.[72] When used alone for hypertension its effects are variable.[72,73]

Adrenergic Neuronal Blocking Agents. Drugs such as guanethidine sulfate (Ismelin) inhibit

Biosynthesis of Norepinephrine and Serotonin

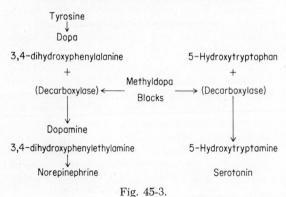

Fig. 45-3.

sympathetic activity at the peripheral nerve terminals by mechanisms involving the release, and depletion of adrenergic affector substances.[74] A "chemical sympathectomy" is produced which avoids the annoying symptoms resulting from parasympathetic blockade. Following intravenous administration, blood pressure rises temporarily, suggesting initial release of norepinephrine stores.[75] For ambulatory patients,[76,77] guanethidine is administered orally beginning with 10 mg once or twice daily, increasing to a total of 400 mg per day; gradual titration to therapeutic levels is mandatory, because significant orthostatic hypotension, particularly when the patient first arises in the morning, often results with little effect on recumbent blood pressure. Responses in blood pressure are noted at variable dosage levels independent of the severity of the hypertension.[76,77] Similarly, such unpleasant symptoms as dizziness, fainting, weakness, fatigue, abdominal discomfort, nausea, and loss of ejaculation are not strictly dose-related.

Because postural hypotension is regularly created, caution is observed when cerebral or coronary arteriosclerosis or renal disease is evident. In view of its marked orthostatic effects upon blood pressure and the incidence of its disagreeable effects, guanethidine would appear to have definite but limited utility in the treatment of the severely hypertensive patient.[76,78] Potentiation of its action is noted from the addition of either diuretic compounds or hydralazine.[79]

Bretylium tosylate (Darenthin),[80] introduced concurrently with guanethidine, blocks sympathetic nervous system activity. The drug has not demonstrated particular potency, nor is its action augmented by other compounds, including anticholinergics, *Rauwolfia*, and thiazides. It causes significant undesirable effects such as orthostatic hypotension, exertional syncope, parotid gland and chest pain, epigastric distress, nasal stuffiness, diarrhea, and weakness. Tolerance to the drug develops as treatment continues. Bretylium tosylate now has been discarded as an antihypertensive compound.

Methyldopa (Aldomet). This is a compound capable of blocking the decarboxylase enzyme system which converts dopa (3, 4-dihydroxyphenylalanine) to dopamine (3, 4-dihydroxyphenylethylamine),[81] the immediate precursor of norepinephrine, and to 5-hydroxytryptophan, the precursor of serotonin (Fig. 45-3). Activity of methyldopa in hypertension, which lies in the levorotary isomer, is not correlated with degree of decarboxylase inhibition and may be mediated by amine metabolites of the compound.[82] The exact mechanism of action is unknown, but sympathetic blockade, centrally or peripherally, reduced peripheral arteriolar resistance, and depletion of tissue sores of catecholamine have been suggested. [51] Hemodynamically there is little change in cardiac output, but renal blood flow may be normal or increased.[83]

Methyldopa is customarily prescribed orally, 250 mg three or four times daily increasing to 500 mg four times daily after several weeks. If satisfactory lowering of the blood pressure is not achieved, an oral diuretic is added to the regimen. The diuretic greatly enhances the hypotensive effects of methyldopa and avoids increasing symptoms which appear when larger daily doses, 3.0 to 4.0 Gm, of the drug are given. Intravenous administration of 250 mg to 1.0 Gm has a pronounced hypotensive effect after a delay of 1 to 3 hr, but the effect may last 12 to 18 hr.[84,85] Symptoms commonly encountered in ambulatory patients include dry mouth and sedation, with less frequent gastrointestinal irritation, weakness, depression, headache, arthralgia, weight gain, and acute febrile episodes with chills and aching. Alterations in liver function tests,[85,86] including bromsulphalein excretion, thymol turbidity, cephalin flocculation, phosphatase, lactic dehydrogenase (LDH), and glutamic transaminase (SGOT), have been observed, but the exact incidence is unknown. Hepatic function tests and routine blood counts should be performed initially and repeated at 8-week periods during therapy. The appearance of a febrile episode demands an immediate check by these tests. This drug is contraindicated in depressive states and in liver disease. Caution has been suggested in the presence of angina pectoris or congestive heart failure.[85]

Hypotensive effects of the drug, mild in the average patients, somewhat greater in orthostatic than in recumbent position, are appreciably increased by the addition of diuretic agents (Fig. 45-4). Enthusiasm has been expressed for its use in patients who exhibit mild to malignant hypertension and even renal insufficiency.[83,85,87]

Monoamine Oxidase Inhibitors. The monoamine

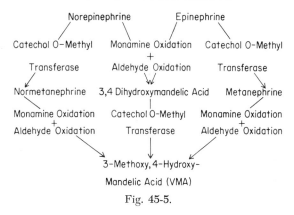

Degradation of Catecholamines

Fig. 45-5.

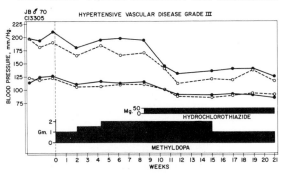

Fig. 45-4. The little effect from oral methyldopa administered alone. An excellent blood pressure response followed the addition of hydrochlorothiazide and permitted reduction in the dose of methyldopa.

oxidase inhibitors have been used primarily as mood elevators for depressive states. Recently, interest has been aroused in their use for hypertension.[88,89] These compounds oppose the degradation of catecholamines (Fig. 45-5). The exact mode of antihypertensive action is unknown, but interference with release of norepinephrine at the neuroeffector junction has been suggested. Neither central depression of sympathetic activity nor adrenergic blockade is regarded as important. Perhaps the monoamine oxidase inhibitors decrease blood pressure by sympathetic ganglion blockade.[90] This group includes both hydrazine and nonhydrazine derivatives.

A serious caution in the use of monoamine oxidase inhibitors is indicated in the light of unequivocal evidence that when they are used in combination with other drugs and unsuspected constituents of diet, extremely severe hypertensive and hyperthermic crises can develop.[91,92] Fatal intracranial hemorrhage and pulmonary edema have been reported. Cheddar cheese, and drugs such as amphetamines have caused hypertensive crises. Meperidine hydrochloride (Demerol hydrochloride) may induce hypotensive crises. Hyperthermic crises may occur when imipramine hydrochloride (Tofranil) and similar drugs are given to patients recieving monoamine oxidose inhibitors. In the light of rapidly accumulating evidence in this field, the use of monoamine oxidase inhibitors for the treatment of hypertension at the present time offers more risks than advantages and should be avoided until more is known of the possible complications.

Drug Combinations. In the management of mild to moderate grades of hypertensive disease, single compounds such as a *Rauwolfia* derivative or a diuretic administered alone may result in normotension. For the more severe hypertensive states it is fundamental to attack the hypertensive mechanisms at multiple sites using various combinations of several drugs, each possessing different pharmacologic actions. Each drug should be administered as a separate tablet and titrated gradually to nearly maximally tolerated doses before other drugs are added. When satisfactory hypotensive response is achieved or when significant side effects occur, the dose of one drug or more may be reduced or discontinued. Smaller yet effective doses of several drugs can be used in combination, and thus unpleasant or serious reactions may be reduced or abolished. Until the effective and tolerated dose of each drug is established, multiple drugs in a single tablet or capsule should not be prescribed, because the dose of one ingredient cannot be altered without changing the dose of others in the combination.

The physician must avoid the prevalent temptation of surrendering too easily or switching from one drug to another before the effectiveness or tolerance of each prescribed drug is firmly established. Often symptoms, unpleasant at first, gradually diminish and disappear as subjective tolerance develops without appreciable change in drug dosage.

Excellent results have been achieved with various combinations of drugs, but the most useful and effective one has not yet been established for all or most hypertensive patients[93-96] (Table 45-6).

Table 45-6. DRUG COMBINATIONS

1. Diuretic
   Rauwolfia   } plus { Guanethidine
   Hydralazine   or
                              Ganglionic blocking
                                 agent

2. Guanethidine   plus { Diuretic
                            Hydralazine

3. Ganglionic blocking   { *Rauwolfia*
       agent   } plus   { Diuretic
                                 { Hydralazine

4. Methyldopa   plus   Diuretic

When contemplating drugs for use in combination, it is well to remember that the *Rauwolfia* derivatives often ameliorate the unpleasant symptoms from, and reinforce the hypotensive activity of, other drugs, e.g., diuretics, hydralazine, and ganglionic blocking agents. The oral diuretics have enhanced the hypotensive activity of each antihypertensive compound with which they have been combined, e.g., *Rauwolfia*, hydralazine, guanethidine, ganglionic blocking agents, methyldopa, and pargyline. Because of salt loss such enhancement, particularly with guanethidine and the ganglionic blocking agents, may be entirely orthostatic and result in postural syncope. This reaction must be anticipated to prevent potentially tragic

injury. Hydralazine hydrochloride has augmented the effects of *Rauwolfia*, diuretics, anticholinergics, and guanethidine. Since *Rauwolfia* compounds and guanethidine both deplete the peripheral stores of catecholamine, this combination is illogical.

For most hypertensive individuals it is simpler to begin therapy with an oral diuretic agent, adding first a *Rauwolfia* compound and later hydralazine hydrochloride if needed. This combination is well tolerated and usually effective. Guanethidine and ganglionic blocking agents drugs are rarely necessary in mild to moderate grades of hypertension, groups I and II, and should be added to drug programs last. For patients suffering from renal disease, hydralazine and methyldopa are potentially the drugs of choice. However, in more severe hypertensive states, when it appears from the outset that intensive therapy will be needed for good blood pressure control, treatment may be initiated with guanethidine; an oral diuretic and then hydralazine can be added by careful titration. If guanethidine is poorly tolerated, a ganglionic blocking agent such as pentolinium may be substituted adding *Rauwolfia*, a diuretic, and hydralazine in this or similar sequence.

The activity of methyldopa, reportedly useful in all grades of hypertension from mild to malignant, with and without renal insufficiency, is certainly augmented by the addition of oral diuretics. Further studies of possible hepatic toxicity are needed before accepting this simple drug combination for widespread application to hypertensive patients. Satisfactory observations on the effects of methyldopa employed in conjunction with *Rauwolfia*, guanethidine, hydralazine, and the ganglionic blocking agents are not yet available.

Patients presenting mild to moderate hypertension, groups I and II, offer no therapeutic difficulties in blood pressure control unless they exhibit multiple drug sensitivities, which fortunately plague only a few individuals. However, patients suffering from the advanced or accelerated phases of hypertension, groups III and IV, are often ill. Prognosis depends to a large extent upon integrity of renal function. When moderate azotemia is present (nonprotein nitrogen above 60 mg per 100 ml of plasma) due to renal failure, the survival time is generally brief.[97] Lowering of blood pressure may produce further renal impairment and a rising blood-nitrogen level.[98] Therapeutic programs are best initiated in the hospital, where rigid control of diet and drugs is monitored by taking blood pressure every few hours with the patient recumbent and standing. When oral medication seems momentarily contraindicated because of nausea, vomiting, renal insufficiency, or irregular drug absorption or when immediate action seems urgently needed, parenteral

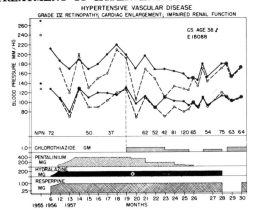

Fig. 45-6. This case, in which the patient was treated entirely as an outpatient, emphasizes the need of extreme care in drug titration when renal insufficiency is present. Although chlorothiazide may have contributed, the fluctuations in NPN were related primarily to excessive lowering of both recumbent and standing blood pressure levels.

administration of the ganglionic blocking agents, *Rauwolfia*, or methyldopa, is particularly desirable along with low-sodium, low-protein, or modified rice-fruit diet for short periods. As the patient's condition permits, drugs are administered orally, and parenteral therapy is withdrawn. Blood pressure should be restored toward normal gradually, since abrupt falls in blood pressure may lead to collapse, irreversible shock, coma, and uremia (Fig. 45-6). Retinopathy, including hemorrhages, exudates, and papilledema, can regress quickly when blood pressure is lowered by drugs and by rigid dietary restriction. It should be emphasized that oral diuretics may lead rapidly to electrolyte depletion when sodium is restricted to 500 mg per day or below, especially when renal function is impaired. Rapid adjustments in diet and drugs after good blood pressure control then may allow even the severe hypertensive patient to delete from his program all save mild salt restriction and one or two antihypertensive drugs.

Treatment regimens should be individualized to each patient's needs and to his abilities to follow various physical, dietary, and drug programs. A simple outline of therapeutic suggestions which are relevant to varying degrees of severity of hypertension is presented in Table 45-7.

Hypertensive Emergencies. As one of many medical emergencies, acute hypertensive crises[98-100] may arise and present an abrupt threat to a patient's life. Such emergencies include hypertensive encephalopathy usually associated with excessive diastolic levels, above 140 mm Hg, increased cerebrovascular resistance, cerebral edema, and elevated spinal fluid pressure. They complicate the

Table 45-7. THERAPEUTIC PROGRAMS

Group I.   Mild labile hypertension (B.P. 140/90–180/110 mm Hg): sedation, *Rauwolfia*, diuretic, methyldopa

Group II.   Moderate hypertension (B.P. 180/110–200/120 mm Hg with or without minor degrees of tissue damage): *Rauwolfia*, diuretic, hydralazine hydrochloride, methyldopa; sodium restriction if needed

Group III. Severe sustained hypertension (B.P. above 200/120 mm Hg with variable tissue alterations in brain, fundi, heart, kidney): *Rauwolfia*, diuretic, hydralazine, methyldopa, guanethidine, or ganglionic blocking agents; low-sodium diet; low-protein diet for azotemia

Group IV.   Accelerated phase (malignant hypertension; diastolic B.P. 140 mm Hg or above, grade IV fundi): oral or parenteral ganglionic blocking agents, guanethidine, diuretic, hydralazine *Rauwolfia*, methyldopa; low-sodium, modified, or rice-fruit diet

course of primary hypertension or the acute forms of hypertension secondary to renal infarction, toxemia of pregnancy, or glomerulonephritis (Fig. 45-7). In these situations it is mandatory to administer hypotensive agents in parenteral form in order to obtain the maximum effect from each milligram of drug and to achieve optimum reduction in blood pressure. For an acute emergency, the drug selected should possess a predictable therapeutic action of known intensity and duration without undesirable side effects.

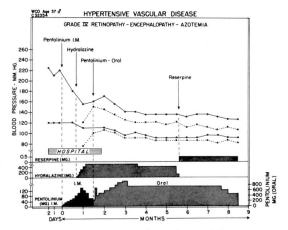

Fig. 45-7. Acute accelerated (malignant) hypertension developed following renal infarction. Blood pressure was reduced first with intramuscular pentolinium; oral hydralazine was added; as the patient's status improved, pentolinium was transferred to oral form. Later, reserpine was substituted for hydralazine and the dose of oral pentolinium reduced.

The simplest compound for general use is reserpine administered intramuscularly in 1.0- to 3.0-mg doses every 2 to 12 hr. Further injections to provide maintenance therapy depend on the duration of each response, which generally ranges from 4 to 12 hr. Such moderate and gradual reduction of blood pressure is of particular utility in the accelerated phase of hypertension presenting headache, vomiting, confusion, papilledema, convulsions, cerebral edema, elevated spinal fluid pressure, and variable reduction in renal function, wherein abrupt lowering of blood pressure can be disastrous, inducing irreversible shock, coma, and uremia.

Similarly, methyldopa, 250 mg to 1.0 Gm administered intravenously, can produce satisfactory blood pressure responses appearing in 1 to 3 hr and lasting 12 to 18 hr. The favorable hemodynamic action of methyldopa recommends its use in renal insufficiency. Also, hydralazine hydrochloride may be injected intramuscularly or intravenously, 5.0 to 20 mg or more every 4 to 6 hr, or by continuous intravenous drip for acute hypertensive disease associated with renal insufficiency, toxemia of pregnancy, or glomerulonephritis.

Pentolinium may be given intramuscularly beginning with 2.0 to 5.0 mg and followed at intervals of 30 min by doses ascending to 50 mg, depending upon blood pressure response. Intravenously, repetitive single doses of 1.0 mg at intervals of 15 min or continuous drip in concentrations of 10 mg per 100 ml may be administered according to degree of blood pressure control. Prominent side effects secondary to parasympathetic ganglion blockade are frequent and potentially serious, involving principally bladder and intestinal paralysis. Effects may last for 4 to 6 hr or longer. The decreased peripheral resistance with lowered arterial and venous pressure is singularly useful for acute pulmonary edema.

Trimethaphan camphorsulfonate (Arfonad), a tertiary amine ganglionic blocking agent, has a shorter duration of action than pentolinium. It is administered in concentrations of 0.1 to 1.0 mg per ml intravenously at a rate of 3.0 to 4.0 mg per min. Hypotension is achieved within minutes, and upon discontinuance of the drug blood pressure rises rapidly. The rapid onset and brief duration of its action offers advantages both for immediate depression of blood pressure when needed and for continuous regulation of blood pressure at desired levels.

The veratrum viride alkaloids (veraloid) and protoveratrines A and B, (Veralba) are potent parenteral compounds but difficult to use and too often associated with nausea and vomiting. One derivative, cryptenamine, has found use in toxemias of pregnancy.

In general, reserpine intramuscularly and methyldopa intravenously are probably the simplest and safest drugs of choice. However, pentolinium and trimethaphan are preferred when conditions, e.g., pulmonary edema or dissecting aneurysm of aorta, demand immediate lowering of pressure.

The treatment of hypertensive emergencies require considerable skill on the part of the physician based on a background of knowledge regarding the physiologic disturbances involved, the status of the kidneys, brain, and heart, and a practical pharmacologic familiarity with effective hypotensive drugs.

Surgical Therapy

Sympathectomy, introduced three decades ago as a new surgical procedure for hypertension, was received with enthusiasm. Successive alterations in surgical approach involving more extensive procedures then followed in an effort to denervate larger areas of the vascular bed, reduce vasoconstrictor reflexes and vascular resistance, and thus lower blood pressure (Table 45-8). Benefits both sub-

Table 45-8. SURGICAL THERAPY: SYMPATHECTOMY

Adson: Subdiaphragmatic splanchnicectomy, celiac ganglionectomy, L_1 and L_2 (1932)

Peet: Supradiaphragmatic splanchnicectomy and lower dorsal ganglionectomy T_{10}–T_{12} (1933)

Smithwick: Thoracolumbar sympathectomy T_6–L_2 (1938)

Poppen: Thoracolumbar sympathectomy T_4–L_2 (1947)

Grimson: Subtotal to total paravertebral sympathectomy, stellate ganglions, T_1–L_1 (1940)

jective and objective were reported from each procedure. Blood pressure was reduced satisfactorily in one-third to one-half of patients with dramatic results in a few.[101–103] In general it was felt that lowering of the blood pressure was directly proportional to the extent of the sympathectomy and inversely proportional to the severity of the disease.[101]

Sympathectomy produces predominant orthostatic reduction in blood pressure, which may be temporarily disabling while recumbent pressure is little affected. Postoperative morbidity, e.g., postural hypotension, neuritic pain, patchy sweating in undenervated areas, impaired ejaculation in the male, nasal congestion if stellate ganglions are excised, is high, although mortality is low (3.9 per cent).[102] Mortality and survival rates from thoracolumbar sympathectomy were regarded as superior to medical controls in all four groups of hypertension (Smithwick classification); best results were noted for groups II and III.[104] However, when 100 surgically treated patients were compared 10 years after operation with matched, medically treated controls, there was little difference in mortality (40 per cent surgical, 46 per cent control) or postoperative survival of patients who died (46 months compared to 45 months in the control). There were greater blood pressure reduction, more significant improvement in both cardiac status and retinopathy, and fewer disabling complications in the surgical survivors than in the medical controls.[105] The best surgical procedure for hypertensive patients is not defined, nor is it possible to select or predict those patients for whom a dramatic or even a good result is reasonably certain.

During the past 15 years the introduction of the newer hypotensive drugs has swung the pendulum of therapy away from surgical treatment, and now sympathectomy is rarely performed. It is noteworthy that the blood pressure becomes more responsive to drugs after sympathectomy (Fig. 45-8). At present, those for whom sympathectomy would be indicated would include the younger hypertensive patient, preferably below the age of fifty and possessing satisfactory renal function, who has failed to respond to adequate medical management or who is unable to follow an effective medical program because of multiple drug sensitivities, economic or geographic considerations, or low level of intellectual function.

With the advent of adequate hormonal replacement therapy and the realization of the possible role of adrenal cortical hormones in the pathogenesis of hypertension, total adrenalectomy was advocated for severe hypertensive states. Mortality is high, and a near-Addisonian state is needed for blood pressure reduction. Blood pressure tends to

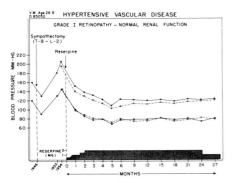

Fig. 45-8. The occasional dramatic effect noted from oral reserpine administered alone. Blood pressure was controlled at normotensive levels in this previously sympathectomized young woman exhibiting recurrence of high diastolic pressure levels but normal renal function.

rise with replacement therapy, which becomes a lifetime obligation. Neither adrenalectomy nor its combination with subdiaphragmatic sympathectomy[106] have received widespread acceptance.

SECONDARY (NONESSENTIAL) HYPERTENSION

Acute Glomerulonephritis

The pathophysiologic alterations in acute glomerulonephritis involve primarily decrease in effective renal blood flow and glomerular filtration rate, followed by retention of salt and water, edema, generalized arteriolar spasm, hypertension, and occasionally encephalopathy. Cardiac output, circulation time, and atrioventricular (A-V) oxygen differences remain essentially normal, but blood- and extracellular-fluid volumes are increased.

Hypertension and edema are common presenting manifestations of acute nephritis but may be absent in mild cases. Hypertension has been attributed to vasospasm from neurogenic or hormonal influences and to expansion of the extracellular and intravascular fluid volumes. Usually the blood pressure is only moderately elevated, in the range of 140 to 160 mm Hg systolic and 90 to 110 mm Hg diastolic. Few patients exhibit rises in diastolic pressure higher than 115 mm Hg; blood pressures above 200/120 mm Hg are unusual.[107] Although glomerulonephritis is more common in children, hypertension occurs with approximately the same frequency and severity as in older age groups.

Slight elevations in blood pressure do not influence the clinical course of the disease and do not require treatment. If the diastolic pressure is below 90 mm Hg and oliguria is absent, rest and sedation are all that is indicated. Oliguria and edema may be present, however, without hypertension. When blood pressures rise above 100 mm Hg diastolic, even without signs of either cardiac or cerebral involvement, more active antihypertensive therapy should be instituted. In children basic therapy should begin with salt restriction and the use of reserpine, 80 to 150 μg per kg given intramuscularly once every 12 to 24 hr. In more resistant cases, hydralazine 100 μg per kg, may be added. For adults the parenteral doses are 1.0 to 3.0 mg for reserpine and 5.0 to 20 mg for hydralazine hydrochloride. Effects appear in 30 min and persist for 12 hr or longer. Hypotensive therapy usually is needed only for brief periods, and drug toxicity does not present a problem.

In more severe form, when the diastolic pressure exceeds 120 mm Hg and cerebral symptoms of hypertensive encephalopathy appear, a life-threatening emergency exists which must be controlled by appropriate therapy. Although thiazide drugs can be given orally or intravenously (20 to 500 mg chlorothiazide in 20 ml distilled water or in 5 per cent glucose solution) to promote salt and water excretion, and drugs (reserpine, hydralazine, and methyldopa) can be used to lower blood pressure, magnesium sulfate is still a useful drug to control hypertension and encephalopathy. It increases effective renal blood flow, glomerular filtration rate, and urinary output within 5 to 15 min, and may raise urinary excretion of sodium fivefold.[108,109] Magnesium sulfate, 200 to 250 mg per kg, is administered as a 3 per cent solution in distilled water intravenously over a period of 60 to 75 min.° This "priming dose" may be repeated every 6 hr intravenously if the patient is urinating, but only two doses should be given if the patient is anuric, the second one cautiously. Calcium gluconate, 10 per cent solution, or calcium chloride, 5 per cent solution, should be held ready for intravenous use, 5.0 to 10 Gm, as an antidote. Although extinction of the knee jerks has been used as a point of toxicity, these reflexes may disappear before an effective level of magnesium, 5.6 mEq per liter, is reached. The toxic level for respiratory depression is approximately 16.6 mEq per liter. Some investigators regard the margin between reflex suppression and respiratory depression as sufficiently narrow to conclude that the newer antihypertensive agents have rendered magnesium sulfate therapy obsolete.[110] In severe cases with complications, however, the newer drugs sometimes fail to control the problem, and intravenous magnesium sulfate is indicated. In addtion to hypotensive agents other signs of central nervous system dysfunction may be combatted by the administration of sedatives, phenobarbital, and anticonvulsants (Dilantin sodium).

Chronic Glomerulonephritis

Chronic glomerulonephritis is conventionally associated with gradual deterioration in renal function and the development of renal insufficiency, azotemia, and hypertension. The majority have significant reduction in both glomerular filtration rate and renal plasma flow.[111] Therapeutic maneuvers designed to lower blood pressure in the presence of renal insufficiency present special hazards which deserve emphasis. Measures, notably drug therapy with the exception of hydralazine and methyldopa, generally reduce cardiac output, renal blood flow, and glomerular filtration; renal function becomes further impaired, and the patient's condition may

° A sufficient amount for the average patient can be prepared by diluting 30 ml of a 25 per cent (Lilly) or 15 ml of a 50 per cent (Parke-Davis) magnesium sulfate solution to a total of 250 ml with distilled water.

seriously deteriorate as a result. This is particularly true of the ganglionic blocking agents, which, depending upon the kidney for their excretion, offer the additional danger of cumulative toxicity, since the potent compound cannot be satisfactorily excreted.[112] Shock, oliguria, uremia, and death may result. Patients suffering from renal insufficiency seem particularly sensitive to depressor therapy. Reserpine in oral doses of 0.25 to 1.0 mg daily is a mild, safe, hypotensive agent for treatment of glomerulonephritis which may be combined with hydralazine. Methyldopa also has been advocated for renal insufficiency.[87] Salt restriction may lead to salt depletion, hyponatremia, acidosis, azotemia, and hyperkalemia, particularly if there is vomiting, diarrhea, obligatory salt wasting, or concomitant exposure to diuretic compounds. Thiazide derivatives may be used when nephritis is complicated by hypertension and edema, but their exhibition in the presence of renal insufficiency can lead to irreversible hyponatremia.

The mild and asymptomatic hypertension which usually accompanies chronic glomerulonephritis needs no therapy. However, significant hypertension adds to the gravity of the prognosis in renal disease. Resting high diastolic pressures, 120 mm Hg or above, retinopathy, encephalopathy, or cardiovascular disease all represent unquestioned indications for aggressive treatment. One must carefully balance lowering of blood pressure against the status of renal function, azotemia, and general well-being of the patient. The dangers are particularly real when frank uremia complicates severe hypertension.

The primary aim of treatment is gradual reduction of blood pressure by means of rest, diet, and drugs. Protein is restricted to levels of 20 to 40 Gm per day depending upon the degree of nitrogen retention. Rigid sodium restriction should be imposed with caution because of possible salt wasting and consequent serum-electrolyte depletion. Such depletion correlates more closely with depression of phenolsulfonphthalein excretion than with the level of azotemia.[37] If sodium is restricted to 500 mg or less per day or the rice-fruit diet is instituted, diuretic compounds must be rigidly avoided. The drugs of choice alone or in combination appear to be reserpine, hydralazine, and methyldopa.

If convulsions occur with uremia and hypertension, intravenous Sodium Amytal is administered, and efforts are made to lower the blood pressure rapidly by parenteral medication, either reserpine or hydralazine. The prognosis in general depends upon the degree of renal insufficiency and the level of azotemia. The role of repetitive dialysis in the management of chronic glomerulonephritis with chronic renal failure is not clearly defined at this time, but the procedure is gaining favor. Homotransplantation is still experimental in spite of successes with renal transplantation in identical twins.

The treatment of unilateral renal disease is discussed in Chap. 42. The treatment of pheochromocytoma is discussed in Chap. 43. The treatment of aldosteroma is discussed in Chap. 44.

REFERENCES

1. Hoobler, S. W. (ed.): Proceedings of the Conference on Basic Mechanisms of Arterial Hypertension, Circulation, **17**:641, 1958.
2. Page, I. H.: The Nature of Arterial Hypertension, *Arch. Int. Med.* 3:103, 1963.
3. Conway, J.: Current Concepts Concerning the Etiology of Essential Hypertension, *Am. Heart J.,* **66**:409, 1963.
4. Insurance Statistics, Society of Actuaries: "Build and Blood Pressure Study," Chicago, vol. 1, 1959; vol. 2, 1960.
5. Benford, D. M.: Blood Pressure and Longevity, *Am. Heart J.,* **63**:433, 1962.
6. Gubner, S.: Systolic Hypertension: A Pathogenetic Entity. Significance and Therapeutic Considerations, *Am. J. Cardiol.,* **9**:773, 1962.
7. Mathisen, H. S., Jensen, D., Löken, E., and Löken, H.: The Prognosis in Essential Hypertension, *Am. Heart J.,* **57**:371, 1959.
8. Burch, G. E., and Phillips, J. H.: Hypertension and Arteriosclerosis, *Am. Heart J.,* **60**:163, 1960.
9. Stamler, J.: Interrelationships between the Two Diseases, Hypertension and Atherosclerosis, *Am. J. Cardiol.,* **9**:743, 1962.
10. Kannel, W. B., Dawber, T. R., Kagan, A., Revotskie, N., and Stokes, J., III: Factors of Risk in the Development of Coronary Heart Disease: Six Year Follow-up Experience, *Ann. Int. Med.,* **55**:33, 1961.
11. Newborg, B., and Kempner, W.: Analysis of 177 Cases of Hypertensive Vascular Disease with Papilledema, *Am. J. Med.,* **19**:33, 1955.
12. Dustan, H. P., Schneckloth, R. E., Corcoran, A. C., and Page, I. H.: The Effectiveness of Long-term Treatment of Malignant Hypertension, *Circulation,* **18**:644, 1958.
13. Leishman, A. W. D.: Hypertension—Treated and Untreated: A Study of 400 Cases, *Brit. M. J.,* **1**:1361, 1959.
14. Sokolow, M., and Perloff, D.: Five Year Survival of Consecutive Patients with Malignant Hypertension Treated with Antihypertensive Agents, *Am. J. Cardiol.,* **6**:858, 1960.
15. Hodge, J. V., McQueen, E. G., and Smirk, H.: Results of Hypotensive Therapy in Arterial Hypertension: Based on Experience with 497 Patients Treated and 156 Controls, Observed for Periods from 1 to 8 Years, *Brit. M. J.,* **1**:1, 1961.
16. Farmer, R. G., Gifford, R. W., Jr., and Hines, E. A., Jr.: Effect of Medical Treatment of Severe Hypertension: A Follow-up Study of 161 Patients with Group 3 and Group 4 Hypertension, *Arch. Int. Med.,* **112**:118, 1963.
17. Kinsey, D., Whitelaw, G. P., Walther, R. J., Theophilis, C. A., and Smithwick, R. H.: The Long-term Follow-up of Malignant Hypertension, *J.A.M.A.,* **181**:571, 1962.
18. Page, I. H., and Dustan, H. P.: Persistence of Normal Blood Pressure after Discontinuing Treatment in Hypertensive Patients, *Circulation,* **25**:433, 1962.
19. Freis, E. D.: Current Concepts in Therapy: Antihypertensive Agents: I, II, and III, *New England J. Med.,* **266**:507, 607, 775, 1962.
20. Hoobler, S. W., and Conway, J.: Selection of Patients and Principles of Treatment in Essential Hypertension, *M. Clin. North America,* **45**:349, 1961.
21. Smirk, F. H.: Rationale for Antihypertensive Therapy, in A. N. Brest and J. H. Moyer (eds.), "Hypertension: Recent Advances: The Second Hahnemann Symposium on Hypertensive Disease," Lea & Febiger, Philadelphia, 1961, p. 475.
22. Perera, G. A.: Antihypertensive Drug versus Symptomatic Treatment in Primary Hypertension: Effect on Survival, *J.A.M.A.,* **173**:11, 1960.
23. Perera, G. A.: Hypertensive Vascular Disease: Description and Natural History, *J. Chron. Dis.,* **1**:33, 1955.
24. Burgess, A. M.: Benign Essential Hypertension: Follow-up of 100 Patients under Observation for from 18 to 34 Years, *Ann. Int. Med.,* **43**:740, 1955.
25. Keith, N. M., Wagner, H. P., and Barker, N. W.: Some Different Types of Essential Hypertension: Their Course and Prognosis, *Am. J. M. Sc.,* **197**:332, 1939.
26. Palmer, R. S., Loofbourow, D. G., and Doering, G. R.: Prognosis in Essential Hypertension: 8 Year Follow-up Study of 430 Patients on Conventional Medical Treatment, *New England J. Med.,* **239**:990, 1948.
27. Griep, A. H., Barry, G. R., Hall, W. C., and Hoobler, S. W.: The Prognosis in Arterial Hypertension: Report on 117 Patients under 53 Years of Age Followed 8 to 10 Years, *Am. J. M. Sc.,* **221**:239, 1951.
28. Sokolow, M., and Perloff, D.: The Prognosis of Essential Hypertension Treated Conservatively, *Circulation,* **23**:697, 1961.
29. Smirk, F. H.: Some Principles of Hypotensive Therapy Considered in Relationship to the Pathogenesis of Essential Hypertension, *Am. J. Cardiol.,* **9**:90, 1962.
30. Wolf, S.: Psychosomatic Aspects of Hypertension, *M. Clin. North America,* **45**:339, 1961.
31. Metropolitan Life Insurance Company: "Overweight: Its Prevention and Significance," *Stat. Bull.,* pp. 9–12, 1960.
32. Fregley, M. J. (ed.): Seminar on the Role of Salt

in Cardiovascular Hypertension: I, II, and III, *Am. J. Cardiol.*, 8:526, 684, 863, 1961.

33. Grollman, A., Harrison, T., Mason, M., Baxter, J., Crampton, J., and Reichsman, F.: Sodium Restriction in the Diet for Hypertension, *J.A.M.A.*, 129: 533, 1945.

34. Kempner, W.: Treatment of Hypertensive Vascular Disease with Rice Diet, *Am. J. Med.*, 4:545, 1948.

35. Corcoran, A. C., Taylor, R. D., and Page, I. H.: Controlled Observations on the Effect of Low Sodium Dietotherapy in Essential Hypertension, *Circulation*, 3:1, 1951.

36. Orgain, E. S.: Cation Exchange Resins in Congestive Heart Failure, *M. Clin. North America*, 38: 419, 1954.

37. Peschel, E., and Peschel, R. L.: Electrolyte Metabolism during Rice Diet. II. Serum Electrolytes in Patients with Severe Primary or Secondary Renal Disease, *A.M.A. Arch. Int. Med.*, 91:296, 1953.

38. Gibbons, J. E., Muller, J. C., Pryor, W. W., and Orgain, E. S.: Newer Drugs in the Treatment of Hypertension, III. Experience with *Rauwolfia* Drugs and Protoveratrine, *J.A.M.A.*, 162:92, 1956.

39. Paton, W. D. M., and Zaimis, E. J.: The Methonium Compounds, *Pharmacol. Rev.*, 4:219, 1952.

40. Harington, M.: Ganglion-blocking Agents in Hypertension, *M. Clin. North America*, 45:395, 1961.

41. Sieber, H. A., Grimson, K. S., and Orgain, E. S.: Newer Drugs in the Treatment of Hypertension. I. Use of Hexamethonium Salts, *Circulation*, 8:840, 1953.

42. Grimson, K. S., Tarazi, A. K., and Frazer, J. W., Jr.: A New Orally Active Quaternary Ammonium, Ganglion Blocking Drug Capable of Reducing Blood Pressure, SU-3088, *Circulation*, 11:733, 1955.

43. Freis, E. D., and Wilson, I. M.: Mecamylamine: A New, Orally Effective, Hypotensive Agent. *A.M.A. Arch. Int. Med.*, 97:551, 1956.

44. Stone, C. A., Torchiana, M. L., Navarro, A., and Beyer, K. H.: Ganglionic Blocking Properties of 3-Methylaminoisocamphane Hydrochloride (Mecamylamine): A Secondary Amine, *J. Pharmacol. & Exper. Therap.*, 117:169, 1956.

45. Schneckloth, R. E., Corcoran, A. C., Dustan, H. P., and Page, I. H.: Mecamylamine in Treatment of Hypertensive Disease: Observations on an Unusual Neuromuscular Complication, *J.A.M.A.*, 162: 868, 1956.

46. Freis, E. D., Partenope, E. A., Lilienfield, L. S., and Rose, J. C.: A Clinical Appraisal of Pentapyrrolidinium (M&B 2050) in Hypertensive Patients, *Circulation*, 9:540, 1954.

47. Smith, J. R., Agrest, A., and Hoobler, S. W.: The Effect of Acute and Chronic Administration of Pentilinium Tartrate on Blood Pressure and Cardiac Output of Hypertensive Patients, *Circulation*, 12:777, 1955.

48. Perry, H. M., Jr., and Schroeder, H. A.: The Use of Pentilinium Tartrate with and without Hydralazine in the Treatment of Severe Hypertension, *New England J. Med.*, 252:1057, 1955.

49. Harington, M., Kincaid-Smith, P., and Milne, M. D.: Pharmacology and Clinical Use of Pempidine in Treatment of Hypertension, *Lancet*, 2:6, 1958.

50. Perkins, H. T., Jr., Bogdonoff, M. D., and Black, M.: The Treatment of Hypertension with Trimethidinium Methosulfate in an Outpatient Clinic Group, *South. M. J.*, 53:224, 1960.

51. Wolf, R. L., Mendlowitz, M., Naftchi, N. E., and Gitlow, S. E.: Current Treatment of Hypertension with Drugs, *Am. Heart J.*, 66:414, 1963.

52. Schroeder, H. A.: The Effect of 1-Hydrazinophthalazine in Hypertension, *Circulation*, 5:28, 1952.

53. Schirger, A., and Spittell, J. A.: Pharmacology and Clinical Use of Hydralazine in the Treatment of Diastolic Hypertension, *Am. J. Cardiol.*, 9:854, 1962.

54. Dustan, H. P., Taylor, R. D., Corcoran, A. C., and Page, I. H.: Rheumatic and Febrile Syndrome during Prolonged Hydralazine Treatment, *J.A.M.A.*, 154:23, 1954.

55. Muller, J. C., Rast, C. L., Jr., Pryor, W. W., and Orgain, E. S.: Late Systemic Complications of Hydralazine (Apresoline) Therapy, *J.A.M.A.*, 157: 894, 1955.

56. Hildreth, E. A., Biro, C. E., and McCreary, T. A.: Persistence of the Hydralazine Syndrome: A Follow-up Study of Eleven Cases, *J.A.M.A.*, 173:657, 1960.

57. Bendersky, G., and Ramirez, C.: Hydralazine Poisoning: Review of the Literature and Autopsy Study of a Person with Massive Intestinal Bleeding, *J.A.M.A.*, 173:1789, 1960.

58. Wilkins, R. W., and Judson, W. E.: The Use of *Rauwolfia serpentina* in Hypertensive Patients, *New England J. Med.*, 248, 48: 1953.

59. Bein, H. J.: The Pharmacology of *Rauwolfiia*, *Pharmacol. Rev.*, 8:435, 1956.

60. Plummer, A. J.: Effect of *Rauwolfia* Compounds on Catecholamine Release, In A. N. Brest and J. H. Moyer (eds.), "Hypertension: Recent Advances: The Second Hahnemann Symposium on Hypertensive Disease," Lea & Febiger, Philadelphia, 1961, p. 399.

61. Moyer, J. H., Dennis, E., and Ford, R.: Drug Therapy (*Rauwolfia*) of Hypertension, *A.M.A. Arch. Int. Med.*, 96:530, 1955.

62. Shelburne, P. F., and Orgain, E. S.: Comparison of Syrosingopine and Reserpine in the Treatment of Ambulatory Hypertensive Patients, *Am. J. M. Sc.*, 245:304, 1963.

63. Muller, J. C., Pryor, W. W., Gibbons, J. E., and Orgain, E. S.: Depression and Anxiety Occurring during *Rauwolfia* Therapy, *J.A.M.A.*, 159:836, 1955.

64. Katz, R. L., Weintraub, H. D., and Pepper, E.

M.: Anesthesia, Surgery, and *Rauwolfia, Anesthesiology,* 25:142, 1964.

65. Hollander, W., and Wilkins, R. W.: Chlorothiazide: A New Type of Drug for the Treatment of Arterial Hypertension, *Boston M. Quart.,* 8:69, 1957.

66. Laragh, J. H.: The Mode of Action and Use of Chlorothiazide and Related Compounds, *Circulation,* 26:121, 1962.

67. Conway, J., and Lauwers, P.: Hemodynamic and Hypotensive Effects of Long Term Therapy with Chlorothiazide, *Circulation,* 21:21, 1960.

68. Swartz, C., Seller, R., Fuchs, M., Brest, A. N., and Moyer, J. H.: Five Years' Experience with the Evaluation of Diuretic Agents, *Circulation,* 28:1042, 1963.

69. Schwab, R. H., Perloff, J. K., and Porus, R. L.: Chlorothiazide-induced Gout Diabetes, *A.M.A. Arch. Int. Med.,* 111:465, 1963.

70. Bryant, J. M., Schvartz, N., Torosdag, S., Fletcher, L., Jr., Fertig, H., Schwartz, M. S., Quan, R. B. F., McDermott, J. J., and Spencer, T. B.: The Antihypertensive Effects of Chlorthalidone: A Comparative Analysis with Benzothiazide Compounds, *Circulation,* 25:522, 1962.

71. Finnerty, F. A., Jr., Kakaviatos, N., Tuckman, J., and Magill, J.: Clinical Evaluation of Diazoxide: A New Treatment for Acute Hypertension, *Circulation,* 28:203, 1963.

72. Hollander, W.: Aldosterone Antagonists in Arterial Hypertension, *Heart Bull.,* 12:108, 1963.

73. Georgopoulos, A. J., Dustan, H., and Page, I. H.: Spironolactone in Hypertensive Patients, *A.M.A. Arch. Int. Med.,* 108:389, 1961.

74. Maxwell, R. A., Plummer, A. J., Schneider, F., Povlaski, H., and Daniel, A. I.: Pharmacology of (2-(octahydro-1-azocinyl)-ethyl) Guanethidine Sulfate (SU 5864), *J. Pharmacol. & Exper. Therap.,* 128:22, 1960.

75. Cohn, J. N., Liptak, T. E., and Freis, E. D.: Hemodynamic Effects of Guanethidine in Man, *Circulation Res.,* 12:298, 1963.

76. Eagan, J. T., and Orgain, E. S.: A Study of 38 Patients and Their Responses to Guanethidine: A New Antihypertensive Agent, *J.A.M.A.,* 175:550, 1961.

77. Page, I. H., Hurley, R. E., and Dustan, H. P.: The Prolonged Treatment of Hypertension with Guanethidine, *J.A.M.A.,* 175:543, 1961.

78. Fertig, H., Fletcher, L., Jr., Schvartz, N., Torosdag, S., Spencer, T. B., and Bryant, J. M.: Clinical Experiences with Guanethidine in Ambulatory Hypertensive Subjects, *New England J. Med.,* 265:268, 1961.

79. Shelburne, P. F., Sassen, F. A., and Orgain, E. S.: Guanethidine in Combination with Hydralazine and with Hydrochlorothiazide in Hypertension, *Am. J. M. Sc.,* 247:307, 1964.

80. Boura, A. L. A., Green, A. F., McCoubrey, A., Laurence, D. R., Moulton, R., and Rosenheim,

M. L.: Darenthin: Hypotensive Agent of New Type, *Lancet,* 2:17, 1959.

81. Blaschko, H.: The Development of Current Concepts of Catecholamine Formation, *Pharmacol. Rev.,* 11:307, 1959.

82. Sjoerdsma, A., Vendsalu, A., and Engelman, K.: Studies on the Metabolism and Mechanism of Action of Methyldopa, *Circulation,* 28:492, 1963.

83. Weil, M. H., Barbour, B. H., and Chesne, R. B.: Alpha-Methyl Dopa for the Treatment of Hypertension: Clinical and Pharmacodynamic Studies, *Circulation,* 28:165, 1963.

84. Kirkendall, W. M., and Wilson, W. R.: Pharmacodynamics and Clinical Use of Guanethidine, Bretylium and Methyldopa, *Am. J. Cardiol.,* 9:107, 1962.

85. Sheps, S. G., Schirger, A., Osmundson, P. J., and Fairbairn, J. F., II: Methyldopa for Treatment of Hypertension, *J.A.M.A.,* 184:616, 1963.

86. Colwill, J. M., Dutton, A. M., Morrissey, J., and Yu, P. N.: Alpha-Methyldopa and Hydrochlorothiazide. A Controlled Study of Their Comparative Effectiveness as Antihypertensive Agents, *New England J. Med.,* 271:696, 1964.

87. Cannon, P. J., Whitlock, R. T., Morris, R. C., Angers, M., and Laragh, J. H.: Effect of Alpha-Methyl Dopa in Severe and Malignant Hypertension, *J.A.M.A.,* 179:673, 1962.

88. Gillespie, L., Jr., and Sjoerdsma, A.: Monoamine Oxidase and Decarboxylase Inhibitors as Antihypertensive Agents, *M. Clin. North America,* 45:421, 1961.

89. Onesti, G., Brest, A. N., and Moyer, J. H.: Clinical Application of Monoamine Oxidase Inhibitors, in A. N. Brest and J. H. Moyer (eds.), "Hypertension: Recent Advances: The Second Hahnemann Symposium on Hypertensive Disease," Lea & Febiger, Philadelphia, 1961, p. 412.

90. Zbinden, G.: The Antihypertensive Effect of Monoamine Oxidase Inhibitors: Mechanism of Action, in A. N. Brest and J. H. Moyer (eds.), "Hypertension: Recent Advances: The Second Hahnemann Symposium on Hypertensive Disease," Lea & Febiger, Philadelphia, 1961, p. 407.

91. Goldberg, L. I.: Monoamine Oxidase Inhibitors. Adverse Reactions and Possible Mechanisms, *J.A.M.A.,* 190:132, 1964.

92. Blackwell, B.: Hypertensive Crises Due to Monoamine Oxidase Inhibitors, *Lancet,* 2:849, 1963.

93. Rast, C. L., and Orgain, E. S.: Newer Drugs in the Treatment of Hypertension. II. Use of Hexamethonium in Combination with Hydralazine, *Circulation,* 12:361, 1955.

94. Orgain, E. S., Munroe, C. A., and Donnelly, G. L.: Newer Drugs in the Treatment of Hypertension. IV. Use of Reserpine, Hydralazine, and Pentolinium in Various Combinations, *J.A.M.A.,* 166:2103, 1958.

95. Smith, W. M., Damato, A. N., Galluzzi, N. J., Garfield, C. F., Hanowell, E. G., Stimson, W. H.,

Thurm, R. H., Walsh, J. J., and Bromer, L.: The Evaluation of Antihypertensive Therapy. Cooperative Clinical Trial Method. I. Double-blind Control Comparison of Chlorothiazide, *Rauwolfia Serpentina,* and Hydralazine, *Ann. Int. Med.,* **61:** 829, 1964.

96. Veterans Administration: Cooperative Study on Antihypertensive Agents: A Double Blind Control Study of Antihypertensive Agents. I. Comparative Effectiveness of Reserpine, Reserpine and Hydralazine and Three Ganglionic Blocking Agents, Chlorisondamine, Mecamylamine and Pentolinium Tartrate, *A.M.A. Arch. Int. Med.,* **108:**81, 1960; II. Further Report on the Comparative Effectiveness of Reserpine, Reserpine and Hydralazine, and Three Ganglion Blocking Agents, Chlorisondamine, Mecamylamine, and Pentolinium Tartrate, III. Chlorothiazide Alone and in Combination with Other Agents: Preliminary Results, *A.M.A. Arch. Int. Med.,* **110:**222, 230, 1962.

97. Perry, H. M., Jr., Caloyeropoulos, A., and Moore-Jones, D.: Therapy of Severe Hypertension Complicated by Renal Failure, *Am. J. Cardiol.,* **9:**908, 1962.

98. Brest, A. N., and Moyer, J. H.: Current Status of Drug Therapy and Choice of Drugs in the Treatment of Hypertension, *Progr. Cardiovas. Dis.,* **3:** 350, 1961.

99. Gifford, R. W., Jr.: The Treatment of Hypertensive Emergencies, *Am. J. Cardiol.,* **9:**880, 1962.

100. Freis, E. D.: Hypertensive Emergencies, *M. Clin. North America,* **46:**353, 1962.

101. Grimson, K. S.: The Surgical Treatment of Hypertension: Collective Review, *Internat. Abstr. Surg.* (*Surg. Gynec. & Obst.*), **75:**421, 1942.

102. Grimson, K. S.: The Surgical Treatment of Hypertension, *Advances Int. Med.,* **2:**173, 1947.

103. Grimson, K. S., Orgain, E. S., Anderson, B., Broome, R. A., Jr., and Longino, F. H.: Results of Treatment of Patients with Hypertension by Total Thoracic and Partial to Total Lumbar Sympathectomy, Splanchnicectomy and Celiac Ganglionectomy, *Ann. Surg.,* **129:**850, 1949.

104. Smithwick, R. H., and Thompson, J. E.: Splanchnicectomy for Essential Hypertension: Results in 1266 Cases, *J.A.M.A.,* **152:**1501, 1953.

105. Evelyn, K. A., Singh, M. M., Chapman, W. P., Perera, G. A., and Thaler, H.: Effect of Thoracolumbar Sympathectomy on Clinical Course of Primary (Essential) Hypertension: A Ten-year Study of 100 Sympathectomized Patients Compared with Individually Matched, Symptomatically Treated Control Subjects, *Am. J. Med.,* **28:**188, 1960.

106. Blakemore, W. S., Zintel, H. A., Jeffers, W. A., Sellers, A. M., Sutnick, A. I., and Lindauer, M. A.: A Comparison of Thoracolumbar Sympathectomy and Adrenalectomy with Adson Sympathectomy in the Treatment of Severe Arterial Hypertension: A Three-to-seven-year Follow-up Report, *Surgery,* **43:**102, 1958.

107. Schwartz, W. B., and Kassirer, J. P.: Clinical Aspects of Acute glomerulonephritis, in M. B. Strauss and L. G. Welt (eds.), "Diseases of the Kidney," Little, Brown and Company, Boston, 1963, p. 274.

108. Harris, J. S., and DeMaria, W. J. A.: Effect of Magnesium Sulfate on Renal Dynamics in Acute Glomerulonephritis in Children, *Pediatrics,* **11:**191, 1953.

109. DeMaria, W. J. A.: Management of Acute Nephritis, *South. M. J.,* **50:**1504, 1957.

110. Kassirer, J. P., and Schwartz, W. B.: Acute Glomerulonephritis, *New England J. Med.,* **265:**736, 1961.

111. Kirkendall, W.: The Management of the Hypertensive Patient with Renal Insufficiency, in A. N. Brest and J. H. Moyer (eds.), "Hypertension: Recent Advances: The Second Hahnemann Symposium on Hypertensive Disease," Lea & Febiger, Philadelphia, 1961, p. 554.

112. Seldin, D. W., Carter, N. W., and Rector, F. C., Jr.: Consequences of Renal Failure and Their Management, in M. B. Strauss and L. G. Welt (eds.), "Diseases of the Kidney," Little, Brown and Company, Boston, 1963, p. 207.

SUGGESTED READING

Books

Brest, A. N., and Moyer, J. H. (eds.): "Hypertension: Recent Advances: The Second Hahnemann Symposium on Hypertensive Disease," Lea & Febiger, Philadelphia, 1961.

Burch, G. E., and DePasquale, N. P.: "Primer of Clinical Measurement of Blood Pressure," The C. V. Mosby Company, St. Louis, 1962.

Edwards, J. C.: "Management of Hypertensive Disease," The C. V. Mosby Company, St. Louis, 1960.

Hoobler, S. W.: "Hypertensive Disease: Diagnosis and Treatment," Hoeber Medical Division, Harper & Row, Publishers, Incorporated, New York, 1959.

Moyer, J. H. (ed.): "Hypertension: The First Hahnemann Symposium on Hypertensive Disease," W. B. Saunders Company, Philadelphia, 1959.

Pickering, G. W., Cranston, W. I., and Pears, M. A.: "The Treatment of Hypertension," Charles C Thomas, Publisher, Springfield, Ill., 1961.

Reubi, F. C.: "Essential Hypertension (an International Symposium)," Springer-Verlag OHG, Berlin, 1960.

Smirk, F. H.: "High Arterial Pressure," Charles C Thomas, Publisher, Springfield, Ill., 1957.

Strauss, M. B., and Welt, L. G. (eds.): "Diseases of the Kidney," Little, Brown and Company, Boston, 1963.

Conferences, Seminars, and Symposia

Buckley, J. P.: Pharmacology of Antihypertensive Compounds, *J. Pharmacol. Sc.,* **50:**539, 1961.

Grollman, A. (ed.): New Diuretics and Antihypertensive Agents, *Ann. New York Acad. Sc.,* **88:**771, 1960.

Moyer, J. H. (ed.): Symposium on Hypertension: I. Etiology and Pathologic Physiology, *Am. J. Cardiol.,* **9:**651–820, 1962.

Moyer, J. H. (ed.): Symposium on Hypertension: II. Therapy, *Am. J. Cardiol.,* **9:**821–920, 1962.

Page, I. H. (ed.): Hypertension and Its Treatment, *M. Clin. North America,* **45:**233, 1961.

Rodbard, S. (ed.): Hypertension: Vasoactive Mechanisms, Proc. Council for High Blood Pressure Res., Am. Heart A., *Circulation Res.,* **12:**525, 1963.

Segal, D. (ed.): Symposium: Management of Patients with Primary (Essential) Hypertension, *J. Chron. Dis.,* **1:**471, 1955.

Shapiro, A.: Hypertension: Current Management, *Disease-A-Month,* March, 1963.

Skelton, F. R. (ed.): Hypertension: Chemical and Hormonal Factors, *Circulation Res.,* **9:**715, 1961.

Skelton, F. R. (ed.): Hypertension: Neural and Renal Mechanisms, Proc. Council for High Blood Pressure Res., Am. Heart A., *Circulation Res.,* **11:**131, 1962.

Smirk, F. H.: Recent Developments in Hypertensive Therapy, *Am. Heart J.,* **61:**272, 1961.

Studies on Hypertension, *Am. J. Cardiol.,* **9:**90–155, 1962.

Wood, J. E., and Ahlquist, R. P. (eds.): Symposium on Angiotensin, *Circulation,* **25:**167, 1962.

Section E: Heart Disease Secondary to Disease of the Lungs and Pulmonary Arteries

46 CHRONIC COR PULMONALE

Peter C. Gazes, M.D.

Chronic cor pulmonale is defined as hypertrophy of the right ventricle with or without failure resulting from certain disease states affecting the function and/or structure of the lungs. This does not include pulmonary changes occurring in diseases primarily affecting the left side of the heart or associated with congenital heart disease. The common factor preceding right ventricular hypertrophy is always pulmonary hypertension, and a comparison is often made with systemic hypertension.[1] The term pulmonary hypertensive *vascular* disease is applicable prior to the progression to right ventricular hypertrophy or dilatation and failure, and pulmonary hypertensive *cardiovascular* disease is used once these develop. Even though the right ventricular changes are emphasized, frequently the total heart is affected.

Incidence

Cor pulmonale is not properly identified, and the routine mortality statistics compiled according to the International Classification of Diseases[2] cannot provide adequate information about its frequency. Data indicating the frequency of the disease can be derived from autopsies and hospital admissions, but there are large differences in its reported prev-

alence. Autopsy series report a range of from 0.9 per cent of all cardiac autopsies in Massachusetts to 54 per cent in Arizona, while the frequency of hospital admissions ranges from 16 to 38 per cent in Belgrade, Delhi, Prague, and Sheffield.[2,3] In Buenos Aires cor pulmonale constituted 3.3 per cent of the general admissions to a cardiac clinic.[4] In Jaipur 16 per cent of all cases of heart disease and 23 per cent of all cases with heart failure were due to cor pulmonale.[5] In most series, the cause is attributed to pulmonary emphysema in more than 50 per cent of the cases. A review of 801 consecutive autopsied cases of heart disease of all types from the files of the Medical College Hospital of South Carolina reveals 77 (9.2 per cent) cases of cor pulmonale. It is impossible at present to give a realistic figure, but it probably ranges from 5 to 10 per cent of all cases of organic heart disease. Cor pulmonale is at least five times more common in men than in women, and about 75 per cent of the patients are over fifty years of age.[6]

Pathogenesis

There are four important factors which increase the work of the heart or affect the myocardium: (1) generalized alveolar hypoventilation, (2) reduction in the pulmonary vascular bed, (3) intrapulmonary vascular shunts, and (4) myocardial factors.

Generalized Alveolar Hypoventilation

Alveolar hypoventilation produces hypoxia and eventually hypercapnia and is more frequently encountered in chronic obstructive emphysema. Hypoxia, by its local effect on vessels and by stimulation of neurohumoral mechanisms, increases pulmonary vascular resistance by an actual reduction in the caliber of the pulmonary vessels, thereby producing pulmonary hypertension. Aviado et al.[7] has demonstrated that the pulmonary vascular constriction is due to activation of a reflex initiated by stimulation of the carotid and aortic bodies. The efferent arc runs in the thoracic sympathetic nerves. The site of this vasoconstriction is not known, but it may be in the pulmonary arterioles, capillaries, or venules.[8,9] Pulmonary vascular constriction can produce bronchoconstriction and increase alveolar surface tension.[10,11] Recent investigators have confirmed the fundamental observations of von Neergaard[12] that the major retractive force within the lung is not the elastic recoil [13–15] but that surface tension is equally important. In addition to the alveolar membrane and capillary membrane, Clements[11] has described a surface-active material which lines the alveoli and lowers the surface tension markedly on expiration, preventing collapse of smaller alveoli. This surface-active material has been extracted and found to be a lipoprotein. It is possible with pulmonary vascular constriction that this surface-active material is not formed or is inactivated and so nonobstructive atelectasis (alveolar deflation) develops because of the high surface tension. The increased alveolar musculature observed in patients with pulmonary hypertension also predisposes to further "contraction atelectasis," [16] which is another form of nonobstructive alveolar collapse. With atelectasis, compliance is reduced, and the lungs become more rigid, contributing to the pulmonary hypertension. Hypoxia produces polycythemia with hypervolemia, increased venous return with an increased cardiac output, increased viscosity with

increased resistance to pulmonary blood flow, and resultant pulmonary hypertension. Pulmonary hypertension eventually leads to right ventricular hypertrophy and failure. The effects of hypoxia are illustrated in Fig. 46-1.

Reduction in the Pulmonary Vascular Bed

If this were the only factor involved, more than 50 per cent of the pulmonary vascular bed would have to be eliminated, since pneumonectomy does not produce cor pulmonale. Destruction is gradual, usually occurring in extensive fibrotic diseases of the lung. Emphasis has been placed on the physiologic factors such as hypoxia in emphysema, due to the diffuse nature of the emphysematous change, but a critical compromise of the total capillary bed also appears to be an important factor. The intraalveolar pressure is markedly elevated (because of the great degree of air trapping and the very prolonged expiratory phase), with the result that the pulmonary capillary bed, already damaged through alveolar wall fenestration, is further compromised by the transmitted extramural pressure.[17] Microthromboembolic complications in the lungs cause further loss of function.[18] Regardless of the type of lung disease, through destruction of the pulmonary vascular bed, shrinkage secondary to necrosis and scars, pressure effects, and thromboembolic complications, the pulmonary vascular resistance is increased with resulting pulmonary hypertension, right ventricular hypertrophy, and failure.

Intrapulmonary Vascular Shunts

Large and numerous precapillary shunts develop between the bronchial and pulmonary arteries in chronic lung disease producing an increased pulmonary blood flow, which in the presence of a restricted vascular bed adds to the pulmonary hypertension and right ventricular hypertrophy.[19,20] Anastomoses between the bronchopulmonary veins and pulmonary veins[21,22] also become more prominent, and the flow in the expanded channels may actually reverse from the bronchopulmonary veins to the pulmonary veins. This produces pollution of systemic arterial blood by desaturated, at times hypercapnic, venous blood. This furnishes an important contribution of venous blood to that already existing from the physiologic pulmonary artery–to–pulmonary vein shunt (when the alveolus is not ventilated or its membranes are so thick that diffusion is prevented).

Myocardial Factors

In cor pulmonale the entire heart is affected and not just the right ventricle. The importance of

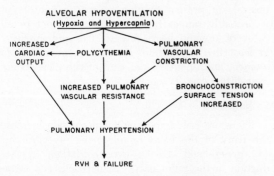

Fig. 46-1. The role of hypoxia secondary to alveolar hypoventilation in the production of cor pulmonale.

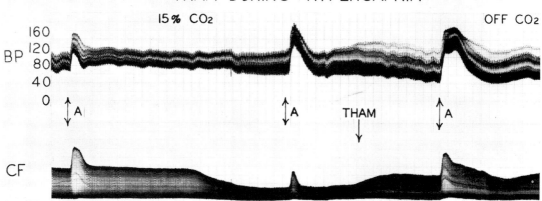

Fig. 46-2. Myocardial depression in the animal produced by carbon dioxide inhalation and its correction by THAM. A = injections of 1 mg per kg levarterenol bitartrate. CF = contractile force measured by a strain-gauge arch attached to the right ventricle. (*Modified from T. D. Darby, E. E. Aldinger, R. H. Gadsden, and W. B. Thrower: Effects of Metabolic Acidosis on Ventricular Isometric Systolic Tension and the Response to Epinephrine and Levarterenol, Circulation Res. vol. 8, November, 1960. By permission of the authors and the American Heart Association, Inc.*)

these factors is emphasized, since in many instances of congenital heart disease the pulmonary artery pressure can be 100 mm or more without heart failure, yet with emphysema heart failure occurs with much lower pulmonary artery pressures. Myocardial factors include the following:

1. Low myocardial oxygen tension. This, occurring in the face of underlying coronary atherosclerosis, undetected clinically but found at autopsy,[23,24] can aggravate right ventricular failure and produce associated left ventricular failure. Hypoxia increases cardiac output equally in both ventricles because of increased flow.[25] Pulmonary disease with hypoxia may place a great burden on the right ventricle, primarily because of increased pulmonary vascular pressure, and on the left ventricle entirely because of increased flow. The right ventricle tolerates poorly the increased load caused by elevation in pressure, while the left ventricle is affected more by increases in flow.[26]

2. High CO_2 tension. In addition to producing a flow load on both ventricles, high CO_2 tension depresses myocardial contractility.[27–29] This effect on contractility is illustrated in Fig. 46-2.

3. Intrapulmonary vascular shunts. The burden on the right ventricle produced by shunts has already been described. Collateral channels between bronchial and pulmonary arteries and anastomoses with flow from the bronchopulmonary veins to pulmonary veins produce a flow load on the left side of the heart with left ventricular enlargement. In severe cases, the amount of blood flowing through these shunts has been estimated at over one-third of the cardiac output.[30] Michel-

son[31] found biventricular hypertrophy in 32 autopsied patients who had had chronic lung disease with no evidence of congenital defects, valvular incompetence, coronary disease, nephrosclerosis, systemic hypertension, or any entity known to cause left ventricular hypertrophy. On a percentage basis, the hypertrophy was greater in the right ventricle. The author has reviewed 97 autopsied cases of cor pulmonale and has found that 83 had biventricular hypertrophy. Thirty-six of these had a significant degree of coronary atherosclerosis but no other cause for left ventricular enlargement.

Functional Classification

Classification is not merely academic but of practical import in terms of instituting appropriate therapy. It is based on whether alveolar hypoventilation or the reduction in pulmonary vascular bed is the more prominent feature. This classification is illustrated in Fig. 46-3. Pulmonary diseases, according to the alterations which produce

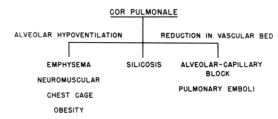

Fig. 46-3. Functional classification of causes of cor pulmonale.

the chronic alveolar hypoventilation syndrome, can be subdivided as follows:

1. Anatomic changes in the lung. Chronic diffuse obstructive emphysema is by far the most common cause in this country. Chronic bronchitis, bronchial asthma, chronic pulmonary tuberculosis, sarcoidosis, pneumoconiosis and mucoviscidosis (fibrocystic disease of the pancreas) can also produce obstructive emphysema and lead to cor pulmonale. The advisory committee in its recent report to the Surgeon General of the Public Health Service concluded that cigarette smoking is the most important of the causes of chronic bronchitis and that a relationship exists between pulmonary emphysema and cigarette smoking. However, it has not been established that this relationship is causal.

2. Defective function of chest bellows. Chronic neuromuscular disorders, massive bilateral pleural thickening, kyphoscoliosis, and obesity have been implicated. In neuromuscular disorders such as poliomyelitis, muscular dystrophies, myasthenia gravis, and amyotrophic lateral sclerosis the muscles of respiration are often too weak to perform their function adequately.[32,33] Changes in the lung or vessels are minor or secondary. Severe kyphoscoliosis with its structural deformity of the chest cage frequently produces chronic cor pulmonale.[34] Bellows restriction is most important in these patients; however, they also develop recurrent pulmonary infections and abnormalities of obstructive emphysema.[35] In certain obese people a cardiopulmonary syndrome (Pickwickian syndrome) may be present. Although the ultimate mechanisms are not well understood, it is agreed that the exogenous obesity plays a large role. This is demonstrated by the fact that weight loss initiates a reversal of the syndrome. The lungs themselves appear normal, but there may be increased need for gas exchange as well as increased resistance to ventilation as a result of the masses of fat.[36–39] Recently Fadell and others[40] reported an autopsied case of the Pickwickian syndrome with marked infiltration of the respiratory musculature by fat in sufficient magnitude to interfere with normal respiratory mechanisms and produce alveolar hypoventilation.

3. Diminished ventilatory drive. Central nervous system lesions that lead to depression of the respiratory center are rare. In these cases the chest bellows and lung are normal, but there is a diminished ventilatory drive because of a damaged respiratory center.[41–43]

Pulmonary diseases that produce cor pulmonale by reduction of the pulmonary vascular bed in contrast to those seen with alveolar hypoventilation are characterized by the development of cor pulmonale in the late stages of the disease and pulmonary hypertension which is usually irreversible. These diseases, according to the pathologic changes, can be subdivided into intraluminal and extraluminal. *Intraluminal* diseases include multiple or massive pulmonary emboli,[44] primary pulmonary hypertension,[45] thrombosis of pulmonary arteries, sickle-cell anemia,[46] and schistosomiasis,[47] which are some of the causes of a reduced vascular bed. Many causes of *extraluminal* diseases are classified under the category of alveolar capillary block syndromes[48,49] and are characterized by impaired pulmonary oxygen diffusion. This syndrome has been described in a variety of conditions with fibrous, granulomatous, inflammatory, or neoplastic involvement of the lung, including berylliosis, sarcoidosis, pulmonary scleroderma, silicosis, radiation fibrosis, histiocytosis X, eosinophilic pneumonitis, miliary tuberculosis, diffuse interstitial fibrosis (Hamman-Rich syndrome), carcinomatosis, and other granulomatoses and fibroses of undetermined cause. Neither alveolar hypoventilation nor reduction in pulmonary vascular bed appear often in pure form, but there are usually combinations such as silicosis combined with emphysema.[50]

Pathology

The pathologic features in the categories of alveolar hypoventilation (primarily chronic obstructive emphysema) and reduction in pulmonary vascular bed (primarily alveolar capillary diffusion defects) will be described.

In patients with emphysema, cor pulmonale will develop only in those who have hypoxia and hypercapnia as a result of severe alveolar respiratory insufficiency. This alveolar hypoventilation stems from bronchiolar obstruction, decreased lung elasticity (not less elastic tissue), and fixation of the chest cage, which combine to interfere with gas distribution to the lungs. When arterial oxygen saturation at rest falls below 80 volumes per cent and carbon dioxide tension rises, one or more of the following appear: a rise in cardiac output, pulmonary hypertension, and an elevated hematocrit. Although the exact mechanisms whereby hypoxia elicits the changes are not fully clarified, there is little doubt that it is the main offender, and with its relief comes an improvement in the circulatory function. In some cases there may be normal-appearing pulmonary arteries, even though cor pulmonale has been present for many years.[51] The reduction of the pulmonary vascular bed in emphysema may play a contributory role, especially when the patient is under such stress as exercise or hypoxia. Pulmonary vascular resistance is increased because of vascular deformity due to pressure by emphysematous spaces, destruction of vascular bed, and intimal fibrosis of the pulmonary arterioles. Newer techniques[52-60] have provided considerable information pertaining to our understanding the morphologic changes in emphysema. Most investigators outline a clinical pathologic classification of emphysema by beginning with a consideration of the secondary lobule, which is described as the smallest functioning unit of lung tissue enveloped by connective tissue septums. Its terminal bronchiole ends in the middle of the lobule, and distal respiratory bronchioles branch outward in a radial fashion with their alveoli outpouchings. Also there can be seen in such a unit a terminal pulmonary arteriole which eventually forms the fine capillaries which drain into the paralobular veins located in the connective tissue septums at the periphery of the secondary lobule.[61,17] On the basis of pathologic studies, centrilobular emphysema has been described as a special anatomic form in which the main lesion is a selective and progressive dilatation and destruction of the respiratory bronchiole occurring initially in the center of the secondary lobule.[59,62,63] A second type of emphysema, equally as frequent, has been identified as panlobular emphysema[64-66] because of its uniform widespread air membrane distension and destruction throughout the secondary lobule and nonlobulated pulmonary tissue. The centrilobular emphysema is often situated at a vital point where the artery supplying the secondary lobule bifurcates, so that the emphysematous space is situated in the fork formed by the two branches and their lumens are narrowed and irregular. This produces increased resistance to blood flow in the whole area of the lobule, even though there may be little parenchymal destruction. In emphysema, especially during expiration, there is a markedly positive intraalveolar pressure which can cause compression of smaller branches of the pulmonary artery. Although this may be intermittent, the prolonged expiratory phase may subject the vessels to extramural pressure for considerable lengths of time.[67] Wyatt et al.[17] emphasized that panlobular emphysema affects the pulmonary vascular bed and compromises the total capillary bed through alveolar wall fenestration and transmitted extramural pressure. Color Plate 6 depicts the vascular deformity and destruction in the secondary lobule associated with panlobular and centrilobular emphysema.[68]

As indicated previously, other factors in the development of cor pulmonale are pathologic shunts from artery to vein, bronchopulmonary shunting, particularly in emphysema with fibrosis, and a decompensating portal azygos–pulmonary vein system. Intimal fibrosis of the pulmonary arterioles

and thromboembolic phenomena are considered to be of minor importance.

In patients with alveolar capillary diffusion defects, the lungs are often found shrunken and fibrotic, showing extensive degrees of interstitial fibrosis, smooth muscle hypertrophy, cystic areas, and bronchiectasis. Herbert et al.[69] described such changes in 19 cases of chronic interstitial pulmonary fibrosis and Rubin and Lubliner[70] in 15 cases of the Hamman-Rich syndrome with a more acute clinical course. There is interference with diffusion of oxygen across a thickened alveolar capillary membrane. Since carbon dioxide is approximately twenty times as diffusible as oxygen, impaired transfer is seldom a problem except in the very late stages of the disease. As a result of the fibrosis and shrinkage of the lungs, there is destruction of alveoli and pulmonary capillaries and thickening of interalveolar septums causing a reduction of the vascular bed, pulmonary hypertension, and eventually cor pulmonale.

Diagnosis

Type of Pulmonary Disease

It is essential to determine the type of pulmonary disease that has precipitated the cor pulmonale in order to institute proper therapy. The diseases that produce alveolar hypoventilation, primarily chronic obstructive emphysema, must be differentiated from those that produce alveolar capillary diffusion defects.

Clinically, patients with obstructive emphysema have a chronic cough, bouts of bronchitis, and exertional dyspnea for a period of 5 to 10 years prior to development of cardiac disability. On examination they are dyspneic, orthopneic, and cyanotic; they cough ineffectually; and their eyes are protuberant, injected, and chemotic. Neck veins of many such patients without heart failure are distended as a consequence of the marked changes in intrapleural pressure. Retrograde filling may aid in distinguishing those with elevated venous pressure. The chest resembles a rectangle with manubrium upward and forward, and their backs have a rounded appearance. In the presence of CO_2 retention, Cheyne-Stokes breathing is rarely encountered. Papilledema may appear, probably the result of a combination of right-sided failure, hypercapnia, and hypoxemia associated with a secondary elevation in cerebral spinal fluid pressure.[71-75] There is no convincing evidence that polycythemia is a factor in producing the papilledema. There is wheezing in the lungs and rhonchi are present. Clubbing of the digits and pulmonary hypertrophic osteoarthropathy may occur, but these are more often seen if there is associated bronchiectasis.

In contrast, the patient with alveolar capillary block has dyspnea with tachypnea and hyperventilation and may be cyanotic, especially after exercise. The configuration of the chest may be normal. Fine rales are present at the lung bases, and there is no evidence of bronchial obstruction. The tachypnea is probably related to the decreased compliance of the lungs, for it has been shown that in this situation rapid, shallow breathing is the most economical in terms of respiratory work.[76]

Pulmonary diseases can also be differentiated by tests of pulmonary function. Ventilation, diffusion, and blood flow (perfusion) are involved in delivering oxygen and removing CO_2 from the pulmonary capillary bed. Ventilation is primarily studied by the total and timed vital capacity and maximum breathing capacity. Diffusion is determined by the uptake of carbon monoxide and of oxygen by blood at different alveolar partial pressures and pulmonary blood flow by heart catheterization. These tests of diffusion and blood flow are costly and time-consuming, and require specialized equipment and technical aid. They are usually performed in medical centers that have special cardiopulmonary laboratories. In actual clinical practice, after careful history taking and physical and roentgenologic examinations of the chest sufficient knowledge of pulmonary function may be obtained by performing the ventilatory test and measurement of the arterial blood gases with very simple apparatus.

Ventilatory Studies. The timed vital capacity is more informative than the total vital capacity (which is measured after a maximal inspiration). It is a dynamic measurement relating the percentage of the total vital capacity expired to time, normally 85 per cent for the first second, 90 per cent for 2 seconds, and 95 per cent for 3 seconds. The degree of reversible bronchospasm can be determined by repeating the test after the administration of a bronchodilator. In chronic obstructive emphysema the total vital capacity may or may not be reduced, while the timed vital capacity and maximum breathing capacity are significantly altered.[77,78] Ventilatory studies may be normal in the alveolar capillary block syndromes in spite of marked impairment of diffusion.

Arterial Gas Studies. These measurements are not only significant as aids in diagnosis but should be performed at intervals as a guide to therapy. Since the advent of the newer instrumentation, pH, O_2 saturation, and pCO_2 (carbon dioxide tension) can be readily measured in a brief period with only 5 ml arterial blood.[79] In emphysema, CO_2 may increase very rapidly, so that it may be impossible for available base to unite with a sufficient amount of CO_2 to maintain the pH within normal range. The pCO_2 will rise considerably, yet the CO_2 content (bicarbonate concentration) may rise only slightly. A serious retention of CO_2 occurs in body cells. The pCO_2 depicts the exchange limits between cells and blood, information which cannot be acquired from knowledge of the CO_2 content.[80] It is directly proportional to the actual amount of dissolved carbonic acid. Therefore, pCO_2 is much more valuable in evaluating the degree and direction of primary respiratory disturbances, especially with reference to acidosis and to therapeutic response. Figure 46-4 compares the ventilatory test and arterial gas studies in emphysema and alveolar capillary diffusion defects. In alveolar capillary block there is no CO_2 retention, in spite of the diffusion difficulty, since CO_2 diffuses twenty times as readily as O_2 through the alveolar capillary membrane. Oxygen breathing in such cases usually produces a normal arterial oxygen saturation, except in a few instances where this will not occur because of physiologic shunts or venous admixture (when perfusion of capillaries is adequate but alveoli are underventilated or membranes are so thick that diffusion is prevented).[81]

Clinical Features

The primary problem is first to recognize the type of pulmonary disease and then to determine if cor pulmonale is present. It is very difficult to

	VENTILATORY TEST VC–MBC	ARTERIAL O_2 SATURATION			ARTERIAL CO_2 TENSION	ARTERIAL pH
		REST	EXERCISE	O_2 BREATHING		
ALVEOLAR HYPOVENTILATION (emphysema)	IMPAIRMENT	LOW	LOWER	NORMAL	HIGH	LOW
ALVEOLAR CAP. BLOCK	NORMAL	NORMAL or LOW	LOWER	NORMAL	NORMAL or LOW	NORMAL

Fig. 46.4. Comparison of ventilatory test and arterial gas studies in emphysema and alveolar capillary block.

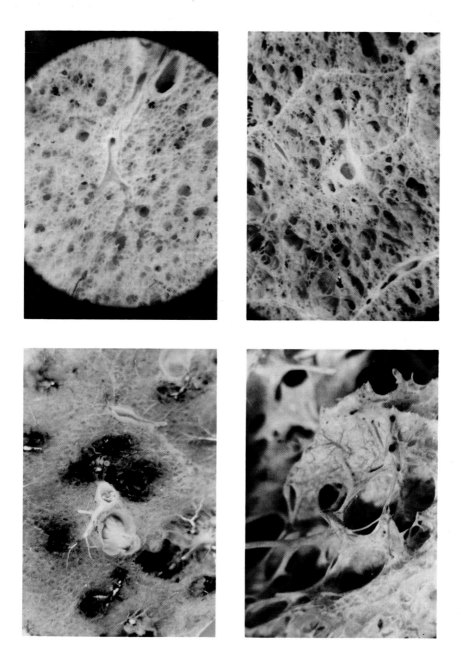

Plate 6. Thin (5-mm) lung sections impregnated with barium sulfate depicting secondary lobules; pulmonary arterioles and capillaries injected with red latex and paralobular veins with blue latex. *Upper left.* Normal lung. Two terminal bronchioles with respiratory bronchioles branching out radially are seen in the center. Pulmonary capillaries give this section a uniform blush appearance, and the paralobular veins are situated at the periphery in the connective tissue septums. *Upper right.* Early panlobular emphysema. Note cavitations and less uniform redness of the tissue, especially on the right where many capillaries are destroyed. *Lower left.* Centrilobular emphysema. Note cavitations near the midpoint affecting the pulmonary arteriole at the entrance into the secondary lobule, with the right branch absent because of pressure and destruction. *Lower right.* Severe mixed type emphysema. Note that the normal architecture is disrupted. A small artery can be seen relatively devoid of branches. (*From unpublished data of S. Appel, F. A. McIver, and R. A. Harley, Department of Pathology, Medical College of South Carolina.*)

make a clinical diagnosis of cor pulmonale prior to the development of heart failure, since right ventricular hypertrophy is almost impossible to detect early. It is also difficult to decide whether failure of the right side of the heart is present or symptoms and findings are due entirely to the emphysema. Heart failure may be very insidious and appear as further impairment of pulmonary function, as though the emphysema were becoming more severe. The usual findings of early congestive failure are often masked by those of the advanced emphysema. Cough, dyspnea, orthopnea, peripheral edema due to inactivity and venous stasis, and a palpable liver because of a low diaphragm may be present in emphysema without heart failure. The neck veins may be distended without congestive failure but usually are more congested on expiration and collapse on inspiration.

In emphysema, once cor pulmonale is present, the following physical signs are noted: The patient may be cyanosed, confused, somnolent, or even comatose. In the early stages, the pulse is usually bounding and regular, and the arms, legs, ears, and nose are warm. The blood pressure may be elevated, with a wide pulse pressure. These findings are due to the peripheral vasodilation often associated even with early CO_2 retention and the increased cardiac output.[82-85] At a later stage the cardiac output can be normal or low.[86] The apex beat cannot be localized because of distension of the overlying lung, but a systolic thrust of the right ventricle may lift the sternum, and the hypertrophied right ventricle can often be felt protruding beneath the xiphosternum on palpation in the epigastric area. A right ventricular diastolic gallop with inspiratory accentuation may be audible near the sternum or in the epigastrium and the pulmonic second sound accentuated, suggesting the presence of pulmonary hypertension. When heart failure is present, the jugular venous pressure is usually elevated, as noted when the patient is lying at an angle of 45° from the horizontal. Its level may be difficult to determine because of fluctuations produced from the great variations in intrapleural pressure due to respiratory effort. Retrograde filling will aid in recognizing true elevation of venous pressure. Cheyne-Stokes respiration is rarely seen with CO_2 retention, and hydrothorax from heart failure due to emphysema is rare.[87,88] The liver will be enlarged (not just displaced downward) and tender. Dependent edema is a common feature, and ascites can occur. If treatment is not effective, increasing respiratory depression and worsening of cardiac failure will ensue with deepening coma and cyanosis, a rising pulse rate, falling blood pressure, and increasing peripheral vasoconstriction recognizable by the develop-

ment of cold extremities. These findings indicate a falling cardiac output and are grave prognostic features. Pulmonary emboli and acute coronary thrombosis are complications which may produce a similar terminal picture. These, rather than terminal cor pulmonale, should be suspected in a patient with pulmonary emphysema and cyanosis when there is no significant CO_2 retention.

In addition to masking failure of the right side of the heart, emphysema often presents findings suggestive of left ventricular failure. The problem is further accentuated when a patient with senile emphysema and failure of the left side of the heart has to be differentiated from obstructive pulmonary emphysema. Differentiation is extremely important, especially with regard to therapeutic considerations. The history is of great importance. Orthopnea, paroxysmal nocturnal dyspnea, pulsus alternans, and frothy sputum, especially with very little wheezing, are features which suggest left ventricular failure, whereas repeated bouts of bronchitis and progressive dyspnea for many years suggest pulmonary disease. A palpable apical impulse, protodiastolic gallop, and pulsus alternans favor left ventricular failure. Chest x-rays and electrocardiograms may be of aid, especially if they clearly demonstrate either right or left ventricular hypertrophy. Circulation time is often prolonged in failure of the left side of the heart. Arterial gas studies will indicate emphysema if there is CO_2 retention and a low arterial pH. Therapeutic tests may be dangerous; however, when in doubt it is usually safe to administer aminophylline, which is of therapeutic value in both.

Since bronchial obstruction produces greater than normal increase of intrathoracic negative pressure during inspiration, patients with pulmonary emphysema may have a paradoxical pulse, which introduces the problem of differentiation from pericardial effusion with tamponade or constrictive pericarditis, since both may have distended neck veins, hepatomegaly, diminished heart sound, and low ECG voltage.

In the alveolar capillary diffusion defects the cardiac output may be normal or low; therefore, these patients are not very warm and do not have bounding pulses. A right ventricular lift is easier to detect than in emphysema, since there is usually less increase in the posteroanterior (PA) diameter of the chest. At times the pulmonary pressure can be very high, producing a diastolic pulmonic insufficiency murmur, systolic murmur of tricuspid insufficiency, a pulmonary systolic click, and a prominent venous jugular A wave. Pulmonary hypertension and right ventricular enlargement may precede the development of even moderate anoxia. Heart failure occurs when there is severe anoxia

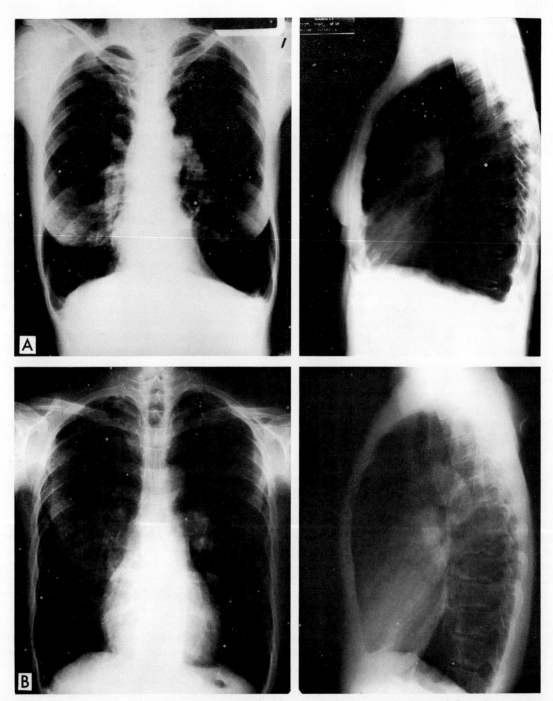

Fig. 46-5. Posteroanterior and lateral x-ray views of the chest in two patients with chronic diffuse obstructive emphysema and chronic cor pulmonale. *A.* In the PA view of this female patient, the pulmonary artery and hilar vessels are prominent, and the heart does not appear enlarged in its transverse diameter. Observe in the lateral view that the right ventricle is enlarged and encroaches on the retrosternal space. *B.* In this male patient the heart is larger, especially the right ventricle, as is seen in the lateral view.

and is usually terminal and seldom reversible, as is seen at times with obstructive emphysema. In both categories, a rising hematocrit reading and blood gas changes should suggest impending failure of the right side of the heart.

X-rays

Roentgenographic studies are of aid in determining the underlying type of pulmonary disease. The heart may be very large or appear to be normal. The enlargement which occurs is confined to the pulmonary arteries, right ventricle, and right atrium, and is best seen in the lateral projections (Fig. 46-5). In the emphysematous patient the small vertical heart may be dilated but without apparent increase in size, and only by comparison with previous films can this be detected. If other films are not available, then after recovery from failure cardiomegaly can be suspected if the heart returns to its previous small size. The marked changes in the heart size as a patient goes in and out of failure suggest that dilatation may be more important than hypertrophy.[88] Cor pulmonale secondary to severe kyphoscoliosis is illustrated in Fig. 46-6. The marked distortion of the thoracic contents make x-ray interpretation very difficult, and it is impossible to determine specific cardiac chamber enlargement.

Electrocardiogram

The electrocardiographic signs in chronic cor pulmonale have been well described.[89-91] The outstanding patterns with their approximate percentages have been described by Armen et al.[92] In 16 per cent the P-wave axis is greater than plus 60°, resulting in tall, peaked P waves in leads II, III, and AVF, which are often associated with prominent Ta waves, which produces a downward displacement of the P-R segment. The heart is usually vertical with extreme clockwise rotation and right axis deviation, with low QRS voltage and rS or QS complexes in all the precordial leads. Often with emphysema these findings are simply due to positional changes of the heart due to the chest deformity. Hecht[93] did not consider the P-wave findings as indicative of right atrial hypertrophy, since they may regress to normal on digitalis therapy. Other writers[94,95] believe that these P-wave changes may result from right atrial enlargement, dilatation, and/or hypertrophy. Twenty-seven per cent have the pattern of right ventricular hypertrophy with a tall R wave in the V_1 or V_3R positions. This is unusual in the cases of cor pulmonale secondary to emphysema and is more often seen in those with alveolar capillary block, which produces more of a resistant load on the right ventricle.

Right bundle branch block occurs in 27 per cent, and in another 8 per cent the QRS duration is 0.12 sec or longer. In 12 per cent the prominent feature was T-wave inversion in leads V_1, V_2, and V_3 in the right side of the chest without R-wave changes. The final 10 per cent have miscellaneous patterns such as left axis deviation and patterns suggestive of anteroseptal, anterior, anterolateral, and diaphragmatic infarctions.[96,97] Abnormal left axis deviation in the range of minus 90° has been considered to be due to abnormal transmission of electric potentials,[98] associated left ventricular enlargement, conduction disturbance,[99] marked right axis deviation,[95] or even an axis illusion phenomenon.[90,99] As mentioned previously, several myocardial factors may affect the whole heart and actually cause associated left ventricular enlargement. Chronic arrhythmias are not frequent, but acute anoxic periods even in the absence of heart failure will produce paroxysmal arrhythmias, primarily atrial in origin, such as atrial tachycardia, atrial flutter, atrial fibrillation, and tachycardia with block. These may disappear with improvement of the anoxic state. A normal tracing may be observed in well-advanced cases of cor pulmonale; therefore, the absence of electrocardiographic evidence of right ventricular disease does not exclude this lesion. In summary, the main positive electrocar-

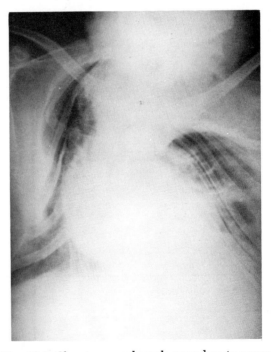

Fig. 46-6. Chronic cor pulmonale secondary to severe kyphoscoliosis. The marked structural deformity of the thoracic cage obscures the cardiac and pulmonary findings.

diographic signs of cor pulmonale are right axis deviation greater than 110°, conduction defects producing an *r*SR′ complex in the right precordial leads, and classic right ventricular hypertrophy in V_1 or V_3R with dominant R waves (R*s*, R, QR, *q*R*s*, and *q*R).

Treatment

Pulmonary Failure

The first object of therapy is to institute vigorous treatment for the pulmonary insufficiency. Lee's findings[100] stress early treatment, since rapidly ensuing death in patients with acute or chronic lung disease is often due to cor pulmonale superimposed upon acute respiratory failure, whether or not infection is present. The following is an outline of therapy for alveolar hypoventilation, particularly that associated with emphysema.

Smoking. The patient with chronic bronchitis and emphysema should omit smoking permanently. The recent Surgeon General's report[101] supports this point of view. Considerable evidence is available suggesting that smoking results in histologic changes in the lung parenchyma as well as in the bronchial epithelium and glands in the bronchial tubes.[102]

Oxygen Therapy. Carbon dioxide, oxygen, and hydrogen concentrations (pH) are paramount factors in the control of respiration. Although CO_2 is the primary stimulant, anoxemia may stimulate the respiratory center reflexly through the chemoreceptors located in the carotid and aortic bodies. In advanced obstructive emphysema a patient is unable to eliminate CO_2, and increased arterial pCO_2 and respiratory acidosis develop. As a result of CO_2 retention, the hydrogen ion concentration is decreased,[103] depressing the respiratory center and leaving anoxemia as its only stimulant. Removal of this hypoxemic stimulus by giving oxygen improperly my result in apnea, further CO_2 retention, coma, and death. Recently there has been some debate as to whether or not there is impaired sensitivity of the respiratory center to CO_2 in emphysema. Cherniak[104] and others have suggested that mechanical limitation of the chest bellows is responsible for the decreased ventilatory reaction to CO_2. Many patients with such a condition can tolerate oxygen without adverse effects if given in lower concentrations, especially with a mechanical respirator. The oxygen-hemoglobin dissociation curve[105] (Fig. 46-7) shows how anoxia can be sufficiently relieved with increase in O_2 saturation, yet not influence oxygen tension to the degree of removing the stimulus to ventilation (low oxygen tension) on aortic chemoreceptors. The S-shaped curve is a distinct advantage to the patient, since oxygen can be given carefully, maintaining up to 94 per cent saturation, yet not increasing O_2 tension above 80 mm Hg, which would remove the stimulus to ventilation. As long as oxygen tension remains below 80 mm Hg, ventilation is increasingly stimulated, but beyond this point a 30-mm rise in O_2 tension is necessary to achieve an increase of 4 per cent saturation. At the bend of the curve a 30-mm rise would give an increase of 34 per cent saturation. During oxygen administration there should be careful clinical observation of the patient and frequent measurements of arterial blood gases.

Mechanical Assistance. Respirators[106,107] may be required to increase alveolar ventilation and aid in CO_2 elimination and oxygenation. Some patients, because of stupor and thick secretions in the airway, will not benefit unless an early elective tracheostomy of the cuffed type or tracheal fenestration is performed.[108,109] Accordingly, the anatomic dead space is decreased with increase in alveolar ventilation, removal of secretions, and establishment of proper humidification and liquefaction. The administration of oxygen by intermittent positive pressure machines is usually quite effective. Although sometimes lifesaving, this may be hazardous in emphysematous patients in respiratory failure if not used cautiously. In patients with severe air trapping from emphysema, the persistent rise in intrathoracic pressure that may occur with

OXYGEN-HEMOGLOBIN DISSOCIATION CURVE

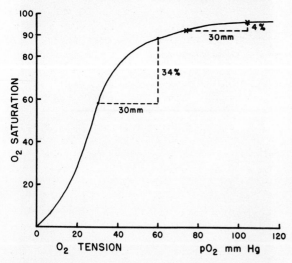

Fig. 46-7. Oxygen-hemoglobin dissociation curve. The curve is given for 37° and a blood pH of 7.4. (*Modified from J. H. Comroe, Jr., R. E. Forster, II, A. B. Dubois, W. A. Briscoe, and E. Carlsen: "The Lung: Clinical Physiology and Pulmonary Function Tests," The Year Book Medical Publishers, Inc., Chicago, 1955. With permission of the authors and publisher.*)

intermittent positive pressure can seriously impede venous return to the heart, with a marked drop in cardiac output and sudden death.[100] These circulatory hazards may be partly avoided by using intermittent positive pressure with a rapidly increasing pressure. during inspiration and a very slow pump frequency, allowing for a long expiratory period, equal to or exceeding inspiratory time with a rapid early drop in mean mask pressure during the expiratory period to near atmospheric pressure.[110,111] Positive-negative pressure, which does not impede venous return to a great degree, may be more appropriate in certain instances, especially when there is an ineffective cough reflex. With any type of respirator the concentration of oxygen should not be higher than 40 per cent, since the hazard of removing the anoxic stimulus to breathing is always present. Studies with volume-controlled ventilation utilizing the Engstrom respirator to relieve the patient completely of respiratory work appear to be promising.[112]

Bronchodilators. Vaporized bronchodilators used with or without a positive pressure apparatus are often quite effective in alleviating bronchospasm and mucosal edema. The removal of tracheobronchial secretions by tracheobronchial aspiration is of utmost importance. The patient should be taught the technique of postural drainage. The advantage of the aerosols now in use is that small doses are effective without side reactions. Isoproterenol hydrochloride (Isuprel hydrochloride), in addition to its bronchodilator action, is capable of altering the pulmonary vascular bed of resting and exercising emphysematous patients so that increases in pulmonary blood flow are associated with a fall in pulmonary artery pressure and a significant decrease in calculated pulmonary vascular resistance.[113] Excessive use of isoproterenol hydrochloride may result in headaches, tremors, sinus tachycardia or arrhythmias. Aminophylline by suppository or slow infusion is often effective in relieving extreme bronchospasm.

Antibiotics. The patient with an acute exacerbation of chronic lung disease often has pulmonary infection, at times without a febrile or leukocyte response. It is very difficult to isolate the responsible bacteria, so treatment must be empirical. Penicillin or a broad spectrum antibiotic can be used unless cultures reveal an organism which is more sensitive to a specific antibiotic.

Drugs Which Counteract the Respiratory Acidosis. Continuous stimulation of ventilation has been tried with aminophylline, Coramine, and salicylates,[114] and more recently with vanillic diethyl amide (Ethamivan).[115,116] Improvement in ventilation has been noted and demonstrated by significant decrease in CO_2 tension. In some patients these drugs may not be of value, because the alveolar hypoventilation is due to the increased work of breathing produced by the abnormal mechanics of the bellows system, rather than to an insensitive or depressed respiratory center. The respiratory center may be discharging a normal quantity of efferent impulses to the respiratory muscles, which in turn are producing a normal work output for a given CO_2 stimulus. Increasing the ventilatory rate in the presence of severe air-flow obstruction may increase the mechanical work and the metabolic cost of breathing so markedly that the resultant production of CO_2 rapidly exceeds the rate of its elimination, resulting in further CO_2 retention and hypoxemia.[117-119]

The carbonic anhydrase inhibitor acetazoleamide (Diamox) has been used as a diuretic. It also promotes elimination of CO_2 by improving ventilation through stimulation of the respiratory center by the excretion of bicarbonate and bicarbonate-bound base. Since this drug produces a metabolic acidosis, it should be used cautiously, and only in patients who are improving as a result of other measures but who continue to manifest hypercapnia. A significant experimental advance in the treatment of chronic CO_2 retention has been the use of the amine buffer THAM (2-amino-2-hydroxymethyl-1,3-propanediol).[120-122] Figure 46-2 illustrates that forced CO_2 ventilation resulted in a marked depression of myocardial contractility and of the response to levarterenol bitartrate. Correction of the respiratory acidosis by the administration of THAM, which increased the CO_2-carrying capacity of the blood, resulted in an immediate improvement in contractility and in levarterenol bitartrate response.[28] However, when ventilation is not assisted, THAM may decrease ventilation and produce severe aggravation of hypoxemia,[123] since it is a respiratory depressant through its direct effect on the respiratory center or its effect on pH. It may produce hypoglycemia and should be administered with glucose. Another problem with this approach is the great amount of carbonic acid that is produced as compared to the relatively small amount of hydrogen ion that is excreted by the kidney. Thus, improving ventilation is more beneficial than an attempt to increase renal excretion of hydrogen ion by means of buffer administration.[124]

Avoidance of Sedation. It is obvious that the use of morphine and other narcotics are contraindicated because of the further respiratory depression which may be produced. Barbiturates and tranquilizers may also be harmful. If sedation is absolutely necessary, chloral hydrate can be administered by mouth or rectum.

Steriods. A trial of adrenal corticosteroids is indicated at times, with careful evaluation of the results and continuation in those who show a satisfactory response.[125] Long-term steroid therapy is much more controversial and cannot be recommended generally in patients with emphysema, because of the lack of efficacy and the potential complications. Results of most studies have shown that prolonged use of steroids produces only minor changes in pulmonary function, although some patients obtain a certain degree of symptomatic relief. Patients should be observed carefully, since gastroduodenal ulcers occur frequently in patients with emphysema[126,127] and can be reactivated. A recent necropsy study demonstrated a significant association between pulmonary emphysema and adrenocortical hyperplasia, and between emphysema and peptic ulceration.[128]

Acid-Base Regulation. Hypokalemia and systemic alkalosis may develop because of diuretics, steroids, and removal of large volumes of carbon dioxide from the lung with respirators without concomitant removal of bicarbonate by the kidneys.[129] Cochran[130] reported two cases of severe chronic pulmonary insufficiency and hypercapnia complicated by systemic alkalosis related to hypokalemia secondary to diuretics and chronic inanition, anoxia, and acidosis. Robin[124] obtained acid-base measurements in 156 patients with primary lung disease without any evidence of other metabolic or renal disease and concluded that such patients with hypercapnia may have alkalotic rather than acidotic values of plasma pH. The possible mechanisms for this paradox include rapid mobilization of carbon dioxide by forced hyperventilation, hypochloremia and body chloride depletion, and alkalizing therapy. Carbonic anhydrase inhibitors may produce bicarbonate diuresis without a concomitant increase in alveolar ventilation resulting in severe metabolic acidosis. It is obvious that in addition to frequent determination of blood gases, there should also be electrolyte evaluations.

Surgical Treatment. Besides tracheostomy in certain cases, surgical removal or obliteration of large bullae may be of value.

The necessity of a balanced approach in the treatment of emphysema, especially with respiratory acidosis, should be emphasized. Overtreatment or attempts to correct any individual chemical factor may result in a more serious problem which can be potentially fatal.

Many of the therapeutic measures mentioned in emphysema should be tried in alveolar capillary diffusion defects, especially oxygen and antibiotics. There is no known direct therapy for the primary pulmonary disease. In the granulomas, the use of adrenal corticosteroids has offered some hope of limiting the cellular proliferation causing the al-

veolar capillary block syndrome. However, it is not always possible to control the degree of pulmonary fibrosis, and there are many steroid side reactions.

Cardiac Failure

Pulmonary hypertension, hypoxia, and hypercapnia can be aggravated by associated heart failure. However, the pulmonary insufficiency must be controlled first, so that effective ventilation, increased oxygenation, and lowering of CO_2 will reduce the load on the heart and allow a better therapeutic response.

Digitalis. Kim and Aviado[131] have shown in the anesthetized dog that intravenous acetylstrophanthidin produces an increase in pulmonary vascular resistance. The situation in the lung of the normal human being is uncertain. Digitalization in patients with cor pulmonale produces variable effects on the pulmonary circulation, but the majority show a reduction in calculated vascular resistance with an increase in cardiac output.[132] This reduction is probably a passive response to the increase in flow, and to improved function of the left ventricle with resulting decrease in pulmonary venous pressure. Pulmonary pressure may increase in the initial phase of digitalization and then subsequently fall to prior levels or lower with improvement of the general circulation. These physiologic changes suggest the need for slow and cautious digitalization. Even though the response is not optimal, digitalization is indicated, since several myocardial factors are implicated, as previously mentioned, and there often are concomitant coronary arteriosclerotic changes with total heart failure. Digitalis intoxication frequently occurs in the management of emphysema. There is a tendency to increase digitalis dosage in an attempt to control edema and reduce dyspnea (which is usually due to the the lung disease) and also to rely solely on the heart rate as an index of full digitalization. Patients often have a rapid heart rate, not only because of failure, but also as a result of anoxia. Adequate digitalization may reduce the rate very little, and if increased further in an attempt to control the rate, digitalis arrhythmias may ensue. During respiratory acidosis, hydrogen ions displace intracellular potassium ions, which diffuse out and produce elevation of extracellular potassium.[133] This hyperkalemia may obscure the action of digitalis with subsequent increase in dosage. If this is reversed rapidly by treatment such as with intravenous sodium or glucose, adrenal steroids, diuretics, and removal of large volumes of carbon dioxide by respirators, sudden hypokalemia and systemic alkalosis may develop with concomitant digitalis toxicity. Goldberg et al.[134] observed that patients with cor pulmonale are more prone to paroxysmal atrial tachycardia with block.

Diuretics. As in other forms of congestive failure, mercurial diuretics, thiazide derivatives, and acetazoleamide may be employed. These should be used cautiously, as they may increase hemoconcentration and viscosity and produce tenacious sputum and loss of potassium with resulting hypokalemia.

Phlebotomy. Polycythemia is a compensatory mechanism associated with increased production of hemoglobin and red cells, so that more oxygen can be carried to the tissues in a given time. Difficulty arises after optimal compensation is established and the regulatory thermostat, which may be erythropoietin stimulated by hypoxemia, fails to act and the benefits of increased oxygen-carrying capacity are overcome. Too many erythrocytes are produced, with resultant high blood viscosity and increased venous return, which may overburden the already decompensated heart. The relationship of specific viscosity of the blood to the hematocrit values is depicted in Fig. 46-8.[135–137] Note that the viscosity increases abruptly between hematocrit values of 60 and 70 per cent, with impediment to blood flow, increased stickiness, decreased delivery of oxygen to tissues, and increased burden on the heart. This suggests that patients with secondary polycythemia should be bled gradually and slowly to the point where the hematocrit values are below 55 volumes per cent, since patients with emphysema do distinctly better with hematocrit values at about this level. The phlebotomies should be done slowly, with removal of small volumes of venous blood (200 to 300 ml) every 2 or 3 days, until the hematocrit reaches the desired level. Ratto et al.[138] and more recently Vanier et al.[139] pointed out that some patients with severe emphysema may have polycythemia, but this is unusual. They postulate that the polycythemic response is inhibited by chronic and acute infections, carbon dioxide retention, and slight decrease in red cell survival. Results of studies by Lertzman and associates show that secondary polycythemia developed proportionately to the degree of hypoxia and may be significantly elevated even though the hematocrit is normal.[140]

Thyroid Ablation. Radioactive iodine for functional ablation of the thyroid to lower the metabolic demands of the body has not proved to be useful.[141]

Once compensation has been regained, maintenance therapy is similar to that for any patient with congestive heart failure, that is, limited activity, maintenance digitalis, sodium restriction, and diuretics (especially acetazoleamide). It is also important to keep pulmonary function as high

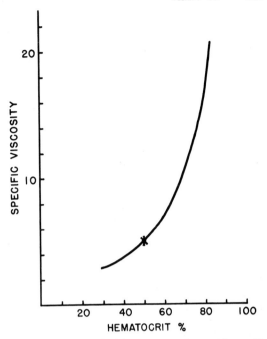

Fig. 46-8. Correlation of hematocrit values with specific viscosity of the blood. (*Modified from A. Nadas: Pediatric Cardiology, 2d ed., W. B. Saunders Company, Philadelphia, 1963. With permission of the authors, publisher, and the American Academy of Pediatrics.*)

as possible. It is imperative to prevent episodes of prolonged severe dyspnea by limiting activities, treating asthmatic episodes and pulmonary infections with the use of bronchodilators, expectorants, antibiotics, and in some cases steroids for continuous wheezing to reduce allergic edema and bronchospasm. Patients should be urged to discontinue cigarette smoking, especially in view of evidence which suggests that it may result in histologic changes in the lung parenchyma as well as in bronchial epithelium and glands in the bronchial tubes.[102] Arterial gases should be measured to detect impending pulmonary failure. Congestive failure, as well as infections, can precipitate acute pulmonary insufficiency in patients with chronic cor pulmonale.

REFERENCES

1. Mack, I., Anderson, M. W., Goldberg, H., and Mattingly, T. W.: Chronic Cor Pulmonale, *Dis. Chest,* **41**:477–488, 1962.
2. Chronic Cor Pulmonale: Report of an Expert Committee of the World Health Organization, *Circulation,* **27**:594–615, 1963.
3. Padmavati, S., and Joshi, B.: Incidence and Etiology of Chronic Cor Pulmonale in Delhi, *Dis. Chest,* **46**:457–463, 1964.

4. McMichael, J.: Emphysema Heart, *Prog. Cardiovas. Dis.*, **1**:446–456, 1959.

5. Sanghvi, L. M., and Kotia, K. C.: Heart Failure in Patients with Chronic Pulmonary Emphysema, *Dis. Chest*, **44**:67–78, 1963.

6. Spain, D. M., and Handler, B. J.: Chronic Cor Pulmonale: Sixty Cases Studied at Necropsy, *A.M.A. Arch. Int. Med.*, **77**:37–65, 1946.

7. Aviado, D. M., Jr., Ling, J. S., and Schmidt, C. F.: Effects of Anoxia on Pulmonary Circulation: Reflex Pulmonary Vasoconstriction, *Am. J. Physiol.*, **189**:253–262, 1957.

8. Cournand, A.: Pulmonary Circulation: Its Control in Man, with Some Remarks on Methodology, *Science*, **125**:1231–1235, 1957.

9. Nisell, O. I.: The Action of Oxygen and Carbon Dioxide on the Bronchioles and Vessels of the Isolated Perfused Lungs, *Acta physiol. scandinav.*, **21** (Suppl. 73), 1950.

10. Comroe, J. H., Jr.: Pulmonary Arterial Blood Flow: Effects of Brief and Permanent Arrest, *Am. Rev. Resp. Dis.*, **85**:179–190, 1962.

11. Clements, J. A.: Surface Phenomena in Relation to Pulmonary Function, *Physiologist*, **5**:11–28, 1962.

12. von Neergaard, K.: Neue Auffassungen über einem Grundbegriff der Atem-mechanik: Die Retraktionskraft der Lunge, abhänging von der Oberflächenspannung in den Alveolen, *Ztschr. ges. exper. Med.*, **66**:373–394, 1929.

13. McIlroy, M. B., and Christie, R. V.: A Postmortem Study of the Viscoelastic Properties of the Lungs in Emphysema, *Thorax*, **7**:295–298, 1952.

14. Macklin, C. C.: The Pulmonary Alveolar Mucoid Film and the Pneumocytes, *Lancet*, **1**:1099–1104, 1954.

15. Mead, J., Whittenberger, J. L., and Radford, E. P., Jr.: Surface Tension as a Factor in Pulmonary Volume-Pressure Hysteresis, *J. Appl. Physiol.*, **10**:191–196, 1957.

16. Corssen, G.: Changing Concepts of the Mechanism of Pulmonary Atelectasis, *J.A.M.A.*, **183**:314–317, 1963.

17. Wyatt, J. P., Fischer, V. W., and Sweet, H. C.: Panlobular Emphysema: Anatomy and Pathodynamics, *Dis. Chest*, **41**:239–259, 1962.

18. Luisada, A. A., *et al.*: Colloquium on Therapy of Right Heart Failure. *Dis. Chest*, **41**:260–280, 1962.

19. Liebow, A. A., Hales, M. R., and Lindskog, G. E.: Enlargement of the Bronchial Arteries and Their Anastomoses with the Pulmonary Arteries in Bronchiectasis, *Am. J. Path.*, **25**:211–231, 1949.

20. Nakamura, T., Katori, R., Miyazawa, K., Ohtomo, S., Watanabe, Tatsuzo, Watanabe, Tetsuya, Miura, Y., and Takiazawa, T.: Bronchial Blood Flow in Patients with Chronic Pulmonary Disease and Its Influences upon Respiration and Circulation, *Dis. Chest*, **39**:193–206, 1961.

21. Liebow, A. A.: The Bronchopulmonary Venous Collateral Circulation, with Special Reference to Emphysema, *Am. J. Path.*, **29**:251–289, 1953.

22. Liebow, A. A.: Pulmonary Emphysema, with Special Reference to Vascular Changes, *Am. Rev. Resp. Dis.*, **80**:67–93 (part 2), 1959.

23. Herrmann, G. R., and Shields, A. H.: Heart Disease of Pulmonary Origin, *Dis. Chest*, **33**:52–63, 1958.

24. Thomas, A. J.: Coronary Heart Disease in the Presence of Pulmonary Disease, *Brit. Heart J.*, **20**:83–91, 1958.

25. Altschule, M. D.: Cor Pulmonale: A Disease of the Whole Heart, *Dis. Chest*, **41**:398–403, 1962.

26. Rushmer, R. F.: Work of the Heart, *Mod. Concepts Cardiovas. Dis.*, **27**:473–477, 1958.

27. Boniface, K. J., and Brown, J. M.: Effect of Carbon Dioxide Excess on Contractile Force of the Heart, in Situ, *Am. J. Physiol.*, **172**:752–756, 1953.

28. Darby, T. D., Aldinger, E. E., Gadsden, R. H., and Thrower, W. B.: Effects of Metabolic Acidosis on Ventricular Isometric Systolic Tension and the Response to Epinephrine and Levarterenol, *Circulation Res.*, **8**:1242–1253, 1960.

29. Boniface, K. J., Brodie, O. J., and Walton, R. P.: Resistance Strain Gauge Arches for Direct Measurement of Heart Contractile Force in Animals, *Proc. Soc. Exper. Biol. & Med.*, **84**:263–266, 1953.

30. Roosenburg, J. G., and Deenstra, H.: Bronchial-Pulmonary Vascular Shunts in Chronic Pulmonary Affections, *Dis. Chest*, **26**:664–671, 1954.

31. Michelson, N.: Bilateral Ventricular Hypertrophy Due to Chronic Pulmonary Disease, *Dis. Chest*, **38**:435–446, 1960.

32. Cherniack, R. M., Ewart, W. B., and Hildes, J. A.: Polycythemia Secondary to Respiratory Disturbance in Poliomyelitis, *Am. Int. Med.*, **46**:720–727, 1957.

33. Lukas, D. S., and Plum, F.: Pulmonary Function in Patients Convalescing from Acute Poliomyelitis with Respiratory Paralysis, *Am. J. Med.*, **12**:388–396, 1952.

34. Bergofsky, E. H., Turino, G. M., and Fishman, A. P.: Cardiorespiratory Failure in Kyphoscoliosis, *Medicine*, **38**:263–317, 1959.

35. Mack, I., and Snider, G. L.: Respiratory Insufficiency and Chronic Cor Pulmonale, *Circulation*, **13**:419–447, 1956.

36. Burwell, C. S., Robin, E. D., Whaley, R. D., and Bickelmann, A. G.: Extreme Obesity Associated with Alveolar Hypoventilation: A Pickwickian Syndrome, *Am. J. Med.*, **21**:811–818, 1956.

37. Lillington, G. A., Anderson, M. W., and Brandenburg, R. O.: The Cardiorespiratory Syndrome of Obesity, *Dis. Chest*, **32**:1–20, 1957.

38. Alexander, J. K., Amad, K. H., and Cole, V. M.: Observations on Some Clinical Features of Extreme Obesity, with Particular Reference to Cardiorespiratory Effects, *Am. J. Med.*, **32**:512–524, 1962.

39. Cullen, J. H., and Formel, P. F.: The Respiratory Defects in Extreme Obesity, *Am. J. Med.,* **32:** 525–531, 1962.

40. Fadell, E. J., Richman, A. D., Ward, W. W., and Hendon, J. R.: Fatty Infiltration of Respiratory Muscles in the Pickwickian Syndrome, *New England J. Med.,* **266:**861–863, 1962.

41. Paré, P., and Lowenstein, L.: Polycythemia Associated with Disturbed Function of the Respiratory Center, *Blood,* **11:**1077–1084, 1956.

42. Richter, T., West, J. R., and Fishman, A. P.: The Syndrome of Alveolar Hypoventilation and Diminished Sensitivity of the Respiratory Center, *New England J. Med.,* **256:**1165–1170, 1957.

43. Rodman, T., and Close, H. P.: The Primary Hypoventilation Syndrome, *Am. J. Med.,* **26:**808–817, 1959.

44. Owen, W. R., Thomas, W. A., Castleman, B., and Bland, E. F.: Unrecognized Emboli to the Lungs with Subsequent Cor Pulmonale, *New England J. Med.,* **249:**919–926, 1953.

45. Dresdale, D. T., Schultz, M., and Michtom, R. J.: Primary Pulmonary Hypertension, *Am. J. Med.,* **11:**686–705, 1951.

46. Moser, K. M., and Shea, J. G.: The Relationship between Pulmonary Infarction, Cor Pulmonale, and the Sickle States, *Am. J. Med.,* **22:**561–579, 1957.

47. Girgis, B.: Pulmonary Heart Disease Due to Bilharzia: The Bilharzial Cor Pulmonale, *Am. Heart J.,* **43:**606–614, 1952.

48. Eldridge, F.: The Alveolar-Capillary Block Syndrome, *A.M.A. Arch. Int. Med.,* **105:**665–667, 1960.

49. Austrian, R., McClement, J. H., Renzetti, A. D., Jr., Donald, K. W., Riley, R. L., and Cournand, A.: Clinical and Physiologic Features of Some Types of Pulmonary Diseases with Impairment of Alveolar-Capillary Diffusion: The Syndrome of "Alveolar-Capillary Block," *Am. J. Med.,* **11:**667–685, 1951.

50. James, W. R. L., and Thomas, A. J.: Cardiac Hypertrophy in Coalworkers' Pneumoconiosis, *Brit. J. Indust. Med.,* **13:**24–29, 1956.

51. Heath, D., Norris, R. M., and Davison, P.: Observations on the Pulmonary Vasculature in a Case of Centri-lobular Emphysema with Hemosiderosis, *Circulation,* **28:**444–450, 1963.

52. Gough, J.: The Pathological Diagnosis of Emphysema, *Proc. Roy. Soc. Med.,* **45:**576–577, 1952.

53. Gough, J., and Wentworth, J. E.: Use of Thin Sections of Entire Organs in Morbid Anatomical Studies, *J. Roy. Microscop. Soc.,* **69:**231–235, 1949.

54. Gough, J.: Correlation of Roentgenological and Pathological Changes in Some Diseases of the Lung, *Harvey Lect.,* **53:**171–181, 1957–1958.

55. Hartroft, W. S., and Macklin, C. C.: Intrabronchial Fixation of the Human Lung for Purposes of Alveolar Measurement, Using 25/μ Microsections

56. Hartroft, W. S.: The Microscopic Diagnosis of Pulmonary Emphysema, *Am. J. Path.,* **21:**889–899, 1945.

57. Heppleston, A. G.: The Pathogenesis of Simple Pneumokoniosis in Coal Workers, *J. Path. & Bact.,* **67:**51–63, 1954.

58. McLean, K. H.: The Pathogenesis of Pulmonary Emphysema, *Am. J. Med.,* **25:**62–74, 1958.

59. Heard, B. E.: A Pathological Study of Emphysema of the Lungs with Chronic Bronchitis, *Thorax,* **13:**136–149, 1958.

60. Heard, B. E.: Pathology of Pulmonary Emphysema: Methods of Study, *Am. Rev. Resp. Dis.,* **82:**792–799, 1960.

61. Boren, H. G.: Pulmonary Emphysema, *M. Clin. North America,* **43:**33–52, 1959.

62. Leopold, J. G., and Gough, J.: The Centrilobular Form of Hypertrophic Emphysema and Its Relation to Chronic Bronchitis, *Thorax,* **12:**219–235, 1957.

63. Wyatt, J. P., Fischer, V. W., and Sweet, H.: Centrilobular Emphysema, *Lab. Invest.,* **10:**159–177, 1961.

64. Wyatt, J. P.: Macrosection and Injection Studies of Emphysema, *Am. Rev. Resp. Dis.,* **80:**94–103 (part 2), 1959.

65. Wyatt, J. P., and Sweet, H.: The Morphogenesis of Panlobular Emphysema, *Am. Rev. Resp. Dis.,* **83:**426–431, 1961.

66. Ciba Guest Symposium, C. M. Fletcher, (ed.), Terminology, Definitions, and Classification of Chronic Pulmonary Emphysema, and Related Conditions, *Thorax,* **14:**286–299, 1959.

67. Dunnill, M. S.: An Assessment of the Anatomical Factor in Cor Pulmonale in Emphysema, *J. Clin. Path.,* **14:**246–258, 1961.

68. Appel, S., McIver, F. A., and Harley, R. A.: Unpublished data, 1963.

69. Herbert, F. A., Nahmias, B. B., Gaensler, E. A., and MacMahan, H. E.: Pathophysiology of Interstitial Pulmonary Fibrosis, *Arch. Int. Med.,* **110:** 629–648, 1962.

70. Rubin, E. H., and Lubliner, R.: The Hamman-Rich Syndrome: Review of the Literature and Analysis of 15 Cases, *Medicine,* **36:**397–463, 1957.

71. Simpson, T.: Papilloedema in Emphysema, *Brit. M. J.,* **2:**639–641, 1948.

72. Westlake, E. K., and Kaye, M.: Raised Intracranial Pressure in Emphysema, *Brit. M. J.,* **1:**302–304, 1954.

73. Mithoefer, J. C.: Increased Intracranial Pressure in Emphysema Caused by Oxygen Inhalation, *J.A.M.A.,* **149:**1116–1120, 1952.

74. Friedfeld, L., and Fishberg, A. M.: The Relationship of Cerebrospinal and Venous Pressures in Heart Failure, *J. Clin. Invest.,* **13:**495–501, 1934.

75. Stevens, P. M., Austen, K. F., and Knowles, J. H.: Prognostic Significance of Papilledema in the

Made Therefrom, *Tr. Roy. Soc. Canada* (*sec. V, Biol. Sc.*), **37:**75–78, 1943.

Course of Respiratory Insufficiency, *J.A.M.A.*, **183**: 161–164, 1963.

76. McIlroy, M. B.: Dyspnea and the Work of Breathing in Diseases of the Heart and Lungs, *Progr. Cardiovas. Dis.*, **1**:284–297, 1959.

77. Gaensler, E. A.: Analysis of the Ventilatory Defect by Timed Capacity Measurements, *Am. Rev. Tuberc.*, **64**:256–278, 1951.

78. Curtis, J. K., Rasmussen, H. K., and Cree, E.: Clinical Evaluation of Pulmonary Function Tests, *M. Clin. North America*, **43**:17–32, 1959.

79. Severinghaus, J. W., and Bradley, A. F.: Electrodes for Blood pO_2 and pCO_2 Determination, *J. Appl. Physiol.*, **13**:515–520, 1958.

80. Farber, S. M., and Wilson, R. H. L.: Pulmonary Emphysema, *Ciba Clin. Symposia*, **10**:171–205, 1958.

81. Marks, A., Cugell, D. W., Cadigan, J. B., and Gaensler, E. A.: Clinical Determination of the Diffusion Capacity of the Lungs, *Am. J. Med.*, **22**: 51–73, 1957.

82. Howarth, S., McMichael, J., and Sharpey-Schafer, E. P.: Effects of Oxygen, Venesection and Digitalis in Chronic Heart Failure from Disease of the Lungs, *Clin. Sc.*, **6**:187–196, 1947.

83. Dexter, L., Wittenberger, J. L., Gorlin, R., Lewis, B. M., Haynes, F. W., and Spiegl, R. J.: The Effect of Chronic Pulmonary Diseases (Cor Pulmonale and Hypoxia) on the Dynamics of the Circulation in Man, *Tr. A. Am. Physicians*, **64**: 226–236, 1951.

84. Fowler, N. O., Westcott, R. N., Scott, R. C., and Hess, E.: The Cardiac Output in Chronic Cor Pulmonale, *Circulation*, **6**:888–893, 1952.

85. Harvey, R. M., Ferrer, M. I., Richards, D. W., Jr., and Cournand, A.: Influence of Chronic Pulmonary Disease on the Heart and Circulation, *Am. J. Med.*, **10**:719–738, 1951.

86. Wade, O. L., and Bishop, J. M.: "Cardiac Output and Regional Blood Flow," Blackwell Scientific Publications, Oxford, 1962, p. 150.

87. "Clinical Cardiopulmonary Physiology," Sponsored by the American College of Chest Physicians, 2d ed., Grune & Stratton, Inc., New York, 1960.

88. Harvey, R. M., and Ferrer, I.: A Clinical Consideration of Cor Pulmonale, *Circulation*, **21**:236–255, 1960.

89. Zuckerman, R., Cabrera, E., Fishleder, B. L., and Sodi-Pollares, D.: Electrocardiogram in Chronic Cor Pulmonale, *Am. Heart J.*, **35**:421–437, 1948.

90. Littmann, D.: The Electrocardiographic Findings in Pulmonary Emphysema, *Am. J. Cardiol.*, **5**:339–348, 1960.

91. Scott, R. C.: The Electrocardiogram in Pulmonary Emphysema and Chronic Cor Pulmonale, *Am. Heart J.*, **61**:843–845, 1961.

92. Armen, R. N., Kanton, M., and Weiser, N. J.: Pulmonary Heart Disease: With Emphasis on Electrocardiographic Diagnosis, *Circulation*, **17**: 164–175, 1958.

93. Hecht, H. H.: Heart Failure and Lung Disease, *Circulation*, **14**:265–290, 1956.

94. Wood, P.: Electrocardiographic Appearance in Acute and Chronic Pulmonary Heart Disease, *Brit. Heart J.*, **10**:87, 1948.

95. Wasserburger, R. H., Kelly, J. R., Rasmussen, H. K., and Juhl, J. H.: The Electrocardiographic Pentalogy of Pulmonary Emphysema, *Circulation*, **20**:831–841, 1959.

96. Sodi-Pollares, D., and Calder, R. M.: "New Bases of Electrocardiography," The C. V. Mosby Company, St. Louis, 1956.

97. Myers, G. B.: QRS-T Patterns in Multiple Precordial Leads That May Be Mistaken for Myocardial Infarction. II. Right Ventricular Hypertrophy and Dilatation, *Circulation*, **1**:860–877, 1950.

98. Grant, R. P.: "Clinical Electrocardiography: The Spatial Vector Approach," McGraw-Hill Book Company, New York, 1957.

99. Spodick, D. H.: Electrocardiographic Studies in Pulmonary Disease. 1. Electrocardiographic Abnormalities in Diffuse Lung Disease, *Circulation*, **20**:1067–1072, 1960.

100. Lee, G. de J.: The Circulatory Effects of Acute Respiratory Failure: With Special Reference to Acute Cor Pulmonale, *Postgrad. M. J.*, **37**:31–42, 1961.

101. "Smoking and Health." Report of the Advisory Committee to the Surgeon General of the Public Health Service, U.S. Department of Health, Education, and Welfare, Public Health Service Publication no. 1103, 1964.

102. Auerbach, O., Stout, A. P., Hammond, E. C., and Garfinkel, L.: Smoking Habits and Age in Relation to Pulmonary Changes, *New England J. Med.*, **269**:1045–1054, 1963.

103. Motley, H. L.: The Use of Pulmonary Function Tests with Special Reference to Anesthesia, *Current Res. in Anesth. & Analg.*, **34**:281–289, 1955.

104. Cherniack, R. M.: The Physical Properties of the Lung in Chronic Obstructive Pulmonary Emphysema, *J. Clin. Invest.*, **35**:394–404, 1956.

105. Comroe, J. H., Jr., Forster, R. E. II, Dubois, A. B., Briscoe, W. A., and Carlsen, E.: "The Lung," The Year Book Medical Publishers, Inc., Chicago, 1955, p. 98.

106. Jameson, A. G., Ferrer, M. I., and Harvey, R. M.: Some Effects of Mechanical Respirators upon Respiratory Gas Exchange and Ventilation in Chronic Pulmonary Emphysema, *Am. Rev. Resp. Dis.*, **80**:510–521, 1959.

107. Marks, A., Bocles, J., and Morganti, L.: A New Ventilatory Assister for Patients with Respiratory Acidosis, *New England J. Med.*, **268**:61–68, 1964.

108. Rockey, E. E., Blazsik, C. F., Thompson, S. A., and Virabutr, S.: Four and One-half Years' Experience in the Treatment of Emphysema and Other Respiratory Insufficiencies by Tracheal Fenestration, *Dis. Chest*, **39**:117–128, 1961.

109. Cullen, J. H.: An Evaluation of Tracheostomy in Pulmonary Emphysema, *Ann. Int. Med.*, **58**:953–960, 1963.

110. Motley, H. L., Werko, L., Cournand, A., and Richards, D. W., Jr.: Observations on the Clinical Use of Intermittent Positive Pressure, *J. Aviation Med.*, **18**:417–435, 1947.

111. Cournand, A., Motley, H. L., Werko, L., and Richards, D. W., Jr.: Physiological Studies of the Effects of Intermittent Positive Pressures on Cardiac Output in Man, *Am. J. Physiol.*, **152**:162–174, 1948.

112. Norlander, O. P., Björk, V. O., Crafoord, C., Friberg, O., Holmdahl, M., Swensson, A., and Widman, B.: Controlled Ventilation in Medical Practice, *Anaesthesia*, **16**:285–307, 1961.

113. Williams, J. F., Jr., White, D. H., Jr., and Behnke, R. H.: Changes in Pulmonary Hemodynamics Produced by Isoproterenol Infusion in Emphysematous Patients, *Circulation*, **28**:396–403, 1963.

114. Hecht, H. H., and Jager, B. V.: Circulatory Adjustments During Treatment with Large Doses of Sodium Salicylate or Acetylsalicylic Acid, *J. Clin. Invest.*, **25**:926, 1946.

115. Silipo, S., Hagedorn, C., Rosenstein, I. N., and Baum, G. L.: Experiences with Ethamivan, a New Respiratory Stimulant and Analeptic Agent, *J.A.M.A.*, **177**:378–380, 1961.

116. Rodman, T., Fennelly, J. F., Kraft, A. J., and Close, H. P.: Effect of Ethamivan on Alveolar Ventilation in Patients with Chronic Lung Disease, *New England J. Med.*, **267**:1279–1285, 1962.

117. Hickam, J. D., and Ross, J. C.: Respiratory Acidosis in Chronic Pulmonary Heart Disease: Pathogenesis, Clinical Features, and Management, *Progr. Cardiovas. Dis.*, **1**:309–325, 1958.

118. Riley, R. L.: The Work of Breathing and Its Relation to Respiratory Acidosis, *Ann. Int. Med.*, **41**:172–176, 1954.

119. Samet, P., Fierer, E. M., and Bernstein, W. H.: The Effect of Respiratory Tract Obstruction upon the Ventilatory Response to Inhaled Carbon Dioxide in Normal Subjects, *Dis. Chest*, **39**:388–402, 1961.

120. Nahas, G. G.: Use of an Organic Carbon Dioxide Buffer in Vivo, *Science*, **129**:782–783, 1959.

121. Luchsinger, P. C.: Use of 2-Amino-2-hydroxymethyl-1, 3-propanediol in the Management of Respiratory Acidosis, *Ann. New York Acad. Sc.*, **92**:743–750, 1961.

122. Sieker, H. O., Merwarth, C. R., Saltzman, H. A., and Manfredi, F.: Use of 2-Amino-2-hydroxymethyl-1, 3-propanediol in Severe Carbon Dioxide Intoxications, *Ann. New York Acad. Sc.*, **92**:783–793, 1961.

123. Massaro, D. J., Katz, S., and Luchsinger, P. C.: Use of Carbon Dioxide Buffer (Trishydroxymethylaminomethane) in Treatment of Respiratory Acidosis, *Am. Rev. Resp. Dis.*, **86**:353–359, 1962.

124. Robin, E. D.: Abnormalities of Acid-Base Regulation in Chronic Pulmonary Disease, with Special Reference to Hypercapnia and Extracellular Alkalosis, *New England J. Med.*, **268**:917–922, 1963.

125. Beerel, F., Hershel, J., and Tyler, J. M.: A Controlled Study of the Effect of Prednisone on Airflow Obstruction in Severe Pulmonary Emphysema, *New England J. Med.*, **268**:226–230, 1963.

126. Silen, W., Brown, W. H., and Eiseman, B.: Peptic Ulcer and Pulmonary Emphysema, *A.M.A. Arch. Surg.*, **78**:897–903, 1959.

127. Kroeker, E. J., and Leon, A. S.: The Association of Diffuse Obstructive Pulmonary Emphysema and Chronic Gastroduodenal Ulceration, *Dis. Chest*, **42**:413–421, 1962.

128. Williams, M. J., and Mendel, J. L.: Pulmonary Emphysema, Adrenocortical Hyperplasia and Peptic Ulceration, *Dis. Chest*, **44**:303–305, 1963.

129. Refsum, H. E.: Hypokalemic Alkalosis with Paradoxical Aciduria during Artificial Ventilation of Patients with Pulmonary Insufficiency and High Plasma Bicarbonate Concentration, *Scandinav. J. Clin. & Lab. Invest.*, **13**:481–488, 1961.

130. Cochran, R. T.: Pulmonary Insufficiency and Hypercapnia Complicated by Potassium-responsive Alkalosis, *New England J. Med.*, **268**:521–525, 1963.

131. Kim, Y. S., and Aviado, D. M.: Digitalis and the Pulmonary Circulation, *Am. Heart J.*, **62**:680–686, 1961.

132. Aviado, D. M.: The Pharmacology of the Pulmonary Circulation, *Pharmacol. Rev.*, **12**:159–239, 1960.

133. Miller, W. F.: Chronic Inflammatory Bronchopulmonary Disorders, *Arch. Int. Med.*, **107**:589–605, 1961.

134. Goldberg, L. M., Bristow, J. D., Parker, B. M., and Ritzmann, L. W.: Paroxysmal Atrial Tachycardia with Atrioventricular Block: Its Frequent Association with Chronic Pulmonary Diseases, *Circulation*, **21**:499–504, 1960.

135. Rudolph, A. M., Nadas, A. S., and Borges, W. H.: Hematologic Adjustments to Cyanotic Congenital Heart Disease, *Pediatrics*, **11**:454–464, 1953.

136. Nadas, A. S.: "Pediatric Cardiology," 2d ed., W. B. Saunders Company, Philadelphia, 1963.

137. Bedell, G. N., Sheets, R. F., Fischer, H. W., and Theilen, E. O.: Polycythemia: A Manifestation of Heart Disease, Lung Disease or a Primary Blood Dyscrasia, *Circulation*, **18**:107–116, 1958.

138. Ratto, O., Brisco, W. A., Morton, J. W., and Comroe, J. H., Jr.: Anoxemia Secondary to Polycythemia and Polycythemia Secondary to Anoxemia, *Am. J. Med.*, **19**:958–965, 1955.

139. Vanier, T., Dulfano, M. J., Wu, C., and Desforges, J. F.: Emphysema, Hypoxia and the Polycythemic Response, *New England. J. Med.*, **269**:169–178, 1963.

140. Lertzman, M., Israels, L. G., and Cherniak, R. M.:

Erythropoiesis and Ferrokinetics in Chronic Respiratory Disease, *Ann. Int. Med.,* **56:**821–833, 1962.

141. Hurst, A., Levine, M. H., and Rich, D. R.: Radioactive Iodine in the Management of Patients with Severe Pulmonary Emphysema, *Ann. Allergy,* **13:** 393–397, 1955.

47 PULMONARY EMBOLISM AND ACUTE COR PULMONALE

Lewis Dexter, M.D.

It is generally considered that pulmonary embolism is the most common form of acute pulmonary disease in the adult hospital population. It is the most common immediate cause of death at the Peter Bent Brigham Hospital. It is potentially curable surgically, and prevention of further attacks is highly successful, but these therapeutic measures cannot be introduced unless a diagnosis can be made. Diagnosis is notoriously difficult.

Incidence of Pulmonary Embolism

Frequency

Pulmonary emboli are found in approximately 10 per cent of all autopsies in general hospitals and in about 25 per cent in hospitals giving custodial care. In patients dying in congestive heart failure, postmortem data indicate an incidence of 30 to 50 per cent. No figures exist regarding frequency of nonfatal pulmonary embolism because of difficulties in its recognition during life.

Age and Sex

The incidence of pulmonary embolism increases with age, being rare under twenty and infrequent under thirty. It becomes progressively more common with advancing years. There is no sex or race predilection.

Origin of Thrombi

In over 90 per cent of cases, the site of formation of venous thrombi is in the calves of the legs. The thrombi propagate upward as a bland thrombus without inflammatory reaction (phlebothrombosis), or there may be an inflammatory (nonbacterial) reaction, in which case it is referred to as *thrombophlebitis.* In either event, it propagates up the vein and may break off to become an embolus at any time. The volume of embolic material liberated depends on the extent of its propagation and the point from which it breaks loose. A clot extending from calf to iliac vein has a volume of approximately 100 ml. Another site of origin of clots is the pelvis, but here the venous volume is much smaller than that of the legs except in the case of the uterine veins postpartum. How often emboli originate in the right atrium of patients with atrial fibrillation and congestive heart failure is not known. The incidence has been reported in the literature as 5, 20, and 40 per cent. However, irrespective of precise incidence, the legs are usually the site of origin and from a therapeutic viewpoint should be considered as the source.

Factors Predisposing to Venous Thrombosis and Embolism

In 1856 Virchow[1] suggested three possible causes of venous thrombosis: stasis of blood, abnormality of venous wall, and abnormal state of coagulation. Since that time little progress has been made in further identification of fundamental causes.

Stasis results from bed rest (e.g., in poliomyelitis, fractures, operations, debilitating diseases of all types), pregnancy, obesity, varicose veins, and congestive heart failure, the latter being by far the most important disease predisposing to thromboembolism.

Abnormality of venous wall occurs from trauma, surgical procedures, phlebosclerosis, which is common in older people, inflammatory diseases of veins (Buerger's disease, typhoid fever, arterial insufficiency, and gangrene), and degenerative lesions (atherosclerosis, diabetes mellitus).

Abnormalities of the clotting mechanism include thrombocytosis (postoperative, postpartum, postsplenectomy, idiopathic thrombocythemia); sickle-cell anemia; and the presence of cold agglutinins, cryoglobulins, cryofibrinogens, and macroglobulins. Raised levels of circulating fibrinogens, or thromboplastin, platelet "stickiness," sludging, and the presence of certain types of carcinoma (pancreas, stomach, ovaries) have all been implicated as causes of intravascular thrombosis, but their role is neither clear nor constant.

Pathogenesis of Embolism

When a clot breaks loose, it travels up the vein without hindrance into the right side of the heart. It may pass unchanged through the right ventricle into the pulmonary artery, or it may become enmeshed in the chordae tendinae and be delayed for some time in its passage into the pulmonary artery. Most frequently it is broken up into multiple small particles by the churning and pumping action of the right ventricle and then passes into the pulmonary arterial system. Its distribution in the lungs follows closely the distribution of blood flow. Thus, the distribution is mainly the lower lobes and to a lesser extent the upper lobes. The rising pulmonary arterial pressure may pound them farther down the vascular system. Circulating fibrinolysin lyses intravascular clots. Little is known of the rate of lysis of embolic material. Fragmentation of a clot into a myriad of small pieces by the right ventricle presents a much larger surface area of clot on which the lytic process may act, but how effective the process of lysis actually is, is at present obscure.

The immediate cause of embolism is usually not apparent, but sometimes it occurs on arising from bed, straining at stool, exertion, or hyperventilation, all of which maneuvers result in distension of veins of the legs, thereby promoting the breaking off of clot.

Response of the Lung to Emboli

When embolism is sufficiently massive, two types of reaction may occur—pulmonary infarction and acute cor pulmonale.

In pulmonary infarction, the circulation is so compromised that the pulmonary parenchyma is destroyed, but the bronchial collateral circulation is sufficient to maintain the viability of fibrous tissue. Septic embolism may give rise to a pulmonary abscess wherein both pulmonary tissue and fibrous tissue are destroyed. This is now seen almost exclusively in unclean manipulations in the evacuation of the pregnant uterus.

Acute cor pulmonale refers to pulmonary and right ventricular hypertension as a result of embolic plugging of the pulmonary arterial system with resultant circulatory obstruction. This results in a rise of pressure in right ventricle and pulmonary artery proximal to the obstruction, and a reduction of blood flow (cardiac output) through the lung.

Pathologic Physiology

Pulmonary Infarction

The lung has two circulations, the pulmonary and the bronchial. The pulmonary artery subserves the purpose of gas exchange. The bronchial circulation supplies the pulmonary structures down to, but not including, the alveoli.

The pulmonary artery rises from the right ventricle, divides into two main branches, which further divide into lobar branches. These and the next division extend out almost to the pleural surface, as shown in Fig. 47-1. Subsequent branches are short, resembling twigs on a tree. The number and sizes of the various divisions are

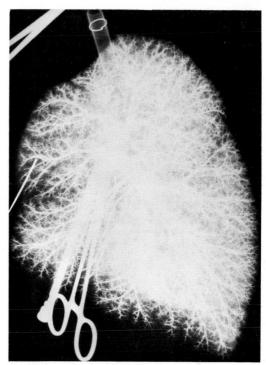

Fig. 47-1. A postmortem pulmonary arteriogram of a normal lung from a sixteen-year-old boy. The pulmonary artery has been injected with a radiopaque mass. There is complete generalized peripheral filling of the smallest muscular arteries close to the pleural surface. This injection mass does not pass into capillaries and in the normal lung requires approximately 55 to 62 ml per m² body surface to fill the arterial system. (*From Dexter, L., Haynes, F., and Smith, G. T.: Physiologic Changes in the Pulmonary Circulation with Age, in L. Cander and J. Moyer (eds.), "Aging of the Lung," Grune & Stratton, New York, 1965, with permission of authors, editors, and publisher.*)

shown in Table 47-1. The pulmonary capillaries are large, surround the alveoli as a mesh, and are extensively anastomotic among themselves. The capillaries empty into venules and then into larger and larger veins, finally culminating in four main venous trunks emptying into the left atrium.

The bronchial arteries arise from the aorta or one of the first two intercostal arteries. They supply the trachea, bronchi, and mediastinal structures. They also supply the vasa vasorum of the pulmonary artery. In the dog, about two-thirds of the bronchial venous blood empties into the pulmonary veins and one-third into the azygos, hemiazygos, and intercostal veins of the systemic system.

Pulmonary and bronchial arterial systems are anastomotic in three regions. There is a potential, if not actual, connection between bronchial artery

Table 47-1. NUMBER OF EMBOLI REQUIRED TO PRODUCE PULMONARY HYPERTENSION

Artery	Diameter of artery and emboli, mm	Number of arteries	Number of emboli
Lobar	5.0	8	7
1st order	4.0	12	28
2nd order	2.3	43	60
3rd order	1.0	1,021	1,600
Lobular	0.3	16,000	20,000
Atrial	0.17	64,000	90,000

SOURCE: Dexter, L., and Smith, G. T.: Quantitative Studies of Pulmonary Embolism, in "Transactions of the American Clinical and Climatological Association," 75:72, Waverly Press, Inc., Baltimore, 1964, with permission of authors, recorder, and publisher.

and pulmonary artery, especially in various pulmonary disease conditions. Liebow[2] found anastomoses at the level of the fourth- to fifth-order branches of the segmental bronchi, which at times were greater than 1 mm in diameter. There is normally an extensive anastomosis between bronchial capillaries and pulmonary capillaries and between bronchial veins and pulmonary veins.

Flow from bronchial vessels to pulmonary vessels is normally less than 1 per cent of the cardiac output. Increase of bronchial collateral flow occurs following pulmonary arterial occlusion by ligation or embolism, in tumors, and in inflammatory lesions of all sorts, particularly bronchiectasis.

Pulmonary infarction cannot be produced experimentally in animals by ligation of the right or left main branch of the pulmonary artery or by microembolization. Ligation of a lobar branch rarely produces infarction, provided that the remainder of the circulation is normal. The collateral circulation is sufficient to maintain the viability of the pulmonary parenchyma. Pulmonary infarction regularly takes place on occlusion of pulmonary arteries ranging in size from lobar arteries down to vessels about 2 mm in diameter if the collateral flow from bronchial arteries is interfered with by ligation of the bronchial arteries, pulmonary veins, or lobar veins, by compression from pleural effusion, or by lowering the systemic (bronchial arterial) blood pressure. In other words, pulmonary infarction seems to occur when two sets of conditions coexist: first, when middle-sized pulmonary arteries are occluded and, second, when the collateral circulation from bronchial arteries is compromised by pulmonary venous hypertension or systemic hypotension.

Pulmonary infarction in man appears to occur as it does in the experimental animal. It occurs as a result of embolization of middle-sized vessels when bronchial collateral circulation is interfered with by pulmonary congestion from heart failure or by systemic hypotension. It rarely occurs in patients who have otherwise normal lungs, hearts, and circulation. A curious and unexplained finding is that only about 10 per cent of occlusions of middle-sized vessels result in pulmonary infarction. This is true both in the experimental animal and in man. Thus, pulmonary infarction radiologically and histologically represents the exception rather than the rule when middle-sized vessels are occluded with embolic material. Infarcts occur in the lower lobes rather than in the upper lobes for two reasons: first, flow to the lower lobes is greater than that to the upper lobes, at least in the upright position, so that the lower lobes receive more embolic material; secondly, the lower lobes in the upright position are more congested than are the upper lobes.

Circulatory Obstruction (Acute Cor Pulmonale)

The lung is a high-flow, low-pressure organ. All the cardiac output passes through the lung. Under basal conditions this amounts to 3.1 liters/min/m² body surface. This flow may be increased about threefold without any appreciable change in pulmonary arterial pressure. Table 47-2 compares the

Table 47-2. PRESSURES (MM HG) AND RESISTANCES (DYNES-SEC-CM⁻⁵) IN NORMAL MAN

Pressures:		Pressures:	
Systemic vein	5	Pulmonary vein	7
Right atrium	0	Left atrium	5
Right ventricle	25/0	Left ventricle	120/5
Pulmonary artery	25/9 (15)	Aorta	120/80 (95)
Pulmonary capillaries	9	Systemic capillaries	25
Resistance:		Resistance:	
Pulmonary vascular	70	Systemic vascular	1,200

low pressures that exist in the normal lung with the relatively high pressures that exist in the systemic circuit. The lung is a low-resistance organ. Its resistance is only about one-fifteenth that of the systemic circuit. There is an enormous pulmonary vascular reserve. The cross-sectional area of the pulmonary vasculature both in dogs and in man must be reduced by over one-half before any change in pressure or flow through the organ can be detected. Pneumonectomy does not result in pulmonary hypertension provided the opposite lung is normal. The amount of embolic material required to produce a 5 to 10 mm Hg rise of pressure in the pulmonary artery in an 8-kg dog, this being the first sign of circulatory embarrassment, is shown in

Table 47-1, where the size and number of embolic particles are compared with the size and number of different branches of the pulmonary artery. A small number of large particles and increasing numbers of small particles are required to produce incipient pulmonary hypertension. At the pre-capillary level, 22 million *Lycopodium* spores are required.

There has been a controversy over the years regarding the presence or absence of reflex vasoconstriction as a result of thromboembolism. It has been postulated that the powerful pulmonary vasoconstrictor serotonin might be released from platelet thrombi and thus give rise to pulmonary hypertension on a vasoconstrictor basis, in addition to the mechanical plugging by the emboli. Such a mechanism has not yet been proved. There is good experimental evidence that diffuse pulmonary vasoconstriction occurs as a result of embolization of *arterioles* in the lung but not as a result of *arterial* occlusion. Thromboemboli occlude mainly arteries, not arterioles (Table 47-3). Furthermore,

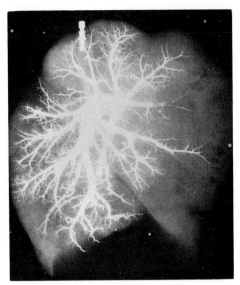

Fig. 47-2. A postmortem pulmonary arteriogram from a patient who died of pulmonary embolism. Note the larger avascular parenchymal areas due to thromboembolic occlusion of medium and small muscular arteries. The volume of injection mass required to fill the pulmonary arterial vasculature in this lung has been reduced by two-thirds. (*From Smith, G. T., Dammin, G. J., and Dexter, L.: Postmortem Arteriographic Studies of the Human Lung in Pulmonary Embolization, J.A.M.A., 188:143, 1964, with permission of the authors, editor, and publisher.*)

Table 47-3. LOCATION OF EMBOLI IN 34 HUMAN LUNGS

Arteries	Size, mm	No. of cases	Frequency
Elastic	>1.0	8	Few
Muscular	0.1–1.0	34	Common
Arterioles	0.03–0.1	13	Rare

SOURCE: Dexter, L., and Smith, G. T.: Quantitative Studies of Pulmonary Embolism, *Am. J. Med. Sci.,* **247**:37, 1946, with permission of authors, editor, and publisher.

the amount of thromboembolic material in the lungs of patients dying of pulmonary embolism is uniformly of such magnitude as to account for the circulatory changes on the basis of simple mechanical obstruction (Table 47-4 and Fig. 47-2). Reports of a single small embolus producing death have not been confirmed by more recent studies utilizing postmortem arteriography. Other types of embolic material (fat, air, amniotic fluid) do occlude arterioles, and it may well be that there is an element of diffuse vasoconstriction in these unusual types of embolism.

With reduction of more than 50 to 60 per cent of the cross-sectional area of the pulmonary arteries, circulatory, and respiratory changes appear. Pressure becomes elevated in the pulmonary artery proximal to the obstruction and in the right ventricle. The systolic pressure may rise to 70 or 80 mm Hg and may return to normal in the course of 30 to 60 min or longer. This fall of pressure may

be due to several factors: (1) partial lysis of clot by circulating fibrinolysin; (2) slippage of the embolic material further down the pulmonary arterial system where the cross-sectional area is larger; or (3) opening up of new vessels which were previously closed in the upper lobes. An abrupt rise of pressure may be so disadvantageous to the right ventricle as to result in acute dilatation, a rise in its diastolic pressure, and a corresponding

Table 47-4. ARTERIAL VOLUME OF HUMAN LUNGS

	No. of cases	Arterial volume, ml/m²
Normal:		
Right	12	62 ± 3.3
Left	14	55 ± 4.0
Embolized:		
Right	10	21 ± 9.8
Left	26	22 ± 11.6

SOURCE: Dexter, L., and Smith, G. T.: Quantitative Studies of Pulmonary Embolism, *Am. J. Med. Sci.,* **247**:37, 1964, with permission of authors, editor and publisher.

rise in systemic venous pressure (right ventricular failure). The cardiac output falls, pulse rate usually rises, and peripheral circulatory failure may appear. Manifestations may be syncope, collapse, or frank shock. Coronary blood flow may become reduced because of the low systemic (coronary arterial) blood pressure and the high right atrial (coronary sinus) pressure. The existence of a pulmonary-coronary reflex is controversial. Hyperventilation occurs regularly. Breathing is one of two types: it is either rapid and shallow or deep and gasping. Arterial oxygen unsaturation occurs regularly for reasons that are not entirely clear.[3] Cyanosis is usually present and is due in part to this mechanism and in part to the low cardiac output (stasis cyanosis).

Clinical Picture

Minor degrees of embolism probably occur frequently, but since they produce no circulatory or respiratory disturbance, they go completely unnoticed. Virtually no information is available concerning the fate of such emboli. It is presumed that lysis of such clots can be handled effectively under normal circumstances.

Pulmonary Infarction

The time elapsing between embolic occlusion and manifestations of pulmonary infarction must vary considerably. It has been reported to occur anywhere from 2½ to 79 hr following wedging of a cardiac catheter into a branch of the pulmonary artery for the measurement of pulmonary capillary wedge pressure in man. Pulmonary infarction causes some disability, never death. Death from embolism is due to circulatory obstruction (acute cor pulmonale). Pulmonary infarction may be looked upon as a fortuitous event in that it draws the physician's attention to the fact that embolism has occurred. It is of great diagnostic importance. It must be emphasized, however, that infarction is inconstantly present even though embolism has occurred. Furthermore, the manifestations of pulmonary infarction may be mimicked by a variety of other pulmonary diseases. The symptoms are often but not always abrupt in onset, vary in severity, and follow the pattern shown in Table 47-5.

Symptoms and Signs. The common manifestations of pulmonary infarction are a rise of temperature, pulse, and respiration. This triad has been emphasized for many years by surgeons. It is seen just as commonly in medical patients, particularly patients with cardiac disease. It is one of the important clues to the presence of pulmonary infarction. Temperature rises characteristically to

Table 47-5. SYMPTOMS AND SIGNS OF PULMONARY INFARCTION (97 CASES)

	Number	Per cent
Tachypnea	87	90
Tachycardia	85	88
Fever	77	79
Pleurisy	71	73
Cough	56	58
Friction rub	44	45
Hemoptysis	38	39
Icterus	22	23
Chill	3	3

101 or 102°F, occasionally higher. A rise to 104° accompanied by a shaking chill suggests a septic infarct, although this is not invariably the case. The pulse rate rises characteristically to about 120 but depends in part on the presence of associated heart disease and in part on associated pleural pain. It is sometimes accompanied by an arrhythmia, either atrial (fibrillation or flutter) or ventricular (premature beats), in which case the pulse rate may become extremely rapid. Tachypnea tends to follow the course of the fever as well as that of the pleural pain.

Pleuritic pain is the next most common manifestation of pulmonary infarction. It may be transient, or it may last for a number of days. It is most commonly located over the lower chest, but with irritation of the diaphragm there may be radiation to the shoulder regions. There may be tenderness of the overlying chest wall.

Cough is frequent, may be dry, or may be productive of sputum.

Hemoptysis occurs in over one-third of cases. The blood may be dark or bright red, or it may be mixed with sputum. Hemoptysis should always suggest pulmonary infarction to the physician. It may, of course, occur as a result of heart disease alone or as a result of a variety of other diseases of the lung.

Icterus is a common but not constant finding in patients with pulmonary infarction. It has been attributed to breakdown of hemoglobin in the infarcted area which cannot be adequately taken care of by the liver that is poorly functioning as a result of chronic passive congestion. Icterus is rare in patients with cardiac disease with the exception of constrictive pericarditis and tricuspid disease. Therefore, its presence in patients with other types of heart disease is strong presumptive evidence of pulmonary infarction.

A friction rub may be heard transiently over the infarcted area. Its presence is of great diagnostic significance. Both pain and friction rub may disappear with the development of an effusion.

Pleural effusions in association with infarction are characteristically bloody but are at times serous.

Laboratory Findings. Characteristically the white cell count rises to 10,000 or 15,000, and occasionally higher. There is usually a modest preponderance of polymorphonuclear cells.

In the serum, there is characteristically a rise of lactic dehydrogenase (LDH) activity and in about two-thirds of cases no rise of activity of glutamic oxalacetic transaminase (SGOT). The serum-bilirubin level rises in about half of the cases. A rise of LDH and of bilirubin level in the face of a normal SGOT is considered by some to be almost diagnostic of pulmonary embolism.

Characteristic radiologic findings of pulmonary infarction are best seen 12 to 24 hr after embolization. These findings consist of an area of consolidation somewhere in the periphery of the lung, usually the lower lobes. There is a rounded profile facing the hilus. The shadow extends out to the pleural surface. Such a picture is found in 15 to 30 per cent of cases. In another 15 to 30 per cent, shadows suggesting patchy pneumonitis or pulmonary edema may be present, pleural fluid may appear, and there may be elevation of the diaphragm and diminished diaphragmatic excursions on the affected side. In perhaps 50 per cent of cases the x-ray picture is either normal or unhelpful. On some occasions a small pneumothorax may occur at the site of infarction.

Pulmonary infarction produces no electrocardiographic findings. Changes that are seen are due to circulatory obstruction.

Angiography can demonstrate embolic occlusion of large vessels but currently is not capable of revealing emboli in the muscular arteries (0.1 to 1.0 mm in diameter), which are the site of the great majority of embolic occlusions (Table 47-3). This is due to the lack of detail in structures this small where injection of contrast material is made intravenously or selectively through a catheter in a branch of the pulmonary artery. Disadvantages of angiography are toxicity of contrast material in patients who are acutely ill and of venous catheterization if angiography is performed selectively.

Lung scanning consists of the intravenous injection of I^{131}-tagged human serum albumin which by appropriate heating, acidification, and agitation consists of aggregates or particles of approximately 50 to 150 μ in size. Many of these particles are caught in the lung and remain there for a period of 2 hr or more. External scanning of the normal lung reveals homogeneous dissemination of radioactive particles. Large embolic occlusions result in areas of absent radioactivity. At this writing this is a new technique which appears promising for the detection of large emboli and has the distinct advantage of not requiring instrumentation or other hazards for the severely ill patient.

Circulatory Obstruction (Acute Cor Pulmonale)

Manifestations of circulatory obstruction are on the basis of hyperventilation, pulmonary hypertension, and reduced cardiac output.

Respiration. Pulmonary embolism results in hyperventilation. The breathing is either shallow and rapid, which is thought to occur as a result of plugging of smaller pulmonary arterial branches, or deep and gasping when major vessels are occluded. This is not entirely accurate, however, because either type of breathing may occur with small- or large-branch occlusion. Respiratory distress may appear in transient episodes lasting only a few minutes; more commonly it persists for about 48 hr. It is frequently associated with orthopnea and dry cough.

Pulmonary Hypertension and Right Ventricular Failure. The rise of pressure in the pulmonary artery is of course generated by the right ventricle and occurs with great rapidity, i.e., in the course of a few beats. The sudden strain put on the right ventricle results in its dilatation and rise of its diastolic filling pressure, right atrial pressure, and systemic venous pressures. Venous distension and hepatic enlargement and tenderness ensue. Tachycardia is the rule. The pulmonic component of the second sound may become accentuated and even palpable. A systolic murmur may appear in the pulmonic area; it may have a scratchy quality suggesting a pericardial friction rub. A holosystolic murmur occasionally appears along the left lower sternal border, increasing a grade or two on inspiration as a result of functional tricuspid regurgitation from right ventricular dilatation. Rarely a systolic murmur may be heard over the lung at the site of obstruction. The venous pulse may exhibit large A waves if cardiac rhythm is normal sinus rhythm. There may also be large V waves as a result of tricuspid incompetence. Arrhythmias of all sorts may occur. Not rarely atrial fibrillation or atrial flutter suddenly appear. Ventricular premature beats, ventricular tachycardia, and even ventricular fibrillation with sudden death can occur as a result of pulmonary embolism. Both atrial and ventricular diastolic gallop rhythm are occasionally observed.

Reduction of Cardiac Output. *Syncope and Shock.* Pulmonary embolism may produce transient dizziness or actual syncope lasting for only a few minutes. With massive embolism a typical shock picture supervenes. The patient is cold, clammy, and sweaty, and the blood pressure is low or unobtainable by cuff method. The patient is weak and pale. The pulse is rapid, small, and thready. This circulatory collapse may persist for hours.

Anginal Pain. Crushing substernal pain indistinguishable from that of an acute coronary occlusion with myocardial infarction may occur as a result of massive embolism and is attributable to the reduction of coronary blood flow because of low aortic pressure in the face of a high right ventricular work load because of pulmonary and right ventricular hypertension. This pain, together with heart failure and shock, and the electrocardiogram may be indistinguishable at the onset from the picture of posterior myocardial infarction. Sometimes it takes several days for the pattern of one or the other to evolve. Fortunately medical treatment of these two conditions does not differ basically.

Left Ventricular Failure. It is not quite clear why the left ventricle should fail in this condition, since it is located distal to the circulatory obstruction and its work load in terms of pressure and flow is reduced. The normal heart does not fail in shock except perhaps terminally. Left ventricular failure as a result of pulmonary embolism is seen almost exclusively in patients with underlying disease of the left ventricle. It is assumed that the failure of the left ventricle is the result of diminished coronary blood flow, tachycardia, which by shortening diastole reduces the period during which the restoration of contractile energy takes place, and arterial oxygen unsaturation resulting in myocardial hypoxia. In any event, pulmonary edema in these individuals is a common complication. Thus, the manifestations of global heart failure with pulmonary edema and hepatomegaly and venous distension may occur as a result of embolism.

Other Manifestations. Cyanosis is common and may occur as a fleeting episode or may be present for a number of days. Usually clinically detectable cyanosis is accompanied by an arterial oxygen saturation less than 85 per cent.

Apprehension is a common symptom and is similar to that seen in association with coronary occlusion. It is a sensation of impending disaster. The symptom is usually observed after the embolism has occurred, and in retrospect it sometimes turns out to be the initial manifestation of embolism, there being no other symptom or signs to account for the patient's anxiety.

Radiologic findings may consist of an area of translucency essentially devoid of vascular markings in an area distal to the obstruction of a major vessel, or the vascular markings in one lobe or even in one lung may be considerably diminished as compared with those of the opposite lung. Another finding is dilatation of the main trunk of

the pulmonary artery, the right ventricle, right atrium, and superior vena cava and a regression toward normal in ensuing days. Heart size may change temporarily because of dilatation of the right ventricle and of the main trunk of the pulmonary artery. All these changes occur immediately following embolic occlusion. The frequency with which such findings are detected depend on the size and location of the embolus, the degree of pulmonary hypertension that ensues, the care with which the x-rays are interpreted, and comparison of sequential films.

Electrocardiographic changes of acute pulmonary embolism are diagnostic in only about 7 per cent of cases and are best observed immediately after the embolic event. Changes can consist of right axis deviation, S-1, Q-3 pattern, depressed ST-1 and ST-2, flat or inverted T-2 and T-3, and P-pulmonale in the standard leads. In the precordial leads, there may be clockwise rotation of the heart, upright R waves with inverted S-T segments over the right precordium, or an RSR' configuration in V_1 suggesting incomplete right bundle branch block. Posterior myocardial infarction may be confused electrocardiographically with acute pulmonary embolism because of the presence of Q waves and inverted T waves in leads II, III, and AVF. Vectorcardiography has not increased diagnostic precision. Other changes which have no diagnostic implications consist of nonspecific T-wave changes, and these are found in about 75 per cent of cases. Posterior rotation of the mean T vector with inverted T waves in the right precordial leads may be noted.

Combination of Pulmonary Infarction and Acute Cor Pulmonale

The manifestations of acute cor pulmonale usually precede those of infarction. However, the clinical picture may be only that of infarction without any evidence of a preceding acute cor pulmonale, or acute cor pulmonale may occur without any evidence of subsequent infarction. Frequently, however, the two occur together. Keeping the two syndromes clearly in mind may be helpful in recognition and interpretation of the sequence of clinical events.

Chronic Recurrent Pulmonary Embolism and Chronic Cor Pulmonale

Repeated episodes of pulmonary embolism may eventually lead to sustained pulmonary hypertension, right ventricular hypertrophy, chronic right ventricular failure, and death. Shortness of breath is the presenting symptom, followed by easy fatigability and eventually abdominal distension.

There may or may not be clear-cut symptoms of embolic episodes or of phlebitis. Physical signs may include venous distension with prominent *a* waves and *v* waves, a sternal lift denoting right ventricular hypertrophy, an accentuated pulmonic component of the second sound, occasionally a pulmonic systolic murmur, a holosystolic murmur in the lower parasternal area due to tricuspid incompetence, an enlarged liver, ankle edema, but rarely ascites. The electrocardiogram characteristically is indicative of right ventricular hypertrophy. X-ray of the heart shows enlargement of the right ventricle, main trunk of the pulmonary artery, and hilar vessels. The proximal branches of the pulmonary artery may be dilated, whereas the peripheral branches are constricted, giving the comma sign. Peripheral lung fields are oligemic.

Definitive treatment should be instituted, because individuals with these conditions are thrombophilic and the disorder is life-threatening. Many recommend vein ligation (bilateral common femorals or inferior vena cava) plus anticoagulants for 2 or 3 months postoperatively.

Differentiation from so-called primary pulmonary hypertension may be impossible during life, the latter being a postmortem diagnosis. Patients suspected of having primary pulmonary hypertension should be considered to have recurrent pulmonary embolism and treated accordingly.

Diagnosis

Diagnosis is rarely easy and straightforward. It is frequently possible only tentatively and by the prepared mind in the proper clinical setting because of the masking of pulmonary infarction by an adequate bronchial collateral circulation and of acute cor pulmonale by the large pulmonary vascular reserve which normally exists. From the foregoing description it is apparent that embolism must be massive before any symptoms whatsoever appear and then they may not be sufficiently characteristic to be pathognomonic of the condition.

Pulmonary infarction may be easily confused with bronchitis, bronchopneumonia, neoplasm, pleurisy of other cause, atelectasis, or fever of unknown origin. Acute cor pulmonale may present as a simple syncopal attack, circulatory collapse, an accentuation of preexisting heart failure, acute pulmonary edema, episodic atrial or ventricular arrhythmia, myocardial infarction, hemoptysis, or pleurisy. The diagnosis should not be overlooked because of normal legs, x-ray, and electrocardiogram when other manifestations are characteristic.

There are a number of clinical clues which are helpful although not diagnostic. If any of the following are present, one must think in terms of pulmonary embolism but at the same time realize that other possibilities exist: (1) any pulmonary or cardiac abnormality in the presence of deep phlebitis of the legs; (2) congestive heart failure without obvious cause; (3) jaundice in the presence of congestive heart failure; (4) blood-streaked or grossly bloody sputum; (5) pleurisy; (6) bloody pleural effusion; (7) unexplained rise of temperature and more rapid pulse and respiration; (8) unexplained apprehension; (9) serum-enzyme changes as described above.

Mortality and Prognosis

The mortality of each episode of embolism of a size sufficient to produce symptoms lies between 20 and 38 per cent. Between one-third and one-half the patients have subsequent episodes of embolism, and 19 per cent are thought to have a fatal embolus subsequently.

Treatment

Treatment or prophylaxis should be instituted when there is a "generous suspicion" that embolism has occurred, because of the likelihood of further episodes, the high mortality of each episode, and the efficacy of prophylaxis. Treatment is directed toward supportive measures during the acute episode, surgical removal of the clot, and prevention of subsequent episodes.

Treatment of Attack

Treatment is symptomatic. For apprehension, pain, and respiratory distress, morphine sulfate, 10 to 15 mg intramuscularly (IM), may be required. Meperidine hydrochloride (Demerol), 50 to 75 mg IM, is less effective. For control of pleuritic pain, strapping the chest may be more efficacious than morphine. Oxygen should be administered by nasal catheter or oxygen mask. Hypotension and shock may require an intravenous infusion of phenylephrine hydrochloride (Neo-synephrine hydrochloride), 4 ml 1 per cent solution in 500 ml dextrose in water, or the more potent l-norepinephrine bitartrate (Levophed), 2 ml 0.2 per cent in 500 ml of 5 per cent dextrose in water. The rate of infusion is determined by the response of the blood pressure. Theophyllin ethylenediamine (aminophyllin), 250 to 500 mg in 200 ml 5 per cent dextrose in water intravenously (IV), is beneficial for bronchoconstriction and heart failure.

For either shock or heart failure, rapid digitalization is indicated but with due caution because of hypoxemia, which predisposes to myocardial irritability. In patients who have not been previously digitalized, digoxin, 1.0 mg IM followed in 1 hr by 0.5 mg, is recommended.

Antibiotics are indicated to prevent secondary infection.

There are no good pulmonary vasodilators that do not have an even greater action on systemic vessels, and all drugs producing systemic vasodilatation are clearly contraindicated. Furthermore, there is no good evidence for widespread vasoconstriction in thromboembolism. Thrombolytic agents should theoretically be of great value. Unfortunately they are still too toxic in their side effects to warrant usage.

Embolectomy

Embolectomy (Trendelenburg operation) was introduced at the turn of the century but met with only occasional success. However, several recent reports have shown the feasibility of putting the lung on bypass and aspirating fresh clot from the pulmonary vasculature. This promises to be done in the future with greater frequency than in the past provided an accurate diagnosis can be made. Accurate diagnosis is currently the bottleneck for widespread use of this approach. Furthermore, the risk of riding out the embolic event medically must be weighed against the risk of the surgical procedure.

Prevention of Another Attack

Prevention of another embolic episode requires recognition of the first one and then consists of general measures, anticoagulants, and/or vein ligation.

General Measures. These measures consist of elevation of the legs in order to collapse the veins; use of elastic stockings or Ace bandages in an effort to maintain superficial venous collapse and increased velocity of flow in deep veins; avoidance of pressure points that obstruct venous return; and leg exercises consisting of pressing the feet against the foot of the bed 80 to 100 times on five or six occasions during the day.

Anticoagulants. If the clotting time of blood is normal, heparin in doses of 5,000 to 7,000 units (e.g., Liquaemin, 50 to 70 mg) is given intramuscularly and repeated at 6-hour intervals for 48 hr. If prothrombin time is normal, a coumarin preparation is given by mouth at the same time, e.g., warfarin (Coumadin), 50 mg, with subsequent doses to be determined by periodic measurements of prothrombin time. Anticoagulant treatment must be maintained at a high level for at least 3 weeks.

Anticoagulants are contraindicated in patients who are potential bleeders, e.g., those who have had peptic ulcers, esophageal varices, any hemorrhagic diathesis, severe liver disease, intracranial disease, or severe renal disease. Those who are potential candidates for surgical treatment should be maintained on heparin instead of warfarin, since the clotting defect of heparin can be reversed immediately with proatamine in contrast to the slower effect of vitamin K on the clotting defect produced by warfarin.

Vein Ligation. Veins may be ligated at the level of the common femorals or above, i.e., the iliacs or the inferior vena cava below the renal veins. Collateral circulation is best at the level of the vena cava, poorest at the iliac level, and intermediate at the femorals. For this reason, iliac ligation is not favored. Femoral ligation is a simple procedure with virtually no mortality. It can be carried out in very ill patients using local anesthesia. Vena cava ligation requires an abdominal incision, carries with it an operative mortality of approximately 5 per cent in otherwise normal patients, of 20 per cent in patients with compensated heart disease but with a past history of heart failure, and of 40 per cent in patients in heart failure. Vena cava ligation is more definitive than femoral ligation and entails fewer leg sequelae. If the venous clot extends above the level of the common femoral veins, vena cava ligation should be performed. Postoperative pain, tenderness, and swelling of legs occurs in about half the patients following vena cava ligation. These symptoms usually disappear within 3 or 4 months.

Vein ligation is more definitive than anticoagulation but likewise carries with it a greater morbidity. Vein ligation is indicated (1) when embolism occurs in patients receiving anticoagulants, (2) when anticoagulants are contraindicated, (3) when diseases predisposing to venous thrombosis and pulmonary embolism are prominent and persistent, and (4) when septic embolism occurs.

Special Types of Embolism

Fat Embolism

The entrance of free globules of fat into systemic veins occurs after fractures of long bones, especially the tibia or femur. Also, it is found in nontraumatic conditions such as tissue necrosis, burns, alcoholism, fatty metamorphosis of the liver, intoxications, decompression sickness, sickle-cell infarcts of bone, nephritis, and various infections and following blood transfusions. It is common after external cardiac massage and sternal splitting incisions for surgical procedures on the heart. There is no doubt that some of the fatty emboli are the result of release of depot fat from traumatized tissue, since myeloid tissue can occasionally be identified within pulmonary vessels. On the other hand, there is an increasing body of evidence to suggest that embolic fat is derived also from circulating blood lipids as a result of physicochemical alterations that produce colloidal instability of blood lipids and aggregation into fat globules.

Fat droplets are of varied size and obstruct branches of the pulmonary artery of all different sizes including arterioles and capillaries. Some fat traverses the capillaries, reaches the systemic circulation, and blocks arterioles and capillaries of brain, skin, heart, kidney, and other organs.

There is usually a latent period of 6 hr to several days after the fracture before the appearance of the clinical features of fat embolism. These features are attributable to embolic lesions in lungs and brain.

The clinical manifestations are those of pulmonary embolism already described. In addition, cerebral symptoms simultaneously with or after the pulmonary symptomatology include somnolence, disorientation, convulsions, delirium, and paralyses; fat emboli may be seen in retinal vessels; red petechial hemorrhages may appear in the skin; protein, red blood cells, and oil droplets may be found in urine. Cotton wool shadows scattered throughout the lungs may be seen by x-ray.

Death may be immediate or may not occur for 2 or 3 days. The patient may recover completely in 48 hr or more.

There is no specific treatment, but the measures described for thromboembolism in the discussion under Treatment should be instituted. Cooling of the patient (30 to 35°C) until neurologic improvement appears has been recently advocated, the rationale being the reduction of tissue metabolism.

Air Embolism

Air may enter the venous system in the course of intravenous infusions, tubal insufflation, pneumoperitoneum, knee-chest position in the puerperium, uterine douches, surgical treatment of the neck, retroperitoneal air injection, irrigation of nasal sinuses, and rapid decompression. The lethal dose varies with the rapidity of entry and varies between 5 and 15 ml per kg. Death is a result of either air lock in the right ventricle or embolism to the lung. Air is said not to traverse the pulmonary capillaries.[4] The clinical manifestations are those of a mill-wheel murmur, which is a loud churning noise over the precordium due to air and blood in the right ventricle, and cyanosis, pallor, dyspnea, and shock from circulatory obstruction produced by the air lock and embolic plugging of pulmonary vessels.

Treatment is correction of the cause, turning the patient on the left side in an effort to trap the air in the superior portion of the right atrium, aspiration of air through a needle inserted into the right ventricle, and administration of artificial respiration and oxygen.

Amniotic Fluid Embolism

First described by Meyer in 1926,[5] Steiner and Lushbaugh[6] described this disorder in detail in 1941. Predisposing factors are uterine tetany, intrauterine fetal death, oversized baby, vigorous labor, and premature separation of the placenta. There is a defect in the myometrium or decidua across which pass amniotic contents consisting of meconium, cells, lipids, mucin, and lanugo hair. It is the solid contents which produce the embolic manifestations. The amniotic fluid itself produces no embolic reaction when injected into animals. On the other hand, amniotic fluid does have thromboplastic activity. Cases have been reported wherein the lung and other organs are the site of diffuse deposition of fibrin. It has been postulated that the thromboplastin released in amniotic fluid produces intravascular deposition of fibrin with resulting depletion of fibrinogen and finally a hemorrhagic tendency. Several abnormalities of the maternal clotting mechanism are sufficiently frequent that copious vaginal bleeding occurs in about 60 per cent of reported cases.

The clinical picture is that of typical acute pulmonary embolism as described for thromboembolism. The diagnosis should be suspected with the occurrence of sudden collapse, dyspnea, and distended neck veins during labor, delivery, or soon thereafter and vaginal hemorrhage.

Treatment is supportive, as described for thromboembolism, and hemorrhage is controlled by transfusion of fresh whole blood and fibrinogen if available.

Tumor Emboli*

In addition to usual forms of pulmonary metastases resulting from the dessemination of malignancies, acute and subacute cor pulmonale may be produced by emboli of malignant tissue cells to the pulmonary arteries and capillaries. These emboli may originate from the primary site of the tumor or from other sites, such as the liver or inferior vena cava, to which the tumor has spread. Tumor emboli occur with virtually any type of malignancy, and their frequency is surely higher than the rarity of reported cases would indicate. Tumor emboli are relatively more common in patients with renal carcinoma, primary hepatic carcinoma, gastric carcinoma, and trophoblastic tumors (chorioepithelioma). Since trophoblastic tumors, even with extensive pulmonary metastases, may respond well to therapy with folic acid and purine antagonists, it

* This section on Tumor Emboli was prepared by Dr. Robert Schlant.

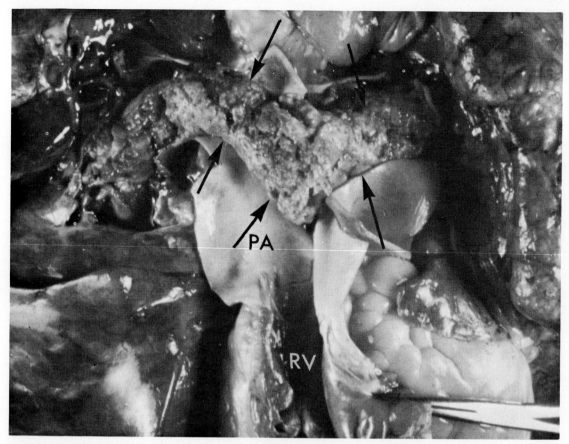

Fig. 47-3. Occlusion of the main pulmonary artery and main branches by chorioepithelioma: the heart, pulmonary arteries and lungs of a thirty-one-year-old woman with history and physical findings compatible with pulmonary hypertension and pulmonary emboli. She had a history of an uneventful pregnancy and delivery 2 years previously followed by "persistent, dark brown vaginal discharge and irregular spotting." Arrows identify the mass of chorioepithelioma nearly occluding the main pulmonary artery and its branches. No tumor could be found in the uterus or pelvis. (*Reproduced through the courtesy of Dr. John T. Ellis, Professor & Chairman, Department of Pathology, Emory University School of Medicine.*)

is imperative to consider this diagnosis whenever a female patent has either symptoms of acute dyspnea, pleurisy, cough, or hemoptysis or unexplained signs of pulmonary hypertension following a hydatidiform mole, an abortion, or a normal pregnancy. Occasionally, the pulmonary emboli may not occur until several years after the initiating pregnancy, and the patient may be asymptomatic in the interval, although usually there is amenorrhea, excessive bleeding or discharge, or other disturbances of menses (Fig. 47-3). Since uterine curettage is often negative, diagnosis is best established by estimations of urinary gonadotropin excretion. The radiologic changes in the lungs resulting from metastasis by trophoblastic tumors may take one or more of the following forms: (1) discrete, usually well-defined, and rounded opacities; (2) snowstorm patterns with multiple, small, less well-defined opac-

ities; and (3) changes resulting from embolic occlusion of the pulmonary arteries without invasion of the lung parenchyma.

REFERENCES

1. Virchow, R. L. K.: "Gesammelte Abhandlungen zur wissentschaffichen Medizin," von Meidinger Sohn u. Comp., Frankfurt-a-M., 1856.
2. Liebow, A. A., Hales, M. R., and Lindskog, G. E.: Enlargement of Bronchial Arteries and Their Anastomoses with Pulmonary Arteries in Bronchiectasis, *Am. J. Path.*, 25:211, 1949.
3. Robin, E. D.: Some Aspects of the Physiologic Disturbances Associated with Pulmonary Embolism, *M. Clin. North America*, 44:1269, 1960.
4. Curtillet, E.: L'embolie gazeuse artérielle, *J. chir.*, 53:461, 1939.

5. Meyer, J. R.: Embolia pulmonar amnio-caseosa, *Brasil-méd.*, **2**:301, 1926.
6. Steiner, P. E., and Lushbaugh, C. C.: Maternal Pulmonary Embolism by Amniotic Fluid as Cause of Obstetric Shock and Unexpected Deaths in Obstetrics, *J.A.M.A.*, **117**:1245, 1941.

SUGGESTED READING

General

Dexter, L., Dock, D. S., McGuire, L. B., Hyland, J. W., and Haynes, F. W.: Pulmonary Embolism, *M. Clin. North America*, **44**:1251, 1960.

Gorham, L. W.: A Study of Pulmonary Embolism, *Arch. Int. Med.*, **108**:8, 189, 418, 1961.

Israel, H. L., and Goldstein, F.: The Varied Clinical Manifestations of Pulmonary Embolism, *Ann. Int. Med.*, **47**:202, 1957.

Price, K. C., Hata, D., and Smith, J. R.: Pulmonary Vasomotion Resulting from Military Embolism of Lungs, *Am. J. Physiol.*, **182**:183, 1955.

Sasahaia, A. A., and Stein, M. (eds.): "Pulmonary Embolic Disease," Grune & Stratton, Inc., New York, 1965, p. 312.

Towbin, A.: Pulmonary Embolism: Incidence and Significance, *J.A.M.A.*, **156**:209, 1954.

Pathogenesis

Bauer, G.: A Venographic Study of Thrombo-embolic Problems, *Acta chir. scandinav.*, **84**: (Suppl. 61), 1, 1940.

Hyland, J. W., Smith, G. T., McGuire, L. B., Harrison, D. C., Haynes, F. W., and Dexter, L.: Effect of Selective Embolization of Various Sized Pulmonary Arteries in Dogs, *Am. J. Physiol.*, **204**:619, 1963.

Smith, G. T., Dammin, G. T., and Dexter, L.: Postmortem Arteriographic Studies of the Human Lung in Pulmonary Embolization, *J.A.M.A.*, **188**:143, 1964.

Laboratory Findings

Fleischner, F. G.: Pulmonary Embolism, *Canad. M.A.J.*, **78**:653, 1958.

Fleischner, F. G.: Unilateral Pulmonary Embolism, *Acta radiol.*, **19**:357, 1938.

Hampton, A. O., and Castleman, B.: Correlation of Postmortem Chest Teleroentgenograms with Autopsy Findings, with Special Reference to Pulmonary Embolism and Infarction, *Am. J. Roentgenol.*, **43**:305, 1940.

Wacker, W. E., Rosenthal, M., Snodgrass, P. J. and Amador, E.: A Triad for the Diagnosis of Pulmonary Embolism and Infarction, *J.A.M.A.*, **178**:8, 1961.

Wagner, H. N., Jr., Sabiston, D., Eoiio, M., Meyer, J., and Langan, J.: Regional Pulmonary Blood Flow in Man by Radio-isotope Scanning, *J.A.M.A.*, **187**:601, 1964.

Wolff, L.: The Electrocardiogram in Pulmonary Embolism, *Heart Bull.*, **8**:111, 1959.

Treatment

Bowers, R. F.: Vena Cava Ligation: Advantages vs. Disadvantages, *Am. Surgeon*, **22**:359, 1956.

Cooley, D. A., and Beall, A. C., Jr.: A Technic of Pulmonary Embolectomy Using Temporary Cardiopulmonary Bypass: Clinical and Experimental Considerations, *J. Cardiovas. Surg.*, **2**:469, 1961.

DeBakey, M. E.: Critical Evaluation of Problem of Thromboembolism, *Surg. Gynec. & Obst.*, **107**:214, 1958.

Edwards, E. A., Dexter, L., and Donahue, W. C.: Recurrent Pulmonary Embolism as a Remediable Cause of Heart Failure, *Geriatrics*, **16**:423, 1961.

Steenburg, R. W., Warren, R., Wilson, R. E., and Rudolf, L. E.: A New Look at Embolectomy, *Surg. Gynec. & Obst.*, **107**:214, 1958.

Wilkins, R. W., and Stanton, J. R.: Elastic Stockings in Prevention of Pulmonary Embolism, *New England J. Med.*, **248**:1087, 1953.

Fat Embolism

Adkins, R. B., and Foster, J. H.: Experimental Study of the Genesis of Fat Embolism, *Ann. Surg.*, **156**:515, 1962.

Aladjemoff, L., Weinberg, H., and Alkalay, I.: Fat Embolism Treatment with Lytic Cocktail and Surface Cooling, *Lancet*, **2**:13, 1963.

LeQuire, V. S., Shapiro, J. L., LeQuire, C. B., Cobb, C. A., Jr., and Fleet, W. F.: A Study of the Pathogenesis of Fat Embolism Based on Human Necropsy Material and Animal Experiments, *Am. J. Path.*, **35**:999, 1959.

Taquini, A. C., Roncoroni, A. J. and Aramendía, P.: Fat Embolism of the Lungs, *Am. Heart J.*, **51**:468, 1956.

Air Embolism

Oppenheimer, M. J., Durant, T. M., and Lynch, P.: Body Position in Relation to Venous Air Embolism and the Associated Cardio-vascular-respiratory Changes, *Am. J. M. Sc.*, **225**:362, 1953.

Wolffe, J. B., and Robertson, H. F.: Experimental Air Embolism, *Ann. Int. Med.*, **9**:162, 1935.

Amniotic Fluid Embolism

Scott, M. M.: Cardiopulmonary Considerations in Nonfatal Amniotic Fluid Embolism, *J.A.M.A.*, **183**:989, 1963.

Tuller, M. A.: Amniotic Fluid Embolism, Afibrinogenemia, and Disseminated Fibrin Thrombosis: Case Report and Review of Literature, *Am. J. Obst. & Gynec.*, **73**:273, 1957.

Tumor Emboli

Bagshawe, K. D., and Brooks, W. D. W.: Subacute Pulmonary Hypertension Due to Chorionepithelioma, *Lancet*, **1**:653, 1959.

Bagshawe, K. D., and Garnett, E. S.: Radiological Changes in the Lungs with Trophoblastic Tumors, *Brit. J. Radiol.*, 36:673, 1963.

Durham, J. R., Ashley, P. F., and Dorencamp, D.: Cor Pulmonale Due to Tumor Emboli: Review of Literature and Report of a Case, *J.A.M.A.*, 175: 757, 1961.

Storey, P. B., and Goldstein, W.: Pulmonary Embolization From Primary Hepatic Carcinoma, *Arch. Int. Med.*, 110:262, 1962.

Storstein, O.: Circulatory Failure in Metastatic Carcinoma of Lung: A Physiologic and Pathologic Study of Its Pathogenesis, *Circulation*, 4:913, 1951.

48 PULMONARY HYPERTENSION

S. Gilbert Blount, Jr., M.D., and Robert F. Grover, Ph.D., M.D.

The Normal Pulmonary Circulation

In the unexpanded fetal lung, the pulmonary vascular resistance is high and the pulmonary blood flow is low. Vessel kinking and other mechanical factors[1] may contribute to the high resistance. However, Dawes[2] has shown active pulmonary vasoconstriction to be the dominant factor determining pulmonary vascular resistance in the fetal lamb. He significantly increased blood flow through the unexpanded lung by increasing the oxygenation of fetal arterial blood or by infusing the vasodilator acetylcholine. Conversely, fetal hypoxemia caused increased pulmonary vascular resistance and decreased pulmonary blood flow. This evidence strongly suggests that fetal pulmonary circulation is regulated by hypoxia.

The first breaths following birth transform the lung from a collapsed, fluid-filled, underperfused organ to its expanded, air-filled, fully perfused postnatal state. With the first inspiration, the lung is subjected to powerful negative distending pressures, as air enters the previously fluid-filled alveoli. Concomitantly, capillaries in the alveolar walls become dilated with blood; a mechanism of capillary erection has been postulated[3] to assist in alveolar expansion. However, study of the pulmonary surfactant, which determines surface tension properties of the fluid film lining the airways, suggests that the pulmonary capillaries may indeed be pulled open by surface forces within the alveoli.[4] More detailed knowledge of the spatial geometry of the alveoli and capillaries is necessary before this intriguing possibility is accepted.

Pulmonary vascular resistance falls as the lung expands and the alveoli are aerated. Pulmonary blood flow increases rapidly, and the lung functions to oxygenate blood and remove carbon dioxide for the infant beginning extrauterine life. The

pulmonary arterial pressure then falls to below aortic pressure; unless the ductus arteriosus closes, blood flows from systemic to pulmonary circulation, producing a left-to-right shunt. The ductus arteriosus may open and close intermittently during the first few days of life. Hemodynamic studies of normal human infants in the first hours of life frequently demonstrate a large left-to-right shunt through a patent ductus arteriosus.[5] Right-to-left shunting of blood has also been demonstrated,[6] indicating that significant fluctuations in pulmonary vascular resistance may occur after birth. However, by the end of the first week of life, the normal ductus arteriosus is functionally closed, and the postnatal pulmonary circulation pattern becomes established.

The most striking histologic feature of the fetal pulmonary vascular bed is the thick muscular media of the small muscular pulmonary arteries. These vessel walls appear thinner with vascular dilatation in the postnatal period. It is widely accepted[7] that this thinning process represents an actual decrease in muscle mass within the media of the vessels. The development of increased pulmonary vascular resistance and pulmonary hypertension after birth has been largely attributed to failure of this decrease in vascular musculature; this may indeed be true. However, the authors believe that existence of a greater muscle mass in the fetal lung than in the normal infant lung has not been definitely established; the thickness of the fetal vessels may merely represent vasoconstriction. Thinning of the pulmonary vessel walls continues during the first year and a half of life, resulting in the normal adult vessel structure. This normal involution of pulmonary arterial smooth muscle occurs as long as no abnormal stimulus produces pulmonary vasoconstriction.[8,9]

Once the structural transition in the pulmonary vascular bed has been completed, the pulmonary circulation assumes its familiar hemodynamic characteristics of low pressure, low resistance, and high compliance. These features can be examined directly by well-established techniques of catheterization of the right side of the heart. Average pulmonary blood flow during several minutes is most accurately determined by the direct Fick method;[10] pulmonary arterial pressure is measured directly at the tip of a cardiac catheter positioned in one of the major branches of the pulmonary artery. The normal resting supine man at sea level has a mean pulmonary arterial pressure, i.e., the average pressure throughout the cardiac cycle and during several respiratory cycles of 12 mm Hg; there is no significant variation over the age range of four to seventy years.[11,12]

The change in pulmonary arterial pressure in the normal lung due to increased pulmonary blood

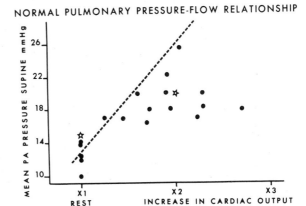

NORMAL PULMONARY PRESSURE-FLOW RELATIONSHIP

Fig. 48-1. If a twofold increase in blood flow produced a twofold increase in pressure, the pressure would rise along the dotted line. Multiple observations reported by several writers (solid dots) indicate that pressure rises less than flow. Therefore, a high pulmonary blood flow through a normal adult pulmonary vascular bed will not produce significant pulmonary hypertension. Similar results are obtained by balloon occlusion of the right pulmonary artery (open stars).

flow has been studied by two different methods. One method diverts the total right ventricular output through the left lung by inflating an occluding balloon within the lumen of the artery to the right lung. Blood flow is approximately doubled in the left lung, without change in cardiac output or other major circulatory adjustments. This maneuver produces a small but consistent rise in pulmonary arterial pressure (Fig. 48-1) of 5 mm Hg.[13,14] The second and more complex method is more physiologic. A supine subject exercises by pumping a bicycle ergometer with his legs. Moderate exercise may double the cardiac output, but very heavy exercise is required to produce a threefold increase in the cardiac output. While this exercise serves to increase the total pulmonary blood flow, associated alterations in respiratory dynamics and cardiac function may also influence the pulmonary circulation. Under the above circumstances, mean pulmonary arterial pressure may increase as much as 15 mm Hg (Fig. 48-1).[11,15] These modest elevations of pulmonary arterial pressure in response to increased blood flow through the normal lung must be borne in mind in evaluating the hemodynamics of left-to-right shunts.

Conditions Leading to Pulmonary Hypertension

The term *pulmonary hypertension* implies an elevation of the pulmonary arterial pressure to levels above the accepted limit of normal, i.e., 35/15 mm Hg. The maintenance of a normal pulmonary arterial blood pressure is dependent upon a physiologic relationship between the volume of pulmonary arterial blood flow per unit of time and the resistance to that flow. The most important and best-understood factors responsible for elevation of pulmonary arterial blood pressure include (1) elevation of pulmonary capillary and/or left atrial pressure, (2) decrease in cross-sectional area of the total pulmonary vascular bed, and (3) significant increase in pulmonary arterial blood flow. Pulmonary blood volume, blood viscosity, bronchopulmonary arterial anastomoses, intrapulmonary

pressure, and intrathoracic pressures may play some part in the development of pulmonary hypertension; however, these mechanisms are probably of minor importance. Pulmonary hypertension may result when one or more of these mechanisms are involved; if it is of sufficient severity and duration, pathologic changes are produced within the pulmonary vascular bed which initiate or further the obstructive element and heighten the pulmonary vascular resistance. Elevated pressure within a muscular structure tends to stimulate a vasoconstrictive response, further decreasing the cross-sectional area of the pulmonary vascular bed and further increasing the pulmonary arterial resistance.

Elevation of Pulmonary Capillary Pressure and/or Left Atrial Pressure

Elevation of Pulmonary Capillary Pressure. The elevation of pulmonary capillary pressure usually results from obstruction to pulmonary venous blood flow. This obstruction may be as distal as the left ventricle or as proximal as the pulmonary vein, encompassing many forms of obstruction at sites in between.

Normal mean left atrial pressure ranges between 2 and 12 mm Hg. A recent study of the components of the normal left atrial pressure tracing[22] revealed the A wave to have an average mean pressure of 10 mm Hg (range, 4 to 16 mm Hg) and the V wave to average 13 mm Hg (range, 6 to 21 mm Hg). The normal mean pulmonary arterial pressure of about 13 to 18 mm Hg thus produces a gradient of 6 to 11 mm Hg across the pulmonary vascular bed. The left atrial and pulmonary capillary pressure may become elevated in the normal individual during severe exercise or with other conditions resulting in greatly increased pulmonary arterial blood flow. Experimental conditions producing pulmonary capillary pressure elevation include the rapid intravenous injection of saline solution[23] and the use of norepinephrine or other potent systemic vasoconstrictive substances.[24] Any other situation causing redistribution of blood into the pulmonary vascular bed could also produce elevation of the left atrial and pulmonary capillary pressures. This would suggest that the mechanism is a passive increase in volume, distending the pulmonary venous and capillary systems and increasing the transmural pressure. A recent study in man[25] has suggested that the pulmonary blood vessels are affected by both active and passive mechanisms and that alterations in pulmonary vascular resistance are not necessarily directly related to change in vessel size.

Variations in intrapulmonary and intrathoracic pressure must also be considered as contributing to the elevation of pulmonary capillary pressure. Although probably of little significance, it seems feasible that increased alveolar pressure might be transmitted to the pulmonary capillary bed; if widespread, it might affect the pulmonary arterial pressure.[26] Variations in intrathoracic pressure may affect the pulmonary capillary pressure and thereby the pulmonary arterial pressure, but this mechanism too is probably of minor significance.

Conditions associated with obstruction to venous flow elevate the pulmonary arterial pressure in a retrograde and passive manner; they will be considered next.

Increase in Resistance to Left Ventricular Filling. Increase in the residual diastolic blood volume in the failing left ventricle results in an increased resistance to left ventricular filling. The left ventricular failure may result from an obstructive defect, such as systemic hypertension or obstruction to left ventricular outflow, or it may be due to myocardial inadequacy secondary to coronary artery disease or primary or secondary myocardial disease. The pulmonary hypertension secondary to such conditions is due to the retrograde transmission of the elevated pulmonary venous pressure across the capillary bed and is usually of moderate degree. The occasional further rise of pulmonary arterial pressure is suggestive of a reflex vasoconstrictive element in the pulmonary hypertension;[27] it produces an increase in the gradient between the pulmonary arterial and left atrial pressure. Constrictive pericarditis, marked myocardial fibrosis, and restrictive endocarditis may also effect this change; in these conditions, there is rarely a vasoconstrictive element, and the gradient across the capillary bed is normal or modestly increased. The pulmonary arterial systolic pressure is usually between 40 and 60 mm Hg.

Mitral Valvular Disease. Left atrial pressure rises when the mitral valve orifice is decreased beyond a critical area. As there are no valves in the left atrial-pulmonary venous-capillary system, a rise in left atrial pressure is transmitted to and across the pulmonary capillary bed, elevating the pulmonary arterial pressure. With mild degrees of mitral valve stenosis, the pulmonary hypertension may be purely passive in nature, with preservation of a normal pressure gradient across the pulmonary vascular bed.

However, in certain individuals with mitral stenosis of such severity as to elevate the left atrial pressure to 25 mm Hg or higher, the pulmonary arterial pressure may rise out of proportion to the left atrial pressure. This varies considerably among individuals and is considered a manifestation of individual variability of pulmonary vascular reactivity. This rise in pulmonary arterial pressure is in excess of that which can be accounted for by retrograde pressure transmission. The increased pressure gradient results from the additive factor of an elevated pulmonary vascular resistance, further raising the pulmonary arterial pressure. The mechanism of this increase in pulmonary vascular resistance remains controversial. Some investigators consider this an active form of pulmonary hypertension mediated by a reflex response to a critical level of pulmonary venous pressure.[27,28] As noted above, this mechanism may vary considerably from one individual to the next; it is rarely noted with slight or moderate left atrial pressure elevation, as seen with left ventricular failure or myocardial disease. Supporting evidence for a reflex vasoconstrictive mechanism for pulmonary hypertension in patients with severe mitral stenosis is the sudden, dramatic fall in pulmonary arterial pressure within a few weeks after successful mitral valvotomy.[29]

The studies of Wood [17] also suggest a vasoconstrictive element; he reported a fall in pulmonary arterial pressure and resistance and a rise in cardiac output and left atrial pressure following acetylcholine injection into the pulmonary artery of patients with mitral stenosis and marked pulmonary hypertension. The acetylcholine is inactivated in the lungs and produces no direct effect on the systemic circulation. In the authors' laboratory a similar response has been noted following the intrapulmonary arterial administration of tolazoline hydrochloride. The study of Sanger et al.[27] adds evidence supporting the presence of a reflex vasoconstrictive mechanism; such studies, though suggestive, are not conclusive in substantiating a vasoconstrictor effect.

It is also possible that no vasoconstrictive element need be postulated; a sudden, significant rise in pulmonary arterial pressure may occur when a critical area of the pressure-volume curve of the pulmonary vascular bed is reached.

Obstruction Proximal to the Mitral Valve. Several rarer abnormalities may also produce an elevated pulmonary arterial pressure by a mechanism similar to that previously described. Such conditions include supramitral valvular obstruction, cor triatriatum, congenital stenosis of pulmonary veins as they enter the left atrium, mediastinitis involving the pulmonary veins, and total anomalous pulmonary venous connections with a long and narrow common venous trunk.

Decrease in Total Cross-sectional Area of the Pulmonary Vascular Bed

Structural changes reducing the total cross-sectional area of the pulmonary vascular bed result in increased resistance to pulmonary arterial blood flow. However, the remarkable distensibility of the pulmonary vasculature provides a considerable compensatory reserve;[11,13] the total area of the pulmonary vascular bed must be reduced by more than 50 per cent before a significant elevation of pulmonary arterial pressure results.[34,35] It is well recognized that patients do not develop pulmonary hypertension following pneumonectomy if the remaining lung is normal.[8] Recent studies involving selective lobectomy in animals have suggested that the distensibility of the lower lobes may not be as great as that of the upper lobes.[35] Hence, not only the volume (mass) of lung tissue removed but also its anatomic location may be an important determinant of the resultant change in pulmonary vascular resistance.

Significant compromise of the pulmonary vascular bed may result from compression of the pulmonary vessels as seen with extensive parenchymal fibrosis of the lung, it may be secondary to reduction of the vessel lumen produced by primary infectious or granulomatous involvement of the vessel wall, or it may stem from great hypertrophy of the musculature of the media. Obstruction may also occur from within, as is the case in widespread miliary emboli or thrombosis involving the small pulmonary arterial vessels; the total pulmonary bed is so reduced as to result in severe pulmonary hypertension.

Pulmonary Emboli. Pulmonary hypertension may occur with widespread obstruction and obliteration of the pulmonary vasculature. The clinical picture of pulmonary embolization may vary considerably; catastrophic, sudden, massive pulmonary embolization resulting in acute right ventricular failure is familiar to all. However, recurrent episodes of pulmonary embolism involving lesser areas of the pulmonary vascular bed may present entirely different and perplexing clinical syndromes.

The so-called primary or essential pulmonary hypertension presents a difficult problem in differential diagnosis. The pathogenesis of essential pulmonary hypertension is not clear; many writers

doubt its existence as a specific entity and consider the changes in the pulmonary vasculature to be secondary to recurrent miliary embolization; some data obtained from animal experiments tends to substantiate this view. The difference between pulmonary hypertension caused by clinically evident recurrent episodes of pulmonary embolism and the more silent clinical picture of so-called primary pulmonary hypertension may be only a function of the size and localization of the emboli. In the former condition, larger emboli occlude vessels of greater size, whereas in so-called primary pulmonary hypertension the emboli are situated more peripherally in vessels of 0.1 to 1.0 mm diameter.

Experimental and clinical studies have indicated the difficulty of determining whether pulmonary vascular changes in patients with pulmonary hypertension represent thrombus formation due to primary vessel disease or whether they represent the vascular reaction to multiple pulmonary emboli. Recurrent miliary pulmonary emboli can effect changes within small pulmonary vessels which are morphologically indistinguishable from the sub-intimal thickening noted in patients with idiopathic pulmonary hypertension;[36] it is entirely possible that patients now considered to have primary or idiopathic pulmonary hypertension may indeed represent cases of recurrent miliary pulmonary emboli. The source of the miliary emboli is not always clear, although silent thrombi are not infrequently found at careful routine postmortem examination. The fact that young women are the most frequently afflicted might suggest a disorder of blood clotting related to the menstrual cycle.

Most likely a multiplicity of disease processes may result in the clinical picture of idiopathic pulmonary hypertension. At the present time, idiopathic pulmonary hypertension probably represents a polyglot group of conditions presenting a similar clinical picture and course.[37]

Medial Hypertrophy. Diffuse thickening of the walls of the small muscular pulmonary arteries may be due to medial hypertrophy or to vasoconstriction. When these processes are of sufficient severity to reduce the vascular lumen to the point where vascular resistance is greatly increased, pulmonary hypertension results. The apparent thickening of the vessel wall has been designated as medial hypertrophy; however, an increased wall-to-lumen ratio can be caused by lumen reduction as well as by increased thickness of the vessel wall. Thus, medial hypertrophy may indicate hypertrophy or vasoconstriction or a combination of the two.

Increased pressure within a vessel is the stimulus for vasoconstriction, which then leads to increased work of the media and, in turn, to further hypertrophy. While this vasoconstriction may be reversible in an early phase, at a later stage it may become fixed because of the persistent shortening of the elastic and muscular coats of the artery. This phenomenon has been designated as arterial contracture;[38] its appearance may be a limiting factor in the regression of the vascular changes described above. Constriction of small muscular arteries with hypertrophied media accounts, in part, for the pulmonary hypertension normally observed in the infant in the immediate postnatal period. If this medial hypertrophy does not regress in a normal manner, increased pulmonary vascular resistance persists; this occurs in certain patients with large ventricular septal defects and other comparable lesions. The resultant pulmonary hypertension apparently traumatizes the pulmonary arteries. With the passage of time, constriction and later contracture, intimal proliferation, fibrosis, thrombosis, and atherosclerosis may make their appearance, further reducing the lumen of the small pulmonary vessels. Their effect is not always additive, however, for as the obstructive lesions become more extensive, there frequently is a concomitant decrease in the extent of medial hypertrophy. Consequently, the magnitude of the increased pulmonary vascular resistance may change little over long periods of time, despite an alteration in the nature of the vascular obstruction.[39]

The authors have been interested in the effect of the vasodilating agent tolazoline on pulmonary vascular resistance, particularly in patients with ventricular septal defects and pulmonary hypertension.[40] Tolazoline, a drug of complex action, produces vasodilatation by several mechanisms,[41] one of which is a direct nonadrenergic relaxant action upon vascular smooth muscle; this is probably the most important factor in vasodilatation produced in man. The authors' studies of children with severe pulmonary hypertension demonstrated that tolazoline reduced pulmonary arterial pressure; this was often associated with an increase, and never with a decrease, in pulmonary arterial blood flow (Fig. 48-5). The authors believe that a vasodilator such as tolazoline is most effective when the increased pulmonary vascular resistance is primarily a consequence of generalized constriction of hypertophied small muscular arteries; when the smooth muscle relaxes, vasodilation can occur. This responsive situation is found most frequently in the first years of life. When pulmonary hypertension has been present for years, obliterative changes such as intimal proliferation and fibrosis, thrombosis, and atherosclerosis may be present in the smaller pulmonary arteries.[39] If these lesions are widespread and account for a large portion of the increased pulmonary vascular resistance, a vasodilator cannot be expected to lower pulmonary vascular resistance appreciably. However, both the magnitude and duration of increased pulmonary vascular resistance are probably important in determining the age at which a given patient will lose his responsiveness to tolazoline.[39] The authors have found the response to tolazoline of help in predicting preoperatively which children with high pulmonary vascular resistance would show a decrease in pulmonary arterial pressure and resistance following closure of the ventricular septal defect (Fig. 48-5).[42]

"Functional" Reduction of the Pulmonary Vascular Bed. Constriction of the small muscular pulmonary arteries (less than 100 μ in diameter) increases the resistance to pulmonary blood flow. Alveolar hypoxia frequently provides the stimulus for such vasoconstriction. Patients with marked alveolar hypoventilation[43] associated with pulmonary parenchymal disease, such as chronic bronchitis, often have a significant element of hypoxic vasoconstriction. Central nervous system disease, paralytic states, or obesity are also associated with hypoventilation leading to pulmonary hypertension. Normal man is exposed to increasing alveolar hypoxia as he ascends to high altitude and is subjected to lowered total atmospheric pressure. This hypoxia, if marked and prolonged, produces marked pulmonary hypertension,[15] as is seen in the Indian populations living above 14,000 feet in the Andes. However, no elevation of pulmonary arterial pressure is seen in the residents of Bogotá, Colombia, at an elevation of 8,300 feet,[44] or at lower altitudes. Whether or not pulmonary hypertension will develop at a given altitude is therefore dependent upon the degree of hypoxia. Also of importance, however, is the pulmonary vascular reactivity of the population involved. Recent work from the authors' laboratory revealed a remarkable degree of pulmonary hypertension in certain individuals living in Colorado at the modest altitude of 10,200 feet.[19] These pressure elevations were much greater than would have been predicted from studies of Peruvian Indians living at similar altitudes in the Andes.[15] Further investigation of these population differences is indicated.

Pulmonary hypertension at high altitude results from increased resistance to blood flow through the lung. Since the pressure elevation is immediately lowered by oxygen administration, hypoxic vasoconstriction is implied. The pulmonary vascular resistance is so grossly elevated that one would expect obvious medial hypertrophy of the small muscular pulmonary arteries. However, histologic examination of the lungs of these adult high-altitude dwellers has been surprisingly unremarkable; only with quantitative techniques has a subtle increase in vascular smooth muscle been demonstrated.[45] The general normality of these pulmonary arteries suggests some other form of structural alteration, such as loss of compliance or contracture.[38]

When an individual is born in a hypoxic environment at high altitude, the muscular fetal pulmonary arteries do not undergo the usual rapid regression; the hypoxia continues to influence the pulmonary circulation significantly, just as it normally does before birth. Hypoxic pulmonary hypertension may therefore be considered a residual phenomenon from intrauterine life. These observations broaden our interpretation of the significance of pulmonary hypertension. In most normal individuals living at high altitude, the moderate pulmonary hypertension produces no symptoms, no decrease in exercise tolerance, and no apparent adverse effects later in life;[15,19] this pulmonary hypertension may well be completely reversible.[15]

Much effort has been devoted to investigating the mechanism by which alveolar hypoxia produces pulmonary hypertension. Most writers believe that pulmonary vascular resistance is increased at the precapillary level. The small muscular pulmonary arteries show muscular thickening, and presumably these are the vessels which constrict in response to hypoxia. Alveolar hypoxia lowers the oxygen tension of the pulmonary capillary blood. Since pulmonary blood flow is pulsatile, with significant reversal of flow during ventricular diastole[46] this hypoxemic capillary blood could easily reflux into the precapillary vessels, thereby exposing the vessel walls to hypoxia from the lumen. The distal airways and pulmonary artery branches are side by side, with less than 100 μ of tissue separating air from blood;[47] gases can and do diffuse across this thin barrier.[48] This anatomic arrangement provides an alternative explanation for exposure of the precapillary arterial vessels to hypoxia from the outside. The mechanism by which hypoxia causes constriction of the pulmonary vascular smooth muscle remains unclear. Recent work in man has shown that the rise of pulmonary arterial pressure during acute hypoxia is determined by the blood pH; it is abolished by alkalosis.[49] This lends support to the hypothesis put forth nearly twenty years ago by von Euler and Liljestrand that hypoxia causes local acidosis (lactic acid), which in turn stimulates vasoconstriction.[50,51]

Increase in Pulmonary Arterial Blood Flow

Increased pulmonary arterial blood flow rarely causes elevated pulmonary arterial blood pressure when it occurs after the normal regression of the so-called fetal pulmonary vascular pattern.[8] The capacious normal pulmonary vascular bed has a great reserve; blood flow is rarely of such magnitude as to produce significant disproportion between the volume of flow and the overall cross-sectional area of the pulmonary vascular bed. Treadmill-exercise studies performed in the authors' laboratory on normal individuals revealed that increases of cardiac output to 16 to 18 liters per min[52] produced pulmonary arterial systolic pressures of only 35 to 40 mm Hg. Furthermore, many patients with atrial septal defects catheterized in the authors' laboratory had normal pulmonary arterial pressures in the presence of pulmonary artery blood flows of approximately 15 liters per min. When significant pulmonary hypertension exists in the presence of elevated pulmonary arterial blood flow, it would appear certain that there is a coexistent decrease in the cross-sectional area of the pulmonary vascular bed. Thus, increased pulmonary arterial blood flow can be significant in the presence of a decreased pulmonary vascular bed; this combination produces a significant increase of pulmonary vascular resistance with resulting pulmonary hypertension. This is the usual situation in patients with intracardiac septal defects and large left-to-right shunts who have significantly increased pulmonary arterial blood pressure.

However, quite a different situation results if pulmonary blood flow is greater than normal from the time of birth. This occurs as an "experiment of nature" in patients with congenital absence of one pulmonary artery as an isolated defect. One lung receives the entire output of the right ventricle, and, from the time of birth, blood flow through this lung is twice normal. The incidence of pulmonary hypertension was 19 per cent[8] in the 32 reported cases of this isolated anomaly. The mechanism of production of pulmonary hypertension in this situation has been postulated as follows:[9] A basic property of smooth muscle is that it will contract in response to the stimulus of stretch. The fetal small pulmonary arteries have a thick media of smooth muscle; these arteries increase in diameter at birth to accept the normal increase in pulmonary blood flow following expansion of the lung. If the pulmonary blood flow is excessive, these muscular arteries may be stretched to the point where they react by constriction. A cycle of stretch-constriction is established, and the increased resistance presented by the constricted vessels results in pulmonary hypertension. The elevated intraluminal pressure also tends to stretch the arteries and acts as an added stimulus to augment the vasoconstriction, perpetuate the hypertension, and lead to contracture, a fixed state.

The fundamental difference in reactivity between the neonatal and adult pulmonary vascular bed has been confirmed experimentally in the authors' laboratory.[8,9] Ligation of the left pulmonary artery in the adult dog produces no significant pulmonary hypertension, whereas the same procedure in the newborn puppy produces right ventricular hypertrophy and failure of the right side of the heart, implying the existence of severe pulmonary hypertension.[8] When pulmonary artery ligation is performed in the newborn calf, pulmonary arterial pressure fails to decrease to adult levels; severe pulmonary hypertension develops after a few weeks.[9] An excessive increase in pulmonary blood flow present from the time of birth may therefore play an important etiologic role in the genesis of pulmonary hypertension. This concept is relevant in understanding the hemodynamics of direct communication between the pulmonary and the systemic circulations, as through a large ventricular septal defect. Here, the shunting of blood from the left side of the heart, added to the right ventricular output, produces excessive pulmonary blood flow. At birth, the muscular pulmonary arteries begin to dilate; however, the more they open, the greater the pulmonary flow becomes. These vessels are stretched until they are stimulated to constrict. Constriction increases pulmonary vascular resistance, and pulmonary hypertension results. This is the mechanism described by Wood for the so-called Eisenmenger reaction.[53]

This implies that an initially normal hyperreactive neonatal pulmonary vascular bed responds to an abnormal stimulus by widespread pulmonary vasoconstriction. The usual medial smooth muscle involution is prevented, and the persisting medial "hypertrophy" maintains the pulmonary vascular resistance at a high level. If the abnormal stimulus were removed, the vascular media would presumably undergo "disuse atrophy," and the pulmonary arteries would become normal. The high intraluminal pressure is apparently traumatic to the pulmonary arteries, for with the passage of time secondary vascular changes develop: intimal proliferation and thickening, atherosclerosis, thrombosis, and extensive vascular occlusion. Once this vascular damage has occurred, the pulmonary hypertension is probably irreversible.

Pulmonary hypertension increases the risk involved in surgical intervention. In patients with pulmonary hypertension who have had successful ventricular septal defect closure, the elevated pulmonary vascular resistance regressed toward normal when medial hypertrophy was the only vascular abnormality. Only an occasional patient surviving surgical treatment has demonstrated regression of pulmonary vascular resistance when additional vascular lesions were present. This is true even with pulmonary vascular resistance equal to systemic resistance, with bidirectional shunting and cyanosis. It is not generally recognized that such cases of the Eisenmenger reaction may be operable if detected at an early age when medial hypertrophy is the only pulmonary vascular abnormality.

Acute Pulmonary Edema of High Altitude with Pulmonary Hypertension

Significant pulmonary hypertension occurs in patients developing so-called acute high-altitude pulmonary edema.[30] Significant elevation of the mean pulmonary arterial pressure to levels of 120 mm Hg has been demonstrated at catheterization of the right side of the heart during the acute illness. The pulmonary hypertension in patients with acute pulmonary edema was originally considered to be due to acute left ventricular failure, resulting in an elevated left atrial pressure and pulmonary edema; pulmonary hypertension was thought to be produced in a passive retrograde manner.

However, during cardiac catheterization studies on a physician during an episode of acute pulmonary edema of high altitude,[31] the catheter fortuitously passed through a foramen ovale; the left atrial pressure was found to be normal in the presence of an elevated pulmonary arterial pressure. This unexpected finding led the writers to postulate that pulmonary venoconstriction produced capillary pressure elevation and resultant pulmonary edema. Recent studies[30] of five patients with acute pulmonary edema of high altitude in the Peruvian Andes (altitude 12,300 feet) have revealed normal pulmonary arterial wedge pressures in all patients. Administration of 100 per cent oxygen resulted in a prompt fall in pulmonary arterial pressure, without significant change in the pulmonary arterial wedge pressure; the fall in pulmonary arterial pressure was rapid, about 80 per cent of the fall occurring within 2 min after oxygen administration. However, the finding of a normal pulmonary wedge pressure does not necessarily indicate that pulmonary capillary and venous pressures are normal in all areas of the lung.

Thus, the available studies are perplexing. At present, there is no completely adequate explanation for the pulmonary edema and pulmonary hypertension of high altitude in man. There is, however, evidence for pulmonary venoconstriction in cattle.[32] An average pressure gradient of 14.6 ± 1.6 mm Hg between the pulmonary arterial wedge pressure and the left ventricular enddiastolic pressure was demonstrated in four animals in heart failure due to Brisket disease. The pulmonary veins of the bovine species have a thick muscular coat,[33] providing a basis for the hypothesis that the obstruction is due to pulmonary venoconstriction. The pulmonary veins of man, on the other hand, have a poorly developed muscular coat; thus, it would be difficult to imagine any significant degree of pulmonary venoconstriction in man.

Individual Variability of Pulmonary Vascular Reactivity

Only recently has consideration been given to the possibility of difference in pulmonary vascular reactivity between individuals of the same species and individuals of different species. A given stimulus often provokes a spectrum of responses, varying in magnitude from one individual to the next; this inherent difference in reactivity is indeed a characteristic of biologic systems. Unfortunately, this well-known concept has only infrequently been considered in discussion of the pulmonary circulation. This variability is apparent when one evaluates the response of the pulmonary vascular bed to such stimuli as elevation of pulmonary venous pressure, increased blood flow, or hypoxia. Wood [16] observed that only 25 to 30 per cent of patients with severe mitral stenosis developed severe pulmonary hypertension. Another group with equal diminution of the mitral valve area and comparable elevation of left atrial and pulmonary venous pressures had no significant increase in precapillary vascular resistance. Thus, a definite difference in individual response is seen to stimuli of the same order.[17] Similar variability in response

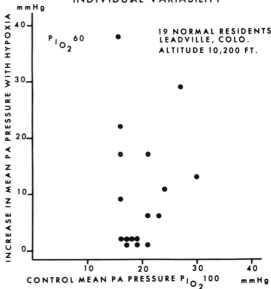

Fig. 48-3. When normal high-altitude residents are made hypoxic acutely by lowering the inspired oxygen tension ($P_{I_{O_2}}$) from 100 down to 60 mm Hg, some individuals have virtually no increase in mean pulmonary arterial pressure (hyporeactors), while other individuals have a marked pressure increase of 15 to 40 mm Hg (hyperreactors).

has been noted in individuals with increased pulmonary arterial blood flow, as seen with a ventricular septal defect. In the past, a direct relationship was thought to exist between the size of the defect and the elevation of the pulmonary arterial pressure. Recently, Lucas and associates[18] analyzed a group of patients with large ventricular septal defects and found a wide range of pulmonary arterial pressures; the hemodynamic stress appeared similar in these patients, and the variation in pulmonary vascular reactivity between individuals was considered responsible for the range of pressure produced. The authors' studies corroborate these findings.

Chronic hypoxia tends to accentuate latent differences of pulmonary vascular reactivity among normal individuals. In a recent study at the authors' laboratory, 28 normal high school students, who resided at an altitude of 10,200 feet, had catheterization of the right side of the heart; in about 25 per cent severe pulmonary hypertension developed during exercise[19] (Fig. 48-2) or when the students were breathing 13 per cent oxygen (Fig. 48-3).[19] In contrast to these hyperreactors, another group demonstrated virtually no rise in pulmonary arterial pressure when breathing 13 per cent oxygen and only a modest rise during exercise.

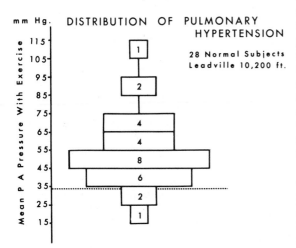

Fig. 48-2. During vigorous supine exercise at sea level, the upper limit reached by the mean pulmonary arterial pressure is less than 35 mm Hg, as indicated by the dotted line (see also Fig. 48-1). However, among normal residents at high altitude, such exercise frequently produces moderate to marked pulmonary hypertension.

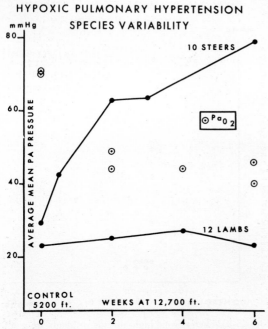

Fig. 48-4. When normal lambs and steers were taken to high altitude, the arterial oxygen tension ($P_{A_{O_2}}$) decreased from 70 to 40 to 45 mm Hg (open circles), indicating that both species were equally hypoxic. However, only the steers developed significant pulmonary hypertension.

Variable degrees of pulmonary vascular reactivity also occur in animals. Recent experiments from the authors' laboratory revealed that cattle develop marked pulmonary hypertension under the hypoxic stress of exposure to an altitude of 12,700 feet;[20] however, lambs exposed to the same altitude retained normal pulmonary arterial pressures[21] (Fig. 48-4). This species difference was also demonstrated when the stimulus for pulmonary hypertension was increased pulmonary blood flow from the time of birth.[9] Thus, as a species, cattle are hyperreactors, and sheep tend to be hyporeactors.

This individual variability relative to pulmonary vascular reactivity is an important feature in understanding the problems of pulmonary hypertension.

Clinical Recognition of Pulmonary Hypertension

The causes of pulmonary hypertension are varied, but the clinical picture in the fully developed state is essentially the same; minor variations are dependent upon the specific cause for the pulmonary hypertension. The purest example is probably *primary (essential) pulmonary hypertension,* frequently designated as *idiopathic pulmonary hypertension.* Its cause is not known, and patients at present in this category will probably ultimately be proved to have disease of polyglot origin. However, the authors believe the cause in many of these patients will eventually be demonstrated to be recurrent miliary embolization to the lung.

The patient with idiopathic pulmonary hypertension is frequently a young woman with symptoms of recent origin who presents the clinical findings of severe pulmonary hypertension. While exertional dyspnea and fatigue are the most common presenting complaints, the initial symptom is not infrequently a syncopal episode. Advanced pulmonary hypertension in a patient with relatively mild symptomatology of recent onset should immediately suggest the diagnosis of primary pulmonary hypertension. Patients with advanced pulmonary hypertension of specified cause will usually report symptoms of greater severity and duration.

Physical examination of the patient with idiopathic pulmonary hypertension reveals either no cyanosis or evidence of peripheral cyanosis. Central cyanosis, although rarely noted, may be due to shunting of blood through a patent foramen ovale; this should suggest a cause of the pulmonary hypertension such as the Eisenmenger reaction. Prominent A waves in the deep jugular veins should also strongly suggest the diagnosis of idiopathic pulmonary hypertension, as this finding usually reflects an intact ventricular septum and right ventricular pressure in excess of left; thus, this is the picture of great hypertrophy of the right ventricle with increased resistance to filling. The precordium is quiet, reflecting a normal or decreased cardiac output. Palpation reveals a forceful, sustained thrust along the left sternal border and thrust and shock in the second left intercostal space. Auscultation usually reveals no murmur of significance, although soft systolic and, at times, diastolic murmurs may be audible in the pulmonary area. A systolic ejection click may be present in the pulmonary area, followed by a single or finely split second heart sound of greatly increased intensity. A fourth heart sound is at times audible along the lower left sternal border and is transmitted toward the apex; this is a reflection of the hypertrophied right atrium, forcefully filling the right ventricle with atrial systole. In the more advanced stage, characterized by dilatation and failure, a murmur of tricuspid insufficiency, a right ventricular gallop, and evidence of fluid retention may be present.

The electrocardiogram reveals right ventricular hypertrophy of varying severity depending upon the stage of the disease process; marked right ventricular hypertrophy is frequently present. Abnormalities reflecting right atrial hypertrophy are common. The radiologic examination reveals a prominent main pulmonary artery and primary pulmonary branches, but the peripheral lung fields usually appear normal or show a slight decrease in vascular markings (Fig. 48-5). There are no findings suggestive of primary pulmonary parenchymal disease. The aorta is not unusual in appearance. The overall heart size may be slightly enlarged with a configuration suggesting slight right atrial and right ventricular hypertrophy; right ventricular hypertrophy is a difficult radiographic diagnosis, and more dependable information about right ventricular hypertrophy is obtainable from the electrocardiogram. Late in the course of the disease, with the development of congestive heart failure, the heart dilates and may greatly increase in size; the main pulmonary artery then actually appears less prominent because of dilatation of the outflow tract of the right ventricle.

The natural history of primary pulmonary hypertension terminates with development of congestive heart failure, which becomes increasingly refractory to therapy. Death is usual within 5 years after onset of symptoms, although the course may terminate abruptly at any time with sudden death.

Recognition of *secondary forms of pulmonary hypertension* is most important, as mitral valve disease or another remediable lesion must always be considered as a cause of the clinical picture. Rheumatic mitral stenosis may present as severe pulmonary hypertension with subtle findings to indicate the presence of mitral valve obstruction. The symptoms are those of low cardiac output, rather than the usual symptoms associated with mitral stenosis, which reflect elevated pulmonary capillary pressure: severe exertional dyspnea, orthopnea, exertional cough, acute paroxysmal pulmonary edema, and hemoptysis. On auscultation, the murmur of mitral stenosis may not readily be detected because of the low cardiac output and the rotation of the heart due to right ventricular hypertrophy. The murmur of mitral stenosis may at times not even be evident after careful evaluation with the possible diagnosis of mitral stenosis in mind. Radiologic examination may reveal only a prominent main pulmonary artery and right-sided enlargement, with little or no evidence of left atrial enlargement. Cardiac catheterization may demonstrate only a high pulmonary artery pressure and low cardiac output, with minimal elevation of pulmonary capillary pressure; in fact, the latter may, on rare occasions, be within normal limits.

Careful radiologic evaluation, including fluoroscopy, may be helpful in suggesting the underlying lesion. An even slightly enlarged left atrium should raise the suspicion of mitral stenosis; the B lines of Kerley, if present, are helpful; and careful search should be made for calcification in the area of the mitral valve, as its presence is tanta-

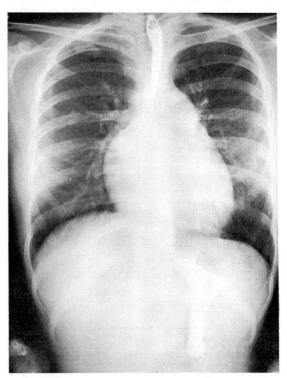

Fig. 48-5. Posteroanterior x-ray of the chest of a patient with primary pulmonary hypertension. There is minimal overall cardiac enlargement, but the silhouette indicates enlargement of the right atrium and configuration compatible with right ventricular hypertrophy. The main pulmonary artery is prominent; the aorta is small and the superior vena cava rather prominent, but the periphery of the lung fields actually appears somewhat clear.

mount to the diagnosis of mitral valve disease until proved otherwise. P waves compatible with left atrial enlargement are a helpful electrocardiographic abnormality suggesting the diagnosis of mitral valve disease. Catheterization of the left side of the heart, however, may be the only method by which mitral stenosis is ruled out and the diagnosis of primary pulmonary hypertension established with reasonable certainty. Admittedly, there is a risk at cardiac catheterization in patients with severe pulmonary hypertension and a relatively low fixed cardiac output; nevertheless, this procedure is justified if performed with care to rule out a possible correctable lesion.

Patients with severe pulmonary hypertension, particularly when central cyanosis is present, should be suspected of having an intracardiac or intervascular shunt. Patients with the Eisenmenger reaction may have a clinical picture indistinguishable from that of primary pulmonary hypertension, although they usually present a history of cardiovascular involvement over many years, if not for life. Cardiac catheterization is again essential in ruling out a small left-to-right shunt or in establishing the presence and level of the right-to-left shunt (Fig. 48-6).

Diseases of the pulmonary parenchyma must also be ruled out by careful evaluation of the clinical picture and radiologic findings. If this evaluation is carefully performed, pulmonary function tests should but rarely have to be resorted to in establishing the presence of parenchymal disease. Pulmonary artery pressure elevation of the order observed in patients with primary pulmonary hypertension is but rarely encountered in pulmonary parenchymal disease; even moderate pulmonary artery pressure elevation appears late in the course of the disease, well after the clinical picture has suggested primary pulmonary parenchymal disease for many years.

Finally, diseases involving the pulmonary vasculature, either primarily or as the result of widespread systemic disease with pulmonary involvement, must be considered in the differential diagnosis of primary pulmonary hypertension. Any patient presenting findings of significant pulmonary hypertension should be carefully evaluated for the presence of a systemic disease process.

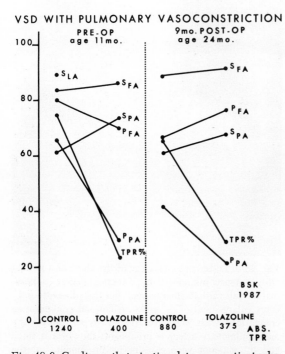

Fig. 48-6. Cardiac catheterization data on a patient who had a large ventricular septal defect. Preoperatively, he had pulmonary hypertension with a mean pulmonary arterial pressure (P_{PA}) approaching the mean femoral arterial pressure (P_{FA}). There was little left-to-right shunt, and the pulmonary blood flow was not increased, since the oxygen saturation in $PA(S_{PA})$ was only 62 per cent. A right-to-left shunt was present, with the systemic arterial saturation (S_{F_A}) of 83 per cent lower than left atrial saturation (S_{L_A}) obtained through a probe-patent foramen ovale. Total pulmonary resistance (TPR per cent) was elevated to 75 per cent of systemic resistance, with an absolute value (ABS·TPR) of 1,240 dynes-sec-cm^{-5}-m^2. Tolazoline hydrochloride selectively reduced the TPR per cent to 23 per cent of systemic resistance, permitting an increase in pulmonary blood flow (S_{PA} 74 per cent), a decrease in right-to-left shunt (S_{F_A} 86 per cent), and a 30 mm Hg decrease in P_{PA}.

Nine months postoperatively, the bidirectional shunts had been eliminated, the pulmonary hypertension was significantly reduced (P_{PA} 42 mm Hg); but the ABS· TPR was still twice normal (880). Tolazoline again reduced the P_{PA} and TPR to normal, indicating some persisting pulmonary vasoconstriction which is potentially reversible.

REFERENCES

1. Reynolds, S. R. M.: Circulatory Adaptation at Birth: Physiologic and Morphologic Correlations, *New York J. Med.*, **56**:1809, 1956.
2. Dawes, G. S.: Vasodilatation in the Unexpended Foetal Lung, in R. F. Grover (ed.), "Progress in Research in Emphysema and Chronic Bronchitis," S. Karger A. G., Basel, 1963, p. 153.
3. Jaykka, S.: Capillary Erection and the Structural Appearance of Fetal and Neonatal Lungs, *Acta paediat.*, **47**:484, 1958.
4. Polgar, G.: The First Breath, *Clin. Pediat.*, **2**:562, 1963.
5. Adams, F. H., and Lind, J.: Physiologic Studies on the Cardiovascular Status of Normal Newborn Infants (with Special Reference to the Ductus Arteriosus), *Pediatrics*, **19**:431, 1957.
6. Assali, N. S., Morris, J. A., Smith, R. W., and Munson, W. A.: Studies on Ductus Arteriosus Circulation, *Circulation Res.*, **13**:478, 1963.
7. Wagenvoort, C. A., Neufeld, N. N., and Edwards, J. E.: The Structure of the Pulmonary Arterial Tree in Fetal and Early Postnatal Life, *Lab. Invest.*, **10**:751, 1961.
8. Pool, P. E., Vogel, J. H. K., and Blount, S. G., Jr.: Congenital Unilateral Absence of a Pulmonary Artery: The Importance of Flow in Pulmonary Hypertension, *Am. J. Cardiol.*, **10**:706, 1962.
9. Vogel, J. H. K., Averill, K. H., Pool, P. E., and Blount, S. G., Jr.: Experimental Pulmonary Arterial Hypertension in the Newborn Calf, *Circulation Res.*, **13**:557, 1963.
10. Reeves, J. T., Grover, R. F., Filley, G. F., and Blount, S. G., Jr.: Cardiac Output of Normal Resting Man, *J. Appl. Physiol.*, **16**:276, 1961.
11. Bevegard, S., Holmgren, A., and Jonsson, B.: The Effect of Body Position on the Circulation at Rest

and during Exercise, with Special Reference to the Influence on the Stroke Volume, *Acta physiol. scandinav.*, 49:279, 1960.

12. Granath, A., Jonsson, B., and Strandell, T.: Circulation in Healthy Old Men, Studied by Right Heart Catheterization at Rest and during Exercise in Supine and Sitting Position, *Acta med. Scandinav.*, 1964 (In press).

13. Brofman, B. L., Charms, B. L., Kohn, P. M., Elder, J., Newman, R., and Rizika, M.: Unilateral Pulmonary Artery Occlusion in Man. I. Control Studies, *J. Thoracic Surg.*, **34**:206, 1957.

14. Charms, B. L., Brofman, B. L., Elder, J. C., and Kohn, P. M.: Unilateral Pulmonary Artery Occlusion in Man. II. Studies in Patients with Chronic Pulmonary Disease, *J. Thoracic Surg.*, **35**:316, 1958.

15. Penaloza, D., Sime, F., Banchero, N., Gamboa, R., Cruz, J., and Marticorena, E.: Pulmonary Hypertension in Healthy Men Born and Living at High Altitudes, *Am. J. Cardiol.*, **11**:150, 1963.

16. Wood, P.: "Diseases of the Heart and Circulation," 2d ed., Eyre & Spottiswoode, Ltd., London, 1957, p. 541.

17. Wood, P.: The Vasoconstrictive Factor in Pulmonary Hypertension, in W. R. Adams and I. Veith (eds.), "Pulmonary Circulation," Grune & Stratton, Inc., New York, 1959, p. 294.

18. Lucas, R. V., Jr., Adams, P., Jr., Anderson, R. C., Meyne, N. G., Lillehei, C. W., and Varco, R. C.: The Natural History of Isolated Ventricular Septal Defect, *Circulation*, **24**:1372, 1961.

19. Vogel, J. H. K., Weaver, W. F., Rose, R. L., Blount, S. G., Jr., and Grover, R. F.: Pulmonary Hypertension on Exertion in Normal Man Living at 10,150 Feet (Leadville, Colorado), in R. F. Grover (ed.), "Progress in Research in Emphysema and Chronic Bronchitis," S. Karger A. G, Basel, 1963, p. 269.

20. Grover, R. F., Reeves, J. T., Will, D. H., and Blount, S. G., Jr.: Pulmonary Vasoconstriction in Steers at High Altitude, *J. Appl. Physiol.*, **18**:567, 1963.

21. Reeves, J. T., Grover, E. B., and Grover, R. F.: Pulmonary Circulation and Oxygen Transport in Lambs at High Altitude, *J. Appl. Physiol.*, **18**:560, 1963.

22. Braunwald, E., Brockenbrough, E. C., Frahm, C. J., and Ross, J., Jr.: Left Atrial and Left Ventricular Pressures in Subjects without Cardiovascular Disease, *Circulation*, **24**:267, 1961.

23. Eliakim, M., Stern, S., and Nathan, H.: Site of Action of Hypertonic Saline in the Pulmonary Circulation, *Circulation Res.*, **9**:327, 1961.

24. Patel, D. J., Mallos, A. J., and DeFreitas, F. M.: Importance of Transmural Pressure and Lung Volume in Evaluating Drug Effect on Pulmonary Vascular Tone, *Circulation Res.*, **9**:1217, 1961.

25. Oakley, C., Glick, G., Luria, M. N., Schreiner, B. F., Jr., and Yu, P. N.: Some Regulatory Mechanisms of the Human Pulmonary Vascular Bed, *Circulation*, **26**:917, 1962.

26. Permutt, S., and Riley, R. L.: Hemodynamics of Collapsible Vessels with Tone: The Vascular Waterfall, *J. Appl. Physiol.*, **18**:924, 1963.

27. Sanger, P. W., Robicsek, F., Taylor, F. H., Magistro, R., and Foti, E.: Observations on Pulmonary Vasomotor Reflexes, *J. Thoracic Surg.*, **37**:774, 1959.

28. Van Bogaret, A., and Tosetti, R.: Experimental Pulmonary Hypertension, *Brit. Heart J.*, **25**:771, 1963.

29. Merrill, J. M., Gobbel, W. G., Jr., and France, R.: The Course of the Total Pulmonary Resistance in Mitral Stenosis Following Mitral Valvulotomy, *Acta med. Scandinav.*, **169**:105, 1961.

30. Hultgren, H. N., Lopez, C. E., Lundberg, E., and Miller, H.: Physiologic Studies of Pulmonary Edema at High Altitude, *Circulation*, **29**:393, 1964.

31. Fred, H. L., Schmidt, A. M., Bates, T., and Hecht, H. H.: Acute Pulmonary Edema of Altitude, Clinical and Physiologic Observations, *Circulation*, **25**: 929, 1962.

32. Kuida, H., Tsagaris, T. J., and Hecht, H. H.: Evidence for Pulmonary Venoconstriction in Brisket Disease, *Circulation Res.*, **12**:182, 1963.

33. Alexander, A. F.: Normal Structure of Bovine Pulmonary Vasculature, *Am. J. Vet. Res.*, **24**:1083, 1963.

34. Downing, S. E., Pursel, S. E., Vidone, R. A., Brandt, H. M., and Liebow, A. A.: Studies on Pulmonary Hypertension with Special Reference to Pressure-Flow Relationships in Chronically Distended and Undistended Lobes, in R. F. Grover (ed.), "Progress in Research in Emphysema and Chronic Bronchitis," S. Karger A. G., Basel, 1963, p. 76.

35. Lategola, M. T., Massion, W., and Schilling, J. A.: The Effect of Bilateral Pulmonary Resection on Total Oxygen Uptake and Total Pulmonary Hemodynamics in the Dog, *J. Thoracic Surg.*, **37**:606, 1959.

36. Berthrong, M., and Cochran, T. H.: Pathological Findings in Nine Children with "Primary" Pulmonary Hypertension, *Bull. Johns Hopkins Hosp.*, **97**: 69, 1955.

37. Berthrong, M.: Discussion, R. F. Grover (ed.), "Progress in Research in Emphysema and Chronic Bronchitis," S. Karger A. G, Basel, 1963, p. 239.

38. Short, D. S.: The Problem of Medial Hypertrophy in Pulmonary Hypertension, in R. F. Grover (ed.), "Progress in Research in Emphysema and Chronic Bronchitis," S. Karger A. G, Basel, 1963, p. 219.

39. Vogel, J. H. K., Grover, R. F., and Blount, S. G., Jr.: Progressive Pulmonary Hypertension in Ventricular Septal Defect, *Clin. Res.*, **11**:100, 1963.

40. Grover, R. F., Reeves, J. T., and Blount, S. G., Jr.: Tolazoline Hydrochloride (Priscoline). An Effective Pulmonary Vasodilator, *Am. Heart J.*, **61**:5, 1961.

41. Nickerson, M.: The Pharmacology of Adrenergic Blockade, *Pharmacol. Rev.*, **1**:27, 1949.

42. Blount, S. G., Jr., and Woodwark, G. M.: Considerations Involved in the Selection for Surgery of

Patients with Ventricular Septal Defects, *Am. J. Cardiol.,* **5**:223, 1960.

43. Williams, M. H.: Alveolar Hypoventilation with Normal Lungs, *Ann. New York Acad. Sc.,* 1964 (In press).

44. Ordonez, J. H., and del Portillo,: Caracteristicas fisiológicas a 2600 metros de altura, *Memorias V congreso de la Asociación latinoamericana de ciencias fisiológicas,* Caracas, 1963 (In press).

45. Arias-Stella, J., and Saldana, M.: The Muscular Pulmonary Arteries in People Native to High Altitude, in R. F. Grover (ed.), "Progress in Research in Emphysema and Chronic Bronchitis," S. Karger A. G, Basel, 1963, p. 292.

46. Shaw, D. B.: Reflux of Blood in the Pulmonary Trunk and Major Pulmonary Arteries during Diastole, *Fed. Proc.,* **22**:454, 1963.

47. Staub, N.: The Interdependence of Pulmonary Structure and Function, *Anesthesiol.* **24**:831, 1963.

48. Sobol, B. J., Bottex, G., Emirgil, C., and Gissen, H.: Gaseous Diffusion from Alveoli to Pulmonary Vessels of Considerable Size, *Circulation Res.,* **13**: 71, 1963.

49. Enson, Y.: Effects of Acidosis on Respiratory Function, *Ann. New York Acad. Sc.,* **121**:674, 1965.

50. Euler, U. S. von, and Liljestrand, G.: Observations on the Pulmonary Arterial Blood Pressure in the Cat, *Acta physiol. scandinav.,* **12**:301, 1946.

51. Liljestrand, G.: Chemical Control of the Distribution of Pulmonary Blood Flow, *Acta physiol. scandinav.,* **44**:216, 1958.

52. Reeves, J. T., Grover, R. F., Blount, S. G., Jr., and Filley, G. F.: Cardiac Output Response to Standing and Treadmill Walking, *J. Appl. Physiol.,* **16**: 283, 1961.

53. Wood, P.: Pulmonary Hypertension, with Special Reference to the Vasoconstrictive Factor, *Brit. Heart J.,* **20**:557, 1958.

Section F: Diseases of the Pericardium

49 PERICARDIAL DISEASE

Noble O. Fowler, M.D.

PATHOLOGIC PHYSIOLOGY

Functions of the Normal Pericardium

It can be readily shown that the pericardium is not essential to life. Removal of both the parietal and visceral pericardium in patients who have chronic constrictive pericarditis or acute inflammatory disease of the pericardium is followed by no recognizable disability. Yet, the pericardium has been found to have certain protective functions. Since the heart dilates more readily without the pericardium, insufficiency of the tricuspid and mitral valves develops more easily when the heart is subjected to increased filling pressure after removal of the pericardium.[1] The pericardium may offer protection against pulmonary edema by limiting right ventricular filling when the left ventricle is dilated.[1] Similarly, the pericardium has been shown to limit cardiac expansion in hypervolemia.[2] The paradoxical pulse which develops in some patients with dilated and failing hearts may be related to restriction of cardiac expansion by the normal pericardium.[3] Decline of intrapericardial pressure during ventricular systole may aid atrial filling. The pericardium is believed to protect the heart from infections of the lungs and pleural space. It has been stated that the lung is protected by the pericardium from the trauma of the beating heart and that the pericardium helps to keep the heart in an optimum functional position. Following removal of the pericardium, roentgen studies of the chest usually reveal that the heart appears somewhat larger than before such an operation. Patients with congenital pericardial deficiency may have a nearly normal life span without disability. However, in two patients with pericardial defects reported by Ellis and associates,[4] there was unexplained chest pain which was conceivably related to increased stress on the anchoring structures of the cardiac base or to cardiopleural adhesions. Partial absence of the parietal pericardium often simulates other varieties of congenital heart disease with pulmonary arterial enlargement.[5] It may be a threat to life if a portion of the heart herniates through the pericardial defect and becomes strangulated.

Pain of Pericarditis

The pain of acute pericarditis is one of the features of major clinical interest. Nearly all patients with recognized acute nonspecific pericarditis have chest pain. In this disorder chest pain is often severe and may resemble that of myocardial infarction. Capps has shown that only the lower portion of the external surface of the parietal pericardium is pain-sensitive,[6] and presumably much of the pain in acute pericarditis is caused by inflammation of the adjoining diaphragmatic pleura. Hence, it is common for the pain of acute pericarditis to be referred to the left supraclavicular area. The characteristic increase of pericardial pain by deep inspiration or by rotating the trunk has been explained by the theory that pain fibers from the pericardium are carried in the left phrenic nerve. More recently it has been shown that the pain of acute pericarditis can be relieved by left stellate ganglion block.[7] This observation casts some doubt upon the earlier theory that the phrenic nerve carries the pain pathways from the pericardium.

Cardiac Tamponade; Paradoxical Pulse

A second major feature of pericardial disease is compression of the heart either by fibrosis or by pericardial fluid. When the heart is thus compressed, it is unable to fill completely. Systemic and pulmonary venous pressures rise, and systemic blood pressure falls. Eventually cardiac output declines, and syncope may occur if these events transpire quickly. When the heart is compressed more gradually over a period of weeks, months, or years, peripheral edema may develop. This sequence of events is called *cardiac tamponade*, or *cardiac compression* if the cardiac restriction results from fibrosis rather than fluid.

Many patients with cardiac tamponade or with cardiac constriction by fibrosis develop an interesting physical finding called the *paradoxical pulse*. The paradoxical pulse is an abnormal inspiratory fall in systemic blood pressure. It is difficult to draw a sharp line between health and disease, because there is normally an inspiratory decline of a few millimeters of mercury in systolic blood pressure. Experimental studies in the author's laboratory suggests that this normal decline is caused by two factors:[8] First, during inspiration there is a transmission of the increased negativity of intrathoracic pressure to the heart and great vessels. Second, inspiration is known to increase filling and output of the right side of the heart. Because of the transit time in the lungs, this increase in the output of the right side of the heart does not increase the output of the left side until nearly the beginning of expiration. When the blood pressure declines more than 8 or 10 mm Hg during normal breathing, the inspiratory decline of systemic blood pressure is considered to be abnormal, and thus a paradoxical pulse is present. It should be pointed out that pericardial disease is not the most common cause of a paradoxical pulse. The most common cause is obstruction to breathing associated with bronchial asthma or pulmonary emphysema. With obstruction to respiration the author has been able to show experimentally that the abnormal inspiratory decline of blood pressure is caused by transmission of the unusually great fluctuations of intrathoracic pressure to the heart and great vessels.[8] There have been a number of theories concerning the paradoxical pulse of pericardial disease. Katz and Gauchat showed in 1924 that with cardiac tamponade intrapericardial pressure did not fall during inspiration.[9] As a result, pulmonary venous pressure should fall more during inspiration than left atrial pressure, thus tending to decrease filling of the left side of the heart during inspiration. Later workers have confirmed this observation, but the interpretation of the data is in dispute. Dock believed that inspiratory traction by the diaphragm and mediastinum upon the taut pericardium further increased intrapericardial pressure, thus interfering with cardiac filling.[10] Dornhorst et al. thought that the normal inspiratory increase in filling of the right side of the heart persisted during cardiac tamponade, thus raising intrapericardial pressure and interfering with left ventricular filling during inspiration.[11] The author has investigated this problem in experimental animals. His studies confirm the postulates of Dornhorst. The author has been able to show that there is indeed a persistence of the normal inspiratory increase of filling of the right side of the heart during cardiac tamponade. If this is prevented, paradoxical pulse does not develop no matter how severe the cardiac tamponade. Furthermore, the paradoxical pulse can be simulated by increasing filling of the right side of the heart in other ways in apneic animals with cardiac tamponade.[12]

ETIOLOGY OF PERICARDITIS

The clinician should remember that few diseases affect the pericardium alone. Hence, the discovery of pericarditis may be the first clue to such systemic illness as uremia, lupus erythematosus, tuberculosis, or previously unsuspected neoplastic disease. The more important causes of pericarditis can be listed in two groups: First are those which are most commonly seen today at the Cincinnati General Hospital, and second are those which are of interest because we have had experience with them only in recent years. There seems to be little question that the most common variety of acute pericarditis is the disease called *acute idiopathic, acute benign, or acute nonspecific pericarditis*. None of these names is free from objection, since the disorder is now known occasionally to be complicated by congestive heart failure or by constrictive pericarditis. Thus the term *benign* is hardly applicable in all instances. In epidemics acute non-specific pericarditis can be shown to be caused by Coxsackie A or B virus, influenza A or B virus, or chickenpox. However, investigation of sporadic cases seldom demonstrates the cause.

At this time it is probably desirable to name two other disorders which affect principally the pericardium and which have clinical features somewhat similar to those of idiopathic benign pericarditis. One of these is the postcardiotomy syndrome, and the other is the post-myocardial-infarction syndrome. Rheumatic pericarditis is not commonly found in adults but is not rare in children. The pericardium may be involved by malignant metastatic tumors, the two most common being carcinoma of the lung in males and carcinoma of the breast in females. Malignant melanoma is known to involve the pericardium fairly frequently, and lymphomas and leukemia affect the pericardium rather commonly. Primary tumors of the pericardium, such as mesothelioma, are quite rare.[14] Uremic pericarditis may occur in the terminal few weeks of life in patients dying of renal failure but may also develop in patients who have reversible tubulorrhexis, or lower nephron nephrosis. Pericarditis may occur in disseminated lupus erythematosus in as many as 48 per cent of instances.[15] Pericarditis may result from specific acute bacterial infections, such as pneumococcal pneumonia or septicemia of varied cause. Rarely, a myocardial abscess complicating bacterial endocarditis may cause pericarditis. Amebic abscesses of the liver may burrow through the diaphragm into the pericardial space. Dissecting aneurysm involving the aortic root may produce a pericardial friction rub and the electrocardiographic changes of acute pericarditis even without frank rupture into the pericardial space.

Traumatic pericarditis as the result of gunshot and stab wounds is familiar to all of us. More recently it has been learned that traumatic pericarditis may result from indirect trauma to the heart without penetration. It has also been learned that pericardial bleeding caused by either direct or indirect trauma may be followed by constrictive pericarditis.[16] At the Cincinnati General Hospital there was a recent example of this in a twenty-year-old man who was stabbed in the heart. A few weeks after discharge from the hospital he was admitted again with acute pericarditis, which was followed within a matter of 6 weeks by the syndrome of cardiac compression. At thoracotomy he was found to have striking pericardial thickening. Rheumatoid arthritis has been recently emphasized as a cause of pericarditis in adults, although it has been recognized as a cause of pericarditis in children for over 60 years. The author has observed three pa-tients with pericarditis associated with rheumatoid arthritis. In one instance, constrictive pericarditis developed, and pericardial resection was necessary.[17] X-irradiation of the mediastinum may be associated with pericarditis which on occasion may lead to cardiac constriction.[18] Of note is the latent period following radiation therapy, which may be as much as 4 to 6 weeks. Radiation pneumonitis may or may not occur. Histoplasmosis may affect the pericardium.[19] Recently several instances of acute pericarditis with effusion and with rising complement fixation titers for histoplasmosis have been observed at the Cincinnati General Hospital. Actinomycosis may affect the pericardium and may closely simulate tuberculous pericarditis.[13] Cultures of the fluid and biopsy of the pericardium or lung are needed to make the distinction. Rarely drugs, such as hydralazine hydrochloride, which can produce a lupus-like syndrome, and psicofuranine, may be associated with pericarditis.

ACUTE PERICARDITIS

History

If the patient with acute pericarditis has a complaint related specifically to the pericarditis, it is usually that of chest pain. Not infrequently, patients with acute pericarditis come to the physician complaining of other manifestations of the systemic illness which causes the pericarditis, such as fever, joint disease, skin disease, fatigue, or the symptoms of uremia. The chest pain of acute pericarditis is often quite characteristic and at other times not. The pain may be of very sudden onset. It may begin over the sternum and radiate to the neck and down the left upper extremity, and mimic very closely the pain of acute myocardial infarction.[20] This syndrome seems to be more common in patients with acute nonspecific pericarditis than in those with other forms of pericarditis. Especially when it occurs in a middle-aged or older man, an erroneous diagnosis of myocardial infarction may be made. The two disorders can often be distinguished by a careful history. In acute pericarditis the pain is usually increased by deep breathing or by rotating the thorax and may be somewhat relieved when the patient sits up and leans forward. In acute myocardial infarction the pain is usually not increased by breathing or by rotation of the thorax. Pain may occur in acute pericarditis caused by tuberculosis or rheumatic fever but is usually less severe. Uremic pericarditis is often found to be associated with pain if specific inquiry is made. Pain usually accompanies pericarditis of the postcardiotomy syndrome and the post-myocardial-infarction syndrome.

Physical Examination

Pericardial Friction Rub

The characteristic pathognomonic finding of pericarditis is the pericardial friction rub, although it is not always present. The pericardial friction rub should be searched for with the patient in various positions including sitting upright, leaning forward with the breath expelled, and on his hands and knees in bed. A pericardial rub occurs as the heart moves. The heart moves with atrial systole, ventricular systole, and ventricular diastole. Accordingly there may be three components to the pericardial rub, one during each of these phases of the cardiac cycle. Each component is a short, scratchy sound. When three components are heard, it is quite diagnostic of pericardial rub. There may be only two components to the rub, one during ventricular systole and one during ventricular diastole. In such a case the to-and-fro sound usually indicates a pericardial friction rub. A pericardial friction rub may be heard only in systole. Under such circumstances it is difficult to be certain that one is not dealing with a murmur or an extracardiac sound. The question can usually be settled by frequent obseration, since a pericardial friction rub will become a to-and-fro sound or disappear within a few days. A pleuropericardial rub is usually louder at the cardiac apex and is often associated with a left pleural friction rub and markedly affected by breathing. Contrary to common belief, a pericardial friction rub may be heard when there is considerable pericardial effusion.

Pericardial Effusion

The other features characteristic of acute pericarditis are the signs of pericardial effusion, which may or may not be found. The circulatory effects of acute pericardial effusion depend upon its rate of accumulation. If pericardial fluid accumulates very suddenly, a few hundred milliliters can cause cardiac compression and cardiac tamponade, with elevation of the venous pressure, decrease of systemic blood pressure, and perhaps syncope or sudden death. On the other hand, a more gradual accumulation of pericardial fluid often fails to produce these symptoms and signs even when the pericardial space contains a liter or more of fluid. In patients with suspected pericardial effusion, it is important to locate the cardiac apex impulse. If the apex impulse is in normal position in the fifth left intercostal space at or inside the midclavicular line and there is percussion dullness beyond this point, pericardial effusion can be suspected. This sign is difficult to evaluate when there is left pleural effusion.

When there is rapid accumulation of pericardial fluid and rising venous pressure, a paradoxical pulse may be found. When this finding is pronounced, the radial pulse will become attenuated or disappear during inspiration. When this sign is less pronounced, it is important to search for it with a blood pressure cuff and a stethoscope when acute or chronic pericarditis is suspected. The patient should breathe normally. The examiner should observe the level of systolic blood pressure at which arterial sounds are heard in expiration only, and then the pressure at which the sounds are heard throughout the cardiac cycle. The difference between the two indicates the magnitude of the paradoxical pulse. A value exceeding 8 to 10 mm Hg in a patient who has normal nonobstructed breathing is strongly suggestive of cardiac compression. However, an occasional patient with congestive heart failure, especially when caused by chronic myocardial disease and myocardial fibrosis, may demonstrate pulsus paradoxus.[21]

When the venous pressure is elevated in pericarditis, the cervical veins may become more distended during inspiration, which is the reverse of the normal situation. This finding is called Kussmaul's sign. This sign is not invariably present and is not diagnostic of acute pericarditis. It may be found in vena caval obstruction and in some patients with congestive heart failure caused by myocardial or valvular disease.

Other Physical Findings

Some patients who have acute pericarditis with effusion may demonstrate Ewart's sign, an area of percussion dullness and bronchial breathing beneath the angle of the left scapula. This sign has not been helpful in the author's experience. It is also found in patients with dilatation of the heart. It is frequently absent in patients with pericardial effusion. An occasional patient with pericardial effusion may demonstrate an early diastolic sound, or pericardial knock sound, between 0.06 and 0.12 sec after the onset of the second heart sound. This sound may be difficult to distinguish from an early ventricular gallop rhythm at the cardiac apex. Other findings in these patients are usually those of the underlying illness. Fever is common, as is tachycardia. Cardiac murmurs are usually difficult to evaluate when there is a pericardial friction rub.

Laboratory Tests

Electrocardiography

The characteristic electrocardiogram of acute pericarditis is not found in all instances. Typically in the first few days after the onset of chest pain there is elevation of the S-T segments in two or three of the limb leads without reciprocal depres-

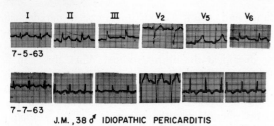

7-5-63

7-7-63

J.M., 38 ♂ IDIOPATHIC PERICARDITIS

Fig. 49-1. Serial electrocardiographic changes in a thirty-eight-year-old man with acute nonspecific pericarditis. The record of July 5, 1963, demonstrates S-T segment elevation without reciprocal depression. Two days later the elevated S-T segments have returned to the isoelectric line, and the T waves are negative. There are no pathologic Q waves.

sion (Fig. 49-1). The precordial leads often show elevated S-T segments in most leads. Depressed S-T segments are found as a rule only in lead V_1 and in lead AVR. There are rare exceptions to this statement. After a few days or a week, the S-T segments tend to return to the base line, and then the T waves become negative as the disorder enters its subacute phase (Fig. 49-1). There may be some diminution of QRS voltage. It is important that the electrocardiogram be distinguished from that of acute myocardial infarction (Fig. 49-2). The most distinctive feature is the development of pathologic Q waves in myocardial infarction; these do not appear in patients with acute pericarditis. In the first few days of the attack, the absence of reciprocal S-T segment depression in the limb leads is usually a reliable indication of pericarditis. Characteristically, the T waves become negative in acute pericarditis only after the S-T segments return to the isoelectric line. In acute myocardial infarction the T waves often become negative while the S-T segments are still elevated. This differential feature is less reliable.

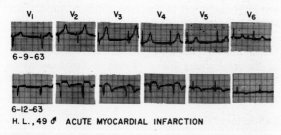

6-9-63

6-12-63

H.L., 49 ♂ ACUTE MYOCARDIAL INFARCTION

Fig. 49-2. Serial electrocardiographic changes in a forty-nine-year-old man with acute myocardial infarction. The record of June 9, 1963, the first day of chest pain, demonstrates S-T segment elevation and tall T waves. Three days later, there are pathologic Q waves; the T waves are now negative, while the S-T segments are still elevated.

Radiologic Studies

In many patients with acute pericarditis routine chest x-ray and cardiac fluoroscopy studies are normal. A few hundred milliliters of pericardial effusion does not necessarily produce a detectable radiologic change. The study of cardiac pulsations by routine fluoroscopy is an unreliable way of detecting pericardial effusion. When there are several hundred milliliters of fluid in the pericardial space, then the cardiac silhouette will be increased in size. Characteristically, the lungs are less congested than in patients with congestive heart failure, and this may be a valuable sign, since at times the clinical features of cardiac dilatation may resemble those of pericardial effusion. Patients who have acute benign pericarditis often show additional pleural effusion and small areas of pneumonitis. There are similar radiologic findings in patients with postcardiotomy or post-myocardial-infarction syndrome.

Image-intensifier cardiac fluoroscopy may be useful in detecting pericardial effusion if the epicardial fat line can be shown as an area of decreased density inside the pericardial fluid. Radiologic demonstration of pericardial fluid or thickening is more reliable, however, if contrast media are employed.

Cardiac scanning, following the injection of radioactive iodinated serum albumin, is free of hazard and discomfort to the patient (Fig. 49-3).[22] This method is less sensitive than the use of iodine containing contrast medium or carbon dioxide. Durant has shown that the injection of 50 to 100 ml carbon dioxide into the antecubital vein of a patient lying on his left side will often demonstrate pericardial thickening or effusion (Fig. 49-4).[23] Errors may

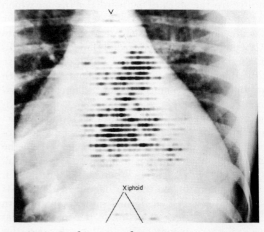

Xiphoid

Fig. 49-3. Cardiac scan demonstrating extensive pericardial effusion. The black dots indicate the blood within the heart chambers and great vessels; the white radiopaque area indicates the extent of the pericardial effusion.

result if there is right pleural effusion or disease of the adjacent right middle lobe.

Angiocardiography, carried out with the patient in the sitting posture, is usually an effective way of detecting pericardial thickening or fluid accumulation in the pericardial space. The distance from the lateral right border of the contrast to the lateral border of the cardiopericardial silhouette should not exceed 3 to 5 mm. It must be remembered that this space includes the right atrial wall, pleura, and visceral and parietal pericardium, as well as any fluid or fibrosis.

Other Tests

The white blood cell count is often increased in acute benign pericarditis but may be within normal limits. The serum glutamic oxalacetic transaminase may be slightly increased.

Differential Diagnosis

In the patient with acute and severe chest pain, the differential diagnosis from acute myocardial infarction, pleurisy, spontaneous pneumothorax, or mediastinal emphysema must be made. Characteristically the pain of acute pericarditis is increased by deep breathing or by rotating the thorax, whereas that of acute myocardial infarction is not. If one hears a pericardial friction rub in a patient within 24 hr of the onset of chest pain, acute pericarditis is more likely than acute myocardial infarction. Characteristic electrocardiographic changes are usually sufficient to make the distinction. The serum glutamic oxalacetic transaminase is nearly always increased in acute myocardial infarction. It is increased in some patients with acute pericarditis. Therefore, a normal transaminase value is more consistent with pericarditis than with acute myocardial infarction. It is of utmost importance that acute pericarditis not be mistaken for acute myocardial infarction. The use of anticoagulants in patients with acute pericarditis may be extremely hazardous. The author has observed three instances of severe pericardial bleeding in patients with nonspecific pericarditis who received anticoagulants. Two patients died, and one required surgical relief of cardiac tamponade.

In acute pleurisy there is only a pleural friction rub, and the characteristic electrocardiographic features of acute pericarditis are missing. Since the two disorders may coexist, roentgen demonstration of fluid in the pericardial space may be necessary for the distinction. In spontaneous pneumothorax, sudden onset of chest pain and dyspnea often occur. Percussion hyperresonance and decreased or absent breath sounds confirm the diagnosis, but these signs are absent when the air collection is small, and chest roentgenograms are

required. Occasional patients with left pneumothorax demonstrate a crunching or bubbling to-and-fro sound over the precordium.[24] A similar sound may be heard in acute spontaneous mediastinal emphysema, which also must be considered in the differential diagnosis of chest pain.[25] Crepitus in the soft tissues of the lower anterior neck and roentgen demonstration of mediastinal air will establish the diagnosis.

Etiologic Diagnosis

Acute Idiopathic Pericarditis. Most of the features of the most common variety of acute pericarditis, acute idiopathic, acute benign, or acute nonspecific pericarditis, have already been discussed. There is an antecedent upper respiratory infection a few weeks before the illness in approximately 28 per cent of patients.[26] Changes in viral antibody titers in acute and convalescent serum may on occasion give support to the possibility of a viral cause. Rarely, pain is absent. Often pericardial effusion is not recognizable but in some instances is great enough to be detectable radiologically and may produce cardiac tamponade. The pericardial fluid is at times bloody. Radiologic examination of the chest often demonstrates associated pleural effusion and transient areas of pulmonary infiltration.[27] The patient is usually febrile. The fever is often greatest on the first day of illness and may last for a few days to as much as 3 to 6 weeks. There are recurrences in about 23 per cent

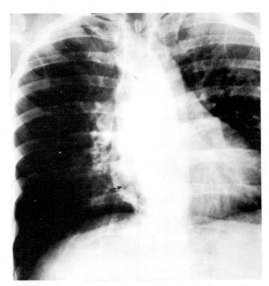

Fig. 49-4. Demonstration of pericardial effusion by injection of carbon dioxide into a peripheral vein. The patient is lying on the left side. The arrow tip indicates carbon dioxide within the right atrium, and the increased pericardial thickness may be seen just above the head of the arrow.

of patients.[26] The differential diagnosis from tuberculous pericarditis presents a significant problem.

Tuberculous Pericarditis. Although patients with tuberculous pericarditis may have underlying miliary tuberculosis or radiologically detectable areas of pulmonary involvement, in the majority of instances in adults the disorder is clinically primary and originates from tuberculosis of the mediastinal nodes. Thus, the clinical evidence of tuberculosis is not readily discernible. Very large amounts of pericardial effusion, a history of previous tuberculosis, a history of weight loss, or fever which persists beyond 3 weeks usually suggest that the possibility of tuberculosis should be thoroughly investigated. If both first- and second-strength PPD skin tests are negative, tuberculosis is unlikely. Aspiration of pericardial fluid, followed by guinea pig inoculation and culture, will reveal tubercle bacilli in about 50 per cent of patients who have tuberculous pericarditis with effusion. Unfortunately the 6-week waiting period for the results of this test is unacceptable to most physicians. The author's policy has been, if the patient continues to be quite ill, with a fever after 3 weeks, to perform a pericardial biopsy at thoracotomy after 1 or 2 weeks' preliminary treatment with isoniazid and paraamino salicylic acid or streptomycin. If the pericarditis is caused by tuberculosis, tubercle bacilli are still demonstrable histologically after this amount of treatment. If the biopsy specimen shows changes indicative of some other disorder, such as rheumatoid nodules, metastatic neoplasm, or fungus disease, then the therapy would be altered accordingly. If the specimen shows caseation necrosis and no acid-fast or other organisms, the antituberculosis therapy should be continued. Difficulty arises if the specimen shows only nonspecific changes of inflammation. In this event, one's decision will have to rest upon judgment based upon clinical evaluation of the entire picture. If tuberculosis still seems a reasonable possibility, then the therapy should be continued.

Other Varieties of Pericarditis. A syndrome like that of acute nonspecific pericarditis, which begins within a period of 10 days to 2 or 3 months following cardiac surgical treatment, direct or indirect cardiac trauma, or myocardial infarction, is very likely related to the antecedent event. At the University of Cincinnati Hospitals, a postcardiotomy syndrome was found in 13.7 per cent of patients subjected to mitral valvotomy.[28] This complication is apparently even more common in some hospitals. When a patient has had an acute myocardial infarction, a recurrence of chest pain within 10 days to a few months may indicate the post-myocardial-infarction syndrome rather than a fresh myocardial infarction.[29] Increase of the pain by breathing, radiologic demonstration of pulmonary infiltration, and electrocardiographic changes of pericarditis rather than myocardial infarction should make the diagnosis clear. This has been a rare complication in the experience of the author, who has seen only two instances. In both post-myocardial-infarction syndrome and postcardiotomy syndrome, recurrent attacks over a period of several years may take place.

Patients who have acute pericarditis caused by rheumatic fever almost always have underlying endocarditis and myocarditis. The absence of cardiac murmurs is strong evidence against rheumatic fever as the cause of acute pericarditis. Patients who have pericarditis associated with lupus erythematosus almost invariably have other manifestations of the illness, such as anemia, leukopenia, thrombocytopenia, skin rash, fever, arthritis, and nephritis. A positive test for lupus erythematosus cells will clarify the diagnosis. In patients with uremic pericarditis, renal failure is usually obvious. Uremic pericarditis is usually fibrinous but occasionally produces a few hundred milliliters of pericardial effusion and even less commonly causes a massive bloody effusion. It is important to know of a history of previous x-irradiation of the mediastinum in order that postradiation pericarditis not be overlooked. Rheumatoid arthritis is readily apparent from the physical examination. One should not forget to inquire into the history of drug ingestion, particularly hydralazine hydrochloride. In patients with persistent pericarditis of obscure cause one should not neglect the possibility of fungus disease, especially histoplasmosis and actinomycosis. It may be necessary to culture a pericardial biopsy specimen to arrive at a satisfactory diagnosis.

Aspiration of the pericardial effusion may be helpful in diagnosis when the causative organism can be identified in the fluid either directly or on culture, or by animal inoculation. The quality of the fluid is usually not too helpful, except when there is an acute pyogenic pericarditis, which may complicate septicemia or result from left empyema, trauma, or mediastinitis. Sanguineous pericardial effusion may be found in a variety of disorders. It may be found in tuberculosis, carcinoma, lupus erythematosus, idiopathic benign pericarditis, rheumatoid arthritis, and even occasionally in rheumatic fever. A grossly bloody pericardial effusion, however, is very suggestive either of neoplastic invasion or of tuberculosis. In the author's experience, a slow leak from aneurysm of the aortic root over a period of several days may also produce grossly bloody pericardial effusion. At times occult bronchogenic carcinoma may produce massive hemorrhagic pericarditis. The primary lesion may be too minute to be detected radiologically. Identification of tumor cells in pericardial fluid may confirm a neoplastic cause; however, expert cytologic examination is necessary to differentiate these cells from normal mesothelial cells. It should be pointed out that even experts may disagree in the interpretation of cells found in the pericardial fluid. Myxedema may induce pericardial effusion (see Chap. 61). Chylopericardium due to anomalous lymphatic drainage into the pericardium may occur. Cholesterol pericarditis with deposits of cholesterol may occur.

Treatment

The treatment of acute pericarditis consists of relief of symptoms and the treatment of the underlying systemic illness. In idiopathic benign pericarditis, reassurance, bed rest as long as fever and pain persist, and aspirin for relief of pain are usually all that is required. Although adrenal steroids have been shown to relieve the discomfort of this disorder,[26] the possibility of tuberculous pericarditis can seldom be dismissed. Thus one feels hesitant to use these drugs in an illness which usually follows a benign course. When the diagnosis is clearly nontuberculous and pain is unrelieved by salicylates, the administration of corticosteroids may produce dramatic results. The treatment of rheumatic pericarditis is that of the underlying rheumatic fever and usually requires a period of bed rest. Therapeutic doses of penicillin for 10 days to 2 weeks and prophylactic penicillin thereafter are recommended. Since there are underlying myocarditis and endocarditis, the use of adrenal steroids for 6 to 12 weeks should be strongly considered.

Tuberculous pericarditis should be treated by bed rest as long as the patient is febrile. Isoniazid, 300 mg a day orally, and paraaminosalicylic acid, 10 to 12 Gm daily, are administered. This therapy is continued for 1 to 2 years. If the patient cannot tolerate paraaminosalicylic acid, streptomycin, 1 Gm a day intramuscularly, is used in its stead. Streptomycin is continued in this dosage until the patient becomes afebrile and for at least 3 months. The streptomycin dosage is then reduced to 1 Gm twice weekly and continued for 1 year. The isoniazid is continued for 2 years. The patient should be closely observed for the development of constrictive pericarditis.

Patients who have acute cardiac tamponade following direct trauma to the heart from stab or gunshot wounds must be treated as emergencies. A rise in intrapericardial pressure interferes with cardiac filling, and cardiac output rapidly becomes inadequate to sustain life. Intravenous infusion of blood or other fluid may temporarily improve blood pressure until cardiac tamponade can be relieved.

It is the policy at the Cincinnati General Hospital to treat the patient by one or two needle aspirations of the pericardial space. If the symptoms of cardiac tamponade are not relieved by needle aspiration or return after a second aspiration, then thoracotomy is required in order to suture the lacerated myocardium or blood vessel.

The treatment of uremic pericarditis is usually hopeless unless the patient has reversible renal disease. In such patients the use of hemodialysis may lead to eventual recovery.

When specific infectious pericarditis related to disease of the left pleural space or to septicemia is treated by the appropriate antibiotics, surgical drainage may or may not be necessary. If response is poor, however, surgical therapy must not be delayed.

Pericarditis in lupus erythematosus usually responds to adrenal steroid therapy, although occasionally cardiac tamponade develops and pericardial aspiration is required.

Postthoracotomy and post-myocardial-infarction syndromes should be managed in the same way as acute benign pericarditis. In all three disorders recurrences are common. In the event of numerous recurrences surgical resection of the pericardium may be considered.

Pericardial effusion due to certain types of neoplastic disease may be treated by instillation of nitrogen mustard into the pericardial space; however, surgical resection of the pericardium may be needed.

Pericardial effusion due to myxedema rarely produces cardiac tamponade and responds to thyroid medication.

Needle Aspiration of the Pericardial Space

Needle aspiration of the pericardial space may be performed in patients with acute pericarditis for one of two major purposes: one is to confirm the diagnosis and to attempt to establish the underlying cause; a second is to relieve acute cardiac tamponade. Needle aspiration of the pericardial space is a major procedure. Laceration of a coronary artery or of the myocardium may cause death from cardiac tamponade. Either ventricular fibrillation or vagovagal arrest is another complication. Needle aspiration of the pericardium is performed with the patient in the sitting posture. The needle is inserted preferably in one of two places:[30] One may employ the subxiphoid approach with the needle inserted in the angle between the left costal margin and the xiphoid and directed toward the right shoulder. A second choice is near the cardiac apex about 2 cm inside the left border of cardiac dullness with the needle directed toward the fourth vertebra. The needle should have a short bevel in order to minimize the danger of laceration. One may use the electrocardiogram to recognize that the aspirating needle is touching the myocardium. The precordial lead wire of the electrocardiograph is attached to the aspirating needle by alligator clips and wire as described by Bishop, Estes, and McIntosh.[31] Elevation of the S-T segment or P-Q segment indicates that the needle tip has reached the myocardium, producing a localized current of injury. If the needle is then withdrawn a few millimeters, the danger of myocardial laceration is minimized. If a grossly bloody fluid is obtained, its hematocrit should be compared with the patient's blood hematocrit to be certain that the needle is not in the cardiac chambers. Failure of the bloody fluid to clot offers further assurance that bloody fluid is not obtained from within the heart. The author has seen fatality result from injection of air into a cardiac chamber when injection into the pericardial space was intended. The injection of air into the pericardial space may demonstrate the size of the heart, the thickness of the parietal pericardium, and the amount of pericardial effusion. Patients with benign pericarditis more commonly have a thin pericardium, but it may become thickened. Patients with tuberculous or neoplastic pericarditis more commonly have a thickened pericardium. In many hospitals it is the practice to have aspiration of the pericardium performed by a thoracic surgeon, in order that he may be available to deal with any emergency which may arise. During the procedure the electrocardiogram should be monitored, as well as blood pressure and venous pressure. A cardiac defibrillator and apparatus for artificial respiration should be at hand. Immediate decline of venous pressure and rise of systemic blood pressure following pericardial aspiration offer convincing proof of cardiac tamponade. If repeated aspirations are needed for the relief of cardiac tamponade, prompt surgical resection of the pericardium is indicated.

CHRONIC PERICARDITIS

The principal symptomatic variety of chronic pericarditis is chronic constrictive pericarditis. Many patients with chronic pericarditis are asymptomatic. Some have chonic pericardial effusion of unknown cause. If the fluid accumulates slowly, unsuspected enlargement of the cardiac silhouette may be discovered on routine radiologic examination of the chest. In such patients, tuberculosis, neoplastic disease, or scleroderma, in addition to asymptomatic idiopathic pericarditis, should be considered in the differential diagnosis.

In many instances, the cause of chronic and asymptomatic pericardial effusion cannot be estab-

lished. The physician should remember that myxedema may produce considerable pericardial effusion. In other patients with chronic pericarditis radiologic examination reveals calcification of the pericardium. Such patients are often asymptomatic and without significant cardiac constriction. Other patients are discovered to have pericardial adhesions or thickening at autopsy after death from an unrelated illness. External adhesions which bind the pericardium to the chest wall are no longer believed to cause cardiac enlargement or embarrassment of cardiac function.

Our discussion of chronic pericarditis will deal principally with cardiac constriction. In such patients the complaints are usually similar to those of congestive heart failure except that they begin very gradually. There is a tendency to develop ascites relatively early. Exertional dyspnea is a common complaint but may be inconspicuous in the presence of edema and ascites. Orthopnea and nocturnal dyspnea are unusual in contrast to the ordinary forms of congestive heart failure. Chest pain is absent as a rule. There are, however, patients who pursue a course intermediate between acute pericarditis and chronic constrictive pericarditis. Such patients develop a rather acute pericarditis caused by tuberculosis, rheumatoid arthritis, acute idiopathic pericarditis, or trauma, for example, and then progress to cardiac constriction in a matter of a few weeks or months. In recent years, this form of constrictive pericarditis has been more common at the University of Cincinnati Hospitals than the classic variety of chronic constrictive pericarditis which develops slowly over several or many years. Chronic constrictive pericarditis is a rare disease, and in most major hospitals only a few instances are seen in a year.[32] At the Mayo Clinic, 79 instances were observed during a 10-year period.[26]

Cause of Chronic Constrictive Pericarditis

The cause of chronic constrictive pericarditis remains in doubt in many patients. It can be shown by histologic examination of the removed pericardium that approximately 17 per cent of instances are caused by tuberculosis.[32] It has been learned in recent years that idiopathic pericarditis can be followed by constrictive pericarditis,[26] and two instances of this have been observed at the University of Cincinnati Hospitals. Cardiac trauma followed by bleeding into the pericardial space may be followed by constrictive pericarditis.[16] At the Cincinnati General Hospital one instance of constrictive pericarditis following tularemic pericarditis was observed. Constrictive pericarditis may follow irradiation pneumonitis and pericarditis;[18] it may follow rheumatoid arthritis[17] and may be associated with neoplastic invasion of the pericardium.[33] Histoplasmosis may be followed by constrictive pericarditis.[34] Rheumatic fever may be followed by adhesive pericarditis and pericardial calcification but seldom, if ever, by constrictive pericarditis.

Physical Examination

The physical examination of a patient with constrictive pericarditis reveals the signs of cardiac compression which were described earlier in this chapter. However, the arterial pulse pressure is often normal. An important and almost invariable sign is elevation of the venous pressure as best judged by distension of the neck veins with the patient at a 45° angle from the horizontal. The cervical venous pulse characteristically shows a deep Y trough. Kussmaul's sign may be present, namely, inspiratory swelling of the neck veins. This sign is not diagnostic of constrictive pericarditis. A paradoxical pulse is found in a minority of patients.[35] The method of examination for this sign was discussed earlier in this chapter. The heart sounds are often distant but not invariably so. The pericardial knock sound may be heard at the cardiac apex.[36] This sound follows the second heart sound by 0.06 to 0.12 sec. It sounds much like a gallop at the cardiac apex but occurs somewhat earlier in diastole. Cardiac murmurs are usually absent. The heart size is usually normal or moderately enlarged. The apex impulse is felt with difficulty. Pulmonary rales are uncommon. The liver is usually enlarged and may be firmer than normal. Cardiac cirrhosis is a common complication. Ascites is a common finding. Some dependent edema may be present but is often absent. There is usually no pericardial friction rub, but one may be heard on rare occasions. Rarely the nephrotic syndrome may occur.

Laboratory Data

Electrocardiogram of Constrictive Pericarditis

The electrocardiogram is often abnormal but is usually not diagnostic. Characteristic changes are low voltage of the QRS complexes, especially in the limb leads (Fig. 49-5). Atrial fibrillation is present in one-fourth to one-third of these patients. Atrial flutter is found in a few patients. Some patients have an electrocardiographic pattern which resembles right ventricular hypertrophy.

Radiologic Studies

Radiologic studies characteristically demonstrate clear lung fields. The heart may be small but occasionally is seen to be slightly enlarged on radiologic

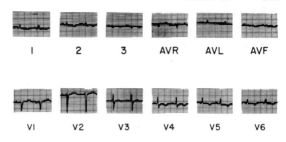

T.D. CONSTRICTIVE PERICARDITIS

Fig. 49-5. Electrocardiogram of a patient with chronic constrictive pericarditis. Note the low voltage of QRS complexes and negative T waves.

study. In more acute cardiac constriction, the cardiac silhouette may be quite large because of a combination of pericardial thickening and pericardial fluid.[37] Calcification of the pericardium is found in 40 to 50 per cent of instances but is not diagnostic of constrictive pericarditis. Calcification of the pericardium may occur in patients who have adhesive pericarditis without cardiac constriction as a result of rheumatic fever and other illnesses. Strangely enough, cardiac fluoroscopy may reveal fairly normal cardiac pulsations in patients with constrictive pericarditis and is not invariably reliable in this respect. Angiocardiography is of much greater value and will demonstrate thickening of the pericardium beyond the normal limit of 3 to 5 mm in patients with constrictive pericarditis.

Cardiac Catheterization

Cardiac catheterization studies are of interest in patients with constrictive pericarditis, but the abnormalities are not specific for the disorder. Characteristic findings at cardiac catheterization are elevation of the mean right atrial pressure, an M pattern of the right atrial pressure pulse, and an early diastolic dip in both right and left ventricles with an elevated end-diastolic pressure in both ventricles (Fig. 49-6). Burwell and Robin have pointed out that the characteristic finding is a pressure plateau in which the pulmonary wedge pressure, pulmonary artery diastolic pressure, right ventricular end-diastolic pressure, mean right atrial pressure, and superior vena cava pressure all tend to be identical in constrictive pericarditis.[38] However, three of six patients with myocardial fibrosis showed the same variety of pressure plateau.[39] Thus, patients with infiltrative disease of the myocardium, including amyloidosis, subendocardial fibroelastosis, and myocardial fibrosis may demonstrate a pressure pattern similar to that of constrictive pericarditis. Patients with biventricular heart failure also have elevated ventricular dias-

CARDIAC PRESSURES IN MYOCARDIAL AND PERICARDIAL DISEASE

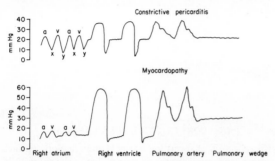

Fig. 49-6. Diagram of pressures of the right side of the heart in constrictive pericarditis as contrasted with those of myocardial disease with heart failure. Note the "M pattern" in the right atrial pressure pulse and the early diastolic dip in the right ventricular pressure pulse of constrictive pericarditis. The systolic right ventricular and pulmonary arterial pressures are lower in constrictive pericarditis than in myocardopathy. In myocardopathy, the wedge pressure exceeds the mean right atrial pressure; the two pressures are approximately equal in constrictive pericarditis.

tolic pressures, but as a rule the pulmonary wedge pressure exceeds the right atrial pressure by more than 10 mm Hg.[40] In patients with constrictive pericarditis, the pressures tend to be the same or the pulmonary wedge pressure no more than 6 mm higher than the right atrial mean pressure. The hemodynamics of pericardial disease are contrasted with those of myocardial disease in Figs. 49-6 and 49-7.

Differential Diagnosis

The diagnosis of constrictive pericarditis should be strongly considered in every patient who has exertional dyspnea with or without edema, when there is persistent elevation of venous pressure after treatment for heart failure, and when there is no readily apparent variety of heart disease. The demonstration of a paradoxical pulse, clear lung fields on fluoroscopy, and a normal or moderately enlarged heart makes the diagnosis virtually certain. As already pointed out, certain patients with myocardial diseases, especially those with myocardial fibrosis and amyloidosis, may present similar findings, although the heart is usually larger. If the venous pressure remains elevated after maximum treatment, the use of angiocardiography to determine the thickness of the pericardium may be of critical value in making a decision as to the diagnosis. The differential diagnosis of myocardial and pericardial disease has been well presented by Burch and Phillips.[41] In an occasional patient the distinction cannot be made, and it is necessary to resort to surgical exploration of the pericardium.

Treatment

The treatment of constrictive pericarditis is pericardial resection if the patient has progressive dyspnea or fatigue. If the patient is believed to have tuberculous pericarditis, the surgical resection should be preceded by several weeks of antituberculous therapy. Although the mortality rate for surgical resection was formerly stated to be 25 per cent, it would appear that in recent years the

HEMODYNAMICS OF MYOCARDIAL AND PERICARDIAL DISEASE

		Constrictive Pericarditis	Myocardopathy
1.	Left Atrial Pressure	Tends to equal RAP	10 to 20 m Hg $>$ RAP
2.	Right Atrial Pressure	Usually $>$ 15 mm Hg with prominent Y trough	Usually $<$ 15 mm Hg: normal if wedge pressure normal
3.	Cardiac Output	Tends to normal with normal A-V difference	Usually low with increased A-V difference
4.	Right Ventricular Pressure	Consistent early diastolic dip	Early diastolic dip may disappear with therapy
5.	Diastolic Right Ventricular Pressure	Tends to equal or exceed 1/3 of systolic pressure	Usually does not equal 1/3 of systolic pressure
6.	Pulmonary Artery Pressure	Systolic pressure usually $<$ 40 mm Hg	Systolic pressure often 45 to 65 mm Hg
7.	Respiratory Variation in Pressures	Tends to be absent	Usually present
8.	Diastolic Pressure Plateau	RAP=RVDP=PADP=PWP	PWP $>$ RAP

Fig. 49-7. RAP = right atrial pressure; A-V = arteriovenous; RVDP = right ventricular diastolic pressure; PADP = pulmonary arterial diastolic pressure; PWP = pulmonary wedge pressure.

figure has been less than this. In Wood's series, the operative mortality was 11 per cent.[35]

REFERENCES

1. Berglund, E., Sarnoff, S. J., and Isaacs, J. P.: Ventricular Function: Role of the Pericardium in Regulation of Cardiovascular Dynamics, *Circulation Res.* 3:133, 1955.
2. Holt, J. P., Rhode, E. A., and Kines, H.: Pericardial and Ventricular Pressure, *Circulation Res.,* 8: 1171, 1960.
3. Shabetai, R., Fowler, N. O., Fenton, J., and Masangkay, M.: The Mechanism of Pulsus Paradoxus in Acute Cardiac Tamponade. (Submitted for publication.)
4. Ellis, K., Leeds, N. E., and Himmelstein, A.: Congenital Deficiencies in the Parietal Pericardium: A Review of 2 New Cases Including Successful Diagnosis by Plain Roentgenography, *Am. J. Roentgenol.,* 82:125, 1959.
5. Fowler, N. O.: Congenital Defect of the Pericardium: Its Resemblance to Pulmonary Artery Enlargement, *Circulation,* 26:114, 1962.
6. Capps, J. A.: Pain from Pleura and Pericardium, *Proc. A. Res. Nerv. & Ment. Dis.,* 23:263, 1943.
7. Weissbein, A. S., and Heller, F. N.: Method of Treatment of Pericardial Pain, *Circulation,* 24:607, 1961.
8. Shabetai, R., Fowler, N. O., and Gueron, M.: The Effects of Respiration on Aortic Pressure and Flow, *Am. Heart J.,* 65:525, 1963.
9. Katz, L. N., and Gauchat, H. W.: Observations on Pulsus Paradoxus (with Special Reference to Pericardial Effusions), *Arch. Int. Med.,* 33:350, 1924.
10. Dock, W.: Inspiratory Traction on the Pericardium: The Cause of Pulsus Paradoxus in Pericardial Disease, *A.M.A. Arch. Int. Med.,* 108:837, 1961.
11. Dornhorst, A., Howard, P., and Leathart, G. C.: Pulsus Paradoxus, *Lancet,* 1:746, 1952.
12. Shabetai, R., Fowler, N. O., and Fenton, J. C.: Respiratory Variation in Blood Pressure, *Circulation,* 28:802, 1963.
13. Wolff, L., and Grunfeld, O.: Pericarditis, *New England J. Med.,* 268:419, 1963.
14. Clincopathologic Conference: Pericardial Disease with Effusion, Systemic Involvement and Pulmonary Edema, *Am. J. Med.,* 33:442, 1962.
15. Harvey, A. M., Shulman, L. E., Tumulty, P. A., Conley, C. L., and Schoenrich, E. H.: Systemic Lupus Erythematosus: Review of the Literature and Clinical Analysis of 138 Cases, *Medicine,* 33:291, 1954.
16. Schaffer, A. I.: Case of Traumatic Pericarditis with Chronic Tamponade and Constriction, *Am. J. Cardiol.,* 7:125, 1961.
17. Keith, T. A., 3d: Chronic Constrictive Pericarditis in Association with Rheumatoid Disease, *Circulation,* 25:477, 1962.
18. Jones, A., and Wedgwood, J.: Effects of Radiations on the Heart, *Brit. J. Radiol.,* 33:138, 1960.
19. Kaplan, M. M., and Sherwood, L. M.: Acute Pericarditis Due to Histoplasma Capsulatum, *Ann. Int. Med.,* 58:862, 1963.
20. Barnes, A. R., and Burchell, H. B.: Acute Pericarditis Simulating Acute Coronary Occlusion: A Report of Fourteen Cases, *Am. Heart J.,* 23:247, 1942.
21. Fowler, N. O., Gueron, M., and Rowlands, D. T.: Primary Myocardial Disease, *Circulation,* 23:498, 1961.
22. Wagner, H. N., McAfee, J. G., and Mosley, J. M.: Medical Radioisotope Scanning, *J.A.M.A.,* 174:162, 1960.
23. Durant, T. M.: Negative (Gas) Contrast Angiocardiography, *Am. Heart J.,* 61:1, 1961.
24. Semple, T., and Lancaster, W. M.: Noisy Pneumothorax: Observations Based on 24 Cases, *Brit. M. J.,* 1:1342, 1961.
25. Hamman, L.: Spontaneous Mediastinal Emphysema, *Bull. Johns Hopkins Hosp.,* 64:1, 1939.
26. Connolly, D. C., and Burchell, H. B.: Pericarditis: A Ten Year Survey, *Am. J. Cardiol.,* 7:7, 1961.
27. McGuire, J., Kotte, J. H., and Helm, R. A.: Acute Pericarditis, *Circulation,* 9:425, 1954.
28. Keith, T. A., Fowler, N. O., Helmsworth, J. A., and Gralnick, H.: The Course of Surgically Modified Mitral Stenosis: Study of Ninety-four Patients with Emphasis on the Problem of Restenosis, *Am. J. Med.,* 34:308, 1963.
29. Dressler, W.: The Post-myocardial-infarction Syndrome: A Report on Forty-four Cases, *A.M.A. Arch. Int. Med.,* 103:28, 1959.
30. Kotte, J. H., and McGuire, J.: Pericardial Paracentesis, *Mod. Concepts Cardiovas. Dis.,* 20, no. 7, 1951.
31. Bishop, L. H., Jr., Estes, E. H., Jr., and McIntosh, H. D.: The Electrocardiogram as a Safeguard in Pericardiocentesis, *J.A.M.A.,* 162:264, 1956.
32. Paul, O., Castleman, B., and White, P. D.: Chronic Constrictive Pericarditis: A Study of 53 Cases, *Am. J. M. Sc.,* 216:361, 1948.
33. Slater, S. R., Kroop, I. G., and Zuckerman, S.: Constrictive Pericarditis Caused by Solitary Metastatic Carcinosis of the Pericardium and Complicated by Radiation Fibrosis of the Mediastinum, *Am. Heart J.,* 43:401, 1952.
34. Wooley, C. F., and Hosier, D. M.: Constrictive Pericarditis Due to Histoplasma Capsulatum, *New England J. Med.,* 264:1230, 1961.
35. Wood, P.: Chronic Constrictive Pericarditis, *Am. J. Cardiol.,* 7:48, 1961.
36. Harvey, W. P.: Auscultatory Findings in Diseases of the Pericardium, *Am. J. Cardiol.,* 7:15, 1961.
37. Fowler, N. O.: "Physical Diagnosis of Heart Disease," The Macmillan Company, New York, 1962.
38. Burwell, C. S.: Some Effects of Pericardial Disease on the Pulmonary Circulation, *Tr. A. Am. Physicians,* 64:74, 1951.

39. Burwell, C. S., and Robin, E. D.: Some Points in the Diagnosis of Myocardial Fibrosis, *Tr. A. Am. Physicians,* **67:**67, 1954.

40. Dye, C. L., Genovese, P. D., Daly, W. J., and Behnke, R. H.: Primary Myocardial Disease. Part II. Hemodynamic Alterations, *Ann. Int. Med.,* **58:** 442, 1963.

41. Burch, G. E., and Phillips, J. H.: Methods in Diagnostic Differentiation of Myocardial Dilatation from Pericardial Effusion, *Am. Heart J.,* **64:**266, 1962.

50 MYOCARDIAL DISEASE

A. Calhoun Witham, M.D.

There are a large number of patients with heart disease in whom mechanical overloading due to valvular, congenital, hypertensive, and pulmonary pathology can be excluded as a cause. The hallmarks of myocardial ischemia are also absent. Such hearts presumably enlarge or function improperly as a result of "muscle failure." The pathogenesis in the majority is, at the moment, highly speculative.

The term *primary myocardial disease* (PMD) has gained wide acceptance, for it accurately locates the basic difficulty in the muscle itself. It is also vague enough to cover numerous diseases of unknown cause. Further justification for the term is found in the clinical similarity of patients, for myocardial insufficiency is reflected by congestive failure, regardless of cause. Unless active myocarditis is present or the telltale histologic evidence of a well-known systemic process, such as sarcoid, is found, the similarity often extends into both gross and microscopic pathologic features.

There are, however, several groups of diseases which fit comfortably into the category of primary afflictions of the myocardium but are very different in their clinical and pathologic manifestations. The first is manifest mainly by striking cardiac dilatation. Unless quickly fatal, the myocardium reacts to *myocarditis* in this manner. There is, additionally, a large group of patients with similar manifestations which, however, many physicians are loath to label myocarditis in the absence of evidence of an inflammatory origin. All sorts of awkward labels have been invented as substitutes, e.g., *noncoronary myocardial degeneration, uncommon form of myocardial disease, primary myocardial degeneration, idiopathic myocardopathy (or cardiomyopathy)*, and *idiopathic myocardial hypertrophy*. Others have doggedly used *chronic myocarditis, Fiedler's myocarditis*, etc., either loosely or with the conviction that most such cases are a late stage of myocarditis—which may indeed be correct. The designation *myocardosis* has the virtue of brevity and avoids the assumption of an unproved link with myocardial inflammation.[1]

Another group of primary myocardial diseases is characterized mainly by a *concentric hypertrophy*, dilatation being only a late and presumably secondary phenomenon. It is often familial, and sudden death is common. Congestive heart failure, an early and prominent feature of the myocarditis and

myocardosis groups, is a late and rather uncommon finding. Sometimes the hypertrophy is peculiarly asymmetrical, and ventricular *outflow tract obstruction* is the most dramatic effect. This feature justifies a separate category for clinical classification but not necessarily for an etiologic or pathologic one.

The clinician is occasionally confronted with still another type of presentation of myocardial disease. The clinical findings suggest constrictive pericarditis. High venous pressure, extraordinary edema, and venous and intraventricular pulses point to *inflow tract obstruction*. The modest enlargement of the cardiac silhouette and the low electrocardiographic voltages complete the mimicry. The common denominator of these cases is a stiffening of the myocardium due to invasion with fibrous tissue or other inelastic material which creates the filling difficulty.

To the author, it appears that the term PMD must be badly stretched to encompass myocardial maladies associated with noninfectious systemic diseases such as sarcoid or amyloid, for the cardiac involvement is certainly not in this sense primary but only part of the multisystem involvement. It seems more natural to refer to them as *secondary myocardial diseases* (SMD). For obvious reasons, some are occasionally grouped as *metabolic* and others as *infiltrative*.

As generic terms, then, both PMD and SMD are satisfactory if defined. In this chapter they will be used as indicated. PMD is inconsistently used in the literature, and there is an abundance of synonyms and near synonyms. The classification below is basically clinical and reflects the several patterns of primary myocardial disease that the physician may encounter. Interrelationships among the five types of PMD will be established in the detailed discussion.

1. Primary myocardial disease (PMD)
   a. Myocarditis. Term restricted to cases in which there is reasonable evidence of an inflammatory reaction in the heart. Evidence may be direct (histopathologic) or, less conclusively, indirect (historical, bacteriologic, serologic).
   b. Myocardosis. Clinically indistinguishable from chronic cardiopathy following myocarditis, but the above links to etiologic agents are absent. Cardiac dilatation, congestive failure, and embolization are the key clinical features. Numerous causes are suggested.

   c. Idiopathic concentric hypertrophy. Dilatation and heart failure are late features. Sudden death and a familial incidence are frequent.

   d. Obstructive cardiomyopathy (functional hypertrophic subaortic stenosis). Also called *asymmetrical* hypertrophy because of its early disproportionate septal involvement creating outflow tract obstruction. Usually simulates aortic stenosis. Probably a variant of *c* above.

   e. Constrictive cardiomyopathy. Clinical features of inflow tract obstruction as in constrictive pericarditis. Several causes identified.

2. Secondary myocardial disease (SMD). Myocardial disease associated with noninfectious systemic disease. The terms infiltrative and metabolic have been applied to some entities.

a. Collagen diseases	*g.* Anemia
b. Amyloid	*h.* Endocrinopathy
c. Sarcoid	*i.* Systemic muscular
d. Carcinomatosis	and neurologic
e. Hemochromatosis	diseases
f. Glycogen storage	

PRIMARY MYOCARDIAL DISEASE (PMD)

Myocarditis

Myocarditis may be the most common of all heart diseases. This statement is supported by both pathologic and clinical studies. Evidence of old inflammation is reported in 10 per cent of routine autopsies,[2] and electrocardiographic studies suggest transient cardiac involvement in 5 to 15 per cent of common infectious diseases.[3] It appears to be even higher in a few such as diphtheria, rickettsial diseases, poliomyelitis, and Chagas's disease.[4-7] The reputation for rarity, of course, exists because the vast majority recover spontaneously without overt signs.

The diagnosis is not difficult if one is aware of the association with almost every known bacterial, viral, rickettsial, and parasitic disease. From 1 to 3 weeks after the illness begins, the patient may complain of breathlessness or palpitations. Pulse rate may be disproportionately elevated. Examination will reveal some of the following: small pulse, cardiomegaly, basilar rales, diastolic gallop rhythm, systolic murmurs of mitral or tricuspid insufficiency. The electrocardiogram will show multiple premature beats, T-wave inversion, prolonged Q-T_c interval, or atrioventricular (A-V) blocks. Low voltage is not particularly common. X-rays will show some globular cardiomegaly and hilar pulmonary congestion. From this point, the illness may take several paths: usually steady improvement occurs over a period of a month or two, but

electrocardiographic effects may persist much longer, even permanently. Chronic myocardial insufficiency may result with death months or even several years later due to intractible heart failure, pulmonary or cerebral emboli, or arrhythmias. The possibilities may be summarized:

$$
\text{Acute myocarditis}
\begin{cases}
\text{Rapid recovery} \\
\text{Sudden death} \\
\text{Subacute illness}
\begin{cases}
\text{with recovery} \\
\text{with relapses}
\end{cases} \\
\text{Chronic heart disease}
\end{cases}
$$

If death occurs within a few days, heart weight is little increased, but various degrees of acute dilatation are present. Focal and/or diffuse accumulations of inflammatory cells are present, usually located interstitially. At times the cellular reaction is minimal. Muscle fibers may appear normal, or there may be scattered loss of cross striations and degenerative changes. If the organism is a pus former like the staphylococcus, myocardial abscesses may be found.

Diphtheritic myocarditis presents a somewhat different picture: cellular reaction is scant and apparently secondary to degenerating muscle fibers injured directly by the toxin.[8]

If the patient survives a month or more, the cellular reaction persists, but histiocytes, mononuclear cells, and fibroblasts are more apparent. The subacute forms with death in a few weeks were those described by Fiedler. The term Fiedler's myocarditis should be confined to such cases of unknown cause; one of his specimens showed accumulations of giant cells, either of muscular origin or of the Langhans type, now thought to be a type of reaction to injury and sometimes designated as *giant cell* or *granulomatous*.[9,10] Occasionally, particularly if associated with allergy, the eosinophil may predominate.[11] Rarely, the basophilic cell predominates.[12] Peculiarly localized involvement of the atria, the conducting system, or the right ventricle has been described.[13,14] Some patients may date the onset of chronic heart failure to an acute febrile illness several years before death. The heart, quite surprisingly, may show a histologic picture similar to that of acute myocarditis, except perhaps for a higher percentage of round cells and of the nonspecific findings described under Myocardosis in the outline above. These conditions warrant the label chronic myocarditis.[9] Generalized dilatation and hypertrophy and a high incidence of mural thrombi are to be expected.

The clinical diagnosis of myocarditis rests on linking the onset of the cardiac illness with an infectious process. It is helpful if a recent prior examination has revealed a normal heart. The history of antecedent illness is elicited in about three-fourths of cases.[15] The diagnosis is more certain if the recent presence of infection can be established by the observation of a characteristic clinical picture, by the isolation of an agent, or by serologic means. Histologic findings of inflammation in the myocardium, however, are the only unassailable evidence. There are several reasons why it is difficult to prove or disprove a specific cause:[15]

1. Rising titers of antibody to a ubiquitous virus do not conclusively indicate an etiologic link. They may represent only an intercurrent, unrelated infection.[16]

2. Negative studies, cultural and serologic, may not disprove a viral cause but only that the guilty agent was not, or could not be, sought for.[17]

3. Negative cultures from the heart do not disprove viral myocarditis, as the agent may not be recovered even when known by other means.[18] The analogy with the inability to culture the streptococcus from the heart in acute rheumatic fever is obvious.

4. Even the culture of a virus directly from the heart in a fatal case does not prove that myocardial invasion has taken place, as it may have been passively transported to the heart during viremia.

The mechanisms by which an infectious agent may damage the heart appear to be both more numerous and more complex than they were formerly considered to be.[19] It may, of course, directly invade the heart and even form abscesses, as in staphylococcal septicemia. It may liberate a toxin which secondarily damages cardiac muscle cells, as in diphtheria. It may modify the antigenic properties of cardiac muscle so that the patient forms antibodies against it. A fourth possible mechanism has been described, at least with the streptococcus: a protein component of this bacterium is apparently so similar antigenically to a constituent of cardiac myofibers that the antibodies stimulated by the streptococcus cross-react with cardiac muscle.[20]

The role of immune mechanisms in myocarditis is almost certainly important but not entirely clear. Circulating anti-heart antibodies have been demonstrated in acute rheumatic fever, postcommissurotomy syndrome, and myocardial infarction, as well as in suspected chronic myocarditis but are thought to be the result rather than cause of cardiac damage.[19] Clinical features suggest an immune reaction also—e.g., the 7- to 10-day delay between onset of the infection and cardiac manifestations, and the often mild or nonexistent symptoms of the initiating illness followed by the severe cardiac reaction.

Myocarditis Associated with Specific Viruses

Clinical evidence of myocarditis is very rare in mumps, rubella, rubeola, rabies, infectious hepatitis, varicella, and infectious mononucleosis, but electrocardiographic evidence, consisting of changes in the T wave and Q-T and P-R intervals, may occur in from 5 to 15 per cent of cases.[21–27] Clinical myocarditis in these diseases may follow any of the courses mentioned above. Partial or complete heart block, transient or permanent, has also been described.[22,23] Fatal myocarditis has been reported several times following vaccination for smallpox.[28]

Saphir has reported three human beings with the onset of encephalitis, sudden death, and autopsy evidence of acute interstitial myocarditis. He has pointed out the similarity of the Columbia SK and MM virus to the virus of encephalomyocarditis, which is a disease of apes, mice, and hamsters. Striking clinical and pathologic similarity exists between these human and animal infections.[29]

The influenza viruses have long been under suspicion as a cause of myocarditis. Investigation of this association has yielded several facts of broader interest as well. For example, during epidemics an asymptomatic infection (proved by serologic methods) may result in a "delayed" type of myocarditis as its only manifestation.[30] This might well occur with other viruses and explain myocarditis without a preceding history of infection. Furthermore, chronic heart disease has developed after an influenzal infection. This fact supports the hypothesis that chronic heart disease of unknown cause (or myocardosis) might have a similar viral origin. A final general point is that two time sequences have been reported in influenzal myocarditis. The majority of cases occur from 1 to 4 weeks after the onset of the illness, but myocarditis has also been found in rapidly fatal infections.[18] This, of course, suggests that viruses may act either by direct invasion or through an antigen-antibody mechanism.

In some epidemics of poliomyelitis the incidence of focal myocarditis in fatal cases may approach 100 per cent, but in others the rate is nearer 20 per cent.[6] The cardiac lesion appears to be clinically significant in a much smaller number of cases. In these patients, however, the usual signs and symptoms of the rapidly fatal type of myocarditis are noted. These include cyanosis, dyspnea, tachycardia, and vascular collapse. The cardiac manifestations occur 2 to 5 days after onset as a rule and are apparently due to direct invasion.[31] The virus has been recovered from the heart.[32] Cor pulmonale may also develop in patients with severe respiratory paralysis.[33]

The Coxsackie B virus deserves special mention.

Although implicated in older children and adults with either myocarditis or pericarditis,[34] its most frequently described picture is of an epidemic form in infants (myocarditis neonatorum). In some outbreaks meningoencephalitic symptoms predominate, and in others cardiac manifestations are more prominent.[35] Usually both are present. One clinical syndrome described is that of a biphasic illness. Diarrhea developed in infants of five to seventeen days of age; these infants recovered for 3 to 4 days, then were affected by lethargy, cyanosis, tachycardia, and collapse; the mortality rate was about 60 per cent. The T waves were sharply inverted on the ECG, but death or recovery usually ensued before much cardiomegaly was evident. Focal collections of inflammatory cells were found throughout the myocardium.[36] This illness apparently always occurs within 3 weeks of birth. A maternal respiratory infection is frequently present about the time of delivery, and some infections may begin in utero.[37] The virus can be recovered from the heart in concentrations so high as to leave little doubt of its invasion of the myocardium.[35]

It must be emphasized that most cases of clinical myocarditis are associated with unidentified respiratory or grippe-like illnesses or with no history of antecedent infection at all. These patients are frequently labeled as Fiedler's or isolated idiopathic myocarditis.[38] Even elaborate virologic studies with current techniques are rarely rewarding. Occasional presumptive evidence of a viral cause is furnished by rises in antibody titers against Coxsackie B, influenza A or B, psittacosis, ECHO, or mumps viruses or less commonly known agents.[15] Because of the association of myocarditis with primary atypical pneumonia, the Eaton agent has also been implicated.[19]

Myocarditis Associated with Bacteria and Allergy

In fatal bacterial endocarditis focal myocarditis and degenerative changes are common.[39] Evidence of their importance is furnished by patients with heart failure who respond promptly to control of the infection without improvement in the mechanical (valvular) lesions. Myocardial dysfunction may play a critical role in the survival of severely ill patients. Myocardial abscesses, particularly due to the staphylococcus, are also well known.

The influence of hemolytic streptococcal infections upon the myocardium is, of course, best known in relation to classic acute rheumatic fever, which follows 2 to 3 per cent of such illnesses. Electrocardiographic changes, however, principally of the P-R and Q-T intervals and T wave occur about five times as frequently, usually after defervescence.[3] The relationship to acute rheumatic fever is unknown. A 70 per cent incidence of acute interstitial myocarditis in no way different from that following other infections has been found in fatal scarlet fever.[40] The streptococcus apparently may affect the myocardium by either of two distinct processes.

Although diphtheria is rare in the United States today, its complicating myocarditis is justly feared. The incidence is usually put at from 10 to 25 per cent but approaches 50 per cent in fatal cases.[4] Classically, myocarditis is said to appear during recovery, although in fulminant infections it may appear by the second or third day. In smoldering infections, it may appear 4 to 5 weeks after the beginning of the illness. It is suspected that specific antitoxin therapy, not without its own dangers, may eliminate, modify, or greatly delay the onset. Mortality rate is said to be about 50 per cent; prognosis is worsened if the patient is less than five years of age and if myocarditis appears early.

The syndrome of heart failure may occur independently of, or be preceded by, conduction disturbances. The most common electrocardiographic changes, however, are in the T waves. Heart block may come and go but is one of the most striking and frequently fatal features. A second cardiovascular complication is vasomotor collapse. This is part of the diphtheritic polyneuritis; the site of action is the vascular myoneural junction and often precedes myocarditis. It is probably the immediate cause of death in most overwhelming infections. Intracardiac thrombosis with death from pulmonary or cerebral embolism has been reported.

Aside from supportive therapy, especially antitoxin, there has been little to offer these patients. Digitalis is probably contraindicated in view of the high incidence of complete heart block. Newer methods of treatment such as artificial pacemakers have arrived too late for adequate evaluation in this country but would seem to warrant trial.

While the majority of cases who survive the acute episode appear to recover completely, there has accumulated fairly impressive evidence of permanent electrocardiographic abnormalities, including A-V blocks, and even smoldering heart failure years after the infection.[41,42] The history of diphtheria in childhood is also said to be found nearly ten times as often as expected in a group of adults in whom the usual causes of A-V block have been excluded.[43]

Trichinosis and typhoid fever have been occasionally reported as causes of myocarditis;[44,45] however, *Trichinella* is rarely found in the myocardium of the former, and it is likely that the myocarditis has an allergic origin.

Allergic Myocarditis

There are several allergic reactions in which the myocardium takes part in greater or lesser degree. In half of a series of patients with serum sickness severe enough to require hospitalization electrocardiographic changes developed. Although the majority were ST-T wave abnormalities, the evolution of an acute pericarditis was noted in one instance and of an acute myocardial infarction in another.[46] When serum therapy, particularly for pneumococcal and meningococcal infection was popular, a predominantly eosinophilic myocarditis, as well as periarteritic lesions, were occasionally found at autopsy in these patients.[47] Both have been reproduced experimentally by rabbit and horse serum.[48] Transient cardiac decompensation and complete heart block have also been described in anaphylactoid purpura.[49]

Of particular interest is the occurrence of smoldering myocarditis and late death following penicillin reaction[50] and the high incidence of mainly eosinophilic interstitial myocarditis found at autopsy in patients who received sulfonamides during their terminal illness.[51]

Mixed with reports of myocarditis occurring during allergic reactions is the occasional case of acute myocardial infarction occurring at the height of an allergic reaction. These have been reported during serum sickness, after wasp stings, and after tetanus antitoxin therapy.[46,52,53] They are presumably due to an allergic vasculitis involving the coronary arteries.

Myocardosis

This form of primary myocardial disease is clinically several times as common in adults as myocarditis and many other better-known entities, such as constrictive pericarditis and some congenital complexes. It constitutes about 1 per cent of all hearts of over 500 Gm.[54] The incidence seems to be slowly increasing. The average age of patients is probably in the late thirties, about 80 per cent falling between thirty and fifty years.[55] All series show a heavy predilection for males, and most for Negroes. Manual workers also seem to predominate.[56] Cardiomegaly may have been identified several months or years before symptoms.[16,57] The usual presenting complaint is dyspnea on exertion. Acute pulmonary edema and even nocturnal dyspnea are surprisingly rare. Unlike other forms of PMD, syncope and early sudden death are very unusual.[57] Hemoptysis or paralysis due to embolization may be presenting complaints.

The positive findings on physical examination are limited to the cardiovascular system. The jugular venous pressure may be elevated, and if so the wave form will often suggest tricuspid incompetence. Giant A waves, presumably due to splinting of the interventricular septum by left ventricular hypertrophy, are also occasionally noted.[57] Mild diastolic hypertension is noted in about half, but pulse pressure is usually normal or rather low. Pulsus alternans is found reasonably frequently if carefully sought with the pressure cuff. The heart is variably, sometimes massively, enlarged; the apex beat is palpable and displaced downward and outward. There may be no murmurs, but a prominent diastolic gallop is heard in the majority. The murmurs of relative tricuspid or mitral insufficiency are usually heard sooner or later and are frequently transient. The closely consecutive third and fourth heart sounds may cause a low-pitched diastolic rumble resembling mitral stenosis.[56] A transient murmur of pulmonary incompetence has also been noted but must be very rare.[58] The lungs are ordinarily surprisingly clear upon auscultation, but edema and hepatomegaly are prominent. Atrial fibrillation is not uncommon, particularly in older patients. The frequency and magnitude of these signs depends on the stage of the disease when the patient is examined.

The x-rays are not distinctive but usually show enlargement of all chambers, the left ventricle being most prominent. Pleural effusions or scars from pulmonary infarction may be seen. The aorta frequently appears hypoplastic. The minimal or absent hilar congestion is striking in view of the heart size.[16]

The ECG is invariably abnormal and shows one or more of the following features: low-voltage limb leads which may become normal with alleviation of edema; increased left ventricular voltage; complete or incomplete left bundle branch block, left axis deviation; or balanced precordial voltages of combined hypertrophy. Right bundle branch block is rare. The P wave is also abnormal in about two-thirds of cases. Fairly distinctive are bifid P waves with a biphasic, prolonged, secondary negative deflection in lead V_1.[54] Evidence of right atrial enlargement is, however, very common also. P-R prolongation is often seen but may be related to digitalis. Certain features sometimes suggest previous myocardial infarction (Fig. 50-1). The most common of these are Q-S complexes in leads V_1 to V_3 or V_4, or faulty R-wave progression in the same leads. These are probably related to one or more of the following: left ventricular hypertrophy, septal fibrosis, or incomplete left bundle branch block. The last has not been emphasized but is found in nearly half of the author's cases and is much more frequent than the complete variety. A rough correlation has been noted between the

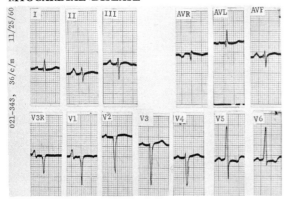

11/25/60 36/c/m 021–343,

Fig. 50-1. Tracing is that of a Negro man, age thirty-six, in chronic heart failure for 2 years. Electrocardiogram illustrates many of the features found in myocardosis. The tracing exhibits left axis deviation, initial right-to-left forces suggesting incomplete left bundle branch block, and faulty R-wave progression in the precordial leads. The P waves are also abnormal. Autopsy revealed gross dilatation hypertrophy and scattered fibrosis. Coronary vessels were normal.

heart weight and the QRS duration.[57] If the patient survives repeated pulmonary emboli, some of the electrocardiographic features of cor pulmonale may modify the above picture.

Hemodynamic studies usually reflect the clinical state. Ordinarily the cardiac index is low (about 1.5 or less). Unless pulmonary emboli have occurred, the pulmonary vascular resistance is nearly normal in contrast to most cases of left ventricular valvular disease and coronary artery disease.[59]

The early history of this disease is not well known. It may even begin in childhood.[16,60] After symptoms begin, however, the outcome is predictable. About half the patients are dead within 1 year and about two-thirds within 2 years.[56] Unusual cases of survival, however, for 5 years or more are known.[54,59] Death rarely occurs with the first bout of decompensation. Poor prognosis seems related to repeated heart failure, heart size, and intraventricular blocks. The cause of death is heart failure, cerebral or pulmonary embolization, or terminal ventricular arrhythmia.

At postmortem the heart is greatly dilated, suggesting that this is the primary pathologic feature (Fig. 50-2). Heart weights, however, indicate advanced hypertrophy also. Mural thrombi are found enmeshed in the trabeculae carnae of one or both ventricles in the majority of patients. Microscopically about three-fourths show increased fibrous tissue.[61] This is scattered focally, interstitially, and particularly in the subendocardium. It is especially prominent beneath mural thrombi, probably a result of Thebesian vein thrombosis.[62] Some of the circumscribed patches of fibrosis appear to be mi-

croinfarcts due to thrombosis of small intramural arteries (Fig. 50-3). Intercellular edema and hypertrophy of muscle fibers are almost constant findings. In general, muscle fibers appear healthy, but in some sections hyalinization, fragmentation, opacification, and loss of striation are seen. Actual necrosis is rare, and inflammatory exudate is not seen. The above changes are nonspecific and rarely are severe enough to explain satisfactorily the failure of the cardiac pump. In about one-fourth of cases, the muscle fibers appear normal except for hypertrophy, and fibrosis is virtually absent.[13] Recently, in 11 of 13 cases chronic inflammatory changes were found in the pericardium. This has been cited as evidence in favor of an infectious origin of most cases.[63]

Treatment is unsatisfactory and is based primarily on attempts to prevent the deleterious effects of dilatation, extensive secondary fibrosis, and mural thrombosis. Digitalis, assisted by diuretics, is usually very rewarding during the first bout of decompensation (Fig. 50-4). Heart size and ECG changes, however, do not return completely to normal, and with succeeding attacks therapeutic efforts become decreasingly effective.

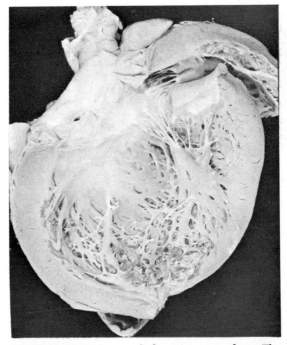

Fig. 50-2. Typical gross findings in myocardosis. The modest hypertrophy of the left ventricular wall is overshadowed by the striking dilatation of the chamber. The trabeculae are flattened. An extensive antemortem clot is enmeshed in the trabeculae at the apex of the left ventricle. Clot was also present in the right ventricle and atrium. (A-1491, *Department of Pathology, Medical College of Georgia, courtesy of Dr. J. Robert Teabeaut.*)

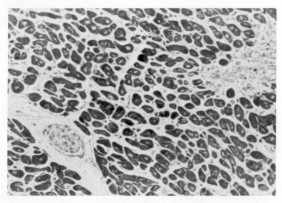

Fig. 50-3. Section of myocardium from a patient who died after 2 years of chronic heart failure. At the lower left is an intramural artery completely occluded by an organizing thrombus which is partially recanalized. At the upper right is a localized area of fibrous tissue representing a microinfarct. (A-775, *Department of Pathology, Medical College of Georgia, courtesy of Dr. J. Robert Teabeaut.*)

Digitalis should be taken continuously, but the margin between therapeutic and toxic dosage narrows as time goes by. The findings of mural thrombosis in three-fourths of autopsies and the frequent and often fatal embolization appear to be adequate indications for permanent anticoagulation. Prolonged bed rest, even sanatorium-like care for many months, would seem to be sound in a further effort to decrease cardiac work and hence dilatation. The only apparent reversals of the inexorable course have been obtained with this regimen.[64]

The differential diagnosis usually involves six entities:

1. Pericardial effusion may be suspected because of a huge cardiac shadow, rapid changes in size, ascites, and other features of right-sided failure. Pulsus alternans, changing murmurs of functional A-V valvular incompetence, diastolic gallop, x-ray evidence of dominant left ventricular enlargement with a distinctively small cardiac waist, and the previously discussed electrocardiographic findings of myocardosis should indicate PMD in the majority. If there is still doubt, a broadened pericardial shadow may be excluded by coiling the catheter against the right atrial wall or by contrast medium injected into this chamber. Pericardial paracentesis under electrocardiographic control should rarely be necessary but is acceptably safe under these circumstances.

2. Rheumatic heart disease may be suggested principally by the systolic murmurs of A-V valvular incompetence, a low-pitched apical rumble, or pseudomurmurs of the third or fourth heart sound. Occasionally, even Kerley's lines and apparent dis-

proportionate left atrial enlargement can be noted on the x-ray.[61,56] Mitralization of the P wave has already been commented upon. Surgical exploration for mitral stenosis or myxoma has occurred. This degree of confusion should, however, be rare. In chronic valvular disease, isolated chamber rather than diffuse enlargement is the rule, the murmurs in myocardosis tend to disappear rather than grow louder with better compensation, and valvular calcification is not seen.

3. Coronary artery disease is often suspected in older patients with this diease, particularly with atrial fibrillation and an ECG compatible with old infarction. There is no history of angina or infarction pain, however, and it is most uncommon for such advanced disease of coronary origin not to have more distinctive features.

4. Chronic myocarditis is almost impossible to exclude with finality, as the course may be indistinguishable. Generally, however, there is no clear-cut history of onset following an infectious disease, fever, or toxicity, and the ECG changes of acute myocarditis are not found at the onset of failure.

5. Recurrent pulmonary embolization may so dominate the picture that one may suspect it to be the primary cause of the chronic, mainly right-sided failure. Evidence of severe left ventricular disease should eliminate this possibility, even if thrombophlebitis is present. As in any type of chronic heart failure, the latter may, of course, occur.

6. Lastly, secondary myocardial disease (SMD) is always assiduously sought in an effort to provide a cause. Careful history, physical examination, and

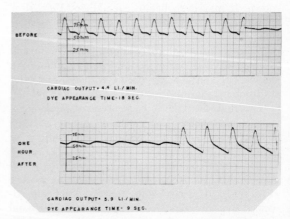

Fig. 50-4. Effect of rapid digitalization on pulse rate, pulse pressure, circulation time, stroke volume, and minute output. Determinations by the Stewart-Hamilton dye-dilution method with Evans blue dye. Patient was a twenty-three-year-old Negro man who developed acute congestive failure following an unidentified lower respiratory tract infection. There was gradual, apparently complete recovery in 4 months.

routine laboratory screening almost always provide a clue to systemic disease. Stated another way, these diseases rarely present as isolated myocardial failure.

Etiology of Myocardosis

Numerous causes have been suggested, such as injury to myocardial muscle from myocarditis, autoimmunity, alcohol, malnutrition, unknown toxins, and the postpartum state. Most appealing is the hypothesis that myocardosis is a nonspecific end result of any acute injury. The toxic agent, however, is rarely identifiable.

This theory supposes that acute cardiac dilatation, such as follows acute myocarditis, may under some circumstances initiate a vicious cycle. This is based primarily on Laplace's law, by which it can be shown that tension on the endocardium must vary with the cube of the radius of the ventricular chamber.[65,66] If the radius is doubled through dilatation, tension will not increase by two but eight times. A ninefold increase in work will be necessary to deliver a given stroke volume, if other factors remain the same. Myocardial efficiency, therefore, declines alarmingly with cardiac dilatation. If the patient survives, heart failure ensues, and hypertrophy appears as a response to increased tension and work. Whereas the muscle cells are then larger, do more work, and thus need a better metabolic exchange, the number of capillaries remains the same. The distance from the capillary to the muscle nuclei is therefore increased, and diffusion is more difficult. Intercellular edema further impairs exchange. The usefulness of the papillary muscles and trabeculae carnae in controlling internal radius gradually declines also as these structures are flattened and effaced with advanced dilatation. Acute muscle injury, therefore, may initiate a self-perpetuating cycle of dilatation, hypertrophy, nutritional injury, fibrosis, failure, more dilatation, etc.

A model for the above sequence of events is probably seen in the natural history of thiamine deficiency. The hyperkinetic circulatory state of beriberi is unusual in the Occident, and a low-output type of heart disease, particularly involving the left ventricle, is found. Response to thiamine is complete when treatment is prompt. If the disease has been present for some months before therapy, the response is incomplete, and residual cardiomegaly may remain. Finally, at a later stage, the process seems irreversible. Patients in the later stages seem indistinguishable, clinically and pathologically, from those with myocardosis.[67] A disease ascribed to diverse nutritional deficiencies among Bantus also seems similar.[68]

Certainly some cases of postinfectious myocarditis follow an identical pathway. The evidence that myocarditis, especially viral, may cause the picture of myocardosis has, until recently, been mainly by analogy; it is known that acute myocarditis may occur without an obvious clinical infection, that it may assume a chronic form, that such cases may not show evidence of inflammation at postmortem, and finally that cases of insidious onset, which might clinically be labeled myocardosis, have shown evidence of inflammation at postmortem. Recently, it has been suggested that viral damage to myocardial muscle may be in the form of subtle biochemical change, so that the contractile efficiency is diminished. This could conceivably occur by direct alteration in structure of contractile protein or by interference with the contractile process caused by autoimmune antibodies bound to muscle cells. The first suggestion is as yet unsupported, but the finding of circulating anti-heart antibodies and, more importantly, of fluorescein-labeled antibody (gamma-globulin) bound to heart muscle in patients dying with the myocardosis syndrome constitutes important evidence.[69]

The role of alcohol in the pathogenesis of PMD is controversial, and "alcoholic myocarditis" is apparently more widely accepted in England than in the United States. A typical clinical profile is described: The patients are invariably men, usually from thirty to fifty, particularly wealthy bachelors or those with ready access to alcoholic beverages, such as bartenders. The patients are either heavy beer or bottle-a-day whisky drinkers. Nutrition is characteristically excellent. They usually lose little time from work, are not "binge" drinkers, but constantly consume large quantities of alcoholic beverages. The unexplained onset of auricular flutter or fibrillation may be the presenting symptoms. Palpitations may be due to premature ventricular beats, often multifocal, in the presence of sinus tachycardia. Breathlessness with little exertion is also common. The heart, in this stage, will be slightly enlarged. Various specific T-wave changes (cleft, cloven, etc.) are described.[70] At this point, the disease is completely reversible by abstinence, balanced diet, etc. Untreated, it merges with the familiar picture of myocardosis and becomes irreversible. Pathologic features do not seem distinctive.

Part of the difference between British and American reports may be only in labels. United States reports rarely describe "alcoholic myocarditis" but series of "idiopathic hypertrophy, myocardosis," etc., usually include patients with a history of heavy alcohol ingestion in from 20 to 60 per cent. The main objection to the diagnosis has been lack of experimental proof that alcohol can directly damage the myocardium. Recent observations, however, tend to support this view.

Alcohol infused into dogs in mildly intoxicating dosages caused a release of potassium, phosphate, and transaminase into the coronary sinus blood and a striking decrease in uptake of free fatty acid, which is the major cardiac substrate. In addition, ventricular function curves showed significant deterioration, and cardiac work was increased in the face of a lower coronary flow.[71,72]

Primary myocardial disease in alcoholics may then be due to an unrelated disease of unknown origin, to the repeated insults of alcohol itself, to thiamine deficiency, or to less well-understood qualitative dietary imbalance, particularly derivation of most calories from carbohydrate. The therapeutic implications are obvious.

The peculiar occurrence of heart failure in the puerperium has excited interest for many years, but the mechanism remains obscure. The term post-partum myocarditis is most frequently used to describe it, but the pathologic findings ordinarily do not suggest an inflammatory lesion, although an occasional case has been due to the fortuitous postpartum appearance of acute infectious myocarditis. There are sufficient specific features to justify its consideration as a separate clinical entity or special form of myocardosis. The occurrence rate varies from 1 in 1,300 to 4,000 deliveries and most often occurs in multiparous Negroes, with a higher incidence of toxemia, anemia, poor nutrition, and desultory prenatal care.[73,74] The incidence of twin births is unusually high. Recurrence in subsequent pregnancies is frequent. Mild, particularly diastolic hypertension is often present, but disappears on successful therapy. In most series of myocardosis, principally a disease of males, the frequency with which failure in the puerperium developed in the few females included is impressive. There may be a suggestion of mild decompensation in the third trimester which disappears but returns dramatically 2 to 10 weeks after delivery.[75] Pulmonary embolism is frequent, probably about 25 per cent, and hemoptysis may even be the presenting complaint. Hull's triad of diastolic gallop, anasarca, and small pulse pressure is found in severe cases.[76] X-rays show generalized enlargement, pleural effusions, or evidence of pulmonary infarction (Fig. 50-5). Electrocardiographic voltages tend to be low, probably due to extrinsic edema. T waves are sometimes initially sharply inverted, as in acute myocarditis. Digitalization and diuresis result in dramatic improvement in the majority. The early prognosis is excellent, and about 30 per cent of patients seem to recover completely. Late morbidity and mortality, however, is high. About 30 per cent die of chronic congestive heart failure or embolization months or years later, and the remaining are left with either x-ray changes, ECG abnormalities, or some disability.[73] Pathologic changes are nonspecific and as previously described for this group in general.

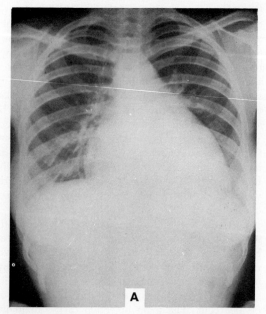 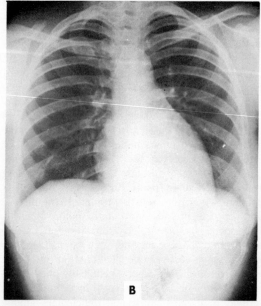

Fig. 50-5. A. Chest x-ray on a young multiparous patient admitted 8 weeks after delivery with hemoptysis, dependent edema, and probable pulmonary infarction. There is moderate pulmonary enlargement and congestion. B. One year later the heart size has greatly decreased, but there is residual left ventricular hypertrophy.

In no other type of PMD should the implications of Laplace's theorem be more conscientiously applied to therapy since vigorous, early, and prolonged treatment, particularly with digitalis, may well prevent the irreversible type of myocardosis. The routine use of anticoagulants has been criticized because of the occasional finding of spontaneous intramyocardial hemorrhage. It is the author's opinion, however, that they should be given until heart size is nearly normal. Steroids are worthless.

An important question arises as to the risk of subsequent pregnancies. The categorical answer cannot be found, but the author's opinion, derived from personal experience modified by the reports of others, is that the risk of recurrence is about 25 per cent and is additive with succeeding pregnancies.[73] Recurrence may skip a pregnancy or even two and is more likely to occur if the patient has not completely recovered. The mortality and morbidity are probably higher on a second occurrence. These figures would appear to furnish adequate medicolegal grounds for sterilization.

Idiopathic Concentric Hypertrophy

In addition to the syndromes of myocarditis and myocardosis there are patients with PMD who present in quite a different manner. They are rare and are seen first in childhood or young adulthood. Because of their infrequency in patients beyond the age of thirty, the long-term survival seems less optimistic. The distinguishing feature from myocardosis is that massive dilatation is not present until very late. X-rays at first show only moderate increases in cardiac transverse diameter, but the features of concentric hypertrophy are present and are amply confirmed by electrocardiogram. The patient may complain of angina or less well-defined chest pain or of mild breathlessness on exertion, or be relatively asymptomatic. The history of syncope, palpitation, tachycardia, or arrhythmias is often present. Careful inquiries may uncover a high frequency of heart disease and sudden death among forebears and siblings. There are no characteristic murmurs, but triple rhythm is common.

Isolated cases occur, but the familial incidence is so high that *familial cardiomegaly* has gained the status of an acceptable clinical diagnosis. The cases reported under this label, unfortunately, do not constitute a homogeneous group clinically or pathologically. It has been suggested that there are "probably as many types of familial heart disease as there are neurological disorders."[57] At least three such groupings may be identified: (1) concentric hypertrophy, sudden death, and gross intraventricular and atrioventricular conduction disturbances;[77] (2) types similar to those in (1) but

without the conduction disturbances and their sequelae;[78] (3) prolonged heart failure with a large element of cardiac dilatation, in no way different from the picture of myocardosis or chronic myocarditis.[79] The third group is the least common but sometimes develops from the first two. There is, then, an overlap between the illnesses classified in this chapter as myocardosis and those labeled idiopathic concentric hypertrophy. The latter also has many features in common with obstructive cardiomyopathy, such as angina, A-V and interventricular blocks, sudden death, and familial incidence. This entity is discussed in detail in Chap. 25. Familial incidence has also been reported in postpartum myocardosis and in chronic myocarditis.[80,81] The single constant pathologic feature is the hypertrophied muscle cell. Vacuolization is sometimes seen. Fibrosis is variable but at times so extensive that some have considered it a distinguishing feature. Unlike myocardosis, mural thrombosis and embolization is an unusual rather than an expected finding.

The familial occurrence of myocardial disease, principally of the concentric hypertrophy type, is well established. Birth rank is not a factor. It is probably a Mendelian dominant and affects both sexes but is transmitted only through the female.[57] Fetal myoglobin, similar to that of progressive muscular dystrophy, has been found in the myocardium of the members of one family.[82] Analogy has also been made between idiopathic concentric hypertrophy and ocular myopathy, which occurs in progressive muscular dystrophy, but also rarely as an isolated entity.[83] Another link is the family described by Kiloh and Nevin in which pseudohypertrophic muscular dystrophy affected some members and cardiomegaly others, and in one a combination of the two occurred.[84] Nadas has described cases of PMD in which muscular dystrophy was not apparent but identified only by muscle biopsy.[82] The similarity of the heart disease of certain hereditary neurologic diseases, such as Friedreich's ataxia, is also notable. Of great interest is the family reported by Roth in which ataxia affected some and heart disease of this type others.[85]

It has been suggested that familial cardiomegaly, at least that confined to a single generation, might be a residuum of a family epidemic of myocarditis. Generally, however, the clinical profile is not that of healed myocarditis with lingering disability. Toxoplasmosis or some other germ cell infection has been suggested but with little evidence.

Electrocardiographic findings vary but also tend to have familial similarities. Evidence of left ventricular hypertrophy is very common, and in children right ventricular hypertrophy is occasionally found. The Wolff-Parkinson-White anomaly is also sometimes a feature.[82] Myocardial infarction is sometimes suggested. Atrioventricular and interventricular conduction disturbances, including left axis deviation, are very common in some families.

Constrictive Cardiomyopathy

The patient who presents the findings of high venous pressure, severe right-sided failure, and clear lung fields, with only modest cardiomegaly immediately suggests constrictive pericarditis. Deep x and y waves in the jugular venous pulse, an inspiratory rise in jugular venous pressure, small paradoxical arterial pulse, and a triple rhythm offer supportive evidence. Cardiac catheterization may confirm the analysis of the venous pulse and reveals the sharp early diastolic dip and high plateau typical of constrictive pericarditis. Nonetheless, the pericardium may be perfectly normal. A number of such patients have come to autopsy.[86,87] There is extensive fibrosis scattered throughout the deep layers of the myocardium, especially in the subendocardium. Endocardial fibrosis is prominent but variable. In some hearts there is evidence of inflammatory disease, and the findings are apparently one end result of acute myocarditis. In others there are no such clues to causes. The clinical separation of this type of patient from the myocardosis group is not absolute. Some patients with large dilated hearts have additional evidence suggesting an element of inflow obstruction. Others have shown, in the course of time, a transition between the myocardosis and constrictive pictures, presumably due to gradually increasing fibroplastic proliferation.[88] Occasionally extensive fibrosis due to coronary arteriosclerosis will be reflected in a similar manner. Endocardial fibroelastosis in children and extensive amyloid infiltration are also proved causes.

In brief, the clinical picture of constrictive cardiomyopathy is a nonspecific hemodynamic pattern of diverse causation. The task of the physician is to distinguish the surgically curable lesion of constrictive pericarditis from the untreatable PMD. There are several aids. Although pulsus paradoxus may be a feature of both, pulsus alternans is strong evidence of a myocardial fault. The gallop sound of PMD is usually lower-pitched, is heard later, and lacks the snapping quality of pericardial "knock." The x-ray will not show pericardial calcification. The ECG tends to exhibit more left ventricular voltage in PMD. Cardiac catheterization may also show some differential features: there is a tendency toward a high A wave in the right atrial tracing in PMD but a sharp X descent in pericarditis. The left atrial pressure usually exceeds the right by 12 mm or more in PMD, but atrial pressures are nearly equal in constrictive pericarditis. In PMD the cardiac output tends to be very low, with a wide A-V oxygen difference, while in pericarditis the output is usually normal with a small A-V oxygen difference. The pulmonary vascular resistance is usually slightly elevated in PMD and normal in pericarditis.[59,89] None of these features is absolute, and biopsy of the pericardium or myocardium or surgical exploration may be necessary.

SECONDARY MYOCARDIAL DISEASE (SMD)

Of the numerous systemic diseases involving the myocardium, only the collagenoses, sarcoid, and amyloid will be mentioned here. The rest are discussed elsewhere (see Chaps. 36, 55, and 61).

Congestive heart failure is rarely, if ever, the only manifestation of collagen disease. In disseminated lupus erythematosus, for example, there is almost always rash, arthralgia, arthritis, effusions into pleural, joint, or pericardial cavities, renal abnormalities, or fever to suggest this entity. Nevertheless, focal myocarditis, fine scarring, and even fibrinoid necrosis are found in the majority of patients at autopsy.[99] The ECG is not distinctive. Clinical similarity to acute rheumatic fever may be striking. Heart failure may be a late feature of the disease. Cardiomegaly, however, is more often due to pericardial effusion than to myocardial involvement or Libman-Sacks endocarditis.

Weiss et al. pointed out that cardiac manifestations, such as orthopnea, dyspnea, cardiomegaly, and ST-T wave changes in the ECG were common manifestations in advanced scleroderma.[91] The pathologic condition is characterized by diffuse scarring or infiltration with granulation tissue. Death due to heart failure is rare but has been recorded. The scarring apparently does not prevent considerable dilatation in some cases. It may, in others, be sufficient to cause hemodynamic evidence of inflow obstruction, electrocardiographic changes similar to myocardial infarction, or complete heart block. Heart weights are usually little increased.[92]

Pathologic changes consisting mainly of interstitial collections of lymphocytes and minimal patchy muscular degeneration have been described in dermatomyositis, but the author knows of no cardiac disability unequivocally linked to this disease.[93] The lesions in the myocardium sometimes found in periarteritis nodosa are usually the result of the arteritis rather than myocarditis.

Amyloid heart has more characteristic features and, unlike the collagen diseases, may present primarily as a myocardial problem (Fig. 50-6). It should be suspected in any patient, middle-aged or older, with ascites, anasarca, elevated venous pressure, and a heart only moderately enlarged. Any of the diseases in which secondary amyloidosis is liable to occur, such as severe rheumatoid arthritis or multiple myeloma, should alert the physician. Features of the nephrotic syndrome are also suspicious. There are a number of other suggestive signs and symptoms, which includes purpura, macroglossia, splenomegaly, hepatomegaly, bilateral carpal tunnel syndrome, skin deposits, and polyneuropathy. The ECGs are also unusual, exhibiting low voltage, left or right axis deviation, atypical left and/or right bundle branch block, and at times focal loss of precordial electromotive force suggesting myocardial infarction. Multiple myeloma and primary amyloidosis are so closely related that results of diagnostic laboratory tests for the former are found frequently in the latter.[94] These include Bence-Jones proteinuria, myeloma cells in bone marrow, skeletal lesions, and high gamma or M peaks in the electrophoretic pattern. The Congo red test is occasionally positive.

The cardiac silhouette on x-ray is not very large, and heart weights are usually from 400 to 600 Gm.[57] Atrial arrhythmias are common and are correlated with widespread deposits of amyloid in the walls of these chambers. Classic angina pectoris is probably related to extensive infiltration into the walls of small arteries, although the lumen is usually fairly well preserved. A diffusion defect is possibly at fault and enhanced by the amyloid material encasing individual muscle fibers. Amyloid infiltration is another process which may cause the constrictive cardiomyopathy hemodynamic pattern.[95] Definitive premortem diagnosis is established most firmly by biopsy. Various sites are favored: rectal or buccal mucosa, tongue, kidney, or liver.

There are five clinical manifestations of cardiovascular sarcoid. The most common is that of cor pulmonale secondary to advanced pulmonary sarcoidosis. On rare occasions, congestive heart failure, due solely to extensive myocardial infiltration, may take place. To make this diagnosis, one must be able to exclude cor pulmonale. This can usually be done on clinical grounds. The ECG and chest x-ray are usually adequate laboratory aids but may be fortified by cardiac catheterization and pulmonary function studies. The most common and most distinctive evidence of myocardial sarcoidosis is complete heart block with Stokes-Adams seizures. It is present in about a third of cases where this is proved at necropsy. The evidence of sarcoid elsewhere in the body is occasionally scanty, but this is not usually true.[96] Arrhythmias are the second most common manifestation of myocardial infiltration, ventricular tachycardia being the most serious one. Sudden death may apparently be due to either heart block or arrhythmia. Finally, one might list

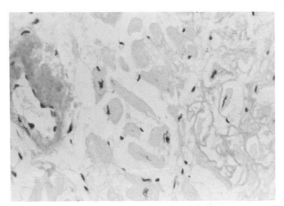

Fig. 50-6. Section through the myocardium of a seventy-two-year-old Negro woman who died from primary amyloidosis. Typical angina pectoris was present. An intramural artery whose wall is heavily infiltrated with amyloid is seen on the extreme left. In the center are relatively normal muscle fibers. On the right muscle fibers have largely disappeared. Their shrunken and distorted outlines are formed by strands of amyloid. A few atrophied fibers completely surrounded by amyloid are still visible. (A-1158, *Department of Pathology, Medical College of Georgia, courtesy of Dr. J. Robert Teabeaut.*)

the occasional ECG in sarcoid which seems diagnostic of anterior or anterolateral infarction.[97]

In view of the frequency of sudden death in myocardial sarcoidosis, ECGs should be taken frequently and steroid therapy instituted at the first hint of cardiac involvement. A remarkable disappearance of the infarction picture following steroids has been recorded.[97] The author has seen complete heart block disappear also, but this complication carries such a poor prognosis with medical therapy that one wonders if an artificial pacemaker should not be implanted as soon as it is recognized.

REFERENCES

1. Blankenhorn, M. A., and Gall, E. A.: Myocarditis and Myocardosis: A Clinicopathological Appraisal, *Circulation,* 13:217–223, 1956.
2. de la Chapelle, C., and Kossman, C. E.: Myocarditis, *Circulation,* 10:747–765, 1954.
3. Weinstein, L.: Cardiovascular Manifestations in Some of the Common Infectious Diseases, *Mod. Concepts Cardiovas. Dis.,* 23:229–233, 1954.
4. Wesselhoeft, C.: Cardiovascular Disease in Diphtheria: Report on Medical Progress, Communicable Diseases, *New England J. Med.,* 223:57–66, 1940.
5. Gould, S. E.: "Pathology of the Heart," 2d ed. Charles C Thomas, Publisher, Springfield, Ill., 1960, p. 813.
6. Teloh, H. A.: Myocarditis in Poliomyelitis, *A.M.A. Arch. Path.,* 55:408–411, 1953.

7. Rosenbaum, M. B., and Alvarez, A. I.: The Electrocardiogram in Chronic Chagasic Myocarditis, *Am. Heart J.,* **50:**492–527, 1955.

8. Wesselhoeft, C.: Cardiovascular Disease in Diphtheria, *New England J. Med.;* **223:**785, 1940.

9. Kline, I. K., and Saphir, O.: Chronic Pernicious Myocarditis, *Am. Heart J.,* **59:**681–697, 1960.

10. Long, W. H.: Granulamatous (Fiedler's) Myocarditis with Extracardiac Involvement: A Case Report with Sudden Death, *J.A.M.A.,* **177:**184–186, 1961.

11. French, A. J., and Wellen, C. V.: Interstitial Myocarditis Following the Clinical and Experimental Use of Sulfonamide Drugs, *Am. J. Path.,* **18:**109–121, 1942.

12. Grosberg, S. J., and Gerstl, B.: Basophilic Myocarditis: Report of a Case, *Arch. Int. Med.,* **108:**599–605, 1961.

13. Tlusty, T.: Idiopathic Myocarditis Involving the Bundle of His, *Brit. Heart J.,* **21:**145–148, 1959.

14. Hayes, J. A.: Isolated Myocarditis of the Right Ventricle, *Brit. Heart J.,* **23:**473–476, 1961.

15. Silber, E. N.: Respiratory Viruses and Heart Disease, *Ann. Int. Med.,* **48:**228–241, 1958.

16. Haskin, M. E., Kricheff, I., Sackner, M. A., and Widman, B. P.: Idiopathic Myocardial Hypertrophy, *Am. J. Roentgenol.,* **86:**1073–1082, 1961.

17. Freundlich, E., Berkowitz, M., Elkon, A., and Wilder, A.: Primary Interstitial Myocarditis: Report of an Epidemic Outbreak, *A.M.A. Am. J. Dis. Child.,* **96:**43–50, 1958.

18. Oseasohn, R., Adelson, L., and Kaji, M.: Clinicopathologic Study of 33 Fatal Cases of Asian Influenza, *New England J. Med.,* **260:**509–518, 1959.

19. Sanders, V.: Viro Myocarditis, *Am. Heart J.,* **66:**707–713, 1963.

20. Kaplan, M. H.: Studies of an Antigen in Cell Walls of Group A Streptococci Possessing an Immunologic Relationship to Human Heart, *J. Clin. Invest.,* **41:**1370, 1962 (Abstract).

21. Felknor, G. E., and Pullen, R. L.: Mumps Myocarditis: Review of Literature and Report of a Case, *Am. Heart J.,* **31:**238–241, 1946.

22. Guistra, F. X., and Nilsson, D. C.: Myocarditis Following Measles, *A.M.A. Am. J. Dis. Child.,* **79:**487–490, 1950.

23. Logue, R. B., Hanson, J. F.: Complete Heart Block in German Measles, *Am. Heart J.,* **30:**205–207, 1945.

24. Ross, E., and Armentrout, S. A.: Myocarditis Associated with Rabies: Report of a Case, *New England J. Med.,* **266:**1087–1089, 1962.

25. Woodward, T. E., McCrumb, F. R., Jr., Carey, T. N., and Togo, Y.: Viral and Rickettsial Causes of Cardiac Disease Including the Coxsackie Virus Etiology of Pericarditis and Myocarditis, *Ann. Int. Med.,* **53:**1130–1150, 1960.

26. Sprague, H. B., Clark, W. H.: Varicella and Heart Failure in an Adult, *New England J. Med.,* **268:**488–494, 1963.

27. Fish, M., and Barton, H. R.: Heart Involvement in Infectious Mononucleosis, *A.M.A. Arch. Int. Med.,* **101:**636–644, 1958.

28. Finlay-Jones, L. R.: Fatal Myocarditis after Vaccination against Smallpox, *New England J. Med.,* **270:**41–42, 1964.

29. Saphir, O.: Encephalomyocarditis, *Circulation,* **6:**843–850, 1952.

30. Coltman, C. A., Jr.: Influenza Myocarditis: Report of a Case with Observations on Serum Glutamic Oxaloacetic Transaminase, *J.A.M.A.,* **180:**204–208, 1962.

31. Dolgopol, V. B., and Cragan, M. D.: Myocardial Changes in Poliomyelitis, *A.M.A. Arch. Path.,* **46:**202–211, 1948.

32. Jungeblut, C. W., and Edwards, J. E.: Isolation of Poliomyelitis Virus from Heart in Fatal Cases, *Am. J. Clin. Path.,* **21:**601–623, 1951.

33. Angelini, F., Marioni, R., and Ugolini, A.: ECG Signs of Myocardial Damage. Right Atrial Strain and Ventricular Strain in Poliomyelitis, *Aggiorn. pediat.* 11/12:739–746, 1960, Abstracted in *Excerpta Med., Cardiovasc. Dis.,* **6:**719, 1962.

34. Glajchen, D.: Myocarditis Due to Coxsackie Virus Infection in an Adult, *Brit. M. J.,* **2:**870–871, 1961.

35. Domok, I., and Molnar, E.: An Outbreak of Meningoencephalomyocarditis among Newborn Infants during Epidemic of Bornholm Disease of 1958 in Hungary: Aetiological Findings, *Ann. paediat.,* **194:**102–104, 1960.

36. Javett, S. N., Heymann, S., Mundel, B., Pepler, W. J., Lurie, H. I., Gear, J., Measrock, V., and Kirsch, Z.: Myocarditis in the Newborn Infant: A Study of an Outbreak Associated with Coxsackie Group B Virus Infections in a Maternity Home in Johannesburg, *J. Pediat.,* **48:**1–22, 1956.

37. Kibrick, S. and Benirschke, K.: Severe Generalized Disease (Encephalohepatomyocarditis) Occurring in the Newborn Period and Due to Infection with Coxsackie Virus, Group B, *Pediatrics,* **22:**857–875, 1958.

38. Saphir, O.: Isolated Myocarditis, *Am. Heart J.,* **24:**167–181, 1942.

39. Saphir, O.: Myocardial Lesions in Subacute Bacterial Endocarditis, *Am. J. Path.,* **11:**143–156, 1935.

40. Brody, H., and Smith, L. W.: Visceral Pathology in Scarlet Fever and Related Streptococcus Infections, *Am. J. Path.,* **12:**373–394, 1936.

41. Claman, H. N.: Progressive Myocardial Damage Following Recovery from Diphtheria: A Case Showing Development of Complete Heart Block, *Am. J. Cardiol.,* **9:**790–794, 1962.

42. Hoel, J., and Berg, A. H.: Persistent Diphtheritic Heart Disorders: A Follow-up Investigation, *Acta med. scandinav.,* **145:**393–405, 1953.

43. Butler, S., and Levine, S. A.: Diphtheria as a Cause of Late Heart Block, *Am. Heart J.,* **5:**592–598, 1930.

44. Gray, D. F., Moore, B. S., and Phillips, W. F.: Trichinosis with Neurologic and Cardiac Involve-

ment: Review of Literature and Report of Three Cases, *Ann. Int. Med.*, **57**:230–244, 1962.

45. Mainzer, F.: Electrocardiographic Study of Typhoid Myocarditis, *Brit. Heart J.*, **9**:145–153, 1947.

46. Contro, S., and Mond, E.: Electrocardiogram in Hypersensitivity Reactions, *Am. Heart J.*, **52**:510–520, 1956.

47. Rich, A. R.: The Role of Hypersensitivity in Periarteritis Nodosa, *Johns Hopkins Hosp. Bull.*, **71**: 123, 1942.

48. Rich, A. R., and Gregory, J. E.: Experimental Anaphylactic Lesions of the Coronary Arteries of the "Sclerotic" Type, Commonly Associated with Rheumatic Fever and Disseminated Lupus Erythematosis, *Johns Hopkins Hosp. Bull.*, **81**:312, 1947.

49. MacGregor, G. A., and Vallance-Owen, J.: Cardiac Involvement in Anaphylactoid Purpura, *Lancet*, **2**: 572, 1957.

50. Felder, S. L., and Felder, L.: Unusual Reaction to Penicillin, *J.A.M.A.*, **143**:361–362, 1950.

51. French, A. J., and Weller, C. V.: Interstitial Myocarditis Following the Clinical and Experimental Use of Sulfonamide Drugs, *Am. J. Path.*, **18**:109–118, 1942.

52. Roussak, N. J.: Myocardial Infarction during Serum Sickness, *Brit. Heart J.*, **16**:218–223, 1954.

53. Milne, M. D.: Unusual Case of Coronary Thrombosis, *Brit. M. J.*, **1**:1123, 1949.

54. Sackner, M. A., Lewis, D. H., Robinson, M. J., and Beller, S.: Idiopathic Myocardial Hypertrophy: A Review, *Am. J. Cardiol.*, **7**:714–723, 1961.

55. Elster, S. K., Horn, H., and Tuchman, L. R.: Cardiac Hypertrophy and Insufficiency of Unknown Etiology, *Am. J. Med.*, **18**:900–922, 1955.

56. Spodick, D. H., and Littmann, D.: Idiopathic Myocardial Hypertrophy, *Am. J. Cardiol.*, **1**: p. 610–623, 1958.

57. Brogden, W. W.: Cardiomyopathies, Lancet, **2**: 1179, 1243, 1957.

58. Fowler, N. O., Gueron, M., and Rowlands, D. T., Jr.: Primary Myocardial Disease, *Circulation*, **23**: 498–508, 1961.

59. Dye, C. L., Rosenbaum, D., Lowe, J. C., Behnke, R. H., and Genovese, P. D.: Primary Myocardial Disease: Hemodynamic Alterations, *Ann. Int. Med.*, **58**:442–453, 1963.

60. Bloomfield, D. K., and Liebman, J.: Idiopathic Cardiomyopathy in Children, *Circulation*, **27**:1071–1078, 1963.

61. Fowler, N. O., Gueron, M., and Rowlands, D. T., Jr.: Primary Myocardial Disease, *Dis. Chest*, **41**: 593–602, 1963.

62. Flynn, J. E., and Mann, F. D.: The Presence and Pathogenesis of Endocardial and Subendocardial Degeneration, Mural Thrombi and Thromboses of the Thespian Veins in Cardiac Failure from Causes Other than Myocardial Infarction, *Am. Heart J.*, **31**: 757–768, 1946.

63. Sanders, V.: Idiopathic Disease of the Myocardium, *Arch. Int. Med.*, **112**:661–676, 1963.

64. Burch, G. E., Walsh, J. J., and Black, W. L.: Value of Prolonged Bed Rest in Management of Cardiomegaly, *J.A.M.A.*, **183**:81–87, 1963.

65. Black-Schaffer, B.: Infantile Endocardial Fibroelastosis: A Suggested Etiology, *A.M.A. Arch. Path.*, **63**:281–306, 1957.

66. Burch, G. E., Ray, C. T., and Cronvich, J. A.: Certain Mechanical Peculiarities of the Human Cardiac Pump in Normal and Diseased States, *Circulation*, **5**:504–513, 1952.

67. Benchimol, A. B., and Schlesinger, P.: Beriberi Heart Disease, *Am. Heart J.*, **46**:245–263, 1953.

68. Higginson, J., Gillanders, A. D., and Murray, J. F.: The Heart in Chronic Malnutrition, *Brit. Heart J.*, **14**:213–223, 1952.

69. Sanders, C. V.: Primary Myocardial Disease: The Presence of Bound Gamma Globulin in Ventricular Muscle, *Circulation*, **28**:797, 1963 (Abstract).

70. Evans, W.: Alcoholic Cardiomyopathy, *Am. Heart J.*, **61**:556–567, 1961.

71. Regan, T. J., Moschos, C. B., and Hellems, H. K.: Ethanol-induced Alteration of Myocardial Metabolism and Function, *Circulation*, **28**:788, 1963 (Abstract).

72. Degerli, I. U., and Webb, W. R.: Ethyl Alcohol: Its Effect on Coronary Flow and Myocardial Capacity, *Circulation*, **28**:709, 1963 (Abstract).

73. Meadows, W. R.: Idiopathic Myocardial Failure in the Last Trimester of Pregnancy and the Puerperium, *Circulation*, **15**:903–914, 1957.

74. Burch, G. E., and Walsh, J. J.: Myocarditis, Postpartal Heart Disease (Editorial), *Arch. Int. Med.*, **108**:817–822, 1961.

75. Benchimol, A. B., Carneiro, R. D., and Schlesinger, P.: Post Partum Heart Disease, *Brit. Heart J.*, **21**: 89–100, 1959.

76. Hull, E., and Hidden, E.: Postpartal Heart Failure, *South. M. J.*, **31**:265–275, 1938.

77. Evans, W.: Familial Cardiomegaly, *Brit. Heart J.*, **11**:68–82, 1949.

78. Whitfield, A. G.: Familial Cardiomyopathy, *Quart. J. Med.*, **30**:119–134, 1961.

79. Beasley, O. C., Jr.: Familial Myocardial Disease: A Report of Three Siblings and a Review of the Literature, *Am. J. Med.*, **29**:476–485, 1960.

80. Pierce, J. A., Price, B. O., and Joyce, J. W.: Familial Occurrence of Postpartal Heart Failure, *Arch. Int. Med.*, **111**:651–655, 1963.

81. Nikkilä, E. A., and Pelkonen, R.: Isolated (Fiedler's) Myocarditis and Idiopathic Cardiac Hypertrophy, *Acta med. scandinav.*, **165**:421–430, 1959.

82. Nadas, A.: "Pediatric Cardiology," 2d ed., W. B. Saunders, Philadelphia, 1963, p. 289.

83. Battersby, E. J., and Glenner, G. G.: Familial Cardiomyopathy, *Am. J. Med.*, **30**:382–391, 1961.

84. Kiloh, L. G., and Nevin, S.: Pseudohypertrophic Muscular Dystrophy with Cardiomegaly, *Proc. Roy. Soc. Med.*, **44**:694, 1951.

85. Roth, M.: On a Possible Relationship between He-

reditary Ataxia and Peroneal Muscular Atrophy, *Brain*, 71:416–433, 1948.

86. Balchum, O. J., McCord, M. C., and Blount, S. G.: The Clinical and Hemodynamic Pattern in Nonspecific Myocarditis: A Comparison with Other Entities also Impairing Myocardial Efficiency, *Am. Heart J.*, 52:430–443, 1956.

87. Wiener, M. J., and Knights, E. M., Jr.: Loffler's Endocarditis Parietalis Fibroplastica with Eosinophilia, *Am. Heart J.*, 53:157–161, 1957.

88. Goodwin, J. F., Gordon, H., Hollman, A., and Bishop, M. B.: Clinical Aspects of Cardiomyopathy, *Brit. M. J.*, 1:69–79, 1961.

89. Robin, E. D., and Burwell, C. S.: Hemodynamic Aspects of Diffuse Myocardial Fibrosis, *Circulation*, 16:730–735, 1957.

90. Taubenhaus, M., Eisenstein, B., and Pick, A.: Cardiovascular Manifestation of Collagen Diseases, *Circulation*, 12:903–920, 1955.

91. Weiss, S., Stead, E. A., Jr., Warren, J. V., and Bailey, O. T.: Scleroderma Heart Disease with Considerations of Certain Other Visceral Manifestations of Scleroderma, *A.M.A. Arch. Int. Med.*, 71:749–776, 1943.

92. East, T., and Oram, S.: The Heart in Scleroderma, *Brit. Heart J.*, 9:167–174, 1947.

93. Kinney, T. D., and Maher, M. M.: Dermatomyositis: A Study of Five Cases, *Am. J. Path.*, 16:561–594, 1940.

94. Kyle, R. A., and Bayrd, E. D.: Primary Amyloidosis and Myeloma: Discussion of Relationship and Review of 81 Cases, *Arch. Int. Med.*, 107:344–353, 1961.

95. Gunnar, R., Dillon, R. F., Wallyn, R. J., and Elisberg, E.: The Physiological and Clinical Similarity between Primary Amyloid of the Heart and Constrictive Pericarditis, *Circulation*, 12:827–832, 1955.

96. O'Phinney, A. O.: Sarcoid of the Myocardial Septum with Complete Heart Block: Report of Two Cases, *Am. Heart J.*, 62:270–276, 1961.

97. Porter, G. H.: Sarcoid Heart Disease, *New England J. Med.*, 263:1350–1357, 1960.

51 ENDOCARDITIS

Edward R. Dorney, M. D.

The endocardium and heart valves may be affected by a variety of diseases, congenital, infectious, immunologic, and endocrine. The pathologic spectrum includes ulceration, overgrowth of tissue, shortening or rupture of chordae tendineae and valves, and verrucus formation. Three entities, (1) bacterial endocarditis, (2) nonbacterial thrombotic endocarditis, and (3) Libman-Sacks endocarditis, are discussed in this chapter.

BACTERIAL ENDOCARDITIS

In the preantibiotic era, the course of bacterial endocarditis was one of unswerving progression to an inevitable conclusion. The natural history of the disease which presented a predictable sequence of signs and symptoms was exhaustively studied and accurately cataloged.[1-4] With the introduction of effective antibiotic therapy by Loewe et al. in 1944,[5] however, this pattern was interrupted, and early recognition, before the classic picture developed, became necessary. In addition to adequate therapy, the innovation of intracardiac surgical procedures in the past decade has further altered the picture of the disease, so that the classic clinical descriptions, classifications, and prognoses of the preantibiotic era no longer pertain.

Before treatment was available, the clinical distinction between acute and subacute bacterial endocarditis was primarily made by the survival time of the patient. Those surviving after 8 weeks were said to be subacute,[6] while those succumbing in less than 8 weeks were said to have been acute. Today, with adequate treatment, a survival of 65 to 80 per cent of all cases of endocarditis is expected in modern hospitals.[7-9] It is still possible to classify certain cases as acute because of fulminating onset or rapid progression, but it is not possible to predict which of the seemingly indolent cases will suddenly result in valve ulceration or crippling cerebral embolization.[10] One cannot consistently predict the severity of the disease from the type of bacteria involved.[8] In view of these facts, the distinction between acute and subacute bacterial endocarditis loses its clinical significance, since all cases should be considered imminently lethal and full therapy instituted as soon as the diagnosis is made.

Pathology

The basic lesion of bacterial endocarditis is a friable, verrucous vegetation which is engrafted on the surface of a heart valve, the endocardial lining of a heart chamber, or the endothelium of a blood vessel.[11] These vegetations usually are located in areas altered by rheumatic, congenital, or syphilitic heart disease but may also be found on apparently normal surfaces.[12,13]

The active vegetations are composed of three layers: The first or innermost layer is usually the thickest and accounts for three-fourths to seven-eighths of the entire vegetation. This layer is made up of platelets, fibrin, white blood cells, red blood cells, some bacteria, strands of collagen, and varying amounts of necrosis. The middle layer is primarily bacteria and the outer layer mostly fibrin with varying amounts of bacteria present.[11] As healing progresses there is a covering of the exposed areas of the vegetation with fibrous tissue, invasion and phagocytosis of the bacterial layer by leukocytes, calcification of some of the bacterial areas, and hyalinization and calcification of the necrotic innermost core of the vegetation.[14]

In the preantibiotic era the pathologic distinction between acute and subacute bacterial endocarditis was made by the size of the vegetation, the amount of necrosis present, and the presence or absence of prior endocardial disease, but the distinction was not always certain.[15] The use of potent antibiotics has made the differentiation even more tenuous because of the changes introduced by healing.[14,15]

Previous rheumatic endocarditis is the most common substrate for bacterial endocarditis. The mitral valve is the site most frequently involved, followed by the aortic, tricuspid, and pulmonic valves, in that order.[16] Involvement of these valves may result in perforation of the leaflets or in secondary spread of the infection to the chordae tendineae or papillary muscles with consequent necrosis and rupture. Vegetations large enough to cause obstruction to a valve orifice have been noted.[17] Extension into the aortic valve ring with abscess formation may result in fistulas between the aorta and the right ventricle or with either of the atria.

In congenital heart disease, the ventricular septal defect is the single defect most often involved and accounts for approximately 50 per cent of the cases. It is followed in frequency by the patent ductus arteriosus, pulmonic stenosis, and aortic stenosis.[5-7] Tetralogy of Fallot, before or after shunting procedures, is the most commonly involved of the cyanotic lesions and in some series ranks second only to the ventricular septal defect.[18-20] Atrial septal defects are seldom involved, and when endocarditis has been reported with this lesion, the vegetations are seen on the pulmonic and tricuspid valves.[21]

Postoperative endocarditis following finger fracture[22] of a valve, insertion of a plastic patch or valve leaflet, a stitch in the endocardium, or a Starr valve or other prosthesis has been reported.[22-25] Elek has shown that the presence of silk suture material reduces by 10,000 times the size of a bacterial inoculum needed to produce infection.[26]

Endocarditis has also been reported in association with coarctation of the aorta,[18] peripheral arteriovenous fistula,[27] aneurysm of the aorta,[28] and postinfarction mural thrombosis.[29] Cardiac lesions other than valvular or endocardial vegetations, such as valve ring abscess, myocarditis, or mural abscess, are less commonly seen. Myocarditis has taken the form of perivascular collections of lymphocytes,[30]

miliary infarctions,[31] or focal inflammatory reaction in the interstitial tissue[32] and is second in frequency only to the endocardial lesion. Valve ring abscess is easily overlooked at postmortem as stressed by Sheldon and Golden and may be more common than is actually reported.[33] It should be suspected in any case of continuing sepsis or recurrent disease despite adequate treatment. Pericardial involvement is rare and when present is usually the result of external rupture of a mural or valve ring abscess or secondary to uremia.[33a] Gross myocardial infarction due to embolization of a major coronary artery has been reported.[34]

The Bracht-Wächter body has been interpreted as being pathognomic of bacterial endocarditis. This is a collection of lymphocytes in the myocardium and is not specific for the disease.[15]

The Osler node, a painful, red, indurated area appearing usually in the pads of the fingers or toes and lasting for several hours to several days, is made up of an endothelial swelling and perivasculitis of the small vessels just below the Malpighian layer of the skin. These lesions are of uncertain origin, do not ulcerate, and are considered to be nonbacterial.[35] Janeway's lesion is a painless, hemorrhagic nodular lesion found in the palm of the hand and on the soles of the feet. These lesions show a definite tendency to ulceration, and biopsy material has demonstrated polymorphonuclear infiltration of the capillaries surrounding tissues with marked necrosis. Bacteria have been cultured from the area of these lesions which were identical to those found in the blood.[35]

Because of the central location in the circulation of the primary lesion and the friable structural characteristics of the endocardial vegetations, peripheral arterial embolism is a common finding in bacterial endocarditis. Embolization may continue for several months after bacteriologic cure.[7] Bland and septic infarction and abscess formation have been reported in all the organs of the body and are most commonly recognized in the kidney, brain, and spleen.

Bacterial embolization to the walls of small arteries may result in mycotic aneurysms ranging in size from 1 to 2 millimeters to several centimeters.[35] These lesions may destroy a vital organ such as the brain by hemorrhage or may cause death by exsanguination.[8]

In addition to gross renal infarction secondary to embolization of a major branch of a renal artery, glomerulitis most likely due to microembolization of bacteria and also glomerulonephritis indistinguishable from acute glomerulonephritis were common findings in the preantibiotic era.[36] They are seen today in long-standing untreated cases of endocarditis and in those which have been inadequately treated. Bell's feeling that the microembolic nephritis results from bacterial embolization and capillary breakdown rather than from thrombotic embolization is supported by the finding of this type of lesion in bacterial endocarditis with involvement of the right side of the heart alone.[36]

Pathogenesis

The question of why endocarditis develops in certain patients with rheumatic valvular or congenital cardiovascular disease while in others with similar lesions it does not is largely unanswered. It does seem, from the experimental work of Highman and Altland,[37] which demonstrated increased susceptibility to endocarditis in rats subjected to high altitudes in a pressure chamber, the similar

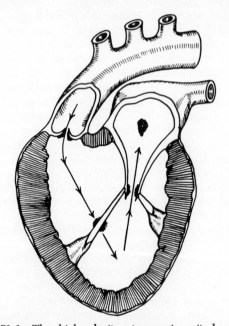

Fig. 51-1. The high-velocity streams in mitral and aortic insufficiency and sites of endocarditic lesions. The arrow at the left indicates a high arterial pressure that generates regurgitant flow from aorta to ventricle. The vena contracta and the endocarditins lesions appear at the ventricular surface of the aortic valves. The stream through the incompetent aortic valve may produce lesions on the chordae tendineae of the aortic leaf of the mitral valve. If the mitral valves cannot seat properly during ventricular systole, the regurgitant stream (arrow at right) will pass to the sink of the left atrium, and endocarditis will tend to become engrafted on the atrial surface of the mitral valve. The atrial endocardium in line with the regurgitant jet stream may show a fibrous reaction. (*Reproduced by permission of the author and the American Heart Association, Inc., from Rodbard, S.: Blood Velocity and Endocarditis, Circulation, 27:18, 1963.*)

experiences of Nedzel[38] with the use of Pitressin, and the observations of Allen and Sirota[39] and those of Angrist and Marquiss,[40] that many factors in addition to bacteremia and cardiac deformities are involved. Lillehei has shown that the creation of a large peripheral arteriovenous fistula will lead to valvular endocarditis in 75 per cent of dogs surviving for 4 weeks.[41] Chronic impairment of cardiac lymphatic flow has been recently demonstrated to make the dog particularly susceptible to the development of endocarditis after injection of staphylococci.[42]

There is good evidence to show that transient bacteremia is a common day-to-day occurrence.[43] Various writers have attempted to establish a possible source of bacteremia in bacterial endocarditis with about a 40 per cent result in the series studied. Bacteremia secondary to tooth extraction, cleaning, and filling has been frequently noted.[44,44a] Bacteremia has been reported with genitourinary manipulations[45-47] such as prostatic massage, catheterization, or cystoscopy or after normal obstetrical deliveries,[48] with upper respiratory infections, and with pyoderma. In recent years bacteremia following cardiac surgical procedure or cardiac catheterization has also become important. The self-administration of narcotics by the intravenous route is a common precipitating cause in endocarditis, particularly that of the variety restricted to the right side of the heart.[49,49a]

Areas of localization of vegetations within the heart are remarkably constant and have been the basis for the main theories concerning the pathogenesis of the disease itself. The lesions are found on the ventricular surface of the aortic valve in aortic insufficiency with satellite lesions in the anteromedial leaflet of the mitral valve, the chordae tendineae, and papillary muscles. They are found on the coapting surfaces of the mitral valve on the atrial side in mitral insufficiency with some extension to the atrial wall where the regurgitant jet impinges. In ventricular septal defects, they may be on the defect itself but frequently involve the area of the jet lesion on the right ventricular wall or the septal leaflet of the tricuspid valve (Fig. 51-1).

There have been many theories advanced to explain this localization of lesions. It has been suggested that trauma in the area of impingement of the valves with the increased pressure applied to the surfaces forces bacteria into the endothelium,[16] or that exposure to a greater volume impact of the bloodstream against the damaged valve may be responsible.[50] There are other suggestions well described elsewhere that have merit in individual cases but do not explain the majority of instances.[15]

Recently Rodbard has proposed that a high-velocity flow from an area of increased pressure through a narrowed orifice into a low-pressure area results in the destruction of laminar flow just distal to the orifice.[51] This results in disruption of the endothelial nutrition in the area and at the same time increases the local bacterial count, thereby setting the stage for infection. He has devised an ingenious set of experiments which lends considerable credence to his theory. His model would also explain the endocarditis on the aortic valve in syphilitic disease when the pathologic lesion is in the valve ring and localization of the bacterial implants in congenital heart disease such as bicuspid aortic valve when the valve surfaces remain intact (Fig. 51-2).

Organisms Involved

Bacterial endocarditis is not a reportable disease, and the overall incidence cannot be accurately estimated. Reports from several large institutions as tabulated by Kerr and others show a variation of from 1 in 1,000 admissions to 1 in 6,000 admissions.[52,10]

Actually this disease should no longer be termed bacterial endocarditis, since it has now been proved due to various forms of fungi and to *Rickettsia*[53-62] as well as bacteria. It would be more descriptive to use the term endocarditis preceded by the name of the appropriate microorganism.

Thayer[63] in 1931 reported a representative series of 536 cases of proved bacterial endocarditis. His statistics showed a 62.5 per cent incidence of streptococci (all types), 14.7 per cent due to pneumococcus, 12.5 per cent due to staphylococcus, and 6.9 per cent due to gonococcus. With the advent of antibiotics and the reduction of the mortality rate from 98 per cent plus to 30 per cent, the comparative incidence of bacteria has been difficult to tabulate, since postmortem studies are no longer representative of the disease as a clinical entity. In addition, during this period most writers have reported under the heading of *subacute* bacterial endocarditis, thereby weighing the frequency of organism occurrence toward the less virulent streptococcus viridans.[10,64] Several recent reports tabulating both clinical and pathologic material and including all infectious endocarditis seen at various teaching hospitals are now available.[8,13,65-69] All these series obtained during the antibiotic era have shown a marked reduction in the occurrence of the pneumococcus and gonococcus as compared to that of Thayer[63] with a concomitant increase in the frequency of staphylococcal infection. Several of these writers[7,8,69] have also shown that the streptococcus faecalis has become the third most common organism, exceeded only by the streptococcus viridans and staphylococci. This increase in frequency of

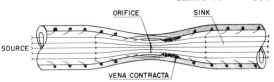

Fig. 51-2. Flow through a permeable tube. A high-pressure source (at left) drives fluid through an orifice into a low-pressure sink. The curved arrows leaving the stream and entering the wall in the upstream segment represent the normal perfusion of the lining layer. Velocity is maximal, and perfusing pressure is low immediately beyond the orifice where the momentum of the stream converges the streamlines to form a vena contracta. The low pressure in this segment results in reduced perfusion and may cause a retrograde flow from the deeper layers of the vessel into the flowing stream. (*Reproduced by permission of the author and the American Heart Association, Inc., from Rodgard, S.: Blood Velocity and Endocarditis, Circulation* 27:18, 1963.)

the streptococcus faecalis has also been noted by others.[45,52,70] Although the streptococcus faecalis has a tendency to produce green hemolysis on blood agar, it can be differentiated from the streptococcus viridans by its ability to grow in 6.5 per cent saline agar. Despite this fact, the streptococcus faecalis has been included in the streptococcus viridans group by many writers, among them Thayer[63] and Wilson.[65] It should, however, be considered as a separate entity because of its growth characteristics in culture, its resistance to antibiotics, and the clinical picture which it produces.

The increasing importance of the group with consistently negative blood cultures but with clinical and pathologic evidence of bacterial endocarditis has been recently emphasized.[7,8,66,71] This group accounted for 13 per cent of the series of Vogler, Dorney, and Bridges[8] and 16 per cent of Morgan and Bland.[7]

Wilson,[65] Kerr,[52] and Afremow[10] have noted the overall decrease in the frequency of bacterial endocarditis since the introduction of antibiotics. The reasons for this decrease in occurrence and the change in bacteria involved are multiple. Adequate antibiotic prophylaxis following genitourinary, obstetric, and gynecologic procedures and during dental manipulations has undoubtedly cut down on bacteremia and implantation of the more sensitive streptococci.[44a,48] It may be that the decrease in rheumatic endocarditis noted during the same period is responsible for the reduction of streptococcus viridans endocarditis, since it represents the common substrate for this particular organism. Penicillin therapy of pneumonia has reduced the frequency and severity of pneumococcal infections and has also afforded control of the gonococcus. At the same time the indiscriminate use of antibiotics has encouraged the emergence of antibiotic-resistant strains, the overgrowth of Gram-negative bacteria,[25,72] and the development of fungi. The aging population with the increasing frequency of long hospitalizations and genitourinary manipulations has favored the development of endocarditis on normal heart valves by the more invasive organisms such as staphylococcus and streptococcus faecalis.[45,52,73,74]

The introduction of cardiac surgical procedures has undoubtedly affected the prevalence of some organisms. Hoffman has estimated that the occurrence of endocarditis after finger fracture of the mitral or aortic valve would average about 1 per cent and the organism involved is most often staphylococcus.[22] Open-heart surgical procedure with placement of prosthetic valves, suture material, or endocardial patches results in a still higher percentage of infection than the closed techniques. Geraci et al. have recently estimated that the incidence of infection is about 10 per cent of the patients having had partial or total prosthetic valve replacement.[24] *Pseudomonas aeruginosa*,[24,25] *Staphylococcus*[24] *aureus*, and *S. albus* and a variety of fungi[24,55] are prevalent on the postoperative-pump group. Bacteria usually considered to be nonpathogenic (*Achromobacter*[75] and *S. albus*) have also been reported in this circumstance. Streptococcus viridans is rarely encountered in postoperative material.

Clinical Picture

The similarity of bacterial endocarditis to other diseases, severe and insignificant, together with the lack of definitive signs and symptoms early in the disease, makes the diagnosis difficult. Friedberg has found the diagnosis of virus infection or influenza made commonly in the first few weeks of illness.[76] To this should be added the group of bacterial endocarditis presenting with signs of other catastrophic illnesses such as stroke, peripheral vascular occlusion, hemorrhage, congestive heart failure, or uremia in which the attention is directed away from the true cause of the disease and toward one of its manifestations.

Classically, bacterial endocarditis has been described as a disease in which a patient presents with an organic heart murmur, fever, splenomegaly, petechiae, and peripheral embolic manifestations. In a recent series of 148 cases collected by the author from the teaching hospitals of Emory University, 74 per cent had no evidence of embolization on admission, 60 per cent had no petechiae, 61 per cent had no splenomegaly, and 88 per cent had no clubbing of the fingers. Four per cent had no heart murmur.[8]

It would be better to think of bacterial endocarditis as a group of syndromes rather than a single stereotyped entity. The disease is caused by a variety of microorganisms, so that fever will be present to a greater or lesser degree depending upon the virulence of the particular organism and the quantity present in the blood at any given time.[77] In some there will be afebrile periods. Shaking chills and profuse sweats may be present, or there may be a feeling of lassitude and anorexia with no awareness of fever. A murmur is not always present early in the disease, and there are no infallible criteria which will distinguish the "functional," or "innocent," murmur from the sound caused by an organic deformity.[12,78–80] Arthralgias are common and septic arthritis has been seen.[81] Clubbing of the fingers is rare in cases which are treated early but may be found in as many as 25 per cent of patients later in the course of the disease.[67] In recent years Osler's nodes and Janeway's lesions have become relatively rare. Osler's nodes were seen only once in the author's series of cases, and Janeway's lesions were never seen.[8] Petechiae are found more frequently and tend to be located in the mucous membranes of the mouth, in the conjunctiva, in the necklace area, or about the wrists and ankles.[8,67] Splinter hemorrhages and small red to black streaks under the fingernails may be seen but are not diagnostic of the disease.[82] For example, these may be secondary to trauma, trichinosis, rheumatic fever, infectious mononucleosis, or cryoglobulinemia or may be without obvious cause. Roth's spots are hemorrhagic areas with a white center which are seen in the retina and the conjunctiva. These are seen late in the disease and are also seen in various forms of anemia and leukemia and in scurvy.[83]

Since the bacterial vegetations are located in the center of the circulation in left-sided endocarditis, embolic episodes may occur to any systemic artery. Abscess formation, hemorrhage, or infarction of various organs will again alter the clinical picture according to the organ involved and the type of involvement.

Neurologic Syndromes

Bacterial endocarditis may present as meningitis, subarachnoid hemorrhage, hemiplegia, coma, convulsions, or toxic psychosis, particularly in the older groups.[12,84] Particularly suspicious is sudden hemiplegia in young adults, brain abscesses in the presence of cyanotic congenital heart disease, or subarachnoid hemorrhage in a patient with a heart murmur. In pneumococcal pneumonia with meningitis, endocarditis of the aortic valve should be sought. It may occur in 25 to 30 per cent of cases.[85] Chorea has been reported.[86]

Hematologic Syndromes

A normochromic, normocytic anemia occurs in 60 to 70 per cent of cases of bacterial endocarditis.[87] Fever, anemia, and murmur should always suggest bacterial endocarditis. Murmur may be absent or "due to anemia." Blood cultures may be sterile or fever may be absent as a result of the indiscriminate use of antibiotics. The combination of fever, anemia, petechiae, and splenomegaly does not always mean primary hematologic disease, and when these signs are present, blood cultures should be taken.[88,89] Phagocytic monocytes may appear in the peripheral blood in great numbers in bacterial endocarditis.[87,90] Anemia, fever, and monocytes in the peripheral blood may suggest bacterial endocarditis rather than leukemia. Cultures are frequently negative when these cells are present.[91]

Peripheral Vascular Disease

The sudden onset of peripheral gangrene in a patient with fever and/or murmur may be due to bacterial endocarditis. Small emboli may lodge in terminal arterioles and produce gangrenous infarctions of various acral portions of the body (i.e., tip of the nose, pinna of the ear, fingers, and toes).[92] Larger emboli may present as peripheral vascular occlusions and simulate atherosclerotic occlusive disease.[93] When large emboli occur, it is wise to consider the possibility of endocarditis due to fungi.

Renal Involvement

The kidney is second only to the spleen in frequency of embolic involvement in bacterial endocarditis.[35,70] When renal infarction occurs in the presence of a heart murmur or fever, bacterial endocarditis should be suspected. Persistent hematuria is a helpful diagnostic point in the evaluation of fever and murmur. In the aged, the appearance of a syndrome simulating acute glomerulonephritis should start the search for a heart murmur or bacteremia.[78,94] Embolic glomerulonephritis may present with pyuria and hematuria and may be mistaken for pyelonephritis.

Splenic Infarction

The spleen is the most common site of embolic infarction in bacterial endocarditis.[70] Pain in the left upper quadrant with radiation to the left shoulder is the usual complaint. There may be local tenderness, abdominal rigidity, and friction rub. Rupture of the spleen may also occur.[8]

Cardiovascular Syndromes

The literature on bacterial endocarditis has referred to "changing murmurs" as a part of the diagnosis of this disease. It does not mean a change in the intensity of an already present murmur but the appearance of a new organic murmur such as that due to aortic insufficiency or mitral regurgitation. This is virtually diagnostic of bacterial endocarditis if it occurs with evidenc of acute sepsis.[78] In the presence of fever, rupture of a chorda tendinea or papillary muscle with the characteristic associated murmur or the appearance of a continuous murmur of aortic–right ventricular fistula has the same significance. Acute myocardial infarction occurring during a prolonged fever is strongly suggestive of bacterial endocarditis. The sudden appearance of congestive heart failure in a previously well-compensated case of rheumatic or congenital disease should suggest the need for blood cultures.

Pericarditis

Pericarditis is said to be rare in bacterial endocarditis.[95] It may occur, however, with staphylococcal infection, embolism to a coronary artery with myocardial infarction, uremic pericarditis, rupture of the mycotic aneurysm into the pericardial sac, and coexistent rheumatic carditis.

Right-sided Bacterial Endocarditis

When bacterial endocarditis is localized to the right side of the heart, murmurs are less common and are seen in only 35 per cent of cases.[96,97] Pulmonary symptoms such as cough and pleuritic pain are common, as are findings of consolidation, pleural friction rub, or pleural fluid.[97] Peripheral embolization is rare. Blood cultures will be positive as in left-sided endocarditis.[49a] Right-sided bacterial endocarditis should be suspected in narcotic addicts with septicemia and fever,[49,97] in infants with fever following septic skin lesions,[98] and in fever following cardiac surgical treatment.[99] A triad of heroin addiction, bacteremia, and pulmonary infarction in the absence of obvious cause is strongly suggestive of staphylococcal tricuspid endocarditis.[96]

Bacterial Endocarditis following Cardiac Surgical Procedure

Bacterial endocarditis following cardiac surgical treatment does not resemble the usual disease. Petechiae, peripheral emboli, and splenomegaly are rare. Anemia may be difficult to evaluate in the postsurgical state, and murmurs seldom change. Bacterial endocarditis should be suspected if fever persists, unexplained, after 5 to 7 days in the postoperative period or if it recurs 4 to 6 weeks after discharge from the hospital.[24,100,101] A syndrome of fever, lymphocytosis, and splenomegaly of unknown cause may rarely occur following open-heart surgical procedures using bypass techniques, and this may cause confusion with endocarditis.

Bacterial Endocarditis following Gynecologic and Genitourinary Procedures

Bacterial endocarditis should be suspected in any patient who sustains a persistent fever following a genitourinary or gynecologic procedure. The bacteria involved in these areas frequently attack normal valves, and a murmur may not be present initially.[12,45] The responsible organism is frequently the enterococcus. The occurrence of peripheral arterial occlusion in a postoperative patient with fever should direct attention to the possibility of bacterial endocarditis.[12] Unexplained persistent fever in the postpartum patient with a murmur suggests the need for blood cultures.

Chronic Disease

Fever occurring during the course of lymphoma, metastatic malignant disease, or myelofibrosis may be due to endocarditis.[12] The appearance of a new murmur, particularly of aortic insufficiency, along with fever is doubly significant.

Diagnosis

The single, most important factor in the diagnosis of bacterial endocarditis is a high index of suspicion. Once suspicion has been aroused, the next step in diagnosis is the procuring of blood cultures. When clinical findings suggest the disease, blood cultures should be drawn. Blood is best obtained from the antecubital vein, since it is easily available and since it has been shown that the bacterial yield of the venous blood from this source closely approximates that of arterial blood.[102–104] An occasional case will show a positive marrow culture when both venous and arterial blood are sterile.[102,105] Blood or marrow should be incubated in aerobic and anaerobic mediums for bacteria, and special culture techniques should also be carried out for fungi. Cultures should not be discarded before 3 weeks to allow for growth of some of the slower organisms such as the *Bacteroides* group, which might otherwise be overlooked.[106] Cultures are positive in bacterial endocarditis in from 60 to 90 per cent of cases reported depending upon the adequacy of the laboratory and the prior use of antibiotics. It has been demonstrated that the first four blood cultures will provide over 90 per cent of the positive returns and that usually all cultures or no cultures will be positive.[64,79,107] If antibiotics have been given prior to obtaining blood cultures, then more cultures will be required over a period of 2 to 3 days.[104] Penicillinase incorporated in the culture mediums will sometimes increase the yield of positive cultures.[44] Bacteremia in this disease is relatively constant, so that the time of the culture is not significant unless chills are occurring regularly.[104] In this case the bacteremia is usually heaviest approximately 1 hr prior to the chill.[46,104]

With the exception of the positive blood culture, the laboratory is of little aid in the diagnosis of bacterial endocarditis. Anemia may be found in up to 70 per cent of cases. The white blood cell count may be normal, low, or elevated. Normal counts are just as prevalent as elevated counts.[79] Sedimentation rate is elevated in 90 per cent of cases but is of no differential aid in the work-up of fever of unknown origin. Considerable attention has been given to the presence of phagocytic monocytes in the peripheral blood. These cells were first described by Van Nuys[108] and associated with bacterial endocarditis by Leede and Suntheim.[90] The cells are about 20 to 30 μ in diameter and have an abundant, finely reticulated cytoplasm and one or two large, oval nuclei. The cytoplasm may contain bacteria or red blood corpuscles in various stages of degeneration. They may be seen in the fingertip blood but are best obtained by ear lobe punctures.[90] According to Hill and Baird, these cells are most commonly seen in cases of endocarditis with negative blood cultures.[91] They are not diagnostic, however, and have been reported in septicemia without endocarditis, tuberculosis, rheumatic fever, or many other conditions.[90]

Since bacterial endocarditis may present in so many disguises and since blood cultures are not always positive, criteria must be set up for treatment without bacterial proof. Friedberg has said that "unexplained fever for more than a week or ten days in a patient with significant cardiac murmur should form the basis of a presumptive diagnosis of bacterial endocarditis."[76] He cautions against the overenthusiastic application of this principle, particularly in children, adolescents, and young adults. Such a decision to treat should not be made lightly, nor should the hunt for another cause of symptoms be abandoned because treatment for endocarditis has been decided upon. Once therapy is instituted, however, it should be carried out for its full duration unless it becomes obvious that the diagnosis of endocarditis is in error.

Treatment[66,109,110]

The treatment of bacterial endocarditis should be directed toward the immediate and total eradication of the infecting organism. To this end, killing doses of specific antibiotics should be given promptly and continued sufficiently long to ensure complete elimination of the bacteria without dependence on host factors.[111] Several principles should be kept in mind when approaching the problem:

1. Bactericidal agents should be used.[70] In this disease the morphologic structure of the vegetation

is such that the bacteria are inaccessible to the leukocytes which would ordinarily be expected to destroy them once growth had been inhibited by bacteriostatic agents.[77,112] When bacteriostatic wide-spectrum antibiotics are used, the bloodstream may be temporarily sterilized, but the colonies of bacteria remain deep within the vegetations and begin to multiply shortly after the treatment is discontinued. There is no place for the exclusive use of bacteriostatic agents in the treatment of bacterial endocarditis regardless of the in vitro sensitivity tests.[78,111]

2. The dose of antibiotics should be sufficiently high to effect a serum concentration at least four times greater than the concentration needed to kill the causative bacteria in vitro.[113] This may be tested by making serial dilutions of the patient's serum inoculated with approximately 50,000 organisms of a fresh young culture of his own bacteria. After 24 hr of incubation in a 5 per cent carbon dioxide atmosphere, the clear tubes are subcultured for 48 hr on semisolid thioglycolate medium.[113] This type of test is particularly helpful, since it has been demonstrated that there may be a total lack of correlation between the usual in vitro antibiotic-sensitivity tests and the results of therapy.[70,111,112,114] Sensitivity tests provide an optimal condition for the interaction of the drug and organism which does not exist in the patient. The end point of these tests may indicate bactericidal activity or merely inhibition of growth. These may be differentiated by subculturing the apparently clear tubes. This method may be used as a general index of the sensitivity of a particular organism. In most cases it is possible to predict by experience the dosage of penicillin or other antibiotic needed in the treatment of a specific organism once its sensitivity is known.[77] The adequacy of the dosage may then be evaluated by the clinical response and the serum inhibition tests.[114]

3. The drug used should be able to penetrate fibrin.[111,112] In this disease the bacteria are deep within the vegetation and must be reached by the antibiotics if cure is to take place. The excellent results seen with penicillin therapy may be in part related to its ability to penetrate fibrin in contrast to a drug such as polymyxin which is potent in the test tube but disappointing in vivo and has only limited fibrin-penetrating ability.

4. Treatment should be continued long enough to effect a cure. The trend today seems to be toward shorter courses of treatment. While this has been successful with the streptococcus viridans group,[113] it has not been so for the streptococcus faecalis (the enterococcus) or staphylococcus, except with some of the newer antibacterial agents.[77,113,115]

5. Once adequate serum levels have been demonstrated and clinical response in the form of a feeling of well-being is experienced by the patient, treatment should not be abandoned if fever or petechiae reappear or embolization should occur. Fever is not uncommonly caused by the penicillin itself during treatment, and this may respond to the use of Benadryl hydrochloride (diphenhydramine hydrochloride).[8] Fever may also be due to phlebitis at the site of intravenous infusion or sterile abscess formation if the intramuscular route is used. Petechiae and peripheral emboli may occur for many weeks after the disease is totally eradicated.[35] If the dosage of penicillin is found to be inadequate as indicated by serum-dilution tests, it is better to double the dose than to increase in small increments. This is a potentially lethal disease which demands early aggressive treatment if disability and/or death is to be prevented. It is far better to overtreat than to undertreat.

Penicillin G or one of the newer penicillinase-resistant varieties, alone or in combination with other bactericidal antibiotics, remains the backbone of therapy in bacterial endocarditis.

Various methods of administration of penicillin have been suggested.[111] Initially, intermittent intramuscular dosage was employed with injections given at 2-, 3-, or 4-hr intervals. More recently, a continuous intravenous drip through a No. 25 pediatric scalp vein needle inserted in a small vein of the hand or arm has been employed.[8] Heparin, 25 mg per 1,000 ml 5 per cent dextrose and water, is added to minimize the tendency of local phlebitis formation which occurs with high dosages of penicillin. A polyethylene catheter may be inserted into the vena cava in selected cases where peripheral veins are not adequate. The experimental work of Eagle, which demonstrated the superiority of intermittent over continuous doses of penicillin in controlling infection in animals,[112] has not proved to be a significant factor in the treatment of bacterial endocarditis.

Oral penicillin treatment of endocarditis has been advocated from time to time, but the variability of the absorption of penicillin from the gastrointestinal tract of the same patient and from patient to patient makes this an unsatisfactory method of treatment for this disease.[70,111,116] This unreliability of absorption also holds true for the newer penicillinase-resistant penicillins,[117] and these drugs are not recommended at this time.

In addition to antibiotics, other medications have been employed as adjuvants in the treatment of bacterial endocarditis such as the anticoagulants and fibrinolytic enzymes. These agents have been used for the purpose of either preventing formation of the vegetations or breaking down the already formed verrucae to allow better penetration of the antimicrobial drugs. Anticoagulants have been abandoned because of the increased danger of bleeding following embolization[118] and are now used only in the treatment of thrombophlebitis and pulmonary emboli occurring during the course of left-sided bacterial endocarditis. Fibrinolytic enzymes have been used in experimental animals with no clear-cut indication of therapeutic value,[119] and in addition they may produce toxic reactions.

Benemid (probenecid) has been recommended by many writers.[111,116,117,120,121] This drug given in doses of 0.5 Gm every 6 hr by mouth will increase the penicillin level of the blood about four times and will prolong the duration of effect of an individual injection to about 12 hr.[121,122] This drug may not be necessary, since any desired level of penicillin may be maintained by intravenous administration as described previously. Nausea and vomiting are seen in 7 per cent of cases.[122]

When penicillin is used in high concentrations, it must be remembered that the sodium salt contains 40 mg sodium per million units and the potassium salt contains 65 mg potassium. This could be a significant factor in patients with congestive heart failure or renal insufficiency.

In the author's experience, penicillin reactions have not constituted a great problem. If a history of previous penicillin sensitivity in the form of rash or itching is obtained, the usual dose is started intravenously with 50 mg Benadryl hydrochloride added to the infusion. Ephinephrine and Solu-Cortef and equipment for providing an airway are held immediately available when the infusion is started. The author has seen no anaphylactic reactions. Other writers have recommended penicillin desensitization,[114] concomitant use of adrenal steroids,[123] or the use of antibiotics other than penicillin.[124] Penicillin desensitization in itself is hazardous and may provide no protection[124] against subsequent anaphylactic reaction. In those cases where itching and rash become a problem despite Benadryl hydrochloride, prednisone has been used orally to control this reaction. The author has found it necessary to discontinue treatment in only one case because of uncontrolled reaction to the penicillin. Previous anaphylactic-type reaction would constitute an indication for the use of another antibiotic.

After treatment is completed, blood cultures should be drawn at 2, 4, and 6 weeks and a close check kept on temperature during this period. Physical activity during treatment is limited according to the individual situation. Bed rest is employed with heart failure or other evidence of myocarditis during treatment, whereas in uncom-

plicated cases the patient is allowed such freedom as can be permitted by a mobile infusion stand. The duration of disability following treatment is also dictated by the stage of compensation of the individual patient. Strenuous exercise should be restricted for several weeks following treatment.

Streptococcus Viridans

In most cases of streptococcus viridans endocarditis, the minimum inhibiting dose of penicillin as measured by tube dilution is less than 0.1 unit per ml.[70,116,125] It has been demonstrated by Tompsett et al.[125] and by Geraci[113,116] that this group of bacteria may be treated with a combination of 1 million units of aqueous procaine penicillin G intramuscularly every 12 hr, 1 Gm streptomycin, and 1 Gm dihydrostreptomycin given alternately every 12 hr, and 0.5 Gm Benemid given orally every 6 hr. The treatment is continued for 14 days. It should be noted that this short-term therapy is recommended only for the most sensitive of the viridans group, those inhibited by 0.1 unit of penicillin per ml or less. Tompsett et al., using a schedule of 500,000 units of penicillin G intramuscularly every 2 hours plus 0.5 Gm dihydrostreptomycin every 6 hr or 1 Gm every 12 hr intramuscularly, obtained a 91 per cent cure rate with 33 cases of streptococcus viridans endocarditis which had sensitivities of 0.4 unit per ml or less.[125] It is interesting that 7 of his 33 cases had a resistance greater than 0.1 unit per ml, but in each of these there was also a bacteriologic cure on this regimen. Since there is a small percentage of cases with streptococcus viridans which are not controlled by the 2-week regimen, it would seem logical to extend the duration of the treatment in an attempt to include these cases.[125] *The suggested treatment for streptococcus viridans endocarditis is 10 million units of aqueous crystalline penicillin G given as a continuous intravenous infusion in 5 per cent dextrose and water with 25 mg heparin added to each 1,000 ml. In addition 1 Gm streptomycin should be given each day intramuscularly. This dosage should be continued for 3 weeks.* Geraci has reported that a 25 per cent incidence of vestibular involvement occurred with 2 Gm streptomycin given each day, whereas, the alternating of dihydrostreptomycin, 1 Gm, and streptomycin, 1 Gm, for 2 weeks has resulted in a 2 per cent incidence of toxicity.[113] At the present time, however, we use only streptomycin and limit the dose to 1 Gm daily. It should be noted that on the 2-week therapy program all the medications, penicillin, streptomycin, and Benemid, are necessary, and if someone cannot be maintained on the dosage described, then the short course of therapy should be abandoned. The newer penicillinase-resistant penicillins, oxacillin and methicillin, should not be used in the treatment of streptococcus viridans.[117,126]

Streptococcus Faecalis (Enterococcus)

The best therapy at the present time for enterococcal infection remains a combination of penicillin G and streptomycin given in a high dosage for a prolonged period of time.[113,127] The suggested method of treatment is 20 million units of penicillin each day given as a continuous intravenous drip supplemented with 1 Gm streptomycin. Treatment should be continued for 4 weeks. Once therapy is established, the efficacy of the dosage should be tested by serum-inhibition studies done about 2 hr after a dose of streptomycin. If the serum is not lethal for the patient's bacteria at a 1:4 dilution, the penicillin is increased to 40 million units. This will usually suffice, but the serum inhibition should again be tested. If for any reason streptomycin must be discontinued, then therapy with vancomycin (Vancocin)[113] or ristocetin (Spontin)[115] should be substituted. Vancomycin is given in a dosage of 1 Gm intravenously every 8 to 12 hr and continued for 4 weeks. It is administered by dissolving 1 Gm in 100 to 200 ml 5 per cent dextrose in water and giving this as an intravenous clysis over a period of 15 to 20 min.[113] Serum-bactericidal levels should be done to ascertain the effectiveness of the dosage. Ototoxicity and elevation of the blood-urea nitrogen have been seen. Ristocetin (Spontin) may be given intramuscularly in a total dosage of 25 mg per kg per day. The treatment with this drug is suggested for 14 days. It is given by dissolving 1 Gm ristocetin in 50 to 100 ml 5 per cent glucose in water and administering one-half of the total dose every 12 hr as a 20- to 30-min intravenous infusion.[115] Toxicity in the form of phlebitis, leukopenia,[128] skin rash, and fever are common.[115] Some writers have reported disappointing experiences with this drug and question whether it is bacteriostatic or bactericidal.[113] It should be used if conventional therapy in the form of penicillin and streptomycin is unsuccessful or cannot be tolerated.

Staphylococcus

The treatment of staphylococcus endocarditis depends upon the resistance of the organism and its ability to produce penicillinase. Sensitivity of the organism should be established by the tube dilution method and the absence of penicillinase production demonstrated by the techniques of Haight.[129] Penicillin G sensitive S. *aureus* or S. *albus* should be treated with 50 million units of aqueous, crystalline penicillin G in a 24-hr intravenous drip and in addition 0.5 Gm streptomycin

intramuscularly every 12 hr. Benemid, 0.5 Gm by mouth every 6 hr, may be used to enhance penicillin levels. If this combination fails to provide a clinical response within 2 or 3 days or if the serum-bactericidal levels are less than a 1:4 dilution of the patient's serum, then the dose of penicillin should be doubled or treatment changed to vancomycin or cephalothin (Keflin).[129a,b] Treatment with penicillin and streptomycin should be carried out for at least 4 weeks. Recurrence of fever during treatment may mean the emergence of a penicillinase-producing resistant staphylococcus, and cultures should be repeated.[126] The duration of the treatment has not been established with certainty for vancomycin or cephalothin, but 4 weeks is probably necessary with this particular type of bacteria. Staphylococci which are more resistant than usual to penicillin but which do not produce penicillinase should also be treated with penicillin G and streptomycin, vancomycin, cephalothin, or ristocetin. Methicillin (Staphcillin) or oxacillin (Prostaphlin) are not as effective against non-penicillinase-producing staphylococci as is penicillin G and should not be used with these bacteria.[126]

For resistant penicillinase producing staphylococci, one of the newer penicillinase-resistant varieties of penicillin is the treatment of choice.[113,114,117,126] For practical purposes, resistance in a clinically identified staphylococcus is synonymous with penicillinase production.[117,126] Treatment for resistant, penicillinase-producing staphylococci is 12 to 24 Gm methicillin or 6 to 12 Gm oxacillin given each day and continued for a period of 4 weeks. This may be given by the intramuscular route in divided doses every 4 hr or preferably by a 24-hr continuous infusion as previously described.[126,130] The antibiotic potency of methicillin declines rapidly in solutions of normal saline or 5 per cent dextrose in water, so that the mixture must be completely used within 4 hr. Unless the preparation of methicillin is specifically buffered, it is useful to add 6 to 7 mEq per liter of bicarbonate solution in order to slow the deterioration.[130] Toxicity to methicillin has been low, but bone marrow depression has been reported.[117,131] Nafcillin (Unipen),[132] 6 to 12 Gm given intramuscularly with Benemid over a 6-week period, has been successfully employed in the treatment of staphylococcal endocarditis. Serum-inhibition tests will be helpful in establishing the proper dosage of the newer antibiotics. Benemid may be used to increase the serum levels of nafcillin, methicillin, or oxacillin.[117] The serum levels will also rise with renal insufficiency. Vancomycin,[133,134] cephalothin,[129a,b] lincomycin (Lincocin),[129c] and gentamycin[129d] may also be used for penicillinase-producing staphylococci. Kanamycin (Kantrex) has been used as a last resort by some writers,[113] as has ristocetin. There is no potentiation of methicillin or oxacillin by other antibiotics such as chloramphenicol (Chloromycetin), erythromycin (Erythrocin), or streptomycin, and, if anything, the bactericidal properties may be somewhat weakened by these combinations.[113] Penicillin G and methicillin give a simple additive response.[117] Resistance to methicillin and oxacillin have been reported.[117,126,135]

Endocarditis with Negative Blood Culture[66,71]

For those cases of bacterial endocarditis in which the diagnosis is clinically certain but bacteriologically unproved, the usual starting therapy is 25 million units of aqueous, crystalline penicillin G given as a 24-hr intravenous drip with 1 Gm streptomycin intramuscularly. Benemid, 0.5 Gm every 6 hr, may be added to this regimen. If there is no clinical response in 2 to 3 days, the penicillin dose is doubled. If again there is no response in a few days, vancomycin, or cephalothin, should be used.

In those cases in which immediate antibacterial therapy is deemed necessary because of rapidly progressing disease before cultures can be returned, treatment should consist of 50 million units of penicillin G given as a continuous intravenous drip with the addition of 2 Gm methicillin or oxacillin given in the tubing every 4 hr if staphlococcus is suspected. Before this is started, three to four blood cultures should be drawn at approximately 15-min intervals. Therapy can be altered as indicated when the cultures are returned.

Postoperative Endocarditis

The treatment of bacterial endocarditis following cardiac surgical treatment presents a different problem from that of the usual case. In this situation there is a nidus of infection; often at the site is a silk suture which ordinarily cannot be reached or eradicated by the usual antibiotic regimen.[136] The individual case should be treated for 4 to 6 weeks with the antibiotic indicated by the causative organism. If the infection recurs after this time, reoperation with removal of the infected stitch, valve, or patch becomes mandatory.[113,136,137] If the patient's condition is such that operation is not feasible, the antibiotics should be continued until such a time as operation can be performed.[113,136]

Gram-negative Endocarditis[138]

The treatment of endocarditis caused by the Gram-negative bacteria has not been satisfactorily deliniated. These bacteria are a rare cause of the disease in the absence of suture material or prosthetic valves, and no large body of experience in their treatment is available. *Salmonella, Shigella, Pseudomonas, Klebsiella,* and *Escherichia coli* have been shown to be sensitive to colistin (Coly-mycin) in vitro.[139] The suggested dosage is 150 mg intramuscularly every 12 hr for adults and 5 to 10 mg per kg every day in three divided doses for children. Neuro- and nephrotoxicity have been reported with this drug, but neither has been serious or persistent. The dose should be reduced to one-half in patients with uremia. Kanamycin, 0.5 Gm given intramuscularly every 6 hr, has been used successfully in the treatment of S. Panama.[140] This drug may produce deafness. Toxicity is related to the total dosage, but with careful evaluation of the serum inhibition it can be used safely.[140] Polymyxin B sulfate (Aerosporin) shows a bacterial spectrum of activity similar to colistin in vitro but also has been shown to have a poor penetrating power for fibrin clots.[23,139] Combinations of streptomycin and tetracycline, although active in vitro, have been for the most part unsatisfactory in treatment of patients.[140] Ampicillin (Polycillin) has shown activity in vitro against *E. coli, Salmonella, Shigella,* and *Proteus mirabilis* organisms with good cure rates in urinary and enteric infections and merits a try in the difficult case of Gram-negative endocarditis.[117,126] Its action may be potentiated by Benemid. It has been ineffective against *Pseudomonas* or *Klebsiella* organisms.[117] Gentamycin[129d] and cephalothin[129a,b] are effective against certain Gram-negative bacteria, and massive doses of penicillin G have also been successfully employed in the treatment of S. *typhimurium* endocarditis.[140a]

Fungal Endocarditis

Amphotericin B is the drug of choice for endocarditis caused by *Histoplasma,*[56,141] *Candida,*[55,142] *Rhodotorula,*[148] and *Blastomycosis.* The optimal dosage has not been decided at present, but cures have been elicited by starting with a dose of 0.25 mg per kg body weight and gradually increasing to a maximal tolerated daily dose, usually 75 to 80 mg per day, which is then continued for a period of 6 months.[56,113] Nephrotoxicity, nausea, and vomiting are the limiting factors with this drug.[56] One case of *Rhodotorula* superinfection has been successfully treated with amphotericin B concomitantly with massive doses of penicillin for treatment of staphylococcus endocarditis.[143]

Miscellaneous Organisms

Endocarditis due to *Rickettsia burnetii* has not been successfully treated. Tetracycline and chloramphenicol have been suggested as therapy.[113] *Bacteroides,*[144] gonococcus, β-hemolytic streptococcus, and pneumococcus should be treated with

20 million units of penicillin G by continuous intravenous drip for a period of 4 weeks.

Prognosis

The prognosis of the patient who has undergone successful antibacterial treatment depends upon several factors, the most important of which is the residual valvular damage. Recent studies have shown that valvular damage in the form of valve perforations or increased insufficiency, particularly of the aortic valve, is responsible for the greatest morbidity and mortality in the posttreatment period.[7,8,145–152] Such patients are frequently candidates for corrective valve surgical procedures. Robinson and Ruedy,[145] in studying autopsy material of bacterial endocarditis, have also noted this increased tendency to valvular perforations and congestive heart failure in their fatal cases. Uremia secondary to acquired nephritis of bacterial endocarditis is no longer a common cause of death during or after treatment.[7,8,147,148] Cerebral vascular accidents[7,148] and coronary embolization[7] in the posttreatment period have been recorded as occasional causes of death. It is difficult to assess the functional importance of the myocarditis which occurs with bacterial endocarditis, since the cases demonstrating severe congestive heart failure have also invariably had severe valvular lesions. Some writers have felt that the myocarditis produced during bacterial endocarditis was the primary factor in congestive heart failure.[111,147] Robinson and Ruedy[145] have noticed the coincidence of valvular perforations and congestive heart failure in their autopsy series and, in reviewing charts, were able to correlate the onset of failure with the appearance of clinical signs of perforation. They also felt that the morphologic changes in the myocardium could not explain the frequency of heart failure, since they were present in equal frequency in patients with and without congestive heart failure.[145]

In general the fate of survivors has been good.[7,8,151,152] In the author's series from Emory University, 82 per cent survived for 5 years.[8] All but 1 of the 10 deaths which occurred after treatment came within the first 5 years after discharge from the hospital. Four occurred within the first year. Morgan and Bland reported a 69 per cent 5-year survival and a 49 per cent 10-year survival in their patients.[7] Eleven of their seventeen deaths occurred within 25 months after discharge from the hospital.

Relapse following treatment is less common today than when smaller doses of antibiotics were used and now occurs in about 5 to 10 per cent of cases. Relapse almost invariably occurs within 6 to 8 weeks after therapy.[64,146] Reinfection is estimated by several writers to occur in about 2 to 4 per cent of patients.[8,64]

Prophylaxis

It has been demonstrated that significant bacteremia may occur in patients with oral sepsis with or without dental manipulations,[153,154] following tooth extraction,[44] transurethral prostatic resection,[47] urethral catheterization,[46] normal pregnancy,[48] tonsillectomy,[155,156] or skin infection,[98] and in many other clinical situations. Since bacteremia plus valvular damage or congenital cardiac deformity may result in bacterial endocarditis, an attempt should be made either to control bacteremia or to prevent implantation and multiplication of the bacteria in the epithelium of the heart.

Studies of bacteremia before and after the use of antibiotics in the procedures mentioned show that bacteremia cannot be eliminated but can be substantially reduced.[44,157] This effect plus the inhibiting action of the drug before the bacteria can be established in the heart valves can logically be assumed to prevent bacterial endocarditis, although statistical proof of this fact is not available.[111]

All patients with rheumatic or syphilitic valvular disease or congenital cardiac abnormalities should be given antibiotic prophylaxis in the following situations:

Dental

Instruction of the patient with valvular or congenital heart disease in meticulous oral hygiene and care of the teeth and gums is the first step in prophylaxis against bacterial endocarditis.

Any dental procedure—filling, cleaning,[44a] extractions, root canal work, or installation of a bridge—may result in bacteremia. Multiple extractions particularly should be avoided in the presence of dental sepsis because of the increase in intensity of the bacteremia in this situation. Bacteremia usually persists for less than 30 min following extractions.[154] Streptococcus viridans is the organism present in the bacteremia in over 90 per cent of the cases.[44,154] Preliminary use of penicillin for several days before extraction may result in the emergence of resistant strains of streptococci.

Prophylaxis should be given as follows: 600,000 units of procaine penicillin given intramuscularly 1 hr prior to the procedure and repeated on 2 subsequent days. Phenoxymethyl penicillin (penicillin V), 500,000 units every 6 hr by mouth, may be substituted for the two daily doses of procaine penicillin on the days following the procedure. Erythromycin, 250 mg taken orally every 6 hr beginning 1 hr before the procedure and continued for 3 days after, should be used in those patients who are sensitive to penicillin. Tetracycline, 250 mg taken every 6 hr orally for 3 days in a similar schedule, also may be used in this situation.[157]

Necessary dental work in the patient with endocarditis should be accomplished during the course of therapy.

Genitourinary

Streptococcus faecalis (enterococcus) is the chief group of bacteria found after genitourinary manipulation or surgical treatment.[45,48] Procaine penicillin, 1.2 million units, and 1 Gm streptomycin should be given intramuscularly 1 hr before the procedure and repeated every 12 hr thereafter for 3 days.[157]

In Pregnancy

Treatment should start with the onset of labor with 1.2 million units of procaine penicillin plus 1 Gm streptomycin intramuscularly and should be continued for 3 days in the postpartum period.[161]

Gastrointestinal Tract

Procedures likely to cause trauma to soft tissues, particularly if infection is present, should be treated with prophylactic antibiotics as outlined for genitourinary disease.[157] If staphylococcal infection is suspected, methicillin, 1 Gm intramuscularly, should be given about 2 hr before the procedure and continued for 2 days at 4-hr intervals.

Tonsillectomy

Patients undergoing tonsillectomy should be given prophylaxis in the same manner as those undergoing dental procedures.

Cardiac Surgical Procedures

Since the advent of intracardiac surgical procedures, endocarditis in the postoperative period has become a pressing problem.[24,157] The routine postoperative antibiotic regimens have afforded no protection, since the usual invader is a penicillin-resistant staphylococcus.[24,158,159] Several writers have suggested that methicillin used alone would constitute the best possible prophylaxis if employed for a short period of time.[24,157,158] Methicillin could be given in a dosage of 1 Gm intramuscularly every 4 hr beginning with the day of surgical treatment and continuing for a total of 7 days into the postoperative period. Sufficient trial has not been given to this regimen to document its efficiency. Since the methicillin is not potent against other Gram-positive cocci, it would be less likely to result in a general change in body flora which would favor the emergence of fungi or Gram-negative bacteria, as has been the case with the usual postoperative regiments including penicillin

G, streptomycin, and broad spectrum antibiotics. Occasional cases of Pseudomonas endocarditis have been reported following cardiac surgical treatment and in most instances have been the result of inadequate sterilization of equipment.[24,160] Proper preparation and sterilization of equipment is the first step in prophylaxis.

NONBACTERIAL THROMBOTIC ENDOCARDITIS

Nonbacterial thrombotic endocarditis (terminal endocarditis, marantic endocarditis, cachexic endocarditis, endocarditis simplex, degenerative verrucal endocarditis) was first described by Ziegler[161] in 1888 and was distinguished from other forms of endocarditis by Libman[162] in 1923. The present nomenclature was applied by Gross and Friedberg in 1936.[161] Except for a prediction by Libman[163] this disease was considered by most writers to be a terminal occurrence[161,162] with no clinical significance until Allen and Sirota[39] suggested that it might actually be the first step in the formation of bacterial endocarditis. Angrist and Marquiss agreed with this idea and suggested that in addition the nonbacterial lesions might also represent a healed form of bacterial endocarditis and could be the cause of postcure embolization.[40] Several studies are now available which show that these lesions are indeed responsible for peripheral arterial embolization and may be a cause of death.[34,163–166]

The lesions appear in five types: (1) a small univerrucous lesion, barely visible, consisting of a single nodule up to 3 mm high seen along the line of closure of the valves; (2) a large univerrucous nodule which is more firmly adherent to the valve proper and which may be smooth or shaggy in appearance and up to 7 mm in size; (3) a small multiverrucous lesion composed of as many as three nodules firmly attached to the valve and spread along the line of valve closure like a beaded ridge, grossly resembling the verrucae of acute rheumatic fever; (4) a large multiverrucous lesion consisting of a friable, granular mass up to 7 mm high spread for several centimeters along the area of closure of the valve[39] (this may be loosely attached to the valve and would be prone to produce emboli); (5) lesions of the healed type which take the form of a fibrous tab or nodule resembling valve tissue at the valve margin, particularly at the corpora Arranti (Lamblian excrescences), and may occur on normal or diseased valves and appear to be the result of collagen degeneration within the valve leaflet which has provided a nidus for thrombosis.[39,164,165]

This disease is not restricted to patients with prolonged disease states or cachexia but may be found in disease of 1 day's to several years' duration.[39,164,165]

Various malignancies, usually with metastasis, are the most common accompanying lesion, but the verrucae may be found with acute pneumonia, pulmonary emboli, peritonitis secondary to perforated viscus, ruptured abdominal aneurysm, and many other acute diseases; in addition, two cases have been reported in patients with organic psychoses.[164,165] Males and females are about equally affected, and the ages reported have been from eighteen to ninety years. Murmurs are present in about one-third of the cases, are usually systolic, and are related to previous rheumatic or arteriosclerotic disease. The valves on the left side of the heart are most commonly affected with only an occasional report of tricuspid or pulmonic involvement.[39,165]

The importance of these lesions lies in their ability to cause peripheral arterial embolization and to mimic the clinical findings of bacterial endocarditis, particularly if fever is present from some other cause. It may be, as suggested by some writers, that these lesions do form a site for implantation of bacteria and may account for some of the bacterial endocarditis seen on previously normal valves.[39]

At the present time there is no definite therapy for these lesions, although anticoagulation may have some place in prevention of repeated embolic episodes.

LIBMAN-SACKS ENDOCARDITIS

Libman-Sacks endocarditis refers to the verrucous lesions which are found in the endocardium of patients dying of lupus erythematosis disseminatus. They were originally described by Libman and Sacks in 1924 [167] but were not recognized as being part of the generalized disease until the dissertation of Klemperer et al. in 1941.[168]

The lesions are verrucous in appearance, dry and granular, and pink or tawny. They may vary from pinhead size to 3 to 4 mm, may be single or multiple, and are capable of forming mulberry-like clusters which may spread down along the chordae tendineae.[168] They are found anywhere in the endocardial surface but are most common in the angles of the atrioventricular (A-V) valves and on the underside of the mitral valve at its base. The affected valves show areas of altered collagen formation not in proximity to these lesions. The lesions themselves usually contain granular, basophilic masses of cellular debris and some basophilic fragments of cytoplasm to make up the characteristic "hematoxylin bodies." [169]

These lesions are found in 30 to 40 per cent of autopsied cases of systemic lupus erythematosis.[167-171] Systolic murmurs are heard in over half of the cases of lupus erythematosis, but there is no correlation at autopsy between the presence of a murmur and the occurrence of the verrucous lesions.[170-175] These murmurs are most likely due to a combination of anemia and fever. Diastolic murmurs have been reported by two writers. In one case the murmur was found to be the result of rheumatic mitral stenosis,[175] and in the other report the findings at postmortem were insufficient to explain its presence.[170]

It is not certain whether or not these lesions make the heart more susceptible to bacterial endocarditis. In four large series, two cases of bacterial endocarditis were identified.[169-171,173] In another series of 35 autopsied cases in the preantibiotic era, 4 cases of bacterial endocarditis were found.[168] Bunim has reported an autopsied case of valvular endocarditis, but the Libman-Sacks verrucae were not involved,[172] although bacteria were found deep in the valve substance at a distance from the verrucae.

The diagnosis of Libman-Sacks endocarditis is made at autopsy, since there are no characteristic physical findings.[170,173,174]

REFERENCES

1. Horder, T.: Infective Endocarditis, with an Analysis of 150 Cases and with Special Reference to the Chronic Form of the Disease, *Quart. J. Med.,* **2**:290, 1909.
2. Libman, E., and Celler, H.: The Etiology of Subacute Infective Endocarditis, *Am. J. M. Sc.,* **140**:516, 1910.
3. Osler, W.: Chronic Infective Endocarditis, *Quart. J. Med.,* **2**:219, 1909.
4. Osler, W.: Gulstonian Lectures on Malignant Endocarditis, *Lancet,* **1**:415–418, 459–464, 505–508, 1885.
5. Loewe, L., Rosenblatt, P., Greene, H., and Russell, M.: Combined Penicillin and Heparin Therapy of Subacute Bacterial Endocarditis: Report of Seven Consecutive Successfully Treated Patients, *J.A.M.A.,* **124**:144, 1944.
6. White, P.: "Heart Disease," 3d ed., The Macmillan Company, New York, 1947.
7. Morgan, W., and Bland, E.: Bacterial Endocarditis in the Antibiotic Era, *Circulation,* **19**:753, 1959.
8. Vogler, R., Dorney, E., and Bridges, H.: Bacterial Endocarditis, *Am. J. Med.,* **32**:910, 1962.
9. Blumenthal, S., Griffiths, S., and Morgan, B.: Bacterial Endocarditis in Children with Heart Disease, *Pediatrics,* **26**:993, 1960.
10. Afremow, M.: A Review of 202 Cases of Bacterial Endocarditis, 1948–1952, *Illinois M. J.,* **107**:67, 1955.
11. Allen, A.: Nature of Vegetations of Bacterial Endocarditis, *A.M.A. Arch. Pathol.,* **27**:661, 1939.

12. Vogler, R., and Dorney, E.: Bacterial Endocarditis in the Normal Heart, *Bull. Emory Univ. Clin.*, 1: 21, 1961.

13. Wilson, L.: Pathology of Fatal Bacterial Endocarditis before and since the Introduction of Antibiotics, *Ann. Int. Med.*, 58:84, 1963.

14. Moore, R. A.: The Cellular Mechanism of Recovery after Treatment with Penicillin, *J. Lab. & Clin. Med.*, 31:1279, 1946.

15. Gould, S.: "Pathology of the Heart," 2d ed. Charles C Thomas, Publisher, Springfield, Ill., 1960.

16. Lepeschkin, E.: On the Relation between the Site of Valvular Involvement in Endocarditis and the Blood Pressure Resting on the Valve, *Am. J. Med. Sc.*, 224:318, 1952.

17. Libman, E.: A Study of the Endocardial Lesions of Subacute Bacterial Endocarditis, *Am. J. Med.*, 13:544, 1952.

18. Vogler, R., and Dorney, E.: Bacterial Endocarditis in Congenital Heart Disease, *Am. Heart J.*, 64: 198, 1962.

19. Gelfman, R., and Levine, S.: The Incidence of Acute and Subacute Bacterial Endocarditis in Congenital Heart Disease, *Am. J. M. Sc.*, 204:324, 1943.

20. Nadas, A.: "Pediatric Cardiology," 2d ed., W. B. Saunders Company, Philadelphia, 1963.

21. Griffith, S.: Bacterial Endocarditis Associated with Atrial Septal Defect of the Ostium Secundum Type, *Am. Heart J.*, 61:543, 1961.

22. Hoffman, F., Zimmerman, S., Bradley, E., and Lapidus, B.: Bacterial Endocarditis after Surgery for Acquired Heart Disease, *New England J. Med.*, 260:152, 1959.

23. Teitel, M., and Florman, A.: Postoperative Endocarditis Due to *Pseudomonas aeruginosa*, *J.A.M.A.*, 172:329, 1960.

24. Geraci, J., Dale, A., and McGoon, D. P.: Bacterial Endocarditis and Endarteritis Following Cardiac Operations: Addendum, *Wisconsin M. J.*, 62:302, 1963.

25. Sykes, C., Beckwith, J., Muller, W., and Wood, J.: Postoperative Endoauriculitis Due to *Pseudomonas aeruginosa* Cured by a Second Operation, *Arch. Int. Med.*, 110:113, 1962.

26. Elek, S.: Experimental Staphylococcal Infections in the Skin of Man, *Ann. N. Y. Acad. Sc.*, 65:85, 1956.

27. Hook, E., Wainer, H., McGee, T., and Sellers T., Jr.: Acquired Arteriovenous Fistula with Bacterial Endarteritis and Endocarditis, *J.A.M.A.*, 164:1450, 1957.

28. Zak, F., Strauss, L., and Saphra, I.: Rupture of Diseased Large Arteries in the Course of Endobacterial (Salmonella) Infections, *New England J. Med.*, 258:824, 1958.

29. Tedeschi, C., Stevenson, T., and Levenson, A.: Abscess Formation in Myocardial Infarction, *New England J. Med.*, 243:1024, 50.

30. Thayer, W.: Studies on Bacterial (Infective) Endocarditis, *Johns Hopkins Hosp. Rep.*, 22:1, 1926.

31. Perry, E., Fleming, R., and Edwards, J.: Myocardial Lesions in Subacute Bacterial Endocarditis, *Ann. Int. Med.*, 36:126, 1952.

32. Saphir, O., Katz, L., and Gore, I.: The Myocardium in Subacute Bacterial Endocarditis, *Circulation*, 1:1155, 1950.

33. Sheldon, W., and Golden, A.: Valve Ring Abscess of the Heart, a Frequent but Not Well Recognized Complication of Acute Bacterial Endocarditis, *A.M.A. Arch. Int. Med.*, 4:1, 1951.

33a. Schneider, G., Patterson, P., and Parnley, L.: Bacterial Endocarditis in an Infant Presenting as Acute Cardiac Tamponade, *Pediatrics*, 27:1010, 1961.

34. Wenger, N., and Bauer, S.: Coronary Embolism, *Am. J. Med.*, 25:549, 1958.

35. Kerr, A.: "Subacute Bacterial Endocarditis," Charles C Thomas, Publisher, Springfield, Ill., 1955.

36. Bell, E.: Glomerular Lesions Associated with Endocarditis, *Am. J. Path.*, 8:639, 1932.

37. Highman, B., and Altland, P.: Effect of Altitude and Cobalt Polycythemia, Hypoxia, and Cortisone on Susceptibility of Rats to Endocarditis, *Circulation Res.*, 3:351, 1955.

38. Nedzel, A.: Experimental Endocarditis, *A.M.A. Arch. Path.*, 24:143, 1937.

39. Allen, A., and Sirota, J.: The Morphogenesis and Significance of Degenerative Verrucal Endocarditis, (Terminal Endocarditis, Endocarditis Simplex, Nonbacterial Thrombotic Endocarditis), *Am. J. Path.*, 20:1025, 1944.

40. Angrist, A., and Marquiss, J.: The Changing Morphologic Picture of Endocarditis Since the Advent of Chemotherapy and Antibiotic Agents, *Am. J. Path.*, 30:39, 1954.

41. Lillehei, C., Robb, J., and Visscher, M.: The Occurrence of Endocarditis with Valvular Deformities in Dogs with Arterio-venous Fistulas, *Ann. Surg.*, 132:577, 1950.

42. Miller, A., Pick, R., and Katz, L.: Susceptibility of Dogs with Chronic Impairment of Cardiac Lymph Flow to Staphylococcal Endocarditis, *Circulation*, 28:769, 1963.

43. Reith, A., and Squier, T.: Blood Cultures of Apparently Healthy Persons, *J. Infect. Dis.*, 51:336, 1932.

44. Glaser, R., Dankner, A., Mathes, S., and Harford, C.: Effect of Penicillin on the Bacteremia Following Dental Extractions, *Am. J. Med.*, 4:55, 1948.

44a. Harvey, W., and Capone, M.: Bacterial Endocarditis Related to Cleaning and Filling Teeth, *Am. J. Cardiol.*, 7:793, 1961.

45. Koenig, M., and Kaye, D.: Enterococcal Endocarditis, *New England J. Med.*, 264:257, 1961.

46. Barrington, F., and Wright, H.: Bacteremia Following Operations in the Urethra, *J. Path. & Bact.*, 33:871, 1930.

47. Merritt, W.: Bacterial Endocarditis as a Complication of Transurethral Prostatic Resection, *J. Urol.*, **65**:100, 1951.

48. Redleaf, P., and Fadell, E.: Bacteremia during Parturition, *J.A.M.A.*, **169**:1284, 1959.

49. Hussey, H., and Katz, S.: Infections Resulting from Narcotic Addiction: Report of 102 Cases, *Am. J. Med.*, **9**:186, 1950.

49a. Bain, R., Edwards, J., Scheifley, C., and Geraci, J.: Right-sided Endocarditis and Endarteritis: A Clinical and Pathological Study, *Am. J. Med.*, **24**:98, 1958.

50. Allen, A.: Mechanism of Localization of Vegetations of Bacterial Endocarditis, *A.M.A. Arch. Path.*, **27**:399, 1939.

51. Rodbard, S.: Blood Velocity and Endocarditis, *Circulation*, **27**:18, 1963.

52. Kerr, A.: Bacterial Endocarditis—revisited, *Mod. Concepts Cardiovas. Dis.*, **33**:831, 1963.

53. Andriole, V., Kravetz, H., Roberts, W., and Utz, J.: Candida Endocarditis: Clinical and Pathologic Studies, *Am. J. Med.*, **32**:251, 1962.

54. Beamer, P., Reinhard, E., and Goodaf, I.: Vegetative Endocarditis Caused by Higher Bacteria and Fungi, *Am. Heart J.*, **29**:99, 1945.

55. Sanger, P., Taylor, F., Robicsek, F., Germuth, F., Senterfit, L., and McKinnon, G.: Candida Infections as a Complication of Heart Surgery, *J.A.M.A.*, **181**:88, 1962.

56. Palmer, R., Geraci, J., and Thomas, B.: Histoplasmin Endocarditis, *Arch. Int. Med.*, **110**:359, 1962.

57. Pearl, M., and Sidransky, H.: Candida Endocarditis, *Am. Heart J.*, **60**:345, 1960.

58. Merchant, R., Louria, D., Geisler, P., Edgcomb, J., and Utz, J.: Fungal Endocarditis: Review of the Literature and Report of Three Cases, *Ann. Int. Med.*, **48**:242, 1958.

59. Smith, W., and Evans, A.: Chronic Q Fever with Mitral Valve Endocarditis, *Lancet*, **2**:846, 1960.

60. McMichael, J.: An Unusual Case of Endocarditis, *Brit. M. J.*, **1**:1143, 1963.

61. Evans, A.: Rickettsia Endocarditis, *Brit. M. J.*, **1**: 1613, 1963.

62. Grist, N.: Rickettsia Endocarditis, *Brit. M. J.*, **1**: 540, 1963.

63. Thayer, W.: Bacterial or Infective Endocarditis, *Edinburgh M. J.*, **38**:237, 1931.

64. Cates, J., and Christie, R.: Subacute Bacterial Endocarditis, *Quart. J. Med.*, **20**.93, 1951.

65. Wilson, L.: Etiology of Bacterial Endocarditis, *Ann. Int. Med.*, **58**:946, 1963.

66. Blount, J.: Bacterial Endocarditis, *Am. J. Med.*, **38**:909, 1965.

67. Pankey, G.: Subacute Bacterial Endocarditis at the University of Minnesota Hospital, 1939 through 1959, *Ann. Int. Med.*, **55**:550, 1961.

68. Pankey, G.: Acute Bacterial Endocarditis at the University of Minnesota Hospital, 1939 through 1959, *Am. Heart J.*, **64**:583, 1962.

69. Jackson, J., and Allison, F.: Bacterial Endocarditis, *South. M. J.*, **54**:1331, 1961.

70. Hunter, T., and Patterson, P.: Bacterial Endocarditis, *Disease-A-Month*, Nov., 1956, pp. 1–48.

71. Pellegrino, E.: Diognostic Difficulties in Bacterial Endocarditis, *Kentucky State M. A. J.*, **60**:953, 1962.

72. Hodges, R., and de Alvarez, R.: Puerperal Septicemia and Endocarditis Caused by *Pseudomonas aeruginosa*, *J.A.M.A.*, **173**:1081, 1960.

73. Guze, L., and Pearce, M.: Hospital Acquired Bacterial Endocarditis, *Arch. Int. Med.*, **112**:56, 1963.

74. Friedberg, C., Goldman, H., and Field, L.: Study of Bacterial Endocarditis *Arch. Int. Med.*, **107**:6, 1961.

75. Linde, L., and Heins, H.: Bacterial Endocarditis Following Surgery for Congenital Heart Disease, *New England J. Med.*, **263**:65, 1960.

76. Friedberg, C.: "Diseases of the Heart," 2d ed., W. B. Saunders Company, Philadelphia, 1956.

77. Tumulty, P.: The Management of Bacterial Endocarditis, *A.M.A. Arch. Int. Med.*, **105**:126, 1960.

78. Segal, B., Likoff, W., and Moyer, J.: "The Theory and Practice of Auscultation," F. A. Davis Company, Philadelphia, 1964, p. 313.

79. Dormer, A.: Bacterial Endocarditis: Survey of Patients Treated between 1945 and 1956, *Brit. M. J.*, **1**:63, 1958.

80. MacGregor, G.: Murmurless Bacterial Endocarditis, *Brit. M. J.*, **1**:1011, 1956.

81. Hollander, J. L.: "Comroe's Arthritis," 5th ed., Lea & Febiger, Philadelphia, 1953.

82. Gross, N., and Tall, R.: Clinical Significance of Splinter Hemorrhages, *Brit. M. J.*, **2**:1496, 1963.

83. Hughes, W.: "Office Management of Ocular Disease," The Year Book Publishers, Inc., Chicago, 1953.

84. Antel, J., Rome, H., Geraci, J., and Sayre, G.: Toxic Organic Psychosis as a Presenting Feature in Bacterial Endocarditis, *Proc. Staff Meet. Mayo Clin.*, **30**:45, 1955.

85. Austrian, R.: The Syndrome of Pneumococcal Endocarditis, Meningitis, and Rupture of the Aortic Valve, *Tr. Am. Clin. & Climatol. A.*, **68**: 40, 1956.

86. Medley, D.: Chorea and Bacterial Endocarditis, *Brit. M. J.*, **1**:861, 1963.

87. Parsons, W., Cooper, T., and Scheifley, C.: Anemia in Bacterial Endocarditis, *J.A.M.A.*, **153**:14, 1953.

88. Weber, F.: Chronic Purpura of Two Years Duration Connected with Malignant Endocarditis Wrongly Suspected to Be Connected with Splenic Anemia, *Brit. J. Dermat.*, **12**:37, 1910.

89. Osler, W.: Chronic Infectious Endocarditis with an Early History Like Splenic Anemia, *Interstate M. J.*, **19**:103, 1912.

90. Engle, R., and Kaprowska, I.: The Appearance of Histiocytes in the Blood in Subacute Bacterial Endocarditis, *Am. J. Med.*, **26**:985, 1959.

91. Hill, R., and Bayrd, E.: Phagocytic RE Cells in

Subacute Bacterial Endocarditis with Negative Cultures, *Ann. Int. Med.*, **52**:310, 1960.

92. Finland, M., and Davis, D.: An Unusual Distribution of Peripheral Gangrene in a Case of Subacute Bacterial Endocarditis, *New England J. Med.*, **199**:1019, 1928.

93. Musser, J.: Subacute Bacterial Endocarditis, *Ann. Int. Med.*, **7**:714, 1933–1934.

94. Hunter, W.: A Study of Diagnostic Errors in Clinical Pathological Conferences at the Massachusetts General Hospital during a 25 Year Period, *Permanente Found. M. Bull.*, **10**:306, 1952.

95. Tykot, H., and Relkin, R.: Massive Pericardial Effusion in Subacute Bacterial Endocarditis, *J.A.M.A.*, **184**:898, 1963.

96. Olssen, R., and Romansky, M.: Staphylococcal Tricuspid Endocarditis in Heroin Addicts, *Ann. Int. Med.*, **57**:755, 1962.

97. Wilder, R.: Staphylococcus Bacterial Endocarditis, *Am. J. Med.*, **23**:325, 1957.

98. McCaulay, D.: Acute Endocarditis in Infancy and Early Childhood, *A.M.A. Am. J. Dis. Child.*, **88**:715, 1954.

99. Little, C., and Reed, W.: Antibiotics and Extracorporeal Circulation, *J. Thoracic & Cardiovas. Surg.*, **41**:34, 1961.

100. Lisan, P., Uricchio, J., Marino, D., Deshmukh, M., and Likoff, W.: Staphylococcal Endocarditis, *Am. Heart J.*, **59**:184, 1960.

101. Denton, C., Pappas, E., Uricchio, J., Goldberg, H., and Likoff, H.: Bacterial Endocarditis Following Cardiac Surgery, *Circulation*, **15**:525, 1957.

102. Bennett, I.: Bacteremia, *Veterans Admin. Tech. Bull.*, **2**, 1954.

103. Beeson, P., Brannon, E., and Warren, J.: Observations on the Site of Removal of Bacteria from the Blood of Patients with Bacterial Endocarditis, *J. Exper. Med.*, **81**:9, 1945.

104. Bennett, I., and Beeson, P.: Bacteremia: A Consideration of Some Experimental and Clinical Aspects, *Yale J. Biol. & Med.*, **26**:241, 1953–1954.

105. Mallen, M., Hube, E., and Brenes, A.: Comparative Study of Blood Cultures Made from Artery, Vein, and Bone Marrow in Patients with Subacute Bacterial Endocarditis, *Am. Heart J.*, **33**:692, 1947.

106. Martin, C., Wellman, W., and Martin, W.: Bacteremia Due to Bacteroides, *Arch. Int. Med.*, **107**:572, 1961.

107. Belli, J., and Waisbren, B.: The Number of Blood Cultures Necessary to Diagnose More Cases of Bacterial Endocarditis, *Am. J. M. Sc.*, **232**:284, 1956.

108. Van Nuys, F.: An Extraordinary Blood: Presence of Atypical Phagocytic Cells, *Boston M. & Sc. J.*, **156**:390, 1907.

109. Geftea, W., Pastor, B., and Myerson, R.: "Synopsis of Cardiology," C. V. Mosby Company, St. Louis, 1965.

110. Barritt, D., and Gillespie, W.: Subacute Bacterial Endocarditis, *Brit. M. J.*, **1**:1235, 1961.

111. Finland, M.: Treatment of Bacterial Endocarditis, *New England J. Med.*, **250**:372, 419, 1954.

112. Eagle, H.: Experimental Approach to the Problem of Treatment Failure with Penicillin, *Am. J. Med.*, **13**:389, 1952.

113. Geraci, J.: Antibiotic Therapy of Bacterial Endocarditis, *Heart Bull.*, **12**:90, 1963.

114. Glaser, R., and Ripkind, D.: The Diagnosis and Treatment of Bacterial Endocarditis, *M. Clin. North America*, **47**:1285, 1963.

115. Romansky, M., Foulke, C., Olson, R., and Holmes, J.: Ristocetin in Bacterial Endocarditis, *Arch. Int. Med.*, **107**:480, 1961.

116. Geraci, J.: The Antibiotic Therapy of Bacterial Endocarditis, *M. Clin. North America*, **42**:1107, 1958.

117. Klein, J., and Finland, M.: The New Penicillins, *New England J. Med.*, **269**:1074, 1963.

118. Cohen, S.: Massive Cerebral Hemorrhage Following Heparin Therapy in Subacute Bacterial Endocarditis, *J. Mt. Sinai Hosp. New York*, **16**:214, 1949.

119. Parker, B., Andresen, D., Thomas, W., and Smith, J.: Effect of Intravenous Fibrolytic Enzymes on the Vegetation of Experimental Bacterial Endocarditis, *J. Lab. & Clin. Med.*, **52**:588, 1958.

120. Beckman, H.: "PHARMACOLOGY, The Nature, Action and Use of Drugs," 2d. ed, W. B. Saunders Co., Philadelphia and London, 1961.

121. Bunnell, J., and Kirby, W.: Effect of Benemid on Serum Penicillin Levels, *J. Clin. Invest.*, **30**:697, 1951.

122. Boger, W., and Strickland, S.: Probenicid, *A.M.A. Arch. Int. Med.*, **95**:83, 1955.

123. Theobold, T., and Grace, W.: Treatment of Subacute Bacterial Endocarditis in Patients Allergic to Penicillin, *Am. J. Cardiol.*, **10**:575, 1962.

124. Grieco, M., Dubin, M., Robinson, J., and Schwartz, M.: Penicillin Hypersensitivity in Patients with Bacterial Endocarditis, *Ann. Int. Med.*, **60**:204, 1964.

125. Tompsett, R., Robbins, W., and Berntsen, C.: Short-term Penicillin and Dihydrostreptomycin Therapy of Streptococcal Endocarditis, *Am. J. Med.*, **24**:57, 1958.

126. Hewitt, W.: The Penicillins. A Review of Strategy and Tactics, *J.A.M.A.*, **185**:264, 1963.

127. Tompsett, R., and Pizette, M.: Enterococcal Endocarditis, *Arch. Int. Med.*, **109**:146, 1962.

128. Gangrosa, E., Johnson, T., and Ramos, H.: Ristocetin Induced Thrombocytopenia: Site and Mechanism of Action, *A.M.A. Arch. Int. Med.*, **105**:83, 1960.

129. Haight, T., and Finland, M.: Modified Gots Test for Penicillinase Production, *Am. J. Clin. Pathol.*, **22**:806, 1952.

129a. Griffith, R., and Black, H.: Cephalothin–A New Antibiotic, *J.A.M.A.*, **189**:823, 1964.

129b. Weinstein, L., Kaplan, K., and Chang, T-W.:

Treatment of Infections in Man with Cephalothin, *J.A.M.A.*, **189**:829, 1964.

129c. Walters, E., Romansky, M., and Johnson, A.: Lincomycin: Laboratory and Clinical Studies, *Antimicrobial Agents and Chemotherapy*, pp. 210–215, 1963.

129d. Jao, R., and Jackson, G.: Gentamycin Sulfate, New Antibiotic against Gram-negative Bacilli, *J.A.M.A.*, **189**:817, 1964.

130. Allen, J., Roberts, C., and Kirby, W.: Staphylococcal Septicemia Treated with Methicillin, *New England J. Med.*, **266**:111, 1962.

131. McElfresh, A., and Huang, N.: Bone Marrow Depression Resulting from the Administration of Methicillin, *New England J. Med.*, **266**:246, 1962.

132. Rosenman, S., and Warren, G.: Comparative in Vitro Activity of Semisynthetic Penicillins, Nafcillin and Oxacillin, *Antimicrobial Agents & Chemotherapy*, 2nd Conference, 1962, 369–378.

133. Geraci, J., Nichols, D., and Wellman, W.: Vancomycin in Serious Staphylococcal Infections, *Arch. Int. Med.*, **109**:53, 1962.

134. Kirby, W., Perry, D., and Bauer, A.: Treatment of Staphylococcal Septicemia with Vancomycin, *New England J. Med.*, **262**:49, 1960.

135. Daikos, G., and Kontomichalou, P.: Persistence of Staphylococcus to Methicillin and Oxacillin, *Arch. Int. Med.*, **111**:719, 1963.

136. Bahnson, H., Spencer, F., and Bennett, I.: Staphylococcal Infections of the Heart and Great Vessels Due to Silk Sutures, *Ann. Surg.*, **146**:399, 1957.

137. Kelsch, J., and Thomson, N.: Bacterial Endocarditis Complicating Repair of a Ventricular Septal Defect, *New England J. Med.*, **265**:1245, 1961.

138. Atuk, N., Mosca, A., and Kunin, C.: The Use of Potentially Nephrotoxic Antibiotics in the Treatment of Gram-negative Infections in Uremic Patients, *Ann. Int. Med.*, **60**:28, 1964.

139. Fekety, F., Norman, P., and Cluf, L.: The Treatment of Gram-negative Bacillary Infections with Colistin, *Ann. Int. Med.*, **57**:214, 1962.

140. Geraci, J., and Dearing, W.: *Salmonella Panama* Endocarditis Cured with Kanamycin Therapy, *Proc. Staff Meet. Mayo Clin.*, **37**:552, 1962.

140a. Weinstein, L., Lerner, P., and Chew, W.: Clinical and Bacteriologic Studies of the Effect of "Massive" Doses of Penicillin G on Infections Caused by Gram-negative Bacilli, *New England J.M.* **271**: 525, 1964.

141. Derby, B., Coolidge, K., and Rogers, D.: *Histoplasma capsulatum* Endocarditis with Major Arterial Embolism, *Arch. Int. Med.*, **110**:101, 1962.

142. Koroetz, F., Leonard, J., and Everett, C.: *Candida albicans* Endocarditis Successfully Treated with Amphotericin B, *New England J. Med.*, **266**:592, 1962.

143. Shelburne, P., and Carey, R.: *Rhodotorula fungemia* Complicating Staphylococcal Endocarditis, *J.A.M.A.*, **180**:118, 1962.

144. Fisher, A., and McKusick, V.: Bacteroides Infections: Clinical Bacteriological and Therapeutic Features of Fourteen Cases, *Am. J. M. Sc.*, **225**: 253, 1953.

145. Robinson, M., and Ruedy, J.: Sequelae of Bacterial Endocarditis, *Am. J. Med.*, **32**:922, 1962.

146. Hunter, T.: Bacterial Endocarditis, *Am. Heart J.*, **42**:472, 1951.

147. Gorlin, R., Cutting, B., and Emery, F.: Long Term Follow-up Study of Penicillin Treated Subacute Bacterial Endocarditis, *New England J. Med.*, **242**: 995, 1950.

148. Pillsbury, P., and Fiese, M.: Subacute Bacterial Endocarditis, *A.M.A. Arch. Int. Med.*, **85**:675, 1950.

149. Pearce, M., and Guze, L.: Some Factors Affecting Progress in Bacterial Endocarditis, *Ann. Int. Med.*, **55**:270, 1961.

150. Cohen, L., and Freedman, L.: Damage to the Aortic Valve as a Cause of Death in Bacterial Endocarditis, *Ann. Int. Med.*, **55**:562, 1961.

151. Hall, B.: Long Term Follow-up of Patients with Healed Bacterial Endocarditis, *Ann. Int. Med.*, **47**:880, 1957.

152. Mendelson, C., Cahue, A., Katz, L., and Brams, W.: Long Term Outlook for Healed Subacute Bacterial Endocarditis, *J.A.M.A.*, **160**:437, 1956.

153. Round, H., Kirkpatrick, H., and Hails, B.: Further Investigation of Bacterial Infections of the Mouth, *Proc. Roy. Soc. Med.*, **29**:1552, 1936.

154. Okell, C., and Elliott, S.: Bacteremia and Oral Sepsis with Special Reference to the Etiology of Subacute Endocarditis, *Lancet*, **2**:869, 1935.

155. Fischer, L., and Gottdenker, F.: Transient Bacteremia Following Tonsillectomies: Experimental, Bacteriological and Clinical Studies, *Laryngoscope*, **51**:271, 1941.

156. Rhoads, P., Sibley, J., and Billings, C.: Bacteremia Following Tonsillectomy, *J.A.M.A.*, **157**:877, 1955.

157. Hook, E., and Kaye, D.: Prophylaxis of Bacterial Endocarditis, *J. Chron. Dis.*, **15**:635, 1962.

158. Holswade, G., Dineen, P., Redo, S., and Goldsmith, E.: Prophylactic Antibiotic Therapy in Open Heart Operations, *Circulation*, **28**:739, 1963.

159. Keown, K., Gilman, R., and Bailey, C.: Open Heart Surgery, *J.A.M.A.*, **165**:781, 1957.

160. Boake, W.: Staphylococcal Endocarditis in an Australian Hospital, *Circulation*, **28**:692, 1963.

161. Gross, L., and Friedberg, C.: Non-bacterial Thrombotic Endocarditis, *A.M.A. Arch. Int. Med.*, **58**:620, 1936.

162. Libman, E.: Characterization of Various Forms of Endocarditis, *J.A.M.A.*, **80**:813, 1923.

163. Libman, E.: The Varieties of Endocarditis and Their Clinical Significance, *Tr. A. Am. Physicians*, **53**:345, 1938.

164. Barry, W., and Scarpelli, D.: Non-bacterial Thrombotic Endocarditis, *Arch. Int. Med.*, **109**: 79, 1962.

165. MacDonald, R., and Robbins, S.: The Significance of Non-bacterial Thrombotic Endocarditis: An

Autopsy and Clinical Study of 78 Cases, *Ann. Int. Med.*, **46**:255, 1957.

166. Boas, N., and Barnett, R.: Coronary Embolism with Myocardial Infarction: Complication of Verrucous Endocarditis, *J.A.M.A.*, **170**:1804, 1959.

167. Libman, E., and Sacks, B.: A Hitherto Undescribed Form of Valvular and Mural Endocarditis, *A.M.A. Arch. Int. Med.*, **33**:701, 1924.

168. Klemperer, P., Pollack, A., and Baehr, G.: Pathology of Disseminated Lupus Erythematosus, *A.M.A. Arch. Path.*, **32**:569, 1941.

169. Harvey, A., Shulman, L., Tumulty, P., Conley, C., and Schoenrich, E.: Systemic Lupus Erythematosus: Review of the Literature and Clinical Analysis of 138 Cases, *Medicine*, **33**:291, 1954.

170. Shearn, M., and Pirofsky, B.: Disseminated Lupus Erythematosus, *A.M.A. Arch. Int. Med.*, **90**:790, 1952.

171. Dubois, E.: The Effect of the L.E. Test on the Clinical Picture of Systemic Lupus Erythematosus, *Ann. Int. Med.*, **38**:1205, 1953.

172. Bunim, J.: Lupus Erythematosus Disseminatus, *Ann. Int. Med.*, **13**:1399, 1940.

173. Kong, T., Kellum, R., and Hasenck, J.: Clinical Diagrams of Cardiac Involvement in Systemic L.E., *Circulation*, **26**:7, 1962.

174. Jarcho, S.: The Clinical Features of Systemic Lupus Erythematosus, *J. Mt. Sinai Hosp. New York*, **26**:278, 1959.

175. Griffith, G., and Vural, I.: Acute and Subacute Disseminated Lupus Erythematosus, *Circulation*, **3**:492, 1951.

52 TRAUMATIC HEART DISEASE

Loren F. Parmley, Jr., M.D., and Thomas W. Mattingly, M.D.

Traumatic injuries continue to constitute one of the major causes of mortality and morbidity in our present society. When cardiac trauma occurs, there are usually associated injuries, and the more overt manifestations of cerebral, abdominal, or musculoskeletal trauma often dominate the clinical picture. Under these circumstances the more subtle aspects of injury to the cardiovascular system remain unnoticed, occasionally becoming manifest in a catastrophic manner either in the immediate post-injury period or as a delayed manifestation hours, days, or even months after the injury. Consequently only the more serious injuries of the heart and great vessels may be clearly evident initially and unless sought out by appropriate clinical evaluation of the injured patient the diagnosis may be frequently overlooked. Obviously, then, an awareness of possible cardiac injury in every traumatized individual is a prerequisite to early diagnosis and treatment.

The most common cause of traumatic heart disease is mechanical injury produced by physical force. These injuries may be classified as penetrating or nonpenetrating. A penetrating injury requires a vector for the physical force—that is, an object such as a knife or metallic fragment that penetrates the heart or great vessels by traversing the body surface or a needle that migrates through the wall of an adjacent organ like the esophagus, or the object may be a missile fragment that is embolic to the heart from a distant intravascular location. Nonpenetrating injuries, on the other hand, are cardiovascular lesions resulting from physical forces acting externally upon the body. These forces act through any one or a combination of several of the following six mechanisms:[1-5] (1) unidirectional force against the chest; (2) bidirectional or compressive force against the thorax; (3) indirect forces—i.e., compression of the abdomen and lower extremities resulting in marked increase in intravascular pressure; (4) decelerative forces, particularly when imparting differential deceleration to the heart and great vessels; (5) blast forces when of great magnitude; and, finally, (6) concussive force, which is an empirical category indicating a jarring force that interferes with cardiac rhythm yet is not of a magnitude to produce a significant anatomic lesion. However, even these definitions are not exact, as a high-velocity missile that passes adjacent to the heart may result in a contusive injury to the myocardium due to the shock wave in the tissues and, contrariwise, nonpenetrating trauma may cause a penetrating injury to the heart due to puncture by a fractured rib.

There is a subgroup of these mechanical injuries that is becoming increasingly important as the diagnostic and therapeutic techniques in the management of heart disease become more complex and refined. This is the iatrogenic trauma group comprising the complications of vigorous cardiopulmonary resuscitative procedures[6,7] resulting in nonpenetrating contusive injuries of the pericardium and myocardium, the diagnostic procedures of cardiac catheterization[8,9] and regional angiocardiography[10] (Fig. 52-1) that may produce penetrating cardiac injuries, and the associated injuries and sequelae of surgical treatment of congenital and acquired heart disease.[11]

There are two additional categories of heart trauma that are not due to mechanical injury yet are sufficiently distinctive to warrant separate classification. The first category encompasses cardiac injuries due to ionizing radiation which predominantly causes pericarditis but may also result

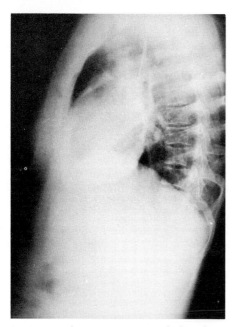

Fig. 52-1. Lateral roentgenogram of the chest of a thirty-four-year-old woman showing accumulation of contrast material in the pericardial cavity producing cardiac tamponade as the result of inadvertent perforation of the left atrium during transeptal regional angiocardiographic study. The contrast material was removed by pericardiotomy; the patient recovered completely.

in myocardial injury.[12] The second includes the group of cardiac injuries due to electric current, which most often produces either atrial or ventricular arrhythmias but may also cause burns of the heart and great vessels.

The incidence of traumatic heart disease is difficult to establish. Some penetrating injuries and the majority of nonpenetrating injuries of the heart are well tolerated, as clinical and experimental studies[13–17] have indicated. Consequently the majority of these lesions are infrequently diagnosed, since their initial clinical manifestations may be relatively minimal and the lesion overlooked unless specific studies are undertaken.[14] For this reason and because only the more severe injuries are reflected in autopsy studies,[15,18,19] the relatively high incidence of traumatic heart disease is not appreciated.

PENETRATING WOUNDS

Two to four per cent of penetrating wounds of the thoracoabdominal region involve the heart.[1,20–22] Even though the site of the penetrating wound may not involve the precordium, the possibility of cardiac injury must always receive serious consideration, particularly if a missile wound has oc-

curred. To deny the possibility of heart and great-vessel injury because of a presumed remote location of the wound may result in a false sense of security. The delayed appearance of serious clinical manifestations of penetrating heart wounds is well known.[23] The rapidity of death from the onset of symptoms, particularly when cardiac tamponade is due to hemorrhage, is often swift.[24] Therefore all patients who might have incurred a penetrating heart wound should be kept under close medical and surgical observation for several days.

Almost half of the individuals who have incurred stab wounds of the heart may be expected to survive for a sufficient time to reach medical treatment.[23] Gunshot or other missile injury carries with it a much more serious outlook, and only 10 to 15 per cent of these injured individuals would fall in the salvageable category.

The variety of objects[23,25] that may produce penetrating heart wounds is legion, including such diverse objects as pieces of glass, needles, toothpicks, parts of dental plates, coins, and even the spine of a stingray. Obviously penetration of the heart may occur as a result of erosion by a foreign body from an adjacent organ or cavity as well as migration of a foreign body from a more distant site.[23]

There are a multiplicity of heart and great-vessel lesions that may be produced by penetrating wounds, as indicated in Table 52-1. Lacerating or penetrating wounds immediately result in hemorrhage of varying magnitude. The severity of the hemorrhage and whether it is intra- or extrapericardial determine the clinical picture and dictate the requirements of treatment.[24] When there is intrapericardial hemorrhage, cardiac tamponade is the major threat. Paradoxically this may be the mechanism that permits temporary survival,[27] but death then follows quickly unless relief is afforded. The management of penetrating wounds should be based primarily on prompt diagnosis with appropriate emergency resuscitative procedures and surgical treatment as indicated. The immediate treatment of these lesions has been a matter of controversy between proponents of immediate surgical treatment[26–29] and a group who prefer the conservative approach[30–32] utilizing repeated pericardiocentesis when needed and relying on surgical treatment only if clots or other factors prevent adequate relief of the tamponade or if there is rapidly recurring tamponade. Both schools of therapeutic thought have reported a low mortality in the range of 10 to 20 per cent. In favor of an immediate surgical approach are the propensity of these lesions to produce a treacherous and delayed hemorrhage, the possibility of coronary artery laceration in every penetrating heart wound,

Table 52-1. CARDIAC LESIONS PRODUCED
BY PENETRATING WOUNDS

I. Pericardial injury
   A. Laceration
   B. Hemopericardium
      1. Cardiac tamponade
   C. Effusion, fibrinous pericarditis
      1. Recurrent effusion
   D. Pneumopericardium
   E. Suppurative pericarditis
      1. Pericardial abscess
   F. Constrictive pericarditis
II. Myocardial injury
   A. Laceration
   B. Penetration or perforation
   C. Rupture
   D. Retained foreign body
      1. Abscess
   E. Structural defects
      1. Aneurysm formation
      2. Septal defects
      3. Aorticocardiac fistula
III. Valvular injury
   A. Leaflet injury
   B. Papillary muscle or chordae tendineae laceration
      or rupture
IV. Coronary artery injury
   A. Thrombosis or laceration, with or without myo-
      cardial infarction
   B. Arteriovenous fistula
V. Embolism
   A. Foreign body
   B. Thrombus
      1. Septic
      2. Sterile
VI. Bacterial endocarditis
VII. Rhythm or conduction disturbances

and the infrequent though documented late development of constrictive pericarditis[24] secondary
to retained hemopericardium. Consequently gunshot wounds are best managed surgically because
of the extensive damage that this type of injury
produces.[33] Similarly if there is extensive extrapericardial hemorrhage producing shock or if the
hemorrhage is progressive in nature, a surgical
approach is necessary.

There are many sequelae of penetrating lesions,
encompassing primarily the complications of infection, embolism, arrhythmias and the creation of
structural defects (Table 52-1). Appropriate medical and surgical treatment has been developed for
most of these complications of penetrating wounds.
The techniques of extracorporeal circulation are
now utilized for the correction of hemodynamically
significant structural lesions such as interventricular
septal defects[34] and aorticocardiac fistulas.[35]

Foreign bodies retained in the myocardium are
often well tolerated. Although removal of these

foreign bodies has been simplified by surgical
methods utilizing extracorporeal circulation techniques, in many instances surgical treatment is
unnecessary unless the foreign body is producing
recurrent pericardial effusions, is a threat from the
standpoint of erosion or migration particularly into
the cardiac cavities, or is serving as a nidus for
thrombus formation or infection.

The phenomenon of recurrent pericardial effusion (Fig. 52-2) that may complicate a penetrating
heart wound in approximately 22 per cent of the
cases has been compared to the postcardiotomy
syndrome following surgical treatment of the
heart.[36] The medical management is primarily
symptomatic, unless cardiac tamponade or other
sequelae develop that require surgical treatment.

Coronary artery laceration usually results in
cardiac tamponade, and surgical treatment is required. Rarely is myocardial infarction produced [37]
in the absence of surgical ligation of the lacerated
vessel; however, survival in these patients is dependent on repair of the vessel (Fig. 52-3).

Embolism of thrombi, which may be septic,
developing at the site of cardiac injury or subsequent to aneurysm formation,[38] produces the typical clinical consequences dependent upon the size
and site of origin and termination of the thrombo-
embolus.[23] The embolism of a foreign body caught
within the heart or intravascular structures is a
fascinating study in variability of action.[39] If caught

Table 52-2. NONPENETRATING TRAUMA

I. Pericardial injury
   A. Hemopericardium
   B. Rupture or laceration
   C. Serofibrinous or suppurative pericarditis
   D. Constrictive pericarditis
   E. Recurrent pericarditis with effusion
II. Myocardial injury
   A. Contusion
      1. Anginal syndrome
      2. Aneurysm
      3. Delayed rupture
      4. Thromboembolism
      5. Myocarditis with or without failure
   B. Laceration
   C. Rupture, including septal rupture
III. Coronary artery injury
   A. Laceration or thrombosis with or without myo-
      cardial infarction
IV. Valvular injury
   A. Laceration, rupture, contusion
   B. Papillary muscle or chordae tendineae injury
V. Disturbances of rhythm or conduction
VI. Great vessel injury
   A. Laceration, rupture
   B. Aneurysm formation
   C. Thrombotic occlusion

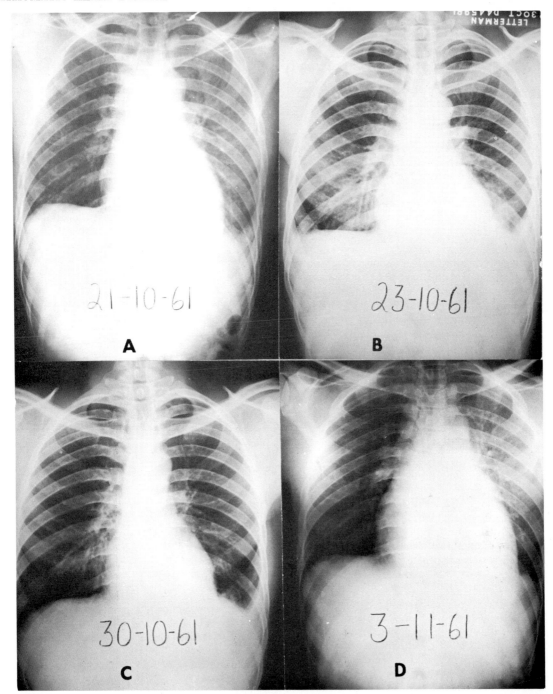

Fig. 52-2. Series of chest roentgenograms of a thirty-nine-year old man who incurred a penetrating stab wound of the heart on October 20, 1961. Initial films October 21 (A) and October 23 (B) reveal hemopericardium and the development of bilateral hemothorax on October 23, both clearing on conservative treatment by October 30 (C) after repeated left thoracenteses. Increasing symptoms of pericarditis, spiking temperatures to 104°F, and increasing size of the cardiac silhouette, with hazy infiltration of left mid-lung, led to pericardiocentesis on November 3, 1961 (D) with removal of 300 ml sterile serosanguinous fluid. Subsequently there was prompt clinical improvement and no recurrence of pericardial effusion.

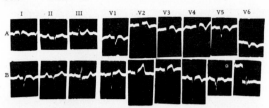

Fig. 52-3. Electrocardiagrams from a soldier who received an injury to the left ventricle resulting in a laceration and ligation of the anterior descending branch of the left coronary artery. The ECG findings (A) 4 months after injury and (B) 7 months after injury are indistinguishable from the usual abnormalities of anterior wall infarction from other causes. Recovery was good, and death occurred by drowning 5 years later.

in the large venous channels embolization may occur to the heart[40] and pulmonary arteries,[41] and, in fact, the embolus may pass back and forth within these structures.[42] Similarly a foreign body may become embolic in a retrograde fashion, passing from an initial site in the right side of the heart to the peripheral veins[43] or from the pulmonary artery or vein to either the right or left side of the heart, respectively.[23] Embolism of a foreign body from the left side of the heart to the systemic arterial system is often of serious consequence, depending on the site of arterial obstruction. A foreign body in the left side of the heart that is potentially embolic or one that has become an embolus to the systemic circulation should be surgically removed without delay.

Besides the obvious result of either prompt or delayed hemorrhage, a penetrating wound of the great vessels may also result in the formation of a false aneurysm, particularly should the aorta be involved.[23] Subsequent rupture of the aneurysm is then a constant threat. If adjacent large venous and arterial vessels are penetrated, an arteriovenous fistula may develop,[44–46] producing either immediate or latent congestive heart failure (see Chap. 54). An arteriovenous fistula of this type, especially if it be an iatrogenic lesion secondary to intervertebral disk surgical procedure, may result in surreptitious heart failure that may be overlooked.[46] Traumatic arteriovenous fistulas are occasionally complicated by the development of bacterial endarteritis and endocarditis,[47,48] which provide additional problems in medical and surgical management.

NONPENETRATING INJURIES

The forces that produce nonpenetrating lesions of the heart and great vessels are of such a nature that external evidence of injury is meager or not detectable in almost a third of the traumatized

individuals.[15] This lack of evidence of chest injury and the frequent preoccupation of the physician with more obvious bodily injuries is the most frequent cause of failure to diagnose cardiovascular lesions of this type.

There are a wide variety of injuries produced by nonpenetrating trauma as summarized in Table 52-2. Although minor insignificant myocardial contusion of the right ventricle is the most frequently occurring lesion, by far the most common fatal lesion is that of myocardial rupture, as has been demonstrated by necropsy study (Table 52-3). Myocardial rupture can rarely be treated successfully because of the rapid demise of the patient, and, in fact, very often when traumatic cardiac rupture occurs, it is only one of many severe bodily injuries, any one of which would be fatal.[15] Although most instances of cardiac rupture of the walls of the ventricular chambers are not amenable to therapy, rupture of the atrium[23] or of the interventricular septum[49,50] is not always fatal, and surgical repair[51,52] may be feasible by employing surgical techniques utilizing extracorporeal circulation.

Myocardial contusion is often asymptomatic, or its manifestations are masked by symptoms of the usual associated injuries. Often chest pain may appear following a latent period of several hours or days.[53] An anginal syndrome may also be initiated by the contusion[13,54] but is usually transient unless there is concomitant coronary artery injury or, more likely, antecedent atherosclerotic coronary artery disease. Rarely is coronary thrombosis produced solely on the basis of nonpenetrating trauma,[15] as is demonstrated by the fact that in a series of 546 necropsy cases of nonpenetrating cardiac trauma (Table 52-3) not a single instance of coronary thrombosis was found despite instances

Table 52-3. PREDOMINANT INJURY IN 546 CASES OF FATAL NONPENETRATING CARDIAC TRAUMA

Predominant type of injury	No. of cases
Myocardial rupture, including septum	353
Myocardial contusion and/or laceration	129
Pericardial laceration	36
Hemopericardium	25
Valvular laceration	1 (6*)
Papillary muscle laceration and/or rupture	1 (23*)
Coronary artery laceration and/or rupture	1 (9*)
Coronary artery thrombosis	0
Total	546

* Combined with other serious cardiac injury.

SOURCE: Modified, with permission of the authors and the American Heart Association, Inc., from L. F. Parmley, W. C. Manion, and T. W. Mattingly: Nonpenetrating Traumatic Injury of the Heart, *Circulation*, **18**: 372, Table I, 1958.

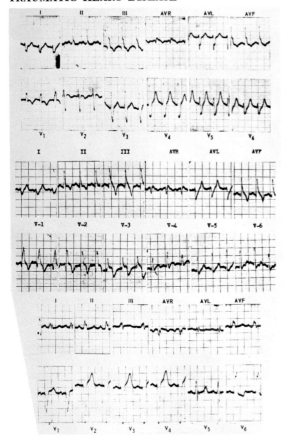

Fig. 52-4. *Top:* Electrocardiogram of a patient demonstrating right bundle branch block as a result of interventricular septal necroses due to nonpenetrating trauma. *Middle:* Electrocardiogram of another patient demonstrating right bundle branch block and suggesting anteroseptal necroses in a patient with an interventricular septal defect due to nonpenetrating chest trauma. *Bottom:* Electrocardiogram demonstrating left bundle branch block in a twenty-seven-year-old man in whom a traumatic interventricular septal defect developed as a result of nonpenetrating injury incurred in an automobile accident. (*Reproduced by permission of the authors and the American Heart Association, Inc., from L. F. Parmley, W. C. Manion, and T. W. Mattingly: Nonpenetrating Traumatic Injury of the Heart, Circulation,* 18:371, 1958.)

sis may occur, leading to rupture, to the formation of an aneurysm which also may subsequently rupture,[55] to mural thrombosis and embolism, and, in rare instances, to diffuse necrosis and fibrosis with congestive heart failure.[56] Also localized areas of necrosis or hemorrhage involving the cardiac conduction system may produce varying degrees of atrioventricular (A-V) block or any of the different types of intraventricular conduction defects (Fig. 52-4).[15,54,57]

Electrocardiographic studies may be the only clinical clue[13,15,54,58] that myocardial contusion has occurred, but the nonspecific ST-T abnormalities produced may be caused by so many different factors[59] that their value is not so much that of establishing the diagnosis as it is of alerting one to the possibility of cardiac contusion. Similarly elevated serum-enzyme-level studies may be suggestive of cardiac injury, but serum-enzyme levels are also elevated by other bodily trauma and are of questionable diagnostic usefulness.[58] When there is more extensive contusion, the electrocardiographic abnormalities may be more persistent, and, indeed, changes similar to that produced by myocardial infarction may develop. Atrial as well as ventricular arrhythmias of all types[15,60] may also be produced, and undoubtedly ventricular tachycardia and fibrillation may be the cause of death in some contusive injuries.

Because of the complications of myocardial contusion, patients with this lesion should be treated by bed rest or restricted activity for several weeks. Otherwise the treatment is symptomatic, with conventional management of associated abnormalities, such as arrhythmias.

Valvular laceration is an infrequent result of nonpenetrating injury primarily involving the A-V valves but usually occurring in the presence of severe cardiac trauma.[15] However, the aortic valve has been most commonly involved in the surviving patient, characteristically leading to the rapid development of congestive heart failure secondary to aortic insufficiency.[61,62] Mitral valvular lacerations may have similar severe hemodynamic consequences, but this lesion is rarely encountered clinically, as it is usually associated with other severe myocardial injury incompatible with life. Papillary muscle (Fig. 52-5) or chordae tendineae rupture and laceration occur more frequently than valvular lacerations (Table 52-3), but, as in the latter, the outcome is dependent upon whether the structures involved are on the left side of the heart, where the high-pressure system leads to serious hemodynamic consequences. The murmurs produced by these lesions are in the main typical of valvular insufficiency murmurs, but unusually high-pitched diastolic and systolic murmurs of variable intensity

where extensive contusion and hemorrhage surrounded a major coronary artery. More frequently laceration of the coronary artery results from nonpenetrating injury producing cardiac tamponade.[15]

Though myocardial contusion is primarily manifest pathologically by hemorrhage within the myocardium, various degrees of necrosis do occur. Usually this is minimal, and healing is complete with little or no obvious scar or impairment of myocardial function. Nevertheless, extensive necro-

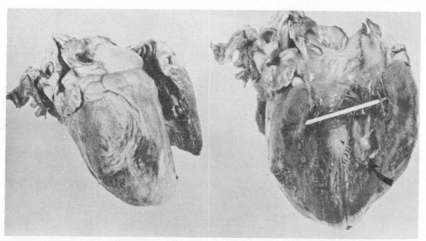

Fig. 52-5. *Left:* Heart showing area of ecchymosis and contusion of the myocardium in the region of the lacerated branch of the anterior descending left coronary artery. *Right:* Heart opened, revealing laceration of the posterior papillary muscle of the mitral valve (arrow) and areas of contusion in the anterior and posterior walls of the left ventricular myocardium. (*Reproduced by permission of the authors and the American Heart Association, Inc, from L. F. Parmley, W. C. Manion, and T. W. Mattingly: Nonpenetrating Traumatic Injury of the Heart, Circulation,* **18**:371, 1958.)

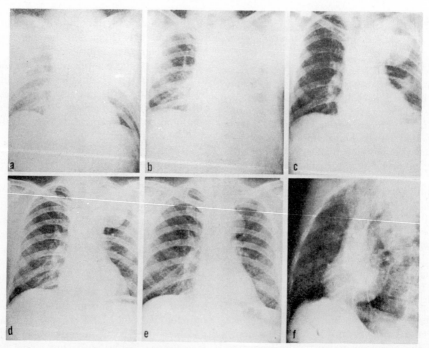

Fig. 52-6. Series of posteroanterior chest roentgenograms demonstrating the development of a false aneurysm of the isthmus region of the aorta following chest trauma. A. Immediately after accident. B. Five days later, a rounded mass becomes evident. C. Seventeen days after injury. D. Five weeks after injury. E,F. Venous angiocardiogram demonstrating the aneurysm just distal to the left subclavian artery. The aneurysm was successfully removed 18 months after injury. (*Reproduced by permission of the authors and the American Heart Association, Inc., from L. F. Parmley, T. W. Mattingly, W. C. Manion, and E. J. Jahnke, Jr.: Nonpenetrating Traumatic Injury of the Aoarta, Circulation,* **17**:1086, 1958.)

may result. Prompt and correct diagnosis is important, as operative techniques employing extracorporeal circulation are now available for the surgical correction of these lesions.

Pericardial lesions are common and are clinically similar to those of myocardial contusion, often being overlooked and healing without incident. However, hemopericardium may occur, and if hemorrhage is severe, cardiac tamponade will occur rapidly. If there is a slow oozing of blood, often evoking a pericardial reaction and an associated effusion, tremendous dilatation of the pericardial sac may develop over an extended period of time. Symptomatology and signs of traumatic pericarditis are similar to those of pericarditis produced by a wide variety of causes. Also the syndrome of recurrent pericarditis,[15,36] which is similar to the postmyocardial infarction syndrome, may develop, but this is a less frequent occurrence than in the penetrating cardiac injuries. In the presence of pericardial laceration, herniation of the heart may occur. This rarely leads to serious consequences and death.[63]

Although great-vessel rupture and laceration result in serious hemorrhage that may be stemmed by thrombus formation, there is always the probability that the thrombus will be dislodged. The most representative and important nonpenetrating traumatic lesion of the great vessels is that of aortic laceration and rupture. The classic sites of aortic rupture and aneurysm formation is at the isthmus region just below the origin of the left subclavian artery, presumably the result of differ-

ential rates of deceleration of the aorta at this relatively fixed point. Fracture or displacement of a thoracolumbar vertebra may also be a factor in the causation of aortic rupture. Ruptures of the ascending aorta and arch are about half as frequent as isthmus ruptures and are associated with a much higher incidence of cardiac injury. Thoracic and abdominal aorta ruptures are much less common. Considering the extent of the lesion which frequently transects the aorta, it is amazing that at least 15 per cent of the individuals so injured survive—some only for a few hours but others for days, weeks, and even many years.[64] Survival initially is due to the formation of a false aneurysm by the periaortic structures (Fig. 52-6). The hemorrhage into the mediastinal structures tamponades the lesion and permits continuity of the circulation until the aneurysm has formed. Roentgen signs of a widened mediastinum,[64] (Fig. 52-7) evidence of persistent thoracoabdominal hemorrhage,[64] and, particularly, the appearance of hemothorax[64] hours after the initial injury are clinical findings that are highly suggestive of recent aortic rupture. Surgical treatment can now be effectively carried out for the acute lesion including ruptures of the ascending aorta.[65] A false aortic aneurysm is often discovered months or years after the injury[64,65] and, in fact, may even be partially calcified (Fig. 52-8). However, rupture of the aneurysm may occur at any time after its formation.[64] Rarely the complications of dissection,[66] peripheral embolism of a thrombus contained in the aneurysm,[64] or the development of bacterial endaortitis[67] may

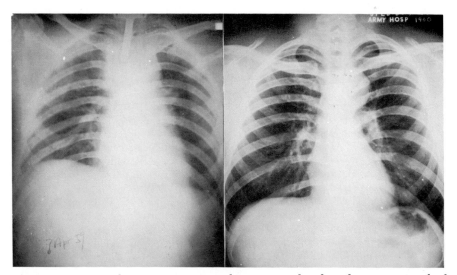

Fig. 52-7. *Left:* Posteroanterior chest roentgenograms showing a widened mediastinum typical of aortic rupture in a twenty-two-year-old man who also suffered chest contusion, concussion, and a fractured left tibia and femur in an automobile accident in April, 1959. *Right:* The typical appearance of a traumatic aortic aneurysm 11 months later.

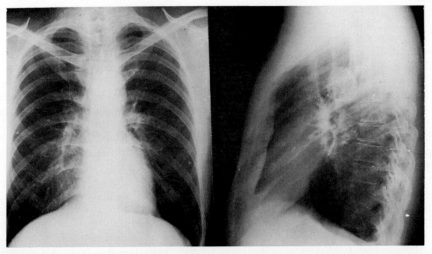

Fig. 52-8. Posteroanterior and left lateral chest roentgenogram showing a typical traumatic aneurysm just below the left subclavian artery. Note partial calcification of the aneurysm evident in the left lateral view. This forty-three-year-old man was involved in an automobile accident in 1941, suffering multiple injuries and requiring 6 months' hospitalization. An abnormality was first discovered on the patient's x-ray in 1957. The diagnosis of traumatic aortic aneurysm was not made until 1959. By utilizing partial arterial blood bypass from the left atrium to the left femoral artery the aneurysm was surgically resected and a Teflon graft inserted to preserve aortic continuity.

occur. Because of the relative instability of these aneurysms and the complications as cited, surgical correction is the treatment of choice.

REFERENCES

1. Kahn, M. H., and Kahn, S.: Cardiovascular Lesions Following Injury to the Chest, Ann. Int. Med., 2: 1013, 1929.
2. Beck, C. S.: Contusions of the Heart, J.A.M.A., 104:109, 1935.
3. Beck, C. S., and Bright, E. F.: Changes in the Heart and Pericardium Brought about by Compression of the Legs and Abdomen, J. Thoracic Surg., 2:616, 1933.
4. Wilson, J. V.: The Pathology of Closed Injuries of the Chest, Brit. M. J., 1:470, 1943.
5. Hass, G. M.: Types of Internal Injuries of Personnel Involved in Aircraft Accidents, J. Aviation Med., 15:77, 1944.
6. Guevara, V., Greenberg, H., and Hertzog, A. J.: Traumatic Damage to the Heart from Cardiac Massage, Anesth. & Analg., 41:639, 1962.
7. Reiff, T. R., Oppenheimer, J., and Fergusson, G.: Cardiac Injury Presumably Due to Use of the External Electric Cardiac Pacemaker in Stokes-Adams Disease, Am. Heart J., 54:437, 1957.
8. Lurie, P. R., and Grajo, M. Z.: Accidental Cardiac Puncture during Right Heart Catheterization, Pediatrics, 29:283, 1962.
9. Adrouny, Z. A., Sutherland, D. W., Griswold, H. E., and Ritzmann, L. W.: Complications with Left Heart Catheterization, Am. Heart J., 65:327, 1963.
10. Doppman, J. L., Shapiro, R., Wilson, G. L., Mattie, L. R., and Carter, M. G.: Perforation of the Right Ventricle during Selective Angiography: Report of a Case, J. Thoracic & Cardiovas. Surg., 39:500, 1960.
11. Lilly, E. J., Macmillan, R. D., Dent, S. J., and Stephen, C. R.: Iatrogenic Acute Cardiac Tamponade, J.A.M.A., 176:8, 1961.
12. Catterall, M., and Evans, W.: Myocardial Injury from Therapeutic Irradiation, Brit. Heart J., 22:168, 1960.
13. Sigler, L. H.: Traumatic Injury of the Heart, Am. Heart J., 30:459, 1945.
14. Arenberg, H.: Traumatic Heart Disease: A Clinical Study of 250 Cases of Nonpenetrating Chest Injuries and Their Relation to Cardiac Disability, Ann. Int. Med., 19:326, 1943.
15. Parmley, L. F., Manion, W. C., and Mattingly, T. W.: Nonpenetrating Traumatic Injury of the Heart, Circulation, 18:371, 1958.
16. Moritz, A. R., and Atkins, J. P.: Cardiac Contusion: An Experimental and Pathologic Study, A.M.A. Arch. Path., 25:445, 1938.
17. Kissane, R. W., Fidler, R. S., and Koons, R. A.: Electrocardiographic Changes Following External Chest Injury to Dogs, Ann. Int. Med., 11:907, 1937.
18. Osborn, G. R.: Findings in 262 Fatal Accidents, Lancet, 2:277, 1943.
19. Leinoff, H. D.: Direct Nonpenetrating Injuries of the Heart, Ann. Int. Med., 14:653, 1940.
20. Samson, P. C.: Battle Wounds and Injuries of the Heart and Pericardium: Experiences in Forward Hospitals, Ann. Surg., 127:1127, 1948.
21. Elkin, D. C.: The Diagnosis and Treatment of

Wounds of the Heart, *J.A.M.A.*, 111:1750, 1938.

22. Valle, A. R.: War Injuries of the Heart and Mediastinum, *A.M.A. Arch. Surg.*, 70:398, 1955.

23. Parmley, L. F., Mattingly, T. W., and Manion, W. C.: Penetrating Wounds of the Heart and Aorta, *Circulation*, 17:953, 1958.

24. Isaacs, J. P.: Sixty Penetrating Wounds of the Heart, *Surgery*, 45:696, 1959.

25. Decker, H. R.: Foreign Bodies in the Heart and Pericardium—Should They Be Removed? *J. Thoracic Surg.*, 9:62, 1939.

26. Smyth, N. P. D., Hughes, R. K., and Cornwell, E. E.: Stab Wounds of the Heart, *M. Ann. District of Columbia*, 31:146, 1962.

27. Elkan, W.: The Surgical Repair of Injuries to the Heart: Report of 21 Cases with 19 Survivals, *J. Internat. Coll. Surgeons*, 37:323, 1962.

28. Naclerio, E. A., Maynard, A. DeL., and Cordice, J. W. V., Jr.: Personal Experience with Ten Consecutive Cases of Heart Wounds Treated Successfully by Pericardiotomy and Cardiorrhaphy with Reference to 74 Earlier Cases, 54 Surgically Treated at Harlem Hospital, *J. Thoracic Surg.*, 25:448, 1963.

29. von Berg, V. J., Moggi, L., Jacobson, L. F., Jordan, P., Jr., and Johnston, C. G.: Ten Years' Experience with Penetrating Injuries of the Heart, *J. Trauma*, 1:186, 1961.

30. Elkin, D. C., and Campbell, R. E.: Cardiac Tamponade: Treatment by Aspiration, *Ann. Surg.*, 133:623, 1951.

31. Wilkinson, A. H., Jr., Buttram, T. L., Reid, W. A., and Howard, J. M.: Cardiac Injuries: An Evaluation of Immediate and Long Range Results of Treatment, *Ann. Surg.*, 147:347, 1958.

32. Cooley, D. A., Dunn, J. R., Brockman, H. LeR., and DeBakey, M. E.: Treatment of Penetrating Wounds of the Heart: Experimental and Clinical Observations, *Surgery*, 37:882, 1955.

33. Ransdell, H. T., Jr., and Glass, H., Jr.: Gunshot Wounds of the Heart: Review of 20 Cases, *Am. J. Surg.*, 99:788, 1960.

34. Beall, A. C., Jr., Morris, G. C., Jr., and Cooley, D. A.: Temporary Cardiopulmonary Bypass in the Management of Penetrating Wounds of the Heart, *Surgery*, 52:330, 1962.

35. King, H., and Shumacker, H. B., Jr.: Surgical Repair of a Traumatic Aortic–Right Ventricular Fistula, *J. Thoracic Surg.*, 35:734, 1958.

36. Tabatznik, B., and Isaacs, J. P.: Postpericardiotomy Syndrome Following Traumatic Hemopericardium, *Am. J. Cardiol.*, 7:83, 1961.

37. Heitzman, E. J., and Heitzman, G. C.: Myocardial Infarction Following Penetrating Wounds of the Heart, *Am. J. Cardiol.*, 7:283, 1961.

38. Lyons, C., and Perkins, R.: Resection of a Left Ventricular Aneurysm Secondary to Cardiac Stab Wound, *Ann. Surg.*, 147:256, 1958.

39. Harken, D. E., and Williams, A. C.: Foreign Bodies in, and in Relation to, the Thoracic Blood Vessels

and Heart. II. Migratory Foreign Bodies within the Blood Vascular System, *Am. J. Surg.*, 72:80, 1946.

40. Samson, P. C.: Two Unusual Cases of War Wounds of the Heart, *Surgery*, 20:373, 1946.

41. Straus, R.: Pulmonary Embolism Caused by a Lead Bullet Following a Gunshot Wound of the Abdomen, *A.M.A. Arch. Path.*, 33:63, 1942.

42. Davey, W. W., and Parker, G. E.: The Surgical Pursuit and Removal of a Metallic Foreign Body from the Systemic Venous Circulation, *Brit. J. Surg.*, 34:392, 1946–1947.

43. Robertson, R. W.: Penetrating Heart Wound, *Surgery*, 21:597, 1947.

44. Meredith, J. H., and Bradshaw, H. H.: Fistula between Aorta and Superior Vena Cava: Report of a Traumatic Case with Surgical Repair, *J. Thoracic Surg.*, 34:278, 1957.

45. Pemberton, J. deJ., Seefeld, P. H., and Barker, N. W.: Traumatic Arteriovenous Fistula Involving the Abdominal Aorta and Inferior Vena Cava, *Ann. Surg.*, 123:580, 1946.

46. Smith, V. M., Hughes, C. W., Sapp, O., Joy, R. J. T., and Mattingly, T. W.: High-output Circulatory Failure Due to Arteriovenous Fistula, *A.M.A. Arch. Int. Med.*, 100:883, 1957.

47. Hook, E. W., Jr., Wainer, H. S., McGee, T. J., and Sellers, T. F., Jr.: Acquired Arteriovenous Fistula with Bacterial Endarteritis and Endocarditis, *J.A.M.A.*, 164:1450, 1957.

48. Parmley, L. F., Orbison, J. A., Hughes, C. W., and Mattingly, T. W.: Acquired Arteriovenous Fistulas Complicated by Endarteritis and Endocarditis Lenta Due to *Streptococcus Faecalis*, *New England J. Med.*, 250:305, 1954.

49. Pollock, B. E., Markley, R. A., and Shuey, H. E.: Isolated Traumatic Rupture of the Interventricular Septum Due to Blunt Force, *Am. Heart J.*, 43:273, 1952.

50. Cary, F. H., Hurst, J. W., and Arentzen, W. R.: Acquired Interventricular Defect Secondary to Trauma: Report of Four Cases, *New England J. Med.*, 258:355, 1958.

51. Desforges, G., Ridder, W. P., and Lenoci, R. J.: Successful Suture of Ruptured Myocardium after Nonpenetrating Injury, *New England J. Med.*, 252:567, 1955.

52. Peirce, E. C., II, Dabbs, C. H., and Rawson, F. L.: Isolated Rupture of the Ventricular Septum Due to Nonpenetrating Trauma: Report of a Case Treated by Open Cardiotomy under Simple Hypothermia, *A.M.A. Arch. Surg.*, 77:87, 1958.

53. Kissane, R. W.: Traumatic Heart Disease: Nonpenetrating Injuries, *Circulation*, 6:421, 1952.

54. Warburg, E.: Myocardial and Pericardial Lesions Due to Nonpenetrating Injury, *Brit. Heart J.*, 2:271, 1940.

55. Pitts, H. H., and Purvis, G. S.: Ruptured Traumatic Aneurysm in a Child, *Canad. M. A. J.*, 57:165, 1947.

56. Barber, H., and Osborn, G. R.: A Fatal Case of

Myocardial Contusion, *Brit. Heart J.*, 3:127, 1941.

57. Rankin, T. J., and Patterson, J. W.: Transient Intraventricular Block in Cardiac Contusion, *Am. Heart J.*, 43:103, 1952.

58. Watson, J. H., and Bartholomae, W. M.: Cardiac Injury Due to Nonpenetrating Chest Trauma, *Ann. Int. Med.*, 52:871, 1960.

59. Kissane, R. W., Fidler, R. S., and Koons, R. A.: Electrocardiographic Changes Following External Chest Injury to Dogs, *Ann. Int. Med.*, 11:907, 1937.

60. Taylor, H. B.: Transient Cardiac Arrhythmia Induced by Nonpenetrating Trauma to the Chest, *Am. Heart J.*, 46:557, 1953.

61. Leonard, J. J., Harvey, W. P., and Hufnagel, C. A.: Rupture of Aortic Valve: A Therapeutic Approach, *New England J. Med.*, 252:208, 1955.

62. Kissane, R. W., Koons, R. A., and Clark, T. E.: Traumatic Rupture of Aortic Valve, *Am. J. Med.*, 4:606, 1948.

63. Munchow, O. B. G., Carter, R., Vannix, R. S., and Anderson, F. S.: Cardiac Arrest Due to Ventricular Herniation: Report of a Case of Two Successful Cardiac Resuscitations, *J.A.M.A.*, 173:1350, 1960.

64. Parmley, L. F., Mattingly, T. W., Manion, W. C., and Jahnke, E. J., Jr.: Nonpenetrating Traumatic Injury of the Aorta, *Circulation*, 17:1086, 1958.

65. Jahnke, E. J., Jr., Fisher, G. W., and Jones, R. C.: Acute Traumatic Rupture of the Thoracic Aorta: A Report of Six Consecutive Cases of Successful Early Repair, *J. Thoracic & Cardiovas. Surg.*, 48:61, 1964.

66. Samson, P. C.: Dissecting Aneurysms of the Aorta, Including Traumatic Type: Three Case Reports, *Ann. Int. Med.*, 5:117, 1931.

67. Stryker, W. A.: Traumatic Saccular Aneurysms of the Thoracic Aorta, *Am. J. Clin. Path.*, 18:152, 1948.

53 SYPHILIS AND THE CARDIO-VASCULAR SYSTEM

C. Thorpe Ray, M.D.

It is regrettable that modern texts need to include more than interesting historical notes about cardiovascular syphilis, one of the few truly preventable forms of heart disease. The incidence of cardiovascular syphilis has been decreasing for two to three decades, so that now the disease is uncommon even in geographic areas where the incidence was previously quite high. This radical change in the incidence of cardiovascular syphilis forms the basis of interesting speculation.

Certainly, penicillin is effective and has made the treatment of early syphilis much easier and cheaper than the older regimens of arsenical,

bismuth, and iodide treatment. With modern penicillin treatment of early syphilis there is little likelihood of the incomplete course which was so frequent in the prolonged treatment periods prior to the advent of penicillin. However, it should be emphasized that the incidence of cardiovascular syphilis was decreasing rapidly before penicillin was available for widespread use in civilian practice. Since the stages of cardiovascular syphilis which are symptomatic and diagnosable usually occur from 10 to 30 years after the chancre, changes in incidence of this disease attributable to the use of penicillin would have been expected only after 1956. The clearly evident decrease in incidence prior to 1955 may be attributed to natural changes in the chronic epidemic of syphilis and especially to the efforts of the public health services. The control of syphilis has been quite successful, but the increasing incidence of new infections in the last 3 years would seem to indicate that cardiovascular syphilis will continue to occur but in reduced incidence.

Syphilitic Aortitis

The fundamental lesion of cardiovascular syphilis is aortitis, one of the most common of syphilitic lesions. Localization of the spirochetes in the wall of the aorta occurs quite early after the primary infection. It is first in the adventitia and then spreads into the media by way of the perivascular lymphatics surrounding the vasa vasorum.[1] The vasa vasorum undergo an obliterative endarteritis with subsequent necrosis of the media. The elastic and connective tissues are destroyed and replaced by scar tissue. Active inflammation continues for many years, and virulent *Treponema* has been isolated from the wall of the aorta in untreated cases as long as 25 years after infection.[2] The intima overlying the necrotic areas in the media is thickened. In the late stages the intima appears pitted and scarred with wrinkling of the intervening tissue, an appearance which has been likened to the bark of a tree.

The incidence and severity of the syphilitic aortitis is greatest in the ascending aorta, next in the transverse portion, and least in descending and abdominal portions of the aorta. This distribution of the lesions of syphilitic aortitis has been attributed to the rich supply of lymphatics in the ascending and transverse portions of the arch.[3] The tendency to develop more severe lesions in the first portion of the aorta leads to involvement of the coronary ostiums and the base of the aortic valve leaflets.

The incidence of aortitis in cases of untreated syphilis has been estimated to be as high as 70 to 80 per cent.[4,5] This is in striking contrast to the incidence of the complications of aortitis (aortic insufficiency, aneurysm, and ostial disease) which occur in 9 to 10 per cent.[6,7] The significance of uncomplicated aortitis is that this lesion forms the basis for the symptomatic and lethal forms of cardiovascular syphilis. Furthermore, adequate treatment in the stage of uncomplicated aortitis should arrest the disease and prevent progression to the more serious complication.[6,8,9] The longer treatment is delayed following the primary infection, the greater is the likelihood of the development of more serious lesions.

The diagnosis of uncomplicated syphilitic aortitis has been debated at great length. The diagnostic criteria which have been suggested consist of dilatation of the ascending aorta, a tambour aortic second sound in the absence of hypertension and atherosclerosis, a systolic aortic murmur, burning retrosternal pain, breathlessness, etc. Since the incidence of aortitis is high in untreated syphilis, these criteria might seem to have validity when applied only to known cases of syphilis in large syphilis clinics, but attempts to employ these criteria in a general clinic have met with complete failure. A more reliable indication of syphilitic aortitis is the finding of calcification in the ascending aorta which may be present in the late stages but is of no aid in the diagnosis of early syphilitic aortitis. The incidence of calcification of the ascending aorta has been estimated to occur in about 20 per cent of such patients.[10,11] In one study, approximately two-thirds of patients with calcification of the ascending aorta had positive serologic evidence of syphilis.[12] The tendency for calcification of atherosclerosis to occur along the medial side of the ascending arch and for the calcification to occur also along the anterolateral wall in syphilitic aortitis offers some aid in differentiating the calcification due to these two disorders.[13]

From the foregoing statements it is apparent that a certain diagnosis of early uncomplicated syphilitic aortitis is not possible, since it produces neither signs nor symptoms. However, such a diagnosis in an established case of untreated syphilis is a reasonably sound statistical accusation, and the patient should be treated accordingly with the idea of preventing progression to the serious complications: *aortic insufficiency, aortic aneurysm,* and *coronary ostial disease.*

Aortic Insufficiency

Aortic valvular insufficiency is the most frequent of the complications of syphilitic aortitis.[6] The mesaortitis in the first portion of the aorta results in dilatation of the aortic valve ring, so that the commissures are widened and coaptation of the valve cusps no longer occurs. Thickening and rolling of the edge of the cusp may be present.[1] The result of these pathologic changes is free aortic regurgitation without stenosis. Calcification in the valve cusps does not occur unless there is concomitant rheumatic or atherosclerotic disease. Depending upon the degree and duration of the aortic regurgitation, variable amounts of left ventricular dilatation and hypertrophy occur. The endocardium over the septum may show a thickened plaque in the area of the regurgitant jet. The other complications of syphilitic aortitis may coexist with aortic valvular insufficiency. Disease of the coronary ostiums is present in approximately 20 per cent of cases of aortic insufficiency.[3] Aortic aneurysm may coexist with aortic valvular insufficiency but in much less frequency than ostial disease. After free aortic regurgitation is present, aneurysms do not tend to develop; however, the presence of an aneurysm does not protect against subsequent development of aortic insufficiency.[3] Aortic insufficiency is more common among Negroes than whites (3:1) and more common in males than females (4:1).[6] Aortic insufficiency is most commonly manifest between ages thirty-five and fifty-five years, or 10 to 25 years after the primary lesion. In most cases diagnosis is made after symptoms have appeared.[3]

The diagnosis of syphilitic aortic insufficiency is usually not difficult. Demonstration of a murmur of aortic insufficiency along with evidence of syphilis constitutes a reasonable basis for diagnosis. Evidence of syphilis consists of a history of infection and/or serologic evidences of syphilis and/or evidence of syphilis elsewhere in the body. The serologic tests for syphilis in the blood are positive in approximately three-fourths of the cases of aortic insufficiency and in the spinal fluid in about one-half of the cases.[6]

The clinical manifestations of aortic insufficiency are discussed in detail in Chap. 25. A brief discussion is presented here for the purpose of emphasis and convenience. Slight aortic insufficiency may be present without producing any additional circulatory abnormality. At times, an abnormality of the arterial pulse contour may be detected even though the systemic diastolic blood pressure remains normal. The ascending limb of the arterial pulse is steep, and the crest of the wave is brief in such cases. With more severe aortic insufficiency the diastolic blood pressure becomes low, the pulse pressure wide, and the arterial pulse contour grossly abnormal. When heart failure ensues, the diastolic blood pressure may gradually rise until a normal level is reached. The classic signs include (1) Traube's sign, a pistol-shot sound over the peripheral arteries, (2) Duroziez's sign, a diastolic murmur proximal to constriction of peripheral arteries, (3) de Musset's sign, a systolic nodding of the head, (4) Corrigan's pulse, a water-hammer or collapsing arterial pulse, (5) Quincke's capillary pulse, an alternate flushing and blanching of capillary beds, and (6) Hill's sign, an increase in femoral artery pressure over brachial artery pressure of more than the normal difference of 20 mm Hg. These findings are interesting but are not really helpful. No one misses aortic insufficiency that is severe enough to produce these signs, but many miss the faint murmur that is unassociated with such signs.

The murmur of aortic insufficiency is high-pitched and heard best with the diaphragm of the stethoscope applied with firm pressure. The murmur is usually heard in the second right interspace adjacent to the sternum, along the left sternal border, and at the apex. As a rule, it is louder along the left sternal border. It is louder in early diastole and decreases in intensity during diastole (decrescendo). It is useful to listen to the heart while the patient is leaning forward and holding the breath in expiration. Occasionally, the intensity of the murmur may be accentuated by having the patient lie on the stethoscope (the diaphragm being applied along the left sternal border). On occasion the diastolic murmur may have a musical character, which suggests erosion of perforation of a valve cusp. In syphilitic aortic regurgitation the musical murmur is ascribed to erosion of a cusp which may be permanent or may come and go.

Harvey and associates[14] have pointed out that diseases of the aortic root such as syphilitic aortitis, dissecting aneurysm, aneurysm of a sinus of Valsalva, dilatation of the aorta due to hypertension, and rheumatoid aortitis may produce aortic regurgitation that is heard with maximum intensity along the right sternal border. The technique is to compare the intensity of the murmur as heard in the third right interspace near the sternum with the intensity of the murmur as heard in the third left interspace near the sternum. When the murmur is louder on the right, consider aortic root disease.

The murmur of mild aortic insufficiency may be similar to the murmur of pulmonary insufficiency. The location of the two murmurs may be identical, and when the pulse pressure is normal, the two murmurs may be difficult to separate. When the murmur is louder along the right sternal border, it is usually due to aortic insufficiency. When there is prompt intensification of the murmur with inspiration, it is likely to be pulmonary insufficiency. When there is definite mitral stenosis due to rheumatic fever, the high-pitched murmur along the left sternal border may be due to either aortic insufficiency or pulmonary insufficiency (Steell [15]).

Statistically, while either or both can occur, most are due to aortic insufficiency.[16] When aortic insufficiency is severe, it may be associated with a loud systolic murmur heard best in the second and third right interspaces adjacent to the sternum. This murmur may simulate the murmur of aortic stenosis and may be accompanied by a thrill. A wide pulse pressure and pulsus bisferiens indicate that aortic insufficiency is the major problem in confusing cases.

Mitral insufficiency may be present when there is left ventricular dilatation, and tricuspid insufficiency may be present when heart failure develops.

Virtually all patients with moderate aortic insufficiency associated with a wide pulse pressure will exhibit a ventricular diastolic gallop at the apex. Many patients with severe aortic regurgitation have diastolic rumbles at the apex (Flint[17]). The Flint rumble was originally described in patients with aortic insufficiency due to syphilis but may be secondary to aortic regurgitation of any cause. The differential problem becomes the following: does the patient have aortic insufficiency as the major or only abnormality and a Flint rumble, or does the patient have rheumatic mitral stenosis and aortic insufficiency? The Flint rumble usually occurs in mid-diastole, but there may be presystolic accentuation. The presence of an opening snap and loud first sound indicates mitral stenosis. The P-R interval is often long in patients with aortic insufficiency, and the first heart sound may be faint. The finding of a loud first heart sound despite a long P-R interval favors the diagnosis of mitral stenosis. Occasionally, there is a loud aortic ejection click in patients with aortic regurgitation that may be mistaken for a loud first sound. Atrial fibrillation occurs with greater frequency in patients with mitral stenosis. An abnormal systolic and diastolic thrust is palpable at the apex when aortic regurgitation is present. These pulsations do not occur when there is pure mitral stenosis. The presence of such pulsations does not rule out mitral stenosis but does suggest that aortic regurgitation is the dominant lesion. Calcification of the mitral or aortic valve cusps not only indicates mitral valve disease but signifies a rheumatic cause. Calcifications of the early portion of the aorta suggest a syphilitic cause.

The prognosis of syphilitic aortic insufficiency is generally poor. Only 30 to 40 per cent survive 10 years after the diagnosis is made.[18] The presence of congestive heart failure is the most important determinant of longevity in this disease. Of the patients who remained free of heart failure, 56 per cent survived 15 years, but of those who had heart failure at the time of diagnosis, less than 20 per cent survived 5 years, and less than 6 per cent survived 10 years. The average duration of life from the onset of heart failure is about 3 years. In syphilitic aortic insufficiency with heart failure, sudden death is fairly common. There are exceptional patients who have survived 15 to 20 years after the onset of heart failure. At the other end of the spectrum are those patients who experience a sudden onset of heart failure and who, in spite of the most rigorous treatment, progress inexorably downhill and die during the first hospital admission.

There are several important factors which influence longevity in aortic insufficiency. The degree of regurgitation and the diastolic blood pressure are important. Low diastolic pressure makes for a limited coronary blood flow. The pressure and degree of ostial narrowing are equally important. It is interesting to note that those patients who survive 10 to 15 years after the onset of heart failure usually have only minimal narrowing of the coronary ostiums and those patients who arrive only a short time after onset of failure usually have more severe degrees of ostial disease. The appearance of anginal pain with heart failure indicates a poorer prognosis. Under these circumstances the anginal pain is usually attributed to coronary ostial narrowing, but angina may occur in the absence of significant ostial disease when the regurgitation is severe and the diastolic pressure is low. In either event, the outlook is poorer when coronary blood flow is inadequate. The presence of other diseases, such as coronary artery atherosclerosis, hypertension, or anemia, adds a further burden to an already failing heart. Excessive physical activity may shorten life expectancy in syphilitic aortic insufficiency, and the onset of heart failure may appear quite suddenly for the first time following strenuous exertion.

The treatment of syphilitic aortic insufficiency should first be directed at heart failure if this is present. There is no particular urgency to begin penicillin at this stage of the disease, since the disaster is almost complete. Once the heart failure is controlled, penicillin therapy may be started. The risk of Jarisch-Herxheimer reaction is extremely small, and no particular precautions are necessary.[19] Adequate penicillin therapy is achieved by 6 to 10 million units of procaine penicillin with 2 per cent aluminum monostearate given over a 10-day period, or benzathine penicillin G may be administered in 3-million-unit doses at 7-day intervals for a total of three doses.[20]

The medical management of severe syphilitic aortic insufficiency leaves much to be desired. The continuing physiologic burden of severe regurgitation along with poor coronary blood flow makes for a limited response to the usual measures employed in the treatment of heart failure. Surgical correction of the regurgitation utilizing the Starr-Edwards prosthesis to replace the aortic valve has been successfully employed (see Chap. 26). The presence of coronary ostial disease and the more advanced age of many of these patients are limiting factors to successful surgical approaches to this problem, although endarterectomy has been successfully employed.

Aneurysm

Aneurysm of the aorta is a late complication of syphilitic aortitis, usually occurring from 15 to 30 years after the initial infection. Aneurysms occur about one-third as frequently as aortic insufficiency, but the same race and sex incidence is found for both lesions.[6,21] As a result of damage from aortitis, the aorta may undergo generalized dilatation to form a fusiform aneurysm or a more localized dilatation to form a saccular aneurysm. In the latter, the communication with the aortic lumen may be quite large or only a centimeter in diameter. The aneurysmal sac may contain a laminated clot with the older portion nearest the lumen of the aorta and the newer clot next to the aneurysmal wall where the additional growth occurs. The walls of large aneurysms are composed largely of fibrous tissue, and identification of remnants of the original wall of the aorta may be impossible. Approximately 50 per cent of syphilitic aneurysms occur in the ascending aorta, 30 to 40 per cent in the transverse arch, 15 per cent in the descending aorta, and less than 5 per cent in the abdominal aorta.[22] Frequently, more than one aneurysm exists in the same patient.

Since the signs and symptoms of aneurysms result largely from compression of adjacent structures, one would expect different clinical manifestations from aneurysms in various portions of the aorta. For example, aneurysms of the ascending aorta may compress the pulmonary artery, superior vena cava, or the right main bronchus with predictable results from involvement of each structure. However, aneurysms in this location may enlarge in an anterolateral direction and achieve considerable size before giving rise to symptoms from impingement upon adjacent structures. The close anatomic relationship of the transverse arch to the esophagus, trachea, bronchi, recurrent laryngeal nerve, and vertebrae makes for compression of vital structures with much smaller aneurysmal sacs. Dysphagia, dyspnea, stridor, cough, hemoptysis, hoarseness, and pain are frequently encountered in aneurysms of the transverse arch. Involvement of the orifices of the great vessels results in unequal pulses in the arms, and compression of the left stellate ganglion results in unequal pupils. Atelectasis, infection, and lung abscess are frequent results of compression of the bronchi and lungs. The descending aorta has more space for dilatation and may undergo considerable enlargement before symptoms occur from compression of lung or erosion of vertebrae and impingement upon sensitive nerve roots. Aneurysms in this location may erode ribs and present a pulsatile mass in the left side of the chest posteriorly. Aneurysms of the abdominal aorta often present a pulsating epigastric mass and pain in the abdomen and back.

There is always danger of rupture of syphilitic aneurysms. In the thorax, perforation is most commonly into the pericardial cavity, pleural cavities, bronchial tree, and esophagus.[23] Aneurysms of the ascending aorta tend to perforate into the pericavity and right pleural spaces. Infrequently, there is perforation into the pulmonary artery which causes a sudden appearance of a continuous murmur and right ventricular strain.[23]

The diagnosis of syphilitic aortic aneurysm is made by the demonstration of the characteristic structural changes in the aorta with a history of syphilis and/or serologic evidence of syphilis and/or evidences of syphilis elsewhere in the body. To be sure that the mass in question is an aneurysm, it must be shown to be a part of the aorta in all views. Expansile pulsation in a mass is helpful if present, but not all aneurysms demonstrate expansile pulsations, particularly those containing laminated clots and very large aneurysms. A solid tissue mass located adjacent to the aorta may reveal systolic movement which is transmitted from the aorta. The presence of linear calcification extending along the wall of the aorta and into the wall of the mass is helpful in establishing the mass as an aneurysm. If the aorta is displaced to either side, there is disease of the aorta. The aorta is never displaced by extravascular solid tumor masses such as neoplasms, lymphadenopathy, dermoid cysts, substernal goiter, or enlarged thymus. Differentiation of aneurysms from such extravascular tumors is usually not too difficult, but if any doubt remains, the issue is settled by aortography.

Other diseases of the aorta which result in dilatation must be differentiated from syphilitic aneurysm. Traumatic aneurysm occurs in the region of the isthmus; the serologic tests for syphilis are negative, and there is usually a history of trauma. Coarctation of the aorta, dissecting aneurysm, Marfan's syndrome, aortic stenosis with poststenotic dilatation, and atherosclerosis may produce a dilated aorta and aortic valvular insufficiency. These various diseases have rather diagnostic characteristics of their own which allow differentiation from syphilis. The dilatation and elongation of the aorta with atherosclerosis forms a simple smooth arc from ascending aorta to the aortic knob. Syphilitic changes in this portion of the aorta result in more than one arc in this segment.

The prognosis of syphilitic aortic aneurysms is grave. After the onset of symptoms, the average duration of life is measured in months. In a series of 188 cases, only 18 patients were alive at the end of 2 years; of the 170 who died, the average duration of life was about 6 months.[21] There are many aneurysms which are diagnosed radiologically before the onset of symptoms, and the duration of life in the asymptomatic patients might be expected to be longer than in those presenting symptoms of compression of some vital organ.

Once the aorta has dilated in either saccular or fusiform manner, the hydraulic principles are such that this weakened segment is subjected to a greater sheering force per unit length than is the adjacent aorta of normal diameter. The total force acting along the wall of the aorta is greatly increased by an increase in diameter of the aorta. The aneurysm usually continues to grow unless the lumen is filled with a large clot which may tend to protect against further disruption of the wall.

The treatment in syphilitic aortic aneurysm is often symptomatic and directed at complications of the aneurysm such as atelectasis, infection, lung abscess, and the control of pain. Penicillin is recommended in the same dosage schedule as in aortic insufficiency. That antisyphilitic therapy will prolong life at this stage of the disease is questionable, since the aortic defect is now a mechanical one with hydraulic reasons for progression. At the present time the preferred treatment is surgical excision of the aneurysm with restoration of the continuity of the aorta (see Chap. 59).

Coronary Ostial Disease

Involvement of the ostiums of the coronary arteries in syphilitic aortitis results in a gradual, progressive narrowing. The coronary ostiums may be so nearly occluded that one is impressed by the ability of extracoronary collateral vessels to maintain life. Because of the slowness of the occlusive process, myocardial infarction is rare; however, small areas of fibrosis throughout the myocardium are common. The incidence of ostial narrowing without other complications of aortitis is difficult to determine from published autopsy data, but the association of aortic insufficiency and coronary ostial disease is quite common.[3,18,21]

The presence of coronary ostial narrowing is suspected when angina pectoris occurs in patients with syphilitic aortic insufficiency, but it must be remembered that angina may occur with aortic regurgitation alone. In the absence of aortic insufficiency, a diagnosis of syphilitic ostial disease as a cause of angina pectoris can be made only by coronary arteriography.

The outlook of coronary ostial disease is poor.[18]

It is often associated with aortic insufficiency, and the low diastolic pressure plus the narrowing of the ostiums provides an inadequate blood flow to an overloaded heart. Sudden death due to ventricular fibrillation secondary to myocardial ischemia is common in this group of patients, and they are extremely poor risks for surgical treatment or any maneuver which impairs effective coronary perfusion. Treatment of coronary ostial disease consists of the usual management of angina and heart failure, plus the same antisyphilitic regimen of penicillin as for aortic insufficiency. Occasionally, the anginal syndrome may disappear after antisyphilitic therapy. Initial experience with coronary ostial endarterectomy offers hope of future surgical correction.

Gumma of the Myocardium

Involvement of the myocardium by gumma formation is unusual. The manifestations of an isolated gumma are determined by its location. In instances of high septal involvement, bundle branch block and atrioventricular block may occur. When areas of the free wall of the ventricle are replaced by gummatous tissue, the electrocardiogram resembles that of myocardial infarction. In most instances the diagnosis of myocardial gumma is made post mortem.

Other Vascular Manifestations of Syphilis

Syphilis is a widespread disease and commonly involves blood vessels other than the aorta. The formation of a gumma anywhere in the body depends primarily on changes in blood vessels. The changes in the central nervous system in syphilis result from an obliterative arteritis of the cerebral vessels. Syphilis primarily in the central nervous system may give rise to secondary systemic vascular disorders such as the postural hypotension seen in tabes dorsalis.[24,25]

REFERENCES

1. Boyd, W.: "The Pathology of Internal Diseases," 4th ed., Lea & Febiger, Philadelphia, 1945.
2. Reynolds, F. W., and Moore, J. E.: Syphilis. A Review of the Recent Literature, *A.M.A. Arch. Int. Med.*, 80:655–690, 1947.
3. Kampmeier, R. H., and Morgan, H. J.: The Specific Treatment of Syphilitic Aortitis, *Circulation*, 5:771–778, 1952.
4. Warthin, A. S.: The Lesions of Latent Syphilis, *South. M. J.*, 24:273–278, 1931.
5. Langer, E.: Die Taufigkeit der leutischen Organveranderungen insbesondere der Aortitis luetica, *München. med. Wchnschr.*, 73:1782–1785, 1926.
6. Cole, H. N., et al.: Cooperative Clinical Studies in the Treatment of Syphilis, *J.A.M.A.*, 108:1861–1866, 1937.
7. Turner, T. B.: The Race and Sex Distribution of the Lesions of Syphilis in Ten Thousand Cases, *Bull. Johns Hopkins Hosp.*, 46:159–184, 1930.
8. Kemp, J. E., and Cochems, K. D.: Studies in Cardiovascular Syphilis. IV. The Influence of the Treatment of Early Syphilis upon the Incidence of Cardiovascular Syphilis, *Am. J. Syphilis*, 21:625–633, 1937.
9. Stokes, J. H., Beerman, H., and Ingraham, N. R.: "Modern Clinical Syphilology," 3d ed., W. B. Saunders Company, Philadelphia, 1944.
10. Jackman, J., and Lubert, M.: Significance of Calcification in the Ascending Aorta as Observed Roentgenologically, *Am. J. Roentgenol.*, 53:432–438, 1945.
11. Thorner, M. C., Carter, R. A., and Griffith, G. C.: Calcification as a Diagnostic Sign of Syphilitic Aortitis, *Am. Heart J.*, 38:641–653, 1949.
12. Leighton, R. S.: Calcification of the Ascending Aorta as a Sign of Syphilitic Aortitis, *Radiology*, 51:527–529, 1948.
13. Lodwick, G. S., and Gladstone, W. S.: Correlation of Anatomic and Roentgen Changes in Arteriosclerosis and Syphilis of the Ascending Aorta, *Radiology*, 60:70–78, 1957.
14. Harvey, W. P., Corrado, M., and Perloff, J. K.: Right-sided Murmur of Aortic Insufficiency (Diastolic Murmur Better Heard to the Right of the Sternum Rather than the Left), *Am. J. M. Sc.*, 245:533–543, 1963.
15. Steell, G.: Murmur of High Pressure in the Pulmonary Artery, *M. Chronicle*, 9:182–188, 1888–1889.
16. Brest, A. N., Udhoji, V., and Likoff, W.: A Reevaluation of the Graham-Steell Murmur, *New England J. Med.*, 263:1229–1231, 1960.
17. Flint, A.: On Cardiac Murmurs, *Am. J. M. Sc.*, 44:29–54, 1862.
18. Webster, B., Rich, C., Jr., Dense, P. M., Moore, J. E., Nicol, C. S., and Padget, P.: Studies in Cardiovascular Syphilis. III. The Natural History of Syphilitic Aortic Insufficiency, *Am. Heart J.*, 46:117–145, 1953.
19. Moore, J. E., Farmer, T. W., and Hoekenga, M. T.: Penicillin and the Jarisch-Herxheimer Reaction in Early Cardiovascular and Neurosyphilis, *Tr. A. Am. Physicians*, 61:176–183, 1948.
20. "Syphilis: Modern Diagnosis and Management," U.S. Public Health Service Publication no. 743, 1961.
21. Kampmeier, R. H., and Combs, S. R.: The Prognosis in Syphilitic Aortic Insufficiency: An evaluation of Factors Other than Antisyphilitic Treatment, *Am. J. Syphilis*, 24:578–589, 1940.
22. Boyd, L. J.: A Study of Four Thousand Reported Cases of Aneurysms of the Thoracic Aorta, *Am. J. M. Sc.*, 168:654–668, 1924.
23. Nicholson, R. E.: Syndrome of Rupture of Aortic Aneurysm into Pulmonary Artery: Review of the

Literature with Report of Two Cases, *Ann. Int. Med.,* **19**:286–325, 1943.

24. Spingarn, C. L. and Hitzig, W. M.: Orthostatic Circulatory Insufficiency: Its Occurrence in Tabes Dorsalis and Addison's Disease, *A.M.A. Arch. Int. Med.,* **69**:23–40, 1942.

25. Ellis, L. B., and Haynes, F. W.: Postural Hypotension with Particular Reference to Its Occurrence in Diseases of the Central Nervous System, *A.M.A. Arch. Int. Med.,* **58**:773–798, 1936.

54 HIGH-CARDIAC-OUTPUT STATES

Noble O. Fowler, M.D.

The disorders discussed in this chapter are those in which the resting cardiac output is increased beyond the accepted normal range of 2.3 to 3.9 liters per m² per min.[1] In order to understand the mechanism of an increased resting cardiac output, it is well to consider the several means by which the cardiac output is controlled. Important factors are:

1. The necessity for maintaining a normal blood pressure, when peripheral resistance is altered.[2]

2. The tissue needs for oxygen.

3. The cardiac filling pressure.

4. The effects of normally produced hormones and of hormones or chemical substances produced by certain neoplasms, such as pheochromocytoma or carcinoid tumors, upon cardiac output.

5. The effect of the sympathetic nervous system upon cardiac output.[3]

6. Alterations in blood viscosity.

7. Body temperature. The circulation time is known to be decreased and the cardiac output increased with fever.

In most of the hyperkinetic, or high-output, states increased cardiac filling pressure is not a factor in the elevated cardiac output. Decrease of peripheral vascular resistance will, of necessity, cause the cardiac output to rise in order to maintain a normal blood pressure, so that the tissues may receive the oxygen which they require. Decrease of peripheral vascular resistance is an important factor in systemic arteriovenous fistulas and probably contributes to the increased cardiac output of thyrotoxicosis, anemia, and beriberi heart disease, and the increased cardiac output in warm, humid environments. In hypoxic states such as chronic cor pulmonale and anemia, cardiac output must rise in order that the tissues receive an adequate supply of oxygen. In hypoxia, increased secretion

of epinephrine by the adrenal medulla is a factor in the increase of cardiac output, but a direct effect upon the central nervous system which causes increasing sympathetic outflow to the heart and local effects upon small arteries is more important. In patients with pheochromocytoma or carcinoid tumors the chemical substances released by the neoplasms act upon the heart to increase cardiac output. In the increased cardiac output of anxiety and that which occurs with exercise, increased sympathetic outflow to the heart is of major importance.

Increase of the resting cardiac output may be accomplished by increasing the heart rate, by increasing the cardiac stroke volume, or by both mechanisms. When the cardiac stroke volume is increased in response to a decrease of peripheral resistance, there are usually clinical signs related to this phenomenon. These include increase of the systemic pulse pressure, bounding carotid, radial, and femoral pulses, and in some instances pistol-shot sounds over the peripheral arteries. "Capillary pulses," systolic bruits over large arteries, and pulmonary systolic murmurs are common.

THYROTOXICOSIS

Pathologic Physiology

There are several factors involved in the increased cardiac output associated with thyrotoxicosis. Among these are the increased oxygen consumption and the tachycardia which are usually found in this disorder. In addition, there is often an increased cardiac stroke volume.[4] There are at least three major factors which may contribute to the increased cardiac stroke volume of thyrotoxicosis: It has been shown that there is probably a direct action of thyroid hormone upon the isolated heart which causes it to beat more strongly. It has been demonstrated that in thyrotoxicosis there is increased sensitivity to circulating epinephrine and norepinephrine.[5] This tends to increase cardiac stroke volume. Finally, in thyrotoxicosis there is evidence of decreased peripheral vascular resistance, which tends to increase cardiac output.[4]

Physical Findings

Most patients with thyrotoxicosis have evidence of increased cardiac output without congestive heart failure. Congestive heart failure is rare in hyperthyroidism unless the patient is in the older age group. It is postulated that most patients who have congestive heart failure with thyrotoxicosis have additional underlying heart disease, but in many instances neither the heart disease nor its nature can be established. In patients under the age of thirty-five one occasionally observes cardiac decompensation without evident additional heart disease.[4] Most patients with thyrotoxicosis demonstrate the usual physical features of stare, exophthalmos, enlarged and firm thyroid with or without nodule formation, fine tremor of the outstretched hands, warm, moist skin of salmon hue, and tachycardia. If the metabolic rate is considerably increased, there is usually a loud cervical venous hum. In the author's experience, continuous murmurs over the thyroid gland in thyrotoxic patients have been caused by a cervical venous hum rather than by dilated arteries within the gland.[6] Others have found occasional continuous murmurs over the thyroid gland which are distince from the venous hum. In thyrotoxicosis without heart failure, the cardiac rhythm is usually of normal sinus origin, although 20 to 25 per cent of patients have atrial fibrillation. On the other hand, in patients with heart failure, primarily those of the older age groups, atrial fibrillation is found in perhaps 90 per cent of instances. There is characteristically an increase of systolic blood pressure with a modest decrease of diastolic pressure; thus the pulse pressure is increased, and the peripheral arterial pulse may be quite bounding. The heart itself is usually of normal size, unless there is complicating heart disease or congestive heart failure. The first heart sound is often of increased intensity and may at times suggest an incorrect diagnosis of mitral stenosis. In older patients with thyrotoxicosis and heart disease, the thyrotoxicosis may be masked; that is, the eye signs may be minimal or absent, and the thyroid enlargement and tachycardia may be inconspicuous. The possibility of thyrotoxic heart disease is often suggested by the observation of atrial fibrillation without obvious cause, some widening of the pulse pressure, and unusual alertness in the patient with congestive heart failure. It is desirable that studies for thyrotoxicosis be made in all patients with unexplained atrial fibrillation. Thyrotoxicosis should be considered in patients with atrial fibrillation whose ventricular rate fails to slow with adequate amounts of digitalis. Generalized lymphadenopathy and splenomegaly are found in about 10 per cent of instances.

Laboratory Data

The diagnosis of thyrotoxicosis can be confirmed by demonstrating an increase in the basal metabolic rate, a serum-protein–bound iodine above 8 μg per ml serum, and a determination of radioactive iodine uptake, which usually considerably exceeds 55 per cent in 24 hr. Cardiac catheterization studies characteristically reveal an increased cardiac output and at times an increase of stroke volume with a narrowed arteriovenous oxygen difference below the normal value of 4.5 ± 0.7 * ml

* Standard deviation.

per 100 ml blood.[4] The circulation time is characteristically shortened in the absence of heart failure. With heart failure the circulation time is usually within the normal range, the arm-to-tongue time being 9 to 16 sec measured with Decholin.

Diagnosis and Treatment

The diagnosis of thyrotoxicosis is based upon the characteristic physical findings and laboratory data. Treatment in patients under the age of twenty-five usually consists of subtotal thyroidectomy preceded by adequate preparation with a combination of methimazole and Lugol's solution. In older patients, especially in those with congestive heart failure or recurrent thyrotoxicosis after surgical treatment, the use of radioactive iodine is usually preferred. If there is severe thyrotoxicosis, reserpine may mitigate some of the adverse effects upon the heart until the thyrotoxicosis can be controlled.[7] Guanethidine decreases the cardiac output in induced hyperthyroidism[8] but is not generally employed in the therapy of patients with thyrocardiac disease. The use of guanethidine may aggravate the manifestations of heart failure in euthyroid patients with cardiac decompensation.[9]

BERIBERI HEART DISEASE

Pathologic Physiology

Beriberi heart disease is a rare disorder in the United States, and some have questioned its existence in this country. However, Blankenhorn collected 12 cases during the years 1940 to 1948 from the Cincinnati General Hospital.[10] In his study, patients with beriberi heart disease were almost invariably chronic alcoholics. They demonstrated evidence of either peripheral neuritis, with calf tenderness, decreased or absent vibratory sense in the lower extremities, and loss of knee or ankle reflexes, or of pellagra, with a red, smooth tongue and perhaps skin changes over the face, neck, and upper part of the chest, knees, and elbows. The mechanism of increased cardiac output is obscure. Some patients with beriberi have lesions of the sympathetic nuclei[10] which may decrease the peripheral resistance, thus increasing cardiac work and leading to congestive failure. In addition, thiamine deficiency interferes with myocardial metabolism of pyruvate to active acetate. Patients with beriberi heart disease display the usual findings of biventricular congestive failure. There is elevation of the venous pressure, edema, and hepatic engorgement. There is very commonly an apical systolic murmur of relative mitral insufficiency and a diastolic ventricular gallop rhythm. Characteristically, there are widening of the pulse pressure and bounding peripheral pulses.

Pistol-shot sounds may be heard over the peripheral arteries. The heart is usually dilated.

Laboratory Data

The electrocardiogram in patients with beriberi heart disease is usually normal except for sinus tachycardia and perhaps minor nonspecific ST segment and T-wave changes. The circulation time is usually within the normal limits. Rarely is it shorter than normal. An example of the cardiac catheterization data in beriberi heart disease is given in the following case description:

The patient was a twenty-eight-year-old barmaid, who was admitted to the Cincinnati General Hospital on September 18, 1950. There was a history of alcoholism for 3 years. The diet was considered deficient in bread and meat. She complained of dependent edema and numbness of the hands and legs for 4 days before admission.

On examination, blood pressure was 150/70. Heart rate was 106 per min; temperature, 99.8°F. The neck veins were abnormally distended. The skin was warm. The heart was enlarged, with a ventricular gallop. There were fine rales at the lung bases and signs of peripheral neuritis.

Laboratory Data. Hemoglobin was 10.2 Gm. Arm-to-tongue Decholin circulation times were 9.5, 7.5, and 10 sec on three occasions. The electrocardiogram was normal except for very slight decrease of T-wave amplitude.

CATHETERIZATIONS OF THE RIGHT SIDE OF THE HEART

	9/22/50	11/17/50	12/29/50
Pressures, mm Hg:			
Right atrium	10	5*	3
Pulmonary artery	36/25 (32)	25/8 (17)	21/7 (14)
Pulmonary wedge	22	8.5	8
Systemic arterial O_2			
saturation, %	87	93	94
Arteriovenous O_2			
difference	3.4	4.5	3.1
Cardiac index,			
L/min/m²	6.1	4.9	4.5

* Right ventricular end-diastolic pressure.

Comment: This patient was first studied four days after admission, while still in clinical heart failure. The data for catheterization of the right side of the heart were consistent with biventricular failure, showing elevation of both right atrial and pulmonary wedge pressures, together with cardiac output twice the average normal cardiac index of 3.1 liters per min per m²,[11,12] The arteriovenous oxygen difference was decreased. On November 17, 1950, and December 29, 1950, after the patient was treated with rest and thiamine and other vitamins of the B complex, congestive heart failure was no longer present. It may be seen that the right atrial and pulmonary wedge pressures were normal at the time of the second and third studies. The cardiac output had decreased but remained above the normal range (cardiac index 3.1 ± 0.4* liters per min per m²).

Burwell and Dexter[11] showed that recovery from acute beriberi heart disease was associated with a decrease in cardiac output, heart rate, and oxygen consumption, a return of arteriovenous oxygen difference to normal, and a rise of diastolic blood pressure.

Diagnosis

The criteria for the diagnosis of beriberi heart disease were listed by Blankenhorn.[13] They include a history of a thiamine-deficient diet for 3 months or more, absence of another cause of heart disease, elevation of venous pressure, edema, an enlarged heart, minor electrocardiographic changes, evidence of peripheral neuritis or pellagra, and a response to thiamine with a decrease in heart size, or autopsy findings consistent with the diagnosis. Nutritional cirrhosis is found at autopsy in many instances. At the University of Cincinnati Hospitals it is doubted that beriberi leads to a specific anatomic form of chronic myocardial disease or intractable congestive failure.[14] In the author's experience patients with beriberi heart disease either died suddenly in the acute stage or made a complete recovery.

Treatment

Patients with beriberi heart disease should be treated with bed rest. There is a tendency to syncope and sudden death, so that it is important that they receive treatment early. The optimum treatment is thiamine along with remainder of the vitamin B complex. Thiamine may be given parenterally in doses of 50 mg daily. Digitalis apparently is of little benefit.[15] Sodium restriction and diuretics are of some value.

ANEMIA

Pathologic Physiology

Despite many studies of the mechanism of increased cardiac output in anemia, the exact pathologic physiology is not well understood. From studies made in the author's laboratory it is apparent that a decrease of blood viscosity is one factor. However, the relatively small increase in cardiac output achieved makes it unlikely that decreased blood viscosity is responsible alone. It has been shown that the adrenal glands are not necessary

* Standard deviation.

for the increase in cardiac output,[16] nor is the sympathetic nervous system.[17] Increased cardiac filling pressure is not essential to the increased cardiac output of acute experimental anemia.[18] It seems likely that dilitation of small arteries is the most important mechanism, but the manner in which this decreased peripheral resistance is mediated remains uncertain. In man with chronic anemia it has been shown by Brannon and associates[19] that the cardiac output is usually not increased by anemia until the hemoglobin is below 7 Gm per 100 ml blood, or about 50 per cent of normal. In experimental animals ventricular function curves become abnormal when the hematocrit is reduced below 24 per cent, presumably because coronary blood flow can no longer be increased beyond this point to compensate for the effects of severe anemia.[20] Although angina pectoris may be caused by anemia, it is more likely that anemic patients with angina have associated coronary artery disease.[21] Patients who are anemic may have congestive heart failure. As in thyrotoxicosis, most patients with anemia in whom congestive heart failure develops have underlying heart disease, and the anemia serves as an aggravating factor which increases the work of the heart.[21] However, with very severe anemia congestive heart failure may occur from anemia alone. This event is rare in the United States but apparently not uncommon in tropical countries.[22] As a rule, it may be said that cardiac enlargement or congestive heart failure on the basis of chronic anemia is unlikely unless the hemoglobin is below 5 Gm per 100 ml blood. When anemia results from sickle-cell disease, congestive failure may occur at higher hemoglobin levels. This is perhaps a reflection of myocardial and pulmonary arterial disease and an altered oxygen dissociation curve. The increased cardiac output of anemia is produced by both tachycardia and increased cardiac stroke volume. As a result in many patients there is an increase in the systemic pulse pressure. Dyspnea, dependent edema, and reduction in vital capacity may result from anemia alone without added congestive heart failure.[21]

Physical Findings

In patients with severe anemia (hemoglobin below 7 Gm per 100 ml blood) there is pallor of the skin and mucous membranes. Tachycardia is usually present. There is often an increase in systemic pulse pressure which reflects the increase in cardiac stroke volume. The peripheral arterial pulses may be bounding, and there may be Duroziez's sign and pistol-shot sounds over the femoral artery. There may be "capillary" pulsations. There is probably an increase in the frequency of cervical venous hums in these patients. There may be systolic bruits over both carotid arteries. These are usually rather short. There is commonly a pulmonary ejection systolic murmur presumably reflecting the increased blood flow and eddying in this area. With severe anemia, there may be cardiac dilatation with resulting murmurs of mitral and tricuspid insufficiency. Murmurs of aortic insufficiency have been described in patients with severe anemia.[21] This finding is extremely unusual in the author's experience at the University of Cincinnati Hospital.

Patients with sickle-cell anemia may display a variety of cardiac murmurs. The murmurs may suggest mitral stenosis, and as a rule the diagnosis of mitral stenosis should be made with great caution in patients with sickle-cell anemia. In children with sickle-cell anemia, systolic murmurs are found invariably. Most commonly these are in the second left intercostal space and presumably related to increased flow into the pulmonary artery.[23] A prominent third heart sound in mid-diastole is common in sickle-cell anemia. There is a tendency to some exaggeration of the expiratory splitting of the second heart sound.[23] In sickle-cell anemia, cor pulmonale may develop because of pulmonary arterial thrombosis, but this complication is uncommon.[24]

Laboratory Data

In patients with anemia, the circulation time is usually normal or decreased, and this finding may persist during congestive heart failure.[22] Studies made by catheterization of the right side of the heart show an increase of resting cardiac output which is partly the result of tachycardia. There is usually an additional increase of stroke volume.[25] Graettinger et al. have shown that in patients with mild anemia (average hemoglobin 9.4 Gm) the cardiac output is normal at rest but with exercise rises higher than normal.[25] In patients with anemia in whom congestive heart failure develops the cardiac output may fall from the peak value but is still above the normal resting value.[25]

Treatment

The treatment of anemia depends on the underlying cause, whether this be iron deficiency, pernicious anemia, sickle-cell anemia, or anemia related to bone marrow replacement, hemolysis, or blood loss. In patients who have anemia associated with congestive heart failure, it may be necessary to correct the anemia before optimal response of the heart failure can occur. It is generally believed that digitalis is of little or no benefit in congestive heart failure accompanied by severe anemia.[15] However, the author has been able to show that digitalis is effective in anemic heart failure produced in the heart-lung preparation, since it lowers elevated atrial pressures and increases cardiac output.[26] Anemia alone is seldom the cause of heart failure; hence it seems logical to use digitalis. Bed rest, sodium restriction, and diuretics may be used as indicated. The anemia should be corrected gradually. When necessary, slow infusions of ½ unit of packed red cells (125 ml) may be carried out over a period of 3 or 4 hr with careful examination of the patient for dyspnea and auscultation of the lungs for evidences of pulmonary edema. At times it may be necessary to correct anemia quickly in this way in order to obtain satisfactory improvement in congestive heart failure.

SYSTEMIC ARTERIOVENOUS FISTULA

Pathologic Physiology

The decreased systemic vascular resistance associated with large systemic arteriovenous fistulas usually requires that the cardiac output be increased to maintain adequate blood pressure and adequate blood supply to the tissues. Increased cardiac output can be demonstrated as a rule only when there is a large fistula which involves a large artery, such as the aorta, or such major arteries as the subclavian artery, the femoral artery, the common carotid arteries, and the iliac vessels. Pulmonary arteriovenous fistulas involve the low-resistance lesser circulation and seldom, if ever, lead to cardiac enlargement or congestive heart failure. Congenital systemic arteriovenous fistulas are rarely of sufficient size to produce generalized circulatory signs. The mechanism of increased cardiac output in systemic arteriovenous fistula apparently does not involve an increase in cardiac filling pressure. When there is a large arteriovenous fistula, arterialized blood from a high-pressure artery is shunted into a low pressure vein, thus decreasing the arterial blood flow to the tissue beyond the fistula and increasing the venous pressure distal to the fistula. The venous pressure proximal to the fistula and in the right side of the heart are usually normal unless there is congestive heart failure. As a compensatory mechanism, the heart rate and stroke volume increase. The diastolic blood pressure falls, and the cardiac output rises. Obliteration of the arteriovenous fistula by compression results in a fall in cardiac output. There tends to be an increase of plasma volume. Catheterization of the right side of the heart in patients with large systemic arteriovenous fistulas reveals increased oxygenation of venous blood at the site of communication and an increased cardiac output. Intracardiac pressures are normal unless congestive heart failure develops.[12] If heart failure develops, right atrial and peripheral venous pressures rise. The cardiac output is above normal resting levels but fails to increase normally with exercise.[27] Heart failure may develop in patients with hearts which are apparently otherwise normal.[12,27] The following description illustrates some of the hemodynamic features of a large systemic arteriovenous fistula:

The patient was a fifty-seven-year-old man who was admitted to the hospital because of the symptoms of congestive heart failure which had been present for 4 years. Twenty-two years before admission, he had sustained a gunshot wound of the right supraclavicular area. Physical examination revealed signs of a right subclavian arteriovenous fistula. Hemoglobin was 14.5 Gm per 100 ml blood.

CATHETERIZATION OF THE RIGHT SIDE OF THE HEART

	Rest	Exercise
Pressures, mm Hg:		
Right atrium	7	
Pulmonary artery	56/18 (31)	64/28 (43)
Pulmonary wedge	24	
Systemic arterial O_2 saturation, %	92.5	94.4
Arteriovenous O_2 difference	3.3	4.4
O_2 consumption, ml/min	246	386
Cardiac index, L/min/m²	4.4	5.1

Comment: The cardiac catheterization data were consistent with biventricular failure with an elevated resting cardiac output. Both right atrial and pulmonary wedge pressures were above normal. The cardiac index was well above the normal range of 3.1 ± 0.4* liters per min per m². The increased cardiac output was associated with a narrow arteriovenous oxygen difference. Venous blood proximal to the fistula showed a step-up in oxygen content of 3.4 vol per 100 ml blood. With exercise, there was a relatively normal increase of cardiac output from 7.6 to 8.8 liters per min. Such response of cardiac output to exercise would be very unusual for patients with low-output heart failure.

Physical Findings

If the examiner finds an increased systemic arterial pulse pressure when there is no evidence of aortic insufficiency, the possibility of a systemic arteriovenous fistula should be considered. If the patient has had an injury or an operation, careful auscultation should be carried out over that site in order to look for the typical continuous murmur of arteriovenous fistula with a systolic accentuation. Manual compression of the fistula tends to produce

* Standard deviation.

slowing of the heart (Branham's sign). The author has recently studied a patient who acquired a large arteriovenous fistula as the result of nephrectomy. Congestive heart failure may develop in patients with large arteriovenous fistulas. The onset of heart failure may be quite delayed. In one instance a thirty-year-old man who was studied at the Cardiac Laboratory of the Cincinnati General Hospital had congestive heart failure in 1951, 7 years following a gunshot wound involving the internal iliac artery and vein.[12] In another instance congestive heart failure developed in a sixty-eight-year-old patient 57 years after a gunshot wound involving the femoral artery and vein.[28] Presumably, in patients like the latter, there is an additional underlying heart disease. However, in such patients repair of the fistula may result in the return of heart size and function to normal.

Diagnosis

The possibility of a systemic arteriovenous fistula should be considered in all patients who have an increase in systemic arterial pulse pressure with bounding arterial pulses. When there is no obvious cause for a wide arterial pulse pressure such as in aortic insufficiency or thyrotoxicosis, careful auscultation should be carried out over any scars, including those of injury or surgical operations. If the characteristic continuous murmur with systolic accentuation is found in an area of trauma or surgical operation, no further studies should be required to establish the diagnosis. In some instances the systemic arteriovenous fistula may become infected so that there is endarteritis. This complication in turn may lead to aortic valve involvement with aortic bacterial endocarditis. In dogs with large experimental arteriovenous fistulas, aortic, mitral, or tricuspid endocarditis may develop with or without infection of the fistula. The treatment of a systemic arteriovenous fistula, when it is large enough to produce increased arterial pulse pressure, cardiac enlargement, or congestive heart failure, should be that of surgical repair or excision of the fistula.

HEPATIC DISEASE

It is known that the resting cardiac output may be increased in patients with liver disease, especially those with nutritional cirrhosis[29] and infectious hepatitis. The increase in patients with nutritional cirrhosis is usually moderate and occurs in approximately one-third of the patients.[29] The mechanism is uncertain but has been attributed to increased blood volume, intrahepatic arteriovenous shunts, mesenteric arteriovenous shunts, and defects in inactivation of a circulating vasodilator.

Some patients with nutritional cirrhosis have anemia or coexisting beriberi. In a few patients with nutritional cirrhosis or infectious hepatitis, the cardiac output may be quite high, with a bounding pulse and wide pulse pressure. Congestive heart failure may develop,[30] but most patients in this group probably die of hepatic failure before heart failure can develop. One authority has described a cardiac output as high as 15 liters per min, or twice the normal, in a patient with infectious hepatitis.[30]

PAGET'S DISEASE OF BONE

In Paget's disease of the bone, there may be an increased systemic arterial pulse pressure and increased cardiac output.[31] In most patients with Paget's disease this is not a prominent finding. Lequime and Denolin found evidence of increased blood flow to limbs involved by Paget's disease, but increase of resting cardiac output was unusual.[32] The cardiac output in patients with extensive bone involvement showed a greater than normal increase with exercise. The increased cardiac output is presumably related to multiple small systemic arteriovenous fistulas in the bones involved by this disorder, especially in the lower extremities. The possibility of Paget's disease of the bone as a cause of an increased systemic arterial pulse pressure must be considered in a middle-aged or older patient who has enlargement of the skull, decreased stature, and bowing of the tibias. Radiologic studies of the skull, pelvis, and bones of the lower extremities will usually confirm the diagnosis. As a rule, the serum alkaline phosphatase is increased.

HYPERKINETIC HEART SYNDROME

Gorlin and associates[33] have described a hyperkinetic syndrome of unknown cause which they found principally in young patients and in those of early middle age. In their report 24 patients were described. The majority of the patients had an increased cardiac output at rest. Others did not but had an increased rate of ventricular ejection. Bounding peripheral pulses were common. Heart failure developed in some patients observed for as long as 16 years. Electrocardiograms usually showed evidence of left ventricular enlargement. Systolic ejection clicks were common. Ejection and apical pansystolic murmurs were found. Gorlin's description of some of these patients is very similar to a description of patients who have idiopathic muscular obstruction of the left ventricular outflow tract.[34] The possibility that a common denominator of increased activity of the sympathetic nervous system exists in these two groups of patients must not be overlooked, since beta-adrenergic receptor blockade may be of value in therapy.

COR PULMONALE

Studies made by Harvey and associates[35] have shown that the resting cardiac output is above normal in some patients with chronic cor pulmonale associated with pulmonary emphysema. This finding apparently is most common when the patient has an acute pulmonary infection and may be in part related to acute hypoxia and hypermetabolism associated with fever and infection. In the author's experience and in that of others increased cardiac output in cor pulmonale associated with emphysema is not found in the majority of patients.[36] In some a tendency to increased cardiac output may be overcome because the pulmonary vascular resistance is greatly elevated or because heart failure is too advanced. The author did find that the cardiac output in patients with cor pulmonale caused by emphysema was on the average higher during heart failure than in patients with hypertensive or coronary artery disease and congestive heart failure.[36]

POLYOSTOTIC FIBROUS DYSPLASIA

In patients with Albright's syndrome, or polyostotic fibrous dysplasia, the cardiac output may be increased above normal. The cardiac index was 3.9 liters per min per m[2] or greater in five of six patients studied by McIntosh and associates.[37] These writers thought that anxiety or increased metabolic demands were not responsible. Biopsy material from involved bones showed numerous thin-walled sinusoidal capillaries. The writers postulated that the lesions of polyostotic fibrous dysplasia act as minute arteriovenous fistulas, thus increasing cardiac output by lowering peripheral resistance.

CARCINOID SYNDROME

Schwarber and Lukas[38] have documented increased resting cardiac output in two patients with metastatic carcinoid tumors. The patients had a narrow arteriovenous oxygen difference and decreased peripheral vascular resistance. Serotonin, known to be elaborated by carcinoid tumors, increases myocardial contractility by direct action. These writers speculate that the increased cardiac output combined with tricuspid or pulmonary valve deformity may explain the high incidence of heart failure in this disease.

WARM AND HUMID ENVIRONMENT

Burch and associates[39] studied 10 subjects during the New Orleans summers of 1957 and 1958. The mean of their cardiac outputs when in an air-conditioned ward was 4.0 liters per min. When exposed to the environmental conditions with a room temperature of 87 to 92° and relative humidity of 58 to 93 per cent, the mean cardiac output rose 43 per cent to 5.7 liters per min. Calculated ventricular work rose in some subjects, suggesting that an air-conditioned ward may reduce the work load of the heart in some patients with heart disease. Brief exposure to dry heat apparently has little effect on cardiac output.[40]

ACUTE GLOMERULONEPHRITIS

In acute glomerulonephritis, the cardiac output at rest may be normal (in other words "relatively high") when the right atrial pressure is elevated, and there are clinical features usually found in heart failure.[41] Such patients have hypervolemia, increased venous pressure, enlargement of the heart, and plumonary edema. Hypertension is common but is not invariably present. Some such patients, when treated with intravenous digoxin, show no decrease of right atrial or venous pressure, no increase of cardiac output, and no sodium or water diuresis.[15] Some patients with edema and increased venous pressure with acute glomerulonephritis do not have heart failure; this state may be referred to as *noncardiac circulatory congestion*. These patients can be recognized clinically by demonstrating that they have a normal circulation time.

POLYCYTHEMIA VERA

Cobb and associates[42] found an increased cardiac index in 5 of 10 patients with polycythemia vera. The cardiac stroke index was uniformly increased, with an average of 39 per cent above normal. The mechanism of increased cardiac output was uncertain but appeared to be correlated with the degree of hypervolemia. Right atrial and pulmonary wedge pressures were not increased.

PREGNANCY

During normal pregnancy the cardiac output increases progressively until the seventh or eighth month.[43] The increase averages 30 to 50 per cent. During the last 4 to 6 weeks of pregnancy, the cardiac output declines toward normal.

REFERENCES

1. Cournand, A., Riley, R. L., Breed, E. S., Baldwin, E. deF., and Richards, D. W., Jr.: Measurement of Cardiac Output in Man Using the Technique of

Catheterization of the Right Auricle or Ventricle, *J. Clin. Invest.*, 24:106, 1945.

2. Hamilton, W. F.: Role of the Starling Concept in Regulation of the Normal Circulation, *Phys. Rev.*, 35:161, 1955.

3. Rushmer, R. F., Smith, O., and Franklin, D.: Mechanisms of Cardiac Control in Exercise, *Circulation Res.*, 7:602, 1959.

4. Graettinger, J. S., Muenster, J. J., Selverstone, L. A., and Campbell, J. A.: A Correlation of Clinical and Hemodynamic Studies in Patients with Hyperthyroidism with and without Congestive Heart Failure, *J. Clin. Invest.*, 38:1316, 1959.

5. Brewster, W. R., Jr., Isaacs, J. P., Osgood, P. F., and King, T. L.: The Hemodynamic and Metabolic Interrelationships in the Activity of Epinephrine, Norepinephrine, and the Thyroid Hormones, *Circulation*, 13:1, 1956.

6. Fowler, N. O.: "Physical Diagnosis of Heart Disease," The Macmillan Company, New York, 1962, p. 478.

7. Canary, J. J., Schaaf, M., Duffy, B. J., Jr., and Kyle, L. H.: Effects of Oral and Intramuscular Administration of Reserpine in Thyrotoxicosis, *New England J. Med.*, 257:435, 1957.

8. Gaffney, T. E., Braunwald, E., and Kahler, R. L.: Effects of Guanethidine on Tri-iodothyronine-induced Hyperthyroidism in Man, *New England J. Med.*, 265:16, 1961.

9. Gaffney, T. E., and Braunwald, E.: The Importance of the Adrenergic Nervous System in Support of Circulatory Function in Patients with Congestive Heart Failure, *Am. J. Med.*, 34:320, 1963.

10. Blankenhorn, M. A.: The Heart in Vitamin Deficiencies, in R. L. Levy (ed.), "Disorders of the Heart and Circulation," Thomas Nelson & Sons, New York, 1951.

11. Burwell, C. S., and Dexter, L.: Beri-beri Heart Disease, *Tr. A. Am. Physicians*, 60:59, 1947.

12. Fowler, N. O.: Cardiac Catheterization in the Diagnosis of Adult Heart Disease, *Ann. Int. Med.*, 38:478, 1953.

13. Blankenhorn, M. A.: Effect of Vitamin Deficiency on the Heart and Circulation, *Circulation*, 11:288, 1955.

14. Rowlands, D. T., and Vilter, C. F.: A Study of Cardiac Stigmata in Prolonged Human Thiamine Deficiency, *Circulation*, 21:4, 1960.

15. Eichna, L. W., Farber, S. J., Berger, A. R., Rader, B., Smith, W. W., and Albert, R. E.: Non-cardiac Circulatory Congestion Simulating Congestive Heart Failure, *Tr. A. Am. Physicians*, 68:72, 1954.

16. Lovegrove, T. D., Gowdey, C. W., and Stevenson, J. A. F.: Sympathoadrenal System and Response of Heart to Acute Exchange Anemia, *Circulation Res.*, 5:659, 1957.

17. Gowdey, C. W.: Anemia-induced Changes in Cardiac Output in Dogs Treated with Dichloroisoproterenol, *Circulation Res.*, 10:354, 1962.

18. Fowler, N. O., Shabetai, R., Anderson, D., and Braunstein, J. R.: Some Circulatory Effects of Experimental Hypovolemic Anemia, *Am. Heart J.*, 60:551, 1960.

19. Brannon, E. S., Merrill, A. J., Warren, J. V., and Stead, E. A., Jr.: The Cardiac Output in Patients with Chronic Anemia as Measured by the Technique of Right Atrial Catheterization, *J. Clin. Invest.*, 24:332, 1945.

20. Case, R. B., Berglund, E., and Sarnoff, S. J.: Ventricular Function. VII. Changes in Coronary Resistance and Ventricular Function Resulting from Acutely Induced Anemia and the Effect Thereon of Coronary Stenosis, *Am. J. Med.*, 18:397, 1955.

21. Porter, W. B., and James, G. W., III: The Heart in Anemia, *Circulation*, 8:111, 1953.

22. Sanghvi, L. M., Sharma, R., and Misra, S. N.: Cardiovascular Disturbances in Chronic Severe Anemia, *Circulation*, 15:373, 1957.

23. Shubin, H., Kaufman, R., Shapiro, M., and Levinson, D. C.: Cardiovascular Findings in Children with Sickle cell anemia, *Am. J. Cardiol.*, 6:875, 1960.

24. Leight, L., Snider, T. H., Clifford, G. O., and Hellems, H. K.: Hemodynamic Studies in Sickle Cell Anemia, *Circulation*, 10:653, 1954.

25. Graettinger, J. S., Parsons, R. L., and Campbell, J. A.: A Correlation of Clinical and Hemodynamic Studies in Patients with Mild and Severe Anemia with and without Congestive Failure, *Ann. Int. Med.*, 58:617, 1963.

26. Fowler, N. O., and Holmes, J. C.: Dextran-exchange Anemia and Blood Viscosity Reduction in the Heart-Lung Preparation: With an Observation upon the Action of Ouabain in Anemic Heart Failure, *Am. Heart J.* 68:204, 1964.

27. Muenster, J., Graettinger, J. S., and Campbell, J. A.: Correlation of Clinical and Hemodynamic Findings in Patients with Systemic Arteriovenous Fistulas, *Circulation*, 20:1079, 1959.

28. Dorney, E. R.: Peripheral A-V Fistula of Fifty-seven Years Duration with Refractory Heart Failure, *Am. Heart J.*, 54:778, 1957.

29. Kowalski, H. J., and Abelmann, W. H.: The Cardiac Output at Rest in Laennec's Cirrhosis, *J. Clin. Invest.*, 32:1025, 1953.

30. Murray, J. F., Dawson, A. M., and Sherlock, S.: Circulatory Changes in Chronic Liver Disease, *Am. J. Med.*, 24:358, 1958.

31. Edholm, O. G., Howarth, S., and McMichael, J.: Heart Failure and Bone Blood Flow in Osteitis Deformans, *Clin. Sc.*, 5:249, 1945.

32. Lequime, J., and Denolin, H.: Circulatory Dynamics in Osteitis Deformans, *Circulation*, 12:215, 1955.

33. Gorlin, R.: The Hyperkinetic Heart Syndrome, *J.A.M.A.*, 182:823, 1962.

34. Braunwald, E., and Aygen, M. M.: Idiopathic Myocardial Hypertrophy without Congestive Heart Failure or Obstruction to Blood Flow, *Am. J. Med.*, 35:7, 1963.

35. Harvey, R. M., Ferrer, M. I., Richards, D. W., and Cournand, A.: Influence of Chronic Pulmonary Disease on the Heart and Circulation, *Am. J. Med.*, **10**:719, 1951.

36. Fowler, N. O., Westcott, R. N., Scott, R. C., and Hess, E.: The Cardiac Output in Chronic Cor Pulmonale, *Circulation*, **6**:888, 1952.

37. McIntosh, H. D., Miller, D. E., Gleason, W. L., and Goldner, J. L.: The Circulatory Dynamics of Polyostotic Fibrous Dysplasia, *Am, J. Med.*, **32**:393, 1962.

38. Schwarber, J. R., and Lukas, D. S.: Hyperkinemia and Cardiac Failure in the Carcinoid Syndrome, *Am. J. Med.*, **32**:846, 1962.

39. Burch, G. E., de Pasquale, N., Hyman, A., and DeGraff, A. C.: Influence of Tropical Weather on Cardiac Output, Work, and Power of Right and Left Ventricles of Man Resting in Hospital, *A.M.A. Arch. Int. Med.*, **104**:553, 1959.

40. Sancetta, S., Kramer, J., and Husni, E.: The Effects of "Dry" Heat on the Circulation of Man. 1. General Hemodynamics, *Am. Heart J.*, **56**:212, 1958.

41. Farber, S. J.: Physiologic Aspects of Glomerulonephritis, *J. Chron. Dis.*, **5**:87, 1957.

42. Cobb, L. A., Kramer, R. J., and Finch, C. A.: Circulatory Effects of Chronic Hypervolemia in Polycythemia Vera, *J. Clin. Invest.*, **39**:1722, 1960.

43. Burwell, C. S., and Metcalfe, J.: "Heart Disease and Pregnancy," Little, Brown and Company, Boston, 1958.

55 RARE CAUSES OF HEART DISEASE

Nanette Kass Wenger, M.D.

The diseases of the myocardium described in Chap. 50 are now being recognized with increasing frequency and can no longer be considered rare. The purpose of this chapter is to highlight the rarer causes of heart disease: rare forms of diffuse myocardial disease, rare forms of endocardial disease, and cardiac tumors. The rarer causes of coronary artery disease have been discussed in Chap. 36.

RARE FORMS OF DIFFUSE MYOCARDIAL DISEASE

Diffuse myocardiopathy occurs with many generalized disease processes; it occasionally causes the predominant symptoms, but more often it is overshadowed by other systemic manifestations of the primary illness.

Diffuse myocardial disease is characterized by

evidence of low-output cardiac failure: weakness, fatigability, exertional dyspnea; by palpitation; and by precordial discomfort. There is episodic remission and relapse, but the congestive heart failure is progressive, and sudden death is not uncommon.

Characteristic physical findings include tachycardia, arrhythmia, a low pulse pressure and often pulsus alternans, cardiomegaly with a diffuse and sustained left ventricular impulse, muffled heart sounds, a ventricular diastolic gallop, cervical venous distension, hepatomegaly, and peripheral edema. Both pulmonary and peripheral embolism occur frequently.

Generalized cardiac enlargement and pulmonary congestion are seen on x-ray examination. The electrocardiographic abnormalities include arrhythmias, conduction defects, diminished QRS voltage, and nonspecific ST-T changes.

The pathologic alterations underlying cardiac failure in diffuse myocardial disease, as described by Robin,[1] include myocardial fiber necrosis, myocardial and interstitial fibrosis, myocardial fiber compression by a diffuse infiltrative process, abnormalities of myocardial metabolism, and necrosis or fibrosis of the conduction system.

Bridgen[2,3] considered the diagnostic problem in diffuse myocardial disease rendered more complex because similar clinical syndromes of myocarditis resulted in widely differing histologic abnormalities; in addition, related etiologic factors produce different histologic patterns. The specific etiologic diagnosis of the myocardiopathy is often dependent on extracardiac manifestations of the disease process, which may remove it from the "wastebasket" of diffuse myocardial disease (Fig. 55-1).[3a]

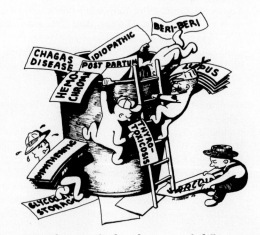

Fig. 55-1. The wastebasket diagnosis of diffuse myocardial disease. The specific etiologic diagnosis is often dependent on extracardiac manifestations of the disease process.

Syphilis

Diffuse miliary interstitial gummatous myocarditis, as described by Virchow[4] in 1858, and localized gumma of the myocardium, first reported by Ricord[5] in 1845, constitute the pathologic manifestations of syphilis in the heart muscle.

Diffuse gummatous myocarditis[6] is characterized by an interstitial infiltrate of fibroblastic or myxomatous tissue and mononuclear cells, associated with muscle fragmentation and vacuolation. As is usual in tertiary syphilis, spirochetes cannot be demonstrated in the myocardium; however, Hinrichsen[7] reported frequent identification of spirochetes in similar lesions of congenital syphilis. Boss et al.[8] suggested that the diffuse myocarditis represented a hypersensitivity response to syphilitic infection. Saphir[9,10] attributed the myocardial changes to syphilitic or atherosclerotic vascular disease; he required a true gumma for the diagnosis of syphilitic myocardial disease. Diffuse syphilitic myocarditis has on occasion presented the clinical and electrocardiographic picture usually associated with myocardial infarction.[6]

Localized myocardial gummas, solitary or multiple, are encountered more frequently, often as unexpected findings at postmortem examination[11] (Fig. 55-2). The gray-white nodule has a central necrotic area, surrounded by granulation tissue, mononuclear cells, fibroblasts, and giant cells[12] (Fig. 55-3). The characteristic location of a gumma in the left ventricular myocardium at the base of the interventricular septum[13] accounts for the clinical manifestations; there may be conduction-system interference with heart block and bundle branch block,[14,15] or symptomatic pseudostenosis of the aortic or pulmonic valves.[16] Fatal rupture of a gummatous aneurysm of the left ventricle has been reported.[17]

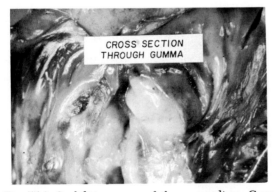

Fig. 55-2. Syphilitic gumma of the myocardium. Cross section through gumma of right ventricular wall. (*Courtesy of Department of Pathology, Emory University School of Medicine.*)

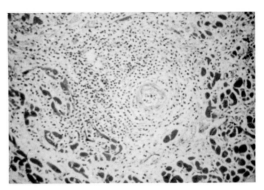

Fig. 55-3. Syphilitic gumma of the myocardium. Perivascular and interstitial inflammatory infiltrate and interstitial fibrosis. (× 150.) (*Courtesy of Department of Pathology, Emory University School of Medicine.*)

Tuberculosis

An arrhythmia occurring in the course of tuberculosis suggests myocardial or coronary artery involvement to Gouley et al.[18] Horn and Saphir[19] list the myocardial manifestations of tuberculosis as (1) large caseous nodules, (2) miliary lesions, and (3) diffuse myocarditis. The tubercle bacilli reach the heart by direct extension or by lymphatic or hematogenous spread.

Myocardial tuberculosis occurs more frequently in children,[20] probably because of their increased incidence of miliary tuberculosis. The miliary lesions often follow the course of the coronary blood vessels. Single or multiple yellow-white tuberculous nodules are most common in the right atrium,[21] usually occurring by direct extension from the hilar lymph nodes. These classic tubercles have central caseation and surrounding granulation tissue with mononuclear and giant cells. As is the case with the syphilitic gumma, the tuberculous nodule may produce symptoms by interfering with cardiac rhythm, conduction, or blood flow;[21,22] it may mimic myocardial infarction.[23] The author has observed a case in which right ventricular outflow-tract obstruction is produced (Fig. 55-4). Rupture of a myocardial tubercle into a cardiac chamber may cause disseminated tuberculosis; fatal rupture of a tuberculous myocardial aneurysm has been reported.[24]

Diffuse tuberculous myocarditis is a curiosity, rarely diagnosed ante mortem. The perivascular and interstitial infiltrate is nonspecific, and diagnosis depends on the identification of tubercle bacilli.[19]

Leptospirosis

Cardiovascular manifestations of leptospirosis—arrhythmias; cardiomegaly, gallop rhythm, and congestive heart failure; and electrocardiographic

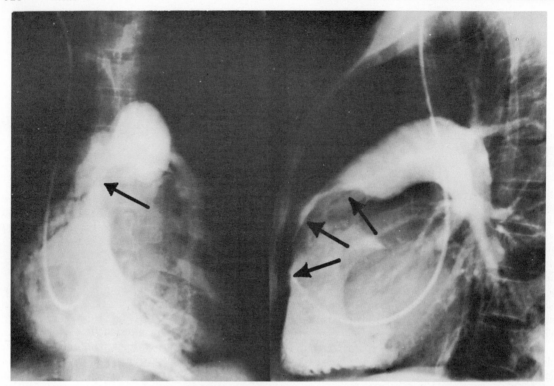

Fig. 55-4. Right ventricular angiocardiogram demonstrating a mass obstructing (arrow) the right ventricular out-flow tract. Upon surgical intervention a lemon-sized mass was found, arising from the right ventricle and containing thick, caseous material. The mass was presumed to be a tuberculoma. (*Courtesy of Dr. Joel Steinberg, Dr. William Rawls, and the Department of Radiology, Emory University School of Medicine.*)

abnormalities—are estimated to occur in about 10 per cent of patients with leptospirosis, predominantly in the second week of illness.[25,26] Myocarditis occurs more commonly with *L. ictero-*

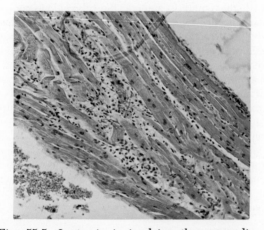

Fig. 55-5. Leptospirosis involving the myocardium. There is a focal interstitial infiltration of mononuclear cells and lymphocytes with fragmentation of muscle substance. ($\times$ 150.) (*Courtesy of Department of Pathology, Emory University School of Medicine.*)

hemorrhagie leptosperosis, but has also been reported with *L. pomona* infection.[26a] Marked bradycardia, complete heart block, and hypotension have an ominous prognosis. Death from parenchymatous and interstitial myocarditis has been reported[27] in a patient with Weil's disease whose hepatic and renal status was improving. The author has recently seen a thirty-eight-year-old man with fatal leptospirosis who, at the end of the first week of illness, developed sinus bradycardia, arrhythmia, terminal congestive heart failure, and shock.

The pathologic myocardial lesion[28] is characterized by focal hemorrhage, pronounced interstitial edema, areas of myocardial degeneration and necrosis, and an inflammatory cell infiltrate (Fig. 55-5). This occurs primarily in the subendocardial region and papillary muscles, frequently involving the conduction system.[29] Rare leptospirae have been demonstrated in the interstitial lesions. Metabolic, allergic, and toxic causes have been suggested for the myocarditis.

Leptospiral endocarditis and pericarditis have also been described, the latter possibly secondary to uremia.[30]

Nonspecific T-wave changes are the most com-

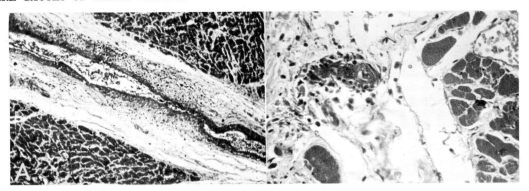

Fig. 55-6. Myocardial involvement in typhus. A. Perivascular inflammatory infiltrate ($\times$ 150). B. Perivascular nodule, with partial obliteration of the vessel lumen. Infiltrate consists of mononuclear cells with occasional polymorphonuclear leukocytes. ($\times$ 350.) (*Courtesy of Department of Pathology, Emory University School of Medicine.*)

mon electrocardiographic abnormalities;[31] sinus bradycardia, premature ventricular contractions, paroxysmal atrial flutter and fibrillation, atrioventricular conduction defects, and prolonged P-R and Q-T intervals are often noted. The electrocardiographic abnormalities are characteristically reversible with convalescence.[25]

Rickettsial Disease: Typhus, Rocky Mountain Spotted Fever, Q Fever

Myocarditis is a common occurrence in rickettsial diseases; Gore and Saphir,[32] in their classification of myocarditis, stated that myocardial involvement was invariably seen and was most severe in scrub typhus (tsutsugamushi disease). There is a focal acute interstitial mononuclear cell infiltrate without myofiber damage;[33] Allen and Spitz[34] believed the disparity between the pathologic severity of scrub typhus myocarditis and the minimal degree of cardiac insufficiency was related to the preservation of myocardial fibers. Endothelial proliferation and perivascular infiltration involve the small blood vessels (Fig. 55-6).

Congestive heart failure, arrhythmias, and nonspecific electrocardiographic changes occur in a considerable proportion of patients in the acute phase of scrub typhus, usually during the second week of illness.[35] The circulatory failure, according to Woodward,[35] is peripheral in origin. There are no residual cardiac symptoms; the few postmortem studies after subsidence of the acute illness show no evidence of permanent myocardial damage.[36]

Minor focal myocardial lesions in epidemic typhus (*Rickettsia prowazeki*) are in part attributable to the coronary arteritis; transient cardiac failure and electrocardiographic abnormalities have been described.[37] There is an acute subendocardial and perivascular interstitial infiltrate, without significant myocardial degenerative changes.[38],[39] Simi-

lar myocardial lesions in Rocky Mountain spotted fever are even less prominent (Fig. 55-7).

Q fever (*R. burnetii*) is not commonly associated with cardiac symptoms in the absence of underlying heart disease;[40] five fatal cases of Q fever endocarditis were reported in patients with diseased heart valves.[41] Pericarditis is not uncommon.[42] Patients with Q fever usually recover, so minimal postmortem evidence is available. Sorel et al.,[43] however, described myocarditis in a fourteen-year-old boy with Q fever, characterized by transient cardiomegaly and electrocardiographic changes of "myopericardial disease." Residual electrocardiographic abnormalities have been described[44] after Q fever myocarditis. Two patients with congestive heart failure and electrocardiographic abnormalities were reported by Tapie et al.,[45] who advocated tetracycline as specific therapy for Q fever.

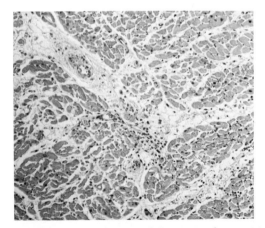

55-7. Rocky Mountain spotted fever. Focal interstitial infiltration of the myocardium with lymphocytes and mononuclear leukocytes. ($\times$ 150.) (*Courtesy of Department of Pathology, Emory University School of Medicine.*)

Mycoses

Actinomycosis

Actinomycotic infection may reach the myocardium both by hematogenous spread via the coronary arteries in generalized actinomycosis[46] and by direct extension from the lungs or pericardium.[47] Edwards[48] described the classic lesion as a necrotizing, suppurative, fibrocaseous myocardial abscess; actinomycotic granules, composed of dense aggregates of branched filamentous organisms, are in the center of the lesion. Symptoms vary, depending upon the extent and distribution of the actinomycotic abscesses; evidence of valve obstruction, arrhythmia, and congestive heart failure occur.

Blastomycosis

The cardiac lesion of blastomycosis is a tubercle; the central caseous area contains *Blastomyces dermatitidis*, as do giant cells in the surrounding granulation tissue.[49,50] Myocardial involvement may be produced by miliary hematogenous spread, by extension from pericardial disease, or by retrograde lymphatic spread from mediastinal lymph nodes.[51] Congestive heart failure may be due to myocardial blastomycosis.[51]

Moniliasis

Systemic moniliasis occurs most frequently in infants and in debilitated adults receiving prolonged antibiotic therapy. The *Candida albicans* organism has a predilection for the brain, heart, and kidney; cardiac symptoms, however, are minimal or absent.[52] Braude and Rock[53] described minute multiple myocardial abscesses; necrotic myocardial cells were seen centrally, with monilial pseudohyphae, yeast forms, and inflammatory cells most prominent at the periphery.[54]

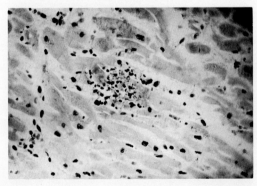

Fig. 55-8. *Aspergillus* abscess of the myocardium, showing fragmented septated hyphae surrounded by polymorphonuclear leukocytes. (× 120.) (*Courtesy of Department of Pathology, Emory University School of Medicine.*)

Aspergillosis

Pulmonary symptoms predominate in aspergillosis, although there is cardiac involvement in the generalized disease. Focal myocardial granulomas contain mycelial and filamentous forms of *Aspergillus*[55] (Fig. 55-8). Rupture of a granulomatous aspergillosis abscess into a cardiac chamber has been reported.[56]

Histoplasmosis

Disseminated histoplasmosis may, on occasion, affect the myocardium, usually without functional impairment;[57] *Histoplasma capsulatum* endocarditis[58] and pericarditis[59] are encountered somewhat more frequently. The microscopic myocardial findings[60,61] consist of focal, minute granulomas; myofiber destruction; and phagocytic cells, glutted with *H. capsulatum*, chiefly perivascular in distribution.

Sporotrichosis

Sporotrichum schenkii produces submiliary necrotic foci with an inflammatory cellular reaction in the myocardium; the organisms are both free and in macrophages.[62] Cardiac symptoms have not been described with disseminated ulcerating sporotrichosis.

Coccidioidomycosis

Forbus and Bestebreurtje[63] described gross and microscopic myocardial lesions in 50 cases of disseminated coccidioidomycosis, but attributed the occasional cardiac symptoms to associated pericarditis. *Coccidioides immitis* spherules are found in the necrotic center of miliary granulomatous myocardial lesions; there are surrounding mononuclear and giant cells.[64] A nonspecific myocarditis with myofiber degeneration and inflammatory-cell interstitial infiltrate has also been reported.[65]

Cryptococcosis

Ventricular tachycardia, congestive heart failure, and sudden death were described in a thirty-one-year-old man with cryptococcosis of the heart.[65a] *Cryptococcus neoformans* were identified in multiple myocardial granulomata.

Parasites

Protozoal

Trypanosomiasis. Chagas' Disease. In an endemic area for *Trypanosoma cruzi*, the young patient with an acquired myocardiopathy, arrhythmia, and a right bundle branch block electrocardiographic pattern most probably has chronic Chagas' disease.[66,66a] It is the most common form of heart disease in some areas of Brazil.

The reservoirs and transmitting vectors for

Chagas' disease are triatomes infected with *T, cruzi,* found mainly in the tropical and subtropical Americas but also encountered in the southwestern United States.[66b,66c] The trypanosomes assume a leishmanial form in the myocardial fiber, where they multiply by binary fission; no myocardial inflammatory response occurs until the myofiber ruptures.

Acute Chagas' disease is most common in the first years of life. This acute parasitic myocarditis presents with tachycardia, cardiomegaly, congestive heart failure, and nonspecific electrocardiographic changes; arrhythmias are notably absent.[67] Recovery from the acute illness, with subsidence of cardiac manifestations, usually occurs within a few months; the patient then appears in good health for the ensuing 10 to 20 years.[68] Postmortem examination during the acute illness shows diffuse myocardial degeneration, *T. cruzi* in the myofibers, and interstitial mononuclear cell and connective tissue proliferation. Patients with chronic Chagas' disease often deny a previous acute illness; thus the initial phase of Chagas' disease must commonly be asymptomatic and unrecognized.

The clinical diagnosis of chronic *T. cruzi* disease[68] depends on recognition of the chronic heart disease, which occurs in about 50 per cent of patients. Confirmatory laboratory evidence includes a positive Machado-Guerreiro complement-fixation reaction and a positive xenodiagnostic study. The predominant cardiac manifestations of chronic Chagas' disease were emphasized by Chagas[69] in his original description of the illness in 1910; he commented on the striking incidence of arrhythmias.

The clinical picture of chronic Chagas' myocarditis is that of insidious, progressive, prolonged congestive heart failure and cardiomegaly. The almost invariable arrhythmias are responsible for syncope and sudden death, which frequently occurs even in the absence of congestive heart failure.[70] There is no known therapy.

The highest incidence of chronic Chagas' disease is in the third and fourth decades of life, with preponderance of males from rural areas.[71] Electrocardiographic abnormalities occur in 87 per cent of patients with chronic Chagas's disease, often as the initial manifestation of illness.[72] Right bundle branch block, with a superiorly oriented Â QRS, is the most common electrocardiographic abnormality, with a greater than 50 per cent incidence.[73] Arrhythmias, atrioventricular (A-V) block, conduction defects, and P- and T-wave abnormalities are common. Complete heart block, premature ventricular contractions, and atrial fibrillation have a grave prognostic significance.[74]

Köberle,[75] in reviewing 100 postmortem cases of chronic Chagas' myocarditis, emphasized the mild cardiac muscle destruction as compared with the severe ganglion and conduction-system damage; he implicated a parasite neurotoxin. Mott and Hagstrom[75a] also described significant inflammation and degeneration of the cardiac nerves and ganglia. All cardiac chambers are hypertrophied; diffuse interstitial myocardial fibrosis and mononuclear cell infiltrate are most prominent in the region of the sinoatrial (S-A) node, the A-V node, the bundle of His, and the subepicardial ganglions. Leishmanial forms of *T. cruzi* are found in degenerated myocardial fibers, especially in the right atrial wall. Endocardial mural thrombosis and resultant pulmonary embolization are often encountered.

Sleeping Sickness. Severe central nervous system disease and relatively asymptomatic cardiac lesions characterize *T. rhodesiense*[76] and *T. gambiense* infections,[77] the former being more severe.

The myocardial lesion in sleeping sickness is an interstitial, perivascular, mononuclear-cell infiltrate, with myocardial edema and myofiber degeneration. Neither arrhythmia nor cardiomegaly was described prior to the report of Manson-Bahr and Charters[78] of two patients with severe congestive heart failure and marked cardiac enlargement, who responded dramatically to therapy for trypanosomiasis. Schyns and Janssen[79] reported a 47 per cent incidence of nonspecific ST-T electrocardiographic changes, more pronounced in the sicker patients.

Toxoplasmosis. In both congenital and acquired toxoplasmosis, hematogenously disseminated *Toxoplasma gondii* invade the myocardial cell without causing myofiber destruction or inflammatory reaction. The protozoa divide by binary fission, filling the myofiber with organisms.[80] With rupture of the parasitized cell, a focal mononuclear inflammatory reaction to the liberated organisms occurs, with associated myofiber necrosis.[81–83]

Callahan et al.[84] described constant pathologic myocardial involvement in toxoplasmosis: frequent nonspecific electrocardiographic abnormalities, unassociated with clinical signs or symptoms, have been noted.[85] Sexton et al.[86] believed that this myocarditis, observed at postmortem examination in all adults with acute toxoplasmosis, explained the invariably observed tachycardia. Most postmortem descriptions of toxoplasma myocarditis do not report clinical cardiac disease,[86a] but occasional patients are cited with cardiac enlargement, arrhythmia,[87,88] congestive heart failure,[89] or nonspecific transient ST-T electrocardiographic abnormalities.[90,90a]

Pyrimethamine and sulfonamides are often effective therapy for toxoplasmosis.

Malaria. No clinical or electrocardiographic indications of cardiac involvement are characteristic of acute malignant tertian malaria (*Plasmodium falciparum*),[91] despite extensive pathologic changes observed at postmortem examination;[92] furthermore, there is little evidence that malaria results in chronic heart disease.[92a,92b]

Spitz[93] reported an 80 per cent incidence of myocardial vessel distension and occlusion with malarial parasites and parasitized red blood cells in falciparum malaria; he described pronounced interstitial edema and a moderate mononuclear-cell infiltrate without associated muscle necrosis or fibrosis. Herrera,[94] however, presented a case of *Pl. vivax* malaria in an eight-year-old boy, with death from congestive heart failure; he described blood vessel occlusion with numerous myocardial microinfarctions and suggested that combined vascular and parenchymal lesions may result in permanent cardiac damage from malaria. Angina pectoris has also been described, presumably secondary to vascular thrombosis.[94a]

Fatty myocardial degeneration and deposition and phagocytosis of pigment are commonly observed in malaria,[95] presumably secondary to the hemolytic anemia.

Leishmaniasis. Minor cardiac symptoms and pathologic changes due to *Leishmania donovani* occur only in the visceral form of kala-azar. Clasmatocytes in the myocardium are heavily laden with Leishman-Donovan bodies; there is associated muscle-cell fragmentation and mononuclear-cell infiltration.[96] These are the lesions presumed responsible for the occasionally observed congestive heart failure and electrocardiographic abnormalities.[96a]

Balantidiasis. Balantidiasis is generally an intestinal infestation, but a case of *Balantidium coli* myocarditis, with death from cardiac failure, has been reported.[97] At postmortem examination there was a granulomatous myocarditis with muscle atrophy; degenerated forms of *B. coli* were found in the small myocardial arteries, and an intact protozoan was identified in the myocardium.

Sarcosporidiosis. Sarcosporidia characteristically invade cardiac and peripheral musculature; the infestations are incidental findings on microscopic tissue examination.[98-100] Sarcocysts have also been described in Purkinje tissue, without clinical evidence of cardiac disease.[100] Each sarcocyst within a muscle fiber contains several hundred basophilic bodies; the involved myocardial fiber is larger than adjacent fibers.

Sarcosporidiosis is differentiated from toxoplasmosis by the large number of parasites within each cyst, by the lack of myocardial degenerative or inflammatory reaction to the protozoan, and by the exclusive localization of Sarcosporidia in muscle.

Helminthic

Trichinosis. Trichinosis is probably the most prevalent helminthic infestation of man; the most common and serious complication is myocarditis, accounting for the reported 5 to 6 per cent mortality.[101]

Circulating *Trichinella spiralis* larvae invade the heart in the acute phase of trichinosis but never encyst in the myocardium; parasites are not found in the myocardium after the second week of illness, and are presumed to have been destroyed or returned to the circulation.[102] A focal acute myocarditis, involving both the parenchyma and interstitial tissue, begins after the second week of illness, attaining its maximum severity in the fourth to eighth week.[103] The myocarditis has been postulated to be a nonspecific inflammatory manifestation of larval invasion of the myocardium, a reaction to the death of the parasite, or a hypersensitivity or toxic response to *T. spiralis*.[104] There are focal areas of muscle necrosis, occasionally containing parasites, and the interstitial connective tissue is diffusely infiltrated with eosinophils and inflammatory cells.

Transient electrocardiographic abnormalities occur in about one-third of cases of trichinosis, often without cardiac symptoms.[104] The electrocardiographic changes parallel the myocarditis, appearing in the second or third week of illness, being most pronounced at about the sixth week, and then gradually disappearing.[105] Gray et al.[103] described nonspecific T-wave changes as the most common electrocardiographic abnormality,[106] with decreased QRS voltage, premature ventricular contractions, and altered conduction also observed [107] (Fig. 55-9).

Clinical evidence of myocarditis—congestive heart failure, cardiomegaly, substernal pain, and arrhythmia—usually appears in the third week of illness, when systemic symptoms are abating.[103] The cardiac manifestations are maximal at about

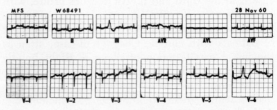

Fig. 55-9. Trichinosis myocarditis. The electrocardiographic abnormalities include sinus tachycardia, premature ventricular contractions, Q-T interval prolongation, and nonspecific ST-T alterations. (*Courtesy of Electrocardiographic Laboratory, Grady Memorial Hospital.*)

the sixth week and subsequently subside. Recovery is the general rule in trichinosis myocarditis, without residual chronic heart disease.[108] The diagnosis of trichinosis should be considered in any patient with periorbital edema, eosinophilia, and marked muscle tenderness, with or without a history of pork ingestion. Skeletal muscle biopsy may be diagnostic. Corticosteroid therapy diminishes the inflammatory response in trichinosis myocarditis and produces striking clinical improvement.[101] Thiabendazole has recently been reported to be effective therapy for trichinosis.[108a]

Echinococcosis. Cardiac echinococcosis, first described by Dévé,[109] is most frequently encountered in sheep-raising areas: Uruguay, Australia, New Zealand, and the Mediterranean countries.[110] Hydatidosis is predominantly a hepatic-pulmonary disease, with 0.5 to 2 per cent cardiac involvement. Most cases occur in the second to fifth decades of life, with men affected more commonly.[111]

Uncomplicated hydatid disease of the heart is characteristically silent and latent[111,112] with rare reports of chest pain, palpitations, tachycardia, murmurs, congestive heart failure, and angina. The first antemortem diagnosis was made about 1925.[117] In an endemic area, the diagnosis of cardiac echinococcosis should be suggested by the presence of echinococcus cysts elsewhere in the body, eosinophilia, a positive intradermal reaction, history of an anaphylactic shock syndrome, a peculiar cardiac murmur, a bizarre and often calcified cardiac shadow on x-ray examination,[113] and electrocardiographic abnormalities. ST-T ischemic changes, particularly in the precordial electrocardiographic leads, may localize the echinococcal cyst.[114] Occasional P-wave changes have been reported with atrial cysts. The electrocardiographic changes may be reversible following excision of a cardiac echinococcal cyst.[115] Angiocardiographic examination delineates the cyst.

Taenia echinococcus is generally believed to invade the myocardium via the coronary circulation, although Jorge and Re[116] have recently proposed a lymphatic spread. Binet and Marchese[115] and Canabal et al.[114] described left ventricular involvement as most common and attributed this to the richer left ventricular coronary artery supply. The cases reviewed by Peters et al.[117] had more frequent right ventricular echinococcal involvement; they explained this as due to a more direct entrance of blood into the right coronary artery. The echinococcus hexacanth forms a pseudocyst in the myocardium with resultant surrounding muscle-compression ischemia, interference with heart valve function, or interference with conduction. Primary echinococcus cysts are always solitary, varying from

pea-size to grapefruit-size. Myocardial density, particularly in the ventricles, limits cyst growth and favors the formation of daughter cysts. The cyst may rupture into a cardiac chamber or into the pericardium,[118] depending on its location and the direction of least resistance.[111]

Echinococcal cyst rupture commonly presents as anaphylaxis, due to sensitization to hydatid protein; the first symptoms often are due to pulmonary or cerebral embolization of daughter cysts.[112] Late complications occur from secondary pericardial echinococcosis or metastatic echinococcosis.

The first successful surgical excision of a cardiac echinococcus cyst was in 1932;[117] successful surgical treatment, both by the closed[119] and open[120] techniques, is reported with increasing frequency. The diagnosis of cardiac hydatid disease must be made in the uncomplicated stage of the illness, prior to cyst rupture; surgical excision is indicated even in an asymptomatic patient, to permit curative surgical treatment.[110,111]

Schistosomiasis. Cardiac manifestations of schistosomiasis are most commonly those of cor pulmonale, secondary to pulmonary schistosomiasis; primary myocardial schistosomiasis is rarely encountered.

Schistosoma japonicum ova,[121] and less commonly, ova of S. *haematobium* and S. *mansoni*, localize in the myocardium. The pathologic lesion, usually an incidental finding at postmortem examination,[122] is a microscopic pseudotubercle with an individual ovum as the center of the tissue reaction.[121] In the report of Zahawi and Shukri[123] of a fatal case of S. *Haematobium* myocarditis, they suggested that the myocardial lesion represented an allergic response to the parasite.

Ascariasis. The larvae of *Ascaris lumbricoides* invade the myocardium via a coronary artery. A verminous myocardial abscess has been described[124] in a twenty-seven-month-old child; an *Ascaris* larva, coiled in the left ventricular muscle, was surrounded by an extensive, necrotizing inflammatory process. Ferreira's[124a] description of a fertilized ascaris ovum in the left ventricular myocardium suggested that its origin was embolic.

Heterophyidiasis. In cases of intestinal heterophyidiasis, the ova of various trematodes enter the general circulation and may lodge in the heart. Africa et al.[125] reported four patients with severe congestive heart failure who, at autopsy, had *Heterophyid* ova in the myocardium. The right ventricle was most prominently involved, with the clinical picture mimicking beriberi. Microscopic examination of these hearts showed marked interstitial edema; ova were found between the myofibers, with surrounding muscle fiber fragmentation. Occlusion of the capillaries and small coronary arteries by *Heterophyid* ova contributed to the myocardial damage. Thickening and calcification of the mitral valve has also been described.[125a]

Filariasis. In an endemic area for filariasis, unexplained congestive heart failure in a patient with eosinophilia suggests filarial myocarditis.[126] Five such cases, due to *Loa loa* infestation, had cardiomegaly and predominant right-sided cardiac failure.[127] The electrocardiographic abnormalities included conduction defects, arrhythmias, and low QRS voltage. Pericardial effusion, myocardial sclerosis with interstitial fibrosis and cellular infiltration, restrictive endocardial fibrosis, and mural thrombi were seen at postmortem examination. Filarial larvae may be seen on histopathologic examination.[128]

Tatibouet[129] described a patient with *L. loa* cardiopathy in whom severe congestive heart failure was not improved by digitalis and diuretic therapy; treatment with corticosteroids effected a complete clinical remission. He suggested that the restrictive endocardial fibrosis, which mimics Loeffler's endocarditis, is an allergic reaction to the filarial parasite.

Severe restrictive filarial endocarditis was demonstrated[130] at cardiac catheterization; this persisted after the congestive heart failure, conduction abnormalities, and systemic allergic manifestations were controlled by corticosteroid therapy.

Paragonimiasis. Cardiac investment, without specific cardiac symptoms, has been described in disseminated visceral infection with *Paragonimus westermani;* adult trematodes were noted at pathologic examination of the myocardium.[130a]

Strongyloidiasis. *Strongyloides stercoralis* infestation of the heart, without cardiac symptoms, has been reported.[131] There were nonspecific T-wave electrocardiographic abnormalities. On microscopic examination of the myocardium, scattered filariform larvae were surrounded by lymphocytes in the interstitial tissue; cardiac muscle fibers were not involved. Thiabendazole has been reported effective against human strongyloidiasis.[131a]

Cysticercosis. Generalized infection with *Taenia solium* may involve the heart.[132] Multiple scolex-containing cysts produce no myocardial damage, and there are usually no cardiac symptoms;[133] however, congestive heart failure has been described. The exudative tissue reaction to *Cysticercus cellulosae* results in fibrous encapsulation of the cyst; the parasite may eventually be resorbed or may calcify.

Visceral Larva Migrans. Patients almost invariably recover from *Toxocara canis* infestation, and there is rarely associated clinical cardiac disease. In a rare fatal case, Brill et al.[134] reported generalized allergic granulomatosis; the scattered myocardial nodules had central fibrinous necrosis and surrounding epithelioid cells, giant cells, and eosinophils. The myocardial fibers were intact. Dent et al.[134a] described a similar pathologic picture in which fragments of the larval parasite were found in the granulomatous lesion.

A case of severe recurrent myocarditis with recovery was described in a child with visceral larva migrans; cortisone therapy resulted in clinical improvement.[134b]

Nutritional Causes

Beriberi

Blankenhorn et al.[135] list seven criteria for the diagnosis of beriberi heart disease: (1) absence of other etiologic factors for heart disease; (2) history of 3 or more months of gross dietary thiamine deficiency; (3) simultaneous evidence of peripheral neuritis or pellagra; (4) cardiomegaly and regular sinus rhythm; (5) edema, increased venous pressure, anemia, and hypoproteinemia; (6) minor, nonspecific electrocardiographic changes usually disappearing after therapy; and (7) response to thiamine therapy by recovery and diminution of heart size, or autopsy proof of the diagnosis.

The cardiac manifestations of beriberi are probably not attributable to anatomic myocardial alterations but to a potentially reversible derangement of carbohydrate metabolism, which results in effects similar to those of hypoxia.[136] Myocardial energy production is impaired because of lack of cocarboxylase. High-output cardiac failure, with decreased myocardial oxygen extraction and consumption, imposes an additional work load on a heart already handicapped by a metabolic defect.

Oriental beriberi,[137,138] usually caused by malnutrition, is characterized by high-output cardiac failure, often associated with syncope, shock, and sudden death; there is predominant right ventricular disease. Occidental[137,139] beriberi, most commonly seen in alcoholic men, presents both right and left ventricular failure, often without evidence of a hyperkinetic circulation; it is not infrequently misdiagnosed as arteriosclerotic heart disease or diffuse myocardial disease of unknown cause.

The presenting symptoms of beriberi heart disease include fatigue, dyspnea, orthopnea, edema, and palpitations. In addition to the neurologic abnormalities, the classic physical findings include sinus tachycardia;[137,141] a full, bounding arterial pulse with an increased pulse pressure; elevated venous pressure with neck vein engorgement; peripheral vasodilatation; cardiomegaly; diminished S-1 and accentuated pulmonic component of S-2; gallop rhythm; hemic systolic murmurs; pulmonary congestion; hepatomegaly; and serous effusions and edema.

Congestive heart failure is most pronounced in patients with minimal neurologic involvement,[142] i.e., those best able to continue at work. Physical exertion precipitated cardiac failure in prisoners of war with beriberi.[143]

Although no characteristic electrocardiographic pattern is described for beriberi, sinus tachycardia and the absence of arrhythmia are worthy of note.[137,142] Nonspecific T-wave changes and diminished QRS voltage have been observed; Q-T interval prolongation has been attributed to hypokalemia. The electrocardiographic abnormalities often disappear after thiamine therapy.[138,144]

There is generalized cardiomegaly on x-ray examination. The circulation time may be rapid or normal, and the arteriovenous oxygen difference is diminished. Burwell and Dexter[145] demonstrated high-output cardiac failure and increased oxygen consumption at cardiac catheterization. Lowered peripheral vascular resistance, which returns to normal after 2 to 3 weeks of thiamine therapy, is responsible for the elevated cardiac output.[145a]

The pathologic myocardial lesions of beriberi[146,147] include biventricular dilatation and hypertrophy, hydropic degeneration of the myocardial fibers and the conduction system, interstitial and intercellular edema, and collagen swelling. Inflammation and necrosis are notably absent. Myocardial fibrosis occurs after prolonged illness.

Therapy[137] consists of thiamine, prolonged rest, adequate diet, vitamins, sodium restriction, and diuretics; digitalis has little effect, as it cannot correct the abnormality in myocardial energy production. Classically, therapy effects a reversal of all symptoms and abnormal clinical and laboratory findings of beriberi.[148] However, Benchimol and Schlesinger[141] noted only 40 per cent regression of cardiomegaly after thiamine therapy, presumably because of irreversible myocardial fibrosis in the later stages of the disease.

Pellagra

The cardiovascular disturbances encountered with pellagra—exertional dyspnea, tachycardia, palpitations, and edema—and the electrocardiographic abnormalities have been attributed both to the nicotinic acid deficiency and to the frequently associated beriberi.[149]

Porter and Higgenbotham[150] and Weiss and Wilkins[151] reported no evidence for heart disease due to pellagra. Cardiac symptoms and electrocardiographic and radiologic abnormalities were noted only in patients with underlying heart disease, and no cardiac lesions attributable to pellagra were demonstrated at postmortem examination.

Electrocardiographic abnormalities are usually associated with the visceral, rather than the dermatologic, manifestations of pellagra. Sinus tachycardia and ST-T changes are observed most commonly, with diminished QRS voltage also described. Nonspecific electrocardiographic changes were encountered in 40 per cent of patients with pellagra;[152] the regression of the electrocardiographic abnormalities paralleled the clinical improvement. Rachmilewitz and Braun[153] demonstrated that the electrocardiographic improvement was due specifically to niacin therapy, rather than to treatment of associated beriberi; they described subsidence of electrocardiographic abnormalities after niacin therapy in patients on thiamine-deficient diets.

Scurvy

Right ventricular hypertrophy has been reported in cases of sudden death in babies with scurvy;[154] the myocardium was described either as normal[155] or as showing fatty degeneration.[156] The cardiac abnormalities are thought to be due to vitamin C deficiency.

Hypervitaminosis D

Gross and microscopic deposits of calcium in the heart, associated with myocardial necrosis and fatty degeneration, are encountered in patients with hypervitaminosis D.[157,158] The electrocardiographic abnormalities[159] associated with hypercalcemia—shortened Q-T interval and ST-T changes—may be present. The ST-T alterations may reflect myocardial damage.

Kwashiorkor

In urbanized South Africa, Bantus on a high-carbohydrate, low-protein diet develop cardiomegaly, low-output cardiac failure, extreme edema, and associated hepatic fibrosis and hemosiderosis.[160] Marked skeletal muscle wasting is particularly prominent in children. The patients respond to bed rest and adequate diet in all but the later stages of the disease and tend to relapse with physical activity and inadequate diet. Pulmonary and peripheral emboli are common, as is sudden death.

Nonspecific ST-T abnormalities were the most frequently encountered electrocardiographic alterations,[161] with sinus bradycardia, low QRS voltage, and V waves also seen.[161a] Arrhythmias are rare. The electrocardiogram becomes normal with clinical improvement.

The pathologic cardiac lesions[162] include biventricular dilatation and hypertrophy, interfibrillary edema, minimal interstitial fibrosis, and ventricular endocardial mural thrombosis; no significant endocardial fibroelastosis or valvular involvement is noted. Atrophic hearts were described in children with kwashiorkor.[163]

Metabolic Causes

Glycogen Storage Disease (Pompe's Disease)

Glycogen storage disease is a familial, non-sex-linked disorder of carbohydrate metabolism, characterized by the accumulation of excessive quan-tities of normal glycogen in cardiac muscle, skeletal muscle, and other tissues.[164] Although McPhie[165] delineated five categories of cardiac glycogenosis, the pattern of inheritance is not yet well defined. The specific metabolic error is an absence of the enzyme alpha-glucosidase.[165a]

The age at onset of symptoms of glycogen storage disease is a diagnostic clue; symptoms usually occur between ages two and six months, and always

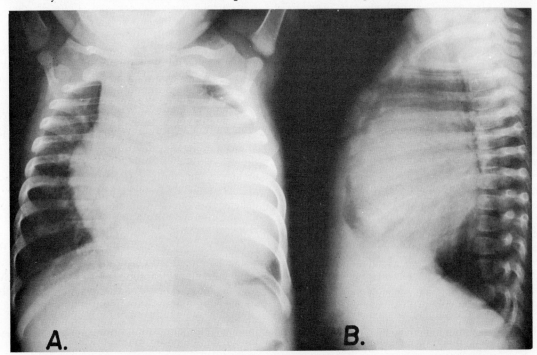

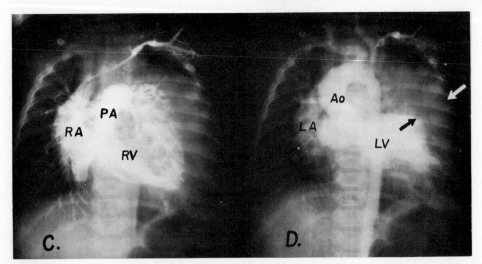

Fig. 55-10. Glycogen storage disease of the heart. *A,B.* Massive generalized cardiomegaly with pulmonary congestion. Normal cardiac pulsations were seen at fluoroscopy. *C,D.* Venous angiocardiogram demonstrating distortion of the right ventricular outflow trace secondary to hypertrophy of the interventricular septum and left ventricle (between arrows). *Courtesy of Department of Radiology, Emory University School of Medicine.*)

before eighteen months. In addition to the generalized muscle weakness, large tongue, areflexia, and other neurologic deficits, the babies present the characteristic findings of feeding difficulty, cyanosis, dyspnea, massive cardiac enlargement, and terminal congestive heart failure. A similar disorder is often described in a sibling. Ehlers and Engle[166] reported a case of glycogen storage disease with massive left ventricular hypertrophy presenting the clinical and hemodynamic picture of functional hypertrophic subaortic stenosis. The author has recently seen a case with massive cardiomegaly and right ventricular preponderance; the angiocardiographic findings were suggestive of a tumor within the right ventricle (Fig. 55-10). Angiocardiography usually demonstrates a massive, thick-walled left ventricle, which appears rigid when there is associated endocardial sclerosis. Sudden death is common,[168] usually in the first year of life. The electrocardiographic pattern is that of left ventricular hypertrophy, with strikingly increased QRS voltage and a shortened P-R interval (Fig. 55-11); Ehlers[164] believed that these electrocardiographic findings distinguished this abnormality from other causes of left ventricular hypertrophy in infancy. Demonstration of increased glycogen content in a skeletal muscle biopsy confirms the diagnosis, as does the absence of alpha-glucosidase activity in skeletal muscle or liver biopsy tissue, or in the blood leukocytes.[168a]

At pathologic examination of the heart, the ventricles are massive and thick-walled (Fig. 55-12), and the atria are normal. The myocardial fibers are enlarged with diffuse and extensive vacuolation, producing a "lacework" pattern; the glycogen-filled vacuoles compress the nuclei, displacing them to the periphery of the cell.[164,169,170]

Di Sant'Agnese[171,172] listed as the four criteria for the diagnosis of cardiac glycogen storage disease (1) marked cardiomegaly, (2) lacework appearance of the myocardium, (3) clinical or his-

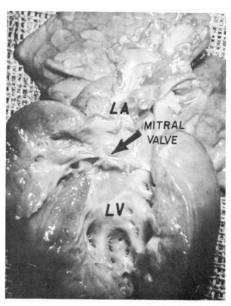

Fig. 55-12. Glycogen storage disease of the heart. Massive thickening of the left ventricular wall and thickening of the left ventricular endocardium. (*Courtesy of Department of Pathology, Emory University School of Medicine.*)

tologic confirmation of the presence of normal glycogen, and (4) death within the first year of life; however, survival has been reported to the age of 34 months.[173] There is at present no specific therapy.

Congenital nodular glycogenic infiltration of the myocardium, previously designated as rhabdomyoma, is commonly seen in children in association with tuberous sclerosis.[174,175] These solitary or multiple "tumors," first described by von Recklinghausen in 1862,[176] are not encapsulated but merge with the surrounding myocardium; the cause is obscure but seems related to a disturbance of glycogen metabolism. The gray-purple nodules are usually incidental findings in the ventricle at postmortem examination,[177] but large glycogenic infiltrates of the interventricular septum may cause arrhythmias[178,179] and A-V block. Sudden death in infancy is not uncommon; 52 per cent fatality was reported in the first year of life and 86 per cent fatality before puberty in cases of rhabdomyoma.[180]

McArdle's Syndrome

McArdle's Syndrome is a metabolic myopathy due to deficient glycogen breakdown in muscle. Ratinov et al.[180a] reported a case with PR interval prolongation, an interventricular conduction delay, increased QRS voltage, and T-wave abnormalities; these electrocardiographic changes are not unlike

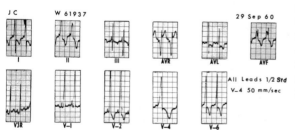

55-11. Three-month-old infant with glycogen storage disease of the heart. There is biventricular hypertrophy with massively increased QRS voltage in the precordial leads and Wolff Parkinson-White conduction. (*Courtesy of Electrocardiographic Laboratory, Grady Memorial Hospital.*)

those encountered in other forms of cardiac glyco-genosis.

Hemochromatosis

The tetrad of liver disease, diabetes mellitus, heart disease, and skin pigmentation comprises hemochromatosis; the disease occurs predominantly in the male and usually in the older age group.[181] Since the advent of insulin therapy for diabetes, cardiac failure has been the single leading cause of death in hemochromatosis,[182] accounting for one-third to one-half of the fatalities listed in recent reviews. Fifteen per cent of patients present with cardiac symptoms, and cardiac disease occurs even in the absence of skin pigmentation and diabetes.[181]

Hemochromatosis is a disease of iron storage with resultant tissue damage, but the genesis of the cardiac insufficiency is unknown. There is lack of correlation between the degree of myocardial iron deposition, the extent of resultant interstitial fibrosis, and the functional cardiac impairment.[183] The rate of iron deposition may be more important than the absolute quantity of iron;[184] interference with an enzyme system or other metabolic abnormality has also been postulated; the pattern of constrictive pericarditis or restrictive cardiopathy found at cardiac catheterization[182,185] implicates a mechanical factor, such as myocardial fibrosis.

The clinical picture[182,185] is that of arrhythmia, A-V block, and rapidly progressive congestive heart failure, responding poorly to digitalis and diuretic therapy. Unexplained precordial pain is occasionally observed. Premature ventricular contractions, paroxysmal atrial tachycardia, and paroxysmal atrial fibrillation are the most frequent arrhythmias. There is diffuse cardiomegaly, dyspnea, stasis cyanosis, edema, and ascites.

Electrocardiographic abnormalities,[181] in addition to arrhythmias, include diminished QRS volt-

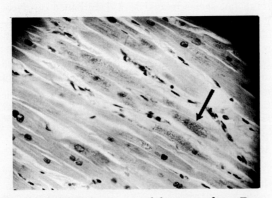

Fig. 55-13. Hemochromatosis of the myocardium. Deposition of hemosiderin granules (arrow) in myocardial fibers. (× 430.) (*Courtesy of Department of Pathology, Emory University School of Medicine.*)

age, conduction disturbances, and nonspecific T-wave changes. The large globular heart with feeble pulsations and biventricular hypertrophy seen at radiologic examination may mimic pericardial effusion, constrictive pericarditis, beriberi, or myxedema heart disease. Confirmatory diagnostic evidence includes the demonstration of excessive iron deposition in a sternal marrow aspirate and/or liver biopsy specimen, and the finding of an elevated serum-iron level.

At postmortem examination[181,182] there are biventricular dilatation and hypertrophy. The myocardial fibers are infiltrated with iron-pigment granules (Fig. 55-13), and there is myofiber fragmentation and atrophy, edema, inflammatory-cell infiltration, and interstitial fibrosis. Extensive deposition of iron pigment and associated tissue damage in the A-V node appear responsible for arrhythmias and heart block.[185a]

Removal of iron by repeated venesection is the accepted therapy.[186] Death usually occurs within a year after onset of cardiac symptoms. One reported patient[187] survived for over 3 years after the onset of cardiac disease; regression of cardiomegaly occurred after repeated phlebotomy, in which about 31 Gm iron was removed.

Porphyria

Despite the absence of cardiac symptoms and clinical cardiovascular abnormalities in porphyria, pigment deposition and myocardial fiber disintegration with loss of nuclei and striations are seen at postmortem examination.[188,189]

Eliaser and Kondo[190] described the development of electrocardiographic abnormalities: diminished QRS voltage, left axis deviation, and S-T segment displacement, during an attack of acute porphyria in a patient with a normal electrocardiogram between attacks; they suggested that coronary artery spasm may produce transient myocardial dysfunction. T-wave abnormalities have also been reported with acute porphyria.[191] Crouch and Herrmann,[192] however, recorded completely normal electrocardiograms in 10 patients with porphyria, 8 recorded during an acute attack.

Gargoylism

Clinical evidence of cardiovascular disease was described in more than 70 per cent of patients with gargoylism (Hurler's syndrome).[193] Gargoylism is an inborn error of metabolism, characterized by the deposition of a complex macromolecular glycoprotein material in the parenchymal cells and supporting connective tissue of most organ systems.[194] Clinical signs and symptoms usually appear between ages 1 and 2, when sufficient stored glyco-

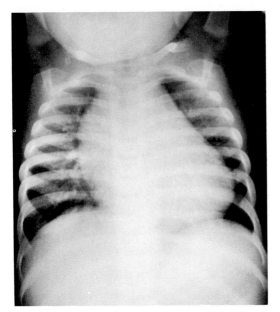

Fig. 55-14. Generalized cardiac enlargement and prominent bronchovascular markings in a child with gargoylism (Hurler's syndrome). (*Courtesy of Department of Radiology, Emory University School of Medicine.*)

protein has accumulated to interfere with tissue growth, structure, and function.

Cardiomegaly and murmurs of valve deformity with resultant congestive heart failure comprise the major cardiac abnormalities.[193] The associated thoracic deformities, pulmonary disease, and anemia contribute to the cardiovascular symptomatology. At radiologic examination there is generalized cardiomegaly (Fig. 55-14); no specific electrocardiographic pattern is noted. Cardiac failure is the cause of death in two-thirds of patients with gargoylism, with death occurring at an average age of 11 years.[195]

At pathologic examination[195] of the heart, the myocardial and connective tissue cells are swollen, hypertrophic, and vacuolated. There is biventricular cardiac hypertrophy; nodulation and thickening of the heart valves, preferentially involving the mitral valve; endocardial sclerosis; and intimal proliferation of the coronary and pulmonary arteries.

The nature of the metabolic error in gargoylism and its pattern of inheritance require further elucidation; there is no known specific therapy.[196]

Primary Xanthomatosis

Patients with familial hypercholesterolemic xanthomatosis have an increased incidence of atherosclerotic coronary artery disease, with coronary occlusion not infrequently seen at an early age. Cardiovascular symptoms are thought to be due to a combination of the ischemic heart disease and the xanthomatous infiltration of the myocardium.

Myocardial disease was described in a patient with hereditary normocholesterolemic xanthomatosis in whom congestive heart failure, arrhythmia, and conduction abnormalities developed.[197] At autopsy the coronary arteries were normal, but the ventricles were hypertrophic with focal yellow-gray patches. The microscopic findings of focal lipid deposition and fibrosis, extensively involving the interventricular septum, probably were responsible for the arrhythmia and conduction abnormalities.

Gout

Urate deposition in the heart may involve the coronary arteries; the valvular endocardium, usually of the mitral valve; the pericardium; and the myocardium per se. A patient with gout was described [198] in whom a mitral valve tophus extended through the myocardium into the epicardium, compressing the left circumflex coronary artery with resultant myocardial infarction. The microscopic appearance was of a classic tophus—central amorphous material, demonstrated to be uric acid and urates, with a rim of fibrous connective tissue containing giant cells and macrophages. Prinzmetal and Kennamer[199] reported bigeminy in a patient with gout, unresponsive to quinidine and Pronestyl hydrochloride but subsiding on several occasions after probenecid therapy; the arrhythmia was presumed due to a gouty deposit. Three cases of probable acute gouty pericarditis were successfully treated with colchicine.[200]

There is no significant increase in the incidence of hypertension or arteriosclerotic coronary artery disease in patients with clinical gout.

Oxalosis

Familial hyperoxaluria, presumed to be a hereditary defect in intermediary metabolism, and secondary hyperoxaluria are characterized by the deposition of calcium oxalate in body tissues.[201] Cardiac arrhythmias and conduction abnormalities have been described in patients with oxalosis.[201–203] At postmortem examination,[202] refractile, yellow, rosette-like calcium oxalate crystals were demonstrated in the myocardial fibers and the interstitial connective tissue of the heart, associated with mononuclear cell infiltration and myofiber degeneration in areas of dense crystal deposition. To date there is no known therapy.

Ochronosis

No clinical cardiovascular disease is associated with either hereditary or exogenous ochronosis, despite the striking pathologic lesions. Areas of gray-blue to purple-black pigmentation occur in the myocardium and coronary arteries; ochronotic pigment granules are deposited preferentially in collagenous and fibrous tissue, without evoking an inflammatory-cell reaction.[204]

Primary Myocardial Calcification

Occlusive coronary artery disease is the most common cause of massive myocardial calcification,[205] although cardiac calcification has been reported secondary to varied vascular, inflammatory, and toxic causes of myofiber necrosis and degeneration. Generalized myocardial calcification was reported [206] in a premature infant with myofiber degenerative changes; right ventricular calcification was described [207] in adults with endomyocardial fibrosis in Uganda. There is no apparent abnormality of calcium metabolism.

Fibrocystic Disease of the Pancreas (Mucoviscidosis)

Cor pulmonale, secondary to chronic pulmonary disease, is the most commonly recognized form of heart disease in patients with fibrocystic disease of the pancreas.

Myocardial fibrosis[208] has been reported in association with fibrocystic disease of the pancreas in infants and young children. The clinical presentation is of cardiac enlargement, arrhythmias, and electrocardiographic abnormalities; the patients usually succumb to congestive heart failure.[209] At postmortem examination there is biventricular dilatation and hypertrophy, with scar tissue replacement of degenerating muscle fibers; there is prominent endocardial fibroelastosis of the atria.[209,210] The suggested cause is a nutritional or metabolic deficiency, probably related either to the steatorrhea or to prolonged antibiotic therapy with alteration of the intestinal flora.[208]

Hypokalemia

Hypokalemia may be due to prolonged diarrhea or vomiting, familial periodic paralysis, primary aldosteronism, potassium-losing nephritis, sprue, gastrointestinal fistula, diabetic acidosis, severe alkalosis, corticosteroid and diuretic therapy, etc.;[211] cardiovascular aberrations are usually associated with a serum-potassium level of less than 3 mEq per liter.

There is usually no significant functional cardiovascular abnormalities, although hypotension, tachycardia, and more rarely congestive heart failure have been reported.[211] The characteristic electrocardiographic pattern[212] consists of Q-U interval prolongation, widening and flattening of the

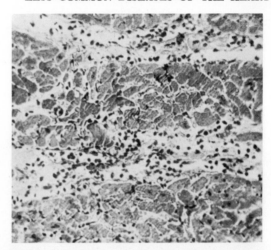

Fig. 55-15. Hypokalemic myocarditis. There is an interstitial inflammatory infiltrate, with myofiber fragmentation. ($\times$ 150.) (*Courtesy of Department of Pathology, Emory University School of Medicine.*)

T-wave, S-T segment displacement, prominent U waves, diminished QRS voltage, and increased A-V conduction time. These abnormalities are probably due to electrophysiologic disturbances rather than anatomic myocardial lesions. Blomberg and Lindquist[212] found no constant relationship between the serum-potassium level and the electrocardiographic changes and suggested that the electrocardiographic changes were dependent upon myocardial potassium concentration; in McAllen's[213] case of hypokalemic myocarditis secondary to steatorrhea, the myocardial potassium concentration was 15 mg per 100 Gm of wet tissue, compared with a normal value of greater than 300 mg. Weaver and Burchell,[214] however, described a specific hypokalemic electrocardiographic pattern which correlated well with the serum-potassium level in stable patients.

The pathologic myocardial lesions of hypokalemia in man are similar to those produced in rats by a potassium-deficient diet.[215] There is loss of muscle striation, myofiber vacuolation and fragmentation, interstitial cellular infiltrate, and varying degrees of myocardial necrosis and fibroblastic proliferation (Fig. 55-15). The lesions are most pronounced in the subendocardial layer of the ventricles and in the papillary muscles.[216,217]

Uremia

Nonspecific pathologic and electrocardiographic abnormalities were described [218,219] in patients with uremia but were attributed to the associated hypertension, anemia, electrolyte abnormalities, and pericarditis.

Hematologic Causes

Leukemia

Cardiovascular involvement with clinical or electrocardiographic abnormalities was described [220] in 25 per cent of patients with leukemia; approximately half of these cardiac manifestations were due to leukemic infiltration of the myocardium, with the remainder attributable to anemia, to myocardial hemorrhage, to pericarditis, and to nonspecific toxic changes. Cardiac infiltration was encountered [221] in 44 per cent of patients with leukemia; this occurred more commonly in lymphatic and stem-cell [222] rather than myelogenous leukemia, and more commonly with the acute than the chronic phase.

The cardiac symptoms and electrocardiographic disturbances are dependent upon the extent and location of leukemic myocardial infiltration according to Aronson and Leroy,[223] who found good correlation between the clinical and pathologic abnormalities. This correlation was not confirmed by Popescu et al.[224]

The pathologic lesion consists of leukemic infiltration of the myocardial capillaries and interstitial tissues, with dense infiltration causing muscle degeneration and necrosis.[225,226]

The predominant clinical features include tachycardia, arrhythmia, cardiac enlargement, and congestive heart failure.[226] Blotner and Sosman[227] described a case of leukemic heart block which disappeared after x-ray therapy. There is no diagnostic electrocardiographic pattern,[223] but tachycardia, premature ventricular contractions, ventricular or atrial excitation abnormalities, and nonspecific ST-T changes are common. Most patients with clinical evidence of leukemic heart disease have abnormal electrocardiograms.

Cardiac invasion and cardiovascular symptoms may occur early in the course of leukemia, particularly in acute leukemia,[228] occasionally as the initial manifestation of the disease.[220] Left atrial rupture due to massive leukemic infiltration has been reported.[229]

Sickle-cell Anemia

Cardiomegaly was reported in 95 per cent of patients with sickle-cell anemia, usually associated with exertional dyspnea and systolic murmurs.[230] The cardiovascular manifestations of sickle-cell disease are due to the chronic anemia; to the pulmonary thromboses, which may lead to cor pulmonale; and to the myocardial disease caused by thrombosis of small cardiac blood vessels.[231]

Although dyspnea is the predominant symptom, classic symptoms and electrocardiographic changes of myocardial ischemia occurred in a twenty-two-year-old man during a sickle-cell crisis; the electrocardiogram reverted to normal after the crisis, and myocardial infarction was not demonstrated at subsequent postmortem examination.[232] Congestive heart failure is a late manifestation.[233]

The frequent pulmonary and mitral systolic murmurs, coupled with the joint symptoms of sickle-cell disease, often lead to the misdiagnosis of rheumatic heart disease. Although there is no predictable electrocardiographic pattern, P-R interval prolongation and nonspecific ST segment and T-wave changes are commonly observed.[230,233,233a]

At postmortem examination there is biventricular dilatation and hypertrophy; muscle fiber hypertrophy; arteritis with proliferation and thrombosis; and resultant myocardial degeneration, necrosis, and secondary fibrosis.[230,232]

Polycythemia Vera

The cardiac manifestations of polycythemia vera are usually those of myocardial infarction, secondary to intravascular thrombosis of the coronary arteries.[234,235] The consensus in the older literature is that coronary thrombosis is a manifestation of the thrombotic tendency seen in polycythemia vera and is unrelated to the degree of coronary atherosclerosis;[235a] however, this problem needs additional study. Associated moderate systemic hypertension may also be implicated as a cause of cardiovascular symptoms.[236]

Essential Thrombophilia

Angina pectoris and electrocardiographic changes of ischemia have been associated with an elevated platelet count in two patients with primary thrombocytosis; therapy with P-32 effected a decrease in angina and concomitant electrocardiographic improvement.[237] Electrocardiographic abnormalities of myocardial infarction have been reported [238] in an eight-year-old girl with essential thrombophilia.

Neurologic Causes

Pseudohypertrophic Muscular Dystrophy

Cardiopathy, occurring in more than 50 per cent of patients with pseudohypertrophic muscular dystrophy,[239] is probably a genetically determined manifestation of this familial disease which more commonly affects the male.[240] Cannon[240] emphasized the lack of correlation between the degree of skeletal muscle disease and the severity of cardiac symptoms and electrocardiographic abnormalities. Cardiac manifestations may, indeed, antedate recognition of the neuromuscular disease,

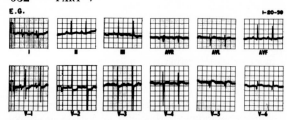

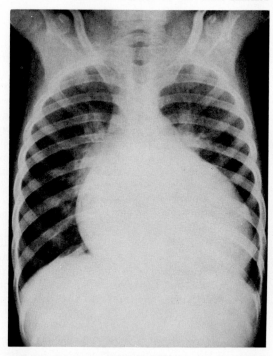

Fig. 55-16. Ten-year-old boy with muscular dystrophy. The electrocardiogram mimics posterolateral wall myocardial infarction. (*Courtesy of Crippled Children's Division, Georgia Department of Public Health.*)

Fig. 55-17. Generalized cardiac enlargement and pulmonary venous congestion in a ten-year-old boy with muscular dystrophy. (*Courtesy of Crippled Children's Division, Georgia Department of Public Health.*)

which is diagnosed by the triad of peculiar gait, large calves, and the "climbing up the legs" phenomenon.[241]

The electrocardiogram is the earliest and most frequent indication of cardiac involvement, being abnormal in 40 to 80 per cent of patients reported in recent series.[242-244] It is generally agreed that no characteristic electrocardiographic pattern occurs, although Wahi[245] described a "specific myopathic" electrocardiogram. Tachycardia, arrhythmias, and P-wave abnormalities are commonly noted; a shortened P-R interval, conduction defects, deep Q waves, and nonspecific T-wave changes are also seen (Fig. 55-16). The ballistocardiogram was thought by Lowenstein et al.[246] to reflect cardiac abnormality even earlier than the electrocardiogram.

Tachycardia is the characteristic clinical finding,[247,248] persisting during sleep,[248a] often associated with arrhythmia and cardiac enlargement (Fig. 55-17). Symptoms of congestive heart failure are generally absent because of the patients' prolonged inactivity and bed rest;[249] arrhythmia or infection tends to precipitate cardiac failure. Incipient congestive heart failure was demonstrated by cardiac catheterization studies.[250] Sudden death is not uncommon in patients with pseudohypertrophic muscular dystrophy.

The cardiac lesion[251-253] consists of fatty and fibrous replacement of the myocardium. There are areas of compensatory myofiber hypertrophy, but most myocardial cells are atrophic with loss of striation, vacuolation, fragmentation, and nuclear degeneration. James[254] noted normal main coronary arteries but described generalized noninflammatory degenerative changes in the small myocardial arteries, including those supplying the sinus and A-V nodes; he suggested this as the pathologic basis for the frequent arrhythmias.

An increase of cardiac output was described in pseudohypertrophic muscular dystrophy; release by the heart muscle of malic acid dehydrogenase and aldolase, which suggests increased permeability of the myocardial cell, was demonstrated.[255]

Friedreich's Ataxia

In his original description of heritable progressive spinocerebellar degeneration, Friedreich[256] noted cardiac involvement—arrhythmia, cardiac enlargement and congestive failure—in five of six patients presented. The cardiac disease of Friedreich's ataxia has been variously attributed to scoliosis or chest deformity causing cor pulmonale, to coronary narrowing or occlusion, to neurogenic or toxic causes, to rheumatic or congenital origin, etc.;[257-259] Boyer et al.[259] believed it to be an example of pleiotropy, that is, a genetically determined disturbance, presumably of a metabolic pathway, having effects on several organs.

Friedreich's ataxia, the most common of the hereditary ataxias, is characterized by the onset in adolescence of progressive skeletal deformities, ataxia, and speech disturbance; death due to congestive heart failure or intercurrent infection usually occurs within 20 years after onset of symptoms.[258] There is evidence of cardiovascular disease in one-third to one-half of the patients, with cardiac symptoms often the initial manifestation of the disease.[260] Palpitations, retrosternal pain, and exertional dyspnea are reported; the classic physical findings are those of arrhythmia, cardiac enlarge-

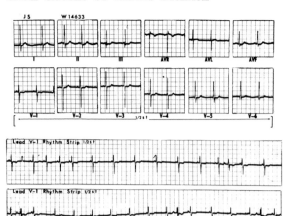

Fig. 55-18. Twenty-one-year-old man with Friedreich's ataxia, congestive heart failure, and recurrent arrhythmias. There is electrocardiographic evidence of biventricular hypertrophy and nonspecific ST-T abnormalities. A wandering supraventricular pacemaker is demonstrated on the rhythm strips. (*Courtesy of Electrocardiographic Laboratory, Grady Memorial Hospital.*)

ment, nonspecific heart murmurs, and congestive heart failure.[261] The congestive heart failure is due to myocardial disease, with or without cor pulmonale.

Electrocardiographic abnormalities (Fig. 55-18) are reported in about 30 per cent of cases of Friedreich's ataxia,[258] occurring more frequently in patients with clinical cardiac disease; Nadas,[262] however, noted T-wave abnormalities suggestive of left ventricular ischemia in all patients with the disease.

ST-T changes of myocardial ischemia, A-V block, and bundle branch block are the most frequently described electrocardiographic disturbances.[263,264] Boyer et al.[259] reported no relationship between the severity of the neurologic disease, the family history of ataxia, and the severity of the heart disease. Evans and Wright[265] found the incidence of electrocardiographic abnormalities unrelated to age, sex, or disease duration but somewhat higher with severe neurologic disease; they described a far more striking association between a family history of Friedreich's ataxia and electrocardiographic disturbances, affected members of the same family tending to show the same electrocardiographic changes. Ivemark and Thorén[265a] described poor correlation between the electrocardiographic abnormalities and the cardiac pathologic changes.

There is cardiac hypertrophy, fatty degeneration, diffuse interstitial fibrosis, and eosinophilic and lymphocytic infiltration. Collagenous tissue replaces the degenerating myofibers, and compensa-

tory hypertrophy of the remaining muscle cells occurs.[261,264] Descriptions of the coronary arteries vary from normal to diffuse atheromatous involvement, with and without obstruction.[261] Involvement of the Purkinje fibers of the A-V node and conducting system by fibrous-tissue infiltration disrupts the normal pathway of excitation; this may be the explanation for the frequent arrhythmias.[261] James and Fisch[266] attributed the cardiopathy to extensive medial degeneration and intimal hyperplasia of the smaller coronary arteries; they believed the arrhythmias may be due to involvement of the S-A and A-V node arteries.

Myotonia Atrophica

Slow muscle relaxation after contraction, muscle atrophy, increased skeletal muscle tone, expressionless face, cataracts, premature baldness, and gonadal atrophy comprise the clinical manifestations of the heredofamilial muscle disorder myotonia atrophica; there are frequently associated abnormalities suggestive or diagnostic of heart disease.[267] Neuromuscular signs discovered during an evaluation of cardiovascular disease may contribute to the earlier diagnosis of myotonia atrophica;[268] Litchfield[269] cited a patient with myotonia atrophica with early severe cardiac involvement who only much later had complaints referable to the neuromuscular system; a similar case was described by Holt.[270] Spillane,[271] on the other hand, stated that the neurologic features of the disease developed earlier and were more readily identified than the cardiac signs.

Evidence of cardiac disease is found most commonly on electrocardiographic examination and is usually a conduction or rhythm disturbance. Miller[272] reported a 60 to 70 per cent incidence of electrocardiographic abnormalities in patients with myotonia atrophica, consisting primarily of P-R interval prolongation, low P-wave voltage, slurred and notched QRS complexes, left axis devi-

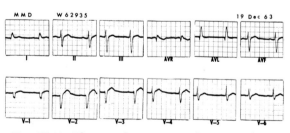

Fig. 55-19. Electrocardiogram mimicking anterolateral myocardial infarction with peri-infarction block. This patient with myotonia atrophica has no symptoms referable to the cardiovascular system. (*Courtesy of Electrocardiographic Laboratory, Grady Memorial Hospital.*)

ation, and bundle branch block. On occasion, the electrocardiographic abnormalities may mimic myocardial infarction (Fig. 55-19). The findings of left axis deviation on the electrocardiogram without associated clinical heart disease in a two-year-old child suggested the diagnosis of myotonia atrophica.[273] Fearrington[274] believed that the conduction defects seen on the electrocardiogram, and the changes in the ventricular activation process on the vectorcardiogram, in 60 per cent of patients with myotonia atrophica were consistent with the autopsy reports of myocardial involvement.

Dyspnea and palpitations are the reported cardiac symptoms. The clinical findings[268,271,272] include arrhythmias, occasionally with Stokes-Adams syncope; a slow, weak pulse; a split S-1 and, at times, an S-4, producing a triple rhythm; and, less commonly, cardiac enlargement and congestive heart failure.

Autopsy reports are rare but usually confirm the description by Fisch and Evans[275] of diffuse myocardial fibrosis, separation of myofibers by fibrous connective tissue, and scattered hypertrophic muscle fibers with large nuclei.[270]

Kilpatrick and Caughey[276] stated that electrocardiographic conduction and rhythm abnormalities constituted the only cardiovascular manifestations of myotonia atrophica; they reported no evidence for significant cardiac symptoms or anatomic alterations and suggested that the cardiac disturbances may be metabolic.

Myasthenia Gravis

Patients with myasthenia gravis have variable generalized weakness following use of voluntary muscles but present no clinical or electrocardiographic evidence of cardiac dysfunction.[277,277a] However, myofiber necrosis with an acute and chronic secondary inflammatory reaction was noted[277-279] at postmortem examination, particularly in cases with associated thymoma; these myocardial abnormalities were not described in the cases reported by Taquini et al.[280]

Chemical Causes

Toxic Conditions

Emetine. Manifestations of cardiovascular toxicity are evident in the majority of patients receiving emetine. Emetine toxicity is most commonly encountered in the therapy of amebiasis, due to the small margin of safety between the effective and toxic drug doses.[281]

Klatskin and Friedman[282] reported electrocardiographic abnormalities, hypotension, tachycardia, dyspnea, and precordial discomfort associated with emetine therapy but believed the electrocardio-

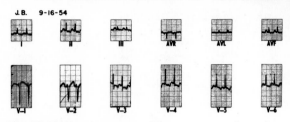

Fig. 55-20. Emetine toxicity. There is sinus tachycardia, Q-T interval prolongation and nonspecific ST-T abnormalities.

graphic abnormalities were the only evidence of myocardial toxicity; they described all other cardiovascular disturbances as transient, subsiding even with continuation of emetine therapy. Most other reports[281] cite the appearance of clinical cardiovascular disturbances as an indication for immediate cessation of emetine therapy, even in the absence of electrocardiographic abnormalities.

Almost invariable T-wave abnormalities and Q-T interval prolongation are noted after the first week of emetine therapy (Fig. 55-20);[283,284] on occasion, electrocardiographic alterations appeared only after the completion of emetine therapy. Tachycardia, P-R interval prolongation, ST-segment displacement, and increased QRS duration have been described, with terminal ventricular fibrillation also recorded. Electrocardiographic abnormalities persist or progress during continued emetine administration but characteristically regress within a month or two after cessation of therapy.[284a] The initial abnormality, precordial T-wave inversion, is usually the last to disappear.[283]

The pathologic changes[285,286] are those of myocardial degeneration (Fig. 55-21); there is myofiber destruction without inflammatory change.

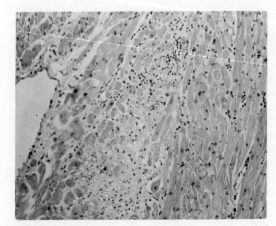

Fig. 55-21. Emetine toxicity. Focal myocytolyses of the myocardium with interstitial and focal perivascular infiltration of lymphocytes.

Dack and Moloshok[281] advocated bed rest during emetine therapy, with frequent evaluation of the symptoms, the physical findings, and the electrocardiogram; they believed emetine therapy was contraindicated in patents with underlying heart disease.

Arsenic. Acute interstitial myocarditis has been reported during arsenical therapy of syphilis, usually in association with an exfoliative arsenical dermatitis.[287–289] An allergic cause was postulated[288,289] for the myocarditis, although the exact nature of the allergen is not apparent. The clinical findings include dyspnea, cardiac enlargement and progressive congestive heart failure.[288,290] Nonspecific T-wave changes and Q-T interval prolongation constitute the electrocardiographic abnormalities.[290,291] The pathologic cardiac lesion[289,292] is an interstitial myocarditis with edema, focal fibrosis, eosinophilic- and mononuclear-cell infiltration, and endocardial thickening with mural thrombosis.

Acute arsenic poisoning, usually due to arsenic trioxide, is probably the most common cause of acute heavy-metal poisoning. Arsenic interferes with the function of respiratory system enzymes and may thus produce myocardial anoxia.[293] There are no cardiac symptoms, and no residual cardiovascular disease is evident in patients who recover.[294] The electrocardiographic changes are those of myocardial ischemia.[293,294] Multiple focal subepicardial hemorrhages occur within the first few hours after poisoning.[293]

Poisoning with arsine gas may terminate fatally as a result of acute myocardial failure. Arsine gas causes red blood cell hemolysis, decreasing the oxygen-carrying capacity of the blood; both the myocardial anoxia and the appreciable amounts of arsenic demonstrated in the heart muscle at autopsy are implicated in the production of the cardiac lesions: subepicardial hemorrhage, myocardial degeneration and fragmentation, and interstitial edema.[295,296] Abnormal T-waves have been noted in the electrocardiogram.[295]

Antimony. Fuadin, tartar emetic, Astiban, and other antimony compounds used to treat schistosomiasis frequently produce myocardial damage. Although fatal hepatic antimony toxicity usually precedes fatal cardiac toxicity, myocardial disturbances may occur early in the course of therapy and even after completion of treatment.[297]

Almost invariably electrocardiographic abnormalities occur by the end of a course of antimony therapy.[298] Cardiovascular symptoms are uncommon, but precordial oppression has been described.[297] Death occurs suddenly, not uncommonly due to arrhythmia, with no constant or significant prior change in heart rate or blood pressure.[297]

Nonspecific ST-T changes and a prolonged Q-T interval constitute the electrocardiographic abnormalities;[298–300] the rare arrhythmias and conduction abnormalities have an ominous prognosis. Electrocardiographic alterations tend to increase as the duration of a course of antimony therapy increases and usually regress after cessation of treatment.[298] Similar electrocardiographic abnormalities have been described with repeated courses of antimony compounds in the same individual.[300]

Ethyl Alcohol. Evans[301] described alcoholic cardiomyopathy as occurring primarily in the middle-aged obese male who regularly drinks to excess; the nutritional state was uniformly good, eliminating the possibility of thiamine or niacin deficiency; there was neither associated anemia nor central nervous system manifestations of disease.

The presenting symptoms of alcoholic cardiomyopathy[301,302] are breathlessness and palpitations, the latter due to arrhythmias. Left ventricular failure occurs later, characterized by cardiomegaly, tachycardia, triple rhythm, edema, and diminished cardiac output. Pericardial effusion may be present. There is excessive sweating, particularly at night. Mild polycythemia is present, and the serum cholesterol level is low.[302a] Distinctive electrocardiographic abnormalities[303] consist of dimpled, cloven, or spinous T waves; arrhythmias such as premature ventricular contractions, atrial fibrillation, or paroxysmal atrial tachycardia; and the conduction disturbances of complete heart block or bundle branch block. Eliaser and Giansiracusa[304] described subsidence of electrocardiographic abnormalities within several days after alcoholic intake was discontinued.

The pathologic changes[301,302] include patchy muscle necrosis with varying amounts of fibrosis and compensatory myocardial hypertrophy. The coronary arteries are usually normal. Mural thrombosis is a frequent occurrence.

Recent physiologic studies[255,305] have demonstrated that ethyl alcohol produces increased myocardial oxygen consumption associated with diminished left ventricular work; this reflects decreased left ventricular efficiency. Decreased left ventricular contractility after ethanol ingestion has been observed in animal experiments.[306] Mitochondrial damage, with abnormalities of the mitochondrial oxidative enzymes, has been demonstrated.[306a,b,c]

l-**Norepinephrine.** Myocarditis, with lesions similar to those seen with pheochromocytoma, has been described following therapy with *l*-norepinephrine. There is focal myocardial necrosis, inflammatory infiltrate, edema, and epicardial hemorrhage.[307] Chest pain has been reported, with electrocardiographic changes of myocardial injury and ischemia.[308] Szakács and Mehlman[309] considered this a toxic myocarditis and suggested that *l*-norepineph-rine dosage should be determined on a milligram per kilogram basis, rather than by blood pressure response to therapy.

Carbon Monoxide. Acute and chronic carbon monoxide poisoning may cause myocardial infarction or myocarditis; increased morbidity is encountered both with acute carbon monoxide poisoning and with higher carbon monoxide blood levels in the chronic illness.[310] The cardiac damage is attributed to anoxemia, as carbon monoxide diminishes the oxygen transport capacity of the blood, and to a direct carbon monoxide toxic effect on myocardial fiber mitochondria.[310,310a]

Clinical manifestations include angina pectoris,[310b] palpitations, and exertional dyspnea.[311] Electrocardiographic alterations are usually transient but may persist for weeks or months;[312] Cosby and Bergeron[313] and others[314,315] described ischemic ST-T changes as occurring most frequently; sinus tachycardia, premature ventricular contractions, and atrial fibrillation were also encountered. Graziani and Rossi[310] reported frequent electrocardiographic evidence of left ventricular hypertrophy in chronic carbon monoxide poisoning, at times associated with incomplete bundle branch block, premature ventricular contractions, and P-wave abnormalities. Carbon monoxide poisoning may produce myocardial infarction in a patient with underlying coronary artery disease.

Hemorrhagic and necrotic lesions, probably anoxemic in origin, have a predilection for the papillary muscles and the subendocardial layer of the left ventricle.[311] Round-cell infiltration occurs in areas of muscle disruption and fragmentation.[316] Rupture of the heart has been reported.[316a]

Phosphorus. Electrocardiographic alterations were described[317] in more than 50 per cent of patients with phosphorus poisoning, apparently related to the amount of phosphorus ingested. Nonspecific ST-T abnormalities and Q-T interval prolongation occurred most commonly, regressing with clinical improvement.[318,319]

Death in the first 12 hr after phosphorus poisoning is usually cardiovascular in origin; the appearance of ventricular fibrillation or peripheral vascular collapse is a grave prognostic sign.[317] Other cardiovascular manifestations are rare. The myocardial lesion is fatty degeneration with myofiber necrosis.[317,319]

Mercury. Dahhan and Orfaly[319a] described ST segment and T-wave abnormalities, Q-T interval prolongation, and occasional arrhythmias in 42 patients with mercury poisoning; a mercury-containing fungicide was inadvertently ingested.

Lead. Pathologic evidence of myocarditis—inter-stitial fibrosis, occasional inflammatory cells and serous exudate—was reported in five patients dying of chronic lead poisoning; tachycardia, gallop rhythm, and pulmonary edema were the clinical manifestations.[320] Kosmider and Petelenz[321] commented on the frequency of "cardiopathy" and electrocardiographic abnormalities in young patients with chronic occupational lead poisoning. Chest pain has also been noted. The electrocardiographic alterations of sinus bradycardia, decreased P-R interval, occasional premature ventricular contractions, and nonspecific ST-T changes subsided after therapy.[322]

Scorpion venom. Poon-King[323] reported 45 cases of myocarditis due to the sting of a scorpion, *Tityus trinitatis*. Heart rate and rhythm disturbances were frequent; transient murmurs were heard; and electrocardiographic alterations—conduction changes, ST-T abnormalities, or Q-T interval prolongation—occurred in 76 per cent of patients. All abnormalities were transient, returning to normal within a week.

Snake venom. Reid et al.[323a] described reversible T-wave electrocardiographic abnormalities due to Malayan viper bites; intravascular clotting was the postulated mechanism. Transient angina pectoris and electrocardiographic changes compatible with myocardial infarction were reported following an adder bite.[323b]

Hypersensitivity

Sulfonamide. Interstitial myocarditis, characterized by mononuclear and eosinophilic perivascular infiltration, was described in patients who had received sulfonamide drugs;[324,325] there were no cardiac symptoms, and only about 50 per cent of the patients had clinical evidence of sulfonamide hypersensitivity. Congestive heart failure was reported as the cause of death in two of three patients with fatal sulfonamide myocarditis.[326] Granulomatous myocardial lesions, myofiber necrosis, and petechial hemorrhages have also been noted.[327,328] Similar fatal myocarditis, due to sulfonylurea antidiabetic therapy, was reported.[329]

Penicillin. Bradycardia and transient ST-T electrocardiographic changes associated with penicillin hypersensitivity are thought to be evidence of myocardial involvement.[330] Granulomatous and diffuse interstitial myocarditis was reported following penicillin hypersensitivity reactions;[331] the patient had no clinical cardiac symptoms or electrocardiographic abnormalities. Classic granulomatous lesions predominated in the papillary muscles; inflammatory arteritis, edema, areas of myofiber necrosis, and eosinophilic and inflammatory cellular exudate were seen on microscopic examination.

Phenylbutazone. A profound interstitial myocarditis, indistinguishable pathologically from other drug-hypersensitivity lesions, has been reported with phenylbutazone therapy.[332] The clinical findings of chest pain, tachycardia, hypotension and heart failure, associated with electrocardiographic changes of myocardial ischemia, have occurred both during and after phenylbutazone therapy in the recommended dosage range.[333] At pathologic examination there were focal perivascular granulomas, muscle necrosis, edema, eosinophilic and acute inflammatory cellular reaction, and fibrinoid collagen degeneration.[333–335]

Smallpox Vaccine. Myocarditis and pericarditis, both presumably due to an antigen-antibody reaction, have been described as occurring 1 to 2 weeks after smallpox vaccination; the time lag suggests that a viremia should not be implicated.[336,337] Although chest pain, rapid heart rate, and electrocardiographic abnormalities have been described preterminally, death has also occurred without premonitory cardiac symptoms.[338,339] The ST-T changes on the electrocardiogram and the occasional arrhythmias disappear in the patients who survive.[336,337,340] There is acute myocardial degeneration, particularly involving the left ventricle, with loss of myofiber striations, myocardial necrosis, edema, and granulocytic infiltration.[338,339]

Aureomycin Hydrochloride. Allergic myocarditis due to Aureomycin hydrochloride hypersensitivity has been described.[341] Fibrinoid necrosis and a diffuse perivascular and interstitial infiltrate of eosinophils, lymphocytes, and Anitschkow myocytes were seen.

Streptomycin. Widespread myofiber necrosis, diffuse eosinophilic- and inflammatory-cell infiltrate, and petechial myocardial hemorrhages were the cardiac lesions in streptomycin allergy.[342] Chest discomfort was the only cardiac abnormality preceding death.

Chlorpromazine. Focal interstitial myocardial necrosis without clinical cardiac disease, presumably due to chlorpromazine therapy, has been reported.[343]

Phenindione. Kerwin[343a] described fatal myocarditis due to sensitivity to phenindione (Danilone).

Miscellaneous Systemic Syndromes

Rheumatoid Disease

Valvular, myocardial, and pericardial disease constitute the cardiac manifestations encountered in patients with rheumatoid disease.[343b]

Granulomata, histologically similar to rheumatoid nodules, occur in the epicardium, myocardium, and at the bases and cusps of the aortic and mitral valves.[343c] There is an associated diffuse arteritis.

Congestive heart failure, disproportionate to the severity of the valvular lesions, is attributed to the associated myocardial disease. Complete heart block with Adams-Stokes syncope has been reported in a case with rheumatoid nodule infiltration of the interventricular septum.[343d]

Reiter's Disease

Pericardial and myocardial involvement has been described in association with the arthritis, urethritis, and conjunctivitis of Reiter's disease.[343e]

The electrocardiographic abnormalities included prolongation of the P-R interval, widening of the QRS complex, and nonspecific ST-T changes. Pericardial friction rubs were encountered, often associated with pericardial pain; apical gallop sounds and apical systolic murmurs were also noted.[343e,343f]

Cogan's Syndrome

About one-third of the reported cases of Cogan's syndrome, nonsyphilitic interstitial keratitis and bilateral deafness, have associated cardiovascular manifestations.[343g] Cardiac enlargement, heart murmurs, and congestive heart failure have been described.

Fibrinoid necrosis, primarily of the aortic valve, produces aortic regurgitation. Angiitis of the myocardial arteries may result in myocardial ischemia and necrosis.

Behcet's Disease

Recurrent oral and genital ulceration with relapsing iritis of unknown etiology constitute Behcet's disease. The reported cardiac manifestations include cardiac enlargement, gallop sounds, pericardial friction rub, arrhythmias, and ST-T electrocardiographic changes.[343h] Corticosteroid therapy has been reported to be effective.

VERY RARE FORMS OF ENDOCARDIAL DISEASE

Carcinoid

In 1952, Biörck et al.[344] described the relationship between heart disease and malignant carcinoid tumors with metastases. Valvular lesions on the right side of the heart[345] are an integral part of the carcinoid syndrome, which also includes episodic cutaneous vasomotor phenomena, telangiectasia, hyperperistalsis, and bronchoconstriction.[346–348] Heart failure is the leading cause of death in metastatic carcinoid disease.[349]

Cardiac involvement occurs late in the course of carcinoid disease, invariably associated with hepatic metastases.[350] The fibrotic cardiac lesions are attributed to the potent concentration of

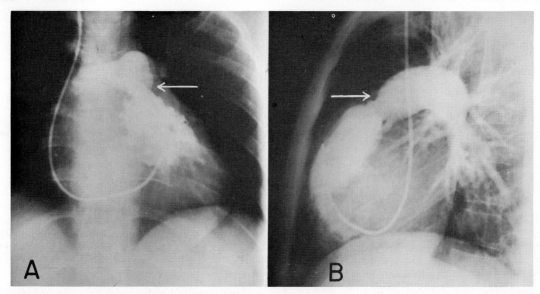

Fig. 55-22. Carcinoid heart disease. Right ventricular angiocardiogram demonstrates moderate pulmonary stenosis. At cardiac catheterization there was a 39 mm Hg systolic gradient across the pulmonary valve. A. One second after injection of contrast material. B. One and one-half seconds after injection of contrast material. (*Courtesy of Department of Radiology, Emory University School of Medicine.*)

5-hydroxytryptamine reaching the right side of the heart;[351,352] serotonin, normally inactivated by the liver, is, in effect, secreted by the hepatic carcinoid metastases.[347] Lung monoamine oxidase inactivates 5-hydroxytryptamine, forming 5-hydroxyindolacetic acid; McKusick[348] believed this explained the rarity of carcinoid lesions on the left side of the heart, which he observed only with a right-to-left intracardiac shunt. However, carcinoid lesions of the left side of the heart were described[353,354] without a right-to-left intracardiac shunt or pulmonary carcinoid tumor. Goble et al.[355] postulated that an elevated serotonin concentration altered the endocardial cellular permeability, allowing deposition of platelets and subsequent fibrosis of the valve cusps.

Cardiac manifestations of the carcinoid syndrome are pulmonic stenosis (Fig. 55-22), tricuspid insufficiency or stenosis, and failure of the right side of the heart. The electrocardiographic pattern may be that of right ventricular hypertrophy. Goble and his associates[355] and others have confirmed the valvular lesions at cardiac catheterization and have documented normal pulmonary vascular resistance. There is often lack of correlation between the severity of the valvular lesions and the severity of the congestive heart failure. Schwaber and Lukas,[356] reported cardiac catheterization findings indicative of hyperkinemia *without* pulmonic or tricuspid valvular disease; he suggested that hyperserotoninemia produced hyperkinemia, which, coupled with the episodic increased cardiac output

associated with flushing, resulted in congestive heart failure. However, increased cardiac output has been noted in patients with the carcinoid syndrome without cardiac involvement.[353]

At postmortem examination,[357,358] there is pearly white thickening of the pulmonic and tricuspid valve cusps and the ventricular endocardium, with retraction of the chordae tendineae (Fig. 55-23). Microscopic examination shows acellular hyalinized collagenous material, devoid of elastic fibers, deposited on an intact endocardial surface, without significant myocardial involvement (Fig. 55-24).

Therapy with serotonin antimetabolites has been ineffective.[348] Wright and Mulder[358] advocated surgical correction of symptomatic valvular lesions.

Endomyocardial Fibrosis

Fibroelastosis of unknown cause, as recognized in the United States during the first few years of life, is discussed in Chap. 20; the adult variety, which seems to be a sequel to many forms of heart disease, is mentioned in Chap. 39.

Endomyocardial fibrosis (see Table 55-1) is reported by Davies[359,360] to account for 15 per cent of congestive heart failure observed in Uganda, without particular age, sex, or racial predilection. The disease process has also been described in Ceylon[361] and in the Sudan.[362] The presenting complaints are dyspnea, palpitations, and edema, with occasional chest pain. The clinical picture[360,363] is of right and left ventricular failure of obscure cause, with mitral insufficiency and tricuspid in-

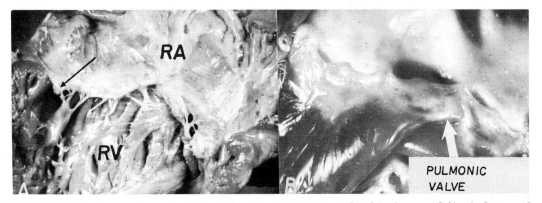

Fig. 55-23. Valvular changes in carcinoid heart disease. A. The tricuspid valve shows nodular thickening along the valve margin (arrow), with scarring and retraction of the valve and the chordae tendineae. B. The pulmonary valve shows thickening and retraction of all leaflets. (*Courtesy of Department of Pathology, Emory University School of Medicine.*)

Table 55-1. VERY RARE FORMS OF ENDOCARDIAL DISEASE

	Endomyocardial fibrosis	Becker's disease	Loeffler's disease
Fibrosis	Characteristic	Inconstant	Inconstant
Elastosis	Rare	Common	Common
A-V valve involvement	+	−	−
Eosinophilia	Inconstant	Inconstant	Characteristic
Emboli	Rare	Characteristic	Characteristic

sufficiency. There are diminished cardiac pulsations and often other signs simulating constrictive pericarditis; pericardial effusion may be present.[363a] An enlarged left atrium with expansile systolic pulsations is seen on x-ray examination. There is no consistent pattern of electrocardiographic abnormalities; but P mitrale, occasional atrial fibrillation, conduction defects, diminished QRS voltage, and nonspecific T-wave changes have been described.[364] Eosinophilia is inconstant. The cardiac catheterization data reported by Shillingford and Somers[365] showed elevated left atrial and pulmonary artery pressures, with the right ventricular pressure pulse resembling that of constrictive pericarditis.

The characteristic pathologic lesion[361,363] is an extensive white rugose endocardial fibrous thickening, affecting predominantly the left ventricular apex and inflow tract. The fibrosis involves the papillary muscles, the chordae tendineae, and the A-V valve cusps, particularly the posterior mitral valve leaflet; the right ventricular apex cavity may be obliterated by fibrosis. Mural thrombi are common, but embolic phenomena are infrequent.[359] There may be fibrosis of the inner one-third of the myocardium, with myofiber atrophy and vacuolation. The coronary arteries are unremarkable.

Histologically, the fibrous tissue is hyaline and avascular, with little or no elastosis.

Both the cause and pathogenesis of endomyocardial fibrosis remain speculative. Lynch and Watt[366] questioned whether there was primary myocardial disease with thrombosis and secondary endocardial disease or whether the endocardial disease was primary, with myocardial anoxia resulting from interference with its blood supply by the thickened endocardium. Lynfield et al.[367] cited the similarity of cardiac catheterization and angiocardiographic data irrespective of the degree of endocardial thickening; they suggested that endocardial fibrosis was a secondary phenomenon which developed in response to left ventricular dilatation which reinforced myocardial contractility.

Crawford[368] implicated excessive amounts of serotonin; he related the incidence of endomyocardial fibrosis to increased consumption of

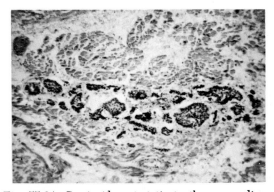

Fig. 55-24. Carcinoid, metastatic to the myocardium. There are nests of small, regular cells, arranged in an organoid pattern. (× 150.) (*Courtesy of Department of Pathology, Emory University School of Medicine.*)

bananas, which are rich in serotonin; the level of 5-hydroxyindolacetic acid excretion in his patients with endomyocardial fibrosis was similar to that seen with carcinoid disease. Other suggested causes[361,366,369,370] include allergy; malnutrition; parasitic, viral, or inflammatory disease; coronary artery disease; and persistence of the infantile form of fibroelastosis.

Thomas et al.[371] delineated three areas of dysfunction related to endocardial thickening: (1) problems of contraction and relaxation, mimicking constrictive pericarditis; (2) interference with proper impulse conduction, manifested by arrhythmias and conduction delays; and (3) deficiency of blood supply to the underlying myocardium, with resultant myocardial anoxia.

Cardiovascular Collagenosis with Parietal Endocardial Thrombosis (Becker's Disease)

In 1953, Becker et al.[372] described 40 cases of an obscure South African cardiopathologic condition which they designated as *cardiovascular collagenosis with parietal endocardial thrombosis* (see Table 55-1). This disease occurred in the robust and the malnourished, without age, sex, or racial predilection.[359] The three major features were[360,372] (1) rapidly fatal congestive heart failure, with an average symptom duration of 6 months; congestive heart failure was the cause of death in all reported cases; (2) bland visceral infarction, solitary or multiple, occurring in over three-fourths of the cases; and (3) characteristic cardiac findings of dilatation with or without hypertrophy, mural thrombosis predominantly in the left ventricle, subendocardial and papillary muscle necrosis and/or fibrosis, focal or diffuse endocardial thickening, and absence of significant lesions in the pericardium, heart valves, coronary arteries, and aorta.

Progressive exertional dyspnea is the initial symptom, with subsequent cough, edema, ascites, chest pain, and hemoptysis. There is tachycardia; tachypnea; severe congestive heart failure with edema, ascites, and effusions; cardiac enlargement with gallop rhythm and nonspecific systolic murmurs; pulmonary congestion; and hepatomegaly.[372] ST-T changes are the most constant electrocardiographic abnormality, with a prolonged Q-T interval and abnormal P waves often seen. Eosinophilia is inconstant. The enlarged heart has poor pulsations at fluoroscopic examination.

The pathologic lesion[360] is endocardial fibrosis and sclerosis, with hyperplasia of elastic tissue. There is involvement of the inner one-third of the myocardium, with myofiber edema and degeneration. An arteritis of the Thebesian and luminal vessels is described.

Viral diseases, toxoplasmosis, hypersensitivity reaction, and nutritional deficiency constitute the suggested causes. The pathogenesis, too, is obscure, but presumably a specific abnormal mural endocardial mucopolysaccharide produces endocardial swelling and fibrinous exudation with subsequent thrombus formation.[360] The intense local tissue anoxia from the mucoid edema produces subendocardial necrosis; blood supply from the heart cavity to the inner one-third of the myocardium is further compromised by thrombus formation, with resultant increased local anoxia and subendocardial necrosis. Fibroelastotic plaques result from organization of the necrotic endocardium and subendocardium and the overlying thrombus.

Fibroplastic Parietal Endocarditis (Loeffler's Disease)

Progressive congestive heart failure, refractory to therapy, with associated eosinophilia, and multiple systemic infarctions due to emboli was reported by Loeffler[373] in 1936 (see Table 55-1); the cardiac lesion was a thickened, scarred endocardium with mural thrombosis.

Patients with Loeffler's endocarditis[374] initially report diminished exercise tolerance, progressing to intractable congestive heart failure over a variable period of months or years. The heart is of normal size or slightly enlarged, with features suggestive of constrictive pericarditis. The murmur of mitral insufficiency is most common, with mitral stenosis and tricuspid insufficiency murmurs also reported. Pleural effusion and evidence of pulmonary and splenic emboli are often encountered. Nonspecific ST-T changes and diminished QRS voltage are the usual electrocardiographic disturbances. Leukocytosis is present with a striking eosinophilia.[375,376]

Pressure patterns from the right side of the heart simulating constrictive pericarditis have been described at cardiac catheterization.[376] The pathophysiologic changes in Loeffler's endocarditis may therefore result from impairment of systolic ejection and restriction of diastolic filling of the ventricle.[376]

In the acute stage of the disease[374] there is an eosinophilic arteritis and inflammatory-cell infiltrate of the heart and other organs; no macroscopic cardiac abnormalities are evident. Chronic fibroplastic parietal endocarditis[374-376] is characterized by a leathery, gray-white, fibrous endocardial scarring, predominantly in the left ventricle, producing an essentially rigid and immobile cavity of almost constant size. The elastic and collagen proliferation and inflammatory infiltrate may extend into the underlying myocardium; the collagenous scarring also deforms the papillary muscles and chordae tendineae, with resultant mitral insufficiency and tricuspid insufficiency. Left ventricular mural thrombi are characteristically described.

Although Loeffler's endocarditis is thought to be a hypersensitivity lesion,[375,377] response to corticosteroid therapy has been unimpressive.[378] Recently a filarial cause[379] has been postulated for fibroplastic parietal endocarditis, because of the dramatic improvement reported with arsenical and Hetrazan therapy.[379a]

CARDIAC TUMORS

In 1783, de Senac stated: "Le coeur est un organe trop noble pour être atteint d'une tumeur primaire." [380] Pritchard,[177] however, noted that cardiac tumors are not disproportionately rare when their incidence is compared with the heart's percentage of total body weight, 0.4 to 0.5 per cent. The paucity of mitotic activity in cardiac muscle is evidenced by the heart's reaction to injury by degenerative rather than regenerative phenomena; this may contribute to the infrequent occurrence of primary cardiac tumors. The low incidence of metastatic disease to the heart has been attributed to (1) strong kneading action of the heart, (2) the metabolic peculiarities of striated muscle, (3) the rapid intracardiac blood flow, and (4) the restricted cardiac lymphatic connections, as metastases to the heart via lymphatic channels spread in a retrograde manner.[177] Cardiac tumors, though still considered medical rarities, are no longer academic curiosities, as surgical cure is possible in some cases.[381]

The first pathologic description of a cardiac tumor has been variously attributed to Columbos[382] in 1559,[383] to Zollicofferus in 1685,[384] to Boneti in 1700,[384,385] and to Morgagni in 1762.[385] Antemortem diagnosis of a primary cardiac tumor was first recorded in 1934 by Barnes, Beaver, and Snell;[386] Rösler, in 1924,[387] is credited with the first in vivo diagnosis of a metastatic cardiac tumor. The dramatic increase in correct antemortem diagnoses of cardiac tumors since 1956 reflects the recent interest in cardiac tumors, concomitant with improved cardiac surgical procedures.[388]

Diagnostic Clues

Tumors of the heart produce no characteristic symptoms unless they interfere with the cardiac mechanism;[386] therefore, only about 5 to 10 per cent of all cardiac neoplasms can be diagnosed clinically.[389] Only minimal cardiac dysfunction may be encountered even with extensive myocardial invasion and destruction.[390] This may be attributed[391] to slow tumor growth, allowing for compensatory cardiac changes, and to the relative resistance of heart valves, conducting tissue, and

arteries to tumor invasion,[392,393] preserving the normal cardiac hemodynamics. Myocardial metabolism is aerobic, requiring lactic acid as its keystone and extracting little glucose from the arterial blood; tumors have a high degree of anaerobic glycolysis, requiring more glucose and less oxygen, and producing more lactate than heart muscle; these two tissues are therefore ideally suited to coexistence, possibly explaining the infrequency of symptoms.[394] Primary cardiac tumors, benign and malignant, and metastatic cardiac tumors may all produce indistinguishable clinical manifestations.

Severe, intractable, rapidly progressive cardiac failure, sudden in onset and without apparent cause, is the hallmark of cardiac neoplasm. Equally supicious[381,391,395,396] are (1) pericardial effusions, particularly if hemorrhagic; (2) rapidly changing arrhythmias, persistent tachycardia, or complete heart block with Stokes-Adams syncope, without other clinical explanation; (3) embolic phenomena with symptoms suggestive of bacterial endocarditis; (4) venous thromboses; (5) congestive heart failure, and (6) the effects of valve blockade. Cardiac tumors often mimic valvular disease, particularly of the mitral and tricuspid valves, but both murmurs and symptoms characteristically vary with position;[396a] the development of pulmonic stenosis is suggestive of a cardiac tumor.[397] Angina pectoris due to cardiac tumor has been described, with electrocardiographic abnormalities simulating myocardial infarction. Sudden death may occur with or without preceding symptoms. Tumor may be detected on microscopic examination of an arterial tumor embolus.[398,399]

The variability of findings at repeated cardiac catheterization studies has been emphasized[388] in patients with cardiac tumors; the catheterization data often correlated poorly with the clinical symptoms. Radiographic clues include an unusual, irregular cardiac silhouette, often without abnormal pulsations; and ectopic or peculiar cardiac calcification. It is important to recognize bizarre, incongruous combinations of symptoms, physical findings, and laboratory studies.[395]

As clinical features are determined primarily by the location of the cardiac tumor, the tumor manifestations will be considered in relation to their anatomic characteristics.

Manifestations of Pericardial Tumors

Tumors of the pericardium are less common than those of the heart.[399] Malignant tumors predominate,[399] with sarcomas encountered most frequently; benign pericardial tumors include mesothelioma, teratoma, lipoma, fibroma, neurofibroma, leiomyoma, and hemangioma.

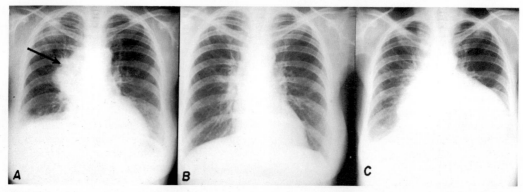

Fig. 55-25. *A.* June 23, 1961: bronchogenic carcinoma with mediastinal extension (arrow). *B.* October 13, 1961: regression of the bronchogenic carcinoma after x-ray therapy. *C.* July 30, 1962: massive pericardial effusion due to pericardial metastases from the bronchogenic carcinoma. (*Courtesy of Department of Radiology, Emory University School of Medicine.*)

The clinical picture is often of acute pericarditis, with precordial pain, a pericardial friction rub, and electrocardiographic ST-T changes of pericarditis. Pericardial effusion (Fig. 55-25), not uncommonly associated with tamponade, may present as cardiac enlargement with decreased cardiac pulsations, pulsus paradoxus, neck vein distension, decreased voltage on the electrocardiogram, and at times a superior vena cava syndrome; the tumor is often initially suspected because of the abnormal cardiac contour on x-ray examination. Constrictive pericarditis due to metastasis is especially common with bronchogenic carcinoma and with carcinoma of the breast.[389]

Hemorrhagic pericardial effusion is the most typical clinical feature, both in benign and malignant pericardial tumors;[178,400] pericardiocentesis provides both symptomatic relief and a diagnosis based on cytologic study of the pericardial fluid. Further aids to diagnosis include pericardial biopsy and the delineation of the tumor mass by angiocardiography and by CO_2 injection into the pericardium.

Pericardial effusion associated with neoplasm tends to reaccumulate rapidly.[401] Radioisotope treatment and chemotherapy may be of little benefit, and pericardial resection is often the treatment of choice.

Manifestations of Myocardial (Mural) Tumors

Myocardial tumors: lipoma, angioma, malignant hemangioendothelioma, rhabdomyoma, sarcoma, mesothelioma, and fibroma may involve the heart wall or heart valves. They occur at all ages and with equal sex incidence. Mural tumors are usually incidental autopsy findings;[400] in the few tumors diagnosed ante mortem, arrhythmia was the observed clinical feature.

Impaired impulse transmission in the conduction system is the most frequent clinical manifestation of myocardial tumor. Atrial fibrillation and flutter, at first transient and later permanent, are often associated with right atrial disease. Tumor invasion of the A-V node or the interventricular septum may produce heart block with Stokes-Adams syncope; this may be the mechanism in otherwise unexplained sudden death. The clinical picture may be of myocardial damage, presenting as cardiac enlargement, congestive heart failure, unexplained tachycardia, and occasionally angina pectoris. There may be associated pericarditis with hemorrhagic effusion.[389]

The numerous electrocardiographic abnormalities include arrhythmias, heart block, bundle branch block, abnormal P waves in cases with atrial disease, nonspecific ST-T variations, and changes mimicking myocardial infarction.

Manifestations of Endocardial (Intracavitary) Tumors

Intracavitary cardiac tumors—myxoma, fibroma, sarcoma—originate almost exclusively in the atria[400] and produce symptoms by acutely or chronically interfering with cardiac filling or ejection. Left atrial tumors produce signs and symptoms of lesser circulation obstruction, whereas right atrial tumors present evidence of inflow stasis. Intracavitary tumors characteristically mimic valvular disease; over 370 reported instances of left atrial tumor or thrombosis have been mistaken for mitral stenosis.[383] Many unsuspected atrial tumors have been found with mitral valve surgical procedures and with the increasing use of angiocardiography.[402]

Acute circulatory failure and acute paroxysmal dyspnea may result from ball-valve blockade of the mitral or tricuspid valve by an atrial tumor. The clinical picture[399,403,404] may be of syncope, epileptiform fits, coma, shock, acute pulmonary edema, cyanosis, gangrene of the nose and toes, or episodes of bizarre behavior.[388,399] Angina pectoris may result from decreased cardiac output, and sudden death is not infrequent, particularly in patients with symptomatic atrial tumors.[402] Murmurs, blood pressure, and symptoms often vary with position.[402] The character of the murmur, as confirmed by phonocardiography, may change on repeated examinations, occasionally being heard as an unusual "whoop";[388] the intensity of the murmur may be disproportionate to the degree of disability.[405] Opening snaps have been recorded in cases of atrial tumor[406] (Fig. 55-26); disparity between the timing of the opening snap and the severity of clinical symptoms is suggestive of an atrial tumor.[388]

Chronic obstruction to the passage of blood through the heart, due to the tumor's maintaining an essentially fixed position in relation to the semilunar valves or pulmonary veins, does not produce the expected positional changes in murmurs and symptoms. Instead, congestive heart failure is seen with exertional dyspnea, paroxysmal nocturnal dyspnea, fatigue, orthopnea, evidence of pulmonary and peripheral embolization, palpitations from atrial fibrillation or other arrhythmias, elevated venous pressure, edema, hepatomegaly, and ascites. Right atrial tumors may mimic constrictive pericarditis, presenting with increased venous pressure, hepatomegaly, pleural effusion, ascites, and edema; they may simulate tricuspid stenosis, producing intractable failure of the right side of the heart by mechanical interference with right ventricular filling; or they may cause superior vena cava obstruction with resultant facial edema, cyanosis, distended neck veins, edema of the upper extremities, and dilated superficial collateral veins.[389,404] Nonspecific systemic manifestations[407] of anemia, low-grade fever, elevated sedimentation rate, weight loss, and clubbing may be encountered with intracavitary tumors.

Kaufmann[408] described marked unilateral shortening of mechanical systole with intraatrial tumors. Semilunar valve closure tended to be premature and A-V valve closure delayed, with resultant decreased mechanical systole of the ventricle on the side of the tumor. With a left atrial tumor, S-1 was fused or paradoxically split, and S-2 was widely split; S-2 was fused and S-1 widely split in cases of right atrial tumor. In addition, Kaufmann noted an exaggerated variation of systolic duration, within a short period of time, both with respiration and with postural changes.

Electrocardiographic clues include unexplained arrhythmias, conduction abnormalities, bundle branch block, and abnormal P waves in the absence of right ventricular hypertrophy, although right

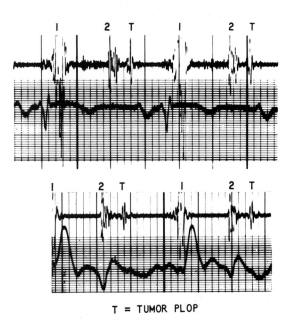

LEFT ATRIAL MYXOMA

T = TUMOR PLOP

Fig. 55-26. "Tumor plop," or opening snap, in a case of left atrial myxoma. (*Courtesy of Dr. B. W. Cobbs, Jr.*)

ventricular hypertrophy is not infrequently present. ST segment changes mimicking myocardial infarction have also been reported.[408a] At cardiac catheterization the atrial pressure is elevated, because of outflow obstruction; the pulmonary capillary pressure may also be increased.[400] An abnormal cardiac silhouette or unusual intracardiac calcification seen on x-ray examination[409] may suggest the presence of an intracavitary tumor (Fig. 55-27), but angiocardiographic demonstration of a filling defect in a cardiac chamber is the definitive method of diagnosis.[400] A venous or right atrial angiocardiogram adequately delineates intracavitary tumors on the right side of the heart; contrast material may be injected into the left atrium via a catheter passed retrograde into the aorta, left ventricle, and through the mitral valve.[410] There are numerous recent reports of successful surgical removal of intracavitary cardiac tumors.[402]

Primary Cardiac Tumors

Benign

Three-fourths of all primary cardiac tumors are benign, and half of these are endocardial in origin. Myxomas and rhabdomyomas account for over one-half of the recorded cases of primary benign cardiac tumors.[393] Fibromas, lipomas, angiomas, papil-

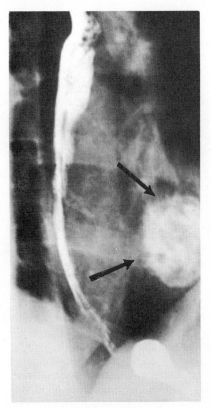

Fig. 55-27. Calcified tumor mass (arrow) in the posterior aspect of the left atrium. At fluoroscopy this mass moved freely in a superior-inferior axis within the cardiac silhouette. The tumor has been known to be present for at least 15 years and is thought to represent a calcified myxoma in a completely asymptomatic patient. (*Courtesy of Department of Radiology, Emory University School of Medicine.*)

lomas, teratomas, leiomyomas, and xanthomas are rare.[393] Primary cardiac tumors in infancy and childhood are almost exclusively benign;[411,412] rhabdomyomas, myxomas, and fibromas are encountered most frequently, with occasional reports of lipomas and teratomas.

Myxoma. Myxomas constitute 35 to 50 per cent[177,393] of all primary cardiac tumors, occurring at all ages and with equal sex incidence.[400] Strouse[413] reported a patient with a 34-year history of intermittent symptoms from an atrial myxoma; death was from an unrelated cause. Over two hundred cases are reported in the literature,[178] and a significant number have been diagnosed ante mortem in recent years.[414] About one hundred reports of successful surgical removal of atrial myxomas appear in the literature.[402]

About 75 per cent of myxomas occur in the left atrium; they are usually solitary and entirely intracavitary, arising on a pedicle from the rim of the

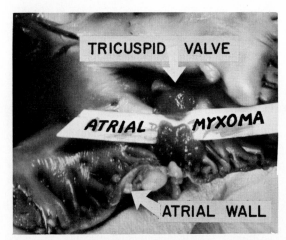

Fig. 55-28. Atrial myxoma. Small, polypoid, gelatinous tumor projecting into the right atrium. (*Courtesy of Department of Pathology, Emory University School of Medicine.*)

interatrial septum near the fossa ovalis. The tumors vary in size from 0.4 to 8.0 cm and are grossly smooth, pale, glistening, and gelatinous,[391] although calcification of myxomas is not infrequent (Fig. 55-28). On microscopic examination the tumor is composed of relatively loose, poorly cellular myxomatous tissue[178] (Fig. 55-29).

The size, situation, and pedunculated nature of the myxoma allows ball-valve blockade of the semilunar valves, simulating mitral (Fig. 55-30) or occasionally tricuspid stenosis.[391] Furthermore, tumor emboli may mimic bacterial endocarditis. Useful features in the differentiation of atrial myxoma from rheumatic mitral stenosis include[393,402] (1) absence of history of rheumatic fever; (2) sudden onset of symptoms; (3) intermittent character of signs and

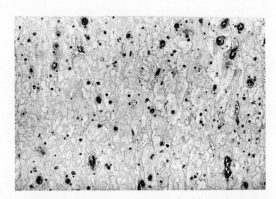

Fig. 55-29. Atrial myxoma composed of loose connective tissue, infiltrated by plasma cells with prominent vascularity and stellate fibroblasts. (× 250.) (*Courtesy of Department of Pathology, Emory University School of Medicine.*)

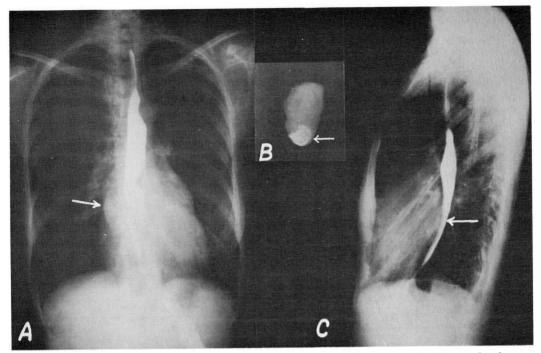

Fig. 55-30. Mitral configuration of the heart due to a calcified left atrial myxoma. *A*. Left atrial enlargement, with visible right border of the left atrium (arrow). *B*. X-ray of surgical specimen, showing calcification of the myxoma (arrow). *C*. Indentation of the esophagus by the enlarged left atrium (arrow). (*Courtesy of Department of Radiology, Emory University School of Medicine.*)

symptoms; (4) lack of correlation between the physical findings, roentgenologic examination, and severity of symptoms; (5) positional variation of murmurs, blood pressure, heart rate, and symptoms; assuming the recumbent position may relieve valve obstruction with dramatic symptomatic improvement; (6) positional syncope; (7) absence of an opening snap or disparity between the timing of the opening snap and the clinical symptoms; and (8) intracardiac calcification not characteristic of mitral valve calcification.

Successful surgical removal was reported [405] of a left atrial myxoma which simulated restenosis of the mitral valve in a patient who had had a mitral commissurotomy 4 years previously. Myxoma of the pulmonary valve has been reported, masquerading as severe pulmonic stenosis in an infant;[415] a myxoma of the right ventricular outflow tract was described which partially obstructed the pulmonary orifice and simulated pulmonic stenosis.[416,416a]

Diagnosis is best made by angiocardiography; surgical excision by the open technique, using inflow stasis and hypothermia or extracorporeal circulation, is advocated.[402]

Fibroma. Fibromas most often arise from the subendothelium of the heart valves, particularly the aortic valve.[177] They are characteristically solitary, small, villous, pedunculated, fibrous masses of acellular, hyaline tissue covered with endothelium.[177,391] Fibromas are usually incidental findings at postmortem examination.[417] However, a fibroma of the interventricular septum was described in an infant, mimicking congenital subaortic stenosis.[418] Electrocardiographic, roentgenologic, and cardiac catheterization data tend to be confusing; the diagnosis is best made by angiocardiography.

Other Benign Primary Cardiac Tumors. *Rhabdomyoma*. See Glycogen Storage Disease, earlier in this chapter.

Angioma. Angiomas occur as clustered, red or white, sessile or polypoid, subendocardial excrescences, usually located on the rim of the foramen ovale and characteristically symptomless. Microscopically, they are endothelial-lined spaces, filled with blood, lymph, and occasional thrombi showing varying organization.[177] The interventricular septum is a comparatively common site of the few symptomatic angiomas, which produce complete heart block, Stokes-Adams syncope, and sudden death.[178,419]

Lipoma. Pritchard[177] suggested that lipomas were possibly variants of myxomas or hamartomas. They are sessile or pedunculated fatty masses,

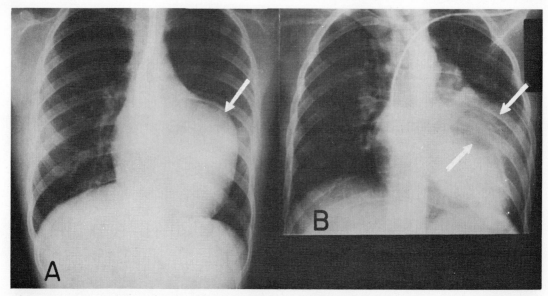

Fig. 55-31. Hamartoma of the myocardium. A. Alteration of the cardiac configuration by a tumor projecting from the border of the left side of the heart (arrow). B. Left-sided opacification following superior vena cava injection of contrast material. A filling defect of the left atrium and left ventricle is produced by encroachment of the tumor mass (arrow). (*Courtesy of Department of Radiology, Emory University School of Medicine.*)

which may be found in any part of the heart.[391] Lipomas have produced valvular insufficiency. Successful surgical removal from the pericardial sac has been described[420] of a 3½-lb lipoma which was attached by a pedicle to the left ventricle.

Hamartoma. Hamartomas are firm, white, unencapsulated nodules, usually in the ventricle (Fig. 55-31), composed of fibrous tissue with varying amounts of fat, elastic tissue, and blood vessels[177] (Fig. 55-32). They are usually silent but occasionally are associated with sudden death.

Teratoma. Teratomas tend to arise near the roots of the great vessels, especially the aorta.[421] They

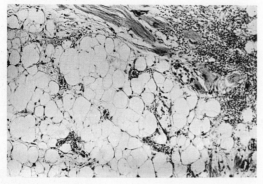

Fig. 55-32. Hamartoma of the heart. There is a haphazard arrangement of fat cells, cardiac muscle cells, and small blood vessels. (× 120.) (*Courtesy of Department of Pathology, Emory University School of Medicine.*)

are usually intrapericardial, producing symptoms of cardiac compression. Beck[422] reported successful surgical removal of an intrapericardial teratoma in 1942. The typical adult type of teratoma contains elements of all three germinal layers.[423]

Leiomyoma. A pericardial leiomyoma has been recorded,[424] causing death by compression of the atrium.

Mesothelioma. A primary mesothelioma of Tawara's node, producing complete heart block, has been described.[425]

Malignant

Primary malignant tumors of the heart are almost exclusively sarcomas;[391] they are extremely rare in infancy and childhood.[411,412,426]

Sarcoma. Sarcomas, the most common primary malignant cardiac tumors, comprise about 21 per cent of all primary tumors of the heart. Pritchard,[177] in 1951, collected 113 cases from the literature; in 1960, Somers and Lothe[427] reviewed 35 cases reported since Whorton's[428] description of 100 cases of primary sarcoma of the heart in 1949. Sarcomas occur at all ages, equally in males and females.[428,429]

There is predominant right-sided occurrence of sarcomas,[430] equally distributed between the atrium and ventricle.[177] Sarcomas originate from the endocardium or pericardium, and very rarely from the myocardium. Endocardial sarcomas tend to be infiltrative or sessile, firm, yellow-gray, mural tumors with intracavitary extension[400] (Fig. 55-33);

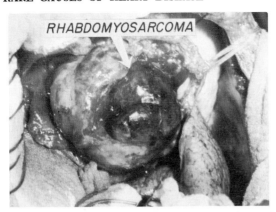

Fig. 55-33. Rhabdomyosarcoma of the left atrium (arrow). There is enlargement of the atrial appendage and distension of the atrium, due to the tumor. (*Courtesy of Dr. Charles R. Hatcher, Jr.*)

they vary in size and appearance. Pericardial sarcomas are diffuse and tend to deform or obliterate the cardiac contour. Many pathologic varieties occur, with preponderance of the round-cell and spindle-cell sarcomas[428] (Fig. 55-34). Over 30 per cent have distant metastases, most commonly to the lung and pleura but also to the mediastinal, tracheobronchial, and retroperitoneal lymph nodes, to the pancreas, to the adrenals, and to the liver and kidneys.[177,400]

The clinical picture[177,391,400,428] is of relentless, unexplained, cardiac failure, with cardiac enlargement, hemopericardium, bizarre cardiac rhythm disturbances, chest pain, and occasionally sudden death. Rapidly progressive superior vena cava or tricuspid valve obstruction is more suggestive of sarcoma, because of its frequency of right atrial localization, than of benign myxoma, which occurs more often on the left.[178,401,429,431] The ball-valve blockade phenomenon is less common with sarcoma than with myxoma. Inferior vena cava obstruction is occasionally seen.[428]

Successful surgical removal was reported[397] of a right ventricular sarcoma which clinically simulated pulmonic stenosis; the development of the murmur of pulmonic stenosis and the appearance of right ventricular hypertrophy on the electrocardiogram, associated with pericardial effusion, syncope, and chest pain, was described[432] in a thirty-two-year-old man who had a primary rhabdomyosarcoma. Temporary symptomatic remission was recorded after surgical removal of a primary sarcoma of the mitral valve; the patient had murmurs of mitral stenosis and mitral insufficiency, recent in onset, associated with hemoptysis and a hemorrhagic pleural effusion.[433] A case of mitral valve fibrosarcoma presented the murmurs of mitral stenosis and mitral insufficiency which gradually increased

in intensity, associated with progressive cardiac enlargement, congestive heart failure, cyanosis, and clubbing.[398]

Sarcomatous invasion and destruction of the conduction system resulted in complete A-V block with Stokes-Adams syncope in two cases.[434]

Sarcomas grow rapidly, producing a rapid change in roentgenographic contour (Fig. 55-35); frequent epicardial involvement produces irregularity of the external surface of the heart, which may be visible by roentgenographic examination or pneumopericardiography.[178,435] Angiocardiography may reveal a filling defect in cases of intracavitary sarcoma.[431]

Mesothelioma. Primary malignant myocardial lymphangioendotheliomas or mesotheliomas selectively involve the conduction system, producing heart block, ventricular fibrillation, Stokes-Adams syncope, and sudden death.[436,437]

About thirty cases of malignant pericardial mesothelioma or coelothelioma appear in the literature.[438] These tumors produce pericarditis, often with hemopericardium and tamponade. They frequently invade the myocardium and tend to metastasize widely.[439,440] Mesotheliomas have few distinctive histologic criteria and are difficult to classify. Pathologic diagnosis depends on exclusion of all other epithelial body structures as a possible source of the tumor.

Teratoma. A malignant teratoma with widespread systemic metastases was described in a two-year-old girl, originating in the interatrial septum and projecting into the right atrial cavity.[441]

Treatment of Malignant Cardiac Tumors. Roentgen therapy and chemotherapy are useful palliative procedures in malignant cardiac tumors.

Secondary (Metastatic) Cardiac Tumors

Metastatic tumor to the heart should be suspected when a patient with malignant disease

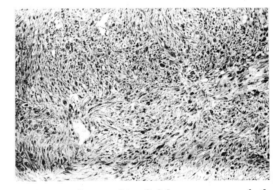

Fig. 55-34. Pleiomorphic rhabdomyosarcoma of the heart. Spindle-cell sarcoma with large pleiomorphic rhabdomyoblasts. ($\times$ 120.) (*Courtesy of Department of Pathology, Emory University School of Medicine.*)

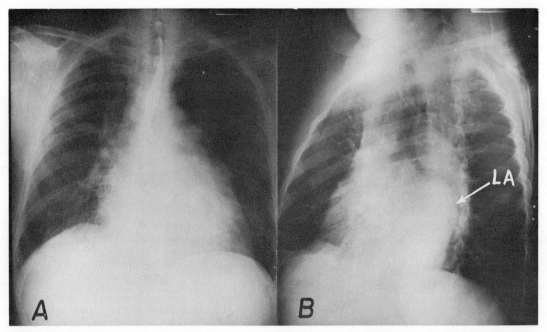

Fig. 55-35. Rhabdomyosarcoma of the left atrium. A. Mitral configuration of the heart with pulmonary congestion. B. Marked left atrial enlargement (arrow) with elevation of the left main bronchus. (*Courtesy of Department of Radiology, Emory University School of Medicine.*)

develops evidence of cardiac dysfunction without apparent cause.[391,442] However, cardiac symptoms occur uncommonly,[442,443] and cardiac metastases are usually not a major factor contributing to death.[444] Bisel et al.[221] reported only an 8.5 per cent incidence of symptoms in patients with cardiac metastases; they found no correlation between the size and extent of cardiac metastases and the clinical manifestations of heart disease. Good correlation was described by Burnett and Shimkin[394] between clinical cardiac findings and the extent of heart metastases found at autopsy; Hanfling[445] stated that symptoms depended more on the location than on the size of the metastases.

Metastatic cardiac tumors occur sixteen[393] to forty[177] times more commonly than primary tumors, with carcinomatous invasion more frequent than sarcomatous.[446] Cardiac metastases are encountered most commonly between the ages of fifty and seventy years, with equal sex incidence.[445,447] Metastatic tumor to the heart has been reported in 0.1 to 6.4 per cent of unselected autopsies and in 1.5 to 20.6 per cent of patients dying of malignancy (see Table 55-2). The increased frequency of diagnosis of secondary cardiac tumors in recent years reflects both a greater interest in the problem and a longer life span of patients with malignancy, due to improved therapy, allowing for increased tumor dissemination.[389,445] Madianos and Sokal,[444] however, found no correlation between disease duration

and cardiac involvement with metastatic disease.

Cardiac metastases are associated with widespread systemic tumor dissemination;[177,221,391] only 18 cases of metastatic tumor limited to the heart or pericardium were reported.[443] Carcinomatous metastases occur most commonly as grossly visible, multiple, discrete, small, white, firm myocardial nodules, microscopically resembling the primary tumor and the metastases in other organs; diffuse infiltration is characteristic of sarcomatous metastases;[177,178,391] necrosis is uncommon.[445]

Cohen et al.[464] described pericardial metastases as occurring more frequently than myocardial; Gassman et al.[443] reported the reverse. There is frequent occurrence of pericardial metastases in cases with primary intrathoracic neoplasm.[445] Willis[392] and others[394,443] stated that all areas of the myocardium were equally prone to neoplastic metastases and were invaded by tumor in proportion to their bulk, with resultant preponderance of left ventricular metastases. Pritchard[177] and others[391,446,456,462,468] reported a greater incidence of right-sided than left-sided heart metastases, presumably because 75 per cent of coronary artery flow returns to the right side of the heart, allowing more embolic tumor cells to lodge there. Herbut and Maisel[460] found equal right and left ventricular metastatic disease. Endocardial or valvular metastatic tumor is most unusual, since these areas are relatively avascular and the spread of metastases

Table 55-2. METASTASES TO THE HEART

Author	Date	No. of autopsies of unselected cases	No. of autopsies of malignancy cases	Cardiac metastases, % unselected cases	Cardiac metastases, % malignancy cases	Total number of cardiac metastases
Pic[448]	1891	......	1,708	....	1.5	25
Bryant[449]	1907	2,492	.....	0.36	.....	9
Karrenstein[450]	1908	6,655	.....	0.29	.....	19
Symmers[451]	1917	5,155	298	0.17	3.1	9
Bardenheuer[452]	1924	......	1,275	....	2.3	30
Morris[453]	1927	3,000	.....	0.17	.....	5
Siegel[454]	1933	592	44	0.5	6.8	3
Burke[455]	1934	......	327	....	4.3	14
Lymburner[456]	1934	8,550	.....	0.61	.....	52
Willis[392]	1934	......	323	....	6.2	20
Helwig[446]	1935	1,000	.....	0.90	.....	9
Pollia[457]	1936	12,000	1,450	0.25	2.0	29
Schnitker[458]	1937	3,570	.....	0.53	.....	19
Scott[442]	1939	11,100	1,082	1.06	10.9	118
Ritchie[459]	1941	3,000	857	1.30	4.5	39
Herbut[460]	1942	4,050	640	0.87	5.5	35
Dimmette[461]	1950	1,815	455	2.11	8.75	38
Pritchard[177]	1951	......	4,375	....	3.4	146
Bisel[221]	1953	......	500	....	21.0	106
De Loach[462]	1953	2,547	980	5.37	13.9	137*
Kahrs[380]	1953	4,915	.....	0.79	.....	39
Burnett[394]	1954	......	288	....	18.4	53
Young[463]	1954	1,400	476†	6.5	19.1	91
Cohen[464]	1955	1,007	315	6.45	20.6	65
Gassman[443]	1955	7,952	4,124	2.73	5.26	217
Goudie[465]	1955	4,687	1,270	2.7	9.9	126
Hanfling[445]	1960	2,652	694	4.8	18.3	127
Lothe[466]	1960	6,644	377	0.39	6.9	26
Clay[467]	1961	1,556	.....	0.83	.....	13
Madianos[444]	1963	......	211 { 170§	....	15.0	25‡
			41¶	....	27.0	11

* Macroscopic malignancies only.
† Tumor deaths less leukemias and brain tumors.
‡ Lymphosarcoma and reticulum cell sarcoma only.
§ Lymphosarcoma.
¶ Reticulum-cell sarcoma.

is primarily hematogenous.[177,394] It is postulated that tumor metastases to the endocardium and heart valves occur by direct implantation,[469] usually on an abnormal or diseased endothelium.[445] Endocardial and valvular metastases may assume a polypoid form, simulating benign myxoma;[470] they may also embolize, mimicking bacterial endocarditis.[445] Metastatic tumors involving the cardiac chambers[445] are probably disseminated via the great veins. Metastases from carcinoma of the kidney and testis reach the right atrium via the inferior vena cava; metastases from bronchogenic carcinoma of the thyroid, and lymphosarcoma invade the right atrium via the superior vena cava; metastases to

the left atrium, via the pulmonary veins, are usually from bronchogenic carcinoma.

Metastatic tumors reach the heart by embolic hematogenous spread, lymphatic spread, or direct invasion, in descending order of frequency.[177,394,445] Gassman et al.[443] described the lymphatic spread of tumors as most common, particularly with carcinoma of the bronchus and the breast; the proximity of the heart to important mediastinal lymphatic channels may explain the high incidence of cardiac metastases when mediastinal structures are involved with tumor.[445] Young and Goldman[463] described primarily pericardial involvement with lymphoma metastases, presumably by direct exten-

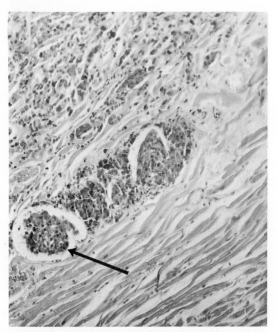

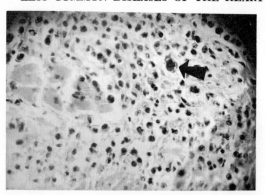

Fig. 55-38. Hodgkin's disease invasion of the myocardium. There is a polymorphic infiltrate composed of plasma cells, eosinophils, and a Reed-Sternberg cell (arrow). (× 250.) (*Courtesy of Department of Pathology, Emory University School of Medicine.*)

Fig. 55-36. Malignant melanoma, metastatic to the heart. There is destruction and replacement of cardiac muscle by neoplastic tissue. A neoplastic deposit is present in a vascular channel (arrow). (× 150.) (*Courtesy of Department of Pathology, Emory University School of Medicine.*)

sion from mediastinal tumors, whereas the finding of Madianos and Sokal[444] of preponderant heart and epicardial involvement in malignant lymphoma suggested hematogenous dissemination. Cardiac metastases have been reported from all types of primary tumors: carcinomas, sarcomas, leukemias, lymphomas, Kaposi's sarcoma,[474] etc. The probability of metastasis[178] to the heart depends both on

the tendency of a specific tumor to metastasize and on the duration of the life of the patient. No particular malignant tumor tends to metastasize to the heart, with the possible exception of malignant melanoma,[178] which involves the myocardium in over 50 per cent of cases[389] (Fig. 55-36). Cardiac metastases occur in one in three cases of bronchogenic carcinoma and of carcinoma of the breast (Fig. 55-37); cardiac infiltration, often microscopic, is seen in one out of two cases of leukemia and one in six cases of lymphoma[221,389] (Fig. 55-38), particularly reticulum-cell sarcoma[444,473] (Fig. 55-39).

The symptomatology[387,399,464] of metastatic cardiac tumors includes progressive intractable cardiac failure; changing cardiac murmurs; pericarditis without apparent cause, especially with a persistent pericardial friction rub; evidence of obstruction to orifices of the great veins; signs of cardiac com-

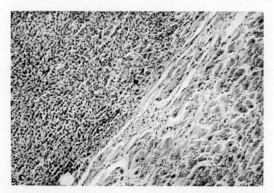

Fig. 55-37. Cystosarcoma phylloides of the breast, metastatic to the heart. The tumor is composed of small spindled sarcoma cells. (× 120.) (*Courtesy of Department of Pathology, Emory University School of Medicine.*)

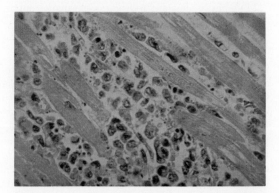

Fig. 55-39. Myocardial invasion by reticulum-cell sarcoma. There is interstitial infiltration of the myocardium by large, atypical reticulum cells. (× 900.) (*Courtesy of Department of Pathology, Emory University School of Medicine.*)

pression; angina pectoris;[476] syncope; and evidence of tumor embolism. Supraventricular arrhythmias, particularly atrial fibrillation or flutter, often resistant to digitalis and quinidine therapy, are seen with tumor involvement of the atria.[477-479] Complete heart block, often with Stokes-Adams syncope, and bundle branch block suggest tumor involvement of the interventricular septum.[480,481] Pericardial effusion,[482] often hemorrhagic, occurs with over one-third of metastatic cardiac tumors.[178] Gassman et al.[443] described pericardial metastases as even more silent than myocardial, usually presenting only as pericardial effusion and infrequently causing constrictive pericarditis.[483,485] Rarely, spontaneous myocardial rupture may result from tumor infiltration.[486,487] Too often, however, symptoms of the primary neoplasm tend to overshadow the cardiac manifestations.

There is no uniformity of electrocardiographic findings in metastatic cardiac tumors,[454] but Bisel et al.[221] described nonspecific electrocardiographic abnormalities in 28.8 per cent of cases, and Young and Goldman[463] in 16 of 23 patients. ST-T alterations occurred most frequently, with atrial arrhythmias, heart block, bundle branch block, abnormal P waves, decreased QRS voltage in cases of pericardial effusion, and changes mimicking myocardial infarction also observed.[476,488] On occasion, electrocardiographic abnormalities may provide a clue to the location of neoplasm in the heart.[489] Roentgenologic demonstration of an altered, bizarre cardiac silhouette or of pericardial effusion aids in the diagnosis of metastatic cardiac tumor,[178] although Bisel et al.[221] reported only a 6 per cent incidence of x-ray abnormalities in patients with cardiac metastases. Angiocardiographic delineation of the lesion confirms the diagnosis. Pericardiocentesis, often required for symptomatic relief,[381,389] provides a cytologic diagnosis by examination of the pericardial fluid[490] (Fig. 55-40); concomitant pneumopericardiography may identify the tumor mass. Examination of embolic material, when available, for tumor cells is advocated.[178]

Therapy of Cardiac Tumors

Surgical excision, if feasible, is the treatment of choice for all benign cardiac tumors; the use of hypothermia and/or extracorporeal circulation is recommended.[388]

Surgical therapy for primary malignant tumors or for metastases to the heart is usually neither possible nor desirable.[178] Palliative radiation with roentgen therapy (Fig. 55-41) or various radioisotope substances, and chemotherapy with compounds such as nitrogen mustards, folic acid antagonists and other antimetabolites, may afford symptomatic relief.[178] Intrapericardial instillation

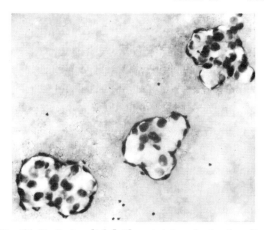

Fig. 55-40. Pericardial fluid containing sheets of malignant cells forming papillary projections. The patient had adenocarcinoma of the breast, metastatic to the heart. (*Courtesy of Dr. Zuher Naib, Department of Pathology, Emory University School of Medicine.*)

of chemotherapeutic and radioisotopic substances produces no predictable results. Disappearance of heart block, presumably due to cardiac metastases, has been reported following x-ray therapy.[227,491] Radiation has also produced regression of pericardial effusion;[445,491] however, pericardiectomy may, at times, be required to prevent cardiac tamponade. Malignant disease of the heart is treated at Grady Memorial Hospital by a combination of high-energy radiation and chemotherapy.[492]

REFERENCES

1. Robin, E. D.: Cardiovascular Disease: Myocardiopathies, *Ann. Rev. Med.,* **12**:55–66, 1961.
2. Bridgen, W.: Uncommon Myocardial Diseases: The Non-coronary Cardiomyopathies, *Lancet,* **2**: 1179–1184, 1957.
3. Bridgen, W.: Uncommon Myocardial Diseases: The Non-coronary Cardiomyopathies (Conclusion), *Lancet,* **2**:1243–1249, 1957.
3a. Primary Myocardial Diseases and the Myocardiopathies, I and II, *Progr. Cardiovascular Diseases,* **7**:1–197, 1964.
4. Virchow, R. V.: Ueber die Natur der constitutionell-syphilitischen Affectionen, *Arch. path. Anat.,* **15**:217–336, 1858.
5. Ricord, P.: [On Syphilis of the Myocardium], *Gaz. des hôp.,* **101**:402, 1845.
6. Reifenstein, E. C.: Acute Gummatous Myocarditis Simulating Acute Myocardial Infarction, *Ann. Int. Med.,* **10**:241–253, 1936/37.
7. Hinrichsen, J.: Cardiovascular Involvement in Congenital Syphilis: A Review of the Literature, *Am. J. Syphilis,* **27**:319–375, 1943.
8. Boss, J. H., Leffkowitz, M., and Freud, M.: Un-

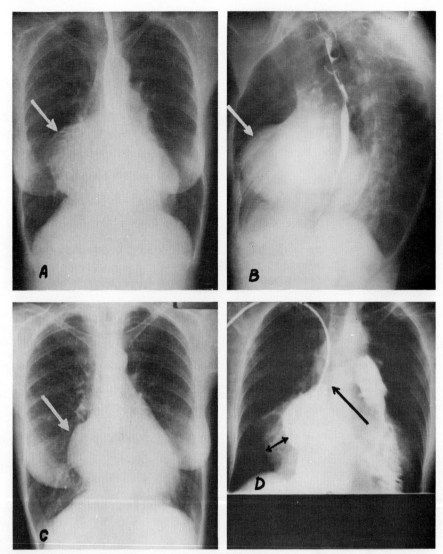

Fig. 55-41. Myocardial metastases from carcinoma of the uterus. *A,B.* November 7, 1960: large tumor mass projecting from the border of the right side of the heart (arrow). *C.* January 3, 1961: Regression of the size of the tumor mass following radiation therapy (arrow). *D.* November 8, 1960: right atrial angiocardiogram showing projection of the tumor mass beyond the opacified right atrium and compression of the right ventricular outflow tract by the tumor mass (arrow). (*Courtesy of Department of Radiology, Emory University School of Medicine.*)

usual Manifestations of Syphilitic Cardiovascular Disease, *Ann. Int. Med.,* **55:**824–831, 1961.

9. Saphir, O.: Syphilitic Myocarditis, *A.M.A. Arch. Path.,* **13:**266–295, 1932.

10. Saphir, O.: Syphilitic Myocarditis (Conclusion), *A.M.A. Arch. Path.,* **13:**436–461, 1932.

11. Clawson, B. J.: Syphilitic Heart Disease, *Urol. & Cutan. Rev.,* **45:**219–225, 1941.

12. Sohval, A. R.: Gumma of the Heart: Report of Two Cases, *A.M.A. Arch. Path.,* **20:**429–444, 1935.

13. Leach, W.: Case Report: Gummatous Myocarditis, *Brit. Heart J.,* **22:**149–152, 1960.

14. Major, R. H.: Stokes-Adams Disease Due to Gumma of the Heart, *A.M.A. Arch. Int. Med.,* **31:** 857–861, 1923.

15. Soscia, J. L., Fusco, J. M., and Grace, W. J.: Complete Heart Block Due to a Solitary Gumma, *Am. J. Cardiol.,* **13:**553–557, 1964.

16. Spain, D. M., and Johannsen, M. W.: Three Cases of Localized Gummatous Myocarditis, *Am. Heart J.,* **24:**689–695, 1942.

17. Rangam, C. M., Bhagwat, R. R., and Bhandari, C. R.: Gumma of the Heart, *J. Indian M. A.,* **35:** 317–318, 1960.

18. Gouley, B. A., Bellet, S., and McMillan, T. M.: Tuberculosis of the Myocardium: Report of Six Cases, with Observations on Involvement of Coronary Arteries, *A.M.A. Arch. Int. Med.*, 51:244–263, 1933.

19. Horn, H., and Saphir, O.: The Involvement of the Myocardium in Tuberculosis: A Review of the Literature and Report of 3 Cases, *Am. Rev. Tuberc.*, 32:492–506, 1935.

20. Auerbach, O., and Guggenheim, A.: Tuberculosis of the Myocardium: A Review of the Literature and a Report of Six New Cases, *Quart. Bull. Sea View Hosp.*, 2:264–283, 1937.

21. Rauchwerger, S. M., and Rogers, R. J.: Tuberculoma of the Myocardium, *Am. Heart J.*, 34:280–283, 1947.

22. Menon, T. B., and Prasada Rao, C. K.: Tuberculosis of the Myocardium Causing Complete Heart Block, *Am. J. Path.*, 21:1193–1197, 1945.

23. Iaroshevskii, A. Ia.: [On Tuberculous Lesions of the Myocardium], *Terapevt. arkh.*, 31:49–52, 1959.

24. Jones, K. P., and Tilden, I. L.: Tuberculous Myocardial Aneurysm, with Rupture and Sudden Death from Tamponade: Review of Literature and Report of Case, *Hawaii M. J.*, 1:295–297, 1942.

25. Bertucci, E. A., Jr.: Leptospirosis, *Am. J. M. Sc.*, 209:86–111, 1945.

26. Klatskin, G.: "Leptospirosis," U.S. Veterans Admin. Tech. Bull. TB10-106, 1955.

26a. Nusynowitz, M. L.: Myocarditis and Heart Failure Due to Leptospira Pomona, *Hawaii Med. J.*, 23:41–44, 1963.

27. Mollaret, P., and Ferroir, J.: A propos de deux observations de spirochétose ictéro-hemorrhagique, dont une avec myocardite mortelle: Contribution á l'étude de la réaction méningée des formes typiques ictérigènes, *Bull. et mém. Soc. méd. hôp. Paris*, 51:1622–1632, 1935.

28. Koppisch, E., and Bond, W. M.: The Morbid Anatomy of Human Leptospirosis, in "Symposium on the Leptospiroses," 11–12 December, 1952, Army Medical Service Graduate School, Walter Reed Army Medical Center, Washington, 1953, pp. 83–115.

29. Aréan, V. M.: Leptospiral Myocarditis, *Lab. Invest.*, 6:462–471, 1957.

30. Edwards, G. A., and Domm, B. M.: Human Leptospirosis, *Medicine*, 39:117–156, 1960.

31. Sodeman, W. A., and Killough, J. H.: The Cardiac Manifestations of Weil's Disease, *Am. J. Trop. Med.*, 31:479–488, 1951.

32. Gore, I., and Saphir, O.: Myocarditis: A Classification of 1402 Cases, *Am. Heart J.*, 34:827–830, 1947.

33. Settle, E. B., Pinkerton, H., and Corbett, A. J.: A Pathologic Study of Tsutsugamushi Disease (Scrub Typhus) with Notes on Clinicopathologic Correlation, *J. Lab. & Clin. Med.*, 30:639–661, 1945.

34. Allen, A. C., and Spitz, S.: A Comparative Study

35. Woodward, T. E., McCrumb, F. R., Jr., Carey, T. N., and Togo, Y.: Viral and Rickettsial Causes of Cardiac Disease, Including the Coxsackie Virus Etiology of Pericarditis and Myocarditis, *Ann. Int. Med.*, 53:1130–1150, 1960.

36. Levine, H. D.: Pathologic Study of Thirty-one Cases of Scrub Typhus Fever with Especial Reference to the Cardiovascular System, *Am. Heart J.*, 31:314–328, 1946.

37. Martin, M., and Bezon, A.: [Curable Acute Primary Carditis Due to *Rickettsia prowazekii*], *Presse méd.*, 68:1253–1254, 1960.

38. Herzog, E., and Rodriguez, H.: Die Beteiligung des Myocards beim Fleckfieber, *Beitr. path. Anat.*, 96:431–442, 1936.

39. Silva, A. G., Hervé, L., and del Solar, A.: Les altérations de l'électrocardiogramme au cours du typhus exanthématique, *Arch. mal. coeur*, 28:265–282, 1935.

40. Huebner, R. J., Jellison, W. L., and Beck, M. D.: Q Fever: A Review of Current Knowledge, *Ann. Int. Med.*, 30:495–509, 1949.

41. Ferguson, I. C., Craik, J. E., and Grist, N. R.: Clinical, Virological and Pathological Findings in a Fatal Case of Q Fever Endocarditis, *J. Clin. Path.*, 15:235–241, 1962.

42. Gadrat, J., Delaude, A., and Cassagneau, J.: [Cardio-rickettsioses: Apropos of Several Cases], *Toulouse méd.*, 62:215–224, 1961.

43. Sorel, R., Dalous, A., Salanova, Martinez, M., and Lazorthes: [Rickettsial Myocarditis (Apropos of a Case)], *Toulouse méd.*, 62:382–383, 1961.

44. Wendt, M. L.: Myokarditis bei Q-fieber, *Ztschr. ges. inn. Med.*, Suppl. 1, 93–115, 1953.

45. Tapie, J., Delaude, A., Cassagneau, J., LeTallec, L., and Fermond: [Rickettsial Myocardiocoronaritis], *Bull. et mém. Soc. méd. Hôp. Paris*, 76:65–72, 1960.

46. Kasper, J. A., and Pinner, M.: Actinomycosis of the Heart: Report of a Case with Actinomycotic Emboli, *A.M.A. Arch. Path.*, 10:687–696, 1930.

47. Letulle, M. M., and Hufnagel, M.: L'actinomycose du coeur, *Bull. Acad. méd.* (Ser. 3), 82:120–147, 1919.

48. Edwards, A. C.: Actinomycosis in Children: A Review of the Literature and Report of Cases, *Am. J. Dis. Child.*, 41:1419–1443, 1931.

49. Coupal, J. F.: Blastomycosis, *Internat. Clin.*, 4:1–14, 1924.

50. Martin, D. S., and Smith, D. T.: Blastomycosis (American Blastomycosis, Gilchrist's Disease). I. A Review of the Literature, *Am. Rev. Tuberc.*, 39:275–304, 1939.

51. Baker, R. D., and Brian, E. W.: Blastomycosis of the Heart: Report of Two Cases, *Am. J. Path.*, 13:139–148, 1937.

52. Brooks, S. E. H., and Young, E. G.: Clinicopatho-

logic Observations on Systemic Moniliasis: A Case Report and Review of the Literature, *Arch. Path.*, 73:383–389, 1962.

53. Braude, A. I., and Rock, J. A.: The Syndrome of Acute Disseminated Moniliasis in Adults, *A.M.A. Arch. Int. Med.*, 104:91–100, 1959.

54. Schaberg, A., Hildes, J. A., and Wilt, J. C.: Disseminated Candidiasis, *A.M.A. Arch. Int. Med.*, 95:112–117, 1955.

55. Grekin, R. H., Cawley, E. P., and Zheuthin, B.: Generalized Aspergillosis: Report of a Case, *A.M.A. Arch. Path.*, 49:387–392, 1950.

56. Cawley, E. P.: Aspergillosis and the Aspergilli: Report of a Unique Case of the Disease, *A.M.A. Arch. Int. Med.*, 80:423–434, 1947.

57. Agress, H., and Gray, S. H.: Histoplasmosis and Reticuloendothelial Hyperplasia, *Am. J. Dis. Child.*, 57:573–589, 1939.

58. Silverman, F. N., Schwarz, J., Lahey, M. E., and Carson, R. P.: Histoplasmosis, *Am. J. Med.*, 19:410–459, 1955.

59. Crawford, S. E., Crook, W. G., Harrison, W. W., and Somervill, B.: Histoplasmosis as a Cause of Acute Myocarditis and Pericarditis: Report of Occurrence in Siblings and a Review of the Literature, *Pediatrics*, 28:92–95, 1961.

60. Humphrey, A. A.: Reticuloendothelial Cytomycosis (Histoplasmosis of Darling), *A.M.A. Arch. Int. Med.*, 65:902–918, 1940.

61. Kuzma, J. F.: Histoplasmosis: The Pathologic and Clinical Findings, *Dis. Chest*, 13:338–344, 1947.

62. Collins, W. T.: Disseminated Ulcerating Sporotrichosis with Widespread Visceral Involvement: Report of a Case, *A.M.A. Arch. Dermat. & Syph.*, 56:523–528, 1947.

63. Forbus, W. D., and Bestebreurtje, A. M.: Coccidioidomycosis: Study of 95 Cases of Disseminated Type with Special Reference to Pathogenesis of Disease, *Mili. Surgeon*, 99:653–719, 1946.

64. Larson, R., and Scherb, R. E.: Coccidioidal Pericarditis, *Circulation*, 7:211–217, 1953.

65. Reingold, I. M.: Myocardial Lesions in Disseminated coccidioidomycosis, *Am. J. Clin. Path.*, 20:1044–1049, 1950.

65a. Jones, I., Nassau, E., and Smith, P.: Cryptococcosis of the Heart, *Brit. Heart J.*, 27:462–464, 1965.

66. Pinto Lima, F. X., Spiritus, O., and Tranchesi, J.: Arrhythmias and Vector Electrocardiographic Analysis of Complete Bundle Branch Block in Chagas' Disease: A Study of 103 Cases, *Am. Heart J.*, 56:501–509, 1958.

66a. Rosenbaum, M. B.: Chagasic Myocardiopathy, *Progr. Cardiovascular Diseases*, 7:199–225, 1965.

66b. Woody, N. C., and Woody, H. B.: I. Clinical and Epidemiologic Background of Chagas' Disease in the United States, *J. Pediat.*, 58:568–580, 1961.

66c. Woody, N. C., De Dianous, N., and Woody, H. B.: II. Current Serologic Studies in Chagas' Disease, *J. Pediat.*, 58:738–745, 1961.

67. Cossio, F.: Some Ideas Concerning Chagas' Myocarditis, *Dia méd.*, 33:1179–1184, 1961.

68. Laranja, F. S., Dias, E., Nobrega, G., and Miranda, A.: Chagas' Disease: A Clinical, Epidemiologic, and Pathologic Study, *Circulation*, 14:1035–1060, 1956.

69. Chagas, C.: Sur les altérations du coeur dans la trypanosomiase américaine (maladie de Chagas), *Arch. mal. coeur*, 21:641–655, 1928.

70. Décourt, L. V., Ramos, J., Jr., Tranchesi, B., Corea, I. A., Dias, J. C., and Tisi, G.: Chronic Heart Involvement in Chagas' Disease, *Am. Heart J.*, 33:697–698, 1947.

71. Lopez, J. E., and Malkett, G. A.: [Chronic Chagasic Myocarditis in Adults: Clinical Description of Pure Cases of Chronic Chagasic Myocarditis without Association with Other Diseases], *Arch. venezolanos de méd. trop.*, 3:107–131, 1960.

72. Rosenbaum, M. B., and Alvarez, A. J.: The Electrocardiogram in Chronic Chagasic Myocarditis, *Am. Heart J.*, 50:492–527,1955.

73. Féhér, J., Pileggi, F., Teixeira, V., Tranchesi, J., Pinto Lima, F. X. P., Spiritus, O., Chansky, M., and Décourt, L. V.: The Vectorcardiogram in Chronic Chagas Myocarditis: An Analysis of the Intraventricular Conduction Delays Associated with a Superiorly Oriented AQRS, *Am. J. Cardiol.*, 5:349–357, 1960.

74. Schabelman, M., Rosenbaum, M. B., and Citrinovitz, A.: [Electrocardiographic Changes of Chagasic Chronic Myocarditis: Studies Carried Out on 100 Cases in the Province of San Juan], *Prensa méd. argent.*, 48:974–979, 1961.

75. Köberle, F.: Die chronische Chagas Kardiopathie, *Arch. path. Anat.*, 330:267–295, 1957.

75a. Mott, K. E., and Hagstrom, J. W. C.: The Pathologic Lesions of the Cardiac Autonomic Nervous System in Chronic Chagas' Myocarditis, *Circulation*, 31:273–286, 1965.

76. Hawking, F., and Greenfield, J. G.: Two Autopsies on Rhodesiense Sleeping Sickness: Visceral Lesions and Significance of Changes in Cerebrospinal Fluid, *Tr. Roy. Soc. Trop. Med. & Hyg.*, 35:155–164, 1941.

77. Lavier, G., and Leroux, R.: Lésions cardiaques dans la maladie du sommeil, *Bul. soc. path. exotique*, 32:927–929, 1939.

78. Manson-Bahr, P. E. C., and Charters, A. D.: Myocarditis in African Trypanosomiasis, *T. Roy. Soc. Trop. Med. & Hyg.*, 57:119–121, 1963.

79. Schyns, C., and Janssen, P.: Recherches électrocardiographiques dans la maladie du sommeil, *Acta cardiol.*, 10:266–278, 1955.

80. Pinkerton, H., and Henderson, R. G.: Adult Toxoplasmosis: A Previously Unrecognized Disease Entity Simulating the Typhus–Spotted Fever Group, *J.A.M.A.*, 116:807–814, 1941.

81. Pinkerton, H., and Weinman, D.: Toxoplasma In-

fection in Man, *A.M.A. Arch. Path.*, **30**:374–392, 1940.

82. Hooper, A. D.: Acquired Toxoplasmosis: Report of a Case with Autopsy Findings, Including a Review of Previously Reported Cases, *A.M.A. Arch. Path.*, 64:1–9, 1957.

83. Hakkila, J., Frick, H. M., and Halonen, P. I.: Pericarditis and Myocarditis Caused by Toxoplasma: Report of a Case and Review of the Literature, *Am. Heart J.*, **55**:758–765, 1958.

84. Callahan, W. P., Jr., Russell, W. O., and Smith, M. G.: Human Toxoplasmosis: A Clinicopathologic Study with Presentation of Five Cases and Review of the Literature, *Medicine,* **25**:343–397, 1946.

85. Korovitskii, L. K., and Litvinenko, A. G.: [On the Problem of Disorders of the Myocardium in Toxoplasmosis], *Klin. med.*, **40**:53–57, 1962.

86. Sexton, R. C., Jr., Eyles, D. E., and Dillman, R. E.: Adult Toxplasmosis, *Am. J. Med.*, **14**:363–377, 1953.

86a. Kass, E. H., Andrus, S. B., Adams, R. D., Turner, F. C., and Feldman, H. A.: Toxoplasmosis in the Human Adult, *Arch. Int. Med.*, **89**:759–782, 1952.

87. Paulley, J. W., Jones, R., Green, W. P. D., and Kane, E. P.: Myocardial Toxoplasmosis, *Brit. Heart J.*, **18**:55–64, 1956.

88. Shee, C. J.: Stokes-Adams Attacks Due to Toxoplasma Myocarditis, *Brit. Heart J.*, **26**:151–153, 1964.

89. Potts, R. E., and Williams, A. A.: Acute Myocardial Toxoplasmosis, *Lancet*, **1**:483–484, 1956.

90. Adams, J. L.: Acute Toxoplasmosis with Involvement of the Heart, *New Zealand M. J.*, **61**:20–24, 1962.

90a. Ström, J.: Toxoplasmosis Due to Laboratory Infection in Two Adults, *Acta med. Scandinav.*, **139**:244–252, 1950–51.

91. Sprague, H. B.: The Effects of Malaria on the Heart, *Am. Heart J.*, **31**:426–430, 1946.

92. Merkel, W. C.: *Plasmodium falciparum* Malaria: The Coronary and Myocardial Lesions Observed at Autopsy in Two Cases of Acute Fulminating *P. falciparum* Infection, *A.M.A. Arch. Path.*, **41**:290–298, 1946.

92a. Rojas, R. A., and Deza, D.: Cardiac Changes in Malarial Patients, *Am. Heart J.*, **33**:702–703, 1947.

92b. Hernberg, C. A.: Myocardial Affection in Malaria Tertiana, *Acta med. scandinav.*, **129**:132–141, 1947–48.

93. Spitz, S.: Pathology of Acute Falciparum Malaria, *Mil. Surgeon,* **99**:555–572, 1946.

94. Herrera, J. M.: [Cardiac Lesions in Vivax Malaria: Study of a Case with Coronary and Myocardial damage], *Arch. Inst. cardiol. México*, **30**:26–36, 1960.

94a. Manohar, K. D., and Khosrawy, K. K.: Anginal Pain in a Case of Malaria, *Indian M. Gaz.*, **73**:151–153, 1938.

95. Dudgeon, L. S., and Clarke, C.: A Contribution to the Microscopical Histology of Malaria, as Occurring in the Salonika Force in 1916, and a Comparison of These Findings with Certain Clinical Phenomena, *Lancet*, **2**:153–156, 1917.

96. Meleney, H. E.: The Histopathology of Kala-azar in the Hamster, Monkey, and Man, *Am. J. Path.*, **1**:147–168, 1925.

96a. Benhamou, E., and Foures, R.: Le coeur dans un cas de kala-azar infantile, *Arch. mal. coeur*, **31**:81–86, 1938.

97. Sidorov, P.: Un cas de balantidiose chez l'homme suivi d'une myocardite granulomateuse, *Ann. anat. path.*, **12**:711–721, 1935.

98. Arai, H. S.: Sarcosporidiosis in 2 Cases with Trichinosis, *J. Mt. Sinai Hosp.* New York, **15**:367–373, 1949.

99. Gilmore, H. R., Jr., Kean, B. H., and Posey, F. M., Jr.: A Case of Sarcosporidiosis with Parasites Found in Heart, *Am. J. Trop. Med.*, **22**:121–125, 1942.

100. Hewitt, J. A.: Sarcosporidiosis in Human Cardiac Muscle, *J. Path. & Bact.*, **36**:133–139, 1933.

101. Segar, L. F., Kashtan, H. A., and Miller, P. B.: Trichinosis with Myocarditis: Report of a Case Treated with ACTH, *New England J. Med.*, **252**:397–398, 1955.

102. Terry, L. L., and Work, J. L.: Trichinosis of the Myocardium, *Am. Heart J.*, **19**:478–485, 1940.

103. Gray, D. F., Morse, B. S., and Phillips, W. F.: Trichinosis with Neurologic and Cardiac Involvement: Review of the Literature and Report of Three Cases, *Ann. Int. Med.*, **57**:230–244, 1962.

104. Spink, W. W.: Cardiovascular Complications of Trichinosis, *A.M.A. Arch. Int. Med.*, **56**:238–249, 1935.

105. Solarz, S. D.: An Electrocardiographic Study of One Hundred Fourteen Consecutive Cases of Trichinosis, *Am. Heart J.*, **34**:230–240, 1947.

106. Cushing, E. H.: Electrocardiographic Changes in Trichinosis, *Am. Heart J.*, **11**:494–496, 1936.

107. Beecher, C. H., and Amidon, E. L.: Electrocardiographic Findings in Forty-four Cases of Trichinosis, *Am. Heart J.*, **16**:219–224, 1938.

108. Roehm, D. C.: Trichinosis: Report of a Case Manifesting Myocarditis, Encephalitis and Radial Neuritis; Response to ACTH; Review of Literature Regarding the Erythrocyte Sedimentation Rate, *Ann. Int. Med.*, **40**:1026–1040, 1954.

108a. Stone, O. J., Stone, C. T., Jr., and Mullins, J. F.: Thiabendazole–Probable Cure for Trichinosis, *J.A.M.A.*, **187**:536–537, 1964.

109. Dévé, F.: Les kystes hydatiques primitifs multiples chez l'homme, *Compt. rend. Soc. biol.*, **80**:859–860, 1917.

110. Heilbrunn, A., Kittle, C. F., and Dunn, M.: Surgical Management of Echinococcal Cysts of the Heart and Pericardium, *Circulation*, **27**:219–228, 1963.

111. Dighiero, J., Canabal, E. J., Aguirre, C. V., Hazan, J., and Horjales, J. O.: Echinococcus Disease of the Heart, *Circulation*, 17:127–132, 1958.

112. Dobrotin, A. N.: Echinococcus of Heart, *Arch. path. Anat.*, 261:575–585, 1926.

113. Attwood, C. J., Sargent, W. H., and Taylor, F.: Echinococcus Cyst of the Heart: Report of a Case, *Ann. Int. Med.*, 15:1109–1115, 1941.

114. Canabal, E. J., Aguirre, C. V., Dighiero, J., Purcallas, J., Baldomir, J. M., and Suzacq, C. V.: Echinococcus Disease of the Left Ventricle: A Clinical, Radiologic and Electrocardiographic Study, *Circulation*, 12:520–529, 1955.

115. Binet, J. P., and Marchese, J. H.: [Cardiac Hydatidosis], *Rev. praticien*, 11:59–62, 1961.

116. Jorge, J. M., and Re, M.: Hidatidosis cardiáca: Vias de infestación, *Arch. internac. hidatidosis*, 6:87, 1946.

117. Peters, J. H., Dexter, L., and Weiss, S.: Clinical and Theoretical Considerations of Involvement of Left Side of the Heart with Echinococcal Cysts: A Review of the Literature with a Report of Five New Cases, Including one observed by the authors, *Am. Heart J.*, 29:143–167, 1945.

118. Di Bello, R., Stanham, J., Rubio, R., and Muxi, F.: Hydatid Cyst of the Left Ventricular Wall with Rupture into the Intrapericardial Space, *J. Thoracic & Cardiovas. Surg.*, 44:268–271, 1962.

119. Houël, J., Raynaud, R., D'Eshougues, J. R., and Morand, P.: 2 New Cases of Cardiac Echinococcosis, *Presse méd.*, 68:2284–2286, 1960.

120. Artucio, H., Roglia, J. L., Di Bello, R., Dubra, J., Gorlero, A., Polera, J., and Urioste, H. A.: Hydatid Cyst of the Interventricular Septum of the Heart with Rupture into the Right Ventricle, *J. Thoracic & Cardiovas. Surg.*, 44:110–114, 1962.

121. Faust, E. C.: An Inquiry into the Ectopic Lesions in Schistosomiasis, *Am. J. Trop. Med.*, 28:175–199, 1948.

122. Africa, C. M., and Santa Cruz, J. Z.: Eggs of *Schistosoma japonicum in the Human Heart*, in "Vol. jubilare pro Sadao Yoshida," Osaka, Japan, 1939, vol. 2, pp. 113–117.

123. Zahawi, S. A., and Shukri, N.: Histopathology of Fatal Myocarditis Due to Ectopic Schistosomiasis, *Tr. Roy. Soc. Trop. Med. & Hyg.*, 50:166–168, 1956.

124. Adelson, L.: Larval Myocardial Ascariasis: Report of a Case, *Ohio M. J.*, 48:723–726, 1952.

124a. Ferreira, A.: Alterações Hepáticas por Ascaris Lumbricoides em um caso de Infestação Maciça dos Intestinos. Localização de Ôva de A. Lumbricoides no Miocárdio, *Rev. Med. Aero.* (*Rio*), 15:35–43, 1963.

125. Africa, C. M., Garcia, E. Y., and de Leon, W.: Intestinal Heterophyidiasis with Cardiac Involvement: A Contribution to the Etiology of Heart Failure, *J. Philippine Islands M. A.*, 15:358–361, 1935 (Abstract).

125a. Africa, C. M., de Leon, W., and Garcia, E. Y.: Visceral Complications in Intestinal Heterophyidiasis of Man, *Acta med. Phillipina*, Monograph series, No. 1, 1940.

126. Fournier, P., Pauchant, M., Voisin, C., and Leduc, M.: Contribution à l'étude anatomo-clinique de l'endocardite pariétale fibroplastique: Ses rapports avec la filariose, *Arch. mal. coeur*, 54:869–876, 1961.

127. Gerbaux, A., Garin, J.-P., and Lenègre, J.: Cardiopathie et filariose, *Bull. et mém. Soc. méd. hôp. Paris*, 73:873–887, 1957.

128. Nagasawa, T.: Histo-pathological Findings of the Human and Canine Hearts in Filariasis, *Tr. Jap. Path. Soc.*, 17:225, 1927.

129. Tatibouet, L., and Eusen, Y.: [Cardiac Insufficiency of Filarial Origin], *Semaine hôp. Paris*, 37:3418–3420, 1961.

130. Giraud, G., Latour, H., Pueck, P., Olivier, G. L., and Hertault, J.: Cardiopathie filarienne: Étude hemodynamique, *Arch. mal. coeur*, 51:546–557, 1958.

130a. Kean, B. H., and Breslau, R. C.: "Parasites of the Human Heart," Grune & Stratton Inc., New York, 1964, pp. 104–106.

131. Kyle, L. H., McKay, D. G., and Sparling, H. J. Jr.: Strongyloidiasis, *Ann. Int. Med.*, 29:1014–1042, 1948.

131a. Franz, K. H.: Clinical Trials with Thiabendazole against Human Strongyloidiasis, *Am. J. Trop. Med. and Hyg.*, 12:211–214, 1963.

132. Khelimskii, A. M.: [Cysticercosis of the Brain, Heart, and Skeletal Muscles], *Med. parazitol. i parazitarnye bolezni*, 31:610–611, 1962.

133. Menon, T. B., and Veliath, G. D.: Tissue Reactions to *Cysticercus cellulosae* in Man, *Tr. Roy. Soc. Trop. Med. & Hyg.*, 33:537–544, 1940.

134. Brill, R., Churg, Jr., and Beaver, P. C.: Allergic granulomatosis with Visceral Larva Migrans: Case Report with Autopsy Findings of Toxocara Infection in a Child, *Am. J. Clin. Path.*, 23:1208–1215, 1953.

134a. Dent, J. H., Nichols, R. L., Beaver, P. C., Carrera, G. M., and Staggers, R. J.: Visceral *Larva Migrans* with a Case Report, *Am. J. Path.*, 32:777–803, 1956.

134b. Friedman, S., and Hervada, A. R.: Severe Myocarditis with Recovery in a Child with Visceral *Larva Migrans*, *J. Pediat.*, 56:91–96, 1960.

135. Blankenhorn, M. A., Vilter, C. F., Scheinker, I. M., and Austin, R. S.: Occidental Beriberi Heart Disease, *J.A.M.A.*, 131:717–726, 1946.

136. Hackel, D. B., Goodale, W. T., and Kleinerman, J:. Effects of Thiamin Deficiency on Myocardial Metabolism in Intact Dogs, *Am. Heart J.*, 46:883–894, 1953.

137. Jones, R. H., Jr.: Beriberi Heart Disease, *Circulation*, 19:275–283, 1959.

138. Epstein, S.: Observations on Beriberi Heart Disease, *Am. Heart J.*, 34:432–440, 1947.

139. Weiss, S.: Occidental Beriberi with Cardiovascular

Manifestations: Its Relation to Thiamin Deficiency, *J.A.M.A.*, **115**:832–839, 1940.

140. Weiss, S., and Wilkins, R. W.: The Nature of the Cardiovascular Disturbances in Nutritional Deficiency States (Beriberi), *Ann. Int. Med.*, **11**:104–148, 1937–1938.

141. Benchimol, A. B., and Schlesinger, P.: Beriberi Heart Disease, *Am. Heart J.*, **46**:245–263, 1953.

142. Keefer, C. S.: The Beriberi Heart, *A.M.A. Arch. Int. Med.*, **45**:1–22, 1930.

143. Alleman, R. J., and Stollerman, G. H.: The Course of Beriberi Heart Disease in American Prisoners-of-war in Japan, *Ann. Int. Med.*, **28**:949–962, 1948.

144. Dustin, C. C., Weyler, H., and Roberts, C. P.: Electrocardiographic Changes in Vitamin B₁ Deficiency, *New England J. Med.*, **220**:15–21, 1939.

145. Burwell, C. S., and Dexter, L.: Beri-beri Heart Disease, *Tr. A. Am. Physicians*, **60**:59–64, 1947.

145a. Wagner, P. I.: Beriberi Heart Disease. Physiologic Data and Difficulties in Diagnosis, *Am. Heart J.*, **69**:200–205, 1965.

146. Robinson, J. J.: Degenerative Heart Disease Resembling Beriberi: Autopsy Findings in 12 Cases from Florida, *South. M. J.*, **53**:1446–1450, 1960.

147. Rowlands, D. T., and Vilter, C. F.: A Study of the Cardiac Stigmata in Prolonged Human Thiamine Deficiency, *Circulation*, **21**:4–12, 1960.

148. Dock, W.: Marked Cardiac Hypertrophy and Mural Thrombosis in Ventricles in Beriberi Heart, *Tr. A. Am. Physicians*, **55**:61–70, 1940.

149. Mainzer, F., and Krause, M.: Electrocardiogram in Pellagra, *Brit. Heart J.*, **2**:85–96, 1940.

150. Porter, W. B., and Higgenbotham, U.: The Heart in Endemic Pellagra, *South. M. J.*, **30**:1–4, 1937.

151. Weiss, S., and Wilkins, R. W.: Disturbance of the Cardiovascular System in Nutritional Deficiency, *J.A.M.A.*, **109**:786–787, 1937.

152. Feil, H.: A Clinical Study of the Electrocardiogram of the Phases of Cardiac Systole in Pellagra, *Am. Heart J.*, **11**:173–184, 1936.

153. Rachmilewitz, M., and Braun, K.: Electrocardiographic Changes and Effect of Niacin Therapy in Pellagra, *Brit. Heart J.*, **7**:72–80, 1945.

154. Erdheim, J.: Ueber das Barlow-Herz, *Wien. klin. Wchnschr.*, **31**:1293–1295, 1918.

155. Follis, R. H., Jr.: Sudden Death in Infants with Scurvy, *J. Pediat.*, **20**:347–351, 1942.

156. Darling, S. T.: The Pathologic Affinities of Beriberi and Scurvy, *J.A.M.A.*, **63**:1290–1294, 1914.

157. Ham, A. W.: Mechanism of Calcification in the Heart and Aorta in Hypervitaminosis D, *A.M.A. Arch. Path.*, **14**:613–626, 1932.

158. Bauer, J. M., and Freyberg, R. H.: Vitamin D Intoxication with Metastatic Calcification, *J.A.M.A.*, **130**:1208–1215, 1946.

159. Colloridi, V.: [Fatal Myocardial Coronary Disease Caused by an Overdosage of Vitamin D₃], *Arch. ital. pediat. e puericoltura*, **20**:386–392, 1960.

160. Gillanders, A. D.: Nutritional Heart Disease, *Brit. Heart J.*, **13**:117–196, 1951.

161. Schyns, C., and Demaeyer, E. M.: Recherches électrocardiographiques dans le kwashiorkor, *Acta cardiol.*, **12**:413–436, 1957.

161a. Swanepoll, A., Smythe, P. M., and Campbell, J. A. H.: The Heart in Kwashiorkor, *Am. Heart J.*, **67**:1–3, 1964.

162. Higginson, J., Gillanders, A. D., and Murray, J. F.: Heart in Chronic Malnutrition, *Brit. Heart J.*, **14**:213–224, 1952.

163. Smythe, P. M., Swanepoel, A., and Campbell, J. A. H.: The Heart in Kwashiorkor, *Brit. M. J.*, **1**:67–73, 1962.

164. Ehlers, K. H., Hagstrom, J. W. C., Lukas, D. S., Redo, S. F., and Engle, M. A.: Glycogen-storage Disease of the Myocardium with Obstruction to Left Ventricular Outflow, *Circulation*, **25**:96–109, 1962.

165. McPhie, J. M.: Cardiac Glycogenosis, *Am. Heart J.*, **60**:836–837, 1960.

165a. Hers, H. G.: α-Glucosidase Deficiency: Generalized Glycogen-storage Disease (Pompe's Disease), *Biochem. J.*, **86**:11–16, 1963.

166. Ehlers, K. H., and Engle, M. A.: Glycogen Storage Disease of the Myocardium, *Am. Heart J.*, **65**:145–147, 1963.

167. Ruttenberg, H. D., Steidl, R. M., Carey, L. S., and Edwards, J. E.: Glycogen-storage Disease of the Heart, *Am. Heart J.*, **67**:469–480, 1964.

168. Gardner, E., and Simpson, K.: Sudden Death from von Gierke's (Glycogen) Disease, *Lancet*, **1**:659–661, 1938.

168a. Huijing, F., van Creveld, S., and Losekoot, G.: Diagnosis of Generalized Glycogen-storage Disease (Pompe's Disease), *J. Pediat.*, **63**:984–987, 1963.

169. Haymond, J. L., and Giordano, A. S.: Glycogen-storage Disease of the Heart, *Am. J. Clin. Path.*, **16**:651–658, 1946.

170. Childs, A. W., Crose, R. F., and Henderson, P. H.: Glycogen Disease of the Heart: Report of Two Cases Occurring in Siblings, *Pediatrics*, **10**:208–217, 1952.

171. di Sant' Agnese, P. A., Anderson, D. H., Mason, H. H., and Bauman, W. A.: Glycogen Storage Disease of the Heart: I. Report of Two Cases in Siblings with Chemical and Pathologic Studies, *Pediatrics*, **6**:402–424, 1950. II. Critical Review of the Literature, *Pediatrics*, **6**:607–624, 1950.

172. di Sant' Agnese, P. A.: Diseases of Glycogen Storage with Special Reference to the Cardiac Type of Generalized Glycogenosis, *Ann. New York Acad. Sc.*, **72**:439–450, 1959.

173. Yamamoto, T., Eguchi, A., Okudaira, M., Suzuki, E., Yokoyama, T., and Tanabe, J.: Glycogen Storage Disease of the Heart: First Case in Japan, *Am. J. Cardiol.*, **5**:556–559, 1960.

174. Kidder, L. A.: Congenital Glycogenic Tumors of the Heart, *A.MA.. Arch. Path.*, **49**:55–62, 1950.

175. Goyer, R. A., and Bowden, D. H.: Endocardial

Fibroelastosis Associated with Glycogen Tumors of the Heart and Tuberose Sclerosis, *Am. Heart J.*, 64:539–542, 1962.

176. von Recklinghausen, F. D.: Ein Herz von einem Neugeborenen, welches mehrere Theils nach aussen, Theils nach dem Höhlen prominirende Tumoren (myomen) Trug, *Monatsschr. Geburtsk. u. Frauenkrankh.*, 20:1–2, 1862.

177. Pritchard, R. W.: Tumors of the Heart, *A.M.A. Arch. Path.*, 51:98–128, 1951.

178. Landing, B. H., and Farber, S.: Tumors of the Cardiovascular System, National Research Council, Committee on Pathology, "Atlas of Tumor Pathology," sec. 3, fasc. 7, Washington, 1956.

179. Sussman, W., and Stasney, J.: Congenital Glycogenic Tumors of the Heart, *Am. Heart J.*, 40:312–315, 1950.

180. Batchelor, T. M., and Maun, M. E.: Congenital Glycogenic Tumors of the Heart, *A.MA.. Arch. Path.*, 39:67–73, 1945.

180a. Ratinov, G., Baker, W. P., and Swaiman, K. F.: McArdle's Syndrome with Previously Unreported Electrocardiographic and Serum Enzyme Abnormalities, *Ann. Int. Med.*, 62:328–335, 1965.

181. Finch, S. C., and Finch, C. A.: Idiopathic Hemochromatosis: An Iron Storage Disease. A. Iron Metabolism in Hemochromatosis, *Medicine*, 34:381–430, 1955.

182. Wasserman, A. J., Richardson, D. W., Baird, C. L., and Wyso, E. M.: Cardiac Hemochromatosis Simulating Constrictive Pericarditis, *Am. J. Med.*, 32:316–323, 1962.

183. Levin, E. B., and Golum, A.: The Heart in Hemochromatosis, *Am. Heart J.*, 45:277–288, 1953.

184. Bothwell, T. H., van Lingen, B., Alper, T., and duPreez, M. L.: The Cardiac Complications of Hemochromatosis, *Am. Heart J.*, 43:333–340, 1952.

185. Faivre, M. G., Gilgenkrantz, J. M., Cherrier, F., Tenette, C., and Gaucher, P.: [Hemochromatosis and Adiastole: Apropos of an Anatomical Case], *Arch. mal. coeur*, 54:935–945, 1961.

185a. James, T. N.: Pathology of the Cardiac Conduction System in Hemochromatosis, *New England J. Med.*, 271:92–94, 1964.

186. Lewis, H. P.: Cardiac Involvement in Hemochromatosis, *Am. J. M. Sc.*, 227:544–558, 1954.

187. Grosberg, S. J.: Hemochromatosis and Heart Failure: Presentation of a Case with Survival after Three Years' Treatment by Repeated Venesection, *Ann. Int. Med.*, 54:550–559, 1961.

188. Goldman, A. M., and Kaplan, M. H.: Acute Porphyria, *Ann. Int. Med.*, 34:415–427, 1951.

189. Saint, E. G., Curnow, D., Paton, R., and Stokes, J. B.: Diagnosis of Acute Porphyria, *Brit. M. J.*, 1:1182–1184, 1954.

190. Eliaser, M., Jr., and Kondo, B. O.: Electrocardiographic Changes Associated with Acute Porphyria, *Am. Heart J.*, 24:696–702, 1942.

191. Eilenberg, M. D., and Scobie, B. A.: Prolonged Neuropsychiatric Disability and Cardiomyopathy in Acute Intermittent Porphyria, *Brit. M. J.*, 1:858–859, 1960.

192. Crouch, R. B., and Herrmann, G. R.: The Electrocardiogram of Acute Porphyria, *Am. Heart J.*, 49:693–695, 1955.

193. Emanuel, R. W.: Gargoylism with Cardiovascular Involvement in Two Brothers, *Brit. Heart J.*, 16:417–422, 1954.

194. Vanace, P. W., Friedman, S., and Wagner, B. M.: Mitral Stenosis in an Atypical Case of Gargoylism: A Case Report with Pathologic and Histochemical studies of Cardiac Tissues, *Circulation*, 21:80–89, 1960.

195. Lindsay, S.: Cardiovascular System in Gargoylism, *Brit. Heart J.*, 12:17–32, 1950.

196. Strauss, L., and Platt, R.: Endocardial Sclerosis in Infancy Associated with Abnormal Storage (Gargoylism): Report of a Case in an Infant Aged Five Months and Review of the Literature, *J. Mt. Sinai Hosp. New York*, 24:1258–1271, 1957.

197. Lyle, W. H., Leonard, B. J., Bowden, W. E., and Miller, D. G.: Normocholesterolemic Xanthomatosis: Report of Case with Myocardial Fibrosis and Myelosclerosis, *Ann. Int. Med.*, 53:1260–1270, 1960.

198. Pund, E. E., Jr., Hawley, R. L., McGee, H. J., and Blount, S. G., Jr.: Gouty Heart, *New England J. Med.*, 263:835–838, 1960.

199. Prinzmetal, M., and Kennamer, R.: Emergency Treatment of Cardiac Arrhythmias, *J.A.MA..*, 154:1049–1054, 1954.

200. Paulley, J. W., Barlow, K. E., Cutting, P. E. J., and Stevens, J.: Acute Gouty Pericarditis, *Lancet*, 1:21–22, 1963.

201. Edwards, D. L.: Idiopathic Familial Oxalosis, *A.M.A. Arch. Path.*, 64:546–555, 1957.

202. Slama, R., Josso, F., and Antoine, B.: [Myocardial Manifestations of Oxalosis], *Arch. mal. coeur*, 53:917–929, 1960.

203. Stauffer, M.: Oxalosis: Report of a Case, with a Review of the Literature and Discussion of the Pathogenesis, *New England J. Med.*, 263:386–390, 1960.

204. Lichtenstein, L., and Kaplan, L.: Hereditary Ochronosis: Pathologic Changes Observed in Two Necropsied Cases, *Am. J. Path.*, 30:99–125, 1954.

205. Brown, C. E., and Evans, W. D.: Primary, Massive Calcification of the Myocardium, *Am. Heart J.*, 19:106–113, 1940.

206. Diamond, M.: Calcification of the Myocardium in a Premature Infant, *A.M.A. Arch. Path.*, 14:137–145, 1932.

207. Somers, K., and Williams, A. W.: Intracardiac Calcification in Endomyocardial Fibrosis, *Brit. Heart J.*, 24:324–328, 1962.

208. Nezelof, C., and Lancret, P.: [Lesions of Myocardial Fibrosis during Fibrocystic Disease of the Pancreas], *Arch. franç. pediat.*, 16:1035–1046, 1959.

209. McGiven, A. R.: Myocardial Fibrosis in Fibro-

cystic Disease of the Pancreas, *Arch. Dis. Child-hood*, **37**:656–660, 1962.

210. Powell, L. W., Jr., Newman, S., and Hooker, J. W.: Cystic Fibrosis of the Pancreas Complicated by Myocardial Fibrosis, *Virginia M. Month.* **84**:178–181, 1957.

211. Perkins, J. G., Petersen, A. B., and Riley, J. A.: Renal and Cardiac Lesions in Potassium Deficiency Due to Chronic Diarrhea, *Am. J. Med.*, **8**:115–123, 1950.

212. Blomberg, L. H., and Lindqvist, T.: Electrocardiogram in Paroxysmal Essential Hypopotassemia (Periodic Paralysis): Report of 2 Cases, *Acta med. scandinav.*, **147**:437–446, 1954.

213. McAllen, P. M.: Myocardial Changes Occurring in Potassium Deficiency, *Brit. Heart J.*, **17**:5–14, 1955.

214. Weaver, W. F., and Burchell, H. B.: Serum Potassium and the Electrocardiogram in Hypokalemia, *Circulation*, **21**:505–521, 1960.

215. Follis, R. H., Jr., Orent-Keiles, E., and McCollum, E. V.: The Production of Cardiac and Renal Lesions in Rats by a Diet Extremely Deficient in Potassium, *Am. J. Path.*, **18**:29–39, 1942.

216. Keye, J. D., Jr.: Death in Potassium Deficiency: Report of a Case Including Morphologic Findings, *Circulation*, **5**:766–770, 1952.

217. Rodriguez, C. E., Wolfe, A. L., and Bergstrom, V. W.: Hypokalemic Myocarditis, *Am. J. Clin. Path.*, **20**:1050–1055, 1950.

218. Gouley, B. A.: The Myocardial Degeneration Associated with Uremia in Advanced Hypertensive Disease and Chronic Glomerular Nephritis, *Am. J. M. Sc.*, **200**:39–49, 1940.

219. Langendorf, R., and Pirani, C. L.: The Heart in Uremia: An Electrocardiographic and Pathologic Study, *Am. Heart J.*, **33**:282–307, 1947.

220. Bregani, P., and Perrotta, P.: The Heart in Leukemia: Clinical and Electrocardiographic Aspects, *Folia cardiol.*, **19**:193–207, 1960.

221. Bisel, H. F., Wróblewski, F., and La Due, J. S.: Incidence and Clinical Manifestations of Cardiac Metastases, *J.A.M.A.*, **153**:712–715, 1953.

222. Bierman, H. R., Perkins, E. K., and Ortega, P.: Pericarditis in Patients with Leukemia, *Am. Heart J.*, **43**:413–422, 1952.

223. Aronson, S. F., and Leroy, E.: Electrocardiographic Findings in Leukemia, *Blood*, **2**:356–362, 1947.

224. Popescu, J., Enescu, V., and Grozea, P.: [Leukemic Heart Changes], *Helvet. med. acta*, **26**:860–875, 1959.

225. Kirchbaum, J. D., and Preuss, F. S.: Leukemia: A Clinical and Pathologic Study of One Hundred and Twenty-three Fatal Cases in a Series of 14,400 Necropsies, *A.M.A. Arch. Int. Med.*, **71**:777–792, 1943.

226. Shekhtman, M. M.: [Cardiac Lesions in Leukemia], *Probl. gematol. i Pereliv. krovi*, **6**:47–51, 1961.

227. Blotner, H., and Sosman, M. C.: X-ray Therapy of the Heart in a Patient with Leukemia, Heart Block and Hypertension: Report of a Case, *New England J. Med.*, **230**:793–796, 1944.

228. Correa-Suárez, R., Cardenas Loaeza, M. E., Bravo, J. L., and Baez Villaseñor, J.: Manifestaciones electrocardiográficas en las leucemias, *Arch. Inst. cardiol. México*, **26**:193–210, 1956.

229. Wintrobe, M. M., and Mitchell, D. M.: Atypical Manifestations of Leukaemia, *Quart. J. Med.*, **9**:67–90, 1940.

230. Winsor, T., and Burch, G. E.: The Electrocardiogram and Cardiac State in Active Sickle-cell Anemia, *Am. Heart J.*, **29**:685–696, 1945.

231. Oliveira, E., and Gómez-Patiño, N.: Falcemic Cardiopathy: Report of a Case, *Am. J. Cardiol.*, **11**:686–688, 1963.

232. Jones, H. L., Jr., Wetzel, F. E., and Black, B. K.: Sickle-cell Anemia with Striking Electrocardiographic Abnormalities and Other Unusual Features, with Autopsy, *Ann. Int. Med.*, **29**:928–935, 1948.

233. Klinefelter, H. F.: The Heart in Sickle Cell Anemia, *Am. J. M. Sc.*, **203**:34–51, 1942.

233a. Uzsoy, N. K.: Cardiovascular Findings in Patients with Sickle-cell Anemia, *Am. J. Cardiol.*, **13**:320–328, 1964.

234. Oppenheimer, B. S.: Vascular Occlusion in Polycythemia Vera, *Tr. A. Am. Physicians*, **44**:338–344, 1929.

235. Boyd, W.: Polycythemia, Duodenal Ulcer and Coronary Thrombosis, *Tr. A. Am. Physicians*, **48**:209–211, 1933.

235a. Miller, H. R.: The Occurrence of Coronary Artery Thrombosis: Polycythemia Vera, *Am. J. M. Sc.*, **198**:323–329, 1939.

236. Tinney, W. S., Hall, B. E., and Giffin, H. Z.: Cardiac Disease and Hypertension in Polycythemia Vera, *Proc. Staff Meet. Mayo Clin.*, **18**:94–96, 1943.

237. Bernstein, A., Simon, F., Rothfeld, E. L., and Cohen, F. B.: Primary Thrombocytosis and Anginal Syndrome, *Am. J. Cardiol.*, **6**:351–354, 1960.

238. Spach, M. S., Howell, D. A., and Harris, J. S.: Myocardial Infarction and Multiple Thromboses in a Child with Primary Thrombocytosis, *Pediatrics*, **31**:268–276, 1963.

239. Berenbaum, A. A., and Horowitz, W.: Heart Involvement in Progressive Muscular Dystrophy: Report of a Case with Sudden Death, *Am. Heart J.*, **51**:622–627, 1956.

240. Cannon, P. J.: The Heart and Lungs in Myotonic Muscular Dystrophy, *Am. J. Med.*, **32**:765–775, 1962.

241. Zatuchni, J., Aegerter, E. E., Molthan, L., and Shuman, C. R.: Heart in Progressive Muscular Dystrophy, *Circulation*, **3**:846–853, 1951.

242. Weisenfeld, S., and Messinger, W. J.: Cardiac Involvement in Progressive Muscular Dystrophy, *Am. Heart J.*, **43**:170–187, 1952.

243. Feruglio, G. A., and Sala, I.: Electrocardiographic Changes in Friedreich's Disease: Presentation of 2 Cases and Review of the Literature, *Minerva med.*, 53:106–109, 1962.

244. Welsh, J. D., Lynn, T. N., Jr., and Haase, G. R.: Cardiac Findings in 73 Patients with Muscular Dystrophy, *Arch. Int. Med.*, 112:199–206, 1963.

245. Wahi, P. L.: Cardiac Changes in Myopathy, *Am. Heart J.*, 66:748–754, 1963.

246. Lowenstein, A. S., Arbeit, S. R., and Rubin, I. L.: Cardiac Involvement in Progressive Muscular Dystrophy, *Am. J. Cardiol.*, 9:528–533, 1962.

247. Levin, S., Baens, G. S., and Weinberg, T.: The Heart in Pseudohypertrophic Muscular Dystrophy, *J. Pediat.*, 55:460–472, 1959.

248. Gilroy, J., Cahalan, J. L., Berman, R., and Newman, M.: Cardiac and Pulmonary Complications in Duchenne's Progressive Muscular Dystrophy, *Circulation*, 27:484–493, 1963.

248a. Hooey, M. A., and Jerry, L. M.: The Cardiomyopathy of Muscular Dystrophy: Report of Two Cases with a Review of the Literature, *Canad. M. A. J.*, 90:771–774, 1964.

249. Rubin, I. L., and Buchberg, A. S.: The Heart in Progressive Muscular Dystrophy, *Am. Heart J.*, 43:161–169, 1952.

250. Gailani, S., Danowski, T. S., and Fisher, D. S.: Muscular Dystrophy; Catheterization Studies Indicating Latent Congestive Heart Failure, *Circulation*, 17:583–588, 1958.

251. Nothacker, W. G., and Netsky, M. G.: Myocardial Lesions in Progressive Muscular Dystrophy, *A.M.A. Arch. Path.*, 50:578–590, 1950.

252. Moore, W. F., Jr.: Cardiac Involvement in Progressive Muscular Dystrophy, *J. Pediat.*, 44:683–687, 1954.

253. Storstein, O., and Austarheim, K.: Progressive Muscular Dystrophy of the Heart, *Acta med. scandinav.*, 150:431–436, 1954–1955.

254. James, T. N.: Observations on the Cardiovascular Involvement, Including the Cardiac Conduction System, in Progressive Muscular Dystrophy, *Am. Heart J.* 63:48–56, 1962.

255. Wendt, V. E., Stock, T. B., Hayden, R. O., Bruce, T. A., Gudbjarnason, S. L., and Bing, R. J.: The Hemodynamics and Cardiac Metabolism in Cardiomyopathies, *M. Clin. North America*, 46:1445–1469, 1962.

256. Friedreich, N.: Ueber degenerative Atrophie der spinalen hinter Stränge, *Arch. path. Anat.*, 26:391–419, 1863.

257. Russell, D. S.: Myocarditis in Friedreich's Ataxia, *J. Path. & Bact.*, 58:739–748, 1946.

258. Gale, H. H.: Friedreich's Ataxia and Its Cardiac Manifestations, *Henry Ford Hosp. M. Bull.*, 7:182–187, 1959.

259. Boyer, S. H., IV, Chisholm, A. W., and McKusick, V. A.: Cardiac Aspects of Friedreich's Ataxia, *Circulation*, 25:493–505, 1962.

260. Manning, G. W.: Cardiac Manifestations in Friedreich's Ataxia, *Am. Heart J.*, 39:799–816, 1950.

261. Schilero, A. J., Antzis, E., and Dunn, J.: Friedreich's Ataxia and Its Cardiac Manifestations, *Am. Heart J.*, 44:805–822, 1952.

262. Nadas, A. S., Alimurung, M. M., and Sieracki, L. A.: Cardiac Manifestations of Friedreich's Ataxia, *New England J. Med.*, 244:239–244, 1951.

263. Lorenz, T. H., Kurtz, C. M., and Shapiro, H. H.: Cardiopathy in Friedreich's Ataxia (Spinal Form of Hereditary Sclerosis): Review of the Literature and Analysis of Cases of Five Siblings, *A.M.A. Arch. Int. Med.*, 86:412–426, 1950.

264. Hartman, J. M., and Booth, R. W.: Friedreich's Ataxia: A Neurocardiac Disease, *Am. Heart J.*, 60:716–720, 1960.

265. Evans, W., and Wright, G.: Electrocardiogram in Friedrich Disease, *Brit. Heart J.*, 4:91–102, 1942.

265a. Ivemark, B., and Thorén, C.: The Pathology of the Heart in Friedreich's Ataxia. Changes in Coronary Arteries and Myocardium, *Acta med. scandinav.*, 175:227–237, 1964.

266. James, T. N., and Fisch, C.: Observations on the Cardiovascular Involvement in Friedreich's Ataxia, *Am. Heart J.*, 66:164–175, 1963.

267. Fisch, C.: The Heart in Dystrophic Myotonica, *Am. Heart J.*, 41:525–538, 1951.

268. Evans, W.: Heart in Myotonia Atrophica, *Brit. Heart J.*, 6:41–47, 1944.

269. Litchfield, J. A.: A-V Dissociation in Dystrophia Myotonica, *Brit. Heart J.*, 15:357–359, 1953.

270. Holt, J. M., and Lambert, E. H. N.: Heart Disease as the Presenting Feature in Myotonia Atrophica, *Brit. Heart J.*, 26:433–436, 1964.

271. Spillane, J. D.: Heart in Myotonia Atrophica, *Brit. Heart J.*, 13:343–347, 1951.

272. Miller, P. B.: Myotonic Dystrophy with Electrocardiographic Abnormalities: Report of a Case, *Am. Heart J.*, 63:704–707, 1962.

273. Payne, C. A., and Greenfield, J. C., Jr.: Electrocardiographic Abnormalities Associated with Myotonic Dystrophy, *Am. Heart J.*, 65:436–440, 1963.

274. Fearrington, E. L., Gibson, T. C., and Churchill, R. E.: Vectorcardiographic and Electrocardiographic Findings in Myotonia Atrophica: A Study Employing the Frank Lead System, *Am. Heart J.*, 67:599–609, 1964.

275. Fisch, C., and Evans, P. V.: The Heart in Dystrophic Myotonica: Report of an Autopsied Case, *New England J. Med.*, 251:527–529, 1954.

276. Kilpatrick, J. A., and Caughey, J. E.: Changes in Heart in Dystrophic Myotonica, *Australasian Ann. Med.*, 4:200–207, 1955.

277. Mendelow, H., and Genkins, G.: Studies in Myasthenia Gravis: Cardiac and Associated Pathology, *J. Mt. Sinai Hosp. New York*, 21:218–225, 1954–1955.

277a. McCrea, P. C., and Jagoe, W. S.: Myocarditis in Myasthenia Gravis with Thymoma, *Irish J. Med. Sci.*, 454:453–457, 1963.

278. Rottino, A., Poppiti, R., and Rao, J.: Myocardial Lesions in Myasthenia Gravis, *A.M.A. Arch. Path.*, 34:557–561, 1942.

279. Russel, D. S.: Histological Changes in the Striped Muscles in Myasthenia Gravis, *J. Path. & Bact.*, **65**:279–289, 1953.

280. Taquini, A. C., Cooke, W. T., and Schwab, R. S.: Observations on the Cardiovascular System in Myasthenia Gravis, *Am. Heart J.*, **20**:611–619, 1940.

281. Dack, S., and Moloshok, R. E.: Cardiac Manifestations of Toxic Action of Emetine Hydrochloride in Amebic Dysentery, *A.M.A. Arch. Int. Med.*, **79**:228–238, 1947.

282. Klatskin, G., and Friedman, H.: Emetine Toxicity in Man: Studies on the Nature of Early Toxic Manifestations, Their Relation to the Dose Level, and Their Significance in Determining Safe Dosage, *Ann. Int. Med.*, **28**:892–915, 1948.

283. de Cossío, A. G.: Electrocardiographic Changes under Emetine Therapy, *Am. Heart J.*, **43**:456–467, 1952.

284. Turner, P. P.: The Effects of Emetine on the Myocardium, *Brit. Heart J.*, **25**:81–88, 1963.

284a. Hardgroove, M., and Smith, E. R.: Effects of Emetine on the Electrocardiogram, *Am. Heart J.*, **28**:752–757, 1944.

285. Kattwinkel, E. E.: Death Due to Cardiac Disease Following the Use of Emetine Hydrochloride in Conditioned-reflex Treatment of Chronic Alcoholism, *New England J. Med.*, **240**:995–997, 1949.

286. Brem, T. H., and Konwaler, B. E.: Fatal Myocarditis Due to Emetine Hydrochloride, *Am. Heart J.*, **50**:476–481, 1955.

287. Sîkl, H.: Eosinophile Myokarditis als idiosynkasisch-allergische Erkrankung, *Frankfurt. Ztschr. Path.*, **49**:283–321, 1936.

288. Brown, C. E., and McNamara, D. H.: Acute Interstitial Myocarditis Following Administration of Arsphenamines, *Arch. Dermat. & Syph.*, **42**:312–321, 1940.

289. Nelson, R. L.: Acute Diffuse Myocarditis Following Exfoliative Dermatitis, *Am. Heart J.*, **9**:813–816, 1933–1934.

290. Robbins, R. L.: Heart Disease in Chronic Arsenic Poisoning: Clinical Report of 2 Cases, *J. Louisiana M. Soc.*, **105**:301–304, 1953.

291. Barry, K. G., and Herndon, E. G., Jr.: Electrocardiographic Changes Associated with Acute Arsenic Poisoning, *M. Ann. District of Columbia*, **31**:25–27, 1962.

292. Edge, J. R.: Myocardial Fibrosis Following Arsenical Therapy: Report of a Case, *Lancet*, **2**:675–677, 1946.

293. Gousios, A. G., and Adelson, L.: Electrocardiographic and Radiographic Findings in Acute Arsenic Poisoning, *Am. J. Med.*, **27**:659–663, 1959.

294. Weinberg, S. L.: The Electrocardiogram in Acute Arsenic Poisoning, *Am. Heart J.*, **60**:971–975, 1960.

295. Josephson, C. J., Pinto, S. S., and Petronella, S. J.: Arsine: Electrocardiographic Changes Produced in Acute Human Poisoning, *Arch. Indust. Hyg.*, **4**:43–52, 1951.

296. McKinstry, W. J., and Hickes, J. M.: Emergency—Arsine Poisoning, *A.M.A. Arch. Int. Med.*, **100**:34–43, 1957.

297. Ch'ien Teh and Liu Yu-K'un: 'Clinical Analysis of One Hundred and Seventy-two Fatal Cases Observed During Antimony Treatment, *Chinese J. Int. Med.*, **5**:524–530, 1957.

298. Honey, M.: The Effects of Sodium Antimony Tartrate on the Myocardium, *Brit. Heart J.*, **22**:601–616, 1960.

299. Somers, K., and Rosanelli, J. D.: Electrocardiographic Effects of Antimony Dimercaptosuccinate ("Astiban"), *Brit. Heart J.*, **24**:187–191, 1962.

300. Tarr, L.: Effect of the Antimony Compounds, Fuadin and Tartar Emetic, on the Electrocardiogram of Man: A Study of the Changes Encountered in 141 Patients Treated for Schistosomiasis, *Ann. Int. Med.*, **27**:970–988, 1947.

301. Evans, W.: Alcoholic Cardiomyopathy, *Am. Heart J.*, **61**:556–567, 1961.

302. Bridgen, W.: Uncommon Myocardial Diseases: The Non-coronary Cardiomyopathies, *Lancet*, **2**:1243–1249, 1957.

302a. Brigden, W., and Robinson, J.: Alcoholic Heart Disease, *Brit. Med. J.*, **2**:1283–1289, 1964.

303. Evans, W.: The Electrocardiogram of Alcoholic Cardiomyopathy, *Brit. Heart J.*, **21**:445–456, 1959.

304. Eliaser, M., Jr., and Giansiracusa, F. T.: The Heart and Alcohol, *California Med.*, **84**:234–236, 1956.

305. Ganz, V.: The Acute Effect of Alcohol on the Circulation and on the Oxygen Metabolism of the Heart, *Am. Heart J.*, **66**:494–497, 1963.

306. Regan, T. J., Moschos, C. B., and Hellems, H. K.: Ethanol-induced Alteration of Myocardial Metabolism and Function, *Circulation*, **28**:788–789, 1963.

306a. Ferrans, V. J., Hibbs, R. G., Weilbaecher, D. G., Black, W. C., Walsh, J. J., and Burch, G. E.: Alcoholic Cardiomyopathy. A Histochemical Study, *Am. Heart J.*, **69**:748–765, 1965.

306b. Hibbs, R. G., Ferrans, V. J., Black, W. C., Weilbaecher, D. G., Walsh, J. J., and Burch, G. E.: Alcoholic Cardiomyopathy, An Electron Microscopic Study, *Am. Heart J.*, **69**:766–779, 1965.

306c. Wendt, V. E., Wu, C., Balcon, R., Doty, G., and Bing, R. J.: Hemodynamic and Metabolic Effects of Chronic Alcoholism in Man, *Am. J. Cardiol.*, **15**:175–184, 1965.

307. Szakács, J. E., and Cannon, A.: 1-Norepinephrine Myocarditis, *Am. J. Clin. Path.*, **30**:425–434, 1958.

308. Mond, E., and Mack, I.: Cardiac Toxicity of Iproniazid (Marsalid): Report of Myocardial Injury in a Patient Receiving Levarterenol, *Am. Heart J.*, **59**:134–139, 1960.

309. Szakács, J. E., and Mehlman, B.: Pathologic Changes Induced by 1-Norepinephrine: Quantitative Aspects, *Am. J. Cardiol.*, **5**:619–627, 1960.

310. Graziani, G., and Rossi, L.: [The Cardiovascular System in Chronic Carbon Monoxide Poisoning], *Folia med.*, **42**:909–923, 1959.

310a. Hayes, J. M., and Hall, G. V.: The Myocardial

Toxicity of Carbon Monoxide, *Med. J. Aust.*, 1: 865–868, 1964.

310b. Shafer, N., Smilay, M. G., and MacMillan, F. P.: Primary Myocardial Disease in Man Resulting from Acute Carbon Monoxide Poisoning, *Am. J. Med.*, 38:316–320, 1965.

311. Beck, H. G., and Suter, G. M.: Role of Carbon Monoxide in the Causation of Myocardial Disease, *J.A.M.A.*, 110:1982–1986, 1938.

312. Middleton, G. D., Ashby, D. W., and Clark, F.: Delayed and Long Lasting Electrocardiographic Changes in Carbon-Monoxide Poisoning, *Lancet*, 1:12–14, 1961.

313. Cosby, R. S., and Bergeron, M.: Electrocardiographic Changes in Carbon Monoxide Poisoning, *Am. J. Cardiol.*, 11:93–96, 1963.

314. Stearns, W. H., Drinker, C. K., and Shaughnessy, T. J.: The Electrocardiographic Changes Found in 22 Cases of Carbon Monoxide (Illuminating Gas) Poisoning, *Am. Heart J.*, 15:434–447, 1938.

315. Bouvrain, Y., Gaultier, M., Gervais, P., and Pasquier, P.: [Delayed Cardiac Complications Caused by Carbon Monoxide], *Semaine hôp. Paris*, 36: 3163–3172, 1960.

316. Beck, H. G., Schulze, W. H., and Suter, G. M.: Carbon Monoxide: A Domestic Hazard, *J.A.M.A.*, 115:1–8, 1940.

316a. Pulvertaft, R. J. V.: Rupture of Heart in Coal-Gas Poisoning, *Lancet*, 2:289–290, 1932.

317. Diaz-Rivera, R. S., Ramos-Morales, F., Garcia-Palmieri, M. R., and Ramirez, E. A.: The Electrocardiographic Changes in Acute Phosphorus Poisoning in Man, *Am. J. M. Sc.*, 241:758–765, 1961.

318. Dathe, R. A., and Nathan, D. A.: Electrocardiographic Changes Resulting from Phosphorus Poisoning, *Am. Heart J.*, 31:98–102, 1946.

319. Newburger, R. A., Beaser, S. B., and Shwachman, H.: Phosphorus Poisoning with Recovery Accompanied by Electrocardiographic Changes, *Am. J. Med.*, 4:927–930, 1948.

319a. Dahhan, S. S., and Orfaly, H.: Electrocardiographic Changes in Mercury Poisoning, *Am. J. Cardiol.*, 14:178–183, 1964.

320. Kline, T. S.: Myocardial Changes in Lead poisoning, *A.M.A. J. Dis. Child.*, 99:48–54, 1960.

321. Kosmider, S., and Petelenz, T.: [Electrocardiographic Studies in Cases of Chronic Occupational Lead Poisoning], *Polskie arch. med. Wewnetrzne*, 31:1349–1357, 1961.

322. Read, J. L., and Williams, J. P.: Lead Myocarditis: Report of a Case, *Am. Heart J.*, 44:797–802, 1952.

323. Poon-King, T.: Myocarditis from Scorpion Stings, *Brit. Heart J.*, 1:374–377, 1963.

323a. Reid, H. A., Thean, P. C., Chan, K. E., and Baharom, A. R.: Clinical Effects of Bites by Malayan Viper (Ancistrodon Rhodostoma), *Lancet*, 1:617–621, 1963.

323b. Brown, R., and Dewar, H. A.: Heart Damage Following Adder Bite in England, *Brit. Heart J.*, 27:144–147, 1965.

324. French, A. J., and Weller, C. V.: Interstitial Myocarditis Following the Clinical and Experimental Use of Sulfonamide Drugs, *Am. J. Path.*, 18:109–121, 1942.

325. French, A. J.: Hypersensitivity in Pathogenesis of Histopathologic Changes Associated with Sulfonamide Chemotherapy, *Am. J. Path.*, 22:679–701, 1946.

326. Blanchard, A. J., and Mertens, G. A.: Hypersensitivity Myocarditis Occurring with Sulfamethoxypyridazine Therapy, *Canad. M. A. J.*, 79:627–630,

327. Wells, A. H., and Sax, S. G.: Isolated Myocarditis Probably of Sulfonamide Origin, *Am. Heart J.*, 30: 522–526, 1945.

328. More, R. H., McMillan, G. C., and Duff, G. L.: Pathology of Sulfonamide Allergy in Man, *Am. J. Path.*, 22:703–735, 1946.

329. Field, J. B., and Federman, D. D.: Sudden Death in a Diabetic Subject during Treatment with BZ-55 (Carbutamide), *Diabetes*, 6:67–70, 1957.

330. Haden, R. F., and Langsjoen, P. H.: Manifestations of Myocardial Involvement in Acute Reactions to Penicillin, *Am. J. Cardiol.*, 8:420–425, 1961.

331. Waugh, D.: Myocarditis, Arteritis, and Focal Hepatic, Splenic and Renal Granulomas Apparently Due to Penicillin Sensitivity, *Am. J. Path.*, 28:437–447, 1952.

332. Engleman, E. P., Krupp, M. A, Rinehart, J. F., Fine, M., Bruck, E. L., Barbour, A. B., Farquhar, J. W., and Jones, R. C.: Uncommon and Serious Reactions to Phenylbutazone: A Clinicopathologic Study, *Ann. Rheumat. Dis.*, 12:351–353, 1953.

333. Hodge, P. R., and Lawrence, J. R.: Two Cases of Myocarditis Associated with Phenylbutazone Therapy, *M. J. Australia*, 1:640–647, 1957.

334. Steinberg, C. L., Bohrod, M. G., and Roodenburg, A. I.: Agranulocytosis Following Phenylbutazone (Butazolidin) Therapy, *J.A.M.A.*, 152:33–36, 1953.

335. MacCarthy, J. M., and Jackson, R. T.: Hepatic Necrosis and Other Visceral Lesions Associated with Phenylbutazone Therapy, *Brit. M. J.*, 2:240–242, 1955.

335a. Edelstein, J. M.: Butazolidin Angiitis and Periangiitis Simulating Aschoff Nodule, *Am. Heart J.*, 69:573, 1965.

336. Cangemi, V. F.: Acute Pericarditis after Smallpox Vaccination, *New England J. Med.*, 258:1257–1259, 1958.

337. MacAdam, D. B., and Whitaker, W.: Cardiac Complications after Vaccination for Smallpox, *Brit. M. J.*, 2:1099–1100, 1962.

338. Dalgaard, J. B.: Fatal Myocarditis Following Smallpox Vaccination, *Am. Heart J.*, 54:156–157, 1957.

339. Finlay-Jones, L. R.: Fatal Myocarditis after Vaccination against Smallpox: Report of a Case, *New England J. Med.*, 270:41–43, 1964.

340. Bengtsson, E., and Lundström, R.: Postvaccinal Myocarditis, *Cardiologia*, 30:1–8, 1957.

341. Kline, I. K., Kline, T. S., and Saphir, O.: Myocarditis in Senescence, *Am. Heart J.*, **65**:446–457, 1963.

342. Chatterjee, S. S., and Thakre, M. W.: Fiedler's Myocarditis: Report of a Fatal Case Following Intramuscular Injection of Streptomycin, *Tubercle*, **39**:240–241, 1958.

343. Campbell, J. E.: Myocardial Lesions and Granulocytopenia Associated with Chlorpromazine Therapy: Liver Necrosis Resulting from Unsuspected Carbon Tetrachloride Poisoning, *Am. J. Clin. Path.*, **34**:133–138, 1960.

343a. Kerwin, A. J.: Fatal Myocarditis Due to Sensitivity to Phenindione, *Canad. M. A. J.*, **90**:1418–1419, 1964.

343b. Cruickshank, B.: Heart Lesions in Rheumatoid Disease, *J. Path. and Bacti.*, **76**:223–240, 1958.

343c. Weintraub, A. M., and Zvaifler, N. J.: The Occurrence of Valvular and Myocardial Disease in Patients with Chronic Joint Deformity, *Am. J. Med.,*. **35**:145–162, 1963.

343d. Gowans, J. D. C.: Complete Heart Block with Stokes-Adams Syndrome Due to Rheumatoid Heart Disease, *New England J. Med.*, **262**:1012–1014, 1960.

343e. Paronen, I.; Reiter's Disease. A Study of 344 Cases Observed in Finland, *Acta med. scandinav.*, **131** (Supp. 212): 1–112, 1948.

343f. Neu, L. T., Reider, R. A., and Mack, R. E.: Cardiac Involvement in Reiter's Disease: Report of a Case with Review of the Literature, *Ann. Intern. Med.*, **53**:215–220, 1960.

343g. Eisenstein, B., and Taubenhaus, M.: Nonsyphilitic Interstitial Keratitis and Bilateral Deafness (Cogan's Syndrome) Associated with Cardiovascular Disease, *New England J. Med.*, **258**:1074–1079, 1958.

343h. Lewis, P. D.: Behcet's Disease and Carditis, *Brit. Med. J.*, **I**:1026–1027, 1964.

344. Biörck, G., Axén, O., and Thorson, A.: Unusual Cyanosis in a Boy with Congenital Pulmonary Stenosis and Tricuspid Insufficiency: Fatal Outcome after Angiocardiography, *Am. Heart J.*, **44**: 143–148, 1952.

345. Spain D. M.: Association of Gastrointestinal Carcinoid Tumors with Cardiovascular Abnormalities, *Am. J. Med.*, **19**:366–369, 1955.

346. Heinmark, J. J., and Parkin, T. W.: Syndrome Associated with Metastatic Carcinoid Tumor: Report of a Case, *Proc. Staff Meet. Mayo Clin.*, **31**:56–61, 1956.

347. Sjoerdsma, A., Weissbach, H., and Udenfriend, S.: Clinical, Physiologic and Biochemical Study of Patients with Malignant Carcinoid (Argentaffinoma), *Am. J. Med.*, **20**:520–532, 1956.

348. McKusick, V. A.: Carcinoid Cardiovascular Disease, *Bull. Johns Hopkins Hosp.*, **98**:13–36, 1956.

349. Thorson, A., Biörck, G., Björckman, G., and Waldenström, J.: Malignant Carcinoid of the Small Intestine with Metastases to the Liver, Valvular Disease of the Right Side of the Heart (Pulmonary Stenosis and Tricuspid Regurgitation without Septal Defects), Peripheral Vasomotor Symptoms, bronchoconstriction, and an Unusual Type of Cyanosis, *Am. Heart J.*, **47**:795–817, 1954.

350. MacDonald, R. A., and Robbins, S. L.: Pathology of the Heart in the Carcinoid Syndrome, *A.M.A. Arch. Path.*, **63**:103–112, 1957.

351. Bean, W. B., Olch, D., and Weinberg, H. B.: The Syndrome of Carcinoid and Acquired Valve Lesions of the Right Side of the Heart, *Circulation*, **12**:1–6, 1955.

352. Savier, C. H.: [Carcinoid Tumors and Their Cardiovascular Lesions], *Coeur et méd. int.*, **1**:211–216, 1962.

353. Roberts, W. C., and Sjoerdsma, A.: The Cardiac Disease Associated with the Carcinoid Syndrome (Carcinoid Heart Disease), *Am. J. Med.*, **36**:5–34, 1964.

354. Schweizer, W., Gloor, F., v. Bertrab, R., and Dubach, U. C.: Carcinoid Heart Disease with Left-sided Lesions, *Circulation*, **29**:253–257, 1964.

355. Goble, A. J., Hay, D. R., Hudson, R., and Sandler, M.: Acquired Heart Disease with Argentaffin Carcinoma, *Brit. Heart J.*, **18**:544–552, 1956.

356. Schwaber, J. R., and Lukas, D. S.: Hyperkinemia and Cardiac Failure in the Carcinoid Syndrome, *Am. J. Med.*, **32**:846–853, 1962.

357. Cosh, J., Cates, J. E., and Pugh, D. W.: Carcinoid Heart Disease, *Brit. Heart J.*, **21**:369–380, 1959.

358. Wright, P. W., and Mulder, D. G.: Carcinoid Heart Disease: Report of a Case Treated by Open Heart Surgery, *Am. J. Cardiol.*, **12**:864–868, 1963.

359. Davies, J. N. P., and Coles, R. M.: Some considerations Regarding Obscure Diseases Affecting the Mural Endocardium, *Am. Heart J.*, **59**:600–631, 1960.

360. Seminar: Some African Cardiopathies: Report of a Joint Seminar of the Departments of Pathology and Medicine of the University of the Witwatersrand, *South African M. J.*, **31**:854–857, 1957.

361. Nagaratnam, N., and Dissanayake, R. V. P.: Endomyocardial Fibrosis in the Ceylonese, *Brit. Heart J.*, **21**:167–173, 1959.

362. O'Brien, W.: Endocardial Fibrosis in the Sudan, *Brit. M. J.*, **2**:899–901, 1954.

363. Ball, J. D., Williams, A. W., and Davies, J. N. P.: Endomyocardial Fibrosis, *Lancet*, **1**:1049–1054, 1954.

363a. Abrahams, D. G., and Parry, E. H. O.: Chronic Pericardial Effusion Complicating Endomyocardial Fibrosis, *Circulation*, **28**:221–231, 1963.

364. Williams, A. W., and Somers, K.: The Electrocardiogram in Endomyocardial Fibrosis, *Brit. Heart J.*, **22**:311–315, 1960.

365. Shillingford, J. P., and Somers, K.: Clinical and Haemodynamic Patterns in Endomyocardial Fibrosis, *Brit. Heart J.*, **23**:433–446, 1961.

366. Lynch, J. B., and Watt, J.: Diffuse Endomyo-cardial Sclerosis, *Brit. Heart J.*, **19**:173–185, 1957.

367. Lynfield, J., Gasul, B. M., Luan, L. L., and Dillon, R. F.: Right and Left Heart Catheterization and Angiocardiographic Findings in Idiopathic Cardiac Hypertrophy with Endocardial Fibroelastosis, *Circulation*, **21**:386–400, 1960.

368. Crawford, M. A.: Endomyocardial Fibrosis and Carcinoidosis: A Common Denominator? *Am. Heart J.*, **66**:273–275, 1963.

369. Fisher, E. R., and Davis, E. R.: Observations Concerning the Pathogenesis of Endocardial Thickening in the Adult Heart, *Am. Heart J.*, **56**:553–561, 1958.

370. Still, W. J. S.: Endocardial Fibroelastosis, *Am. Heart J.*, **61**:579–585, 1961.

371. Thomas, W. A., Randall, R. V., Bland, E. F., and Castleman, B.: Endocardial Fibroelastosis: A Factor in Heart Disease of Obscure Etiology, *New England J. Med.*, **251**:327–338, 1954.

372. Becker, B. J. P., Chatgidakis, C. B., and Van Lingen, B.: Cardiovascular Collagenosis with Parietal Endocardial Thrombosis. A Clinicopathologic Study of Forty Cases, *Circulation*, **7**:345–356, 1953.

373. Löffler, W.: Endocarditis parietalis fibroplastica mit Bluteosinophilie: Ein eigenartiges Krankheitsbild, *Schweiz. med. Wchnschr.*, **66**:817–820, 1936.

374. Brink, A. J., and Weber, H. W.: Fibroplastic Parietal Endocarditis with Eosinophilia: Löffler's Endocarditis, *Am. J. Med.*, **34**:52–70, 1963.

375. Hoffman, F. G., Rosenbaum, D., and Genovese, P. D.: Fibroplastic Endocarditis with Eosinophilia (Löffler's Endocarditis Parietalis Fibroplastica): Case Report and Review of the Literature, *Ann. Int. Med.*, **42**:668–680, 1955.

376. Clark, G. M., Valentine, E., and Blount, S. G., Jr.: Endocardial Fibrosis Simulating Constrictive Pericarditis: Report of a Case with Determinations of Pressure in the Right Side of the Heart and Eosinophilia, *New England J. Med.*, **254**:349–355, 1956.

377. Weiss-Carmine, S.: Die Endocarditis parietalis fibroplastica mit Bluteosinophilie (Löffler) und ihre Stellung im Rahmen der Parietalendokardfibrosen, *Schweiz. med. Wchnschr.*, **87**:890–898, 1957.

378. Wiener, M. J., and Knights, E. M., Jr.: Löffler's Endocarditis Parietalis Fibroplastica with Eosinophilia, *Am. Heart J.*, **53**:157–161, 1957.

379. Vakil, R. J.: Cardiovascular Involvement in Tropical Eosinophilia, *Brit. Heart J.*, **23**:578–586, 1961.

379a. Johny, K. V., and Ananthachari, M. D.: Cardiovascular Changes in Tropical Eosinophila, *Am. Heart J.*, **69**:591–598, 1965.

380. Kahrs, T.: Primary Tumors of Heart: Rhabdolipoma and Rhabdomyosarcoma Cordis, *Acta path. et microbiol. scandinav.*, **33**:151–158, 1953.

381. Mead, J.: Tumors of the Heart, *CA*, **11**:92–96, 1961.

382. Colombus, M. R.: "De re anatomica," libri xv, Paris, 1562, pp. 482–495.

383. Fletcher, F. W.: Primary Cardiac Tumors, *J. Iowa M. Soc.*, **53**:545–550, 1963.

384. Beck, C. S., and Thatcher, H. S.: Spindle Cell Sarcoma of the Heart, *A.M.A. Arch. Int. Med.*, **36**:830–837, 1925.

385. Tedeschi, A.: Beitrag zum Studium der Herzgeschwülste, *Prager med. Wchnschr.*, **18**:121–135, 1893.

386. Barnes, A. R., Beaver, D. C., and Snell, A. M.: Primary Sarcoma of the Heart, *Am. Heart J.*, **9**:480–491, 1934.

387. Doane, J. C., and Pressman, R.: Antemortem Diagnosis of Tumors of the Heart, *Am. J. M. Sc.*, **203**:520–524, 1942.

388. Abbott, O. A., Warshawski, F. E., and Cobbs, B. W., Jr.: Primary Tumors and Pseudotumors of the Heart, *Ann. Surg.*, **155**:855–872, 1962.

389. Hurst, J. W., and Cooper, H. R.: Neoplastic Disease of the Heart, *Am. Heart J.*, **50**:782–802, 1955.

390. Rucks, W. W., Jr., Russell, H. T., and Motley, R. F.: Primary Reticulum Cell Sarcoma of the Heart, *Am. Heart J.*, **66**:97–103, 1963.

391. Yater, W. M.: Tumors of the Heart and Pericardium, *Arch. Int. Med.*, **48**:627–666, 1931.

392. Willis, R. A.: "The Spread of Tumors in the Human Body," J. and A. Churchhill, London, 1934, pp. 259–268.

393. Griffiths, G. C.: Primary Tumors of the Heart, *Clin. Radiol.*, **13**:183–194, 1962.

394. Burnett, R. C., and Shimkin, M. B.: Secondary Neoplasms of the Heart, *A.M.A. Arch. Int. Med.*, **93**:205–218, 1954.

395. Lisa, J. R., Hirschhorn, L., and Hart, C. A.: Tumors of the Heart, *A.M.A. Arch. Int. Med.*, **67**:91–113, 1941.

396. Strauss, R., and Merliss, R.: Primary Tumor of the Heart, *A.M.A. Arch. Path.*, **39**:74–78, 1945.

396a. Griffiths, G. C.: A Review of Primary Tumors of the Heart, *Progr. Cardiovascular Diseases*, **7**:465–479, 1965.

397. Dong, E., Jr., Hurley, E. J., and Shumway, N. E.: Primary Cardiac Sarcoma, *Am. J. Cardiol.*, **10**:871–878, 1962.

398. Woll, E., and Vickery, A. L.: Primary Fibrosarcoma of the Heart with a Vertebral Metastasis, *A.M.A. Arch. Path.*, **43**:244–252, 1947.

399. Mahaim, I.: "Les tumeurs et les polypes du coeur: Étude anatomoclinique," Roth, Lausanne, 1945.

400. Goldberg, H. P., and Steinberg, I.: Primary Tumors of the Heart, *Circulation*, **11**:963–970, 1955.

401. McNalley, M. C., Kelble, D., Pryor, R., and Blount, S. G., Jr.: Angiosarcoma of the Heart, *Am. Heart J.*, **65**:244–252, 1963.

402. Wight, R. P., Jr., McCall, M. M., and Wenger, N. K.: Primary Atrial Tumor: Evaluation of Clinical Findings in Ten Cases and Review of the Literature, *Am. J. Cardiol.*, **11**:790–797, 1963.

403. Kendall, D., and Symonds, B.: Epileptiform At-

tacks Due to Myxoma of Right Auricle, *Brit. Heart J.*, **14**:139–143, 1952.

404. Adams, C. W., Collins, H. A., Dummit, E. S., and Allen, J. H.: Intracardiac Myxomas and Thrombi, *Am. J. Cardiol.*, **7**:176–187, 1961.

405. Deshmukh, M., Nichols, H. T., and Goldberg, H.: Myxoma of the Left Atrium Simulating Restenosis of the Mitral Valve, *Am. Heart J.*, **58**:623–629, 1959.

406. Lefcoe, N. M., Brien, F. S., and Manning, G. W.: An Opening Snap Recorded in a Case of Tumor of the Left Atrium, *New England J. Med.*, **257**:178–180, 1957.

407. Goodwin, J. F.: Diagnosis of Left Atrial Myxoma, *Lancet*, **1**:464–467, 1963.

408. Kaufmann, G., Rutishauser, W., and Hegglin, R.: Heart Sounds in Atrial Tumors, *Am. J. Cardiol.*, **8**:350–357, 1961.

408a. Harris, T. R., Copeland, G. D., and Brody, D. A.: Progressive Injury Current with Metastatic Tumor of the Heart. Case Report and Review of the Literature, *Am. Heart J.*, **69**:392–400, 1965.

409. Belle, M. S.: Right Atrial Myxoma, *Circulation*, **19**:910–917, 1959.

410. Shirey, E. K.: Personal communication, 1964.

411. Bigelow, N. H., Klinger, S., and Wright, A. W.: Primary Tumors of the Heart in Infancy and Early Childhood, *Cancer*, **7**:549–563, 1954.

412. Longino, L. A., and Meeker, I. A., Jr.: Primary Cardiac Tumors in Infancy, *J. Pediat.*, **43**:724–731, 1953.

413. Strouse, S.: Primary Benign Tumor of the Heart of Forty-three Years' Duration, *A.M.A. Arch. Int. Med.*, **62**:401–412, 1938.

414. Goldberg, H. P., Glenn, F., Dotter, C. T., and Steinberg, I.: Myxoma of the Left Atrium: Diagnosis Made during Life with Operative and Postmortem Findings, *Circulation*, **6**:762–767, 1952.

415. Catton, R. W., Guntheroth, W. G., and Reichenbach, D. D.: A Myxoma of the Pulmonary Valve Causing Severe Stenosis in Infancy, *Am. Heart J.*, **66**:248–252, 1963.

416. Gottsegen, G., Wessely, J., Árvay, A., and Temesári, A.: Right Ventricular Myxoma Simulating Pulmonic Stenosis, *Circulation*, **27**:95–97, 1963.

416a. Sakakibara, S., Osawa, N., Konno, S., Hashimoto, A., Gomi, H., Miyamoto, A. N., and Takao, A.: Myxoma of the Right Ventricle of the Heart. Report of a Case with Successful Removal and Review of the Literature, *Am. Heart J.*, **69**:382–391, 1965.

417. Branch, C. F.: Primary Neoplasm of Heart Valve, *Am. J. Path.*, **7**:157–160, 1931.

418. McCue, C. M., Henningar, G. R., Davis, E., and Ray, J.: Congenital Subaortic Stenosis Caused by Fibroma of Left Ventricle, *Pediatrics*, **16**:372–377, 1955.

419. Grant, R. T., and Camp, P. D.: A Case of Complete Heart Block Due to an Arterial Angioma, *Heart*, **16**:137–143, 1931–33.

420. Maurer, E. R.: Successful Removal of Tumor of the Heart, *J. Thoracic Surg.*, **23**:479–485, 1952.

421. Willis, R. A.: An Intrapericardial Teratoma in an Infant, *J. Path. & Bact.*, **58**:284–286, 1946.

422. Beck, C. S.: An Intrapericardial Teratoma and a Tumor of the Heart: Both Removed Operatively, *Ann. Surg.*, **116**:161–174, 1942.

423. Legnami, F. A., and Corwin, R. D.: Intrapericardial Teratoma, *Am. Heart J.*, **65**:674–677, 1963.

424. Brandes, W. W., Gray, J. A. C., and MacLeod, N. W.: Leiomyoma of the Pericardium, *Am. Heart J.*, **23**:426–432, 1942.

425. Mahaim, I.: Le coeolthéliome tawarien bénin: Une tumeur sui generis du noeud de Tawara, *Cardiologia*, **6**:57–82, 1952.

426. Engle, M. A., and Glenn, F.: Primary Malignant Tumor of the Heart, *Pediatrics*, **15**:562–574, 1955.

427. Somers, K., and Lothe, F.: Primary Lymphosarcoma of the Heart, *Cancer*, **13**:449–457, 1960.

428. Whorton, C. M.: Primary Malignant Tumors of the Heart, *Cancer*, **2**:245–260, 1949.

429. Magner, J. W., and Morehan, J. P. A.: A Case of Primary Sarcoma of the Heart, *J. Irish M. A.*, **37**:317–319, 1955.

430. Weir, D. R., and Jones, B. C., Jr.: Primary Sarcoma of the Heart, *Am. Heart J.*, **22**:556–560, 1941.

431. Cheng, T. O., and Sutton, D. C.: Primary Hemangioendotheliosarcoma of Heart Diagnosed by Angiocardiography, *Circulation*, **11**:456–461, 1955.

432. Pund, E. E., Jr., Collier, T. M., Cunningham, J. E., Jr., and Hayes, J. R.: Primary Cardiac Rhabdomyosarcoma Presenting as Pulmonary Stenosis. *Am. Heart J.*, **12**:249–253, 1963.

433. Forker, E. L., January, L. E., and Lawrence, M. S.: Primary Sarcoma of the Mitral Valve, *Am. Heart J.*, **66**:243–247, 1963.

434. Lenegre, J., Moreau, P., and Iris, L.: [2 Cases of Complete Auriculoventricular Block Due to Primary Sarcoma of the Heart], *Arch. mal. coeur*, **56**:361–387, 1963.

435. Lübschitz, K., Lundsteen, E., and Forchhammer, E.: Primary Malignant Heart Tumor Diagnosed in Vivo with the Aid of Artificial Pneumopericardium, *Radiology*, **52**:79–87, 1949.

436. Lloyd, P. C.: Heart Block Due to Primary Lymphangioendothelioma of Atrioventricular node, *Bull. Johns Hopkins Hosp.*, **44**:149–154, 1929.

437. Perry, C. B., and Rogers, H.: Lymphangioendothelioma of the Heart Causing Complete Heart Block, *J. Path. & Bact.*, **39**:281–284, 1934.

438. Bergman, F., and Jacobsson, K.: Primary Pericardial Mesothelioma: Report of a Case, *Acta path. et microbiol. scandinav.*, **42**:235–241, 1958.

439. Brandenburg, R. O., and Edwards, J. E.: Cardiac Clinics. 143. Cardiac Sarcoma: Report of a Case and Comparison with a Case of Metastatic Carcinoma of the Pericardium, *Proc. Staff Meet. Mayo Clin.*, **29**:437–446, 1954.

440. Reals, W. J., Russum, B. C., and Walsh, E. M.:

Primary Mesothelioma of the Pericardium, *A.M.A. Arch. Path.*, **44**:380–384, 1947.

441. Solomon, R. D.: Malignant Teratoma of the Heart, *A.M.A. Arch. Path.*, **52**:561–568, 1951.

442. Scott, R. W., and Garvin, C. F.: Tumors of the Heart and Pericardium, *Am. Heart J.*, **17**:431–436, 1939.

443. Gassman, H. S., Meadows, R., Jr., and Baker, L. A.: Metastatic Tumors of the Heart, *Am. J. Med.*, **19**:357–365, 1955.

444. Madianos, M., and Sokal, J. E.: Cardiac Involvement in Lymphosarcoma and Reticulum Cell Sarcoma, *Am. Heart J.*, **65**:322–326, 1963.

445. Hanfling, S. M.: Metastatic Cancer to the Heart, *Circulation*, **22**:474–483, 1960.

446. Helwig, F. C.: Tumors of Heart, *J. Kansas M. Soc.*, **36**:265–272, 1935.

447. Raven, R. W.: Secondary Malignant Disease of the Heart, *Brit. J. Cancer*, **2**:1–7, 1948.

448. Pic, A., and Bret, J.: Contribution à l'étude du cancer secondaire du coeur, *Rev. méd.*, **11**:1022–1041, 1891.

449. Bryant, C. H.: Primary Sarcoma of the Heart in a Dog, *Bull. Johns Hopkins Hosp.*, **18**:474–476, 1907.

450. Karrenstein: Ein Fall von Fibroelastomyxom des Herzens und Kasuistisches zur Frage der Herzgeschwülste besonders der Myxome, *Arch. path. Anat.*, **194**:127–150, 1908.

451. Symmers, D.: Metastasis of Tumors, *Am. J. M. Sc.*, **154**:225–240, 1917.

452. Bardenheuer, F. H.: Zur Kenntnis der Metastasierung bösartiger Geschwülste im Herzen, *Zentralbl. allg. Path.*, **34**:337–343, 1923–1924.

453. Morris, L. M.: Metastases to the Heart from Malignant Tumors, *Am. Heart J.*, **3**:219–229, 1927–1928.

454. Siegel, M. L., and Young, A. M.: Electrocardiographic Findings in Tumors of the Heart, *Am. Heart J.*, **8**:682–690, 1932–1933.

455. Burke, E. M.: Metastatic Tumors of the Heart, *Am. J. Cancer*, **20**:33–47, 1934.

456. Lymburner, R. M.: Tumors of Heart: Histopathological and Clinical Study, *Canad. M. A. J.*, **30**:368–373, 1934.

457. Pollia, J. A., and Gogol, L. J.: Some Notes on Malignancies of the Heart, *Am. J. Cancer*, **27**:329–333, 1936.

458. Schnitker, M. A., and Bailey, O. T.: Metastatic Tumor of the Heart, *J.A.M.A.*, **108**:1787–1790, 1937.

459. Ritchie, G.: Metastatic Tumors of the Myocardium, *Am. J. Path.*, **17**:483–489, 1941.

460. Herbut, P. A., and Maisel, A. L.: Secondary Tumors of the Heart, *A.M.A. Arch. Path.*, **34**:358–364, 1942.

461. Dimmette, R. M.: The Ante-mortem Diagnosis of Secondary Tumors of the Heart, *U.S. Armed Forces M. J.*, **1**:750–758, 1950.

462. De Loach, J. F., and Haynes, J. W.: Secondary

Tumors of Heart and Pericardium, *A.M.A. Arch. Int. Med.*, **91**:224–249, 1953.

463. Young, J. M., and Goldman, I. R.: Tumor Metastasis to the Heart, *Circulation*, **9**:220-229, 1954.

464. Cohen, G. U., Peery, T. M., and Evans, J. M.: Neoplastic Invasion of the Heart and Pericardium, *Ann. Int. Med.* **42**:1238–1245, 1955.

465. Goudie, R. B.: Secondary Tumors of Heart and Pericardium, *Brit. Heart J.*, **17**:183–188, 1955.

466. Lothe, F., and Somers, K.: Secondary Tumors of the Heart and Pericardium in Uganda Africans, *A.M.A. Arch. Path.*, **69**:158–167, 1960.

467. Clay, A., Dupont, A., Demaille, A., and Adenis, L.: [Origin and Anatomical Aspects of Secondary Tumors of the Heart], *Lille méd.*, **6**:473–487, 1961.

468. Hanbury, W. J.: Secondary Tumors of the Heart, *Brit. J. Cancer*, **14**:23–27, 1960.

469. Coller, F. C., Inkley, J. J., and Moragues, V.: Neoplastic Endocardial Implants, *Am. J. Clin. Path.*, **20**:159–164, 1950.

470. Olsen, S., Bach-Nielsen, P., and Piper, J.: Polypoid Tumors of the Cardiac Auricles, *Acta med. scandinav.*, **171**:637–646, 1962.

471. Watts, R. W. E.: Testicular Teratoma with Extensive Intracardiac Metastases, *Brit. Heart J.*, **9**:175–180, 1947.

472. Rottino, A., and Hoffman, G. T.: Cardiac Involvement in Hodgkins Disease, *Am. Heart J.*, **43**:115–120, 1952.

473. Nabarro, J. D. N.: Cardiac Involvement in Malignant Lymphoma, *A.M.A. Arch. Int. Med.*, **92**:258–264, 1953.

474. Weller, G. L.: The Clinical Aspects of Cardiac Involvement (Right Auricular Tumor) in Idiopathic Hemorrhagic Sarcoma (Kaposi's Disease), *Ann. Int. Med.*, **14**:314–322, 1940–1941.

475. Friedman, B., Simard, E. E., and Schwartz, I.: Unusual Primary Leiomyosarcoma of the Heart, *Am. Heart J.*, **30**:299–308, 1945.

476. Rosenbaum, F. F., Johnston, F. D., and Alzamora, V. V.: Persistent Displacement of the RS-T Segment in a Case of Metastatic Tumor of the Heart, *Am. Heart J.*, **27**:667–675, 1944.

477. Fishberg, A. M.: Auricular Fibrillation and Flutter in Metastatic Growths of the Right Auricle, *Am. J. M. Sc.*, **180**:629–634, 1930.

478. Auerbach, O., Epstein, H., and Gold, H.: Metastatic Carcinoma of the Heart, *Am. Heart J.*, **12**:467–472, 1936.

479. James, T. N., and Carrera, G. M.: Pathogenesis of Arrhythmias Associated with Metastatic Tumors of the Heart, *New England J. Med.*, **260**:869–871, 1959.

480. Reuling, J. R., and Razinsky, L.: Metastatic Bronchogenic Carcinoma of the Heart, *Am. Heart J.*, **21**:470–480, 1941.

481. Dresdale, D. T., Spain, D., and Perez-Pina, F.: Heart Block and Leukemic Cell Infiltration of

Interventricular Septum of Heart, *Am. J. Med.*, **6**: 530–533, 1949.

482. Wendkos, M. H.: Leucemic Pericarditis, *Am. Heart J.*, **22**:417–422, 1941.

483. Wallace, T. J., and Logue, R. B.: Metastatic Carcinoma as a Cause of Constrictive Pericarditis, *Am. Heart J.*, **31**:223–230, 1946.

484. Fischer, J. W.: Neoplastic Involvement of Pericardium Producing the Syndrome of Constrictive Pericarditis, *Am. Heart J.*, **35**:813–819, 1948.

485. Slater, S. R., Kroop, I. G., and Zuckerman, S.: Constructive Pericarditis Caused by Solitary Metastatic Carcinosis of the Pericardium and Complicated by Radiation Fibrosis of the Mediastinum, *Am. Heart J.*, **43**:401–412, 1952.

486. McNamara, W. L., Ducey, E. F., and Baker, L. A.: Cardiac Rupture Associated with Metastases to the Heart from Carcinoma of the Duodenum, *Am. Heart J.*, **13**:108–113, 1937.

487. Keat, E. C. B., and Twyman, V. R.: Cardiac Involvement in Lymphosarcoma with Spontaneous Rupture of the Heart, *Brit. Heart J.*, **17**:563–565, 1955.

488. Pilcher, R. B.: Lymphosarcoma Invading Heart: Report of 3 Cases with Autopsy Findings, *M. J. Australia*, **2**:366–371, 1950.

489. Rothfeld, E. L., and Zirkin, R. M.: Unusual Electrocardiographic Evidence of Metastatic Cardiac Tumor Resembling Atrial Infraction, *Am. J. Cardiol.*, **10**:882–885, 1962.

490. McCandless, F. D., and Faloon, W. W.: The Diagnosis of Metastatic Tumor by Cytological Examination of the Pericardial Fluid: Report of a Case Using Shorr's Stain, *Ann. Int. Med.*, **29**:1157–1168, 1948.

491. Shelburne, S. A., and Aronson, H. S.: Tumors of the Heart. II. Report of a Secondary Tumor of the Heart Involving the Pericardium and the Bundle of His with Remission Following Deep Roentgen-ray Therapy, *Ann. Int. Med.*, **14**:728–736, 1940.

492. Bozzini, M. A.: Personal communication, 1964.

PART VI

Diseases of the Aorta and Peripheral Vessels

Section A: Recognition and Medical Treatment

56 DISEASES OF THE AORTA AND PERIPHERAL VESSELS (ARTERIES AND VEINS)

Ray W. Gifford, Jr., M.D.

DISEASES OF THE AORTA AND PERIPHERAL ARTERIES

Chronic Occlusive Arterial Diseases of the Extremities

Peripheral vascular disease is a term that encompasses a wide variety of conditions affecting the arteries, veins, and lymphatics of the extremities. This term, however, often is erroneously used as a synonym for the chronic occlusive arterial diseases, which, taken as a group, are the most frequently encountered conditions affecting the aorta and peripheral arteries. In this section, only those diseases that produce chronic ischemia due to organic occlusion of the aorta or peripheral arteries will be discussed. Other sections will be devoted to acute arterial occlusion and to conditions that produce ischemia as a result of arterial spasm, instead of organic occlusion.

Etiology

Atherosclerosis of the aorta and/or its branches to the extremities (arteriosclerosis obliterans) is the cause of 95 per cent of cases of chronic occlusive disease. The etiology and the pathogenesis of atherosclerosis are discussed in Chap. 27. It is important to remember that, experimentally and clinically, atherosclerosis behaves differently in different vascular beds, and therefore experimental and epidemiologic data pertaining to coronary atherosclerosis may not be strictly applicable to atherosclerosis of the peripheral arteries.[1,2]

Thromboangiitis obliterans (Buerger's disease), though relatively rare, is the next most common cause for chronic occlusive arterial disease of the extremities. Most authorities agree that the incidence of thromboangiitis obliterans seems to be decreasing, but there are few who share the opinion of Wessler and colleagues[3] that it is not a separate and distinct clinical entity. McKusick and colleagues,[4] as well as Schatz and colleagues,[5] demonstrated the typical pathologic changes described

by Buerger as well as unique angiographic findings in patients with thromboangiitis obliterans. McPherson and colleagues[6] have shown by follow-up studies that clinically thromboangiitis obliterans and arteriosclerosis obliterans have entirely different prognostic implications. The cause of thromboangiitis obliterans is not known, and there may be no single etiologic agent. No infectious agent has been isolated, and presumably the arteritis represents a sterile inflammatory reaction to some unknown agent or agents. Tobacco has been repeatedly implicated, because most victims are heavy smokers and cessation of smoking is usually followed by improvement.

An extremely rare cause for chronic occlusive arterial disease is a nonspecific arteritis affecting predominantly the subclavian and carotid arteries of young women (Takayasu's disease). Ischemic symptoms are confined to the upper extremities and the brain. The cause of Takayasu's disease is not known. In the United States the syndrome of arterial insufficiency of the upper extremities and the brain occurs with greatest frequency in middle-aged and older people, particularly men. In these cases the cause is usually atherosclerosis and not the nonspecific arteritis that has been described as occurring in young women. The terms *aortic arch syndrome* and *pulseless disease* are used to describe the clinical manifestations regardless of cause.[7,8]

The signs and symptoms of chronic occlusive arterial disease are frequently the sequelae to sudden arterial occlusion if the extremity survives the acute insult. Causes for sudden arterial occlusion include arterial embolus, trauma, and simple thrombosis in situ. These will be discussed in detail in the sections on Acute Arterial Occlusion of the Extremities and Arterial Trauma.

Pathology

Histopathologic findings in atherosclerosis are well known and are described elsewhere in this book. In addition to atherosclerotic lesions in the larger arteries of the extremities, arteriolar and capillary lesions consisting of endothelial proliferation and thickening of the basement membrane in diabetic patients have been described.[9]

The pathologic findings in thromboangiitis obliterans are usually distinctly different from those of arteriosclerosis obliterans,[4,5] except in the late stages when old occluding organized thrombus may be seen to fill the lumen of an artery that demonstrates considerable perivascular fibrosis.

In the acute and subacute stages, thromboangiitis obliterans is characterized by an intense inflammatory reaction that, unlike atherosclerosis, involves the veins as well as the arteries. Thromboangiitis obliterans characteristically affects medium-sized and smaller arteries initially, while atherosclerosis usually involves arteries of larger caliber. The visceral arteries rarely are affected by thromboangiitis obliterans, whereas they are commonly the sites of atherosclerosis. Thromboangiitis obliterans is a true panarteritis (or panphlebitis), as all coats of the vessel are affected and the process often extends to the perivascular tissues leading to fibrosis and scarring that firmly binds together the artery, vein, and nerve. Characteristically, the involvement is segmental, with normal segments interspersed between segments of inflammation. Proliferation of the endothelium and invasion of all three coats by lymphocytes and fibroblasts are common characteristics of this disease. Polymorphonuclear leukocytes are present in the acute stage and for this reason are more likely to be seen in veins that can be biopsied easily than in the arteries that are not usually obtained for microscopic study until the disease has reached the chronic stage. Giant cells may be found both in arteries and in veins during the acute stage. The arterial lumen is compromised by proliferation of the endothelium and invasion of the intima by lymphocytes, but final occlusion is usually the result of a thrombus that characteristically is intensely cellular and becomes organized rapidly. Necrosis of the arterial wall does not occur; the internal elastic lamina is preserved, and aneurysm formation as the result of thromboangiitis obliterans is extremely rare.

Pathologic Physiology

The basic pathophysiologic alteration produced by chronic occlusive arterial disease, regardless of its underlying cause, is ischemia of tissues supplied by the obstructed arteries. The severity of the ischemia is dependent not only upon the site and extent of the arterial disease but also on the adequacy of the collateral circulation and the metabolic demands of the tissues involved. In general, tissues usually react to prolonged ischemia by atrophy and fibrosis and, ultimately, if ischemia is severe enough, by necrosis.

Clinical Features

Regardless of the underlying cause, chronic occlusive arterial disease is characterized by (1) objective signs of ischemia, such as absence or diminution of arterial pulsations, pallor on elevation of ischemic extremities, rubor when ischemic extremities are dependent, and various degrees of ischemic changes in the skin and (2) subjective symptoms of ischemia such as intermittent claudication, rest pain, and ischemic neuropathy. The signs and symptoms that are common to all the chronic occlusive arterial diseases will be discussed first, and those which help to identify the specific cause will be discussed subsequently under the heading Differential Diagnosis.

Palpating peripheral pulses is the most important single maneuver in establishing the diagnosis where chronic occlusive arterial disease is suspected (Fig. 56-1). It is perilous to make a diagnosis of chronic occlusive arterial disease when the arterial pulses are all unequivocally normal. On the other hand, the presence of arterial pulsations does not preclude a diagnosis of chronic occlusive arterial disease, for when the occlusion is partial or when complete occlusion involves only a short segment of the terminal aorta or iliac arteries, the distal pulses may be present but dampened. Arterial pulsations may be unimpaired at the wrist and ankle when the occlusive disease is confined to the palmar or plantar arterial arches or to the digital arteries themselves. It is in such unusual circumstances as this that compression tests (Fig. 56-2) and arteriography are useful to confirm or rule out the diagnosis that has been suggested by the history and other findings. It is equally important to recognize that because of anomalies, in about 8 per cent of normal people one or both dorsalis pedis arteries are lacking, or they are so anomalously situated that they are not palpable. Hence the diagnosis of chronic occlusive arterial disease should never depend on the absence of dorsalis pedis pulsations alone.

A systolic bruit over the abdominal aorta, iliac, or femoral arteries, when the patient has been supine for more than 10 min, usually signifies the presence of intimal disease but not necessarily significant occlusion. Conversely, occlusive disease in an artery frequently does not produce a bruit. In the absence of an arteriovenous fistula, bruits that have a diastolic component, whether or not they are continuous through the cardiac cycle, are usually indicative of occlusive arterial disease.[10]

Postural color changes are helpful in evaluating the severity of ischemia but their absence does not rule out chronic occlusive arterial disease. When ischemia is moderately severe, hands or feet blanch when they are elevated (elevation pallor) and become excessively red or cyanotic when they are dependent (dependent rubor). Failure of the color to return within 15 sec after an ischemic extremity

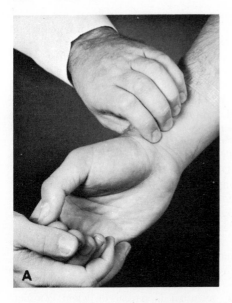

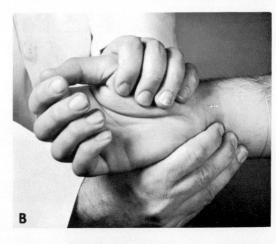

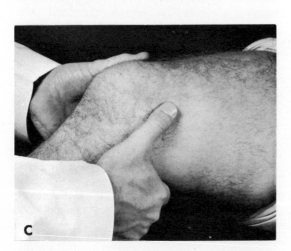

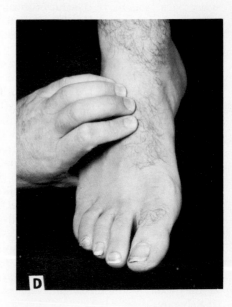

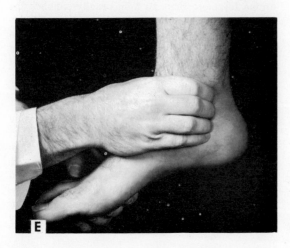

Fig. 56-1. Methods for palpating arteries. *A.* Radial; *B.* ulnar; *C.* popliteal; *D.* dorsalis pedis; *E.* posterior tibial. Palpation of the aorta and peripheral arteries is the single most important maneuver in the examination of patients for chronic occlusive arterial disease.

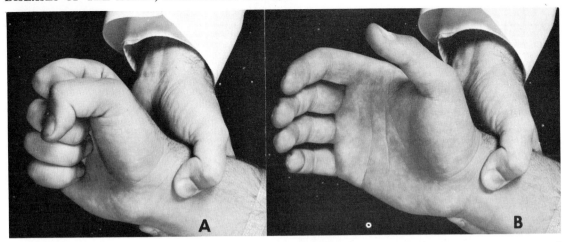

Fig. 56-2. Radial compression test of Allen, which may be employed to test for patency of the ulnar artery and the palmar arterial arch. *A.* While the examiner occludes the radial artery, the patient squeezes the blood out of his hand by making a tight fist. *B.* While radial compression is maintained by the examiner, the patient opens his hand. If color does not return to the hand within 3 sec, occlusion of the ulnar artery or the ulnar side of the palmar arch is usually present. By compressing the ulnar artery and repeating the maneuver it is possible to test for patency of the radial artery and the radial side of the palmar arch. Compression tests are more difficult to perform and give less satisfactory results in the foot than in the hand.

is changed from the elevated to the dependent position is also an indication of moderate to severe ischemia. If the color does not return for 30 sec after the extremity is brought into the dependent position, ischemia usually is severe.

A delay of more than 15 sec in the time required for the veins on the dorsa of the hands or feet to fill after an extremity is changed from the elevated to the dependent position usually is indicative of ischemia (venous filling test). When the venous system is incompetent, retrograde filling occurs promptly and renders the test invalid. As with the postural color test, a normal response to the venous filling test does not rule out chronic occlusive arterial disease, but in general the longer the time for venous filling, the more severe the ischemia.

Nutritional changes, including loss of hair on the dorsum of the foot, trophic changes of the nails, ulceration, and gangrene, represent end stages of ischemia; the diagnosis of chronic occlusive arterial disease should be made before these obvious signs occur. Ischemic ulcerations usually occur first at the tips of the digits, around and under the nails, on the interdigital surfaces, or on the heel (Fig. 56-3). Ischemic ulcers may also occur on the lateral and medial sides of the foot overlying the metatarsal heads. Large, indolent, painless ulcers that occur on the plantar surfaces of the metatarsophalangeal joints usually result from a combination of ischemia, infection, and neuropathy, and are most frequently encountered in diabetic patients (neurotropic ulcer). Ischemic ulcers are usually small

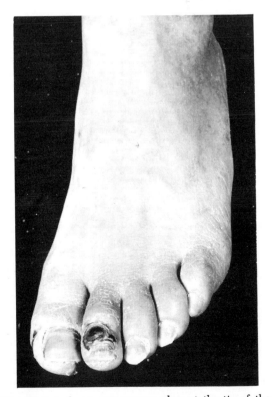

Fig. 56-3. Ischemic gangrenous ulcer at the tip of the second toe of a patient with arteriosclerosis obliterans. Ischemic ulcerations typically occur on toes, whereas stasis ulcers usually occur over or near the malleoli (see Fig. 56-9).

and shallow initially, gradually increasing in size. The base is pale, devoid of granulation tissue, and frequently covered by necrotic debris and crusted exudate (eschar). The rim is indolent, showing no tendency for proliferation and epithelialization of the ulcer. At times the rim is actually necrotic, and the ulcer spreads peripherally in this manner. Stasis ulcers from chronic venous insufficiency tend to occur around the malleoli and lower part of the leg and only rarely occur on the foot and toes. Stasis ulcers are less painful but usually are larger than ischemic ulcers, and their bases are filled with luxuriant granulation tissue. Gangrene is the end stage of chronic occlusive arterial disease. Usually it begins in and around an area of ulceration and at first involves a single digit (Fig. 56-3), from which it spreads to other digits or more proximally onto the foot. If gangrene appears abruptly and involves a large area from the outset, it is virtually certain that trauma and/or sudden arterial occlusion are inciting factors.

Pain is the most frequent presenting complaint of patients with chronic occlusive arterial disease. The characteristics and severity of the pain depend upon the extent of the occlusive arterial disease and the tissues involved. Ischemia of muscle produces intermittent claudication; ischemia of nerves produces ischemic neuropathy; ischemia of skin and subcutaneous tissue produces pretrophic pain and the pain of ulceration and gangrene, and ischemia of bone is a contributing factor in the development of painful osteoporosis.

Intermittent claudication is usually the first symptom of chronic occlusive arterial disease and the one that most frequently brings the patient to the physician. The characteristic feature of intermittent claudication is that it occurs when ischemic muscles are active and is relieved promptly by rest. Most frequently it is induced by walking and may be noted in the foot, calf, thigh, or buttock, depending upon the site of arterial occlusion.[11] The sensation that occurs with walking may be described as a "cramp," "charley horse," "numbness," "ache," or "weakness." Frequently patients will state that it is not a truly painful sensation. Regardless of the description of the discomfort, it occurs only with activity and is relieved promptly within a few minutes by rest. It usually forces the person to stop or slow his pace, but it is not necessary for him to sit down to obtain relief. Once the distress has disappeared, the patient may resume walking again, only to be stopped within a few minutes by the same distress. Patients who have occlusive disease in the subclavian or axillary artery may experience the same type of distress in the muscles of the forearm when writing, typing, washing windows, painting, or engaging in similar types of activity.

The occurrence of pain at rest signifies that ischemia is increasing in severity. Ischemic neuropathy is characterized by severe, lancinating, shooting, or shocklike pains that involve the foot and leg. As is true for other types of ischemic rest pain, pain of ischemic neuropathy is particularly troublesome at night and often requires narcotics for relief.

Pretrophic pain often heralds the onset of necrosis of tissue with ulceration; the pain is steady, boring, and well localized to two or three digits and the adjacent area of the foot which are most ischemic. It is a demoralizing type of pain that causes insomnia, anorexia, and depression, and forces the patient to dangle his foot over the edge of the bed in a dependent position for relief.

The pain of ulceration and gangrene is similar to, but more severe than, pretrophic pain. It occurs in an area of ulceration or gangrene and, like pretrophic pain, is usually relieved somewhat by placing the involved foot in a dependent position.

It is unlikely that ischemia of bone per se can cause pain and osteoporosis, but it is well recognized that in patients with severe ischemia osteoporosis often develops in the ischemic extremity. This is probably due to a combination of ischemia and prolonged disuse because of ischemic pain. The pain of osteoporosis occurs with weight bearing (with or without walking), and tenderness can be elicited by gentle but firm pressure applied to the ischemic foot. This type of pain is similar to that observed in Sudeck's atrophy, which may occur in the presence of normal arterial circulation, and for this reason one may assume that disuse is an important contributing factor to the painful osteoporosis observed in ischemic extremities.

Although chronic occlusive arterial disease can cause pallor or cyanosis and coolness of the skin of the involved extremity, it should be recognized that these are common subjective complaints of neurotic patients, and the diagnosis of chronic occlusive arterial disease should never be made on the basis of these complaints unless there are more specific symptoms and other objective findings. The diagnostic significance of these complaints is much greater if the changes in color and temperature are confined to one extremity or to one or two digits of an extremity. Mottled cyanosis (livedo reticularis) of the arms and legs is not a sign of chronic occlusive arterial disease. Raynaud's phenomenon is occasionally secondary to arteriosclerosis obliterans[12] and, more frequently, may be a symptom of thromboangiitis obliterans[13] when the upper extremities are involved.

When adequate collateral circulation is present, chronic occlusive arterial disease may produce no symptoms, the diagnosis being made on the basis of absence or definite diminution of pulsations in one or more peripheral arteries (exclusive of the dorsalis pedis).

Diagnosis

The diagnosis of chronic occlusive arterial disease can be established with certainty in well over 95 per cent of cases without the aid of special laboratory procedures. Plethysmography, oscillometry, and recordings of skin temperature are not necessary for the diagnosis of chronic occlusive arterial disease; moreover, the results can be misleading if not properly interpreted. Plain roentgenograms may demonstrate evidence of arterial calcification in some cases of atherosclerotic disease, but this is not necessarily an indication that there is obstruction to blood flow. Arteriography is important in the selection of patients for arterial surgical treatment and in helping the surgeon to plan this procedure, but it is essential to diagnosis only in those few cases in which there is a history suggesting chronic occlusive arterial disease but arterial pulsations are normal. The diagnosis of chronic occlusive arterial disease must be considered whenever a patient mentions pain or discomfort in the extremities. If arterial pulsations are normal in the symptomatic extremity, it is highly ·unlikely that the pain is due to ischemia. However, serious diagnostic errors can occur if the physician attributes all types of pain to ischemia just because arterial pulsations are diminished or absent. Chronic occlusive arterial disease is sometimes relatively asymptomatic, and the physician should be aware of the fact that osteoarthritis, peripheral neuropathy, degeneration of lumbar disks, and other types of nonischemic pain in the extremities can occur coincidentally with chronic occlusive arterial disease. Accurate diagnosis depends upon correlation of characteristic ischemic pain with the physical findings of occlusive arterial disease already described.

Differential Diagnosis

Usually the diagnosis of chronic occlusive arterial disease presents less difficulty than the establishment of the specific cause of the arterial obstruction. Trauma, arterial embolus, and acute arterial thrombosis usually can be ruled out on the basis of the history. Symptoms of nonspecific arteritis (Takayasu's disease) are confined to the upper extremities and/or to the brain. Once these uncommon causes for chronic occlusive arterial disease are ruled out, the differential diagnosis between arteriosclerosis obliterans and thromboangiitis obliterans must be made.

When symptoms of chronic occlusive arterial disease appear in persons older than fifty years,

the diagnosis is almost certainly arteriosclerosis obliterans. About 80 per cent of patients with this disease are men,[12,14,15] but the ratio of men to women becomes lower as age increases. The incidence of diabetes among patients with arteriosclerosis obliterans ranges from 20 to 33 per cent.[12,15] When arteriosclerosis obliterans affects men under the age of forty years, the differential diagnosis from thromboangiitis obliterans can be particularly difficult. Usually in this age range the lesions of arteriosclerosis appear first in the aorta or the iliac or femoral arteries, and the first symptom is intermittent claudication of the buttock, thigh, or calf. Pulsations may be diminished or absent in some of the arteries of the upper extremities, but ischemic symptoms of the hands rarely occur as the result of arteriosclerosis obliterans. Hypercholesteremia, diabetes, and roentgenographic evidence of arterial calcification favor the diagnosis of arteriosclerosis obliterans rather than thromboangiitis obliterans.

In contrast, thromboangiitis obliterans is predominantly a disease of young men, symptoms usually appearing before the age of thirty-five years and sometimes before the age of thirty years. Only 1 per cent of patients are women. Ninety-nine per cent of all patients are or have been heavy users of tobacco, usually cigarettes. Superficial thrombophlebitis, which occurs in about 40 per cent of cases, is a helpful diagnostic finding, for its concurrence with arteriosclerosis obliterans is coincidental only and therefore the frequency is low. Lesions of thromboangiitis obliterans characteristically appear first in the tibial arteries, producing intermittent claudication in the arch of the foot or calf. Ischemic symptoms in the upper extremities, especially ulcerations about the fingertips, are strong evidence favoring the diagnosis of thromboangiitis obliterans.

Prognosis

The life expectancy of patients with arteriosclerosis obliterans is compromised because of the high frequency of concomitant atherosclerotic complications in the brain and the heart.[14,16–19] The occlusive disease in the extremities contributes little if at all to the increased mortality. The mortality rate is higher in diabetic patients and in those who have clinical evidence of coexisting cerebral and/or coronary atherosclerosis than in those who do not have these complications.[15–17,19] On the other hand, the life expectancy of patients with thromboangiitis obliterans is not appreciably affected by this disease,[6] and this is an important reason for attempting to make a correct differential diagnosis.

Thromboangiitis obliterans is a greater threat to

limb survival than is arteriosclerosis obliterans. McPherson and colleagues[6] found that 12.6 per cent of patients with thromboangiitis obliterans required amputation of a leg whereas only 6.4 per cent of patients with arteriosclerosis obliterans required major amputation during a 10-year period. Other studies have confirmed the relatively high incidence of major amputations necessary for patients with thromboangiitis obliterans.[20,21] For nondiabetic patients with arteriosclerosis obliterans the incidence of major amputation has been reported to range from 4 to 11 per cent during follow-up periods of from 5 to 10 years.[15–17,19,22] The incidence of amputation for diabetic patients with arteriosclerosis obliterans ranges from 18 to 34 per cent.[15,22] The prognosis for survival of an extremity is better when intermittent claudication is the only symptom than when ischemia is severe enough to produce rest pain, ischemic ulcers, and gangrene.[16,22]

Major amputations of upper extremities are almost never necessary for chronic occlusive arterial disease regardless of the cause.

Treatment

Various surgical methods for revascularizing ischemic limbs have supplemented but have not replaced the more conventional and less glamorous principles of medical management.

Limitations of Surgical Treatment. Surgical treatment of chronic occlusive arterial disease is the subject of another chapter, but it is pertinent to a discussion of medical treatment to consider the limitations and disadvantages of direct arterial surgical procedures. Present surgical techniques are effective only when the occlusive disease is limited to segments of the large arteries; direct surgical attack is not technically feasible on the tibial arteries. A corollary of this is the fact that many patients with severe ischemia who would benefit most from reconstructive operations are not appropriate subjects, because the lesions are too diffuse and they involve the branches of the popliteal arteries, making revascularization procedures on the proximal arteries useless because runoff is inadequate. Segmental obstructive lesions confined to the aorta or the iliac or femoral arteries which are technically feasible to remove or bypass frequently cause intermittent claudication without severe ischemic changes in the skin. Follow-up studies have shown that intermittent claudication usually is not a progressive symptom[19] and does not cause great disability. Consequently only a minority of patients who have operable lesions are subjects for arterial surgical treatment if one uses progressive disability from intermittent claudication as the criterion for operation. Follow-up studies have

already been cited[16,18,19] which indicate that the survival rate of limbs, when intermittent claudication is the only manifestation of ischemia, is extremely good. Although DeWolfe and colleagues[23] have reported follow-up studies that show prognosis for survival of a limb is better after operative treatment than after medical treatment, the amputation rate for their patients not operated on was considerably higher than those reported by most other writers for conservative management. Peripheral arteriosclerosis obliterans is not a fatal disease per se; consequently reconstructive arterial operations do not prolong or preserve life. Furthermore they have no beneficial effect on atherogenesis, either locally or in other arterial beds, and consequently do not ameliorate or prevent atherosclerotic complications in the heart or the brain, or further arterial occlusion in the extremities. Surgical procedures in the aortoiliac region are associated with mortality rates of from 2 to 8 per cent.[24–27] As a matter of fact, the immediate mortality from this type of operation in some series approaches or even exceeds the 5-year amputation rate that can be expected in the natural course of the disease. The frequency of late failures of plastic grafts in the femoropopliteal region is so high that some surgeons no longer advise elective operations for femoropopliteal occlusion.[25,27] Infection at the site of plastic prostheses is an uncommon but disastrous complication that leads to prolonged convalescence and usually requires removal of the septic graft.[28]

Sympathectomy. Regional sympathectomy is indicated when signs and symptoms of ischemia progress despite adequate medical treatment and revascularization procedures are infeasible or inadvisable.

Principles of Medical Management. The goal of medical treatment is to preserve a functional limb, and this objective is accomplished by prophylactic measures to prevent necrosis of the ischemic skin, by preventing progression of the arterial disease whenever possible, by counteracting the discrepancy between metabolic demands and blood supply of ischemic tissue, by local treatment of ischemic ulcers and gangrene when they are already present, and by relief of ischemic pain.

Prophylaxis. There is nothing more important to patients with chronic occlusive arterial disease, regardless of its cause, than careful and detailed instructions concerning the care and hygiene of ischemic extremities. In from 33 to 50 per cent of patients who undergo amputation, the initiating factor that led to gangrene was some avoidable injury.[29,30] It is worthwhile to give each patient with chronic occlusive arterial disease a printed sheet of instructions and to go over them in detail with the patient. The patient must be warned about the dangers of even minor injuries to ischemic hands or feet. Thermal, chemical, and mechanical trauma should be scrupulously avoided. Only comfortable shoes that do not bind or rub should be worn, and new shoes should be broken in gradually by wearing them about an hour daily. Heat should never be applied directly to ischemic extremities, and the immersion of feet in hot water, a common practice among patients with chronic occlusive arterial disease, is to be strictly condemned. Similarly, exposure to cold temperatures should be avoided unless the patient is warmly attired and the ischemic extremity is adequately protected by proper footwear. Toenails should be cut straight across, and corns, calluses, and bunions should not be trimmed or incised except by physicians or podiatrists who are experienced in the management of ischemic extremities. If the skin is excessively dry and tends to crack or scale, hydrous lanolin or cocoa butter should be applied gently every day. Patent medicines for the treatment of corns, calluses, and "athlete's foot" should be avoided, for they may contain chemical irritants that can harm the ischemic skin. Adhesive tape or adhesive plasters should not be applied to the skin of ischemic extremities. Dermatophytosis should be treated promptly, since the fissures that are characteristic of this infection can act as the portal of entry for pathogenic bacteria. In the acute stage, dermatophytosis can be treated by soaking the feet for half an hour twice daily in a 1:10,000 solution of potassium permanganate. In the subacute stage an ointment containing undecylenic acid (Desenex) should be applied to the lesions at bedtime, and a powder containing undecylenic acid should be dusted into the shoes before daytime wear.

Preventing Progression of Arterial Disease. Tobacco in any form should be forbidden to all patients who have chronic occlusive arterial disease. The close relationship between thromboangiitis obliterans and cigarette smoking implicates tobacco as an etiologic agent in this condition, and clinical experience has shown that abstinence from tobacco is the *sine qua non* of treatment, since all other measures usually fail to halt progression of the disease unless the patient abstains totally and permanently from the use of tobacco. Follow-up studies have shown that in both arteriosclerosis obliterans[15,16] and thromboangiitis obliterans,[20,21] the incidence of major amputation is greater for patients who continue to smoke than for those who stop smoking.

The observed relationship between abnormalities of lipid metabolism and atherosclerosis makes it desirable to restrict saturated fat and cholesterol in the diets of patients with arteriosclerosis obliterans, especially when the serum cholesterol value is elevated. A diet containing less than 25 per cent of total calories in the form of saturated fat usually is satisfactory. Unsaturated vegetable oils such as corn oil or cottonseed oil can be used for baking and frying, and certain commercially available margarines, especially prepared to preserve the unsaturated state, are recommended. Anticholesteremic drugs are not used routinely, since none of those currently available are consistently effective and free of untoward or unpleasant side effects. Dietary restrictions are not necessary for patients with thromboangiitis obliterans.

When diabetes is present, it should be adequately controlled to prevent or to ameliorate complications such as infection and neuropathy which add to the problems of the management of arteriosclerosis obliterans.

Decreasing Discrepancy between Metabolic Demands and Blood Supply. When major arterial trunks are obstructed, dilatation of small collateral channels is advisable to increase the arterial blood supply to the ischemic extremity. Although many drugs are advertised as vasodilators, experience has shown that none of them is consistently effective when evaluated objectively in regard to clinical improvement or to measurable increase in blood flow when chronic occlusive arterial disease is present. For these reasons, vasodilating drugs are not routinely prescribed. When ischemia of the skin is becoming progressively worse or when ischemic ulcers are already present, a vasodilating drug such as phenoxybenzamine hydrochloride (Dibenzyline, 0.01 gm four times daily) or cyclandelate (Cyclospasmol, 0.1 or 0.2 gm four times daily) may be prescribed. Ethyl alcohol (30 or 60 ml whiskey three or four times daily) is as good as, and perhaps superior to, any of the vasodilating drugs currently available. In addition, it is an excellent anodyne and sedative, and may be helpful in controlling the pain of the ischemic lesions.

A warm environmental temperature tends to promote vasodilatation, whereas exposure to cold may compromise collateral circulation by direct and reflex vasoconstriction. Blood flow can sometimes be stimulated in ischemic feet by placing a thermostatically controlled heating unit[31] over them. Heat can be injurious to ischemic extremities; it should be used only when there is thermostatic control and when the temperature within the box never exceeds 90°F. This type of therapy should not be used if it makes the pain worse—an indication that heat is increasing the metabolic demands of tissues more than it is increasing the blood supply to the tissues.

The Sanders oscillating bed seems to be helpful in improving circulation for some patients. Patients are placed on this bed for 6 or 8 hr every day. Peripheral edema, uncontrolled infection, and cellulitis are contraindications to the use of the oscillating bed. Its use should be discontinued if it seems to aggravate rather than to alleviate pain. The advantages of this type of therapy are not great enough to encourage patients to purchase an oscillating bed for home use except in unusual circumstances.

Probably the best natural stimulus to the development of collateral circulation is judicious use of the ischemic extremity. Walking is excellent exercise, and patients with chronic occlusive arterial disease of the lower extremities should be encouraged to walk to tolerance several times daily, unless ischemic lesions are present or the patient has severe rest pain or ischemic neuropathy.

Treatment of Ischemic Ulcers and Gangrene. Ischemic ulcers and gangrene are the most feared complications of chronic occlusive arterial disease. Important in the management of these complications are bed rest (with elevation of the head of the bed if edema is not present), relief of pain, eradication of infection, and improvement of the arterial blood supply. Ischemic tissues are particularly susceptible to chemical irritants, so it is wise to use bland applications that are not likely to induce more necrosis.

To eradicate infection, the hand or foot may be soaked in a saturated solution of boric acid three or four times daily. The temperature of solutions applied to ischemic lesions should never exceed 95°F. Moist packs of a solution of boric acid or isotonic saline may be used continuously, provided that maceration of viable tissue is avoided. A 1:10,000 solution of potassium permanganate may be used to soak the foot, especially when active dermatophytosis is present.

Cultures of open lesions should be made, and sensitivity studies should be performed on the isolated organisms. Appropriate antibiotics can be administered orally, as it has been shown that therapeutic concentrations can be achieved in ischemic tissues.[32,33] Frequently the organisms isolated from ischemic ulcers are insensitive to antibiotics that can be administered parenterally with safety; in such cases it is sometimes helpful to use a 0.5 or 1.0 per cent solution or ointment of neomycin locally on the ulcer if boric acid soaks fail to alter the flora favorably.

To remove an adherent, necrotic crust or eschar from an ischemic ulcer, enzymatic debridement using streptokinase and streptodornase (Varidase) as a local application in a solution or in a jelly, or an ointment containing fibrinolysin and deoxyribo-nuclease (Elase) is preferable to surgical debridement, no matter how gentle.

When infection has been reduced to a minimum and the base of the ulcer is clean, application of powdered erythrocytes (Lyocyte powder) often seems to promote healing of ischemic ulcers. The erythrocyte powder is applied to the ulcer and is allowed to remain for several days, during which time it forms a crust; this crust is then removed by soaking the foot in a solution of boric acid. More erythrocyte powder is applied after inspection of the base ensures that the progress of healing is satisfactory.

Relief of Pain. It is fortunate that intermittent claudication produces only mild and transient discomfort, and usually is not a seriously incapacitating symptom, for there is no satisfactory medical treatment for this type of ischemic pain. When intermittent claudication becomes a serious handicap and interferes with the earning of a livelihood, arterial reconstructive surgical treatment should be considered.

Management of ischemic rest pain can be one of the most difficult therapeutic problems. When mild, ischemic pain can usually be controlled by the judicious use of salicylates in conjunction with ethyl alcohol in the form of whiskey, for alcohol is an analgesic as well as a vasodilator. Characteristically, rest pain is worse at night and interferes with sleep. Sometimes it is helpful to use barbiturates and/or chlorpromazine hydrochloride (Thorazine) with alcohol and salicylates. Usually, however, control of rest pain requires use of salicylates in combination with codeine or d-propoxyphene hydrochloride (Darvon), and not infrequently it is necessary to administer narcotics such as morphine sulfate or levorphan tartrate (Levo-Dromoran). The latter, in doses of 2 mg every 4 or 6 hr with or without chlorpromazine hydrochloride, is particularly helpful with minimal risk of addiction. Physicians tend to underestimate the severity of ischemic pain and therefore to undertreat it. This is an error, for if uncontrolled, ischemic pain leads to loss of sleep and appetite and may quickly exhaust and demoralize the patient. Furthermore, the pain of ischemia is frequently less severe if the foot is dependent; hence the tortured victim may resort to sitting in a chair to sleep or to allowing the painful limb to dangle over the edge of the bed. This, in turn, permits accumulation of edema fluid, which further embarrasses the already impoverished circulation. The physician should not hesitate to use enough narcotic to permit the patient to sleep comfortably throughout the night with his legs in the horizontal position.

Individualization of Therapy. In planning therapy for an individual patient, the stage of the disease and the degree of ischemia must be taken into consideration, for not every patient requires all the forms of treatment outlined in the preceding paragraphs. Every patient with chronic occlusive arterial disease should be admonished to stop smoking and should receive explicit instructions in the proper care and hygiene of ischemic extremities. Beyond this, treatment should be individualized for each patient.

When the only symptom is intermittent claudication and when collateral circulation is good as demonstrated by postural color tests, the patient should be encouraged to walk to tolerance several times daily, and to follow a diet restricted in saturated fat if he has hypercholesteremia. Routine use of vasodilating drugs for patients in this category is to be deprecated.

Bed rest is indicated for patients with ischemic rest pain, and the head of the bed should be elevated unless edema is present. Whiskey may be used as a vasodilator and anodyne for periods of 2 or 3 weeks. Other vasodilating procedures outlined previously may be employed. Relief of pain is extremely important, and narcotics should be given if necessary.

When ulceration and gangrene occur, treatment for these complications should be performed as outlined previously, in addition to the measures described in the preceding paragraph.

Direct arterial surgical treatment should be reserved for patients whose intermittent claudication interferes with gainful employment or whose extremities are so severely ischemic that amputation may become necessary in spite of good medical treatment. Sympathectomy is advisable for patients with progressive ischemia who are not subjects for direct arterial surgical treatment. Sympathectomy is of no value in the treatment of intermittent claudication.

Amputation. When all other measures fail to prevent irreversible gangrene or intractable pain, amputation is inevitable and should be performed at the lowest level commensurate with rapid healing. It is desirable to preserve the knee joint when possible, for it is easier to use a prosthesis successfully if the knee joint is intact. On the other hand, it is imprudent to risk nonhealing and a prolonged convalescence to preserve a crippled or a diseased knee joint which would make rehabilitation impossible. Kelly and Janes[34] found that amputation below the knee was justified when sudden arterial occlusion had not occurred recently and when the femoral (but not necessarily the popliteal) pulse was palpable. There should be no ischemic or infected lesions of the skin at the proposed site of amputation, and brisk bleeding at the time of the operation is an encouraging sign. As a matter of fact, the absence of brisk bleeding on incision should lead the surgeon to reconsider his decision to amputate below the knee. Digital and transmetatarsal amputations are more likely to succeed when ischemia is due to thromboangiitis than when it is due to arteriosclerosis.

Acute Arterial Occlusion of the Extremities

When a major artery to an extremity suddenly becomes occluded, survival of the patient as well as of the limb often depends upon prompt and intelligent management.

Etiology

The two most common causes for sudden occlusion of a peripheral artery are embolization and thrombosis in situ. Emboli originate within the cardiac chambers in approximately 96 per cent of cases.[35] Rheumatic mitral valvulitis with subsequent enlargement of the left atrium, acute myocardial infarction, and chronic congestive heart failure from any cause predispose to the formation of mural thrombi within the left ventricle or left atrium, and these may become detached to lodge as emboli in peripheral arteries. The presence of atrial fibrillation enhances the likelihood of formation of mural thrombus but is not an essential prerequisite. Intriguing but rare is the *paradoxical embolus*, which arises from a venous thrombus and is transported to the peripheral arterial circulation through a septal defect with a right-to-left shunt. Usually one or more previous pulmonary emboli have set the stage for the paradoxical embolus by increasing the blood pressure in the pulmonary circuit and right side of the heart, thereby creating a right-to-left shunt through an otherwise asymptomatic atrial septal defect. The most common peripheral site for lodging of an embolus is the bifurcation of the common femoral artery.[35,36]

Sudden local thrombosis in an artery usually occurs at the site of an atherosclerotic plaque. Sometimes sudden arterial thrombosis is the first clinical manifestation of peripheral atherosclerosis, but more often it occurs as an unexpected complication of symptomatic arteriosclerosis obliterans.[23] Acceleration of thromboplastin generation determined by means of a "retarded" thromboplastin-generation test has been demonstrated in approximately 70 per cent of patients with sudden arterial occlusion that complicates arteriosclerosis obliterans,[37] indicating that hypercoagulability of the blood may play an important role in this complication. Thrombosis may occur suddenly in arteries with no intimal disease, presumably because of a hypercoagulable state of the blood, and this type of *primary*, or *simple arterial*, thrombosis may complicate acute infectious diseases, carcinomatosis, chronic ulcerative colitis, or polycythemia vera.

Inadvertent or intentional ligation of an artery during surgical treatment is a rare cause for sudden arterial occlusion. Trauma to arteries may result in laceration, severance, or local thrombosis, any one of which can be responsible for acute ischemia in the extremity distal to the site of interruption. Arterial trauma will be discussed in a separate section of this chapter.

Pathology

Sudden interruption of blood flow through a major artery to an extremity results in acute ischemia of the tissues supplied by the diseased artery. If adequate collateral circulation is present, recovery without permanent residual is possible. In the absence of collateral circulation, however, ischemia may progress to necrosis and gangrene with loss of a portion of the extremity. In the majority of cases of sudden arterial occlusion, the involved limb will survive, but residual ischemic changes will have impaired its function. Ischemic neuropathy is a frequent sequela of sudden arterial occlusion, as is intermittent claudication. Necrosis of the muscles in the anterior compartment of the leg (anterior compartment syndrome) is an uncommon but important residual of sudden arterial occlusion leading to footdrop.[38] When ischemia is severe, venous endothelium is damaged, and the signs and symptoms of ischemic thrombophlebitis appear 2 or 3 days after the acute ischemic insult. When this occurs the extremity becomes swollen, and the resulting pressure on collateral vessels compromises the circulation even further and worsens the prognosis for ultimate recovery.

Pathologic Physiology

When a major arterial trunk to an extremity becomes occluded, the distal tissues must be nourished by collateral vessels, and the adequacy of the collateral circulation determines the eventual outcome. Initially there is usually reflex arterial spasm involving the main trunk proximal and distal to the site of occlusion as well as the small collateral channels. If the spasm is prolonged, endothelial damage occurs in the arterial tree, favoring deposition of thrombus in collateral channels and thereby diminishing the prospects for recovery. However, when the collateral channels remain patent and are reasonably adequate, it is unlikely that irreversible ischemia will occur. Spontaneous improvement with return of pulsations in major arteries shortly after arterial occlusion can occur by one of two mechanisms:

1. Sudden occlusion of a branch of a main arterial channel can give rise reflexly to spasm in the parent artery for a few minutes or hours, giving the clinical impression that a main arterial trunk has been occluded. When the spasm abates, the major arterial pulses can be felt, and the clinical picture improves rapidly, since occlusion of branch arteries or of one of two paired arteries (such as the anterior and posterior tibial and the radial and ulnar arteries) rarely leads to irreversible ischemia and gangrene.

2. Endogenous fibrinolysin may be responsible for dramatic clinical improvement within the first few minutes or hours after sudden arterial occlusion of major arterial trunks. Lysis may permit fragmentation of a large embolus, the resulting fragments being swept by the bloodstream to more distal sites in the extremity. Aterial pulsations in the large arteries suddenly return, and the extent and severity of ischemia diminish rather abruptly.

Clinical Features

Diagnosis of sudden arterial occlusion is usually correctly made in the presence of the typical clinical picture characterized by acute onset of pain, numbness, and hypesthesia of the involved extremity. In half the cases of sudden arterial occlusion, however, pain is not the initial symptom, and the onset is gradual.[39] In 25 per cent of cases, pain is entirely absent. In these cases the only symptoms may be numbness and coldness, and sometimes the only clinical manifestation of sudden arterial occlusion may be the abrupt appearance or worsening of intermittent claudication. Paresis is almost never the presenting complaint, and if it does occur, it usually appears several hours after other symptoms of ischemia have been present. The sudden onset of ischemic symptoms simultaneously in both lower extremities suggests the possibility of an embolus that has lodged at the bifurcation of the aorta (saddle embolus). The most important physical sign in establishing the diagnosis of sudden arterial occlusion is the absence or severe impairment of pulsations in arteries that were known or were assumed previously to have palpable pulsations. The diagnosis of sudden arterial occlusion of a major arterial trunk is untenable if arterial pulsations are normal throughout the extremity. The acutely ischemic extremity appears pale or cyanotic and is cold and hypesthetic or anesthetic, and the superficial veins are collapsed. In the later stages muscular weakness can sometimes be demonstrated.

Diagnosis

When pain, paresthesia, numbness, or coldness, singly or in various combinations, appear either abruptly or over a period of several hours in an extremity with no or diminished arterial pulsations, the diagnosis of sudden arterial occlusion should be made unless there is other obvious cause for the symptoms. The high frequency of atypical and often undramatic symptoms probably explains the observation that the clinical diagnosis of sudden arterial occlusion is suggested in less than half of the patients with this condition.[40] It is advisable routinely to palpate the pulses of any symptomatic extremity. If pulsations are normal, it is safe to assume that symptoms are not due to acute ischemia except in those rare cases where arterial occlusion has occurred distal to the wrists or ankles.

Once the diagnosis of sudden arterial occlusion is established, it is important to determine the level of the occlusion and to differentiate, if possible, between embolus and thrombosis in situ. Emboli usually lodge at bifurcations where the caliber of the artery is suddenly reduced. The site of the occlusion is peripheral to the most distal point at which normal pulsations are noted and proximal to the line at which the temperature of the skin changes from low to normal and to the zone of hypesthesia. Changes in temperature, color, and sensation may be minimal or absent when only one artery of two paired arteries is involved. When sudden arterial occlusion occurs in the presence of overt heart disease and especially if atrial fibrillation is present, it most likely is due to embolization. Recent myocardial infarction should be considered in every patient with acute arterial occlusion; therefore a careful history and an electrocardiogram should be obtained. When arterial occlusion occurs in the course of chronic occlusive arterial disease and in the absence of overt heart disease, it can usually be attributed to thrombosis in situ. When both these predisposing factors are present or when both are absent, an exact etiologic diagnosis may not be possible, but fortunately medical therapy of the ischemic limb is the same, regardless of whether thrombosis or embolism has caused the ischemia.

Differential Diagnosis

It is axiomatic that sudden arterial occlusion per se never produces edema, and this is helpful in differentiating this condition from acute thrombophlebitis. The simultaneous disappearance of arterial pulsations and onset of symptoms of ischemia are helpful in differentiating sudden arterial occlusion from osteoarthritis, peripheral neuropathy, lumbar disk protrusion, and other local conditions that cause pain and/or paresthesia in the extremities. When the status of the peripheral pulsations previous to the onset of symptoms is not definitely known, reliance must be placed upon other signs of acute ischemia, such as pallor or cyanosis of the skin, coolness of the involved extremity, and collapse of the superficial veins.

Prognosis

Without treatment, sudden arterial occlusion results in gangrene in about 50 per cent of cases.[39] Approximately 40 per cent of patients with untreated sudden arterial occlusion die, because most of them have serious cardiovascular disease.[39]

The use of anticoagulant therapy in the management of sudden arterial occlusion has improved the prognosis for survival of involved limbs, and it is now agreed that prompt medical treatment will restore circulation sufficiently to preserve the involved limbs for from 80 to 90 per cent of the patients who survive.[35,40–43] The mortality rate continues to be discouragingly high, however, ranging from 20 to 40 per cent.[40,42–45] It is higher for patients who have arteriosclerotic heart disease as the source for emboli than for those with rheumatic heart disease.[43–45] Although prognosis for limb survival is somewhat worse when sudden arterial occlusion is due to thrombosis than when it is due to embolism,[39] the site of the occlusion has an even greater bearing on the outcome. Prognosis for survival of an upper extremity is far better than that for a lower extremity, and the prognosis for survival of a lower limb is worst when the aorta or common iliac artery is occluded, and the prognosis becomes increasingly better as the site of occlusion becomes more distal.[35,42]

Treatment

Embolectomy, thromboendarterectomy, or bypass graft is the treatment of choice if the site of occlusion is proximal to the popliteal artery, if irreversible ischemic changes have not already taken place and if the condition of the patient is good enough to make the risks acceptable. Unfortunately most of the patients who have embolic arterial occlusion are victims of serious heart disease, and the risk of embolectomy, even under local anesthesia, is considerable. The mortality rate for embolectomy ranges from 36 to 50 per cent.[35,43,46,47] Salvage rates of ischemic limbs by early embolectomy range from 65 to 100 per cent of those patients who survive.[35,36,42–47] Surgical treatment for sudden arterial occlusion is discussed in another chapter.

Although proper medical treatment, instituted within the first 3 to 6 hr, compares favorably with surgical treatment insofar as limb salvage is concerned, there can be little argument that limbs saved by embolectomy or thromboendarterectomy will be less ischemic and therefore more functional than those treated conservatively. However, it is unwise to attempt surgical treatment for a seriously ill patient whose general condition is so precarious that the chance of saving a limb is not much greater than the risk of losing a life.

As soon as the diagnosis of sudden arterial occlusion has been made, heparin sodium should be administered intravenously without delay, unless there are strong contraindications to its use. Even though surgical treatment is being considered, it is advisable to maintain anticoagulation by the injection of heparin until shortly before the operation is started. If the coagulation time is unduly prolonged, the effect of heparin can be neutralized immediately before operation with protamine sulfate. For prompt anticoagulant effect, aqueous heparin (5,000 U.S.P. units, undiluted) should be administered intravenously, and this dose can be repeated every 3 or 4 hr. For those patients who are not subjects for operation, 10,000 or 20,000 U.S.P. units of concentrated aqueous heparin can be administered subcutaneously. The injection should be repeated whenever the coagulation time falls below twice the pretreatment value. If the dosage is properly adjusted, only two to four injections will be required in a 24-hr period. A coumarin anticoagulant can be administered as soon as it is decided that the patient is not to undergo surgical treatment, and the treatment with heparin can be discontinued when the prothrombin time is within the therapeutic range.

In addition to anticoagulation, relief of pain and of arterial spasm are important and urgent considerations in the management of sudden arterial occlusion. Narcotics are often necessary to relieve pain and should be given in adequate doses as often as necessary. To relieve arterial spasm papavarine hydrochloride may be given intravenously or injected directly into the artery proximal to the site of occlusion. The usual dose of 0.032 or 0.065 Gm may be given every 3 to 4 hr as long as the need exists. Instead of papavarine or if papavarine fails to produce vasodilatation, tolazoline hydrochloride (Priscoline hydrochloride) may be given intravenously or intraarterially in doses of 0.025 or 0.05 Gm. Ethyl alcohol is a good vasodilator and should be given, in addition to papavarine or tolazoline hydrochloride, as whiskey, in amounts of 30 or 60 ml every 2 to 4 hr depending on the tolerance of the patient. Warm environmental temperature tends to relieve arterial spasm, so the patient should be placed in a room where it is possible to keep the temperature between 80 and 85°F. In addition it is often advisable to wrap the involved extremity loosely in cotton to preserve body heat and to protect it from trauma.

The blocking of appropriate sympathetic ganglions has been advocated in the treatment of sudden arterial occlusion. This should be done

before heparin is administered and should not be repeated while effective anticoagulation is being maintained, because of the danger of bleeding at the sites of injection. Anticoagulation is more important in the management of sudden arterial occlusion than is regional sympathetic denervation, and for this reason anticoagulant drugs should not be withheld for the purpose of blocking sympathetic ganglions safely.

The head of the bed should be elevated on blocks that are 8 or 10 in. high, so that the feet are in a dependent position and the effect of gravity will augment the flow of blood into the ischemic extremity.

The efficacy of activated fibrinolysin or its activating enzyme (streptokinase) in the treatment of sudden arterial occlusion has not been proved. If these agents are to be employed, they should be used in addition to, and not instead of, conventional anticoagulation therapy.

Refrigeration of an ischemic extremity is contraindicated as long as there is hope for its survival. When amputation is obviously inevitable but the general condition of the patient makes the procedure hazardous, valuable time can be gained, pain can be relieved, and the absorption of toxins stopped by packing the gangrenous extremity in ice. Refrigeration can be maintained for several days while the patient is being prepared for amputation.

It is worth reemphasizing that elevation of an acutely ischemic extremity and the application of heat to it are contraindicated and may hasten the onset of gangrene.

Arterial Trauma

Trauma to arteries may result in laceration, severance, thrombosis, or aneurysm formation. Traumatic aneurysms may be true aneurysms but are more likely to be false aneurysms or arteriovenous aneurysms (arteriovenous fistulas).

Clinical Features

Severance, laceration, or acute traumatic thrombosis of an artery is accompanied by the clinical picture of sudden arterial occlusion previously described. If trauma has been confined to one extremity, the physician's attention will usually be focused upon the region, and the acute arterial insufficiency will be detected. However, if the patient has sustained multiple injuries and, especially, if he is unconscious, arterial trauma may go undetected until irreparable ischemia and gangrene supervene. For this reason it is advisable to palpate the peripheral arteries of all patients who have sustained trauma. If the artery is severed or lacerated, hemorrhage or hematoma will usually direct attention to the involved extremity. False aneurysm formation may occur at the site of arterial laceration, and if an artery and a vein lying in juxtaposition are lacerated, an arteriovenous fistula may result. The latter should be suspected if a continuous thrill can be palpated and a continuous bruit can be heard over the hematoma.

Prognosis

It is interesting that the prognosis for survival of a lower limb after traumatic thrombosis or severance of an artery is worst in the popliteal region and becomes increasingly better as the site of injury becomes more proximal.[48] The opposite is true for spontaneous thrombosis or embolism. Trauma to major arteries of the extremities has resulted in amputation in about 50 per cent of cases without surgical intervention.[49]

Treatment

It is well understood that injuries to the most vital areas should take precedence, for the saving of a life is more important than the saving of a limb. If the patient's general condition permits, operation is usually indicated for traumatic arterial occlusion, laceration, or severance, for in general such patients are young and do not have concomitant cardiovascular disease that makes the risk of surgical treatment great. When arteriorrhaphy or direct anastomosis is not possible, autogenous vein grafts or Dacron prostheses should be used to bridge or bypass the occluded or severed area.[49-51] If surgical intervention is considered too hazardous, medical treatment for traumatic arterial thrombosis is similar to that for arterial embolus or sudden spontaneous thrombosis in situ, except that anticoagulants are contraindicated if trauma has led to hemorrhage.

Arterial Aneurysms

Arterial aneurysms may be classified as true aneurysms, false aneurysms, dissecting aneurysms (dissecting hematomas), and arteriovenous aneurysms (arteriovenous fistulas).

True Aneurysms

True aneurysms are localized dilatations of arteries which result from atrophy of the media; they may be fusiform or saccular.

Etiology. Most arterial aneurysms are arteriosclerotic. Syphilitic aneurysms have seldom been encountered since the advent of penicillin. When they do occur, they are almost always located in the ascending portion or the arch of the thoracic aorta. Mycotic aneurysms are even rarer than syphilitic aneurysms. Trauma sometimes results in true aneurysmal formation, especially in the thoracic aorta, but usually trauma causes false aneurysms rather than true aneurysms. Studies of large series of aneurysms indicated that more than 95 per cent of aneurysms of the abdominal aorta[52] and popliteal artery[53] were arteriosclerotic in origin. Holman has postulated and offered evidence that some aneurysms may represent exaggerated poststenotic dilatations.[54]

Clinical Features. Arteriosclerotic aneurysms occur predominantly in men, usually after the age of fifty years.

The most common site for aneurysm is the abdominal aorta. Abdominal aortic aneurysms may reach tremendous proportions without producing symptoms, and often the diagnosis is first made by palpating the abdomen. When the aneurysm becomes large enough to exert pressure on adjacent structures, pain is usually located in the back, flank, or abdomen and may extend into the thigh and testis. Usually the pain is more noticeable on the left side, since the aneurysm usually is left of the midline. Anteroposterior and lateral roentgenograms of the lumbar spine may show evidence of a soft-tissue mass with a curvilinear rim of calcification on its walls (Fig. 56-4). Frequently, however, the aneurysm is not visible on plain roentgenograms. Aortography is usually not necessary in confirming the diagnosis of abdominal aortic aneurysm and can be misleading if a laminated thrombus fills the aneurysmal sac, leaving a lumen of fairly normal caliber.

Evidence of aneurysms of the thoracic aorta is often discovered on plain roentgenograms of the chest before symptoms occur. Symptoms are due to pressure on contiguous structures and include cough, hoarseness, dysphagia, pain, and venous distension.

Visceral aneurysms are rare and usually asymptomatic until they rupture. Hypertension may be associated with aneurysms of the renal artery, and splenomegaly may be a sign of aneurysm of the splenic artery. The diagnosis may be suggested by plain roentgenograms of the abdomen when thin, ringlike calcifications are visualized. Visceral aneurysms not containing calcium will cast no shadows on the plain roentgenograms. Aortography has led to greater awareness of visceral aneurysms that sometimes are found incidentally when this procedure is carried out for other diagnostic purposes. Splenic aneurysms are the exception to the rule that aneurysms are usually arteriosclerotic and occur predominantly in men. Bedford and Lodge[55] reported that women comprised 70 per cent of their patients with splenic aneurysms, and the underlying pathologic change was medial degeneration.

The most common site for peripheral aneurysms is the popliteal artery. Popliteal aneurysms pro-

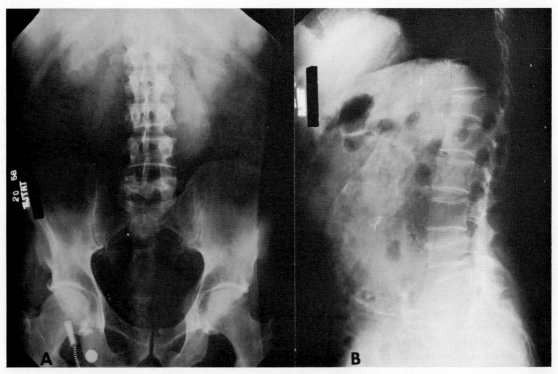

Fig. 56-4. Roentgenograms showing mural calcification of abdominal aortic aneurysm. (*A*). Anteroposterior view with characteristic curvilinear calcification extending to the left of the spine. *B*. Sometimes the aneurysm is seen better in a lateral view.

duce symptoms of acute arterial occlusion if mural thrombus abruptly propagates to occlude the artery or if it gives rise to emboli distally. Popliteal aneurysms also may cause pain in the popliteal region when they become large enough to exert pressure on the medial popliteal nerve and will cause edema and venous distension if the popliteal vein is compressed. The diagnosis usually is made easily by palpating a pulsating, expansile mass in the popliteal space. When thrombosis of the aneurysm has occurred, a firm, nonpulsatile mass may be felt. In doubtful cases, femoral arteriography may be helpful but usually is not necessary. Aneurysms of the iliac artery usually produce no symptoms until they rupture. Diagnosis can be made by palpating an expansile, pulsatile mass in the abdomen above the inguinal ligament. Aneurysms may also occur in the brachiocephalic (innominate), subclavian, femoral, radial, and ulnar arteries. The appearance of pulsatile masses in these regions is a clue to diagnosis.

Prognosis. Estes[52] reported that only 19 per cent of patients with abdominal aortic aneurysms survived for 5 years after the diagnosis was made and that most of the deaths were due to rupture of the aneurysm. Wright and colleagues[56] reported

a higher mortality rate. The prognosis is better for patients with asymptomatic aneurysms that are less than 7.5 cm in diameter than for patients with larger or symptomatic aneurysms.[57,58] Once an abdominal aneurysm (or any aneurysm) becomes symptomatic, rupture is imminent. Five-year survival rate for patients after diagnosis of thoracic aortic aneurysms is less than 10 per cent.[24]

Although Owens and Coffey[59] reported that rupture occurred in 46 per cent of the splenic artery aneurysms reported in the literature, it seems reasonable to assume that reports of aneurysms that ruptured are more likely to be published than are reports of asymptomatic aneurysms. Asymptomatic splenic artery aneurysms have been found in 10.4 per cent of 250 consecutive postmortem examinations without a single instance of rupture.[55] Poutasse[60] has concluded that small asymptomatic calcified aneurysms of the renal artery are not likely to rupture.

Rupture is an uncommon complication of popliteal aneurysms, but these aneurysms often lead to amputation due to arterial occlusion from thrombosis within the aneurysm or distal embolization. In one series of 77 untreated popliteal aneurysms the amputation rate was 23 per cent.[53] Rupture of iliac aneurysms occurred in 16 per cent in one series, with an 80 per cent mortality rate associated with rupture.[61]

Treatment. Surgical extirpation with appropriate arterial reconstruction is the treatment of choice for most aneurysms if the patient's condition is good enough to permit operation. Possible contraindications include small asymptomatic abdominal aortic aneurysms in patients who have coronary or cerebrovascular disease,[57] asymptomatic small calcified renal artery aneurysms in normotensive patients,[60] and asymptomatic aneurysms of the splenic artery.[55] Splenic aneurysms are particularly likely to rupture during the third trimester of pregnancy, and for this reason resection is recommended in women of childbearing age. Resection of abdominal and thoracic aortic aneurysms carries a significant mortality rate, but usually the risk of eventual rupture is even greater.[24] Once rupture has occurred, the risk of surgical treatment is greatly increased.[62] In general the appearance of symptoms heralds the rupture of an aneurysm, and the indications for operation become accordingly urgent. Surgical treatment of aneurysms is discussed in another chapter.

False Aneurysms

False aneurysms result from rupture of true aneurysms or from penetrating trauma to an artery. The clinical manifestations are similar to those of true aneurysm, consisting of an expansile, pulsatile mass. On the basis of clinical history it may be possible to suspect that an aneurysm is false rather than true, but only a pathologic diagnosis can distinguish the two; the distinguishing feature of the false aneurysm is the break in continuity of all three coats of the arterial wall, permitting the extravascular accumulation of blood in adjacent tissues. The wall of the false aneurysmal sac is therefore composed of a mixture of organized blood clot and dense connective tissue. Clinically, the diagnosis and management of false aneurysms are the same as those already described for true aneurysms.

Dissecting Aneurysms (Dissecting Hematomas)

Dissecting aneurysms or dissecting hematomas result when blood gains access to the medial coat of the aorta. The layers of the media are dissected so that a false channel is formed between the adventitia and the intima.

Etiology. The cause of medial necrosis of the aorta, which predisposes to the development of dissecting aneurysm, is not known. Dissecting aneurysm is frequently associated with Marfan's syndrome and occasionally is a complication of pregnancy, but most of the patients are middle-aged or older hypertensive men.

Pathology. It seems likely that the vasa vasorum of the aorta may rupture and allow bleeding to take place into the diseased media. The intima may rupture because of poor medial support, thereby allowing blood to pass from the aortic lumen directly into the media. At times dissection of the aorta occurs without any rent in the intima.[63] Dissection begins at the root of the aorta in 60 per cent of cases and proceeds for various distances around the arch and into the descending thoracic and abdominal aorta.[63] Sometimes the dissection is carried to the bifurcation of the aorta and on into one or both iliac arteries. One or more branches of the aorta may become occluded by the dissecting process.

Clinical Features. Dissecting aneurysm usually produces a dramatic as well as a catastrophic chain of events. Characteristically, dissection is accompanied by the abrupt onset of severe pain in the chest, both anteriorly and posteriorly, radiating into the neck, down one or both arms, into the back, and into both lower extremities. Profuse diaphoresis and ashen-gray pallor in the absence of shock attest to the severity of the pain. If pain is confined to the chest, the differential diagnosis between this condition and acute myocardial infarction may be a difficult one. Absence of one or more peripheral arterial pulsations, especially carotid or brachial, an aortic diastolic murmur that was not present previously, paradoxical pulse (due to cardiac tamponade from rupture of a dissecting aneurysm into the pericardial sac), widening of the mediastinal shadow visible by fluoroscopy or on roentgenograms, and the absence of typical electrocardiographic changes of acute infarction are helpful differential diagnostic clues. Occasionally paraplegia may result from interruption of blood supply to the spinal cord.

It is not widely recognized that dissecting hematoma frequently produces atypical symptoms. Pain was absent in almost half of the patients in one series,[64] and sometimes shock, dyspnea, coma, confusion, or bizarre neurologic defects singly or in various combinations dominate the clinical picture.

Prognosis. Approximately 20 per cent of patients with dissecting aneurysm of the aorta die within 24 hr, and 37 per cent within 48 hr.[63] Although exsanguinating hemorrhage may occur anywhere along the aorta, rupture into the pericardial sac or the left pleural cavity is the most frequent cause of death. At times the dissection terminates spontaneously when the intramural column of blood reenters the natural lumen through a more distal rent in the intima, resulting in a "double-barreled aorta." Only 7 per cent of the patients reported by Hirst, Johns, and Kime[63] survived longer than 1 year.

Treatment. The only satisfactory treatment is surgical intervention before fatal exsanguination occurs. Surgical treatment is discussed in another chapter.

Arteriovenous Aneurysms (Arteriovenous Fistulas)

Arteriovenous fistulas are abnormal direct communications between arteries and veins without the interposition of capillaries; there are two types: acquired and congenital. The hemodynamic effects of peripheral arteriovenous fistulas are discussed in another chapter; consequently, only the peripheral manifestations will be described here.

Acquired Arteriovenous Fistulas. Acquired arteriovenous fistulas result from penetrating trauma or from erosion of an arterial aneurysm into the accompanying vein and usually consist of a single communication between an artery and vein that lie in close proximity. If the arteriovenous fistula is near the surface, a pulsatile mass is palpable.

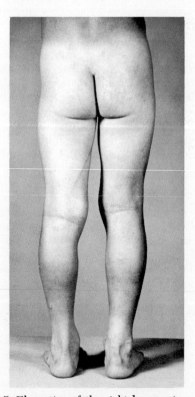

Fig. 56-5. Elongation of the right lower extremity of a 5-year-old boy caused by multiple congenital arteriovenous fistulas.

The diagnostic features of arteriovenous fistula are the continuous thrill and bruit over it. Obliteration of the fistula by manual compression of it or its afferent artery is usually followed promptly by a sharp decrease in pulse rate (Branham's bradycardiac sign). The skin overlying an arteriovenous fistula is unusually warm, and because of increased venous pressure there may be signs of chronic venous insufficiency with incompetent varicose veins in the extremity distal to the fistula. Arterial supply to the extremity may be compromised, and the ipsilateral foot or hand is usually cooler than the opposite normal mate.[65,66] Ischemic ulcers as well as stasis ulcers may occur on the extremity beyond the fistula.

Arteriography is essential for diagnosis only for those fistulas that are situated so deeply that the pulsatile mass, thrill, and bruit cannot be detected.

The only satisfactory treatment is excision of the fistula, with restoration of arterial continuity whenever possible.

Congenital Arteriovenous Fistulas. Congenital arteriovenous fistulas are usually multiple and involve small cutaneous and subcutaneous arteries and veins. Frequently they are accompanied by prominent birthmarks on the skin of the extremity. Congenital fistulas of this type lead to elongation of the long bones of the affected extremity and thus to a measurable lengthening of the entire limb when compared with the uninvolved companion extremity (Fig. 56-5). The skin of the extremity harboring congenital arteriovenous fistulas is frequently warmer than the skin of the opposite extremity. Signs of chronic venous insufficiency including edema, dilated superficial veins, varicosities in atypical locations, and stasis pigmentation with or without stasis ulceration are frequently associated with congenital arteriovenous fistulas because of increased venous pressure. Because the fistulas are small and multiple, thrills and bruits are seldom detected, and there are no localized pulsatile masses.

Arteriography is sometimes helpful in establishing the diagnosis of congenital arteriovenous fistulas. An increased oxygen content of the venous blood from the involved limb as compared with that of the opposite limb is a pathognomonic sign of arteriovenous fistula.

Treatment of congenital arteriovenous fistulas is not satisfactory, since usually it is impossible to eradicate the numerous small abnormal arteriovenous communications. Ligation of arterial branches that lead to the fistulas may give partial relief. The use of an elastic bandage or stocking is advisable to prevent edema and the other complications of chronic venous insufficiency.

Arteriospastic Diseases

Acrocyanosis, livedo reticularis, and Raynaud's phenomenon result from spasm of small arteries and arterioles in the skin and subcutaneous tissues without actual organic occlusion. Although they usually occur separately, two of these conditions and sometimes all three may occur concomitantly.

Etiology

The cause of arteriospasm, which is the common denominator of these three conditions, is unknown. It has been postulated that in Raynaud's disease increased sympathetic tone may be responsible,[67] but it is equally probable that for unexplained reasons the peripheral arteries of patients with this condition are unusually susceptible to normal sympathetic innervation or to a cold environment.[68] Mendlowitz and Naftchi[69] found no evidence of increased sensitivity to the vasconstricting action of norepinephrine in patients with Raynaud's disease and concluded that in some patients with this condition increased vasomotor tone is responsible while in others there is intrinsic vascular disease with normal vasomotor responses. Peacock[70] found abnormally high concentration of norepinephrine in venous blood coming from the hands of patients with Raynaud's disease.

Clinical Features

Typically, the arteriospastic disorders affect young women who are nervous, easily fatigued, emotionally labile, and often unmarried. The clinical manifestations are localized to the skin of the extremities and are characterized by changes in color and temperature. The location, appearance, and duration of the color changes are important in making a differential diagnosis of the arteriospastic disorders.[71] In addition to the typical color changes of the skin, the hands and feet may be chronically cold and often tend to perspire excessively.

Acrocyanosis is the rarest and most innocuous of the arteriospastic disorders. The arteriospasm is persistent and is confined to the hands and/or feet, and as a result they are chronically cyanotic. The cyanosis tends to be less severe in a warm environment, but it usually does not disappear entirely and is a source of embarrassment to the patients, who are usually young ladies. Major arterial pulsations are always palpable, although at times it is necessary to have the patient in a warm environment to demonstrate them. The absence of clubbing and of cyanosis elsewhere, as well as the lack of heart murmurs and of other signs of heart disease, serve to distinguish this benign condition from cyanotic heart disease. The prognosis is excellent, inasmuch as gangrene and other complications of ischemia never occur.

Livedo reticularis is more frequently observed than is acrocyanosis and is characterized by mottled or reticulated cyanotic discoloration of the skin (Fig. 56-6). Livedo reticularis not only involves the hands and feet but may extend onto the arms and legs and, in some cases, is apparent on the buttocks and the trunk. The reticulated or fishnet pattern of cyanosis is more notable when the patients are in a cold environment or are emotionally upset, but it usually can be demonstrated to some degree at all times, except for the evanescent but common condition of cutis marmorata, which is simply intermittent livedo reticularis that appears only when the patient is in a cool environment and disappears when he is warm. Livedo reticularis usually does not cause pain unless ischemic ulceration of the skin occurs. Pulsations are normal in the peripheral arteries, provided that the patient is in a warm environment. Livedo reticularis may be primary, in which case it exists in the absence of any underlying or causative disease, or it may be secondary

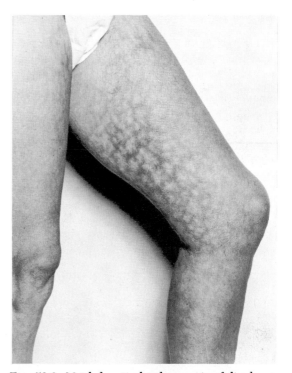

Fig. 56-6. Mottled, reticulated cyanosis of livedo reticularis involving the thigh and to a lesser extent the leg. (*From R. W. Gifford, Jr.: Arteriospastic Disorders of the Extremities, Circulation, 27:970, 1963. Reproduced by permission of the American Heart Association, Inc.*)

to such conditions as systemic lupus erythematosus, periarteritis nodosa, or cryoglobulinemia. Primary, or idiopathic, livedo reticularis infrequently leads to complications and is usually only cosmetically objectionable to the patient. Secondary, or symptomatic, livedo reticularis sometimes results in ischemic ulcerations at the tips of the digits or in the malleolar areas. The ischemic ulcerations resulting from livedo reticularis may be difficult to heal, but amputation is seldom, if ever, necessary.

Raynaud's phenomenon is characterized by intermittent changes in color of the skin of the fingers and/or toes (Fig. 56-7). The change in color persists for only a few minutes at a time. Rarely is the entire hand or foot affected, and often only one or two digits at a time are involved. Typically the affected digits turn dead white (pallor phase), after which they become cyanotic (cyanotic phase). Before normal color returns to the affected parts, they may become excessively hyperemic (rubor phase) because of reactive vasodilatation. Raynaud's phenomenon can occur without the rubor phase, but pallor and/or cyanosis must be present before the diagnosis of Raynaud's phenomenon is. tenable. The color changes of Raynaud's phenomenon are usually induced by exposure of the affected extremity or the entire body to a cool or cold environment. Occasionally the typical color changes occur when the patient is emotionally upset, and sometimes they occur for no obvious reason.

Raynaud's phenomenon is often secondary to some disease or condition that may not be clinically obvious at the time when the vasospastic phenomena first appear.[72] Some of the diseases or conditions that may manifest Raynaud's phenome-

Table 56-1. CAUSES OF SECONDARY RAYNAUD'S PHENOMENON: CONDITIONS TO BE RULED OUT BEFORE DIAGNOSIS OF RAYNAUD'S DISEASE (PRIMARY RAYNAUD'S PHENOMENON) CAN BE MADE

1. Occlusive arterial disease
   a. Arteriosclerosis obliterans (10% of patients demonstrate Raynaud's phenomenon[12])
   b. Thromboangiitis obliterans (30% of patients demonstrate Raynaud's phenomenon[13])
2. Systemic diseases
   a. Systemic scleroderma[73]
   b. Rheumatoid arthritis[74]
   c. Systemic lupus erythematosus[74]
   d. Periarteritis nodosa
3. Trauma
   a. Pneumatic-hammer disease[75]
   b. Raynaud's phenomenon in typists and pianists
   c. Occupational occlusive arterial disease of the hand[76] (mechanics, butchers, creamery workers, gynecologists, farmers, plumbers, etc.)
4. Neurogenic lesions
   a. Thoracic outlet syndromes (scalenus anticus syndrome, hyperabduction syndrome, costoclavicular syndrome)
   b. Diseases of nervous system (multiple sclerosis, peripheral neuropathy, transverse myelitis, syringomyelia, hemiplegia, myelodysplasia, causalgia, and spinal cord tumors)
5. Intoxication
   a. Lead
   b. Arsenic
   c. Ergot
6. Abnormalities of blood
   a. Cryoglobulins
   b. Cold agglutinins
7. Late result of cold injury
   a. Trench foot
   b. Immersion foot
   c. Frostbite

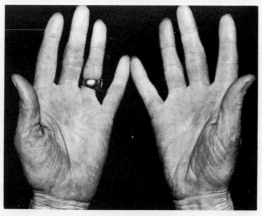

Fig. 56-7. Pallor phase of Raynaud's phenomenon involving the fingers. (*From R. W. Gifford, Jr.: Arteriospastic disorders of the extremities, Circulation, 27:970, 1963. Reproduced by permission of the American Heart Association, Inc.*)

non as a symptom are listed in Table 56-1. Among the most common causes of secondary Raynaud's phenomenon are rheumatoid arthritis, systemic lupus erythematosus, and systemic scleroderma. Indications that Raynaud's phenomenon may be secondary to some underlying disease include onset after the age of fifty years, especially in men; unilateral Raynaud's phenomenon, especially when confined to one or two digits; rapid progression to ulceration shortly after onset of symptoms; extensive ulceration or gangrene; and presence of fever, systemic symptoms, anemia, and elevation of sedimentation rate of erythrocytes. When one or more of the peripheral arterial pulses are reduced in amplitude or are not palpable in the symptomatic extremity or when the Allen compression test is positive (Fig. 56-2), the physician should suspect that Raynaud's phenomenon is secondary to chronic occlusive arterial disease such as arteriosclerosis obliterans,[12] thromboangiitis obliterans,[13] or chronic occupational trauma of the hand.[76]

The diagnosis of primary Raynaud's phenomenon, or Raynaud's disease, cannot be made until the diseases and conditions listed in Table 56-1 have been ruled out. Allen and Brown[77] proposed the following criteria for establishing the diagnosis of primary Raynaud's disease: (1) episodes of Raynaud's phenomenon excited by cold or emotion; (2) bilaterality of Raynaud's phenomenon; (3) absence of gangrene or, if present, its limitation to minimal grades of cutaneous gangrene; (4) presence of normal pulsations in the palpable arteries; (5) absence of any other primary disease that might be causal (see Table 56-1); and (6) duration of symptoms for at least 2 years (to permit any occult underlying disease to become manifest).

Extensive gangrene does not occur as a complication of Raynaud's disease, and major amputations never are necessary. In a large series of patients, fewer than 30 per cent had complications of Raynaud's disease, and less than 1 per cent required amputation of one or more phalanges.[74] The chief complications are sclerodactylia, which refers to sclerodermatous changes that remain confined to the skin of the digits (in contradistinction to progressive involvement of systemic scleroderma), and trophic changes such as ulceration, superficial necrosis, scarring, and fissuring of the tips of the digits, or chronic paronychia.

The prognosis for patients with secondary Raynaud's phenomenon depends upon the underlying disease and may be quite dismal in regard to survival and cutaneous necrosis. The importance and difficulties of correct differential diagnosis are illustrated by the fact that of 220 patients with systemic scleroderma 81 per cent had Raynaud's phenomenon as a symptom and in 32 per cent it was the initial manifestation.[73] Nearly 50 per cent of these patients were dead after an average follow-up period of 9 years, and 40 per cent of them had trophic ulcerations of their fingers as a result of their disease. On the other hand, of 307 women with primary Raynaud's disease whose progress was followed for an average period of 12 years after the diagnosis was established, only 12 died, and none of the deaths was due to Raynaud's disease.[74] In less than 10 per cent of these patients ischemic ulcerations of the fingers developed during the period of follow-up.

Treatment

Most patients with acrocyanosis, livedo reticularis, or Raynaud's disease require no specific treatment other than reassurance that the condition is benign and will not lead to major amputation, as so many of them fear. They should be advised to avoid unnecessary exposure to cold and to wear warm clothing as well as gloves whenever they go out in cool or cold weather. Housewives should avoid defrosting of refrigerators. Patients with Raynaud's disease should avoid mechanical and chemical trauma as much as possible. Repeated exposure of the hands to water and detergents leads to drying and fissuring of the skin. Patients with Raynaud's disease should be advised to apply an emollient such as lanolin to the fingers at least twice daily and oftener if the hands are exposed to water and detergents. These precautions are not so necessary for patients with acrocyanosis and livedo reticularis, since dryness and fissuring of the skin are less likely to occur in these conditions.

Vasodilating drugs are not necessary routinely in the management of any of these diseases. If symptoms are unusually severe, phenoxybenzamine hydrochloride (Dibenzyline) may be administered in doses of 0.01 or 0.02 Gm three or four times daily. Often the side effects of vasodilating drugs are more troublesome than the disease itself. If phenoxybenzamine hydrochloride is not well tolerated, cyclandelate (Cyclospasmol) may be administered in doses of 0.1 or 0.2 Gm three or four times daily.

Sympathectomy may be beneficial in all these conditions. Since acrocyanosis is primarily a cosmetic defect that never leads to complications, sympathectomy is seldom if ever advisable. When livedo reticularis is complicated by ischemic ulcerations, sympathectomy may be helpful in healing them and keeping them healed. Sympathectomy should be advised for patients with Raynaud's disease when conservative measures fail to prevent or to control ischemic ulcerations at the tips of the digits. Experience has shown that less than 25 per cent of patients with Raynaud's disease require sympathectomy and that it is beneficial in about two-thirds of the patients who have this operation.[78] The results are much better in the lower extremities than in the upper, where the disease is usually much more severe. Sympathectomy for secondary Raynaud's phenomenon has yielded such poor results that it should be recommended only in unusual circumstances.[78]

Treatment of ischemic ulcerations secondary to livedo reticularis or Raynaud's disease is similar to that already discussed for ulcerations secondary to chronic occlusive arterial disease. The affected part should be soaked in a lukewarm saturated solution of boric acid for ½ hr three or four times daily. Appropriate antibiotics should be given systemically after cultures of the ulcers have been made and sensitivities determined. Local applications of a 1 per cent solution or ointment of neomycin sulfate may be helpful in eradicating organisms resistant to the usual antibiotics. Enzymatic debridement of adherent crusts and exudates with streptokinase and streptodornase (Varidase), or an ointment containing fibrinolysin and deoxyribonuclease (Elase) is preferable to surgical debridement. When ischemic ulcerations are present, the patient should not be permitted to use the involved hand until after it has healed.

Erythermalgia (Erythromelalgia)

Erythermalgia is probably the rarest of the syndromes included under the general term peripheral vascular disease. In contrast to the arteriospastic diseases, the primary fault in erythermalgia appears to be excessive vasodilatation, occurring in the hands and/or feet.

Etiology

The mechanisms and pathogenesis are poorly understood. During the attacks of pain that characterize this syndrome, the arteries of the involved part are dilated, but whether or not this vasodilatation or abnormal sensitivity of the skin to heat produces the pain is not clear.

Clinical Features

In approximately 60 per cent of patients erythermalgia exists as a primary disease, while in the others it is a symptom of other diseases, notably polycythemia vera and hypertension.[79] Erythermalgia may precede other clinical manifestations of polycythemia vera by as much as 12 years.[79] In contrast to primary erythermalgia, which affects men more often than women and may occur at any age, the secondary form affects the sexes equally and occurs almost invariably after the age of forty years. In primary erythermalgia the distress tends to be more severe, to involve a larger area of the extremity, and to be symmetrical in distribution more often than in the secondary type.[79]

Diagnosis

Clinically erythermalgia is characterized by paroxysms of burning pain in the hands and/or more often the feet. During the painful paroxysms the parts are red and objectively as well as subjectively warm. Relief is obtained by exposing the affected extremities to cold air or by immersing them in cold water. It must be emphasized that erythermalgia is an extremely rare condition, although many people complain of burning pain of the hands or feet. In differentiating between erythermalgia and burning parasthesia of the extremities, which may imitate erythermalgia, the important finding is the presence or absence of *objective* warmth of the affected part during the

episodes of pain. In most cases of burning paresthetic pain, the affected part is actually cool, while in erythermalgia it is definitely warmer than the unaffected parts. In other words, the warmth in erythermalgia is both subjective and objective.

In establishing the diagnosis of erythermalgia, studies of skin temperatures are essential. By using thermocouples on the digits it is possible to establish a *critical* skin temperature, which usually is in the range of 32 to 36°C. When the temperature of the skin is above this critical level, the patient experiences the burning pain; when it is below this level, the pain is absent or rapidly subsides. Burning pain due to other causes is not so definitely related to a critical skin temperature.

Treatment

Patients learn from experience to avoid warm environmental temperatures and to wear perforated shoes or sandals. Treatment should be directed to the underlying disease when erythermalgia is secondary. Salicylates are helpful in controlling the symptoms either of the primary or of secondary types of erythermalgia. For reasons that are not apparent, one dose of aspirin (0.65 Gm) may prevent attacks of pain for several days in some cases. When the pain is resistant to salicylates, ephedrine sulfate (0.024 Gm) may be administered three or four times daily, or isoproterenol hydrochloride (Isuprel hydrochloride), 0.01 Gm sublingually as necessary, may be helpful. Paradoxically, the vasodilating agent phenoxybenzamine hydrochloride (Dibenzyline), 0.01 Gm three or four times daily, or even sympathectomy has been beneficial in alleviating the symptoms of erythermalgia in some cases.

Cold Injury

In addition to the arteriospastic diseases that are aggravated but not necessarily caused by exposure to cold temperatures, there is a group of conditions that can be attributed directly to cold exposure.

Exposure to cold can result in freezing of tissue (frostbite) or in injury without actual freezing (pernio syndromes, immersion foot, trench foot, or mild frostbite). Relatively short exposure to subfreezing temperatures is responsible for freezing injuries; the colder the temperature, the shorter the exposure necessary to produce tissue damage. Relatively prolonged exposure (usually several days) to dampness and cold above the freezing point is necessary for production of immersion foot or trench foot. Although chronic pernio is classified as a nonfreezing injury, exposure to cold need not be prolonged, since patients affected with this syndrome seem to manifest unusual susceptibility to cold.

Freezing of extracellular fluid results in hypertonicity of the extracellular compartment, and this in turn leads to dehydration and destruction of cells.[80] The mechanism of tissue damage in nonfreezing cold injury is not so well understood and may simply be a slow metabolic strangling due to reduced blood flow and direct inhibiting effect of the cold on metabolic processes and exchange of metabolites.[80,81]

Nonfreezing Injury

Chronic pernio is characterized clinically by the development of superficial ulcers that occur in crops over the lower third of the leg and on the ankles, feet, and toes. They begin as small erythematous papules or nodules, which then break down into superficial ulcers with a hemorrhagic base surrounded by a violaceous border. Healing ordinarily is spontaneous in from 3 to 5 weeks, leaving pigmented and often depressed scars, but new lesions may appear as the older ones heal. The lesions result from actual necrosis of the skin, because of a combination of spasm and endothelial proliferation of the arterioles and small arteries. The lesions appear after exposure to cold, although the temperature need not be excessively low nor the exposure prolonged. Apparently individual hypersusceptibility to cold is a major factor. Although at first the lesions occur during the winter months only, eventually in some cases the relation to the seasons may be less pronounced as time goes on. Protection from cold is the most important facet of treatment. When ulcers occur, the patient should be put to bed and treated with applications of local dressings of a saturated solution of boric acid. Vasodilating drugs such as phenoxybenzamine or cyclandelate are sometimes helpful. Sympathectomy may be necessary in intractable cases.

Immobility in the dependent position and dampness are important contributing factors in the development of trench foot and immersion foot, which are characterized by three clinical stages. During the initial stage of exposure the feet become edematous and painful. Later, hypesthesia or even anesthesia may supervene. Violaceous ulcers similar to those of chronic pernio may appear. The second stage occurs after the patient has been removed from the cold and placed in a warm environment. Reactive hyperemia occurs, and the foot becomes red and warm. Swelling increases unless the foot is elevated. Hyperesthesia, and burning, throbbing pain are characteristic. Arterial pulsations are full and bounding, and hemorrhagic blebs, infarcts in the skin, ulcers, and even superficial gangrene may appear. Following this phase, which lasts for several days or weeks, the chronic phase of arterial spasm and ischemia appears. The extremities are chronically cold, cyanotic, and hyperhydrotic. Secondary Raynaud's phenomenon may occur; when severe, this chronic stage may severely handicap the patient, because even mild degrees of cold produce distressing parasthesia and pain.

The use of proper footwear to keep the feet dry and warm will prevent this syndrome or will minimize the chronic disability from it. During the period of exposure it is important to elevate the feet as often as possible to reduce edema. In the hyperemic stage the legs should be elevated and kept at room temperature. Local and systemic measures to prevent infection or to combat it if it is present are indicated. Treatment of the chronic arteriospastic, ischemic phase frequently is ineffective. Protection of the feet from cold is important, as is abstinence from tobacco. Vasolidating drugs, mild heat, light massage, and sympathectomy have been helpful in some cases.

Acute pernio (acute chilblains) is similar to, and sometimes indistinguishable from, first-degree frostbite. Although the inciting exposure is usually to subfreezing temperatures, it is doubtful that the tissues are actually frozen, and hence these two conditions are properly included with the nonfreezing cold injuries. During or immediately after exposure, the exposed parts, usually the hands, nose, ears, or shins, become bluish-red and slightly swollen, and they burn or itch. The injured part is susceptible to infection, and treatment consists of immediate warming to room temperature and prevention of infection by protection of the inflamed skin with sterile dressings and administration of antibiotics.

Freezing Injury

Frostbite may be classified according to the degree of severity: First-degree frostbite has been discussed in the previous paragraph, since it is unlikely that actual freezing of tissue occurs in the mild form. Second-degree frostbite is characterized by the formation of blebs, or vesicles, in the skin of the region affected. Third-degree frostbite results in necrosis of subcutaneous tissue. Fourth-degree frostbite results in gangrene with loss of an extremity or portion of an extremity. Initially, the affected part appears pale or waxy-yellow, is objectively anesthetic, but frequently is subjectively pruritic. Affected parts frequently remain hypersensitive to cold for long periods after the initial insult, and secondary Raynaud's phenomenon may appear. Frostbite is best treated by rapid thawing.[82] Preferably the part should be immersed in a water bath at a temperature between 108 and 112°F (42 to 44°C) for at least 20 min or until all tissues show flushing to the distal nailbed and volar pad. Hexachlorophene may be added to the bath to prevent infection. After thawing, the injured part should be thoroughly but gently cleansed with a mild soap and water. Since infection is the greatest danger during the recovery phase, strict isolation and aseptic nursing care should be carried out until the blebs have dried. The blebs should be allowed to remain intact, since they protect the denuded underlying surface from bacterial invasion. Vasodilating drugs and anticoagulants have not been consistently beneficial. It has been reported that sympathectomy performed during the acute phase hastens resolution of skin lesions and minimizes the frequency and severity of late sequelae.[83] Gangrene from cold injury often is superficial and frequently appears to be worse than it actually is. For this reason decision about amputation should be postponed for several weeks or months until the true extent of necrosis can be adequately evaluated.[82]

DISEASES OF VEINS

Thrombophlebitis

Venous thrombosis (phlebothrombosis) cannot occur without inciting some inflammatory reaction of the venous intima, although at times it is so minimal that it cannot be detected clinically. Likewise, *phlebitis*, or inflammation of a vein, cannot exist very long without inciting thrombus formation on the inflamed endothelium. Consequently the term *thrombophlebitis*, which implies simultaneous existence of thrombosis and inflammation, is preferable to the others, although from the standpoint of clinical behavior it must be recognized that sometimes thrombosis is the initiating factor, whereas inflammation may predominate in other cases.

Etiology

Stasis, hypercoagulability,[84] and injury of the endothelium of the vein are recognized as the three most important factors in the etiology of thrombophlebitis. Venous stasis is an important factor in postoperative, postpartum, and varicose thrombophlebitis as well as in the thrombophlebitis that complicates congestive heart failure or prolonged bed rest for any chronic illness or follows severe trauma that does not involve the vein directly; endothelial injury seems to be the predominant factor in thrombophlebitis associated with thromboangiitis obliterans (Buerger's disease), in septic thrombophlebitis, and in thrombophlebitis resulting from direct trauma to veins; hypercoagulability of the blood may play a major role in thrombophlebitis associated with malignant disease and blood dyscrasias and in idiopathic thrombophlebitis.[85] It is unlikely, however, that a single factor is operative in most cases, even though one seems to be dominant. For instance, direct trauma to veins (endothelial injury) and release of tissue thromboplastin (hypercoagulability) àt the time of laparotomy may conspire with prolonged bed rest, inadequate hydration, and hypotension following surgical treatment (venous stasis) to produce postoperative iliofemoral thrombophlebitis. It should not be forgotten that the majority of instances occur in patients with medical disease including myocardial infarction and chronic congestive heart failure.

Pathology

The histologic findings depend upon the underlying cause and range from extensive panphlebitis with cellular infiltration and fibroblastic proliferation involving the thrombus, the vein wall, and the perivenous tissues (thromboangiitis obliterans) to a long, unorganized, acellular, bland thrombus loosely attached to the endothelial surface of a vein that shows only minimal inflammatory changes localized to the area of attachment (early cases of postoperative thrombophlebitis). The greater the inflammatory reaction of the vein, the sooner the thrombus will become securely attached to the intimal surface and the less chance for embolization. Only the "tail" of fresh thrombus (red thrombus) that wags freely in the bloodstream is likely to become detached and give rise to pulmonary embolism. If it remains in situ, however, this loosely attached friable thrombus will undergo lysis or become organized and firmly adherent to the venous wall (white thrombus), probably within 24 to 48 hr after its formation, thus eliminating the risk of embolization. Propagation of organized or organizing thrombi may occur with deposition of platelets and red cells in a matrix of fibrin, giving rise to another loosely attached tail that once again places the patient in jeopardy of pulmonary embolism.

The term *chronic thrombophlebitis* is a misnomer, since healing inevitably takes place once the acute inflammatory reaction has subsided. Recanalization of the organized thrombus usually occurs, thus restoring patency of the lumen within a period of a few weeks. Chronic venous insufficiency results only if the valves of the major venous channels have been destroyed or rendered incompetent by the fibrosis that occurs during the healing process.

Thrombophlebitis involves veins of the lower extremities most frequently, but any vein of the body can be affected. The inflammatory process may extend for only a few millimeters along the vein or may affect the entire length of the vein and many of its tributaries.

Pathologic Physiology

Because of abundant collateral venous channels, there is usually little functional disturbance as a result of thrombophlebitis unless major venous trunks such as the iliofemoral or axillary and subclavian veins are completely occluded by thrombus. When major veins are obstructed, there is passive congestion with elevation of venous pressure distally in the involved limb. This causes cyanosis and visible distension of veins due to engorgement with blood. The limb becomes swollen, and initially this swelling results almost entirely from increased intravascular volume; hence there is no pitting edema. Eventually the increased venous and capillary pressure leads to increased transudation of fluid into the extravascular compartment with the formation of pitting edema. Usually, arterial blood supply is unaffected, but in rare instances, during the initial phase of extensive and severe iliofemoral thrombophlebitis (phlegmasia cerulea dolens), arterial pulsations may be absent, as the result of either arterial spasm or massive edema. Gangrene may ensue without demonstrable organic occlusion of the arterial tree.[86,87] With this unusual exception, thrombophlebitis does not lead to tissue necrosis.

Clinical Features

The clinical findings in thrombophlebitis vary with the site and extent of the venous involvement. From the standpoint of clinical behavior, prognosis, and therapy, it is helpful to consider superficial thrombophlebitis and deep thrombophlebitis separately (Table 56-2).

Superficial Thrombophlebitis. This can be seen and felt, making the diagnosis easy in most cases. The thrombus and accompanying inflammatory reaction are palpable as a tender, indurated cord that extends for various distances along a superficial subcutaneous vein. During the acute stage, redness, local heat, and tenderness are prominent features. The thrombus usually remains palpable for several days or weeks after the inflammatory component subsides. Fever is minimal or absent, and there is no systemic reaction. The most common cause of superficial thrombophlebitis in the arm is intra-

Table 56-2. SUMMARY OF CLINICAL CHARACTERISTICS OF THROMBOPHLEBITIS

Clinical classification	Usual causes	Usual location	Clinical findings	Edema of extremities	Embolization	Chronic venous insufficiency
Superficial	Varicose veins Direct trauma IV injections Thromboangiitis obliterans Malignant disease Blood dyscrasias Idiopathic	Saphenous veins and their tributaries Forearm	Tender, red, inflamed induration along course of subcutaneous vein (visible and palpable)	Almost never	Almost never	Almost never
Deep: Small veins	Postoperative Postpartum Direct or distant trauma Congestive heart failure Prolonged bed rest Acute febrile disease	Sural, calf Posterior tibial, calf Popliteal Pelvic (see text)	Tenderness to deep pressure Induration of overlying muscle Minimal or no venous distension	Occasional	Always a threat	Usually not
Major venous trunks	Debilitating disease Malignant disease Blood dyscrasias Systemic lupus erythematosus Pressure of tumors on veins Idiopathic Sepsis	Femoral Iliac Inferior or superior vena cava Axillary Subclavian	Swelling Cyanosis Venous distension of limb with mild to moderate pain Tenderness over involved vein (groin or axilla)	Usual	Always a threat	Frequently

venous injection of irritating solutions. The most common cause in the lower extremities is thrombophlebitis involving incompetent saphenous veins or their tributaries. The unexplained appearance of superficial thrombophlebitis in a young man should suggest the possibility of thromboangiitis obliterans, whereas in middle-aged or older persons it should suggest occult malignancy.[88,89] Superficial thrombophlebitis involving longitudinal veins of the anterolateral aspect of the thorax (including the breasts in women) is a benign condition that has been given the eponym of *Mondor's disease*.[90]

Differential diagnosis includes all types of inflammatory nodular lesions that occur in subcutaneous tissues of the extremities. Some of these are erythema nodosum, nodular vasculitis, erythema induratum, periarteritis nodosa, chronic pernio, and nonsuppurative panniculitis. Usually these lesions are globular, and some of them eventually ulcerate. Typically, the lesion of superficial thrombophlebitis is linear, not globular, extends along the course of a subcutaneous vein, and does not ulcerate. Thrombophlebitis that is limited to a varix may be globular rather than linear, but usually its location in the course of a varicose vein is an obvious clue. Thrombophlebitis occurring in a localized varix of the greater saphenous vein near the fossa ovalis may be mistaken for a lymph node or a femoral hernia.

Deep Thrombophlebitis. When thrombophlebitis is confined to small venous channels beneath the subcutaneous tissue or in the pelvis, the lesions are neither visible nor palpable. The sural veins of the calf are the most common site, and this type of thrombophlebitis is usually a postoperative or postpartum complication. Other causes, less common, are listed in Table 56-2. Because symptoms and clinical signs are often minimal, the diagnosis is difficult and is often overlooked. Mild pain in the calf may be the only symptom, and tenderness which is often unimpressive may be the only sign. Characteristically, but for obscure reasons, this tenderness is elicited more consistently by compressing the calf from side to side than by compressing it from the posterior aspect anteriorly. Since there are many collateral channels, edema and venous distension rarely result from sural thrombophlebitis, although the calf muscles may be somewhat indurated. Homans' sign (pain in the calf induced by forcible dorsiflexion of the foot) is not a reliable diagnostic aid. Fever is usually absent or if present is minimal. There is no systemic reaction.

Sural thrombophlebitis often goes unrecognized clinically simply because of the paucity of signs and symptoms. Deep veins of the calf are frequently the source of pulmonary emboli that occur before there are any peripheral signs of thrombophlebitis. Not

uncommonly, proximal propagation of a thrombus arising in the sural veins leads to iliofemoral thrombophlebitis. For these reasons, a presumptive diagnosis of deep-calf thrombophlebitis should be made whenever a patient complains of pain and tenderness in the calf after operation, trauma, or childbirth, or during the course of any severe debilitating illness. The diagnosis is more certain if the signs and symptoms are unilateral. Myositis of the calf is a condition with which deep-calf thrombophlebitis may be easily confused. Patients who have been in stirrups for obstetric, gynecologic, or urologic procedures frequently have painful and tender calf muscles for several days postoperatively. Usually both calves are involved, and the discomfort is noticed immediately after operation, whereas, typically, postoperative thrombophlebitis first appears unilaterally from the fifth to the fourteenth postoperative days. Neurotic women with obese legs (lipedema) usually complain of tenderness when the legs are examined, but the tenderness is bilateral, is not confined to the calf muscles, and has been present for many years.

Thrombophlebitis involving pelvic veins occurs after childbirth and following operative procedures on the pelvic viscera. Except for low-grade fever, symptoms are absent unless pulmonary embolism occurs or unless the thrombus extends to the common iliac vein to produce the clinical findings of iliofemoral thrombophlebitis described below. Although asymptomatic pelvic thrombophlebitis may be the source for some postpartum and postoperative pulmonary emboli that occur in the absence of signs of peripheral thrombophlebitis, the majority of such emboli probably arise in the sural veins. The advent of antibiotics has sharply reduced the incidence of septic thrombophlebitis that rather commonly occurred in the uterine venous plexus after induced abortions or as a complication of parturition.

When deep thrombophlebitis occurs in major venous trunks such as the iliofemoral or axillary and subclavian veins, a typical clinical picture results, due largely to venous obstruction with passive congestion of the extremities. The entire extremity becomes swollen, mildly to moderately painful, and slightly cyanotic over a period of several hours. The skin is warm, superficial veins are distended, and there is tenderness along the course of the involved vein in the groin or axilla. When iliofemoral thrombophlebitis results from extension of sural thrombophlebitis, the calf and popliteal space are tender also. Temperature rarely exceeds 101°F and is usually lower. There may be moderate malaise. Subclavian thrombophlebitis may result from unusual use of the arms, especially involving work overhead (effort thrombophlebitis). Iliofemoral thrombophlebitis is usually a postoperative, postpartum, or post-traumatic complication. When the inferior vena cava is involved, both lower extremities are swollen and cyanotic, and if one or both renal veins are obstructed, the nephrotic syndrome may occur. When the superior vena cava is obstructed, both upper extremities as well as the face and neck become swollen and cyanotic. Bronchogenic carcinoma is the most common cause for superior vena cava obstruction.[91]

Phlegmasia cerulea dolens is an unusually extensive thrombosis of the iliofemoral vein and most of its tributaries which occurs abruptly with sudden, massive swelling and intense cyanosis of the extremity.[86,87] Shock may ensue as a result of trapping of blood in the swollen extremity. Frequently there is arterial spasm initially, and gangrene may ensue.

In the differential diagnosis of iliofemoral and axillary-subclavian thrombophlebitis, acute cellulitis and lymphedema should be considered. Lymphedema usually comes on and progresses slowly, so that for the first few weeks or months edema that appears around the ankle during the day disappears at night. Only later in the course of the disease is the entire extremity swollen. There is no accompanying venous distension, and venous pressure is not elevated. Lymphedema of the upper extremity is usually secondary to malignant involvement, extirpation, or irradiation of axillary lymph nodes. Cellulitis and lymphangiitis are usually accompanied by higher temperature (102°F or higher) and more profound systemic reaction (chills, nausea and vomiting, malaise) than is iliofemoral or axillary-subclavian thrombophlebitis. The extremity may become swollen rather abruptly in both conditions, but the skin is erythematous and not cyanotic, there is more local heat in the involved extremity, and regional lymph nodes may be enlarged and tender when cellulitis and lymphangiitis are present. Iliofemoral thrombophlebitis is sometimes unnecessarily confused with sudden arterial occlusion. Distinguishing features of the latter condition include absence of edema and arterial pulsations, coolness and pallor of the skin, collapsed superficial veins, and various degrees of hypesthesia. Pain accompanying sudden arterial occlusion is usually more prominent and more severe than that produced by iliofemoral thrombophlebitis.

When thrombophlebitis recurs without obvious cause, the physician should rule out occult malignancy[88,89] (often in the pancreas), blood dyscrasias, and systemic lupus erythematosus before making the diagnosis of idiopathic recurrent thrombophlebitis.[92]

Complications

There are three major complications of thrombophlebitis. The most feared because of its lethal potentialities is pulmonary embolism, the manifestations of which are discussed in Chap. 47. It is worth noting that 85 per cent of fatal pulmonary emboli after operation occur without any warning symptoms in the extremities.[93] The majority of nonfatal emboli precede the peripheral manifestations of thrombophlebitis, and it is not uncommon for symptoms of thrombophlebitis not to appear at all following pulmonary embolism.[93] On the other hand, 6.6 per cent of patients with iliofemoral thrombophlebitis died of pulmonary embolism before anticoagulant therapy was available.[93]

Chronic venous insufficiency, a common sequela of deep thrombophlebitis, will be discussed subsequently.

Postphlebitic neurosis is often iatrogenically induced.[94] Most patients in whom this complication develops are apprehensive women who have been kept in bed for unnecessarily long periods for treatment of thrombophlebitis and who, through careless statements or implication on the part of physicians, nurses, or friends, acquire the misconception that their veins harbor "clots" which may suddenly break loose and "go to the heart." The involved extremity remains inordinately painful and tender, and attempts to examine it meet with hysterical withdrawal. They often refuse to bear weight on it or to walk normally, with the result that disuse ensues and augments the pain. Successful treatment depends upon the physician's ability to convince the patient that the danger of embolism is no longer present and to outline a regimen of progressive rehabilitation.

Prophylaxis

Prophylactic measures include avoidance of blood loss, shock, and dehydration during surgical treatment, and early ambulation after surgical treatment. Also helpful are leg exercises and the use of elastic stockings during and after surgical treatment. Prophylactic use of anticoagulants is sometimes justified for patients who are predisposed to the development of thrombophlebitis or following certain operations that carry an unusually high risk of postoperative thrombophlebitis. Patients who have a history of thrombophlebitis and especially those who have evidence of chronic venous insufficiency or varicose veins, elderly patients, and patients who are dehydrated or debilitated or develop infections are unusually susceptible to thrombophlebitis following operation or trauma, or during any protracted illness. Surgical procedures that particularly predispose to the development of postoperative thrombophlebitis include splenectomy, pelvic operations, and extensive resections for carcinoma.[95]

Treatment

Bed rest with elevation of the involved extremity is usually advisable until tenderness and edema subside, but only in unusual circumstances should the patient be kept in bed for more than 14 days. Hot, moist packs are helpful in alleviating pain and hastening resolution of the inflammatory process. Codeine sulfate (0.032 to 0.065 Gm every 4 to 6 hr) or d-propoxyphene hydrochloride (Darvon) (0.032 to 0.065 Gm every 4 to 6 hr) given with salicylates may be necessary to relieve pain during the first 2 or 3 days, but often salicylates alone are adequate. Phenylbutazone (Butazolodin), 0.1 Gm four times daily for 3 to 5 days, is remarkably effective in relieving the pain and hastening the resolution of the inflammatory reaction accompanying superficial thrombophlebitis. It may also be used in management of deep thrombophlebitis if pain is unusually prominent and troublesome.

Anticoagulant drugs are seldom indicated for treatment of superficial thrombophlebitis, because embolism is rarely a complication of this type. Anticoagulant drugs should be employed in the management of most cases of deep thrombophlebitis unless urgent contraindications are present, for their usefulness in preventing fatal pulmonary embolism has been convincingly proved.[41] For sural thrombophlebitis without pulmonary embolism, treatment may be started with a coumarin derivative, such as warfarin sodium (Coumadin), 0.040 Gm initially, adjusting the dose thereafter to keep the Quick one-stage prothrombin time between 1.5 and 2.5 times normal. When pulmonary embolism has already occurred or in the management of acute iliofemoral thrombophlebitis with or without pulmonary embolism, heparin sodium should also be given either intravenously (5,000 units every 4 hr) or subcutaneously (20,000 units every 12 hr) for the first 24 to 48 hr until the coumarin drug has produced a therapeutic deficiency in prothrombin activity. It is a clinical impression that prompt use of heparin, in the management of iliofemoral thrombophlebitis, shortens convalescence and reduces frequency and severity of the late sequelae of chronic venous insufficiency.

The effectiveness of fibrinolysin (Actase or Thrombolysin) or its activator, streptokinase, in the management of thrombophlebitis has not been established, nor has adequate laboratory control of its administration been defined.[96] For these reasons and because the preparations are expensive, this type of treatment is not recommended for routine use.

If edema is present or appears when the patient becomes ambulatory, elastic stockings or elastic bandages should be applied whenever the patient is out of bed. The use of the elastic support can be discontinued whenever the extremity remains free of edema without it. Adequate elastic support is the most important measure to prevent chronic venous insufficiency.

Ligation or plication of veins should be considered only when pulmonary embolism occurs in spite of adequate anticoagulant treatment or when anticoagulation is absolutely contraindicated for a patient who has had one pulmonary embolus. It has already been stated that pulmonary emboli frequently occur in the absence of clinical signs of peripheral thrombophlebitis; moreover, when there are peripheral signs of thrombophlebitis, the embolus may arise from the opposite, asymptomatic extremity.[93] Consequently, any operation should be directed to the inferior vena cava, and plication[97] or creation of a filter[98] seems less likely to produce late sequelae of venous insufficiency than does ligation. Recent claims that thrombectomy in management of iliofemoral thrombophlebitis reduces the frequency and severity of late complications of chronic venous insufficiency[99] are not yet substantiated.

Varicose Veins

Varicose veins, or dilated veins, are commonly encountered in clinical practice. They range in severity from the innocuous but sometimes cosmeti-

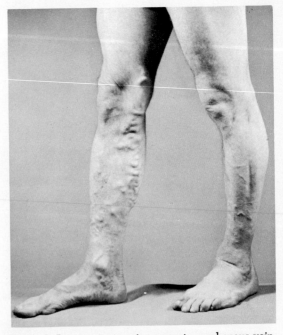

Fig. 56-8. Incompetent varicose greater saphenous vein.

cally objectionable dilatation of superficial cutaneous veins to the huge, serpiginous dilatation of the long saphenous vein (Fig. 56-8) that renders it functionally incompetent and leads to venous stasis and insufficiency. Only rarely are varicose veins found in the upper extremities, and when they do occur in this location, they almost always signify the presence of a congenital vascular anomaly or an acquired arteriovenous fistula.

Etiology

Varicose veins may be primary or secondary. Primary varicose veins appear without antecedent thrombophlebitis and are presumably the result of a congenital weakness of the veins that becomes manifest at puberty or later in life, often during pregnancy. The familial incidence of varicose veins is striking and is evidence of an inherited defect, although this has never been conclusively demonstrated. In addition to pregnancy, obesity and occupations that entail prolonged standing predispose to development of varicose veins.

Secondary varicose veins usually result from previous deep thrombophlebitis with resulting insufficiency of the deep venous system; rarer causes include acquired or congenital arteriovenous fistulas and extrinsic pressure on the inferior vena cava or iliofemoral veins.

Pathology

Characteristically, varicose veins, whether primary or secondary, are dilated and elongated. The thickness of the wall varies considerably, but in general it is thicker than normal as a result of an increase in fibrous connective tissue. There is usually also hypertrophy of the muscular coat and increase in thickness of the intima. As the veins dilate, the valves become incompetent and atrophy.

With the exception of the hemorrhoidal plexus, the most commonly involved veins are the greater and lesser saphenous and their tributaries.

Pathologic Physiology

Venous stasis results when valves in varicose veins are rendered incompetent. The increased venous pressure is transmitted to the capillary bed, promoting the formation of edema, the deposition of hemosiderin, and the proliferation of subcutaneous fibrous tissue. These changes will be considered more in detail in the section on Chronic Venous Insufficiency. Normally, venous pressure in the lower extremities decreases during walking when veins are competent. In the presence of incompetent varicose veins, however, there is less than the normal decrease in venous pressure during walking; thus the capillaries around the ankles are subjected to higher than normal pressures during physical activity.[100]

Clinical Features

Primary varicose veins are almost always bilateral, although they may not appear simultaneously in both extremities. Varicosities of this type appear without antecedent history of thrombophlebitis or other predisposing cause. Women frequently notice them for the first time during pregnancy. Secondary varicose veins on the other hand are not infrequently unilateral, since usually they are the result of deep venous insufficiency from previous iliofemoral thrombophlebitis. The history of previous thrombophlebitis and chronic swelling of the involved extremity are clues that varicose veins are secondary. When varicose veins are present at birth or appear early in life or when they occur in the upper extremity, congenital arteriovenous fistula should be suspected.

Usually varicose veins produce minimal or no symptoms. Hypersensitive patients, especially women, complain of a variety of bizarre pains that are usually located in the varices. When venous insufficiency is present, diffuse dull aching in the leg after prolonged standing or walking is a common complaint. This is usually relieved by a period of elevation of the legs. If the deep veins are competent, orthostatic edema and stasis pigmentation of the ankles and lower legs are usually minimal or absent.

Special Examinations for Venous Competency

Varicose veins are not necessarily incompetent, for in some cases the varicosities may be so localized that they do not interfere with function of the valves. For this reason incompetency of the veins should be established before surgical intervention is considered. The course of the vein can be traced by firmly compressing it with one hand while the fingertips of the other hand feel for the impact above and below the area of compression. If the impulse can be felt for a distance of 20 cm above or below the compression, the vein is usually incompetent. By the application of tourniquets at various levels in the thigh and leg and the observation of the direction and rapidity of filling of superficial veins after the leg has been placed in a dependent position following elevation, it is possible to locate incompetent perforating veins and to determine whether or not the greater and lesser saphenous veins are incompetent.[101,102]

Complications

The most frequent complication of incompetent varicose veins is venous insufficiency manifested by chronic edema, pigmentation, induration, and sometimes ulceration of the lower part of the legs and ankles. This complication is more likely to occur when deep venous insufficiency is also present; it is discussed in the following section of this chapter.

Thrombophlebitis may occur in varicose veins either spontaneously or following trauma, surgical procedures, or parturition. It may occur repeatedly for no apparent reason. Pulmonary embolism from thrombophlebitis in superficial varices is rare.

Rupture of varicose veins with massive bleeding is extremely uncommon, although many patients secretly or otherwise harbor a fear of it.

Treatment

Reassurance is the only treatment necessary for patients with dilated cutaneous capillaries. This is also true for patients with minor and localized varicose veins without incompetency of the saphenous systems.

Adequate elastic support in the form of bandages or stockings should be recommended if the saphenous veins are extensively incompetent and especially if edema occurs when the patient is up. When the deep veins are also incompetent, a heavier support is required to prevent accumulation of edema than when only the superficial veins are involved. Proper elastic support, faithfully worn, will prevent the complications of venous insufficiency in most cases and obviate the need for surgical intervention.

Injections of sclerosing solutions may be helpful if only short segments of small tributary veins are involved. Large and extensive varicosities cannot be successfully treated in this manner, for ultimately the thrombus so induced recanalizes. Injection therapy is sometimes useful in conjunction with surgical stripping when small varicose veins remain after the main channels have been eradicated.

Operation becomes necessary whenever signs and symptoms of chronic venous insufficiency, including stasis ulcer, cannot be controlled by elastic support or the patient refuses to wear the support faithfully. Recurrent thrombophlebitis in varicose veins is another indication for operation, and in some cases it may be justifiable to operate on varicose veins for cosmetic reasons only. It must be remembered that many patients with varicose veins can get along without symptoms or complications for many years with no treatment whatsoever. Stripping of the entire vein as well as careful dissection and evulsion of its incompetent tributaries and resection of all incompetent perforating veins are the procedure of choice when surgical intervention becomes necessary. The late results of extensive stripping operations are much superior to those of simple ligation and injection.[103,104]

Cellulitis and lymphangiitis, systemic diseases, acute thrombophlebitis in deep veins, and arterial insufficiency are contraindications to surgical treatment of varicose veins. Deep venous insufficiency is not a contraindication to stripping superficial veins that are incompetent.[102] However, the patient with deep venous insufficiency should understand before operation that he must continue to wear adequate elastic support after operation, whereas most patients who have competent deep veins can eventually discard the elastic support after successful stripping of incompetent varicose veins.

Chronic Venous Insufficiency

Chronic venous insufficiency is the end result of incompetency of the valves of damaged veins. Most frequently it occurs in the lower extremity following iliofemoral thrombophlebitis with resulting destruction of the valves. Occasionally incompetency of the saphenous system will lead to chronic venous insufficiency even though the deep veins are competent. Rarely, chronic venous insufficiency occurs in the upper extremity following axillary-subclavian thrombophlebitis.

Pathology

Chronic venous insufficiency is characterized by edema and induration of the subcutaneous tissues around the malleoli and in the lower third or more of the leg. The foot is seldom involved to any appreciable degree unless for some reason shoes are not worn regularly. Chronic edema of the subcutaneous tissue leads to fibrosis, inflammation, and induration (chronic indurated cellulitis). The cellulitis is usually a sterile inflammation. The characteristic brownish pigmentation of the distal third of the leg and the malleolar areas is due to deposition

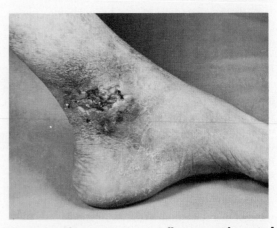

Fig. 56-9. Chronic venous insufficiency with typical pigmentation and stasis ulceration overlying the internal malleolus.

of melanin and hemosiderin. The latter comes from disintegration of erythrocytes that reach the subcutaneous tissues when capillaries rupture. Not infrequently ulcers occur spontaneously or following trauma, and these are characteristically located in the malleolar areas, usually on the internal side (Fig. 56-9). Weeping, eczematoid dermatitis is a frequent occurrence.

Pathologic Physiology

The basic fault is incompetence of the valves of the deep or superficial veins or both. Under these circumstances the usual decrease in venous pressure that results from walking no longer occurs, and consequently the venous capillaries of the lower extremities are subjected to pressures that equal the height of a column of blood extending from the right atrium to the level of the malleoli, whether the patient is walking or standing still.[100] This inevitably leads to increased transudation of fluid into the extravascular compartment with formation of edema.

Clinical Features

Chronic venous insufficiency presents a characteristic clinical picture.

Often only one leg is involved, and it is chronically swollen; the skin and subcutaneous tissue around and above the malleoli are indurated and firm, and the entire area has the typical brownish pigmentation.

Usually a history of iliofemoral thrombophlebitis can be elicited. Occasionally this diagnosis has not been made previously to the patient's knowledge, but the patient can date the onset of swelling from childbirth, operation, or major trauma. Sometimes the chronic swelling does not appear for several years or months after the episode of thrombophlebitis. Chronic venous insufficiency can result from incompetent varicose veins of the long saphenous system without deep venous incompetency, but this is unusual. Incompetency of the long or short saphenous vein or both can usually be demonstrated in patients who have chronic venous insufficiency, but in the majority of cases this is secondary to deep insufficiency.

Stasis or varicose ulcers usually occur after chronic venous insufficiency is well established and the pigmentation and chronic induration have already occurred (Fig. 56-9). The ulcers are rarely very painful, and although they are frequently infected, it is obvious that granulation tissue is abundant unless arterial circulation is also impaired. The ulcers usually occur in the area of, or just above, the internal malleolus. Rarely they occur on the foot or toes, and often in such circumstances it can

be demonstrated that the patients wear slippers or go barefoot instead of using shoes regularly.

Early in the course of chronic venous insufficiency, before induration and pigmentation have occurred, lymphedema must be ruled out. Lymphedema usually occurs in adolescent girls or young women, and there is no history of preceding thrombophlebitis, nor can incompetency of superficial veins be demonstrated. Recording of venous pressure at the ankle during walking is helpful in particularly difficult cases. The venous pressure will decrease when patients with lymphedema walk, since the venous system is competent, whereas the venous pressure will not change when patients with incompetent veins walk.[100]

Prophylaxis

Chronic venous insufficiency can usually be prevented if patients with acute femoral or iliofemoral thrombophlebitis wear an adequate elastic support on the involved leg below the knee as soon as they begin to ambulate. The elastic support, whether it be a stocking or wrap-around bandage, should be strong enough and should be applied firmly enough to prevent the accumulation of edema when the patient is upright. It should be worn whenever the patient is up and around but can be removed when the patient is recumbent. It is reasonable to omit the use of the support for 1 day every 3 or 4 months to see if edema recurs. It can be discarded whenever the leg remains free of edema without it. It is a clinical impression that prompt treatment of acute iliofemoral thrombophlebitis with heparin reduces the frequency and severity of chronic venous insufficiency. Elevation of the involved extremity during the acute episode is also helpful in eliminating or ameliorating this late complication.

Treatment

Once chronic venous insufficiency is well developed, the patient is probably condemned to the use of adequate elastic support for the rest of his life, if he is to avoid disability from recurrent ulcerations and eczematoid dermatitis. If edema is prominent, the patient should be put to bed with the leg elevated in order to reduce the swelling as much as possible. Following this, the leg should be fitted with a good elastic support that will prevent reaccumulation of edema when the patient is ambulatory. Rubber-reinforced elastic bandages usually provide excellent support, but their daily application is a nuisance. If elastic stockings are to be used, they must be constructed well enough to offer the necessary support, and they must be fitted to measurement after edema has been drained from the leg.

Ulcers of chronic venous insufficiency (stasis ulcers) are best treated by bed rest with the involved extremity elevated. Continuous application of dressings moistened with isotonic saline solution or saturated solution of boric acid will help to eliminate infection and stimulate granulation. If specific pathogens are isolated from the ulcers, appropriate antibiotics can be given systemically or applied locally in the form of solution or ointment. When infection is controlled, the application of dried, powdered erythrocytes (Lyocyte powder) may be helpful in promoting healing. When ulcers are large, healing can be hastened by applying skin grafts after the base of the ulcer has become clean and covered with healthy granulation tissue. Stasis ulcers usually heal remarkably rapidly, provided that arterial blood supply is normal. When indurated cellulitis is present and stasis ulcers have healed, recurrence can usually be prevented by applying, under a rubber-reinforced elastic bandage, a foam-rubber pad to the pigmented ulcer-bearing region around and above the internal malleolus. It sometimes becomes necessary to excise incompetent perforating or superficial veins that lead to an area of recurrent or recalcitrant stasis ulceration. If indurated cellulitis is far advanced to the point that subcutaneous tissue has a woody consistency, it is often difficult to prevent recurrent ulceration in spite of adequate elastic support. When this occurs, wide excision of the indurated area followed by application of skin grafts is indicated.[101]

Eczematoid dermatitis (stasis eczema) can be particularly difficult to manage, since the intense pruritis incites scratching, which in turn aggravates and spreads the dermatitis. Patients with active eczematoid dermatitis should be put to bed with the extremity elevated. Continuous application of packs moistened with a 0.5 per cent solution of aluminum subacetate is the treatment of choice when the involved skin is wet and oozing. In the subacute stage an ointment containing 3 per cent Ichthyol in zinc oxide often prevents pruritus and promotes healing.

Patients with chronic venous insufficiency should be instructed carefully about the adverse effect of gravity on venous circulation, and they should be encouraged to elevate their legs on footstools or hassocks when sitting and should be warned to avoid trauma to the skin of the ulcer-bearing areas.

REFERENCES

1. Groom, D.: Population Studies of Atherosclerosis, *Ann. Int. Med.*, **55**:51–62, 1961.
2. Katz, L. N., Pick, R., and Stamler, J.: Athero-
sclerosis, *Mod. Concepts Cardiovas. Dis.*, **23**:239–242, 1954.
3. Wessler, S., Ming, S., Gurewich, V., and Freiman, D. G.: A Critical Evaluation of Thromboangiitis Obliterans: The Case against Buerger's Disease, *New England J. Med.*, **262**:1149–1160, 1960.
4. McKusick, V. A., Harris, W. S., Ottesen, O. E., Goodman, R. M., Shelley, W. M., and Bloodwell, R. D.: Buerger's Disease: A Distinct Clinical and Pathologic Entity, *J.A.M.A.*, **181**:5–12, 1962.
5. Schatz, I. J., Fine, G., and Eyler, W. R.: Thromboangiitis Obliterans, *Brit. Heart J.* (In press.)
6. McPherson, J. R., Juergens, J. L., and Gifford, R. W., Jr.: Thromboangiitis Obliterans and Arteriosclerosis Obliterans: Clinical and Prognostic Differences, *Ann. Int. Med.*, **59**:288–296, 1963.
7. Ross, R. S., and McKusick, V. A.: Aortic Arch Syndromes, *A.M.A. Arch. Int. Med.*, **92**:701–740, 1953.
8. Thurlbeck, W. M., and Currens, J. H.: The Aortic Arch Syndrome (Pulseless Disease): A Report of Ten Cases with Three Autopsies, *Circulation*, **19**:499–510, 1959.
9. Pedersen, J., and Olsen, S.: Small-vessel Disease of the Lower Extremity in Diabetes Mellitus: On the Pathogenesis of the Foot Lesions in Diabetics, *Acta med. scandinav.*, **171**:551–559, (fasc. 5) 1962.
10. Burchell, H. B.: Peripheral Auscultation: Prospecting with a Stethoscope, *Heart Bull.*, **12**:81–85, 1963.
11. Gifford, R. W., Jr., and Hurst, J. W.: A Note on the Location of Intermittent Claudication, *GP*, **16**:89, 1957.
12. Hines, E. A., Jr., and Barker, N. W.: Arteriosclerosis Obliterans: A Clinical and Pathologic Study, *Am. J. Med. Sc.*, **200**:717–730, 1940.
13. Allen, E. V., and Brown, G. E.: Thromboangiitis Obliterans: A Clinical Study of 200 Cases. I. Etiology, Pathology, Symptoms, Diagnosis, *Ann. Int. Med.*, **1**:535–549, 1928.
14. Boyd, A. M.: Natural Course of Arteriosclerosis of Lower Extremities, *Proc. Roy. Soc. Med.*, **55**:591–593, 1962.
15. Silbert, S., and Zazeela, H.: Prognosis in Arteriosclerotic Peripheral Vascular Disease, *J.A.M.A.*, **166**:1816–1821, 1958.
16. Juergens, J. L., Barker, N. W., and Hines, E. A., Jr.: Arteriosclerosis Obliterans: Review of 520 Cases with Special Reference to Pathogenic and Prognostic Factors, *Circulation*, **21**:188–195, 1960.
17. LeFevre, F. A., Corbacioglu, C., Humphries, A. W., and deWolfe, V. G.: Management of Arteriosclerosis Obliterans of the Extremities, *J.A.M.A.*, **170**:656–661, 1959.
18. Massarelli, J. J., and Estes, J. E.: Atherosclerotic Occlusion of the Abdominal Aorta and Iliac Arteries: A Study of 105 Patients, *Ann. Int. Med.*, **47**:1125–1137, 1957.
19. Schadt, D. C., Hines, E. A., Jr., Juergens, J. L.,

and Barker, N. W.: Chronic Atherosclerotic Occlusion of the Femoral Artery, *J.A.M.A.*, **175**:937–940, 1961.

20. Campbell, K. N., Harris, B. M., and Coller, F. A.: A Follow-up Study of Patients with Thromboangiitis Obliterans (Buerger's Disease), *Surgery*, **26**:1003–1013, 1949.

21. Lynn, R. B., and Burt, C. C.: Thrombo-angiitis Obliterans: A Clinical Review, *Edinburgh M. J.*, **56**:422–430, 1949.

22. Cranley, J. J., Krause, R. J., and Strasser, E. S.: Limb Survival with and without Definitive Surgical Treatment in Obliterative Arterial Disease, *Surgery*, **45**:32–40, 1959.

23. DeWolfe, V. G., Humphries, A. W., Young, J. R., and LeFevre, F. A.: A Comparison of the Natural History of Arteriosclerosis Obliterans with the Results of Arterial Reconstruction, *Heart Bull.*, **12**:101–107, 1963.

24. Crawford, E. S., DeBakey, M. E., Cooley, D. A., and Morris, G. C., Jr.: Surgical Considerations of Aneurysms and Atherosclerotic Occlusive Lesions of the Aorta and Major Arteries, *Postgrad. Med.*, **29**:151–163, 1961.

25. Szilagyi, E., Smith, R. F., and Whitcomb, J. G.: The Contribution of Angioplastic Surgery to the Therapy of Peripheral Occlusive Arteriopathy: A Critical Evaluation of Eight Years' Experience, *Ann. Surg.*, **152**:660–677, 1960.

26. Whitman, E. J., and McGoon, D. C.: Surgical Management of Aortoiliac Occlusive Vascular Disease, *J.A.M.A.*, **179**:923–929, 1962.

27. Shucksmith, H. S., and Addison, N. V.: Late Results of Arterial Reconstructive Surgery, *Brit. M. J.*, **5313**:1144–1149, 1962.

28. Shaw, R. S., and Baue, A. E.: Management of Sepsis Complicating Arterial Reconstructive Surgery, *Surgery*, **53**:75–86, 1963.

29. Barker, N. W.: Danger of Gangrene of Toes in Thromboangiitis Obliterans and Arteriosclerosis Obliterans, *J.A.M.A.*, **104**:2147–2149, 1935.

30. Edwards, E. A., McAdams, A. J., and Crane, C.: Events Leading to Major Amputation in Patients with Arteriosclerosis, *New England J. Med.*, **249**:514–519, 1953.

31. Woolling, K. R., and Wilson, C.: Heat Therapy for Ischemia in the Lower Extremities: The Use of a New Thermostatically Controlled Therapeutic Heating Box, *Diabetes*, **4**:389–392, 1955.

32. Spittel, J. A., Jr., Martin, W. J., Heilman, F. R., Janes, J. M., and Shick, R. M.: Concentration of Penicillin in Ischemic Tissue after Intramuscular Injection, *J. Lab. & Clin. Med.*, **54**:599–602, 1959.

33. Spittel, J. A., Jr., Martin, W. J., Shick, R. M., and Janes, J. M.: Concentration of Orally Administered Erythromycin and Tetracycline in Ischemic Tissue, *Proc. Staff Meet. Mayo Clin.*, **36**:118–122, 1961.

34. Kelly, P. J., and Janes, J. M.: Criteria for Determining the Proper Level of Amputation in Occlusive Vascular Disease: A Review of 323 Amputations, *J. Bone & Joint Surg.*, **39-A**:883–891, 1957.

35. Haimovici, H.: Peripheral Arterial ˥mbolism, *Angiology*, **1**:20–45, 1950.

36. McGarity, W. C., Logan, W. D., Jr., and Cooper, F. W., Jr.: Peripheral Arterial Emboli, *Surg. Gynec. & Obst.*, **106**:399–408, 1958.

37. Spittell, J. A., Jr., Pascuzzi, C. A., Thompson, J. H., Jr., and Owen, C. A., Jr.: Accelerated Thromboplastin Generation in Acute Arterial Occlusion Complicating Arteriosclerosis Obliterans, *Ann. Int. Med.*, **55**:765–771, 1961.

38. Mozes, M., Ramon, Y., and Jahr, J.: The Anterior Tibial Syndrome, *J. Bone & Joint Surg.*, **44-A**:730–736, 1962.

39. McKechnie, R. E., and Allen, E. V.: Sudden Occlusion of Arteries of the Extremities: A Study of 100 Cases of Embolism and Thrombosis, *Surg. Gynec. & Obst.*, **63**:231–240, 1936.

40. Wessler, S., Sheps, S. G., Gilbert, M., and Sheps, M. C.: Studies in Peripheral Arterial Occlusive Disease. III. Acute Arterial Occlusion, *Circulation*, **17**:512–525, 1958.

41. Allen, E. V., Hines, E. A., Jr., Kvale, W. F., and Barker, N. W.: The Use of Dicumarol as an Anticoagulant: Experience in 2307 Cases, *Ann. Int. Med.*, **27**:371–381, 1947.

42. Warren, R., Linton, R. R., and Scannell, J. G.: Arterial Embolism: Recent Progress, *Ann. Surg.*, **140**:311–317, 1954.

43. Young, J. R., Humphries, A. W., deWolfe, V. G., and LeFevre, F. A.: Peripheral Arterial Embolism, *J.A.M.A.*, **185**:621–627, 1963.

44. Andrus, W. DeW.: Peripheral Arterial Embolism, with Particular Reference to Evaluation of Conservative Treatment, *Arch. Surg.*, **60**:511–519, 1950.

45. Des Prez, J. D., and Hubay, C. A.: Acute Arterial Embolism, *A.M.A. Arch. Surg.*, **67**:865–874, 1953.

46. Blum, L., and Rosenthal, I.: Embolectomy in Arteries to Extremities, *J.A.M.A.*, **172**:794–798, 1960.

47. Goldowsky, S. J., and Bowen, J. R.: Arterial Embolectomy, *J.A.M.A.*, **172**:799–802, 1960.

48. Spencer, F. C., and Grewe, R. V.: The Management of Arterial Injuries in Battle Casualties, *Ann. Surg.*, **141**:304–313, 1955.

49. McBurney, R. P., and Gegan, E.: Blunt Trauma to the Aorta and Major Arteries, *J.A.M.A.*, **180**:330–332, 1962.

50. Smith, R. F., Szilagyi, D. E., and Pfeifer, J. R.: Arterial Trauma, *Arch. Surg.*, **86**:825–835, 1963.

51. Hershey, F. B., and Spencer, A. D.: Autogenous Vein Grafts for Repair of Arterial Injuries, *Arch. Surg.*, **86**:836–845, 1963.

52. Estes, J. E.: Abdominal Aortic Aneurysm: A Study of 102 Cases, *Circulation*, **2**:258–264, 1950.

53. Gifford, R. W., Jr., Hines, E. A., Jr., and Janes, J. M.: An Analysis and Follow-up Study of 100 Popliteal Aneurysms, *Surgery*, **33**:284–293, 1953.

54. Holman, E.: The Obscure Physiology of Post-stenotic Dilatation: Its Relation to the Development of Aneurysms, *J. Thoracic Surg.*, 28:109–133, 1954.

55. Bedford, P. D., and Lodge, B.: Aneurysm of the Splenic Artery, *Gut*, 1:312–320, 1960.

56. Wright, I. S., Urdaneta, E., Wright, B.: Re-opening the Case of the Abdominal Aortic Aneurysm, *Circulation*, 13:754–768, 1956.

57. Schatz, I. J., Fairbairn, J. F., II, and Juergens, J. L.: Abdominal Aortic Aneurysms: A Reappraisal, *Circulation*, 26:200–205, 1962.

58. Sommerville, R. L., Allen, E. V., and Edwards, J. E.: Bland and Infected Arteriosclerotic Abdominal Aortic Aneurysms: A Clinicopathologic Study, *Medicine*, 38:207–221, 1959.

59. Owens, J. C., and Coffey, R. J.: Collective Review: Aneurysm of the Splenic Artery, Including a Report of 6 Additional Cases, *Internat. Abstr. Surg.*, 97:313–335, 1953.

60. Poutasse, E. F.: Renal Artery Aneurysm: Report of 12 Cases, Two Treated by Excision of the Aneurysm and Repair of Renal Artery, *J. Urol.*, 77:697–708, 1957.

61. Markowitz, A. M., and Norman, J. C.: Aneurysms of the Iliac Artery, *Ann. Surg.*, 154:777–787, 1961.

62. Gryska, P. F., Wheeler, C. G., and Linton, R. R.: A Review of Seven Years' Experience with Excision and Graft Replacement in 150 Ruptured and Unruptured Aneurysms of the Abdominal Aorta, *New England J. Med.*, 264:639–641, 1961.

63. Hirst, A. E., Jr., Johns, V. J., Jr., and Kime, S. W., Jr.: Dissecting Aneurysm of the Aorta: A Review of 505 Cases, *Medicine*, 37:217–279, 1958.

64. Baer, S.: Varied Manifestations of Dissecting Aneurysm of the Aorta, *J.A.M.A.*, 161:689–692, 1956.

65. Elkins, D. C., and Warren, J. V.: Arteriovenous Fistulas; Their Effect on the Circulation, *J.A.M.A.*, 134:1524–1528, 1947.

66. Wakim, K. G., and Janes, J. M.: Influence of Arteriovenous Fistula on the Distal Circulation in the Involved Extremity, *Arch. Phys. Med. & Rehabil.*, 39:431–434, 1958.

67. Adson, A. W., and Brown, G. E.: The Treatment of Raynaud's Disease by Resection of the Upper Thoracic and Lumbar Sympathetic Ganglia and Trunks, *Surg. Gynec. & Obst.*, 48:577–603, 1929.

68. Lewis, T.: "Vascular Disorders of the Limbs Described for Practitioners and Students," The Macmillan Company, New York, 1936.

69. Mendlowitz, M., and Naftchi, N.: The Digital Circulation in Raynaud's Disease, *Am. J. Cardiol.*, 4:580–584, 1959.

70. Peacock, J. H.: Peripheral Venous Blood Concentrations of Epinephrine and Norepinephrine in Primary Raynaud's Disease, *Circulation Res.*, 7:821–827, 1959.

71. Gifford, R. W., Jr.: Arteriospastic Disorders of the Extremities, *Circulation*, 27:970–975, 1963.

72. Gifford, R. W., Jr.: The Clinical Significance of Raynaud's Phenomenon and Raynaud's Disease, *M. Clin. North America*, 42:963–970, 1958.

73. Farmer, R. G., Gifford, R. W., Jr., and Hines, E. A., Jr.: Prognostic Significance of Raynaud's Phenomenon and Other Clinical Characteristics of Systemic Scleroderma, *Circulation*, 21:1088–1095, 1960.

74. Gifford, R. W., Jr., and Hines, E. A., Jr.: Raynaud's Disease among Women and Girls, *Circulation*, 16:1012–1021, 1957.

75. Hardgrove, M. A. F., and Barker, N. W.: Pneumatic Hammer Disease: A Vasospastic Disturbance of the Hands in Stone-cutters, *Proc. Staff Meet. Mayo Clin.*, 8:345–349, 1933.

76. Schatz, I. J.: Occlusive Arterial Disease in the Hands Due to Occupational Trauma, *New England J. Med.*, 268:281–284, 1963.

77. Allen, E. V., and Brown, G. E.: Raynaud's Disease Affecting Men, *Ann. Int. Med.*, 5:1384–1386, 1932.

78. Gifford, R. W., Jr., Hines, E. A., Jr., and Craig, W. McK.: Sympathectomy for Raynaud's Phenomenon: Follow-up Study of 70 Women with Raynaud's Disease and 54 Women with Secondary Raynaud's Phenomenon, *Circulation*, 17:5–13, 1958.

79. Babb, R. R., Alarcón-Segovia, D., and Fairbairn, J. F., II: Erythermalgia: Review of 51 Cases, *Circulation*, 29:136–141, 1964.

80. Merryman, H. T.: Tissue Freezing and Local Cold Injury, *Physiol. Rev.*, 37:233–251, 1957.

81. Montgomery, H.: Experimental Immersion Foot: Review of Physiopathology, *Physiol. Rev.*, 34:127–137, 1954.

82. Washburn, B.: Frostbite: What It Is, How to Prevent It, Emergency Treatment, *New England J. Med.*, 266:974–989, 1962.

83. Golding, M. R., deJong, P., Sawyer, P. N., Hennigar, G. R., and Wesolowski, S. A.: Protection from Early and Late Sequelae of Frostbite by Regional Sympathectomy: Mechanism of "Cold Sensitivity" Following Frostbite, *Surgery*, 53:303–308, 1963.

84. Alexander, B.: Blood Coagulation and Thrombotic Disease, *Circulation*, 25:872–890, 1962.

85. Spittell, J. A., Jr.: Blood Coagulation and Intravascular Thrombosis, *M. Clin. North America*, 46:947–954, 1962.

86. Ross, J. V., Jr., Baggenstoss, A. H., and Juergens, J. L.: Gangrene of Lower Extremity Secondary to Extensive Venous Occlusion, *Circulation*, 24:549–556, 1961.

87. Boyd, D. P., and Clarke, F. M.: Phlegmasia Cerulea Dolens, *Surgery*, 51:19–25, 1962.

88. Woolling, K. R., and Shick, R. M.: Thrombophlebitis: A Possible Clue to Cryptic Malignant Lesions, *Proc. Staff Meet. Mayo Clin.*, 31:227–233, 1956.

89. Lieberman, J. S., Borrero, J., Urdaneta, E., and

Wright, I. S.: Thrombophlebitis and Cancer, *J.A.M.A.*, **177**:542–545, 1961.

90. Bircher, J., Schirger, A., Clagett, O. T., and Harrison, E. G., Jr.: Mondor's Disease: A Vascular Rarity, *Proc. Staff Meet. Mayo Clin.*, **37**:651–656, 1962.

91. Effler, D. B., and Groves, L. K.: Superior Vena Caval Obstruction, *J. Thoracic & Cardiovas. Surg.*, **43**:574–584, 1962.

92. Ackerman, R. F., and Estes, J. E.: Prognosis in Idiopathic Thrombophlebitis, *Ann. Int. Med.*, **34**: 902–910, 1951.

93. Barker, N. W., Nygaard, K. K., Walters, W., and Priestley, J. T.: A Statistical Study of Postoperative Venous Thrombosis and Pulmonary Embolism. IV. Location of Thrombosis: Relation of Thrombosis and Embolism, *Proc. Staff Meet. Mayo Clin.*, **16**: 33–37, 1941.

94. Schatz, I. J., Allen, E. V., Allen, C. V., and Litin, E. M.: Disability after Real or Alleged Venous Thrombosis, *Postgrad. Med.*, **31**:358–363, 1962.

95. Barker, N. W., Nygaard, K. K., Walters, W., and Priestley, J. T.: A Statistical Study of Postoperative Venous Thrombosis and Pulmonary Embolism. I. Incidence in Various Types of Operations, *Proc. Staff Meet. Mayo Clin.*, **15**:769–773, 1940.

96. Sandy, J. T., and Perrett, T. S.: Fibrinolysin Therapy of Thrombophlebitis and Pulmonary Embolism: A Double-blind Study, *Canad. M.A.J.*, **88**: 1139–1146, 1963.

97. Spencer, F. C., Quattlebaum, J. K., Quattlebaum, J. K., Jr., Sharp, E. H., and Jude, J. R.: Plication of the Inferior Vena Cava for Pulmonary Embolism: A Report of 20 Cases, *Ann. Surg.*, **155**:827–837, 1962.

98. De Weese, M. S., and Hunter, D. C., Jr.: A Vena Cava Filter for the Prevention of Pulmonary Embolism: A Five Year Clinical Experience, *Arch. Surg.*, **86**:852–868, 1963.

99. Haller, J. A.: Thrombectomy for Deep Thrombophlebitis of the Leg, *New England J. Med.*, **267**: 65–68, 1962.

100. Pollack, A. A., Taylor, B. E., Myers, T. T., and Wood, E. H.: The Effect of Exercise and Body Position on the Venous Pressure at the Ankle in Patients Having Venous Valvular Defects, *J. Clin. Invest.*, **28**:559–563, 1949.

101. de Takats, G.: Postphlebitic Syndrome, *J.A.M.A.*, **164**:1861–1867, 1957.

102. Myers, T. T., and Cooley, J. C.: Varicose Vein Surgery in the Management of the Postphlebitic Limb, *Surg. Gynec. & Obst.*, **99**:733–744, 1954.

103. Lofgren, K. A., Ribisi, A. P., and Myers, T. T.: An Evaluation of Stripping versus Ligation for Varicose Veins, *A.M.A. Arch. Surg.*, **76**:310–316, 1958.

104. Højensgård, I. C.: Treatment of Varicose Veins of the Lower Extremities, *Acta chir. scandinav.*, **125**: 395–404, 1963.

57 THE NEUROLOGIC MANIFESTATIONS OF CARDIOVASCULAR DISEASE

Herbert R. Karp, M.D.

Neurologic signs and symptoms are often seen as a prominent manifestation of diseases of the cardiovascular system. The correct interpretation of these neurologic findings frequently provides the clinician with important clues as to the nature and extent of the primary disease process. It is the purpose of this chapter to discuss the major cardiovascular diseases in which the nervous system may be significantly involved and to relate the neurologic manifestation to the pathophysiology of the underlying cardiovascular disease.

In many of the diseases to be discussed the involvement of the nervous system is mediated by the cerebral vessels. The neurologic deficit which results from such involvement is referred to as a focal deficit, by which is implied a disturbance in nervous system function which can be related to a lesion in the distribution of a particular cerebral vessel. This *focal nature of the neurologic deficit,* along with its *sudden onset* and the *clinical setting* in which it occurs, constitutes the major clinical features of the diseases of the cerebral vessels. Therefore, in order to recognize the manifestation of diseases affecting the cerebral vessels, it is essential to have an understanding of the distribution of the principal cerebral arteries and the nature of the neurologic deficit produced by their occlusion or stenosis. An outline of these basic anatomic relationships is given in Table 57-9.

Neurologic Manifestations of Myocardial and Valvular Disease

The most frequent neurologic manifestation of disease of the heart or its valves is cerebral embolization. The clinical presentation of cerebral embolism is dominated by the sudden onset of a focal neurologic deficit. Although there are usually no premonitory symptoms such as those seen in cerebral thrombosis, Wells[1] and Fisher[2] call attention to the fact that such symptoms occasionally do occur in patients with cerebral emboli. Headache is the most common prodromal complaint and is thought to be due to stretching and disortion of the artery as the embolic particle first becomes lodged in a proximal segment. Perhaps as the vessel dilates, the embolus becomes dislodged only to occlude the more distal branches and produce an acute, persistent neurologic deficit. Often the headache clears as the neurologic deficit appears. Other patients experience more focal prodromal symptoms suggesting either multiple emboli in the same vascular distribution or an embolus advancing from a proximal segment in which collateral vessels can compensate for the occlusion to more distal segments where the available collateral flow is inadequate to prevent ischemia. Unfortunately, premonitory symptoms are rare, and the interval between them and the onset of the neurologic deficit is so short that one is unable to institute any therapy which might modify the subsequent ischemia.

The nature of the focal neurologic deficit is of course dependent on the vessel which is occluded and the extent of the ischemia which follows. Any cerebral vessel may be involved, and reliable figures as to the distribution of cerebral emboli are not available.

In the author's experience, cerebral emboli occur in decreasing order of frequency in the territory of the middle cerebral artery, the posterior cerebral artery, the superficial branches of the vertebral artery, particularly involving the inferior surfaces of the cerebellum, and least frequently in the territory of the anterior cerebral artery and the vessels supplying the more medial aspects of the brain stem. Although there is no predilection for the right or left side of the brain, one is impressed by the frequency with which recurrent emboli in a given patient are seen to involve one side to the almost complete exclusion of the other. The vessel which becomes occluded is a function of the size of the embolic particle in relation to the cross-sectional area of the arterial lumen. As most emboli are small, it then follows that very frequently the smaller arborizations are occluded, often leading to ischemia in the terminal distribution of the arteries. Consequently, discrete neurologic deficit such as an isolated aphasia, weakness or sensory loss limited to one hand, or a homonymous visual defect without other neurologic findings may be encountered. The incidence of seizures as early or late sequelae is greater in embolic than in thrombotic occlusion of cerebral arteries, related in part to the higher incidence of small cortical infarctions in cerebral embolism.[3]

Arterial embolization can be encountered in any myocardial or valvular disease in which there is a thrombus in the left side of the heart. The major causes of the formation of intracardiac thrombi are rheumatic heart disease, atherosclerotic heart disease, and bacterial endocarditis. Less frequent cardiac sources of emboli include endocardial fibroelastosis, thyrotoxic heart disease with atrial fibrillation, cardiac myxoma, and idiopathic myocarditis. In patients under the age of fifty, the most frequent cause of cerebral embolization is rheumatic heart disease, particularly in association with

either chronic atrial fibrillation, mitral valvular disease, or both. According to the data of Askey,[4] patients with rheumatic heart disease with normal sinus rhythm and no previously recognized embolus have only a 10 per cent chance of having a left atrial thrombus. Those patients with atrial fibrillation with or without previous history of embolus and with or without valvular lesions have a 50 per cent chance of having a thrombus in the left auricular appendage or the body of the left atrium. When atrial fibrillation was seen with mitral stenosis with or without previous history of embolus, 87 per cent were found to have a left auricular thrombus with a 50 per cent chance of eventually having peripheral embolization.

In the age group over fifty the incidence of cerebral embolism of cardiac origin is highest in patients with arteriosclerotic heart disease. The likelihood of left ventricular thrombus formation and peripheral embolization is greatest in the acute stages of myocardial infarction, especially in infarctions which involve a large area of myocardium, and in infarction of the anterior wall of the left ventricle.[5,6] Cerebral emboli occurring in the later stages of myocardial infarction are usually associated with a ventricular aneurysm.[7] Coexisting aortic valvular disease appears not to influence mural thrombus formation except insofar as it increases the probability of congestive heart failure.[8] Mitral stenosis even in the absence of atrial fibrillation may lead to left auricular thrombus formation and cerebral embolus. Atrial fibrillation due to arteriosclerotic heart disease, as in rheumatic heart disease, predisposes to left auricular thrombi.[9]

The immediate treatment of cerebral embolism is based primarily on anticoagulant therapy, since the surgical removal of the embolus is possible only if an embolus is lodged in an accessible portion of the cervical arteries. Uncontrolled, retrospective studies present data which suggest a statistical advantage in the immediate use of anticoagulants.[10,11] Whereas cerebral thrombosis results in a pale infarction, cerebral embolization may produce either pale or hemorrhagic infarction[12] (Fig. 57-1). In view of the frequency with which hemorrhagic infarction is seen in cerebral embolism, the decision to use anticoagulants should take into consideration the risk of increasing the amount of hemorrhage in the cerebral infarct versus the likelihood of permitting recurrent emboli or extension of the vascular occlusion if anticoagulants are withheld. In experimental embolic infarction in dogs, Whisnant et al.[13] have shown a higher morbidity and mortality in animals receiving anticoagulants immediately after infarction, probably because of an increase in the hemorrhagic component of the cerebral infarct. When anticoagulation was delayed 36 to 48 hr after the infarction, there was no significant difference in clinical or pathologic findings between the treated and control groups. Though a similar deleterious effect has not been firmly documented in man, the author's practice is to regard an increase in the extent of hemorrhage as a potential risk and to use a slower-acting anticoagulant, such as bishydroxycoumarin, rather than more rapidly acting forms, such as warfarin or heparin. These patients usually reach levels of 20 to 25 per cent prothrombin activity in 48 hr, and this level is maintained for the duration of therapy. The rationale for this form of therapy is to prevent repeated emboli rather than to attempt to modify the accomplished embolic infarction.

The prophylactic aspects of the treatment of cerebral embolism consist of long-term anticoagulant therapy, prophylaxis for bacterial endocarditis, the surgical correction of the lesions predisposing to the formation of thrombi of the left side of the heart, and the proper management of cardiac arrhythmias.

The neurologic findings in bacterial endocarditis are usually the same as those seen in other forms of cerebral embolization. Because of the occurrence of multiple embolization by small particles, the patient may exhibit signs of diffuse cerebral involvement, such as agitated confusion (delirium) or depressed consciousness. Some may only have signs of meningitis. Focal signs when present may be quite discrete. Mycotic cerebral aneurysms can result in intracranial bleeding with the characteristics of either intracerebral or primary subarachnoid hemorrhage. When the infective organism is a pyogenic one, such as staphylococcus, the occurrence of an episode of cerebral embolism followed by progressive worsening of the neurologic deficit and increasing intracranial pressure suggests the presence of a cerebral abscess.

The treatment of the cerebral complications of bacterial endocarditis is primarily directed at the eradication of the bacterial infection. The occasional occurrence of an episode of brain embolism after the bloodstream is sterile raises the question of the concomitant use of anticoagulants, particularly in the later phases of therapy. Most of the recorded instances of catastrophic intracranial hemorrhage attributed to anticoagulant therapy in bacterial endocarditis occurred in the preantibiotic era, when the sulfonamide drugs were the only available antimicrobial agent. This suggests that continuing infection was as significant a factor as the anticoagulants in the production of the hemorrhage. In spite of this possibility, it is still generally held that anticoagulants are contraindicated in either early or late phases of the treatment of bacterial endocarditis.

Nonbacterial thrombotic endocarditis in associa-

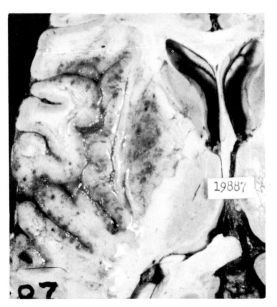

Fig. 57-1. Hemorrhagic infarction resulting from embolic occlusion of the middle cerebral artery. Note the relative preservation of neural architecture and predominance of hemorrhage in depths of the sulci and deep gray matter.

tion with cancer or other debilitating diseases, frequently referred to as *marantic endocarditis,* has been regarded as a rare cause of peripheral embolization. This condition has been shown to be a more frequent cause of cerebral embolism than had been previously suspected. Barron et al.[14] presented autopsy data from a hospital with a large service for the treatment of terminal cases of malignant neoplasm. These workers found that 85 per cent of the cases of nonbacterial thrombotic endocarditis were associated with cancer, these vegetations of the cardiac valves accounting for 10 per cent of all the autopsied cases of cerebral emboli. MacDonald and Robbins[15] in an analysis of 18,486 cases, found 78 instances of nonbacterial thrombotic endocarditis, 14 per cent of which had resulted in arterial emboli. Clinically, there was a frequent association with thrombophlebitis. Thus, the acute onset of a focal neurologic deficit in a patient with suspected or known cancer seen in association with thrombophlebitis should suggest cerebral embolization from nonbacterial thrombotic endocarditis. The recognition of this clinical picture is important in preventing the erroneous diagnosis of cerebral metastasis, since an otherwise operable neoplasm may not receive adequate treatment because of the inaccurate conclusion that the cerebral symptoms indicate that the lesion has become dessiminated. Adams[16] cites instances in which cerebral embolism was the first evidence of neoplasm and states that an apoplectic event in a patient with cancer is more likely due to nonbacterial endocarditis than either tumor embolus or cerebral metastasis.

The nonembolic neurologic aspects of myocardial and valvular disease consist primarily of syncope and are discussed in Chap. 17.

Neurologic Complications of Cardiac Surgery

Central nervous system emboli constitute a significant complication of cardiac surgery. Valvotomy for the correction of mitral stenosis, whether transatrial or transventricular, carries the risk of peripheral embolization either by calcific valve fragments or as a result of accidental dislodgment of thrombotic material in the left atrium. Wood, quoted in a personal communication by Emanuel,[17] states that in mitral stenosis uncomplicated by valve calcification the risk of arterial embolization at operation is between 5 and 8 per cent. However, when stenosis is accompanied by incompetence and calcification of the valve, the risk of emboli increases to 13 per cent. In open-heart surgical procedures employing extracorporeal circulation, the risk of cerebral embolization is theoretically greater than it is with closed procedures. Here, along with embolization by calcium plaques, there are the added hazards of air emboli as well as systemic emboli by thrombi, silicon, and fat. In an excellent review of this subject, Allen[18] reports an incidence of 18 embolic episodes in 500 cases of bypass surgical procedures performed at the Vancouver General Hospital. Air emboli were the most frequently encountered, occurring most often in the repair of mitral and aortic valves and to a lesser degree during the closure of atrial septal defects of the ostium secundum and primum types. Calcium emboli were seen in calific lesions of the aortic or mitral valves. Thrombotic emboli were less frequent and were usually encountered during active attempts to remove a left atrial thrombus rather than occurring by accidental dislodgement at the time of operation. Thrombotic emboli were also seen in resection of postinfarction myocardial aneurysms in which friable thrombi were dislodged during the resection of the aneurysmal sac. Silicon emboli, though infrequent, may be seen in systems using Antifoam as a defoaming agent and are more likely to occur during procedures requiring high-volume perfusion over an extended period during which the silicon may be washed from the oxygenator into the arterial system.

The neurologic manifestations of central nervous system (CNS) emboli in surgical treatment of the heart are highly variable. The early manifestations, such as slowness to respond after anesthesia, persistently depressed consciousness, generalized seizures, and the absence of focal neurologic signs, sug-

gest a generalized disorder and are likely to be due to air, silicon, or fat emboli. An intermediate group also thought to be due to air or silicon is characterized by a normal response for the first 12 to 24 hr followed by depressed consciousness and frequently generalized seizures. The third clinical picture is dominated by focal signs (either focal neurologic deficits or focal seizures) with or without impaired consciousness and is seen immediately postoperatively. This picture is more likely due to calcific or thrombotic emboli. Focal CNS manifestations appearing 48 hr or later are most likely due to embolization from thrombi forming on operative suture lines.

Comparatively little is written about fat embolization during cardiotomy and cardiopulmonary bypass. Caugin and Carter,[19] reporting on 93 bypass operations, noted an occasional patient who exhibited a wide variety of vague neurologic signs and symptoms, usually appearing between the third and seventh postoperative day. The neurologic features ranged from mild confusion and amnesia to a picture resembling delirium tremens which responded to sedation. Focal signs were minimal, and all patients recovered without apparent residual deficits. Petechiae were not encountered in any patients. None of the patients developing delirium gave a history of significant alcohol consumption. Although hypoxia could not be ruled out, the electroencephalograms done during the operation were normal in all patients, and none had undue respiratory symptoms.

Because of the similarity of these symptoms to those seen in some patients with multiple fractures, fat embolization was suspected as a cause. Subsequently, evidence of fat embolization was looked for routinely, and significant lipuria was found in 10 of 45 patients, 8 of whom demonstrated these neurologic events. Fat globules were demonstrated in the cerebrospinal fluid of one patient who also had lesions in his retinal arterioles consistent with fat emboli. There was no correlation with the type of thoracotomy, the surgical procedure, or the duration of the bypass.

The writers noted that the symptoms seem to occur only in patients in whom the blood overflowed from the cardiac chambers into the pericardial sac or the pleural space and was then returned to the bypass circuit via the coronary suction apparatus. Fat globules could be seen on the surface of the blood pooled in these cavities. Sudan III stains on the pooled blood were positive, whereas venous blood drawn simultaneously was negative for free fat. This suggests that the source of the fat was the marrow of the ribs and sternum or other surfaces cut during the operative procedure. In subsequent operations on 56 patients, recirculation of the blood in the pericardial sac was avoided if possible. In one patient in whom technical problems necessitated return of pericardial blood neurologic signs and severe lipuria developed. In two others mild lipuria developed without neurologic findings. These patients differ in some respects from the instances of fat embolization after trauma reported by Sevitt,[20] who emphasizes a characteristic petechial rash over the anterior chest and shoulders as a prominent and reliable sign. Sevitt also regards the examination of the urine to be unreliable, though he apparently examined only random specimens rather than 24-hr pooled specimens as done in Caguin's study.

There is no explanation for the delayed appearance of the neurologic symptoms in these cases. This time sequence is reminiscent of the biphasic course seen in patients with carbon monoxide intoxication and reported by Plum et al.[21] in patients with cerebral anoxia from a variety of other causes. The close relationship between the appearance of lipuria and the development of neurologic symptoms in Caguin's cases favor fat embolization as being the primary pathogenetic factor. Fromm[22] regards a "free interval" of 12 to 48 hr between the trauma and the onset of cerebral symptoms as charactreistic of cerebral fat embolization.

A classification of the neurologic complications of open-heart surgical procedure with cardiopulmonary bypass is presented in Table 57-1. This classification, although inadequate, provides the clinician with a reasonable basis for establishing the source of emboli associated with open-heart surgical procedures. No single group of observers has had sufficient experience with postoperative emboli to formulate more definite criteria. In addition, the problem is compounded by such factors as unrecognized fat emboli, hypoxia, hemoconcentration, and hypoglycemia possibly related to the use of stored, whole blood. Similarly, the neuropathologic data on autopsy cases is frequently incomplete because of failure to use appropriate histologic techniques, as silicon and fat emboli are dissolved by the usual solvents used in routine histologic preparation.

The study by Brierly[23] provides excellent clinicopathologic correlation in 11 patients who died after open-heart surgical operation. These patients include two in whom cardiopulmonary bypass was not used but in whom there was deliberate circulatory arrest under mild hypothermia, and nine patients in whom cardiopulmonary bypass with a pump oxygenator was used along with mild hypothermia. The predominant pathologic lesions were multifocal, perivascular, irregular areas of ischemic changes involving the cortex and underlying white matter, seen predominantly in the dependent portions of the brain (posterior portion of the middle cerebral artery territory, occipital lobes, and cerebellum). These lesions had neither the histologic features nor the distribution characteristic of diffuse cerebral anoxia. Brierly postulates that these lesions are due either to severely reduced cerebral blood flow or to air embolism. The predominance of lesions in the posterior portions of the brain suggests that a gravitational pooling may have occurred in this region in patients lying in the supine position. The resulting congestion of the dependent portion of the vascular bed might delay the resumption of normal pulsatile blood flow when normal cardiac function is resumed and thus lead to ischemia.

Neurologic Complications of Congenital Heart Disease

Tyler and Clark[24,25] reviewed the neurologic complications of congenital heart disease and found evidence of neurologic involvement in 25 per cent of 1,875 patients of the cardiac clinic at the Harriett Lane Home of the Johns Hopkins Hospital. Those patients with congenital heart disease in whom the major physiologic defects were decreased pulmonary flow or transposition (e.g., tetralogy of Fallot, truncus arteriosus with de-

Table 57-1. CLINICAL FEATURES OF EMBOLIC COMPLICATIONS OF CARDIAC SURGICAL TREATMENT

Time of onset	Clinical findings	Probable type of emboli
Immediate or 12–24 hr postoperatively	(1) Failure to respond after surgical treatment; persistently depressed consciousness; possibly generalized seizures; no focal signs.	Air, fat, or silicon. Generalized petechiae and hematuria favor silicon or fat.
	(2) Prominent focal signs; neurologic defect and/or focal seizures	Calcific fragments or intracardiac thrombi.
Delayed—48 hr or later postoperatively	(1) Prominent focal signs	Thrombotic from thrombi on suture lines.
	(2) Confusion, stupor, delirium tremens-like picture usually without focal signs; significant lipuria	Fat.

creased flow, transposition) had a high incidence of episodic loss of consciousness. This clinical picture consists of loss of consciousness lasting from minutes to 2 to 3 hr, characteristically brought on by increased physical activity and preceded in most patients by severe cyanosis and dyspnea. Based on the history of cyanosis and dyspnea preceding the loss of consciousness or convulsions, the writers conclude that these episodes are caused by a sudden shift of hemodynamics in which more venous blood enters the systemic circulation. In this study there were 27 cases of cerebral abscess, all occurring in patients with cardiac defects which allowed the passage of venous blood directly into systemic circulation, bypassing the pulmonary circuit. Abscesses were significantly more frequent in patients with tetralogy of Fallot (1.4 per cent), transposition (1.7 per cent), and septal defects (0.7 per cent). No abscesses were seen in association with patent ductus arteriosus. It is interesting that in this series cerebral abscesses were not seen in patients under the age of two years. Instances of mental retardation were seen in a wide variety of cardiac malformations and were related to associated developmental abnormalities of the brain rather than to the severity of the cardiac lesion.

Cerebral vascular accidents were more frequent in patients with transposition of the great vessels, tricuspid atresia, and other forms of congenital heart disease which produced a high degree of cyanosis and hypoxia in the first two years of life. The majority of cerebral vascular accidents (74 per cent) occurred in the first twenty months of life, decreasing in frequency up to age six and then recurring in the mid-teens. On postmortem examination all infarctions were in the distribution of the middle cerebral arteries, but in only 3 of 14 autopsied cases was an actual thrombosis demonstrated. No embolic origin was demonstrated in any patient in this series. Determinations of red blood cell count and oxygen saturation at the time of the cerebrovascular accident suggest to these writers that in the younger group anoxia is a major factor in the pathogenesis of cerebral lesions, whereas in the older group polycythemia appears to be of greater pathogenetic importance. The frequency with which these events were associated with acute illness suggests that fever and dehydration were contributing factors.

Neurologic Manifestations of Atherosclerosis

The principal mechanisms by which atherosclerosis affects the nervous system are (1) direct involvement of the intracranial arteries, (2) stenosis or occlusion of the cervicobrachial arteries, and (3) embolization of the cerebral vessels from atheromatous deposits in the thoracic aorta and the cervical arteries. The cerebral arterial circulation is involved by atherosclerosis in a manner that tends to parallel the atherosclerotic process in other systemic arteries. The earliest and most frequently involved segment is the proximal internal carotid and the carotid sinus. The common carotid artery may be involved but to a much lesser degree. Significant narrowing of the cervical portion of the vertebral artery is less than that seen in the carotid and tends to be concentrated in its proximal 2 cm. Examinations of the entire length of the vertebral arteries have shown atheromatous changes to be more widely distributed, in many instances bearing a relationship to distortion of the vessel by osteoarthritis of the cervical spine.[26]

Maximum involvement of the intracranial arteries is seen at the carotid siphon, at the trifurcation of the internal carotid, at the first bifurcation of the middle cerebral artery, in the basilar artery at its bifurcation, at the proximal segment of the posterior cerebral artery as it passes around the cerebral peduncles, and at the anterior cerebral artery in its course over the genu of the corpus callosum. Hypertension and diabetes increase the severity of the atherosclerotic process in both the extra- and intracranial arteries and in addition is associated with atheromatous changes in smaller vessels, such as the meningeal arteries and the perforating branches originating from the main stem of the middle cerebral, basilar, and posterior cerebral arteries.

In 100 consecutive autopsies of patients over the age of fifty years, Martin et al.[27] found 40 per cent of the cases to have stenosis of at least one major cervical artery to a degree of 50 per cent or greater. However, only 17 of these 40 patients had symptoms of cerebral ischemia during life. The only significant difference between the symptomatic and asymptomatic patients was a greater degree of atherosclerosis of the intracranial arteries in the symptomatic group. There was also a close relationship between atherosclerosis of the cervical arteries and coronary artery disease, both tending to reach their maximum extent in the same age group. The peak incidence of significant atherosclerosis of the intracranial arteries occurred some 10 years later. These data suggest that although a large segment of the population over fifty has significant atherosclerosis of the cervical arteries, most are asymptomatic. The occurrence of symptoms of ischemia depends on other factors, one of which is concomitant involvement of the intracranial arteries. Other recognized factors predisposing to symptoms of ischemia include anemia, hypoxia, hemoconcentration, decreased perfusion pressure (on the basis of either decreased arterial pressure, increased venous pressure, or increased intracranial pressure), and inadequacy of collateral channels due to congenital variations in the distribution and size of the major cerebral arteries (Fig. 57-2).

The clinical features of atherosclerosis of the cerebral vessels with thrombosis are more varied than those of cerebral embolism. There is, however, a central core of signs and symptoms which can be of assistance in arriving at a diagnosis of cerebral thrombosis. The clinical manifestations may develop in one of several forms. There may be a single event on awakening; there may be a stuttering progression, with the full deficit appearing over several hours or even days; or severe paralysis may clear within hours or a day only to be followed by persistent paralysis.

Many patients with cerebral thrombosis have a history of one or more transient episodes of neurologic deficit that preceded the accomplished infarction. Such episodes do not precede intracranial hemorrhage and are uncommon in cerebral embolism. These episodes, referred to as *transient ischemic attacks* (TIA), consist of recurrent, transient episodes of neurologic dysfunction. They may be considered a reversible fragment of the stroke which is often imminent. Onset is usually sudden, most often when the patient is active, and the attack may last from a few seconds to several hours. The attack usually ends as suddenly as it began, clearing without significant residual deficit. The successive attacks are usually of the same pattern, although somewhat different in detail. The neurologic features depend on the distribution of the artery involved.

In the carotid system the episodes commonly take the form of unilateral numbness and weakness of the side of the body opposite the involved vessel. It is to be emphasized that monocular blindness and associated symptoms that affect the opposite side of the body are virtually pathognomonic of involvement of the carotid artery on the same side as the blindness. Diminished or absent pulsations in the carotid artery in the neck or pharynx, reduced retinal artery pressure, and a bruit over the carotid artery or the orbit suggest narrowing or occlusion of the carotid artery. These features are summarized in Table 57-2.

Table 57-2. COMMON SIGNS AND SYMPTOMS OF TRANSIENT ISCHEMIC ATTACKS IN THE DISTRIBUTION OF THE INTERNAL CAROTID ARTERY

1. Unilateral weakness and numbness on side opposite involved vessel
2. Aphasia (when dominant hemisphere involved)
3. Monocular blindness with sensory or motor symptoms affecting opposite side of body
4. Reduced pulsations in carotid artery
5. Reduced central retinal artery pressure
6. Neck or cranial bruit

The characteristic features in the vertebral-basilar system are more varied and are summarized in Table 57-3.

Table 57-3. COMMON SIGNS AND SYMPTOMS OF TRANSIENT ISCHEMIC ATTACKS INVOLVING THE VERTEBRAL-BASILAR ARTERY SYSTEM

1. Weakness, numbness of one or both sides of the body	6. Dysarthria or speechlessness
2. "Crossed symptoms," such as one side of the face and the opposite body half	7. Dysphagia
	8. Staggering
	9. Peculiar head and face sensations
3. Dizziness	10. Hiccupping
4. Diplopia	11. "Apparent" unconsciousness
5. Partial or complete blindness	

In differential diagnosis the following conditions must be considered: cerebral seizures, Ménière's syndrome and other forms of aural vertigo, paralytic migraine, Stokes-Adams attacks and hyperactive carotid sinus reflexes, and cerebral embolism.

The differentiation of cerebral seizures is outlined in Table 57-4. Although motor convulsions do not occur in TIA, patients may frequently report feelings of distortion or contortion of the extremities. Paralysis is, of course, frequent in TIA. In seizure, however, paralysis is a postictal phenomenon occurring after a frank motor convulsion. Sensory seizures are much more difficult to differentiate from TIA than are motor convulsions. As a rule, the sensory march in cerebral seizure is extremely rapid, whereas in TIA the rate of spread is much slower, extending over a period of several minutes.

Dizziness is one of the most frequent neurologic

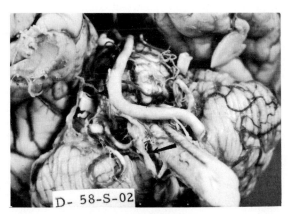

D- 58-S-02

57-2. Anomalous vertebral-basilar artery system with an atretic right vertebral artery (arrow). The patient had recurrent TIA in the distribution of the vertebral artery.

Table 57-4. DIFFERENTIAL DIAGNOSIS OF CEREBRAL SEIZURES AND TRANSIENT ISCHEMIC ATTACKS

Symptoms	Seizures	TIA
Frank motor convulsion	+	−
Paralysis as only manifestation	−	+
Numbness, paresthesias, scintillating scotoma, sensory march	+	+
Associated phenomena, such as monocular blindness, diplopia, dizziness	−	+
Unconsciousness, incontinence, residual drowsiness, myalgia	+	−

symptoms in the older age group and poses a difficult diagnostic problem. There are no characteristics of the dizziness itself which make it possible to determine whether the complaint is of aural origin or that it represents a manifestation of brain stem ischemia. Only by careful search for signs of disturbance of function of other structures that are innervated by the brain stem can this differentiation be made (Table 57-5).

Table 57-5. DIFFERENTIAL DIAGNOSIS OF MÉNIÈRE'S SYNDROME AND TRANSIENT ISCHEMIC ATTACKS

Symptoms	Ménière's syndrome	TIA
Dizziness	+	+
Dizziness, tinnitus, deafness in "isolation"	+	−
Other evidence of brain stem involvement, such as diplopia, facial numbness, and dysarthria	−	+

Differential diagnosis between "paralytic" migraine and TIA is difficult, because both states may consist of focal sensory or motor phenomena with attendant headache of a vascular nature. A history of such symptoms from early life suggests migraine (Table 57-6).

Table 57-6. DIFFERENTIAL DIAGNOSIS OF "PARALYTIC" MIGRAINE AND TRANSIENT ISCHEMIC ATTACKS

Symptoms	Paralytic migraine	TIA
Visual, sensory, motor phenomena	+	+
Headache	+	−
History beginning in early life	+	−

If only one episode of transient neurologic disturbance has occurred, it is virtually impossible to differentiate between cerebral embolism and TIA. When there have been several attacks of similar character, the most likely diagnosis is TIA, since it would be highly unlikely that successive showers of embolic particles would always find their way to the same cerebral vessel.

Stokes-Adams attacks and hyperactive carotid sinus reflexes as a rule produce syncopal symptoms and are not associated with focal sensory or motor disturbances. An electrocardiogram and gentle massage of the carotid sinus are of help in differential diagnosis.

The pathophysiology of transient ischemic attacks remains obscure. Whatever their exact mechanism, they are closely related to cerebral atherosclerosis. The observed effect of anticoagulants of reducing the frequency of attacks, the finding in some patients of fibrin or cholesterol emboli (Plate-7) in the retinal arterioles during an attack, and the arteriographic evidence of significant stenosis of the cervical arteries in many patients with TIA all suggest that in some instances recurrent emboli from cervical arterial atheroma may precipitate the episodes. On the other hand, the stereotyped nature of successive attacks could be explained only by embolic particles entering the same arterial segment. Although this could happen on the basis of the pattern of arterial flow in a given patient, it seems statistically unlikely. An alternative explanation is based on the supposition that the area of brain from which the symptoms arise is one in which collateral blood flow is marginal, being adequate only under basal conditions. The added limitations imposed by stenosis of the cervical arteries and other factors, such as a minimal reduction in blood pressure or a mild degree of hypoxia, might then be sufficient to render the area ischemic. This theory is more compatible with the stereotyped nature of the recurrent attacks but is less tenable when one considers how infrequently TIA can be precipitated in these patients by artificially inducing hypotension or anoxia.

While it is true that many patients with cerebral thrombosis do have an antecedent history of transient ischemic attacks, it does not necessarily follow that these episodes invariably lead to a cerebral infarction with persistent neurologic deficit. In fact, recent observations of patients with transient ischemic attacks alone have shown that the majority of the patients did not progress to cerebral infarction within the 2- to 3-year observation period[28] (Table 57-7). These data suggest that there may be a group of patients in whom transient ischemic attacks do not portend an impending stroke. However, in the absence of clinical criteria by which to recognize this group, it remains important to regard transient ischemic attacks as

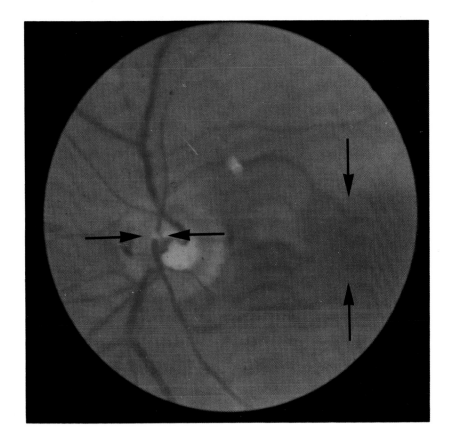

Plate 7. Retinal photograph showing a cholesterol crystal in the superior temporal artery as it courses over the optic disk. The dark red area in the temporal retina is the resulting infarction. (*Courtesy of Wm. S. Hagler, M.D., Department of Ophthalmology, Emory University School of Medicine.*)

Table 57-7. PROGNOSIS OF UNTREATED TRANSIENT
ISCHEMIC ATTACKS (24- TO 41-MONTH FOLLOW-UP)

	Patients with TIA	Patients developing cerebral infarction	Deaths from cerebral infarction	Deaths from other causes
PHS cooperative study[29]	20	4	1	1
VA cooperative study[30]	15	0	0	0
N. J. David and A. Heyman[31]	8	3	3	1
Total	43	7	4	2

SOURCE: *Modified from J. L. Patterson and A. Heyman.*[28]

"warning episodes," in order that appropriate diagnostic procedures and therapy may be instituted before a permanent neurologic deficit occurs.

In the absence of effective means of modifying the process of atherosclerosis, the treatment of cerebral atherosclerosis is twofold: (1) the long-term use of anticoagulants and (2) surgical maneuvers designed to bypass or excise areas of obstruction of the cervicobrachial portion of cerebral circulation. The role of anticoagulant drugs has not yet been fully established. Earlier reports suggested that this form of therapy in patients with transient ischemic attacks reduced the number and frequency of attacks and postponed or prevented cerebral infarction. It was also held that anticoagulants favorably influenced the course of an advancing cerebral thrombosis. More recent results of several controlled, cooperative studies of the effects of anticoagulant drugs have failed to demonstrate any statistically significant reduction of either the incidence of cerebral infarction or the mortality rate in patients with transient ischemic attacks.[29,30] There was, however, a reduction in the number of ischemic attacks, this effect being most prominent in the first 3 to 4 months of the observation period. The suggestive benefit of anticoagulants in patients with advancing thrombosis was offset by the high incidence of hemorrhagic complication in the treated group. These studies conclusively demonstrated that there is no advantage in the use of anticoagulant drugs in the accomplished cerebral infarction.

Comparable controlled studies in the surgical management of cerebral atherosclerosis are not available. Published reports of uncontrolled studies suggest that carotid endarterectomy or similar procedures have a favorable influence on the course of patients with transient ischemic attacks. The surgical aspects of treatment are discussed in Chap. 59. Based on personal experience and the interpretation of the available data, the author's practice is to limit the use of anticoagulant drugs to patients

with transient ischemic attacks or an advancing stroke who do not have a surgically accessible lesion or in whom coexisting illness precludes subjecting them to arteriography or surgical treatment.

Other Forms of Cervicobrachial Circulation Disease with Cerebral Symptoms

Other forms of disease of the cervical and brachial arteries producing cerebral symptoms include kinking of the carotid arteries, obstruction in the brachiocephalic or subclavian arteries, and the various forms of the aortic arch syndrome. Kinking of the cervical arteries has been attributed to the effects of hypertension and atherosclerosis or to the persistence of fetal configuration of the carotid artery. Examples of kinking have been found in every decade from the first to the ninth, frequently without relationship to hypertension or atherosclerosis. Metz et al.[32] found no greater incidence of cerebral manifestation in patients with severe kinking when compared with patients of similar age without this abnormality. They were able to produce vague cerebral symptoms in 4 of 24 patients by rotation of the neck. In spite of the lack of firm clinical correlation, one is justified in carefully considering the surgical excision of an area of kinking in a patient who clearly has recurrent cerebrovascular episodes related to turning of the neck and in whom no other adequate cause can be demonstrated.

Occlusion or stenosis of the subclavian or innominate artery can lead to symptoms which in most instances are referable to the distribution of the vertebral-basilar artery. This condition should be considered when there is a significant difference in the blood pressure in each arm or a bruit which is maximal over the supraclavicular area. Occasionally symptoms may be precipitated by exercise of the homolateral arm leading to retrograde collateral flow to the arm at the expense of the vertebral-basilar system. This syndrome has been designated as the *subclavian steal* [33] syndrome (Fig. 57-3).

Cerebral symptoms are frequently seen in the various forms of the aortic arch syndrome, in which there is obliteration of the large arteries arising from the convexity of the aorta. Causes of such involvement include atherosclerosis, syphilitic aortitis, Takayasu's arteritis of young females, trauma, neoplasm, and congenital malformation. The neurologic manifestations are dependent on the relative degree of involvement of the major vessels and may include findings such as those described in conjunction with the carotid or vertebral-basilar arteries.

The association between coarctation of the aorta and aneurysms of the intracranial arteries is well known. Reifenstein et al.[36] found that subarachnoid hemorrhage from a berry aneurysm accounted for

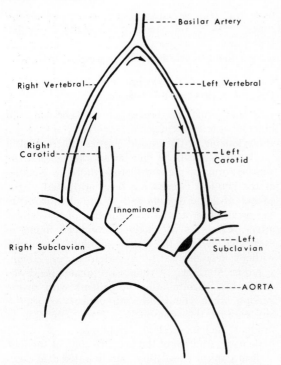

Fig. 57-3. Retrograde flow in the left vertebral artery bypassing a stenotic area in the left subclavian artery, as seen in the subclavian steal syndrome.

10.6 per cent of deaths in their series of cases. In addition they report three cases of cerebral embolism from bacterial endocarditis arising from associated congenital valvular malformation.

Aortic Disease Involving the Spinal Cord

The spinal cord is frequently cited as being that portion of the central nervous system less likely to be affected by vascular disease. This statement is in general valid with regard to atherosclerotic involvement of the intrinsic arteries of the cord. However, the spinal cord may be significantly involved in several types of aortic disease. The most familiar of these is dissecting aortic aneurysm, in which the spinal cord may be rendered ischemic by virtue of the dissection occluding the ostia of the intercostal and lumbar arteries. Occlusion of the abdominal aorta by atherosclerosis or embolus may lead to dysfunction of the spinal cord. Cook[34] has reported findings suggesting anterior spinal artery occlusion in such patients. The clinical picture was characterized by the acute onset of paraparesis of a varying degree with signs pointing to the seventh to ninth thoracic segment consisting of altered pinprick response below this level with relative or absolute preservation of the response to light-touch and proprioception. There was a bilat-

eral extensor plantar response and impaired sphincter control. Some patients experienced radicular-type pain in the lower extremities. Plain spine x-rays and lumbar puncture with bilateral jugular vein compression and myelograph were negative. Cook found that alteration in one of the major arterial pulses was frequently the only evidence of involvement of the circulation to the skin and lower extremities, this being one means of differentiation of this syndrome from that of aortic dissection. Aortography proved to be the most reliable means of establishing the correct diagnosis.

Coarctation of the aorta may affect the spinal cord as a result of hypertrophy of the anterior spinal artery as it participates in the collateral circulation to the trunk and lower limbs. Such hypertrophy may lead to the formation of a false aneurysm which can act as an extramedullary compressive lesion.[35]

Hypertension and the Nervous System

The major central nervous system manifestations of hypertension are (1) spontaneous intracerebral hemorrhage, (2) hypertensive encephalopathy, (3) cerebral atherosclerosis as modified and accelerated by hypertension.

The spontaneous or hypertensive intracerebral hemorrhage is one of the most frequent nervous system concomitants of hypertension. It occurs almost without exception in patients who have significant and persistent elevation of blood pressure or who have evidence of hypertension in the past as manifested by changes in the retinal arterioles, cardiomegaly, left ventricular hypertrophy pattern on ECG, etc. The hemorrhages arise in one of several sites: the putamen, the thalamus and subthalamic region, the external capsule, the tegmentum of the pons, or the cerebellum. Although apparently unrelated, these areas have in common the fact that they are in the distribution of the short, penetrating arteries which originate from major arterial trunks and pass immediately into cerebral substance. The hemorrhage appears to originate within deep nuclear masses, e.g., the putamen, the thalamus, or the dentate nucleus of the cerebellum, and then dissect through and compress surrounding white matter.

Using the putaminal hemorrhage as the paradigm of a hypertensive intracerebral hemorrhage, the clinical events are as follows: The onset is abrupt while the patient is active and is not preceded by recurrent prodromal symptoms such as are seen in cerebral thrombosis. The patient usually complains of an abnormal head sensation, which is frequently, though not invariably, a severe headache. Initially there may be no localizing signs, but as the adja-

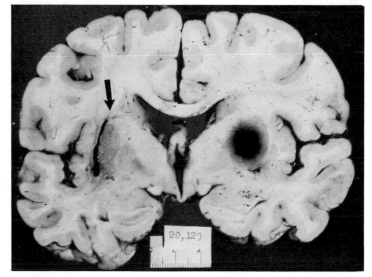

Fig. 57-4. Nonfatal hypertensive intracerebral hemorrhage. Slit hemorrhage in the left putamen and external capsule (arrow) is the residuum of an episode that occurred 12 months previously. Ball hemorrhage on the right is of 2 days' duration. The patient died of a hemorrhage in the tegmentum of the pons.

cent internal capsule is compressed, a contralateral hemiparesis and sensory deficit develop. As the process extends anteriorly, there may be paralysis or weakness of gaze to the opposite side, often with the eyes conjugately deviated to the side of the hemorrhage. If the dominant hemisphere is involved, there may be aphasia; in the nondominant hemisphere, the syndrome of apractognosia may be seen. Gradually, the hemiparesis worsens, and the patient becomes more stuporous. In its severest forms the hemorrhage ruptures into the lateral ventricle. The involved hemisphere is shifted medially under the falx and tentorium, producing compression of the midbrain. Coma deepens and bilateral signs appear, respiration becomes irregular, and there is decerebrate posturing, with fixed miotic pupils and death in a few hours. It is to be emphasized, however, that not all cases take this form. An estimated 10 to 15 per cent of patients survive, sometimes with amazing return of neurologic function (Fig. 57-4). Others survive for 5 to 10 days, gradually losing ground each day, reflecting either slow continued bleeding or progressive swelling of the brain in response to the original bleeding. Though it was previously believed that coma was invariably seen when the blood entered the ventricular system, there are well-documented cases of patients with grossly bloody cerebrospinal fluid and massive hemiplegia and hemisensory deficits who are sufficiently alert to respond to commands. The most difficult problem in differential diagnosis is posed by the patient who has a massive intracerebral hemorrhage which does not extend into the ventricular system and who, as a consequence, does not have blood in the cerebrospinal fluid. In general, however, a safe clinical rule is that the existence of a massive hemiplegia in the

presence of a well-preserved state of consciousness speaks in favor of occlusive rather than hemorrhagic disease.

The general criteria in Table 57-8 based on

Table 57-8. CRITERIA HELPFUL IN ESTABLISHING THE CLINICAL DIAGNOSIS OF HYPERTENSIVE INTRACEREBRAL HEMORRHAGE

1. Hypertension or corollary evidence of hypertension present
2. Recurrent prodromal attacks not seen
3. Onset during activity rather than in sleep
4. Severe unilateral headache at onset
5. Moderately rapid progression of neurologic deficit which may extend beyond the distribution of a given cerebral artery
6. Rapid progression to come
7. Absence of rapid fluctuation in clinical course or rapid reversal of signs and symptoms
8. Displacement of pineal gland early in the episode
9. Blood in the cerebrospinal fluid in most instances
10. Probably no late rebleeding from the same site

those originally proposed by Fisher[37,38] are useful in establishing the clinical diagnosis of hypertensive intracerebral hemorrhage.

The clinical differentiation as to the site of hemorrhage can be made using the following summary:

1. Putaminal hemorrhage. Contralateral hemiparesis usually extensive; hemianopsia *usually* present, but some degree of sensory loss *always* present. Cortical signs such as aphasia or apractognosia found if patient sufficiently alert to permit examination; deepening coma along with evidence of brain stem compression as late event.

2. Thalamic hemorrhage. Extensive contralateral sensory loss—hemiplegia may be of lesser degree; prominent ocular signs primarily involving vertical gaze, i.e., elements of Parinaud's syndrome; contralateral hemianopsia; less frequently fatal than

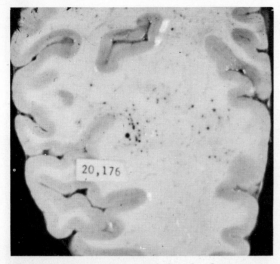

Fig. 57-5. Hypertensive encephalopathy demonstrating cerebral edema and multiple petechial hemorrhages.

putaminal hemorrhage; coma and brain stem compression if extensive.

3. Cerebellar hemorrhage. Onset, if sufficiently slow, with ataxia and inability to maintain upright position; frank motor paralysis not present; conjugate paralysis of gaze to side of hemorrhage from extension into, or compression of, pontine center for lateral gaze. Coma usually rapid; if patient survives, may have late appearance of raised intracranial pressure secondary to compression of fourth ventricle or cerebral aqueduct.

4. Pontine hemorrhage. Usually produces coma in minutes; bilateral signs present initially; pupils characteristically miotic and unreactive; frequently total paralysis of conjugate eye movement; decerebrate rigidity early—may disappear as condition worsens.

The association between intracerebral hemorrhage and hypertension has been recognized for over a century, but the basic pathogenesis of these lesions has not yet been elucidated. For a historical presentation of the various theories as to the cause of hypertensive hemorrhage, the reader is referred to an article by Adams and vander Eecken,[39] Russell,[40] using a radiographic technique, has recently reported the results of a survey of changes in the small arteries in brains from elderly normotensive and hypertensive subjects without intracerebral hemorrhage. The smaller penetrating arteries showed an increase in thickness of the wall and a narrowing of the lumen. In addition, Russell demonstrated miliary aneurysms arising from these small vessels. The aneurysms were more numerous in the hypertensive group and were located most commonly in the basal ganglions and thalamus. He concludes from his findings that

the combination of age and hypertension produces degenerative changes in the muscular and elastic coats of the small penetrating arteries; these changes lead to the formation of multiple miliary aneurysms. The aneurysms frequently showed evidence of minor hemorrhage, suggesting that at some point in their development, perhaps before the stage of intimal thickening, there may exist a potential for massive hemorrhages.

The term *hypertensive encephalopathy* has been erroneously applied to virtually any form of neurologic illness occurring in a patient with hypertension. More correctly, hypertensive encephalopathy designates a specific clinical entity appearing in an acute or subacute manner in a patient with hypertension and is characterized by headache, impaired consciousness, convulsions, and evidence of elevated intracranial pressure. Focal neurologic findings are rare and when present are frequently the result of other forms of cerebral vascular disease, such as cerebral thrombosis or embolus. Often there is impaired renal function and congestive heart failure. Another frequent, though not invariable, feature of hypertensive encephalopathy is improvement of the neurologic status when the blood pressure is lowered. The neuropathologic findings are brain swelling, and in severe cases, hemorrhages of petechial or larger size (Fig. 57-5). Microscopically, the smaller arteries show fibrinoid degeneration, occasionally with frank necrosis. These vessels are surrounded by areas of fibrin deposition and small aggregations of glial cells which have been referred to as microinfarcts (Fig. 57-6). Gross areas of infarction are infrequent and are usually related to incidental vascular disease. The clinical and pathologic aspects of hypertensive encephalopathy have been reproduced by Byrom[41] in experimental hypertension in the

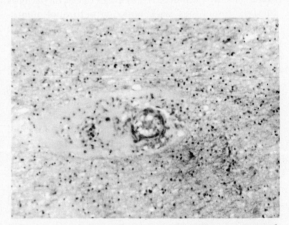

57-6. Hypertensive encephalopathy. Photomicrograph showing fibrinoid necrosis of an arteriole, perivascular fibrin deposit, and microinfarction.

rat. He presents evidence that the clinical events are related to widespread vascular spasm, which leads to transient disturbances of function, progressing in more severe instances to increased capillary permeability with focal edema and local necrosis of both the arterial wall and the tissue supplied by the involved vessel. Furthermore, he was able to reduce or abolish the arterial spasm by lowering the blood pressure.

As previously mentioned in the discussion of atherosclerosis of the brain, hypertension not only accelerates the atheromatous process at the usual sites but also predisposes the smaller penetrating arteries to the development of atheromatous changes. These changes in vessels which supply deep medial structures lead to multiple small lacunar infarcts in the deep gray and white matter. Such lesions in the cerebral hemispheres are most numerous in the region of the basal ganglions and internal capsule and produce a clinical picture characterized by bilateral pyramidal tract signs with rigidity and increased reflexes. The patient's gait is one of small mincing steps (marche-à-petit-pas). There is also evidence of pseudobulbar palsy, emotional lability, and varying degrees of dementia. This picture has been erroneously referred to as arteriosclerotic Parkinsonism. Lesions in the median and paramedian area of the brain stem are less frequent but may produce predominantly motor signs or defects in medial gaze (internuclear ophthalmoplegia, frequently unilateral).

It is obvious from a consideration of the relationship of the brain to chronic elevation of blood pressure that it is to the patient's advantage to detect significant hypertension early and control it as effectively as possible. However, there is considerable controversy regarding the use of antihypertensive therapy once clinically apparent cerebrovascular disease is present. In the management of the acute hypertensive intracerebral hemorrhage, there is no evidence that lowering of blood pressure has any favorable effect on prognosis for survival or recovery of function. If hypotensive therapy is used, there should be a concomitant attempt to lower the cerebral metabolic requirements by such methods as hypothermia. This combined approach has not been extensively evaluated, however. In a patient with evidence of cerebral atherosclerosis, the dangers of inadvertent, drastic lowering of blood pressure outweigh any postulated benefit of antihypertensive therapy on vascular changes which are by this time fixed. Evidence to the contrary is presented by Marshall[42] in a study of patients with nonembolic cerebral infarction with diastolic blood pressures of 110 mm Hg or higher. The aim was to reduce the blood pressure to 100 to 110 mm Hg (an estimated mean reduction of 19.4 mm in men

and 18.7 mm in women) rather than to a level considered desirable in a young patient with severe hypertension. In this series, using a wide variety of antihypertensive drugs, there was no instance of transient ischemic episodes appearing after therapy was begun, nor were cerebrovascular incidents precipitated by unusually low blood pressures. Marshall concludes that there was a significant reduction in the incidence of further cerebrovascular accidents in the treated group. The beneficial effect was more significant in men than in women. In the author's experience, reduction of blood pressure to the degree reported in Marshall's series can frequently be achieved by simple measures such as weight reduction, sodium restriction, mild sedation, and the use of thiazide diuretics, thus sparing the patient the potential hazards of medication which might predispose to the development of orthostatic hypotension.

Miscellaneous Conditions Affecting Nervous System and Vessels

The inflammatory vasculities of periarteritis nodosa tends to involve small and medium-sized arteries and produces neurologic symptoms in approximately one-third of the cases. The most frequent neurologic manifestation is mononeuropathy multiplex. Involvement of the central nervous system is less common and may result in focal neurologic deficits or seizures as a result of thrombosis of small arteries. Subarachnoid hemorrhage or intracerebral hemorrhage is said to occur in rare instances. Lupus erythematosus involves small arteries and may be associated with polyneuropathy or a wide variety of central nervous system manifestations, such as dementia, seizures, and focal neurologic deficits. Involvement of the nervous system in scleroderma and dermatomyositis is less frequent and usually consists of a peripheral neuropathy.[43] Giant-cell arteritis (temporal arteritis) may, in addition to blindness, be associated with ocular palsies[44] or focal neurologic deficits which result from the involvement of larger arteries, such as the carotid or vertebral artery, and their major branches.[45]

Involvement of the central nervous system in rheumatic fever is most frequently the result of cerebral embolism. Changes in cerebral vessels and brain parenchyma have been described as related to rheumatic fever, but their pathologic and clinical significance is still open to question. Acute (Sydenham's) chorea and chorea gravidarum are well recognized neurologic accompaniments of rheumatic fever. The pathology and pathogenesis of chorea and rheumatic fever are still undetermined, and to date there is no recognized cerebral lesion to account for this syndrome.

There are several neurologic diseases which may have prominent cardiovascular manifestations. These include muscular dystrophy and Friedreich's ataxia. The incidence of cardiac involvement in muscular dystrophy is unknown but is perhaps seen more frequently in myotonic dystrophy. The most prominent cardiovascular symptoms are related to cardiac arrhythmias.[46] The myocardial lesions consist of multiple areas of scarring, which tend to divide the muscle fibers into fasciculi of various sizes. Individual muscle fibers may show vacuolization and fragmentation.[47]

It is of interest that Friedreich described fatty degeneration in hypertrophy of the myocardium in some of his original cases of spinocerebellar degeneration,[48] though he failed to relate the two findings. Since this original observation, approximately one hundred cases of Friedreich's ataxia with heart disease have been reported. The features of the heart disease include arrhythmias, palpitations, retrosternal pain, pericardial effusion, and cardiac decompensation.[49,50] James and Fisch[51] have reported the autopsy findings of a young male with Friedreich's ataxia who died of intractable atrial arrhythmias and cardiac failure. There was evidence of widespread arteriopathy involving the small vessels of the myocardium including the arteries supplying the cardiac conduction system. A similar process was present in the lungs. These writers suggest that these changes in the small coronary arteries result in progressive myocardial degeneration and fibrosis which leads ultimately to cardiac failure. The disease in the nutrient arteries of the sinus nodes and AV nodes was postulated as being responsible for the atrial arrhythmias, heart block, and sudden death which have been reported in patients with Friedreich's ataxia. An abnormal electrocardiogram in a patient with a cerebellar disorder is strong evidence in favor of the diagnosis of Friedreich's ataxia. The disorder of movement related to the spinocerebellar degeneration may be confused with chorea and may lead to the erroneous diagnosis of rheumatic fever. In both muscular dystrophy and Friedreich's ataxia, the limitations of activity imposed by the cardiac findings may be so great as to make the neurologic manifestations less apparent.

Table 57-9. DISTRIBUTION OF MAJOR CEREBRAL ARTERIES IN RELATION TO THE NATURE OF THE NEUROLOGIC DEFICIT PRODUCED BY THEIR OCCLUSION

I. Anterior (carotid) circulation.
  A. Internal carotid artery.
    1. Supplies:
      a. The optic nerve and retina via the ophthalmic artery.
      b. Major portion of the cerebral hemispheres via the anterior and middle cerebral arteries.
    2. Signs and symptoms of ischemia:
      a. Homolateral blindness.
      b. Contralateral motor and/or sensory manifestations, usually referable to the distribution of the middle cerebral artery. May have minor evidence of involvement of anterior cerebral artery territory as well.
  B. Middle cerebral artery. (Lesions in superficial distribution can result in discrete deficit due to the fact that representation of various regions of the body is spread out over a large area of brain. In contrast, lesions in the deep branches may produce widespread neurologic deficit as a reflection of the fact that descending and ascending tracts are in a compact bundle in the internal capsule.)
    1. Superficial (cortical) branches
      a. Supply lateral surface of cerebral hemisphere except for frontal pole and strip along the superiomedial aspect. This area includes centers for contraversive head and eye movements, sensory and motor cortical representation, and major part of optic radiations. In hemisphere dominant for speech it includes those regions concerned with the sensory and motor aspects of language. In nondominant hemisphere it includes the regions concerned with spatial orientation and body image.
      b. Signs and symptoms of ischemia (all or part of the following):
        (1) Either hemisphere.
          (a) Motor and/or sensory impairment of opposite side of the body affecting the arm and face more than the leg.
          (b) Contralateral homonymous visual field defect.
          (c) Impairment of conjugate gaze to the opposite side.
        (2) Additional findings dependent on the hemisphere involved.
          (a) Dominant hemisphere: (i) motor and/or sensory aphasia; (ii) Gerstmann's syndrome (inability to recognize and use fingers, defects in calculating and writing, right-left disorientation; (iii) perseveration.
          (b) Nondominant hemisphere: (i) apractognosia (denial of neurologic deficit, neglect of opposite body half, dressing apraxia, loss of topographic memory); (ii) motor impersistence.
    2. Deep branches.
      a. Supply basal ganglions, posterior limb of internal capsule, and corona radiata.

b. Signs and symptoms of ischemia:
  (1) Motor and sensory impairment of contralateral face, arm, and leg, frequently with equal involvement.
  (2) No detectable signs of dysfunction of basal ganglions.
  (3) No visual field loss.
  (4) Occasionally aphasia, the basis of which remains unexplained.

C. Anterior cerebral artery. (Aphasia and visual field loss not usually seen. Infrequently involved in occlusive disease probably because of rich cross vascularization and anastomosis by way of anterior communicating artery. Therefore, findings referable to anterior cerebral artery suggest stenosis or occlusion in internal carotid artery *or* a cause other than ischemia.)
1. Superficial branches.
  a. Supply the anterior four-fifths of the medial surface of the cerebral hemisphere, medial part of the orbital surface of the frontal lobe, the frontal poles, and the majority of the corpus callosum. This includes areas of cortical representation of leg, bladder, and shoulder girdle.
  b. Signs and symptoms of ischemia:
    (1) Unilateral lesion.
      (a) Motor and/or sensory loss of contralateral leg and, to a lesser extent, shoulder, frequently sparing face and distal upper extremity.
      (b) Mental changes, e.g., forgetfulness.
      (c) Prominent grasp and sucking reflexes.
      (d) Apraxia (inability to use a limb to execute movements even though there is no significant weakness, sensory loss, or incoordination).
    (2) Bilateral involvement.
      (a) Quadriparesis with limbs in flexion.
      (b) Akinetic mutism (lack of spontaneous movement or speech).
      (c) Profound mental changes.
2. Deep branches. Syndrome of ischemia in distribution of penetrating branches of anterior cerebral artery has not been recognized clinically.

II. Posterior (vertebral-basilar) circulation.
A. Vertebral and basilar arteries. Supply medulla and pons which contain cranial nerve nuclei in close association with major ascending and descending tracts. Also supply cerebellar hemispheres, their nuclei and tracts.
1. Superficial (lateral) branches.
  a. Supply cerebellum and lateral portion of pons and medulla.
  b. Signs and symptoms of occlusion:

    (1) Incoordination, particularly in lesions affecting the medulla.
    (2) Impaired pain and temperature sensation over same side of face and opposite body half.
    (3) Disturbed sympathetic function on the same side (Horner's syndrome).
    (4) Involvement of visceral and branchial motor nuclei (fifth, seventh, ninth, tenth, eleventh cranial nerves), along with special sensory nuclei (eighth).
    (5) Does not produce corticospinal tract signs or impairment of proprioception and light touch to body.
2. Deep (median) branches. (Lesions in distribution of these vessels characterized by involvement of one or more cranial nerve nuclei, cerebellar incoordination, and motor and sensory findings which may involve both sides of body in a symmetrical or "crossed" distribution, i.e., one side of face and opposite body half. Localization of brain stem lesions in longitudinal axis (segmental level) is determined on basis of involved cranial nerve; e.g., ophthalmoplegia (third and fourth cranial nerves) indicates midbrain lesion; paralysis of muscles of mastication (motor, fifth), a midpontine lesion; peripheral-type facial paralysis (seventh), a lesion at the pontomedullary junction; palatal paralysis and dysphagia (nucleus ambiguous, ninth and tenth), midmedullary lesion; paralysis of tongue (twelfth), low-medullary lesion.)
  a. Supply median and paramedian regions of medulla and pons.
  b. Signs and symptoms of occlusion:
    (1) Involvement of somatic motor nuclei (third, fourth, sixth, twelfth cranial nerves).
    (2) Paralysis of medial gaze with sparing of other functions of third nerve due to involvement of medial longitudinal fasciculas (internuclear ophthalmoplegia).
    (3) Weakness of opposite body half due to involvement of descending motor fibers.
    (4) May have impaired light-touch response and proprioception on opposite body half with sparing of pain and temperature response (involvement of medial lemniscus).

B. Posterior cerebral artery.
1. Cortical branches.
  a. Supply inferior and medial surface of temporal lobe and the entire occipital lobe including the visual cortex.
  b. Signs and symptoms of occlusion:
    (1) Unilateral.
      (a) May have only contralateral ho-

monymous visual field deficit, frequently with macular sparing.

  (*b*) On dominant hemisphere may have difficulty reading or other disturbances of higher level of integration of visual image.

  (2) Bilateral.

    (*a*) Cortical blindness (blindness with intact pupillary reflex to light, no optic atrophy, and frequently denial of blindness).

    (*b*) Profound memory deficit (bilateral involvement of hippocampal formation of temporal lobes).

2. Deep branches.

  a. Supply midbrain subthalamic nucleus, cerebral peduncles, third nerve nucleus, reticular formation, thalamus including lateral geniculate bodies, i.e., sensory or "optic" thalamus.

  b. Signs and symptoms of occlusion:

    (1) Thalamic syndrome (Dejerine-Roussy) —loss of all sensory modalities from opposite body half including vision— frequently followed by severe spontaneous pain. Motor loss mild or absent.

    (2) Weber syndrome—homolateral third nerve paralysis and contralateral paralysis of face, arm, and leg.

    (3) Hemichorea of contralateral limbs.

    (4) Peduncular hallucinosis—visual hallucinations, usually vivid, colorful scenes. Not alarming to patient.

    (5) Extensive infarction can lead to quadriplegia and profound coma.

REFERENCES

1. Wells, C. E.: Premonitory Symptoms of Cerebral Embolism, *Arch. Neurol.,* **5**:490–496, 1961.

2. Fisher, C. M.: Neurologic Aspects of Cerebral Vascular Diseases and Therapeutic Approach, in I. S. Wright and E. H. Luckey (eds.), "Cerebral Vascular Diseases," Grune & Stratton, Inc., New York, 1955, p. 93.

3. Dodge, P. R., Richardson, E. P., Jr., and Victor, M.: Recurrent Convulsive Seizures as a Sequel to Cerebral Infarction: A Clinical and Pathological Study, *Brain,* **77**:610–638, 1959.

4. Askey, J. M.: "Systemic Arterial Embolization," Modern Medical Monographs, 14, Grune & Stratton, Inc., New York, 1957, p. 43.

5. Garvin, C. F.: Mural Thrombi in the Heart, *Am. Heart J.,* **21**:713–719, 1941.

6. Jordon, R. A., Miller, R. D., Edwards, J. F., and Parker, R. L.: I. Intracardiac Mural Thrombosis: Thromboembolism in Acute and in Healed Myocardial Infarction, *Circulation,* **6**:1–15, 1952.

7. Schlichter, J., Hellerstein, H. K., and Katz, L. N.:

8. Kumpfe, C. W., and Bean, W. B.: Aortic Stenosis: A Study of the Clinical and Pathologic Aspects of 107 Proved Cases, *Medicine,* **27**:139, 1948.

9. Wright, I. S., Marple, C. D., and Beck, D. F.: "Myocardial Infarction: Its Clinical Manifestations and Treatment with Anticoagulants," Grune & Stratton, Inc., New York, 1954, p. 249.

10. Wells, C. E.: Cerebral Embolism: Natural History, Prognostic Signs and Effects of Anticoagulation, *A.M.A. Arch. Neurol. & Psychiat.,* **81**:667–677, 1959.

11. Carter, A. B.: The Immediate Treatment of Cerebral Embolism, *Quart. J. Med.,* n.s., **26**:335–348, 1957.

12. Fisher, C. M., and Adams, R. D.: Observation on Brain Hemorrhage with Special Reference to the Mechanism of Hemorrhagic Infarction, *J. Neuropath. & Exper. Neurol.,* **10**:92–93, 1950.

13. Whisnant, J. P., Millikan, C. H., Sayre, G. P., and Wakim, K. G.: Effect of Anticoagulants on Experimental Cerebral Infarction: Clinical Implications, *Circulation,* **20**:56–65, 1959.

14. Barron, K. D., Siqueira, E., and Hirano, A.: Cerebral Embolism Caused by Nonbacterial Thrombotic Endocarditis, *Neurology,* **10**:391–397, 1960.

15. MacDonald, R. A., and Robbins, S. L.: The Significance of Nonbacterial Thrombotic Endocarditis: An Autopsy and Clinical Study of 78 Cases, *Ann. Int. Med.,* **46**:255–273, 1957.

16. Adams, R. D.: Case Records of Massachusetts General Hospital, Case 41491, *New England J. Med.,* **253**:1031–1036, 1955.

17. Emanuel, R.: Valvotomy in Mitral Stenosis with Extreme Pulmonary Vascular Resistance, *Brit. Heart J.,* **25**:119–125, 1963.

18. Allen, P.: Central Nervous System Emboli in Open Heart Surgery, *Canad. J. Surg.,* **6**:332–337, 1963.

19. Caguin, F., and Carter, M. G.: Fat Embolization with Cardiotomy with the Use of Cardiopulmonary Bypass, *J. Thoracic & Cardiovas. Surg.,* **5**:665–671, 1963.

20. Sevitt, S.: The Significance and Classification of Fat Embolism, *Lancet,* **2**:825–828, 1960.

21. Plum, F., Posner, J. B., and Hain, R. F.: Delayed Neurological Deterioration after Anoxia, *Arch. Int. Med.,* **110**:18–25, 1962.

22. Fromm, von Hartnut: Zur Differentialdiagnose und Prognose der cerebralen Fettembolie, *Nervenarzt,* **33**:430–436, 1962.

23. Brierly, J. B.: Neuropathologic Findings in Patients Dying after Open-heart Surgery, *Thorax,* **18**:291–304, 1963.

24. Tyler, H. R., and Clark, D. B.: Incidence of Neurological Complication in Congenital Heart Disease, *A.M.A. Arch. Neurol. & Psychiat.,* **77**:17–22, 1957.

25. Tyler, H. R., and Clark, D. B. Cerebrovascular Accidents in Patients with Congenital Heart Disease, *A.M.A. Arch. Neurol. & Psychiat.,* **77**:438–489, 1957.

Aneurysms of the Heart: A Correlative Study of 102 Proved Cases, *Medicine,* **33**:43–86, 1954.

26. Yates, P. O., and Hutchinson, E. C.: "The Role of Stenosis of the Extracranial Cerebral Arteries," Special Report Series, Medical Research Council, no. 300, London, 1961.

27. Martin, M. J., Whisnant, J. P., and Sayre, G. P.: Occlusive Vascular Disease in the Extracranial Cerebral Circulation, *Arch. Neurol.*, 3:530–538, 1960.

28. Patterson, J. L., and Heyman, A.: Cerebral Vascular Insufficiency, *Disease-A-Month*, July, 1963.

29. Baker, R. N., Broward, J. A., Fang, H. C., Fisher, C. M., Groch, S. N., Heyman, A., Karp, H. R., McDevitt, E., Schwartz, W., and Toole, J. F.: Anticoagulant Therapy in Cerebral Infarction: Report on Cooperative Study, *Neurology*, 12:823–835, 1962.

30. Baker, R. N.: An Evaluation of Anticoagulant Therapy in the Treatment of Cerebrovascular Disease: Report of the Veterans Administration Cooperative Study of Atherosclerosis, Neurology Section, *Neurology*, 11(Suppl.):132–138, 1961.

31. David, N. J., and Heyman, A.: Factors Influencing the Prognosis of Cerebral Thrombosis and Infarction Due to Atherosclerosis, *J. Chron. Dis.*, 11:394–404, 1960.

32. Metz, H., Murray-Leslie, R. M., Bannister, R. G., Bull, J., and Marshall, J.: Kinking of the Internal Carotid Artery in Relation to Cerebrovascular Disease, *Lancet*, 1:424–426, 1961.

33. Reivich, M., Holling, H. E., Roberts, B., and Toole, J. F.: Reversal of Blood Flow through the Vertebral Artery and Its Effect on the Cerebral Circulation, *New England J. Med.*, 265:878–885, 1961.

34. Cook, A. W.: Occlusion of the Abdominal Aorta and Dysfunction of the Spinal Cord: A Clinical Syndrome, *Bull. New York Acad. Med.*, 35:480–489, 1959.

35. Blackwood, W., McMenemey, W. H., Meyer, A., Norman, R. M., and Russell, D. S.: Vascular Disease of the Central Nervous System, in "Greenfield's Neuropathology," The William & Wilkins Company, Baltimore, 1963, p. 133.

36. Reifenstein, G. H., Levine, S. A., and Gross, R. E.: Coarctation of the Aorta, *Am. Heart J.*, 33:146–163, 1947.

37. Fisher, C. M.: Clinical Syndromes in Cerebral Hemorrhage, in W. S. Fields (ed.), "Pathogenesis and Treatment of Cerebrovascular Disease," Charles C Thomas, Publisher, Springfield, Ill., 1961, pp. 318–342.

38. Fisher, C. M.: The Pathology of Intracerebral Hemorrhage, in W. S. Fields (ed.), "Pathogenesis and Treatment of Cerebrovascular Disease," Charles C Thomas, Publisher, Springfield, Ill., 1961, pp. 295–317.

39. Adams, R. A., and vander Eecken, H. M.: Vascular Diseases of the Brain, *Ann. Rev. Med.*, 4:213–252, 1953.

40. Russell, R. W. R.: Observation on Intracerebral Aneurysms, *Brain*, 86:425–442, 1963.

41. Byrom, F. B.: The Pathogenesis of Hypertensive Encephalopathy and Its Relation to the Malignant Phase of Hypertension: Experimental Evidence from the Hypertensive Rat, *Lancet*, 2:201–211, 1954.

42. Marshall, J.: A Trial of Long Term Hypotensive Therapy in Cerebrovascular Disease, *Lancet*, 1:10–14, 1964.

43. Kibler, R. F., and Rose, F. C.: Peripheral Neuropathy in the "Collagen Diseases": A Case of Scleroderma Neuropathy, *Brit. M. J.*, 1:1781–1784, 1960.

44. Ferber, C. M.: Ocular Palsy in Temporal Arteritis, *Minnesota Med.*, 42:1258–1268, 1959.

45. Hollenhorst, R. W., Brown, J. R., Wagener, H. P., and Shick, R. M.: Neurologic Aspects of Temporal Arteritis, *Neurology*, 10:490–498, 1960.

46. Zatuchni, J., Aegerter, E. E., Molthan, L., and Shuman, C. R.: The Heart in Progressive Muscular Dystrophy, *Circulation*, 3:846–853, 1951.

47. Nothacker, W. G., and Netsky, M. G.: Myocardial Lesions in Progressive Muscular Dystrophy, *A.M.A. Arch. Path.*, 50:578–590, 1950.

48. Friedreich, N.: Ueber degenerative Atrophie der spinalen Hinterstrange, *Arch. path. Anat.*, 26:391, 423, 1863.

49. Nadas, A. S., Alimurung, M. M., and Sieracki, L. A.: Cardiac Manifestations of Friedreich's Ataxia, *New England J. Med.*, 244:239–244, 1951.

50. Thilenius, O. G., and Grossman, B. J.: Friedreich's Ataxia with Heart Disease in Children, *Pediatrics*, 27:246–254, 1961.

51. James, T. N., and Fisch, C.: Observations on the Cardiovascular Involvement in Friedreich's Ataxia, *Am. Heart J.*, 66:164, 1963.

58 VASCULAR DISEASES OF THE ABDOMINAL VISCERA

John T. Galambos, M.D.

The clinical study of the vasculature of the abdominal viscera was made possible by only recently developed roentgenographic techniques. Therefore, our knowledge and understanding of vascular diseases of the abdominal viscera are still embryonic. It is anticipated that the rapid accumulation of valid information on vascular lesions in the abdomen will result in revision and enlargement of this chapter in subsequent editions of this book.

Primary vascular lesions can affect the function of the abdominal viscera. The diseases may involve (1) the arteries, (2) the arterioles, or (3) the veins.

Occlusion of the mesenteric arteries may be associated with three types of clinical responses: (1) a dramatic abdominal crisis, (2) a difficult diagnostic problem of an abdominal disease in which pain is usually an outstanding feature, and (3) no symptoms at all.

Acute Occlusion of the Superior Mesenteric Artery

This is a sudden, catastrophic, usually fatally terminating event due to ischemia and gangrene of the intestine. Such an event may be precipitated by either an embolus or thrombosis. Embolic occlusion of the celiac axis is rare, and that of the inferior mesenteric artery usually does not result in bowel necrosis if the superior mesenteric artery is patent, because of the efficient collateral circulation. Successful embolectomies have been reported.[1] Embolic occlusion of smaller branches may cause no bowel ischemia unless progressive thrombosis involves the arcades where the usually rich mesenteric arterial anastomosis does not exist.[2] Vasospasm may be associated with mesenteric arterial occlusion; splanchnic nerve block may reverse the ischemic changes.[3] Thrombosis of the superior mesenteric artery may result in sudden infarction of the intestine. It is usually associated with arteriosclerotic narrowing of the vessel and previous occlusion of the celiac and inferior mesenteric arteries.

Gradual occlusion of the mesenteric arterial inflow may cause abdominal angina. This is characterized by postprandial abdominal pain and may be accompanied by nausea, vomiting, flatulence, diarrhea, or constipation. The pain may last for several hours, and in some cases it radiates to the back.[4] It is thought to be caused by ischemia of the intestine secondary to arteriosclerotic narrowing of the artery. The severity of symptoms may depend on the size of meal. Indeed, patients may forgo food to avoid the pain, and consequently weight loss may become an outstanding problem.[5-8] Some of these patients also have malabsorption.[9] In addition to the nonspecific abdominal tenderness, one of the outstanding diagnostic findings is a bruit[4,5,7,8] heard best in the epigastrum or mid-abdomen. The patient should be turned during auscultation, because the bruit may change as the position of the mesentery shifts about. Usually arteriosclerosis of other vessels is also evident. In some cases hypomotility of the intestine has been demonstrated roentgenographically.[10,11] Occult blood in the stool has been found in some,[7,10,11] but its source is not known. When both the superior mesenteric and celiac arteries are occluded, the blood flow to the liver is reduced enough to be a diagnostic clue.[7] Unexplained malabsorption may be another diagnostic hint.[9] In abdominal angina the superior mesenteric artery is always involved (Fig. 58-1) together with the celiac artery and/or the inferior mesenteric artery.[12] Because of the extensive collateral circulation between the branches of the celiac axis, the superior and inferior mesenteric

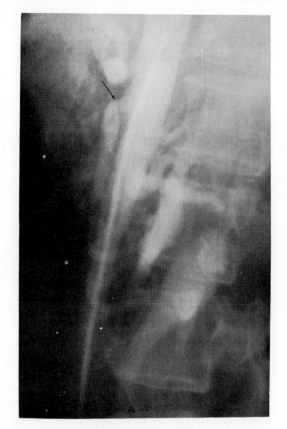

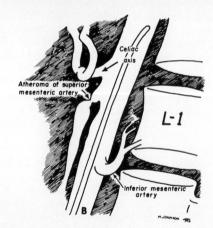

Fig. 58-1. *A.* Lateral abdominal aortogram. The plastic radiopaque catheter is seen in the aorta with its tip in front of T₁₂. A narrowing is seen in the superior mesenteric artery at 1 cm from its aortic ostium. *B.* An atheromatous plaque was found in this location at subsequent surgical treatment. A selective superior mesenteric arteriogram was also performed in this patient. The area of narrowing was not detected by this selective angiogram, because the positioning of the catheter tip permitted the injection of contrast material across the narrowed portion without detection of the lesion in the proximal 1 cm of the artery.

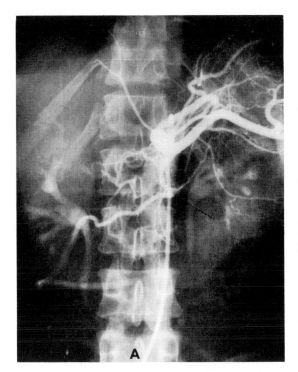

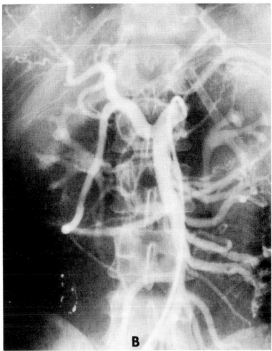

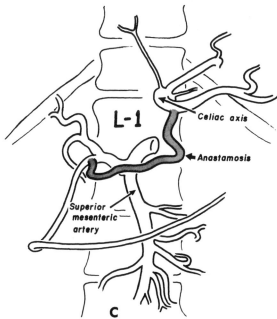

Fig. 58-2. A large anastomotic vessel between the celiac axis and superior mesenteric artery. Such readily demonstrable anastomosis occurs so frequently that it is considered normal. A. Selective celiac arteriogram. The splenic and left gastric arteries are opacified, but the hepatic artery is not seen. A large artery pursues a tortuous course, traveling down over L_1 medially from the catheter, which is in the aorta; it crosses to the right of the spine at the L_1-L_2 interspace and over the top of L_2 and turns sharply down over the right uretro-pelvic junction; after a sharp turn to the right it crosses over L_3 as the right gastroepiploic artery. Note the characteristic course of this vessel to the right of the spine, and compare it with that seen in B. B. Selective superior mesenteric arteriogram. The x-ray tube was moved caudad for this exposure from that seen in A. The most proximal branch of the superior mesenteric artery is the hepatic artery. Note that the first branch of the hepatic artery runs the same characteristic course and ends at the right gastroepiploic artery, as was seen on A. The density of this artery is less than that of the hepatic distal to the bifurcation, because the radiopaque contrast material was diluted with blood entering from the collateral vessel from the celiac artery. This collateral artery across the spine did not opacify, confirming that the direction of flow was from the celiac toward the superior mesenteric arterial system. C. A composite drawing of A and B illustrating the large collateral artery connecting the celiac with the superior mesenteric arterial system, which is a normal variation.

arteries,[13,14] abdominal angina is usually absent when the superior mesenteric artery alone is occluded at or near its origin, though it has been observed.[15] Large collateral vessels may be seen on selective celiac or mesenteric angiograms[16] even in the absence of arterial narrowing or occlusion (Fig. 58-2). The potential of adequate collateral circulation is so great that both the inferior mesenteric and the celiac arteries have been ligated in men without incident.[17] Significant occlusion of at least two of these three major arteries is usually present when symptoms are produced.[7,14,18] However, if extensive anastomosis does not exist, occlusion of a major branch of the mesenteric arteries may result in bowel ischemia and infarction (Fig. 58-3).

Abdominal angina is rarely caused by arterial disease other than atherosclerosis.[17,19] The lesions involve either the ostiums of the arteries at the aorta[5] or a proximal segment of the vessel.[7] The diagnosis is established and the extent of the arterial disease is defined only by angiography. This can be done either by aortography with lateral

exposures[7] (Fig. 58-1) or by selective angiography of the vessels in question (Fig. 58-3). The latter procedure gives better details, while the former can identify lesions at the orifice of the vessels. During operation decreased or absent pulsation of these vessels and their branches can be overlooked, and unless these are deliberately palpated, the diagnosis may be easily missed.[4,17]

The principle of surgical therapy is to establish flow in the superior mesenteric artery. Correction of flow in the celiac or inferior mesenteric arteries is not essential to give relief but may provide the additional safeguard against future ischemia. A by-pass seems to be preferred to thromboendarter-

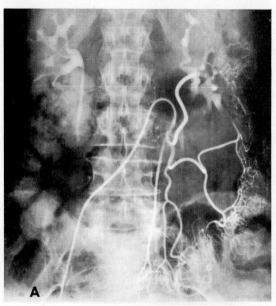

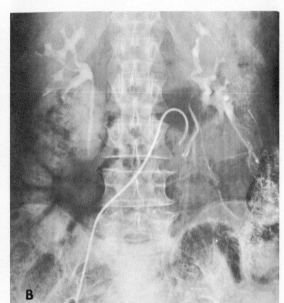

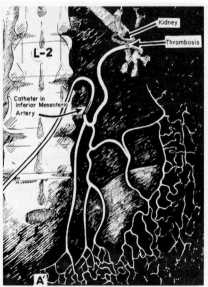

Fig. 58-3. Selective inferior mesenteric arteriogram. The most proximal branch of the inferior mesenteric artery is occluded just prior to its bifurcation. (The occlusion overlies the opacified left renal pelvis.) Ischemia of the splenic flexure and proximal descending colon was due to the lack of adequate collateral blood flow through Riolan's arc from the superior mesenteric artery. *A.* Note the increased density and wider diameter of the occluded branch of the inferior mesenteric artery. The landmarks of this roentgenogram are accentuated in the illustration (*A'*). Note the extensive anastomosis among the branches of the inferior mesenteric artery after the tertiary bifurcations. Such an extensive anastomotic network also characterizes the branches of the superior mesenteric artery. *B.* The thrombosed vessel remained opacified during the venous phase when none of the normal arterial branches contained visible contrast material.

ectomy.[4,7,20] If viability of the intestine is in doubt, a second look in 24 hr is advocated. Postoperatively, malabsorption may occur for a period.[17] Occlusion of the mesenteric arteries or their branches occurs more often without intestinal infarction than with it.[21] When ischemic injury does occur, resection of the ischemic intestine is usually required. However, at times adequate healing may take place with tubular stenosis of the bowel.[18,22]

Intestinal infarction without mesenteric vascular occlusion is rare. When it does occur, it is often associated with heart disease. The infarction is said to be massive when it is associated with aortic insufficiency[23] in contrast to its segmental distribution.[24] The author has recently seen two cases of segmental ischemic infarction of the intestine at autopsy without organic vascular occlusion. Both patients were in shock and were treated with sympathomimetic amines prior to death. Infarction of the intestine without vascular occlusion may be due to a combination of reduced cardiac output and local vascular forces such as spasm.[23] An alternative mechanism was suggested by the production of intestinal infarction following the intraarterial injection of Forssman antiserum.[25]

Gastrointestinal bleeding, jaundice, or abdominal pain may complicate aneurysms of the hepatic artery. Aneurysms of the visceral arteries are often unsuspected clinically. Aneurysmal rupture may cause death by intraabdominal bleeding.[26]

Small Vessels

Ulceration of the intestine due to necrotizing arteritis has been described in malignant hypertension.[27] After surgical correction of coarctation of the aorta, mesenteric arteritis with medial necrosis and fibrinoid changes may develop and can be severe enough to cause intestinal infarction.[28]

Periarteritis nodosa involves the gastrointestinal tract in about half of the patients. The most common manifestation is abdominal pain. The segmental destruction of the arteriolar wall associated with small aneurysmal dilatation and ischemia may result in focal ulcerations, bleeding, or at times perforation of the viscera. Gastrointestinal bleeding may occur, but it is rarely severe.[29,30] Although involvement of hepatic or cystic arterial or the portal venous radicals are common, clinical manifestations of liver disease develop before the terminal episode in only an occasional patient. Nevertheless, in some patients with periarteritis nodosa the hepatic lesions dominate the clinical picture, and such patients are thought to have primary liver disease.[30] Periarteritis may produce hepatic infarctions.

In patients with lupus erythematosus, small-vessel involvement of the abdominal viscera may be associated with abdominal symptoms severe enough to simulate an acute surgical condition.[31] The abdominal catastrophe may be associated with vasculitis of the bowel or of the pancreas. The peritoneum may be involved with polyserositis, giving the symptoms of peritonitis. Ileus involving the duodenum and/or the jejunum may be seen.[32]

The gastrointestinal tract may be involved with angiomas: (1) the hereditary hemorrhagic telangiectasia with or without cutaneous or nasopharyngeal involvement or (2) angiomas associated with hypertrophy of one or both limbs.[33] Angiomas may be the source of occult gastrointestinal bleeding, which may be severe and is often recurrent.

Exclusive vascular involvement of the abdominal viscera is more conspicuous in primary than in secondary amyloidosis.[34] In 47 patients with hepatic amyloidosis, the amyloid was deposited exclusively in the blood vessels in 34 per cent of the patients. In one-fourth of these, the involvement was confined exclusively to the hepatic arterioles.[34] In an extensive review of primary amyloidosis, vascular involvement of the gastrointestinal tract was found in 70 per cent of cases, and the liver was involved in 35 per cent of cases.[35]

Pseudoxanthoma elasticum is commonly associated with vascular lesions. These vascular lesions may occur in the mesentery and in the pancreas and may be associated with massive gastrointestinal hemorrhage.[36] Mesenteric vessels may be involved in thromboangitis obliterans.[37]

Arteritis with fibrinoid changes and with perivascular inflammation involving medium-sized and small peripheral arteries and arterioles has been described in acute rheumatic fever.[38] Abdominal pain on occasion has been the presenting symptom of acute rheumatic fever, and it has been confused with acute appendicitis. At operation mesenteric lymphadenitis, peritoneal hyperemia, and increased amount of peritoneal fluid were found.

The Venous System

Inadequate drainage of the hepatic vein can significantly impair liver function. Congestive heart failure with or without recognizable pulmonary emboli may cause intermittent jaundice. Though heart failure is associated occasionally with centrolobular necrosis, it is a rare cause of cirrhosis. Hepatic vein occlusion can involve either the major or the small hepatic veins. The former may be due to a primary lesion of the vein itself, may be associated with polycythemia, or may be secondary to infection or tumor. The veno-occlusive disease of hepatic venules is secondary to *Senecio* or *Crotolaria* toxicity.[39] Shock, for whatever reason, may result in massive hemorrhagic necrosis along the distribution of the hepatic veins.

Portal or mesenteric venous thrombosis causes

hemorrhagic necrosis of the intestine unless the rate of occlusion is slow enough to allow the development of adequate collaterals. Early diagnosis and resection of necrotic bowel is essential for survival in the acute cases. Surgical ligation of the portal vein in man is feasible. It results in transient engorgement of the intestine and fall of the blood pressure.[40] The catastrophic events which follow the sudden thrombosis of the portal vein in man are most likely due to the simultaneous thrombosis of the mesenteric and splenic veins which, as a rule, accompany spontaneous portal vein thrombosis. Slow occlusion of the portal vein results in portal hypertension. Cavernomatous transformation of the vein develops when the thrombus becomes recanalized.

Acute hemorrhage and necrosis of the bowel has followed the administration of high doses of digitalis. Neither mesenteric arterial lesions nor congestive heart failure were factors. Splanchnic venous congestion appeared to be the mechanism. This was probably precipitated by hepatic vein or hepatic sinusoidal sphincter constriction.[41]

REFERENCES

1. Atwell, R. B.: Superior Mesenteric Artery Embolectomy, *Surg. Gynec. & Obst.*, **112**:257, 1961.
2. Maingot, R.: "Abdominal Operations," 4th ed., Appleton-Century-Crofts, Inc., New York, 1961.
3. Orr, T. G., Jr., Lorhan, P. H., and Kaul, P. G.: Mesenteric Vascular Occlusion, *J.A.M.A.*, **155**:648, 1954.
4. Heard, G., Setteries, J. D., and Peters, D. K.: Chronic Intestinal Ischemia, *Lancet*, **2**:975, 1963.
5. Derrick, J. R., Pollard, H. S., and Moore, R. M.: The Pattern of Arteriosclerotic Narrowing of the Celiac and Superior Mesenteric Arteries, *Ann. Surg.*, **149**:684, 1959.
6. Mavor, G. E.: Stenosis of the Superior Mesenteric Artery, *Postgrad. M. J.*, **35**:558, 1959.
7. Morris, G. C., Crawford, E. S., Cooley, D. A., and DeBakey, M. E.: Revascularization of the Celiac and Superior Mesenteric Arteries, *Arch. Surg.*, **84**:95, 1962.
8. Ranger, I., and Spence, M. P.: Superior Mesenteric Artery Occlusion Treated by Ileo-colic Aortic Anastomosis, *Brit. M. J.*, **2**:95, 1962.
9. Shaw, R. W., and Maynard, E. P.: Acute and Chronic Thrombosis of the Mesenteric Arteries Associated with Malabsorption, *New England J. Med.*, **258**:874, 1958.
10. Keeley, F. X., Misanik, L. F., and Wirts, C. W.: Abdominal Angina Syndrome, *Gastroenterology*, **37**:480, 1959.
11. Mandell, H. N.: Abdominal Angina, *New England J. Med.*, **257**:1035, 1957.
12. Mikkelsen, W. P.: Intestinal Angina, *Am. J. Surg.*, **94**:262, 1957.
13. Reiner, L., Rodriguez, F. L., Platt, R., and Schlesinger, M. J.: Injection Studies on the Mesenteric Arterial Circulation, *Surgery*, **45**:820, 1959.
14. Reiner, L.: Chronic Vascular Insufficiency of the Gastrointestinal Tract, Presented at the American Gastroenterological Association Meeting, 1963. (Unpublished data.)
15. Clinical Pathology Conference, The Patient with Abdominal Pain, *Proc. Staff Meet. Mayo Clin.*, **39**:118, 1964.
16. Acker, J. J., Galambos, J. T., and Weens, H. S.: Selective Celiac Angiography, *Am. J. Med.*, **37**:417, 1964.
17. Maynard, E. P.: Intestinal Angina, in Gordon McHardy (ed.), "Current Gastroenterology," Hoeber Medical Division, Harper & Row, Publishers, Incorporated, New York, 1962.
18. Mikkelsen, W. P., and Zaro, J. A.: Intestinal Angina, *New England J. Med.*, **260**:912, 1959.
19. Schwartz, C. J., Acheson, E. D., and Webster, C. V.: Chronic Mid-gut Ischemia with Steatorrhea in Polycythemia Rubra Vera, *Am. J. Med.*, **32**:950, 1962.
20. Mavor, G. E., and Lyall, A. D.: Superior Mesenteric Artery Stenosis Treated by Iliac Mesenteric Arterial Bypass, *Lancet*, **2**:1143, 1962.
21. Reiner, L., Rodriguez, F. L., Jiming, F. A., and Platt, R.: Injection Studies on Mesenteric Arterial Occlusion, III, *Arch. Path.*, **73**:461, 1962.
22. Wolf, B. S., and Marshak, R. H.: Segmental Infarction of the Small Bowel, *Radiology*, **66**:701, 1956.
23. Hoffman, F. G., Zimmerman, S. L., and Cardwell, E. S., Jr.: Massive Intestinal Infarction without Vascular Occlusion Associated with Aortic Insufficiency, *New England J. Med.*, **263**:436, 1960.
24. Eude, N.: Infarction of the Bowel in Cardiac Failure, *New England J. Med.*, **258**:879, 1958.
25. Levine, S., and Warren, B.: Intestinal Infarction Produced by Fossman Antibodies, *A.M.A. Arch. Path.*, **68**:119, 1959.
26. Allen, E. B., Barker, N. W., and Hines, E. A.: "Peripheral Vascular Disease," 3d ed. W. B. Saunders Company, Philadelphia, 1962.
27. DeNavasquez, S., and French, E. B.: Intestinal Ulceration Due to Arterial Necrosis, *Guy's Hosp. Rep.*, **96**:85, 1947.
28. Benson, W. R., and Sealy, W. C.: Arterial Necrosis Following Resection of Coarctation of Aorta, *Lab. Invest.*, **5**:359, 1956.
29. Wold, E., and Baggenstoss, A. H.: Gastrointestinal Lesions of Periarteritis Nodosa, *Proc. Staff Meet. Mayo Clin.*, **24**:28, 1949.
30. Mowrey, F. H., and Lundberg, E. A.: Clinical Manifestations of Essential Polyangitis (Periarteritis Nodosa) with Emphasis on Hepatic Manifestations, *Ann. Int. Med.*, **41**:1145, 1954.
31. Muehrcke, R. C., Pirani, C. L., and Steck, I. E.:

Systemic Lupus Erythematosus Simulating Acute Surgical Conditions of the Abdomen, *New England J. Med.*, **259**:258, 1958.

32. Brown, C. H., Shirey, E. K., and Hasserick, J. R.: Gastrointestinal Manifestations of Systemic Lupus Erythematosus, *Gastroenterology*, **31**:649, 1956.

33. Shepherd, J. A.: Angiomatous Conditions of the Gastrointestinal Tract, *Brit. J. Surg.*, **40**:409, 1953.

34. Levine, R. A.: Amyloid Disease of the Liver, *Am. J. Med.*, **33**:349, 1962.

35. Symmers, W. St. C.: Primary Amyloidosis, *J. Clin. Path.*, **9**:187, 1956.

36. Whitecomb, F. F., and Brown, C. H.: Pseudoxanthoma Elasticum, *Ann. Int. Med.*, **56**:834, 1962.

37. de Takats, G.: "Vascular Surgery," W. B. Saunders Company, Philadelphia, 1959.

38. Von Glahn, W. C., and Pappenheimer, A. M.: Specific Lesions of Peripheral Blood Vessels in Rheumatism, *Am. J. Path.*, **2**:235, 1926.

39. Bras, G., Berry, D. M., and Gyorgy, P.: Plants as Etiological Factors in Veno-occlusive Disease of the Liver, *Lancet*, **1**:960, 1957.

40. Child, C. G.: "The Hepatic Circulation and Portal Hypertension," 3d ed., W. B. Saunders Company, Philadelphia, 1954.

41. Gazes, P. C., Holmes, C. R., Moseley, V., and Pratt-Thomas, N. R.: Acute Hemorrhage and Necrosis of the Intestines Associated with Digitalization, *Circulation*, **23**:358, 1961.

Section B: Surgical Treatment

59 SURGICAL TREATMENT OF DISEASES OF THE AORTA AND MAJOR ARTERIES

Michael E. De Bakey, M.D.

Arterial diseases, especially those of arteriosclerotic origin, have consistently ranked among the most common ailments of the Western world and now account for more deaths than all other diseases combined. Although the cause of most of these diseases remains undetermined, great progress has been made in recent years toward a better understanding of their nature and better methods for their treatment. This striking progress has been influenced by a number of factors, most important among these having been, first, the development of relatively safe and readily applied methods of angiography, which by providing roentgenographic visualization of the arterial tree permit precise delineation of the location and extent of the diseased area as well as its hemodynamic disturbances, and, second, the development of highly successful methods of vascular surgical procedures including the use of vascular replacements which may be applied to correct both the pathologic and hemodynamic disturbances of the lesion.

Still another important factor responsible for this progress has been the great intensification of experimental and clinical investigations in this field of endeavor. As a consequence of these studies and

surgical experience, certain conceptual changes have evolved concerning diseases of the aorta and major arteries that provide the basis for rational and more effective therapy. Most important among these has been the emphasis placed upon the anatomic-pathologic characteristics of the lesion itself and its hemodynamic effects rather than upon its causation. The concept has thus evolved that regardless of cause the lesion in many forms of aortic and arterial disease may be well localized and segmental in nature with a relatively normal patent proximal and distal arterial bed. The great significance of this important concept lies in the fact that it provides the basis for corrective surgical therapy designed to eliminate the pathologic and hemodynamic disturbance of the lesion and to restore normal circulation.

To achieve this objective four basic principles of surgical therapy may be employed: excision with graft replacement, the bypass procedure, thromboendarterectomy, and patch-graft angioplasty. The application of each of these procedures or, in some instances, their combined use is dependent upon the nature, location, and extent of the lesion.

Most, if not all, arterial diseases may be classified in two major categories: aneurysms and occlusive lesions.

The lesions in both categories may be of congenital, acquired, or traumatic origin, but from a practical therapeutic standpoint their etiologic considerations are much less significant than their nature and location or the hemodynamic disturbances that they produce. The most significant fact about aneurysms of the aorta, for example, is that all types, if untreated, have the same ultimately disabling and even fatal course and that they may be cured by the same surgical techniques. Actually, aneurysms and occlusive lesions may have the same basic cause, arteriosclerosis being the most common cause of both.

ANEURYSMS

Aneurysm is a word derived from the Greek *aneurynein* meaning "to widen or dilate" and is a hollow tumor or sac directly connected with the lumen of an artery and filled with liquid or coagu-

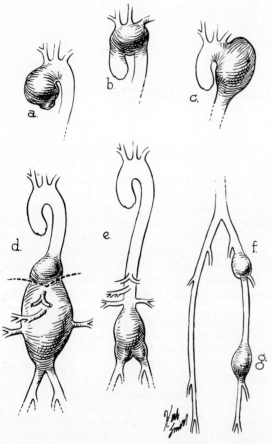

Fig. 59-1. Most frequent sites of aneurysms of the aorta and major arteries. *a.* Fusiform aneurysm of the ascending aorta. *b.* Fusiform aneurysm of the aortic arch involving the innominate, carotid, and subclavian arteries. *c.* Fusiform aneurysm of the descending portion of the aortic arch. *d.* Large fusiform thoraco-abdominal aneurysm involving the celiac, superior mesenteric, and renal arteries. *e.* Fusiform aneurysm of the abdominal aorta and iliac arteries. *f.* Fusiform aneurysm of the femoral artery. *g.* Fusiform aneurysm of the popliteal artery.

lated blood. Aneurysms may be classified in numerous ways according to the nature and cause of the lesion. For our purposes, however, we shall classify them morphologically as sacciform, fusiform, and dissecting, and subsequently they will be classified by location.

Sacciform aneurysms are pouchlike with a relatively narrow neck constituting the orifice from the side of the artery to which the sac is connected. Fusiform aneurysms are more spindle-shaped and involve the entire circumference of the parent artery. Dissecting aneurysms are a marked entity and will be dealt with separately.

Once an aneurysmal lesion has formed through weakening and destruction of the media, it tends to progress and to produce serious and ultimately lethal complications from compression of surrounding structures or from rupture with possible fatal hemorrhage. In the past, treatment of aneurysm of the aorta was directed toward obliteration of the aneurysm by inducing thrombosis within the lesion or by reinforcing the wall to forestall perforation. Such procedures proved to be inadequate and may now be considered obsolete. The only effective treatment consists of obliteration or preferably extirpation of the aneurysm with restoration of normal aortic continuity and function. This may be accomplished by one of several methods depending upon the type and location of the lesion. In sacciform aneurysms, for example, it may be possible to apply an occluding clamp across the relatively narrow neck of the lesion and in this way to perform tangential excision of the aneurysm with repair by lateral aortorrhaphy or patch-graft angioplasty. In fusiform aneurysms the entire segment of aorta involved by the aneurysm must be removed and replaced by a graft. A flexible, knitted, seamless Dacron tube has been proved to be the most satisfactory vascular replacement for this purpose. Under some circumstances a fusiform aneurysm may preferably be obliterated by endoaneurysmorrhaphy and circulation restored by means of a bypass graft attached end to side above and below the obliterated segment.

The site and extent of the aneurysmal lesion also have great influence upon operability and method of operation. Aneurysms of the aorta and major arteries may accordingly be usefully classified by their location, as follows (Fig. 59-1):

1. Aneurysms of the aortic arch (Fig. 59-1A and B)

2. Aneurysms of the descending thoracic aorta (Fig. 59-1C)

3. Aneurysms of the thoracoabdominal segment of aorta (Fig. 59-1D)

4. Aneurysms of the abdominal aorta distal to the renal arteries (Fig. 59-1E)

5. Aneurysms of the major peripheral arteries (Fig. 59-1F and G)

The risk of operation may be considered greatest in the first category and least in the last two, because in applying surgical treatment circulation is necessarily arrested temporarily through the segment to be resected and replaced with a graft. The potentially hazardous consequences of this procedure are, first, resultant increased vascular resistance upon the heart with left ventricular strain and, second, possible ischemic damage to the tissues distal to the occlusion. These problems assume significance for the first three categories only, since temporary arrest of aortic circulation below the renal arteries is well tolerated (Fig. 59-2).

Several methods have been devised to overcome problems arising from temporary arrest of aortic circulation. For aneurysms of the aortic arch two methods are available, depending upon whether or not the lesion involves the proximal portion of the ascending aorta. When such involvement is present, cardiopulmonary bypass with the artificial heart-lung machine becomes necessary (Fig. 59-3A). In the absence of such involvement, the temporary bypass principle may be employed (Fig. 59-3B). This principle is also applicable to aneurysms involving the thoracoabdominal segment (Fig. 59-4). For aneurysms of the descending thoracic aorta, the pump-bypass method is employed in which blood is removed from the left auricle or the left subclavian artery and pumped through a plastic cannula into the left femoral artery (Figs. 59-3C and 59-5).

At the Baylor University College of Medicine these methods of surgical treatment have been used in more than two thousand patients, and analysis of the results is most encouraging. The risk of operation varies in accordance with a number of factors, including particularly the type and location of the lesion, the presence or absence of rupture, heart disease, and hypertension, and the age of the patient. The total operative mortality for aneurysms of the descending thoracic aorta is about 15 per cent, but for aneurysms of the abdominal aorta it is less than 7 per cent. Rupture is very significant, operative mortality for ruptured aneurysms of the abdominal aorta being about 33 per cent. For nonruptured aneurysms it is only a little over 4 per cent. The influence of heart disease may be illustrated by the fact that operative mortality for aneurysms of the abdominal aorta in patients with heart disease is 13 per cent whereas in patients without heart disease it is less than 2 per cent.

Follow-up studies on these patients for periods ranging up to 10 years provide evidence of maintenance of good results with long-term survival. The

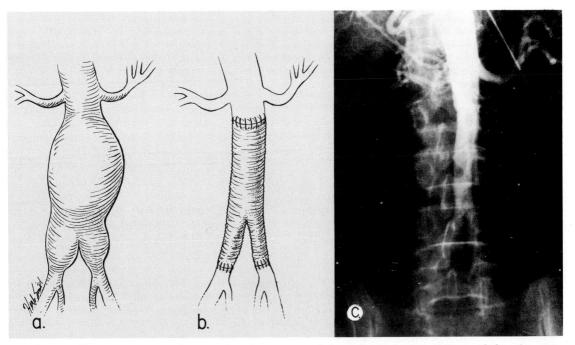

Fig. 59-2. *a.* Characteristic type of arteriosclerotic aneurysm of the abdominal aorta arising just below the origin of the renal arteries, treated by (*b*) resection and replacement with a bifurcation Dacron graft. *c.* Aortogram made 5 years after operation showing the restoration of normal circulation.

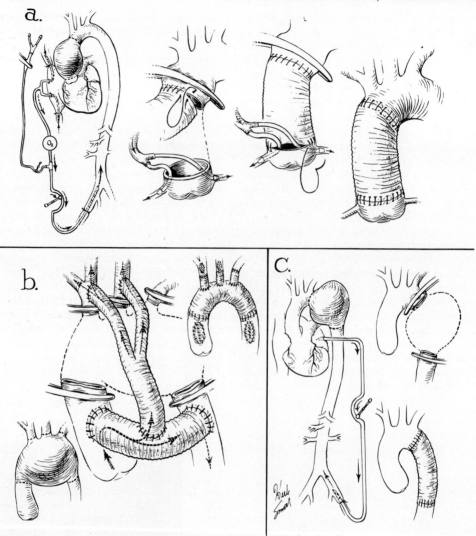

Fig. 59-3. Types of surgical treatment for aneurysms of the thoracic aorta. *a.* Method of resection and graft replacement of aneurysm of the ascending aorta with cardiopulmonary bypass. *b.* Method of resection and graft replacement of aneurysm of the arch involving the major vessels, using a temporary bypass of Dacron to maintain aortic and cerebral circulation during the procedure. *c.* Method of resection and graft replacement of aneurysm of the descending portion of the aortic arch using a left atrium–femoral artery pump bypass.

5- to 10-year survival rate, for example, for patients operated upon for aneurysms of the abdominal aorta closely parallels that for comparable age groups in the normal population.

Dissecting Aneurysm

Dissecting aneurysm of the aorta is a distinct clinical and pathologic entity characterized by hemorrhagic intramural separation of the medial layer of the aortic wall usually communicating with the normal lumen by an intimal tear. The cause is unknown, but the underlying predominant lesion appears to be degeneration of the elements of the media in the form of cystic medionecrosis. Certain factors have been considered to have a causal relationship to dissecting aneurysm owing to their frequent association with its occurrence. These include Marfan's syndrome, pregnancy, hypertension, coarctation, and idiopathic kyphoscoliosis. Men are affected about twice as often as women, with the highest age incidence in the fourth to seventh decades. The prognosis in untreated cases is extremely grave with a fatal termination in about half the cases within the first 24 hr after onset and in about three-fourths of the cases within the first week after onset.

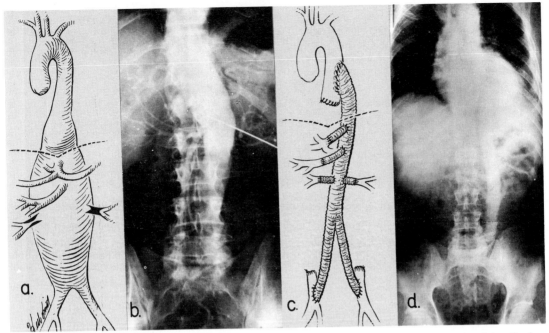

Fig. 59-4. Drawing (*a*) and aortogram (*b*) showing the extent of a large fusiform aneurysm involving the lower segment of the descending thoracic aorta and the entire abdominal aorta associated with occlusive lesions involving the origin of both renal arteries and producing incomplete occlusion of the right renal and complete occlusion of the left renal artery in a thirty-eight-year-old white man with manifestations of severe hypertension and abdominal pain. *c*. Method of surgical treatment consisting of resection of the aneurysm and replacement with a Dacron graft. *d*. Postoperative aortogram showing restoration of normal circulation through a Dacron graft to the lower extremities, as well as to both renal arteries and the celiac and superior mesenteric arteries. The patient was able to resume normal activities after the operation.

On the basis of both anatomic and pathologic patterns of the lesions and their respective methods of surgical treatment, dissecting aneurysms may be classified into three basic types, as follows (Fig. 59-6): type I, in which the dissecting process arises in the ascending aorta and extends distally, often into the abdominal aorta; type II, in which the dissecting process is limited to the ascending aorta and is characterized by a transverse tear in the intima just above the aortic valves; and type III, in which the dissecting process arises in the descending thoracic aorta at, or just distal to, the origin of the left subclavian artery and extends distally for a varying distance, sometimes being limited to the descending thoracic aorta but more often extending into the abdominal aorta (Fig. 59-7).

Surgical treatment for type I aneurysms consists of transection of the ascending aorta using cardiopulmonary bypass, obliteration of the false lumen by approximation of the inner and outer walls of the dissecting process by a continuous suture proximally and distally, and end-to-end anastomosis of the transected aorta (Fig. 59-6). In instances in which this method of direct repair is inapplicable, it may be necessary to resect the proximal segment and restore vascular continuity by means of a Dacron patch or tube graft. In some cases aortic valve incompetence is encountered and may be corrected by suture approximation of the inner and outer layers of the dissecting process.

Surgical treatment for type II aneurysms consists essentially of resection and graft replacement of the entire ascending aorta using cardiopulmonary bypass (Fig. 59-6). Aortic valve incompetence is more often encountered in this type than in type I and in most instances can be corrected in the same manner. Sometimes, however, it is necessary to use annuloplasty or even valve replacement.

Surgical treatment for type III aneurysms consists in resection of the descending thoracic aorta above the level of the origin of the dissecting process usually at, or just below, the origin of the left subclavian artery, obliteration of the distal false passage by suture closure of the inner and outer layers, and replacement of the excised segment with an aortic graft (Figs. 59-6 and 59-7).

Analysis of the author's experience with about

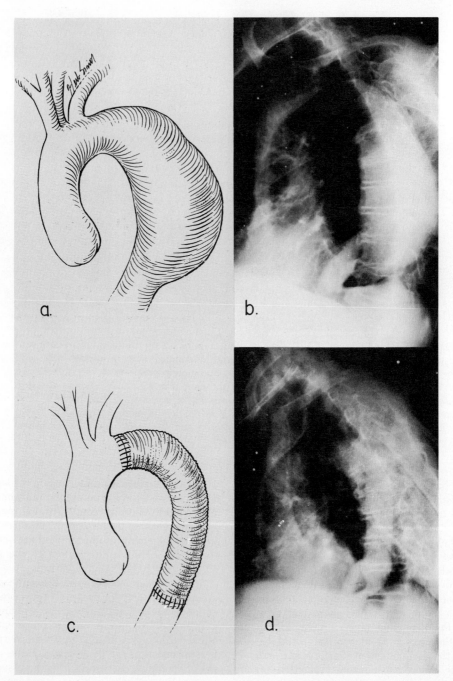

Fig. 59-5. Drawing (*a*) and preoperative aortogram (*b*) showing a large fusiform aneurysm of the descending aorta in a sixty-seven-year-old white woman. *c*. Method of surgical treatment consisting of resection of an aneurysm and replacement with a Dacron graft. *d*. Postoperative aortogram made 5 years after operation shows restoration of normal aortic continuity and function.

150 cases in which these methods of surgical treatment have been applied reveal gratifying results with an operative mortality of about 25 per cent. Follow-up observations extending over 5 years reveal maintenance of good functional activity.

OCCLUSIVE LESIONS

Occlusive lesions of the aorta and major arteries may be of congenital or acquired origins. The former are represented largely by coarctation and the latter predominantly by arteriosclerosis or ather-

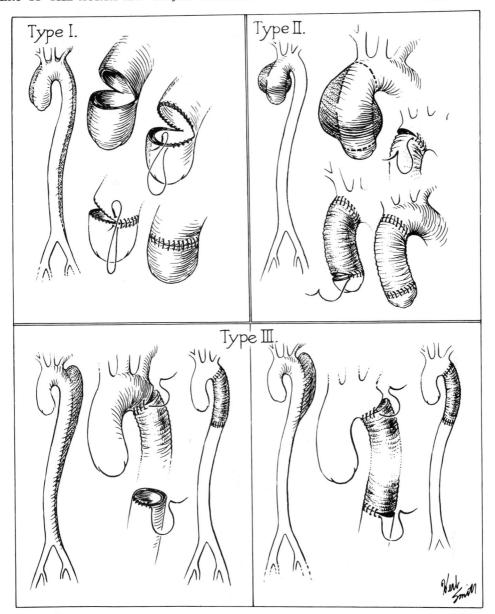

Fig. 59-6. Surgical classification of dissecting aneurysms of the aorta based on anatomic and pathologic patterns of the lesions and their respective methods of surgical treatment.

osclerosis, although in a small proportion of cases they may be due to nonspecific forms of arteritis or to embolic phenomena. Acquired forms of arterial occlusive lesions are by far the most common. Except for those associated with embolic episodes, their characteristic patterns of involvement and manifestations of arterial insufficiency may be classified into three major catagories, each of which may also be classified into two subgroups: (1) lesions involving the major branches of the aortic arch, (2) lesions involving the visceral branches of the abdominal aorta, and (3) lesions involving the termi-

nal abdominal aorta and its major branches (Fig. 59-8).

Coarctation of the Aorta

Coarctation of the aorta is a congenital disease characterized by narrowing or complete obstruction of the aortic lumen usually occurring in the distal segment of the aortic arch but occasionally in the descending thoracic or abdominal aorta.

The most satisfactory classification of the forms of coarctation is based on two factors: (1) relationship of the coarctation to the ductus arteriosus

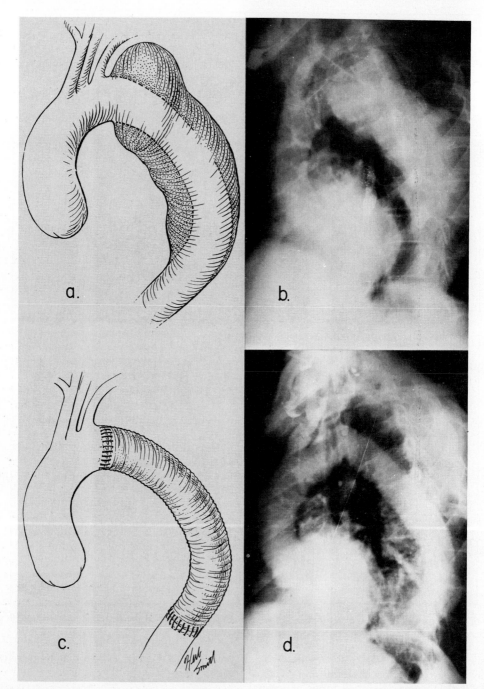

Fig. 59-7. Drawing (*a*) and preoperative aortogram (*b*) showing extensive dissecting aneurysm arising just distal to the left subclavian artery and involving the entire descending thoracic aorta in a fifty-four-year-old white man. *c.* Operative procedure consisting of resection of a dissecting aneurysm and replacement with a Dacron graft. *d.* Postoperative aortogram showing restoration of normal continuity and function of the thoracic aorta.

(preductile or postductile) and (2) patency of the ductus arteriosus.

The coarctation is usually located close to, and just distal to, the aortic insertion of the ligamentum arteriosum. Occasionally the areas of narrowing may lie more proximally to involve the segment between the left common carotid and left subclavian arteries, or they may be located in the distal portion of the

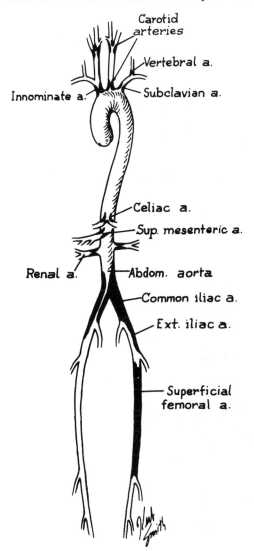

Fig. 59-8. Typical patterns of location and extent of occlusive disease of the aorta and its major branches.

descending thoracic aorta, extending down to involve even the upper segment of the abdominal aorta.

Other congenital anomalies involving the cardiovascular system are associated with coarctation in a significant proportion of cases. Patent ductus arteriosus, for instance, occurs in about 15 per cent of patients surviving to adulthood. Other associated anomalies include aortic valve deformity, interventricular or interatrial septal defects, mitral valve deformity, pulmonary stenosis, and subendocardial fibroelastosis.

Most cases of coarctation, particularly of the postductal type, may be treated by surgical removal of the coarcted segment with restoration of aortic continuity by end-to-end anastomosis. Occasionally,

wedge resection laterally with direct repair is a satisfactory procedure for young patients with very short isthmic coarctations. This type of suture repair is similar to end-to-end anastomosis except that the posteromedial wall of the aorta in the stenotic area is not resected and forms one segment of the aortic wall opposite the suture line. In cases associated with aneurysm formation or in which a longer segment is involved, it may be necessary to replace the resected portion with a graft. Graft repair minimizes necessary dissection of the distal aortic segment, since a suitable curved vascular clamp may be used to control this segment and exclude the origin of the intercostal vessels. Occasionally, particularly in older or poor-risk patients, the preferred method of treatment consists of insertion of a bypass graft (Fig. 59-9).

Results of surgical treatment are gratifying, with low mortality and morbidity rates. Symptoms are usually relieved, and blood pressure in the extremities is restored to normal levels.

Arterial Emboli

Peripheral arterial emboli usually are associated with atherosclerotic or rheumatic heart disease. They may originate from within the left atrium in the presence of atrial fibrillation, from the ventricular endocardial surface following myocardial infarction, or from the mitral or aortic valve in association with valvular heart disease. Embolization usually is associated with a change in heart rate or rhythm, and diagnosis and localization of the embolus often is possible on the basis of clinical findings alone. Occasionally, arteriography is helpful in exact localization (Fig. 59-10A and B).

Delay in embolectomy may result in varying degrees of distal thrombosis, and the embolus should be removed surgically as soon as feasible. The artery first is exposed in the region of the proximal extent of the embolus, the embolus extracted through a small arteriotomy, and the artery repaired (Fig. 59-10C, D, and E). Occasionally, a second more distal arteriotomy is necessary. Prior to repair the artery should be flushed proximally and free distal backflow obtained in order to insure against retained thrombotic material. In patients with peripheral arterial embolization secondary to rheumatic heart disease with mitral stenosis, concomitant definitive valve surgical treatment should be considered at the same time as embolectomy.

Lesions Involving the Major Branches of the Aortic Arch

These lesions may be classified as *proximal* or *distal*. Proximal occlusive lesions are located near the origin of the brachiocephalic, left common carotid, and left subclavian arteries (Fig. 59-11).

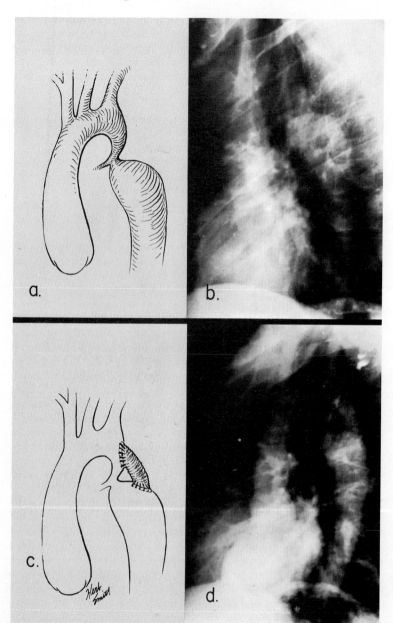

Fig. 59-9. Drawing (*a*) and preoperative aortogram (*b*) showing typical coarctation of the aorta in a thirty-six-year-old white man. *c*. Application of the bypass principle employing a Dacron graft attached by end-to-side anastomosis to the left subclavian artery above and to the descending thoracic aorta below the coarcted segment. *d*. Postoperative aortogram showing restoration of normal aortic circulation through the bypass graft. The patient remained asymptomatic after the operation, with normal blood pressure in both upper and lower extremities.

These lesions may produce complete or incomplete occlusion and are usually multiple, but they are predominantly segmental in nature and therefore operable. Characteristic sites of involvement in the distal form are the vertebral arteries at their origin from the subclavian arteries, the common carotid arteries at their bifurcation, and the internal carotid arteries at their origin (Fig. 59-12). In this type of case also, the occlusive process may be complete or incomplete and is often multiple. Incomplete occlusions are usually segmental and therefore operable, whereas complete occlusions of long duration are rarely amenable to surgical repair. Depending upon the location and extent of the lesion, the clinical manifestations vary considerably, the proximal type being associated with symptoms of ischemia of the cerebrum and upper extremities and the distal type with episodes of cerebrovascular insufficiency which may be transient, progressive, or apoplectic in nature. Arteriography is mandatory to establish the diagnosis with certainty and to determine the precise location and extent of the occlusive lesions in order to facilitate application of proper surgical treatment.

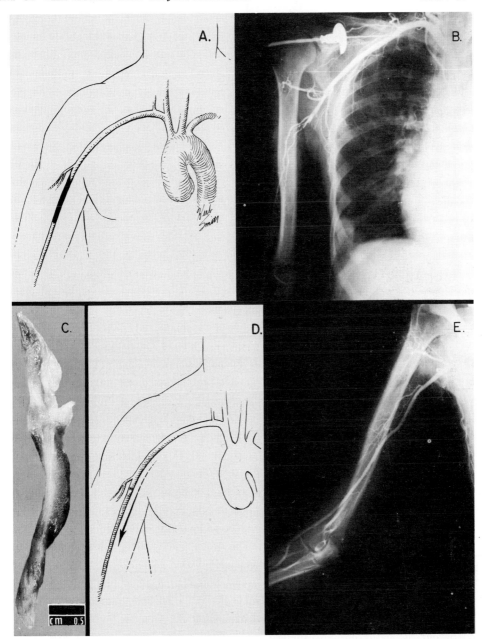

Fig. 59-10. Right brachial artery embolism following myocardial infarction. *a.* Location of an embolus. *b.* Right subclavian arteriogram demonstrating occlusion of the brachial artery at the junction of the upper and middle thirds. *c.* Embolus following removal. *d.* Completed operation. *e.* Right subclavian arteriograms following an operation demonstrating patency of brachial artery.

Lesions Involving the Visceral Branches of the Abdominal Aorta

This category includes lesions (1) which produce abdominal or intestinal angina or (2) which produce renovascular hypertension. The occlusive lesions in group 1 are located in the celiac axis and superior mesenteric artery near their origins from the aorta and are usually caused by atherosclerosis. They may be complete or incomplete but are usually well localized and segmental in nature and therefore are surgically correctible. These lesions, producing the syndrome of abdominal or intestinal angina, are characterized by manifestations of abdominal pain occurring after meals, disturbances

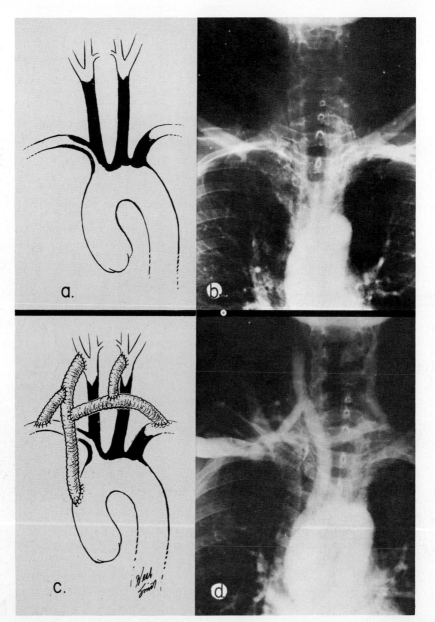

Fig. 59-11. Drawing (*a*) and preoperative arteriogram (*b*) showing complete occlusion of both carotid and sub-clavian arteries and partial occlusion of the brachiocephalic artery in a forty-six-year-old white woman. *c.* Operative procedure employed consisting of Dacron bypass grafts from the ascending aorta to the brachiocephalic, both common carotid, and the subclavian arteries. *d.* Postoperative arteriogram showing restoration of normal circulation.

in bowel rhythm and function, bulky stools, nutritional disturbances, and weight loss. Lumbar aortography, performed in the lateral position rather than the usual prone, is essential to establish the diagnosis and to determine proper surgical treatment.

Occlusive lesions in group 2 involve the renal arteries. In this group also the occlusive process tends to be fairly well localized in the main renal artery, usually near its origin from the aorta (Fig. 59-13). In the great majority of cases the lesion is atherosclerotic, but occasionally, most often in

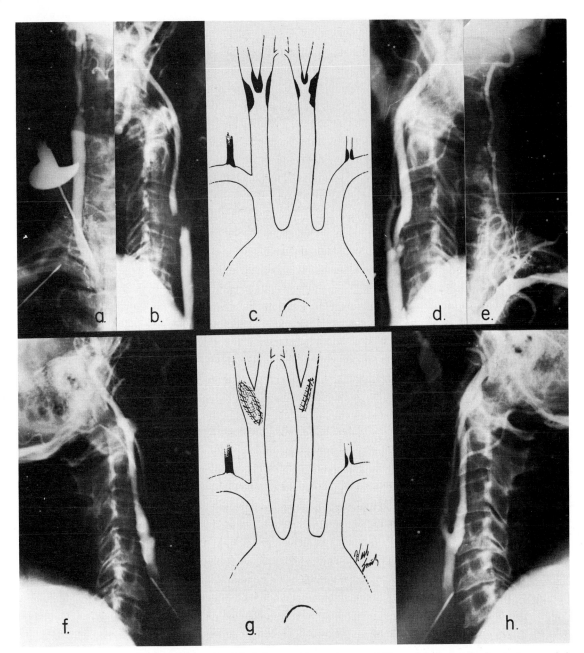

Fig. 59-12. Right carotid arteriograms (*a, b*), left carotid arteriogram (*d*), and left vertebral arteriogram (*e*) in a sixty-seven-year-old man with partial occlusion of both common carotid arteries at the bifurcation, involving the origin of internal and external carotid arteries and with complete occlusion of the right vertebral and severe stenosis of the left vertebral arteries producing severe manifestations of cerebrovascular insufficiency, as depicted in *c*. Operative procedure consists of endarterectomy with patch-graft angioplasty in the right carotid and endarterectomy with primary closure in the left carotid (*g*). Postoperative right (*f*) and left (*h*) arteriograms made 2 years after operation demonstrate restoration of normal blood flow. The patient has remained asymptomatic.

young women, the pathologic features of the lesion may be described as fibromuscular hyperplasia. Apparently, no distinctive clinical features in history or physical examination distinguish this type of renovascular hypertension from essential hypertension, and the definitive diagnosis of this form of hypertension can be established only by means of properly performed aortography.

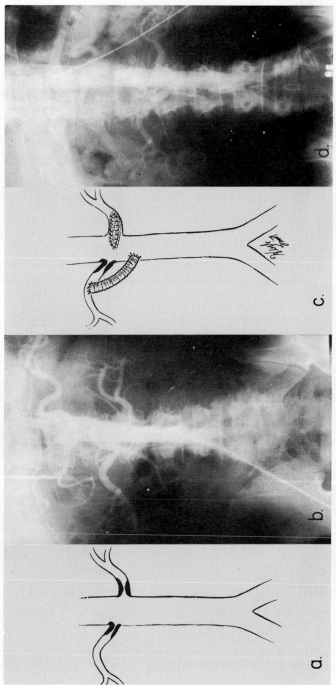

Fig. 59-13. Drawing (*a*) and preoperative aortogram (*b*) showing well-localized and severe stenotic lesions involving both renal arteries at their origin in a forty-six-year-old white man with manifestations of severe hypertension (blood pressure 220/130 mm Hg). *c*. Method of surgical treatment consisting of insertion of a Dacron bypass graft from the abdominal aorta to the right renal artery distal to the occlusive lesion, and endarterectomy and patch-graft angioplasty of the left renal artery. Postoperative aortogram (*d*) shows restoration of normal circulation to both renal arteries.

Lesions Involving the Terminal Abdominal Aorta and Its Major Branches

There are two main groups: proximal, or aortoiliac, occlusions and distal, or femoropopliteal, occlusions. Variation in the nature, extent, and pathologic features of the occlusive process is often encountered. In general, however, proximal lesions with complete occlusion tend to be well localized to the terminal abdominal aorta and bifurcation and common iliac arteries, whereas those with incomplete occlusion are more frequently associated with occlusive disease of the superficial femoral arteries (Figs. 59-14 and 59-15). Combinations of both proximal and distal types of involvement are not uncommon (Fig. 59-15). The distal forms of occlusion seem to be more often associated with diffuse involvement, particularly when diabetes is also present.

No matter how extensive the pattern of occlusive disease, effective therapy most often depends upon the presence of a patent distal arterial bed, particularly in cases involving segments and branches of the popliteal artery. For this reason arteriographic visualization of the aortoiliac and femoropopliteal arterial circulation is absolutely essential. The diagnosis can usually be made from clinical manifestations of arterial insufficiency of the lower extremities, and with experience one can even be fairly sure of the location and pattern of the occlusive process, but in order to determine the proper surgical procedure to employ, it is necessary to ascertain precisely by arteriography the full extent and location of the occlusive process.

Experience with these major categories of arterial occlusive disease has disclosed that they may occur in various combinations in the same patient. This should not be an unexpected finding, since the predominant underlying pathologic lesion in these forms of occlusive disease is atherosclerosis, which has a predilection for involving and blocking the origin or bifurcations of major arteries. Patients have been observed who have such combinations of

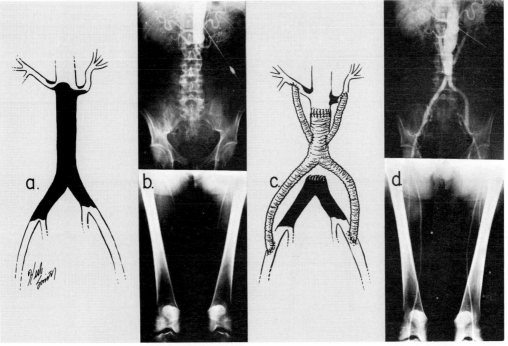

Fig. 59-14. Drawing (a) and aortogram (b) showing complete occlusion of the abdominal aorta arising at the level of the renal arteries and extending down to involve the bifurcation and both common iliac arteries. Well-localized stenotic lesions involve the origin of both renal arteries in this sixty-one-year-old white man who had severe manifestations of intermittent claudication of the lower extremities and hypertension (blood pressure 230/130 mm Hg). c. Operative procedure employed in this patient consisting of excision of abdominal aorta and replacement with a Dacron bifurcation graft, with bypass to both renal arteries distal to the occlusive lesion and to both external iliac arteries distal to the occlusive process. d. Aortogram made 2 years after operation shows restoration of normal circulation through a graft to both arteries and to the lower extremities. The patient's blood pressure at this time was 120/80 mm Hg, and he was completely relieved of his previous symptoms of intermittent claudication.

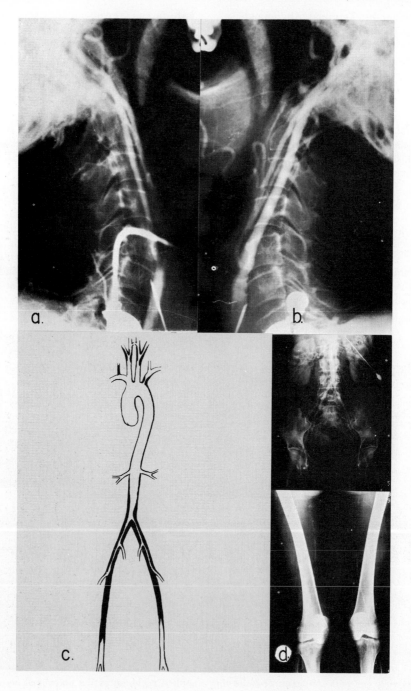

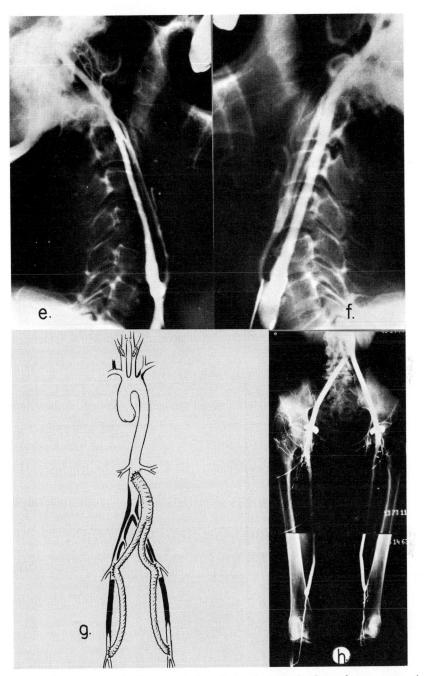

Fig. 59-15. Location and extent of multiple segmental occlusive lesions of atherosclerotic origin (*c*) in a sixty-year-old white woman with manifestations of cerebrovascular insufficiency indicative primarily of basilar artery insufficiency and severe intermittent claudication of the lower extremities. Preoperative right carotid (*a*) and left carotid (*b*) arteriograms showing well-localized segmental occlusive lesions of the internal carotid arteries near their origins. There was complete occlusion of the right vertebral artery and marked stenosis of the left subclavian artery. *d.* Preoperative lumbar aortogram showing extensive incomplete occlusive disease of the lower abdominal aorta and common iliac arteries and bilateral complete segmental occlusive lesions of superficial femoral arteries. *g.* Operative procedures employed. Right (*e*) and left (*f*) carotid arteriograms and aortogram (*h*) made 3 years after operation, showing restoration of normal circulation.

the three major categories as cerebrovascular insufficiency with renovascular hypertension or with arterial insufficiency of the lower extremities, and sometimes these clinical patterns may also be associated with aneurysms of the aorta or major arteries (Figs. 59-14–59-16).

Four basic principles of surgical therapy have been developed for occlusive diseases: thrombo-

endarterectomy, excision with graft replacement, bypass graft, and patch-graft angioplasty. The application of each of these procedures, and in some instances their combined use, is dependent upon a number of factors, including particularly the nature, extent, and site of involvement of the occlusive lesions.

Lesions located in the internal carotid and verte-

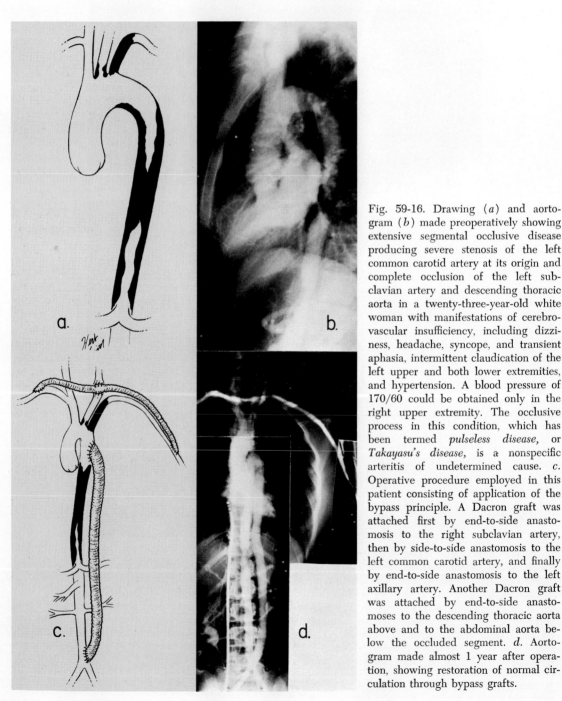

Fig. 59-16. Drawing (*a*) and aortogram (*b*) made preoperatively showing extensive segmental occlusive disease producing severe stenosis of the left common carotid artery at its origin and complete occlusion of the left subclavian artery and descending thoracic aorta in a twenty-three-year-old white woman with manifestations of cerebrovascular insufficiency, including dizziness, headache, syncope, and transient aphasia, intermittent claudication of the left upper and both lower extremities, and hypertension. A blood pressure of 170/60 could be obtained only in the right upper extremity. The occlusive process in this condition, which has been termed *pulseless disease,* or *Takayasu's disease,* is a nonspecific arteritis of undetermined cause. *c.* Operative procedure employed in this patient consisting of application of the bypass principle. A Dacron graft was attached first by end-to-side anastomosis to the right subclavian artery, then by side-to-side anastomosis to the left common carotid artery, and finally by end-to-side anastomosis to the left axillary artery. Another Dacron graft was attached by end-to-side anastomoses to the descending thoracic aorta above and to the abdominal aorta below the occluded segment. *d.* Aortogram made almost 1 year after operation, showing restoration of normal circulation through bypass grafts.

bral arteries are treated by endarterectomy and patch-graft angioplasty (Fig. 59-12). The involved arterial segment is exposed, and temporary arterial clamps are placed proximally and distally. A longitudinal incision is made through the involved segment, and the diseased intima is removed by dissection through a well-defined cleavage plane. The arterial incision is then closed by inserting a patch graft, the edges of which are sutured circumferentially to the arterial wound edges.

Occlusions of the great vessels arising from the aortic arch are preferably treated by end-to-side bypass graft, because lesions at this level are usually more extensive and involve long segments of vessel (Fig. 59-11). The proximal end of the graft is attached to the side of the ascending aorta, and the distal end or ends of the graft are attached to the patent arterial segments in the neck or supraclavicular region distal to the occlusion. The ascending aorta is exposed through a second or third right anterior intercostal incision. Using a partial occlusion clamp and end-to-side anastomosis, the proximal end of the graft is attached to the aorta. The patent distal arterial segments are exposed through separate incisions in the neck and supraclavicular regions. The other end of the graft is drawn retrosternally through a tunnel made by blunt dissection and attached to the side of the patent distal segment. In the presence of multiple occlusions, the appropriate limbs are attached to the side of this graft in the neck, and the other ends of the limbs are attached to the sides of the other patent arterial segments. Knitted Dacron tubes 8 to 10 mm in diameter are used for this purpose.

Operation in cases of abdominal angina may consist of endarterectomy, excision and graft replacement, or bypass graft, the latter procedure being preferable in most instances. The abdominal aorta is exposed between the renal and the common iliac arteries. The proximal end of the graft is attached to the side of the abdominal aorta in this region, and the other end of the graft is carried behind the transverse mesocolon and stomach and sutured to the side of the normal hepatic or splenic artery. Since the trifurcation of the celiac artery usually is uninvolved by the occlusive process, attachment of the graft to the hepatic or splenic artery provides complete revascularization of the celiac distribution. One end of a second tube is sutured to the side of the graft, and the other end is carried through a tunnel in the small bowel mesentery under the duodenum and attached to the side of the superior mesenteric artery distal to the site of the occlusive lesion. Knitted Dacron tubes 8 mm in diameter have been employed in all the author's cases.

Treatment for renovascular hypertension is di-rected toward correction of renal ischemia. Well-localized lesions may be treated by endarterectomy and patch-graft angioplasty. For more extensive segmental lesions the end-to-side bypass principle is preferred. The proximal end of an 8-mm Dacron graft is attached to the abdominal aorta below the origin of the renal arteries, and the distal end of the graft is attached to the side of the renal artery distal to the obstruction (Figs. 59-13 and 59-14). Bifurcation grafts are, of course, required in the treatment of bilateral lesions when this method is employed. The bypass graft method has been found particularly effective in restoring normal circulation to both the kidneys and the lower extremities in patients with combined lesions of the aorta, iliac arteries, and renal arteries. The proximal end of the renal artery graft is attached to the side of the aortic segment of the aortoiliac bypass graft in these cases. Reconstructive operation is impossible in a small number of cases because of both location and extent of the disease. Nephrectomy or partial nephrectomy may be required in these cases.

In cases of aortoiliac occlusion the method of reconstruction is selected at the time of operation on the basis of extent of the disease and the characteristics of the outer layers of the arterial wall. Thromboendarterectomy is employed when the occlusive process is well confined to the intima of the distal aorta and common iliac arteries. This operation is performed through separate longitudinal incisions placed in the common iliac arteries and the aorta, exposing both the proximal and distal extent of the lesion. The proper cleavage plane between the diseased intima and more normal outer layers is entered, and the occlusive process is removed using sharp and blunt dissection. In larger vessels vascular continuity is restored by simple closure of the arterial incisions. In smaller vessels, to avoid arterial constriction, the incisions are closed by inserting patch grafts made of knitted Dacron fabric, the edges of which are sutured circumferentially to the arterial wound edges by simple over-and-over suture.

Excision and graft replacement is employed when the occlusive process is associated with destructive changes of the entire vessel wall (Fig. 59-14). This procedure consists simply of excising the involved segment and replacing it with a bifurcation Dacron graft. The aortic end of the graft is attached to the proximal cut end of the aorta. Afterward the end of one iliac limb of the graft and then the other is attached to the distal end of the appropriate common or external iliac or femoral artery.

In cases in which the external iliac arteries are involved, the entire aortoiliac segment must be considered. The end-to-side bypass-graft procedure, using a flexible knitted Dacron graft, is the preferable treatment. One end of the graft is attached to the side of the uninvolved abdominal aorta above the obstruction, and the other end of the graft is drawn through a tunnel made behind the peritoneum and attached to the side of the distal patent segment either in the external iliac artery or in the common femoral artery opposite the origin of the profunda femoris artery in the groin (Fig. 59-15).

The type of procedure employed for occlusive lesions involving the superficial femoral and popliteal arteries depends upon the location and extent of occlusion. Lesions localized to a short segment of vessel, 15 cm or less, are well suited to endarterectomy and patch-graft angioplasty. The involved segment of artery is exposed, and temporary occluding clamps are placed across the uninvolved vessel above and below the obstruction, as well as on all branches arising from the occluded segment. A longitudinal incision is made through the region of obstruction, and under direct vision the diseased intima is removed both from the main central channel and from the orifices of the arterial branches arising from this segment. The arterial incision is then closed by inserting a patch graft with simple sutures.

More extensive lesions are usually treated by end-to-side bypass-graft technique (Fig. 59-15). Through a small incision in the groin one end of an 8-mm Dacron graft is attached by simple over-and-over suture to the side of the common femoral artery, and the other end of the graft is drawn through a subcutaneous tunnel made by blunt dissection into a second incision employed to expose the distal patent segment usually located in the popliteal artery. This end of the graft is then sutured to the side of the distal patent segment. By temporarily releasing the proximal clamp before the latter anastomosis is completed, blood is allowed to flow through the graft momentarily to flush out thrombi which may have formed in the graft during its insertion.

Analysis of experience with these methods of therapy at the Baylor University College of Medicine in more than five thousand patients with arterial occlusive disease reveals highly gratifying results. Although the incidence of successful results is not uniform in the various categories of occlusive disease because of the differences in location, nature, and extent of involvement of the occlusive process, the figures for successful restoration of normal circulation range from about 85 per cent to more than 95 per cent of cases treated. In patients with occlusive disease of the major branches of the aortic arch, for example, successful restoration of normal circulation was obtained in

about 85 per cent of those with distal occlusions and in virtually all those with proximal occlusions. Similarly, in patients with renovascular hypertension, successful restoration of normal circulation and normotension were obtained in 86 per cent of our cases. Even better results were obtained in the category involving the terminal abdominal aorta and its major branches, successful restoration of normal circulation being obtained in 97 per cent of patients with aortoiliac occlusions and in 90 per cent of those with femoropopliteal occlusions. Follow-up observations in these patients extending over 5 years, and up to 10 years in some, have provided evidence of maintenance of good long-term results with a relatively low recurrence rate of about 5 per cent in the proximal type of occlusion and about 20 per cent in the distal form.

SUGGESTED READING

Abbott, M. E.: Coarctation of Aorta of Adult Type: A Statistical Study and Historical Retrospect of 200 Recorded Cases, with Autopsy, of Stenosis, or Obliteration, of the Descending Arch in Subjects above the Age of Two Years, *Am. Heart J.*, 3:574–618, 1928.

Austin, D. J., and Thompson, J. E.: Excision and Arterial Grafting in the Surgical Management of Popliteal Aneurysms, *South. M. J.*, 51:43–48, 1958.

Baer, S.: Dissecting Aneurysm of the Aorta, *Mod. Concepts Cardiovas. Dis.*, 23:214–216, 1954.

Bahnson, H. T.: Definitive Treatment of Saccular Aneurysms of the Aorta with Excision of Sac and Aortic Suture, *Surg. Gynec. & Obst.*, 96:383–402, 1953.

Bazy, L., Huguier, J., Reboul, H., and Laubry, P.: Technique des "endartériectomies" pour artéries oblitérantes chroniques des membres inférieurs, des iliaques et de l'aorte abdominale inférieure, *J. chir.*, 65:196–210, 1949.

Beaconsfield, P., and Kunlin, J.: Insidious Thrombosis of the Aortic Bifurcation: Report of 35 Cases, *A.M.A. Arch. Surg.*, 66:356–364, 1953.

Beall, A. C., Jr., Cooley, D. A., Morris, G. C., Jr., and De Bakey, M. E.: Perforation of Arteriosclerotic Aneurysms into the Inferior Vena Cava, *Arch. Surg.*, 86: 809–818, 1963.

Beall, A. C., Jr., Crawford, E. S., Cooley, D. A., and De Bakey, M. E.: Extracranial Aneurysms of the Carotid Artery: Report of Seven Cases, *Postgrad. Med.*, 32:93–102, 1962.

Beall, A. C., Jr., Henly, W. S., Morris, G. C., Jr., Crawford, E. S., Cooley, D. A., and De Bakey, M. E.: Translumbar Aortography: A Simple, Safe Technic, *Ann. Surg.*, 157:882–893, 1963.

Beall, A. C., Jr., Morris, G. C., Jr., Crawford, E. S., Cooley, D. A., and De Bakey, M. E.: Translumbar Aortography: Re-evaluation, *Surgery*, 49:772–778, 1961.

Bean, W. B., and Ponseti, IV.: Dissecting Aneurysm

Produced by Diet, *Circulation,* 12:185–192, 1955.

Bing, R. J., Handelsman, J. C., Campbell, J. A., Griswold, H. E., and Blalock, A.: The Surgical Treatment and the Physiopathology of Coarctation of Aorta, *Ann. Surg.,* 128:803–824, 1948.

Blackford, L. M.: Coarctation of the Aorta, *A.M.A. Arch. Int. Med.,* 41:702–735, 1928.

Blalock, A., and Park, E. A.: Surgical Treatment of Experimental Coarctation (Atresia) of Aorta, *Ann. Surg.,* 119:445–456, 1944.

Bonnet, L. M.: Sur la lésion dite stenose congénitale de l'aorte dans la région de l'isthme, *Rev. méd.,* 23:108, 1903.

Bramwell, C.: Coarctation of the Aorta: II. Clinical Features, *Brit. Heart J.,* 9:100–127, 1947.

Bramwell, C., and Jones, A. M.: Coarctation of the Aorta: The Collateral Circulation, *Brit. Heart J.,* 3:205–227, 1941.

Broadbent, W. H.: Absence of Pulsation in Both Radial Arteries, Vessels Being Full of Blood, *Tr. Clin. Soc. London,* 8:165–168, 1875.

Burchell, H. B.: Aortic Dissection (Dissecting Hemotoma; Dissecting Aneurysm of the Aorta), *Circulation,* 12:1068–1079, 1955.

Clagett, O. T., Kirklin, J. W., and Edwards, J. E.: Anatomic Variations and Pathologic Changes in Coarctation of the Aorta: A Study of 124 Cases, *Surg. Gynec. & Obst.,* 98:103–114, 1954.

Cooley, D. A., and De Bakey, M. E.: Surgical Considerations of Intrathoracic Aneurysms of the Aorta and Great Vessels, *Tr. South. S. A.,* 63:91–111, 1951; also *Ann Surg.,* 135:660–680, 1952.

Cooley, D. A., and De Bakey, M. E.: Surgical Considerations of Excisional Therapy for Aortic Aneurysms, *Surgery,* 34:1005–1020, 1953.

Cooley, D. A., and De Bakey, M. E.: Ruptured Aneurysms of Abdominal Aorta: Excision and Homograft Replacement, *Postgrad. Med.,* 16:334–342, 1954.

Cooley, D. A., and De Bakey, M. E.: Resection of the Thoracic Aorta with Replacement by Homograft for Aneurysms and Constrictive Lesions, *J. Thoracic Surg.,* 29:66–104, 1955.

Cooley, D. A., and De Bakey, M. E.: Resection of Entire Ascending Aorta in Fusiform Aneurysm Using Cardiac Bypass, *J.A.M.A.,* 162:1158–1159, 1956.

Cooley, D. A., De Bakey, M. E., and Morris, G. C., Jr.: Controlled Extracorporeal Circulation in Surgical Treatment of Aortic Aneurysm, *Ann. Surg.,* 146:473–485, 1957.

Crafoord, C., and Nylin, G.: Congenital Coarctation of Aorta and Its Surgical Treatment, *J. Thoracic Surg.,* 14:347–361, 1945.

Crawford, E. S., Beall, A. C., Jr., Moyer, J. H., and De Bakey, M. E.: Complications of Aortography: Critical Analysis of Experience with 300 Cases and Review of the Literature, *Surg. Gynec. & Obst.,* 104:129–141, 1957.

Crawford, E. S., Beall, A. C., Jr., Ellis, P. R., Jr., and

De Bakey, M. E.: A Technic Permitting Operation upon Small Arteries, *S. Forum,* 10:671–675, 1960.

Crawford, E. S., and De Bakey, M. E.: The Bypass Operation in the Treatment of Arteriosclerotic Occlusive Disease of the Lower Extremities, *Surg. Gynec. & Obst.,* 101:529–535, 1955.

Crawford, E. S., and De Bakey, M. E.: Surgery for Strokes, in I. H. Page, "Strokes," E. P. Dutton & Co., Inc., New York, 1961, pp. 132–153.

Crawford, E. S., and De Bakey, M. E.: Surgical Treatment of Stroke by Arterial Reconstructive Operation, *Clin. Neurosurg.,* 9:150–162, 1963.

Crawford, E. S., De Bakey, M. E., and Blaisdell, F. W.: Simplified Treatment of Large, Sacciform Aortic Aneurysms with Patch Grafts: Experiences with Five Cases, *J. Thoracic & Cardiovas. Surg.,* 41:479–491, 1961.

Crawford, E. S., De Bakey, M. E., Blaisdell, F. W., Morris, G. C., Jr., and Fields, W. S.: Hemodynamic Alterations in Patients with Cerebral Arterial Insufficiency before and after Operation, *Surgery,* 48:76–94, 109–110, 1960.

Crawford, E. S., De Bakey, M. E., and Cooley, D. A.: Clinical Use of Synthetic Arterial Substitutes in 317 Patients, *A.M.A. Arch. Surg.,* 76:261–270, 1958.

Crawford, E. S., De Bakey, M. E., and Cooley, D. A.: Surgical Considerations of Peripheral Arterial Aneurysms: Analysis of 107 Cases, *A.M.A. Arch. Surg.,* 78:226–238, Feb. 1959.

Crawford, E. S., De Bakey, M. E., Cooley, D. A., and Morris, G. C., Jr.: Use of Crimped, Knitted Dacron Grafts in Patients with Occlusive Disease of the Aorta and of the Iliac, Femoral and Popliteal Arteries, in S. A. Wesolowski and C. Dennis, "Fundamentals of Vascular Grafting," McGraw-Hill Book Company, New York, 1963, pp. 356–364.

Crawford, E. S., De Bakey, M. E., Morris, G. C., Jr., and Cooley, D. A.: Thrombo-obliterative Disease of the Great Vessels Arising from the Aortic Arch, *J. Thoracic & Cardiovas. Surg.,* 43:38–53, 1962.

Crawford, E. S., Edwards, W. H., De Bakey, M. E., Cooley, D. A., and Morris, G. C., Jr.: Peripheral Arteriosclerotic Aneurysm, *J. Am. Geriat. Soc.,* 9:1–15, 1961.

Creech, O., Jr., De Bakey, M. E., Cooley, D. A., and Self, M. M.: Preparation and Use of Freeze-dried Arterial Homografts, *Ann. Surg.,* 140:35–43, 1954.

Davis, J. B., Grove, W. J., and Julian, O. C.: Thrombic Occlusion of Branches of Aortic Arch, Martorell's Syndrome: Report of a Case Treated Surgically, *Ann. Surg.,* 144:124–126, 1956.

De Bakey, M. E.: Changing Concepts in Thoracic Vascular Surgery, *J. Thoracic & Cardiovas. Surg.,* 38:145–165, 1959.

De Bakey, M. E.: Changing Concepts in Vascular Surgery, *J. Cardiovas. Surg.,* 1:3–44, 1960.

De Bakey, M. E.: Basic Concepts of Therapy in Arterial Disease, *Bull. New York Acad. Med.,* 39:704–749, 1963.

De Bakey, M. E.: Basic Concepts of Therapy in Arterial Disease, *J.A.M.A.*, **186**:484–498, 1963.

De Bakey, M. E.: Diseases of the Arterial Wall: Concepts of Therapy, *Mal. cardiovas.* 4:377–414, 1963.

De Bakey, M. E.: Concepts Underlying Surgical Treatment of Cerebrovascular Insufficiency, *Clin. Neurosurg.*, **10**:310–340, 1963.

De Bakey, M. E., and Cooley, D. A.: Successful Resection of Aneurysm of Thoracic Aorta and Replacement by Graft, *J.A.M.A.*, **152**:673–676, 1953.

De Bakey, M. E., and Cooley, D. A.: Surgical Treatment of Aneurysm of Abdominal Aorta by Resection and Restoration of Continuity with Homograft, *Surg. Gynec. & Obst.*, **97**:257–266, 1953.

De Bakey, M. E., and Cooley, D. A.: Surgical Considerations of Acquired Diseases of the Aorta, *Ann. Surg.*, **139**:763–777, 1954.

De Bakey, M. E., and Cooley, D. A.: Successful Resection of Aneurysm of Distal Aortic Arch and Replacement by Graft, *J.A.M.A.*, **155**:1398–1403, 1954.

De Bakey, M. E., Cooley, D. A., Crawford, E. S., and Morris, G. C., Jr.: Aneurysms of the Thoracic Aorta: Analysis of 179 Patients Treated by Resection, *J. Thoracic Surg.*, **36**:393–420, 1958.

De Bakey, M. E., Cooley, D. A., Crawford, E. S., and Morris, G. C., Jr.: Clinical Application of a New Flexible Knitted Dacron Arterial Substitute, *A.M.A. Arch. Surg.*, **77**:713–724, 1958.

De Bakey, M. E., Cooley, D. A., and Creech, O., Jr.: Surgical Considerations of Dissecting Aneurysm of the Aorta, *Ann. Surg.*, **142**:586–612, 1955.

De Bakey, M. E., Cooley, D. A., and Creech, O., Jr.: Surgery of the Aorta, *Clin. Symposia*, **8**:45–75, 1956.

De Bakey, M. E., Cooley, D. A., and Creech, O., Jr.: Surgical Treatment of Dissecting Aneurysm, *J.A.M.A.*, **162**:1654–1657, 1956.

De Bakey, M. E., Cooley, D. A., and Creech, O., Jr.: Aneurysm of the Aorta Treated by Resection: Analysis of 313 Cases, *J.A.M.A.*, **163**:1439–1443, 1957.

De Bakey, M. E., Cooley, D. A., Morris, G. C., Jr., Crawford, E. S., and Beall, A. C., Jr.: Surgery of Congenital Cardiovascular Disease, in W. H. Cole and R. M. Zollinger, "Textbook of Surgery," 8th ed., Appleton-Century-Crofts, Inc., New York, 1963, pp. 914–970.

De Bakey, M. E., Cooley, D. A., Morris, G. C., Jr., Crawford, E. S., and Beall, A. C., Jr.: Surgery of Acquired Cardiovascular Disease, in W. H. Cole and R. M. Zollinger, "Textbook of Surgery," 8th ed., Appleton-Century-Crofts, Inc., New York, 1963, pp. 971–1065.

De Bakey, M. E., and Crawford, E. S.: Surgical Considerations of Acquired Diseases of the Aorta and Major Peripheral Arteries. I. Aortic Aneurysms, *Mod. Concepts Cardiovas. Dis.*, **28**:557–561, 1959.

De Bakey, M. E., and Crawford, E. S.: Surgical Considerations of Acquired Diseases of the Aorta and Major Peripheral Arteries. II. Dissecting Aneurysms of the Aorta, *Mod. Concepts Cardiovas. Dis.*, **28**:563–564, 1959.

De Bakey, M. E., and Crawford, E. S.: Surgical Considerations of Acquired Diseases of the Aorta and Major Peripheral Arteries. III. Atherosclerotic Occlusive Vascular Disease, *Mod. Concepts Cardiovas. Dis.*, **29**:571–576, 1960.

De Bakey, M. E., Crawford, E. S., and Cooley, D. A.: Chronic Arterial Insufficiency of the Lower Extremities, *Disease-A-Month*, 3–45, 1957.

De Bakey, M. E., Crawford, E. S., Cooley, D. A., and Morris, G. C., Jr.: Successful Resection of Fusiform Aneurysm of Aortic Arch with Replacement by Homograft. *Surg. Gynec. & Obst.*, **105**:657–664, 1957.

De Bakey, M. E., Crawford, E. S., Cooley, D. A., and Morris, G. C., Jr.: Surgical Considerations of Occlusive Disease of the Abdominal Aorta and Iliac and Femoral Arteries: Analysis of 803 Cases, *Ann. Surg.*, **148**:306–324, 1958.

De Bakey, M. E., Crawford, E. S., Cooley, D. A., and Morris, G. C., Jr.: Surgical Considerations of Occlusive Disease of Innominate, Carotid, Subclavian and Vertebral Arteries, *Ann. Surg.*, **149**:690–710, 1959.

De Bakey, M. E., Crawford, E. S., Creech, O., Jr., and Cooley, D. A.: Arterial Homografts for Peripheral Arteriosclerotic Occlusive Disease, *Circulation*, **15**:21–30, 1957.

De Bakey, M. E., Crawford, E. S., and Fields, W. S.: Surgical Treatment of Lesions Producing Arterial Insufficiency of the Internal Carotid, Common Carotid, Vertebral, Innominate and Subclavian Arteries, *Ann. Int. Med.*, **51**:436–448, 1959.

De Bakey, M. E., Crawford, E. S., and Fields, W. S.: Surgical Treatment of Patients with Cerebral Arterial Insufficiency Associated with Extracranial Arterial Occlusive Lesions, *Neurology*, **11**:145–149, 1961.

De Bakey, M. E., Crawford, E. S., Morris, G. C., Jr., and Cooley, D. A.: Surgical Considerations of Occlusive Disease of the Innominate, Carotid, Subclavian, and Vertebral Arteries, *Ann. Surg.*, **154**:698–725, 1961.

De Bakey, M. E., Crawford, E. S., Morris, G. C., Jr., and Cooley, D. A.: Arterial Reconstructive Operations for Cerebrovascular Insufficiency Due to Extracranial Arterial Occlusive Disease, *J. Cardiovas. Surg.*, 3:12–25, 1962.

De Bakey, M. E., Crawford, E. S., Morris, G. C., Jr., and Cooley, D. A.: Patch Graft Angioplasty in Vascular Surgery, *J. Cardiovas. Surg.*, 3:106–141, 1962.

De Bakey, M. E., Creech, O., Jr., and Cooley, D. A.: Occlusive Disease of the Aorta and Its Treatment by Resection and Homograft Replacement, *Ann. Surg.*, **140**:290–310, 1954.

De Bakey, M. E., Creech, O., Jr., Cooley, D. A., and Halpert, B.: Structural Changes in Human Aortic

Homografts: Study of 10 Cases, *A.M.A. Arch. Surg.*, 69:472–482, 1954.

De Bakey, M. E., Creech, O., Jr., and Cooley, D. A.: The Leriche Syndrome and Its Surgical Treatment by Resection and Homograft Replacement, *Lyon chir.*, 52:402–411, 1956.

De Bakey, M. E., Creech, O., Jr., and Morris, G. C., Jr.: Aneurysm of Thoracoabdominal Aorta Involving the Celiac, Superior Mesenteric, and Renal Arteries: Report of Four Cases Treated by Resection and Homograft Replacement, *Ann. Surg.*, 144:549–573, 1956.

De Bakey, M. E., Henly, W. S., Cooley, D. A., Crawford, E. S., and Morris, G. C., Jr.: Surgical Treatment of Dissecting Aneurysm of the Aorta: Analysis of 72 Cases, *Circulation*, 24:290–303, 1961.

De Bakey, M. E., Morris, G. C., Jr., Crawford, E. S., and Cooley, D. A.: Surgical Considerations of Renal Hypertension, *J. Cardiovas. Surg.*, 2:435–448, 1961.

De Bakey, M. E., Morris, G. C., Jr., Jordan, G. L., Jr., and Cooley, D. A.: Segmental Thrombo-obliterative Disease of Branches of Aortic Arch: Successful Surgical Treatment, *J.A.M.A.*, 166:998–1003, 1958.

De Camp, P. T., and Birchall, R.: Recognition and Treatment of Renal Arterial Stenosis Associated with Hypertension, *Surgery*, 43:134–151, 1958.

De Wolfe, V. G., LeFevre, F. A., Humphries, A. W., Shaw, M. B., and Phalen, G. S.: Intermittent Claudication of the Hip and the Syndrome of Chronic Aorto-iliac Thrombosis, *Circulation*, 9:1–16, 1954.

Dissecting Aneurysm of the Aorta, *Pfizer Spectrum*, 6:5–7, 1958.

Dos Santos, J. C.: Sur la désobstruction des thromboses artérielles anciennes, *Mém. Acad. chir.*, 73:409–411, 1947.

Dubost, C., Allary, M., and Oeconomos, N.: Resection of an Aneurysm of the Abdominal Aorta: Reestablishment of the Continuity by a Preserved Human Arterial Graft, with Result after Five Months, *A.M.A. Arch. Surg.*, 64:405–408, 1952.

Edwards, C., and Rob, C.: Relief of Neurological Symptoms and Signs by Reconstruction of a Stenosed Internal Carotid Artery, *Brit. M. J.*, 2:1265–1267, 1956.

Elkin, D. C., and Cooper, F. W., Jr.: Surgical Treatment of Insidious Thrombosis of the Aorta: Report of Ten Cases, *Ann. Surg.*, 130:417–427, 1949.

Estes, J. E., Jr.: Abdominal Aortic Aneurysm: A Study of 102 Cases, *Circulation*, 2:258–264, 1950.

Friedman, M., Selzer, A., and Rosenblum, H.: The Renal Blood Flow in Coarctation of the Aorta, *J. Clin. Invest.*, 20:107–111, 1941.

Gerbode, F., Braimbridge, M., Osborn, J. J., Hood, M., and French, S.: Traumatic Thoracic Aneurysms: Treatment by Resection and Grafting with the Use of an Extracorporeal Bypass, *Surgery*, 42:975–985, 1957.

Gifford, R. W., Jr., Hines, E. A., Jr., and Janes, J. M.: An Analysis and Follow-up Study of 100 Popliteal Aneurysms, *Surgery*, 33:284–293, 1953.

Glendy, R. E., Castleman, B., and White, P. D.: Dissecting Aneurysm of Aorta: Clinical and Anatomical Analysis of 19 Cases (13 Acute) with Notes on Differential Diagnosis, *Am. Heart J.*, 13:129–162, 1937.

Glenn, F., Keefer, E. B. C., Speer, D. S., and Dotter, C. T.: Coarctation of the Lower Thoracic and Abdominal Aorta Immediately Proximal to Celiac Axis, *Surg. Gynec. & Obst.*, 94:561–569, 1952.

Golden, A., and Weens, H. S.: The Diagnosis of Dissecting Aneurysm of the Aorta by Angiocardiography: Report of a Case, *Am. Heart J.*, 37:114–118, 1949.

Goodson, W. H., Jr.: Coarctation of the Aorta: A Report of Two Unusual Cases, *New England J. Med.*, 216:339–345, 1937.

Gore, I., and Seiwert, V. J.: Dissecting Aneurysm of the Aorta: Pathological Aspects. An Analysis of 85 Fatal Cases, *A.M.A. Arch. Path.*, 53:121–141, 1952.

Greenfield, I.: Thrombosis and Embolism of the Abdominal Aorta, *Ann. Int. Med.*, 19:656–668, 1943.

Gross, H., and Philips, B.: Complete Occlusion of the Abdominal Aorta: A Review of Seven Cases, *Am. J. M. Sc.*, 200:203–208, 1940.

Gross, R. E.: Coarctation of the Aorta, *Circulation*, 7:757–768, 1953.

Gross, R. E., and Hufnagel, C. A.: Coarctation of the Aorta: Experimental Studies Regarding Its Surgical Correction, *New England J. Med.*, 233:287–293, 1945.

Hallenbeck, G. A., Wood, E. H., Burchell, H. B., and Clagett, O. T.: Coarctation of the Aorta: The Relationship of Clinical Results to Cardiovascular Dynamics Studied before, during, and after Surgical Treatment, *Surg. Gynec. & Obst.* 92:75–80, 1951.

Halpert, B., and Brown, C. A.: Dissecting Aneurysms of the Aorta: Study of 12 Cases, *A.M.A. Arch. Path.*, 60:378–386, 1955.

Halpert, B., Erickson, E. E., De Bakey, M. E., Creech, O., Jr., and Cooley, D. A.: Occlusive Disease of the Abdominal Aorta: Structural Alterations, *A.M.A. Arch. Path.*, 65:158–165, 1958.

Hirst, A. E., Jr., Johns, V. J., Jr., and Kime, S. W., Jr.: Dissecting Aneurysm of the Aorta: A Review of 505 Cases, *Medicine*, 37:217–279, 1958.

Howard, J. E., Berthrong, M., Gould, D. M., and Yendt, E. R.: Hypertension Resulting from Unilateral Renal Vascular Disease and Its Relief by Nephrectomy, *Bull. Johns Hopkins Hosp.*, 94:51–85, 1954.

Johnson, A. L., Ferencz, C., Wiglesworth, F. W., and McRae, D. L.: Coarctation of the Aorta Complicated by Patency of the Ductus Arteriosus: Physiologic Considerations in the Classification of Coarctation of the Aorta, *Circulation*, 4:242–250, 1951.

Julian, O. C., Dye, W. S., Javid, H., and Grove, W. J.:

The Use of Vessel Grafts in the Treatment of Popliteal Aneurysms, *Surgery*, 38:970–980, 1955.

Julian, O. C., Dye, W. S., Olwin, J. H., and Jordan, P. H.: Direct Surgery of Arteriosclerosis, *Ann. Surg.*, 136:459–474, 1952.

Julian, O. C., Grove, W. J., Dye, W. S., Olwin, J. H., and Sadove, M. S.: Direct Surgery of Arteriosclerosis: Resection of Abdominal Aorta with Homologous Aortic Graft Replacement, *Ann. Surg.*, 138:387–399, 1953.

Kalmansohn, R. B., and Kalmansohn, R. W.: Thrombotic Obliteration of Branches of Aortic Arch, *Circulation*, 15:237–244, 1957.

Kampmeier, R. H.: Saccular Aneurysm of the Thoracic Aorta: A Clinical Study of 633 Cases, *Ann. Int. Med.*, 12:624–651, 1938.

Keeley, F. X., Misanik, L. F., and Wirts, C. W.: Abdominal Angina Syndrome, *Gastroenterology*, 37:480–482, 1959.

Kekwick, A., McDonald, L., and Semple, R.: Obliterative Disease of the Abdominal Aorta and Iliac Arteries with Intermittent Claudication, *Quart. J. Med.*, 21:185–200, 1952.

Kunlin, J.: Le traitement de l'ischémie artéritique par le greffe veineuse longue, *Rev. chir.*, 70:206, 1951.

Leriche, R.: Des oblitérations artérielles hautes (oblitération de la terminaison de l'aorte) comme cause des insuffisances circulatoires des membres inférieurs, *Bull. et mém. Soc. chir.*, 49:1404, 1923.

Leriche, R.: De la résection du carrefour aortoiliaque avec double sympathectomie lombaire pour thrombose artéritique de l'aorte: Le syndrome de l'oblitération termino-aortique par artérite. *Presse méd.*, 48:601–604, 1940.

Leriche, R., and Morel, A.: The Syndrome of Thrombotic Obliteration of the Aortic Bifurcation, *Ann. Surg.*, 127:193–206, 1948.

Levinson, D. C., Edmeades, D. T., and Griffith, G. C.: Dissecting Aneurysm of Aorta: Its Clinical, Electrocardiographic and Laboratory Features. Report of 58 Autopsied Cases, *Circulation*, 1:360–387, 1950.

Linton, R. R.: The Arteriosclerotic Popliteal Aneurysm: Report of 14 Patients Treated by Preliminary Lumbar Sympathetic Ganglionectomy and Aneurysmectomy, *Surgery*, 26:41–58, 1949.

Lueth, H. C.: Thrombosis of the Abdominal Aorta: A Report of Four Cases Showing the Variability of Symptoms, *Ann. Int. Med.*, 13:1167–1173, 1940.

Luke, J. C., and Levitan, B. A.: Revascularization of the Kidney in Hypertension Due to Renal Artery Stenosis, *A.M.A. Arch. Surg.*, 79:269–275, 1959.

Lyons, C., and Galbraith, G.: Surgical Treatment of Atherosclerotic Occlusion of the Internal Carotid Artery, *Ann. Surg.*, 146:487–496, 1957.

McGeachy, T. E., and Paullin, J. E.: Dissecting Aneurysm of the Aorta, *J.A.M.A.*, 108:1690–1698, 1937.

McKusick, V. A.: The Cardiovascular Aspects of Marfan's Syndrome: A Heritable Disorder of Connective Tissue, *Circulation*, 11:321–342, 1955.

Maniglia, R., and Gregory, J. E.: Increasing Incidence of Arteriosclerotic Aortic Aneurysms: Analysis of 6,000 Autopsies, *A.M.A. Arch. Path.*, 54:298–305, 1952.

March, H. W., Hultgren, H. N., and Gerbode, F.: Immediate and Remote Effects of Resection on Hypertension in Coarctation of Aorta, *Brit. Heart J.*, 22:361–373, 1960.

Marston, E. L., Bradshaw, H. H., and Meredith, J. H.: Agenesis of the Aortic Isthmus: A Case Report, Discussion of Different Factors, and Reclassification of Coarctations, *Surgery*, 42:352–363, 1957.

Matas, R.: An Operation for the Radical Cure of Aneurism Based upon Arteriorrhaphy, *Ann. Surg.*, 37:161–196, 1903.

Matas, R.: Surgery of the Vascular System, in W. W. Keen (ed.), "Surgery: Its Principles and Practice." W. B. Saunders Company, Philadelphia, 1914, vol. 5, chap. 70.

Moersch, F. P., and Sayre, G. P.: Neurologic Manifestations Associated with Dissecting Aneurysm of the Aorta, *J.A.M.A.*, 144:1141–1148, 1950.

Morris, G. C., Jr., Cooley, D. A., Crawford, E. S., Berry, W. B., and De Bakey, M. E.: Renal Revascularization for Hypertension: Clinical and Physiologic Studies in 32 Cases, *Surgery*, 48:95–110, 1960.

Morris, G. C., Jr., Cooley, D. A., De Bakey, M. E., and Crawford, E. S.: Coarctation of the Aorta with Particular Emphasis upon Improved Techniques of Surgical Repair, *J. Thoracic & Cardiovas. Surg.*, 40:705–722, 1960.

Morris, G. C., Jr., Crawford, E. S., Cooley, D. A., and De Bakey, M. E.: Revascularization of the Celiac and Superior Mesenteric Arteries, *Arch. Surg.*, 84:95–107, 1962.

Morris, G. C., Jr., Crawford, E. S., Cooley, D. A., Selzman, H. M., and De Bakey, M. E.: Renovascular Hypertension: Experience with Renal Artery Reconstruction in 115 Patients, *Am. J. Cardiol.*, 9:141–150, 1962.

Morris, G. C., Jr., and De Bakey, M. E.: Abdominal Angina: Diagnosis and Surgical Treatment, *J.A.M.A.*, 176:89–92, 1961.

Morris, G. C., Jr., and De Bakey, M. E.: Diagnosis of Renal Vascular Disease, *Am. J. Cardiol.*, 9:756–759, 1962.

Morris, G. C., Jr., and De Bakey, M. E.: Treatment of Hypertension Associated with Renal Arterial Occlusive Disease, *Am. J. Cardiol.*, 9:916–919, 1962.

Morris, G. C., Jr., and De Bakey, M. E.: Aortic Aneurysms and Occlusive Diseases of the Aorta, *Am. J. Cardiol.*, 12:303–308, 1963.

Morris, G. C., Jr., De Bakey, M. E., Cooley, D. A., and Crawford, E. S.: Arterial Bypass below the Knee, *Surg. Gynec. & Obst.*, 108:321–332, 1959.

Morris, G. C., Jr., De Bakey, M. E., Cooley, D. A., and Crawford, E. S.: Surgical Treatment of Renal Hypertension, *Ann. Surg.*, 151:854–866, 1960.

Morris, G. C., Jr., De Bakey, M. E., Cooley, D. A., and Crawford, E. S.: Experience with 200 Renal Artery

Reconstructive Procedures for Hypertension or Renal Failure, *Circulation*, 27:346–350, 1963.

Morris, G. C., Jr., De Bakey, M. E., Cooley, D. A., and Crawford, E. S.: Surgical Aspects of Renovascular Hypertension, *Heart Bull.*, 12:51–53, 1963.

Morris, G. C., Jr., De Bakey, M. E., Crawford, E. S., and Cooley, D. A.: Surgical Treatment of Renovascular Hypertension, *A.M.A. Arch. Surg.*, 82:723–734, 1961.

Morris, G. C., Jr., Edwards, W. H., Cooley, D. A., Crawford, E. S., and De Bakey, M. E.: Surgical Importance of Profunda Femoris Artery: Analysis of 102 Cases with Combined Aortoiliac and Femoropopliteal Occlusive Disease Treated by Revascularization of Deep Femoral Artery, *Arch. Surg.*, 82:32–37, 1961.

Morris, G. C., Jr., Henly, W. S., and De Bakey, M. E.: Correction of Acute Dissecting Aneurysm of Aorta with Valvular Insufficiency, *J.A.M.A.*, 184:63–64, 1963.

Morris, G. C., Jr., Wheeler, C. G., Crawford, E. S., Cooley, D. A., and De Bakey, M. E.: Restorative Vascular Surgery in the Presence of Impending and Overt Gangrene of the Extremities, *Surgery*, 51:50–57, 1962.

Mote, C. D., and Carr, J. L.: Dissecting Aneurysm of Aorta, *Am. Heart J.*, 24:69–87, 1942.

Oudot, J.: La greffe vasculaire dans les thromboses du carrefour aortique, *Presse méd.*, 59:234–236, 1951.

Oudot, J.: Greffe de la bifurcation aortique depuis les artères rénales jusqu'aux artères iliaques externes pour thrombose artéritique, *Mém. Acad. chir.*, 77:642–644, 1951.

Oudot, J., and Beaconsfield, P.: Thrombosis of the Aortic Bifurcation Treated by Resection and Homograft Replacement: Report of Five Cases, *A.M.A. Arch. Surg.*, 66:365–374, 1953.

Paullin, J. E., and James, D. F.: Dissecting Aneurysm of Aorta, *Postgrad. Med.*, 4:291–299, 1948.

Poutasse, E. F.: Surgical Treatment of Renal Hypertension: Results in Patients with Occlusive Lesions of Renal Arteries, *J. Urol.*, 82:403–411, 1959.

Railsback, O. C., and Dock, W.: Erosion of the Ribs Due to Stenosis of the Isthmus (Coarctation) of the Aorta, *Radiology*, 12:58–61, 1929.

Reboul, H., and Laubry, P.: Endarteriectomy in the Treatment of Chronic Endarteritis Obliterans of the Limbs and Abdominal Aorta, *Proc. Roy. Soc. Med.*, 43:547–552, 1950.

Reifenstein, G. H., Levine, S. A., and Gross, R. E.: Coarctation of the Aorta: Review of 104 Autopsied Cases of "Adult Type," Two Years of Age or Older, *Am. Heart J.*, 33:146–168, 1947.

Ritvo, M., and Votta, P. J.: Clinical and Roentgen Manifestations of Dissecting Aneurysm of Aorta, *Am. J. Roentgenol.*, 52:583–594, 1944.

Rob, C. G., and Eastcott, H. H. G.: Arterial Grafting, in *British Surgical Progress*, Vol. 3, Supplement to *British Surgical Practice*, Butterworth & Co., (Publishers), Ltd., London, 1953, p. 1.

Ross, R. S., and McKusick, V. A.: Aortic Arch Syndromes: Diminished or Absent Pulses in Arteries Arising from Arch of Aorta, *A.M.A. Arch. Int. Med.*, 92:701–740, 1953.

Sailer, S.: Dissecting aneurysm of aorta, *A.M.A. Arch. Path.*, 33:704–730, 1942.

Schnitker, M. A., and Bayer, C. A.: Dissecting Aneurysm of the Aorta in Young Individuals, Particularly in Association with Pregnancy, with Report of a Case, *Ann. Int. Med.*, 20:486–511, 1944.

Schuster, S. R., and Gross, R. E.: Surgery for Coarctation of the Aorta: A Review of 500 Cases, *J. Thoracic & Cardiovas. Surg.*, 43:54–70, 1962.

Scott, H. W., Jr., Collins, H. A., Langa, A. M., and Olsen, N. S.: Additional Observations Concerning the Physiology of the Hypertension Associated with Experimental Coarctation of the Aorta, *Surgery*, 36:445–459, 1954.

Scott, W. G., and Bottom, D. S.: Laminagraphic Studies of Aorta: Their Advantages and Limitations, *Am. J. Roentgenol.*, 51:18–28, 1944.

Shaw, R. S., and Maynard, E. P., III: Acute and Chronic Thrombosis of the Mesenteric Arteries Associated with Malabsorption: Report of Two Cases Successfully Treated by Thromboendarterectomy, *New England J. Med.*, 258:874–878, 1958.

Shennan, T.: "Dissecting Aneurysm," Medical Research Council Special Report Series no. 193, London, 1934.

Shimizu, K., and Sano, K.: Pulseless Disease, *J. Neuropath. & Clin. Neurol.*, 1:37–47, 1951.

Siegel, M. L., and Garvin, C. F.: Thrombosis and Embolism of the Abdominal Aorta: Report of a Case with Obstruction of the Renal Arteries, *Ohio M. J.*, 37:750–751, 1941.

Steele, J. M., and Cohn, A. E.: The Nature of Hypertension in Coarctation of the Aorta, *J. Clin. Invest.*, 17:514, 1938.

Surgical Treatment of Coarctation of the Aorta (Report of Section on Cardiovascular Surgery, American College of Chest Physicians), *Dis. Chest*, 31:468–478, 1957.

Symposium on Coarctation of the Aorta. II, *Proc. Staff Meet. Mayo Clin.*, 23:321–360, 1948.

Takayasu, M.: Case of Queer Changes in Central Blood Vessels of Retina, *Acta Soc. ophth. Jap.*, 12:554, 1908.

Taussig, H. B.: "Congenital Malformations of the Heart" The Commonwealth Fund, New York, 1947.

Tuffier, T.: Intervention chirurgicale directe pour un anévrysme de la crosse de l'aorte, ligature du sac, *Presse méd.*, 1:267–271, 1902; also *Bull. Acad. méd. Paris*, 85:586, 1921.

Warren, W. D., Beckwith, J., and Muller, W. H., Jr.: Problems in Surgical Management of Acute Dissecting Aneurysm of Aorta, *Ann. Surg.*, 144:530–548, 1956.

Weiss, S., Kinney, T. D., and Maher, M. M.: Dissecting Aneurysm of the Aorta with Experimental Atherosclerosis, *Am. J. M. Sc.*, 200:192–203, 1940.

Welch, W. H.: Embolism and Thrombosis of the Abdominal Aorta, in T. C. Allbutt and H. D. Roleston, "System of Medicine," Macmillan & Co., Ltd., London, 1909, vol. 6, p. 809.

Winter, C. C., Maxwell, M. H., Rockney, R. E., and Kleeman, C. R.: Results of Radioisotope Renogram and Comparison with Other Kidney Tests among Hypertensive Persons, *J. Urol.*, **82**:674–680, 1959.

Wood, F. C., Pendergrass, E. P., and Ostrum, H. W.: Dissecting Aneurysm of the Aorta, with Special Reference to Its Roentgenographic Features, *Am. J. Roentgenol.*, **28**:437–465, 1932.

Wright, I. S., Urdaneta, E., and Wright, B.: Reopening the Case of the Abdominal Aortic Aneurysm, *Tr. Am. Clin. & Climatol. A.*, **67**:213–232, 1955; also *Circulation*, **13**:754–768, 1956.

Wright, J. L., Burchell, H. B., Wood, E. H., Hines, E. A., Jr., and Clagett, O. T.: Hemodynamic and Clinical Appraisal of Coarctation Four to Seven Years after Resection and End-to-end Anastomosis of Aorta, *Circulation*, **14**:806–814, 1956.

Wylie, E. J., and McGuinness, J. S.: The Recognition and Treatment of Arteriosclerotic Stenosis of Major Arteries, *Surg. Gynec. & Obst.*, **97**:425–433, 1953.

60 SURGICAL TREATMENT OF DISEASES OF THE VENOUS SYSTEM

Arthur C. Beall, Jr., M.D., and Michael E. De Bakey, M.D.

While advances in arterial reconstructive surgery recently have progressed at a phenomenal rate, most diseases of the venous system continue partially or completely to elude surgical correction. Operative techniques employed successfully in the arterial system, where blood flow at high pressure is dependent upon cardiac action, have found little application in the venous system, where propulsion of blood at low pressure is brought about by the combined action of valves within the lumen and external muscular compression. Not only has replacement of venous valves been wholly unsuccessful, but grafts in the venous system rarely have remained patent. Even if early thrombosis is prevented by meticulous surgical technique and vigorous use of anticoagulants, most venous grafts are doomed to late fibrous tissue occlusion because of the low-pressure system involved. In a few diseases of the venous system, however, surgical therapy may be quite helpful and occasionally lifesaving.

Varicose Veins

Varicosities of the saphenous system may occur primarily or secondarily to involvement of the deep venous system. When varicose veins occur primarily and are associated with symptoms, surgical extirpation may prove quite helpful. When they develop secondarily to deep venous insufficiency, surgical therapy is far less applicable. However, judiciously applied operative intervention occasionally may be indicated even in this latter category of varicose veins, especially if associated with skin ulceration. Techniques of surgical therapy for varicose veins now have become rather standardized and are described in detail in most textbooks of surgery. In many instances, however, varicose veins can be controlled quite adequately by well-fitted elastic supports and avoidance of prolonged ambulation.

Thrombosis of the Deep Venous System

A precise knowledge of the causes and pathogenesis of deep venous thrombosis is lacking. Little has been added to Virchow's original hypothesis that damage to the vessel wall, increased coagulability of the blood, and stasis of the venous circulation are the basic mechanisms involved in venous thrombus formation. Predisposing factors in the development of venous thrombosis include congestive heart failure, trauma, immobility, surgical procedures, pregnancy, polycythemia, malignancy, and varicose veins.

Complications of deep venous thrombosis can be divided into those occurring acutely and those of the postphlebitic state. During the acute phase signs and symptoms may vary from almost total absence, phlebothrombosis, to the acute fulminating illness seen with phlegmasia cerulea dolens. In the former category dangers of pulmonary embolism always exist, whereas the massive reaction associated with iliofemoral thrombosis in the latter category may progress from loss of a portion of the extremity to death of the patient. With subsidence of the acute phase of deep venous thrombosis varying degrees of recannulization occur, but the patient frequently is left with chronic venous insufficiency and numerous postphlebitic sequelae.

Anticoagulant therapy has been used extensively in patients with deep venous thrombosis and in many instances probably has resulted in functional salvage of varying portions of the deep venous system. In recent years considerable interest has developed in direct surgical removal of the venous thrombus through single or multiple venotomies, particularly in the acutely ill patient with phlegmasia cerulea dolens. With increasing experience these techniques have been applied successfully to patients with lesser degrees of deep venous thrombosis in an effort to prevent development of chronic venous insufficiency.

Operative techniques employed are not dissimilar to those used for embolectomy in the arterial system. Venography often is quite helpful in determining the location and extent of venous thrombosis, thereby aiding in planning the surgical approach. The common femoral vein first is exposed through an incision in the groin, and in many instances complete extirpation of the thrombus is possible through this incision alone. When involvement is more extensive, such as in patients with phlegmasia cerulea dolens secondary to iliofemoral thrombosis, an abdominal incision also may be necessary in order to expose the inferior vena cava and allow complete removal of the thrombus while preventing possible pulmonary embolization (Fig. 60-1). During such procedures heparinization has been quite helpful in preventing recurrence of thrombosis, and many investigators advise continued anticoagulation for a period of days to

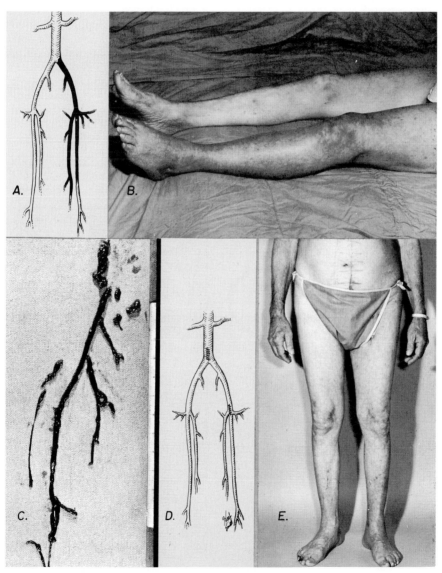

Fig. 60-1. Iliofemoral thrombectomy for phlegmasia cerulea dolens. *A.* Location and extent of iliofemoral thrombosis. *B.* Patient with left iliofemoral thrombosis demonstrating a swollen, cyanotic leg. *C.* Thrombi removed at operation. *D.* Completed operation with inferior vena cava and left common femoral venotomies repaired. *E.* Patient prior to discharge from the hospital demonstrating normal appearance of the left leg following iliofemoral thrombectomy.

weeks. Results of these procedures have been quite encouraging, and with the passage of time operative intervention probably will be employed in an increasing number of patients with deep venous thrombosis.

Pulmonary Embolism

Even less clearly understood than other diseases of the venous system, and often with far more devastating results, is pulmonary embolism. Although numerous historical and statistical reviews of venous thromboembolic phenomena have done much to increase recognition of these occurrences, few conditions in medicine have been subjected to so much analysis with so little elucidation. Not only is the cause unknown, the true incidence in doubt, and the diagnosis frequently questionable, but methods of treatment are highly arguable.

Most pulmonary emboli are small, and treatment is aimed toward prevention of further embolic episodes. The patient is put to bed with the legs wrapped and elevated, and most physicians place heavy reliance on anticoagulation therapy. When these measures are unsuccessful in preventing further pulmonary emboli, some form of venous ligation should be considered, either alone or in conjunction with anticoagulant therapy. Ligation of the superficial femoral veins for prevention of fatal pulmonary embolism has been used extensively; however, most surgeons now believe that ligation at this level is inadequate. Thrombus formation often has extended proximally beyond the femoral vessels, or emboli have originated in the pelvic or prostatic venous plexuses, and higher ligation is required.

When venous interruption is indicated in patients with pulmonary embolism, this should be done at the level of the inferior vena cava. Occurrence of venous insufficiency following inferior vena cava ligation varies greatly and depends to a great extent on the underlying disease rather than caval ligation per se. In an effort to avoid unfavorable sequelae of inferior vena cava ligation, several ingenious procedures have been devised to prevent

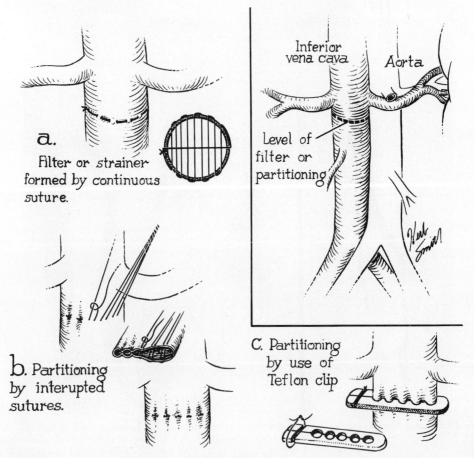

Fig. 60-2. Operative procedures designed to prevent passage of pulmonary emboli of significant size through inferior vena cava without complete interruption of blood flow.

fatal pulmonary embolism without permanent interruption of blood flow. These include insertion of a "filter" into the inferior vena cava using small vascular sutures (Fig. 60-2A), the use of suture techniques to partition the inferior vena cava into several channels large enough to allow flow of blood but small enough to prevent passage of pulmonary emboli of significant size (Fig. 60-2B), and the use of a serrated Teflon clip to accomplish similar partitioning (Fig. 60-2C). These modifications of vena cava ligation are relatively new, and additional experience is necessary to evaluate accurately whether or not these procedures are superior to ligation.

In some patients with pulmonary embolism the magnitude of obstruction to pulmonary arterial flow precludes long-term survival. Although death in such a patient occasionally is almost instantaneous, the majority live for varying periods of time following embolization. For these patients Trendelenburg advocated immediate embolectomy, but because of numerous technical difficulties this procedure never became popular. Development of the pump oxygenator for temporary cardiopulmonary bypass and widespread use of this technique provided a logical means of pulmonary embolectomy under more favorable circumstances, and success-

ful surgical treatment of acute massive pulmonary embolism using temporary cardiopulmonary bypass was reported from Baylor University College of Medicine in 1961. Subsequently, the feasibility and advantages of such a technique of pulmonary embolectomy have been demonstrated on numerous occasions.

Diagnosis of acute massive pulmonary embolism usually can be made on clinical grounds alone. Occasionally, pulmonary arteriography is helpful in a questionable case (Fig. 60-3A and B). The technique of pulmonary embolectomy employing temporary cardiopulmonary bypass is not complicated and is facilitated by immediate availability of cardiopulmonary bypass using plastic disposable oxygenators primed with 5 per cent dextrose in distilled water. General endotracheal anesthesia with only minimal amounts of depressant drugs should be used. A median sternotomy incision provides excellent exposure of the main pulmonary artery. Standard cannulations for total cardiopulmonary bypass are employed, and a longitudinal arteriotomy is made in the anterior wall of the main pulmonary artery. Both pleural spaces are entered, and the lungs are vigorously compressed toward the hilus until only liquid blood is obtained. During this maneuver, suction and

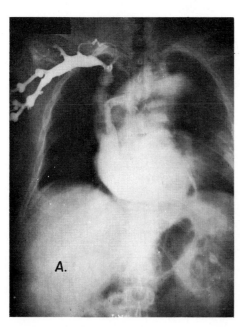
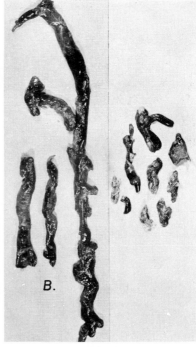

Fig. 60-3. Patient with acute massive pulmonary embolism. A. Pulmonary arteriogram prior to operation showing the right side of the heart distended, almost no opacification of pulmonary arterial tree, and minimal amounts of contrast material passing through the lesser circulation into aorta. B. Numerous thrombi removed at operation.

curved sponge forceps are used to extract emboli once they have been dislodged from the peripheral portions of the pulmonary arterial tree into the main pulmonary arteries (Fig. 60-4). On completion of embolectomy, the pulmonary arteriotomy is repaired, and cardiopulmonary bypass is discontinued once the patient's own cardiorespiratory system is able to maintain satisfactory function.

Increasing experience with pulmonary embolectomy using cardiopulmonary bypass has demonstrated clearly that many lives which would otherwise be lost may be salvaged by an aggressive surgical approach. Pulmonary embolectomy by this technique should be considered in the management of every patient with pulmonary embolism in order that it may be available for those who will require such a procedure for survival and in order that the indications for pulmonary embolectomy may be defined further. Additional improvements in the technical aspect of pulmonary embolectomy are foreseeable, and extensions of the procedure into

other areas of pulmonary embolism should be forthcoming.

SUGGESTED READING

Beall, A. C., Jr., and Cooley, D. A.: Surgical Treatment of Pulmonary Embolism, *Heart Bull.*, **13**:41–43, 1964.

Beall, A. C., Jr., and Fred, H. L.: Pulmonary Embolectomy Using Temporary Cardiopulmonary Bypass in a Patient with Previous Pulmonary Infarction, *Cardiovas. Res. Center Bull.*, **2**:15–22, 1963.

Beall, A. C., Jr., Fred, H. L., and Cooley, D. A.: Pulmonary Embolism, *Current Probl. Surg.*, **1**:1–47, 1964.

Cooley, D. A., and Beall, A. C., Jr.: A Technic of Pulmonary Embolectomy Using Temporary Cardiopulmonary Bypass, *J. Cardiovas. Surg.*, **2**:469–476, 1961.

Cooley, D. A., Beall, A. C., Jr., and Alexander, J. K.: Acute Massive Pulmonary Embolism: Successful

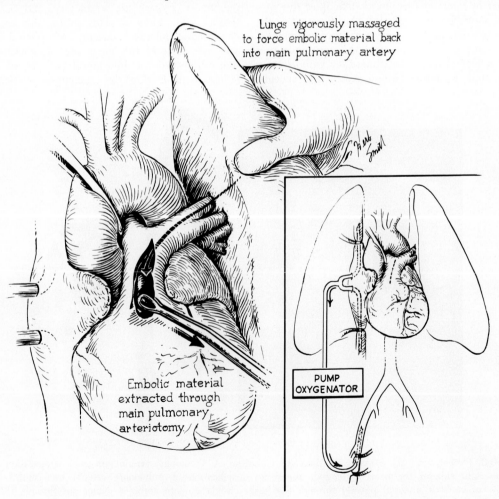

Lungs vigorously massaged to force embolic material back into main pulmonary artery

Embolic material extracted through main pulmonary arteriotomy

PUMP OXYGENATOR

Fig. 60-4. Technique of pulmonary embolectomy using a temporary cardiopulmonary bypass.

Surgical Treatment Using Temporary Cardiopulmonary Bypass, *J.A.M.A.,* **177**:283–286, 1961.

Cooley, D. A., Beall, A. C., Jr., and Grondin, P.: Open-heart Operations with Disposable Oxygenators, 5 Per Cent Dextrose Prime, and Normothermia, *Surgery,* **52**:713–719, 1962.

Cole, W. H., and Zollinger, R. M.: "Textbook of Surgery," 8th ed., Appleton-Century-Crofts, Inc., New York, 1963.

Collins, H. A., Burrus, G., and De Bakey, M. E.: Experimental Evaluation of Grafts in the Canine Inferior Vena Cava, *Am. J. Surg.,* **99**:40–44, 1960.

De Bakey, M. E.: A Critical Evaluation of the Problem of Thromboembolism, *Surg. Gynec. & Obst.,* **98**:1–27, 1954.

De Bakey, M. E., and Ochsner, A.: Phlegmasia Cerulea Dolens and Gangrene Associated with Thrombophlebitis, *Surgery,* **25**:16–29, 1949.

DeWeese, M. S., and Hunter, D. C., Jr.: A Vena Cava Filter for the Prevention of Pulmonary Embolism: A Five-year Clinical Experience, *Arch. Surg.,* **86**: 852–866, 1963.

Fogarty, T. J., Cranley, J. J., Krause, R. J., Strasser, E. S., and Hafner, C. D.: Surgical Management of Phlegmasia Cerulea Dolens, *Arch. Surg.,* **86**: 256–263, 1963.

Haller, J. A., Jr.: Thrombectomy for Acute Iliofemoral Venous Thrombosis, *Arch. Surg.,* **83**:448–453, 1961.

Haller, J. A., Jr.: Thrombectomy for Deep Thrombophlebitis of the Leg, *New England J. Med.,* **267**: 65–68, 1962.

Matas, R.: Postoperative Thrombosis and Pulmonary Embolism before and after Lister: A Retrospect and Prospect, *Univ. Toronto M. Bull.,* **10**:1–32, 1932.

Ochsner, A.: Indications for and Results of Inferior Vena Caval Ligation for Thromboembolic Disease, *Postgrad. Med.,* **27**:193–196, 1960.

Spencer, F. C., Quattlebaum, J. K., Quattlebaum, J. K., Jr., Sharp, E. H., and Jude, J. R.: Plication of the Inferior Vena Cava for Pulmonary Embolism: A Report of 20 Cases, *Ann. Surg.,* **155**:827–835, 1962.

Trendelenburg, F.: Ueber die operative Behandlung der Embolie der Lungerarterie, *Arch. klin. Chir.,* **86**: 686–700, 1908.

PART VII

Miscellaneous Problems Affecting the Cardiovascular System

Section A: Certain Medical Considerations

61 THE EFFECTS OF ENDO-CRINE DYSFUNCTION AND METABOLIC DISORDERS ON THE HEART

E. Garland Herndon, Jr., M.D., and Nanette Kass Wenger, M.D.

Virtually all hormones secreted by major endocrine glands have a direct or indirect effect on the cardiovascular system.

THE THYROID AND THE HEART

Thyrotoxicosis and the Heart

The occurrence of heart disease in thyrotoxicosis is well recognized, although the precise relationship between excessive amounts of thyroid hormone and thyrotoxic heart disease has not been defined. Parry, in 1825,[1] first described cardiac involvement in thyrotoxicosis consisting of palpitations, irregularity of the pulse, edema, and cardiac enlargement; more detailed descriptions by Graves[2] and others[3-5] were recorded in subsequent years. Some writers described thyrotoxic heart disease as a distinct entity,[6-8] whereas others[9-15] claimed that antecedent or concomitant primary heart disease was always present in thyrotoxic patients in whom heart disease developed. Schlesinger and Benchimol[16] stated that pure thyrotoxic heart disease did occur, although it was a relatively uncommon condition. There is a progressive increase in the incidence of cardiac involvement in thyrotoxicosis with increasing age,[8,12,17-19] in patients with and without underlying heart disease. Thyroid heart disease is unusual prior to the age of forty years.[6,20] The sex distribution is similar in thyrotoxic patients with and without cardiac complications.

Younger thyrotoxic patients more commonly present evidence of catecholamine excess: tachycardia, warm flushed skin due to vasodilatation and accelerated blood flow, moist palms, and elevation of systolic and lowering of diastolic blood pressure with resultant widening of the pulse pressure. The young thyrotoxic patient usually has exophthalmos and diffuse thyroid enlargement, with a bruit audible over the thyroid gland. In the older patient, clinical evidence of thyrotoxicosis is commonly more subtle: unexplained atrial fibrillation, particularly when unresponsive to digitalis; unexplained sinus tachycardia; congestive heart failure without other evidence of heart disease, often with a normal circulation time; congestive heart failure which responds poorly to therapy; thyrotoxic myopathy; unexplained weight loss; or episodes of alternating diarrhea and constipation. Furthermore, in the older age group, eye signs are less frequent, and the thyroid gland is not as significantly enlarged as in the young patient with classic Graves' disease.[21]

Older patients with thyrotoxicosis have an increased incidence of primary heart disease; thus the occurrence of true thyrotoxic heart disease in the absence of underlying anatomic changes in the coronary arteries, myocardium, or heart valves remains debatable. Thyrotoxicosis superimposed on primary heart disease may make the underlying disease clinically apparent; recognition and therapy of thyrotoxicosis will return the patient toward his previous cardiovascular status.

Effects of Thyroid Hormone

The widespread metabolic effects of thyroxin indicate that thyroxin probably stimulates a basic energy-producing reaction common to most tissues.[22a] There is a time lag following the administration of thyroxin before detectable changes occur, suggesting that thyroxin is not the active form of thyroid hormone. Thyroxin acts directly on the heart[23] and most other tissues to stimulate the metabolic rate and increase oxygen consumption; however, thyroxin depresses oxygen consumption in the anterior pituitary gland, probably due to depression of thyrotropin synthesis and release.[24]

The metabolic action of thyroxin, in vitro, is to effect an uncoupling of oxidative phosphorylation, causing wasteful heat production instead of formation of "high-energy" phosphate bonds;[25] this may explain the hypermetabolism of hyperthyroidism. However, other substances[26] which actively uncouple oxidative phosphorylation and cause increased oxygen consumption cannot reproduce most effects of thyroid hormone. Thyroid hormone causes mitochondrial swelling[27] related to alterations in mitochondrial oxidation-reduction and to high-energy phosphate (ATP) production.

The primary action of thyroid hormone is stimulation of oxygen consumption. The increased metabolism caused by thyroid hormone becomes apparent after a latent period of about 6 hr and is most marked in cardiac tissue. Triiodothyronine causes a more prompt, but briefer, elevation of basal metabolic rate. The thyroxin-deficient individual is hypersensitive to thyroxin in that his calorigenic response to a given dose of thyroxin exceeds that seen in the normal person; the thyrotoxic individual shows a subnormal response.[22a]

Both thyroxin and growth hormone seem necessary for normal growth and development. Thyroxin is probably not vital during the first 15 weeks of fetal development,[28] but thyroxin deficiency after this time causes cretinism. Thyroid hormone is required for the normal development of the anterior pituitary cells which produce growth hormone, and thyroxin enables growth hormone to produce its full effects. Thyroxin sensitizes cardiac muscle to the effects of growth hormone, possibly explaining the cardiac hypertrophy encountered in thyrotoxicosis.[29]

Thyroxin causes significant urinary loss of extracellular sodium and water in the myxedematous patient[30] and a similar but lesser effect in the euthyroid patient.

The increased glomerular filtration rate and increased renal plasma flow in thyrotoxicosis are secondary to the elevation of cardiac output; however, triiodothyronine apparently has a direct effect on the renal tubular capacity for PAH.[31] Large doses of thyroxin effect a water diuresis associated with potassium rather than sodium loss, suggesting an intracellular origin of water, probably related to protein catabolism. The potassium loss in hyperthyroidism can be accounted for by the loss of lean-tissue cell mass.[32] Triiodothyronine may regulate phosphorus loss[33] by the kidney. Another renal effect of thyroxin is significant calcium loss in the urine; markedly negative calcium balance may occur in the absence of a negative protein balance.[32]

Thyrotoxicosis induces a change from preponderant carbohydrate metabolism to preponderant fatty acid utilization. Normally glucose, lactate, pyruvate, etc., provide most of the energy for cardiac muscle, but no biochemical abnormality of energy liberation or conservation is evident in cardiac muscle in thyrotoxicosis;[34] the cardiac carbohydrate metabolism is apparently normal.[35] Thyroxin, however, inhibits enzymes which catalyze the anaerobic synthesis of high-energy phosphate compounds, causing cardiac metabolism to be aerobic and thus increasing cardiac oxygen consumption.[36]

Thyroxin excess impairs the conversion of creatine to creatinine,[37] impairs phosphocreatine formation, and produces creatinuria.[38,39] Phosphocreatine is the principal source of muscle energy, and its deficiency causes weakness and myopathy of variable severity; the myocardium may be affected by this myopathy.[22a] Thyroxin excess significantly reduces the tension developed by myocardial muscle bundles, probably reflecting phosphocreatine deficiency.[40]

The increased cutaneous circulation with decreased peripheral resistance in thyrotoxicosis functionally simulates an arteriovenous shunt and causes increased cardiac work. Arteriovenous shunting within the hyperactive goiter per se has been thought to contribute to the high-output cardiac failure; however, Fowler[41] considers the continuous murmur in the neck of thyrotoxic patients to be a cervical venous hum rather than a bruit originating in the gland itself.

The vascular effects of the pressor amines, epinephrine and norepinephrine,[42,43] are greatly enhanced by thyroxin. Excessive thyroxin secretion increases cardiac sensitivity to sympathetic stimulation and decreases its sensitivity to vagal stimulation, explaining in part the tachycardia of thyrotoxicosis.[44,45] Intravenous epinephrine causes a significantly greater increase in oxygen consumption, blood pressure, and heart rate in the thyrotoxic patient than in the normal individual.[46] Many epinephrine effects on the cardiovascular and nervous systems and on oxygen consumption are similar to the effects of thyroxin, although of much shorter duration; the similarity led to the use of sympathetic blocking agents in the treatment of thyrotoxic crisis.[22a] Thyroxin decreases epinephrine and norepinephrine degradation by inhibiting amine oxidase and/or other enzymes involved in catecholamine deactivation; epinephrine, however, cannot mimic thyroxin action in increasing oxygen consumption in thyroidectomized animals.

Histopathology of the Myocardium

Cardiac hypertrophy is uncommon in uncomplicated hyperthyroidism; it is frequently encountered in thyrotoxic patients with atrial fibrillation and congestive heart failure, and is almost invariably attributable to complicating heart disease or hypertension.[14]

There is a divergence of opinion regarding the histopathologic effects of thyrotoxicosis on the myocardium.[47] Experimental thyrotoxicosis in animals produces myofibril degeneration, myocardial edema, focal necrosis, cellular infiltration, and myocardial fibrosis.[48-50] Focal necrosis and interstitial myocarditis have been described [51,52] in fatal cases of thyrotoxicosis. At autopsy, patients with long-sustained, severe thyrotoxicosis have had swollen myofibers with indistinct striations and more advanced myocardial fat changes than nonthyrotoxic individuals of the same age.[9] Weller et al.[53] described increased myocardial fibrosis in thyrotoxicosis unrelated to vascular obliteration and associated with endocardial sclerosis and cellular infiltration.

The increased work demand on the heart has been thought to produce mild to moderate cardiac dilatation and hypertrophy and to render the heart more susceptible to secondary noxious influences.[54-56] Hurxthal[12] believed that a specific excitatory effect of thyroxin on the heart, rather than increased work from the circulatory demand, produced heart failure. Many studies demonstrated no relationship between atrial fibrillation or the duration of clinical hyperthyroidism and structural changes in the myocardium; congestive heart failure has been reported in thyrotoxic patients with apparently normal hearts at necropsy.[53,55,57,58] All evidence to date refutes a specific pathologic change in the myocardium associated with thyrotoxicosis. The thyrotoxic heart seems physiologically hyperactive, with an increased heart rate and increased oxygen consumption, but with no pathologic alteration; however, longstanding hyperthyroidism may cause moderate cardiac hypertrophy.[59] The cardiac phenomena of hyperthyroidism cannot be attributed to structural changes in the heart muscle, and metabolic and functional myocardial changes must be studied.[58]

Cardiovascular Pathophysiology

Excessive amounts of thyroxin may directly impair the function of cardiac muscle[40] by interfering with creatine-phosphocreatine metabolism.

Experimental evidence indicates that thyroxin acts directly on the heart muscle rather than on nerve elements,[60] possibly by some metabolic alteration,[36] to cause increased rate and force of contraction. However, neither the atrial fibrillation nor the congestive heart failure of clinical hyperthyroidism can be attributed to a direct cardiac effect of thyroxin.

The heart shares in the general tissue hypermetabolism, and its oxygen requirement is augmented;[61] the heart muscle glycogen depletion occurring in experimental hyperthyroidism[36,62] has been attributed to relative hypoxia.[63] Cardiac muscle glycogen depletion in thyrotoxicosis has been ascribed to increased physiologic cardiac activity and has been thought to render the heart susceptible to nonspecific injury.[55] However, neither cardiac failure nor cardiac arrhythmias appear related to the presence or absence of myocardial glycogen.[64] Cardiac catheterization studies in thyrotoxic patients[35,66-67] have demonstrated an increase in heart rate, in cardiac output, in the left ventricular work, in coronary blood flow, and in myocardial oxygen consumption. Coronary arteriolar dilatation in thyrotoxicosis is proportional to the tachycardia and the increased cardiac work. Increased coronary blood flow is due to a decrease in coronary vascular resistance and an increase in cardiac output; coronary vascular resistance increases after treatment of the thyrotoxicosis. Pulmonary vascular resistance remains unchanged, causing the pulmonary blood flow to increase with the increase in cardiac output; there is an associated increase in systolic pressure in the right ventricle and pulmonary artery,[68] attributable to the normal blood viscosity and the absence of pulmonary vasodilatation.[69] Myocardial hypermetabolism imposes an added burden on the increased cardiac output and cardiac work caused by the hypermetabolism of the body as a whole.[35] The increased cardiac work required to maintain the increased peripheral blood flow is necessitated both by the augmented tissue oxygen demand and by the augmented need for heat dissipation.[70]

The cardiac disturbances in hyperthyroidism have been attributed to excessive sympathetic stimulation, as thyroxin sensitizes the sympathetic nervous system to the action of epinephrine and norepinephrine.[43,44] The metabolic and hemodynamic effects of thyrotoxicosis can be abolished in animals by a total sympathetic block, indicating that the physiologic effects of thyrotoxicosis result from the combined action of thyroid hormone and epinephrine and norepinephrine.[71] McGee et al.[72] suggested that "apathetic hyperthyroidism" in the human being might be explained by a lack of sympathetic response. However, isolated sympathetic stimulation produces vasoconstriction, whereas cutaneous vasodilatation is characteristic of hyperthyroidism; and although epinephrine not uncommonly causes ventricular fibrillation, it rarely produces atrial fibrillation.

Excessive amounts of thyroxin elevate the basal metabolic rate and increase oxygen consumption. The increased tissue oxygen requirement is met by a 25 to 100 per cent increase in cardiac output, rather than by increased tissue oxygen utilization; the arteriovenous oxygen difference is diminished in hyperthyroidism.[73] Tachycardia[66,74] was, in the past, believed to account for the increased cardiac output in Graves' disease, as no significant stroke-volume alteration was demonstrated. However, more recent studies[75-77] have documented both tachycardia and an increase in stroke volume in thyrotoxicosis. The acute administration of *Rauwolfia* alkaloids in thyrotoxicosis unequivocally slows the pulse rate but does not decrease cardiac output; thus the increased stroke volume maintains the metabolic demands of hyperthyroidism, with a resultant marked increase in left ventricular stroke work. Significant increases in stroke volume are encountered primarily in those patients with a greatly augmented cardiac output.[68] Guanethidine has been shown[77a] to effect a reduction in left ventricular work and pressure time; it may thus prove an effective adjunct in the management of the thyrotoxic patient with severe congestive heart failure.

The thyrotoxic tachycardia alone is not of sufficient severity to produce congestive heart failure in the normal heart. The cardiac output and oxygen consumption during exercise were shown to increase to a greater extent in the hyperthyroid than in the normal individual,[78] with a greater increase in stroke volume, pulmonary artery pressure, and right ventricular work also observed in the thyrotoxic patient.[75] This increased cardiac output, associated with tachycardia, may adversely affect patients with underlying coronary atherosclerosis, valvular disease, or idiopathic myocarditis.[70,79]

The increased cardiac output has been attributed to increased venous return. The increase in heat production and increase in tissue metabolites due to the elevated metabolic rate in thyrotoxicosis produce peripheral vasodilatation and arteriovenous shunting. This peripheral vasodilatation with decreased peripheral resistance results in increased peripheral blood flow and increased venous return to the heart.[80] The increased peripheral blood flow in hyperthyroidism is obtained both by shunting of blood from the interior of the body and by an actual increase in blood volume.[56] The increase in blood volume correlates well with the increase in cardiac output.[77] There also occurs a significant increase in the total red-cell mass, presumably in response to increased oxygen demand.[81] The 30 to 70 per cent acceleration of circulatory velocity parallels the elevation of the basal metabolic rate and results in a diminished circulation time.[82,83]

The increased cardiac output[84] is due primarily to the increased velocity of blood flow. The rate and depth of respiration are also increased, aiding the venous return of blood to the heart.[74]

Williams[22a] reported thiamine deficiency in 75 per cent of unselected patients with thyrotoxicosis; the role of thiamine deficiency in the congestive heart failure of thyrotoxicosis remains speculative.

Adequate oxygenation of the heart muscle is critical in hyperthyroidism, both because of the increased metabolic demands of the heart and because of the increased cardiac work in the hypermetabolic patient. Therefore, associated diminution of oxygen supply due to coronary sclerosis and increased myocardial oxygen requirement due to ventricular hypertrophy predispose the thyrotoxic patient to cardiac failure. Some underlying pathologic cardiac condition seems requisite in the majority of patients in whom congestive heart failure develops as a complication of thyrotoxicosis.

Clinical Cardiac Manifestations

Cardiac and circulatory alterations occur in thyrotoxicosis in the absence of heart disease. There is evidence of cardiac hyperactivity and peripheral vasodilatation: sinus tachycardia is present at rest; the pulse pressure is increased, with full and bounding arterial pulsations mimicking the water-hammer pulse of aortic insufficiency; there are prominent carotid artery pulsations; the cardiac apex impulse is brisk and slapping; S-1 is loud and snapping; and systolic murmurs at the apex and in the pulmonic area may result from accelerated blood flow and pulmonary artery dilatation. Left sternal border "scratch" and/or pericardial rub have been described, possibly related to pulmonary conus dilatation and increased blood flow.[85,86]

The cardiovascular complications of thyrotoxicosis are primarily those of atrial fibrillation, cardiac enlargement, and congestive heart failure; angina pectoris and disorders of rhythm are also encountered. The possibility of occult thyrotoxicosis should be investigated in any patient with atrial fibrillation or congestive heart failure unresponsive to the usual therapy.[87,88]

The younger the patient, the more classic the hyperthyroidism is apt to be, particularly in the female. Palpitation is extremely common and is usually due to the increased rate and strength of cardiac contraction rather than to arrhythmia. Exertional dyspnea is reported even in the absence of pulmonary congestion; the most likely explanations for the exertional dyspnea are thyrotoxic myopathy involving the chest wall muscles[89] and increased pulmonary blood flow.[82] Increased sweating,[90] increased appetite, hyperkineticism, emotional lability, weight loss, and myopathy occur more regularly in the younger age group.

In the older patient, the clinical manifestations may be more subtle, often presenting predominantly the cardiac signs of atrial fibrillation, unexplained tachycardia, or congestive heart failure. Palpitations and dyspnea are frequently the presenting complaints. Angina pectoris occurs commonly[8,91,92] and has been ascribed to the increased work demanded of a heart with underlying coronary sclerosis or other disease.[93] Somerville and Levine[91] found no correlation between the severity of the angina pectoris and the severity of the thyrotoxicosis. Decreased coronary perfusion, due both to the lowered diastolic blood pressure and to the decreased diastolic duration which occur with tachycardia, probably contributes to the occurrence of angina pectoris. Myocardial infarction is unusual in active thyrotoxicosis[94,95] but has occurred after remission of the thyrotoxicosis; it may be related to elevation of the serum lipid levels. The rarity of myocardial infarction may reflect the decrease in calories available for storage as fat or may be attributed to a hypolipemic effect of thyroid hormone. However, Burstein et al.[96] have challenged the apparent nonsusceptibility of thyrotoxic patients to myocardial infarction.

The older patient may also report profound muscle weakness, unexplained weight loss, anorexia, alternating constipation and diarrhea, peripheral neuropathy, depression, or dementia. On careful examination the patient is often noted to be unusually alert and hyperactive; there is tachycardia and a widened pulse pressure; the skin is warm and moist; a slight stare is usual; and the thyroid gland may be slightly enlarged.

The progressive increase in *incidence of thyrotoxic heart disease* with advance in age is well recognized, and several studies indicate that neither the duration nor the severity of the thyrotoxicosis appears significant in the production of thyrocardiac disease.[6,20,79] However, Griswold and Keating[8] suggested that the duration of the thyrotoxicosis and the age and sex of the patient were all determinants of cardiac complications; they found that thyrocardiac patients tended to be older, that men were more likely to become thyrocardiac patients, and that the longer the hyperthyroidism proceeded unchecked, the more probable was the development of cardiac signs and symptoms. The pathologic state of the thyroid gland, adenomatous or diffuse, cannot be correlated with the development of cardiac manifestations.[8] Diffuse thyroid enlargement predominates in the younger patients without heart disease, but nodular goiter is not specifically associated with cardiac complications.

The *resting heart rate* in thyrotoxicosis varies from 90 to 125 beats per minute and may increase with exercise and excitement.[36] Assessment of the sleeping pulse is important in clinically confirming the diagnosis of thyrotoxicosis and in following the patient after therapy has been instituted, as there is little reduction in the heart rate in thyrotoxicosis with sleep. Particularly in the older thyrotoxic patient, the minimum sleeping pulse rate averages 30 beats per minute higher than that of the normal individual (89 versus 53 to 58 per minute).[97] A sleeping pulse rate of over 80 beats per minute makes the diagnosis of thyrotoxicosis highly probable, but no consistent correlation exists between the sleeping pulse rate and the severity of the thyrotoxicosis.[98] The pulse is bounding, as a result of increased cardiac output and peripheral vasodilatation.

Most patients with thyrotoxicosis have normal sinus rhythm with a rapid heart rate.[99,100] Atrial fibrillation is the only characteristic rhythm disturbance; however, atrial flutter, nodal tachycardia, atrial tachycardia, and premature contractions have been described.

Atrial fibrillation is common in patients with thyrotoxicosis and its incidence increases progressively with increase in age.[6] Ernstene[101] described atrial fibrillation as more common in patients over age forty-five, occurring somewhat more frequently with increased duration of the thyrotoxicosis, and more often encountered with adenomatous than diffuse goiter. Atrial fibrillation in thyrotoxicosis was invariably reported [13] with coexistent organic heart disease and seemed the most important factor in the production of congestive heart failure.[101] Thyrotoxic atrial fibrillation is more likely to be transient or paroxysmal than atrial fibrillation due to other causes.[102] The occurrence of atrial fibrillation has been attributed to increased excitability of the atrial musculature and possibly to its increased sensitivity to epinephrine and other vasopressor substances. Atrial fibrillation adds to the burden of the heart[8] and favors the development of congestive heart failure; in all age groups, the incidence of congestive heart failure is greater in patients with atrial fibrillation. Reversion of the atrial fibrillation occurs spontaneously in over half of the patients following correction of the thyrotoxicosis[102] and greatly improves the prognosis of congestive heart failure.

The incidence of atrial fibrillation is most prominently influenced by the presence of underlying cardiac disease;[12,101] the degree of basal metabolic rate elevation appears to have no effect.[101] Griswold and Keating[8] reported that neither the severity of the hyperthyroidism nor the type of goiter predictably disposes to the development of atrial fibrillation, which occurs predominantly in the older age group. Ten to twenty per cent of all hyperthyroid patients have transient atrial fibrillation before or after surgical treatment,[12,101] with permanent atrial fibrillation reported with even greater frequency.[101]

A 30 to 50 per cent incidence of *cardiac enlargement* or hypertrophy has been reported in thyrotoxicosis. The most pronounced cardiac enlargement is associated with congestive heart failure, usually with atrial fibrillation or underlying heart disease.[14] It occurs most frequently in the older patient.

The systolic *blood pressure* in thyrotoxicosis[99] is slightly to moderately elevated, and the diastolic blood pressure is normal or slightly lowered, with a resultant increase in the pulse pressure. These changes are physiologic responses to thyrotoxicosis and return to normal with normalization of the basal metabolic rate. The diagnosis of thyrotoxicosis should be entertained in cases of unexplained systolic hypertension,[103] as hyperthyroidism appears to precipitate or exaggerate labile essential hypertension. The systolic and mean blood pressure elevations occur in the periphery, the right ventricle, and the pulmonary artery;[104] the elevated pulmonary blood flow is associated with a normal pulmonary vascular resistance, so the cause of the pressure increase is unknown[104] but may be due to pulmonary vascular engorgement.

The average age of development of congestive heart failure in thyrotoxicosis is over fifty years, so that both age and coexistent cardiovascular changes are significant in the production of congestive heart failure.[12] The increased circulatory load of thyrotoxicosis causes congestive heart failure when myocardial function is reduced by heart disease of other causes, when thyrotoxicosis transiently causes inadequate myocardial function, or when the excessive circulatory load apparently overcomes the reserve capacity of an otherwise normal heart.[70]

A clue suggestive of hyperthyroidism is congestive heart failure with a normal or rapid circulation time.[83] The venous pressure usually remains normal[82] until severe congestive heart failure develops. The increased cardiac output of thyrotoxicosis decreases somewhat with the onset of congestive heart failure but often remains above normal levels.[75,67]

Likoff and Levine[7] believed that thyrotoxicosis was not infrequently the sole cause of congestive heart failure; this congestive heart failure was more common in the female, with increase in age, with longer duration of the thyrotoxicosis, and with

associated atrial fibrillation. They described 21 thyrotoxic patients without primary heart disease who developed congestive heart failure; there was no recurrence of heart failure after thyroidectomy, which suggests that the prognosis of congestive heart failure in thyrotoxicosis is favorable after therapy. Lahey[11] reviewed 303 thyrotoxic patients with cardiac involvement, 216 of whom had congestive heart failure; only 1.5 per cent had significant symptomatic heart disease 5 years after thyroidectomy. Andrus[62] described congestive heart failure in 18.5 per cent of patients with hyperthyroidism, particularly related to increased symptom duration, increased age of the patient, and associated heart disease.

Sandler and Wilson[79] reported that over 50 per cent of the thyrocardiac patients treated with radioactive iodine were free of congestive heart failure after therapy; the prognosis for the congestive heart failure was more favorable if regular sinus rhythm was restored, but congestive heart failure tended to adversely affect the reversion rate of the atrial fibrillation.

It is not difficult to diagnose cardiac disease in thyrotoxicosis when the patient presents a classic picture of hyperthyroidism and there is confirmatory evidence of an elevated radioactive iodine uptake and elevated serum-protein-bound iodine level. The diagnostic problems are cases with predominant cardiac manifestations and subtle signs of thyrotoxicosis[72] (Fig. 61-1). Correct diagnosis will be made in these latter cases only if the diagnosis of hyperthyroidism is considered in all patients with

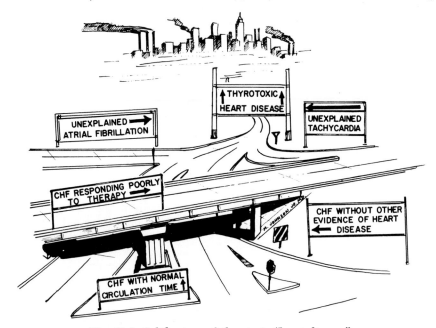

Fig. 61-1. Subtle signs of thyrotoxic "heart disease."

unexplained sinus tachycardia or atrial fibrillation, cardiac enlargement or congestive heart failure of obscure cause, digitalis toxicity prior to cardiac compensation and slowing of the heart rate, and dissociation between the apparent clinical well-being of the patient and the severity of the congestive heart failure.[105] Once the diagnosis of thyrotoxicosis is considered, many clinical manifestations compatible with thyrotoxicosis are often noted in the "masked," or "apathetic," hyperthyroid patient.

Laboratory Diagnosis of Thyrotoxicosis

The laboratory investigation of hyperthyroidism often shows slight anemia and leukopenia with a relative lymphocytosis; the total serum-cholesterol level is normal or somewhat depressed, and creatinuria is common. The basal metabolism rate is elevated, the serum-protein-bound iodine level usually exceeds 8 μg per 100 ml, and the radioactive iodine uptake is usually in excess of 45 per cent in 24 hr. If the results of these latter studies are equivocal, the butanol-extractable iodine, resin-sponge test (T_3), and/or red-cell uptake should be determined.

Radiologic Findings in Thyrotoxic Heart Disease

The usual radiologic appearance of the thyrotoxic heart in the absence of atrial fibrillation, congestive heart failure, or primary heart disease is not grossly abnormal. Dilatation and increased pulsation of the pulmonary artery have been attributed to the hemodynamic effects of an arteriovenous shunt, causing enlargement of the right ventricular outflow tract and pulmonary artery dilatation.[106]

Cardiac fluoroscopy reveals increased activity of cardiac contraction and prominence and increased pulsation of the pulmonary artery.[107] The prominent pulmonary artery in thyrotoxicosis may straighten the left cardiac silhouette, mimicking mitral stenosis, but there is no left atrial enlargement in thyrotoxicosis in the absence of significant congestive heart failure. The pulmonary artery abnormalities regress following control of the hyperthyroidism.

However, moderate generalized cardiac enlargement has also been described in uncomplicated thyrotoxicosis,[107] and its incidence seems unrelated to age. Evans[108] described prominence of the pulmonary artery, left ventricle, and right atrium, giving a "hamlike" configuration to the heart in the posteroanterior projection. Cardiac enlargement demonstrable by x-ray examination rarely regresses to normal following subsidence of the thyrotoxicosis This contrasts with the electocardiographic evidence of left ventricular hypertrophy, which, in the absence of radiographic evidence of left ventricular hypertrophy, usually reverts to normal following therapy for hyperthyroidism.[91]

When congestive heart failure supervenes, the cardiac silhouette assumes a globular appearance. The lung fields are often remarkably clear despite clinical evidence of congestive heart failure, probably related to rapid pulmonary blood flow and rapid circulation time.

Electrocardiographic Findings

There are no distinctive electrocardiographic features of thyrotoxicosis. Both sinus tachycardia and atrial fibrillation, paroxysmal or fixed, are common. P-R interval prolongation has been described,[109,110] and shortening of the Q-T interval was noted.[111] High voltage P and T waves have been ascribed to increased sympathetic tone. Increased QRS complex duration, changes of left ventricular hypertrophy, and other electrocardiographic abnormalities have been reported to disappear after therapy for thyrotoxicosis.[91,112] The majority of electrocardiographic abnormalities are probably associated with underlying coronary atherosclerosis, myocardial disease, or valvular heart disease rather than specifically related to the thyrotoxicosis.

Treatment of Thyrotoxic Heart Disease

The initial object of therapy in the patient with heart disease and thyrotoxicosis is control of the hypermetabolism. The patient with severe congestive heart failure or rapid atrial fibrillation who does not respond to digitalization, diuretic therapy, sodium restriction, and bed rest should be treated with appropriate antithyroid drugs, such as propylthiouracil or methimazole (Tapazole). The rapid ventricular rate of thyrotoxic atrial fibrillation may be resistant to therapy with the usual dose of digitalis until the hypermetabolism is corrected. Braunwald et al.[112a] have shown that larger doses of digitalis are required to slow the ventricular rate in atrial fibrillation in the hyperthyroid patient than in the euthyroid patient. As the onset of action of propylthiouracil and methimazole is delayed from 5 to 7 days, the addition of iodide therapy may be necessary in the severely ill thyrocardiac patient.

Therapy for the severely ill thyrocardiac patient should include methimazole, 10 to 15 mg every 6 hr; 5 drops of a saturated solution of potassium iodide every 6 hr; and reserpine, 0.25 mg every 12 hr. Beneficial effects of iodide therapy become evident during the first 24 hr, whereas reserpine action is cumulative and does not become clinically apparent for 48 to 72 hr. Reserpine decreases vascular responsiveness to catecholamines as evidenced by slowing of the pulse, decrease in systolic blood pressure, and narrowing of the pulse pressure.

Methimazole prevents synthesis of thyroid hormone by the thyroid gland; hormone depletion in the thyroid gland is followed by a decrease in circulating thyroid hormone with a resultant decrease in oxygen consumption and improvement of the cardiac status. Maximum control of congestive heart failure and/or atrial fibrillation with the above regimen occurs in 3 to 6 weeks; decision regarding definitive therapy for the hyperthyroidism can then be made.

Three alternatives for definitive therapy of thyrotoxicosis[113] include (1) cessation of iodide and reserpine therapy and the chronic administration of methimazole or another antithyroid drug; (2) cessation of iodide and reserpine therapy, continuation of methimazole for 2 or 3 weeks more, followed by therapy with radioactive iodine; and (3) continuation of iodide and methimazole therapy, cessation of reserpine therapy, and planning for thyroidectomy after 2 to 3 weeks or longer.

The simplest and most effective therapy in the thyrocardiac patient is medical control of the thyrotoxicosis and congestive heart failure followed by radioactive iodine therapy. Often the elderly patients have a normal or small-sized thyroid gland, which may render surgical treatment technically difficult. However, prior to the advent of radioactive iodine therapy, even patients with significant cardiac decompensation tolerated thyroidectomy relatively well; this was because, postoperatively, the metabolic load on the heart was decreased, and sinus rhythm was often restored.[11] In the majority of thyrocardiac patients, it is unnecessary to add iodide to methimazole and reserpine therapy to control the thyrotoxicosis. Iodide omission is advantageous when radioactive iodine therapy is planned, as the thyroid gland will not have become saturated with iodine.

The hyperthyroid thyroid gland is hyperplastic and thus has a greater avidity for radioactive iodine than does the normal thyroid gland. The usual hyperplastic thyroid gland weighs 35 to 45 Gm; 3.5 to 4.5 mc radioactive iodine (I^{131}) delivered to the gland will render the patient euthyroid. Ten to twelve millicuries of radioactive iodine (I^{131}) is often required for control of the thyrotoxicosis in a thyroid gland weighing over 70 Gm. However, the thyroid gland much larger than 70 Gm often presents obstructive symptoms; surgical intervention, with appropriate preoperative preparation, is then the recommended management.

Radiation thyroiditis following I^{131} therapy may, on rare occasions, increase the level of circulating thyroid hormone and temporarily increase the incidence and severity of angina pectoris.[36] The complete response to radioactive iodine therapy may be delayed from 2 to 4 months, and this may present a problem in the acutely ill thyrocardiac patient.[114] The response to radioactive iodine therapy can be documented by a progressive decrease in the serum-protein-bound iodine level.

After control of the thyrotoxicosis and improvement of congestive heart failure, direct current reversion of atrial fibrillation to regular sinus rhythm should be planned, if it has not occurred spontaneously. The direct current reversion of atrial fibrillation to normal sinus rhythm prior to therapy for thyrotoxicosis is possible, but recurrence of atrial fibrillation is frequent; greater permanent regularization of rhythm occurs after control of the thyrotoxicosis. Quinidine should be administered preparatory to direct current defibrillation and should be continued for several weeks after the reestablishment of normal sinus rhythm.

With lowering of the basal metabolic rate, the velocity of blood flow is slowed.[82] There is a return to normal of the cardiac output, cardiac work, coronary blood flow, and myocardial oxygen consumption, and an increase in coronary vascular resistance.[66] The pulmonary artery and right ventricular systolic pressures concomitantly decrease.[68] Almost complete relief of angina pectoris and uncomplicated atrial fibrillation has been reported following control of thyrotoxicosis.[93,115]

Myxedema and the Heart

Since Zondek's description in 1918 [116] of the clinical cardiac features of myxedema—cardiac chamber dilatation, electrocardiographic abnormalities, and changes in the blood pressure and pulse pressure—it has been debated whether or not myxedema causes heart failure. Although about three-fourths of untreated patients with myxedema manifest cardiac enlargement, poor myocardial contractility, electrocardiographic abnormalities, and other evidences of cardiac dysfunction, all of which are usually reversible with thyroid hormone therapy,[117,118] no specific pathologic myocardial lesion has been delineated in myxedema. Myxedema appears to predispose to coronary atherosclerosis,[119] which may be asymptomatic until thyroid replacement therapy is initiated; the resultant increase in metabolism may cause relative coronary insufficiency to become apparent.[120,121] The occurrence of pericardial effusion has been emphasized,[122,123] but myxedema is not generally thought to cause congestive heart failure; however, heart failure has been considered a complication of long-standing myxedema.[124] Conversely, it is recognized that patients with intractable cardiac failure may improve if made mildly myxedematous,[125] as cardiac work is decreased both at rest and with exercise in hypothyroidism; however, the value of thyroidectomy in the control of congestive heart failure has been questioned.[126]

Effects of Lack of Thyroid Hormone

Most bodily activities and functions are slowed in myxedema, and the reduction in basal metabolic rate is associated with a diminution in tissue oxygen consumption. Diminution of myocardial oxygen consumption has been demonstrated in animals.[23] The myocardial sensitivity to epinephrine and norepinephrine is diminished in hypothyroidism,[42,44] accounting for the bradycardia and rarity of arrhythmias.

Histopathology of the Myocardium

Available pathologic data do not delineate a specific histologic myocardial lesion associated with myxedema. Swollen myofibers and increased interstitial fluid with an excessive mucin content are encountered in a dilated, pale, and flabby heart. The homogeneous mucoid myocardial infiltrate in cases of untreated myxedema is a histochemically distinct mucoprotein from the myxedematous skin and tongue infiltrate.[127] Myocardial necrosis, hydropic muscle degeneration, and fibrosis have also been described.[128–130]

Higgins[131] asserted that heart disease in myxedema was a distinct clinical and pathologic entity. He described a mucoid myocardial infiltrate in the early stages of the disease which was reversible with thyroid therapy. Later in the disease, he described myocardial degenerative changes, cardiac enlargement and fibrosis, and coronary sclerosis, which were usually not reversible.

Pathologic and clinical evidence of atherosclerosis are frequent concomitants of myxedema,[128,131] but there is only suggestive evidence that the hypercholesterolemia and lipid abnormalities of myxedema predispose the female to premature advanced coronary atherosclerosis or increase the incidence of coronary artery disease in the male.[132,133]

Myxedematous pericardial effusion is common and is primarily responsible for the enlargement of the cardiac silhouette seen in myxedema;[134–136] the pericardial effusion is attributable to increased capillary permeability.[121,122,137] True cardiac dilatation and hypertrophy have been reported but probably occurred secondary to underlying heart disease.

Cardiovascular Pathophysiology

The *diminished cardiac output* in myxedema is compatible with the absence of congestive heart failure as long as it parallels the reduced oxygen consumption of the body.[35] This decrease in cardiac output in the presence of a normal or slightly increased arterial pressure indicates a generalized increase of vascular resistance.[138] The reduced cardiac output in myxedema is an adjustment to the increase in peripheral resistance and reflects decreased venous return secondary to diminished peripheral blood flow.[67,84]

The *diminished peripheral blood flow* in myxedema[139] reflects a reduction in metabolism, diminished vasodilating metabolite production, and decreased heat production. In general, the circulatory changes parallel the reduction of oxygen consumption.[140] The peripheral vasoconstriction, coupled with the decreased cardiac output, produces the cool, dry skin of myxedema.[80] These circulatory disturbances are compensatory mechanisms to adjust to reduced tissue oxygen requirements and maintain a stable body temperature despite diminished heat production.

Bradycardia is common in severe myxedema. It may be due to diminished venous return or may represent a change in sensitivity of the adrenergic and cholinergic cardiac effectors to their respective neurotransmitters.[44] The degree of bradycardia parallels the decrease in basal metabolic rate and peripheral blood flow.[139] By administering atropine to hypothyroid dogs, Scott et al. demonstrated that the capacity to increase heart rate was unimpaired.[141] The decreased cardiac output is due both to bradycardia and to diminished stroke output. The association of bradycardia and low stroke output is unusual, as slowing of the heart rate is usually accompanied by greater ventricular filling and increased cardiac output per beat.

Cardiac catheterization[67,140,142] of myxedematous patients has documented a normal increase in cardiac output during exercise, without an increase in intracardiac pressures or pulmonary resistance. This is evidence that cardiac failure is not present. Normal intracardiac pressures were documented even in the presence of cardiac enlargement and electrocardiographic abnormalities.[35]

The *circulatory slowing* in myxedema with prolongation of the circulation time[143] is related to the reduction of basal metabolism, the diminished oxygen consumption, the decreased cardiac output, and the slowing of peripheral blood flow.[140,144] The venous pressure is usually normal, and there is a diminution of circulating blood volume and circulating erythrocyte mass, proportional to the severity of the hypometabolism;[81,145,146] this occurs despite an increase in total body water and extracellular fluid.

The *arterial blood pressure* in myxedema is usually normal; the mean arterial blood pressure may be slightly increased, but the pulse pressure is below normal. The occasional hypertension, particularly of the diastolic type, described in myxedema returns toward normal following administration of thyroid extract; this suggests a relationship between myxedema and hypertension, the mechanism of which is not understood.[135,147,148]

The arteriovenous oxygen difference is greater than normal in myxedema, reflecting greater oxygen utilization by the tissues.[144] However, Bakker et al.[149] reported apparent glycolysis in cardiac muscle with normal myocardial oxygen consumption in a patient with hypothyroidism. The heart in myxedema appears more efficient than normal, as the diminution of cardiac work is greater than the decrease in oxygen consumption; cardiac reserve is apparently adequate in that cardiovascular function can return to normal following therapy with thyroid hormone.[150a]

Clinical Cardiac Manifestations

Clinical changes occur slowly in myxedema; the manifestations are often quite subtle, and the diagnosis may be missed for several years. The average interval between onset of symptoms and diagnostic recognition is 6 years.[151] Myxedema affects women predominantly, usually following Hashimoto's struma; it must be differentiated from hypopituitarism causing secondary thyroid failure.

Patients with myxedema have weakness; dry, coarse, cool skin; decreased sweating; cold intolerance; slow, awkward movements; pallor; and a lemon-yellow tint to the skin. Lethargy, slowness and hoarseness of speech, weight gain, constipation, slow cerebration, and personality changes are common. There may be precordial pain, eyelid and facial edema, thickness of the tongue, loss of hair, peripheral neuropathy, and slowness of deep-tendon-reflex relaxation.

Cardiac symptoms are rare, and there is considerable doubt that congestive heart failure occurs in myxedema in the absence of underlying heart disease; exertional dyspnea, unusual fatigue, orthopnea, and angina pectoris have been reported. It is difficult to differentiate the changes of congestive heart failure in advanced myxedema from the changes of myxedema per se. The combination of facial and peripheral edema; pericardial, pleural, and peritoneal effusion; weight gain; dyspnea; palpitation; cardiac enlargement with weak and distant heart sounds; sluggish cardiac action; and an abnormal venous pulse curve[119] may *simulate congestive heart failure.*[108,152]

The origin of the *peripheral edema* and serous effusions in myxedema is probably increased capillary permeability, as confirmed by the high protein content of the effusions;[153,154] the edema and serous effusions of true congestive heart failure are associated with little or no change in capillary permea-

bility. Hypoproteinemia occasionally occurs in myxedema but is less common than in advanced congestive heart failure with generalized anasarca. The venous pressure is usually normal and the blood pressure diminished in myxedema, whereas in congestive heart failure both the venous pressure and the blood volume are significantly increased.[134,145] The pulmonary artery and right ventricular pressures are normal in myxedema, and the cardiac output increases in response to exercise without an increase in pulmonary artery or systemic venous pressure; this is not seen in congestive heart failure.[150a] At fluoroscopic examination, there is no evidence of pulmonary congestion in myxedematous patients with cardiac enlargement and serous effusions, while pulmonary congestion is characteristic of congestive heart failure. The peripheral edema and serous effusions in myxedema do not respond to digitalis and diuretic therapy as do these manifestations in congestive heart failure; replacement of thyroid hormone may be necessary for regression of the myxedematous edema and effusions.[155]

The Valsalva maneuver permits differentiation of true cardiac failure from its simulators.[156] This distinction is of importance in the management of myxedematous patients with clinical features suggesting cardiac failure, as patients with myxedema and true congestive heart failure usually have primary cardiac disease; the heart failure may increase with elevation of the metabolic rate after thyroid hormone treatment. A Valsalva maneuver was performed by patients with long-standing unequivocal myxedema, some of whom had cardiac enlargement, edema, and elevation of the venous pressure; the stroke output fell as the filling pressure was reduced, indicating the absence of congestive heart failure; there was no detectable paradox in the arterial tracing. All evidence of cardiac abnormality subsided after thyroid therapy. In the one patient who demonstrated the heart failure response to the Valsalva maneuver, thyroid hormone therapy caused deterioration and death from cardiac failure, indicative of underlying heart disease aggravated by the increase in metabolic rate.

There is generalized *cardiac enlargement* in most cases of advanced myxedema,[136] primarily due to pericardial effusion; significant and often massive pericardial effusions have been demonstrated during life and at autopsy, even in the absence of congestive heart failure.[122,157,158] The slight increase of right atrial and pulmonary artery pressure, associated with a diastolic dip in the right ventricular pressure tracing of myxedematous patients, implicates pericardial effusion rather than cardiac dilatation as the cause of the cardiac enlargement.[142] Kern et al.[134] described pericardial effusion as a constant early major cardiac finding in myxedema and believed it accounted for most electrocardiographic and radiologic abnormalities in myxedema. Pulsus paradoxus and evidence of cardiac tamponade are generally absent, because the pericardial fluid accumulates slowly, allowing the pericardial sac to be distended without significantly increasing the intrapericardial pressure.[159] The bradycardia probably prevents some degree of cardiac dysfunction from the pericardial effusion. The pulse is slow and weak, reflecting a diminution of cardiac output, the heart sounds are feeble, and the precordium is quiet with a barely perceptible apical impulse.

However, cardiac dilatation and hypertrophy and myxedematous myocardial changes may contribute to the cardiac enlargement. Cardiac dilatation may affect the atrioventricular valves, producing the murmurs of relative mitral insufficiency and tricuspid insuffiicency. Indeed, some studies emphasize the infrequency of pericardial effusion and suggest that cardiac chamber dilatation is primarily responsible for the globular shape of the heart.[160,161]

The regression of cardiac enlargement soon after the institution of therapy with thyroid hormone and its reappearance with cessation of hormone therapy suggest a direct relationship between thyroid hormone and the myocardium.[124]

An increased incidence of *angina pectoris and coronary thrombosis*[162] has been reported in patients with myxedema, presumably related to the hypercholesterolemia, although some contradictory studies are worthy of note;[163,164] atherosclerosis has been noted prominently in those cases of myxedema which are complicated by hypertension and cardiac hypertrophy.[165] Nikkilä and Karlsson[166] found no difference in thyroid status between a "coronary" and "noncoronary" group of patients, but in patients with myxedema, coronary artery disease was reported as frequently in the female as in the male.[36] Since myxedema is characteristically a disease of females and angina pectoris and coronary thrombosis are encountered predominantly in males, the occurrence of coronary artery disease in myxedema is unexpected. However, the lipid patterns differ in coronary artery disease and in hypothyroidism; the serum cholesterol is markedly elevated in hypothyroidism, with relatively normal triglyceride levels, whereas in coronary artery disease abnormal elevation of triglycerides occurs more commonly than increase in cholesterol.[150b]

Degeneration and rupture of the aorta have been reported in induced myxedema for therapy of hypertension; it is not known whether the precipitating factor was the hypothyroidism, the hypertension, or both.[167]

Laboratory Diagnosis of Myxedema

Most cases of myxedema do not present a problem in diagnosis; the most frequent error is not suspecting the disease, particularly in an elderly patient.

There may be slight anemia and occasionally slight leukopenia; the sedimentation rate may be elevated. The basal metabolic rate is low, usually between −30 and −40. In primary myxedema, the total cholesterol, cholesterol esters, and plasma phospholipids are usually increased but may be normal in secondary myxedema. It is of interest that the coronary atherosclerosis and cardiac hypertrophy described with primary myxedema were not encountered in pituitary myxedema.[128] The serum-carotene level is often elevated because of decreased conversion of carotene to vitamin A.

Determination of the serum-protein-bound iodine level is one of the most reliable tests in myxedema. The value is usually below 3.0 μg per 100 ml; this small amount of protein-bound iodine is present even though the patient may have had no thyroid tissue for many years, as tissues other than the thyroid can synthesize thyroxin at a very slow rate. The I^{131} uptake in patients with myxedema is usually below 10 per cent; the 24-hr urinary excretion is greater than in euthyroid or hyperthyroid patients.

Radiologic Findings
in Myxedema Heart Disease

The cardiac silhouette in primary myxedema is invariably enlarged, and the abnormal globular cardiac contour is more suggestive of pericardial effusion than of true cardiac enlargement (Fig. 61-2*A* and *B*). However, with minimal increase in cardiac size, an erroneous diagnosis of cardiac failure may be made.

Fluoroscopy may help differentiate true cardiac enlargement from pericardial effusion. With pericardial effusion, the cardiac pulsations are decreased and sluggish, and the absence of pulmonary congestion contrasts with the marked enlargement of the cardiac shadow.[161] The fat-pad lines of the left apical area are characteristically within the lateral extension of the cardiac shadow, confirming the presence of pericardial effusion.

Serous effusions in the pleural and peritoneal cavities[168] and anasarca, due to increased capillary permeability, are not uncommon in myxedema,[122,169] even in the absence of heart failure; they characteristically regress with thyroid therapy.

Electrocardiographic Findings in Myxedema

Significant electrocardiographic abnormalities often occur in the absence of congestive heart failure.[136]

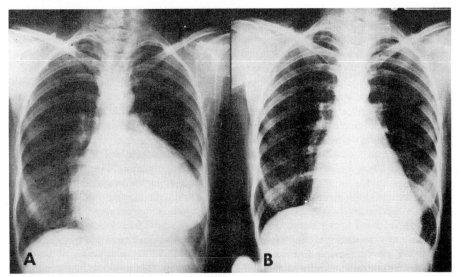

Fig. 61-2. *A.* Chest x-ray of a fifty-year-old woman with myxedema. There is marked cardiac enlargement due to pericardial effusion. *B.* Chest x-ray 4 months after adequate thyroid replacement therapy. There is a marked decrease in transcardiac diameter.

There is sinus bradycardia and low voltage of all electrocardiographic complexes,[32,170] but particularly of the P and T waves, as reported by Zondek[116] in his early cases. The low voltage has been attributed both to pericardial effusion and to a myxedematous infiltrate in the myocardium. T-wave flattening or inversion has been commonly noted.[135,152,171] The P-R interval is frequently slightly prolonged.[172]

Improvement of arrhythmias[173] and heart block[174] has been reported after thyroid therapy; however, arrhythmias are rare. Return to normal of T-wave direction, decrease in P-R interval duration, and increase in QRS-complex voltage occurs following therapy with thyroid hormone.[175,176]

The genesis of the electrocardiographic abnormalities is unknown, but their regression with thyroid therapy suggests a direct relationship to the effects of myxedema on the heart.[124] The rapid effects of thyroid hormone on the electrocardiographic abnormalities[177] suggests a primary action of thyroid hormone on the cardiocirculatory system, independent of the metabolic effects of thyroid hormone. Electrocardiographic abnormalities may regress after thyroid therapy before changes occur in the basal metabolic rate or serum-protein-bound iodine level; this suggests that potentiation of epinephrine effect on the heart is produced by thyroid hormone before there is general elevation of the basal metabolism rate.[178]

The electrocardiographic changes have been postulated to result not from myocardial electrical conductivity changes but from the pericardial effusion encountered so frequently in myxedema.[157]

Predictable disappearance of electrocardiographic abnormalities has been observed after pericardiocentesis.[15] However, repolarization abnormalities (T wave) have been thought to be due to cellular metabolic derangements.[179]

Treatment of Myxedema Heart Disease

Thyroid hormone reverses most abnormalities encountered in myxedema heart disease, but replacement therapy must be administered cautiously in the presence of underlying organic heart disease.[120,180,181] Angina pectoris, myocardial infarction, or severe congestive heart failure may develop if the thyroid dosage is increased too rapidly, imposing too abruptly an increased demand on the heart and increasing the sensitivity of the myocardium to catecholamine effects.[121,182,183] There is also increased sensitivity of myxedematous patients to morphine and other drugs. The complications seem more related to initial vigorous thyroid therapy than to the total dosage of thyroid hormone.[184] The results of thyroid therapy in myxedema heart disease depend on the relationship between the increase in myocardial blood flow and the increased cardiac work associated with augmentation of body metabolism.[36]

The usual therapeutic dose is 30 mg thyroid extract daily for 7 to 10 days, with a 30-mg weekly dose increase until the patient is receiving 60 to 90 mg thyroid extract daily. In the elderly patient with underlying heart disease, 15 mg thyroid extract daily should be administered initially with gradual increments of 15 mg every 2 to 4 weeks; 6 or 8 weeks of therapy are usually required to reach a satisfactory dosage level, which may be 30 to 60 mg daily.[113]

Rapidly acting triiodothyronine therapy is the logical choice for the myxedematous patient with underlying cardiac disease. Five micrograms a day may be given initially, with a slow dose increase depending on the patient's clinical response. The advantages of triiodothyronine are rapidity of onset of action and rapidity of decrease in metabolic effect once therapy has been discontinued; nevertheless, the rapid onset of action can precipitate cardiac complications when an excessive dose is administered.[148]

The daily maintenance dose of thyroid hormone should be based predominantly on the clinical response, rather than on values for laboratory tests. Gibson[185] suggested electrocardiographic monitoring for evaluating dose increase, as excessive doses commonly produce electrocardiographic abnormalities.

Therapy with thyroid hormone increases cardiac contractility, heart rate, and cardiac output; causes absorption of serous effusions; effects a return to normal of the heart size[135,144] and the electrocardiographic pattern; and lowers the serum-cholesterol level. Thyroid therapy causes this cardiovascular normalization by increasing cardiac muscle tone and by decreasing both the myocardial interstitial edema and the pericardial effusion.[135]

THE PITUITARY AND THE HEART

From the cardiovascular standpoint, the two anterior pituitary trophic hormones which warrant special consideration are the adrenocorticotropic (ACTH) and the somatotropic (growth) hormones.

Theories of Mechanism of Action of Trophic Hormones

Adrenocorticotropic Hormone

Corticotropin (ACTH) is the pituitary hormone which controls cortisol secretion by the adrenal cortex. In the past, crude pituitary extracts proved effective in restoring adrenal function after hypophysectomy; the principal corticotropin peptides have recently been characterized.[186,187]

Corticotropin is not stored in the pituitary and is presumed to be rapidly synthesized in response to stress. A "feedback" mechanism controls cortisol secretion by the adrenal cortex. Plasma-cortisol concentration falls in response to a tissue need; the neurohypophysis stimulates the pituitary to synthesize and release ACTH, which then stimulates the adrenal cortex to increase its release and/or synthesis of cortisol. As the increased

cortisol level satisfies the tissue need, the anterior pituitary secretion of ACTH ceases.

In addition to stimulating the release of cortisol, ACTH acts on the adrenal cortex to produce an increase of oxidative phosphorylation, an acceleration of glycolysis,[188] an alteration of lipid metabolism as evidenced by depletion of adrenocortical cholesterol and lipid, an increase in protein synthesis, and a depletion of adrenocortical ascorbic acid.[22b]

In adrenalectomized animals, ACTH affects fat metabolism by mobilizing nonesterified fatty acids and neutral fats from fat depots and increasing fat oxidation with a lowering of the respiratory quotient and enhancement of ketogenesis. Carbohydrate-metabolism changes include the production of hyperglycemia and an increase in muscle glycogen.[22b]

Somatotropic Hormone

Somatotropic, or growth, hormone has differences in molecular structure among the variant species; of interest is the smaller molecular size of primate growth hormone as compared with the larger molecular size of bovine hormone. Growth-hormone activity is species-specific; hence enzymatic digestion of bovine hormone, making it active in man, would be an important advance. Li[186] removed 24 per cent of amino acids from bovine growth hormone without loss of biologic activity, but further enzymatic digestion resulted in hormone inactivation; in the molecularly smaller human growth hormone only 10 per cent of amino acids could be removed before biologic activity was lost.[22b]

The human anterior pituitary is rich in growth hormone, and little change in growth-hormone content occurs with age. Levels of circulating growth hormone have been recently measured;[189] children have 85 to 570 μg growth hormone per ml plasma, a value similar to that found in adults. Increased levels of growth hormone have been documented in acromegaly.[189] The anterior pituitary produces about 4 mg growth hormone daily, the average amount required to treat hypopituitarism in the human being adequately.[186]

Growth hormone affects numerous metabolic activities of most body tissues.[22b] Growth-hormone administration to pituitary dwarfs causes growth to begin within a few days; the preponderant changes in body composition are increase of protein and decrease of body fat. Marked decrease occurs in serum and urinary urea levels and in the rate of conversion of amino acids to blood urea; growth hormone accelerates amino acid entrance into the cell and may thus stimulate protein synthesis. Growth hormone induces important alterations in fat metabolism in the pituitary-deficient patient. Fat mobilization occurs[190] from peripheral depots to the liver; there is increased fat metabolism, with lowering of the respiratory quotient and increased ketogenesis. Growth hormone probably decreases amino acid utilization for catabolic purposes by increasing fat oxidation; protein synthesis results. Carbohydrate-metabolism abnormalities following hypophysectomy include fasting hypoglycemia and decreased muscle and liver glycogen; the hypoglycemic action of insulin is greatly enhanced by hypopituitarism. Carbohydrate-metabolism disturbances result from both growth-hormone and ACTH deficiency; cortisol restores normal blood-glucose levels and increases liver glycogen, but abnormal insulin sensitivity persists, indicating an important role of pituitary growth hormone. Hypoglycemia may stimulate growth-hormone release by the anterior pituitary; growth hormone may therefore be more important in the homeostatic control of blood glucose than has been previously recognized.

Hyperpituitarism and the Heart

Two forms of anterior pituitary hyperactivity affect the cardiovascular system: Cushing's syndrome (pituitary basophilism) and acromegaly (pituitary eosinophilism).

Cushing's Syndrome (Pituitary Basophilism)

In pituitary basophilism, the basophilic cells of the anterior pituitary secrete excessive ACTH in an uncontrolled fashion; the adrenal cortex responds by bilateral hyperplasia, producing the clinical syndrome described by Cushing in 1932.[191] Increased ACTH secretion may be due to a basophilic adenoma; this tumor is characteristically small, uncommonly erodes the dorsum sellae,[192] and therefore rarely produces secondary pituitary failure or visual disturbances.

Cardiovascular and renal abnormalities are important features of Cushing's syndrome; of the 12 original cases reported by Cushing,[191] hypertension occurred in 9 and cardiac hypertrophy in 4. Hypertension is the most frequent and significant cardiovascular derangement;[192-195] it is often severe and associated with cardiac enlargement, cerebral hemorrhage, and renal insufficiency. Prior to present-day therapy, congestive heart failure, cerebral hemorrhage, and chronic uremia were the most common causes of death in Cushing's syndrome. Hypertension tends to be more severe in the patient with bilateral adrenal hyperplasia than in the patient with Cushing's syndrome due to adrenal adenoma or carcinoma.

Cardiovascular Pathology. The morphologic changes in the systemic arterioles of hypertensive patients with Cushing's syndrome consist of subendothelial accumulation of a homogeneous eosinophilic material, medial hypertrophy, increase in the number and size of smooth muscle cells, and increased intracellular collagen in the media. The histopathologic features do not differ from those encountered in essential hypertension.[195] In the malignant phase of hypertension in Cushing's disease, the degenerative arteriolar changes progress rapidly, and acute hyaline necrosis with obliteration of the lumen may occur. Patients with malignant hypertension complicating Cushing's syndrome demonstrate the same vascular abnormalities as those with idiopathic malignant hypertension.[196] Two patients with malignant hypertension complicating Cushing's syndrome whom the authors studied at our Clinical Research Center[30] (Emory University School of Medicine) were found to have arteriosclerotic changes in the arterioles on adrenocortical biopsy at surgery.

Scholz et al.[195] described significant hypertension in 17 young-to-middle-aged patients with Cushing's syndrome. Cardiac enlargement was present in 15, the largest hearts being associated with the most severe hypertension of longest duration; the 3 patients who died of cardiac failure had severe hypertension with pronounced cardiac enlargement. At autopsy, the systemic arteriolar changes did not differ from those of so-called essential hypertension.

Cardiovascular Pathophysiology. The mechanism of blood pressure elevation in Cushing's syndrome remains obscure, although the hypertension and most other manifestations of spontaneous Cushing's syndrome have been observed in patients receiving prolonged cortisol or ACTH therapy. The mild mineralocorticoid effect of cortisol causes increased renal retention of sodium and water. Experimentally, cortisol and sodium administration fail to produce hypertensive vascular complications; however, the addition of desoxycorticosterone predictably causes both hypertension and vascular lesions.

In the authors' series[30] of 23 patients with Cushing's syndrome, 21 had mild hypertension, and 2 had malignant hypertension. With the exception of these latter two, the blood pressure returned to normal following treatment of the Cushing's syndrome. The two patients with malignant hypertension reverted to the essential benign variety but required antihypertensive therapy, which suggested that the hypertension was so advanced that complete remission was impossible.

Clinical Manifestations; Laboratory, Radiologic, and Electrocardiographic Findings. See the section on the Adrenal Cortex and the Heart, below.

Treatment. Laboratory studies permit differentiation between bilateral adrenocortical hyperplasia and adrenal adenoma or carcinoma.[197–199] Pituitary irradiation, rather than bilateral adrenalectomy, is the treatment of choice for adrenal hyperplasia, since bilateral adrenalectomy necessitates prolonged continuous hormone-replacement therapy. Anterior pituitary hyperactivity, rather than primary adrenal disease, accounts for about 60 per cent of cases of Cushing's syndrome.

The author's five patients[30] treated with pituitary irradiation had a 2- to 7-year remission without recurrence to the present time; the three hypertensive patients are now normotensive, and the two with malignant hypertension have benign essential hypertension. The author's patients with Cushing's syndrome treated by adrenalectomy prior to the advent of high-voltage irradiation all had benign hypertension and are now all normotensive.

Acromegaly (*Pituitary Eosinophilism*)

Excessive anterior pituitary growth-hormone secretion, usually due to a chromophobe or eosinophilic pituitary tumor, produces acromegaly. When the tumor develops before puberty, pituitary gigantism results; if, as occurs more commonly, the tumor develops in the third or fourth decades, acral rather than linear growth occurs, producing the clinical features of acromegaly.

Cardiac enlargement in acromegaly was first described by Huchard in 1895[200] and congestive heart failure by Fournier in 1896.[201]

Pathology of the Heart in Acromegaly. Pronounced cardiac hypertrophy, particularly of the left ventricle, excessively disproportionate to the enlargement of other viscera,[202] is a most impressive physical and radiologic finding in acromegaly.[203] The heart often weighs more than 500 Gm, occasionally weighing over 1,000 Gm. In addition to the cardiomegaly, pronounced coronary artery and major vessel arteriosclerosis commonly occur and are associated with myocardial infarction and fibrosis.

Postmortem examination of the acromegalic heart confirms the myocardial hypertrophy and advanced arteriosclerotic changes. There is no specific myocardial alteration in acromegaly.[202] Microscopically, there is hypertrophy of individual muscle bundles. The diffuse interstitial myocardial fibrosis is often extensive enough to produce gross scarring and is probably secondary both to the hypertrophy and to the coronary arteriosclerosis with chronic low-grade hypoxia.[204,205]

Cardiovascular Pathophysiology. Excessive growth-hormone secretion by a pituitary tumor causes growth of skeletal parts, viscera, and endocrine glands. The cardiac enlargement may reflect a direct pituitary-hormone action on the heart, an increased work demand on the heart, and possibly the effect of thyrotoxicosis, diabetes, and/or hypertension.[206] Growth hormone increases muscle mass, as evidenced by the striking retention of nitrogen, magnesium, potassium, phosphate, iodine, and calcium. Excessive growth hormone produces cardiac enlargement in the adult; the prepubertal individual exposed to excessive growth hormone becomes a giant but does not develop cardiac enlargement.[108] The supernormal strength claimed by some acromegalic patients soon disappears, being replaced by progressive weakness and associated decrease in skeletal muscle mass with fibrous tissue replacement; animal studies have shown the degree and duration of muscle contraction to be decreased with growth-hormone excess.[207]

The mechanism of the arteriosclerosis and cardiac hypertrophy in acromegaly is not completely understood; growth-hormone excess, the commonly associated diabetes, and the frequently encountered hypertension may contribute to the cardiomegaly. The incidence of hypertension is not increased in acromegaly, but hypertension when present is poorly tolerated.[205]

The chronic congestive heart failure is presumed secondary to myocardial hypertrophy with malfunctioning hypertrophied fibers, impaired contraction and impulse transmission due to fibrosis, and the frequently associated coronary arteriosclerosis. The myocardial hypertrophy probably reflects both the generalized organomegaly and the excessive cardiac work required to supply blood to an enlarged body.[202]

Clinical Manifestations. The clinical manifestations of acromegaly are related to the expanding lesion within the pituitary fossa, to growth-hormone excess, and to other hormone disturbances.

Sella turcica enlargement, severe headache, and visual impairment are common. Continued tumor growth may produce hypopituitarism by destruction of surrounding normal pituitary tissue. Growth-hormone excess causes weight gain, hypermetabolism and associated hyperhidrosis, and visceromegaly. Growth of acral parts occurs in all adults with excessive growth-hormone secretion, prognathism and osteoporosis are common, and arthritic complaints are related to specific joint changes.[208] The progressive facial and acral changes are so gradual that only advanced abnormalities may be recognizable.

Cardiac enlargement, hypertension, and congestive heart failure are the major cardiovascular manifestations of acromegaly.[202,205,209] Disproportionate cardiac enlargement is almost universal. The reported frequency of hypertension varies, although Hamwi et al.[209] described sustained diastolic hypertension in over one-third of patients with active acromegaly. Significant cardiac failure is encountered in about one-fourth of cases. Dyspnea is the most prominent cardiac symptom;[209] kyphoscoliosis, secondary to progressive degenerative joint disease and osteoporosis, is often accompanied by exertional dyspnea even in the absence of congestive heart failure. Weakness, palpitation, and syncope are also encountered.

Laboratory and Radiologic Diagnosis. The red blood cell count and hemoglobin are high-normal or slightly elevated. Serum–inorganic phosphate and alkaline phosphatase levels are commonly increased, and about one-third of acromegalic patients have a diabetic glucose-tolerance curve.

The serum-protein-bound iodine level, 24-hr I^{131} thyroidal uptake, and urinary excretion of 17-hydroxysteroids and 17-ketosteroids are all slightly elevated, particularly during the active growth phase. However, both this increased thyroid hormone secretion and increased adrenocortical hormone secretion are considered normal for the acromegalic patient with a large body mass and increased thyroid and adrenal gland weight.

X-ray examination of the skull characteristically reveals enlargement of the sella turcica, erosion of the clinoids, and widening of the acral parts with prominence of the mandible and prognathism. There is generalized cardiac enlargement on radiologic examination; the chest is likewise massively enlarged, but the heart size appears to have increased disproportionately to somatic growth. There are degenerative joint changes and osteoporosis of the spine with dorsal kyphoscoliosis.

Electrocardiographic Findings. The electrocardiographic abnormalities encountered in acromegaly are not diagnostic. Left axis deviation, left ventricular hypertrophy, and nonspecific QRS-complex and T-wave abnormalities have been reported.[202,205,206] These derangements occur late in the course of the disease, suggesting that anterior pituitary insufficiency may have developed, producing electrocardiographic alterations in part attributable to pituitary myxedema.

Treatment. Therapy for the cardiovascular disease associated with acromegaly is directed toward control of excessive growth-hormone secretion. Current management of active acromegaly consists of pituitary irradiation; in patients with tumor encroachment on the optic chiasm, neurosurgical removal of the tumor is indicated.

Hypopituitarism

Hypopituitarism may be due to tumor, to necrosis, or to inflammation.[210] Anterior pituitary failure causes failure of gonadal, adrenal cortical, and thyroid function because of the absence of trophic hormones to stimulate these glands, with target-gland failure usually presenting in the following order: gonadal, adrenal, and thyroid. There is associated hyperinsulinism.

Anterior pituitary failure usually develops slowly; there is occasional sudden occurrence as in Sheehan's syndrome complicating pregnancy. Postpartum pituitary necrosis (Sheehan's syndrome) is characterized by severe asthenia and labile blood-sugar levels, but by only minor salt- and water-metabolism disturbances.

The pituitary cachexia described by Simmonds is uncommon today, and most patients with anterior pituitary insufficiency appear well nourished.

Pathophysiology

The pathophysiologic alterations in hypopituitarism depend on the extent of target-gland failure.

There may be inappropriate antidiuretic hormone secretion and the clinical syndrome of water intoxication; lethargy, hyponatremia, increased urinary sodium excretion, and widening of the pulse pressure suggestive of increased extracellular fluid volume occur. Judicious water restriction and cortisol administration constitute the recommended therapy.

Pituitary insufficiency may produce cardiac changes similar to those of myxedema or of Addison's disease. Cardiac atrophy with myofiber degeneration is seen on microscopic examination of the heart. Many cardiac effects of Simmonds's disease are similar to those of Addison's disease, suggesting that they are due to adrenal deficiency induced by the pituitary lesion.[108]

Clinical Manifestations

Hypopituitarism occurs more commonly in the female. The clinical findings are dependent on the degree of target-gland failure. Patients most commonly have predominant manifestations of myxedema; adrenal cortical failure produces few recognizable clinical abnormalities in the presence of pituitary myxedema. Addisonian crisis and severe electrolyte disturbances are uncommon. Inadequate response to stress in the absence of pigmentation and associated with hypothyroidism and hypogonadism are suggestive of pituitary ACTH deficiency.

There is asthenia, anorexia, and weight loss in hypopituitarism; there may be anemia, with pallor of the skin, mucous membranes, and nail beds. As in primary myxedema, the skin is thickened, pale, and yellowish; the deep-tendon reflexes often have a prolonged relaxation phase. Evidence of hypogonadism is usually present.

The blood pressure is often low and the heart size small, although both blood pressure and heart size may be normal. Pericardial effusion does not occur as commonly in secondary myxedema as in the primary variety; this is surprising, as other cardinal manifestations of myxedema are similar in both primary and secondary thyroid failure; however, true congestive heart failure has been described[211] in secondary myxedema. Arteriosclerosis is characteristically absent.

Laboratory and Radiologic Diagnosis

A normochromic normocytic anemia and eosinophilia are not uncommon. Occasional hyposthenuria or isosthenuria is recorded on routine urinalysis. Serum-electrolyte and blood-urea-nitrogen levels are usually normal. The blood-glucose level is normal to low, with an abnormal glucose-tolerance curve and insulin hypersensitivity.[210] The serum-protein-bound iodine level and 24-hr I[131] thyroidal uptake are low, and TSH stimulation causes an increase in the 24-hr I[131] thyroidal uptake.

The serum-cholesterol level is normal in most patients with secondary myxedema; therefore, a normal serum-cholesterol level in a myxedematous patient should raise the suspicion of underlying hypopituitarism.

There is no specific cardiac radiologic abnormality in hypopituitarism, as changes are usually those of secondary myxedema. Radiologic alterations in the skull are uncommon except for those cases due to expanding tumors.

Electrocardiographic Findings

Electrocardiographic changes compatible with myxedema predominate in hypopituitarism, generalized low voltage being the classic abnormality. On rare occasions, with severe stress, the patient with hypopituitarism may manifest electrocardiographic changes of hyperkalemia: peaking of the T wave, widening of the QRS complex, and disappearance of the P wave. P-R interval prolongation has been attributed to inadequate quantities of cortisol.[212]

Treatment

The treatment of hypopituitarism consists of target-gland-hormone replacement in the order in which the glands fail: testosterone and/or estrogen, cortisol, and then thyroxin. Theoretically, acute adrenal crisis can be precipitated by correcting the thyroid deficiency before the cortisol deficiency. Less thyroxin is required to correct pituitary myxedema than primary hypothyroidism; 60 to 90 mg of desiccated thyroid daily is adequate replacement therapy. Five milligrams of cortisol three times daily is adequate therapy for the patient with hypopituitarism, less than the requirement in Addison's disease. In the hypopituitary patient treated with digitalis for congestive heart failure, digitalis intoxication may occur following cortisol-

replacement therapy with the ensuing potassium diuresis.

THE ADRENAL CORTEX AND THE HEART

Action of Adrenal Cortical Hormones

Adrenal steroid hormones affect inorganic and organic metabolism. Sodium retention and potassium excretion are influenced primarily by the mineralocorticoid aldosterone, whereas organic metabolism is controlled by the glucocorticoids cortisol and corticosterone. Considerable overlap and probably functional interaction occurs between the effects of aldosterone and cortisol.[213] Some 17-ketosteroids are anabolic and weakly androgenic. Small amounts of weakly active estrogen are produced in the adrenal.

Cortisol effects a centripetal redistribution of fat, increasing body fat at the expense of protein; chronic cortisol excess causes hyperlipemia and hypercholesterolemia, associated with a predisposition to atherosclerosis. Cortisol and cortisone help maintain extracellular fluid volume and enhance water diuresis. Cortisol may raise the blood pressure; it increases angiotensin production, which stimulates aldosterone production, thus further elevating the blood pressure.[214] Cortisol sensitizes the arterioles to the effects of epinephrine and norepinephrine;[42] this explains the occasional restoration of blood pressure by large doses of cortisol in patients with shock who are unresponsive to norepinephrine alone.[22c]

Aldosterone causes sodium retention and urinary potassium loss. Adrenal cortical extract lowers the blood-potassium level in adrenalectomized animals, protecting them from otherwise fatal amounts of administered potassium.[215] With excessive amounts of aldosterone, the serum-sodium level rises, the serum-potassium level falls, and hypochloremic alkalosis with a greater than normal extracellular fluid volume is established.[216] Aldosterone lack results in sodium loss, potassium retention, dehydration, and hypovolemic shock, as seen in the patient with Addison's disease.

Cushing's Syndrome

In 1932, Cushing[191] first described glucocorticoid excess associated with a basophilic pituitary adenoma and bilateral adrenal cortical hyperplasia; he suggested that pituitary hyperactivity was the cause of this syndrome. About 65 to 80 per cent of cases of Cushing's syndrome have bilateral adrenal hyperplasia secondary to hyperpituitarism; of the remainder, the majority are due to adrenal cortical adenoma and, more rarely, to carcinoma. Modern techniques[198] often enable differentiation between the pituitary and adrenal cortical origin of Cushing's syndrome. Tumors of the bronchus, pancreas, and thymus have also been described in association with Cushing's syndrome;[217] these tumors apparently secrete an ACTH-like substance.

Cushing's syndrome is a rare entity, occurring approximately once in 1,000 autopsies, predominantly in the female. The peak incidence is in the third to fourth decades, particularly following pregnancy.[22c]

The systemic changes in Cushing's syndrome[191] include obesity, hirsutism, marked osteoporosis, generalized muscle wasting, amenorrhea, disappearance of elastic fibers causing striae and marked thinning of the skin, hypercholesterolemia and hyperglycemia with severe progressive atherosclerosis of the larger blood vessels, hypertension, polycythemia, nephrosclerosis, and at times renal calcinosis; the ovaries are small and sclerotic, and the pancreas may show fatty necrosis and beta-cell hyperplasia.

Cardiac Histopathology

The heart in Cushing's syndrome is characteristically hypertrophied with advanced atherosclerotic coronary artery changes. These abnormalities are generally attributed to the hypertension, the hypercholesterolemia, and the diabetes mellitus[196] but may be due to a direct cortisol effect on blood lipids.[218,219]

Pathophysiology

The pathophysiologic alterations in Cushing's syndrome are secondary to excessive adrenal cortical hormone secretion; the altered physiologic state depends upon which of the cortical hormones is secreted in excess.

With mineralocorticoid excess, major cardiovascular complications occur, including hypertensive cardiovascular disease, cerebrovascular accident, and chronic renal failure. The catabolic effect of excessive cortisol causes a prominent decrease in extremity muscle mass, accompanied by profound weakness. There is hypercholesterolemia with an abnormal distribution of body fat. The mineralocorticoid activity of cortisol may cause renal retention of sodium with resultant hypervolemia.

If androgen secretion predominates, the muscle mass increases, and muscle fibers increase in volume and size with intracellular retention of nitrogen, phosphorus, and potassium. Virilism is evident in the female.

Excessive estrogen secretion is difficult to detect in the female, but gynecomastia, testicular atrophy, and impotence are common in the male. Estrogen excess is usually indicative of adrenal adeno-

carcinoma, as it rarely occurs with benign adenoma or bilateral adrenal hyperplasia.

Clinical Manifestations

The clinical signs and symptoms of Cushing's syndrome also depend on the relative excess secretion of cortisol, aldosterone, androgen, and estrogen. The primary cardiovascular complications include hypertension, cardiac enlargement, cardiovascular hypertrophy, and congestive heart failure.[195,220]

If cortisol secretion predominates, mooning of the face, plethora, buffalo hump, truncal obesity, thinning of the skin, easy bruising, osteoporosis, muscular weakness, hypertension, cardiomegaly, and atherosclerosis are evident. If androgen secretion is predominant, masculinization and obesity may be the presenting findings in the female. If aldosterone secretion predominates, the patient may present primarily with hypertension, hypernatremia, hypokalemia, hypochloremic alkalosis, hyposthenuria, alkaline urine, and decreased total body potassium, associated with kaliopenic nephropathy (see Chap. 44). If estrogen secretion predominates, the presenting findings in the male may be gynecomastia, decline in libido, and softening of the testicles.

The combination of cortisol and aldosterone excess produces far more severe cardiovascular disturbances—hypertension and atherosclerotic changes—than occur with estrogen or androgen predominance. Hypertension occurs in 75 to 90 per cent of patients with Cushing's syndrome,[221,222] with elevation of both the systolic and diastolic blood pressure. The hypertension of bilateral adrenal hyperplasia, similar to that of pituitary basophilism, may not regress completely after therapy for Cushing's syndrome.[192,194] The hypertension of Cushing's syndrome is severe and is related to the duration of the disease; prior to recent advances in therapy it was commonly complicated by cerebrovascular accident, congestive heart failure, and chronic renal failure.[221] The arteriolar lesions of cortisol excess resemble those of essential or malignant hypertension.

Congestive heart failure occurs in about one-fourth of patients with Cushing's syndrome of significant duration.[221] Patients with Cushing's syndrome who develop congestive heart failure respond poorly to digitalization, sodium restriction, and diuretic therapy; thiazide diuretics are particularly to be avoided, as they produce a potassium diuresis, increasing the metabolic alkalosis and augmenting the profound weakness.

Arteriosclerosis and atherosclerosis are associated with increased duration of Cushing's syndrome and increased severity and duration of the hypertension.[210b]

The onset of Cushing's syndrome is often insidious. Symptoms may occasionally appear rapidly during the last trimester of pregnancy and may be misinterpreted as toxemia of pregnancy; however, the manifestations do not disappear postpartum. Cushing's syndrome is often characterized by remissions and exacerbations, but the patient becomes increasingly weak and finally bedridden because of loss of muscle strength and multiple vertebral fractures. There is an increased susceptibility to infection. The untreated disease progresses to general debility, cerebrovascular accident, or congestive heart failure within an average of 5 years.[22c]

Laboratory and Radiologic Diagnosis

Leukocytosis, lymphopenia, mild polycythemia, mild to moderate metabolic alkalosis, sodium retention, hypochloremia, excessive urinary potassium loss, and hyperglycemia occur in Cushing's syndrome. Electrolyte abnormalities are not as common as in adrenal hypofunction,[223] with alkalosis noted most frequently. Kaliopenic nephropathy is frequently complicated by pyelonephritis.

Cushing's syndrome, irrespective of cause, is characterized by an increase in urinary excretion of 17-hydroxysteroids, 17-ketogenic steroids, and 17-ketosteroids. Differentiation between pituitary and adrenal origin of the hyperfunctioning state and between adrenal hyperplasia and tumor may be accomplished by special studies using dexamethasone, methopryapone (SU-4885), and ACTH.[197–199]

Prominent cardiac enlargement with left ventricular preponderance and pulmonary congestion is seen on radiologic examination of the chest. The skull x-ray is important in the hyperpigmented patient with Cushing's syndrome, as pituitary tumor is more common in the presence of hyperpigmentation; however, the sella turcica usually appears normal. Pseudofractures and osteoporosis may be seen in the ribs, skull, and pelvis. A suprarenal tumor may be demonstrated by abdominal tomography. Depression of the left kidney shadow should be sought, as most adrenal tumors occur on the left. Oppenheimer and Silver[224] advocated retroperitoneal pneumography to delineate the adrenal gland, but this procedure has not been particularly helpful in the authors' hands. Aortography may identify a tumor by demonstrating an excessive vascular bed in the suprarenal area.

Electrocardiographic Findings

The P-R interval is short in Cushing's syndrome because of excessive amounts of adrenal cortical hormone; the atrioventricular (A-V) conduction time correlates well with the 17-ketosteroid urinary excretion.[212] Left ventricular hypertrophy is secondary to the hypertension.[108]

Treatment

Most patients with Cushing's syndrome have hyperpituitarism, with excessive ACTH secretion causing bilateral adrenal hyperplasia and excessive cortisol secretion.

If an adrenal cortical tumor can be excluded as the etiologic factor for Cushing's syndrome, pituitary irradiation with high-voltage therapy or cobalt[60] is the treatment of choice. It seems preferable to reduce excessive ACTH secretion by irradiation than by surgical removal of the adrenal glands; the latter converts a patient with Cushing's syndrome into one with Addison's disease, subsequently requiring lifelong hormone-replacement therapy.

Pituitary irradiation produces some symptomatic remission within 3 or 4 months but may require up to 6 months before the remission is impressive. The authors' five patients treated with pituitary irradiation have continued in remission from 2 to 7 years without repeated irradiation or surgical intervention.

Surgical intervention with bilateral adrenal exploration is recommended for patients with presumed adrenal tumor; the treatment of choice for adrenal adenocarcinoma with metastases is excision of the primary tumor followed by therapeutic doses of *o,p'*-dichlorodiphenyldichloroethane (*o,p'*-DDD).[225]

Addison's Disease

Addison's disease, first described in 1855,[226] is not an uncommon clinical syndrome. It occurs with equal frequency in the male and female, predominantly in the third and fourth decades of life.[227]

Primary adrenocortical insufficiency may result from adrenal cortical destruction by infection, hemorrhage, trauma, vascular lesions, or tumor;[228] in a patient with marginal adrenocortical reserve from prior disease or steroid therapy, adrenocortical insufficiency may occur after surgical treatment, anesthesia, or other stress. An occasional case of Addison's disease secondary to adrenal hemorrhage has been reported in patients receiving anticoagulant therapy.

The authors recently studied a patient in whom acute adrenal insufficiency developed during heparin therapy for thrombophlebitis. There occurred dull bilateral flank pain, a progressive fall in blood pressure, narrowing of the pulse pressure, orthostatic tachycardia, weakness, pigmentation of the extremities, and increased renal sodium excretion with decreased serum-sodium levels. All signs and symptoms disappeared with adrenocortical hormone replacement therapy; subsequent study revealed a failure of response to exogenous ACTH.

Histopathology

In past years, tuberculosis was the most common cause of Addison's disease;[229,230] the most common cause today is primary idiopathic atrophy of the adrenal cortex,[231] possibly resulting from an autoimmune reaction similar to that producing Hashimoto's struma of the thyroid.[230]

The heart is atrophic and flabby without specific myocardial abnormality except for an increase in hemofuscin pigment, the so-called brown atrophy.[227,228] The decreased cardiac size may reflect body-weight loss, decreased cardiac work, systemic hypotension, or hypovolemia.

Pathophysiology

The pathophysiologic alterations in Addison's disease are due to excessive ACTH secretion by the anterior pituitary and to inadequate cortisol and aldosterone secretion by the adrenal cortex. Glucocorticoid (cortisol) deficiency causes impairment of carbohydrate metabolism and resultant hypoglycemia.[230] Cortisol deficiency is associated with hypocholesterolemia and loss of body fat.

The hypotension is due to hypovolemia, secondary to mineralocorticoid inadequacy, resulting in excessive sodium and water loss, and to decreased vascular sensitivity to the pressor amines, with failure of vasoconstriction. The reduced blood volume primarily determines the decrease in heart size in Addison's disease. Some investigators have also documented an absolute decrease in myocardial mass with decrease in myocardial fiber and bundle size, possibly related to potassium and water loss from the myocardium. The melanin-stimulating effect of ACTH or excessive secretion of melanin-stimulating hormone (MSH) produces diffuse pigmentation, primarily on the exposed surfaces of the skin, the buccal mucous membranes, and the pressure points.

Clinical Manifestations

The onset of Addison's disease is usually insidious, although occasionally it appears suddenly.

It is characterized by striking asthenia, hypotension, anorexia, weight loss and dehydration, gastrointestinal disturbances, hypoglycemic manifestations, dyspnea and palpitations, skin and mucous membrane pigmentation, and nervous and mental symptoms. The cardiocirculatory manifestations include arterial hypotension, postural hypotension, and small heart size, consistent with Addison's original description[226] of the feebleness of the heart action. Acute episodic crises are precipitated by stress and characterized by hypovolemia, hyponatremia, and electrocardiographic abnormalities.[227] The retention of normal gonadal function and secondary sex characteristics help differentiate primary hypoadrenocorticism from that due to anterior pituitary failure.

Hypotension is one of the most constant physical findings in Addison's disease.[108] The actual blood pressure level is dependent on the level prior to the disease onset, but the systolic pressure is usually below 100 mm Hg. A normotensive patient in whom Addison's disease develops may have profound hypotension late in the disease, whereas a patient with preexisting hypertension may have classic Addison's disease with a normal blood pressure. Increased duration and severity of Addison's disease are associated with more profound hypotension. The dehydration, decreased plasma volume, hypotension, and small heart size predispose to dizziness and syncopal attacks. Muscular weakness and limitation of muscular activity probably accentuate the postural hypotension.

Cardiac damage in Addison's disease[232] is attributable to the combined effects of inadequate dietary intake, vitamin B_1 deficiency, hemoconcentration, diminution of cardiac glycogen reserve, and alterations of electrolyte potential across the myocardial cell membrane. However, congestive heart failure is unusual in Addison's disease prior to therapy, probably because of the minimal activity of these debilitated patients.

Addison's disease should be suspected in all patients with systolic blood pressure levels consistently below 100 mm Hg who have asthenia, weight loss, gastrointestinal manifestations, progressive pigmentation, and marked emotional lability. Any patient receiving prolonged corticoid or ACTH therapy must be considered to have potential Addison's disease when subjected to the stress of surgical treatment, trauma, infection, etc.

Laboratory Diagnosis

Hemoconcentration often conceals a normochromic normocytic anemia; moderate neutropenia with relative lymphocytosis is common. There is a low urine specific gravity. About 50 per cent of patients with Addison's disease have gastric achlorhydria.[227] The total serum-protein level is normal, probably because of hemoconcentration; the hypoproteinemia, probably due to poor dietary intake, becomes evident with rehydration.[22c]

Impairment of water diuresis is common in Addison's disease and may be demonstrated by the water test of Soffer and Gabrilove;[233] cortisol therapy before water ingestion produces a normal water diuresis. Marked reduction in 24-hr urinary excretion of 17-hydroxycorticoids, 17-ketosteroids, and 17-ketogenic steroids is characteristic of Addison's disease and is unchanged by intravenous ACTH administration; corticotropin (ACTH) also fails to produce the expected eosinopenia.[234]

Serum-sodium levels of less than 142 mEq per liter and serum-potassium levels over 4.5 mEq per liter are characteristic of Addison's disease; there is a slight diminution in the serum-chloride and bicarbonate levels.[223] However, hemoconcentration may mask the hyponatremia, and only an elevated serum-potassium level may be observed. Hypercalcemia[235] has been reported as frequently as hyponatremia in adrenalectomized dogs; however, data is lacking for human beings.

There are increased blood levels of cholesterol and blood-urea nitrogen. Hypoglycemia may be due to decreased carbohydrate intake, decreased intestinal absorption of carbohydrate, and/or abnormalities in the storage, formation, and utilization of carbohydrate,[227] or to increased sensitivity to insulin.

Radiologic Findings

The heart is small and hypodynamic in Addison's disease (Figs. 61-3A and 61-4A), heart size tending to parallel the severity of the disease. McGavack[236] described a 32 per cent average reduction in heart volume with Addisonian crisis and a 16 per cent reduction in Addison's disease without crisis. The cardiac silhouette enlarges following treatment with sodium and mineralocorticoids (Figs. 61-3B and 61-4B).

Adrenal calcification is suggestive of Addison's disease. Skull x-ray may reveal a chromophobe adenoma causing secondary adrenocortical insufficiency; however, marked reduction in cardiac size is unusual in secondary adrenocortical failure.

Electrocardiographic Findings

The electrocardiographic abnormalities encountered in Addison's disease are nonspecific and probably reflect a decrease in carbohydrate regulating factor, intracellular and extracellular electrolyte imbalance, changes in extracellular fluid volume, diminution of the basal metabolic rate, anatomic changes in the myocardium, etc.[237]

Bradycardia, generalized low voltage, ST-segment and T-wave abnormalities, and prolonged P-R and Q-T intervals have been reported in about 60 per cent of untreated Addisonian patients; these alterations often regress with therapy.[212,227,229,238] Electrocardiographic evidence of hyperkalemia may occur during Addisonian crisis.

Following treatment with mineralocorticoids and sodium, the voltage of all electrocardiographic complexes increases, similarly to the results observed following thyroid therapy for myxedema. Paradoxically, mineralocorticoid therapy may be followed by electrocardiographic changes of pro-

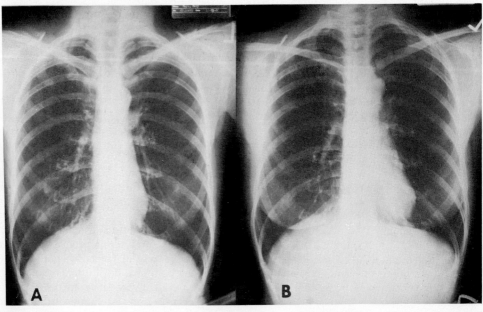

Fig. 61-3. *A.* Chest x-ray of a forty-two-year-old woman with Addison's disease. The small heart shadow (transcardiac diameter 7.4 cm) is characteristic of this disorder. *B.* Repeat chest x-ray 6 months after all symptoms of Addison's disease have subsided in response to therapy with cortisol, α-fluorohydrocortisone, and added salt. The transcardiac diameter measures 10.0 cm.

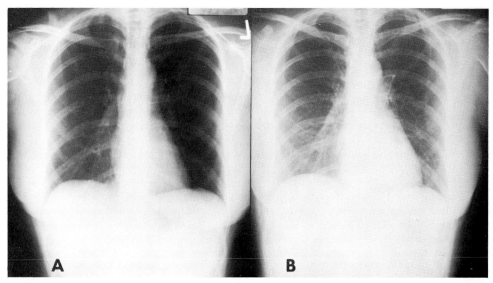

Fig. 61-4. *A.* Chest x-ray of a thirty-eight-year-old woman with Addison's disease with only moderate decrease in transcardiac diameter (10.0 cm.). *B.* Repeat chest x-ray 3 months after adequate replacement therapy. The transcardiac diameter measures 13.0 cm.

gressive myocardial damage, possibly related to the sudden increase in cardiac work;[229] high, peaked T waves occur and have been attributed to hyperkalemia.[239] The prolonged P-R and Q-T intervals are presumed secondary to inadequate cortisol, as replacement therapy tends to shorten these intervals.[212]

Excessive mineralocorticoid therapy may result in prominent U waves and other electrocardiographic evidence of hypokalemia.[227,237] The electrocardiogram, however, may demonstrate no significant change following hormone-replacement therapy.

Treatment

Adequate mineralocorticoid and sodium therapy can reestablish a normal blood volume in Addison's disease by increasing sodium and water retention with resultant return toward normal of the blood pressure and cardiac size; measurement of cardiac size may serve to measure therapeutic efficacy.[236] The blood pressure often does not return to normal levels with hormone and sodium therapy, despite general clinical improvement.[108] Adequate therapy consists of 15 to 30 mg cortisol daily, supplemented by a sodium-retaining hormone and increased dietary sodium. Daily administration of 0.05 to 0.2 mg 9-α-fluorohydrocortisone, a sodium-retaining hormone, will obviate orthostatic hypotension.

Excessive mineralocorticoid administration may produce severe hypertension, angina pectoris, cardiac enlargement, and congestive heart failure due to sodium and water retention,[229,240] particularly in a patient who has previously been hypertensive; the congestive heart failure is attributable to increased cardiac work, due both to the increased blood volume and the hypertension. Hypokalemia with weakness, cardiac arrhythmias, and electrocardiographic changes are also encountered.[229, 239, 241] Excessive sodium and water intake and/or diminished potassium intake may produce the same abnormalities.

The cardiac failure is attributable both to the excessive sodium and water retention and to the hypokalemic myocardiopathy.[240] As regards hypokalemic myocardiopathy, there is a difference of opinion as to whether potassium depletion per se, direct steroid effect, or a combination of electrolyte-steroid disorders causes the myocardial necrosis.[242, 243]

MISCELLANEOUS METABOLIC DISORDERS AND THE HEART

In many metabolic disorders, alteration in the composition of the extracellular fluid may cause electrocardiographic abnormalities; clinical cardiovascular abnormalities are also described. Some metabolic myocardial diseases are discussed in Chap. 55.

Parathyroid Disorders

Hyperparathyroidism

Hypertension, congestive heart failure and electrocardiographic abnormalities constitute the car-

diovascular alterations encountered in hyperparathyroidism. Hypertension is constant in about 50
per cent of patients with hyperparathyroidism,
often persisting after parathyroidectomy; the occurrence and severity of the hypertension seem
related to the degree of impairment of renal function.[244]

An abnormally short Q-T interval, due to hypercalcemia, is present on the electrocardiogram; the
S-T segment seems to fuse with the upstroke of
the T wave.[245] However, the Q-T interval shortening is not sufficiently pronounced to be of diagnostic value.[246]

Myocardial and arterial calcification may occur
secondary to the hypercalcemia.[108]

Long-standing hypercalcemia, with associated
hypercalcemic nephropathy, secondary pyelonephritis, polyuria, and hypovolemia may predispose to
orthostatic hypotension.

Hypoparathyroidism

Cardiovascular manifestations are uncommon in
hypoparathyroidism and usually are confined to
electrocardiographic alterations resulting from the
hypocalcemia. Most commonly, hypocalcemia produces prolongation of the Q-T interval,[247] primarily due to prolongation of the S-T segment; lengthening of the P-R interval, nonspecific T-wave abnormalities, and changes in QRS duration have
also been recorded.[245] The Q-T interval prolongation returns to normal with correction of the hypocalcemia.[248]

Hypocalcemia sensitizes the heart to the effects
of epinephrine and may trigger the mechanism for
arrhythmia, angina pectoris, or sudden death.[249]

Cardiac decompensation, without associated organic heart disease, has been reported in hypoparathyroidism; improvement followed the return
to normal of the serum-calcium level.[250]

Pseudohypoparathyroidism

Q-T interval prolongation in pseudohypoparathyroidism is attributable to the decrease of ion-
ized calcium; the Q-T interval returns toward
normal and tetany subsides as the serum-calcium
concentration increases.[251, 252]

Idiopathic Hypercalcemia of Infancy

Infants with idiopathic hypercalcemia have a
significant incidence of cardiac enlargement, hypertension, and heart murmurs.[253] The origin of
the hypertension is probably the associated severe
renal disease. The heart murmurs are presumed
due to pathologic changes in the myocardium and
heart valves. Myocardial and endocardial calcification and coronary artery calcification are often extensive. Despite the hypercalcemia, the Q-T in-

terval of the electrocardiogram is usually normal.[253]

Paget's Disease (Osteitis Deformans)

Vascular changes in osteitis deformans were first
described by Paget in 1877.[254] There is a marked
increase in peripheral blood flow in the affected
bones, causing an increase in cardiac output.[255]
The circulatory changes resemble those of an arteriovenous fistula;[256] an abnormal increase in cardiac output occurs with exercise, but the increase
in blood flow is not sufficient to cause an increase
in cardiac output at rest.[257] The circulation time is
diminished, the pulse is collapsing in character,
and orthostatic hypotension is present. With over
one-third of the skeleton involved, high-output cardiac failure may occur.[256]

Sornberger and Smedal[258] described an increased incidence of severe atherosclerosis and cardiac enlargement in extensive Paget's disease; this,
associated with the chest deformities and the relatively frequent hypertension, predisposes patients
with Paget's disease to congestive heart failure.

Harrison and Lennox[259] described heart block in
Paget's disease, secondary to calcification of the
interventricular septum.

Hyperinsulinism and Hypoglycemia

Hypoglycemic shock due to an insulinoma may
have a deleterious effect on patients with underlying cardiovascular disease, particularly disease of
the coronary arteries. Myocardial anoxia may result in tachycardia, cardiac arrhythmia, angina pectoris, or myocardial infarction.[260]

Insulin hypoglycemia in the diabetic patient similarly increases cardiac work and may produce cardiac dysfunction; angina pectoris or myocardial
infarction may be precipitated in the patient with
underlying coronary artery disease.[261]

Miscellaneous Endocrine Syndromes Associated with Congenital Heart Disease

Gonadal Dysgenesis

Forty-four per cent of patients with gonadal
dysgenesis, in a recent series, were reported to have
associated cardiovascular abnormalities.[262] Coarctation of the aorta, subaortic stenosis, and pulmonic stenosis constitute the most frequently encountered forms of congenital heart disease in
these patients.[262,263]

Laurence-Moon-Biedl Syndrome

The Laurence-Moon-Biedl syndrome, occurring
more commonly in the male and with a familial
tendency, consists of hypogenitalism, obesity, poly-
dactylism, retinitis pigmentosa, and mental retarda-

tion. Associated congenital heart disease has been described,[264] with a recent report of pulmonic stenosis and ventricular septal defect.[265]

Ellis–van Creveld Syndrome

Chondrodysplasia, ectodermal dysplasia, polydactyly, and congenital heart disease constitute the Ellis–van Creveld syndrome.[266] A review of the literature shows that congenital heart disease is present in more than 50 per cent of cases and is usually the cause of death. There is an unusually high incidence of complex cardiac abnormalities; the occurrence of associated septal defects is common.[267-269]

Electrolyte Disorders

Electrocardiographic abnormalities may be associated with alterations and interactions of intracellular and extracellular fluid electrolytes. Alteration in the composition of the extracellular fluid surrounding cardiac muscle fibers may affect the centers of impulse initiation, the conduction system, or the repolarization process, producing cardiac arrhythmias, conduction abnormalities, etc.

The electrolyte levels in the fluid surrounding the myocardium may be altered before those of the blood; the electrocardiogram might therefore be presumed to be a more sensitive index of electrolyte imbalance than the serum-electrolyte levels. However, many other factors may produce significant electrocardiographic alterations; the function of the electrocardiogram in electrolyte disorders, therefore, is not to make an unequivocal diagnosis but to alert the physician to the possibility of electrolyte imbalance.[270] When electrolyte disturbances are expected, careful electrocardiographic monitoring often reveals the earliest manifestation of the anticipated change.

Sodium and potassium are the main substances responsible for altered myocardial electrical activity. Myocardial fiber potential is dependent on the high potassium and low sodium concentration in the resting myofiber and on the intracellular-to-extracellular gradient of these ions.[271] Alkalosis, insulin activity, and the level of serum glucose and serum calcium also exert an effect on the myocardium.

Hyperkalemia

The possibility of hyperkalemia and its cardiac complications should be considered in (1) untreated diabetic ketoacidosis, (2) adrenal cortical insufficiency, especially Addison's disease, (3) acute renal tubular necrosis (lower nephron nephrosis), (4) acute and chronic glomerulonephritis, (5) chronic pyelonephritis,[270] (6) potassium iodide or other potassium therapy, (7) extra-renal insufficiency of multiple causation, and (8) therapy with diuretic drugs such as spironolactone, triampterene, etc.

The earliest electrocardiographic manifestation of hyperkalemia is increased voltage and peaking of the T wave. This has been attributed to an absolute increase in extracellular potassium concentration but is probably more dependent upon the relationship of potassium and sodium ions. In the presence of a normal serum sodium, electrocardiographic evidence of hyperkalemia is extremely rare at serum-potassium levels below 7 mEq per liter; electrocardiographic alterations occur at lower levels of serum potassium when the serum-sodium concentration is low. Conversely, with high serum-sodium levels, the serum-potassium level may reach 7.5 mEq per liter before electrocardiographic changes of hyperkalemia appear. The lowered serum-sodium content often associated with severe acidosis augments the electrocardiographic abnormalities of hyperkalemia; hypocalcemia also accentuates the effect of hyperkalemia. Intravenous administration of saline, bicarbonate, glucose, insulin, or calcium tends to reverse the electrocardiographic abnormalities of hyperkalemia.

The usual electrocardiographic sequence in hyperkalemia[273-275] begins with increased amplitude and peaking of the T wave, seen at a potassium level of 7 to 9 mEq per liter; the T-wave amplitude often exceeds that of the R wave. With increased hyperkalemia, hyponatremia, or associated acidosis, there is widening of the QRS complex, due to abnormal intraventricular conduction. The combination of tall, symmetrical, peaked T waves, a wide QRS complex, and an S wave in the left precordial leads is characteristic of hyperkalemia.[270] At potassium levels greater than 9 mEq per liter, the P-R interval becomes prolonged, with loss or blending of the P wave into the preceding T wave; S-T segment changes occur; and there is progressive QRS widening, ending in a smooth, biphasic QRS-T wave. Rhythm disturbances such as supraventricular tachycardia, premature ventricular contractions, or atrial fibrillation may occur; there may be periods of sinus arrest with nodal or ventricular escape beats. The ventricular complexes next become abnormal, frequently resembling bundle branch block; by this time, atrial activity is usually absent. The ventricular rhythm may display periods of slow irregularity and of tachycardia, with and without further aberration in the ventricular complexes. With progression of the hyperkalemia beyond 10.5 mEq per liter, complete A-V dissociation, ventricular fibrillation, or cardiac arrest in diastole and death ensue.[276,277]

Hypokalemia

Significant lowering of the total body potassium may result from inadequate potassium intake; excessive loss from prolonged vomiting and diarrhea; attacks of familial periodic paralysis; and, rarely, renal loss in chronic nephritis. Therapy of diabetic ketoacidosis may cause hypokalemia,[278,279] as may overtreatment with desoxycorticosterone.[242,243,280]

Weakness, tachycardia, arrhythmia, hypotension, cardiac dilatation, hypoperistalsis, polyuria, kaliopenic nephropathy, and complicating pyelonephritis are encountered with a significant total body-potassium deficit; electrocardiographic abnormalities constitute the most common cardiovascular manifestations. The anatomic myocardial abnormalities of hypokalemia are described in Chap. 55.

The electrocardiographic changes of diminished extracellular fluid potassium concentration are probably due to electrolyte abnormality rather than to a pathologic degenerative lesion in the myocardium, as most electrocardiographic alterations are reversible with the administration of potassium.[281] Schwartz et al.,[282] however, found the electrocardiographic abnormalities in hypokalemia related neither to the total potassium deficit nor to the serum-potassium concentration. The electrocardiographic abnormalities of hypokalemia resemble those of so-called digitalis effect except that the Q-U interval is significantly prolonged in hypokalemia.[281] However, mechanical systole, as timed by phonocardiography, is either normal or shortened.[248]

Electrocardiographic abnormalities are common with a serum-potassium concentration below 3 mEq per liter[275] but do not occur predictably; the electrocardiogram is of diagnostic value primarily in advanced hypokalemia.[270] There is depression of the RS-T segment, with flattened or inverted T waves;[248] prominent U waves are common, occurring in about 40 per cent of cases.[283] The P-R interval may be prolonged, the P-wave amplitude increased, and the QRS complex increased in amplitude and duration in advanced hypokalemia.[270]

Hypokalemia may cause atrial and ventricular extrasystoles, paroxysmal tachycardia, atrial fibrillation or flutter, and disturbances of intraventricular and atrioventricular (A-V) conduction,[270] all of which subside with correction of the hypokalemia. Digitalis toxicity is more common in the presence of hypokalemia.

Hypercalcemia

Hypercalcemia is present in hyperparathyroidism, multiple myeloma, sarcoidosis, milk-alkali syndrome, hypervitaminosis D, etc. The serum-calcium level plays an important role in the regulation of cardiac excitability and cardiac contractility;[284] increased serum-calcium concentration causes increased myocardial contractility[285] with shortening of ventricular systole.[270]

In hypercalcemia, the shortening of the Q-T interval of the electrocardiogram is almost invariably present when the serum-calcium level is greater than 13 mg per 100 ml.[285]

Animal experiments have demonstrated T-wave changes and changes in A-V conduction at calcium levels of 15 to 65 mg per 100 ml, with increased automaticity often ending in ventricular fibrillation at levels of 25 to 90 mg per 100 ml; in animals surviving the increased automaticity phase, there is generalized depression with cardiac arrest at calcium levels of 70 to 190 mg per 100 ml.[286] These elevated calcium levels do not occur in clinical practice.

Hypocalcemia

Hypocalcemia may be encountered in hypoparathyroidism, intestinal malabsorption syndromes, uremia, acute pancreatitis, etc. Hypocalcemia causes diminished cardiac contractility.[287]

The most common electrocardiographic manifestation of hypocalcemia is prolongation of the Q-T interval;[247] this is, more specifically, S-T interval prolongation with a normal T-wave width, whereas in hypokalemia there is Q-U interval prolongation. The Q-T interval prolongation usually occurs with a serum-calcium level of less than 6 mg per 100 ml;[285] the prolongation is proportional to the degree of hypocalcemia and is of diagnostic value in the recognition of hypocalcemia. Mechanical systole, as measured by phonocardiography, is also prolonged, but not as much as the Q-T interval duration.[248] The R-R interval is shortened.[288]

Hypocalcemia may attenuate digitalis effect.[289] Hypokalemia may mask the signs and symptoms of hypocalcemic tetany; the tetanic manifestations correlate well with the serum-potassium level. With combined hypokalemia and hypocalcemia, the electrocardiographic abnormalities are characteristic of hypokalemia and are abolished by potassium rather than calcium administration.[290]

Hypermagnesemia

Vasodilatation with a rise in skin temperature, hypotension, decreased myocardial contractility, and decreased cardiac output occur in hypermagnesemia in animal experiments,[291] but the severe cardiotoxic effects of magnesium occur at serum levels incompatible with spontaneous respiration.[276] Magnesium depresses myocardial conduction and irritability.[292]

Studies in dogs have demonstrated tachycardia at a magnesium level of 2 to 5 mEq per liter, with the initial tachycardia progressing to bradycardia; at magnesium levels of 5 to 10 mEq per liter, the P-R interval is prolonged, and there is widening of the QRS complex. Sinoatrial (S-A) and A-V block appear with magnesium levels above 15 mEq per liter. Respiratory depression occurs at 17 to 27 mEq per liter, with cardiac arrest almost constant subsequent to the respiratory arrest, occurring at magnesium levels of 27 to 44 mEq per liter.[293]

Hypermagnesemia suppresses ventricular extrasytoles and other arrhythmias in animals and in man; this occurs in arrhythmias both related to and unrelated to digitalis toxicity. The clinical use of magnesium is limited by its transient action and its undesirable side effects.[292,294]

The heart has an unusual concentrating ability for magnesium[28] as compared with skeletal muscle, particularly in the area of the interventricular septum; the significance of this is as yet unknown.[295] In general, no clearly defined electrocardiographic abnormalities are encountered in hypermagnesemia within the range encountered in clinical situations in man.[270,275]

Hypomagnesemia

There are no distinctive electrocardiographic alterations in hypomagnesemia.[275]

Animal experiments show lipid deposition and atherogenesis to increase with magnesium deficiency and to decrease with high dietary levels of magnesium.[296,297] Although most studies are in animals, magnesium deficiency seems associated with an increased serum cholesterol, increased β-lipoproteins, and decreased α-lipoproteins.[298] There is an apparent inverse relationship in man between the serum-magnesium level and serum-cholesterol level; magnesium administration effects a return toward normal of an abnormal lipoprotein pattern.[299]

ATHEROSCLEROSIS AND ENDOCRINE DISEASE

Hormones may affect coronary artery disease by altering cholesterol and lipid metabolism, by altering vasomotor tone, by altering vascular tissue metabolism, and by changing vascular permeability.[300,301]

Diabetes Mellitus

Severe and premature atherosclerosis is encountered with unusual frequency in patients with diabetes mellitus.[302]

In diabetic patients over age forty coronary sclerosis, angina pectoris, and death from coronary artery disease is as common in women as in men.

Fatal myocardial infarction and coronary artery disease occur at least twice as commonly in diabetic as in nondiabetic men and three times as frequently in diabetic as in nondiabetic women.[303–305] Diabetes mellitus accelerates coronary atherosclerosis, with a more pronounced effect in the female than in the male.[303] A diabetic patient over age forty of either sex can be assumed to have significant coronary sclerosis, particularly if the diabetes is of long duration or associated with hypertension.[306–308] There is almost invariable atherosclerosis in patients with diabetes mellitus of over 5 years' duration.[301] Warren[309] described more severe atherosclerosis in the diabetic patient, with atherosclerotic lesions developing 10 to 12 years earlier than in nondiabetic persons. Significant symptomatic coronary atherosclerosis is not uncommon among young diabetic patients.[301]

Coronary artery disease, cerebrovascular disease, and peripheral vascular disease have constituted the main causes of death in diabetic patients since the advent of insulin therapy. The mortality rate from acute myocardial infarction is disproportionately high in diabetic patients, particularly in diabetic women; long-term survival after myocardial infarction is also decreased among diabetic patients.[310]

Hypertension, secondary to renal lesions, is frequently encountered among diabetic patients, particularly with disease of long duration. The congestive heart failure in diabetic patients probably results from both atherosclerotic heart disease and hypertensive cardiovascular disease.

Myxedema

Hypercholesterolemia, cardiac enlargement, and coronary atherosclerosis are frequently encountered in myxedema, but myxedema has its highest incidence at the age when atherosclerosis is most common. However, the significant atherosclerosis documented in young patients with endemic cretinism and goiter is suggestive of a relationship between thyroxin deficiency and atherosclerosis.[301]

Angina pectoris is uncommon in patients with untreated myxedema, but often appears at the onset of therapy. Cautious thyroid-hormone replacement is advocated in the myxedematous patient who develops angina pectoris during therapy, as myocardial infarction may supervene.[183]

Atherosclerosis can be produced or accelerated in animals by the induction of hypothyroidism and the feeding of excessive cholesterol;[36] this requires further study in the human being.[311]

d-Thyroxin administration to euthyroid men produces a variable, but significant reduction in serum-cholesterol levels; however, angina pectoris may occur, and the eventual effect on atherogenesis requires further study.[312] Desiccated thyroid hormone administration has a similar hypolipemic effect.[37,313,314]

Acromegaly

Myocardial hypertrophy in acromegaly is attributable both to excessive growth hormone and to hypertension; coronary atherosclerosis is a frequent complication.[204]

Cushing's Syndrome

Generalized vascular sclerosis and coronary artery disease are commonly encountered in Cushing's syndrome, even among young patients. Animal studies indicate that adrenal cortical hormones have a role in the regulation of serum-lipid and lipoprotein levels.[315] It remains questionable whether the atherosclerosis in man is a direct result of excessive adrenal steroid hormone secretion or whether it is related to the frequently associated diabetes mellitus, hypertension, and depression of thyroid function.[231]

Hydrocortisone, in physiologic doses, has a hypolipemic effect in man; the relationship to atherogenesis requires further study.[313,314]

Pheochromocytoma

Angina pectoris, cardiac hypertrophy, hypertension, and coronary atherosclerosis have been described in pheochromocytoma.[316] Cardiac enlargement is probably secondary to the hypertension, which may persist for a considerable period of time after the removal of the tumor.[317]

Primary Aldosteronism

Cardiac hypertrophy and severe atherosclerosis have been described in primary aldosteronism, but the cardiac complications of aldosteronism require further study.

Estrogen and Androgen

Most experimental data indicate that estrogen secretion is a major factor in the resistance of the premenopausal female to coronary atherosclerosis;[318,302] although several hormones apparently play a role in human atherogenesis, Kurland and Freedberg[311] believe that the evidence for the role of estrogen is the strongest. The incidence of clinical coronary artery disease in women is low before the menopause and increases rapidly thereafter;[301] surgically induced menopause accelerates the development of atherosclerosis.[319] However, Ritterband et al.[320] found no difference in the prevalence of atherosclerotic heart disease between oophorectomized women and a control group who had undergone hysterectomy; they suggested that factors other than ovarian function were responsible for the relative freedom of women from coronary heart disease.

Estrogen administration lowers the plasma-cholesterol level, the cholesterol/phospholipid ratio, and the β-lipoprotein fraction and increases the α-lipoprotein fraction; testosterone administration produces the reverse effects.[321,322] The effects of the sex hormones on serum-cholesterol levels are probably direct effects, not mediated by the thyroid.[323] The male preponderance in atherosclerosis is believed due both to a difference in lipid metabolism between the male and female and to the preventive effects of estrogen in the female. Castration in the female results in increased levels of plasma cholesterol.[301]

Synthetic estrogen compounds can alter serum-lipid and lipoprotein levels in man;[324] it has not yet been determined whether this prevents atherosclerosis.[325] No change in the clinical incidence of chest pain or in the electrocardiographic abnormalities was observed in hypercholesterolemic men with coronary artery disease treated with estrogenic substances.[321] There is no evidence to date to support the use of estrogen therapy in the management of clinical coronary artery disease.[326,327]

Coronary heart disease is uncommon in feeble-minded male castrates.[301,328] Eunuchs with androgen deficiency have hypotension and bradycardia, probably secondary to depression of the basal metabolic rate; they have a greater than normal increase in heart rate with exercise, probably secondary to their decrease in physical stamina.[210c]

Progeria

The Hutchinson-Gilford syndrome (childhood progeria), usually occurs at about the age of 1 year in a previously healthy infant; it is characterized by dwarfism, loss of hair and subcutaneous fat, and the precocious development of atherosclerosis.[329] The generalized arteriosclerosis is associated with hypertension, angina pectoris, myocardial infarction, cerebrovascular catastrophies, and early death.

Werner's syndrome (progeria of the adult) is characterized by premature senescence and diminished body growth (dwarfism). There are marked skin changes, cataracts, osteoporosis, and a variety of glandular dysfunctions, particularly hypogonadism. Severe generalized arteriosclerosis is present, with thickening, calcification, and occlusion of the coronary arteries, myocardial infarction, and cerebrovascular accidents. Electrocardiographic abnormalities are those associated with atherosclerotic heart disease and myocardial infarction.[330-333]

REFERENCES

1. Parry, C. H.: "Collections From the Unpublished Medical Writings of the Late Caleb H. Parry, M.D., vol. 2, Underwood, London, 1825, p. 111.

2. Graves, R. J.: Clinical Lectures, *London M. & S. J.*, **7**:516, 1835.

3. Von Basedow, C. A.: Exophthalmos durch Hypertrophie des Zellgewebes in der Augenhöhle, *Wchnschr. ges. Heilk.*, **6**:197, 220, 1840.

4. Lockridge, J. E.: On Graves' Disease or Cardiac Exophthalmic Goiter, *Am. Practitioner*, **19**:287–301, 1879.

5. Möbius, P. J.: "Die Basedow'sche Krankheit: Nothnagel's System," *Spec. Path. u. Therap.*, **22**:1, Alfred Hölder, Weiss, 1896.

6. Magee, H. R., and Smith, H. L.: Auricular Fibrillation in Hyperthyroidism: The Influence of Age, *Am. J. M. Sc.*, **189**:683–690, 1935.

7. Likoff, W. B., and Levine, S. A.: Thyrotoxicosis as the Sole Cause of Heart Failure, *Am. J. M. Sc.*, **206**:425–434, 1943.

8. Griswold, D., and Keating, J. H., Jr.: Cardiac Dysfunction in Hyperthyroidism: A Study of 810 Cases, *Am. Heart J.*, **38**:813–822, 1949.

9. Willius, F. A., Boothby, W. M., and Wilson, L. B.: The Behavior of the Heart in Exophthalmic Goiter and Adenomatous Goiter with Hyperthyroidism, *Tr. A. Am. Physicians*, **38**:137–145, 1923; and *M. Clin. North America*, **7**:189–219, 1923.

10. Lahey, F. H., and Hamilton, B. E.: Thyrocardiacs: Their Diagnostic Difficulties, Their Surgical Treatment. A Relatively New Field for Surgery, *Surg. Gynec. & Obst.*, **39**:10–14, 1924.

11. Lahey, F. H.: Thyroid Operations in Cardiac Disease, *S. Clin. North America*, **14**:1225–1234, 1934.

12. Hurxthal, L. M.: Heart Failure and Hyperthyroidism, with Special Reference to Etiology, *Am. Heart J.*, **4**:103–108, 1928–1929.

13. Maher, C. C., and Sittler, W. W.: The Cardiovascular State in Thyrotoxicosis, *J.A.M.A.*, **106**:1546–1557, 1936.

14. Friedberg, C. K., and Sohval, A. R.: The Occurrence and the Pathogenesis of Cardiac Hypertrophy in Graves' Disease, *Am. Heart J.*, **13**:599–618, 1937.

15. Logue, R. B.: Personal communication.

16. Schlesinger, P., and Benchimol, A. B.: The Pure Form of Thyrotoxic Heart Disease: A Clinical and Pathological Study, *Am. J. Cardiol.*, **2**:430–440, 1958.

17. Read, J. M.: Cardiac Status after Prolonged Thyrotoxicosis, *Am. Heart J.*, **8**:84–90, 1932–1933.

18. Summers, V. K., and Surtess, S. J.: Thyrotoxicosis and Heart Disease, *Acta med. scandinav.*, **169**:661–671, 1961.

19. McPhedran, H.: Cardiovascular Changes in Toxic Goiter, *Canad. M. A. J.*, **46**:471–474, 1942.

20. Andrus, E. C.: Heart Failure with Hyperthyroidism, *New York J. Med.*, **29**:661–662, 1929.

21. Hamilton, B. E.: Heart Failure of the Congestive Type Caused by Hyperthyroidism, *J.A.M.A.*, **83**:405–410, 1924.

22. Williams, R. H.: "Textbook of Endocrinology," 3d ed., W. B. Saunders Company, Philadelphia, 1962, (*a*) chap. 4; (*b*) chap. 2; (*c*) chap. 5.

23. Goh, K., and Dallam, R. D.: Oxygen Consumption of the Auricles, Right and Left Ventricles of the Normal, Hypothyroid and Hyperthyroid Rat Heart, *Am. J. Physiol.*, **188**:514–518, 1957.

24. Levey, H. A., and Roberts, S.: Influence of Thyroid Function on the Metabolism of the Anterior Pituitary Gland, *Am. J. Physiol.*, **189**:86–90, 1957.

25. Hoch, F. L., and Lipmann, F.: Uncoupling of Respiration and Phosphorylation by Thyroid Hormones, *Proc. Nat. Acad. Sc.*, **40**:909, 1954.

26. Austen, F. K., Rubini, M. E., Meroney, W. H., and Wolff, J.: Salicylates and Thyroid Function. I. Depression of Thyroid Function, *J. Clin. Invest.*, **37**:1131–1143, 1958.

27. Lehninger, A. L.: Thyroxine and the Swelling and Contraction Cycle in Mitochondria, *Ann. New York Acad. Sc.*, **86**:484–493, 1960.

28. Osorio, C., and Myant, N. B.: The Passage of Thyroid Hormone from Mother to Foetus and Its Relation to Foetal Development, *Brit. M. Bull.*, **16**:159–164, 1960.

29. Beznak, M., and Hajdu, J.: Über den Einfluss der Schilddrüse auf die Rolle der Hypophysein den Veränderungen des Herzmasse, *Schweiz. med. Wchnschr.*, **76**:390, 1946.

30. Herndon, E. G., Jr.: Unpublished data.

31. Ford, R. V., Owens, J. C., Curd, G. W., Moyer, J. H., and Spurr, C. L.: Kidney Function in Various Thyroid States, *J. Clin. Endocrinol.*, **21**:548–553, 1961.

32. Wayne, E. J.: Clinical and Metabolic Studies in Thyroid Disease, *Brit. M. J.*, **1**:78–90, 1960.

33. Rubini, M. E.: Personal communication.

34. Olson, R. E., and Piatnek, D. A.: Conservation of Energy in Cardiac Muscle, *Ann. New York Acad. Sc.*, **72**:466–479, 1959.

35. Leiter, L.: Metabolic Heart Disease, *Mod. Concepts Cardiovas. Dis.*, **26**:403–409, 1957.

36. Andrus, E. C.: The Thyroid and the Circulation, *Circulation*, **7**:437–444, 1953.

37. Moses, C., Sunder, J. H., Vester, J. W., and Danowski, T. S.: Hydrocortisone and/or Desiccated Thyroid in Physiologic Dosage. XI. Effects of Thyroid Hormone Excesses on Lipids and Other Blood and Serum Solutes, *Metabolism*, **13**:717–728, 1964.

38. Danowski, T. S., Rodnan, G. P., Sarver, M. E., and Moses, C.: Hydrocortisone and/or Desiccated Thyroid in Physiologic Dosage. XII. Effects of Thyroid Hormone Excesses on Urinary Solutes and Steroids, *Metabolism*, **13**:729–738, 1964.

39. Richardson, H. B., and Wolff, H. G.: The Nature of the Muscular Weakness in Graves' Disease, *J. Clin. Invest.*, **12**:966–967, 1933.

40. Whitehorn, W. V., Ullrick, W. C., and Andersen, B. R.: Properties of Hyperthyroid Rat Myocardium, *Circulation Res.*, **7**:250–255, 1959.

41. Fowler, N. O.: "Physical Diagnosis of Heart Dis-

ease," The Macmillan Company, New York, 1962, p. 478.

42. Schneckloth, R. E., Kurland, G. S., and Freedberg, A. S.: Effect of Variation in Thyroid Function on the Pressor Response to Norepinephrine in Man, *Metabolism*, 2:546–555, 1953.

43. Wiswell, J. G., Hurwitz, G. E., Coronho, V., Bing, O. H. L., and Child, D. L.: Urinary Catechol Amines and Their Metabolites in Hyperthyroidism and Hypothyroidism, *J. Clin. Endocrinol.*, **23**: 1102–1106, 1963.

44. Hoffmann, F., Hoffmann, E. J., and Talesnik, J.: Influence of the Thyroid Hormone on the Effector Systems of the Mammalian Heart, *Am. J. Physiol.*, **148**:689–699, 1947.

45. Danowski, T. S., Heineman, A. C., Jr., Bonessi, J. V., and Moses, C.: Hydrocortisone and/or Desiccated Thyroid in Physiologic Dosage. XIV. Effects of Thyroid Hormone Excesses on Pressor Activity and Epinephrine Responses, *Metabolism*, **13**:747–752, 1964.

46. Murray, J. F., and Kelly, J. J.: The Relation of Thyroidal Hormone Level to Epinephrine Response: A Diagnostic Test for Hyperthyroidism, *Ann. Int. Med.*, **51**:309–321, 1959.

47. Saphir, O.: Myocarditis: A General Review, with an Analysis of Two Hundred and Forty Cases, *A.M.A. Arch. Path.*, **33**:88–137, 1942.

48. Goodpasture, E. W.: The Influence of Thyroid Products on the Production of Myocardial Necrosis, *J. Exper. Med.*, **34**:407–423, 1921.

49. Hashimoto, H.: The Heart in Experimental Hyperthyroidism, with Special Reference to Its Histology, *Endocrinology*, **5**:579, 1921.

50. Nora, E. D., and Flaxman, N.: The Heart in Experimental Thyrotoxicosis, *J. Lab. & Clin. Med.*, **28**:797–808, 1942–1943.

51. Fahr, T.: Histologische Befunde am Kropfherzen, *Zentralbl. allg. Path.*, **27**:1–5, 1916.

52. Lewis, W.: The Question of a Specific Myocardial Lesion in Hyperthyroidism (Basedow's Disease), *Am. J. Path.*, **8**:255–261, 1932.

53. Weller, C. V., Wanstrom, R. C., Gordon, H., and Bugher, J. C.: Cardiac Histopathology in Thyroid Disease: Preliminary Report, *Am. Heart J.*, **8**:8–18, 1932–1933.

54. Lewis, W.: Hyperthyroidism and Associated Pathology, *Am. J. M. Sc.*, **181**:65–74, 1931.

55. Rake, G., and McEachern, D.: A Study of the Heart in Hyperthyroidism, *Am. Heart J.*, **8**:19–23, 1932–1933.

56. Keeton, R. W.: The Heart and Circulation in Patients with Hyperthyroidism, *Surgery*, **16**:657–667, 1944.

57. Rake, G., and McEachern, D.: Experimental Hyperthyroidism and Its Effect upon the Myocardium in Guinea Pigs and Rabbits, *J. Exper. Med.*, **54**: 23–30, 1931.

58. McEachern, D., and Rake, G.: A Study of the

Morbid Anatomy of Hearts from Patients Dying with Hyperthyroidism, *Bull. Johns Hopkins Hosp.*, **48**:273–314, 1931.

59. Gould, S. E.: "Pathology of the Heart," 2d ed., Charles C Thomas, Publisher, Springfield, Ill., 1960, pp. 524–525.

60. Markowitz, C., and Yater, W. M.: Response of Explanted Cardiac Muscle to Thyroxine, *Am. J. Physiol.*, **100**:162–166, 1932.

61. Bing, R. J.: Metabolic Activity of the Intact Heart, *Am. J. Med.*, **30**:679–691, 1961.

62. Andrus, E. C.: The Heart in Hyperthyroidism: A Clinical and Experimental Study, *Am. Heart J.*, **8**: 66–74, 1932–1933.

63. Moses, L. E.: Mechanism of the Effect of Hyperthyroidism on Cardiac Glycogen, *Am. J. Physiol.*, **142**:686–699, 1944.

64. McDonald, C. H., Boyle, R. W., and DeGroat, A. F.: Hyperthyroidism and Cardiac Glycogen, *Am. J. Physiol.*, **124**:742–749, 1938.

65. Rowe, G., Huston, J. H., Weinstein, A. B., and Crumpton, C. W.: Coronary Blood Flow, Cardiac Work, and Myocardial Metabolism in Thyrotoxicosis Before and After Treatment, *J. Lab. & Clin. Med.*, **44**:921, 1954.

66. Rowe, G. G., Huston, J. H., Weinstein, A. B., Tuchman, H., Brown, J. F., Crumpton, C. W., Peterson, A., Welch, B., and Fosshage, P.: The Hemodynamics of Thyrotoxicosis in Man, with Special Reference to Coronary Blood Flow and Myocardial Oxygen Metabolism, *J. Clin. Invest.*, **35**:272–276, 1956.

67. Graettinger, J. S., Muenster, J. J., Checchia, C. S., and Campbell, J. A.: Correlation of Clinical and Hemodynamic Studies in Patients with Thyroid Disease, *Clin. Res. Proc.*, **4**:120, 1956.

68. Humerfelt, S., Müller, O., and Storstein, O.: The Circulation in Hyperthyroidism: A Cardiac Catheterization Study Before and After Treatment, *Am. Heart J.*, **56**:87–94, 1958.

69. Judson, W. E.: Cardiovascular Renal Regulation in the Hyperkinetic States, *Progr. Cardiovas. Dis.*, **4**:65–87, 1961–1962.

70. Graettinger, J. S., Muenster, J. J., Selverstone, L. A., and Campbell, J. A.: A Correlation of Clinical and Hemodynamic Studies in Patients with Hyperthyroidism with and without Congestive Heart Failure, *J. Clin. Invest.*, **38**:1316–1327, 1959.

71. Brewster, W. R., Jr., James, P. I., Osgood, A. B., and King, T. L.: The Hemodynamic and Metabolic Interrelationships in the Activity of Epinephrine, Norepinephrine and the Thyroid Hormones, *Circulation*, **13**:1–20, 1956.

72. McGee, R. R., Whittaker, R. L., and Tullis, I. F.: Apathetic Thyroidism: Review of the Literature and Report of Four Cases, *Ann. Int. Med.*, **50**: 1418–1432, 1959.

73. Liljestrand, G., and Stenstrom, N.: Clinical Studies on the Work of the Heart During Rest. I. Blood

Flow and Blood Pressure in Exophthalmic Goiter, *Acta med. scandinav.*, 63:99–129, 1925–1926.

74. Yater, W. M.: Symposium on the Thyroid Heart, *Am. Heart J.*, 8:1–7, 1932–1933.

75. Bishop, J. M., Donald, K. W., and Wade, O. L.: Circulatory Dynamics at Rest and on Exercise in the Hyperkinetic States, *Clin. Sc.*, 14:329–360, 1955.

76. DeGroot, W. J., Leonard, J. J., Paley, H. W., and Warren, J. V.: Observations on Stroke Volume and Ventricular Dynamics in Hyperthyroidism and Their Modification by Reserpine Administration, *J. Lab. & Clin. Med.*, 56:803, 1960.

77. Abrahamsen, A. M., Haarstad, J., and Oulie, C.: Haemodynamic Studies in Thyrotoxicosis Before and After Treatment, *Acta med. scandinav.*, 174:463–467, 1963.

77a. Goldstein, S., and Killip, T.: Catecholamine Depletion in Thyrotoxicosis. Effect of Guanethidine on Cardiovascular Dynamics, *Circulation*, 31:219–227, 1965.

78. Boothby, W. M., and Rynearson, E. H.: Increase in Circulation Rate Produced by Exophthalmic Goiter, *A.M.A. Arch. Int. Med.*, 55:547–557, 1935.

79. Sandler, G., and Wilson, G. M.: The Nature and Prognosis of Heart Disease in Thyrotoxicosis: A Review of 150 Patients Treated with I[131], *Quart. J. Med.*, n.s., 28:347–369, 1959.

80. Eichna, L. W., and Wilkins, R. W.: Blood Flow to the Forearm and Calf. IV. Thyroid Activity: Observations on the Relation of Blood Flow to Basal Metabolic Rate, *Bull. Johns Hopkins Hosp.*, 68:512–521, 1941.

81. Muldowney, F. P., Crooks, J., and Wayne, E. J.: The Total Red Cell Mass in Thyrotoxicosis and Myxoedema, *Clin. Sc.*, 16:309–314, 1957.

82. Blumgart, H. L., Gargill, S. L., and Gilligan, D. R.: The Circulatory Response to Thyrotoxicosis, *J. Clin. Invest.*, 9:69–89, 1930–1931.

83. Stewart, H. J., and Evans, W. F.: The Peripheral Blood Flow in Ten Women Exhibiting Graves' Disease, *J. Mt. Sinai Hosp. New York*, 8:1051–1059, 1941–1942.

84. Thomas, H. M., Jr.: Effect of Thyroid Hormone on Circulation, *J.A.M.A.*, 163:337–341, 1957.

85. Strong, J. A.: Thyrotoxicosis with Ophthalmoplegia, Myopathy, Wolff-Parkinson-White Syndrome, and Pericardial Friction Rub, *Lancet*, 1:959–961, 1949.

86. Lerman, J., and Means, J. H.: Cardiovascular Symptomatology in Exophthalmic Goiter, *Am. Heart J.*, 8:55–65, 1932–1933.

87. Allison, H. W., and Bliss, T. L.: Protein-bound Blood Iodine in Cardiovascular Disease, *Ann. Int. Med.*, 39:326–332, 1953.

88. Bortin, M. M., Silver, S., and Yohalem, S. B.: Diagnosis of Masked Hyperthyroidism in Cardiac Patients with Auricular Fibrillation, *Am. J. Med.*, 11:40–43, 1951.

89. Schorr, E., Richardson, H. B., and Wolff, H. G.: Endogenous Glycine Formation in Myopathies and Graves' Disease, *Proc. Soc. Exper. Biol. & Med.*, 31:207–209, 1933.

90. Peters, J. P.: Water Exchange, *Physiol. Rev.*, 24:491–531, 1944.

91. Somerville, W., and Levine, S. A.: Angina Pectoris and Thyrotoxicosis, *Brit. Heart J.*, 12:245–257, 1950.

92. Kuševelvskji, B. P., and Gurova, A. M.: Anginal Syndrome in Thyrotoxicosis, *Abstr. World Med.*, 27:48, 1960.

93. Lev, M. W., and Hamburger, W. W.: Studies in Thyroid Heart Disease. II. Angina Pectoris and Hyperthyroidism, *Am. Heart J.*, 8:109–113, 1932–1933.

94. Littman, D. S., Jeffers, W. A., and Rose, E.: The Infrequency of Myocardial Infarction in Patients with Thyrotoxicosis, *Am. J. M. Sc.*, 233:10–15, 1957.

95. Grytting, G., and Salvesen, H. A.: Thyrotoxicosis and Myocardial Infarction, *Acta med. scandinav.*, 157:169–171, 1957.

96. Burstein, J., Lamberg, B. A., and Erämaa, E.: Myocardial Infarction in Thyrotoxicosis, *Acta med. scandinav.*, 166:379–393, 1960.

97. Boas, E. P.: The Heart Rate During Sleep in Graves' Disease and in Neurogenic Sinus Tachycardia, *Am. Heart J.*, 8:24–28, 1932–1933.

98. Crooks, J., and Murray, I. P. C.: The Sleeping Pulse Rate in Thyrotoxicosis, *Scot. M. J.*, 3:120–122, 1958.

99. Danowski, T. S., Sarver, M. E., D'Ambrosia, R. D., and Moses, C.: Hydrocortisone and/or Desiccated Thyroid in Physiologic Dosage. X. Effects of Thyroid Hormone Excesses on Clinical Status and Thyroid Indices, *Metabolism*, 13:702–716, 1964.

100. Berteau, B. A., Engstrom, W. W., and Engbring, N. H.: Cardiac Complications in Patients with Nontoxic and Toxic Nodular Goiter and with Graves' Disease, *J. Lab. & Clin. Med.*, 52:687–693, 1958.

101. Ernstene, A. C.: The Cardiovascular Complications of Hyperthyroidism, *Am. J. M. Sc.*, 195:248–256, 1938.

102. Barker, P. S., Bohning, A. L., and Wilson, F. N.: Auricular Fibrillation in Graves' Disease, *Am. Heart J.*, 8:121–127, 1932–1933.

103. Bisgard, J. D.: Relation of Hyperthyroidism to Hypertension, *A.M.A. Arch. Int. Med.*, 63:497–503, 1939.

104. Myers, J. D., Brannon, E. S., and Holland, B. C.: A Correlative Study of the Cardiac Output and the Hepatic Circulation in Hyperthyroidism, *J. Clin. Invest.*, 29:1069–1077, 1950.

105. Selenkow, H. A., and Marcus, F. I.: Masked Hyperthyroidism and Heart Disease, *M. Clin. North America*, 44:1305–1322, 1960.

106. Greenberg, S. U., Rosenkrantz, J. A., and Beranbaum, S. L.: Prominence of the Left Mid-cardiac

Segment in Thyrotoxicosis as Visualized by Roentgen Studies, *Am. J. M. Sc.*, **224**:559–564, 1952.

107. Margolies, A., Rose, E., and Wood, F. C.: The Heart in Thyroid Disease. I. The Effect of Thyroidectomy on the Orthodiagram, *J. Clin. Invest.*, **14**:483–496, 1935.

108. Evans, W.: The Heart in Endocrine Disease, *Proc. Roy. Soc. Med.*, **42**:331–342, 1949.

109. Blizzard, J. J., and Rupp, J. J.: Prolongation of the P-R Interval as a Manifestation of Thyrotoxicosis, *J.A.M.A.*, **173**:1845, 1960.

110. Rosenblum, R., and Delman, A. J.: First-degree Heart Block Associated with Thyrotoxicosis, *Arch. Int. Med.*, **112**:488–490, 1963.

111. Hoffman, I., and Lowrey, R. D.: The Electrocardiogram in Thyrotoxicosis, *Am. J. Cardiol.*, **6**: 893–904, 1960.

112. Sandler, G.: The Effect of Thyrotoxicosis on the Electrocardiogram, *Brit. Heart J.*, **21**:111–116, 1959.

112*a*. Braunwald, E., Mason, D. T., and Ross, J., Jr.: Studies on the Cardiocirculatory Actions of Digitalis, *Medicine*, **44**:233–248, 1965.

113. Stanbury, J. B.: The Thyroid Gland in Relation to Heart Disease, *Mod. Concepts Cardiovas. Dis.*, **21**: 134–137, 1952.

114. Maloof, F., and Chapman, E. M.: Responses to Radioactive Iodine Therapy in Hyperthyroidism, with Special Reference to Cardiac Problems, *J. Clin. Endocrinol.*, **11**:1296–1322, 1951.

115. Delit, C., Silver, S., Yohalem, S. B., and Segal, R. L.: Thyrocardiac Disease and Its Management with Radioactive Iodine I131, *J.A.M.A.*, **176**:262–267, 1961.

116. Zondek, H.: Das Myxödemherz, *München. med. Wchnschr.*, **65**:1180–1182, 1918.

117. Fahr, G.: Myxedema Heart, *J.A.M.A.*, **84**:345–349, 1925.

118. Fahr, G.: Myxedema Heart: A Report Based upon a Study of 17 Cases of Myxedema, *Am. Heart J.*, **8**:91–101, 1932–1933.

119. Zondek, H.: Association of Myxedema Heart and Arteriosclerotic Heart Disease, *J.A.M.A.*, **170**:1920–1921, 1959.

120. Means, J. H., White, P. D., and Krantz, C. I.: Observations on the Heart in Myxedema, with Special Reference to Dilatation and Angina Pectoris, *Boston M. & S. J.*, **195**:455–460, 1926.

121. McGavack, T. H., Lange, K., and Schwimmer, D.: Management of the Myxedematous Patient with Symptoms of Cardiovascular Disease, *Am. Heart J.*, **29**:421–439, 1945.

122. Marks, P. A., and Roof, B. S.: Pericardial Effusion Associated with Myxedema, *Ann. Int. Med.*, **39**: 230–240, 1953.

123. Gordon, A. H.: Pericardial Effusion in Myxedema, *Tr. A. Am. Physicians*, **50**:272–277, 1935.

124. Hallock, P.: The Heart in Myxedema, with a Report of Two Cases, *Am. Heart J.*, **9**:196–211, 1933–1934.

125. Blumgart, H. L., Freedberg, A. S., and Kurland, G. S.: Treatment of Incapacitated Euthyroid Cardiac Patients with Radioactive Iodine, *J.A.M.A.*, **157**:1–4, 1955.

126. Sul'e, E. V.: The Functional State of the Thyroid Gland in Cases of Cardiovascular Insufficiency, *Abstr. World Med.*, **21**:118, 1957.

127. Brewer, D. B.: Myxedema: An Autopsy Report with Histochemical Observations on the Nature of the Mucoid Infiltrations, *J. Path. & Bact.*, **63**:503–512, 1951.

128. Douglass, R. C., and Jacobson, S. D.: Pathologic Changes in Adult Myxedema: Survey of 10 Necropsies, *J. Endocrinol. & Metab.*, **17**:1354–1364, 1957.

129. Lufkin, N. H.: Pathologic Changes in the Heart in Myxedema, *The Journal Lancet* **60**:41, 1940 (Abstract).

130. La Due, J. S.: Myxedema Heart: A Pathological and Therapeutic Study, *Ann. Int. Med.*, **18**:332–344, 1943.

131. Higgins, W. H.: The Heart in Myxedema: Correlation of Physical and Postmortem Findings, *Am. J. M. Sc.*, **191**:80–88, 1936.

132. Malmros, H., and Swahn, B.: Lipid Metabolism in Myxedema, *Acta med. scandinav.*, **145**:361–365, 1953.

133. Bartels, E. C., and Bell, G.: Myxedema and Coronary Sclerotic Heart Disease, *Tr. Am. A. Study of Goiter*, 5–15, 1939.

134. Kern, R. A., Soloff, L. A., Snape, W. J., and Bello, C. T.: Pericardial Effusion: A Constant, Early and Major Factor in the Cardiac Syndrome of Hypothyroidism (Myxedema Heart), *Am. J. M. Sc.*, **217**:609–618, 1949.

135. Lerman, J., Clark, R. J., and Means, J. H.: The Heart in Myxedema: Electrocardiograms and Roentgen-ray Measurements before and after Therapy, *Ann. Int. Med.*, **6**:1251–1271, 1933.

136. Lerman, J., Clark, R. J., and Means, J. H.: Further Observations on the Heart in Myxedema, *Ann. Int. Med.*, **8**:82–84, 1934–1935.

137. Lange, K.: Capillary Permeability in Myxedema, *Am. J. M. Sc.*, **208**:5–15, 1944.

138. Scheinberg, P., Stead, E. A., Jr., Brannon, E. S., and Warren, J. V.: Correlative Observations on Cerebral Metabolism and Cardiac Output in Myxedema, *J. Clin. Invest.*, **29**:1139–1146, 1950.

139. Stewart, H. J., and Evans, W. F.: The Peripheral Blood Flow in Myxedema as Compared with That in Hyperthyroidism, *Am. Heart J.*, **23**:175–184, 1942.

140. Ellis, L. B., Mebane, J. G., Maresh, G., Hultgren, H. N., and Bloomfield, R. A.: The Effect of Myxedema on the Cardiovascular System, *Am. Heart J.*, **43**:341–356, 1952.

141. Scott, J. C., Balourdas, T. A., and Croll, M. N.: The Effect of Experimental Hypothyroidism on Coronary Blood Flow and Hemodynamic Factors, *Am. J. Cardiol.*, **7**:690–693, 1961.

142. Graettinger, J. S., Muenster, J. J., Checchia, C. S., Grissom, R. L., and Campbell, J. A.: A Correlation of Clinical and Hemodynamic Studies in Patients with Hypothyroidism, *J. Clin. Invest.*, **37**:502–510, 1958.

143. Macy, J. W., Claiborne, S., and Hurxthal, L. M.: The Circulation Rate in Relation to Metabolism in Thyroid and Pituitary States (Decholin Method), *J. Clin. Invest.*, **15**:37–40, 1936.

144. Stewart, H. J., Dietrick, J. E., and Crane, N. F.: Studies of the Circulation in Patients Suffering from Spontaneous Myxedema, *J. Clin. Invest.*, **17**:237–248, 1938.

145. Thompson, W. O.: Studies in Blood Volume. I. The Blood Volume in Myxedema, with a Comparison of Plasma Volume Changes in Myxedema and Cardiac Edema, *J. Clin. Invest.*, **2**:477–520, 1925–1926.

146. Gibson, J. G., and Harris, A. W.: Clinical Studies of the Blood Volume. V. Hyperthyroidism and Myxedema, *J. Clin. Invest.*, **18**:59–65, 1939.

147. Barnes, B. O.: A New Approach to Hypertension and Arteriosclerosis, *Fed. Proc.*, **18**:8, 1959.

148. King, W. E.: Medical Aspects of Thyroid Disease, *M. J. Australia*, **2**:821–823, 1958.

149. Bakker, P. B. D., Sundermeyer, J. F., Wendt, V. C., Salhaney, M., Gudbjarnason, S., and Bing, R. J.: Myocardial Metabolism in a Patient with Hashimoto's Thyroiditis and Hypothyroidism, *Am. J. Med.*, **34**:822–826, 1962.

150. Werner, S. C.: "The Thyroid," 2d ed., Harper & Row, Publishers, Incorporated, New York, 1962, (*a*) chap. 42; (*b*) chap. 14.

151. Dorney, E. R.: Personal communication.

152. Howell, L. P.: The Heart in Myxedema: Report of a Case, *Proc. Staff Meet. Mayo Clin.*, **20**:250–256, 1945.

153. Watson, C. J., Graig, D., and Beach, N.: Myxedematous Ascites, *New Internat. Clin.*, **4**:176–182, 1941.

154. Harrell, G. T., and Johnston, C.: Pericardial Effusion in Myxedema, *Am. Heart J.*, **25**:505–511, 1943.

155. Weyher, R. F.: Myxedema Heart: Advanced Failure with Rapid Recovery, *J.A.M.A.*, **153**:639–642, 1953.

156. McBrien, D. J., and Hindle, W.: Myxoedema and Heart Failure, *Lancet*, **1**:1066–1068, 1963.

157. Schnitzer, R., and Gutmann, D.: Myxoedema with Pericardial Effusion, *Brit. Heart J.*, **8**:25–28, 1946.

158. Marzullo, E. R., and Franco, S.: Myxedema with Multiple Serous Effusions and Cardiac Involvement (Myxedema Heart), *Am. Heart J.*, **17**:368–374, 1939.

159. Feasby, W. R.: Pericardial Effusion in Myxedema: Report of a Case in Which the Intrapericardial Pressure Was Measured, *Am. Heart J.*, **19**:749–754, 1940.

160. Hamilton, J. D., and Greenwood, W. F.: Myxedema Heart Disease, *Circulation*, **15**:442–447, 1957.

161. Schmidt, S.: Pericardial Effusion in Myxoedema (Myxoedema Heart), *Brit. J. Radiol.*, **25**:389–390, 1952.

162. Bruger, M., and Rosenkrantz, J. A.: Arteriosclerosis and Hypothyroidism: Observations on Their Possible Interrelationship, *J. Clin. Endocrinol.*, **2**:176–180, 1942.

163. Blumgart, H. L., Freedberg, A. S., and Kurland, G. S.: Hypercholesterolemia, Myxedema, and Arteriosclerosis, *Tr. A. Am. Physicians*, **65**:114–120, 1952.

164. Hamolsky, M. W., Kurland, G. S., and Freedberg, A. S.: The Heart in Hypothyroidism, *J. Chron. Dis.*, **14**:558–569, 1961.

165. Baker, S. M., and Hamilton, J. D.: Capillary Changes in Myxedema, *Lab. Invest.*, **6**:218–226, 1957.

166. Nikkilä, E. A., and Karlsson, K.: Thyroid Function and Clinical Coronary Heart Disease, *Acta med. scandinav.*, **166**:195–203, 1960.

167. Kountz, W. B., and Hempelmann, L. H.: Chromatrophic Degeneration and Rupture of the Aorta Following Thyroidectomy in Cases of Hypertension, *Am. Heart J.*, **20**:599–610, 1940.

168. Levine, H. J., and Levine, S. A.: Myxedema Ascites: Report of Two Cases, *Am. Heart J.*, **60**:456–463, 1960.

169. Ferayorni, R. R., and Sprague, R. G.: Myxedema with Ascites and Hydrothorax: Report of Case, *Proc. Staff Meet. Mayo Clin.*, **27**:25–28, 1952.

170. Kurland, G. S., Schneckloth, R. E., and Freedberg, A. S.: The Heart in I[131]-induced Myxedema: Comparison of the Roentgenographic and Electrocardiographic Findings before and after the Induction of Myxedema, *New England J. Med.*, **249**:215–222, 1953.

171. Reid, W. D., and Kenway, F. L.: Electrocardiographic Signs Associated with Low Basal Metabolism, *Endocrinology*, **13**:191–204, 1929.

172. Aber, C. P., and Thompson, G. S.: Factors Associated with Cardiac Enlargement in Myxedema, *Brit. Heart J.*, **25**:421–424, 1963.

173. Hansen, J. E.: Paroxysmal Ventricular Tachycardia Associated with Myxedema: A Case Report, *Am. Heart J.*, **61**:692–697, 1961.

174. Lee, J. K., and Lewis, J. A.: Myxoedema with Complete AV Block and Adams-Stokes Disease Abolished with Thyroid Medication, *Brit. Heart J.*, **24**:253–256, 1962.

175. Schlesinger, B., and Landtman, B.: Electrocardiographic Studies in Cretins, *Brit. Heart J.*, **11**:237–248, 1949.

176. Ljung, O.: Mild Hypothyreosis Causing Electrocardiographic Changes Suggesting Coronary Insufficiency, *Acta med. scandinav.*, **137**:120–129, 1950.

177. Zondek, H.: The Electrocardiogram in Myxoedema, *Brit. Heart J.*, **26**:227–232, 1964.

178. Starr, P., and Liebhold-Schueck, R.: The Effect

of Levothyroxine, Dextrothyroxine and Levo-tri-iodo-thyronine on the Electrocardiogram in Myxedema: Preliminary Report, *Ann. Int. Med.*, **42**:595–606, 1955.

179. Urschel, D. L., and Gates, G. E.: Mean Spatial Vectorcardiography: The T Vector Changes in Hypothyroidism, *Am. Heart J.*, **45**:611–622, 1953.

180. Peel, A. A. F.: Anginal Pain in Myxoedema, *Brit. Heart J.*, **5**:89–96, 1943.

181. Keating, F. R., Jr., Parkin, T. W., Selby, J. B., and Dickinson, L. S.: Treatment of Heart Disease Associated with Myxedema, *Progr. Cardiovas. Dis.*, **3**:364–381, 1960–1961.

182. Bjerkelund, C. J.: Hjerteinfarkt under Thyroxinbehandling AV Myxodem, *Nord. med.*, **47**:827–828, 1952.

183. Smyth, C. H.: Angina Pectoris and Myocardial Infarction as Complications of Myxedema, with Especial Reference to the Danger of Treatment with Thyroid Preparations, *Am. Heart J.*, **15**:652–660, 1938.

184. Wallach, E. E., Lubash, G. D., Cohen, B. D., and Rubin, A. L.: Cardiac Disease and Hypothyroidism: Complications Induced by Initial Thyroid Therapy, *J.A.M.A.*, **167**:1921–1924, 1958.

185. Gibson, P. C.: Control of Treatment in Myxoedema by Electrocardiography, *Lancet*, **1**:128–131, 1958.

186. Li, C. H.: Studies on Human Pituitary Growth and Gonadotropic Hormones, in "Human Pituitary Hormones," Ciba Foundation Colloquia on Endocrinology, 13, 1960, pp. 46–67.

187. Wilhelmi, A. E.: Personal communication.

188. Haynes, R. C., and Berthet, L.: Studies on the Mechanism of Action of the Adrenocorticotropic Hormone, *J. Biol. Chem.*, **225**:115–124, 1957.

189. Read, C. H., and Bryan, G. T.: Immunological Studies of Human Growth Hormone, in "Human Pituitary Hormones," Ciba Foundation Colloquia on Endocrinology, 13, 1960, pp. 68–88.

190. Raben, M. S., and Hollenberg, C. H.: Growth Hormone and the Mobilization of Fatty Acids, in "Human Pituitary Hormones," Ciba Foundation Colloquia on Endocrinology, 13, 1960, pp. 89–105.

191. Cushing, H.: The Basophil Adenomas of the Pituitary Body and Their Clinical Manifestations (Pituitary Basophilism), *Bull. Johns Hopkins Hosp.*, **50**:137–195, 1932.

192. Sprague, R. G., Randall, R. V., Salassa, R. M., Scholz, D. A., Priestley, J. T., Walters, W., and Bulbulian, A. H.: Cushing's Syndrome, a Progressive and Often Fatal Disease: A Review of 100 Cases Seen Between July 1945 and July 1954 (Scientific Exhibit), *A.M.A. Arch. Int. Med.*, **98**:389–397, 1956.

193. Eisenhardt, L., and Thompson, K. W.: A Brief Consideration of the Present Status of So-called Pituitary Basophilism, with a Tabulation of Verified Cases, *Yale J. Biol. & Med.*, **11**:507–522, 1938–1939.

194. Cope, O., and Raker, J. W.: Cushing's Disease: The Surgical Experience in the Care of 46 Cases, *New England J. Med.*, **253**:119–127, 1955.

195. Scholz, D. A., Sprague, R. G., and Kernohan, J. W.: Cardiovascular and Renal Complications of Cushing's Syndrome: A Clinical and Pathological Study of Seventeen Cases, *New England J. Med.*, **256**:833–837, 1957.

196. MacMahon, H. E., Close, H. G., and Hass, G.: Cardiovascular Renal Changes Associated with Basophil Adenoma of the Anterior Lobe of the Pituitary (Cushing's Syndrome), *Am. J. Path.*, **10**:177–191, 1934.

197. Liddle, G. W., Estep, H. L., Kendall, J. W., Williams, W. C., Jr., and Townes, A. W.: Clinical Application of a New Test of Pituitary Reserve, *J. Clin. Endocrinol.*, **19**:875–894, 1959.

198. Liddle, G. W.: Tests of Pituitary-Adrenal Suppressibility in the Diagnosis of Cushing's Syndrome, *J. Clin. Endocrinol.*, **20**:1539–1560, 1960.

199. Gold, E. M., Kent, J. R., and Forsham, P. H.: Clinical Use of a New Diagnostic Agent, Methopyrapone (SU-4885), in Pituitary and Adrenocortical Disorders, *Ann. Int. Med.*, **54**:175–188, 1961.

200. Huchard, H.: Anatomie pathologique, lésions et troubles cardiovasculaires de l'acromégalie, *J. praticiens*, **9**:249, 1895.

201. Fournier, J. B. C.: "Acromégalie et troubles cardiovasculaires," Thesis, Paris, no. 111, 1896.

202. Courville, C., and Mason, V. R.: The Heart in Acromegaly, *A.M.A. Arch. Int. Med.*, **61**:704–713, 1938.

203. Humphry, L., and Dixon, W. E.: A Case of Acromegaly with Hypertrophied Heart: Pressor Substances in the Urine, *Brit. M. J.*, **2**:1047–1049, 1910.

204. Cushing, H., and Davidoff, L. M.: "The Pathological Findings in Four Autopsied Cases of Acromegaly, with a Discussion of Their Significance," Rockefeller Institute for Medical Research, Monograph 22, New York, 1927.

205. Hejtmancik, M. R., Bradfield, J. Y., Jr., and Herrmann, G. R.: Acromegaly and the Heart: A Clinical and Pathologic Study, *Ann. Int. Med.*, **34**:1445–1456, 1951.

206. Herrmann, G. R., and Hejtmancik, M. R.: The Heart in Acromegaly: A Clinical and Pathologic Study, *Acta med. scandinav.*, Suppl. 256–36:171–180, 1951.

207. Bigland, B., and Jehring, B.: Muscle performance in Rats, Normal and Treated with Growth Hormone, *J. Physiol.*, **116**:129–136, 1952.

200. Kellgren, J. H., Ball, J., and Tutton, G. K.: The Articular and Other Limb Changes in Acromegaly: A Clinical and Pathological Study of 25 Cases, *Quart. J. Med.*, **45**:405–424, 1952.

209. Hamwi, G. J., Skillman, T. G., and Tufts, K. C.: Acromegaly, *Am. J. Med.*, **29**:690–699, 1960.

210. Soffer, L. J.: "Diseases of the Endocrine Glands,"

2d ed., Lea & Febiger, Philadelphia, 1956, (*a*) chap. 4; (*b*) chap. 11; (*c*) chap. 17.

211. Cluxton, H. E., Jr., Bennett, W. A., and Kepler, E. J.: Anterior Pituitary Insufficiency (Panhypopituitarism—Simmonds' Disease), Pituitary Myxedema and Congestive Heart Failure (Myxedema Heart): Report of Case and Findings at Necropsy, *Ann. Int. Med.,* **29:**732–745, 1948.

212. Lown, B., Arons, W. L., Ganong, W. F., Vazifdar, J. P., and Levine, S. A.: Adrenal Steroids and Auriculoventricular Conduction, *Am. Heart J.,* **50:** 760–769, 1955.

213. August, J. T., Nelson, D. H., and Thorn, G. W.: Aldosterone, *New England J. Med.,* **259:**917–923, 967–971, 1958.

214. Laragh, J. H.: The Role of Aldosterone in Man: Evidence for Regulation of Electrolyte Balance and Arterial Pressure by a Renal-Adrenal System Which May Be Involved in Malignant Hypertension, *J.A.M.A.,* **174:**293–295, 1960.

215. Zwemer, R. L., and Truszkowski, R.: The Importance of Cortico-Adrenal Regulation of Potassium Metabolism, *Endocrinology,* **21:**40–49, 1937.

216. Conn, J. W.: Part II. Primary Aldosteronism, a New Clinical Syndrome, *J. Lab. & Clin. Med.,* **45:**6–17, 1955.

217. Bornstein, P., Nolan, J. P., and Bernanke, D.: Adrenocortical Hyperfunction in Association with Anaplastic Carcinoma of the Respiratory Tract, *New England J. Med.,* **264:**363–371, 1961.

218. Adlersberg, D., Schaefer, L. E., and Dritch, R.: Adrenal Cortex and Lipid Metabolism: Effects of Cortisone and Adrenocorticotropin (ACTH) on Serum Lipids in Man, *Proc. Soc. Exper. Biol. & Med.,* **74:**877–879, 1950.

219. Adlersberg, D., Schaefer, L. E., and Wang, C. I.: Adrenal Cortex, Lipid Metabolism, and Atherosclerosis: Experimental Studies in the Rabbit, *Science,* **120:**319–320, 1954.

220. Russell, D. S., Evans, H., and Crooke, A. C.: Two Cases of Basophil Adenoma of the Pituitary Gland, *Lancet,* **2:**240–246, 1934.

221. Plotz, C. M., Knowlton, A. I., and Ragan, C.: The Natural History of Cushing's Syndrome, *Am. J. Med.,* **13:**597–614, 1952.

222. Hurxthal, L. M., and O'Sullivan, J. B.: Cushing's Syndrome: Clinical Differential Diagnosis and Complications, *Ann. Int. Med.,* **51:**1–16, 1959.

223. Knowlton, A. I.: Electrolyte Disturbances in Adrenal Diseases, *Am. J. Med.,* **15:**771–776, 1953.

224. Oppenheimer, B. S., and Silver, S.: The Variability in the Pathological Findings in Cushing's Syndrome: Report of Six Cases, *Tr. A. Am. Physicians,* **52:**146–163, 1937.

225. Bergenstal, D. M., Lipsett, M. B., May, R. H., and Hertz, R.: Regression of Adrenal Cancer and Suppression of Adrenal Function in Man by O,P'-DDD, in G. Pincus and E. R. Vollmer, (eds.), "Biological Activities of Steroids in Relation to Cancer," Academic Press, Inc., New York, 1960, p. 463.

226. Addison, T.: "On the Constitutional and Local Effects of Disease of the Suprarenal Capsules," S. Hyghley, London, 1855; reprinted in *Medical Classics,* **2:**244, 1937.

227. Sorkin, S. Z.: Addison's Disease, *Medicine,* **28:**371–425, 1949.

228. Guttman, P. H.: Addison's Disease: A Statistical Analysis of Five Hundred and Sixty-six Cases with a Study of the Pathology, *A.M.A. Arch. Path.,* **10:** 742–785, 895–935, 1930.

229. Thorn, G. W., Dorrance, S. S., and Day, E.: Addison's Disease: Evaluation of Synthetic Desoxycorticosterone Acetate Therapy in 158 Patients, *Ann. Int. Med.,* **16:**1053–1096, 1942.

230. Dunlop, S. D.: Eighty-six Cases of Addison's Disease, *Brit. M. J.,* **2:**887–891, 1963.

231. Friedman, N. B.: The Pathology of the Adrenal Gland in Addison's Disease, with Special Reference to Adrenocortical Contraction, *Endocrinology,* **42:**181–200, 1948.

232. McGavack, T. H.: Some Pitfalls in the Treatment of Addison's Disease, *J. Clin. Endocrinol.,* **1:**68–75, 1941.

233. Soffer, L. J., and Gabrilove, J. L.: A Simplified Water-loading Test for the Diagnosis of Addison's Disease, *Metabolism,* **1:**504–510, 1952.

234. Thorn, G. W., Forsham, P. H., Prunty, F. T. G., and Hills, A. G.: Test for Adrenal Cortical Insufficiency, *J.A.M.A.,* **137:**1005–1009, 1948.

235. Walser, M., Robinson, B. H. B., and Duckett, J. W.: The Hypercalcemia of Adrenal Insufficiency, *J. Clin. Invest.,* **42:**456–465, 1963.

236. McGavack, T. H.: Changes in Heart Volume in Addison's Disease and Their Significance, *Am. Heart J.,* **21:**1–16, 1941.

237. Somerville, W., Levine, H. D., and Thorn, G. W.: The Electrocardiogram in Addison's Disease, *Medicine,* **30:**43–79, 1951.

238. Wilson, G. M., and Miller, H.: Exchangeable Sodium in Addison's Disease in Relation to the Electrocardiogram and the Action of Cortisone, *Clin. Sc.,* **12:**113–129, 1953.

239. Currens, J. H., and White, P. D.: Congestive Heart Failure and Electrocardiographic Abnormalities Resulting from Excessive Desoxycorticosterone Acetate Therapy in the Treatment of Addison's Disease, *Am. Heart J.,* **28:**611–620, 1944.

240. Goodof, I. I., and MacBryde, C. M.: Heart Failure in Addison's Disease with Myocardial Changes of Potassium Deficiency, *J. Clin. Endocrinol.,* **4:**30–34, 1944.

241. Soffer, L. J., Engel, F. L., and Oppenheimer, B. S.: Treatment of Addison's Disease with Desoxycorticosterone Acetate, *J.A.M.A.,* **115:**1860–1866, 1940.

242. Nickerson, M., Karr, G. W., and Dresel, P. E.: Pathogenesis of "Electrolyte-steroid-cardiopathy," *Clin. Res.,* **9:**209–217, 1961.

243. Prioreschi, P.: Role of Potassium in the Patho-

genesis of the "Electrolyte-steroid-cardiopathy with necrosis," *Clin. Res.,* **10**:782–785, 1962.

244. Hellstrom, J., Birke, G., and Edvall, C. A.: Hypertension in Hyperparathyroidism, *Brit. J. Urol.,* 30:13–24, 1958.

245. Bradlow, B. A., and Segel, N.: Acute Hyperparathyroidism with Electrocardiographic Changes, *Brit. M. J.,* 2:197–200, 1956.

246. Kellogg; F., and Kerr, W. J.: Electrocardiographic Changes in Hyperparathyroidism, *Am. Heart J.,* 12:346–351, 1936.

247. Barker, P. S., Johnston, F. D., and Wilson, F. N.: The Duration of Systole in Hypocalcemia, *Am. Heart J.,* 14:82–86, 1937.

248. Surawicz, B., and Lepeschkin, E.: The Electrocardiographic Pattern of Hypopotassemia with and without Hypocalcemia, *Circulation,* 8:801–828, 1953.

249. Raab, W.: Adreno-sympathogenic Heart Disease (Neurohormonal Factors in Pathogenesis and Treatment), *Ann. Int. Med.,* 28:1010–1039, 1948.

250. Schulman, J. L., and Ratner, H.: Idiopathic Hypoparathyroidism with Bony Demineralization and Cardiac Decompensation, *Pediatrics,* 16:848–856, 1955.

251. Peterman, M. G., and Garvey, J. L.: Pseudohypoparathyroidism: Case Report, *Pediatrics,* 4:790–797, 1949.

252. Elrick, H., Albright, F., Barter, F. C., Forbes, A. P., and Reeves, J. D.: Further Studies on Pseudo-hypoparathyroidism: Report of Four New Cases, *Acta endocrinol.,* 5:199–225, 1950.

253. Rashkind, W. J., Golinko, R., and Areasoy, M.: Cardiac Findings in Idiopathic Hypercalcemia of Infancy, *J. Pediat.,* 58:464–469, 1961.

254. Paget, J.: On a Form of Chronic Inflammation of Bones (Osteitis Deformans), *Tr. M. & S. Soc. London,* 60:37, 1877.

255. Edholm, O. G., and Howarth, S.: Studies on the Peripheral Circulation in Osteitis Deformans, *Clin. Sc.,* 12:277–292, 1953.

256. Howarth, S.: Cardiac Output in Osteitis Deformans, *Clin. Sc.,* 12:271–275, 1953.

257. Lequime, J., and Denolin, H.: Circulatory Dynamics in Osteitis Deformans, *Circulation,* 12:215–219, 1955.

258. Sornberger, C. F., and Smedal, M. I.: The Mechanism and Incidence of Cardiovascular Changes in Paget's Disease (Osteitis Deformans): A Critical Review of the Literature with Case Studies, *Circulation,* 6:711–726, 1952.

259. Harrison, C. V., and Lennox, B.: Heart Block in Osteitis Deformans, *Brit. Heart J.,* 10:167–176, 1948.

260. Turner, K. B.: Insulin Shock as the Cause of Cardiac Pain: Case Report, *Am. Heart J.,* 5:671–672, 1929–1930.

261. Blotner, H.: Coronary Disease in Diabetes Mellitus, *New England J. Med.,* 203:709–713, 1930.

262. Rainier-Pope, C. R., Cunningham, R. D., Nadas, A. S., and Crigler, J. F., Jr.: Cardiovascular Malformations in Turner's Syndrome, *Pediatrics,* 33:919–925, 1964.

263. Haddad, H. M., and Wilkins, L.: Congenital Anomalies Associated with Gonadal Aplasia, *Pediatrics,* 23:885–902, 1959.

264. Cockayne, E. A., Krestin, D., and Sorsby, A.: Obesity, Hypogenitalism, Mental Retardation, Polydactyly, and Retinal Pigmentation: The Laurence-Moon-Biedl Syndrome, *Quart. J. Med., n.s.,* 4:93–120, 1935.

265. Blumel, J., and Kniker, W. T.: Laurence-Moon-Bardet-Biedl Syndrome: Review of the Literature and a Report of Five Cases Including a Family Group with Three Affected Males, *Texas Rep. Biol. & Med.,* 17:391–410, 1959.

266. Ellis, R. W. B., and Creveld, S. van: A Syndrome Characterized by Ectodermal Dysplasia, Polydactyly, Chondro-Dysplasia and Congenital Morbus Cordis, *Arch. Dis. Childhood,* 15:65–84, 1940.

267. Keizer, D. P. R., and Schilder, J. H.: Ectodermal dysplasia, Achondrodysplasia, and Congenital Morbus Cordis, *A.M.A. Am. J. Dis. Child.,* 82:341–344, 1951.

268. Smith, H. L., and Hand, A. M.: Chondroectodermal Dysplasia (Ellis-van Creveld Syndrome): Report of Two Cases, *Pediatrics,* 21:298–307, 1958.

269. Husson, G. S., and Parkman, P.: Chondroectodermal Dysplasia (Ellis-van Creveld Syndrome) with a Complex Cardiac Malformation, *Pediatrics,* 28:285–291, 1961.

270. Surawicz, B.: Electrolytes and the Electrocardiogram, *Mod. Concepts Cardiovas. Dis.,* 33:875–880, 1964.

271. Sampson, J. J.: Relationship of Potassium to Cardiac Disease, *Dis. Chest,* 42:330–333, 1962.

272. Keith, N. M., Burchell, H. B., and Baggenstoss, A. H.: Electrocardiographic Changes in Uremia Associated with a High Concentration of Serum Potassium: Report of Three Cases, *Am. Heart J.,* 27:817–844, 1944.

273. Levine, H. D., Merrill, J. P., and Somerville, W.: Advanced Disturbances of the Cardiac Mechanism in Potassium Intoxication in Man, *Circulation,* 3:889–905, 1951.

274. Pearson, C. M., and O'Mera, M. P.: An Electrocardiographic Log of Recurrent Hyperkalemia in a Severely Wounded Man, *Ann. Int. Med.,* 43:601–615, 1955.

275. Merrill, A. J.: The Significance of the Electrocardiogram in Electrolyte Disturbances, *Am. Heart J.,* 43:634–639, 1952.

276. Winkler, A. W., Hoff, H. E., and Smith, P. K.: Cardiovascular Effects of Potassium, Calcium, Magnesium, and Barium: An Experimental Study of Toxicity and Rationale of Use in Therapeutics, *Yale J. Biol. & Med.,* 13:123–132, 1940–1941.

277. Finch, C. A., and Marchand, J. F.: Cardiac Arrest by the Action of Potassium, *Am. J. M. Sc.,* **206**:507–520, 1943.

278. Henderson, C. B.: Potassium and the Cardiographic Changes in Diabetic Acidosis, *Brit. Heart J.*, **15**:87–94, 1953.

279. Holler, J. W.: Potassium Deficiency Occurring During the Treatment of Diabetic Acidosis, *J.A.M.A.*, **131**:1186–1189, 1946.

280. Darrow, D. C., and Miller, H. C.: The Production of Cardiac Lesions by Repeated Injections of Desoxycorticosterone Acetate, *J. Clin. Invest.*, **21**:601–611, 1942.

281. Lepeschkin, E., and Surawicz, B.: The Measurement of the QT Interval of the Electrocardiogram, *Circulation*, **6**:378–388, 1952.

282. Schwartz, W. B., Levine, H. D., and Relman, A. S.: The Electrocardiogram in Potassium Depletion: Its Relation to the Total Potassium Deficit and the Serum Concentration, *Am. J. Med.*, **16**:395–403, 1954.

283. Bellet, S., Steiger, W. A., Nadler, C. S., and Gazes, P. C.: Electrocardiographic Patterns in Hypopotassemia: Observations of 79 Patients, *Am. J. M. Sc.*, **219**:542–558, 1950.

284. Mayler, W. G.: The Significance of Calcium Iions in Cardiac Excitation and Contraction, *Am. Heart J.*, **65**:404–411, 1963.

285. Yu, P. N. G.: The Electrocardiographic Changes Associated with Hypercalcemia and Hypocalcemia, *J. M. Sc.*, **224**:413–423, 1952.

286. Hoff, H. E., Smith, P. K., and Winkler, A. W.: Electrocardiographic Changes and Concentration of Calcium in Serum Following Intravenous Injection of Calcium Chloride, *Am. J. Physiol.*, **125**:162–171, 1939.

287. Niedergerke, R.: The Rate of Action of Calcium Ions on the Contraction of the Heart, *J. Physiol.*, **138**:506–515, 1958.

288. Bechtel, J. T., White, J. E., and Estes, E. H., Jr.: The Electrocardiographic Effects of Hypocalcemia Induced in Normal Subjects with Edathamil Disodium, *Circulation*, **13**:837–842, 1956.

289. Brothers, M. J., and Kabakow, B.: Effects of Induced Hypocalcemia upon the Electrocardiographic Manifestations of Digitalis, *Circulation*, **16**:864, 1957.

290. Engel, F. L., Martin, S. P., and Taylor, H.: On the Relation of Potassium to the Neurological Manifestations of Hypocalcemic Tetany, *Bull. Johns Hopkins Hosp.*, **84**:285–301, 1949.

291. Hoff, H. E., Smith, P. K., and Winkler, A. W.: The Relation of Blood Pressure and Concentration in Serum of Potassium, Calcium and Magnesium, *Am. J. Physiol.*, **127**:722–730, 1939.

292. Szekely, P. and Wynne, N. A.: The Effects of Magnesium on Cardiac Arrhythmias Caused by Digitalis, *Clin. Sc.*, **10**:241–253, 1951.

293. Smith, P. K., Winkler, A. W., and Hoff, H. E.: Electrocardiographic Changes and Concentration of Magnesium in Serum Following Intravenous Injection of Magnesium Salts, *Am. J. Physiol.*, **126**:720–730, 1939.

294. Enselberg, C. D., Simmons, H. G., and Mintz, A. A.: The Effects of Magnesium upon Cardiac Arrhythmias, *Am. Heart J.*, **39**:703–712, 1950.

295. Glaser, W., and Brandt, J. L.: Localization of Magnesium-28 in the Myocardium, *Am. J. Physiol.*, **196**:375–376, 1959.

296. Hellerstein, E. E., Vitale, J. J., White, P. D., Hegsted, D. M., and Nakamura, M.: Influence of Dietary-magnesium on Cardiac and Renal Lesions of Young Rats Fed an Atherogenic Diet, *J. Exper. Med.*, **106**:767–775, 1957.

297. Vitale, J. J., Hellerstein, E. E., Hegsted, D. M., Nakamura, M., and Farbman, A.: Studies on the Interrelationships Between Dietary Magnesium and Calcium in Atherogenesis and Renal Lesions, *Am. J. Clin. Nutrition*, **7**:13–22, 1959.

298. Krehl, W. A., and Barboriak, J. J.: Influence of Magnesium Deficiency on Serum Cholesterol Levels in the Rat, *Am. J. Physiol.*, **194**:387–389, 1958.

299. Bersohn, I., and Oelofse, P. J.: Correlation of Serum-magnesium and Serum-cholesterol Levels in South African Bantu and European Subjects, *Lancet*, **1**:1020–1021, 1957.

300. Stamler, J., Pick, R., and Katz, L. N.: Influence of Thyroid, Pancreatic, and Adrenal Hormones on Lipid Metabolism and Atherosclerosis in Experimental Animals, in G. Pincus (ed.), "Hormones and Atherosclerosis," Academic Press, Inc., New York, 1959, pp. 173–195.

301. Oliver, M. F., and Boyd, G. S.: Hormonal Aspects of Coronary Artery Disease, *Vitamins & Hormones*, **16**:147–178, 1958.

302. Katz, L. N., Stamler, J., and Pick, R.: Research Approach to Atherosclerosis: Guest Editorial, *J.A.M.A.*, **161**:536–538, 1956.

303. Clawson, B. J., and Bell, E. T.: Incidence of Fatal Coronary Disease in Nondiabetic and in Diabetic Persons, *A.M.A. Arch. Path.*, **48**:105–106, 1949.

304. Feldman, M., and Feldman, M., Jr.: The Association of Coronary Occlusion and Infarction with Diabetes Mellitus: A Necropsy Study, *Am. J. M. Sc.*, **228**:53–56, 1954.

305. Thomas, W. A., Lee, K. T., and Rabin, E. R.: Fatal Acute Myocardial Infarction in Diabetic Patients, *A.M.A. Arch. Int. Med.*, **98**:489–494, 1956.

306. Liebow, I. M., Hellerstein, H. K., and Miller, M.: Arteriosclerotic Heart Disease in Diabetes Mellitus: A Clinical Study of 383 Patients, *Am. J. Med.*, **18**:438–447, 1955.

307. Stearns, S., Schlesinger, M. J., and Rudy, A.: Incidence and Clinical Significance of Coronary Artery Disease in Diabetes Mellitus, *A.M.A. Arch. Int. Med.*, **80**:463–474, 1947.

308. Nathanson, M. H.: Coronary Disease in 100 Autopsied Diabetics, *Am. J. M. Sc.*, **183**:495–502, 1932.

309. Warren, S.: "The Pathology of Diabetes Mellitus," 2d ed., Lea & Febiger, Philadelphia, 1938.

310. Bradley, R. F., and Bryfogle, J. W.: Survival of Diabetic Patients after Myocardial Infarction, *Am. J. Med.*, 20:207–216, 1956.

311. Kurland, G. S., and Freedberg, A. S.: Hormones, Cholesterol, and Coronary Atherosclerosis, *Circulation*, 22:464–473, 1960.

312. Oliver, M. F., and Bóyd, G. S.: Reduction of Serum-cholesterol by Dextrothyroxine in Men with Coronary Heart Disease, *Lancet*, 1:783–785, 1961.

313. Danowski, T. S., and Moses, C.: Symposium: Hydrocortisone and/or Desiccated Thyroid in Physiologic Dosage. I. Introduction to Studies of Hypolipemic and Other Effects Including Relationships to the Aging Process, *Metabolism*, 11:648–652, 1962.

314. Moses, C., Jablonski, J. R., Sunder, J. H., Greenman, J. H., and Danowski, T. S.: Symposium: Hydrocortisone and/or Desiccated Thyroid in Physiologic Dosage. II. Hypolipemic Effects, *Metabolism*, 11:653–663, 1962.

315. Adlersberg, D.: Adrenocortical Hormones and Experimental Atherosclerosis, in G. Pincus (ed.) "Hormones and Atherosclerosis," Academic Press, Inc., New York, 1959, pp. 197–204.

316. Kremer, D. N.: Medullary Tumor of the Adrenal Glands with Hypertension and Juvenile Arteriosclerosis, *A.M.A. Arch. Int. Med.*, 57:999–1007, 1936.

317. Goldenberg, M., Aranow, H., Jr., Smith, A. A., and Faber, M.: Pheochromocytoma and Essential Hypertensive Vascular Disease, *A.M.A. Arch. Int. Med.*, 86:823–836, 1950.

318. Pick, R., Stamler, J., and Katz, L. N.: Influence of Estrogens on Lipids and Atherosclerosis in Experimental Animals, in G. Pincus (ed.) "Hormones and Atherosclerosis," Academic Press, Inc., New York, 1959, pp. 229–245.

319. Wuest, J. H., Jr., Dry, T. J., and Edwards, J. E.: The .Degree of Coronary Atherosclerosis in Bilaterally Oophorectomized Women, *Circulation*, 7:801–809, 1953.

320. Ritterband, A. B., Jaffe, I. A., Densen, P. M., Magagna, J. F., and Reed, E.: Gonadal Function and the Development of Coronary Heart Disease, *Circulation*, 27:237–251, 1963.

321. Steiner, A., Payson, H., and Kendall, F. E.: Effect of .Estrogenic Hormone on Serum Lipids in Patients with Coronary Arteriosclerosis, *Circulation*, 11:784–788, 1955.

322. Oliver, M. F., and Boyd, G. S.: Endocrine Aspects of Coronary Sclerosis, *Lancet*, 2:1273–1276, 1956.

323. Rall, J. E., Robbins, J., and Federman, D. D.: Methyltestosterone and the Thyroid, in G. Pincus (ed.), "Hormones and Atherosclerosis," Academic Press, Inc., New York, 1959, pp. 89–101.

324. Barr, D. P., Russ, E. M., and Eder, H. A.: Influence of Estrogens on Lipoproteins in Atherosclerosis, *Tr. A. Am. Physicians*, 65:102–113, 1952.

325. Eder, H. A.: The Effect of Sex Hormones on Serum Lipids and Lipoprotein, in G. Pincus (ed.), "Hormones and Atherosclerosis," Academic Press, Inc., New York, 1959, pp. 335–348.

326. Stamler, J., Pick, R., Katz, L. N., Pick, A., and Kaplan, B. M.: Interim Report on Clinical Experiences with Long-term Estrogen Administration to Middle-aged Men with Coronary Heart Disease, in G. Pincus (ed.), "Hormones and Atherosclerosis," Academic Press, Inc., New York, 1959, pp. 423–442.

327. Meissener, G. F., and Moehring, C. M.: Synthetic Estrogens in Treatment of Atherosclerosis: A Study of Prostatic Cancer Patients, *Arch. Int. Med.*, 110:467–471, 1962.

328. White, P. D.: Cited in D. P. Barr, E. M. Russ, and H. A. Eder, Influence of Estrogens on Lipoproteins in Atherosclerosis, *Tr. A. Am. Physicians*, 65:112, 1952.

329. Talbot, N. B., Butler, A. M., Pratt, E. L., MacLachlan, E. A., and Tannheimer, J.: Progeria: Clinical, Metabolic and Pathologic Studies on a Patient, *Am. J. Dis. Child.*, 69:267–279, 1945.

330. Jacobson, H. G., Rifkin, H., and Zucker-Franklin, D.: Werner's Syndrome: A Clinical-roentgen Entity, *Radiology*, 74:373–385, 1960.

331. Thannhauser, S. J.: Werner's Syndrome (Progeria of the Adult) and Rothmunds' Syndrome: Two Types of Closely Related Heredofamilial Atrophic Dermatoses with Juvenile Cataracts and Endocrine Features: A Critical Study with Five New Cases, *Ann. Int. Med.*, 23:559–626, 1945.

332. Boyd, M. W. J., and Grant, A. P.: Werner's Syndrome (Progeria of the Adult): Further Pathological and Biochemical Observations, *Brit. M. J.*, 2:920–925, 1959.

333. Mitchell, E. C., and Goltman, D. W.: Progeria: Report of a Classic Case with a Review of the Literature since 1929, *Am. J. Dis. Child.*, 59:379–385, 1940.

62 THE HEART AND PREGNANCY

James Metcalfe, M.D., and Kent Ueland, M.D.

Pregnancies are dangerous to some women with heart disease. Heart disease is the leading cause of maternal death in some large American clinics.[1] For maximum success in managing a cardiac patient through pregnancy, the obstetrician and cardiologist must know the stresses which pregnancy places upon the maternal heart. On the basis of this knowledge and an understanding of their patient, they must construct a program which the patient accepts and can follow. They must form a working professional relationship in which clear advice is given to their patient and from which she derives optimum psychic as well as physical benefits. Following pregnancy a continuing, flexible life plan should be developed for each patient in which the desirability and timing of future pregnancies is carefully discussed, the continuance of prophylactic measures against subacute bacterial endocarditis and rheumatic fever is emphasized, and appointments are made for sustained cardiologic care.

Most maternal cardiovascular defects which are important in connection with childbearing exist before pregnancy: pregnancy is superimposed upon them. These women have valvular disease resulting from rheumatic fever, syphilis, or bacterial endocarditis, or congenital defects of the heart or great vessels. Other heart diseases such as coronary insufficiency and hypertensive heart disease are so rare in women of childbearing age that their consideration is left to specialized texts.[2] In addition to these preexisting maternal cardiovascular defects, a few circulatory diseases have their origin in pregnancy. These include pulmonary hypertension on the basis of multiple pulmonary emboli (of blood clots, fibrin, or air); the supine hypotensive syndrome of pregnancy, which, while not an example of heart disease, often excites cardiac consultation; pulmonary congestion, which may occasionally occur as the result of hypervolemia in pregnant women with normal hearts; and the vague, perhaps disappearing, syndrome called *postpartum myocardial degeneration*.[3] There appears to be increased danger of dissecting aneurysm of the aorta during pregnancy,[4] and paroxysmal atrial tachycardia is more common during pregnancy. Finally, the climate in which the fetal organism develops is dependent upon the environmental milieu provided by the mother. In this sense congenital defects, including heart defects, begin during pregnancy.

HEART DISEASE IN THE MOTHER

Incidence of Heart Disease in Pregnancy

Heart disease exists in from 1.2[5] to 3.7 per cent[1] of American women entering pregnancy. Rheumatic heart disease accounts for 80 per cent or more of the total incidence. Congenital cardiovascular defects in the mother appear to be relatively more common in the Scandinavian and German experience.[6,7] From the declining incidence and severity of rheumatic fever, we may expect a relative increase in congenital heart disease in American obstetric practice.[8]

The frequency with which circulatory disease begins during pregnancy on the basis of multiple pulmonary emboli, dissection of the aorta, or postpartum myocardial degeneration is impossible to estimate at the present time, but these disorders are probably uncommon causes of heart disease. Recent evidence leads experienced observers[9] to doubt that the hypertensive toxemias of pregnancy cause permanent hypertensive disease.

Congenital heart disease is found in between 1 and 2 infants per 1,000 born to a "normal" population. It occurs more often in children born to women with congenital heart disease.

Maternal Circulatory Physiology during Pregnancy

To understand the effects of pregnancy upon preexisting maternal heart disease, a knowledge of the circulatory adjustments which occur during normal pregnancy is essential. The changes in cardiac output, plasma volume, and heart rate which accompany pregnancy are of outstanding importance to patients with valvular heart disease, particularly rheumatic mitral stenosis.

Figure 62-1 shows a graph of the heart rate during successive months of pregnancy as related to the average value during the postpartum period. The observations were made in a small group of patients under strictly standardized basal conditions. The heart rate rises early in pregnancy, reaches its highest point 8 to 12 weeks before delivery, then declines, and after delivery returns to the value which represents that of nonpregnant women. Measurements of cardiac output during pregnancy have repeatedly shown maximum increases of 30 to 50 per cent above the nonpregnant level. This maximum is reached, as in the case of the heart rate, not at term but approximately 8 to 12 weeks before delivery; then, as shown in Fig. 62-2, it declines toward its nonpregnant value in the last weeks of pregnancy. The change in cardiac output is proportionately greater than the accompanying increase in pulse rate, the difference being accomplished by an augmented stroke volume. The increased cardiac output during pregnancy expresses the integral of a series of changing patterns of distribution of maternal blood flow. Renal plasma flow[10] is increased by 30 to 80 per cent early in pregnancy and declines toward or below normal values as term approaches. Late in pregnancy blood flow to the hands is increased, apparently reflecting the need of the metabolically active but encysted fetus to lose heat through its mother's skin. As term approaches a progressively greater proportion of the increased maternal cardiac output is diverted to the pregnant uterus and probably to the engorging breasts of the mother. Figure 62-3 shows the changes in blood volume and its components which occur during pregnancy.

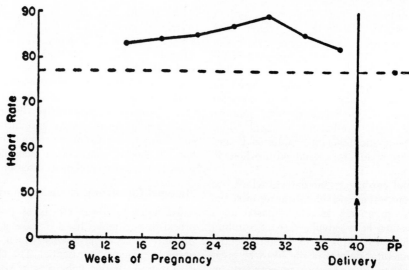

Fig. 62-1. Heart rate during successive months of pregnancy (solid line) as related to the average value during the postpartum period (dotted line).

Again the familiar dromedary curve is seen with a peak approximately 8 weeks before delivery. This increment in blood volume is brought about by increases in both plasma volume and red-cell volume.[11] The increase in plasma volume is greater than the increase in red-cell mass, so the hematocrit and hemoglobin percentage values are lowered during pregnancy. Adams[12] documented an increase in plasma volume which reached an average maximum of 22 per cent above the nonpregnant level between the thirty-second and thirty-fourth weeks of pregnancy. Hytten and Paintin[13] demonstrated that the magnitude of plasma volume increase during pregnancy correlates better with the subsequent birth weight of the fetus than with the

weight of the mother. In the final weeks before delivery, plasma volume decreases while the red-cell volume continues to rise. Thus, the point of maximum hemodilution occurs at the time of maximum cardiac output, pulse rate, and plasma volume, at about the thirty-second week of pregnancy.

With the information presently available a precise description of the distribution of the blood-volume increment accompanying pregnancy is not possible. At term, a substantial amount is probably contained in the placenta and the uterine vessels. X-rays of the lungs during pregnancy may show "increased vascular markings" in normal women, and Adams,[12] using the dye-dilution technique, has presented evidence of increased pulmonary

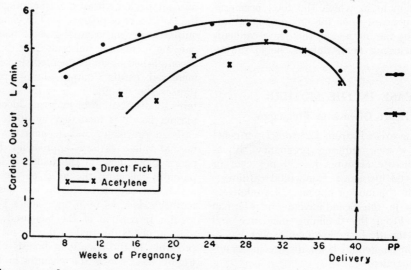

Fig. 62-2. Cardiac output during successive months of pregnancy.

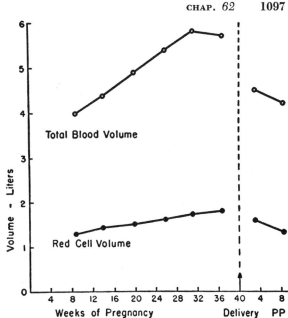

Fig. 62-3. The changes in blood volume and its components during pregnancy.

blood volume during pregnancy, greatest in the period of maximum cardiac output and blood volume. In addition to these changes in pulse rate, cardiac output, and blood volume, there is a decrease in mean maternal arterial blood pressure. This fall in blood pressure accompanying the increased cardiac output led Burwell et al.[14] to postulate that the placenta acts as an area of low vascular resistance and functions hemodynamically (though not metabolically) as an arteriovenous fistula in the maternal circulation. This hypothesis is supported by subsequent measurements of uterine blood flow and is teleologically appealing as ensuring adequate maternal blood flow to satisfy the metabolic needs of the mammalian fetus. The mechanism by which the low vascular resistance is established and maintained is unclear.

Labor itself is accompanied by a series of complicated cardiovascular changes which continue into the puerperium. Adams[15] demonstrated a 20 per cent increase in cardiac output (due to an increased pulse rate) at the height of each uterine contraction during labor and an increased pulmonary blood volume of similar magnitude at the acme of each uterine contraction. Presumably this increase in central blood volume is due to blood "squeezed out" of the contracting uterus. In the immediate postpartum period the cardiac output is increased over the prepartum level:[15] the elevation is of less magnitude than that observed during pregnancy and persists for about 1 week after delivery. Brown et al.[16] demonstrated a transient decrease in plasma volume at the time of delivery and a subsequent reentry of fluid into the vascular compartment for several days of the early postpartum period. These changes were attributed to the removal of the placental arteriovenous shunt at the time of delivery and have been partly confirmed by the detailed studies of Landesman and Miller.[17]

In addition to these well-documented changes in maternal hemodynamics which occur in association with pregnancy, clinical observations suggest that important structural changes occur in the walls of maternal blood vessels. The appearance of spider angiomas early in pregnancy is well known. Rupture of aneurysms of the splenic artery occurring before the age of forty-five are more common in females than in males, and the majority occur during pregnancy, usually between the seventh and ninth months. Sudden and striking growth of pre-existing arteriovenous fistulas in an extremity have been reported during pregnancy,[2] and Schnitker and Bayer[4] have presented evidence for an increased incidence of dissecting aneurysm of the aorta in association with pregnancy. The mechanisms by which these structural changes are produced are not known. Neither are the myocardial alterations which lead to an increased incidence of paroxysmal atrial tachycardia during pregnancy.[18] As noted above, a relative resting tachycardia occurs in all women as part of pregnancy. Under the circulatory demands of normal pregnancy, atrial fibrillation may begin in some patients with mitral stenosis. Disturbances of cardiac rate and rhythm are important to health to the degree that they interfere with the heart's action as a pump either by decreasing the cardiac output or, in patients with mitral stenosis, by leading to pulmonary congestion.

The tumor of pregnancy may itself lead to cardiovascular derangements. In some pregnant women near term, the assumption of the supine position allows pressure by the enlarged uterus upon the inferior vena cava and a consequent decrease in venous return and cardiac output. The resulting syncope[19] is quickly reversed by rolling the patient on her side, and many pregnant women learn to avoid the supine position during the final weeks of pregnancy. Bruce and Johnson[20] have documented the occurrence of dyspnea and fatigue on exertion during pregnancy in a thirty-seven-year-old woman without evidence of heart disease. Wrapping the legs with Ace bandages to prevent venous pooling in the upright position caused immediate symptomatic and objective improvement in exercise tolerance; this suggested that the gravid uterus caused venous obstruction and limited cardiac output. Such venous pooling in the final days of pregnancy and the early postpartum period may be frightening in patients who experience the supine hypotensive syndrome; it may be mortally dangerous to a few patients with congenital heart disease whose continued survival depends upon the maintenance of adequate venous return to the right side of the heart. These include patients with septal defects, patent ductus arteriosus, primary pulmonary hypertension,[20] and pulmonary stenosis.

Clinical Correlations

The circulatory changes which accompany pregnancy have effects which are important to the patient with heart disease and to her physician. The patient with a normal heart may develop systolic murmurs of low intensity which accompany the hyperdynamic circulation characteristic of pregnancy. The heart sounds may be accentuated, and moderate tachycardia may develop. A third heart sound in early diastole may occasionally be heard during pregnancy in a patient with a normal heart but does not in itself indicate heart disease. The venous pressure is elevated in the lower extremities, and in normal patients on unrestricted sodium diets edema of the lower extremities is very common. Diaphragmatic compression by the enlarging uterus may lead to transient rales in the lung bases and an awareness of the necessity for hyperventilation (sometimes called dyspnea) often occurs in pregnant women. Hurst et al.[21] described two types of extracardiac murmurs that may develop during the last few months of pregnancy: a systolic bruit that originates in branches of the mammary artery and a continuous murmur that originates in the veins of the breast. Roentgenologic and electrocardiographic evidence of elevation and rotation of the normal heart due to pressure upward from the enlarging uterus accompanies normal pregnancy. An awareness of these confusing changes should enable the physician to make several important decisions early in pregnancy: first, a persistent diastolic murmur, an abnormal heart rhythm, or clear cardiomegaly is indicative of heart disease even during pregnancy, and such patients need extra attention for maximum safety; second, soft systolic murmurs of low intensity (grade I or II) are not significant in the absence of cardiomegaly, and such patients are not helped by continuous cardiologic consultation. The cardiologist may properly request another opportunity for evaluation after pregnancy, but he must minimize the crippling concern about their circulatory adequacy which many patients date to pregnancy.

Heart disease in women of the childbearing age is overwhelmingly of rheumatic origin. Of these, the great majority have mitral stenosis as their sole or predominant valve lesion. Mendelson[22] found that 75 per cent of his pregnant rheumatic patients had mitral stenosis as the only clinically recognizable lesion; another 10 to 15 per cent had combined mitral and aortic lesions. Szekely and Snaith[23] record an experience with 845 pregnancies in 594 patients with rheumatic heart disease. Of these, 90 per cent had pure or predominant mitral stenosis. Furthermore, the physiology of mitral stenosis makes it especially dangerous in young people. The hemodynamic effects of mitral stenosis will be reviewed here only for the sake of continuity in discussion. The primary defect is obstruction to the flow of blood during diastole from the left atrium to the left ventricle. Such obstruction is hemodynamically insignificant until the valve orifice is diminished to a critical value or the rate of blood flow through the constricted orifice during diastole is increased above a certain critical value. *Critical* may be defined as that value which leads to an increase of pressure within the left atrium. Such increases in left atrial pressure are accompanied by pressure changes of similar magnitude in the pulmonary veins and pulmonary capillaries; their magnitude may be minimized in some patients (at the expense of increasing right ventricular work) by pulmonary arteriolar constriction. At some value near 25 mm Hg, pulmonary capillary tension exceeds the opposing forces of colloid osmotic pressure and lung tissue tension, and transudation into the alveolar walls and alveoli occurs. This may be transient when precipitated by an increased cardiac output accompanying exercise or momentary fright or pain, but in pregnancy the hemodynamic effects are persistent and compound.

The increase in pulse rate which accompanies pregnancy is accomplished at the expense of diastolic time per minute. This diminution in time available for blood to flow from left atrium to left ventricle necessitates a higher rate of flow for maintenance of cardiac output. The rate of flow is further accelerated by the increase in peripheral blood flow (cardiac output) which accompanies normal pregnancy. In the face of significant mitral stenosis these increases in flow rate across the mitral valve orifice can be accomplished only by an increase of pressure within the left atrium, the pulmonary veins, and pulmonary capillaries. In addition, there is evidence that the pulmonary blood volume is increased in normal pregnancy. The suggestion has been made that this increased volume of blood within the lungs leaves less elasticity for further distension in the presence of significant mitral stenosis. However the hemodynamic details are arranged, it is clear that the series of circulatory changes which accompany pregnancy tend to increase pulmonary capillary pressure and distension in women with mitral stenosis of severe degree. This pulmonary hypertension, which may lead to pulmonary edema, is due to mechanical obstruction to blood flow and not to ventricular myocardial failure. In the authors' experience, death due to myocardial failure seldom occurs during pregnancy; patients whose rheumatic lesions are predominantly mitral valve incompetence or aortic stenosis or incompetence seldom experience pulmonary congestion during pregnancy despite the increased work load upon the left ventricle which pregnancy imposes.

For evidence that the circulatory physiologic changes do integrate logically to produce an increased danger of disability and death during pregnancy, consider Fig. 62-4. The greatest incidence of pulmonary congestion during pregnancy occurs at the time of maximum cardiac output and blood volume. Patients who pass the seventh month of pregnancy without evidence of pulmonary congestion rarely experience it in the remaining weeks on continued careful management.

In the experience of most observers,[8,23] pulmonary congestion and maternal death are less common in patients with congenital than with rheumatic heart disease. Nevertheless, specific hazards exist in some such patients. In patients with pulmonary stenosis, septal defects, patent ductus arteriosus, and primary pulmonary hypertension the danger period (in contrast to patients with mitral stenosis) is at term and postpartum. At these times they are subject to syncope, hypotension, and sudden death.[24] These episodes are frequently accompanied by cyanosis. The mechanism of their production is unclear. Some observers[22] speak of "postpartum venoarterial shunting." The authors' hypothesis is that when venous return is impeded by the pressure of the uterus on the inferior vena cava, or by muscular paralysis from spinal anesthesia, or by pooling of blood in distensible veins surrounded by flaccid muscles of the lower extremities upon standing upright in the postpartum

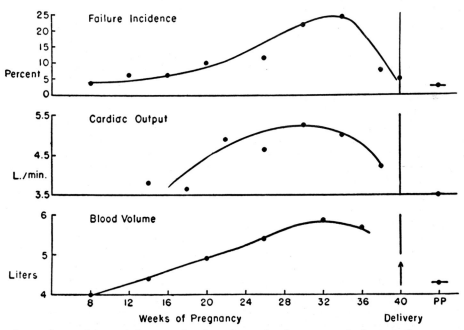

Fig. 62-4. The incidence of heart failure as related to the weeks of pregnancy is shown in the upper part of the figure. Note that the increase in incidence of failure occurs at the time of maximum cardiac output and blood volume.

period, right ventricular output is suddenly decreased. In patients with septal defects or patent ductus arteriosus this leads to diversion of left ventricular output into the pulmonary circuit and a consequent fall in peripheral cardiac output. In patients without shunting the fall in left ventricular output follows inexorably upon decreased right ventricular output. The decrease in peripheral blood flow leads to syncope: cyanosis is produced by a decrease in peripheral blood flow rather than by "venoarterial shunting." As evidence for this hypothesis, the authors have observed reversal of this syndrome by elevation of the legs in a patient with ventricular septal defect who became hypotensive following delivery.

Schnitker and Bayer[4] pointed out that 50 per cent of the reported instances of aortic dissection in women under forty occurred during pregnancy and concluded that pregnancy is a time of increased danger from this catastrophe. Goodwin[25] reviewed the recorded experience with pregnancy in women with coarctation of the aorta. As in normal patients, the mean arterial blood pressure tends to decline in pregnancy, especially in the middle trimester, and arterial blood pressure does not rise in labor. In support of these physiologic observations, pregnancy and labor cannot be shown to be periods of increased danger of aortic dissection or rupture, or of cerebral vascular accidents from rupture of intracranial aneurysms in patients with uncomplicated coarctation. At the childbearing ages, heart failure in a patient with coarctation almost always indicates the presence of an associated cardiac lesion such as aortic valve incompetence, patent ductus arteriosus, or ventricular septal defect. In such patients failure may originate or be aggravated during the cardiovascular burden of pregnancy.

Women with organic heart disease are liable to subacute bacterial endocarditis. Although recent evidence suggests that bacteremia is unusual during labor and delivery,[2,26] prophylaxis at this time against the establishment of subacute bacterial endocarditis is still recommended.

The Management of Maternal Heart Disease during Pregnancy

Patients with mitral stenosis comprise the great bulk of cardiovascular concern during pregnancy. The danger to them is of pulmonary congestion and edema. Several British writers[27,23] have emphasized the occurrence of acute pulmonary edema, often unanticipated and frequently fatal, tending to occur in relatively young women with a regular heart rhythm and only slight cardiac enlargement. These women are said to have often been unlimited by symptoms before pregnancy and may not have

tight mitral stenosis. Their pulmonary vascular resistance is usually not greatly increased, and episodes of pulmonary edema can occur and recur on good medical management. The British writers separate this group of patients from those with chronic or subacute pulmonary congestion occurring during pregnancy, but the authors of this chapter have not been impressed by this dichotomy in performance. In the latter's experience, pulmonary congestion and edema is predictable upon the basis of an imbalance between cardiac capacity (expressed as an inverse function of mitral valve orifice size) and cardiac demand (the sum of all metabolic requirements on the maternal heart). This oversimplification is useful as a basis for discussing methods of management of heart disease during pregnancy. To restore a safe balance in which cardiac capacity exceeds the demand on the maternal heart, the total cardiac demand must be limited to levels of tolerance, or the total cardiac capacity must be increased.

Obstetric Considerations

Interruption of pregnancy is one method of reducing the total cardiac burden in pregnant women. It has been of lifesaving value in some patients with heart disease, but with increasing medical understanding and surgical skill the necessity for its use is diminishing. It is unacceptable to some women on moral grounds and disabling to the morale of many more. It should be performed before the twelfth week of pregnancy for maximum safety, almost never after the sixteenth week of pregnancy (by then a major surgical procedure is necessary) and, in the authors' opinion, never in the presence of pulmonary congestion. It does not lead to an immediate reversal of the circulatory effects of pregnancy.

It should be emphasized that the major service of the cardiologist is to bring the cardiac patient to term without pulmonary congestion. If this is achieved, the danger of pulmonary congestion and death during delivery is slight. Abundant experience demonstrates that maternal heart disease is not an indication for premature delivery or Cesarean section. Indeed, the weight of clinical evidence suggests that premature delivery imposes increased hazards to the woman with heart disease who is in danger of pulmonary congestion. In other words, a term vaginal delivery in a carefully controlled cardiac patient is the best solution to the problems presented by the combination of maternal heart disease and pregnancy. On the other hand, maternal heart disease, even when symptomatic, should not be regarded as a contraindication to obstetrically indicated Cesarean section, although surgical intervention should be delayed, if possible, until the maximum cardiac burden of pregnancy has been passed.

The authors have been impressed by the desirability and importance of adequate analgesia for pain relief during labor in the cardiac patient. They agree with Mendelson[22] that "The choice of anesthetic technique and agents depends not only upon the maternal and fetal states, but also largely upon the training and competency of the anesthesiologist. The functions and responsibilities of the anesthesiologist cannot be assumed safely by the obstetrician or by unqualified persons." Spinal anesthesia poses some hazards consequent upon the pooling of blood in the flaccid extremities and should, in the authors' opinion, be avoided in patients with a liability toward vascular collapse at delivery. The authors have been impressed by the safety and adequacy of local nerve block in skilled hands.

In all pregnant patients who are susceptible to sudden death, the possibility of performing a postmortem Cesarean section should be recognized.[28]

A few other points regarding obstetric management in the postpartum period are worthy of mention. Synthetic Pitocin, which is free of contamination by pressor agents, is preferable to the natural product in the cardiac patient. Mendelson[22] recommends the omission of ergonovine or methylergonovine tartrate (which tend to raise the venous pressure) in cardiac patients. Intravenous fluid administration has obvious hazards to the cardiac patient and should be avoided or used with caution. Since the incidence of thromboembolic phenomena is increased by both the postpartum state and the existence of heart disease, early ambulation is strongly recommended but should not be strenuously employed. Finally, the postpartum period is an optimum point for designing with the patient and obstetric and surgical consultants a flexible life plan for the woman with heart disease. The desirability and timing of future pregnancies should be carefully and frankly discussed. The authors believe that contraception, because it is reversible, is more desirable than sterilization.

Medical Considerations

The basis of medical management of the cardiac patient during pregnancy is expressed by Burwell:[29] ". . . we attempt to make a place in the patient's cardiac budget for the expenditures of pregnancy by eliminating equivalent amounts of other expenditures." The principle is to reduce the total cardiac demand of the pregnant woman to levels of tolerance within her cardiac capacity. Let us consider first those factors which increase cardiac demand.

Pregnancy itself must head the list in this discussion, but the demands of pregnancy are not unique or isolated. Changes in cardiac output and plasma volume during pregnancy can be limited by sodium restriction and the use of diuretics without jeopardizing fetal health. The use of chlorothiazide should be accompanied by recognition of the hazards of potassium depletion, particularly when digitalis is being used concurrently. Furthermore, changes in blood volume induced by chlorothiazide derivatives may accentuate or precipitate postural hypotension.

Activity exacts a price in cardiac output and tachycardia. In a recent discussion of the cardiologic problems of pregnancy, Eastman[30] commented, "The most important factor in the reduction of maternal mortality in the past thirty years is the employment of prolonged bed rest in the hospital. Indeed, by and large the best management of desperate heart disease in pregnancy is not therapeutic abortion or valvotomy but hospitalization throughout pregnancy usually with complete bed rest." This statement is justified by the evidence. The excellent results reported by Gorenberg and Chesley[31] were based upon recognition of the importance of restriction of physical activity. Hours and intensity of rest and sleep should be evaluated along with hours and intensity of physical activity. Most pregnant cardiac patients need little or no restriction of activity to keep their cardiac demand within safe limits for their cardiac capacity; some need moderate restriction; a few need hospitalization (at least at the period of peak load) to survive and succeed in pregnancy. For some patients strict bed rest is less restful than hospital confinement with carefully regulated ambulation.

Infections of the upper respiratory tract and especially influenzal pneumonia impose dangerous burdens upon the heart in pregnancy. Pregnant cardiac patients should be especially protected. Pyelonephritis is more common during pregnancy and the postpartum period than at other times and should be avoided by discouraging catheterization and teaching careful hygiene.

Disorders of the heartbeat are important to the degree that they interfere with the function of the heart as a pump. In women with mitral stenosis tachycardia of any type is important. Pregnancy causes a relative sinus tachycardia and increases the susceptibility to paroxysmal atrial tachycardia. In a few women with mitral stenosis, atrial fibrillation begins during pregnancy. The authors attempt reversion in all cases. Quinidine is used during pregnancy and, in the authors' experience, has not led to obstetric difficulties.

Anemia should be avoided by the use of iron supplements in all pregnant women. Anemia appearing in the face of iron administration should be investigated promptly and specific therapy instituted at once. If transfusion is necessary, packed red cells are preferable to whole blood in patients with pulmonary congestion. Any intravenous fluid should be given slowly.

Obesity imposes a cardiac burden which should be reversed as soon as the diagnosis is made. With careful supplementation by vitamins and minerals weight loss can safely occur during pregnancy.

Anxiety is expensive in terms of heart work. The authors have seen pulmonary edema precipitated by emotional trauma. Less obvious but perhaps more important are the (often iatrogenically imposed) fears of death or disaster which take their toll over weeks, months, and years. Careful, firm support is more rewarding to the patient and her physician than indecision, conflicting opinions, or scolding.

Pain, in some patients, accompanies labor and delivery. Some of these patients have mitral stenosis, and pain may cause pulmonary congestion, probably because of tachycardia. Relief of pain is especially important in these patients.

Hyperthyroidism may coexist with pregnancy, although its diagnosis is more difficult in the face of the normal hypermetabolism of pregnancy.

In the management of patients with heart disease during pregnancy the obstetrician and cardiologist will recognize that the cardiovascular burden reaches its maximum at the thirtieth to thirty-fourth week. Maximum restrictive and supportive measures are employed at this time with judicious preliminary preparation, reassurance, and understanding.

These, then, are the factors which the authors recognize as important in constituting the total cardiac burden of the pregnant woman. They are important to the degree that they can be altered to restore a favorable balance of cardiac demand in the patient with heart disease. Such alterations of total cardiac demand are the basis of successful medical management. Less important in the authors' experience are measures for increasing cardiac capacity. The first of these to be discussed is the use of digitalis. Although the authors employ it in the treatment of pulmonary edema in patients with mitral stenosis, they are not convinced of its efficacy except when it slows the pulse rate. It is, of course, indicated in patients with myocardial failure secondary to acquired or congenital defects causing ventricular overwork. The authors have not employed prophylactic digitalization during pregnancy because of their belief that such therapeutic interference will, in most cases, only complicate an already complicated situation. Recently the cardiac capacity for work has become subject to

surgical alterations. This great advance will now be considered.

Cardiovascular Surgery

Great advances in cardiovascular surgery have occurred in the past 15 years. Their relevance to the management of heart disease during pregnancy is difficult to assess because of conflicting statistics.

Mitral valvotomy, in the authors' opinion, has a small but established role to play in the management of women with mitral stenosis during pregnancy. The earliest reports of this operation in pregnancy appeared in 1952. Brock,[32] Cooley and Chapman,[33] Logan and Turner,[34] and Mason[35] reported a total of 11 cases of mitral valvotomy with one maternal death and one premature delivery. By 1961, Harken and Taylor[36] were able to collect 394 cases from the literature with a total of 7 maternal deaths (1.8 per cent maternal mortality rate) and 35 fetal deaths (9 per cent fetal mortality rate). When these results are compared with those achieved by medical management alone, they lie between the maternal and fetal mortality rates recorded for all patients with heart disease in pregnancy and the higher rates experienced in patients with class III and IV functional disability. However, in some series the mortality of surgical treatment is not so low. Gilchrist[27] reported an overall operative mortality from valvotomy (in nonpregnant individuals) of approximately 4 per cent. He quoted Soulié et al.[37] as having tabulated an operative mortality from mitral valvotomy during pregnancy of 5 per cent. Even Harken and Taylor,[36] whose maternal mortality figure is lower than that reported by others in nonpregnant patients, express the view that valvotomy is not justified during pregnancy in patients with functional class I or II heart disease. Unfortunately, the operative mortality mounts with age and with severity of functional classification, just as does the maternal mortality associated with pregnancy itself. It seems unlikely that the cardiovascular stresses of pregnancy would be associated with a lower operative mortality. Most writers agree that nonoperative management of the cardiac patient is preferred when possible and that surgical intervention should be reserved for those patients with proved mitral stenosis who show progressive cardiac disability, especially in the first two trimesters of pregnancy. The operative mortality to be expected in these severely ill patients is not clear. Gilchrist[27] recorded a 5 per cent operative mortality in class III heart disease and a 20 per cent operative mortality in class IV patients. These figures are for nonpregnant cardiac patients. They are considerably higher than the recorded mortality during pregnancy in some series handled with medical management alone[2] in these same functional classes. At the present time the authors are guided by the following general principles:

1. The question to be answered is not whether mitral valve surgical procedures can be performed during pregnancy but whether such procedures will improve the chances of survival of mother and infant through pregnancy and the years subsequent to pregnancy.

2. The safest time for cardiac surgical treatment, judged by mortality and subsequent hemodynamic improvement, is the time of greatest cardiac reserve. Pregnancy lowers the cardiac reserve[38] in patients with heart disease.

3. In some patients, open-heart surgical treatment is necessary for optimum relief of mitral stenosis. Extracorporeal circulation carries a very high fetal mortality, giving a considerable risk of abortion (with its associated physical and psychic trauma) in the postoperative period. Once the decision for surgical intervention is made, the best operation for that patient must be performed. Reoperation is difficult and dangerous, and a poor operation is often worse than none at all.

4. Mitral valvotomy is, in almost all cases, a palliative rather than a curative procedure.[39,27] The benefits of valvotomy are often of limited duration. Operation should be timed for maximum effectiveness and not performed on inadequate or transient evidence. In the authors' experience[2] valvotomy, even in the best hands, cannot be counted upon to remove the danger of pulmonary congestion in current or subsequent pregnancies in every patient.

With these principles in mind, the authors would advise mitral valvotomy during pregnancy only in the rare patient with disabling mitral stenosis (documented by catheterization of the left side of the heart) in whom pulmonary congestion or dangerous hemoptysis persists despite several weeks of intensive medical care under hospital conditions and to whom interruption of pregnancy is not acceptable. The authors believe that the decision for surgical intervention should, whenever possible, be made before the twentieth week of pregnancy and that such intervention is not advisable after the twenty-fourth week of pregnancy. It is only by a judicious selection of patients for valvotomy that we can hope to arrive at the ultimate goal, which is to decrease maternal and fetal mortality. Gilchrist[27] achieved a maternal mortality rate of less than 1 per cent in 592 patients with heart disease. Mitral valvotomy was performed 11 times in that large series. Elective sterilization is not advisable in any patient with surgically correctable cardiac disease. Mortensen and Ellsworth[40] studied 62 couples sterilized before the wife's cardiac surgical treatment.

Of these, 38 women (61 per cent) improved sufficiently so that (in the cited authors' opinion) pregnancy could have been undertaken safely.

Surgical treatment for congenital heart disease is seldom necessary during pregnancy for maternal survival. From their experience with 372 pregnancies in 125 women with congenital heart disease, Copeland and coworkers[41] reached the conclusion that ". . . the effect of pregnancy in congenital heart disease is not sufficient to indicate cardiac operation in the gravid state." In their extensive series only one patient died (from bacterial endocarditis following a dental extraction). Similarly, Cannell and Vernon[8] observed 61 pregnancies in women with congenital heart disease without a maternal death. Although multiple reports indicate that surgical correction of congenital defects can be achieved successfully during pregnancy[1,7,8,23, 32,36,40,42-44] and that even prolonged hypothermia is consistent with fetal survival,[45,46] extracorporeal circulation during open-heart surgical treatment has been associated with a high incidence of fetal death and deformity.[47-50] Since current trends in cardiac surgical treatment favor the increased use of open-heart techniques and extracorporeal circulation, the authors consider that careful corrective cardiac surgical treatment is best done under basal conditions which do not obtain during pregnancy.

There is adequate evidence that judiciously planned surgical treatment for congenital defects should be carried out as soon as the diagnosis is made, and certainly before pregnancy occurs. Early surgical intervention will prevent the pulmonary vascular complications of patent ductus arteriosus and septal defects, the hazards of infection, heart failure, and aortic rupture in coarctation of the aorta, and the myocardial burdens of stenosis of the outflow tracts.

Harken and Taylor[36] have said, "Ideally the management of cardiac disease in women of child-bearing age is prevention of conception, surgical correction and subsequent pregnancy." Clearly, corrective surgical treatment before the childbearing age is even more desirable. However, since the present authors believe mitral valvotomy to be palliative rather than corrective, they believe that its proper use must be timed to coincide with maximum need. Gilchrist[27] summarizes our point:

A well-timed valvotomy can break this sequence [of progressive deterioration with succeeding pregnancies in women with disabling mitral stenosis], and perhaps allow a woman to have a child for whom the burden might otherwise be too great. The benefits of valvotomy are often of limited duration, and as increasing age is an adverse factor for the cardiac woman, pregnancy after a successful operation should not be long delayed.

The authors recognize, above all, that for maximum maternal and fetal health, heart disease must be recognized early, corrected at once when possible, and otherwise managed with careful weighing of the obstetric, medical, and surgical opportunities and responsibilities.

Pregnancy in patients who have had previous cardiac surgical treatment must be evaluated on an individual basis. With progress in cardiovascular surgical techniques such patients will require an increasing percentage of our cardiologic concern. Patients who have been subjected to palliative procedures such as mitral valvotomy must be assessed on the basis of their functional capacity before advice concerning pregnancy is given. All such patients should be under continued long-term management and should be schooled in planning their lives (including pregnancy) for maximum enjoyment and accomplishment. Patients who have undergone corrective surgical treatment, such as correction of a patent ductus arteriosus with successful results, can approach pregnancy as normal individuals. In patients with coarctation of the aorta, extra medical attention should be given because of the likelihood of associated cardiac or vascular anomalies.

Experience with pregnancy in patients with valvular prosthesis is limited. Four patients[8,51-53] successfully completed pregnancies with Hufnagel valves in place for correction of aortic insufficiency. Only one of these patients experienced congestive failure. The authors have followed two patients in their clinic who have had Starr-Edwards aortic valve prosthetic replacements. Both delivered uneventfully at term and have remained free of cardiovascular symptoms.

The majority of evidence indicates that pregnancy, if survived, does not shorten the life or permanently decrease the cardiac competence of the mother.[54] Donzelot and coworkers[54] have presented evidence of increased maternal disability following pregnancy, but their conclusions find little support from other writers. Indeed, Miller and Metcalfe suggest on the basis of a 4-year follow-up of 106 patients with heart disease seen during pregnancy that this group constitutes a better than average risk for survival and health in the years of motherhood.[55]

HEART DISEASE AND THE FETUS

An increased fetal mortality associated with symptomatic maternal heart disease has repeatedly been demonstrated.[2] In mothers with functional class I heart disease during pregnancy, the fetal and neonatal death rate is the same as in women without heart disease. It is insignificantly elevated in mothers with functional class II heart disease but reaches 12 per cent (twice the class I rate) in patients of functional class III and 31 per cent in mothers who are symptomatic at rest, this is, with class IV heart disease. When the functional severity of maternal heart disease is improved by medical or surgical management, the fetal prognosis for survival is demonstrably improved.

Despite the increased incidence of fetal and neonatal mortality in symptomatic patients with rheumatic heart disease, there is no evidence that the surviving children of such mothers have a higher incidence of congenital deformity.

In women with congenital heart disease who become pregnant, the fetus seems to suffer both genetic and environmental handicaps in utero. Neill and Swanson[56] have recently expanded the data relevant to the genetic transmission of congenital heart disease. In 508 pregnancies in which one parent had congenital heart disease, there was a 1.8 per cent incidence of congenital heart disease in the children. This is six times the "normal" incidence of congenital heart disease. Pregnancies in cyanotic mothers have an extremely high incidence of spontaneous abortion (greater than 60 per cent), and live-born children of such mothers are small when contrasted with the offspring of cyanotic fathers. This suggests that the intrauterine environment may be at fault in cyanotic women. The limiting defect is probably an abnormally poor supply of oxygen to the fetus. Because of the demonstrated teratogenic effect of hypoxia it can be postulated that cyanosis of the mother from any cause will be associated with a high incidence of fetal loss and deformity. Copeland and coworkers[41] noted a high fetal loss in patients with congenital heart disease causing cyanosis or accompanied by pulmonary hypertension. In a discussion of a paper by Cannell and Vernon,[8] Dr. Alan C. Barnes of Baltimore reported an association in mothers with cyanotic congenital heart disease between the hematocrit level and the prognosis of pregnancy. In cyanotic mothers with a hematocrit greater than 60, twelve pregnancies ended in 10 abortions and 2 premature births. One premature baby died. In cyanotic mothers with hematocrits between 48 and 60, sixteen pregnancies yielded 6 abortions, 9 premature deliveries, and 1 term delivery, 3 of whom died; and in cyanotic mothers with hematocrits less than 48, twenty-six pregnancies resulted in 4 abortions, 11 premature births, and 11 term infants, 2 of whom died. This experience gives added weight and urgency to the prompt diagnosis and correction of congenital heart disease early in life, preferably prior to pregnancy.

REFERENCES

1. Mendelson, C. L.: "Cardiac Disease in Pregnancy: Medical Care, Cardiovascular Surgery and Obstetric Management as Related to Maternal and Fetal Welfare," F. A. Davis Company, Philadelphia, 1960.
2. Burwell, C. S., and Metcalfe, J.: "Heart Disease and Pregnancy: Physiology and Management," Little, Brown and Company, Boston, 1958.
3. Metcalfe, J.: The Maternal Heart in the Postpartum Period, Am. J. Cardiol., 12:439–440, 1963.
4. Schnitker, M. A., and Bayer, C. A.: Dissecting Aneurysm of the Aorta in Young Individuals, Particularly in Association with Pregnancy: With Report of a Case, Ann. Int. Med., 20:486–511, 1944.
5. Gorenberg, H., and McGleary, J.: Rheumatic Heart Disease in Pregnancy, Am. J. Obst. & Gynec., 41: 44–52, 1941.
6. Berger, J., and Haenel, L.: Schwangerschaft und Geburt bei organischem Herzfehler, Schweiz. med. Wchnschr., 93:453–459, 1963.
7. Buemann, B., and E. Kragelund: Clinical Assessment of Heart Disease During Pregnancy, Acta obst. et gynec. scandinav., 41:57–79, 1962.
8. Cannell, D. E., and Vernon, C. P.: Congenital Heart Disease and Pregnancy, Am. J. Obst. & Gynec., 85:744–753, 1963.
9. Chesley, L. C., Cosgrove, R. A., and Annitto, J. E.: A Follow-up Study of Eclamptic Women, Am. J. Obst. & Gynec., 83:1360–1372, 1962.
10. de Alvarez, R. R., and Bratvold, G. E.: Renal Glomerulotubular Mechanisms During Normal Pregnancy, Am. J. Obst. & Gynec., 75:931–944, 1958.
11. Pritchard, J. A., and Adams, R. H.: Erythrocyte Production and Destruction During Pregnancy, Am. J. Obst. & Gynec., 79:750–757, 1960.
12. Adams, J. Q.: Cardiovascular physiology in normal pregnancy: Studies with the Dye Dilution Technique, Am. J. Obst. & Gynec., 67:741–759, 1954.
13. Hytten, F. E., and Paintin, D. B.: Increase in Plasma Volume During Normal Pregnancy, J. Obst. & Gynaec. Brit. Commonw., 70:402–407, 1963.
14. Burwell, C. S., Strayhorn, W. D., Flickinger, D., Corlette, M. B., Bowerman, E. P., and Kennedy, J. A.: Circulation during Pregnancy, Arch. Int. Med., 62:979–1003, 1938.
15. Adams, J. Q., and Alexander, A. M., Jr.: Alterations in Cardiovascular Physiology during Labor, Obst. & Gynec., 12:542–549, 1958.
16. Brown, E., Sampson, J. J., Wheeler, E. O., Gundelfinger, B. F., and Giansiracusa, J. E.: Physiologic Changes in the Circulation during and after Obstetric Labor, Am. Heart J., 34:311–333, 1947.
17. Landesman, R., and Miller, M. M.: Blood Volume Changes during the Immediate Postpartum Period, Obst. & Gynec., 21:40–48, 1963.
18. Szekely, P., and Snaith, L.: Paroxysmal Tachycardia in Pregnancy, Brit. Heart J., 15:195–198, 1953.
19. Howard, B. K., Goodson, J. H., and Mengert, W. F.: Supine Hypotensive Syndrome in Late Pregnancy, Obst. & Gynec., 1:371–377, 1953.
20. Bruce, R. A., and Johnson, W. P.: Exercise Tolerance in Pregnant Cardiac Patients, Clin. Obst. & Gynec., 4:665–676, 1961.
21. Hurst, J. W., Staton, J., and Hubbard, D.: Precordial Murmurs during Pregnancy and Lactation, New England J. Med., 259:515–517, 1958.
22. Mendelson, C. L.: Heart Disease and Pregnancy, Clin. Obst. & Gynec., 4:603–629, 1961.
23. Szekely, P., and Snaith, L.: The Place of Cardiac Surgery in the Management of the Pregnant Woman with Heart Disease, J. Obst. & Gynaec. Brit. Commonw., 70:69–77, 1963.
24. Jewett, J. F.: Pulmonary Hypertension in Pregnancy, Clin. Obst. & Gynec., 4:630–644, 1961.
25. Goodwin, J. F.: Pregnancy and Coarctation of the Aorta, Clin. Obst. & Gynec., 4:645–664, 1961.
26. Redleaf, T. D., and Fadell, E. J.: Bacteremia during Parturition, J.A.M.A., 169:1284–1285, 1959.
27. Gilchrist, A. R.: Cardiological Problems in Younger Women: Including Those of Pregnancy and the Puerperium, Brit. M. J., 1:209–216, 1963.
28. Leonard, M. W. E., and Stone, M. L.: Postmortem Cesarean Section, Obst. & Gynec., 12:344–345, 1958.
29. Burwell, C. S.: The Management of Heart Disease in Pregnant Women, Bull. Johns Hopkins Hosp., 95: 130–143, 1954.
30. Eastman, W. J.: Editorial Comment, Obst. & Gynec. Surv., 18:569–570, 1963.
31. Gorenberg, H., and Chesley, L. C.: Rheumatic Heart Disease in Pregnancy: Immediate and Remote Prognosis, Obst. & Gynec., 1:15–25, 1953.
32. Brock, R. C.: Valvotomy in Pregnancy, Proc. Roy. Soc. Med., 45:538–540, 1952.
33. Cooley, D. A., and Chapman, D. W.: Mitral Commissurotomy during Pregnancy, J.A.M.A., 150:1113–1114, 1952.
34. Logan, A., and Turner, R. W. D.: Mitral Valvulotomy in Pregnancy, Lancet, 1:1286, 1952.
35. Mason, J.: In Discussion of F. E. Stabler and P. Szekely, J. Obst. & Gynaec. Brit. Emp., 59:567, 1952.
36. Harken, D. E., and Taylor, W. J.: Cardiac Surgery during Pregnancy, Clin. Obst. & Gynec., 4:697–709, 1961.
37. Soulié, P., Acar, J., Degeorges, M., and Barrillon, A.: Commissurotomie mitrale au cour de la grossesse, Arch. mal. coeur, 54:361–376, 1961.
38. Robbe, H.: Physical Working Capacity, Blood Volume and Heart Volume in Cardiac Patients during and after Pregnancy, Acta obst. et gynec. scandinav., 38:1–39, 1959.
39. Ellis, L. B., and Adler, L. N.: Criteria for Surgery in Mitral Valvular Disease, Am. J. Cardiol., 12:17–29, 1963.
40. Mortensen, J. D., and Ellsworth, H. S.: Pregnancy and Cardiac Surgery, Circulation, 28:773, 1963.

41. Copeland, W. E., Wooley, C. F., Ryan, J. M., Runco, V., and Levin, H. S.: Pregnancy and Congenital Heart Disease, *Am. J. Obst. & Gynec.*, **86:** 107–110, 1963.

42. Baker, J. L., Russell, C. S., Grainger, R. G., Taylor, D. G., Thornton, J. A., and Verel, D.: Closed Pulmonary Valvotomy in the Management of Fallot's Tetralogy Complicated by Pregnancy, *J. Obst. & Gynaec. Brit. Commonw.*, **70:**154–157, 1963.

43. Kirklin, J. W., Weidman, W. H., Burroughs, J. T., Burchell, H. B., and Wood, E. H.: The Hemodynamic Results of Surgical Correction of Atrial Septal Defects: A Report of Thirty-three Cases, *Circulation*, **13:**825–833, 1956.

44. Reid, J. M., Berger, R. L., and Stevenson, J. G.: Transventricular Mitral Valvotomy during Pregnancy, *Brit. M. J.*, **2:**1197–1199, 1960.

45. Daley, R., Harrison, G. K., and McMillan, I. K. R.: Direct-vision Pulmonary Valvotomy during Pregnancy, *Lancet*, **2:**875–876, 1957.

46. Rowbotham, G. F., Bell, K., Akenhead, J., and Cairns, A.: A Serious Head Injury in a Pregnant Woman Treated by Hypothermia, *Lancet*, **1:**1016–1019, 1957.

47. Dubourg, G., Broustet, P., Bricand, H., Fontan, F., Trarieux, M., and Fontanille, P.: Correction complète d'une triade de Fallot, en circulation extracorporelle, chez une femme enceinte, *Arch. mal. coeur,* **52:**1389–1391, 1959.

48. Kay, C. F., and Smith, K.: Surgery in the Pregnant Cardiac Patient, *Am. J. Cardiol.*, **12:**293–295, 1963.

49. Lee, W. H., and Pate, J. W.: Surgical Aspects of Heart Disease in Pregnancy, *GP*, **28:**78–83, 1963.

50. Leyse, R., Ofstun, M., Dillard, D. H., and Merendino, K. A.: Congenital Aortic Stenosis in Pregnancy, Corrected by Extracorporeal Circulation, *J.A.M.A.*, **176:**1009–1012, 1961.

51. Canfield, M. C., Edgar, A. L., and Kimball, A. P.: Successful Completion of Pregnancy in a Patient with a Hufnagel Valve, *California Med.*, **88:**54–55, 1958.

52. Crockett, J. E., Kittle, C. F., and Dimond, E. G.: Relief of Angina and Congestive Heart Failure by Hufnagel Valve: Subsequent Term Pregnancy, *Am. Heart J.*, **57:**144–148, 1959.

53. Gorman, J. F.: Pregnancy and Aortic Insufficiency: Term Pregnancy in a Patient with a Hufnagel Valve, *Obst. & Gynec.*, **20:**238–242, 1962.

54. Donzelot, E., De Balsac, R. H., and David, A.: Aggravation of Mitral Heart Disease Following Pregnancy: A Statistical Study of 233 Cases, *Am. J. Cardiol.*, **1:**51–56, 1958.

55. Miller, M. D., and Metcalfe, J.: Effect of Pregnancy on the Course of Heart Disease: Re-evaluation of 106 Cardiac Patients Three to Five Years after Pregnancy, *Circulation*, **13:**481–488, 1956.

56. Neill, C. A., and Swanson, S.: Outcome of Pregnancy in Congenital Heart Disease, *Circulation*, **24:** 1003, 1961.

Section B: Emotional and Environmental Factors

63 CARDIOVASCULAR DISEASE, CARDIOVASCULAR SYMPTOMS, AND EMOTIONAL STRESS

Edwin O. Wheeler, M.D.

Men have been aware of the cardiovascular effects of emotions throughout recorded history. The relation of such phenomenon as palpitation, blushing, pallor, and fainting to emotional stress and their increased occurrence in nervous or emotional persons has been well recognized. It has become clear that emotional stimuli may profoundly influence the cardiovascular system through their effects on the system's autonomic nervous control. Sympathetic or adrenergic activity accelerates the heart, elevates the blood pressure, and strengthens the heartbeat, while parasympathetic or cholinergic activity slows the pulse, lowers the blood pressure, and weakens the heartbeat.

Experimental work in man and animals has demonstrated that temporary cardiovascular changes can be induced by stimulation of many areas of the brain, but the direction of the effects has varied, depending on the techniques employed, and has often been unpredictable. Thus, stimulation of areas of the hypothalamus has produced effects similar to either sympathetic or parasympathetic stimulation.[1] Studies of the effects of emotions on cardiovascular function in man have produced somewhat variable results, in part because of the use of varying and sometimes inadequate physiologic techniques and in part because of the varying reactions which may be encountered in the same subject at different times. From a number of careful studies, several patterns of cardiovascular response to acute emotional stress or anxiety have emerged.[2-6] The usual reaction to emotion-provoking stimuli, such as stressful interviews, mental arithmetic, preexamination anxiety, criticism, or pain, has been an increase in heart rate, blood pressure, oxygen consumption, and cardiac output with little change in, or a decrease in, total peripheral resistance. Less frequently, the rise in heart rate and blood pressure is associated with an increase in total peripheral resistance and a decrease in cardiac output. Brod et al.[5] points out that there is no basic difference between these two types of response, which in any case overlap. In both, the emotional stress produces vasoconstriction in the kidneys and splanchnic area, and vasodilatation in the muscles. Thus, the change in total peripheral resistance depends on a balance between visceral vasoconstriction and muscular vasodilatation. This hemodynamic response is nonspecific and resembles that occurring with muscular exercise.

Another type of hemodynamic response to emotional stress has been observed less frequently and less predictably. This consists of circulatory collapse with a profound fall in heart rate, arterial pressure, and total peripheral resistance without much change in cardiac output.[7] This type of response, which is familiar to all physicians, has typically been observed just preceding venesection (Chap. 17).

The suggestion has been made that specific types of cardiovascular response may follow specific alterations in emotions or affect.[8-10] Other studies have failed to support these findings.[5,6] It does seem probable that there is a quantitative relation between the degree of emotion that is provoked and the magnitude of the cardiovascular response.[6,11]

Such studies have been concerned with the transient effects of acute emotional stress. The physiologic effects of prolonged, chronic, or repetitious emotional stress have not been adequately studied.

EMOTIONAL STRESS AND CARDIOVASCULAR DISEASE

The obvious relation between emotion and cardiovascular function has naturally led to speculation and study of the possible role of emotions as causative or aggravating factors in cardiovascular disease, a field of study which unfortunately has too often been concerned with fancy rather than fact. Most studies in this area attempt to demonstrate one or more of the following: (1) the presence of a specific type of personality in association with a specific disease, (2) a correlation between emotional stress or events in the past and the onset or aggravation of a specific disease, (3) a different physiologic or biochemical reaction, in persons with a specific disease, to experimental emotional stress, and (4) the development of a specific disease in animals in response to experimental emotional stress. These studies have been hampered by problems in defining and measuring personality, emotions, emotional stress, experimental neuroses, etc. In addition, the retrospective technique involving historical data of uncertain reliability, the frequent use of physiologic techniques of questionable validity such as the ballistocardiograph or radioactive diodrast for the determination of cardiac outputs, and the use of certain psychologic techniques such as psychoanalysis, Rorschach tests, and dream analysis make it difficult to draw conclusions from many studies. Finally, many studies are uncontrolled and are obviously biased. In spite of these problems, the clinical impression is strong that emotional stress does play a role in cardiovascular disease, and many attempts have been made to study the relationship.

Hypertension

The fact that transient elevations of blood pressure can be produced by acute emotional stress[5,6,11] plus the observation that in persons exhibiting "transient hypertension" sustained hypertension often develops in later life[12] have suggested that emotional stress might play a role in the development of hypertension. A number of studies have attempted to demonstrate a correlation between the onset, the worsening, or the improvement of hypertension and certain events in the life of the patient.[13-15] These are largely retrospective and anecdotal studies. Although it is evident, both clinically and experimentally, that the blood pressure in patients with hypertension is increased by emotional stress, these studies do not provide evidence that the course of the disease is altered with regard to mortality or involvement of the heart, kidney, or brain. A few studies of large groups of persons exposed to stress have been made. In one, 27 per cent of soldiers were found to have diastolic pressures above 100 mg Hg 1 to 2 months after combat,[16] while in another 56 per cent of 180 persons had diastolic pressures above 95 mm Hg 1 to 2 weeks after the Texas City explosion.[17] The stress in these instances was complex, and there were no data to indicate that sustained hypertension appeared. In a 20-year follow-up study of 173 patients with neurocirculatory asthenia, that is, patients generally considered to be "anxious," there was no increase in the prevalence of hypertension.[18]

Some writers have concluded that patients with hypertension have a specific type of personality, although there is no agreement on just what type is found.[19-21] Saslow,[22] in a study of personality factors, concluded that there was significant positive correlation with "obsessive-compulsive behavior" and "subnormal assertiveness." However, he states that this association does not imply an etiologic relationship. This association between personality factors and hypertension was present regardless of the type of hypertension—renal or essential.

It has been suggested that cardiovascular responses to emotional stress were qualitatively different in persons with hypertension.[9,23] Wolf and Wolff [23] observed that the blood pressure may increase in one of two ways during a stressful interview: either the cardiac output increases while total peripheral vascular resistance does not change or even decreases, or there is a rise in total peripheral vascular resistance with an unchanged or falling cardiac output. They concluded that the "resistance" type characterizes subjects with suppressed hostility and occurs more frequently among hypertensives. However, others have been unable to confirm these observations.[5,11] Brod et al.[5] noted that the stress of mental arithmetic produced a blood pressure rise but that the hemodynamic pattern was the same in normotensive and hypertensive persons. The above patterns were seen in varying degrees in both groups. Quantitatively, however, the hemodynamic response was of greater magnitude and lasted longer in the hypertensive person.

Finally, there have been studies on the development of hypertension in animals exposed to various noxious stimuli or by the technique of conditioned reflexes.[24] The relation of such hypertension to human disease or of such stimuli to emotional stress in man is not known.

Thus, at present, there is no convincing evidence that patients with hypertension have different personalities, have been exposed to different or greater emotional stress, or physiologically react in a qualitatively different way than normotensive persons.

Coronary Heart Disease

Attempts to establish a relationship between emotional stress and coronary disease have been based on studies purporting to show a coronary-prone personality, unusual life stress in persons with coronary disease, unusual emotional stress preceding acute coronary thrombosis, and elevations of blood lipids as a result of emotional stress. Studies of personality in coronary disease have failed to agree on a specific personality type.[21,25,26] Miles and associates[27] compared the personalities of 46 young men with coronary disease and 49 healthy young men. Only 11 of the coronary patients and 5 of the controls showed a consistent tendency toward compulsive striving, hard work, self-discipline, and a need to get to the top, features which have been said to characterize the coronary personality.[21] They note that even this slight difference

was due to the larger proportion of Jewish men in the coronary group (16:6) and suggest that ethnic, social, and educational backgrounds may have biased previous uncontrolled studies. It has been suggested without evidence that acute coronary disease is often precipitated by an emotionally stressful incident or that chronic emotional stress somehow results in coronary atherosclerosis.[28-30] Other studies have suggested that persons engaged in stressful occupations, such as certain types of physicians, dentists, lawyers, and accountants,[31,32] have a high incidence of coronary disease. Studies of executives versus nonexecutives and of persons in various types of industrial occupations have not confirmed this finding.[33,34] There is a tendency to ascribe the high prevalence of coronary disease in some Western civilizations in part to emotional stress as well as to diet, although there is no evidence that men in "civilized" Western countries are exposed to more or less emotional stress than people living in underdeveloped countries. However interesting such studies may be, they are uncontrolled in regard to many factors of possible significance, so that one can only speculate about their significance.

There has been recent interest in studies showing a rise of blood-cholesterol level at times of emotional stress, such as in students prior to examinations[35,36] or accountants during preparation of yearly tax returns.[32] These observations suggest a possible mechanism by which emotions and the development of coronary disease might be connected. Whether the observed changes are the result of emotional stress per se or due to other factors, such as change in diet, physical activity, sleep, or amount of smoking, is not known.

There is abundant evidence to indicate that angina pectoris, a complication of coronary atherosclerosis, may be precipitated and aggravated by emotional stress (Part IV, Section C). The types of emotions involved may vary from intense anger (which may be obvious to an outside observer) to carefully concealed stressful thoughts on the part of the patient. The thoughts may be pleasant or unpleasant.

The cause of coronary atherosclerosis is not known. It is likely that the cause is multifactored, and therefore it is not possible at the present time to identify the relationships of emotional stress to the total problem. It is clear that emotional stress may aggravate and precipitate angina pectoris in patients with coronary atherosclerosis.

Cardiac Arrhythmias

Palpitation and tachycardia are among the most widely recognized effects of emotional stress, and perhaps because of this emotional stress is commonly thought to be a cause or precipitating factor in cardiac arrhythmias. Stimulation of various parts of the brain or autonomic nervous system and the administration of adrenergic and cholinergic drugs have given rise to various arrhythmias. In view of this, the paucity of reports supporting this relationship is surprising. There are a few individual case reports[37-39] and some retrospective, anecdotal studies[40,41] which claim that such an association may occur.

The development of electronic equipment that permits the continuous monitoring of the electrocardiogram over a period of many hours may yield information concerning the relation of emotions to cardiac arrhythmias.

Congestive Heart Failure

Acute emotional upsets may precipitate acute left ventricular failure or pulmonary edema in patients with coronary, hypertensive, or rheumatic heart disease. The known physiologic effects of emotional stress, which are very similar to those of exertion, are sufficient to account for this in patients with advanced heart disease. However, it has been suggested that chronic emotional stress may aggravate or precipitate congestive heart failure in some unexplained way.[42,43] More recently, it has been claimed that emotional upsets may alter the excretion of water and electrolytes, aggravating or precipitating congestive heart failure by retention of sodium and water,[44,45] and that different alterations of affect are associated with different patterns of electrolyte and water excretion. These recent studies were not sufficiently controlled to allow valid conclusions but suggest interesting approaches for further study. In any case, the majority of physicians would agree on the benefit of a tranquil existence in a patient with congestive failure, but whether the ill effects of chronic emotional stress are the result of some autonomic nervous system effect on the kidneys, heart, or peripheral circulation or the result of changes in activity and diet is not clear.

Electrocardiogram

Electrocardiographic abnormalities have been noted for a number of years in persons with neurocirculatory asthenia, psychoneurosis, and emotional lability.[46-49] In such individuals the abnormalities have usually been limited to inversions of the T waves, most frequently in leads II, III, and AVF but occasionally involving leads I, AVL, and V_4, V_5, and V_6. These abnormalities tend to vary from time to time and with factors such as standing, lying, exercise, hyperventilation, breath holding, and drugs.[50-52] Although such lability of the T waves has generally been reported in anxious pa-

tients, they have occasionally been seen in stable, healthy persons. Whether they occur more frequently in neurotic persons cannot be ascertained from the literature. Studies comparing the electrocardiograms of persons with neurocirculatory asthenia and healthy controls have shown no difference in the frequency of T-wave abnormalities.[53,54] Whatever the cause of these T-wave abnormalities, it is extremely important for physicians to be aware of their existence, since misinterpretation of such findings to a psychoneurotic anxious patient may aggravate his condition.

PSYCHIATRIC DISEASE AND CARDIOVASCULAR SYMPTOMS

Cardiovascular symptoms, such as palpitation, chest pain, shortness of breath or faintness, commonly occur in patients who have no heart disease. The majority of persons who have such symptoms are found to have one of a group of disorders generally considered to be psychiatric in nature. Anxiety neurosis (neurocirculatory asthenia), depression, and hysteria are the most common disorders found in these patients, although some are difficult to classify in a helpful diagnostic category. The recognition of these disorders and their differentiation from cardiac disease is of great importance. An incorrect diagnosis of heart disease may aggravate the symptoms of the preexisting nervous disorder and lead to invalidism.

"Cardiovascular Symptoms" and Anxiety Neurosis (Neurocirculatory Asthenia)

Anxiety neurosis is a syndrome characterized by palpitation, chest pain, fatigue, and nervousness. A number of names have been given to this disorder, often reflecting the interests or theories of the particular writer or the situation under which the disorder was studied. Among those which have been commonly used are neurasthenia, Da Costa's syndrome, irritable heart, soldier's heart, effort syndrome, anxiety neurosis, cardiac neurosis, and neurocirculatory asthenia. The last term is frequently used in the American literature. An analysis of the symptoms and signs of patients described under these various labels suggests that these patients had the same disorder.[55] In this chapter the term *anxiety neurosis* will be used.

Prevalence

The prevalence of this disorder in the population as a whole cannot be accurately determined for several reasons: there is no way in which mild cases can be clearly differentiated from normal persons, the symptoms may come and go, and differences in diagnostic criteria and terminology make estimates in the literature difficult to compare. It is a common disorder, however, as indicated by a number of studies. White, in an analysis of civilian patients in a private cardiology practice, found 12 per cent of 3,000 patients so affected in one study (White and Jones[56]) and 13.7 per cent of 5,000 patients in another (White[57]). Wheeler et al.[58] found a prevalence of 4.7 per cent in a series of 365 working persons. The Framingham Epidemiologic Study[54] revealed a prevalence of 11.6 per cent in 1,214 persons.

There has been renewed interest in this disorder in time of war. It was first described from the British campaign in India[59] and in the Union armies[60] during the War between the States and rediscovered as a common military problem in World Wars I and II.[61–64, 89] The dimension of this problem in military service is emphasized by the fact that the British army hospitalized 70,000 patients for this disorder in World War I.[65] The apparent decrease in prevalence of this disorder in World War II was undoubtedly due to the use of different diagnostic terms. The increased importance of this syndrome in time of war may result from the presence in increased degree of factors which commonly aggravate the disorder, such as physical work, emotional strains, and infections, and from the fact that complaining about the disorder may lead to a medical discharge and pension for disability.

Etiology

The anxiety state (neurocirculatory asthenia) is considered to be a psychiatric disorder. The reasons why symptoms develop that refer to the cardiovascular system—such as dyspnea, chest pain, palpitation, and exhaustion—rather than symptoms referring to some other body system are not clear. At times it is easy to identify an emotional problem that has greatly aggravated the basic disorder, but it is often difficult to determine the cause of the preexisting disorder. The apparent psychiatric nature of this syndrome does not relieve the internist or cardiologist of his responsibility for the correct diagnosis and management of this syndrome. In fact, for various reasons, the nonpsychiatrist must manage most of these patients.

Age

This is primarily a disorder of young adults. The average age of onset is about twenty-five years.[66] This by no means indicates that the syndrome is rare at middle life. If the patient's symptoms first occur in the later decades of life, it is wise to consider the more serious psychiatric disorders or to

search carefully for a previously unrecognized medical disease.

Sex

Although more women than men with this disorder are seen by physicians,[18,67] there is little data concerning the relative frequency in the sexes. In the epidemiologic study at Framingham,[54] neurocirculatory asthenia was diagnosed in 15.7 per cent of the women but in only 4.6 per cent of the men. There was, however, no evidence of sex linkage in a genetic study by Cohen et al.[68]

Family History

A high familial prevalence of this syndrome has been noted by many investigators.[61,63,68–70] Wheeler et al.[58] found that 48.6 per cent of the children of affected parents had the same disorder. Whether this high familial prevalence is due to heredity or to environmental factors is not known.

Aggravating Factors

Patients describe a large number of factors which they believe aggravate symptoms, cause recurrences, or precede the onset of this disorder. Among the most common are emotion-provoking situations, illness, hard physical work, pregnancy, and military service. The fact that military service includes many of these factors plus the fact that complaining of the disorder frequently resulted in discharge from military service have probably played a large role in the prevalence and severity of this disorder in armies at war.

Clinical Picture

The symptoms of this disorder are multiple, and there are few signs. While a patient may complain of only two or three symptoms, a large number will generally be found if a careful history is taken. This is not a monosymptomatic disorder. The chief complaint, however, commonly determines the type of specialist who eventually sees the patient. Patients with predominant complaints of headache, dizziness, and faintness are likely to see neuropsychiatrists, whereas those with palpitation, dyspnea, and chest pain are often seen by cardiologists. Chest pain is a common complaint in patients with anxiety neurosis, and it must be differentiated from the discomfort associated with organic disease—especially that of ischemic heart disease (Chap. 32). The chest discomfort of anxiety neurosis may be characterized either as "sticks and stabs" of a fleeting nature, or "dull and aching" of prolonged duration. An individual may have both types of chest pain. This discomfort is usually located near the cardiac apex and is rarely located in the substernal area. The painful area is usually quite small; often it is no larger than a 25-cent piece. The pain sometimes radiates into the arm, axilla, or scapula. The patient may relate the pain to exertion, but on more detailed questioning it is generally found that the pain comes on after exertion—often hours after—and is associated with fatigue rather than with effort. Tenderness of the chest wall over the area of the pain is a common finding.

Breathing difficulties are found in almost all patients with neurocirculatory asthenia. In addition to shortness of breath on exertion, the patient may have complaints such as "I can't get enough oxygen" or "I can't get a full breath." Sighing respirations are quite characteristic and may be noted by the physician when the patient is unaware of them. Choking sensations or smothering feelings are commonly noted, especially in crowded places.

Palpitation is for the most part an awareness of the heartbeat of sinus origin, although arrhythmias, commonly premature beats, may aggravate the patient's consciousness of this symptom.

Faint feelings, "dizzy" spells or lightheadedness, unsteadiness, and nervous spells are common. These vary from giddy sensations when walking or standing, causing the patient to steady himself against a wall or chair, to characteristic anxiety attacks with choking, palpitation, hyperventilation, trembling, and fear of fainting or dying. These are especially prone to occur in crowded places and may make it difficult for the patient to ride in trains or buses, shop in crowded stores, attend church, or go to the theater. At the theater the patient commonly prefers an aisle seat. It should be noted that similar anxiety attacks may occur in other disorders such as manic-depressive disease and hysteria.

Exhaustion, fatigue, or lack of pep are common complaints. The patient may "feel tired all the time" regardless of activity or rest. He begins the day exhausted. Nervousness and irritability are generally present. Insomnia is frequent.

There are no characteristic signs of this disorder. Tachycardia, tachypnea, sighing, tremor, moist cold palms, and brisk tendon reflexes are often observed but are inconstant and often found in nervous patients without this disorder.

This clinical picture is usually quite different from the symptom complexes of organic heart disease. It may, of course, coexist with heart disease or, more commonly, confuse the picture of angina pectoris, arrhythmias, or congestive heart failure. It may be the major cause of disability in the patient with organic heart disease. It has also been mistaken for other medical disorders such as thyrotoxicosis, tuberculosis, and brucellosis.

Laboratory Findings

A large number of clinical and experimental laboratory studies have been made of patients with this disorder. These have not produced information or techniques which are of much help in diagnosis. However, certain of these studies are of practical as well as theoretical interest.

Electrocardiographic abnormalities thought to be due to, or associated with, anxiety neurosis have been reported by a large number of investigators,[46,49,67,71,72] but others have not confirmed this. Logue et al.,[73] in a study of 150 soldiers with this disorder, found a number of variations from the normal but concluded that there was no characteristic electrocardiogram. White et al.,[53] in a study of civilians and soldiers with this disorder, concluded that the variations from normal were associated with factors such as body build, pulse rate, posture, and the effects of previous illness. A recent study by Kannel et al.[54] of 203 cases of this syndrome and 757 control subjects free of cardiovascular disease revealed the same kinds and frequencies of electrocardiographic abnormalities in the two groups. The electrocardiogram is thus of little help in the diagnosis.

The heart size was reported to be small by Master,[71] probably because he limited his study to patients of asthenic build. This has not been borne out by other studies. The routine clinical laboratory studies, blood chemical determinations, and indices of thyroid function have been normal.

In various research studies abnormalities have been found in fingernail capillaries,[74] in oxygen consumption,[75,76] in blood lactate,[75,77] in palmar sweat,[78] on psychologic testing,[66] during muscular work,[66,75,79] and with painful stimuli.[80]

Of particular interest are the studies of respiration, oxygen consumption, and blood-lactate production in response to exercise. It was found that during a standard exercise test patients with this syndrome had a lower oxygen consumption and greater rise in blood lactate than normal controls.[75,77] Cohen and White[66] concluded that these abnormalities ". . . are consistent with the hypothesis that aerobic metabolism is abnormal in these patients." Whether these findings apply specifically to patients with anxiety neurosis or whether they are general signs of poor health or poor conditioning is not known. Attempts to alter these abnormalities by physical training by Cohen and his associates were unsuccessful, since the patients could not or would not follow the prescribed training program. Holmgren et al.,[81,82] in a small series of patients, noted an increase in "physical working capacity" following a period of systematic physical training. Future studies may help elucidate the significance of these and other abnormalities found in this disorder.

Course and Prognosis

The condition tends to persist for years; periods with remission and exacerbation are common. A small number of patients with typical symptoms may recover entirely. In a 20-year follow-up study[18] of 173 patients seen in a private practice, 12 per cent recovered and remained free of the symptoms of this disorder, but the remainder continued to have symptoms of varying severity. Thirty-five per cent noted continuing symptoms but no disability. Thirty-eight per cent had symptoms and intermittent disability, while only fifteen per cent were completely disabled. It is of interest that the only men in this study who were totally disabled and unable to work were veterans receiving a pension. The incidence of disability has been reported to be much higher in veterans. In follow-up studies of military personnel from England[83] and from Australia,[84] 50.6 per cent and 35 per cent respectively were in poor health and disabled. This suggests that disability pensions are one factor which may aggravate the complaints of this disorder.

There have been three long-term studies of mortality in this disorder. Grant[83] reported in 1925 that a follow-up study of 600 veterans of World War I showed an excess of mortality due to tuberculosis. Another study of 107 veterans of World War I with this disorder showed an excess of mortality from all causes.[85] In a 20-year follow-up study[18] of patients seen in a private practice, there was no excess mortality. Furthermore, there was no increase in the prevalence of peptic ulcer, ulcerative colitis, asthma, thyrotoxicosis, hypertension, coronary disease, or other diseases which are often labeled psychosomatic.

Management

Reassurance is the most important measure in the management of most patients with this syndrome. This cannot be done well unless other disorders can be excluded to the satisfaction of both the physician and patient. Thus, certain basic studies, such as chest x-rays, electrocardiograms, or thyroid function tests, may be necessary, though the physician may be satisfied as to the diagnosis on the basis of the history and physical examination alone. Patients frequently have enough medical knowledge to feel that heart disease cannot be excluded without an electrocardiogram, thyroid disease without a metabolism test, or mental disease without an electroencephalogram. Since worry concerning the presence or development of such disorders may play an important role in aggravating anxiety, their careful exclusion may be as important in treatment as in diagnosis. Reassurance should not stop with the exclusion of other diseases but should include an emphasis on the favorable aspects of the disorder, its good prognosis for life expectancy, and the low incidence of disability (in civilian life). An incorrect diagnosis, scary words, and restriction of activity can undoubtedly aggravate the symptoms. It is just as wrong to ascribe this disorder to "nerves" or "imagination" as it is to regard it as a dangerous or serious condition. Time spent in sympathetic explanation and reassurance about this disorder early in its course may be worth more than any amount of prolonged psychotherapy at a later time.

An attempt should be made to identify factors which may aggravate the patient's symptoms. Some of these—especially certain chronic emotion-provoking situations (mother-in-law problems, conflicts with children, etc.)—may be amenable to some alterations which make them more bearable. Long hours of work, boredom, unpleasant tasks, and fears of various sorts may play a role and often can be modified. In some cases an extra vacation, a period of rest, a change of scene, an increase in social life (visiting friends, regular nights out), or a regular program of physical activity may be of great help.

Drugs do not have an important role in the management of this condition. Their symptomatic use for extreme nervousness, insomnia, and headache may be helpful for short periods of time but should not be continued for long. This tends to be a chronic disorder with remittances and exacerbations of symptoms regardless of the drugs employed. Drugs such as sedatives, tranquilizers, and sleeping pills may help alleviate acute exacerbations of symptoms but are not helpful in the long-term management of this disorder.

Intensive psychotherapy or psychoanalysis has been used in the treatment of this disorder. The published results do not support the view that this is any better than simple reassurance, simple drug therapy, and advice about aggravating factors.[18]

Depression and Hysteria

Depression and hysteria are two rather well-defined psychiatric disorders often accompanied by cardiac symptoms which may be confused with heart disease. Patients with manic-depressive disorder, particularly older depressed men, often note cardiac symptoms similar to those just described. In some instances these accompany anxiety attacks which may be a part of the disorder, but often these symptoms are more chronic and associated with a fear of heart disease or an abnormal conviction that such exists. It has been noted that this disease is frequently confused with medical or surgical disorders, such as hypertension, coronary heart disease, menopause, cholelithiasis, and ulcers.[86] Anxiety attacks, i.e., spells with fear, apprehension, palpitation, breathlessness, tremor, and sweating, were noted to occur in 33 of 100 patients with depression whose medical symptoms were recorded.[87] These symptoms are often quite similar to those of simple anxiety neurosis and the two conditions may be confused unless the symptoms of depression are noted. Symptoms such as feeling blue, inability to concentrate, irritableness, early morning insomnia, loss of interest in family, friends, and work, anorexia, weight loss, and suicidal thoughts or attempts help to distinguish the two disorders. Since a depression may be aggravated by an incorrect diagnosis of heart disease, since its management may require psychiatric help, and since the risk of suicide is present, physicians must be acquainted with the symptoms of this disorder. Depressive disorders commonly coexist with heart disease, adding to the problems of their diagnosis and management. Reserpine has been thought to precipitate or aggravate depressed states, so its use should be avoided in these patients.

Hysteria is less commonly confused with cardiac disease, although patients with this disorder may complain of dyspnea, palpitation, and other symptoms of anxiety attacks.[88] In this disorder, which occurs almost exclusively in women, a number of symptoms are found which are uncommon in heart disease and anxiety neurosis. A history of fainting or "blackouts," loss of voice, blindness, painful menstrual periods, dyspareunia, and multiple surgical procedures is common. In addition, the complaints are often bizarre and dramatically presented. Schizophrenia is often overlooked in some of these patients. A carefully taken medical history will usually make obvious the true nature of the patient's complaints.

While the management of these and other psychiatric disorders may, in certain instances, require the services of a psychiatrist, the recognition of these disorders and their differentiation from heart disease is the responsibility of the general physician and cardiologist.

REFERENCES

1. Rushmer, R. F., and Smith, O. A., Jr.: Cardiac Control, *Physiol. Rev.*, **39**:41, 1959.
2. Grollman, A.: The Effect of Psychic Disturbances on the Cardiac Output, Pulse Rate, Blood Pressure and Oxygen Consumption of Man, *Am. J. Physiol.*, **89**:366, 1929.
3. Stead, E. A., Jr., Warren, J. V., Merrill, A. J., and Brannon, E. S.: The Cardiac Output in Male Subjects as Measured by the Technique of Right Atrial Catheterization: Normal Values with Observations on the Effect of Anxiety and Tilting, *J. Clin. Invest.*, **24**:326, 1945.
4. Hickam, J. B., Cargill, W. H., and Golden, A.: Cardiovascular Reactions to Emotional Stimuli: Effect on the Cardiac Output, Arteriovenous Oxygen Difference, Arterial Pressure, and Peripheral Resistance, *J. Clin. Invest.*, **27**:290, 1948.
5. Brod, J., Fencl, V., Hejl, Z., and Jirka, J.: Circulatory Changes Underlying Blood Pressure Elevation during Acute Emotional Stress (Mental Arithmetic) in Normotensive and Hypertensive Subjects, *Clin. Sc.*, **18**:269, 1959.
6. Bogdonoff, M. D., Combs, J. J., Jr., Bryant, G. D. N., and Warren, J. V.: Cardiovascular Responses in Experimentally Induced Alterations of Affect, *Circulation*, **20**:353, 1959.
7. Warren, J. V., Brannon, E. S., Stead, E. A., Jr., and Merrill, A. J.: The Effect of Venesection and the Pooling of Blood in the Extremities on the Atrial Pressure and Cardiac Output in Normal Subjects with Observations on Acute Circulatory Collapse in Three Instances, *J. Clin. Invest.*, **24**:337, 1945.
8. Adsett, C. A., Schottstaedt, W. W., and Wolf, S. G.: Changes in Coronary Blood Flow and Other Hemodynamic Indicators Induced by Stressful Interviews, *Psychosom. Med.*, **24**:331, 1962.
9. Stevenson, I. P., Duncan, C. H., Flynn, J. T., and Wolf, S.: Hypertension as a Reaction Pattern to Stress: Correlation of Circulatory Hemodynamics with Changes in the Attitude of Emotional State, *Am. J. M. Sc.*, **224**:286, 1952.
10. Ax, A. F.: Physiologic Differentiation between Fear and Anger in Humans, *Psychosom. Med.*, **15**:433, 1953.
11. Schacter, J.: Pain, Fear and Anger in Hypertensives and Normotensives, *Psychosom. Med.*, **19**:17, 1957.
12. Hillman, C. C., Levy, R. L., Stroud, W. D., and White, P. D.: Studies of Blood Pressure in Army Officers: Observations Based on an Analysis of the Medical Records of 22,741 Officers of the U.S. Army, *J.A.M.A.*, **125**:699, 1944.
13. Reiser, M. F., Brust, A. A., and Ferris, E. B.: Life Situations, Emotions and Course of Patients with Arterial Hypertension, *Psychosom. Med.*, **13**:133, 1951.
14. Reiser, M. F., Rosenbaum, M., and Ferris, E. B.: Psychologic Mechanisms in Malignant Hypertension, *Psychosom. Med.*, **13**:147, 1951.
15. Moses, L., Daniels, C. E., and Nickerson, J. L.: Psychogenic Factors in Essential Hypertension: Methodology and Preliminary Report, *Psychosom. Med.*, **18**:476, 1956.
16. Graham, J. D. P.: High Blood Pressure after Battle, *Lancet*, **1**:239, 1945.
17. Ruskin, A., Beard, D. W., and Schaffer, R. L.: Blast Hypertension: Elevated Arterial Pressure in Victims of the Texas City Disaster, *Am. J. Med.*, **4**:228, 1948.

18. Wheeler, E. O., White, P. D., Reed, E. W., and Cohen, M. E.: Neurocirculatory Asthenia (Anxiety Neurosis, Effort Syndrome, Neurasthenia): A Twenty Year Follow-up Study of 173 Patients, *J.A.M.A.*, **142**:878, 1950.

19. Weiss, E., English, O. S., Fisher, H. K., Kleinbart, M., and Zatuchni, J.: The Emotional Problems of High Blood Pressure, *Ann. Int. Med.*, **37**:677, 1952.

20. Gold, L.: Mental Characteristics Associated with "Essential" Hypertension, *Psychiat. Quart.*, **17**:364, 1943.

21. Dunbar, F.: "Psychosomatic Diagnosis," Hoeber Medical Division, Harper & Row, Publishers, Incorporated, New York, 1943.

22. Saslow, G., Gressel, C. C., Shobe, F. O., Du Bois, P. H., and Schroeder, H. A.: Possible Etiologic Relevance of Personality Factors in Arterial Hypertension, *Psychosom. Med.*, **12**:292, 1950.

23. Wolf, S., and Wolff, H. G.: A Summary of Experimental Evidence Relating Life Stress to the Pathogenesis of Essential Hypertension in Man, in E. Bell (ed.), "Hypertension; a Symposium," The University of Minnesota Press, Minneapolis, 1951, p. 288.

24. Dykman, R. A., and Gant, W. H.: Experimental Psychogenic Hypertension: Blood Pressure Changes Conditioned to Painful Stimuli (Schizokinesis), *Bull. Johns Hopkins Hosp.*, **107**:72, 1960.

25. Arlow, J. A.: Identification Mechanisms in Coronary Occlusion, *Psychosom. Med.*, **7**:195, 1945.

26. Cleveland, S. E., and Johnson, D. L.: Personality Patterns in Young Males with Coronary Disease, *Psychosom. Med.*, **24**:600, 1962.

27. Miles, H. H. W., Waldfogel, S., Barrabe, E. L., and Cobb, S.: Psychosomatic Study of 46 Young Men with Coronary Artery Disease, *Psychosom. Med.*, **16**:455, 1954.

28. Weiss, E., Dlin, B., Rollin, H. R., Fischer, H. D., and Bepler, C. R.: Emotional Factors in Coronary Occlusion: 1. Introduction and General Summary, *A.M.A. Arch. Int. Med.*, **99**:628, 1957.

29. Järvinen, K. A. J.: Can Ward Rounds be a Danger to Patients with Myocardial Infarction? *Brit. M. J.*, **1**:318, 1955.

30. Dreyfuss, F.: Role of Emotional Stress Preceding Coronary Occlusion, *Am. J. Cardiol.*, **3**:590, 1959.

31. Russek, H. I.: Emotional Stress and Coronary Heart Disease in American Physicians, Dentists and Lawyers, *Am. J. M. Sc.*, **243**:716, 1962.

32. Friedman, M., and Rosenman, R. H.: Association of Specific Overt Behavior Pattern with Blood and Cardiovascular Findings: Blood Cholesterol Level, Blood Clotting Time, Incidence of Arcus Senilis and Clinical Coronary Artery Disease, *J.A.M.A.*, **169**:1286, 1959.

33. Lee, R. E., and Schneider, R. F.: Hypertension and Arteriosclerosis in Executive and Nonexecutive Personnel, *J.A.M.A.*, **167**:1447, 1958.

34. Raffle, P. A. B.: Stress as a Factor in Disease, *Lancet*, **2**:839, 1959.

35. Thomas, C. B., and Murphy, E. A.: Further Studies on Cholesterol Levels in the Johns Hopkins Medical Students: The Effect of Stress at Examinations, *J. Chron. Dis.*, **8**:661, 1958.

36. Grundy, S. M., and Griffin, A. C.: Relationship of Periodic Mental Stress to Serum Lipoprotein and Cholesterol Levels, *J.A.M.A.*, **171**:1794, 1959.

37. Harvey, W. P., Levine, S. A.: Paroxysmal Ventricular Tachycardia Due to Emotion, *J.A.M.A.*, **150**:479, 1952.

38. Katz, L. N., Winton, S. S., and Megibow, R. S.: Psychosomatic Aspects of Cardiac Arrhythmias: A Physiological Dynamic Approach, *Ann. Int. Med.*, **27**:261, 1947.

39. Alterman, S. L., and Dick, M. M.: Bigeminy Due to Autonomic Nervous System Imbalance (in a Recruit), *U.S. Armed Forces M. J.*, **3**:1863, 1952.

40. Duncan, C. H., Stevenson, I. P., and Ripley, H. S.: Life Situations, Emotions and Paroxysmal Auricular Arrhythmias, *Psychosom. Med.*, **12**:23, 1950.

41. Fox, J. R., and McKinlay, C. A.: Major Cardiac Arrhythmias of Apparent Psychogenic Origin Observed in Young Adults, *J.-Lancet*, **71**:425, 1951.

42. Chambers, W. N., and Reiser, M. F.: Emotional Stress in Precipitation of Congestive Failure, *Psychosom. Med.*, **15**:38, 1953.

43. Vernon, C. R., Martin, D. A., and White, K. L.: Psychophysiological Approach to Management of Patients with Congestive Failure, *J.A.M.A.*, **171**:1947, 1959.

44. Schottstaedt, W. W., Grace, W. J., and Wolf, H. G.: Life Situations, Behavior, Attitudes, Emotions and Renal Excretion of Fluid and Electrolytes. IV. Situations Associated with the Retention of Water, Sodium and Potassium, *J. Psychosom. Res.*, **1**:287, 1956.

45. Barnes, R., and Schottstaedt, W. W.: The Relation of Emotional State to Renal Excretion of Water and Electrolytes in Patients with Congestive Heart Failure, *Am. J. Med.*, **29**:217, 1960.

46. Graybiel, A., and White, P. D.: Inversion of the T Waves in Lead I or II of the Electrocardiogram in Young Individuals with Neurocirculatory Asthenia, with Thyrotoxicosis, in Relation to Certain Infections and Following Paroxysmal Ventricular Tachycardia, *Am. Heart J.*, **10**:345, 1935.

47. Wendkos, M. H., and Logue, R. B.: Unstable T Waves in Leads II and III in Persons with Neurocirculatory Asthenia, *Am. Heart J.*, **31**:711, 1946.

48. Magendantz, H., and Shortsleeve, J.: Electrocardiographic Abnormalities in Patients Exhibiting Anxiety, *Am. Heart J.*, **42**:849, 1951.

49. Levander-Lindgren, M.: Studies in Neurocirculatory Asthenia (Da Costa's Syndrome). I. Variations with Regard to Symptoms and Some Pathophysiological Signs, *Acta med. scandinav.*, **172**:665, 1962.

50. Graybiel, A., Hartwell, A. S., Barrett, J. B., and White, P. D.: The Effect of Exercise and Four Commonly Used Drugs on the Normal Human Electrocardiogram with Particular Reference to T

Wave Changes, *J. Clin. Invest.*, **21**:409, 1942.

51. Ljung, O.: Alterations in the Electrocardiogram as a Result of Emotionally Stimulated Respiratory Movements, Especially with Reference to the So-called "Fright Electrocardiogram," *Acta med. scandinav.*, **141**:221, 1951.

52. Wasserburger, R. H., Siebecker, K. L., Jr., and Lewis, W. C.: The Effect of Hyperventilation on the Normal Adult Electrocardiogram, *Circulation*, **13**:850, 1956.

53. White, P. D., Cohen, M. E., and Chapman, W. P.: The Electrocardiogram in Neurocirculatory Asthenia, Anxiety Neurosis, or Effort Syndrome, *Am. Heart J.*, **34**:390, 1947.

54. Kannel, W. B., Dawber, T. R., and Cohen, M. E.: The ECG in Neurocirculatory Asthenia (Anxiety Neurosis or Neurasthenia): A Study of 203 Neurocirculatory Asthenia Patients and 757 Healthy Controls in the Framingham Study, *Ann. Int. Med.*, **49**:1351, 1958.

55. Cohen, M. E., White, P. D., and Johnson, R. E.: Neurocirculatory Asthenia, Anxiety Neurosis or the Effort Syndrome, *Arch. Int. Med.*, **81**:260, 1948.

56. White, P. D., and Jones, T. D.: Heart Disease and Disorders in New England, *Am. Heart J.*, **3**:302, 1928.

57. White, P. D.: "Heart Disease," 4th ed., The Macmillan Company, New York, 1956, p. 582.

58. Wheeler, E. O., White, P. D., Reed, E., and Cohen, M. E.: Familial Incidence of Neurocirculatory Asthenia (Anxiety Neurosis, Effort Syndrome), *J. Clin. Invest.*, **27**:562, 1948.

59. Myers, A. B. R.: "On the Etiology and Prevalence of Diseases of the Heart among Soldiers," J. Churchill and Sons, London, 1870, p. 22.

60. Da Costa, J. M.: On Irritable Heart: A Clinical Study of a Functional Cardiac Disorder and Its Consequences, *Am. J. M. Sc.*, **61**:17, 1871.

61. Oppenheimer, B. S., Levine, S. A., Morison, R. A., Rothschild, M. A., St. Lawrence, W., and Wilson, F. N.: Report on Neurocirculatory Asthenia and Its Management, *Mil. Surgeon*, **42**:409, 1918.

62. Lewis, T.: "The Soldier's Heart and the Effort Syndrome." Paul B. Hoeber, Inc., New York, 1919.

63. Wood, P.: Da Costa's Syndrome (or Effort Syndrome), *Brit. M. J.*, **1**:767, 805, 845, 1941.

64. White, P. D.: The Soldier's Irritable Heart, *J.A.M.A.*, **118**:270, 1942.

65. Lewis, Sir T.: "Soldier's Heart. Effort Syndrome," Shaw and Sons, Ltd., London, 1940.

66. Cohen, M. E., and White, P. D.: Life Situations, Emotions and Neurocirculatory Asthenia (Anxiety Neurosis, Neurasthenia, Effort Syndrome), *Psychosom. Med.*, **13**:335, 1951.

67. Craig, H. R., and White, P. D.: Etiology and Symptoms of Neurocirculatory Asthenia: Analysis of 100 Cases with Comments on Prognosis and Treatment, *A.M.A. Arch. Int. Med.*, **53**:633, 1934.

68. Cohen, M. D., Badal, D., Kilpatrick, A., Reed, E. W., and White, P. D.: The High Familial Prevalence of Neurocirculatory Asthenia (Anxiety Neurosis, Effort Syndrome), *Am. J. Human Genet.*, **3**:126, 1951.

69. Brown, F. W.: Heredity in Psychoneuroses, *Proc. Roy. Soc. Med.*, **35**:785, 1942.

70. Slater, E.: Neurotic Constitution: A Statistical Study of 2000 Neurotic Soldiers, *J. Neurol. & Psychiat.*, **6**:1, 1943.

71. Master, A. M.: Effort Syndrome or Neurocirculatory Asthenia in the Navy, *U.S. Navy M. Bull.*, **41**:666, 1943.

72. Friedman, M.: Studies Concerning the Etiology and Pathogenesis of Neurocirculatory Asthenia. III. The Cardiovascular Manifestations of Neurocirculatory Asthenia, *Am. Heart J.*, **30**:478, 1945.

73. Logue, R. B., Hanson, J. F., and Knight, W. A.: Electrocardiographic Studies in Neurocirculatory Asthenia, *Am. Heart J.*, **28**:574, 1944.

74. Cobb, S., Cohen, M. E., and Badal, D. W.: Capillaries of the Nail Fold in Patients with Neurocirculatory Asthenia (Effort Syndrome, Anxiety Neurosis), *Arch. Neurol. & Psychiat.*, **56**:643, 1946.

75. Jones, M., and Mellersh, V.: A Comparison of the Exercise Response in Various Groups of Neurotic Patients, and a Method of Rapid Determination of Oxygen in Expired Air Using a Catharometer, *Psychosom. Med.*, **8**:192, 1946.

76. Cohen, M. E., Johnson, R. E., Conzolazio, F. C., and White, P. D.: Low Oxygen Consumption and Low Ventilatory Efficiency during Exhausting Work in Patients with Neurocirculatory Asthenia, Effort Syndrome, Anxiety Neurosis, *J. Clin. Invest.*, **25**:292, 1946.

77. Cohen, M. E., Conzalazio, F. C., and Johnson, R. E.: Blood Lactate Response during Moderate Exercise in Neurocirculatory Asthenia, Anxiety Neurosis or Effort Syndrome, *J. Clin. Invest.*, **26**:339, 1947.

78. Cohen, M. E.: Studies of Palmar Hand Sweat in Healthy Subjects and in Patients with Neurocirculatory Asthenia (Anxiety Neurosis, Neurasthenia, Effort Syndrome) with a Description of a Simple Method for Its Quantitative Estimation, *Am. J. M. Sc.*, **220**:496, 1950.

79. Holmgren, A., Jonson, B., Levander, M., Linderholm, H., Sjostrand, T., and Strom, G.: Low Physical Working Capacity in Suspected Heart Cases Due to Inadequate Adjustment of Peripheral Blood Flow (Vasoregulatory Asthenia), *Acta med. scandinav.*, **158**:413, 1957.

80. Chapman, W. P., Cohen, M. E., and Cobb, S.: Measurements Related to Pain in Neurocirculatory Asthenia, Anxiety Neurosis, or Effort Syndrome: Levels of Heat Stimulus Perceived as Painful and Producing Wince and Withdrawal Reaction, *J. Clin. Invest.*, **25**:890, 1946.

81. Holmgren, A., Bengt, J., Levander, M., Linderholm, H., Mossfeldt, F., Sjostrand, T., and Strom, G.: Effect of Physical Training in Vasoregulatory Asthenia, in Da Costa's Syndrome and in Neurosis

without Heart Symptoms, *Acta med. scandinav.*, **165**:89, 1959.

82. Holmgren, A., Jonson, B., Levander, M., Linderholm, H., Mossfeldt, F., Sjostrand, T., and Strom, G.: Physical Training of Patients with Vasoregulatory Asthenia, *Acta med. scandinav.*, **158**:437, 1957.

83. Grant, R. T.: Observations on the After Histories of Men Suffering from the Effort Syndrome, *Heart,* **12**: 121, 1925–1926.

84. Wishaw, R.: A Review of the Physical Condition of 130 Returned Soldiers Suffering from the Effort Syndrome, *M. J. Australia*, **2**:891, 1939.

85. Bryce, J. C., Wanklin, J. W., and Hobbs, G. E.: Long Term Mortality in Cardiac Neuroses, *M. Serv. J. Canada*, **17**:669, 1961.

86. Stone, T. T., and Burris, B. C.: Melancholia: Clinical Study of 50 Cases, *J.A.M.A.*, **142**:165, 1950.

87. Cassidy, W. L., Flanagan, N. B., Spellman, M., and Cohen, M. E.: Clinical Observations in Manic Depressive Disease, *J.A.M.A.*, **164**:1535, 1957.

88. Purtell, J. J., Robins, E., and Cohen, M. E.: Observations on Clinical Aspects of Hysteria: A quantitative Study of 50 Hysteria Patients and 156 Control Subjects, *J.A.M.A.*, **146**:902, 1951.

89. Levine, S. A.: The Origin of the Term Neurocirculatory Asthenia, *New England J. Med.*, **273**:604, 1965.

64 IATROGENIC PROBLEMS AND HEART DISEASE *

J. Willis Hurst, M.D.

The aim of the physician is to help his patient. This he does the vast majority of the time. Despite his best intentions he may play a role in creating certain problems that may be troublesome to his patient. These problems may be organic or psychologic, mild or severe, correctable or noncorrectable, disabling or not disabling, and preventable or not preventable.

The term "iatrogenic heart disease" [1-4] is not a good one. First of all, it points an accusing finger solely at the physician; while this is sometimes justified, it is by no means always justified. Secondly, heart disease may or may not be actually produced in the patient given such a diagnosis; accordingly, the author has chosen to discuss the matter under a broader heading—iatrogenic problems and heart disease.

Iatrogenic problems related to heart disease can be divided into three groups: (1) problems produced as a direct result of procedures, drugs, diet,

* Grateful acknowledgement is made to Dr. Bernard Holland, Professor and Chairman of the Department of Psychiatry of Emory University School of Medicine, for his assistance in the preparation of this chapter.

and altered activity; (2) problems resulting from the misinterpretation of symptoms, signs, and laboratory data; (3) problems resulting from the effect of actions, words, and demeanor of a physician on a susceptible patient.

Iatrogenic Problems Resulting from Procedures, Drugs, Diet, and Altered Activity

There are no harmless procedures and no harmless drugs available for use in the practice of medicine. Even a recommended change in diet or the alteration of activity may cause problems in some patients. Also, if history can teach us, we can anticipate no change in this regard in the future. Accordingly, not all aspects of the new procedures and the new drugs yet to come will be good; with them will come new problems.

Procedures

The complications and risks of cardiac surgical procedures are discussed in Chaps. 21 and 26. Therefore, only a few points will be discussed here. Peripheral emboli may occur during and after aortic and mitral valve surgical procedures. Bacterial endocarditis may develop after intracardiac surgical procedures. Complete heart block may result from closure of an interventricular septal defect. Aortic regurgitation may develop as a complication of surgical treatment for aortic stenosis, and mitral regurgitation may result from the surgical treatment for mitral stenosis. The postmitral commissurotomy and postpericardiotomy syndrome occur in an unpredictable manner. Cardiac arrhythmias may occur after thoracotomy and cardiac surgical procedures. Atelectasis may develop after thoracic surgical procedures. Arteritis may occur after correction of coarctation of the aorta. Surgical ligation of the inferior vena cava may lead to persistent edema and venous insufficiency. Cardiac resuscitation utilizing external cardiac compression may produce contusion of the heart, rib and liver fracture, and fat and marrow emboli to the lungs. The use of defibrillators may lead to cardiac arrhythmias and burns of the skin.

Diagnostic procedures are not always innocuous. The complications of these procedures are discussed in detail in Part II, Section C. Cardiac catheterization may precipitate cardiac arrhythmias. The catheter may penetrate the right or left atrium and produce hemopericardium. A left-to-right atrial fistula may occur as a result of septal puncture in patients with high left atrial pressure associated with mitral valve disease. Rarely endocarditis may occur as a result of cardiac catheterization. Aortography may cause arterial damage. An arterial puncture may also cause arterial damage and may produce an arteriovenous fistula. A venipuncture may lead to thrombophlebitis and even introduce bacteria into the bloodstream.

Drugs

The complications of drug therapy are discussed in detail in Chap. 68. Digitalis may produce anorexia, nausea, diarrhea, and yellow vision. Arrhythmias related to digitalis medication are common. Arrhythmias, especially atrial tachycardia with atrioventricular block, are especially common in patients who receive digitalis and in whom there is a potassium deficit secondary to diuretic therapy. This is very likely to happen when the diuretic is a chlorothiazide derivative. Potassium supplement may not be sufficient to prevent this type of arrhythmia. On the other hand, potassium intoxication may develop when potassium is given in moderate dosage and is continued after a diuretic is no longer effective or has been discontinued. Vigorous diuresis may produce weakness and intravascular clotting. Quinidine sulfate may produce fever, purpura, diarrhea, and cardiac arrhythmias. Morphine sulfate may produce nausea, constipation, respiratory depression, and hypotension and contribute to atrioventricular block. Norepinephrine may produce cardiac arrhythmias and necrosis of skin and subcutaneous tissue near the region of intravenous injection or in a distant location. Epinephrine may produce cardiac arrhythmias. Isopropyl norepinephrine may produce arrhythmias and hypotension. Antihypertensive drugs including chlorothiazide and ganglionic blocking agents may produce postural hypotension and syncope. Nitroglycerin and digitalis may aggravate angina pectoris in patients with functional hypertrophic subaortic stenosis. Anticoagulants may produce hemorrhage, including hemopericardium, in certain circumstances.

A change in diet may produce psychologic problems, electrolyte disturbance, and malnutrition. Frequent determination of serum-cholesterol level in patients on various diets can, at times, lead to much anxiety and unscientific medicine. Fluids administered intravenously may precipitate pulmonary edema.

A recommendation of increased activity may produce cardiac arrhythmias, syncope, angina pectoris, and heart failure, while severe restriction may produce much emotional turmoil, disability, and pulmonary emboli.

This list of problems associated with procedures, drugs, diet, and activity in relationship to heart disease is far from complete. The list serves as a background to point out that there is much overlap of what is called "iatrogenic problems" and what is designated as "complications." This is true because the doctor is usually in control of the diagnostic work-up and therapy. Since virtually all procedures and all drugs are potentially hazardous, how is the doctor to function? If he fails to offer a patient corrective surgical treatment, a proper diagnostic work-up, or the proper drug or diet because he is terrified by the possible *complications,* then he will also fail to offer his patient the *benefits* of procedures, drugs, and diet. The problem is solved in two ways:

1. The physician is obligated to reduce the risk of surgical and diagnostic procedure to the minimum. He does this by assembling the best team that is possible and being cognizant of the complications in order to prevent them if possible. The same approach applies to drug therapy and alterations of the diet. Despite the most careful preparation and execution of a planned program, complications may occur. The obligation of the physician at this point is to recognize the complications and institute the proper therapy when such is available.

2. The physician must always weigh the risk of what he *does* with the associated complications against the risk of what he *does not do* with the associated complications. The physician must ask himself and must answer the following questions: Will the benefit of surgical procedures with its price—the risk—be worthwhile for the patient when compared with his state without surgical treatment? Will the information gained from a diagnostic procedure be of enough value in the care of the patient to justify the risk involved? Will the potential benefit of drug therapy be worth the risk of drug complications in a certain clinical situation?

Iatrogenic Problems Resulting from the Misinterpretation of Symptoms, Signs, and Laboratory Data

The misinterpretation of symptoms, signs, and laboratory data may create iatrogenic problems. Dyspnea due to anxiety or pulmonary disease may be incorrectly attributed to heart disease and treated with digitalis. Chest pain associated with anxiety, gastrointestinal disease, musculoskeletal disease may be misdiagnosed as angina pectoris. Palpitation due to an occasional ectopic contraction may be disabling to a sensitive patient and thought to be ominous by the physician. Edema of the extremities secondary to obesity or venous insufficiency may be wrongly attributed to congestive heart failure. Episodes of hyperventilation may be diagnosed as acute pulmonary edema. Oral hyperthermia or the normal temperature of a child may be thought to be due to rheumatic fever. A diagnosis of essential hypertension may be made and the patient treated accordingly simply because the blood pressure is elevated on a single recording.

Systolic hypertension may be misinterpreted completely and treatment started for diastolic hypertension. Kinking of the carotid artery may be misdiagnosed as an aneurysm of the artery. Innocent murmurs are very common, are often misinterpreted, and are often attributed to heart disease. This is especially true in children, in pregnant females, when fever is present, and in patients with anemia or thyrotoxicosis. Benign arrhythmias, such as sinus arrhythmia, may be diagnosed as a serious abnormality of cardiac rhythm. Edema due to extracardiac conditions may be thought to be due to heart failure.

The normal range of the electrocardiogram is wide and is difficult to learn. Many benign ST-T wave "abnormalities" are unfortunately attributed to heart disease. QRS conduction disturbances are frequently misdiagnosed as myocardial infarction. Occasionally myocardial infarction may be correctly diagnosed by electrocardiography but from a tracing that belongs to someone else! Wilson[5] wrote the following in Lepeschkin's book on electrocardiography:

In the last two decades there has been a tremendous growth of interest in electrocardiographic diagnosis and in the number and variety of electrocardiographs in use. In 1914, there was only one instrument of this kind in the state of Michigan and this was not in operation; there were probably no more than a dozen electrocardiographs in the whole of the United States. Now there is one or more in almost every village of any size, and there are comparatively few people who are not in greater danger of having their peace and happiness destroyed by an erroneous diagnosis of cardiac abnormality based on a faulty interpretation of an electrocardiogram, than of being injured or killed by an atomic bomb. (This paragraph is reprinted here with the permission of Dr. Eugene Lepeschkin and the Williams and Wilkins Company.)

An erroneous diagnosis of cardiac enlargement is often made on examination of the x-ray of the chest when the apparent enlargement is really due to a depressed sternum or an epicardial fat pad. The pulmonary artery may be normally prominent when the heart is vertically placed and may be misinterpreted as an abnormality. Elevation of the serum–glutamic oxalacetic transaminase level by a noncardiac condition may be thought to be due to myocardial infarction. The level of the serum cholesterol is often used in a nonscientific manner. The determination of venous pressure and circulation time may be executed poorly, and the results may be no more than the accurate recording of inaccurate data. Cardiac catheterization data may be misinterpreted.

This is a partial list of symptoms, signs, and laboratory data that may be misinterpreted by the physician. Physicians are human, and the problems of medicine are often very complex. Accordingly, even experts acting with great care may misinterpret clinical data.

The conscientious physician is aware of the impact of erroneous diagnosis on his patient. He therefore makes every effort to minimize these problems by careful study and accurate diagnosis, by asking for consultation when he is uncertain, and by correcting his opinion as soon as possible when new information clarifies the problem.

Iatrogenic Problems Resulting from the Effect of Actions, Words, and Demeanor of a Physician upon a Susceptible Patient[2, 4, 6]

A patient's visit to a physician's office is an emotional experience for all concerned. The patient is influenced by the physician, the nurse, the technician, the maid, the fellow patient, and the entire environment. The effect of these influences on the patient depends upon his emotional status. For example, one patient may be told by his physician that he has a "terrible-looking" electrocardiogram and might respond to the knowledge by saying, "It must not mean too much because I feel fine," whereas another patient may become convinced that he has serious heart disease simply because the physician listened to his heart longer than was anticipated. The first patient may remain asymptomatic and return to work. The second patient, who may have gone to the physician because of sighing, breathing, sticks and stabs of pain near the cardiac apex, palpitation, and exhaustion, now may become disabled from the symptoms despite the reassurances of the physician. In the first case the physician would not be speaking wisely, even though despite the frightening words the patient is not harmed because he is emotionally normal.[4] In the second case the patient would be reacting abnormally to a careful examination because he is emotionally disturbed.

Many people, perhaps the majority, have varying degrees of emotional problems. Accordingly, a few comments regarding the emotional makeup of doctors and the emotional makeup of patients are in order.

The physician may feel insecure and uncertain in his appraisal of a problem. Because of this he hedges in his opinion regarding a medical problem. The patient who complains of dyspnea and "heart pains" related to anxiety frequently tests the doctor. The physician may reassure him in many ways, indicating that his blood pressure is normal, the physical examination and electrocardiogram are normal, and "all seems fine." The patient may seem relieved of his worry regarding heart disease and just as he is leaving the office asks about making a trip, playing golf, etc. When he is advised to "take it easy," he may become firmly convinced that his heart is so bad the doctor wants to keep the bad news from him. This is a simple and obvious example of "opinion hedging." The physician, of course, does not consciously realize that he has contributed to the patient's anxiety.

The physician may be extremely concerned that some seriously ill patient may die while under his care. He advises the patient's family of his concern and transmits to them his own anxiety. He may feel protected in that the family, knowing how grave the situation is, will not blame him if the clinical situation deteriorates and death ensues. He stands to gain if the patient survives under his care despite the great odds that have been pointed out.

The physician may become frustrated because he cannot solve a difficult medical problem and may transmit this frustration to the patient. He may become angry because the patient with emphysema will not stop smoking or the obese patient will not lose weight. He may threaten the patient by suggesting that he cannot take care of him if the patient will not obey his rules.

A patient recovering from a serious illness is frequently very dependent upon the physician. This is as it should be, but at times it is carried to the abnormal degree. If the physician does not recognize this as only one stage of the total rehabilitation process, the patient's progress may remain on a plateau at this level. The insecure physician may have a large share of such patients under his care.

Unless the physician is aware of the problems he can cause by loose, thoughtless talk and his actions and demeanor, he may frighten the susceptible patient. For example, the doctor who whistles or frowns when the blood pressure is noted to be at a high level, who comments that the heart is huge, who uses strange new words such as organic, physiologic, murmur, skipped beats, systole, or diastole in the presence of the patient, who teaches and points out all findings to his students at the bedside, who threatens his patients by saying, "If you don't get your cholesterol down you are going to have a heart attack" is likely to create iatrogenic problems of anxiety. When this sort of environment prevails, it is likely that many medically unqualified personnel may contribute their own anxiety-provoking statements. For example, the electrocardiographic technician not wishing to appear unknowing, may answer a query by the patient with frightening statements.

Physical illness is one of the most fear-producing contingencies of modern man. Living has been made secure in many ways, but physical illness remains as the severe threat. Physical illness happens to the individual, yet many other factors influence the illness. Some of these factors are the personality structure of the patient, his family structure, his work, the degree of financial security, and the nature of his illness.

The personality structure of the patient may influence the patient's illness favorably or unfavorably. There are some patients who exaggerate their illnesses and with minor illnesses become permanent invalids; some patients minimize their illnesses and deny the existence of real danger. The family influences the course of illness; a family may either exaggerate or minimize the medical problem. At times families bring to the patient stories of friends and neighbors who had a similar illness and had an early demise. These stories intensify the patient's anxieties. In addition to their illnesses, many patients have realistic anxieties about their work and financial security and the degree to which illness will affect their present and future work life. Sometimes these fears are realistic and sometimes they are exaggerated. The nature of the illness has a direct bearing on the degree of anxiety. There is much common knowledge among the general populace about illness today. There is some understanding of the nature of heart disease, but this information and misinformation may either add to or diminish the patient's anxiety.

Most patients pass through a usual course of illness. In the beginning, there may be denial of the illness or the seriousness of the illness. In time this is replaced by fear of the illness, which may be considerably exaggerated. This may be followed by a period of regression, clinging, and dependency upon the physician and the nursing staff. Normally this is followed by a period of depression where the patient has periods of low self-esteem, difficulty in sleeping, loss of appetite, loss of usual interest in family and friends. This is usually followed by realistic adaptation to the illness and the limitations of the illness. However, there are many patients who never work through this course. There are some who become anxious about their illnesses and become chronic invalids for the rest of their lives.

The physician has many problems dealing with patients. He must be accurate in his diagnosis of the patient's problem and must teach him realistically to care for his illness. If he has a patient who is overly anxious, without due care he may easily stir up these anxieties by realistic instruction. On the other hand, if the patient denies his illness and will not take realistic care of his problem, then the physician must find a way to deal with the patient's denial, without stirring up undue anxiety.

Iatrogenic problems which are a result of the actions, words, and demeanor of a physician in dealing with a susceptible patient may be minimized by considering the following points:

1. The physician must be aware of the problem under discussion. He must understand that certain anxious patients will visit him and that his words, actions, and demeanor and the entire environment created by him may enhance the patient's fears, worries, and anxiety.

2. The physician must know himself. He cannot manage or prevent anxiety if he does not attempt to analyze his own reactions and emotional make-up.

3. The physician must learn as much as possible about organic disease and try to understand the emotional problems of patients.

4. The physician must understand the stages of rehabilitation through which a patient should go after having a serious illness. His job is to lead him through various stages and to establish a healthy and nondependent physician-patient relationship.

REFERENCES

1. Aurbach, A., and Gliebe, P. A.: Iatrogenic Heart Disease: Common Cardiac Neurosis, *J.A.M.A.*, **129**: 338, 1945.
2. Weinberg, H. B.: Iatrogenic Heart Disease, *Ann. Int. Med.*, **38**:9, 1953.
3. Hart, A. D.: Iatrogenic Cardiac Neurosis: Critique, *J.A.M.A.*, **156**:1133, 1954.
4. Wheeler, E. O., Williamson, C. R., and Cohen, M. E.: Heart Scare, Heart Surveys, and Iatrogenic Heart Disease: Emotional and Symptomatological Effects of Suggesting to 162 Adults That They Might Have Heart Disease, *J.A.M.A.*, **167**:1096, 1958.
5. Wilson, F., in E. Lepeschkin: "Modern Electrocardiography," The Williams & Wilkins Company, Baltimore, 1951, foreword, vol. 1, pp. v–vi.
6. Harrison, T. R., and Reeves, T. J.: The Psychologic Management of Patients with Heart Disease, *Am. Heart J.*, **70**:136, 1965.

65 THE EFFECTS OF TOBACCO ON THE CARDIOVASCULAR SYSTEM

Joseph T. Doyle, M.D.

The smoldering combustion of tobacco evolves, through a series of pyrolyses, distillations, and condensations, numerous highly reactive chemical radicals which combine into at least 270 identifiable organic compounds dispersed as fine droplets in a gaseous phase comprised of nitrogen and its oxides, carbon monoxide, carbon dioxide, and steam. This highly toxic aerosol is promptly rendered relatively innocuous by dilution. Thus, although a puff of cigarette smoke contains about 8 per cent carbon monoxide, the blood–carbon monoxide level of even heavy smokers is only slightly higher than in nonsmokers. Cigarette smoke also contains considerable microscopic debris such as shreds of tobacco and paper, charcoal, and elements of filter tips. This finely particulate matter produces, quite nonspecifically, a small but measurable increase in airway resistance.

All toxicologic and pharmacologic studies have shown that the sole physiologically active ingredient of tobacco smoke is nicotine. This alkaloid has no known function in the plant economy. It is synthesized in the roots and transported to the leaves. The nicotine content of tobacco varies considerably with regional and climatic factors and can be altered by selective breeding. Although cigar and pipe tobaccoes contain considerably larger quantities of nicotine than does cigarette tobacco, their heavy, alkaline smoke is intensely irritating to the respiratory tract and is not usually inhaled. On the other hand, the light, bland smoke of cigarettes is, with practice, readily tolerated by the bronchial tree. Accordingly, nicotine is rapidly and completely absorbed in the lungs by the cigarette smoker, while absorption of nicotine from the buccal mucosa in cigar and pipe smokers and in tobacco chewers is slower and less complete. For all practical purposes, the measurable effects of tobacco smoking relate to cigarettes and are identical with those produced by equivalent doses of nicotine.

A standard cigarette contains about 20 mg nicotine. Considerable amounts of nicotine are destroyed by heat or dispersed in the side-stream smoke, so that the average inhaling cigarette smoker absorbs about 2 mg nicotine. Depending on rate of puffing, depth of inhalation, and length of cigarette the nicotine absorption from a single cigarette in the average adult male is 3 to 6 μg per kg per min. The lethal human oral dose of nicotine is estimated to be 1 mg per kg.

The earliest descriptions of tobacco smoking among South American aborigines repeatedly mention trancelike or unconscious states not usually considered typical of nicotine effect. The novice smoker commonly experiences the toxic effects of nicotine: giddiness, nausea and vomiting, abdominal cramps, cold sweat, and even vasomotor collapse. These symptoms when usually severe have, in the past, been incorrectly construed as evidence of sensitivity to tobacco and may, understandably, deter formation of the smoking habit. The veteran smoker probably does not acquire tolerance to nicotine, inasmuch as all measurable circulatory responses persist without attenuation, but learns to manipulate time-dosage factors so as to avoid poisonous effects. Radioactively labeled nicotine is rapidly degraded after ingestion, but the metabolic pathways are unknown. Approximately 10 per cent of ingested nicotine is excreted unchanged. Chronic administration of nicotine to experimental animals produces no demonstrable tissue damage. The possibility of allergic or hypersensitivity reactions to tobacco or its combustion products has been suggested but not convincingly proved. Acquisition of the tobacco habit is clearly related to social, cultural, and psychologic pressures. It is universally recognized that, once entrenched, the cigarette habit is difficult to break. There is some evidence that parenterally administered nicotine can induce the same feeling of satiety produced by a cigarette. Some but not all heavy smokers derive complete satisfaction from low-nicotine cigarettes. It is unlikely that nicotine is addicting in the same sense as that applied to narcotics.

The pharmacologic and toxic effects of nicotine have been extensively studied in experimental animals for a century and more. The applicability of these observations to human subjects is, however, questionable. Therefore, despite the meagerness of such information, the data to be cited are based primarily on studies in human beings.

In nonsmokers as well as experienced smokers, cigarette smoke and nicotine cause significant increases in heart rate, in systolic, diastolic, and pulse pressures, in cardiac output, and in stroke volume. Indirect observations of human beings indicate that the inhalation of cigarette smoke is followed by shortening of the isometric period of left ventricular contraction. Skin temperature and blood flow are sharply reduced. Muscle blood flow is augmented. Information on coronary blood flow is scanty because of the technical difficulty of measurement. It appears, however, that there is an increase in coronary blood flow after smoking that parallels rises in systemic blood pressure and in left ventricular output. The resultant increase in cardiac work in individuals with overt coronary heart disease is not met by a corresponding increase in coronary arterial flow.

No electrocardiographic changes are associated with smoking which cannot be explained by the increase in heart rate. The striking electrocardiographic abnormalities induced by nicotine and tobacco smoke in animals with artificial coronary arterial obstruction have no counterpart in human subjects with coronary disease. Ballistocardiographic abnormalities induced by cigarette smoking are not reproduced by nicotine. The ballistocardiographic cigarette test, after initial enthusiastic acceptance, has been discarded as adequate evidence of subclinical coronary artery disease.

The circulatory responses to tobacco smoke in subjects both human and animal are accounted for by the mobilization of epinephrine and norepinephrine from chromaffin tissue in and around blood vessels, from ganglions in the myocardium, and from the adrenal medulla itself. Structures activated by the release of acetylcholine are stimulated by nicotine. Such structures include the central nervous system, notably the supraopticohypothalamic system, neuromuscular junctions, and chemoreceptors of the carotid and aortic bodies. A dose of nicotine produces a blood-epinephrine level virtually equivalent to concentrations used therapeutically. In human subjects, urinary epinephrine excretion may increase up to 50 per cent after heavy cigarette smoking. In experimental animals, the effect of nicotine can be blocked by ganglioplegics such as hexamethonium. Depletion of the norepinephrine stores of chromaffin cells by reserpine blocks the response to nicotine, an effect of possible therapeutic significance in vasospastic disorders. Stimulation of the posterior pituitary causes measurable antidiuresis, although the amount of pitressin liberated is quite inadequate to produce coronary arterial constriction.

Substantial quantities of free fatty acids are mobilized in the serum of human subjects by smoking cigarettes or by the injection of nicotine. This metabolic response to sympathetic stimulation can be prevented by ganglionic blockade and is absent in adrenalectomized human subjects. Some data indicate increased serum total-cholesterol levels in heavy cigarette smokers, although other data show no relationship.

An increase in blood sugar has been regularly found in experimental animals after the exhibition of nicotine, but observations in human beings are contradictory. Oxygen consumption in the human subject, furthermore, is not increased by nicotine or by cigarette smoke. Blood clotting is not measurably affected by cigarette smoking.

The use of tobacco has been violently condemned on both moral and hygienic grounds virtually from its first introduction into Europe, but few scientifically acceptable data on the chronic effects of smoking have been available until recently. "Tobacco angina," so often described by clinicians of a previous generation, has disappeared as the clinical definition of coronary heart disease has become more precise. Since Buerger first described thromboangiitis obliterans in 1908, cigarette smoking has been generally considered to be a primary etiologic factor. On the other hand, Wessler has submitted impressive evidence that Buerger's disease is indistinguishable from the ischemic complications of atherosclerosis, arterial embolization, or thrombosis and is not correlated with smoking habit. De Bakey and associates[1] imply similar conclusions based on their large clinical experience.

Chronic toxicity studies in animals have consistently failed to show evidence of tissue damage. Observations of the long-continued effects of tobacco on human subjects are necessarily anecdotal and, interestingly, confined exclusively to males at the time of this writing. Twenty-five years ago Pearl[2] concluded on rather dubious evidence that ". . . the smoking of tobacco is statistically associated with an impairment of life duration, and the amount or degree of this impairment increases as the habitual amount of smoking increases." More recently, Berkson[3] has extended this concept. He holds that tobacco exercises a nonspecific lethal influence on the human organism, since heavy smokers die at an accelerated rate from all causes, most commonly from cardiovascular disease. Large-scale retrospective and prospective studies of the association between tobacco habit and bronchiogenic carcinoma have been accepted by most physicians and statisticians as clearly inculpating cigarettes. A much more striking although incidental observation has been the large excess of cardiovascular deaths in heavy cigarette smokers (Fig. 65-1).[4] The same trends in mortality as well as in morbidity have been witnessed in the pooled data of the Framingham and Albany studies. The consumption of 20 or more cigarettes daily is associated with at least a three times greater hazard of myocardial infarction than is found in nonsmokers or in cigar or pipe smokers.

On the other hand, angina pectoris is no more common in cigarette smokers than in nonsmokers. Similar observations were reported 30 years ago by White and Sharber.[5] This striking difference between angina pectoris and other manifestations of

coronary heart disease is not easily explained. It is tempting to speculate that heavy cigarette smoking, despite the absence of supporting experimental evidence, may predispose toward the acute occlusive complications of coronary atherosclerosis but plays no role whatsover in that form of arterial disease manifested only by angina. This is in no way inconsistent with the frequent clinical observation that angina may be precipitated or aggravated by smoking. In support of such a hypothesis is the observation that the risk of myocardial infarction in the ex-cigarette smoker reverts to that of the nonsmoker or cigar or pipe smoker, suggesting that the effects of cigarette smoke are acute rather than chronic. The little, if any, increased risk of myocardial infarction in cigar and pipe smokers seems most plausibly explained by the smaller amounts of nicotine and other substances inhaled. Observations on the relationship between smoking habit and vascular disease in large groups of women are not yet available.

Although cigarette smoking is regularly associated with an immediate, although transient, rise in arterial blood pressure, the prognostic significance of this response is unclear. Vascular hyperreactors have an excessive pressor response and a striking reduction in retinal arterial caliber after cigarette smoking, but follow-up observations have not been reported. Thomas has found that the sons of hypertensive parents tend to show exaggerated increases in pulse rate, cardiac output, and arterial blood pressure after cigarette smoking, perhaps as a genetic expression. On the other hand, epidemiologic findings are that heavy cigarette smokers tend to have lower blood pressure readings than nonsmokers. Moreover, Blackburn et al.[6] find no significant differences in the pulse rate, the blood pressure, the response to the cold pressor test, or the response to the inhalation of carbon dioxide between smokers and nonsmokers in various male populations. They conclude that smokers show no evidence of impaired cardiovascular "fitness" on work tests, a view supported by limited but careful studies by Karpovich and Hale.[7] Comparable studies on middle-aged populations of heavy smokers are not available. Again, it should be noted that epidemiologic and prognostic studies of the smoking habit in women have not yet been reported.

The therapeutic inferences to be derived from these incomplete pharmacologic and epidemiologic observations are necessarily at present empiric. The acute circulatory responses to smoking are due to the absorption of nicotine and the resultant mobilization of catecholamines. Heart rate, systolic blood pressure, and cardiac output increase. A narrowed coronary arterial tree may not be able

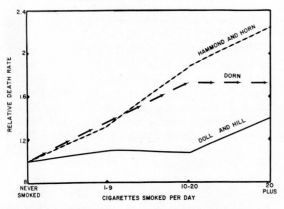

DEATH RATE FROM CORONARY HEART DISEASE
RELATED TO USE OF CIGARETTES

Fig. 65-1. Death rate from coronary heart disease related to the use of cigarettes. (*From E. C. Hammond: The Effects of Smoking, Scient. Am.,* **207**:39, 1962. *Courtesy of E. C. Hammond, Sc.D., and Scientific American.*)

to sustain the increased myocardial work load. In contrast, the sharp decrease in blood flow to the extremities is ill tolerated in advanced obliterative vascular disease. Mortality data in men indicate that heavy cigarette smokers die more rapidly than nonsmokers, while morbidity data, also in men, reveal a threefold greater hazard of myocardial infarction in men who smoke 20 or more cigarettes daily. It is difficult to escape the conclusion that abstention from cigarettes may improve longevity, particularly since the same morbidity data indicate that former cigarette smokers experience little if any greater risk than nonsmokers or pipe or cigar smokers. Moreover, many, though admittedly anecdotal, observations attest to the amelioration of vasospastic and obliterative vascular diseases of the extremities after the discontinuance of smoking. Recently the Surgeon General's Advisory Committee on Smoking and Health[8] has affirmed the significance of the association between cigarette smoking and coronary heart disease. Furthermore, the Committee has unequivocally termed cigarette usage the most important of the causes of chronic bronchitis and significantly related to pulmonary emphysema. Both these conditions can aggravate heart disease of any type and may cause chronic cor pulmonale.

REFERENCES

1. De Bakey, M. E., and Cohen, B. M.: "Buerger's Disease: A Follow-up Study of World War II Army Cases," Charles C Thomas, Publisher, Springfield, Ill., 1963.
2. Pearl, R.: Tobacco Smoking and Longevity, *Science*, **87**:216, 1938.
3. Berkson, J.: Smoking and Cancer of the Lung, *Proc. Staff Meet. Mayo Clin.*, **35**:637, 1960.
4. Hammond, E. C.: The Effects of Smoking, *Scient. Am.*, **207**:39, 1962.
5. White, P. D., and Sharber, T.: Tobacco, Alcohol and Angina Pectoris, *J.A.M.A.*, **102**:655, 1934.
6. Blackburn, H., Brozek, J., and Taylor, H. L.: Common Circulatory Measurements in Smokers and Nonsmokers, *Circulation*, **22**:1112, 1960.
7. Karpovich, P. V., and Hale, C. J.: Tobacco Smoking and Physical Performance, *J. Appl. Physiol.*, **3**:616, 1951.
8. "Smoking and Health: Report of the Advisory Committee to the Surgeon General of the Public Health Service," Public Health Service Publication no. 1103, Washington, 1964.

SUGGESTED READING

Cattell, McK. and Wiggers, C. J., eds.: Cardiovascular Effects of Nicotine and Smoking, *Ann. New York Acad. Sci.*, **90**:1, 1960.
Cusick, P. L., and Herrell, W. E.: Retinal Arteriolar Changes as Part of an Induced General Vasospastic Reaction: Effect of Tobacco and Cold, *A.M.A. Arch. Ophthal.*, **21**:111, 1939.
Doll, R., and Hill, A. B.: Lung Cancer and Other Causes of Death in Relation to Smoking: Second Report on Mortality of British Doctors, *Brit. M. J.*, **2**: 1071, 1956.
Dorn, H. F.: Tobacco Consumption and Mortality from Cancer and Other Diseases, *Pub. Health Rep.*, **74**: 581, 1959.
Doyle, J. T., Dawber, T. R., Kannel, W. B., Kinch, S. H., and Kahn, H. A.: The Relationship of Cigarette Smoking to Coronary Heart Disease: The Second Report of the Combined Experience of the Albany, N.Y., and Framingham, Mass., Studies, *J.A.M.A.*, **190**:886, 1964.
Hammond, E. C., and Horn, D.: Smoking and Death Rates: Report on Forty-four Months of Follow-up of 187,783 Men. I. Total Mortality, *J.A.M.A.*, **166**: 1159, 1958. II. Death Rates by Cause, *J.A.M.A.*, **166**:1294, 1958.
James, G., and Rosenthal, T., eds.: "Tobacco and Health," Charles C Thomas, Publisher, Springfield, Ill., 1962.
Larson, P. S., Haag, H. B., and Silvette, H.: "Tobacco: Experimental and Clinical Studies," The Williams and Wilkins Company, Baltimore, 1961.
Roth, G. M.: "Tobacco and the Cardiovascular System: The Effects of Smoking and Nicotine on Normal Persons," Charles C Thomas, Publisher, Springfield, Ill., 1951.
Thomas, C. B., Bateman, J. L., and Lindberg, E. V.: Observations on the Individual Effects of Smoking on the Blood Pressure, Heart Rate, Stroke Volume and Cardiac Output of Healthy Young Adults, *Ann. Int. Med.*, **44**:874, 1956.
Wessler, S., Ming, S., Gurewich, V., and Freiman, D. G.: A Critical Evaluation of Thromboangiitis Obliterans: The Case against Buerger's Disease, *New England J. Med.*, **262**:1149, 1960.
Wynder, E. L. (ed.): "The Biologic Effects of Tobacco with Emphasis on the Clinical and Experimental Aspects," Little, Brown and Company, Boston, 1955.

Section C: Anesthesia and Surgery

66 THE HEART AND ANESTHESIA

John E. Steinhaus, Ph.D., M.D.

The primary purpose served by the induction of anesthesia is the relief of pain. Related to this main purpose has been the production of unconsciousness, amnesia, and skeletal muscle control. Unfortunately, all known anesthetic agents also have adverse actions which impair both respiration and circulation, and consequently a second and equally important purpose of anesthesia is the establishment and maintenance of the oxygen transport system, which in essence is resuscitation. As the knowledge of respiratory physiology has expanded and developed, inadequate ventilation during anesthesia can be prevented to a very large degree. The maintenance of adequate cardiovascular function is a more difficult problem, and consequently it has come to be an increasingly important concern during the administration of anesthesia. In addition, the cardiovascular effects of anesthetic agents have assumed a greater role in recent years, because the patients scheduled for anesthesia are older and have more serious diseases of the heart. It is not uncommon to encounter a seriously ill patient in which the resuscitative aspect of anesthesia far outweighs the problem of producing pain relief or muscle control.

The circulation of the blood is determined by an interrelation of numerous cardiac and vascular factors. Inadequate vasomotor tone or deficient blood volume, due to disease or blood loss, is frequently an important cause of circulatory failure. Deficient myocardial function may be related to a conduction disturbance, or a depression of myocardial contractility. The cardiovascular system, like many vital organ systems, has a considerable margin of reserve. Attitudes toward the cardiac effects of anesthesia have varied from one extreme that these drugs have no important effect on the heart to the other extreme that hearts stop suddenly and somewhat mysteriously (cardiac arrest) under their influence. A more accurate concept, of course, would be that all anesthetic agents produce some depression of the heart but that the normal cardio-vascular system maintains adequate function over a fairly wide spectrum of drug action.

Changes in cardiovascular function during anesthesia may be due to other factors than the direct effect of anesthetic drugs on the heart. The most important of these factors are changes in ventilation and autonomic nervous system function. Almost all anesthetic agents depress ventilation, and if this is not corrected, the resulting hypoxia and hypercapnia will alter cardiac function. Although the changes in heart rate are variable, severe hypoxia will produce a complete depression of myocardial contraction. An increase in blood pressure, related to the release of catecholamines, commonly occurs during the early phase of hypercapnia. At the same time the increased carbon dioxide depresses myocardial contraction and will add to the cardiac depression produced by hypoxia and drugs. Rapid removal of very high levels of carbon dioxide can produce severe arrhythmias; however, the severe degree of hypercapnia required for this phenomena is almost never encountered clinically. So-called cyclopropane shock would appear to be in part due to the depression of respiration during anesthesia and the resultant hypercapnia. The recovery from anesthesia and the removal of accumulated carbon dioxide apparently functions like the withdrawal of a vasopressor, and a characteristic hypotension may occur. Anesthetic agents have complex actions of both the sympathetic and parasympathetic nervous system, and consequently it is not possible to account for the cardiovascular changes during anesthesia without a careful analysis of the autonomic effects.

Cardiac Rhythm

The role of anesthetic agents in the production of cardiac arrhythmias became a subject of great interest after the introduction of cyclopropane. The most common arrhythmias noted during anesthesia were atrioventricular dissociation and ventricular extra systoles, the latter often occuring as bigeminy.[1] Early studies with cyclopropane revealed that epinephrine could precipitate both ventricular tachycardia and fibrillation.[2] It was also recognized that arrhythmias were more apt to occur with deep cyclopropane anesthesia, and later a relationship was demonstrated between the increased incidence of arrhythmias and an increase in carbon dioxide tension.[3] Hypercapnia appears to produce arrhythmias through the release of catecholamines.[4] Experimental work has shown that epinephrine will produce similar arrhythmias during halothane (Fluothane) anesthesia;[5] however, carefully controlled dosages of epinephrine in clinical studies did not produce serious arrhythmias in patients anesthetized with this halogenated agent.[6] Although it is possible to use epinephrine in restricted dosages with halogenated agents, the hazard of a potentially serious arrhythmia cannot be removed. In deep hypothermia it also appears that cyclopropane and halogenated hydrocarbons are more likely to be associated with serious arrhythmias than other anesthetic agents.[7] In common clinical experience the ventricular extra systole seldom indicates serious trouble and usually disappears with increased ventilation and lighter anesthesia. It appears that the mechanism for the ventricular premature beat commonly encountered may differ from that which produces ventricular fibrillation.[8]

Auxiliary agents which cause changes in rhythm include succinylcholine, which has been found to produce bradycardia and asystole with repeated doses. It is suggested that choline formed from either acetyl- or succinylcholine can sensitize the myocardium to the succeeding doses of the relaxant.[9] This arrhythmia is not frequently encountered in routine anesthesia, because of the blocking action of barbiturate commonly employed for induction. Intravenous atropine has also been reported to precipitate severe arrhythmia.[10]

A more serious problem in cardiac conduction is found in patients with atrioventricular heart block.[11] The hearts of these patients will tolerate only the mildest depressant action of anesthetic agents. It is very important that preanesthetic medication should include a sufficient dose of atropine to block the vagus together with the normal measures (sympathomimetic amine) for controlling Stokes-Adams attacks. Anesthetics with the minimal cardiac depression, such as nitrous oxide, and rapid reversibility, such as cyclopropane, are the least hazardous general anesthetic agents for patients in this precarious state.

Many drugs, such as procaine, diethyl ether, and barbiturate, have been reported as effective measures for reducing the incidence of arrhythmias during cyclopropane anesthesia. As previously mentioned, ventilation and decreasing anesthetic concentrations will usually correct this defect without resorting to a special drug treatment. It should also be noted that spontaneous arrhythmias present in the preanesthetic period commonly disappear with the induction of anesthesia and the maintenance of

adequate ventilation. Serious arrhythmias due to disease or mechanical stimulation may require treatment with antiarrhythmics like quinidine and procaine amide. It should be noted that these drugs impair cardiac contractility and add to the myocardial depression produced by the anesthetic agent. Local anesthetics in general have a quinidine-like action, and lidocaine (Xylocaine) has been used successfully to revert ventricular fibrillation both with and without the use of electroshock.[12] Lidocaine has also been used as a supplement in general anesthesia for its antiarrhythmic action, as shown in Fig. 66-1. A comparison with procaine amide indicated that this local anesthetic gave better control of arrhythmias with less depression of the heart than procaine amide.[13] In routine use local anesthetics are administered for a local analgesia; however, they are absorbed systemically in significant concentration and may frequently produce definite myocardial effects.

Myocardial Contraction

The term *cardiac arrest* has come to be applied to all acute severe depressions of cardiovascular function, because of the early beliefs that the mechanism was similar to the asystole produced by strong vagal stimulation. Although the direct myocardial depressant action of general anesthetic agents has long been recognized, work with the heart-lung preparation[14] and the Walton-Brodie strain gauge[15] has emphasized the importance of this action. It should also be noted that myocardial contraction can become completely ineffective at a time when electrical activity has not failed. This situation is illustrated in Fig. 66-2 in an experimental preparation subjected to coronary occlusion. The use of electrocardiographic monitors which depend upon certain changes in the electric potential represented by the QSR complex may be entirely misleading in these circumstances. All anesthetic agents may decrease the force of myocardial contraction,[15] including the newer agents, such as halothane, which produces a decreased myocardial contractility proportional to its concentration. A comparison of the degree of myocardial depression produced by various anesthetic agents is very difficult, because of the variability of techniques, dosage, and animal species employed. The margin of cardiovascular reserve in most patients is such that potent agents like halothane, cyclopropane, and diethyl ether can be employed with careful management, although adverse effects will make it necessary to change the anesthetic agent or technique in some patients. Nitrous oxide has been shown to cause the least depression of the cardiovascular system, and in usual practice its limited potency makes it almost impossible to pro-

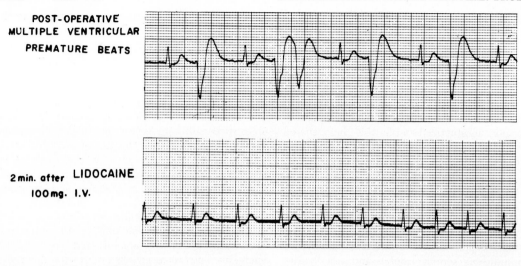

POST-OPERATIVE
MULTIPLE VENTRICULAR
PREMATURE BEATS

2 min. after LIDOCAINE
100 mg. I.V.

B.H.N.   03 - 43 - 93

Fig. 66-1. Electrocardiograms, recorded in the immediate postoperative period, of a patient in whom prosthetic replacement of both the mitral and tricuspid valves had been carried out. Before treatment (above) bigeminal rhythm and multiple premature ventricular systoles are evident. Two minutes after 100 mg lidocaine hydrochloride was administered intravenously, the basic rhythm of atrial fibrillation had been restored. In this instance the duration of the lidocaine hydrochloride effect was 12 min. (*Reproduced by permission of D. C. Harrison et al.: The Antiarrhythmic Properties of Lidocaine and Procaine Amide, Circulation, 28:486, 1963, and The American Heart Association, Inc.*)

duce significant myocardial depression when adequate oxygenation is maintained. On the other hand its lack of potency leads to the need for supplementation, and unfortunately most of these supplements cause significant myocardial depression. Supplementation with succinylcholine is an exception, and

consequently the nitrous oxide–succinylcholine combination is a very advantageous choice when the myocardium is least able to tolerate depression.

When minimal myocardial depression is essential, another possibility would be the use of local or regional anesthesia. The merit of these techniques

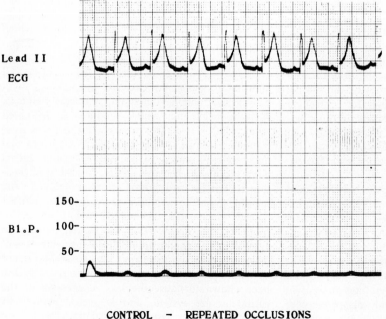

Lead II
ECG

B1.P.

Fig. 66-2. Electrocardiogram and blood pressure tracing in a dog subjected to repeated coronary occlusion. This is demonstration of the failure of myocardial contraction when electrical activity is adequate to produce a good signal on a cardiac monitor.

CONTROL - REPEATED OCCLUSIONS

will depend upon the amount of drug required and the degree of sympathetic nervous system paralysis produced, such as occurs with spinal anesthesia. Although local anesthetics produce their desired effects in a restricted area of the body, they are absorbed systemically. In addition to an antiarrhythmic effect, local anesthetics depress myocardial contractility in a degree approximating their potency.[16] The importance of dosage was demonstrated by the blood levels of local anesthetic found following various routes of administration.[17]

Indirect Cardiac Effects

It is difficult to separate the various components of the cardiovascular action of anesthetic agents. A recent report[18] suggests that the depression of myocardial contractility produced by halothane is due in large degree to the central autonomic effect of this agent. In addition to direct action of anesthetic drugs on the heart, Price et al.[19] lists the circulatory actions of anesthetic agents as being due also to reduced metabolic demands of body tissues and their effects on the autonomic nervous system. The reduction of metabolic demand would be generally beneficial and would offset to some degree the direct depressant effects on the heart. The release of catecholamines during diethyl ether anesthesia[20] counteracts the direct myocardial depressant effect of this agent during the lighter levels of anesthesia. The increased level of sympathomimetic amines during cyclopropane anesthesia counteracts myocardial depression and also causes an increase in the level of blood pressure.[19] Halothane lacks this property of releasing catecholamines, and consequently the depression of myocardial contraction is unopposed.[18]

Another factor which makes it difficult to assess the cardiac effects of anesthetic agents accurately is venous return. Cardiac output and even myocardial contractility[18] are dependent upon venous return. Vasomotor paralysis produced by spinal anesthesia can severely depress cardiac output and cause "cardiac arrest." Any assessment of the effect of anesthesia on the heart must account for all these factors. Maintenance of blood pressure becomes an important practical problem in patients with coronary artery disease. Additional information is needed to evaluate properly the advantage of a generally reduced metabolic demand under general anesthesia as against the disadvantage of a fall in blood pressure which may reduce the level of coronary perfusion.

Prevention and Treatment of Cardiovascular Depression

The preceding discussion would indicate that the cardiovascular changes during anesthesia are complicated and that no simple answer can be supplied for the management of anesthesia in patients who have limited cardiac reserve. Special care is necessary in preoperative preparation as regards the problems of electrolytes and blood volume, as well as the treatment of the heart disease. Previous drug therapy must be considered. For example, corticosteroids may be needed in a patient who has been on this drug previously, and the possible depletion of norepinephrine with reserpine therapy must be considered in the preanesthetic evaluation and preparation of the patient. Prevention of hypoxia and hypercapnia due to airway difficulties or other problems of ventilation is paramount, since the margin of reserve is narrow.

No ideal agent or technique exists, but certain general principles can be applied in the selection of agents and technique. Local anesthetic techniques produce minimal cardiovascular actions if the dosage is low and vasomotor effects are limited. A subcutaneous dose of procaine less than 100 mg in the average patient should produce little cardiovascular effect, whereas 500 mg (50 ml of 1 per cent solution) may have substantial systemic effects. Since a patient's tolerance to drugs can be determined only by trial, rapid reversibility is a highly desirable property of an anesthetic agent selected for patients with impaired cardiovascular reserve. In this regard, inhalation agents have a marked advantage over intravenous agents, because the former can be removed by ventilation. Of the various inhalation agents, nitrous oxide and cyclopropane can be removed most rapidly, and ether and methoxyflurane (Penthrane) are the slowest, with halothane in an intermediate position. On the other hand, intravenous agents provide much smoother inductions which may be important in certain apprehensive patients.

In patients with marginal blood volumes and in patients who require the maintenance of a stable blood pressure, cyclopropane anesthesia has definite advantages. In these patients halothane and spinal anesthesia will generally be the most difficult to manage, and the nitrous oxide and relaxant techniques occupy a middle position. A general anesthesia technique of choice for patients with a severely limited myocardial reserve and in whom muscle relaxation is needed would be nitrous oxide–succinylcholine. The use of thiobarbiturate (Pentothal sodium) in patients with heart disease has the limitations of myocardial depression without the reversibility of the inhalation agents. Nevertheless, this agent should not be eliminated from consideration, particularly in those patients where ventricular arrhythmias are a major problem. The thiobarbiturate techniques are associated with fewer arrhythmias than the other general anesthetics, and they have particular advantages in providing smooth inductions for the anxious, apprehensive patient such as those with a history of myocardial infarctions. Since hypotension is hazardous to these patients, the rate of thiobarbiturate administration must be slow and the total dosage severely limited. As with all choices the advantages and disadvantages must be carefully weighed.

The choice of anesthetic agents is often compromised by surgical requirements which may exclude the use of explosive agents. As in other medical situations the need for the electrocautery must be balanced against the advantages of the explosive anesthetic agent. Mechanical embarrassments of the cardiovascular system are frequently exaggerated in the anesthetized patient because of lack of muscle tone. Particularly serious problems are frequently caused by the "kidney position," extreme Trendelenburg position, pressure of abdominal packs, traction on thoracic vessels, and sudden movement of the patient such as occurs at the end of the procedure.

The treatment of acute failure of cardiovascular output should be directed toward the offending agent or process if it can be determined. Adequate ventilation and removal of the anesthetic agent (if inhalation) should be the first consideration. Sympathomimetic amines ranging in potency from mephenteramine to epinephrine and norepinephrine should be selected for administration, according to the degree of cardiovascular depression. If circulation is severely depressed, these drugs must be administered by intracardiac route unless the circulation is augmented by external cardiac massage. Since irreversible changes occur in the central nervous system in periods of time over 3 or 4 min, immediate institution of cardiac massage is essential if evidences of adequate circulation cannot be obtained. If cardiac action cannot be readily reestablished, the most useful drugs are epinephrine and/or norepinephrine. In hearts which do not respond rapidly, sodium bicarbonate and calcium ion are useful. Ventricular fibrillation requires defibrillation with electroshock. It is important that the heart be well oxygenated before defibrillation is attempted. In difficult cases lidocaine in 100- to 200-mg doses has been found to facilitate defibrillation.

In general, anesthesia introduces some degree of hazard to cardiac function. After a careful appraisal of the patient's general condition and in particular his cardiovascular status, a physician experienced in the use of anesthetic agents and responsible for their administration should select the anesthetic agent and technique. He will need to weigh carefully the advantages and disadvantages of the alternative techniques, although long experience with a given technique may override the reputed pharmacologic advantages of newer, less well-established methods of anesthetic management. With careful attention to ventilation, dosage, and the pharmacologic properties of these agents, the deleterious effect of these drugs can be reduced so that even very sick patients can be managed for the necessary operative and diagnostic procedures.

REFERENCES

1. Dodd, R. B., Sims, W. A., and Bone, D. J.: Cardiac Arrhythmias Observed during Anesthesia and Surgery, *Surgery*, **51**:440–447, 1962.
2. Orth, O. S., Leigh, M. D., Mellish, C. H., and Stutzman, J. W.: Action of Sympathomimetic Amine in Cyclopropane, Ether and Choloroform Anesthesia, *J. Pharmacol. & Exper. Therap.*, **67**:1–16, 1939.
3. Johnstone, M.: Cyclopropane Anaesthesia and Ventricular Arrhythmias, *Brit. Heart J.*, **12**:239–244, 1950.
4. Price, H. L., Lurie, A. A., Jones, R. E., Price, M. L., and Linde, H. W.: Cyclopropane Anesthesia; Epinephrine and Norepinephrine in Initiation of Ventricular Arrhythmias by Carbon Dioxide Inhalation, *Anesthesiology*, **19**:619–630, 1958.
5. Hall, K. D., and Norris, F. H., Jr.: Fluothane Sensitization of Dog Heart to Action of Epinephrine, *Anesthesiology*, **19**:631–641, 1958.
6. Matteo, R. S., Katz, R. L., and Papper, E. M.: The Injection of Epinephrine during General Anesthesia with Halogenated Hydrocarbons and Cyclopropane in Man, *Anesthesiology*, **24**:327–330, 1963.
7. Siebecker, K. L., Kimmery, J. R., Kraemer, R. J., Bamforth, B. J., and Steinhaus, J. E.: The Prevention and Treatment of Cardiac Arrhythmias during Hypothermia, *Anesth. & Analg.*, **42**:527–533, 1963.
8. Dresel, P. E., and Sutter, M. C.: Factors Modifying Cyclopropane Epinephrine Cardiac Arrhythmias, *Circulation Res.*, **9**:1284–1290, 1961.
9. Schoenstadt, D. A., and Whitcher, C. E.: Observations on the Mechanism of Succinyldicholine-induced Cardiac Arrhythmias, *Anesthesiology*, **24**:358–362, 1963.
10. Jones, R. E., Deutsch, S., and Turndoff, H.: Effects of Atropine on Cardiac Rhythm in Conscious and Anesthetized Man., *Anesthesiology*, **22**:67–73, 1961.
11. Vandam, L. D., and McLemore, G. A., Jr.: Circulatory Arrest in Patient with a Complete Heart Block during Anesthesia and Surgery, *Ann. Int. Med.*, **47**:518–532, 1957.
12. Carden, N. L., and Steinhaus, J. E.: Lidocaine in Cardiac Resuscitation from Ventricular Fibrillation, *Circulation Res.*, **4**:680–683, 1956.
13. Harrison, D. C., Sprouse, J. H., and Morrow, A. G.: The Antiarrhythmic Properties of Lidocaine and Procaine Amide, *Circulation*, **28**:486–491, 1963.

14. Price, H. L., and Helrich, M.: The Effect of Cyclo-propane, Diethyl Ether, Nitrous Oxide, Thiopental, and Hydrogen Ion Concentration on the Myocardial Function of the Dog Heart-Lung Preparation, *J. Pharmacol. & Exper. Therap.*, 115:206–216, 1955.

15. Brown, J. M.: Anesthesia and the Contractile Force of the Heart, *Anesth. & Analg.*, 39:487–497, 1960.

16. Stewart, D. M., Rogers, W. P., Mahaffery, J. E., Witherspoon, S., and Woods, E. F.: Effect of Local Anesthetics on the Cardiovascular System of the Dog, *Anesthesiology*, 24:620–624, 1963.

17. Campbell, D., and Adriani, J.: Absorption of Local Anesthetics, *J.A.M.A.*, 168:873–877, 1958.

18. Price, H. L., Linde, H. W., and Morse, H. T.: Central Nervous Actions of Halothane Affecting the Systemic Circulation, *Anesthesiology*, 24:770–778, 1963.

19. Price, H. L.: Circulatory Action of General Anes-thetic Agents and the Homeostatic Roles of Epi-nephrine and Norepinephrine in Man, *Clin. Pharma-col. & Therap.*, 2:163–175, 1961.

20. Brewster, W. R., Jr., Issacs, J. P., and Wains-Andersen, T.: Depressant Effect of Ether on Myo-cardium of Dog and Its Modification by Reflex Release of Epinephrine and Norepinephrine, *Am. J. Physiol.*, 175:399–414, 1953.

67 SURGICAL TREATMENT IN THE PATIENT WITH HEART DISEASE

R. Bruce Logue, M.D.

There are numerous complications involving the cardiovascular system which may occur during surgical treatment or in the postoperative period. These may develop in the presence of a normal cardiovascular system but are more frequent in the presence of heart disease.[1] The incidence and risks associated with such complications are deter-mined by the type and severity of the cardiovascu-lar disease, the magnitude of the surgical proce-dure, and the expertise of the anesthetist and attending physician.

PREOPERATIVE EVALUATION

An evaluation of the patient's status prior to surgical treatment may be obtained relatively simply by analyzing the findings gathered from the history, the physical examination, the electro-cardiogram, the chest x-ray, and the routine exam-ination of the blood and urine. One should deter-mine the following: (1) Is there evidence of heart disease? (2) Is there a history of angina pectoris or myocardial infarction? (3) Is there cardiac en-largement? (4) Are there symptoms or signs of congestive heart failure? (5) Is there significant disturbance of cardiac rhythm such as atrial fibril-lation? (6) Is there significant hypertensive disease or postural hypotension? (7) Is there evidence or symptoms of cerebral vascular disease or syncope? (8) Is there evidence of chronic lung disease? (9) Is there history or evidence of old or recent phle-bitis? (10) Has the patient been on antihyper-tensive or cardiac medication or previously re-ceived corticosteroids? (11) Is there evidence of kidney disease or prostatic obstruction?

The signs and symptoms associated with heart disease are discussed in Chaps. 4 and 5. Although the details will not be repeated here, a few points deserve emphasis.

The *history* must include a careful search for chest discomfort, dyspnea, palpitation, syncope, cough, hemoptysis, wheezing, cerebral ischemia attacks, and calf pain. The *physical examination* may give evidence of cerebral vascular disease by the presence of carotid bruits, diminished or absent carotid pulsations, Hollenhorst plaques in the ret-ina, or significant differences in the blood pressure in the arms. Cardiac enlargement is revealed by the presence of a large, sustained apex impulse of left ventricular hypertrophy or the sustained para-sternal lift of right ventricular hypertrophy. A vis-ible or audible ventricular diastolic gallop may be the clue to presence of myocardial insufficiency with the need for digitalization. Heart murmurs must be specifically sought, since the murmur of mitral stenosis, aortic stenosis, and faint aortic regurgitation are often overlooked. Pulmonary rales may be due to failure of the left side of the heart but are common with chronic lung disease; it is emphasized that failure of the left side of the heart manifested by interstitial edema may be present without rales or ventricular diastolic gallop rhythm and may be detected solely by the roentgeno-gram. Abnormal venous distension or pulsations may indicate failure of the right side of the heart, and pulsus alternans indicates left ventricular myo-cardial failure. The presence of hepatomegaly with-out other signs or symptoms is unreliable evidence of heart failure, since it may be due to the presence of a hyperesthetic build, to emphysema with de-pression of the diaphragms, or to intrinsic liver disease. Edema is a late manifestation of conges-tive heart failure and may be due to noncardiac causes. The rate and rhythm of the heart may fur-nish evidence of cardiac arrhythmia such as atrial fibrillation or complete heart block. Prior to sur-gical treatment one should record the pulses in all extremities, so that possible embolic or thrombotic complications of surgical treatment can be evaluated. In the male it is very wise to know the status of the prostate prior to surgical treatment.

The *electrocardiogram* is commonly misused and may give a false sense of security (see Chaps. 6 and 32). It may be normal when heart failure is present. It may be normal when the patient is having life-threatening angina decubitus, and it is commonly normal 6 months or so following myocardial infarction. It gives no indication of the need for digitalis or of when a patient may be optimally digitalized. It may furnish important evidence of overdigitalization, the presence of atrioventricular (A-V) or bundle branch block or various cardiac arrhythmias. It is useful to have a base-line tracing, so that alterations during or after surgical treatment may be evaluated, particularly since myocardial infarction is often unaccompanied by pain, either because infarction occurred during anesthesia or because it was obscured by opiate administration or normal postoperative discomfort.

A *chest x-ray* is needed for a complete examination, since interstitial pulmonary edema may be the only clue that heart failure is present (see Chap. 14). The film may reveal cardiac enlargement, a diagnostic cardiac contour, and unsuspected lung and aortic disease. Obviously, when the patient is quite ill, a good film is difficult to obtain and the diagnostic value decreases, but it is still useful.

The routine *examination of the blood* may reveal anemia, which may require proper diagnosis and treatment prior to surgical treatment. The margin of safety is not as great in patients with cardiovascular disease, and the degrees of anemia ordinarily tolerated by otherwise healthy persons may not be tolerated by patients with heart disease. When the nature of the surgical procedure suggests that the patient may be on intravenous fluids for some time, when fluid is likely to be removed from the stomach or some other source, or when the patient has a disease that is likely to disturb the electrolytes, it is useful to know the concentration of sodium, potassium, chloride, and carbon dioxide in the serum. The hematocrit, body weight, levels of serum electrolytes, and output of fluid are all necessary information when intravenous fluid replacement must be continued for a long period of time. A fasting blood sugar and blood-urea nitrogen may be needed in the preoperative evaluation of some patients. This especially applies to patients with renal disease, hypertension, or congestive heart failure, and when there is a history of diabetes.

The routine *examination of the urine* may reveal albumin, glucose, red-cell casts, and white-cell casts. These findings may require therapy prior to an elective operative procedure.

The following discussion highlights the unique features associated with each category of heart disease which influence the evaluation and management of the patient undergoing surgical treatment.

Coronary Disease[2–7]

Coronary disease is the major hazard to the adult over the age of forty. The disease may be asymptomatic and totally unsuspected, but in the overwhelming majority it is recognized by a history of angina or previous infarction. Unfortunately, the first evidence may be sudden death. Knapp et al.,[8] in a study of 8,984 males over the age of fifty, found the following incidence of postoperative coronary occlusion: The incidence of postoperative coronary occlusion was 0.7 per cent in the group composed of 8,557 patients who had no preoperative history of coronary occlusion. The mortality in this group was 18 per cent. The incidence of postoperative coronary occlusion was 6 per cent in the group composed of 427 patients who had a history of preoperative coronary occlusion. The mortality in this group was 58 per cent. Forty-six per cent of the patients with a history of preoperative coronary occlusion occurring less than 24 months prior to surgical treatment had a postoperative occlusion. Occasionally, the electrocardiogram may reveal evidence of previously unsuspected infarction; it may demonstrate nondiagnostic changes such as left bundle branch block or ST-T wave abnormalities. It is important to determine whether angina pectoris is stable or whether there has been a recent change in pattern. Does it occur only with strenuous exertion, or does it occur at rest? The risk of anesthesia and major surgical procedure will vary from 1 to 3 per cent in the former and may approach 50 per cent in the latter situation. A history of prior myocardial infarction but good cardiac reserve and no history of angina pectoris may carry only a small risk of 3 to 4 per cent. A history of myocardial infarction within the preceding 2 to 3 months entails greater surgical risk and contraindicates anything but emergency surgical treatment.

When angina pectoris occurs frequently and is precipitated by emotional tension, it is well to give nitroglycerin and adequate sedation before transferring the patient to the operating room in order to minimize emotional influences. A long wait in the corridor or operating room prior to anesthesia should be avoided if possible. Reassurance may be afforded if the physician who knows the patient best accompanies him to the operating room.

Hypertension

Hypertension, even of severe degree, does not appreciably increase the risk of general anesthesia and major surgical treatment, the frequency of symptomatic or asymptomatic associated coronary disease being the major factor. Antihypertensive medication should usually be omitted prior to surgical intervention unless the diastolic pressure rises to 120 or higher. The chlorothiazide drugs may reduce blood volume and produce potassium depletion, which may add to the risk of surgical treatment. *Rauwolfia* derivatives are preferably omitted 2 weeks prior to operation; however, the risks have been overemphasized, and surgical procedures may be carried out in the reserpinized patient.[9] These drugs deplete catecholamines and may be associated with shock resulting in resistance to blood replacement; this can usually be controlled by atropine and catecholamine administration, but it should be noted that there may be a hyperactive response to catechols in this setting. Hypertensive crises during surgical procedure suggest the presence of pheochromocytoma and are best controlled by intravenous phentolamine (Regitine) or dibenzyline. Ganglionic blocking drugs and trenethaphan (Arfonad) are contraindicated in the patient with pheochromocytoma, since they may potentiate the hypertension produced by *l*-epinephrine and *l*-norepinephrine. Similarly atropine and hydrocarbon anesthetics such as cyclopropane, halothane, and trichlorethylene may produce hypercapnia and sensitize the myocardium to the effects of catecholamines with production of ventricular arrhythmias.[10]

Valvular Heart Disease

Aortic stenosis and insufficiency of severe degree pose a small hazard of sudden death due to ventricular fibrillation. Patients with mild or moderate disease tolerate anesthesia satisfactorily. Those with predominant mitral insufficiency who are well compensated run no increased risk. Those with tight mitral stenosis of class III or IV may undergo surgical treatment with slight increase in incidence of pulmonary edema. Even corrective surgical treatment in the form of valvuloplasty in class III patients carries a risk of only 1 to 3 per cent. Care to avoid overloading with blood or saline solution during surgical treatment and during the postoperative period is mandatory.

Congenital Heart Disease

Patients with congenital heart disease with left-to-right shunts but with good cardiac compensation undergo no increase in risks with anesthesia and surgical treatment. Even children with cyanotic heart disease such as tetralogy of Fallot tolerate anesthesia and surgical procedures remarkably well. Patients with rheumatic and congenital heart disease should receive appropriate antibiotics following surgical treatment to minimize the risk of bacterial endocarditis.

Lung Disease

Patients with pulmonary disease have an increased anesthetic risk and are subject to postoperative complications. If the patient is able to walk up several flights of stairs without undue dyspnea, there is little anesthetic risk. Those with chronic bronchitis due to smoking have increased bronchial secretions and bronchospasm and are particularly subject to postoperative atelectasis and pneumonia. Patients with chronic bronchitis and lung disease should omit smoking some days (and preferably several weeks) prior to surgical treatment. At times preoperative preparation of the cardiac patient with chronic lung disease with expectorants, bronchodilators, chest exercises, and the use of aerosol with intermittent positive pressure breathing may be needed to improve vital capacity and clear bronchial secretions. Atropine sulfate and hyoscine should be avoided because of their drying effect on the bronchial mucosa. Preanesthetic medication may induce dangerous respiratory depression in patients with lung disease. For example, serious respiratory depression may occur in patients with emphysema after an average dose of morphine sulfate or barbiturate.

Congestive Heart Failure

The presence of compensated congestive heart failure may produce a modest increase in risk. The cardiac reserve should be estimated by determining whether the patient is able to carry on normal activities without symptoms of congestive heart failure. If the patient develops dyspnea on walking one block or has paroxysmal nocturnal dyspnea, the operative risk is increased. If he can walk up several flights of steps without symptoms, there is little hazard from the standpoint of congestive heart failure. It is useful to classify the function according to the criteria of the New York Heart Association.[11]

Congestive heart failure should be controlled by conventional methods prior to contemplated surgical treatment. It is important to avoid massive diuresis with hemoconcentration and electrolyte depletion. Accordingly, diuretic therapy should be completed several days prior to operation. Digitalis is indicated for congestive heart failure, but it is far better to have the patient underdigitalized than overdigitalized. Digitalis should be given several days prior to surgical treatment when possible in order to judge whether the desired amount has been given and to ascertain that no toxic signs or symptoms have developed. If the surgical procedure is urgently needed, it may be necessary to digitalize the patient rapidly (see Chap. 15). The subtle signs of heart failure are sought, since these are often overlooked. For example, digitalis is indicated when a ventricular gallop is heard. Digitalis is not indicated prior to surgical treatment in the elderly patient with a heart of normal size. The value of digitalizing a patient with an enlarged heart without evidence of heart failure is not known. We now know that it is not as harmful as was formerly believed. Accordingly, if it is not possible to obtain a history that will enable one to estimate cardiac reserve and if the physical examination reveals no sign of heart failure but does reveal a large heart, then digitalis may be given without fear of harm (if the drug is used properly) and with some hope of benefit. Braunwald et al. have demonstrated that digitalization decreases the oxygen consumption of the enlarged heart in the absence of decompensation and suggest that the drug be given to those with cardiac enlargement in the absence of congestive heart failure.[12]

Shock, occurring after induction of anesthesia, may be due to inadequate fluid replacement preoperatively or to excessive diuresis. Also the blood pressure in patients with heart failure may be maintained by vasoconstriction, but with anesthesia and impaired reflexes hypotension may develop.

Arrhythmias and Heart Block

Digitalis should be used to control the ventricular rate of patients with atrial fibrillation or flutter. The heart rate, determined by listening to the apex of the heart or by the electrocardiogram, should be controlled after exercise (see Chap. 16). Digitalis should be given even though the apical rate may be normal prior to digitalis administration, since undue acceleration may occur during anesthesia. It is preferable to know the patient's response to digitalis prior to surgical treatment, since nausea and vomiting occur on occasions and predispose to aspiration of gastric contents. Premature beats,[13] unless multifocal and frequent, require no therapy; they are often due to anxiety. When there is a history of paroxysmal atrial tachycardia, quinidine sulfate, 0.4 gm, may be given intramuscularly 1 hr prior to operation. When complete heart block is present, an indwelling venous catheter pacemaker may furnish an added margin of safety and the heart may be paced throughout the surgical procedure and the postoperative period for periods up to a week. The catheter should not be removed until it is clear that normal cardiac pacemakers have been functioning for several days without

Stokes-Adams attacks. Procaine amide hydrochloride (Pronestyl hydrochloride) and quinidine sulfate are contraindicated for arrhythmias that interrupt complete heart block (see Chap. 16).

General Preoperative Measures

When corticosteroids have been administered within 6 months, it is well to give prednisone, 40 mg, on the day before surgical treatment and for a few days thereafter. Hydrocortisone, 100 mg IV may be given during surgical treatment if hypotension occurs. Anticoagulants may be continued for dental extractions but should be omitted prior to operations, and the prothrombin time should be at, or close to, normal.

When anemia is so severe that transfusion is needed, it is well to avoid whole blood in the patient with congestive heart failure or cardiomegaly but rather to use packed red blood cells in isotomic glucose. Polycythemia predisposes to thrombosis, and phlebotomy may be helpful in minimizing such complications when the hematocrit is higher than 50. Dehydration should be avoided particularly.

Electrolyte depletion should be corrected prior to surgery.[14-16] Hypokalemia predisposes to arrhythmias and sensitizes the myocardium to the toxic effects of digitalis. This effect may be aggravated by the intravenous administration of glucose. It is emphasized that this may occur with a normal serum potassium. Hyponatremia is often associated with a contracted blood volume and predisposes the patient to hypotension during anesthesia.

All too often the patient undergoes a prolonged fast with discomfort and dehydration while waiting for surgical treatment, and when it is known that surgical treatment will not be done until late in the day, this state can be prevented by the administration of isotonic glucose.

THE MANAGEMENT OF THE CARDIAC PATIENT DURING SURGICAL PROCEDURES

With the introduction of cardiac monitoring, cardiac resuscitation by external massage, pulmonary ventilation, and effective defibrillation apparatus, there has been a margin of safety added to anesthesia and surgical procedures in the cardiac and noncardiac patient.

The choice of anesthesia should be left to the anesthesiologist, whose judgment and experience may dictate the type[17-19] (see Chap. 66). All anesthetics produce myocardial depression and impair contractility.[20] Cardiac arrest associated with anesthesia may occur once in every 3,000 patients, once in every 1,000 elderly or poor-risk patients, and once in 5,000 healthy, good-risk patients.[21, 22] All anesthetics reduce pulmonary ventilation and must be used with great care in patients with heart disease and lung disease.[23] Curare-like drugs used to achieve muscle relaxation may also impair pulmonary ventilation. In addition, the accessory muscles of respiration, which may be needed to overcome expiratory airflow resistance, may become inactivated by the anesthetic agent and curare. The secretion of viscid mucus may be stimulated by the anesthetic agent at a time when airway reflexes are depressed. Ventilation may be further impaired by the nonphysiologic positions required for certain surgical procedures.[24] Thiopentobarbital sodium (Pentothal sodium) is often considered a safe anesthetic for short procedures; however, it may produce hypotension, shock, and laryngospasm. Cyclopropane and halothane produce CO_2 retention and predispose to arrhythmias from endogenous or exogenous catecholamines. Nitrous oxide in high concentration reduces arterial oxygen, and supplemental oxygen is needed. A patent airway must be maintained at all times, and this may necessitate the use of an intratracheal tube which may also be used for positive pressure.

A low-spinal anesthetic may be quite satisfactory for surgical treatment in the perineal area. Anesthesia at lumbar level may produce hypotension, which, if uncorrected, may be hazardous to the patient with coronary disease. Local anesthesia may be used at times, but preparations containing epinephrine should be avoided in the coronary patient. Absorption of large amounts of cocaine, procaine, or Xylocaine may produce cerebral excitement and convulsions, and these effects can be lessened by prior administration of barbiturates.

Vagal reflexes may be heightened at induction of anesthesia and on occasion induce cardiac arrest.[22] These may be lessened by the administration of 1 mg atropine sulfate. The oculocardiac reflex brought into play in surgical treatment of the eye may be counteracted by atropine sulfate or retrobulbar injection of Xylocaine. Vagal reflexes may be invoked by tracheal intubation, stimulation of the pleura, spreading the ribs, clamping the vagal nerve endings, passing a bronchoscope or esophagoscope, stimulation of the bronchi, tugging on the mesentery, and stimulating the pharynx.

It is axiomatic to avoid hypoxia and hypercapnia, both of which predispose to arrhythmia, hypotension, and cardiac arrest. Adequate ventilation to ensure CO_2 disposal and adequate oxygenation are important. The development of cyanosis means severe unsaturation, since this may not be noted until O_2 saturation falls to 60 to 70 per cent. An increase in pulse rate may precede the development of cyanosis. The pulse rate may be a sensitive indicator of blood loss and reduction of blood volume; however, the pulse may be slow, and the blood pressure may rise or fall at the onset of hemorrhage. Some of the factors which may cause hypoxia are excessive anesthetic agent, respiratory depression from opiates, or curare-like drugs, inadequate airway, mucus plugs, laryngospasm, inadequate manual support of respirations, atelectasis, pneumothorax, hypercapnia, hemorrhage, arrhythmia, shock, aspiration, myocardial depression, myocardial infarction, and pulmonary edema.

The onset of a cardiac arrhythmia may signal hypoxia or hypercapnia. Frequent extrasystoles may be readily controlled by procaine amide (Pronestyl hydrochloride) or lidocaine hydrochloride (Xylocaine hydrochloride), 1 to 2 mg per kg intravenously. The rapid ventricular rate associated with atrial fibrillation and atrial flutter may be controlled by intravenous digoxin (Lanoxin). Atrial tachycardia may revert to normal with digoxin. Ventricular tachycardia may be reverted to normal with procaine amide (Pronestyl hydrochloride). It is also important to identify and to eliminate the precipitating factors including hypotension and anoxia. Bradycardia often precedes cardiac arrest during anesthesia.

One of the common mistakes when hypotension occurs is to give pressor therapy to maintain the blood pressure and to overlook the need for volume replacement. The hematocrit and red blood cell count do not reflect the acute need for blood or plasma. These measurements may be normal with acute blood loss, and hemodilution may be delayed or not occur, particularly in the presence of increased vasomotor tone, anemia, preexisting hypovolemia, low total-body-water level, or in the debilitated or elderly patient.[15] The need for blood or plasma may be difficult to determine, and when hypotension is otherwise unexplained, a trial administration of 500 ml may stabilize the blood pressure and clearly settle the issue. Measurement of the central venous pressure may give valuable evidence of the need for blood or plasma. Positioning of the patient may influence hypotension. The Trendelenburg position may result in pooling of blood in the lower part of the body. Hypotension may not become apparent until the patient is moved at the termination of anesthesia. Some patients with tight mitral stenosis develop hypotension when placed in the left lateral position. Hypotension may follow myocardial depression with ischemia and is often the initial clue to myocardial infarction. Bradycardia at onset is more common with occlusion of the right coronary artery, and atropine may be needed to lessen vagal suppression of pacemaker function.

Carbon dioxide retention occurs with all anesthetics, but this may be exaggerated with the halothane derivatives. The resultant hypercapnia predisposes the myocardium to the effects of catecholamines and the production of arrhythmia—nodal or ventricular.[25] The lateral position interferes with normal ventilation-perfusion relationships, the dependent lung having decreased ventilation and increased perfusion whereas the opposite is true for the lung that is uppermost. The presence of emphysema or pulmonary fibrosis accentuates the tendency to metabolic acidosis, and airway obstruction or inadequate assisted ventilation increases CO_2 retention. Hypertension or hypotension may occur, and when hypercapnia is advanced, respiratory paralysis and convulsions may occur. The rapid elimination of CO_2 by excessive hyperventilation may induce cardiac arrest.

Transfusion reactions may produce chilling and hypotension. When multiple transfusions (8 to 10) are necessary in 24 hr, there may be a decrease in platelets, fibrinogen, prothrombin, factor VII, and possibly factors V and X, and these may facilitate bleeding. Calcium may be depleted when large amounts of stored blood are used because of the citrate content. Supplemental calcium may be needed when hypotension occurs. The plasma-potassium concentration of blood that has been stored for 2 weeks may increase to 20 mEq per liter. This fact should be noted especially when poor renal function and oliguria are present. Postoperatively, the first urine should be checked for red blood cells, red-cell casts, and hematin casts. Where evidence of transfusion reaction with oliguria is present, intravenous mannitol is given cautiously to enhance urine flow and to prevent renal damage.

THE MANAGEMENT OF THE CARDIAC PATIENT DURING THE POSTOPERATIVE PERIOD

During the postoperative period it is necessary to look for signs of congestive heart failure, hypotension, myocardial infarction,[26] pulmonary infection, pulmonary infarction and atelectasis, cardiac arrhythmias,[27] overhydration, underhydration, and electrolyte disturbances.

The cardiac patient undergoing surgical treatment may show water retention due to decreased urinary output and increased ADH secretion. The serum sodium may decrease while the total body sodium remains unchanged, the so-called sodium paradox. The total body potassium decreases under the influence of increased aldosterone, while the serum potassium remains normal or increases. The greatest diuresis of potassium occurs on the day of operation in spite of a decrease in urinary output. The serum chloride may decrease. Thus parenteral fluid should be restricted to 1,000 to 1,200 ml plus extrarenal loss in the first 24 hr. The hematocrit, central venous pressure, body weight, serum-electrolyte levels, and intake and output determinations are all necessary information to judge the amount and type of fluid and electrolytes that are needed. Where the postoperative total-body-sodium level is low because of preoperative sodium restriction and diuretics and when hyponatremia persists following surgical treatment and signs of hypovolemia occur, one may cautiously give 200 to 300 ml of 3 per cent sodium chloride intravenously.

As emphasized earlier, the incidence of postoperative coronary occlusion is small in patients without a previous symptom of coronary disease but occurs in 6 per cent of patients with a history of preoperative coronary occlusion. A base-line electrocardiogram should be obtained prior to the surgical procedure, and the electrical activity of the heart should be monitored throughout the course of the operative procedure.[28] The monitoring should be continued for several days in patients recognized to be in the high-risk group. Myocardial infarction and cardiac arrhythmias may be recognized with greater facility using this technique. It must be remembered that pain is a symptom in less than half of the cases of postoperative myocardial infarction and that the manifestations are notoriously atypical.[26] In some series one-half of the postoperative infarcts would have been missed without routine postoperative electrocardiograms. An electrocardiogram is indicated to detect myocardial infarction when any of the following conditions are present: (1) unexplained hypotension during or after surgery; (2) development of pulmonary rales, venous distension, or ventricular gallop rhythm; (3) development of arrhythmia, sinus bradycardia or sinus tachycardia; (4) complaints of pain or indigestion in the chest, shoulders, back, or arms; (5) dyspnea, persistent cough, or wheezing; (6) unexplained syncope; and (7) routinely in the postoperative period in the patient with prior history of angina pectoris or myocardial infarction. Because changes may occasionally be delayed 7 to 10 days after onset of infarction, serial tracings may be needed if the initial tracing is normal and there is suspicion of myocardial infarction.

Pulmonary infection in the postoperative period may precipitate congestive heart failure, of which prompt recognition and appropriate therapy is essential. Where thoracotomy has not been done, significant fever in the first few days suggests atelectasis and infection, and bronchoscopy may be needed. Sinus tachycardia and cardiac arrhythmias refractory to conventional therapy may be associated with atelectasis and may respond following bronchoscopy and "tracheal toilet." Unfortunately, this sequence of events is not generally appreciated.

The frequency of pulmonary embolism is decreased by early ambulation after surgical treatment, and this should be done whenever possible. The frequent movement of the lower extremities while in bed is also essential. Many venous clots are laid down during the period of the operation, and, unfortunately, not all pulmonary emboli can be prevented. The first sign may be sudden death. Other clues are sudden dyspnea, hypotension, chest pain, and cardiac arrhythmias. When a pulmonary embolus is recognized during the postoperative course, heparin should be started if the surgeon feels that the danger of hemorrhage has subsided (see Chap. 47). Since the patient is in the hospital and the usual delay should not occur, it is occasionally possible to remove a large pulmonary embolus from the main pulmonary artery.

Surgery of the genitourinary or biliary tract is associated with occasional risk of Gram-negative septicemia and resistant shock, which may simulate myocardial infarction or cerebral vascular accident. Massive steroid therapy in the equivalent of 300 mg cortisone and 60 to 80 million units of penicillin intravenously per 24 hr or antibiotics effective against Gram-negative organisms may be helpful, but even with such therapy the mortality approaches 50 per cent. Lactic acidosis may occur in this as well as other types of shock and requires the administration of sodium bicarbonate.

REFERENCES

1. Wessler, S., and Blumgart, H. L.: Management of the Cardiac Patient Requiring Major Surgery, *Circulation*, 23:121, 1961.
2. Etsten, B. E., Weaver, D. C., Li, T. H., and Friedman, J. B.: Appraisal of the Coronary Patient as an Operative Risk, *New York J. Med.*, 50:2065, 1954.
3. Etsten, B., and Proger, S.: Operative Risk in Patients with Coronary Heart Disease, *J.A.M.A.*, 159:845, 1955.
4. Wasserman, F., Bellet, S., and Saicheck, R. P.: Postoperative Myocardial Infarction, *New England J. Med.*, 252:967, 1955.
5. LaDue, J. S.: Evaluation and Preparation of the Patient with Degenerative Cardiovascular Disease for Major Surgery, *Bull. New York Acad. Med.*, 32:418, 1956.
6. Thompson, G. J., Kelalis, P. P., and Connolly, D. C.: Transurethral Prostatic Resection after Myocardial Infarction, *J.A.M.A.*, 182:110, 1962.
7. Thompson, G. J., Kelalis, P. P., and Connolly, D. C.: Transurethral Prostatic Resection after Myocardial Infarction, *J.A.M.A.*, 182:908, 1962.
8. Knapp, R. B., Topkins, M. J., and Artusio, J. F., Jr.: The Cerebrovascular Accident and Coronary Occlusion in Anesthesia, *J.A.M.A.*, 182:106, 1962.
9. Munson, W. M., and Jenicek, J. A.: Effect of Anesthetic Agents on Patients Receiving Reserpine Therapy, *Anesthesiology*, 23:741, 1962.
10. Crandall, D. L., and Myers, R. T.: Pheochromocytoma: Anesthetic and Surgical Considerations, *J.A.M.A.*, 187:12, 1964.
11. Criteria Committee of The New York Heart Association, Inc.: "Diseases of the Heart and Blood Vessels: Nomenclature and Criteria for Diagnosis," 6th ed., Little, Brown and Company, Boston, 1964.
12. Braunwald, E., Bloodwell, R. D., Goldberg, L. H., and Morrow, A. G.: Studies on Digitalis. IV. Observations in Man on the Effects of Digitalis on the Contractility of the Non-failing Heart and on Total Vascular Resistance, *J. Clin. Invest.*, 40:52, 1961.
13. Lamb, L. E., and Hiss, R. G.: Influence of Exercise on Premature Contractions, *Am. J. Cardiol.*, 10:209, 1962.
14. Moore, F. D.: Common Patterns of Water and Electrolyte Changes in Injury, Surgery and Disease, Medical Progress, *New England J. Med.*, 258:277, 1958.
15. Albert, S. N.: Blood Volume, *Anesthesiology*, 24:231, 1963.
16. Lown, B., Black, H., and Moore, F. D.: Digitalis, Electrolytes and the Surgical Patient, *Am. J. Cardiol.*, 6:309, 1960.
17. Van Dam, L. D., and Burnap, T. K.: Anesthesia in Patients with Heart Disease, *Circulation*, 17:292, 1958.
18. Dripps, R. D., Strong, M. J., and Price, H. L.: The Heart and General Anesthesia, *Mod. Concepts Cardiovas. Dis.*, 32, (No. 7): 805–808, 1963.
19. Beecher, H. K., Bendixen, H. H., Hallowell, P., Pontoppidan, H., and Todd, D. P.: The Anesthetist as a Physician, *J.A.M.A.*, 188:169, 1964.
20. Sprouse, J. H., Galindo, A. H., and Morrow, A. G.: Influence of Various Drugs and Anesthetic Agents on Cardiac Excitability in Man, *Anesthesiology*, 24:141, 1963.
21. Keeley, J. L., Schairer, A. E., and Carroll, J. P.: Cardiac Arrest in Surgical Patients: Prevention, Recognition and Treatment. *S. Clin. North America*, 38:55, 1958.
22. Stephenson, H. E., Jr., Reid, L. C., and Hinton, J. W.: Some Common Denominators in 1200 Cases of Cardiac Arrest, *Ann. Surg.*, 137:731, 1953.
23. Gabbard, J. G., Ross, A., Eastwood, D. E., and Burford, T. H.: The Effect of Ether Anesthesia upon Alveolar Ventilation and Acid-base Balance in Man, *Ann. Surg.*, 136:680, 1952.
24. Rodman, T.: The Effect of Anesthesia and Surgery on Pulmonary and Cardiac Function, *Am. J. Cardiol.*, 12:444, 1963.

25. Catenacci, A. J., DiPalma, J. R., Anderson, J. D., and King, W. E.: Serious Arrhythmias with Vasopressors during Halothane Anesthesia in Man, *J.A.M.A.*, **183**:136, 1963.

26. Driscoll, A., Hobika, J. H., Etsten, B. C., and Proger, S.: Postoperative Myocardial Infarction, *New England J. Med.*, **264**:633, 1961.

27. Buckley, J. J., and Jackson, J. A.: Postoperative Cardiac Arrhythmias, *Anesthesiology*, **22**:723, 1961.

28. Cannard, T. H., Dripps, R. D., Helwig, J., Jr., and Zinsser, H. F.: The Electrocardiogram during Anesthesia and Surgery, *Anesthesiology*, **21**:194, 1960.

Section D: Certain Aspects of Treatment

68 PHARMACOLOGY OF CARDIOVASCULAR DRUGS

Leon I. Goldberg, Ph.D., M.D.

The indications and directions for the use of drugs in specific cardiovascular conditions have been presented in many chapters of this book. The present chapter is designed to supplement the previous presentations and is concerned primarily with the pharmacologic actions of a few of the more important agents.

CARDIAC GLYCOSIDES

Since the classic studies of Withering in 1785,[1] the cardiac glycosides have been extensively used in the therapy of congestive heart failure. The history and use of these agents have been exhaustively reviewed.[2-7]

Source and Chemistry

Cardiac glycosides are found in a large number of plants. The most commonly used preparations are from *Digitalis purpurea* (digitoxin, gitalin, digitalis leaf, U.S.P.), *lanata* (lanatoside C, digoxin) and *Strophanthus gratus* (ouabain). In addition, cardiac glysosides are present in the venom from skin glands of toads; these glycosides contain only a 6-membered lactone ring.

All cardioactive glycosides have two major constituents: a genin, which is a steroid structure to which is attached either a 5- or 6-membered lactone ring, and a sugar molecule. The pharmacologic action resides in the genin, and the sugar molecule is important for the properties of absorption, accumulation, and passage through biologic membranes. Complete synthesis of a cardiac glycoside has not been accomplished, but synthetic derivatives have been prepared by attaching vari-

ous groups to the steroid nucleus (example: acetylstrophanthidin, which has an acetate group at the 3 position).

A comprehensive review of the botanic origin of more than two hundred cardiac glycosides and genins, their chemical structure, and lethal doses in the cat has been published by Hoch.[8] The known relationships of chemical structure to biologic activity of the glycosides has been reviewed by Tamm.[9]

Pharmacologic Actions: Myocardial Effects

Increased Myocardial Contractility (Increased Contractile Force, Positive Inotropic Effect)

It has now been demonstrated in many animal species, including man, that cardiac glycosides increase myocardial contractile force. A classic demonstration of this direct myocardial effect of digitalis was made by Catell and Gold in 1938.[10] These investigators demonstrated that when ouabain and digitoxin were added to a bath containing a failed, electrically driven, isolated, papillary muscle of the cat, restoration of the contractile force of the muscle occurred without changing the resting tension. Since the rate of contraction was constant and since there was no coronary circulation, the positive inotropic action of these glycosides was considered to be a direct myocardial effect. More recent studies of isolated preparations have indicated that the glycosides can produce a positive inotropic effect before any evidence of failure is obtained.[11,12]

The positive inotropic action of cardiac glycosides has also been demonstrated in the nonfailing intact heart of the dog by use of weighted lever systems and electronic-resistance strain-gauge arches sutured to the myocardium.[13,14] Studies of the nonfailing human heart with use of the strain-gauge arch technique during cardiopulmonary by-

ACUTE DIGITALIZATION DURING
EXTRACORPOREAL CIRCULATION

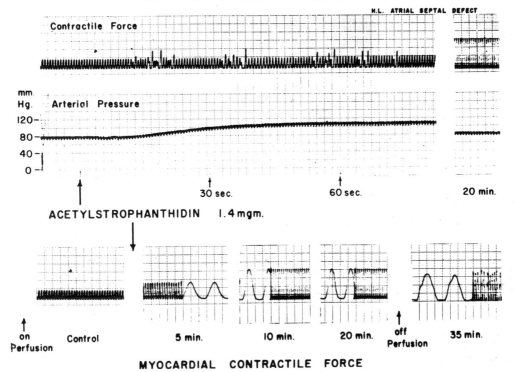

MYOCARDIAL CONTRACTILE FORCE

Fig. 68-1. Contractile force and arterial pressure recordings immediately and 20 min after the injection of 1.4 mg acetylstrophanthidin, in a twenty-eight-year-old woman with an atrial septal defect, are reproduced in the upper tracings. The lower tracings show contractile force recordings before injection and at intervals after acetylstrophanthidin. The final recording was obtained after bypass had been completed, 35 min after administration of the drug. (*From E. Braunwald, R. D. Bloodwell, L. I. Goldberg, and A. G. Morrow: Studies on Digitalis, J. Clin. Invest., 40:52, 1961. By permission of the publishers.*)

pass surgical procedures have indicated that similar increments in contractile force occur after the administration of cardiac glycosides to man (Fig. 68-1).[15] Evidence for a positive inotropic effect of digitalis in the nonoperated, nonfailing human heart has been obtained by Eddleman and associates[16] by means of electrokymography and more recently by Mason and Braunwald[17] by analysis of the rate of change of left ventricular pressure curves (Fig. 68-2).

Effects on Refractory Period and Conduction

Cardiac glycosides preferentially decrease conduction and prolong the functional refractory period of the atrioventricular (A-V) node. These effects have been found to begin at about 30 per cent of the lethal doses of cardiac glycosides in dogs and progress to complete A-V dissociation when about 65 per cent of the lethal dose is administered.[18,19] These effects are sometimes observed in the therapeutic range of digitalis dosage

as may be manifested in patients by prolonged P-R interval.

The increased functional refractory period of the A-V node is related in part to the vagal effect of cardiac glycosides (see below under Extramyocardial Actions) and also possibly to an antiadrenergic effect. The antiadrenergic effect was demonstrated by Méndez and associates,[20] who found that in the adrenalectomized dog with denervated heart a much larger dose of cardiac glycosides was required to produce an increase in the functional refractory period (55 per cent of the lethal dose). In addition to the important influences of the sympathetic and parasympathetic nerves, a direct effect of cardiac glycosides has been demonstrated on the functional refractory period of the A-V node in the chronically denervated, catecholamine-depleted dog heart.[21]

The refractory period of atrial tissue is decreased by cardiac glycosides in the innervated dog heart at about 40 per cent of the lethal dose but is in-

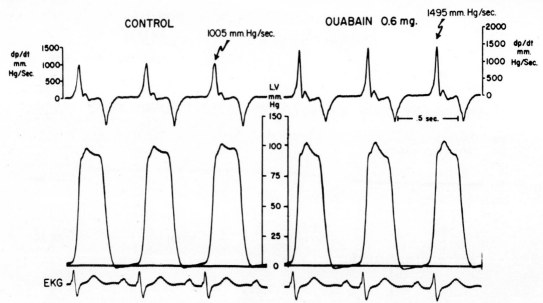

Fig. 68-2. Recordings of left ventricular (LV) pressure and rate of change (*dp/ dt*) before and 30 min after ouabain administration. (*From D. Mason and E. Braunwald: Studies on Digitalis, J. Clin. Invest.,* **42**:1105, 1963. *By permission of the authors and publisher.*)

creased in the denervated heart. The refractory period of ventricular muscle decreases only slightly at doses above 40 per cent of the lethal dose.[18]

Increased Production of Arrhythmias and Conduction Disturbances

Toxic doses of digitalis are demonstrated by increased production of arrhythmias and the appearance of conduction disturbances in both atrial and ventricular muscle. These adverse effects may be produced by several myocardial actions of digitalis, either alone or in combination, including increase in automaticity, depression of excitability,[22] decrease in refractory period, and depression of conduction through the Purkinje system.[23] The vulnerability of the ventricle to fibrillation is definitely enhanced.[24] Depending on the preponderance of the toxic effects, a lethal dose of digitalis may result in ventricular fibrillation or cardiac arrest.

Fundamental Studies of the Mechanism of Action of Cardiac Glycosides

Extensive studies have been carried out in attempts to determine the exact site in the contractile scheme in which cardiac glycosides exert their positive inotropic action, but this is unknown despite these investigations. However, a number of interesting effects of cardiac glycosides have been demonstrated. It is important in reviewing such data to keep two important questions in mind: Is the dose (or concentration) of the cardiac glyco-

sides in the range which is necessary to produce a positive inotropic effect, or is the dose more clearly a "toxic dose"? Secondly, is the effect noted in the biochemical or biophysical experiment the specific result of active cardiac glycosides, or can similar results be demonstrated with physiologically inactive compounds? Another possible objection to many studies of isolated tissues was recently raised by Moran.[25] His studies suggested that cardiac glycosides react with "tissue receptors" only during the phase of contraction and that no reaction occurs in the quiescent ventricle.

Fundamental investigations of the mechanism of action of cardiac glycosides have involved the following areas:

Energy Production and Utilization

A number of studies have indicated that the positive inotropic action of cardiac glycosides is not dependent upon increased substrate production or utilization; i.e., the high-energy phosphates adenosine triphosphate (ATP), adenosine diphosphate (ADP), and creatine phosphate are unchanged.[26–29] Studies of the failed isolated papillary muscles have indicated that a positive inotropic effect can be observed before an increase in oxygen utilization takes place, indicating an increased efficiency of myocardial contraction.[27,30] These studies have demonstrated a fundamental difference between the positive inotropic action of cardiac glycosides and sympathomimetic amines; the latter compounds utilize oxygen and high-energy substrates in parallel with the positive inotropic action.[31] It should be emphasized here that studies in the intact failing heart indicating increased cardiac efficiency with cardiac glycosides[32] may not represent the same phenomenon as is measured in isolated tissues.[33] The oxygen utilization of the intact heart is dependent upon a number of factors such as heart size, peripheral resistance, coronary flow, and heart rate.[34]

Many investigators have demonstrated increased oxygen utilization of toxic concentrations of digitalis on isolated myocardium, and it has been suggested that this effect may be related to uncoupling of oxidative phosphorylation.[30]

Influence of Cations

Potassium. It has been known for a number of years that toxic doses of cardiac glycosides diminish the potassium content of cardiac tissue.[35] This effect has been shown to be the result of inhibition of potassium influx with no effect on potassium efflux.[36] The reduction in intracellular potassium was considered to be the mechanism for the positive inotropic action of the cardiac glycosides.[37] More recent studies, however, contest this hypothesis, since it was demonstrated that the positive inotropic effect of glycosides may occur independently of changes in potassium content and since several lactones produced similar losses of potassium as cardiac glycosides without increasing contractility.[38,39]

Calcium. Calcium ions exert a positive inotropic effect and have a synergistic action when used in combination with cardiac glycosides. Despite extensive studies, the role of this ion in the positive inotropic action of cardiac glycosides is not known.[39-43]

Adenosine Triphosphatase (ATPase). Intimately linked to the concept that cardiac glycosides produce their effects by affecting ion transport across cell membranes has been the demonstration that cardiac glycosides inhibit the activity of the sodium- and potassium-dependent enzyme ATPase, which is responsible for destruction of ATP. Since transport of ions across cell membranes requires energy from ATP, inhibition of ATPase could alter the ionic content of tissues and ionic fluxes. The effects of cardiac glycosides on ATPase has been demonstrated in many types of cells,[44,45] and a relationship has been established between inhibition of ATPase and ion transport in studies of red blood cell ghosts.[46] Again, most of these investigations have been carried out with "toxic" concentrations of the glycosides. More recently Repke[47] has demonstrated that "nontoxic" doses of the glycosides are associated with stimulation of ATPase, and he

suggested that such stimulation may be the basic mechanism of the positive inotropic action.

Effects on Transmembrane Potential

It was hoped that recording of transmembrane action potentials by use of intracellular electrodes would give an indication of the mechanism of action of the positive inotropic action of cardiac glycosides. Earlier studies made by use of this technique indicated alterations of the action potentials of frog[48] and dog ventricular muscle[49] with relatively large concentrations. A more recent study,[50] however, has demonstrated that contractility of the sheep trabeculae carneae can be increased by cardiac glycosides without alteration of the action potentials recorded from Purkinje fibers. Since the form and duration of the action potential are dependent upon the changes in ionic concentration, the results of this study are evidence against a direct relationship of transmembrane permeability and the positive inotropic effect. On the other hand, alterations in action potentials produced by higher concentrations of cardiac glycosides support the concept that their toxic effects are related to ionic changes.

Combination with Contractile Proteins

A number of investigations have dealt with the effects of cardiac glycosides on muscle protein and on the ionic and enzymatic content of the proteins. The rate of polymerization of solutions of globular (G-) actin to form the long-chain (F-) actin was found to be increased by these drugs.[51] Wollenberger,[52] however, demonstrated that inactive cardiac glycosides had similar effects. Robb and Mallov[53] observed that ATP-induced shortening of threads of heart muscle actomyosin increased after addition of ouabain. Kako and Bing[54] found that impaired contractions of actomyosin bands obtained from hearts of patients with congestive heart failure were improved by the addition of digoxin and calcium. More recently the effects of cardiac glycosides have also been found to antagonize an inhibitory substance of actomyosin contraction known as the *relaxing factor*.[30]

Effects on Myocardial Catecholamine Content

The hypothesis that cardiac glycosides produce their cardiac actions by depletion of catecholamines[55,56] has not been confirmed, since these agents produce both their positive inotropic and toxic effects in the dog heart depleted of catecholamines by sympathectomy or reserpine.[21,54] Furthermore, the β-adrenergic blocking agent dichloroisoproterenol (DCI), which blocks the cardiac effects of catecholamines, does not prevent the positive inotropic action of the glycosides.[57,58]

To summarize: At this time the exact mechanism of the positive inotropic action of cardiac glycosides has not been delineated despite a number of attractive hypotheses. The magnitude of the problem and steps necessary for final solution have been presented in a recent symposium[59] and have been the subject of a number of reviews.[23,33,60-62]

Extramyocardial Actions

Augmentation of Vagal Activity

Cardiac glycosides increase the effects of normal vagal activity of the heart. This effect is commonly manifested by bradycardia in experimental animals and in normal human subjects. The vagal action of the bradycardia is verified by the fact that it can be abolished either by vagotomy or by large doses of atropine.[63]

Since vagal fibers are distributed to atrial tissues and to both sinus and A-V nodes, the effects of increased action of acetylcholine must be considered when the actions of digitalis are analyzed. Because of this effect, part of the A-V block produced by digitalis is considered to be the result of vagal stimulation, and the increased rate of atrial fibrillation often observed after administration of glycosides may also be the result of vagal stimulation. (Acetylcholine and vagal stimulation decrease the refractory period and increase conduction in atrial tissue.[24])

Several mechanisms have been evoked for the augmentation of vagal activity by cardiac glycosides. Heymans and his associates[64] considered that the augmentation was an effect mediated through the caroticoaortic barostatic reflexes. Greene and Peeler[65] have emphasized the possibility that the glycosides have a direct action on the vagal nuclei in the medulla. More recently Gaffney and associates[66] demonstrated that cardiac glycosides sensitized the sinoatrial (S-A) and A-V nodes to acetylcholine, thus indicating a possible peripheral site for the vagal augmentation.

Effects on Blood Vessels

Arteries. Direct injection of cardiac glycosides into perfused arteries produces vasoconstriction.[67] This may explain in part the increase in blood pressure which sometimes occurs following intravenous administration of large doses to experimental animals and to man.[68] Studies in man[15] during cardiopulmonary bypass procedures suggest that this arterial vasoconstriction is a transient phenomenon when compared with the more prolonged positive inotropic effect (Fig. 68-1). Similar vasoconstriction has been observed in the coronary arteries of dogs following direct injection of cardiac glyco-

sides.[69] The clinical significance of such vasoconstriction is unknown. In this respect, Gold and associates[70] did not observe an increase in angina pectoris following administration of cardiac glycosides to patients in a well-controlled study.

Veins. The effect of digitalis on the venous system has been the subject of considerable controversy. In 1930 Dock and Tainter[71,72] reported that ouabain caused constriction of the hepatic vein in dogs with resultant pooling of blood in the splanchnic regions. Baschieri and associates[73] suggested that a similar effect occurred in man, since they observed an elevation in hepatic venous wedge pressure and increase in the gradient between the hepatic venous wedge and inferior vena cava pressures and a decline in hepatic blood flow in patients in congestive heart failure after administration of cardiac glycosides. Nadler and associates,[74] on the other hand, were unable to detect an increase in spleen size following digitalis administration in dogs, although intestinal volume increased. More recent studies in the dog, both with intact heart[14] and with heart excluded by cardiopulmonary bypass techniques, have indicated that an increase in capacity of the vascular system takes place after administration of cardiac glycosides.[75] This was demonstrated by the fact that the animal takes up blood from a venous reservoir after administration of the glycoside. Such an increased capacity could be due either to dilatation of all or part of the vascular bed or to constriction of some area of the venous system, with passive dilatation and pooling of blood in the vessels behind it. The site of this increased capacity is not known, but evidence by Ross and associates[75] suggests that it is primarily in the splanchnic bed.

In 1944 McMichael and Sharpey-Schafer[76] considered that reduction of venous pressure after administration of cardiac glycosides was the basis for the increased cardiac output produced in patients in heart failure and postulated that a relaxation of venomotor tone occurred. Later McMichael[77] conceded that this initial interpretation was erroneous and that the cardiac output in most, but not all, patients increased prior to a change in venous pressure. More recently Mason and Braunwald[78] demonstrated by plethysmographic techniques that venous constriction is produced in normal subjects by cardiac glycosides. In patients in congestive heart failure, however, cardiac glycosides were found to produce venous dilatation. It was suggested that these paradoxical results were related to the fact that digitalis itself has a venous constrictor effect, but that in the patient with congestive heart failure improvement in cardiac function resulted in reduction of abnormally elevated sympathetic activity which had produced venous constriction.

Effects on the Gastrointestinal System

Cardiac glycosides produce anorexia, nausea, vomiting, and diarrhea, both by a direct irritant effect on gastrointestinal mucosa[79] and because of a central nervous system action.

Effects on the Central Nervous System

In addition to the effects of cardiac glycosides on the emetic[80] and possibly on the vagal center, a number of central nervous system manifestations have been observed, particularly in toxic doses. Some of these are included in the list of toxic manifestations of digitalis shown in Table 68-1.

Effects on the Kidney

When cardiac glycosides are injected directly into the renal artery of dogs, excretion of sodium and water increases; this suggests a direct tubular effect.[81] This action may be related to the inhibition of ATPase.[45] It is unlikely, however, that a direct tubular action is the mechanism for the diuresis observed following digitalization of patients with congestive heart failure, since a consistent diuretic effect cannot be demonstrated in normal individuals.[82]

Effects of Cardiac Glycosides on the Intact Heart and Circulation

Cardiac Output

The cardiac output of patients with congestive heart failure and low cardiac output is usually increased by cardiac glycosides.[76,83–86] This increase in cardiac output is the basis for the beneficial actions of the drugs according to the "forward-failure" concept. The increase in cardiac output leads to increased emptying of the heart with resultant decrease in atrial, venous, and pulmonary arterial pressures. The renal blood flow and glomerular filtration rate increase, and with the improvement of circulation there may be a reduction in aldosterone secretion.[87] These changes lead to a sodium diuresis which decreases the abnormally elevated circulating blood volume and further reduces heart size. The sodium loss and decreased venous pressure favor the elimination of edema. The studies of Merrill [88] and Eichna and associates[89] have illustrated the complex cardiovascular and renal changes which occur following digitalization of patients in congestive heart failure.

Although cardiac output increases in most patients with congestive heart failure, the cardiac output of normal subjects usually does not change or may even decrease after administration of cardiac glycosides.[68,83,90–94] This apparent paradox in the action of the drug has been offered as evidence to support the concept that they do not increase the contractility of the normal heart. It is most important in this connection to understand that cardiac output is not necessarily an accurate measure of cardiac contractility. Cardiac output is dependent not only upon myocardial contractility, but also upon venous return, heart rate, peripheral resistance, and valvular competence.

The studies in the dog by Cotten and Stopp[14] have provided a possible explanation for the difference in the action of digitalis in the normal subject and the patient in heart failure. These investigators attached a strain-gauge arch to the myocardium and measured cardiac output by use of a Shipley-Wilson flowmeter in the aorta. They observed that when ouabain was administered to the dog, the expected increase in myocardial contractility occurred, but the stroke volume and cardiac output decreased (Fig. 68-3). Accompanying this decrease was a marked reduction in left atrial pressure. When left atrial pressure was maintained (analogous to the failed heart with elevated left atrial pressure), cardiac output and myocardial contractility increased in parallel (Fig. 68-4).

These results suggest that both the increased myocardial contractility and the increased vascular capacity produced by cardiac glycosides are important determinants of the effect on cardiac output. In normal subjects the decreased venous return precludes translation of the increased myocardial contractility into increased cardiac output. In the patient in heart failure, however, with increase in blood volume, elevation of venous and atrial pressures, and dilatation of the heart, the increase in myocardial contractility enables the ventricles to eject larger volumes of blood.

Heart Size

Another controversial question in both clinical and experimental studies is whether the decrease in heart size noted after digitalization in normal and failing hearts is entirely the result of more adequate emptying of the ventricle and/or decrease in venous return or whether cardiac glycosides actually have an effect on diastolic tone. The majority of evidence indicates that decrease in heart size is secondary to the increased cardiac output and decreased venous return.[4,16]

Heart Rate

The influence of cardiac glycosides on heart rate is dependent upon a number of factors including vagal and sympathetic effects, improvement in congestive heart failure, and degree of direct effect of the glycosides on the S-A and A-V nodes. In normal subjects large doses of cardiac glycosides sometimes produce a moderate reduction in heart rate which

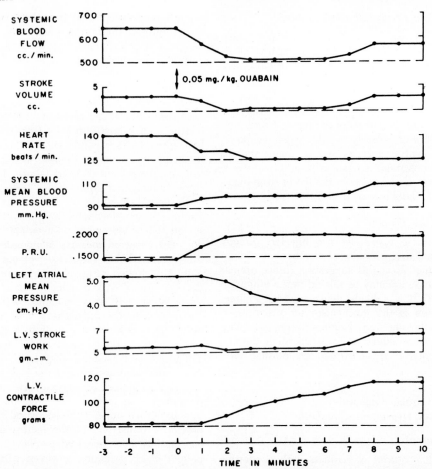

Fig. 68-3. Effects of 0.05 mg per kg ouabain in an anesthetized dog with uncontrolled left atrial pressure. Note the substantial increase in contractile force with only slight changes in systemic flow and stroke work. (*From M. deV. Cotten and P. E. Stopp: Action of Digitalis on the Nonfailing Heart of the Dog, Am. J. Physiol., 192:114, 1958. By permission of the authors and publisher.*)

can be eliminated with atropine, whereas in the patient with heart failure reduction in rate may be more striking.[6]

Electrocardiographic Changes[95,96]

In therapeutic doses there is characteristic scaphoid depression of the S-T segment and decrease in magnitude of the T waves and reduction of the duration of the Q-T interval. In toxic doses premature atrial and ventricular contractions, bigeminal rhythm, runs of ventricular tachycardia, multifocal tachycardia, and ventricular fibrillation may occur. Because of the decreased conduction through the A-V node, there may be prolongation of the P-R interval in therapeutic doses and, with toxicity, varying degrees of heart block. A common but not exclusive manifestation of digitalis intoxication is paroxysmal atrial tachycardia with block (Fig. 68-5).[97] It should be emphasized that cardiac

glycosides can produce any arrhythmia or conduction defect in toxic doses.

Differences in Cardiac Glycosides: Absorption, Doses, Duration of Action

Despite enthusiastic claims, there is no good evidence that there are any differences in therapeutic index (arrhythmic dose/positive inotropic dose) among the various glycosides. The glycosides differ only in the percentage of oral dose absorbed, their speed of action, and the duration of effect. In respect to absorption, it may be noted that lanatoside C, for example, is only about 10 per cent absorbed whereas digitoxin is 100 per cent absorbed. Speed of action varies from 5 to 10 min intravenously for acetylstrophanthidin to about 1 hr for digitoxin. The duration of effects appears to be related to the time of onset. It should be mentioned that differences in therapeutic index have occasionally been made in studies which did not consider the differences in speed of action of two compounds or did not compare the glycosides at equivalent biologic doses.[4]

Additional information concerning the absorption, distribution, and excretion of cardiac glycosides has been obtained by studies of radioactive glycosides.[98,99] In addition, new techniques for measuring the cardiac action of the drugs may also eventually expand our knowledge in this area.[100]

Digitalization and Maintenance Doses

Although a number of dosage schedules are available for the cardiac glycosides, dosage must still be adjusted on purely clinical grounds. In general, arrhythmias develop with smaller doses in older individuals and those with more severe myocardial disease. Furthermore, in these days in which chlorothiazide derivatives are widely used and potassium depletion is common, great care must be exercised to prevent toxicity. The commonly recommended doses for a few of the more frequently used glycosides are presented in Chap. 15. Pediatric doses are

available in the papers of Nadas and Hauck[101] and Engle[102] and are presented in Chap. 20.

Clinical Applications

Congestive Heart Failure

Clinical evidence has suggested that digitalis is more effective in low-output congestive heart failure related to hypertensive and atherosclerotic heart disease, less effective in valvular heart disease, and least effective where there is widespread myocarditis or myocardial degeneration. It has been successfully used in the treatment of congestive heart failure accompanying acute myocardial infarction. Digitalis is considered to be less effective in the treatment of high-output cardiac failure as in arteriovenous fistulas, beriberi heart disease, and thyrotoxic heart disease.

Atrial Fibrillation

Digitalis is used to decrease the ventricular rate in atrial fibrillation and at the same time to increase the force of ventricular contraction. Although the

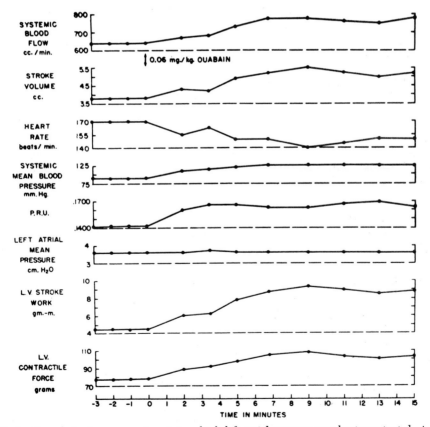

Fig. 68-4. Effects of ouabain in an experiment in which left atrial pressure was kept constant during its actions. Infusion of 100 ml whole blood was necessary to keep the left atrial pressure constant during the period of observation. Compare with the results shown in Fig. 68-3. (*From M. deV. Cotten and P. E. Stopp: Action of Digitalis on the Nonfailing Heart of the Dog, Am. J. Physiol.,* **192:**114, *1958. By permission of the authors and publisher.*)

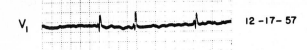

V₁   12 –17– 57

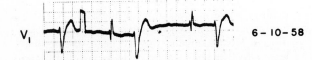

V₁   6 – 10– 58

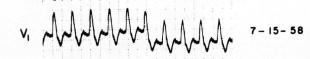

V₁   7 – 15– 58

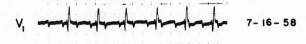

V₁   7– 16 – 58

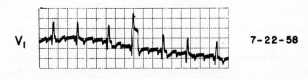

V₁   7-22-58

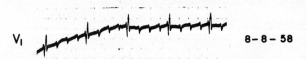

V₁   8- 8 – 58

Fig. 68-5. Electrocardiographic manifestations of digitalis intoxication in a forty-one-year-old patient with rheumatic heart disease. In the first record, December 17, 1957, atrial fibrillation is present. In the second record, June 10, 1958, bigeminal rhythm due to ventricular ectopic beats is present. On July 15, 1958, regular supraventricular rhythm is noted with aberrant QRS conduction. On July 16, 1958, the tracing shows atrial tachycardia with block. On July 22, 1958, the atrial rate is increased, and the ventricular rate shows more obvious variations in regularity. By August 8, 1958, the atrial rate is approximately 280, and the ventricular rate has slowed to 65. (*From "Electrocardiographic Interpretation," J. W. Hurst and N. Wenger* (eds.), *McGraw-Hill, Book Company, Blakiston Division, New York, 1963, p. 134.*)

vagal action of cardiac glycosides would tend to perpetuate fibrillation,[24] conversion of the arrhythmia frequently takes place after digitalis administration, presumably because of improved oxygenation of the myocardium.

Paroxysmal Atrial Tachycardia

Paroxysmal atrial tachycardia which does not respond to other methods of vagal stimulation will frequently respond to administration of digitalis either alone or in combination with the vagal stimulation.

Prophylactic Digitalization

Although it has previously been considered harmful to digitalize a patient without evidence of congestive heart failure, more recent studies have demonstrated that digitalization has no deleterious

effects on normal subjects.[91–94] These studies indicated that cardiovascular responses to exercise did not change in normal subjects after large doses of digitalis. Such evidence and demonstration of a positive inotropic effect in normal subjects has suggested to surgeons that digitalization may be beneficial prior to open-heart surgery.[15] It is important to remember in this respect that although no useful effect of digitalization occurs in normal subjects, marked improvement has been demonstrated in patients with latent, but not overt, congestive heart failure.[103,104] The question of prophylactic digitalization is a controversial subject, with arguments for and against each viewpoint.

Contraindications

An absolute contraindication for the use of cardiac glycosides is obviously digitalis intoxication.

Relative contraindications are incomplete heart block and hypertrophic subaortic stenosis.[105]

Digitalis Intoxication

The toxic effects of digitalis were well described by Withering[1] and have been the subject of several reviews.[106–110] Table 68-1 lists a number of the common toxic manifestations.

Table 68-1. MANIFESTATIONS OF DIGITALIS INTOXICATION

Arrhythmias	Anorexia	Weakness and fatigue
Atrial	Nausea	Yellow vision
Nodal	Vomiting	Scotomas
Ventricular	Diarrhea	Delirium
A-V block		
S-A block		

The incidence of digitalis intoxication is not known. Rodensky and Wasserman[108] estimate that 20 per cent of digitalized patients in their institutions had cardiotoxicity. This high value may be related to the severity of the cardiac disease in the patients. No estimate of the incidence of toxicity in unselected populations, including outpatients, has been made, but it would probably be a lower incidence.

Several factors will increase the dangers of digitalis intoxication. Most important is electrolyte imbalance, primarily potassium depletion. Since the introduction of the oral thiazide diuretics, the dangers of potassium depletion complicating digitalis therapy have greatly increased. It should be emphasized that all diuretic agents can lower serum-potassium levels with production of digitalis arrhythmias; however, it should be realized that potassium depletion may occur with normal levels of serum potassium. The danger of precipitating digitalis arrhythmias with intravenous administration of calcium has been known for many years.[111] Drugs which may increase the danger of digitalis intoxication are antiarrhythmic agents and antihypertensive agents such as reserpine[112–113] and guanethidine.[114] The mechanism for the arrhythmias reported with the use of reserpine and guanethidine is not known. Although several investigators have suggested that a relationship exists between the catecholamine depletion produced by these agents and digitalis intoxication, this viewpoint is not supported by experimental evidence. It is possible that the increase in toxicity may be related in part to a relative increase in vagal activity.

In most cases of digitalis intoxication the only treatment required is discontinuance of the drug. When serious arrhythmias occur, administration of potassium, preferably orally but when necessary intravenously, may be useful.[107] Potassium adminis-

tration should not be used for any manifestation of digitalis intoxication except increased ectopic activity, and it may be detrimental in the presence of conduction defects.[115] Chelation of calcium by use of EDTA and other chelating agents has also been used with some success.[116] Antiarrhythmic agents such as procaine amide and quinidine may be useful in digitalis-induced ventricular tachycardia, but the danger exists that cardiac arrest or ventricular fibrillation may result from such therapy. Accordingly, when these drugs are used, an electrical pacemaker should be available.[117,118] Finally, although digitalis-induced ventricular fibrillation has long been considered to be an irreversible arrhythmia, the use of electric countershock and cardiac massage has resulted in reversion of the arrhythmia and survival.[102]

AMINOPHYLLINE

Aminophylline (theophylline ethylenediamine) may be useful in the treatment of cardiac dyspnea and pulmonary edema. This xanthine derivative has several pharmacologic actions which may explain its beneficial effects. (1) Aminophylline increases myocardial contractility in both the isolated [119] and intact heart.[120] This positive inotropic action is considered to be the basis for the increased cardiac output and reduction in right atrial pressure following intravenous administration of the xanthine to patients with congestive heart failure.[121] The increase in cardiac output is of relatively short duration (20 to 30 min). Cardiac glycosides and aminophylline may be given in succession with summation of their actions on cardiac output.[121] (2) Aminophylline has a direct vasodilating effect on arteries and veins.[122] Its effects as a coronary vasodilator are debatable and of doubtful clinical value.[123–125] (3) Aminophylline is a potent bronchodilator which may be useful in relaxing bronchospasm which frequently accompanies cardiac dyspnea.[122] (4) Aminophylline has a diuretic action both because of its effects of increasing renal blood flow and glomerular filtration rate and because of direct action on the tubules to prevent the reabsorption of sodium.[126,127] (5) Because of a central nervous system action, aminophylline may revert the periodic breathing of Cheyne-Stokes respiration to a more normal pattern.[122,123]

Aminophylline may be administered orally, rectally, or intravenously. The oral route, however, is unsatisfactory because of severe gastrointestinal disturbances which occur when therapeutic doses are used. When administered intravenously, the agent must be infused slowly in a dilute form to prevent the occurrences of cardiac arrhythmias and shock.

MORPHINE

There are two principal indications for the use of morphine and other narcotics in cardiovascular disease: first, for relief of pain and anxiety and, second, for the treatment of cardiac dyspnea and pulmonary edema. The analgesic actions of narcotics have been reviewed extensively and will not be repeated here.[128-130]

The exact mechanism of action of morphine in the treatment of pulmonary edema has not been elucidated. Several actions or presumed effects of morphine have been implicated.

Vasodilator Effect

Morphine has long been known to exert a hypotensive effect both in experimental animals and in man. Studies in the dog in 1933 by Schmidt and Livingston[131] demonstrated that the hypotension was related to dilation of cutaneous and muscular beds by a direct action of the narcotic on the vessels. They did not consider that the hypotension was related to cardiac depression. Studies in normal subjects have demonstrated profound hypotension after morphine when the subjects are tilted to a head-up position.[132] These effects were considered to be due to venous pooling and could be prevented by raising the legs or application of pressure bandages to the legs. If such an effect takes place in the patient in pulmonary edema, the beneficial effects of morphine could be readily explained by a type of 'internal tourniquet." Unfortunately there is no good data to confirm this impression. It should be mentioned that the hypotensive effect of narcotics may sometimes occur with the patient in the supine position, making it mandatory to monitor the blood pressure frequently in patients with myocardial infarction after administration of narcotics.

Reduction of Anxiety and Rate of Respiration

It is difficult to assess the contributions of the sedative effects of morphine to its value in the treatment of pulmonary edema. The beneficial effects of relief of anxiety are evident, whatever means are used, including reassurance. This hypothesis states that because of relief of anxiety, the respiratory rate is decreased with resultant reduction in work of the ventilatory muscles. The direct action of morphine to depress respiration is also included in this concept.

Interference with Reflexes from the Heart and Lungs

Luisada[133] suggested that morphine relieves pulmonary edema by interfering with reflexes which would tend to perpetuate pulmonary edema. There is no direct evidence to support this concept.

Bronchoconstrictor Action

Rodbard[134] suggested that the bronchoconstrictor effect of morphine increases alveolar pressure and thus produces an internal positive pressure mechanism to relieve pulmonary edema. This theory has recently been contested by Sharp and associates,[135] who did not observe bronchoconstriction in patients with pulmonary edema treated with morphine and, furthermore, noted no change in pulmonary compliance after administration of the narcotic.

Adverse Effects

The most important and serious adverse effect of morphine is respiratory depression.[136] This effect is produced by direct action on the respiratory center. An early manifestation of morphine action is reduction of the increased respiratory effort produced by carbon dioxide. Bronchoconstriction (possibly related to histamine release[137]) may occur with morphine, especially in patients known to be asthmatic.

A feature of morphine pharmacology that should never be forgotten is addiction. Cases of morphine addiction have frequently occurred during treatment of cardiac dyspnea. An occasional effect is the occurrence of excitation rather than sedation with morphine. Finally, morphine commonly causes constipation and may produce nausea and vomiting by effects on the chemoreceptive emetic zone.[138]

The respiratory and central nervous system depression produced by morphine and some other narcotics may be antagonized by nalorphine hydrochloride or levallorphan tartrate. Despite claims to the contrary, respiratory depression, addiction, and hypotension occur with all potent narcotics.

MERCURIAL DIURETICS [45,127,139-141]

Chemistry

The mercurial diuretics are organic mercurial compounds with the following basic structure:

$$\begin{array}{ccc} H & OY\ H \\ X-Hg-C-C-C-R \\ H & H\ \ \ H \end{array}$$

X is theophylline sodium in meralluride sodium (Mercuhydrin) and mercumatilin sodium (Cumertilin) and thioacetate sodium in mercaptomerin sodium (Thiomerin). The addition of this group affects solubility, irritation on injection, and cardiotoxicity. The side group OY may be methoxy, ethoxy, or hydroxy and seems to have little effect on diuretic action. The R group is also important for diuretic potency and side effects and is alicyclic in mercaptomerin, heterocyclic in mercumatilin, and acyclic in meralluride.

Pharmacologic Actions

Mercurial diuretics act directly on the kidney to prevent the reabsorption of sodium chloride and water. It was formerly considered that the primary action of the agents was to prevent the tubular reabsorption of chloride, and that water and sodium were passively excreted. More recent evidence, however, favors the concept that the reabsorption of sodium is actively blocked and reabsorption of chloride and water is passive.[142] The greater increase in chloride than sodium excretion, which characteristically occurs with mercurial diuresis, has been explained by a distal tubular exchange of potassium and hydrogen ions for the increased amount of sodium which appears in the distal tubule.[143] This exchange of potassium for sodium may be pronounced in massive diuresis with the resultant production of potassium depletion. The loss of potassium is opposed to some extent by the fact that the secretion of potassium is inhibited by mercurial diuretics.[144] The exact sites of mercurial actions are not known. Stop-flow studies of the dog suggested that these diuretics blocked reabsorption of sodium in the proximal tubule.[145] More recent studies of mercurial diuretics during water diuresis and hydropenia have pointed to a more distal tubular site of action.[146] It is possible, as Orloff and Berliner[45] have suggested, that mercurial diuretics partially inhibit sodium transport throughout most of the nephron.

Mechanism of Action

The exact mechanism of action of mercurial diuretics is also unknown. Because of the great affinity of inorganic mercury for sulfhydryl groups, however, a number of concepts have evolved which consider that mercuric ions, either in free or bound form, combine with essential sulfhydryl enzymes to form inactive mercaptide complexes. These hypotheses have received support from the observation that the dithiol dithiopropanol (BAL), which can remove mercuric ions from sulfhydryl mercurial combinations, interrupts mercurial diuresis.[147] Monothiols do not prevent mercurial diuresis but reduce cardiotoxicity. Evidence against the sulfhydryl-combination hypothesis is the fact that *p*-chloromercuribenzoate, a powerful sulfhydryl inhibitor, is not a diuretic. This evidence has resulted in revised concepts which postulate that in order to be a diuretic, a sulfhydryl inhibitor must have a particular spatial arrangement.

Factors Affecting Mercurial Diuresis

Mercurial diuresis is potentiated by acidosis[148] and inhibited by alkalosis.[149] After repeated diuresis with mercurial diuretics, hypochloremic alkalosis may develop, with great limitation of the diuretic action. Effectiveness may be reestablished by acidification by ammonium chloride or lysine hydrochloride. Other factors which limit mercurial and other diuretics include reduction in glomerular filtration rate, hyponatremia, and increased aldosterone activity. Accordingly, measures which act to increase glomerular filtration rate such as administration of digitalis or aminophylline may potentiate a mercurial diuresis. Concurrent administration of aldosterone antagonists may also facilitate diuresis.

Modes of Administration

Mercurial diuretics are usually administered intramuscularly. Mercaptomerin may also be administered subcutaneously. The use of orally active mercurial diuretics has decreased because of the availability of more effective oral diuretics. Intravenous administration increases the toxic hazards of mercurial diuretics and should be reserved for extremely resistant cases.

Following intramuscular administration the diuretic action of most of the mercurial diuretics begins to be apparent in about 2 hr, reaches a peak in 4 to 6 hr, and lasts up to 24 hr. The mercurial diuretics are rapidly excreted by the kidneys and are mostly excreted in 24 hr. In patients with impaired renal function, however, excretion may be greatly delayed with possibilities of cumulation and resultant toxicity.

Toxicity[127]

The mercurial diuretics have produced a number of fatal reactions immediately following intravenous administration. It is likely that most of these deaths were due to ventricular fibrillation. Hypersensitivity reactions have also been described. Typical mercurialism, with stomatitis, salivation, colitis, and renal damage is relatively rare and usually occurs only in patients with severe renal insufficiency. Chills and fever may rarely occur. Although not exclusively manifestations of mercurial diuretics but relatively common because of their marked potency are the occurrences of electrolyte imbalance, reduced plasma volume with decreased glomerular filtration rate, and thrombotic episodes.

CARBONIC ANHYDRASE INHIBITORS[45,127,139–141,150]

Carbonic anhydrase inhibitors were introduced as diuretics after it was found that sulfanilamide produces metabolic acidosis and increases excretion of an alkaline urine. These effects were found to be related to an inhibition of the enzyme carbonic anhydrase, and agents chemically related to the sulfonamides were synthesized which were far more potent inhibitors of the enzyme. The chemical structure of a commonly used anhydrase inhibitor, acetazoleamide (Diamox), is shown in Fig. 68-6. The diuretic action of carbonic anhydrase inhibitors is due to the fact that carbonic anhydrase accelerates the reaction

$$CO_2 + H_2O \rightleftharpoons H_2CO_3$$

which instantaneously dissociates to $H^+ + HCO_3^-$. The H^+ provided by the reaction is normally exchanged for sodium, and when the enzyme is inhibited, there is an increased excretion of sodium bicarbonate. The loss of sodium bicarbonate results in an alkaline urine and diminished production of ammonia. If the administration of the inhibitors is continued, metabolic hyperchloremic acidosis develops. When pronounced acidosis occurs, the diuretic potency of these agents is lost. In addition to the loss of sodium, carbonic anhydrase inhibitors increase the excretion of potassium, presumably because of increased distal tubular exchange of potassium for sodium and inhibition of hydrogen ion exchange. The principal advantage of carbonic anhydrase inhibitors is that they are orally active. However, they are relatively weak agents when compared to the more potent thiazide diuretics and are, accordingly, no longer extensively used in the treatment of cardiovascular disease. Side effects include anorexia, nausea, vomiting, diarrhea, occasional development of skin rashes, and, rarely, blood dyscrasia. In addition, these agents may produce pronounced hypokalemia.

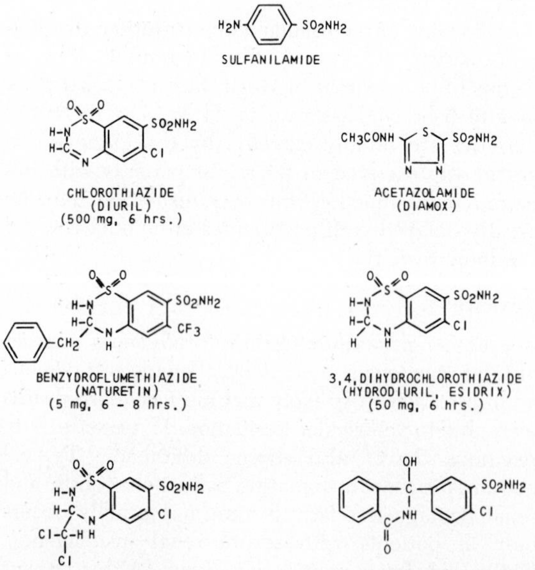

CHLOROTHIAZIDE AND RELATED DIURETICS[45,127,139–141,151,152]

Chlorothiazide (Diuril) was synthesized with the aim of developing a more potent carbonic anhydrase inhibitor.[153] Pharmacologic studies revealed that although the compound exhibited carbonic anhydrase–inhibiting properties, it possessed a far more potent action of increasing the excretion of sodium chloride.

Chemistry

The chemical structures of chlorothiazide and several of the related diuretics are shown in Fig. 68-6. All these agents are chemically similar to the sulfonamides and the carbonic anhydrase inhibitors. The specific requirement for diuretic activity appears to be the sulfamyl group (SO_2NH_2) and adjacent halogen. The thiazide structure present in chlorothiazide and many of its derivatives is not essential for activity and has been replaced, for example, by a phthalimidine group in chlorthalidone and a quinazoline derivative in quinethazone.

Pharmacologic Actions

Chlorothiazide and its derivatives resemble mercurial diuretics in that they act directly on the renal tubules to prevent the reabsorption of sodium, chloride, and water. The thiazide diuretics differ from mercurials in the following respects: (1) Thiazide and mercurial diuretics apparently have a different mechanism of action, for maximal doses of the two types of drugs have been shown to exhibit additive effects. (2) The diuresis produced by chlorothiazide and its derivatives is not affected by acidosis or alkalosis. (3) The thiazide diuretics, under similar experimental conditions, produce a greater excretion of solute and lesser excretion of free water than do mercurials. (4) The thiazide diuretics, unlike mercurial diuretics, do not have an action to inhibit renal tubular secretion of potassium. (5) Chlorothiazide and its derivatives are more effective than orally administered mercurials.

Fig. 68-6. Structural formulas of sulfanilamide, acetazoleamide, chlorothiazide, and several diuretics with action similar to chlorothiazide. In parentheses below the formulas of chlorothiazide and its derivatives, a recommended single oral dosage and its reported duration of action are presented. (J. H. Laragh. The Mode of Action and Use of Chlorothiazide and Related Compounds, Circulation, 26:121, 1962, for additional information.)

There is good evidence for both proximal and distal sites of action for the chlorothiazide-type diuretics. The carbonic anhydrase–inhibiting properties exhibited by chlorothiazide have little importance in its diuretic action and are almost absent in the newer derivatives. Accordingly, this effect can largely be discounted in explaining the increased potassium secretion produced by all thiazide diuretics. The loss of potassium is one of the major disadvantages in the use of chlorothiazide and related compounds. Experimental data suggest that the loss of potassium is not a primary action of these drugs but is the result of the greater load of sodium presented to the distal tubular site for potassium-sodium exchange. If this is the case, then potassium loss is a consequence of the natriuretic potency of these agents and will be present in all effective agents.[152] This has been true for all derivatives synthesized thus far. The danger of potassium depletion is intensified in the presence of sodium depletion and in conditions such as cirrhosis and congestive heart failure where production of aldosterone may be increased.

Chlorothiazide and its derivatives have an antihypertensive action and potentiate the effects of other antihypertensive agents. This use of the diuretics has been described in greater detail in another section. The mechanism of the antihypertensive action was initially considered to be related to the natriuretic effect with concomitant decrease of blood volume, but recently the development of a sodium-retaining thiazide derivative, diazoxide,[154,155] with properties to lower blood pressure by diminution of peripheral resistance, has suggested that part of the antihypertensive action of thiazide diuretics may be related to a direct vascular effect.

Adverse Effects

Prolonged administration of chlorothiazide and derivatives may produce pronounced electrolyte abnormalities with eventual production of hypokalemic, hypochloremic alkalosis. Hyponatremia may also develop with resultant decreased plasma volume, cardiac output, and glomerular filtration rate. Persistent use may therefore result in diminished glomerular filtration rate and elevation of blood-urea-nitrogen level, even in the absence of renal disease. The electrolyte imbalance produced by thiazides may be particularly dangerous in cirrhosis and may precipitate hepatic coma.

The thiazide diuretics depress the urinary excretion of uric acid and commonly produce elevations in serum uric acid, with occasional appearance of gout.[156] In addition, these agents exert a hyperglycemic effect in patients with latent or overt diabetes.[157] This hyperglycemic action may greatly complicate diabetic control in some patients, requiring discontinuance of the diuretic. It is important to emphasize in these respects that thiazide diuretics should be discontinued before diagnostic tests for diabetes mellitus or gouts are carried out. The mechanisms of action for these metabolic disturbances of the thiazide diuretics are under active investigations but are largely unknown.

Side effects and toxicity not related to the diuretic action include skin rashes, thrombopenia, agranulocytosis, and photosensitivity. In addition, a number of cases of pancreatitis have been described.

Administration

All the thiazide derivatives are effective orally and differ primarily in their dosage, time of onset, and duration of action. The dosage, chemical structure, and duration of action of several compounds are shown in Fig. 68-6. Despite enthusiastic claims which heralded the appearance of each new derivative, there is no good evidence that these compounds differ in effectiveness as diuretics or in the tendency to produce hypokalemia and other adverse effects. Therefore, it is important to ensure adequate potassium intake, in the form of supplements, in order to prevent hypokalemia and the associated danger of digitalis intoxication with all chlorothiazide derivatives.

SPIRONOLACTONE (ALDACTONE)[158,159]

In 1957 Kagawa and associates[160,161] reported that a number of newly synthesized steroid lactones had a specific action of competitively antagonizing the effects of aldosterone and deoxycorticosterone. One of these steroids, spironolactone (Aldactone), was found to be the most potent, and it was introduced as a diuretic agent. Clinical studies indicated that it had a natriuretic effect in patients with primary aldosteronism and in patients with secondary aldosteronism due to nephrosis, cirrhosis, congestive heart failure, and malignant hypertension. There was no effect in adrenalectomized patients and only a slight action in normal subjects in whom aldosterone secretion was low. Renal clearance studies in normal subjects demonstrated that the drug had no effect on renal plasma flow or glomerular filtration rate.[162] In addition to increasing sodium excretion, spironolactones were found to have a tendency to promote potassium retention and diminish hydrogen excretion.

Spironolactone is generally ineffective when administered as the sole diuretic agent to patients with severe congestive heart failure, possibly because of the low glomerular filtration rate in such patients. However, when spironolactone is administered with mercurial or thiazide diuretics, true synergism occurs, and the potassium loss produced by the more potent diuretics is reduced. It may greatly enhance diuresis when properly used.

Spironolactone appears to have an antihypertensive action similar to that of the thiazide diuretics. In addition, it does not produce hyperuricemia and hyperglycemia and may be a suitable substitute for thiazides in patients in whom these metabolic disturbances are detrimental.

Spironolactone has a relatively slow onset of action and must be continued for at least 3 days for maximum effect. The only adverse effects noted thus far have been occasional reports of drowsiness, mental confusion, skin rash, and rarely the occurrence of gynecomastia.[163] In addition, hyperkalemia may be produced in patients with renal disease.

TRIAMTERENE (DYRENIUM)[163a,163b]

Triamterene is a new pteridine diuretic agent which primarily acts on the distal tubule and appears to be similar to spironolactone in its pharmacologic actions and clinical efficacy. Although triamterene resembles spironolactone in tending to promote potassium retention, the actions of triamterene are not entirely the result of aldosterone antagonism, since a diuretic action is observed in the adrenalectomized animal. Diuresis may be observed with triamterene during the first day of therapy, but frequently maximum effects are not seen for several days. Reversible reductions of creatinine clearance and elevations of blood urea nitrogen have been reported during therapy with triamterene. Therefore, it is advisable to monitor blood urea nitrogen in addition to serum potassium levels of patients receiving this new diuretic. Side effects in some patients have included nausea and vomiting, diarrhea, headache, and weakness. Triamterene has not been reported to elevate serum uric acid or blood glucose levels. Contraindications are severe kidney and hepatic disease.

ETHACRYNIC ACID (EDECRIN)[163c,163d,163e] and FUROSEMIDE (LASIX)[163f,163g,163h]

Ethacrynic acid and furosemide are extremely potent oral diuretics with markedly different chemical structures but with many similarities in pharmacologic action. Ethacrynic acid is a derivative of aryloxyacetic acid, and furosemide is a derivative of anthralinic acid. These agents have had extensive clinical trials and appear to be useful in patients with refractory edema. Their mode of action appears to be different from other diuretic agents, for, in addition to preventing sodium reabsorption at the proximal and possibly distal tubule, they also are considered to prevent sodium

reabsorption at the ascending limb of the loop of Henle. Dose response curves have indicated that maximal doses of these drugs produce greater natriuresis than that produced by maximal doses of thiazide diuretics. From the clinical viewpoint, patients who did not respond to thiazide or mercurial diuretics have responded to these agents; the reverse situation also has occurred. Because of the potency of these agents, hypokalemia and hypochloremic metabolic alkalosis may occur unless adequate potassium and chloride are administered. The occurrence of electrolyte imbalance and severe plasma volume depletion is particularly prone to occur with these drugs since their diuretic action is not limited by alkalosis. Electrolyte imbalance may be minimized by using an intermittent dosage schedule and by concurrent administration of spironolactone. The onset of action of these diuretics is rapid. Accordingly, their intravenous use has been advocated for the treatment of pulmonary edema. The diuretic action of ethacrynic acid and furosemide following oral administration becomes apparent in about 1 hr and lasts from about 4 to 8 hr. Both of these agents have been shown to increase serum uric acid levels, but, as yet, there have not been reports of elevations of blood glucose.

QUINIDINE

The systematic use of cinchona alkaloids for the treatment of cardiac arrhythmias was begun in 1912 by Wenckebach.[164] In 1918 after testing a number of cinchona alkaloids, Frey[165] considered quinidine, the dextrorotary isomer of quinine, the most effective antiarrhythmic agent.

Cardiac Actions[24,117,122,166–168]

1. Quinidine increases the effective refractory period of atrial and ventricular muscle in doses which have little effect upon the refractory period of normal, pacemaker tissue. The total refractory period is not prolonged.

2. Quinidine decreases the excitability of the myocardium. Excitability is defined as the ability of the ventricle to respond to a stimulus.

3. Quinidine decreases conduction in cardiac muscle, Purkinje fibers, and A-V conduction tissue.

4. Quinidine decreases the automaticity of myocardial tissue, which is defined as the property of automatic rhythmic activity of the tissue, independent of innervation.

5. Quinidine depresses myocardial contractility. This effect can be demonstrated both in isolated cardiac tissue[169] and in the intact dog heart.[120,170]

Extracardiac Actions

1. Quinidine decreases vagal activity and the effects of administered acetylcholine.[171] This effect

is similar to that produced by atropine but is less pronounced. This action of quinidine results in decreased effective refractory period of atrial tissue and increased conduction through the A-V node, actions which are opposite to the direct myocardial effects of the drug. Because of the increased conduction through the A-V node, rapid ventricular response may occur during conversion of atrial fibrillation, particularly if atrial flutter intervenes. The atropine-like effect must also be taken into account in the treatment of paroxysmal atrial tachycardia, for if vagal stimulating procedures are to be tried for treatment of this arrhythmia, they should be used before administration of quinidine. The sinus tachycardia which sometimes occurs with quinidine treatment is said to be partly related to reduction of vagal activity. However, it is possible that a more complex mechanism is involved.[172]

2. Quinidine is a potent vasodilator and can produce pronounced hypotension, particularly after large oral doses or parenteral administration.[117] Ferrer and associates[173] have demonstrated that the decrease in blood pressure resulting from a single oral administration of 0.8 Gm quinidine in most cases is related to decreased peripheral resistance rather than to depression of myocardial contractility.

Basis of the Antiarrhythmic Action

Although the depression of excitability, increased refractory period, and decreased conduction produced by quinidine have been used to explain the basis for the effectiveness of quinidine as an antiarrhythmic and antifibrillary agent, such explanations are probably oversimplifications. It is easy to illustrate the possible conversion of a circus movement, or reentry, to normal sinus rhythm by prolongation of the refractory period or to explain that excitability depresses spontaneous firing, but both the origin of the arrhythmias and the action of quinidine are undoubtedly more complicated.[174]

In analyzing the data available concerning the fundamental mechanism of the action of quinidine, the problem again arises as to which studies were carried out with *toxic* concentrations and prolonged periods of contact of quinidine and which could be more reasonably considered as resulting from *therapeutic* concentration of quinidine.

With respect to ionic changes, the administration of relatively large doses of quinidine to experimental animals has been found to increase potassium content of myocardial cells.[175] Studies by Holland and associates[169,176] have demonstrated that a depression in potassium efflux occurs in isolated rabbit atriums which are bathed in relatively high concentrations of quinidine. These investigators considered that this effect may be related to a block of acetylcholine. Weidmann[177]

observed that concentrations of quinidine which were close to those producing conduction block markedly altered the slope and appearance of the intracellularly recorded action potential of sheep or calf Purkinje fibers. He considered that this effect was similar to that produced by local anesthetics and postulated that these changes were the result of a disturbance in transfer of sodium ions to the muscle fiber through the cell membrane during the period of repolarization (based on the Hodgkin-Huxley concept). Johnson and McKinnon[178] in studies of guinea pig atrial tissue concluded that such an explanation did not explain their experimental findings. Vaughan-Williams[179] demonstrated in studies of isolated rabbit atriums bathed in concentrations of quinidine of less than 10 μg per liter that there was great slowing of the rate of rise of the action potential without change of the resting potential. He further observed that there was a decrease in rate of depolarization but that the 50 per cent time of the duration of the action potential was unaffected. He considered that these effects of quinidine accounted for both the prolonged effective refractory period and the decreased excitability. Since the duration of the action potential was not affected, the total refractory period would not be expected to be altered. Hoffmann[180] studied dog Purkinje fibers bathed in concentrations of quinidine of 3 to 6 μg per liter and was unable to find any effect of quinidine on the form of the action potential except for a decrease in the rate of depolarization.

Electrocardiographic Effects

In small doses quinidine may have no effect or may produce nonspecific T-wave alterations. With larger doses, decreased conduction is apparent by both prolongation of the P-R interval and the duration of the QRS complex. From a clinical standpoint, Gold[117] has suggested that in order to avoid severe toxicity, quinidine administration should be discontinued when the QRS complex increases by 50 per cent in patients with normal conduction and 25 per cent in patients with bundle branch block. Despite the antiarrhythmic action of quinidine, ventricular premature contractions, ventricular tachycardia, and ventricular fibrillation may occur. The occurrence of these adverse effects by antiarrhythmic agents has been explained by the interplay of actions of quinidine on refractory period, conduction, and excitability.[24,167,230]

Methods of Administration
and Serum Concentrations[181,182]

It is possible to follow serum concentrations of quinidine by simple chemical procedures.[183] Quinidine is rapidly absorbed orally and in about 15 min can be detected in the serum. In most cases maximum serum levels are reached in from 2 to 4 hr after administration of a single dose. The disappearance of quinidine from the serum follows an exponential decay curve,[184] so that 60 per cent of the initial value remains after 6 hr and 25 per cent after 12 hr. Serum levels increase progressively with each 2-hr dose up to a maximum of five or six doses. After this, no further rise in serum concentration occurs unless the dose is increased. Sokolow[185] found that toxicity never occurred with quinidine serum concentrations below 3 μg per ml and was only 1.6 per cent below 6 μg per ml. At concentrations between 6 and 8 μg per ml toxicity was 12 per cent and with levels over 14 μg per ml the toxicity was 65 per cent. These studies also indicated that marked differences occurred in the serum concentration of quinidine with the same dose administered to different patients. Although serum concentrations correlated well with toxicity, there was frequently little relationship between reversion of arrhythmias and serum concentration.

The dose of quinidine must be individualized and is usually administered at 2 to 4 hr intervals for conversion of atrial fibrillation. Several regimens have been developed which involve periodic increases in quinidine dose until either conversion takes place or signs of toxicity appear.[181,182,185–187] The usual starting dose is 0.2 Gm, although some clinicians give even smaller doses to check for idiosyncrasy or hypersensitivity.

Quinidine may also be administered parenterally in the form of gluconate or lactate. Administration by intramuscular or intravenous routes, however, are considerably more toxic than oral administration and should be avoided if possible. Severe hypotension and shock are more common with intravenous administration, and this route should be reserved for extreme emergencies.

Toxicity[117,122,182]

Cardiovascular Toxicity

Development of S-A or A-V block and serious ventricular arrhythmias may occur. These are considered as extensions of the basic myocardial actions of the drug and usually are seen only with large doses or in patients with severe myocardial damage. These adverse effects can usually be avoided by frequent observation of the electrocardiogram during quinidine administration. Marked hypotension also occurs in some patients.

Idiosyncrasy and Hypersensitivity

Small doses of quinidine may result in severe hypotension, respiratory depression, convulsions, and even death in certain individuals. Thrombo-

cytopenic purpura is not rare, and it appears to be more predominant in elderly females.[188] Bolton found[189] a platelet-quinidine-antibody complex in the gamma-globulin fraction of the plasma which is able to cause platelet agglutination and, in the presence of complement, to destroy both normal platelets and platelets from the patient. Fever may occur as an early or late manifestation of quinidine therapy.

Cinchonism

Cinchonism is a term used for certain adverse effects of cinchona alkaloids and salicylates. The symptoms include anorexia, nausea, vomiting, mild diarrhea, vertigo, tinnitus, headache, and visual disturbance.

Indications

Quinidine is considered to be the most useful drug for the conversion of atrial fibrillation or flutter. Quinidine is also effective in ventricular premature contractions, ventricular tachycardia, and paroxysmal atrial tachycardia. However, other drugs are often used before quinidine in these arrhythmias. This subject is treated elsewhere in this text in greater detail.

Contraindications

The only absolute contraindications to administration of quinidine are idiosyncrasy and hypersensitivity. Relative contraindications include conduction defects and conditions in which conversion of atrial fibrillation to normal sinus rhythm may result in embolism. The administration of quinidine and other antiarrhythmic agents in complete heart block may decrease the automaticity of the ventricular pacemaker and, therefore, should be administered with caution in this condition.

PROCAINE AMIDE

In 1946 Mautz[190] demonstrated that the local anesthetic procaine possessed antiarrhythmic activity. Procaine, however, is rapidly hydrolyzed and thus has a short duration of action and is not orally absorbed. It also has an undesirable central nervous system action. By addition of the amide group as in procaine amide, the antiarrhythmic activity is preserved, and the agent is resistant to hydrolysis and has less central nervous system action.[191] The cardiovascular actions of procaine amide are similar to those of quinidine.[24,117,166,170,192]

Procaine amide may be administered orally, intramuscularly, or intravenously. It is rapidly absorbed from the gastrointestinal tract, and the peak level of the drug is achieved in about 2 hr after oral administration. With intramuscular administration the maximal plasma levels are reached in ½ to 1 hr.[192]

The principal indication for procaine amide is in the treatment of ventricular tachycardia, particularly when intravenous medication is required, since procaine amide appears to be safer and more effective than intravenously administered quinidine. Procaine amide is not considered as effective as quinidine for the treatment of auricular fibrillation. It may be used, however, for this purpose in combination with quinidine[193] in resistant patients and as a substitute for quinidine in patients who have idiosyncrasy or hypersensitivity to quinidine.

The myocardial toxicity of procaine amide is similar to that produced by quinidine. Other side effects and symptoms of toxicity are anorexia, nausea, vomiting, chills, fever, and drug rashes. The development of agranulocytosis has been observed in a few patients. Intravenously, procaine amide may cause hypotension, and this effect appears to be related to rate of infusion. In order to avoid hypotension Kayden[192] suggests that procaine amide be given intravenously at a rate of about 50 to 75 mg per min and that the rate should not exceed 100 to 125 mg per min.

ATROPINE [117,194]

Atropine and other cholinergic blocking agents are used in the treatment of certain arrhythmias and conduction defects because of their ability to block the cardiac actions of the vagus nerve. Because of this vagus-blocking action, atropine increases the rate of the S-A node and the speed of conduction through the A-V node. Accordingly it has some application in treatment of severe sinus bradycardia and partial A-V block when these effects are due to increased vagal actions. Although atropine may also have direct antiarrhythmic effects,[166] it is important to separate such an action from reduction in ectopic activity, which results from increase in rate of the normal pacemaker. Another use for atropine is in combination with morphine to decrease the gastrointestinal effects and to reduce the potential danger of vagal stimulation produced by the narcotic. Atropine has limited clinical application in the cardiovascular system, because in the doses required to block vagal action to the heart, other effects of cholinergic block may be intolerable. These include dryness of mouth and skin, dilatation of the pupil (danger—glaucoma!), and paralysis of accommodation. With large doses and in sensitive individuals marked central nervous system stimulation may occur with hallucinations and hyperpyrexia.

NITRITES AND OTHER DRUGS USED IN THE TREATMENT OF ANGINA PECTORIS

The critical evaluation of drugs for the treatment of angina pectoris is complicated by the fact that angina pectoris is a subjective symptom which is affected by many environmental conditions. Furthermore, the symptoms may be relieved with time, with either improvement or deterioration of the state of the coronary vessels. Many drugs have been introduced for the treatment of angina pectoris, but few have passed tests of prolonged clinical acceptance and rigorous, controlled clinical trials.[195-197]

The nitrites (and organic nitrates) were introduced for the therapy of angina pectoris about a hundred years ago.[198] These agents, especially glyceryl trinitrate (nitroglycerin) have achieved the most prolonged and universal acceptance.

Cardiovascular Action[117,199-201]

The principal pharmacologic effect of nitrites is a direct action to relax smooth muscle, including that in vascular walls. Accordingly, administration of nitrites has been shown experimentally to produce dilatation of arteries, veins, and capillaries. Wilkins and his associates[201] have suggested that the nitrites do not act with equal intensity on all blood vessels and have postulated that the predominant action of the nitrates is on postarteriolar vessels. Vasodilation of coronary arteries by nitrites has been demonstrated repeatedly on hearts of many experimental species[117,199,200] and in the human being by means of coronary arteriography.[202]

Nitrites have no direct effect on myocardial contractility or heart rate. Blood pressure usually decreases when large doses of nitrites are given, particularly when the subject is in an erect position. The reduction in blood pressure results from both decreased venous return and cardiac output and from arteriolar dilatation. Because of the direct effect of the nitrites to dilate blood vessels and thus lower blood pressure, there may be pronounced reflex increases in sympathetic activity in the heart and in peripheral vessels.[120,203]

Basis for the Relief of Angina Produced by Nitrites

Several hypotheses have been advanced to explain the relief of angina pectoris produced by nitrites. Probably the most widely held concept is that nitrites relieve angina by increasing coronary flow and thereby improving the oxygenation of the ischemic myocardium. Gorlin and associates,[204,205] however, observed increments in coronary flow in normal subjects by use of the nitrous oxide method but did not find a reduction in the coronary arteriovenous oxygen differences when coronary venous samples were obtained from the coronary sinus. Of even more importance, these investigators could find no narrowing of the arteriovenous difference in patients with coronary heart disease or myocardial hypertrophy and observed a reduction in coronary flow. Despite this evidence it is possible that localized spasm of coronary arteries may be relaxed by nitrites without appreciably altering the content of oxygen in coronary sinus blood and without affecting measurements of coronary flow by the nitrous oxide method.

A second major concept is that the nitrites improve the oxygenation of the myocardium because of their peripheral vascular actions.[206] Dilatation of veins with pooling of blood in the venous system would produce a reduction in heart size and decrease the diastolic filling pressures of the ventricles, thus reducing oxygen consumption of the myocardium. Peripheral arteriolar dilatation would also reduce ventricular work and oxygen consumption. The relationships of alterations of pressure-work of the myocardium, myocardial tension, and heart size to myocardial oxygen consumption have been demonstrated by a number of experimental techniques.[207–209] It has been suggested that the vasodilating properties of nitrites reduce the oxygen-wasting effects of sympathetic stimulation and catecholamine release.[210] A third hypothesis for the beneficial action of the nitrites is that they improve cardiac oxygenation by alteration of myocardial metabolism.[211–213]

In addition to the relief of angina pectoris, the use of nitrites has been promoted for the stimulation of a development of collateral coronary vessels. Zoll and Norman in 1952 [214] demonstrated that prolonged administration of large doses of nitrites stimulated intraarterial anastomoses in the myocardium of young pigs. More recently Lumb and Hardy,[215] also using pigs, have demonstrated increased collateral vessels after administration of pentaerythritol tetranitrate (Peritrate tetranitrate). It is not known whether such changes take place in patients with coronary heart disease with clinically recommended doses of either nitroglyecrin or long-acting nitrates.

Side Effects[117]

The most common side effect produced by nitrites is the induction of headache. Headache is seen with all actively absorbed nitrites. The mechanism for production of the headache is presumed to be dilatation of the cerebral vessels. Tolerance to the headache develops in most patients, and after repeated use the symptom is less troublesome. The development of tolerance to the vascular action of the nitrites brings up the question as to whether patients no longer attaining relief from nitrites have

not developed tolerance to their beneficial action. The hypotensive effect of even small doses of the nitrites is marked in some individuals and prevents their use. Methemoglobinemia may be produced by large doses of nitrites, but this effect is seen rarely in the use of the compound for the treatment of angina pectoris. Finally, the nitrites increase intraocular pressure and may precipitate glaucoma in susceptible individuals.

Preparations and Modes of Administration

Glyceryl trinitrate may be administered sublingually or by application to the skin in the form of an ointment. This agent is ineffective when administered orally. Volatile nitrites such as amyl nitrite may be administered by inhalation. Numerous organic nitrates are promoted for a sustained action after oral administration. The usefulness of these latter agents for the prophylaxis of angina pectoris is debatable.[197]

Other Agents

A number of other agents have been introduced for the treatment of angina pectoris on the basis of the production of coronary vasodilation in the experimental animal. Aminophylline and khellin, which were once used with great enthusiasm, have not passed the test of prolonged clinical trials. More recently another nonnitrite coronary vasodilator, dipyridamole (Persantin), has been introduced for the treatment of angina pectoris. As with the older agents, a number of uncontrolled studies have resulted in enthusiastic claims of therapeutic success.[216] Also as with older agents, negative results have also been published.[217]

Antihypertensive agents have frequently relieved the symptoms of angina pectoris in patients with hypertension.[218–220] It appears reasonable to assume that judicious use of these compounds can decrease oxygen utilization of the myocardium and thereby result in relief of angina pectoris. On the other hand, pronounced reduction in arterial pressure may result in decreased coronary flow and possibly myocardial infarction. It is also possible that agents which block the sympathetic nervous system may reduce exaggerated cardiovascular responses to exercise, emotion, or ingestion of food and thereby relieve angina pectoris. Such a hypothesis has been evoked to explain the beneficial effects of monoamine oxidase inhibitors in some patients with angina pectoris.[221]

Finally, because of the emotional aspects of angina pectoris, the beneficial use of sedatives must be considered. The treatment of angina pectoris is outlined in greater detail in Chap. 35.

SYMPATHOMIMETIC AMINES

Hundreds of sympathomimetic amines have been synthesized, and an extremely large literature concerning their pharmacologic actions is available.[122,222-224] This presentation is limited to a brief survey of certain of their cardiovascular actions and clinical indications.

Cardiac Actions[61,62,225-228]

Most sympathomimetic amines exert a direct effect on myocardial cells to increase myocardial contractility. The amines vary greatly, however, in the magnitude and duration of their actions on the heart. Table 68-2 lists several commonly used sympathomimetic amines and indicates their effects on myocardial contractility and arterial blood pressure. Norepinephrine (Levophed), epinephrine (Adrenalin), and isoproterenol hydrochloride (Isuprel hydrochloride) produce pronounced increments in myocardial contractility but have a short duration of action. Metaraminol (Aramine), mephentermine (Wyamine), methamphetamine hydrochloride (Methedrine), and ephedrine have more prolonged positive inotropic effects. Methoxamine hydrochloride (Vasoxyl hydrocholride), on the other hand, has virtually no cardiac actions, and phenylephrine hydrochloride (Neo-Synephrine hydrochloride) exerts only a relatively slight effect on the heart. The differences in the actions of these amines have been

Table 68-2. EFFECTS OF SEVERAL SYMPATHOMIMETIC AMINES ON CARDIAC CONTRACTILE FORCE AND BLOOD PRESSURE

Compound	Effect* on cardiac contractile force	Effect on blood pressure
Norepinephrine (Levophed)	↑	↑
Epinephrine (Adrenalin)— large doses	↑	↑
Metaraminol (Aramine)	↑	↑
Mephentermine (Wyamine)	↑	↑
Ephedrine	↑	↑
Methamphetamine hydrochloride (Methedrine)	↑	↑
Epinephrine—small doses	↑	↓
Isoproterenol hydrochloride (Isuprel hydrochloride)	↑	↓
Methoxamine hydrochloride (Vasoxyl hydrochloride)	0	↑
Phenylephrine hydrochloride (Neo-Synephrine hydrochloride)	±	↑

* ↑ = increase; ↓ = decrease.

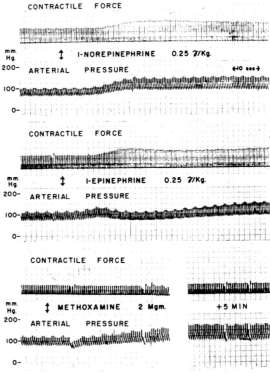

Fig. 68-7. The effects of 0.25 μg per kg norepinephrine and epinephrine and of 2 mg (34 μg per kg) methoxamine on right ventricular contractile force and arterial pressure in a thirty-nine-year-old patient with pulmonary stenosis (*From L. I. Goldberg, R. D. Bloodwell, E. Braunwald, and A. G. Morrow: The Direct Effects of Norepinephrine, Epinephrine, and Methoxamine on Myocardial Contractile Force in Man, Circulation, 22: 1125, fig. 2, 1960. By permission of the American Heart Association, Inc.*)

demonstrated in the isolated and intact animal heart and directly in the human heart by means of a strain-gauge arch sutured to the ventricle prior to cardiac surgical treatment (Fig. 68-7).[229]

Sympathomimetic amines which increase contractility also directly increase the rate of the heart by stimulation of the S-A node, increase conduction through the A-V node, and increase ectopic activity.[24,230] The increase in ectopic activity is particularly evident in the presence of cyclopropane anesthesia and hypoxia.

Peripheral Vascular Effects[225,226]

Sympathomimetic amines may either constrict or dilate blood vessels. All the amines in Table 68-2 constrict arterioles in certain dose levels with the exception of isoproterenol hydrochloride, which has only vasodilating actions. The amines differ considerably in their effects on various vascular beds, and certain amines will constrict one vascular bed and dilate another (alpha and beta action; see Alpha and Beta Receptors, below). As an example of such dual action, intraarterial infusions of certain doses of epinephrine constrict skin and renal arterioles but will dilate the blood vessels to skeletal muscles. Norepinephrine, on the other hand, does not dilate peripheral arterioles in any dose and increases total peripheral resistance. The effects of sympathomimetic amines on coronary arteries are much more difficult to evaluate and depend upon many factors such as myocardial contractility, heart rate, and systemic pressure, in addition to direct action on the vessels.

Cardiac Output[225,226]

As with cardiac glycosides, cardiac output measurements have led to erroneous conclusions concerning the myocardial effects of sympathomimetic amines in man. Consideration of the actions of the amines illustrated in Fig. 68-7 may clarify the confusion concerning the action of these drugs.[229] Epinephrine usually increases cardiac output, whereas norepinephrine and methoxamine either decrease or do not change this function. Therefore, it has been concluded that norepinephrine and methoxamine were similar amines with "pure pressor" actions. Epinephrine, on the other hand, was considered to be a myocardial stimulant. Yet when myocardial contractility is measured directly, it is apparent that different effects on cardiac output produced by epinephrine and norepinephrine are not caused by any dissimilarity in their action on myocardial contractility but are the result of differing effects on the peripheral vascular bed. Differences in cardiac output may be explained as follows: Norepinephrine increases cardiac contractility but at the same time increases peripheral resistance, which by stimulation of baroreceptors tends to result in bradycardia and diminished cardiac output despite the increased contractility. Epinephrine, on the other hand, usually decreases peripheral resistance, and under these circumstances the increased heart rate and myocardial contractility are unopposed, and cardiac output increases. Methoxamine has no cardiac action and raises blood pressure by increasing peripheral resistance. Therefore, although norepinephrine and methoxamine both decrease cardiac output, their actions on the heart are not similar.

Since cardiac output is the resultant of several cardiovascular functions, an amine may have different effects on cardiac output under different experimental or clinical conditions.[231–233] Furthermore, as Li and associates have demonstrated with mephentermine, an amine may exert different effects on cardiac output at different times after ad-

ministration, depending upon the preponderance of the cardiac or peripheral effects.[234]

Alpha and Beta Receptors—Adrenergic Blocking Agents

The ability of sympathomimetic amines to produce excitatory and inhibitory effects in various organ systems suggested to Ahlquist[235] that the actions of sympathomimetic amines could be classified into two types—alpha and beta. According to this classification, blood vessel constriction produced by sympathomimetic amines is the result of action of the amines on alpha receptors; vasodilation and cardiac stimulation are produced by action on beta receptors. Accordingly, methoxamine exerts only an alpha action, isoproterenol only a beta action, and the other amines in Table 68-2 would have mixtures of both actions. This hypothesis has received confirmation by the discovery of specific adrenergic receptor-blocking agents. Phentolamine (Regitine) and phenoxybenzamine hydrochloride (Dibenzyline) block only alpha effects of sympathomimetic amines;[236,237] dichloroisoproterenol (DCI) and nethalide (Alderlin) block only beta effects.[57,238–240]

Phenoxybenzamine is being extensively studied for possible application in the treatment of noncardiac shock,[240a] and the beta-adrenergic blocking agents are being studied for possible application in the treatment of cardiac arrhythmias and angina pectoris. It should be emphasized that the beta-adrenergic blocking agents have other pharmacologic actions in addition to their adrenergic blocking actions, and clinical efficacy may not be related to blockade of beta-receptors.[240b]

Direct and Indirect Actions of Sympathomimetic Amines

In 1958 Burn and Rand[241] demonstrated that sympathomimetic amines may also differ in their effects after administration of reserpine, which in large doses causes depletion of catecholamine stores. It was found that the actions of sympathomimetic amines such as tyramine and mephentermine were partially or totally blocked by prior administration of large doses of reserpine, whereas the effects of norepinephrine were augmented. Therefore, it was postulated that tyramine and mephentermine act indirectly by releasing norepinephrine. Subsequent investigations have classified amines according to whether they have direct or indirect actions or possess a mixture of both effects.[242]

Although most investigations have been carried out in animals and with massive doses of reserpine, there is also evidence that amine action in man can be altered by administration of reserpine[243,244] and other catecholamine depleting agents such as guanethidine (Ismelin).[245] Therefore, it would seem to be inadvisable to depend upon the action of an indirectly acting amine in a patient who had received reserpine or guanethidine for a long period. On the other hand, Burn and Rand [246] have suggested that the hypotension which may occur following withdrawal of prolonged norepinephrine therapy may be reversed by administration of an "indirectly acting" amine.

Indications

Shock

Proper treatment of hypotensive states is complicated by differing causes and lack of precise physiologic data in the individual patient. For want of more specific therapy, sympathomimetic amines are often used to increase blood pressure with the hope of thereby also increasing perfusion pressure to vital organs. In some cases such therapy appears to be lifesaving. However, it is important to remember that blood flow is determined by the ratio pressure/resistance, and a drug which increases pressure by increasing arteriolar resistance may decrease the flow of blood to an organ. Since all commonly used sympathomimetic amines increase arteriolar resistance, it is necessary constantly to evaluate the clinical state of the patient even though the blood pressure has been increased.

The choice of a sympathomimetic amine depends upon the condition for which it is used. Most clinical studies have indicated that sympathomimetic amines with cardiac stimulating and peripheral vasoconstricting properties are more effective than those with vasoconstrictor actions alone. This appears to be particularly true in shock accompanying myocardial infarction.[225,226,247,248] On the other hand, there may be patients in whom cardiac stimulation is not desired and a pure vasoconstrictor agent would be more suitable.[249]

Heart Block[250–253]

Sympathomimetic amines with cardiac stimulating actions are used to increase the rate of nodal and ventricular pacemakers in heart block. Frequently used agents are isoproterenol hydrochloride, epinephrine, and ephedrine.

Paroxysmal Atrial Tachycardia[223,253]

Sympathomimetic amines are sometimes used to treat resistant cases of paroxysmal atrial tachycardia by elevating the blood pressure and thereby stimulating vagal inhibitory reflexes. The amines without cardiac stimulating effects, phenylephrine and methoxamine, would appear to be most suitable for this purpose.

Congestive Heart Failure

Although sympathomimetic amines can increase myocardial contractility as much as, or more than, digitalis, they have been used previously only for treatment of acute cardiac failure. Studies with dopamine, a naturally occurring catecholamine, have demonstrated that it is possible to increase sodium excretion of patients with congestive heart failure with a sympathomimetic amine.[254,255] Therefore, it may be possible eventually to develop amines useful in the treatment of chronic congestive heart failure.

Adverse Effects[225,226]

Adverse effects of sympathomimetic amines usually can be related to extensions of their basic pharmacologic actions. Ischemic necrosis with sloughing of tissues has occurred following extravasation of norepinephrine and metaraminol. This effect can be minimized by administering the agents through polyethylene catheters inserted well into the vein and by local administration of phenotolamine if extravasation does occur. Cardiac arrhythmias may be produced both by direct cardiac actions of sympathomimetic amines and by increased peripheral resistance. Ischemic damage to the heart, liver, kidney, and other organs have been blamed on the action of sympathomimetic amines. Although it is theoretically possible that such changes can be produced by large doses of any vasoconstrictor agent, it is difficult to evaluate the role of sympathomimetic amines in the production of many of these lesions, since the patients were usually moribund prior to the administration of the amine and such changes could be related to the hypotensive state.

Finally, it should be mentioned that prolonged infusions of sympathomimetic amines, primarily norepinephrine, may result in a resistant state which requires ever-increasing amounts of the amine to maintain the blood pressure. Several reasons have been advanced to explain this phenomenon, but none is entirely satisfactory.[226]

REFERENCES

1. Withering, W.: "An Account of the Foxglove and Some of Its Medical Uses: With Practical Remarks on Dropsy and Other Diseases, in F. A. Willius and T. E. Keys (eds.), "Cardiac Classics," The C. V. Mosby Company, St. Louis, 1941, p. 232.
2. Walton, R. P.: "The Cardiac Glycosides, in V. A. Drill (ed.), "Pharmacology in Medicine," 2d ed., McGraw-Hill Book Company, New York, 1958, p. 451.

3. Movitt, E. R.: "Digitalis and Other Cardiotonic Drugs," 2d ed., Oxford University Press, Fair Lawn N.J., 1949.

4. Friend, D. G.: Cardiac Glycosides, *New England J. Med.*, **266**:88, 187, 300, 402, 1962.

5. Lown, B., and Levine, S. A.: "Current Concepts in Digitalis Therapy," Little Brown and Company, Boston, 1954.

6. Modell, W. Clinical Pharmacology of Digitalis Materials, *Clin. Pharmacol. & Therap.*, **2**:177, 1961.

7. Kay, C. F.: The Clinical Use of Digitalis Preparations, *Circulation*, **12**:116, 1955.

7a. Braunwald, E., Mason, D. T., and Ross, J., Jr.: Studies of the Cardio-circulatory Actions of Digitalis, *Medicine*, **44**:233, 1965.

8. Hoch, J. H.: "A Survey of Cardiac Glycosides and Genins," The University of South Carolina Press, Columbia, S.C., 1961.

9. Tamm, C.: The Stereochemistry of the Glycosides in Relation to Biological Activity, in "New Aspects of Cardiac Glycosides: Proceedings of the 1st International Pharmacological Meeting," Pergamon Press, New York, 1963, vol. 3, p. 11.

10. Cattell, M., and Gold, H.: Influence of Digitalis Glucosides on the Force of Contraction of Mammalian Cardiac Muscle, *J. Pharmacol. & Exper. Therap.*, **62**:116, 1938.

11. Sanyal, P. N., and Saunders, P. R.: Action of Quabain upon Normal and Hypodynamic Myocardium, *Proc. Soc. Exper. Biol. & Med.*, **95**:156, 1957.

12. Stewart, G. A.: The Actions of Digitalis Leaf Preparations and of Cardiac Glycosides on the Isolated Right Ventricle of the Guinea Pig, *J. Pharm. & Pharmacol.*, **10**:741, 1958.

13. Walton, R. P., Leary, J. S., and Jones, H. P.: Comparative Increase in Ventricular Contractile Force Produced by Several Cardiac Glycosides, *J. Pharmacol & Exp. Therap.*, **98**:346, 1950.

14. Cotten, M. deV., and Stopp, P. E.: Action of Digitalis on the Nonfailing Heart of the Dog, *Am. J. Physiol.*, **192**:114, 1958.

15. Braunwald, E., Bloodwell, R. D., Goldberg, L. I., and Morrow, A. G.: Studies on Digitalis. IV. Observations in Man on the Effects of Digitalis Preparations on the Contractility of the Non-failing Heart and on Total Vascular Resistance, *J. Clin. Invest.*, **40**:52, 1961.

16. Eddleman, E. E., Jr., Willis, K., Greve, M. J., and Heyer, H. E.: The Effect of Digitoxin on the Apparent Stroke Volume, Posterio-anterior Cardiac Diameter, and the Cardiac Cycle in Normal Subjects as Studied by the Electrokymograph, *Am. Heart J.*, **41**:161, 1951.

17. Mason, D., and Braunwald, E.: Studies on Digitalis. IX. Effects of Ouabain on the Nonfailing Human Heart, *J. Clin. Invest.*, **42**:1105, 1963.

18. Méndez, R., and Méndez, C.: The Action of Cardiac Glycosides on the Refractory Period of Heart Tissues, *J. Pharmacol. & Exper. Therap.*, **107**:24, 1953.

19. Moe, G. K., and Méndez, R.: The Action of Several Cardiac Glycosides on Conduction Velocity and Ventricular Excitability in the Dog Heart, *Circulation*, **4**:729, 1951.

20. Méndez, C., Aceves, J., and Méndez, R.: The Antiadrenergic Action of Digitalis on the Refractory Period of the A-V Transmission System, *J. Pharmacol. & Exper. Therap.*, **131**:199, 1961.

21. Morrow, D. H., Gaffney, T. E., and Braunwald, E.: Studies on Digitalis. VIII. Effect of Autonomic Innervation and of Myocardial Catecholamine Stores upon the Cardiac Action of Ouabain, *J. Pharmacol. & Exper. Therap.*, **140**:236, 1963.

22. Méndez, C., and Méndez, R.: The Action of Cardiac Glycosides on the Excitability and Conduction Velocity of the Mammalian Atrium, *J. Pharmacol. & Exper. Therap.*, **121**:402, 1957.

23. Swain, H. H., and Weidner, C. L.: A Study of Substances Which Alter Intraventricular Conduction in Isolated Dog Heart, *J. Pharmacol. & Exper. Therap.*, **120**:137, 1957.

24. Brooks, C. McC., Hoffman, B. F., Suckling, E. E., and Oriás, O.: "Excitability of the Heart," Grune & Stratton, Inc., New York, 1955, p. 273.

25. Moran, N. C.: Contraction-dependency of the Myocardial Binding and Positive Inotropic Action of Cardiac Glycosides, in New Aspects of Cardiac Glycosides: Proceedings 1st International Pharmacological Meeting, Pergamon Press, New York, 1963, vol. 3, p. 251.

26. Furchgott, R. F., and Gubareff, T. de: The High Energy Phosphate Content of Cardiac Muscle under Various Experimental Conditions Which Alter Contractile Strength, *J. Pharmacol. & Exper. Therap.*, **124**:203, 1958.

27. Lee, K. S.: A New Technique for the Simultaneous Recording of Oxygen Consumption and Contraction of Muscle: The Effect of Ouabain on Cat Papillary Muscle, *J. Pharmacol. & Exp. Therap.*, **109**:304, 1953.

28. Lee, K. S., Yu, D. H., and Burstein, R.: The Effect of Ouabain on the Oxygen Consumption, the High Energy Phosphates and the Contractility of the Cat Papillary Muscle, *J. Pharmacol. & Exper. Therap.*, **129**:115, 1960.

29. Wollenberger, A.: The Energy Metabolism of the Failing Heart and the Metabolic Action of the Cardiac Glycosides, *Pharmacol. Rev.*, **1**:311, 1949.

30. Lee, K. S.: Relation of Cations to the Inotropic and Metabolic Actions of Cardiac Glycosides, in "New Aspects of Cardiac Glycosides," Proceedings 1st International Pharmacological Meeting," Pergamon Press, New York, 1963, vol. 3, p. 185.

31. Lee, K. S.: The Simultaneous Recording of Oxygen Uptake and Contraction of Papillary Muscle as Affected by *L*-epinephrine and *L*-norepinephrine, *J. Pharmacol. & Exper. Therap.*, **109**:313, 1953.

32. Bing, R. J., Maraist, F. M., Dammann, J. F., Jr., Draper, A., Jr., Heimbecker, R., Daley, R., Gerard, R., and Calazel, P.: Effect of Strophanthus on Coronary Blood Flow and Cardiac Oxygen Consumption of Normal and Failing Hearts, *Circulation*, 2:513, 1950.

33. Fawaz, G.: Cardiovascular Pharmacology, *Ann. Rev. Pharmacol.*, 3:57, 1963.

34. Sarnoff, S. J., Braunwald, E., Welch, G. H., Jr., Case, R. B., Stainsby, W. N., and Macruz, R.: Hemodynamic Determinants of Oxygen Consumption of the Heart with Special Reference to Tension-time Index, *Am. J. Physiol.*, 192:148, 1958.

35. Calhoun, J. A., and Harrison, T. R.: Studies in Congestive Heart Failure. IX. The Effect of Digitalis on the Potassium Content of the Cardiac Muscle of Dogs, *J. Clin. Invest.*, 10:139, 1931.

36. Conn, H. L., Jr.: Effects of Digitalis and Hypoxia on Potassium Transfer and Distribution in the Dog Heart, *Am. J. Physiol.*, 184:548, 1956.

37. Hajdu, S.: Mechanism of Staircase and Contracture in Ventricular Muscle, *Am. J. Physiol.*, 174:371, 1953.

38. Vick, R. L.: Effects of Some Steroid and Nonsteroid Lactones on Potassium Exchange and Physiological Properties of the Isolated Perfused Guinea Pig Ventricle, *J. Pharmacol, & Exper. Therap.*, 125:40, 1959.

39. Kahn, J. B., Jr.: Cardiac Glycosides and Ion Transport, in "New Aspects of Cardiac Glycosides: Proceedings of the 1st International Pharmacological Meeting," Pergamon Press, New York, 1963, vol. 3, p. 111.

40. Holland, W. C., and Sekul, A. A.: Effect of Ouabain on Ca^{45} and Cl^{36} Exchange in Isolated Rabbit Atria, *Am. J. Physiol.*, 197:757, 1959.

41. Holland, W. C., and Klein, R. L.: "Chemistry of Heart Failure," Charles C Thomas, Publisher, Springfield, Ill., 1960.

42. Gersmeyer, E. F., and Holland, W. C.: Effect of Heart Rate on Action of Ouabain on Ca Exchange in Guinea Pig Left Atria, *Am. J. Physiol.*, 205:795, 1963.

43. Farah, A., and Witt, P. N.: Cardiac Glycosides and Calcium, in "New Aspects of Cardiac Glycosides: Proceedings of the 1st International Pharmacological Meeting," Pergamon Press, New York, 1963, vol. 3, p. 137.

44. Kahn, J. B., Jr., and Acheson, G. H.: Effects of Cardiac Glycosides and Other Lactones, and of Certain Other Compounds, on Cation Transfer in Human Erythrocytes, *J. Pharmacol. & Exper. Therap.*, 115:305, 1955.

45. Orloff, J., and Berliner, R. W.: Renal Pharmacology, *Ann. Rev. Pharmacol.*, 1:307, 1961.

46. Durham, E. T., and Glynn, I. M.: Adenosinetriphosphatase Activity and the Active Movements of Alkali Metal Ions, *J. Physiol.*, 156:274, 1961.

47. Repke, K.: Metabolism of Cardiac Glycosides, in "New Aspects of Cardiac Glycosides: Proceedings

48. of the 1st International Pharmacological Meeting," Pergamon Press, New York, 1963, vol. 3, p. 47.

48. Woodbury, L. A., and Hecht, H. H.: Effects of Cardiac Glycosides upon the Electrical Activity of Single Ventricular Fibers of the Frog Heart, and Their Relation to the Digitalis Effect of the Electrocardiogram, *Circulation*, 6:172, 1952.

49. Stutz, H., Feigelson, E., Emerson, J., and Bing, R. J.: The Effect of Digitalis (Cedilanid) on the Mechanical and Electrical Activity of Extracted and Non-extracted Heart Muscle Preparations, *Circulation Res.*, 2:555, 1954.

50. Kassebaum, D. G.: Electrophysiological Effects of Strophanthin in the Heart, *J. Pharmacol. & Exper. Therap.*, 140:329, 1963.

51. Snellman, O., and Gelotte, B.: A Reaction between a Deaminase and Heart Actin, and Inhibition of the Effect with Cardiac Glycosides, *Nature*, London, 165:604, 1950.

52. Wollenberger, A.: Non-specificity of the Effect of Cardiac Glycosides on the Polymerization of Actin, *Experientia*, 10:311, 1954.

53. Robb, J. S., and Mallov, S.: Effect of Ouabain on Actomyosin Threads, *J. Pharmacol. & Exper. Therap.*, 108:251, 1953.

54. KaKo, K., and Bing, R. J.: Contractility of Actomyosin Bands Prepared from Normal and Failing Human Hearts, *J. Clin. Invest.*, 37:465, 1958.

55. Tanz, R. D.: The Release of Catecholamines Following Ouabain, *Pharmacologist*, 2:95, 1960.

56. Cairoli, V., Reilly, J., and Roberts, J.: The Effect of Reserpine Pretreatment on the Positive Inotropic Action of Ephedrine and Ouabain, *Fed. Proc.*, 20:122, 1961.

57. Moran, N. C., and Perkins, M. E.: Adrenergic Blockade of the Mammalian Heart by a Dichloro Analogue of Isoproterenol, *J. Pharmacol. & Exper. Therap.*, 124:223, 1958.

58. Yelnosky, J., and Ervin, R.: The Effect of Ouabain on Cardiac Automaticity in Reserpine-pretreated Dogs, *Am. Heart J.*, 62:687, 1961.

59. Wilbrandt, W. (ed.): "New Aspects of Cardiac Glycosides: Proceedings of the 1st International Pharmacological Meeting, Pergamon Press, New York, 1963, vol. 3.

60. Leonard, E., and Hajdu, S.: Action of Electrolytes and Drugs on the Contractile Mechanism of the Cardiac Muscle Cell, in "Handbook of Physiology," sec. 2, *Circulation*, 1:151, 1962.

61. Cotten, M. deV., and Moran, N. C.: Cardiovascular Pharmacology, *Ann. Rev. Pharmacol.*, 1:261, 1961.

62. Cotten, M. deV., and Moran, N. C.: The Effects of Drugs on Myocardial Contractility, in G. H. Bourne (ed.), "The Structure and Function of Muscle," Academic Press, Inc., New York, 1960, vol. 3, p. 482.

63. Eichna, L. W., Taube, H., and DeGraff, A. C.: Serial Determinations of Cardiac Output (Ballistocardiogram) and Electrocardiogram in Normal

Man after the Intravenous Administration of Puri-
fied Cardiac Glycosides, *J. Pharmacol. & Exper.
Therap.*, **78**:22, 1943.

64. Heymans, C., Bouckaert, J. J., and Regnier, P.:
Sur le mécanisme réflexe de la bradycardie pro-
voquée par les digitaliques, *Arch. int. pharmacodyn.*, **44**:31, 1932.

65. Greene, C. W., and Peeler, J. O.. The Central
Action of Digitalis as Tested by the Cardio-inhibi-
tory Center. *J. Pharmacol. & Exper. Therap.*, **7**:
591, 1915.

66. Gaffney, T. E., Kahn, J. B., Jr., Van Maanen, E. F.,
and Acheson, G. H.: A Mechanism of the Vagal
Effect of Cardiac Glycosides, *J. Pharmacol. &
Exper. Therap.*, **122**:423, 1958.

67. Ross, J., Jr., Waldhausen, J. A., and Braunwald,
E.: Studies on Digitalis. I. Direct Effects on Peripheral Vascular Resistance, *J. Clin. Invest.*, **39**:
930, 1960.

68. Williams, M. H., Jr., Zohman, L. R., and Ratner,
A. C.: Hemodynamic Effects of Cardiac Glycosides
on Normal Human Subjects during Rest and
Exercise, *J. Appl. Physiol.*, **13**:417, 1958.

69. Gracey, D. R., and Brandfonbrener, M.: The Effect of Lanatoside C on Coronary Vascular Resistance, *Am. Heart J.*, **66**:88, 1963.

70. Gold, H., Otto, H., Kwit, N. T., and Satchwell, H.:
Does Digitalis Influence the Course of Cardiac
Pain? A Study of 120 Selected Cases of Angina
Pectoris, *J.A.M.A.*, **110**:859, 1938.

71. Dock, W., and Tainter, M. L.: The Circulatory
Changes after Full Therapeutic Doses of Digitalis, with a Critical Discussion of Views on Cardiac Output, *J. Clin. Invest.*, **8**:467, 1930.

72. Tainter, M. L., and Dock, W.: Further Observations on the Circulatory Actions of Digitalis and
Strophanthus, with Special Reference to the Liver,
and Comparisons with Histamine and Epinephrine,
J. Clin. Invest., **8**:485, 1930.

73. Baschieri, L., Ricci, P. D., Mazzuoli, G. F., and
Vassalle, M.: Studi su la portata epatica nell'uomo:
Modificazioni del flusso epatico da digitale, *Cuore
è circolaz.*, **41**:103, 1957.

74. Nadler, J. E., Berger, A. R., and Ballinger, J.:
Action of Ouabain on the Splanchnic Circulation
in the Dog, *J. Lab. & Clin. Med.*, **25**:557, 1940.

75. Ross, J., Jr., Braunwald, E., and Waldhausen,
J. A.: Studies on Digitalis. II. Extracardiac Effects
on Venous Return and on the Capacity of the
Peripheral Vascular Bed, *J. Clin. Invest.*, **39**:937,
1960.

76. McMichael, J., and Sharpey-Schafer, E. P.: The
Action of Intravenous Digoxin in Man, *Quart. J.
Med.*, **37**:123, 1944.

77. McMichael, J.: "Pharmacology of the Failing Human Heart," Charles C Thomas, Publisher, Springfield, Ill., 1950.

78. Mason D. T., and Braunwald, E.: Studies on Digitalis. X. Effects of Ouabain on Forearm Vascular
Resistance and Venous Tone in Normal Subjects

and in Patients in Heart Failure, *J. Clin. Invest.*,
43:532, 1964.

79. Gold, H., Greiner, T., Cattell, M., Modell, W.,
Gluck, J., Marsh, R., Mathes, S., Hudson, D.,
Robertson, D., Warshaw, L., Otto, H., Kwit, N.,
and Kramer, M.: Difference in the Relation of
Cardiac to Emetic Actions in Oral and Parenteral
Digitalization, *Am. J. Med.*, **13**:124, 1952.

80. Borison, H. L., and Wang, S. C.: Physiology and
Pharmacology of Vomiting, *Pharmacol. Rev.*, **5**:
193, 1953.

81. Hyman, A. L., Jaques, W. E., and Hyman, E. S.:
Observation on the Direct Effect of Digoxin on
Renal Excretion of Sodium and Water, *Am. Heart
J.*, **52**:592, 1956.

82. Kellum, E. L.: The Diuretic Effect of Digitalis,
Am. Heart J., **7**:342, 1932.

83. Stewart, H. J., and Cohn, A. E.: Studies on the
Effect of the Action of Digitalis on the Output of
Blood from the Heart: III, part I. The Effect on
the Output in Normal Human Hearts; part II.
The Effect on the Output of the Hearts in Heart
Failure with Congestion in Human Beings, *J. Clin.
Invest.*, **11**:917, 1932.

84. Bloomfield, R. A., Rapoport, B., Milnor, J. P.,
Long, W. K., Mebane, J. G., and Ellis, L. B.: The
Effects of the Cardiac Glycosides upon the Dy-
namics of the Circulation in Congestive Heart
Failure, *J. Clin. Invest.*, **27**:588, 1948.

85. Stead, E. A., Jr., Warren, J. V., and Brannon,
E. S.: Effect of Lanatoside C on the Circulation of
Patients with Congestive Failure, *A.M.A. Arch.
Int. Med.*, **81**:282, 1948.

86. Harvey, R. M., Ferrer, M. I., Cathcart, R. T.,
Richards, D. W., Jr., and Cournand, A.: Some
Effects of Digoxin upon Heart and Circulation in
Man: Digoxin in Left Ventricular Failure, *Am. J.
Med.*, **7**:439, 1949.

87. Davis, J. O.: Mechanisms of Salt and Water Retention in Congestive Heart Failure: The Importance of Aldosterone, *Am. J. Med.*, **29**:486,
1960.

88. Merrill, A. J.: Edema and Decreased Renal Blood
Flow in Patients with Chronic Heart Failure: Evidence of "Forward Failure" as the Primary Cause
of Edema, *J. Clin. Invest.*, **25**:389, 1946.

89. Eichna, L. W., Farber, S. J., Berger, A. R., Earle,
D. P., Rader, B., Pellegrino, E., Albert, R. E.,
Alexander, J. D., Taube, H., and Youngwirth, S.:
Cardiovascular Dynamics, Blood Volumes, Renal
Functions, and Electrolyte Excretions in the Same
Patients during Congestive Heart Failure and after
Recovery of Cardiac Compensation, *Circulation*,
7:674, 1953.

90. Selzer, A., Hultgren, H. N., Ebnother, C. L.,
Bradley, H. W., and Stone, A. O.: Effect of Di-
goxin on the Circulation in Normal Man, *Brit.
Heart J.*, **21**:335, 1959.

91. Goodyer, A. V. N., Chetrick, A., and Huvos, A.:
The Effect of Lanatoside C on the Response of

the Human Cardiac Output to Walking Exercise, *Yale J. Biol. & Med.*, **32**:265, 1960.

92. Rodman, T., Gorczyca, C. A., and Pastor, B. H.: The Effect of Digitalis on the Cardiac Output of the Normal Heart at Rest and during Exercise, *Ann. Int. Med.*, **55**:620, 1961.

93. Schroder, G., Malmcrona, R., Varnauskas, E., and Werko, L.: Hemodynamics during Rest and Exercise before and after Prolonged Digitalization in Normal Subjects, *Clin. Pharm. & Therap.* **3**:425, 1962.

94. Russell, R. O., Jr., and Reeves T. J.: The Effect of Digoxin in Normal Man on the Cardiorespiratory Responses to Severe Effort, *Am. Heart J.*, **66**:381, 1963.

95. Katz, L. N., and Pick, A.: "Clinical Electrocardiography. Part I. The arrhythmias," Lea & Febiger, Philadelphia, 1956.

96. Friedberg, C. K., and Donoso, E.: Arrhythmias and Conduction Disturbances Due to Digitalis, *Progr. Cardiovas. Dis.*, **2**:408, 1960.

97. Lown, B., and Levine, H. D.: "Atrial Arrhythmias, Digitalis and Potassium," Landsberger Medical Books, Inc., New York, 1959.

98. Spratt, J. L., and Okita, G. T.: Protein Binding of Radioactive Digitoxin, *J. Pharmacol. & Exper. Therap.*, **124**:109, 1958.

99. Doherty, J. E., and Perkins, W. H.: Studies with Tritiated Digoxin in Human Subjects after Intravenous Administration, *Am. Heart J.*, **63**:528, 1962.

100. Weissler, A. M., Gamel, W. G., Grode, H. E., Cohen, S., and Schoenfeld, C. D.: The Effects of Digitalis on Ventricular Ejection in Normal Human Subjects, *Circulation*, **29**:721, 1964.

101. Nadas, A. S., and Hauck, A. J.: Pediatric Aspects of Congestive Heart Failure, *Circulation*, **21**:424, 1960.

102. Engle, M. A.: Cardiac Failure in Infancy: Recognition and Management, *Mod. Concepts Cardiovas. Dis.*, **32**:825, 1963.

103. Selzer, A., and Malmborg, R. O.: Hemodynamic Effects of Digoxin in Latent Cardiac Failure, *Circulation*, **25**:695, 1962.

104. Kahler, R. L., Thompson, R. H., Buskirk, E. R., Frye, R. L., and Braunwald, E.: Studies on Digitalis. VI. Reduction of the Oxygen Debt after Exercise with Digoxin in Cardiac Patients without Heart Failure, *Circulation*, **27**:397, 1963.

105. Braunwald, E., Brockenbrough, E. C., and Frye, R. L.: Studies on Digitalis. V. Comparison of the Effects of Ouabain on Left Ventricular Dynamics in Valvular Aortic Stenosis and Hypertrophic Subaortic Stenosis, *Circulation*, **26**:166, 1962.

106. Cohen, B. M.: Digitalis Poisoning and Its Treatment, *New England J. Med.*, **246**:225, 1952.

107. Sodeman, W. A.: The Treatment of Digitalis Toxicity, *Progr. Cardiovas. Dis.*, **3**:309, 1960.

108. Rodensky, P. L., and Wasserman, F.: Observations of Digitalis Intoxication, *Arch. Int. Med.*, **108**:171, 1961.

109. Rosenberg, M. S., and Graettinger, J. S.: Digitalis Intoxication: Management and Prevention, *Disease-A-Month*, Nov. 1962.

110. von Capeller, D., Copeland, G. D., and Stern, T. N.: Digitalis Intoxication: A Clinical Report of 148 Cases, *Ann. Int. Med.*, **50**:869, 1959.

111. Golden, J. S., and Brams, W. A.: Mechanism of the Toxic Effects from Combined Use of Calcium and Digitalis, *Ann. Int. Med.*, **11**:1084, 1938.

112. Lown, B., Ehrlich, L., Lipshultz, B., and Blake, J.: Effect of Digitalis in Patients Receiving Reserpine, *Circulation*, **24**:1185, 1961.

113. Dick, H. L., McCawley, E. L., and Fisher, W. A.: Reserpine-Digitalis Toxicity, *Arch. Int. Med.*, **109**:503, 1962.

114. Dollery, C. T., Emslie-Smith, D., and Milne, M. D.: Clinical and Pharmacological Studies of Guanethicine in the Treatment of Hypertension, *Lancet*, **2**:381, 1960.

115. Fisch, C., Martz, B. L., and Priebe, F. H.: Enhancement of Potassium-induced A-V Block by Toxic Dose of Digitalis Drugs, *J. Clin. Invest.*, **39**:1885, 1960.

116. Cohen, B. D., Spritz, N., Lubash, G. D., and Rubin, A. L.: Use of a Calcium Chelating Agent (NaEDTA) in Cardiac Arrhythmias, *Circulation*, **19**:918, 1959.

117. Gold, H.: "Quinidine in Disorders of the Heart," Hoeber Medical Division, Harper & Row, Publishers, Incorporated, New York, 1950.

118. Goldberg, L. I., and Cotten, M. deV.: Effectiveness of Procaine Amide in Digitalis-induced Ventricular Tachycardia, *Proc. Soc. Exper. Biol. & Med.*, **77**:741, 1951.

119. Hardman, H. F.: Molecular Form of Theophylline Responsible for Positive Inotropic Activity, *Circulation Res.*, **10**:598, 1962.

120. Darby, T. D., Sprouse, J. H., and Walton, R. P.: Evaluation of Sympathetic Reflex Effects on the Inotropic Action of Nitroglycerin, Quinidine, Papaverine, Aminophylline and Isoproterenol, *J. Pharmacol. & Exper. Therap.*, **122**:386, 1958.

121. Howarth, S., McMichael, J., and Sharpey-Schafer, E. P.: The Circulatory Action of Theophylline Ethylene Diamine, *Clin. Sc.*, **6**:125, 1947.

122. Goodman, L. S., and Gilman, A.: "The Pharmacological Basis of Therapeutics," 2d ed., The Macmillan Company, New York, 1955.

123. Boyer, N. H.: Aminophylline and Related Xanthine Derivatives, *J.A.M.A.*, **122**:306, 1943.

124. Foltz, E. L., Rubin, A., Steiger, W. A., and Gazes, P. C.: The Effects of Intravenous Aminophylline upon the Coronary Blood-Oxygen Exchange, *Circulation*, **2**:215, 1950.

125. Maxwell, G. M., White, D. H., Jr., Crumpton, C. W., Rowe, G. G., and Castillo, C. A.: Effects of Intravenous Aminophylline upon Coronary Hemodynamics and Myocardial O_2 and CO_2 Metabolism of Normal and Diseased Hearts, *Circulation*, **18**:757, 1958.

126. Davis, J. O., and Shock, N. W.: The Effect of Theophylline Ethylene Diamine on Renal Function in Control Subjects and in Patients with Congestive Heart Failure, *J. Clin. Invest.*, **28:** 1459, 1949.

127. Pitts, R. F.: "The Physiological Basis of Diuretic Therapy," Charles C Thomas, Publisher, Springfield, Ill., 1959.

128. Wikler, A.: Sites and Mechanisms of Action of Morphine and Related Drugs in the Central Nervous System, *Pharmacol. Rev.*, **2:**435, 1950.

129. Beecher, H. K.: The Measurement of Pain, *Pharmacol. Rev.*, **9:**59, 1957.

130. Murphree, H. B.: Clinical Pharmacology of Potent Analgesics, *Clin. Pharmacol. & Therap.*, **3:**473, 1962.

131. Schmidt, C. F., and Livingston, A. E.: The Action of Morphine on the Mammalian Circulation, *J. Pharmacol. & Exper. Therap.*, **47:**411, 1933.

132. Drew, J. H., Dripps, R. D., and Comroe, J. H., Jr.: Clinical Studies of Morphine. II. The Effects of Morphine upon the Circulation of Man and upon the Circulatory and Respiratory Responses to Tilting, *Anesthesiology*, **7:**44, 1946.

133. Luisada, A.: The Pathogenesis of Paroxysmal Pulmonary Edema, *Medicine*, **19:**475, 1940.

134. Rodbard, S.: Bronchomotor Tone: A Neglected Factor in Regulation of Pulmonary Circulation, *Am. J. Med.*, **15:**356, 1953.

135. Sharp, J. T., Bunnell, I. L., Griffith, G. T., and Greene, D. G.: The Effects of Therapy on Pulmonary Mechanics in Human Pulmonary Edema, *J. Clin. Invest.*, **40:**665, 1961.

136. Eckenhoff, J. E., and Oech, S. R.: The Effects of Narcotics and Antagonists upon Respiration and Circulation in Man: A review, *Clin. Pharmacol. & Therap.*, **1:**483, 1960.

137. Paton, W. D. M.: Histamine Release by Compounds of Simple Chemical Structure, *Pharmacol. Rev.*, **9:**269, 1957.

138. Wang, S. C., and Glaviano, V. V.: Locus of Emetic Action of Morphine and Hydergine in Dogs, *J. Pharmacol. & Exper. Therap.*, **111:**329, 1954.

139. Sprague, J. M.: The Chemistry of Diuretics, *Ann. New York Acad. Sc.*, **71:**328, 1958.

140. Crawford, J. D., and MacGillivray, M. H.: Modern Diuretic Agents. I. Mechanisms of Action and Pharmacologic Considerations, *J. Pediat.*, **62:**413, 1963.

141. Milne, M. D.: Diuretics and Electrolyte Balance, in J. M. Robson and R. S. Stacey, "Recent Advances in Pharmacology," 3d ed., Little, Brown and Company, Boston, 1962, p. 214.

142. Jamison, R. L.: The Action of a Mercurial Diuretic on Active Sodium Transport, Electrical Potential and Permeability to Chloride of the Isolated Toad Bladder, *J. Pharmacol. & Exper. Therap.*, **133:**1, 1961.

143. Berliner, R. W.: Renal Mechanisms for Potassium Excretion, *Harvey Lect.*, **55:**141, 1960.

144. Mudge, G. H., Ames, A., III, Foulks, J., and Gilman, A.: Effects of Drugs on Renal Secretion of Potassium in the Dog, *Am. J. Physiol.*, **161:**151, 1950.

145. Kessler, R. H., Hierholzer, K., Gurd, R. S., and Pitts, R. F.: Localization of Diuretic Action of Chlormerodrin in the Nephron of the Dog, *Am. J. Physiol.*, **194:**540, 1958.

146. Levitt, M. F., and Goldstein, M. H.: Mercurial Diuretics, *Bull. New York Acad. Med.*, **38:**249, 1962.

147. Earle, D. P., Jr., and Berliner, R. W.: Effect of 2, 3-dimercaptopropanol on Diuresis, *Am. J. Physiol.*, **151:**215, 1947.

148. Keith, N. M., Barrier, C. W., and Whelan, M.: The Diuretic Action of Ammonium Chloride and Novasurol, *J.A.M.A.*, **85:**799, 1925.

149. Ethridge, C. B., Myers, D. W., and Fulton, M. N.: Modifying Effects of Various Inorganic Salts on the Diuretic Action of Salyrgan, *Arch. Int. Med.*, **57:**714, 1936.

150. Berliner, R. W., and Orloff, J.: Carbonic Anhydrase Inhibitors, *Pharmacol. Rev.*, **8:**137, 1956.

151. Beyer, K. H., and Baer, J. E.: Physiological Basis for the Action of Newer Diuretic Agents, *Pharmacol. Rev.*, **13:**517, 1961.

152. Laragh, J. H.: The Mode of Action and Use of Chlorothiazide and Related Compounds, *Circulation*, **26:**121, 1962.

153. Novello, F. C., and Sprague, J. M.: Benzothiadiazine Dioxides as Novel Diuretics, *J. Am. Chem. Soc.*, **79:**2028, 1957.

154. Rubin, A. A., Roth, F. E., Taylor, R. M., and Rosenkilde, H.: Pharmacology of Diazoxide, an Antihypertensive, Nondiuretic Benzothiadiazine, *J. Pharmacol. & Exper. Therap.*, **136:**344, 1962.

155. Wilson, W. R., and Okun, R.: The Acute Hemodynamic Effects of Diazoxide in Man, *Circulation*, **28:**89, 1963.

156. Aronoff, A.: Acute Gouty Arthritis Precipitated by Chlorothiazide, *New England J. Med.*, **262:**767, 1960.

157. Runyan, J. W.: Influence of Thiazide Diuretics on Carbohydrate Metabolism in Patients with Mild Diabetes, *New England J. Med.*, **267:**541, 1962.

158. Bartter, F. C. (ed.): "The Clinical Use of Aldosterone Antagonists," Charles C Thomas, Publisher, Springfield, Ill., 1960.

159. Streeter, D. H. P.: Symposium on the Experimental Pharmacology and Clinical Use of Antimetabolites. Part VII. The Spirolactones, *Clin. Pharmacol. & Therap.*, **2:**359, 1961.

160. Kagawa, C. M., Cella, J. A., and Van Arman, C. G.: Action of New Steroids in Blocking Effects of Aldosterone and Deoxycorticosterone on Salt, *Science*, **126:**1015, 1957.

161. Kagawa, C. M., Sturtevant, F. M., and Van Arman, C. G.: Pharmacology of a New Steroid That Blocks Salt Activity of Aldosterone and Desoxycortico-

sterone, *J. Pharmacol. & Exper. Therap.*, **126**:123, 1959.

162. Wiggins, R. A., Hutchin, M. E., Carbone, J., and Doolan, P. D.: Effect of Spirolactone SC 8109 on Renal Function in Normal Human Subjects, *Proc. Soc. Exper. Biol. & Med.*, **100**:625, 1959.

163. Mann, N. M.: Gynecomastia during Therapy with Spironolactone, *J.A.M.A.*, **184**:778, 1963.

163a. Baba, W. J., Tudhope, G. R., and Wilson, G. M.: Triamterene, a New Diuretic Drug, *Brit. M. J.*, **22**:756, 1962.

163b. Sevelius, H., and Colmore, J. P.: Combination of Triamterene and Hydrochlorothiazide in the Treatment of Congestive Heart Failure, *J. New Drugs*, **5**:43, 1965.

163c. Dollery, C. T., Parry, E. H. O., and Young, D. S.: Diuretic and Hypotensive Properties of Ethacrynic Acid: A Comparison with Hydrochlorothiazide, *Lancet*, **1**:947, 1964.

163d. Goldberg, M., McCurdy, K. K., Foltz, E. L., and Bluemle, L. W., Jr.: Effects of Ethacrynic Acid (A New Saluretic Agent) on Renal Diluting and Concentrating Mechanisms: Evidence for Site of Action in the Loop of Henle, *J. Clin. Invest.*, **43**:201, 1964.

163e. Cannon, P. J., Heinemann, H. O., Stason, W. B., and Laragh, J. H.: Ethacrynic Acid: Effectiveness and Mode of Diuretic Action in Man, *Circulation*, **31**:5, 1965.

163f. Timmerman R. J., Springman, F. R., and Thomas, R. K.: Evaluation of Furosemide, A New Diuretic Agent, *Current Therap. Res.*, **6**:88, 1964.

163g. Todays Drugs–Furosemide, *Brit. M. J.*, **2**:164, 1964.

163h. Bencomo, L., Fyvolent, J., Kahana, S., and Kahana, L.: Clinical Experience with a New Diuretic, Furosemide, *Current Therap. Res.*, **7**:339, 1965.

164. Wenckebach, K. F.: "Die unregelmässige Herztätigkeit und ihre klinische Bedeutung," W. Engelmann, Leipzig, 1914.

165. Frey, W.: Weitere Erfahrungen mit Chinidin bei absoluter Herzunregelmassigkeit, *Klin. Wchnschr.*, **55**:849, 1918.

166. Dawes, G. S.: Experimental Cardiac Arrhythmias and Quinidine-like Drugs, *Pharmacol. Rev.*, **4**:43, 1952.

167. DiPalma, J. R., and Schults, J. E.: Antifibrillatory Drugs, *Medicine*, **29**:123, 1950.

168. Bellet, S.: Current Concepts in Therapy: Drug Therapy in Cardiac Arrhythmias, *New England J. Med.*, **262**:769, 979, 1179; **263**:85, 1960.

169. Holland, W. C., and Klein, R. L.: Effects of Temperature, Na and K Concentration and Quinidine on Transmembrane Flux of K^{42} and Incidence of Atrial Fibrillation, *Circulation Res.*, **6**:516, 1958.

170. Angelakos, E. T., and Hastings, E. P.: The Influence of Quinidine and Procaine Amide on Myocardial Contractility in Vivo, *Am. J. Cardiol.*, **5**:791, 1960.

171. Hiatt, E., Brown, D., Quinn, G., and MacDuffie, K.: The Blocking Action of the Cinchona Alkaloids and Certain Related Compounds of the Cardioinhibitory Vagus Endings of the Dog, *J. Pharmacol. & Exper. Therap.*, **85**:55, 1945.

172. Roberts, J., Stadter, R. P., Cairoli, V., and Modell, W.: Relationship between Adrenergic Activity and Cardiac Actions of Quinidine, *Circulation Res.*, **11**:758, 1962.

173. Ferrer, M. I., Harvey, R. M., Werkö, L., Dresdale, D. T., Cournand, A., and Richards, D. W., Jr.: Some Effects of Quinidine Sulfate on the Heart and Circulation in Man, *Am. Heart J.*, **36**:816, 1948.

174. Moe, G. K., and Méndez, C.: Basis of Pharmacotherapy of Cardiac Arrhythmias, *Mod. Concepts cardiovas. Dis.*, **31**:739, 1962.

175. Gertler, M. M., Kream, J., Hylin, J. W., Robinson, H., and Neidle, E. G.: Effect of Digitoxin and Quinidine on Intracellular Electrolytes of the Rabbit Heart, *Proc. Soc. Exper. Biol. & Med.*, **92**:629, 1956.

176. Holland, W. C.: A Possible Mechanism of Action of Quinidine, *Am. J. Physiol.*, **190**:492, 1957.

177. Weidmann, S.: Effects of Calcium Ions and Local Anaesthetics on Electrical Properties of Purkinje Fibers, *J. Physiol.*, **129**:568, 1955.

178. Johnson, E. A., and McKinnon, M. G.: The Differential Effect of Quinidine and Pyrilamine on the Myocardial Action Potential at Various Rates of Stimulation, *J. Pharmacol. & Exper. Therap.*, **120**:460, 1957.

179. Vaughan-Williams, E. M.: The Mode of Action of Quinidine on Isolated Rabbit Atria Interpreted from Intracellular Potential Records, *Brit. J. Pharmacol.*, **13**:276, 1958.

180. Hoffman, B. F.: The Action of Quinidine and Procaine Amide on Single Fibers of Dog Ventricle and Specialized Conducting System. *An. Acad. brasil. cien.*, **29**:365, 1957.

181. Sokolow, M., and Perloff, D. B.: The Clinical Pharmacology and Use of Quinidine in Heart Disease, *Progr. Cardiovas. Dis.*, **3**:316, 1960–1961.

182. Marriott, H. J. L.: Rational Approach to Quinidine Therapy, *Mod. Concepts Cardiovas. Dis.*, **31**:745, 1962.

183. Brodie, B. B., and Udenfriend, S.: Estimation of Quinine in Human Plasma, with Note on Estimation of Quinidine, *J. Pharmacol. & Exper. Therap.*, **78**:154, 1943.

184. Brown, M. G., Holzman, D., and Creelman, E.: Serum Quinidine Concentration in Congestive Heart Failure, *Am. J. Med. Sc.*, **225**:129, 1953.

185. Sokolow, M.: Some Quantitative Aspects of Treatment with Quinidine, *Ann. Int. Med.*, **45**:582, 1956.

186. Yount, E. A., Rosenblum, M., and McMillan, R. L.: Use of Quinidine in Treatment of Chronic Auricular Fibrillation: Results Obtained in a Series

of 155 Cases, *A.M.A. Arch. Int. Med.,* **89**:63, 1952.

187. Weisman, S. A.: Do's and Don'ts in the Treatment of Auricular Fibrillation with Quinidine, *Am. J. Cardiol.,* **3**:333, 1959.

188. Bolton, F. G., and Dameshek, W.: Thrombocytopenic Purpura Due to Quinidine: Clinical Studies, *Blood,* **11**:527, 1956.

189. Bolton, F. G.: Thrombocytopenic Purpura Due to Quinidine. II. Serologic Mechanisms, *Blood,* **11**: 547, 1956.

190. Mautz, F. R.: Reduction of Cardiac Irritability by the Epicardial and Systemic Administration of Drugs as a Protection in Cardiac Surgery, *J. Thoracic Surg.,* **5**:612, 1936.

191. Mark, L. C., Kayden, H. J., Steele, J. M., Cooper, J. R., Berlin, I., Rovenstine, E. A., and Brodie, B. B.: The Physiological Disposition and Cardiac Effects of Procaine Amide, *J. Pharmacol. & Exper. Therap.,* **102**:5, 1951.

192. Kayden, H. J.: The Current Status of Procaine Amide in the Management of Cardiac Arrhythmias, *Progr. cardiovas. Dis.,* **3**:331, 1960–1961.

193. Goldman, M. J.: Combined Quinidine and Procaine Amide Treatment of Chronic Atrial Fibrillation, *Am. Heart J.,* **54**:742, 1957.

194. Averill, K. H., and Lamb, L. E.: Less Commonly Recognized Actions of Atropine on Cardiac Rhythm, *Am. J. M. Sc.,* **237**:304, 1959.

195. Symposium, Multiple Authors: Experimental Methods for the Evaluation of Drugs in Various Disease States. Part II. Angina Pectoris, *Ann. New York Acad. Sc.,* **64**:494, 1956.

196. Gorlin, R.: Drugs and Angina Pectoris, *Am. J. Cardiol.,* **9**:419, 1962.

197. Modell, W.: Clinical Pharmacology of Antianginal Drugs, *Clin. Pharmacol. & Therap.,* **3**:97, 1962.

198. Brunton, T. L.: On the Use of Nitrite of Amyl in Angina Pectoris, *Lancet,* **2**:97, 1867.

199. Wégria, R.: Pharmacology of the Coronary Circulation, *Pharmacol. Rev.,* **3**:197, 1951.

200. Gregg, D. E.: "Coronary Circulation in Health and Disease," Lea & Febiger, Philadelphia, 1950.

201. Wilkins, R. W., Haynes, F. W., and Weiss, S.: The Rôle of Venous System in Circulatory Collapse Induced by Sodium Nitrite, *J. Clin. Invest.,* **16**: 85, 1937.

202. Likoff, W., Kasparian, H., Lehman, J. S., and Segal, B. L.: Evaluation of "Coronary Vasodilators" by Coronary Arteriography, *Am. J. Cardiol.,* **13**:7, 1964.

203. Perloff, J. K., Calvin, J., DeLeon, A., and Bowen, P.: Systemic Hemodynamic Effects of Amyl Nitrite in Normal Man, *Am. Heart J.,* **66**:460, 1963.

204. Brachfeld, N., Bozer, J., and Gorlin, R.: Action of Nitroglycerin on the Coronary Circulation in Normal and in Mild Cardiac Subjects, *Circulation,* **19**:697, 1959.

205. Gorlin, R., Brachfeld, N., MacLeod, C., and Bopp,

P.: Effects of Nitroglycerin on Coronary Circulation in Patients with Coronary Artery Disease or Increased Left Ventricular Work, *Circulation,* **19**,705, 1959.

206. Rowe, G. G., Chelius, C. J., Afonso, S., Gurtner, H. P., and Crumpton, C. W.: Systemic and Coronary Hemodynamic Effects of Erythrol Tetranitrate, *J. Clin. Invest.,* **40**:1217, 1961.

207. Katz, L. N.: The Design of Proper Experiments to Investigate Clinical Angina Pectoris and the Importance of Knowing the Determinants of Coronary Flow in Considering Therapy of Angina Pectoris, *Ann. New York Acad. Sc.,* **64**:505, 1956.

208. Braunwald, E., Sarnoff, S. J., Case, R. B., Stainsby, W. N., and Welch, G. H., Jr.: Hemodynamic Determinants of Coronary Flow: Effect of Changes in Aortic Pressure and Cardiac Output on the Relationship between Myocardial Oxygen Consumption and Coronary Flow, *Am. J. Physiol.,* **192**:157, 1958.

209. Rodbard, S., Williams, C. B., Rodbard, D., and Berglund, E.: Myocardial Tension and Oxygen Uptake, *Circulation Res.,* **14**:139, 1964.

210. Darby, T. D., and Aldinger, E. E.: Further Studies of the Effects on Myocardial Energy Utilization Elicited by Nitroglycerin, *Circulation Res.,* **8**:100, 1960.

211. Honig, C. R., Tenney, S. M., and Gabel, P. V.: The Mechanism of Cardiovascular Action of Nitroglycerine, *Am. J. Med.,* **29**:910, 1960.

212. Raab, W., Van Lith, P., Lepeschkin, E., and Herrlich, H. C.: Catecholamine-induced Myocardial Hypoxia in the Presence of Impaired Coronary Dilatability Independent of External Cardiac Work, *Am. J. Cardiol.,* **9**:455, 1962.

213. Krantz, J. C., Jr., Carr, C. J., and Bryant, H. H.: Alkyl Nitrites. XIV. The Effect of Nitrites and Nitrates on Arterial Adenosine Triphosphatase, *J. Pharmacol. & Exper. Therap.,* **102**:16, 1951.

214. Zoll, P. M., and Norman, L. R.: The Effects of Vasomotor Drugs and of Anemia upon Interarterial Coronary Anastomoses, *Circulation,* **6**:832, 1952.

215. Lumb, G. D., and Hardy, L. B.: Collateral Circulation and Survival Related to Gradual Occlusion of the Right Coronary Artery of the Pig, *Circulation,* **27**:717, 1963.

216. Wirecki, M.: Dipyridamole: Evaluation of Longterm Therapy in Angina Pectoris, *Current Therap. Res.,* **5**:472, 1963.

217. Kinsella, D., Troup, W., and McGregor, M.: Studies with a New Coronary Vasodilator Drug: Persantin, *Am. Heart J.,* **63**:146, 1962.

218. Doyle, A. E., and Kilpatrick, J. A.: Methonium Compounds in the Angina of Hypertension, *Lancet,* **1**:905, 1954.

219. Lewis, B. I., Lubin, R. I., January, L. E., and Wild, J. B.: *Rauwolfia serpentina* in the Treatment of Angina Pectoris, *Circulation,* **14**:227, 1956.

220. Georgopoulos, A. J., Sones, F. M., Jr., and Page,

I. H.: Relationship between Arterial Pressure and Exertional Angina Pectoris in Hypertensive Patients, *Circulation,* **23**:892, 1961.

221. Goldberg, L. I., Horwitz, D., and Sjoerdsma, A.: Attenuation of Cardiovascular Responses to Exercise as a Possible Basis for Effectiveness of Monoamine Oxidase Inhibitors in Angina Pectoris, *J. Pharmacol. & Exper. Therap.,* **137**:39, 1962.

222. Barger, D., and Dale, H. H.: Chemical Structure and Sympathomimetic Action of Amines, *J. Physiol.,* **41**:19, 1910.

223. Ahlquist, R. P.: Adrenergic Drugs, in V. A. Drill (ed.), "Pharmacology in Medicine," McGraw-Hill Book Company, New York, 1958, p. 378.

224. Lands, A. M.: Pharmacological Activity of Epinephrine and Related Dihydroxyphenylalkylamines, *Pharmacol. Rev.,* **1**:279, 1949.

225. Aviado, D. M., Jr.: Cardiovascular Effects of Some Commonly Used Pressor Amines, *Anesthesiology,* **20**:71, 1959.

226. Eckstein, J. W., and Abboud, F. M.: Circulatory Effects of Sympathomimetic Amines, *Am. Heart J.,* **63**:119, 1962.

227. Goldberg, L. I., Cotten, M. deV., Darby, T. D., and Howell, E. V.: Comparative Heart Contractile Force Effects of Equipressor Doses of Several Sympathomimetic Amines, *J. Pharmacol. & Exper. Therap.,* **108**:177, 1953.

228. Brewster, W. R., Jr., Osgood, P. F., Isaacs, J. P., and Goldberg, L. I.: Hemodynamic Effects of a Pressor Amine (Methoxamine) with Predominant Vasoconstrictor Activity, *Circulation Res.,* **8**:980, 1960.

229. Goldberg, L. I., Bloodwell, R. D., Braunwald, E., and Morrow, A. G.: The Direct Effects of Norepinephrine, Epinephrine, and Methoxamine on Myocardial Contractile Force in Man, *Circulation,* **22**: 1125, 1960.

230. Trautwein, W.: Generation and Conduction of Impulses in the Heart as Affected by Drugs, *Pharmacol. Rev.,* **15**:277, 1963.

231. Li, T. H., Shimosato, S., and Etsten, B.: Hemodynamics of Mephentermine in Man, *New England J. Med.,* **267**:180, 1962.

232. Malmcrona, R., Schröder, G., and Werkö, L.: Hemodynamic Effects of Metaraminol. I. Normal Subject, *Am. J. Cardiol.,* **13**:10, 1964.

233. Malmcrona, R., Schröder, G., and Werkö, L.: Hemodynamic Effects of Metaraminol. II. Patients with Acute Myocardial Infarction, *Am. J. Cardiol.,* **13**:15, 1964.

234. Li, T. H., Shimosato, S., Gamble, C. A., and Etsten, B.: Hemodynamics of Mephentermine during Spinal Anesthesia in Man, *Anesthesiology,* **24**: 817, 1963.

235. Ahlquist, R. P.: A Study of Adrenotropic Receptors, *Am. J. Physiol.,* **153**:586, 1948.

236. Nickerson, M.: The Pharmacology of Adrenergic Blockade, *Pharmacol. Rev.,* **1**:27, 1949.

237. Nickerson, M.: Blockade of the Actions of Adrenaline and Noradrenaline, *Pharmacol. Rev.,* **11**: 443, 1959.

238. Black, J. W., and Stephenson, J. S.: Pharmacology of a New Adrenergic Beta-receptor Blocking Compound (Nethalide), *Lancet,* **2**:311, 1962.

239. Moran, N. C.: Adrenergic Receptors within the Cardiovascular System, *Circulation,* **28**:987, 1963.

240. Harrison, D. C., Braunwald, E., Glick, G., Mason, D. T., Chidsey, C. A., and Ross, J., Jr.: Effects of Beta Adrenergic Blockade on the Circulation, with Particular Reference to Observations in Patients with Hypertrophic Subaortic Stenosis, *Circulation,* **29**:84, 1964.

240a. Nickerson, M.: Drug Therapy of Shock, in K. D. Bock (ed.), "Shock, Pathogenesis and Therapy, an International Symposium (Ciba)," Springer Verlag, Berlin, 1962, p. 356.

240b. Lucchesi, B. R.: The Effects of Pronethelol and Its Dextro Isomer upon Experimental Cardiac Arrhythmias, *J. Pharmacol. & Exper. Therap.,* **148**:94, 1965.

241. Burn, J. H., and Rand, M. J.: The Action of Sympathomimetic Amines in Animals Treated with Reserpine, *J. Physiol.,* **144**:314, 1958.

242. Trendelenburg, V.: Supersensitivity and Subsensitivity to Sympathomimetic Amines, *Pharmacol. Rev.,* **15**:225, 1963.

243. Mashford, M. D., and Mahon, W. A.: Impairment of Cardiovascular Response to Tyramine by Reserpine Administration in Man, *J. Clin. Invest.,* **41**: 1382, 1962.

244. Abboud, F. M., and Eckstein, J. W.: Effects of Small Oral Doses of Reserpine on Vascular Responses to Tyramine and Norepinephrine in Man, *Circulation,* **29**:219, 1964.

245. Abboud, F. M., and Eckstein, J. W.: Effects of Guanethidine on the Vasoconstrictor Response to Tyramine in Man, *Fed. Proc.,* **21**:93, 1962.

246. Burn, J. H., and Rand, M. J.: Fall of Blood Pressure after a Noradrenaline Infusion and Its Treatment by Pressor Agents, *Brit. M. J.,* **1**:394, 1959.

247. Gazes, P. C., Goldberg, L. I., and Darby, T. D.: Heart Force Effects of Sympathomimetic Amines as a Basis for Their Use in Shock Accompanying Myocardial Infarction, *Circulation,* **8**:883, 1953.

248. Selzer, A., and Rytard, D. A.: Use of Drugs in Shock Accompanying Myocardial Infarction, *J.A.M.A.,* **168**:762, 1958.

249. Kuhn, L. A.: The Mechanism of Shock in Myocardial Infarction, *J. Mt. Sinai Hosp. New York,* **30**:20, 1963.

250. Nathanson, M. H., and Miller, H.: Action of Norepinephrine, Epinephrine and Isopropyl Norepinephrine on Rhythmic Function of Heart, *Circulation,* **6**:238, 1952.

251. Zoll, P. M., Linenthal, A. J., Gibson, W., Paul, M. H., and Norman, L. R.: Intravenous Drug Therapy of Stokes-Adams Disease: Effects of Sym-

pathomimetic Amines on Ventricular Rhythmicity and Atrioventricular Conduction, *Circulation*, **17:** 325, 1958.

252. Stack, M. F., Rader, B., Sobol, B. J., Farber, S. J., and Eichna, L. W.: Cardiovascular Hemodynamic Functions in Complete Heart Block and Effect of Isopropylnorepinephrine, *Circulation*, **17:**526, 1958.

253. Bellet, S.: Clinical Pharmacology of Antiarrhythmic Drugs, *Clin. Pharmacol. & Therap.*, **2:**345, 1961.

254. Goldberg, L. I., McDonald, R. H., Jr., and Zimmerman, A. M.: Sodium Diuresis Produced by Dopamine in Patients with Congestive Heart Failure, *New England J. Med.*, **269:**1060, 1963.

255. McDonald, R. H., Jr., Goldberg, L. I., McNay, J. L., and Tuttle, E. P., Jr.: Effects of Dopamine in Man: Augmentation of Sodium Excretion, Glomerular Filtration Rate and Renal Plasma Flow, *J. Clin. Invest.*, **43:**1116, 1964.

69 CARDIAC ARREST AND RESUSCITATION

Marvin M. McCall, M.D.

Cardiac arrest is defined as the sudden cessation of cardiac output and includes both ventricular asystole and ventricular fibrillation. It is probable that asystole is the initial occurrence in 70 to 75 per cent of unselected cases of arrest. In cardiac surgical treatment ventricular fibrillation accounts for approximately 70 to 75 per cent. Initial resuscitative procedures are the same in both conditions.

Although Vesalius wrote of cardiac resuscitation in the sixteenth century, it was 1901 before Igelsrud successfully resuscitated an arrested human heart.[1, 2] By 1916 open-chest massage was accepted but not frequently attempted outside the operating room. In 1947 Beck et al. reported successful defibrillation using electric current,[3] and in 1960 Kouwenhouven et al. reported successful closed-chest cardiac massage.[4]

Since Kouwenhouven's reports, the increasing interest in resuscitation is reflected in the rapidly expanding literature on the subject, both in medical and lay publications. All physicians now have the moral and legal responsibility for being familiar with resuscitative procedures and their prompt application.[5] When cardiac arrest occurs, one must decide immediately whether or not resuscitative attempts are advisable. Attempted resuscitation is mandatory when arrest occurs during surgical procedures; conversely, there are many who die from incurable diseases in whom resuscitation should not be attempted. Since a decision regarding advisability must be made, there is no time left for hesitancy regarding proper procedure.

Cardiac Arrest

Etiology

The precise biochemical abnormalities that result in cardiac arrest are the subject of extensive studies currently in progress. There are well-known gross factors, however, that are distinctly related and should be noted, since prevention of arrest is far easier than treatment.

Cardiac arrest has been associated with the use of all anesthetic agents.[6, 7] It is likely that some act directly on the heart while others produce their effect through the autonomic nervous system. The anxious patient who fights anesthetic induction secretes increased amounts of catecholamines, and in the presence of hypoxia, hypercapnia, or hypotension ventricular fibrillation may occur. In addition, stimulation of the glottis, esophagus, peritoneum, bladder, urethra, mesentery, gallbladder, anus, orbital structures, and carotid sheath may result in bradycardia and asystole presumably through vagal stimulation. The use of atropine in adequate doses (1 mg before induction and repeat doses every 90 min during surgical treatment) will prevent many arrests which apparently result from increased vagal tone.

Calcium and potassium have a profound effect upon cardiac activity. Not only are their absolute serum and tissue levels important, but their relationship to one another is equally important; e.g., the patient with renal insufficiency who has hyperkalemia and hypocalcemia is much more likely to have cardiac arrest than is the patient who has either of the two conditions in the absence of the other.

The intravascular administration of many therapeutic and diagnostic agents as well as radiographic contrast mediums has been associated with cardiac arrest, and there are many catastrophes, such as drowning, electrocution, and pulmonary embolism, which do not directly damage the heart but produce death by cardiac arrest.

Diagnosis

Even at surgical operation with a qualified anesthetist in attendance, the exact moment that arrest occurs may be difficult to ascertain unless the heart is under direct observation. Since time is the critical factor, not only for the preservation of brain tissue but also for the ease of resuscitation, multiple diagnostic attempts must be avoided. Examination of the fundi for vascular changes, prolonged ascultation for faint cardiac sounds, attachment of an electrocardiogram, or placement of an endotracheal tube should be avoided. Intravenous or intracardiac injections of stimulants are of little value at this point, and valuable time is wasted in procuring them. If examination of a large artery (aorta, iliac, carotid, femoral) fails to reveal adequate pulsations in a patient who has shown evidence of vascular collapse, resuscitative measures should be instituted immediately. A vigorous blow with the closed fist should be delivered to the precordium; this has sometimes been sufficient to institute effective electrical activity.

Resuscitation

There are two distinct objectives in cardiac resuscitation: the immediate one is the delivery of oxygenated blood to vital organs including the heart; the secondary one is the reestablishment of the heart's own effective contractions. From the beginning adequate oxygenation is of extreme importance. Outside the operating room this is best accomplished by mouth-to-mouth or mouth-to-nose resuscitation by one person while another initiates cardiac massage. It is possible for one operator to do both by alternately giving five or six respiratory exchanges and then compressing the heart for 10 or 12 cycles, but this is obviously extremely fatiguing. In either closed or open massage it is not necessary to know whether the heart has stopped in asystole or in ventricular fibrillation, since effective circulation can be produced under both circumstances.[8,9] Once effective massage and adequate oxygenation have been initiated, one has ample time to call for the equipment necessary for further diagnosis and therapy.

With few exceptions closed-chest massage is the treatment of choice for cardiac arrest. Open-chest cardiac massage is indicated when the chest is already open, when there has been massive hemorrhage and arterial transfusion is indicated, when cardiac tamponade is present, when air embolism is the cause of the arrest, and when back or chest deformity prevents adequate compression of the heart between the sternum and the spine. In addition, external massage must be terminated if the heart is in fibrillation and no external defibrillator is available.

Closed-chest Massage

A closed-chest approach is the method of choice for most patients. It requires no equipment and can be successfully done by personnel who have had only minimal training. It eliminates our natural fear of opening the chest and has been shown to be as effective as direct cardiac massage. It involves the compression of the heart between the sternum and the spine with lateral motion of the

ventricles limited by the pericardium. The most critical factor involved is the location at which sternal pressure is applied. If applied too high, it will be ineffective at best, and multiple rib fractures will occur; if applied too low, laceration of the liver may occur and result in fatal intraperitoneal bleeding. The sternum should be compressed in its lower one-third. The heel of one hand should be placed directly over the sternum, with the heel of the other hand placed on the dorsum of the first. There are three features of compression which one must consider:

1. Rate. About 60 massages per minute is satisfactory.

2. Depth. The sternum should be depressed 3 to 4 cm and allowed to spring back into place by complete rapid removal of the hands from the chest wall.

3. The manner of compression is extremely important; it should not be described as massage, since this gives the impression of a slow, milking action. In order to produce good ejection and palpable carotid and femoral pulses, a vigorous quick compression must be carried out. The patient must be placed on a firm surface which will support the spine and allow the heart to be compressed between it and the sternum. If removal of the patient from the bed to the floor is not feasible, then an ordinary food tray placed under the patient's back gives adequate support to the spine.

External cardiac message and adequate ventilation may immediately reestablish cardiac output, and certainly the promptness with which this is instituted must have a bearing on its success.

Direct Cardiac Massage

In open-chest cardiac massage an incision is made in the fourth or fifth interspace and extended from the edge of the sternum to the midaxillary line; the ribs are retracted, and the heart is given 15 or 20 vigorous massages immediately. The palmar surfaces of the fingers (not the fingertips) compress the heart against the sternum. If cardiac activity does not return, the pericardium must be opened widely for better exposure. This allows the operator to place both hands on the heart, one anteriorly and the other posteriorly, and achieve better compression. Attention must be given to complete cardiac filling after each compression, and for this reason the hands must be quickly and completely removed from the ventricular surfaces after each compression. The rate of compression depends upon the rapidity of filling of the heart, but generally a rate of 60 to 70 massages per minute will be adequate to maintain cerebral circulation. As soon as possible, rib spreaders must be inserted to ease the pressure on the wrists of the operator. Even when good exposure is obtained, fatigue is marked, and more than one physician must alternate in the compression. With direct cardiac massage the physician must be particularly careful not to rupture areas which may be damaged by myocardial infarction, myocarditis, or recent surgical treatment.

Reestablishing the Heartbeat

There are times when an effective heartbeat is not obtained by cardiac massage. Ventricular fibrillation will not be abolished by simple massage and must be treated further. If asystole is the cause of arrest, electrolyte and metabolic abnormalities may prevent adequate myocardial contraction.

Electrical Defibrillation. There are two types of electrical defibrillators available: one delivering alternating current (a-c) and the other delivering direct current (d-c). It should be pointed out that not all a-c defibrillators are suitable for external defibrillation, and one must be certain of the type of a-c defibrillator in use. All of the d-c defibrillators are equipped for both external and internal use. Both a-c and d-c machines are designed to produce complete depolarization of all cardiac muscle, stop the chaotic electrical activity, and allow one of the cardiac pacing areas to stimulate contractions in an effective and rhythmic manner. There are a number of good papers describing in detail the use of both instruments.[10,11] At present the author uses the d-c machine, because it appears to be more effective and is more versatile in the treatment of arrhythmias which may occur following cardiac arrest.

With the a-c machine a charge of 250 to 800 volts is delivered with one electrode at the base and the other at the apex of the heart for a duration of 0.25 sec. Occasionally one must deliver three immediately successive shocks to defibrillate the heart effectively. The average adult requires from 400 to 800 volts. With the d-c instrument the electrodes are placed in the same manner, and a charge of 100 to 400 watt-seconds is delivered in 0.0025 second.

At times, particularly when the electrocardiogram shows "fine" fibrillation waves, defibrillation efforts are unsuccessful. An injection of epinephrine (5 to 10 ml 1:10,000 solution) will result in a more vigorous and coarse fibrillation following which electrical defibrillation may be promptly accomplished.

After defibrillation with either instrument, a rhythmic contraction will usually occur which may be normal sinus rhythm but generally is not. The treatment of these arrhythmias should be carried out as described elsewhere in this book. If the defibrillation produces asystole, treatment should be carried out as outlined for the patient who has arrest in asystole.

Treatment of Asystole. If after 5 to 10 min of massage and ventilation the heart arrested in asystole has not resumed effective contraction, one must initiate drug therapy to stimulate contraction.

Calcium Chloride. Calcium chloride has a direct effect on myocardial contractility, increasing the strength as well as the duration of the contractions. Instead of using the usual 10 per cent solution, 5 to 10 ml diluted 1 per cent solution should be injected directly into the ventricular cavity.[7]

Epinephrine. Epinephrine increases the rate and force of myocardial contractions as well as increasing the peripheral resistance. In a poorly oxygenated heart, however, epinephrine may produce ventricular fibrillation, which should be treated as previously discussed. The dose is 5 to 10 ml 1:10,-000 solution.[7]

Drugs in Treatment of Acidosis. In addition to administering stimulants one must usually treat the metabolic acidosis that inevitably accompanies prolonged attempts at resuscitation. Molar lactate has been used for many years, but it has no real advantage over sodium bicarbonate and does not act as rapidly. Sodium bicarbonate may be needed in doses of 44 mEq intravenously every 20 to 30 min as long as resuscitation attempts are being made.

Other Drugs. Neo-Synephrine hydrochloride (phenylephrine hydrochloride), norepinephrine, barium chloride, caffeine, Isuprel hydrochloride (isoproterenol hydrochloride), and many other agents have been used in the management of cardiac arrest, but none of these agents is superior to those mentioned above. Furthermore, drug therapy should be kept at a minimum, and the resuscitation tray should be kept as simple as possible, not only to avoid errors in drug administration but also to avoid confusion in the selection of drugs to be used.

Subsequent Care

Following successful cardiac resuscitation there is usually a period of varying cardiac arrhythmias, difficulty of maintenance of blood pressure, occasional respiratory distress, and frequently evidence of transient cerebrovascular insufficiency. It may be necessary to use external monitoring and pacing devices, or one may choose to put a cardiac catheter into the right ventricle and pace the heart from that site until stability returns. Hypothermia has been advocated following arrest to keep vital-organ damage at a minimum.

Results of Resuscitaton Reports

The initiating factors responsible for cardiac arrest, the underlying heart disease, the general health of the patient, the promptness with which resuscitation efforts are begun, and the expertness with which they are delivered all play an important part in the salvage of patients who have had cardiac arrest. There will be fewer successful cardiac resuscitations in patients who have severe coronary disease than in healthy individuals who have arrest during anesthetic induction. However, as more physicians become competent in cardiac resuscitation and as patients are better selected for resuscitative attempts, the percentage of successful cases will gradually rise. At present work is being done on complete and partial cardiac bypass, and although this is not yet a standard procedure, the theory is sound, and technical advances in the near future should further increase successful resuscitation of "hearts too good to die." [12]

REFERENCES

1. Willius, F. A., and Dry, T. J.: "A History of the Heart and Circulation," W. B. Saunders Company, Philadelphia, 1948.
2. Keen, W. W.: A Case of Total Laryngectomy (Unsuccessful) and a Case of Abdominal Hysterectomy (Successful), in Both of Which Massage of the Heart for Chloroform Collapse Was Employed, with Notes of 25 Other Cases of Cardiac Massage, *Therap. Gaz.*, **28**:217, 1904.
3. Beck, C. S., Pritchard, W. H., and Feil, H.: Ventricular Fibrillation of Prolonged Duration Abolished by Electric Shock, *J.A.M.A.*, **135**:985, 1947.
4. Kouwenhouven, W. B., Jude, J. R., and Knickerbocker, G. G.: Closed Chest Cardiac Massage, *J.A.M.A.*, **137**:1064, 1960.
5. Hurst, J. W.: "Cardiac Resuscitation," Charles C Thomas, Publisher, Springfield, Ill., 1960.
6. Briggs, B. D., Sheldon, D. B., and Beecher, H. K.: Cardiac Arrest: Study of a 30-year Period of Operating Room Deaths at Massachusetts General Hospital, 1925–54, *J.A.M.A.*, **160**:1439, 1956.
7. Millstein, B. B.: "Cardiac Arrest and Resuscitation," The Year Book Medical Publishers, Inc., Chicago, 1963.
8. Jude, J. R.: Cardiac Resuscitation, *Am. Heart J.*, **62**:286, 1961.
9. Jude, J. R., Kouwenhouven, W. B., and Knickerbocker, G. G.: Cardiac Arrest: Report of Application of External Cardiac Massage on 118 Patients, *J.A.M.A.*, **178**:1063, 1961.
10. Zoll, P. M., Paul, M. H., Lilenthal, A. J., Norman, L. R., and Gibson, W.: The Effects of External Electric Currents on the Heart: Control of Cardiac Rhythm and Induction in Termination of Cardiac Arrhythmias, *Circulation*, **14**:745, 1956.
11. Lown, B., Amarasingham, R., and Neuman, J.: New Method for Terminating Cardiac Arrhythmias: Use of Synchronized Capacitor Discharge, *J.A.M.A.*, **182**:548, 1962.
12. Beck, C. S., and Leighninger, D. S.: Hearts too Good to Die—Our Problem, *Ohio M. J.*, **56**:1221, 1960.

Section E: Certain Nonmedical Considerations

70 INSURANCE PROBLEMS IN HEART DISEASE

Royal S. Schaaf, M.D.

Heart problems in insurance have two main aspects. First, there is the clinical task of detection, diagnosis, and estimation of the severity of any disease or impairments present in each applicant for insurance. Here, clinicians and insurance underwriters are on common ground. Second, and inseparable from the first for insurance purposes, is evaluation of the applicant's long-term prognosis, and it is here that misunderstandings sometimes arise. Many a physician has been astonished to find that a patient he has treated or an applicant he has examined has been charged an increased premium for some condition that the physician regards as of little or no clinical importance.

Why do these differences of opinion arise? For one thing, when a clinician considers the prognosis of a disease entity, he is thinking of a relatively short time—usually not more than 5 or 10 years. Possibilities of accident, additional disease, or a great advance in treatment of the patient's current disease make speculation unprofitable on the future of the individual. An insurance company, however, must take into consideration a much longer period of time, since its contracts often run for 50 years or more. To do this, a company must make predictions based on statistical studies on its own policyholders or on large, multicompany experience like the *Impairment Study, 1951*, made by the Society of Actuaries (see Suggested Reading at the end of this chapter). In such studies the measuring rod is the mortality experienced on standard lives—that is, on individuals without any detectable impairments who were issued insurance at standard premium rates. The mortality rates obtained from these standard lives are applied, age by age and year by year, to whatever group of impaired lives is being studied, to get the "expected deaths"—that is, the number of deaths that would have been expected among the members of the impaired group if they had had no impairment. The number of deaths that actually occurred among the impaired lives is then divided by the number of expected deaths to give a mortality ratio. If, for example, in a particular impairment, 50 deaths are expected and actually 75 occur, the mortality ratio is 150 per cent; if 250 deaths occur, the mortality ratio is 500 per cent. Conversely, if only 45 deaths take place where 50 are expected, the mortality ratio is 90 per cent, that is, lower than standard, a preferred group of risks. The mortality ratio thus arrived at is the basis for calculating the premiums needed to cover the impairment under consideration.

In all fairness, every insurance group must pay its own way. Impaired risks who have been charged an extra premium must, as a group, live up to the life expectancy assumed for them, and this may be a long time indeed. Table 70-1 shows the number of years that applicants with various degrees of impairment would have to live, on the average, for their premiums to be sufficient.

Table 70-1. LIFE EXPECTANCY FOR VARIOUS DEGREES
OF IMPAIRMENT
(In years)

Age at issue	Standard 100%	Impair-ment 150%	Impair-ment 200%	Impair-ment 300%	Impair-ment 400%	Impair-ment 500%
0	71	67	64	60	55	50
10	62	58	55	51	47	43
20	52	49	46	42	38	34
30	43	39	36	33	30	27
40	33	30	27	24	21	18
50	24	22	19	16	14	12
60	17	15	12	10	8	7

It should be emphasized that these figures are averages. Some persons in each rating group must live much longer than the average to offset those in the same group who die early. Further, as medical progress continues, these life expectancy figures will doubtless have to be revised upward.

A mortality ratio of 150 per cent may represent only one or two extra deaths a year out of each 1,000 persons insured. For purposes of clinical

statistics an increase of 0.1 or 0.2 per cent in the annual death rate would be virtually imperceptible and certainly not reason enough to justify alarming a patient. Yet for this small increase in mortality an insurance company must charge an additional premium if it is to cover its claims.

It would be a simple matter actuarially to work out a premium which, varying of course with age and provided everyone took the insurance, would be enough to insure the entire population without regard to physical health or prospects, including the coronary patient, the cancer patient, and the victim of central nervous system disease. Clearly these three groups are the types of people who need insurance the most. Unfortunately, their situation is like that of the man who seeks to buy fire insurance when his house is already in flames. Insurance is designed to help people protect themselves against hazards which are possible in the future but which are not yet in being in the individual. Few people enjoying good health would be willing to pay the very high premiums necessary to cover all, taxing themselves for the benefit of others for whom they bear no personal responsibility. On the other hand, those knowing or believing themselves shortly to die would bend every effort to purchase a maximum amount of insurance. In this way the claims would rise, the premium receipts decrease, and the company trying such a program quickly go under.

Only a system of compulsory inclusion of the healthy with the sick could make a uniform premium plan work, and this is unacceptable to the great majority. Therefore, it becomes necessary to place very high ratings on some policies and to exclude some persons altogether from coverage. Still, the numbers involved are relatively small. Despite all the possible impairments and combinations of impairments to which mankind is heir, slightly over 90 per cent of all life insurance policies are issued at standard rates, about 5 per cent receive some substandard rating, and only about 3 per cent of all applications are rejected.

Another way of looking at mortality ratios is illustrated by Table 70-2. These figures indicate that out of 1,000 men who are standard risks at age thirty-five, only 25 are expected to die over the next 10 years from all causes (disease, accident, suicide); 975 will still be alive at age forty-five. Even if a group of thirty-five-year-old men have an impairment that gives them a mortality ratio of 500 per cent, out of 1,000 such there would still be 830 alive 10 years later. In other words there would be an 83 per cent survival rate. Most clinicians would feel that such a survival rate is little short of ordinary "normal health" in comparison to really serious disease. Yet for insurance purposes the

Table 70-2. PROPORTION OF MEN AGED THIRTY-FIVE
YEARS SURVIVING 10 YEARS AT VARIOUS
MORTALITY RATIOS

Mortality percentage	Proportion surviving 10 years
Standard	0.975
150	0.961
200	0.945
300	0.915
400	0.875
500	0.830

premiums required to cover a mortality ratio of 500 per cent are so high that as a practical matter few people are willing to pay them.

A second cause for misunderstanding between clinician and medical underwriter is a difference in viewpoint. The attention of the attending physician is centered on his patients as individuals, and when adverse action has been taken on one of them by an insurance company, he tends to recall the people he has known with the same impairment who have lived far into old age. Insurance companies see these long-lived individuals, too. There are some in every impaired group, and without them the average future lifetime would be less (and the premium more) than it is. Still, the insurance company must be concerned with the performance of the entire group, the short-lived as well as the long-lived. It is impossible to foresee which individuals will live long and which will die early; this is why people buy insurance. But with large groups of individuals it is possible to predict mortality with sufficient accuracy to cover the death claims; this is why insurance companies can exist.

There is a widespread impression that insurance companies are living in the past, basing their premiums on old statistics with high death rates that have long since become obsolete. This is not true. It is true that the companies take their past experience as a starting point, but they restudy their data at frequent intervals, and if it appears reasonable to assume that a more favorable mortality may be expected in the future, they modify their calculations accordingly. When a modification of existing tables will no longer produce equity among policyholders, a new mortality table is prepared.

A similar procedure is followed on individual medical impairments to bring the companies' action in line with current medical thought. Insurance companies must be wary of accepting too completely the early rosy clinical reports of new therapeutic measures, many of which later prove to have been overoptimistic, but they do not wait years for supporting statistical evidence. Ratings for hypertension, for example, have been reduced where modern methods of treatment have lowered the blood pressure and maintained it at lower levels, although there has not yet been time to accumulate statistical evidence to support such action. It must be remembered, also, that the latest techniques in diagnosis and treatment, used first in the big cities and medical centers, require time to attain widespread use and to lower appreciably the general mortality.

Moreover, old statistics are not always so out of date as one might suppose. While spectacular progress has been made clinically in some fields, in others little has been accomplished. Table 70-3 shows comparative results of two large multicompany studies on heart murmurs: the Impairment Study, 1951, covering the period from 1935 to 1950, and the Medical Impairment Study, 1929, covering the period from 1908 to 1928 (see Suggested Reading). If one is inclined to feel that we are doing so much better now than we were doing in 1935 to 1950 and that all statistics for that period are outmoded, it would be well to reflect that in 1945 we might have thought we were doing greatly better than in 1908 to 1928, but the mortality ratios on some murmurs are virtually the same and on others are actually higher. In each of these studies, moreover, the impaired lives were being measured by the standard mortality rates that were then current. This automatically takes into account the improvement in the general mortality among people living under the same social and economic conditions and in the same era of medicine as the impaired group that is being studied. Impaired groups whose mortality ratios have remained essentially unchanged over the years have done no better than to improve in the same proportion as the standard mortality. Those whose mortality ratios are higher than before have shown less than the general improvement. As might be expected, the increased mortality observed in the classifications in Table 70-3 was preponderantly of cardiovascular causes.

An insurance classification like the one in Table 70-3, in which heart murmurs are classified according to the description of the murmur, may seem inadequate to a clinician. The evaluation of symptoms and physical signs is often difficult and in clinical practice may require extensive study and a considerable period of observation. This is now and should properly remain within the province of the practicing physician. The insurance classification must be based on the findings that are available on all applicants from the insurance examination, which is, because of factors of convenience, cost and the unwillingness of applicants to undergo

Table 70-3. COMPARATIVE RESULTS OF TWO IMPAIRMENT
STUDIES OF MORTALITY RATIOS FOR CERTAIN
HEART MURMURS

Description of heart murmur	1951 study, per cent	1929 study, per cent
Systolic pulmonic, not transmitted	107	102
Systolic at apex, inconstant, not transmitted	111	104
Systolic at apex, constant, not transmitted	139	156
Systolic at apex, constant, transmitted to left	220	224
Systolic at apex, constant, transmitted to left, with history of rheumatic fever or chorea	267	332
Systolic at apex, constant, transmitted to left, with history of streptococcic infection	263	181
Systolic aortic, constant, not transmitted	191	131
Systolic aortic, constant, transmitted upward	491	257

NOTE: This table illustrates the fact that, despite general medical progress, old statistics may still give a substantially accurate prediction of current mortality experience and in some instances may be even more favorable than current experience.

extensive study for insurance purposes, less searching than a clinician's diagnostic study. Of course, when such a study has already been made for clinical purposes, the company will usually try to obtain it from the attending physician and give it full weight in the underwriting decision.

An insurance company action may sometimes appear overly conservative to the clinician for another reason. If the diagnosis is obscure, the company is at a disadvantage as compared with the clinician. The latter can, in such a case, await developments and defer his opinion until the situation becomes clearer. The company, however, must make its decision now, either to decline the application or to enter into a contract that cannot be changed later except in favor of the insured. If subsequent developments show that the company has overestimated the risk, it can reduce the premium and often does. But if it has underestimated the risk, it cannot increase the premium or refuse to accept a premium tendered by the policyholder.

Insurance is a business, of course, but it is also a public trust. Whenever an insurance company accepts an applicant for insurance, it is backing its judgment with money—other people's money. Policyholders place their money in the company's hands, not for speculative purposes or even for "a

businessman's risk," but to guarantee funds to their families after their deaths. The company is required to invest these funds in certain types of high-quality securities that are specified by law. It must show equal conservatism in selecting its risks, a conservatism always tempered, however, by the competition of over one thousand other life insurance companies and by the reluctance, natural to any enterprise, to cause ill will and alarm to its clients by unfavorable action.

Underwriting Cardiovascular Impairments

It is not practical in a single chapter to discuss the underwriting aspects of the full range of cardiovascular impairments. Attention instead will be directed to some of the conditions most frequently encountered in clinical and insurance medicine, illustrating more specifically the way the underwriting approach to individuals must differ from the clinical. Unless otherwise indicated, the figures appearing hereafter derive from the *Impairment Study 1951.* The material for this study was contributed by a group of companies whose business comprises 70 per cent of the insurance in force in the United States and Canada. Overall, the study covered a total of 725,000 policies, of which 18,000 ended in death during the observation period. It is interesting to look first at the experience with persons giving a family history of two or more parents or siblings known to have or to have had cardiovascular-renal disease under the age of sixty. Table 70-4 summarizes this experience in almost fifteen thousand applicants giving such a history.

Table 70-4. FAMILY HISTORY* OF CARDIOVASCULAR-RENAL DISEASE

Age at issue	Actual deaths	Expected deaths	Mortality ratio, per cent
15–29	42	31	136
30–39	140	101	139
40–49	298	190	157
50–64	251	196	128
15–64	731	518	141

* Two or more cases under age sixty. When there are two or more deaths due to cardiovascular-renal disease under the age of sixty in the parents and siblings of an individual, there will be a small but significant increase in mortality ratio.

The number of lives involved minimizes the possibility that these ratios reflect chance fluctuation. Although the increased mortality is not great, it is nonetheless significant as compared with standard ratios. It must be pointed out that these individuals aside from their family history were standard risks, in no case presenting any other impairment requiring a rating.

Congenital Heart Disease

No insurance statistics are available on long-term prognosis of congenital heart disease, because until recently no cases were accepted, and the policies now being issued on relatively mild types and degrees of congenital impairment have not been in force long enough to develop an insurance experience. Enough has been said, however, about the relatively low mortality ratios and long survival periods associated with even highly rated insurance, especially among young persons, to make it evident that the majority of congenital cardiac anomalies are uninsurable. This is especially true, of course, of cyanotic heart disease, in which large numbers of the victims may not even survive to adulthood, but in acyanotic anomalies, as well, the frequency of onset of serious complications in early or middle life leads to mortality ratios beyond the scope of insurance coverage in most cases.

Adults with certain types of unoperated acyanotic congenital heart disease constitute a more favorable group for possible insurance consideration than do children having similar defects. This is for the obvious reason that by simply surviving to age twenty or over, the adults give proof of a lesser degree of severity of impairment or of greater ability to tolerate their disease, or both. Here, when the diagnosis is definite, as proved by catheterization or angiocardiography or as diagnosed clinically by a qualified cardiologist, some companies may be willing to make a substandard insurance offer where there is no significant cardiac enlargement and the electrocardiogram is normal or nearly so. Defects in this category include interventricular septal defects and congenital pulmonic or subaortic stenosis.

Rapid advance in recent years in the techniques and capabilities of cardiovascular surgical treatment is apparently achieving results which may greatly improve the long-range outlook for both morbidity and mortality in congenital cardiac anomalies. Pending the passage of a significant number of years, however, and the accumulation of clinical experience with the operated cases, insurance medicine will have to maintain a conservative and strictly experimental approach to these surgically treated cases. At present only two procedures, both extracardiac, can be considered as established successes for insurance purposes. Most companies would be willing to accept a corrected patent ductus arteriosus. There is a tendency to take more favorable action when the surgical procedure has been carried out early in the patient's life, and when both ligation and division of the ductus rather than ligation alone have been done. Correction of a coarctation of the aorta without use of a graft is also acceptable in many instances after passage of a year or so following operation to give assurance of good healing of the anastomosis and persistent reduction of the blood pressure. Again, patients operated on below age twenty are probably more favorable. A few companies are accepting some corrected interatrial septal defects, usually after some waiting period following surgical treatment.

In summary, insurance medicine approaches the long-term prognosis of untreated or surgically treated congenital cardiac anomalies slowly and cautiously, but the rapid progress in the clinical handling of such cases gives promise of increasingly optimistic insurance action in the future.

Rheumatic Fever without Residual Murmur

From the clinical viewpoint, both the incidence and severity of rheumatic fever have been decreasing in recent decades, and it is gratifying to find that actuarially the experience with acute rheumatic fever is also favorable, as evidenced by Tables 70-5 and 70-6. In both these categories, acute rheumatic fever without complications occurring within 5 years of application and over 5

Table 70-5. ACUTE ARTICULAR RHEUMATISM: ONE ATTACK WITHIN 5 YEARS OF APPLICATION

Age at issue	Actual deaths	Expected deaths	Mortality ratio, per cent
15–29	27	15	182
30–39	26	20	127
40–49	26	28	92
50–64	30	21	142
15–64	109	84	129

Table 70-6. ACUTE ARTICULAR RHEUMATISM: ONE ATTACK OVER 5 YEARS BEFORE APPLICATION

Age at issue	Actual deaths	Expected deaths	Mortality ratio, per cent
15–29	29	28	102
10–39	85	64	134
40–49	106	103	102
50–64	103	82	126
15–64	323	277	116

years prior to application, the mortality ratios are low enough to justify standard issue in most cases. The exceptions are the cases still within a year or two of rheumatic activity. Here a small substandard rating is necessary to cover the occasional patient in whom a cardiac murmur develops only after a latent period following the active inflammatory disease.

Systolic Heart Murmurs, Including Rheumatic

For practical purposes it is impossible to have every applicant with a heart murmur examined by a cardiologist. Instead, most heart murmurs are detected, described, and diagnosed by physicians who have not had extensive training in cardiac auscultation. As a result, in many cases confusion and even contradiction may still remain when the insurance examination has been completed, whether by a single examining physician or with an alternative heart examination by another physician. Largely offsetting this relative lack of full and accurate cardiac evaluation, however, is the fact that the broad groups in which acceptable heart murmurs may be placed are relatively few and the numbers of lives in each group large, so that a certain range of diagnostic uncertainty can be included in each group without materially affecting the overall long-range experience.

The first categories for consideration are the localized apical systolic murmurs, inconstant or constant, as summarized in Tables 70-7 and 70-8. These figures, based on 7,500 and 10,000 lives, respectively, show a generally favorable mortality rate except in the constant murmur in the younger groups. Probably here a few cases of unrecognized rheumatic or other organic disease have led to the very few extra deaths required to give a substantial boost to the mortality ratio at ages fifteen to twenty-nine.

When the apical systolic murmur is constant and also transmitted to the left or is specifically diagnosed as mitral regurgitation, the mortality ratios are sharply increased, as seen in Table 70-9,

Table 70-8. CONSTANT, LOCALIZED APICAL SYSTOLIC MURMURS

Age at issue	Actual deaths	Expected deaths	Mortality ratio, per cent
15–29	52	31	170
30–39	60	43	141
40–49	87	65	134
50–64	70	56	126
15–64	269	195	139

covering almost nineteen thousand lives. When, in addition to being constant and transmitted to the left or diagnosed as mitral regurgitation, the murmur is accompanied by a history of rheumatic fever or chorea or by a history of tonsillitis or other streptococcal infection (not definitely known to have been followed by rheumatic fever or chorea), the mortality ratios climb another significant distance, from the 220 per cent of Table 70-9 to 267 and 263 per cent, respectively (Table 70-3). Most constant, transmitted apical systolic murmurs are of moderate to loud intensity and of harsh or musical quality. However, for underwriting purposes, if a suggestive or definite history of rheumatic fever is present, even the soft, or blowing, apical systolic murmurs, which on auscultation may sound physiologic, may be expected over the long run to give distinctly higher than standard mortality experience and hence require a substandard rating. If cardiac hypertrophy is present, especially as proved by x-ray, or if the electrocardiogram is abnormal in association with an organic apical systolic murmur, the mortality ratios rise beyond the insurable range.

The experience with basal systolic murmurs at the pulmonic area, not transmitted, supports their clinical reputation for being physiologic and harmless. (Table 70-10).

Table 70-7. INCONSTANT APICAL SYSTOLIC MURMURS

Age at issue	Actual deaths	Expected deaths	Mortality ratio, per cent
15–29	27	24	110
30–39	41	41	101
40–49	67	54	125
50–64	41	40	103
15–64	176	159	111

Table 70-9. APICAL SYSTOLIC MURMURS, CONSTANT, TRANSMITTED TO THE LEFT

Age at issue	Actual deaths	Expected deaths	Mortality ratio, per cent
15–29	188	58	325
30–39	178	78	227
40–49	248	118	210
50–64	120	79	152
15–64	734	333	220

Table 70-10. LOCALIZED PULMONIC SYSTOLIC MURMURS

Age at issue	Actual deaths	Expected deaths	Mortality ratio, per cent
15–29	30	30	100
30–39	54	42	129
40–49	26	27	97
50–64	8	11	71
15–64	118	110	107

NOTE: Clinically physiologic pulmonic systolic murmurs have a standard mortality experience.

Basal systolic murmurs at the aortic area, not transmitted, are distinctly more significant, however, and when the aortic systolic murmur is transmitted as well, the mortality ratio approaches the limit of insurability. The number of deaths in these two categories is too small to justify breakdown by ages, because isolated aortic systolic murmurs are not common and most aortic murmurs occur in combination with other clinical features which make the applicant uninsurable. Composite Table 70-11 summarizes the mortality experience of both groups of aortic systolic murmurs.

In general summary, systolic heart murmurs having the characteristics identifying them clinically as organic will not give standard mortality experience, even though x-ray and electrocardiogram may currently be normal, and especially not when there is a history of rheumatic fever or streptococcal infection. Diastolic heart murmurs have long been known to carry greater hazard than systolic murmurs as a class and have generally been considered uninsurable. In recent years some companies have issued highly rated insurance to adults with diastolic murmurs whose heart size has been normal as seen by x-ray and who do not have a history or signs of cardiac failure. Insured cases remain too few and the period of observation too short to provide any reliable experience.

Table 70-11. AORTIC SYSTOLIC MURMURS
(AGE AT ISSUE FIFTEEN TO SIXTY-FOUR)

Murmur	Mortality ratio, per cent
Not transmitted	191
Transmitted upward	491

NOTE: Even localized aortic systolic murmurs show almost twice the standard mortality, and organic aortic systolic murmurs have a mortality ratio of five times standard.

Coronary Artery Disease

Despite its prominent position among the causes of death at the present time, coronary artery disease is not an area on which life insurance experience can throw much light. Again the reason for this is that the mortality is known to be so high that until very recently no company would knowingly issue insurance to an applicant giving a history or showing clinical evidence of a coronary episode or angina pectoris. As with diastolic murmurs, a number of companies have lately been issuing policies to selected coronary patients on a very highly rated, experimental basis, but as yet too few policies have been accepted and have remained in force to build up substantial experience. One study of 1,551 disability claims caused by proved coronary occlusion was reported by Waldron and Constable (see Suggested Reading) from experience of the Mutual Life Insurance Company of New York, and the marked shortening of life expectancy in these cases is easily apparent (Table 70-12).

Table 70-12. AVERAGE LIFE EXPECTANCY AFTER MYOCARDIAL INFARCTION

Age at onset	Expectancy after infarction, years	Normal expectancy, years
30–39	11.5	33.4
40–49	10.5	25.2
50–60	8.5	17.8

Electrocardiography

Electrocardiographic experience on insured lives is sketchy and difficult to evaluate. Most people are insured without benefit of any electrocardiographic study whatever, past or present, and in those cases where tracings may be available, complete details of clinical history and current status are not assured, which makes useful follow-up difficult. Although underwriters in many instances are now making insurance offers in various types of electrocardiographic abnormalities, these actions for the most part must be taken on a cautious, judgment basis, weighing especially the degree to which any particular abnormality may reflect the possible presence of coronary artery disease.

One area of electrocardiographic evaluation in which there tends to be a divergence between clinical and insurance judgments is that of T-wave changes appearing in otherwise normal tracings taken on persons having no history or clinical evidence of cardiac or related impairments. Transient T-wave changes can be brought about in many people by a number of everyday physiologic actions.

As a result, when a clinician encounters a person in whom the only objective finding is a T-wave change, he rightly takes an optimistic view and either makes no mention of the finding to the patient or gives him assurance that it is not a cause for alarm, leaving it to follow-up examinations at later dates to determine whether the finding has long-range significance. Needless to say, the patient is sorely taken aback if an insurance company on the basis of the same electrocardiogram finds it necessary to apply a rating or to decline. Someone must be making a mistake! In an effort to quantitate the qualitative judgment that even isolated T-wave changes often are not standard risks, in 1955 the Prudential Insurance Company undertook a study of the problem based on its own employees. A file was available of about twenty-two thousand electrocardiograms taken in the Employee Health Service since 1933, with full details of all the illnesses, physical examinations, and laboratory studies of each individual on whom a tracing had been taken. The marked job stability of Prudential personnel, together with retirement and death benefit records, made follow-up relatively easy and complete.

Among all the persons in the file, selections were restricted to the men between the ages of forty and sixty-nine, when coronary disease is considered to be most prevalent. From these men four groups were further selected. The normal group was comprised of individuals who had normal electrocardiograms and who appeared normal clinically, with no evidence of organic disease, cardiac or otherwise. Blood pressure readings were consistently below 150/90 in all cases. Contrasting with the normal and serving only as a basis for comparison with the groups being studied were 112 persons who had had a coronary occlusion and survived the acute episode by at least 60 days. In these men the coronary disease was uncomplicated by diabetes, hypertension, valvular heart heart disease, or any other organic impairment. The remaining two groups were those whose electrocardiograms were normal at all times except for showing slight, or minor, T-wave changes (flat or disproportionately low in relation to the QRS) and those showing marked, or major, T-wave changes (diphasic or inverted where one would normally expect an uprigtht T-wave). Again, only those men were included who had normal clinical examination results and case histories, excluding even those with seemingly irrelevant disease such as peptic ulcer or tuberculosis. Table 70-13 shows the results of this study, together with a second one carried out in 1961.

From these figures, certain conclusions seem valid. Although the electrocardiogram may be of very little prognostic value in the individual case, groups of individuals showing T-wave changes, even though slight, will show an increase in mortality. There will be more cardiovascular disease in such groups than in groups not showing similar T-wave changes. Isolated major T-wave changes are rare in clinically normal people but when found carry a sharply raised mortality ratio. (There were, of course, hundreds of examples of major T-wave changes in the file, but almost always in association

Table 70-13. ANALYSIS BY GROUPS OF MEN, AGES FORTY TO SIXTY-NINE, WITH ELECTROCARDIOGRAMS SHOWING T-WAVE CHANGES

Group	Number	Deaths	Per cent actual to expected deaths	Per cent deaths from Cardiovascular causes	Per cent total number subsequently developing coronary occlusion
1955 study:					
Normal	1,388	75	84	47	3.2
Minor T-wave changes	273	29	163	65.5	10.6
Major T-wave changes	43	7	302	71.4	16.3
Previous coronary history	112	40	526	95	
1961 study:					
Normal	1,805	145	78	36	6
Minor T-wave changes	422	65	166	49	12

NOTE: Even minor T-wave abnormalities, unaccompanied by any other electrocardiographic or clinical abnormality, show a significant increase in mortality ratio and in subsequent incidence of coronary occlusion. The period of follow-up observation in these cases averaged about 7 years.

with obvious organic disease.) The more pronounced the isolated T-wave changes, the greater the possibility that they indicate cardiovascular disease, and it is against this possibility that increases in premium rates are required. Furthermore, since the persons in this study were clinically normal, it can reasonably be inferred that if an applicant for life insurance should show other evidence of cardiovascular disease, such as hypertension or a murmur, the T-wave changes, even though slight, may take on even greater significance.

In 1961 a second study was completed on all clinically normal men in the file, ages forty to sixty-nine, having normal electrocardiograms or showing isolated minor T-wave changes. The figures fell closely in line with the earlier study, as shown in the lower part of Table 70-13.

Decision as to whether a T wave is normal or slightly or markedly abnormal is often difficult and may have to be made arbitrarily. However, to the extent that some way might be found to remove borderline instances from a particular group, the remainder of the group may be expected to show a corresponding increase in mortality ratio, and vice versa. Further, the observed mortalities of 84 and 78 per cent on the normal employees in these studies fall distinctly below the standard (100 per cent) mortality of insured lives in general. Accordingly, it is probable that a somewhat higher mortality ratio for isolated T-wave changes may occur among the population at large than was observed in this sheltered population.

Blood Pressure

Blood pressure is a subject on which insurance companies have accumulated a vast experience, which can be only touched on here. In general, as might be predicted clinically, the evidence shows that for any given systolic pressure, the mortality ratio rises as the diastolic pressure rises. Correspondingly, for any given diastolic pressure, the mortality ratio rises as the systolic pressure rises. For this reason it is not possible to give a single specific reading indicating the limit between normal and elevated readings. What is arresting to anyone accustomed to the clinical approach to blood pressure elevation is the evidence that even mild elevations of systolic or diastolic blood pressure, or both, are accompanied by significant rises in mortality ratios. Indeed, by the time an individual exhibits blood pressure readings high enough to call for close follow-up or treatment clinically, he may already be near or beyond the limits of insurability. In other words, a clinically "mild" or "moderate" blood pressure elevation may be "severe" for insurance purposes.

The most recent major blood pressure review from the insurance viewpoint is the *Build and Blood Pressure Study, 1959*, made by the Society of Actuaries (see Suggested Reading). In the blood pressure section of this study there were 3,900,000 entrants, with 102,000 deaths, with an average duration of exposure of a little over 7 years. Tables 70-14 and 70-15 give an indication of the experience developed. In each table builds are normal, and no other significant impairments are involved.

For the same blood pressure readings, mortality ratios are higher among the younger men. Female experience, not quoted here, is more favorable than in the male. These features should be born in mind in attempting to compare clinical hypertensive series with insurance mortality tables. Since the insured lives on which insurance mortality tables are built tend to be about 90 per cent male and clinical hypertensive series tend to have a preponderance of female lives, it is not always possible to make meaningful comparisons between the two.

A final point of interest is how low average blood pressures are, as shown for males of various ages in the figures in Table 70-16 based on 235,000 males,

Table 70-14. MORTALITY RATIOS OF MEN, AGES THIRTY TO THIRTY-NINE, OBSERVATION PERIOD 1935 TO 1954

Systolic pressures	Diastolic pressures 48–67	Diastolic pressures 68–82	Diastolic pressures 83–87	Diastolic pressures 88–92	Diastolic pressures 93–97	Diastolic pressures 98–102
98–127	45%	88%	116%	120%	(113%)	—
128–137	99%	113%	134%	160%	240%	—
138–147	(121%)	140%	176%	221%	249%	277%
148–157	—	171%	246%	201%	261%	498%
158–167	—	—	—	(292%)	(439%)	—

NOTE: Dashes indicate groups in which the number of deaths was less than 10. Parentheses indicate groups in which the number of deaths was between 10 and 34. Altogether there were 20,383 deaths in the thirty-to-thirty-nine age group and 22,850 deaths in the fifty-to-fifty-nine age group.

Clinically mild to insignificant blood pressure readings may give highly significant mortality experience, especially in younger men.

Table 70-15. MORTALITY RATIOS OF MEN, AGES FIFTY TO FIFTY-NINE, OBSERVATION PERIOD 1935 TO 1954

Systolic pressures	Diastolic pressures 48–67	Diastolic pressures 68–82	Diastolic pressures 85–87	Diastolic pressures 88–92	Diastolic pressures 93–97	Diastolic pressures 98–102
98–127	73%	83%	97%	107%	—	—
128–137	109%	107%	116%	112%	163%	(162%)
138–147	165%	142%	145%	153%	199%	201%
148–157	(245%)	158%	193%	195%	208%	196%
158–167	—	202%	201%	219%	270%	336%

NOTE: Dashes indicate groups in which the number of deaths was less than 10. Parentheses indicate groups in which the number of deaths was between 10 and 34. Altogether there were 20,383 deaths in the thirty–to–thirty-nine age group and 22,850 deaths in the fifty–to–fifty-nine age group.

Clinically mild to insignificant blood pressure readings may give highly significant mortality experience, especially in younger men.

a representative sample taken from the larger study. The best mortality ratios are experienced with pressures even lower than these averages.

SUGGESTED READING

Actuarial Society of America and Association of Life Insurance Medical Directors, "Medical Impairment Study, 1929," New York, 1931.

Society of Actuaries, "Impairment Study, 1951," New York, 1954.

Society of Actuaries, "Build and Blood Pressure Study, 1959," Chicago, 1959, 2 vols.

Baum, D.: Life Insurance for the Young Cardiovascular Patient, *J.A.M.A.*, **184**:593, 1963.

Gubner, R. S., and Ungerleider, H. E.: Life Expectancy and Insurability in Heart Disease, *Mod. Concepts Cardiovas. Dis.*, **28**:565M, 1959.

Halliday, J H.: The Differentiation and Assessment of

Table 70-16. AVERAGE BLOOD PRESSURES, MALES

Ages	Systolic	Diastolic
15–19	117	71
20–24	119	73
25–29	121	75
30–34	122	76
35–39	123	77
40–44	124	78
45–49	126	78
50–54	128	79
55–59	130	79
60–64	132	80

NOTE: Average blood pressure remains relatively low at least up to age sixty-five.

Basal Systolic Murmurs, *Tr. A. Life Ins. M. Dir. America*, **38**:24, 1954.

Hutchinson, J. J.: Highlights of the New Build and Blood Pressure Study, *Tr. A. Life Ins. M. Dir. America*, **43**:34, 1959.

Kirkland, H. B.: Prognosis in Heart Disease, *New York J. Med.*, **55**:3443–3452, 1955.

Kirkland, H. B., Kiessling, C. E., and Lyle, A. M.: The Evaluation of Certain Fundamental Electrocardiographic Patterns in the Selection of Insurance Risks, *Tr. A. Life Ins. Dir. America*, **35**:86, 1951.

Kiessling, C. E., Schaaf, R. S., and Lyle, A. M.: A Reevaluation of the T-wave Changes in the Electrocardiograms of Otherwise Normal People, *Tr. A. Life Ins. M. Dir. America*, **45**:70, 1961.

Kiessling, C. E., Schaaf, R. S., and Lyle, A. M.: Mortality Studies of Isolated Electrocardiographic T-wave Changes, *Tr. A. Life Ins. M. Dir. America*, **39**:5, 1956.

Lew, E. A.: Some Implications of Recent Changes in Mortality, *Tr. A. Life Ins. M. Dir. America*, **37**:4, 1953.

Master, A. M., and Rosenfeld, I.: The Master "2-step" Electrocardiographic Test Brought up to Date, *Tr. A. Life Ins. M. Dir. America*, **43**:70, 1959.

Pollack, A. A., McGurl, T. J., and Plucinski, T. E.: Hypertension in Substandard Insurance, *Tr. A. Life Ins. M. Dir. America*, **41**:51, 1957.

Robb, G. P. and Marks, H. H.: The Postexercise Electrocardiogram in the Detection of Coronary Diseases: A Long Term Evaluation, *Tr. A. Life Ins. M. Dir. America*, **45**:81, 1961.

Robb, G. P., Marks, H. H., and Mattingly, T. W.: The Value of the Double Standard Two-step Exercise Test in the Detection of Coronary Disease, *Tr. A. Life Ins. M. Dir. America*, **40**:52, 1956.

Waldron, F. A., and Constable, W. P.: Myocardial Infarction: A Mortality Study, *Tr. A. Life Ins. M. Dir. America*, **34**:69, 1950.

71 MEDICOLEGAL ASPECTS OF HEART DISEASE

Howard B. Sprague, M.D.

Heart disease enters the field of legal medicine through several avenues but in general because it is claimed that a specific event or a continuing environmental influence made it worse. Rarely is it asserted that these influences were the "cause" of heart disease, as the physician understands cause —namely, the etiologic agent. There are some exceptions, as in cor pulmonale secondary to an occupational lung disease, such as silicosis or berylliosis, or in instances of subacute bacterial endocarditis following trauma. In some states, however, laws have been passed defining certain occupations of governmental employees as etiologic in the development of heart disease or hypertension. Chiefly these apply to firemen and policemen.

MEDICAL ASPECTS OF TRAUMATIC HEART DISEASE

It is not intended in this section to discuss in detail direct trauma to the heart. Such injuries are relatively easy to assess and thus amenable to adjudication but may present difficulties involving late effects, such as constrictive pericarditis after pericardial damage or questions of myocardial contusion.

Injuries or unusual work loads or toxic hazards in industry may precipitate cardiac failure or abnormal rhythms in those with cardiac disease. Aneurysms may rupture prematurely during strenuous effort. Rarely, even a valve cusp may give way. Serious states of shock, hemorrhage, or severe pain may induce myocardial ischemia in individuals with narrowed coronary arteries. Chronic impairment of the peripheral circulation may be worsened by injury. Trauma to a foot, for example, may induce gangrene in the presence of old occlusion of leg arteries.

In litigated cases one of the difficulties is the lack of differentiation by the courts of the different cardiovascular conditions. That is to say, a "heart attack" may have been acute coronary failure or thrombosis, pulmonary edema in mitral stenosis, paroxysmal atrial fibrillation, dissecting aneurysm, or pericarditis. There is a great need for definition of terms and determination of facts in these court cases. It is in these matters of fact that the physician's testimony is essential and where his adherence to scientific standards is imperative.

The much broader problem is concerned with coronary artery disease and its relationship to stressful events or to employment.

It is apparently true that coronary artery degeneration has no single cause. Indeed, its increase since 1920 may well be due entirely, as Campbell [1] has demonstrated, to the saving of lives, by improved medical and economic measures, of those who would have died of other disease at an earlier age and to the halving of the death rate from all disease from 1880 to 1920. Many factors, from heredity to diet, have been implicated, but it is popular to attribute the devastation of coronary disease to emotional and physical strains of modern life, chiefly those of employment. The reason that employment pressures are blamed is that this is an area in which financial recompense may be expected—as from Workmen's Compensation payments or special retirement pensions.

There is no good evidence that any occupation predisposes to coronary degeneration. It is ubiquitous and starts in childhood. The circumstances leading to its acceleration in any individual are unknown but are probably genetic. The belief that the emotions have anything to do with it is entirely speculative, and the weight of evidence is against the theory. There may be certain human strains so constituted as to have a susceptible humoral and emotional pattern and in whom coronary disease is more prevalent, but this is again a relationship without causality and is inborn.

Furthermore, there is no reason to suppose our era to be more stressful than any previous one. Stress has been blamed for man's ills during all of recorded history. The first contribution to the American literature of occupational medicine, by Dr. Benjamin McCready [2] in 1837, stated: "The population of the United States is beyond that of other countries, an anxious one. . . . We are an anxious and care-worn people."

It was the hope of defining reasonable criteria of the relationship between strain and trauma, and primarily coronary artery disease, that led to the studies and report of the committee of the American Heart Association on the subject. [3]

It is commonly supposed that some stress is necessary to precipitate a coronary attack, either with sudden death or with coronary failure or what is usually called "coronary thrombosis." This is apparently not true, nor is thrombosis the common finding in abrupt coronary deaths.

Fresh thrombosis is found in less than 20 per cent of cases of sudden coronary death. [4] Osborn, [5] of the Department of Pathology at the University of Sheffield, England, states: "There is a popular, but often erroneous belief, that death takes place because of a sudden or sustained exercise that the heart was not equal to, especially running for a bus or train. Only two, in several thousand, of the deaths I have investigated, were of men who were taking significant exercise at the time they dropped dead." In only 41 of 86 fatal cases diagnosed as "coronary thrombosis" was Osborn able to demonstrate thrombosis by meticulous reconstruction of the coronary system from serial sections.

The medical subcommittee of the American Heart Association Committee on the Effect of Strain and Trauma on the Heart and Great Vessels summarized their conclusions as follows:[3]

1. Coronary atherosclerosis is a progressive process; at any stage, factors, as yet unknown, may precipitate either sudden death or the patterns of myocardial ischemia or necrosis.

2. Physical or emotional activity may, in such individuals, produce coronary insufficiency and this may be fatal. Death may be abrupt without detectable warning, presumably by the mechanism of ventricular fibrillation. These factors also may produce myocardial ischemia of a degree measurable by the electrocardiogram, with disappearance of the electrocardiographic abnormalities on a return to the unstressed state.

3. Acute myocardial infarction with or without antecedent coronary thrombosis, is often a nonfatal process in which the potential molecular substrate for ventricular fibrillation may not be operative to cause immediate death. For the muscle to undergo infarction, there must be a critical degree of ischemia from coronary stenosis or occlusion for a considerable time, even hours. Unlike angina pectoris, it is an unexplained occurrence without demonstrable relationship to any precipitant, except events causing acute lowering of systemic blood pressure, such as shock, hemorrhage, tachycardia, or abnormal heart rhythms.

4. Since the time of onset of the occlusive process in acute coronary thrombosis often cannot be determined without an autopsy study, no precise conclusions can be drawn concerning the relationship between a coronary occlusive attack and the events preceding it, on the basis of clinical data. Even with meticulous necropsy examination, such a temporal relationship is often equivocal.

5. The appearance of clinical symptoms is the only practical guide at present available for even attempting to evaluate the connection between an environmental event and a coronary response (be it angina pectoris, severe myocardial ischemia, or infarction). It seems inevitable, therefore, that such overt evidence must, at this time, remain the criterion for decision.

The single dissenting opinion of Dr. J. C. Paterson[6] stressed the possible role of effort in inducing intimal hemorrhage as a precipitant of acute coronary occlusion. While such hemorrhage seems to be very common in coronary atherosclerosis, the committee could determine no criteria for relating it to any unusual event and considered hemorrhage only an unpredictable part of the disease process.

One may say, therefore, that neither physical nor emotional stress, nor accustomed activity, nor any of the hazards of daily living can be reasonably claimed as precipitants of the type of coronary failure commonly called "coronary thrombosis" or "acute coronary occlusion." There may be rare exceptions to this opinion, but the weight of statistical evidence supports it.

Obviously this does not exclude certain cases of sudden death under a severe emotional stress. John Hunter, the famous British physician who suffered from angina, was aware of his sensitivity to emotional stimuli. As he said, "My life is in the hands of any rascal who chooses to annoy and tease me." But as Aaron[7] points out, Hunter had had angina for 20 years when he died at the age of sixty-five, ". . . no mean achievement 200 years ago."

In summary, an attempt at a strict medical and scientific approach to the problem of the relationship of a specific event to an abrupt death from coronary disease leads to the admission that we must deal with probabilities. One's opinion is based upon judgment of the degree of stress imposed at the moment. The physician is influenced by what would be stressful to himself—by no means always a valid criterion. But for any justification of the relationship of the event to the death they must be clearly connected in time, or with intercalary or bridging symptoms suggesting relationship.[8]

Similarly, the appearance of a nonfatal attack of coronary ischemia (whether or not of sufficient duration to result in myocardial necrosis) during, or directly after, an unusual physical or emotional stimulus can only be explained by the progression of coronary disease to a critical point where spontaneous occlusion might have been expected at any time.

Again, it must be remembered that unexpected, advanced myocarditis may be present in young individuals in apparent good health and without coronary disease who die suddenly without any obvious excess stimulus. This points up the value of autopsy study in all cases of sudden death.

LEGAL ASPECTS OF TRAUMATIC HEART DISEASE

The litigious aspects of heart disease appear because of the assertion that an event, a series of events, or an environmental influence, somewhat in control of the defendant, aggravated or accelerated underlying heart disease or brought death to the plaintiff "sooner than otherwise would have occurred."

Personal Injury

In Biblical times personal injury was recompensed by equal injury to the wrongdoer: "An eye for an eye and a tooth for a tooth." This gave way to a system of satisfying the victim, instead, by granting him money or goods in exchange for his injury.

Such injuries were, in the main, obvious, and the blame could be fixed and quantitated. This is the domain of tort law, or the law of personal injury. "At Common Law there is a cause of action whenever one person did damage to another willfully and intentionally and without just cause and excuse." [9] However, this liability can be incurred by ". . . non-culpable acts or conduct resulting in accidental harm for which, because of hazards involved, the law imposes strict or absolute liability notwithstanding the absence of fault."

In cardiac cases involving personal injury, the element of direct trauma is usually of major importance. This implies "impact," as in trauma to the chest or severe injuries with secondary cardiovascular reactions such as fatal inhibitory cardiac reflexes, shock, abnormal heart rhythms, or embolism. From a legal viewpoint, the facts are usually obtainable, and the damages are a matter for the judge or jury to determine.

Much more difficult to assess, and much more suspect, are the injuries claimed to be related to minor traumatic experiences occurring days, weeks, or months before the appearance of cardiac symptoms, or those attributed to psychic trauma. With the exception of the rare case of traumatic pericarditis,[10] there seems to be no justification for believing that heart failure of any type is related to an event in the remote past unless there are definite bridging symptoms of a nonneurotic type in the intervening period and signs clearly appearing at the time of the injury.

An unfortunate trend is becoming evident through the activities of organized plaintiffs' attorneys to bring into court personal injury cases of dubious merit based, the author believes, on perversions of psychiatric thinking.

Recently an attorney[11] was quoted as saying in an address to physicians: ". . . changes are going to come rapidly now and all over the country. . . . In an age when the teachings of psychiatry have made clear the effects of emotional disturbance, it would be incongruous to hold that we must not allow recovery for such injury because it is hard to measure or because it may be simulated." He suggested that a new legal doctrine is required that

would take into consideration a "pre-existing neurotic personality." The author of this chapter cannot conceive of a more fertile field for barratry.[12]

Pension and Retirement Claims

Government employees are entitled to retirement with pension at certain ages. If the employment contributes to their inability to work, they may be retired earlier for physical disability. If this disability is the result of an accident, the pension provisions may be financially superior to those of the ordinary pension.

In certain states, statutes have been enacted which assert that the development of heart disease or hypertension is an accidental disability and is to be presumed to be due to a specific category of employment, such as that of policeman, fireman, or traffic inspector. These have been called *heart laws*, and their enactment appears to be politically motivated. They represent an example of the determination of a cardiac disease etiologic agent by legislative fiat. Similar laws have been passed defining the occupation of a fireman as the cause of any type of lung disease that he may acquire. Such laws create unjustified inequities in the pension system and are not only scientifically indefensible but are open to extension to other categories of civil employees who may possess sufficient political power. The Supreme Court of North Carolina has found such laws unconstitutional in that state.

Workmen's Compensation[13]

Before the advent of Workmen's Compensation laws, the employee who was injured was required to bring legal action against his employer through a claim of negligence. Under the common law, the employer had certain defences such as "contributory negligence," "scope of employment," and "fellow servant rule."

Workmen's Compensation abolished such actions in exchange for guaranteeing the employee redress for injury ". . . arising out of and in the course of employment." It was a new principle of "liability without fault." Originally the concept of an accident was embodied in the law, but not in all states. However, the definition of an *accident* was much influenced by a decision of the House of Lords in England in 1903, which interpreted the term *by accident* to include the result as well as the cause.

Thus, as Larson[14] says, "The 'by accident' requirement is now deemed satisfied in most jurisdictions either if the cause was of an accidental character or if the effect was the unexpected result of a routine performance of the claimant's duties." In some states the degree of aggravation of preexisting disease by the accident is compensable on the percentage basis attributable to the accident. The present status of heart disease in litigation is admirably covered by Dean Harold McNiece in *Heart Disease and the Law*,[15] an investigation sponsored by the American Heart Association and the National Heart Institute.

There has been a growing trend to include diseases under Workmen's Compensation coverage, and degenerative heart disease is one of the most controversial. Such claims are almost always based on the argument that the employment aggravated an underlying cardiac ailment. Much of the legal dispute hinges on the presence of a "usual" or "unusual" stress. Interpretations of this vary widely in the different states and even within a state at different times. The state of Washington is an example. From 1926 to 1951 a very liberal interpretation prevailed, but in 1952 a complete reversal occurred in the Supreme Court, essentially invalidating its previous pronouncements. This is an example of social and medical pressures affecting the law, since the situation became such that employers feared to hire older workers and even suggested the discharge of this group, since every cardiac disablement was being decided as related to employment.

Recent experience in some of the larger industries indicates a more realistic program in returning the employee, even of the blue-collar type, to his original job after a coronary attack, and this rehabilitation approach has reduced disability claims. It is hoped that this may indicate some appreciation of the fact that regular physical exertion appears to have a protective rather than deleterious effect on the coronary circulation.

As in personal injury cases there is a burgeoning of litigation under Workmen's Compensation that is based on claims of aggravation of coronary disease from emotional factors, anxiety, overwork, frustration, and so on.

Judgments in these cases, as in all others, differ in the various jurisdictions. Three examples may suffice:

During a twenty-minute argument with his supervisor regarding wages, an employee experienced chest pains. An ambulance was summoned, and he was taken to a hospital. The diagnosis was myocardial infarction caused by the excitement during the argument, superimposed on a cardiac condition. . . .

The Supreme Court of New York, Appellate Division, Third Department held . . . [that] the episode neither involved nor induced emotional strain or tension greater than the countless differences and irritations to which all workers are occasionally subjected without untoward results.[16]

In a state of Washington case, the Supreme Court ruled against recovery where a coronary occlusion was claimed to be related to anxiety and worry over a job,

saying that worry over one's duties does not meet the requirements of "proximate cause" of the Occupational Disease Statute. It was not characteristic of the employment concerned, and there was no proof that the attack would not have occurred if the claimant had pursued another calling.[17] Similarly in that state "long hours of work over a period of time are not generally considered basis for recovery."

On the other hand in the District of Columbia in the case of a claims adjuster with a heavy case load, the court ruled in his favor, saying, "It is well known that nervous shock, continual anxiety, and excessive exertion at work under trying circumstances may contribute toward the collapse of persons who are already suffering from hardening of the arteries." [18]

These cases indicate a pressure to make coronary disease occupational, and since everyone can claim emotional stress in the simple acts of living, acceptance of such claims may well lead to endless litigation on the most tenuous bases.

True, job stresses may exist, and so do stresses off the job. Not only is it often impossible to distinguish their relative potencies, but rarely do they approach the stress of being without a job. Emphasis on job stresses may well result in increased unemployment if industry must always be the whipping boy for psychic disorders.

The interpretation of Workmen's Compensation laws has tended to favor the workman on the priciple that this was social legislation intended to be liberally construed and to furnish financial support to those forced out of employment by physical disability. This has often resulted in the acceptance of something less than accurate medical testimony or the disregard of preponderant medical evidence at the whim of a board or court, and appeal boards tend to uphold compensation boards even in the absence of "a single shred" of medical evidence of causal relation. This creates friction between lawyers and physicians and motivates a search for better methods of solving a socioeconomic problem.

Second-injury Funds

In some states special funds exist that recompense the employer for the breakdown or second injury of an employee either retained or hired with a history of previous disability and provides full compensation for the employee in case of a "second injury." These are of some benefit in the employment of persons with cardiac disease but have not been widely used for such purposes, since they were originally intended for individuals with accidental injuries.

Waivers

It might be thought that a workman with a known heart condition could agree not to press a claim for disability arising during his employment, that is, to waive such a claim. However, 25 states rule waivers to be illegal, and in general they are questionable, since it is considered that the injured or disabled workman cannot relinquish the rights to which his heirs might be entitled. The waiver has been of negligible importance in the cardiac field.

Impartial Physicians and Panels

Some states utilize the services of impartial physicians and panels. The latter have been especially effective in Utah and the state of Washington. There is no uniformity of usage of "impartial" physicians, and some lawyers and boards deny that such exist. They appear of value in special situations where cooperation between boards and the medical profession is well developed and professional integrity is of a high order.

Disability Insurance

There is some indication that a form of insurance coverage for disability may develop. In some large companies, this has been secured as a fringe benefit. In 1951 five states had a sickness cash-benefit insurance system, and it obtains under the Railroad Unemployment Insurance Act.

The Legal Subcommittee of the American Heart Association Committee on the Effect of Strain and Trauma on the Heart and Great Vessels offered the following recommendations:[3]

Recommendation One:

> Encourage the interpretation and publication by authoritative medical groups of evidence as to the causative factors in cardiac disease.

> The question whether a cardiac incident was "caused" within the meaning of a compensation statute, by a work-connected event, such as shock, worry, strain or trauma, can only be decided by compensation commissions and courts in the light of the legislative intent and purposes underlying the particular statute involved. "Cause" in this legal sense is by no means necessarily synonymous with "cause" as understood by the average medical practitioner. Yet courts and commissions, in order to decide the legal question of causation intelligently, should have the benefit of the fullest scientific knowledge concerning the factors which bring about the cardiac disability and death. The reported cases show considerable conflict in medical testimony with respect to the causative factors in cardiac disease. The

quality and uniformity of such testimony might well be improved by the availability of authoritative statements made by medical groups of their views concerning the causative factors in cardiac disease. In view of the multitude of factors influencing the constantly changing physical status of a cardiac patient, especially a sufferer from coronary disease, it is recommended that an unusual strain for the given individual be the only acceptable injury recognized as aggravating, or revealing, underlying cardiac disease.

Recommendation Two:

> Disseminate medical information relating to cardiac cases to the general practitioner on a broader scale.

> The court decisions show that the medical man first approached by a workman with cardiac symptoms is usually a general practitioner. The general practitioner frequently testifies before courts and commissions and his testimony is often accorded great weight. To the extent that he can be better informed of the latest developments in cardiology, he should be a better and more accurate witness.

Recommendation Three:

> Educate the medical witness as to his proper role.

> The same words when used in medicine and law often have different meanings. Particularly is this true of such terms as "causation" and "unusual strain." To a physician, the term "causation" is likely to connote causation in the etiological sense, while to an attorney, it may mean something entirely different, such as a slight degree of aggravation. Physicians, and particularly those who are called upon to give testimony, should have at least a rudimentary knowledge of the legal concepts and terminology involved in the case in which they are appearing, as well as of their rights and obligations as a witness. This would held eliminate the common complaint of physicians that they are not allowed to testify fully and completely, and are badgered into giving monosyllabic or otherwise incomplete answers to complex questions.

Recommendation Four:

> Diminish the emphasis by commissions and courts on the language in which medical opinion testimony is couched.

The courts and commissions of a number of states place undue emphasis on the exact phraseology employed by medical witnesses, such as whether they use the word "possibility" or the word "probability" in speaking of causative factors. Since physicians are often unfamiliar with the great importance attached by courts and commissions to the particular wording of testimony, their statements should be examined by these tribunals on an over-all basis to glean the total meaning, rather than in accordance with preconceived verbal formulas.

Recommendation Five:

Encourage wider use of autopsies.

Some states rarely use autopsies in cardiac compensation cases; others use them regularly. On a national basis, there is widespread neglect of the opportunities which the properly conducted autopsy provides for insight into the causative factors of death. Better medical testimony would probably result if autopsies were the rule rather than the exception.

In summary, cardiovascular disease is the chief cause of death in the United States. This is the result of the increasing life span of our population. It is reasonable to expect that situations will arise in which the inevitable hazards of ordinary life will be claimed to have accelerated a degenerative disease, such as coronary atherosclerosis, to a point of disability or death sooner than would have been projected. Where such a stress can be shown to be related to the act of an individual or corporation, there may be the basis for legal redress. The possibilities of cardiac damage in personal injury situations are many, from a simple altercation in the street to hemorrhage from a stab wound. Similarly, in all sorts of employment there are elements of stress which, in the end stages of coronary narrowing, are adduced as the final precipitants of a "heart attack." The physician should recognize that this is what the lawyer calls the *proximate cause* of the attack—namely, the modicum of acceleration which is assumed to have taken place. The dispute, therefore, usually hinges on the opinions of those experts who consider the attack to be an unrelated episode in the natural history of the disease vis-à-vis those who find the last straw sufficiently weighty as to disable the camel.

These disputes will continue, and they will expand in numbers in proportion to the expansion of the view that almost any life experience may be claimed as deleterious. This will in turn obstruct the employment of older workers, in whom old-age diseases are more prevalent. In the author's opinion, there must either be an acceptance of Workmen's Compensation as a form of disability insurance or a holding to the original intent of such laws wherein the element of "accidental injury" existed. That is, an "unusual" event should be required to be followed at once by cardiac disturbance or failure of a recognizable type. Continuance in employment to which a man is accustomed up to the time when a "heart attack" occurs should be ruled as not contributing to the attack; the attack should be considered the natural result of his disease.

It should be agreed that these laws were intended to protect and recompense injured workers and not to cover the hazards of simple aging and chronic disease. Some method of covering such hazards is necessary in our industrial civilization, and it is to be hoped that insurance of some sort may be found practical. The medical profession is in a difficult situation because of the inherent lack of exactness in medical science. Perhaps continued research will clear away some clouds, but the ways of medicine and law are different and should, the author believes, remain so.

These cases will probably be decided in different ways in different courts and often on grounds that seem not medically justified to the physician. But the physician must present facts and opinions that are the best we now have and let the courts interpret the law.

REFERENCES

1. Campbell, M.: Death Rate from Diseases of the Heart, 1876 to 1959, *Brit. M. J.*, 2:528, 1963.
2. Quoted in Sigerist, H. E.: "Civilization and Disease." 1st Phoenix ed., The University of Chicago Press, Chicago, 1962, p. 49.
3. Report of the Committee on the Effect of Strain and Trauma on the Heart and Great Vessels, *Circulation* 26:612, 1962.
4. *Ibid.*, p. 617.
5. Osborn, G. R.: "The Incubation Period of Coronary Thrombosis," Butterworth & Co. (Publishers), Ltd., London, 1963, p. 1.
6. Minority Report of the Committee on the Effect of Strain and Trauma on the Heart and Great Vessels, *Circulation*, 28:268, 1963.
7. Aaron, K.: The Interrelationship between Emotion tion and Cardiac Function, *M. J. Australia*, 2:705, 1959.
8. Sprague, H. B.: The Effect of Trauma and Strain on the Production and Aggravation of Heart Disease, *Bull. New York Acad. Med.*, 23:631, 1947.
9. Marshall, F. W.: "Popular Guide to Modern Legal Principles," Rev. Ed., Wm. H. Wise & Co., Inc., New York, 1949, p. 4.

10. Sprague, H. B.: Heart Diseases—Pericardium, Section on Traumatic Pericarditis, in "Traumatic Medicine and Surgery for the Attorney," Butterworth, Inc., Washington, D.C., 1959.

11. Morris, R. C.: Quoted in *M. Tribune Apr.* 12, 1963.

12. Sprague, H. B.: Emotional Factors in Coronary Heart Disease, *Circulation,* **23:**648, 1961.

13. Sprague, H. B.: Legal Aspects of Coronary Disease, *Circulation,* **22:**627, 1960.

14. Larson, A.: "The Law of Workmen's Compensation," Matthew Bender & Co., 1958 Albany, N.Y., sec. 38–83, p. 566.

15. McNiece, H.: "Heart Disease and the Law," Prentice-Hall, Inc., Englewood Cliffs, N.J., 1961.

16. 223 New York Supplement (2d) 813 (1962) Supreme Court Appelate Division, Third Dept.

17. 53 Washington (2d) 698; 336 (p. 2) 382 (1959).

18. 90 F District of Columbia (2d) 387 (Cir. 1937).

Index

When there are several pages listed for an entry, boldface is used to indicate the more extensive discussion. More than one number is shown in boldface when the discussions are presented from a different point of view. When there are only one or two page references for an entry this distinction is not used.

THE MOSES H. CONE MEMORIAL HOSPITAL
GREENSBORO, NORTH CAROLINA